Canadian drugs identified with a maple-leaf icon

...atric, geriatric, ...other special ...ges included ...ughout

calcium carbonate (Rx) (PO-OTC, Rx)

Acid Free, Alka-Mints, Amitone, Apo-Cal ♣, Calcarb, Calci-Chew, Calci-Mix, Calcite ♣, Cal-Gest, Caltrate, Equaline Calcium, Leader Calcium, Maalox Antacid, Os-Cal 500, Rolaids Extra Strength Soft-chew, Tums, Tums E-X, Walgreens Calcium
Func. class.: Antacid, calcium supplement
Chem. class.: Calcium product

calcium acetate (OTC)
(kal′see-um ass′e-tate)
Calphron, Eliphos, PhosLo
Pregnancy category C

Do not confuse:
Os-Cal/Asacol

ACTION: Neutralizes gastric acidity

Therapeutic outcome: Neutralized gastric acidity; calcium at normal levels

USES: Antacid, calcium supplement; not suitable for chronic therapy, hyperphosphatemia, hypertension in pregnancy, osteoporosis, prevention/treatment of hypocalcemia, hypoparathyroidism

CONTRAINDICATIONS: Hypersensitivity, hypercalcemia, hyperparathyroidism, bone tumors

Precautions: Pregnancy C, breastfeeding, geriatric, fluid retention, decreased GI motility, GI obstruction, dehydration, renal disease

Subheadings indicate various administration routes

DOSAGE AND ROUTES

Nutritional supplement including osteoporosis prophylaxis
Adult ≥51 yr: PO 1000-1500 mg/day elemental calcium (2500-3750 calcium carbonate)
Adult 19-50 yr: PO 1000 mg/day elemental calcium (2500 mg/day calcium carbonate)

Chronic hypocalcemia
Adult: PO 2-4 g/day elemental calcium (5-10 g calcium carbonate) in 3-4 divided doses
Child: PO 45-65 mg/kg/day elemental calcium (112.5-162.5 mg/kg calcium carbonate) in 4 divided doses
Neonate: PO 50-150 mg/kg/day elemental calcium (125-375 mg/kg/day in 4-6 divided doses, max 1 g/day)

Supplementation
Adolescent and child 9-18 yr: PO 1300 mg elemental calcium (3250 mg calcium carbonate)
Child 4-8 yr: PO 800 mg/day elemental calcium (2000 mg calcium carbonate)
Child 1-3 yr: PO 500 mg/day elemental calcium (1250 mg calcium carbonate)
Infant 6-12 mo: PO 270 mg/day elemental calcium based on total intake
Neonate and infant <6 mo: PO 210 mg/day elemental calcium based on total intake

Hyperphosphatemia
Adult: PO Individualized on response

Heartburn, dyspepsia, hyperacidity (OTC)
Adult: PO 1-2 tabs q2hr, max 9 tabs/24 hr (Alka-mints); chew 2-4 tab q1hr prn, max 16 tabs (Tums regular strength); chew 2-4 tab q1hr prn, max 10 tabs (Tums E-X); chew 2-3 tabs q1hr prn, max 10 tabs (Tums Ultra); chew 2 tabs q2-3hr, max 19 tabs/24 hr (Titralac Extra Strength)

Available forms: Calcium carbonate: chewable tabs 350, 420, 450, 500, 750, 1000, 1250 mg; tabs 500, 600, 650, 667, 1000, 1250, 1500 mg; gum 300, 450 500 mg; susp 1250 mg/5 ml; caps 1250 mg; powder 6.5 g/packet; **calcium acetate:** tabs 250 mg (65 mg Ca), 667 mg (169 mg Ca), 668 mg (169 mg Ca), 1 g (250 mg Ca); caps 500 mg (125 mg Ca)

Implementation
PO route
• Administer as antacid 1 hr after meals and at bedtime
• Administer as supplement 1½ hr after meals and at bedtime
• Administer only with regular tablets or capsules; do not give with enteric-coated tablets
• Administer laxatives or stool softeners if constipation occurs

ADVERSE EFFECTS

GI: *Constipation,* anorexia, nausea, vomiting, flatulence, diarrhea, rebound hyperacidity, eructation
GU: Calculi, hypercalciuria

Common and life-threatening adverse effects grouped by body system

♣ Canada only

Adverse effects: *italics* = common; **bold** = life-threatening

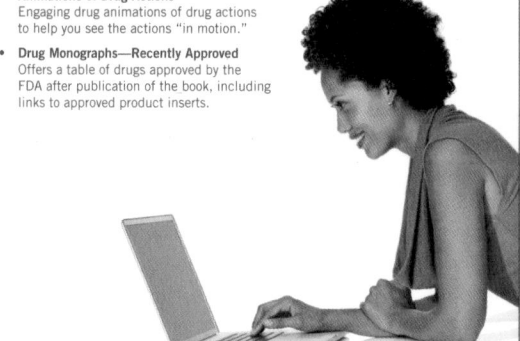

Administer drugs safely, accurately, and professionally.
*Now the MOST trusted book in nursing is
also available electronically!*

Mosby's
DRUG GUIDE
FOR NURSING
STUDENTS

ELEVENTH EDITION

Linda Skidmore-Roth, RN, MSN, NP

Consultant
Littleton, Colorado

Formerly, Nursing Faculty
New Mexico State University
Las Cruces, New Mexico
El Paso Community College
El Paso, Texas

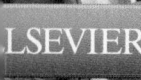

ELSEVIER

http://evolve.elsevier.com

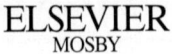

3251 Riverport Lane
St. Louis, Missouri 63043

MOSBY'S DRUG GUIDE FOR NURSING STUDENTS,
ELEVENTH EDITION

ISBN: 978-0-323-17297-4
ISSN: 2213-4409

Notices

Knowledge and best practice in this field are constantly changing. As new research and experience
broaden our understanding, changes in research methods, professional practices, or medical treatment may become necessary.

Practitioners and researchers must always rely on their own experience and knowledge in evaluating
and using any information, methods, compounds, or experiments described herein. In using such information or methods they should be mindful of their own safety and the safety of others, including
parties for whom they have a professional responsibility.

With respect to any drug or pharmaceutical products identified, readers are advised to check the
most current information provided (i) on procedures featured or (ii) by the manufacturer of each
product to be administered, to verify the recommended dose or formula, the method and duration of
administration, and contraindications. It is the responsibility of practitioners, relying on their own experience and knowledge of their patients, to make diagnoses, to determine dosages and the best treatment for each individual patient, and to take all appropriate safety precautions.

To the fullest extent of the law, neither the Publisher nor the authors, contributors, or editors, assume
any liability for any injury and/or damage to persons or property as a matter of products liability, neg-
ligence or otherwise, or from any use or operation of any methods, products, instructions, or ideas
contained in the material herein.

International Standard Book Number: 978-0-323-17297-4

Director, eContent Solutions: Robin Carter
Product Specialist: Shephali Graf
Content Coordinator: Samantha Taylor

Publishing Services Manager: Pat Joiner
Project Manager: Lisa A. P. Bushey
Book Designer: Brian Salisbury

Printed in the United States of America

Last digit is the print number: 9   8   7   6   5   4   3   2   1

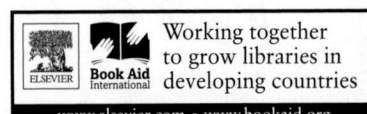

Working together
to grow libraries in
developing countries

www.elsevier.com • www.bookaid.org

Consultants

Timothy L. Brenner, PharmD, BCOP
Clinical Pharmacy Specialist
UPMC Cancer Centers
Pittsburgh, Pennsylvania

David S. Chun, PharmD, BCPS
Pharmacist
Richmond Heights, Missouri

Donna Ciulla, RPh
Faculty
Salem State University
Salem, Massachusetts;
Staff Pharmacist
Lahey Health Systems
Beverly, Massachusetts

Amanda Gross, RPh
Clinical Pharmacist
Atrium Pharmacy
University of Colorado Hospital
Aurora, Colorado

Paul E. Milligan, PharmD
Clinical Lead
BJC Learning Institute
St. Louis, Missouri

Joshua J. Neumiller, PharmD, CDE, CGP, FASCP
Assistant Professor
Washington State University
Spokane, Washington

Kristin Oneail, MSN, RN
Assistant Professor
Lourdes University
Sylvania, Ohio

Sarah R. Pool, RN, MS
Nursing Education Specialist, Cardiac Surgery
Mayo Clinic
Rochester, Minnesota

Sheila Seed, PharmD, MPH, RPh
Associate Professor and Vice Chair of Pharmacy Practice
MCPHS University
Worcester, Massachusetts

Melissa Sellers, MSN, BSN, RN
Nursing Instructor
Jackson State Community College
Jackson, Tennessee

Travis E. Sonnett, PharmD, FASCP
Clinical Pharmacy Specialist
Spokane VA Medical Center
Clinical Assistant Professor
WSU College of Pharmacy
Spokane, Washington

Patricia A. Talbert, RN
Preoperative/Pain Clinic Nurse
Aromatherapist
Herbalist
Horticulturist
Baxter Regional Medical Center
Mountain Home, Arkansas

Shamim Tejani, PharmD
Clinical Pharmacist
Adelante Healthcare
Phoenix, Arizona

Kristine C. Willett, PharmD
Associate Professor of Pharmacy Practice
MCPHS University
Manchester, New Hampshire

Preface

Mosby's Drug Guide for Nursing Students, eleventh edition, is the most in-depth handbook available for nursing students! Since its first publication in 1996, more than 100 U.S. and Canadian pharmacists and consultants have reviewed the book's content closely. Today, *Mosby's Drug Guide for Nursing Students* is more up-to-date than ever—with features that make it easy to find critical information fast!

NEW FEATURES
• Common drugs seen on the NCLEX® examination are highlighted to help in review.
• Over 20 recent FDA-approved drugs for 2015 are located throughout the book and in Appendix A.

NEW FACTS
This edition features thousands of new drug facts, including:
• New drugs and new dosage information
• Newly researched adverse effects
• New Black Box Warnings
• The latest precautions, interactions, and contraindications
• IV therapy updates
• Revised nursing considerations
• Updated patient/family education guidelines
• Updates on key new drug research

ORGANIZATION
This handbook is organized into four main sections:
• Individual drug monographs (in alphabetical order by generic name)
• Drug Categories
• Appendixes
• Illustrated mechanisms and sites of action
The guiding principle behind this book is to provide fast, easy access to drug information and nursing considerations. Every detail—from the cover, binding, and paper to the typeface, four-color design, and appendixes—has been carefully chosen with the user in mind. Here's what you'll find in each section of the handbook:

Individual Drug Monographs
This book includes monographs for more than 4000 generic and trade medications—those most commonly administered by students. Common trade names are given for all drugs regularly used in the United States and Canada, with drugs available only in Canada identified by a maple leaf icon (✤). In addition to the maple leaf icon, we've added a NEW feature to help with your review. Select monographs, important to learn and know for the NCLEX examination, have been identified by a ✲.

Each monograph provides the following information, whenever possible, for safe, effective administration of each drug:

High-alert status: Identifies drugs with the most potential to cause harm to patients if administered incorrectly.

"Tall Man" lettering: Uses the capitalization of distinguishing letters to avoid medication errors and is required by the FDA for drug manufacturers.

Pronunciation: Helps the nurse master complex generic names.

Rx, OTC: Identifies prescription or over-the-counter drugs.

Functional and chemical classifications: Helps the nurse recognize similarities and differences among drugs in the same functional but different chemical classes.

Pregnancy category: Notes FDA pregnancy categories A, B, C, D, and X at the beginning of each monograph, as well as under Precautions or Contraindications, depending on FDA category. Appendix D provides a detailed explanation of each category.

Do not confuse: Presents drug names that might easily be confused within each appropriate monograph.

Action: Describes pharmacologic properties concisely.

Therapeutic outcome: Details all possible results of medication use.

Uses: Lists the conditions the drug is used to treat.

Unlabeled uses: Describes drug uses that may be encountered in practice but are not yet FDA approved.

Dosages and routes: Lists all available and approved dosages and routes for adult, pediatric, and geriatric patients.

Available forms: Includes tablets, capsules, extended release, injectables (IV, IM,

SUBCUT), solutions, creams, ointments, lotions, gels, shampoos, elixirs, suspensions, suppositories, sprays, aerosols, and lozenges.

Adverse effects: Groups these reactions by alphabetical body system, with common side effects *italicized* and life-threatening reactions in **bold, red type** for emphasis.

Contraindications: Lists conditions under which the drug absolutely should not be given, including FDA pregnancy safety categories D and X.

Precautions: Lists conditions that require special consideration when the drug is prescribed, including FDA pregnancy safety categories A, B, and C.

Black Box Warnings: Identifies FDA warnings that highlight serious and life-threatening adverse effects.

Pharmacokinetics/pharmacodynamics: Features a quick-reference chart of concise facts of pharmacokinetics (absorption, distribution, metabolism, excretion, half-life) and pharmacodynamics (onset, peak, duration).

Interactions: Lists confirmed drug, food, herb, and lab test interactions.

Nursing considerations: Identifies key nursing considerations for each step of the nursing process: Assessment, Implementation, Patient/Family Education, and Evaluation, including positive therapeutic outcomes. Instructions for giving drugs by various routes (e.g., **IV**, PO, IM, SUBCUT, topically, rectally) appear under Implementation, with route subheadings in bold.

Compatibilities: Lists syringe, Y-site, and additive compatibilities and incompatibilities. If no compatibilities are listed for a drug, the necessary compatibility testing has not been done and that compatibility information is unknown. To ensure safety, assume that the drug may not be mixed with other drugs unless specifically stated.

Nursing Alert icon ⚠: Highlights situations in which the patient could potentially be at risk.

Treatment of overdose: Lists drugs and treatments for overdoses where appropriate.

Drug Categories
The Drug Categories section, following the individual drug monographs, provides general information about the various functional classes to promote learning about the similarities and differences among drugs in the same functional class. It summarizes action, uses, adverse effects, contraindications, precautions, pharmacokinetics, interactions, and nursing considerations for each functional class.

Appendixes

Selected new drugs: Includes comprehensive information on 25 key drugs approved by the FDA during the last 12 months.

Ophthalmic, nasal, topical, and otic products: Provides essential information for 140 ophthalmic, nasal, topical, and otic products commonly used today, grouped by chemical drug class.

Vaccines and toxoids: Features an easy-to-use table with generic and trade names, uses, dosages and routes, and contraindications for 39 key vaccines and toxoids.

Abbreviations and pregnancy categories: Lists abbreviations alphabetically with their meanings and explains the five FDA pregnancy categories.

Immunization schedule: Recommended childhood and adolescent immunization schedules.

Standard Precautions: Used in the care of all patients regardless of their diagnosis or disease.

Illustrated mechanisms and sites of action: These 13 detailed, full-color illustrations are added to help enhance the understanding of the mechanism or site of action for the following drugs and drug classes:
- Anticholinergic bronchodilators
- Antidepressants
- Antidiabetic agents
- Antifungal agents
- Antiinfective agents
- Antiretroviral agents
- Benzodiazepines
- Diuretics
- Laxatives
- Narcotic agonist-antagonist analgesics
- Narcotic analgesics
- Phenytoin
- Sympatholytics

Photo atlas of drug administration: This practical resource for students and practitioners lists standard precautions and provides more than 20 full-color illustrations depicting the physical landmarks and administration techniques used for IV, IM, SUBCUT, and ID drug delivery.

The following sources were consulted in the preparation of this edition:

Blumenthal M: *The Complete German Commission E Monographs: Therapeutic Guide to Herbal Medicines,* Austin, 1998, American Botanical Council.

Brunton L, Lazo J, Parker K: *Goodman and Gilman's The Pharmacological Basis of Therapeutics,* ed 11, New York, 2006, McGraw-Hill.

Clinical Pharmacology [database online], Tampa, 2014, Gold Standard, Inc. http://www.clinicalpharmacology.com. Updated March 2014.

Gahart BL, Nazareno AR: *Intravenous Medications,* ed 29, St. Louis, 2013, Mosby.

McKenry LM, Tessier E, Hogan MA: *Mosby's Pharmacology in Nursing,* ed 22, St. Louis, 2006, Mosby.

Acknowledgments

I am indebted to the nursing and pharmacology consultants who reviewed the manuscript and pages and thank them for their criticism and encouragement. I would also like to thank Robin Carter and Shephali Graf, my editors, whose active encouragement and enthusiasm have made this book better than it might otherwise have been. I am likewise grateful to Pat Joiner, Lisa Bushey, and Mike Ederer at Graphic World Inc., for the coordination of the production process and assistance with the development of the new edition.

Linda Skidmore-Roth

Contents

INDIVIDUAL DRUG MONOGRAPHS, 1

DRUG CATEGORIES, 1128

APPENDIXES

INDEX, 1241

NEW DRUGS FOR 2016, 1273

EVOLVE WEBSITE CONTENTS
Animations of Drug Actions
Canadian Resources
- Canadian Controlled Substance Chart
- Canadian Recommended Immunization Schedules for Infants and Children
- High Alert Canadian Medications
Content Changes
Drug Monographs—Additional Monographs
Drug Monographs—Recently Approved
Formulas for Drug Calculations
Syringe Compatibility Chart
Weights and Equivalents

abacavir (Rx)

(a-ba-ka'veer)

Ziagen

Func. class.: Antiretroviral

Chem. class.: Nucleoside reverse transcriptase inhibitor (NRTI)

Pregnancy category C

ACTION: Inhibitory action against HIV; inhibits replication of HIV by incorporating into cellular DNA by viral reverse transcriptase, thereby terminating the cellular DNA chain

Therapeutic outcome: Decreased symptoms of HIV

USES: In combination with other antiretroviral agents for HIV-1 infection (not to be used with lamivudine or tenofovir)

CONTRAINDICATIONS:

BLACK BOX WARNING: Hypersensitivity, moderate to severe hepatic disease

Precautions: Pregnancy **C**, breastfeeding, child <3 mo, granulocyte count <1000/mm^3 or Hgb <9.5 g/dl, severe renal disease, impaired hepatic function, HLA B5701 (Black, Caucasian, Asian patients), abrupt discontinuation; Guillain-Barré syndrome, immune reconstitution syndrome, MI, obesity, polymyositis

BLACK BOX WARNING: Lactic acidosis

DOSAGE AND ROUTES

Adult/adolescent ≥16 hr: PO 300 mg bid or 600 mg daily with other antiretrovirals

Adolescent <16 yr/child ≥3 mo: PO 8 mg/kg bid, max 300 mg bid with other antiretrovirals

Hepatic dose

Adult: (Child-Pugh 5-6) PO oral/sol 200 mg bid; severe hepatic disease, do not use

Available forms: Tabs 300 mg; oral sol 20 mg/ml

Implementation

PO route

• May give without regard to food q12hr around the clock

• Give in combination with other antiretrovirals with or without food; do not use triple therapy as a beginning treatment, resistance may occur

• Store in cool environment; protect from light; do not freeze

ADVERSE EFFECTS

CNS: *Fever, headache, malaise, insomnia,* paresthesia

GI: *Nausea, vomiting, diarrhea, anorexia, cramps, abdominal pain, increased AST, ALT,* **hepatotoxicity, hepatomegaly with steatosis**

HEMA: **Granulocytopenia, anemia,** lymphopenia

INTEG: Rash, urticaria, hypersensitivity reactions

META: **Lactic acidosis**

MISC: Increased CPK, **fatal hypersensitivity reactions, fat redistribution, immune reconstitution**

RESP: Dyspnea

Pharmacokinetics

Absorption	Rapid/extensive (PO)
Distribution	50% protein binding, extravascular space, then erythrocytes
Metabolism	To inactive metabolite
Excretion	Kidneys, feces
Half-life	1½-2 hr

Pharmacodynamics

Unknown

INTERACTIONS

Individual drugs

Do not coadminister with abacavir-containing products

Alcohol: increased abacavir levels; do not use with alcohol

Ribavirin: possible lactic acidosis

Methadone: decreased levels of methadone

Tipranavir: decreased abacavir levels

Drug/lab test

Increased: glucose, triglycerides, GGT, LFTs

NURSING CONSIDERATIONS

Assessment

• Assess for symptoms of HIV and possible infection, increased temp

• **Assess for lactic acidosis** (elevated lactate levels, increased liver function tests) and severe hepatomegaly with steatosis; discontinue treatment and do not restart, women are at greater risk for lactic acidosis

BLACK BOX WARNING: Assess for fatal hypersensitivity reactions: fever, rash, nausea, vomiting, fatigue, cough, dyspnea, diarrhea, abdominal discomfort; treatment should be discontinued and not restarted

⚠ Assess for pancreatitis: abdominal pain, nausea, vomiting, elevated liver enzymes; product should be discontinued because condition can be fatal
- Monitor CBC, differential, platelet count qmo; withhold product if WBC is <4000/mm^3 or platelet count is <75,000/mm^3; notify prescriber of results; monitor viral load and CD4 counts during treatment, perform hepatitis B virus (HBr) screening to confirm correct treatment
- Monitor renal function studies; BUN, serum uric acid, urine CCr before, during therapy; these may be elevated throughout treatment
- Monitor temp q4hr; may indicate beginning of infection

BLACK BOX WARNING: Monitor liver function tests before, during therapy (bilirubin, AST, ALT, amylase, alkaline phosphatase, creatine phosphokinase, creatinine prn or qmo)

Patient/family education
- Advise patient to report signs of infection: increased temp, sore throat, flulike symptoms; to avoid crowds and those with known infections, to carry emergency ID with condition, products taken
- Instruct patient to report signs of anemia: fatigue, headache, faintness, shortness of breath, irritability
- Advise patient to report bleeding; avoid use of razors or commercial mouthwash
- Inform patient that product is not a cure but will control symptoms
- Inform patient that major toxicities may necessitate discontinuing product
- **Instruct patient to use contraception during treatment,** that body fat distribution may occur, not to share product
- Caution patient to avoid OTC products or other medications without approval of prescriber
- Caution patient not to have any sexual contact without use of a condom; needles should not be shared; blood from infected individual should not come in contact with another's mucous membranes
- Give Medication Guide and Warning Card; discuss points on guide
- Advise patient to notify prescriber if skin rash, fever, cough, shortness of breath, GI symptoms occur; advise all health care providers that allergic reactions have occurred with this product

Evaluation
Positive therapeutic outcome
- Increased CD4 count
- Decreased viral load

abatacept (Rx)
(ab-a-ta′sept)
Orencia
Func. class.: Antirheumatic agent (disease modifying); immunomodulator
Pregnancy category C

ACTION: A selective costimulation modulator, inhibits production of T-lymphocytes, inhibits tumor necrosis factor (TNF-α), interferon-γ, interleukin-2, which are involved in immune and inflammatory reactions

Therapeutic outcome: Decreased pain, inflammation in joints

USES: Polyarticular juvenile rheumatoid arthritis; acute chronic rheumatoid arthritis that has not responded to other disease-modifying agents; may use in combination with DMARDs; do not use with TNF antagonists (adalimumab, etanercept, infliximab) or anakinra

CONTRAINDICATIONS: Hypersensitivity

Precautions: Pregnancy **C,** breastfeeding, children, geriatric, recurrent infections, COPD, immunosuppression, neoplastic disease, respiratory infection, TB, viral hepatitis

DOSAGE AND ROUTES
Rheumatoid arthritis
Adult: SUBCUT 125 mg within a day after single IV loading dose, then 125 mg weekly, weekly subcut may be initiated without IV loading dose for those unable to receive an infusion; give at 2, 4 wk after first infusion, then q4wk
Adult >100 kg (220 lb): IV INF 1 g over 30 min; give at 2, 4 wk after first infusion, then q4wk
Adult 60-100 kg (132-220 lb): IV INF 750 mg over 30 min; give at 2, 4 wk after first infusion, then q4wk
Adult <60 kg (132 lb): IV INF 500 mg over 30 min; give at 2, 4 wk after first infusion, then q4wk

Juvenile rheumatoid arthritis (JRA)/juvenile idiopathic arthritis (JIA)

Child/adolescent ≥6 yr >100 kg: IV 1000 mg over 30 min q2wk × 2 doses, then 1 g over 30 min q4wk starting at wk 8

Child/adolescent >6 yr >75 kg: IV INF 750 mg over 30 min q2wk × 2 doses, then 750 mg over 30 min q4wk starting at wk 8

Child/adolescent ≥6 yr <75 kg: IV INF 10 mg/kg over 30 min q2wk × 2 doses, then 10 mg/kg q4wk starting at wk 8

Available forms: Lyophilized powder, single-use vials 250 mg, sol for subcut injection 125 mg/ml

Implementation

• Store in refrigerator; do not use expired vials, protect from light, do not freeze

Intermittent IV infusion route

• To **reconstitute,** remove plastic flip top from vial and wipe the top with alcohol wipe; insert syringe needle into vial and direct stream of sterile water for inj on the wall of vial; rotate vial until mixed; vent with needle to rid foam after reconstitution 25 mg/ml; **further dilute** in 100 ml from a 100 ml NS infusion bag/bottle; withdraw the needed volume (2 vials remove 20 ml; 3 vials remove 30 ml, 4 vials remove 40 ml); slowly add the reconstituted Orencia sol from each vial into the infusion bag/bottle using the same disposable syringe supplied; mix gently, discard unused portions of vials; do not use if particulate is present or if discolored; **give** over 30 min; use non–protein binding filter (0.2-1.2 mcg)

• Do not admix with other sol or medications
• Store in refrigerator; do not use expired vials; protect from light

Subcut route

• Use prefilled syringe for subcut only, do not use for IV, only those trained should use this system; allow syringe to warm to room temperature (30-60 min) do not speed up warming process; the amount of liquid should be between the two lines on the barrel, do not use the syringe if there is more or less liquid; use front of thigh, outer area of the upper arm, or abdomen except 2-inch area around the navel, do not inject into tender, bruised area

• Gently pinch skin and hold firmly, insert needle at 45-degree angle, inject full amount in 125 mg syringe, rotate injection sites

ADVERSE EFFECTS

CNS: Headache, asthenia, dizziness
CV: *Hypertension, hypotension*
GI: Abdominal pain, dyspepsia, nausea
INTEG: Rash, *inj site reaction,* flushing, urticaria, pruritus
RESP: *Pharyngitis, cough, URI,* non-URI, *rhinitis,* wheezing
SYST: Anaphylaxis, malignancies, angioedema, serious infections

Pharmacokinetics

Absorption	Unknown
Distribution	Unknown; steady state 60 days
Metabolism	Increased clearance in obesity (subcut); clearance increases with increased body weight
Excretion	Unknown
Half-life	Terminal IV 13 days, subcut 14.3 days; subcut half-life 85 days

Pharmacodynamics

Unknown

INTERACTIONS

Individual drugs

Anakinra: do not use
Atropine, scopolamine, halothane: avoid concurrent use

Drug classifications

Corticosteroids, immunosuppressives: avoid concurrent use, nitrous oxide
TNF antagonists (adalimumab, etanercept, inFLIXimab): do not use
Vaccines: do not give concurrently; immunizations should be brought up to date before treatment

NURSING CONSIDERATIONS

Assessment

• **RA:** Assess for pain, stiffness, ROM, swelling of joints during treatment
• Assess for latent/active TB before beginning treatment
• Assess for inj site pain, swelling
• Monitor patient's overall health on each visit; product should not be given with active infections; parenteral product contains maltose; glucose monitoring must be done with glucose-specific testing
• **Infection:** sinusitis, urinary tract infection, influenza, bronchitis, serious infections have occurred

Patient/family education
• Teach patient that product must be continued for prescribed time to be effective
• Advise patient to use caution when driving; dizziness may occur
• Advise patient not to have vaccinations while taking this product
• Discuss with patient information included in packaging

Evaluation
Positive therapeutic outcome
• Decreased inflammation, pain in joints; decreased erythrocyte sedimentation rate (ESR)

---

abiraterone
Zytiga
(a-bir-a′ter-one)
Func. class.: Androgen inhibitor
Pregnancy category X

ACTION: Converted to abiraterone, which inhibits CYP17, the enzyme required for androgen biosynthesis; androgen-sensitive prostate cancer responds to treatment that decreases androgens

Therapeutic outcome: Decreases spread of malignancy

USES: Metastatic castration-resistant prostate cancer in combination with prednisone in patients who have received prior chemotherapy containing docetaxel

CONTRAINDICATIONS:
Pregnancy (X), women, children

Precautions:
Adrenal insufficiency, cardiac disease, MI, heart failure, hepatic disease, hypertension, hypokalemia, infection, surgery, ventricular dysrhythmia

DOSAGE AND ROUTES
Adult Males: PO 1000 mg q day with predniSONE 5 mg bid

Hepatic dose
Adult Males: (Child-Pugh B, 7-9) **PO** 250 mg q day with predniSONE; (Child-Pugh C, >10) do not use

Available forms: Tab 250 mg

Implementation
PO route
• Give whole, on empty stomach two hrs before or 1 hr after meals with full glass of water

• Women who are pregnant or may become pregnant should not touch tabs without gloves
• Storage of tabs at room temperature

ADVERSE EFFECTS
CV: Angina, **dysrhythmia exacerbation, atrial flutter/fibrillation/tachycardia, AV block,** chest pain, edema, **heart failure, MI,** hypertension, **QT prolongation, sinus tachycardia, supraventricular tachycardia, ventricular tachycardia**
ENDO: Hot flashes
GI: Diarrhea, dyspepsia
GU: Increased urinary frequency, nocturia, urinary tract infection
META: Adrenocortical insufficiency, hyperbilirubinemia, hypertriglyceridemia, hypokalemia, hypophosphatemia
MS: Arthralgia, myalgia
RESP: Cough, upper respiratory infection
SYST: Infection

Pharmacokinetics

Absorption	Food increases effect; give on empty stomach; increased effect in hepatic disease
Distribution	99% protein binding
Metabolism	Converted to abiraterone (active metabolite)
Excretion	88% (feces), 5% (urine)
Half-life	Mean terminal half-life 7-17 hr

Pharmacodynamics

Onset	Unknown
Peak	Unknown
Duration	Unknown

INTERACTIONS
Drug classifications
CYP3A4 inhibitors (clarithromycin, atazanavir, nefazodone, saquinavir, telithromycin, ritonavir, indinavir, nelfinavir, voriconazole, ketoconazole, itraconazole); CYP3A4 inducers (carBAMazepine, phenytoin, rifampin, rifabutin, rifapentine, PHENobarbital): avoid use with this product
CYP2D6 substrate (dextromethorphan, thioridazine): increased action of these products; dose of these products should be reduced

NURSING CONSIDERATIONS
Assessment
• Monitor prostate specific antigen (PSA), serum potassium, serum bilirubin

---

• Monitor liver function tests (AST/ALT) baseline and every 2 wk for 3 mo and monthly thereafter in those with no known hepatic disease; interrupt treatment in patients without known hepatic disease at baseline who develop ALT/AST >5 times ULN or total bilirubin >3 times ULN; in baseline moderate hepatic disease, measure ALT, AST, and bilirubin before the start of treatment, every week for the first month, every 2 weeks for the following 2 months, and monthly thereafter; if elevations in ALT and/or AST >5 times ULN or total bilirubin >3 times ULN occur in patients with baseline moderate hepatic impairment, discontinue and do NOT restart. Measure serum total bilirubin, AST, and ALT if hepatotoxicity is suspected. Elevations of AST, ALT, bilirubin from baseline should prompt more frequent monitoring.
• **Monitor musculoskeletal pain, joint swelling, discomfort**: Arthritis, arthralgia, joint swelling, and joint stiffness, some severe. Muscle discomfort that included muscle spasms, musculoskeletal pain, myalgia, musculoskeletal discomfort, and musculoskeletal stiffness may be relieved with analgesics
• Assess for signs and symptoms of adrenocorticoid insufficiency; monthly for hypertension, hypokalemia, and fluid retention
• Monitor ECG for QT prolongation, ejection fraction in those with cardiac disease, small increases in the QTc interval such as <10 ms have occurred; monitor for arrhythmia exacerbation such as sinus tachycardia, atrial fibrillation, supraventricular tachycardia (SVT), atrial tachycardia, ventricular tachycardia, atrial flutter, bradycardia, AV block complete, conduction disorder, and bradyarrhythmia

Patient/family education
• Teach patient that women must not come in contact with tabs, wear gloves if product needs to be handled, pregnancy (X)
• Instruct patient to report chest pain, swelling of joints, burning/pain when urinating

acarbose (Rx)
(a-kar′bose)
Precose
Func. class.: Oral antidiabetic
Chem. class.: α-Glucosidase inhibitor
Pregnancy category B

Do not confuse:
Precose/PreCare

ACTION: Delays the digestion/absorption of ingested carbohydrates by inhibiting α-glucosidase, results in a smaller rise in blood glucose after meals; does not increase insulin production

Therapeutic outcome: Decreased blood glucose levels in diabetes mellitus

USES: Type 2 diabetes mellitus, alone or in combination with a sulfonylurea, metformin, insulin

CONTRAINDICATIONS:
Hypersensitivity, breastfeeding, diabetic ketoacidosis, cirrhosis, inflammatory bowel disease, ileus, colonic ulceration, partial intestinal obstruction, chronic intestinal disease, serum creatinine >2 mg/dl

Precautions: Pregnancy **B**, children, renal/hepatic disease

DOSAGE AND ROUTES
Initial dose
Adult >60 kg (132 lb): PO 25 mg tid with first bite of meal

Maintenance dose
Adult: PO May be increased to 50-100 mg tid; dosage adjustment at 4-8 wk intervals, individualized
Adult <60 kg (132 lb): PO Max 50 mg tid

Available forms: Tabs 25, 50, 100 mg

Implementation
• Give tid with first bite of each meal
• Provide storage in tight container in cool environment

ADVERSE EFFECTS
GI: *Abdominal pain, diarrhea, flatulence*

Pharmacokinetics

Absorption	Poor systemic
Distribution	Unknown
Metabolism	GI tract
Excretion	Kidneys as intact drug
Half-life	Elimination 2 hr

Pharmacodynamics

Onset	Unknown
Peak	1 hr
Duration	2-4 hr

INTERACTIONS
Individual drugs
Acetaminophen: increased toxicity combined with alcohol

Digoxin: decreased acarbose effect

Phenytoin: increased hypoglycemia

Baclofen, cycloSPORINE, tacrolimus, isoniazid: increased hyperglycemia

Drug classifications
Androgens, quinolones: increased or decreased glycemic control

Corticosteroids, diuretics, estrogens, oral contraceptives, phenothiazines, progestins, sympathomimetics: digestive enzymes, intestinal absorbents, thiazide diuretics, loop diuretics, corticosteroids, protease inhibitors, atypical antipsychotics, carbonic anhydrase inhibitors: increased hyperglycemia, decreased effect of acarbose

MAOIs, salicylates, fibric acid derivatives, bile acid sequestrants, ACE inhibitors, angiotensin II receptor antagonists, β-blockers, sulfonylureas, insulins: increased hypoglycemia

Drug/herb
Chromium, garlic, horse chestnut: increased hypoglycemia

Drug/lab test
Increased: ALT, AST, bilirubin

Decreased: calcium, vit B_6, Hgb , Hct

NURSING CONSIDERATIONS
Assessment
• Assess for hypoglycemia (weakness, hunger, dizziness, tremors, anxiety, tachycardia, sweating), hyperglycemia; even though this product does not cause hypoglycemia, if on a sulfonylurea or insulin, hypoglycemia may be additive; if hypoglycemia occurs, treat with glucose or if severe, **IV** dextrose or IM glucagon

• Monitor 1 hr postprandial glucose for establishing effectiveness, then glycosylated Hgb q3mo, 1 hr PP throughout treatment

• Monitor AST, ALT q3mo $\times$ 1 yr, and periodically thereafter, if elevated dose, may need to be reduced or discontinued, usually increased with doses $\geq$ 300 mg/day; obtain glycosylated Hgb periodically

• Assess for stress, surgery, or other trauma that may require change in dose

Patient/family education
• Teach patient the symptoms of hypoglycemia, hyperglycemia, and what to do about each

• Instruct that medication must be taken as prescribed; explain consequences of discontinuing the medication abruptly; that insulin may need to be used during stress such as trauma, surgery, fever

• Tell patient to avoid OTC medications, herbal products unless approved by prescriber

• Teach patient that diabetes is a lifelong illness; product will not cure condition; that diet and exercise regimen must be followed

• Instruct patient to carry/wear emergency ID as diabetic

• Teach patient to avoid breastfeeding if using acarbose with other antidiabetics

• Inform that GI side effects may occur

Evaluation
Positive therapeutic outcome
• Improved signs, symptoms of diabetes mellitus (decreased polyuria, polydipsia, polyphagia; clear sensorium, absence of dizziness, stable gait)

---

acetaminophen (OTC)
(a-seat-a-mee'noe-fen)
Acephen, Aceta, Aminofen, Apacet, APAP, Apra, Children's Feverall, Equaline Children's Pain Relief, Equaline Infant's Pain Relief, Exdol ✿, Genapap, Good Sense Acetaminophen, Good Sense Children's Pain Relief, Infantaire, Leader Children's Pain Reliever, Mapap, Maranox, Meda, Neopap, Ofirmen, Oraphen-PD, Q-Pap, Q-Pap Children's, Redutemp, Ridenol, Silapap, Tapanol, Tempra, T-Painol, Tylenol, Uni-Ace, Walgreen's Acetaminophen, Walgreen's Non-Aspirin, XS Pain Reliever
Func. class.: Nonopioid analgesic
Chem. class.: Nonsalicylate, paraaminophenol derivative
Pregnancy category B

ACTION: May block pain impulses peripherally that occur in response to inhibition of prostaglandin synthesis; does not possess antiinflammatory properties; antipyretic action results from inhibition of prostaglandins in the CNS (hypothalamic heat-regulating center)

Therapeutic outcome: Decreased pain, fever

USES: Mild to moderate pain or fever; arthralgia, dental pain, dysmenorrhea, headache, myalgia, osteoarthritis

CONTRAINDICATIONS:
Hypersensitivity

Precautions: Pregnancy B; C (IV) breast-feeding, geriatric, anemia, renal/hepatic disease, chronic alcoholism

DOSAGE AND ROUTES
Adult and child >12 yr: PO/RECT 325-650 mg q4-6hr prn, max 4 g/day; weight ≥50 kg IV 1000 mg q6hr or 650 mg q4hr prn, max single dose 1000 mg, minimum dosing interval 4 hr; weight <50 kg IV 15 mg/kg/dose q6hr or 12.5 mg/kg/dose q4hr, max single dose 15 mg/kg minimum dosing interval 4 hr, max 75 mg/kg/day from all sources, ext rel 650-1300 mg q8hr as needed, max 4 g/day
Child ≥2 yr and <50 kg: IV 15 mg/kg/dose q6hr or 12.5 mg/kg/dose q4hr, max single dose 15 mg/kg, minimum dosing interval 4 hr, max 75 mg/kg/day from all sources
Child 1-12 yr: PO 10-15 mg/kg q4-6hr, max 5 doses/24 hr; RECT 10-20 mg/kg/dose q4-6hr
Neonate: RECT 10-15 mg/kg/dose q6-8hr

Available forms: Rectal supp 120, 325, 650 mg; chewable tabs 80 mg; caps 500 mg; elix 120, 160, 325 mg/5 ml; tabs 160, 325, 500, 650 mg; sol for injection 1000 mg/100 ml; disintegrating tab 80, 160 mg; oral drops 80 mg/10.8 ml; liquid 500 mg/5 ml, 160 mg/5 ml, 1000 mg/30 ml, 80 mg/ml; ext rel tabs 650 mg

Implementation
PO route
• Administer to patient crushed or whole; chewable tabs may be chewed; do not crush or chew EXT REL product
• Give with food or milk to decrease gastric symptoms; give 30 min before or 2 hr after meals; absorption may be slowed
• Shake susp well; check all product concentrations carefully; check elixir, liquid, suspension concentration carefully; susp and cups are bioequivalent

Intermittent IV infusion route
• No further dilution needed, do not add other medications to vial or infusion device
• For doses equal to single vial, a vented IV set may be used to deliver directly from vial; for doses less than a single vial, withdraw dose and place in an empty sterile syringe, plastic IV container, or glass bottle, infuse over 15 mins

• Discard unused portion, once seal is broken or vial penetrated or transferred to another container, give within 6 hr

Rectal route
• Store suppositories <80° F (27° C)

ADVERSE EFFECTS
GI: Nausea, vomiting, abdominal pain; **hepatotoxicity, hepatic seizure (overdose), GI bleeding**
GU: **Renal failure** (high, prolonged doses)
HEMA: **Leukopenia, neutropenia, hemolytic anemia** (long-term use)**, thrombocytopenia, pancytopenia**
INTEG: Rash, urticaria
SYST: **Hypersensitivity**
TOXICITY: **Cyanosis, anemia, neutropenia, jaundice, pancytopenia, CNS stimulation, delirium followed by vascular collapse, seizures, coma, death**

Pharmacokinetics

Absorption	Well absorbed (PO), variable (RECT)
Distribution	Widely distributed; crosses placenta in low concentrations
Metabolism	Liver 85%-95%; metabolites are toxic at high levels
Excretion	Kidneys—metabolites, breast milk
Half-life	3-4 hr

Pharmacodynamics

	PO	RECT
Onset	½-1 hr	½-1 hr
Peak	1-3 hr	1-3 hr
Duration	3-4 hr	3-4 hr

INTERACTIONS
Individual drugs
Alcohol, carBAMazepine, diflunisal, imatinib, isoniazid, lamoTRIgine, rifabutin, rifampin, zidovudine: increased hepatotoxicity
Colestipol, cholestyramine: decreased absorption of acetaminophen
Avoid use with salicylates
Warfarin: hypoprothrombinemia; long-term use, high doses of acetaminophen

Drug classifications
Barbiturates, hydantoins: decreased effect; increased hepatotoxicity
NSAIDs, salicylates: increased renal adverse reactions

Adverse effects: *italics* = common; **bold** = life-threatening

Drug/herb
St. John's wort: increased hepatotoxicity due to acetaminophen metabolism

Drug/lab test
Interference: 5-HIAA
Increased: LFTs, potassium, bilirubin, LDH, pro-time
Decreased: Hgb/Hct, WBC, RBC, platelets; albumin, magnesium, phosphate (pediatrics)

NURSING CONSIDERATIONS
Assessment
• Monitor liver function studies: AST, ALT, bilirubin, creatinine before therapy if long-term therapy is anticipated; may cause hepatic toxicity at doses >4 g/day with chronic use
• Monitor renal function studies: BUN, urine creatinine, occult blood; albumin indicates nephritis
• Monitor blood studies: CBC, PT if patient is on long-term therapy
• Check I&O ratio; decreasing output may indicate renal failure (long-term therapy)
• Assess for fever and pain: type of pain, location, intensity, duration, temp, diaphoresis
• **Assess for chronic poisoning:** rapid, weak pulse; dyspnea; cold, clammy extremities; report immediately to prescriber
• **Assess hepatotoxicity:** dark urine, clay-colored stools, yellowing of skin and sclera; itching, abdominal pain, fever, diarrhea if patient is on long-term therapy
• **Assess allergic reactions:** if rash, urticaria occur, product may have to be discontinued

Patient/family education
⚠ Teach patient not to exceed recommended dosage; the elixir, liquid, and suspension come in several concentrations, read label carefully; acute poisoning with liver damage may result; acute toxicity includes symptoms of nausea, vomiting, and abdominal pain; prescriber should be notified immediately
• Inform patient that toxicity may occur when used with other combination products
• Advise patient not to use with alcohol, OTC products, or herbals without prescriber approval
• Teach patient to recognize signs of chronic overdose: bleeding, bruising, malaise, fever, sore throat
• Inform patient that urine may become dark brown as a result of phenacetin (metabolite of acetaminophen)

• Tell patient to notify prescriber for pain or fever lasting more than 3 days, not to be used in <2 yr unless approved by prescriber
• May be used when breastfeeding, short-term

Evaluation
Positive therapeutic outcome
• Decreased pain, use pain scoring
• Decreased fever

TREATMENT OF OVERDOSE:
Product level q4hr, gastric lavage, activated charcoal; administer oral acetylcysteine to prevent hepatic damage (*see acetylcysteine monograph*, p. 11)

---

acetaZOLAMIDE (Rx)
(a-set-a-zole'-a-mide)
Diamox Sequels
Func. class.: Diuretic carbonic anhydrase inhibitor; antiglaucoma agent, antiepileptic
Chem. class.: Sulfonamide derivative
Pregnancy category C

Do not confuse:
acetaZOLAMIDE/acetoHEXAMIDE,
Diamox/Dobutrex/Trimox

ACTION: Decreases the aqueous humor in the eye, which lowers intraocular pressure by the inhibition of carbonic anhydrase; also inhibits carbonic anhydrase activity in proximal renal tubules to decrease reabsorption of water, sodium, potassium, bicarbonate; decreases carbonic anhydrase in CNS, increasing seizure threshold; prevents uric acid or cysteine buildup in the renal system by the decrease in pH, causing increased urine volume and alkaline urine

Therapeutic outcome: Decreased intraocular pressure; control of seizures; prevention and treatment of acute mountain sickness; prevention of uric acid/cysteine renal stones; decreased edema in lung tissue and peripherally; decreased B/P

USES: Open-angle glaucoma, angle closure glaucoma (preoperatively if surgery delayed), seizures (petit mal, grand mal, mixed, absence), edema in CHF, product-induced edema, acute altitude sickness

CONTRAINDICATIONS:
Hypersensitivity to sulfonamides, severe renal/hepatic disease, electrolyte imbalances (hypona-

---

tremia, hypokalemia), hyperchloremic acidosis, Addison's disease, long-term use in closed-angle glaucoma, adrenalcortical insufficiency, metabolic acidosis, acidemia, anuria

Precautions: Pregnancy **C**, breastfeeding, hypercalciuria, COPD, respiratory acidosis, pulmonary obstruction/emphysema

DOSAGE AND ROUTES

Angle closure glaucoma
Adult: PO/**IV** 250 mg q4hr or 250 mg bid, to be used for short-term therapy

Open-angle glaucoma
Adult: PO/**IV** 250 mg/day in divided doses for amounts over 250 mg or 500 mg **EXT REL** bid, max 1 g/day

Edema in CHF
Adult: PO/**IV** 250-375 mg/day or 5 mg/kg in AM, give for 2 days, then 1-2 days drug-free
Child: PO/**IV** 5 mg/kg/day or 150 mg/m² in AM

Seizures
Adult: PO/**IV** 8-30 mg/kg/day in 1-4 divided doses, usual range 375-1000 mg/day; EXT REL not recommended in seizures
Child: PO/**IV** 8-30 mg/kg/day in divided doses tid or qid, or 300-900 mg/m²/day, not to exceed 1 g/day

Altitude sickness
Adult: PO 250 mg q6-12hr; EXT REL 500 mg q12-24hr, start therapy 24-48 hr prior to ascent and ≥48 hr after arrival at high altitude
Geriatric: PO 250 mg bid; use lowest effective dose

Renal dose
Adult: PO/**IV** CCr 50-80 ml/min, give dose ≥6 hr reg rel of IV; CCr 10-50 ml/min, give dose q12hr; CCr <10 ml/min, avoid use

Available forms: Tabs 125, 250 mg; ext rel caps 500 mg; inj 500 mg

Implementation
• Give in AM to avoid interference with sleep
• Administer fluids 2-3 L/day to prevent renal calculi, unless contraindicated
• Potassium replacement if potassium level is <3.0 ml/dl

PO route
• Do not crush or chew ext rel caps; caps may be opened and sprinkled on food
• Give with food; if nausea occurs, crush tabs and mix with sweet substance to counteract bitter taste

IV route
• Do not use solution that is yellow or has a precipitate or crystals
• **Dilute** 500 mg of product/5 ml or more sterile water for inj: use within 24 hr, **give** at 100-500 mg/min

IV, direct route
• Give over 1 min or more

Intermittent IV infusion route
• May be added to NS, D₅W, D₁₀W, 0.45% NaCl; **give** over 15-30 min
• Store in cool, dark area, use reconstituted solution within 24 hr

Additive compatibilities: Cimetidine, ranitidine

Additive incompatibilities: Multivitamins

ADVERSE EFFECTS
CNS: Drowsiness, paresthesia, anxiety, depression, headache, dizziness, confusion, stimulation, fatigue, **seizures**
EENT: Myopia, tinnitus
ENDO: Hyperglycemia, hypoglycemia
GI: Nausea, vomiting, anorexia, diarrhea, melena, weight loss, **hepatic insufficiency, cholestatic jaundice, fulminant hepatic necrosis,** taste alterations, **bleeding**
GU: Frequency, polyuria, **uremia,** glucosuria, hematuria, dysuria, crystalluria, renal calculi
HEMA: Aplastic anemia, **hemolytic anemia, leukopenia, thrombocytopenia purpura, pancytopenia**
INTEG: Rash, pruritus, urticaria, fever, **Stevens-Johnson syndrome,** photosensitivity, flushing, toxic epidermal necrolysis
META: *Hypokalemia, hyperchloremic acidosis,* hyponatremia, sulfonamide-like reactions, metabolic acidosis, growth inhibition in children, hyperuricemia, hypercalcemia

Pharmacokinetics

Absorption	GI tract—65% if fasting, 75% with food; **IV**— complete
Distribution	Crosses placenta; widely distributed
Metabolism	None
Excretion	Kidneys, unchanged (80% within 24 hr); breast milk
Half-life	2½-5½ hr

Pharmacodynamics

	PO	PO—ext rel	IV
Onset	1½ hr	2 hr	2 min
Peak	8-12 hr	3-6 hr	15 min
Duration	8-12 hr	18-24 hr	4-5 hr

INTERACTIONS
Individual drugs
Amphotericin B, corticotropin, ACTH: increased hypokalemia

Arsenic trioxide, levomethadyl: increased cardiac toxicity if hypokalemia develops

CarBAMazepine, ethotoin: increased osteomalacia

CycloSPORINE: increased toxicity

Diflunisal: increased side effects

Lithium: increased excretion of lithium

Methenamine: decreased acetaZOLAMIDE effect

Primidone: decreased primidone level

Topiramate: increased renal stone formation, heat stroke, avoid concurrent use

Drug classifications
Amphetamines: increased action

Anticholinergics, folic acid antagonists: increased action of each product

Cardiac glycosides: increased cardiac toxicity if hypokalemia develops

Corticosteroids: increased hypokalemia

Flecainide, memantine, phenytoin, procainamide, quiNIDine, mecamylamine, mexiletine: increased effect of each product

Salicylates: increased toxicity

Drug/lab test
Increased: glucose, bilirubin, calcium, uric acid

Decreased: thyroid iodine uptake

False positive: urinary protein, 17-hydroxysteroids

NURSING CONSIDERATIONS
Assessment
• Assess patient for tinnitus, hearing loss, ear pain; periodic testing of hearing is needed when high doses of this product are given by **IV** route

• **Assess for seizures:** type, location, duration; provide seizure precautions

• Assess fluid volume status: I&O ratio and record, count or weigh diapers as appropriate, distended neck veins, crackles in lung, color, quality, and specific gravity of urine, skin turgor, adequacy of pulses, moist mucous membranes, bilateral lung sounds, peripheral pitting edema; dehydration symptoms of decreasing output, thirst, hypotension, dry mouth, and mucous membranes should be reported

• Monitor electrolytes: potassium, sodium, calcium, magnesium; also include BUN, blood pH, ABGs, uric acid, CBC, blood glucose

• Assess B/P before and during therapy with patient lying, standing, and sitting as appropriate; orthostatic hypotension can occur rapidly

• Monitor blood, urine glucose in diabetic patients; glucose levels may be increased

• Assess for eye pain, change in vision when using product for intraocular pressure

• Assess neurologic status when using product for seizures

• **Assess for decreased symptoms of acute mountain sickness:** headache, nausea, vomiting, dizziness, fatigue, drowsiness, shortness of breath, insomnia

• Assess for cross-sensitivity between other sulfonamides and this product

Patient/family education
• Teach patient to take the medication early in the day to prevent nocturia

• Instruct patient to take with food or milk if GI symptoms of nausea and anorexia occur

• Teach patient to maintain a record of weight on a weekly basis and notify prescriber of weight loss of >5 lb

• Caution patient that this product causes a loss of potassium, so food rich in potassium should be added to the diet; refer to a dietitian for assistance in planning

• Advise patient to wear protective clothing and sunscreen in the sun to prevent photosensitivity

• Teach patient not to use alcohol or any OTC medications without prescriber's approval; serious product reactions may occur

• Emphasize the need to contact prescriber immediately if muscle cramps, weakness, nausea, dizziness, or numbness, rapid weight changes, change in stools, rash, sore throat, bleeding/bruising, Stevens-Johnson syndrome, toxic epidermal necrolysis (red rash that spreads, blistering) occur

• Avoid prolonged sun exposure

• Teach patient to take own B/P and pulse and record

• Teach patient to continue taking medication even if feeling better; this product controls symptoms but does not cure the condition

• Teach patient to see ophthalmologist periodically; glaucoma is a slow process

• Advise patient to increase fluids to 2-3 L/day if not contraindicated

Evaluation
Positive therapeutic outcome
• Decreased intraocular pressure (glaucoma)

- Decreased edema in feet, legs, sacral area daily (CHF)
- Decreased frequency of seizures
- Prevention of altitude sickness

TREATMENT OF OVERDOSE:
Lavage if taken orally, monitor electrolytes, administer dextrose in saline, monitor hydration, CV, renal status

acetylcholine ophthalmic
See Appendix B

acetylcysteine (Rx)
(a-se-teel-sis'tay-een)
Acetadote, Mucomyst ✤
Func. class.: Mucolytic; antidote—acetaminophen
Chem. class.: Amino acid L-cysteine
Pregnancy category B

Do not confuse:
acetylcysteine/acetylcholine,
Mucomyst/Mucinex

ACTION: Decreases viscosity of secretions in respiratory tract by breaking disulfide links of mucoproteins; serves as a substrate of glutathione, which is necessary to inactivate toxic metabolites in acetaminophen overdose

Therapeutic outcome: Decreased hepatotoxicity from acetaminophen overdose (PO); decreased viscosity of mucus in respiratory disorders (inh)

USES: Acetaminophen toxicity, bronchitis, cystic fibrosis, COPD, atelectasis

CONTRAINDICATIONS:
Hypersensitivity, increased intracranial pressure, status asthmaticus

Precautions: Pregnancy **B**, breastfeeding, hypothyroidism, Addison's disease, CNS depression, brain tumor, asthma, renal/hepatic disease, COPD, psychosis, alcoholism, seizure disorders, bronchospasms, asthma, anaphylactoid reactions, fluid restriction, weight <40 kg

DOSAGE AND ROUTES
Mucolytic
Adult and child: Instill 1-20 ml (10%-20% sol) q6-8hr prn, or 3-5 ml (20% sol) or 6-10 ml (10% sol) tid or qid; nebulization (face, mask, mouthpiece, tracheostomy) 1-10 ml

of a 20% sol or 2-20 ml of a 10% sol q2-6hr; nebulization (tent, croupette) may require large dose, up to 300 ml/treatment

Acetaminophen toxicity
Adult and child: PO 140 mg/kg, then 70 mg/kg q4hr × 17 doses to total 1330 mg/kg; **IV** loading dose 150 mg/kg over 60 min (dilution 150 mg/kg in 200 ml of D_5); maintenance dose 1:50 mg/kg over 4 hr (dilution 50 mg/kg in 500 ml D_5); maintenance dose 2:100 mg/kg over 16 hr (dilution 100 mg/kg in 1000 ml D_5)

Available forms: Oral sol 10%, 20%; inj 20% (200 mg/ml)

Implementation
- Give decreased dosage to geriatric patients; their metabolism may be slowed; give gum, hard candy, frequent rinsing of mouth for dryness of oral cavity
- Use only if suction machine is available
PO route (Antidotal use)
- Give within 24 hr; dilute 10% or 20% sol to a 5% sol with diet soda; may use water if giving via gastric tube; dilution of 10% sol 1:1, 20% sol 1:3; use within 1 hr, store open undiluted solution refrigerated ≤96 hr
Direct intratracheal INSTILL
- Use ½-1 hr before meals for better absorption, to decrease nausea; only after patient clears airway by deep breathing, coughing
- Give by syringe 2-3 doses of 1-2 ml of 10%-20% sol up to q1hr; 20% sol diluted with NS or water for injection; may give 10% sol undiluted
- Store in refrigerator: use within 96 hr of opening
- Provide assistance with inhaled dose: bronchodilator if bronchospasm occurs; wash face and rinse mouth after use to remove sticky feeling
- Use decreased dose in geriatric, metabolism may be slowed
- Use mechanical suction if cough insufficient to remove excess bronchial secretions
- Store in refrigerator; use within 96 hr of opening

IV route
21-hr regimen:
- **Loading dose:** dilute 150 mg/kg in 200 ml D_5W; maintenance dose no. 1 **dilute** 50 mg/kg in 500 ml D_5W; maintenance dose no. 2 **dilute** 100 mg/kg in 1000 ml D_5W
- **Give** loading over 15 min; **give** maintenance dose no. 1 over 4 hr; **give** maintenance dose no. 2 over 16 hr; **give** sequentially without time between doses

Incompatibilities: Rubber, metals, stability with other products unknown

ADVERSE EFFECTS
CNS: Chills, *dizziness, drowsiness,* fever, headache
CV: Flushing, hypotension, tachycardia
EENT: *Rhinorrhea,* tooth damage
GI: Anorexia, constipation, diarrhea, **hepatotoxicity,** *nausea,* stomatitis, vomiting
INTEG: Clamminess, fever, pruritus, rash, urticaria
MISC: **Anaphylaxis, angioedema**
RESP: **Bronchospasm,** burning, chest tightness, cough, **hemoptysis,** dyspnea

Pharmacokinetics

Absorption	Extensive (PO), locally (inh)
Distribution	Protein binding 83%
Metabolism	Liver
Excretion	Kidneys
Half-life	5.6 hr (adult), 11 hr (newborn)

Pharmacodynamics

	PO	Inh
Onset	Unknown	5-10 min
Peak	1-2 hr (antidote)	10 min
Duration	Up to 4 hr (antidote)	1 hr

INTERACTIONS
Individual drugs
Iron, copper, nickel, activated charcoal, rubber: do not use with acetylcysteine

Drug classifications
Nitrates: increased effect

NURSING CONSIDERATIONS
Assessment
Mucolytic use
• **Assess cough:** type, frequency, character, including sputum
• **Assess characteristics, rate, rhythm of respirations,** increased dyspnea, sputum; discontinue if bronchospasm occurs; ABGs for increased CO_2 retention in asthma patients
• Monitor VS, cardiac status including checking for dysrhythmias, increased rate, palpitations
Antidotal use
• Assess liver function tests, acetaminophen levels, PT, glucose, electrolytes, BUN, creatinine; inform prescriber if dose is vomited or vomiting is persistent; provide adequate hydration; decrease dosage in hepatic encephalopathy
• Assess for nausea, vomiting, rash; notify prescriber if these occur

Patient/family education
Mucolytic use
• Tell patient to avoid driving or other hazardous activities until patient is stabilized on this medication; avoid alcohol, other CNS depressants; will enhance sedating properties of this product
• Inform patient that foul odor and smell may be unpleasant
• Instruct patient to clear airway for inhalation; that discoloration of solution after bottle is opened does not impair its effectiveness; avoid smoking, smoke-filled rooms, perfume, dust, environmental pollutants, cleaners
• Teach patient to report vomiting, as dose may need to be repeated

Evaluation
Positive therapeutic outcome
• Absence of purulent secretions when coughing (mucolytic use)
• Clear lung sounds bilaterally (mucolytic use)
• Absence of hepatic damage (acetaminophen toxicity)
• Decreasing blood toxicology (acetaminophen toxicity)

acyclovir (Rx)
(ay-sye′kloe-veer)
Zovirax
Func. class.: Antiviral
Chem. class.: Acyclic purine nucleoside analog
Pregnancy category B

Do not confuse:
Zovirax/Zyvox/Valtrex/Zostrix

ACTION: Interferes with DNA synthesis by conversion to acyclovir triphosphate, causing decreased viral replication

Therapeutic outcome: Decreased amount and time of healing of lesions

USES: Mucocutaneous herpes simplex virus, herpes genitalis (HSV-1, HSV-2), varicella infections, herpes zoster, herpes simplex encephalitis

CONTRAINDICATIONS:
Hypersensitivity to this product or valacyclovir

Precautions: Pregnancy **B**, breastfeeding, renal/hepatic disease, electrolyte imbalance, dehydration, neurologic disease; hypersensitivity to famciclovir, ganciclovir, penciclovir, valganciclovir

DOSAGE AND ROUTES
Renal dose
Adult and child: PO/IV CCr >50 ml/min 100% dose q8hr; CCr 25-50 ml/min 100% dose q12hr; CCr 10-24 ml/min 100% dose q24hr; CCr 0-10 ml/min 50% of dose q24hr

Herpes simplex
Adult: PO 400 mg 3 ×/day for 5 days or 200 mg 5 ×/day × 5 days
Adult and child >12 yr (use ideal weight in obesity): IV INF 5 mg/kg over 1 hr q8hr × 5 days
Infant >3 mo/child <12 yr: IV INF 250 mg/m² or 30 mg/kg/day divided q8hr over 1 hr × 5 days

Genital herpes
Adult: PO 200 mg q4hr (5 times a day while awake) × 5 days to 6 mo depending on whether initial, recurrent, or chronic; IV 5 mg/kg q8hr × 5 days

Genital herpes, initial limited, mucocutaneous HSV in immuno-compromised patients, non-life-threatening
Adult and child ≥12 yr: TOP cover lesions q3hr 6 times/day

Herpes simplex encephalitis
Adult: IV 10 mg/kg over 1 hr q8hr × 10 days
Child 3 mo-12 yr: IV 20 mg/kg q8hr × 10 days
Child birth-3 mo: IV 10 mg/kg q8hr × 10 days

Herpes labialis, recurrent
Adult and child ≥12 yr: TOP apply cream 5 times a day × 4 days, start as soon as symptoms appear

Herpes zoster (shingles): immuno-compromised patients
Adult and adolescent: PO 800 mg q4hr 5 times/day × 7-10 days; IV 10 mg/kg q8hr × 7 days
Child ≥12 yr: IV 10 mg/kg q8hr × 7 days
Infant and child <12 yr: IV 20 mg/kg q8hr × 7-10 days

Herpes zoster (shingles): immuno-competent patient
Adult: PO 800 mg q4hr 5 times/day × 7-10 days; start within 48-72 hr of rash onset

Varicella (chickenpox): immuno-competent patient
Adult, adolescent, and child >40 kg: PO 800 mg 4 times/day × 5 days
Child ≥2 yr and ≤40 kg: PO 20 mg/kg (max 800 mg) PO 4 times per day × 5 days

Mucosal/cutaneous herpes simplex infections in immunosup-pressed patients
Adult and child >12 yr: IV 5 mg/kg q8hr × 7 days
Infant >3 mo/child <12 yr: IV 10 mg/kg q8hr × 7 days

Recurrent ocular herpes, prevention (unlabeled)
Adult and child ≥12 yr: PO 600-800 mg/day × 8-12 mo

Available forms: Caps 200 mg; tabs 400, 800 mg; powder for inj 500, 1000 mg; sol for inj 50 mg/ml; oral susp 200 mg/5 ml; ointment/cream 5%

Implementation
PO route
• Do not break, crush, or chew caps
• Give with food to lessen GI symptoms; may give without regard to meals with 8 oz of water
• Store at room temperature in dry place
• May be taken orally before infection occurs or when itching or pain occurs, usually before eruptions
• Must be taken at equal intervals around the clock
• Shake susp before use

IV route
• Provide increased fluids to 3 L/day to decrease crystalluria, most critical during first 2 hr after IV infusion
Intermittent IV infusion route
• Reconstitute with 10 ml sterile water for injection/500 mg of product (50 mg/ml); shake; **further dilute** in 50-125 ml compatible sol, use within 12 hr; **give** over at least 1 hr (constant rate) by infusion pump to prevent nephrotoxicity; do not reconstitute with sol containing benzyl alcohol or parabens; check infusion site for redness, pain, induration; rotate sites
• Lower dosage in acute or chronic renal failure
• Store at room temp for up to 12 hr after reconstitution; if refrigerated, sol may show a precipitate that clears at room temperature; yellow discoloration does not affect potency

Topical route
- Use finger cot or glove to cover all lesions completely, do not get in eye, wash hands after use

Y-site compatibilities: Alemtazumab, allopurinol, amikacin, aminophylline, amphotericin B cholesteryl, amphotericin B liposome, ampicillin, anidulafungin, argatroban, atracurium, bivalirudin, buprenorphine, busulfan, butorphanol, calcium chloride/gluconate, CARBOplatin, ceFAZolin, cefonicid, cefoperazone, cefotaxime, cefOXitin, cefTAZidime, ceftizoxime, cefTRIAXone, cefuroxime, cephapirin, chloramphenicol, chlolesteryl sulfate compex, cimetidine, clindamycin, dexamethasone sodium phosphate, dimenhyDRINATE, DOXOrubicin, doxycycline, erythromycin, famotidine, filgrastim, fluconazole, gentamicin, granisetron, heparin, hydrocortisone sodium succinate, HYDROmorphone, imipenem-cilastatin, LORazepam, magnesium sulfate, melphalan, methylPREDNISolone sodium succinate, metoclopramide, metroNIDAZOLE, multivitamin, nafcillin, oxacillin, PACLitaxel, penicillin G potassium, PENTobarbital, perphenazine, piperacillin, potassium chloride, propofol, ranitidine, remifentanil, sodium bicarbonate, teniposide, theophylline, thiotepa, ticarcillin, tobramycin, trimethoprim-sulfamethoxazole, vancomycin, vasopressin, voriconazole, zidovudine

Y-site incompatibilities: DOBUTamine, DOPamine, ondansetron, verapamil

ADVERSE EFFECTS
CNS: Tremors, confusion, lethargy, hallucinations, **seizures,** *dizziness, headache,* encephalopathic changes
EENT: Gingival hyperplasia
GI: Nausea, vomiting, diarrhea, increased ALT, AST, abdominal pain, glossitis, colitis
GU: **Oliguria, proteinuria, hematuria,** vaginitis, moniliasis, **glomerulonephritis, acute renal failure,** changes in menses, polydipsia
HEMA: **Thrombotic thrombocytopenia purpura, hemolytic uremic syndrome** (immunocompromised patient)
INTEG: Rash, urticaria, pruritus, pain or phlebitis at **IV** site, unusual sweating, alopecia, **Stevens-Johnson syndrome**
MS: Joint pain, leg pain, muscle cramps

Pharmacokinetics

Absorption	Minimal (PO)
Distribution	Widely distributed, crosses placenta; CSF concentration 50% plasma; protein binding 9%-33%
Metabolism	Liver, minimal
Excretion	Kidneys, 95% unchanged
Half-life	2.0-3.5 hr, increased in renal disease

Pharmacodynamics

	PO	IV
Onset	Unknown	Rapid
Peak	2.5-3.3 hr	Infusion's end
Duration	Unknown	Unknown

INTERACTIONS
Individual drugs
Aminoglycosides: increased nephrotoxicity
Entecavir, PEMEtrexed, tenofovir: increased concentration of each product
Probenecid: increased neurotoxicity, nephrotoxicity
Valproic acid: decreased action of valproic acid
Zidovudine, IT methotrexate: increased CNS side effects

Drug classifications
Hydantoins: decreased actions of hydantoins

NURSING CONSIDERATIONS
Assessment
- **Monitor for signs of infection,** type of lesions, area of body covered, purulent drainage
- Check I&O ratio; report hematuria, oliguria, fatigue, weakness; may indicate nephrotoxicity; check for protein in urine during treatment
- **Toxicity:** monitor any patient with compromised renal system, since product is excreted slowly in poor renal system function; toxicity may occur rapidly
- Monitor liver studies: AST, ALT
- Monitor renal studies: urinalysis, protein, BUN, creatinine, CCr; increased BUN, creatinine indicates renal failure and **nephrotoxicity**
- Monitor bowel pattern before, during treatment; if severe abdominal pain with bleeding occurs, product should be discontinued
- Assess allergies before treatment, reaction of each medication; place allergies on chart in bright red letters; allergic reaction: burning, stinging, swelling, redness, rash, vulvitis, pruritus
- Assess neurologic status in herpes encephalitis

Patient/family education
PO route
• Teach patient that product may be taken orally before infection occurs or when itching or pain occur, usually before eruptions; that partners need to be told that patient has herpes; they can become infected, so condoms must be worn to prevent reinfections

⚠ **Tell patient to report sore throat, fever, fatigue; may indicate superinfection; that product must be taken at equal intervals around the clock to maintain blood levels for duration of therapy**

• Tell patient to notify prescriber of side effects: bruising, bleeding, fatigue, malaise; may indicate blood dyscrasias
• Adequate intake of fluids (2 L) to prevent deposits in kidneys, more likely to occur with rapid administration or in dehydration
• Tell patient to seek dental care during treatment to prevent gingival hyperplasia
• Teach female patients with genital herpes to have regular Pap smears to prevent undetected cervical cancer

Evaluation
Positive therapeutic outcome
• Absence of itching, painful lesions
• Crusting and healed lesions

TREATMENT OF OVERDOSE:
Discontinue product, hemodialysis, resuscitate if needed

acyclovir topical
See Appendix B

adalimumab (Rx)
(add-a-lim'yu-mab)
Humira
Func. class.: Antirheumatic agent (disease modifying), immunomodulator, anti-TNF
Pregnancy category B

Do not confuse:
Humira/Humalin/Humalog

ACTION: A form of human IgG1 monoclonal antibody specific for human tumor necrosis factor (TNF); elevated levels of TNF are found in patients with rheumatoid arthritis

Therapeutic outcome: Decreased pain, inflammation in joints, better ROM

USES: Reduction in signs and symptoms and inhibiting progression of structural damage in patients with moderate to severe active rheumatoid arthritis in patients ≥18 years of age who have not responded to other disease-modifying agents, JRA, psoriatic arthritis, Crohn's disease, moderate-severe plaque psoriasis, ankylosing spondylitis

CONTRAINDICATIONS:
Hypersensitivity

Precautions: Pregnancy **B**, breastfeeding, children, geriatric, CNS demyelinating disease, lymphoma, latent TB, CHF, hepatitis B carriers, manitol hypersensitivity, latex allergy, neoplastic disease

> **BLACK BOX WARNING:** Active infections, risk of lymphomas/leukemias, TB

DOSAGE AND ROUTES
Rheumatoid arthritis, ankylosing spondylitis, psoriatic arthritis
Adult: SUBCUT 40 mg every other wk or every week if not combined with methotrexate

Juvenile rheumatoid arthritis (JRA)
Child ≥4 yr/adolescent ≥30 kg: SUBCUT 40 mg every other wk
Child ≥4 yr/adolescent ≥15 kg to <30 kg: SUBCUT 20 mg every other wk
Child ≥4 yr/adolescent <15 kg: SUBCUT 24 mg/m² BSA (up to 40 mg total) every other wk, then 20 mg every other wk

Crohn's disease
Adult: SUBCUT 160 mg given as 4 inj on day 1, or 2 inj on days 1 and 2, then 80 mg at wk 2 and 40 mg every other wk, starting at wk 4

Plaque psoriasis
Adult: SUBCUT 80 mg baseline as 2 inj, then 40 mg every other week starting 1 wk after initial dose × 16 wk

Available forms: Inj 40 mg/0.8 ml; 20 mg/0.4 ml (pediatric)

Implementation
SUBCUT route
• Do not admix with other sol or medications, do not use filter, protect from light

ADVERSE EFFECTS
CNS: Headache, **Guillain-Barré syndrome**
CV: Hypertension, CHF
EENT: Sinusitis

Adverse effects: *italics* = common; **bold** = life-threatening

GI: Abdominal pain, nausea, hepatic damage, **GI bleeding**
HEMA: **Leukopenia, pancytopenia, aplastic anemia, agranulocytopenia, thrombocytopenia**
INTEG: Rash, *inj site reaction*
MISC: Flulike symptoms, UTI, hypertension, back pain, lupuslike syndrome, risk of cancer, antibody development to this drug, **risk of infection (TB, invasive fungal infections, other opportunistic infections); may be fatal, Stevens-Johnson syndrome,** anaphylaxis
RESP: *URI,* **pulmonary fibrosis,** bronchitis

Pharmacokinetics

Absorption	Unknown
Distribution	Unknown
Metabolism	Unknown
Excretion	Unknown
Half-life	Terminal 2 wk

Pharmacodynamics

Unknown

INTERACTIONS

Individual drugs
Anakinra: do not use together, serious infections may occur
Rilonacept: increase serious infections

Drug classifications
Vaccines: do not give concurrently; immunization should be brought up to date before treatment
Other TNF blockers: increased serious infections

Drug/lab test
Increased: ALT, cholesterol

NURSING CONSIDERATIONS

Assessment
• Rheumatoid arthritis: assess for pain, stiffness, ROM, swelling of joints during treatment
• Check for inj site pain, swelling, redness; usually occur after 2 inj (4-5 days) use cold compress to relieve pain/swelling

> **BLACK BOX WARNING:** Check for infections, fever, flulike symptoms, dyspnea, change in urination, redness/swelling around wounds, stop treatment if present, some serious infections, including sepsis, may occur; patients with active infections should not be started on this product

• May reactivate hepatitis B in chronic carriers, may be fatal

> **BLACK BOX WARNING:** Assess for latent TB prior to therapy; treat before starting this product

• Assess for anaphylaxis, latex allergic; stop therapy if lupuslike syndrome develops
• Assess for blood dyscrasias: CBC, differential periodically

> **BLACK BOX WARNING:** Assess for neoplastic disease (lymphomas/leukemia); in children, adolescents, hepatosplenic T-cell lymphoma is more likely in adolescent males with Crohn's disease or ulcerative colitis

Patient/family education
• Teach patient about self-administration if appropriate: inj should be made in thigh, abdomen, upper arm; rotate sites at least 1 inch from old site; do not inject in areas that are bruised, red, hard
• Advise patient that if medication is not taken when due, inject next dose as soon as remembered and inject next dose as scheduled
• Advise patient not to take any live-virus vaccines during treatment
⚠ **Instruct patient to report signs of infection, allergic reactions, lupuslike syndrome, immediately**

Evaluation
Positive therapeutic outcome
• Decreased inflammation, pain in joints, decreased joint destruction

---

adefovir (Rx)
(add-ee-foh´veer)
Hepsera
Func. class.: Antiviral
Pregnancy category C

ACTION: Inhibits hepatitis B virus DNA polymerase by competing with natural substrates and by causing DNA termination after its incorporation into viral DNA; causes viral DNA death

Therapeutic outcome: Improving liver function tests, lessening symptoms of chronic hepatitis B

USES: Chronic hepatitis B

CONTRAINDICATIONS:
Hypersensitivity

Precautions: Pregnancy **C,** breastfeeding, children, geriatric, dialysis, females, labor, obesity, organ transplant

---

BLACK BOX WARNING: Severe renal disease, impaired hepatic disease, lactic acidosis, HIV

DOSAGE AND ROUTES
Adult/adolescent: PO 10 mg daily, optimal duration unknown

Renal dose
Adult: PO CCr $\geq$50 ml/min 10 mg q24hr; CCr 30-49 ml/min 10 mg q48hr; CCr 10-29 ml/min 10 mg q72hr; hemodialysis 10 mg q7 days following dialysis

Available forms: Tabs 10 mg

Implementation
• Give by mouth without regard to food
• Store in cool environment; protect from light
• Take with full glass of water

ADVERSE EFFECTS
CNS: *Headache*
GI: *Dyspepsia,* abdominal pain, nausea, vomiting, diarrhea, hepatomegaly, flatulence, **pancreatitis**
GU: Hematuria, glycosuria, **nephrotoxicity, Fanconi syndrome, renal failure**
MISC: Fever, rash, weight loss, cough

Pharmacokinetics

Absorption	Rapidly from GI tract
Distribution	Unknown
Metabolism	Unknown
Excretion	Kidneys 45%
Half-life	7.48 hr

Pharmacodynamics

Onset	Unknown
Peak	1¾ hr
Duration	Unknown

INTERACTIONS
Individual drugs
AMILoride, cimetidine, cycloSPORINE, digoxin, dofetilide, efavirenz, emtricitabine, memantine, metformin, midodrine, morphine, PEMEtrexed, procainamide, quiNIDine, quinine, ranitidine, tacrolimus, tenofovir, triamterene, trospium, vancomycin: increased serum concentrations, toxicity
Do not use in combination with emtricitabine/tenofovir, emtricitabine/rilpivirine, emtricitabine/efavirenz/tenofovir

Drug classifications
Benzodiazepines, nucleoside analogs (experimental), NSAIDs, sulfonamides: increased serum concentrations, toxicity

BLACK BOX WARNING: Lactic acidosis, severe hepatomegaly, NNRTIs, NRTIs, antiretroviral protease-inhibitors, aminoglycosides

Drug/lab test
Increased: ALT, AST, amylase, creatine kinase

NURSING CONSIDERATIONS
Assessment

BLACK BOX WARNING: Assess **nephrotoxicity:** increasing CCr, BUN

BLACK BOX WARNING: Assess for HIV antibody testing before beginning treatment because HIV resistance may occur in chronic hepatitis B patients

BLACK BOX WARNING: Assess **lactic acidosis,** severe hepatomegaly with stenosis, more common in females, obesity, and prolonged nucleoside use

• Assess geriatric patients more carefully; may develop renal, cardiac symptoms more rapidly

BLACK BOX WARNING: Assess exacerbations of **hepatitis** after discontinuing treatment, monitor liver function tests, hepatitis B serology

• Pregnancy: If planned or suspected; if pregnant call the Pregnancy Registry 800-258-4263

Patient/family education
• Advise patient that optimal duration of treatment is unknown, that drug is not a cure; transmission may still occur
• Advise patient to avoid use with other medications unless approved by prescriber
• Advise patient to notify prescriber of decreased urinary output
• Teach patient not to stop abruptly unless directed, worsening of hepatitis may occur
• Teach patient to report immediately dyspnea, nausea, vomiting, abdominal pain, weakness, dizziness, cold extremities
• Teach patient to notify prescriber if pregnancy is planned or suspected, avoid breastfeeding

Evaluation
Positive therapeutic outcome
• Decreased symptoms of chronic hepatitis B, improving liver function tests

> ⚠️ **HIGH ALERT**

adenosine (Rx)
(ah-den'oh-seen)
Func. class.: Antidysrhythmic—
miscellaneous
Chem. class.: Endogenous nucleoside
Pregnancy category C

ACTION: Slows conduction through AV node, can interrupt reentry pathways through AV node, and can restore normal sinus rhythm in patients with paroxysmal supraventricular tachycardia (PSVT), decreases cardiac oxygen demand decreasing hypoxia

Therapeutic outcome: Normal sinus rhythm in patients diagnosed with SVT or diagnosis of perfusion defect

USES: PSVT, as a diagnostic aid to assess myocardial perfusion defects in CAD; Wolff-Parkinson-White (WPW) syndrome

CONTRAINDICATIONS:
Hypersensitivity, 2nd- or 3rd-degree heart block, AV block, sick sinus syndrome

Precautions: Pregnancy **C,** breastfeeding, children, geriatric, asthma, atrial flutter, atrial fibrillation, ventricular tachycardia, bronchospastic lung disease, symptomatic bradycardia, bundle branch block, heart transplant, unstable angina, COPD, hypotension, hypovolemia, vascular heart disease, CV disease

DOSAGE AND ROUTES
Antidysrhythmic
Adult and child >50 kg: **IV** BOL 6 mg; if conversion to normal sinus rhythm does not occur within 1-2 min, give 12 mg by rapid **IV** BOL; may repeat 12 mg dose again in 1-2 min
Infant and child <50 kg: **IV** BOL 0.05 mg/kg; if not effective, increase dose by 0.05-0.1 mg/kg q2min to a max of 0.3 mg/kg/dose
Neonate: **IV** BOL: 0.05 mg/kg by rapid **IV** BOL, may increase by 0.05 mg/kg q2min, max 0.3 mg/kg/dose

Implementation
IV, direct (bolus) route
• Give **IV** BOL undiluted; give 6 mg or less by rapid inj; if using an **IV** line, use port near insertion site, flush with 0.9% NaCl (20 ml), then elevate arm
• Store at room temperature; sol should be clear; discard unused product

Solution compatibilities: D$_5$LR, D$_5$W, LR, 0.9% NaCl

ADVERSE EFFECTS
CNS: Light-headedness, dizziness, arm tingling, numbness, headache
CV: Chest pain/pressure, **atrial tachydysrhythmias,** sweating, palpitations, hypotension, *facial flushing,* **AV block, cardiac arrest, ventricular dysrhythmias, atrial fibrillation**
GI: *Nausea,* metallic taste
RESP: *Dyspnea, chest pressure,* hyperventilation, **bronchospasm (asthmatics)**

Pharmacokinetics

Absorption	Complete bioavailability
Distribution	Erythrocytes, cardiovascular endothelium
Metabolism	Liver, converted to inosine and adenosine monophosphate
Excretion	Kidneys
Half-life	10 sec

Pharmacodynamics

Onset	Rapid
Peak	Unknown
Duration	1-2 min

INTERACTIONS
Individual drugs
Caffeine, theophylline: decreased effects of adenosine
CarBAMazepine: increased heart block
Digoxin, verapamil: increased ventricular fibrillation
Dipyridamole: increased effects of adenosine
Smoking: increased tachycardia

Drug/herb
Ginger: increased effect
Green tea, guarana: decreased effect

NURSING CONSIDERATIONS
Assessment
• **Assess cardiopulmonary status:** pulse, respiration, ECG intervals (PR, QRS, QT); check for transient dysrhythmias (PVCs, PACs, sinus tachycardia, AV block)
• Assess respiratory status: rate, rhythm, lung fields for crackles, watch for respiratory depression; bilateral crackles may occur in CHF patient; if increased respiration, increased pulse occurs, product should be discontinued

---

• Assess CNS effects: dizziness, confusion, paresthesias; product should be discontinued

Patient/family education
• Tell patient to report facial flushing, dizziness, sweating, palpitations, chest pain

Evaluation
Positive therapeutic outcome
• Normal sinus rhythm
• Diagnosis of perfusion defect

---

albumin, human 5% (Rx)
(al-byoo'min)
Albumarc, Albuminar-5, Albutein 5%, Buminate 5%, Plasbumin-5
albumin, human 25% (Rx)
Albuminar-25, Albutein 25%, Buminate 25%, Plasbumin-25
Func. class.: Blood derivative—plasma volume expander
Pregnancy category C

ACTION: Exerts colloidal oncotic pressure, which expands volume of circulating blood by pulling fluid from extravascular to intravascular spaces, and maintains cardiac output

Therapeutic outcome: Increased B/P, decreased edema, increased serum albumin levels, increased plasma protein

USES: Restores plasma volume in burns, hyperbilirubinemia, shock, hypoproteinemia, prevention of cerebral edema, cardiopulmonary bypass procedures, ARDS, hemorrhage; also replacement in nephrotic syndrome

CONTRAINDICATIONS:
Hypersensitivity, CHF, severe anemia, renal insufficiency, pulmonary edema

Precautions: Pregnancy C, decreased salt intake, decreased cardiac reserve, lack of albumin deficiency, renal/hepatic disease, chronic anemia

DOSAGE AND ROUTES
Burns
Adult: **IV** dose to maintain plasma albumin at 3-4 mg/dl

Hypovolemic shock
Adult: **IV** Rapidly give 5% sol; when close to normal, infuse at ≤2-4 ml/min; 25% sol ≤1 ml/min
Child: 0.5-1 g/kg/dose, 5% sol, may repeat as needed; max 6 g/kg/day

Nephrotic syndrome
Adult: **IV** 100-200 mg of 25% and loop diuretic × 7-10 days

Hypoproteinemia
Adult: **IV** 25 g, may repeat in 15-30 min, or 50-75 g of 25% albumin infused at ≤2 ml/min
Child/infant: **IV** 0.5-1 g/kg/dose over 2-4 hr, may repeat q1-2days

Hyperbilirubinemia/erythroblastosis fetalis
Infant: **IV** 1 g/kg 1-2 hr before transfusion

Available forms: Inj 50, 250 mg/ml (5%, 25%)

Implementation
IV route
• Check type of albumin; some are stored at room temperature, some need to be refrigerated; use only amber-colored sol without precipitate; solution should be clear, use within 4 hr of opening
• Give **IV** slowly to prevent fluid overload; 5% sol may be given undiluted; 25% sol may be given diluted (D₅W, 0.9% NaCl) or undiluted; give over 4 hr, use infusion pump
• Provide adequate hydration before, during administration; whole blood may need to be given to prevent anemia; monitor hydration during treatment
• 5% sol may be used in hypovolemic/intravascular depletion
• 25% sol may be used in sodium/fluid restriction

Y-site compatibilities: Diltiazem

Solution compatibilities: LR, NaCl, Ringer's, D₅W, D₁₀W, D₂½W, dextrose/saline, dextran₆ D₅, dextran₆ NaCl 0.9%, dextrose/Ringer's, dextrose/LR

ADVERSE EFFECTS
CNS: Fever, chills, flushing, headache
CV: Fluid overload, hypotension, erratic pulse, tachycardia
GI: Nausea, vomiting, increased salivation
INTEG: Rash, urticaria
RESP: Altered respirations, **pulmonary edema**

Pharmacokinetics

Absorption	Complete bioavailability
Distribution	Intravascular spaces
Metabolism	Liver
Excretion	Unknown
Half-life	Terminal, 21 days

Pharmacodynamics

Onset	15-30 min
Peak	Unknown
Duration	Unknown

INTERACTIONS
Drug/lab test
Increased: alkaline phosphatase

NURSING CONSIDERATIONS
Assessment
• Monitor blood studies: Hct, Hgb; if serum protein declines, dyspnea, hypoxemia can result; check for decreasing B/P, erratic pulse, respiration

• Adequate hydration before, during administration

• Check type of albumin; some stored at room temp, some need to be refrigerated, use within 4 hr of opening

⚠ **Monitor CVP: pulmonary wedge pressure will increase if overload occurs; I&O ratio: urinary output may decrease; CVP reading: distended neck veins indicate circulatory overload; shortness of breath, anxiety, insomnia, expiratory crackles, frothy blood-tinged sputum, cough, cyanosis indicate pulmonary overload**

• Assess for allergy: fever, rash, itching, chills, flushing, urticaria, nausea, vomiting, hypotension; requires discontinuation of infusion, use of new lot if therapy reinstituted; premedicate with diphenhydrAMINE

Patient/family education
• Explain use, reason for albumin; provide information on what to report to prescriber (hypersensitivity, fluid overload)

Evaluation
Positive therapeutic outcome
• Increased B/P, decreased edema (shock, burns)

• Increased serum albumin levels

• Increased plasma protein (hypoproteinemia)

albuterol (Rx)
(al-byoo'ter-ole)
**AccuNeb, Gen-Salbutamol ✦,
Airomir, Apo-Salvent ✦, Proair HFA,
Proventil, Proventil HFA, Relion,
Ventolin HFA, Vospire ER**
Func. class.: Bronchodilator
Chem. class.: Adrenergic β_2-agonist, sympathomimetic, bronchodilator
Pregnancy category C

Do not confuse:
albuterol/atenolol/Albutein, **Proventil**/Prinivil, **Ventolin**/Vantin

ACTION: Causes bronchodilatation by action on β_2 (pulmonary) receptors by increasing levels of cyclic AMP, which relaxes smooth muscle; produces bronchodilatation; CNS, cardiac stimulation, increased diuresis, and increased gastric acid secretion; longer acting than isoproterenol

Therapeutic outcome: Increased ability to breathe because of bronchodilatation

USES: Prevention of exercise-induced asthma, acute bronchospasm, bronchitis, emphysema, bronchiectasis, reversible airway obstruction

Unlabeled uses: Hyperkalemia in dialysis patients

CONTRAINDICATIONS:
Hypersensitivity to sympathomimetics, tachydysrhythmias, severe cardiac disease, heart block

Precautions: Pregnancy **C**, breastfeeding, exercise-induced bronchospasm (aerosol) in children <12 yr, cardiac/renal disease, hyperthyroidism, diabetes mellitus, hypertension, prostatic hypertrophy, closed-angle glaucoma, seizures, hypoglycemia

DOSAGE AND ROUTES
Bronchospasm
Adult and child ≥4 yr: INH (metered dose inhaler) 2 puffs q4-6hr prn

Other respiratory conditions
Adult and child ≥12 yr: INH (metered dose inhaler) 1 puff q4-6hr; PO 2-4 mg tid-qid, max 32 mg/day, depending on formulation; NEB/IPPB 2.5 mg tid-qid
Geriatric: PO 2 mg tid-qid, may increase gradually to 8 mg tid-qid

Child 2-12 yr: INH (metered dose inhaler) 0.1 mg/kg tid (max 2.5 mg tid-qid); NEB/IPPB 0.1-0.15 mg/kg/dose tid-qid or 1.25 mg tid-qid for child 10-15 kg or 2.5 mg tid-qid >15 kg

Available forms: Aerosol 90 mcg/actuation; tabs 2, 4 mg; oral syr 2 mg/5 ml; ext rel 4, 8 mg; inh sol 0.5, 0.83, 1, 2, 5 mg/ml; powder for inh (Ventodisk) 200, 400 mcg; inh caps 200 mcg; 100 mcg/spray, 80 inh/canister, 200 inh/canister

Implementation
PO route
- Do not break, crush, or chew ext rel tabs
- Give PO with meals to decrease gastric irritation; oral sol for children (no alcohol, sugar)
- In geriatric patients, a spacing device is advised

Aerosol route
- Give after shaking metered dose inhaler; have patient exhale and place mouthpiece in mouth, inhale slowly while depressing inhaler, hold breath, remove inhaler, exhale slowly; allow at least 1 min between inhalations; avoid using near flames or source of heat
- Track number of inhalations used and discard when labeled inhalations have been used
- Store in light-resistant container; do not expose to temperatures >86° F (30° C)

Nebulizer/IPPB route
- **Dilute** 5 mg/ml sol/2.5 ml 0.9% NaCl for inhalation; other solutions do not require dilution for nebulizer O_2 flow or compressed air 6-10 L/min

ADVERSE EFFECTS
CNS: *Tremors, anxiety,* insomnia, headache, dizziness, stimulation, *restlessness,* hallucinations, flushing, irritability
CV: *Palpitations, tachycardia, hypertension,* angina, hypotension, dysrhythmias
EENT: Dry nose, irritation of nose and throat
GI: *Heartburn, nausea, vomiting*
MISC: Flushing, sweating, anorexia, bad taste/smell changes, hypokalemia
MS: Muscle cramps
RESP: Cough, wheezing, dyspnea, **bronchospasm,** dry throat

Pharmacokinetics

Absorption	Well absorbed (PO)
Distribution	Unknown
Metabolism	Liver extensively, tissues
Excretion	Unknown, breast milk
Half-life	3-4 hr

Pharmacodynamics

	PO	PO—ext rel	INH
Onset	½ hr	½ hr	5-15 min
Peak	2½ hr	2-3 hr	1-1½ hr
Duration	4-6 hr	12 hr	4-6 hr

INTERACTIONS
Individual drugs
Atomoxetine, selegiline: increased CV effects
Digoxin: increased digoxin level

Drug classifications
Adrenergics: increased action of albuterol; do not use together
β-Adrenergic blockers: block therapeutic effect
Bronchodilators (aerosol): increased action of bronchodilator
CNS stimulants: increased CNS stimulation
Diuretics (potassium-losing): increased ECG changes/hypokalemia
MAOIs, tricyclics: increased chance of hypertensive crisis; do not use together
Other drugs that increase QT prolongation: increased QTc prolongation
Oxytocics: severe hypotension; do not use together
Theophylline: toxicity

Drug/herb
Black tea, green tea, kola nut, guarana, yerba maté: increased stimulation

Drug/food
Caffeine products, chocolate: increased stimulation

Drug/lab test
Decreased: potassium

NURSING CONSIDERATIONS
Assessment
- Assess respiratory function: vital capacity, forced expiratory volume, ABGs, lung sounds; heart rate, rhythm; B/P, sputum (baseline and during therapy)
- Determine that patient has not received theophylline therapy before giving dose, to prevent additive effect; client's ability to self-medicate
- Monitor for evidence of allergic reactions; paradoxic bronchospasm; withhold dose; notify prescriber if bronchospasm occurs

Patient/family education
- Tell patient not to use OTC medications before consulting prescriber; excess stimulation may occur; instruct patient to use this medication before other medications and allow at least 5 min between each to prevent overstimulation; to

limit caffeine products such as chocolate, coffee, tea, and cola
- Teach patient to use inhaler; review package insert with patient; to avoid getting aerosol in eyes or blurring may result; to wash inhaler in warm water and dry daily; to rinse mouth after using; to avoid smoking, smoke-filled rooms, persons with respiratory infections

⚠ Teach patient that if paradoxic broncho-spasm occurs to stop product immediately and notify prescriber
- Instruct patient on administration of dose, not to use more than prescribed; serious side effects may occur; if taking PO regularly and dose is missed, take when remembered; space other doses on new time schedule; do not double doses
- In geriatric patients, a spacing device is advised

Evaluation
Positive therapeutic outcome
- Absence of dyspnea and wheezing after 1 hr
- Improved airway exchange
- Improved ABGs

TREATMENT OF OVERDOSE:
Administer a β_1-adrenergic blocker, **IV** fluids

---

alendronate (Rx)
(al-en′droe-nate)
Apo-Alendronate ✦, CO Alendronate, Fosamax, Fosamax plus D
Func. class.: Bone-resorption inhibitor
Chem. class.: Bisphosphonate
Pregnancy category C   ✳

Do not confuse:
Fosamax/Flomax

ACTION: Decreases rate of bone resorption and may directly block dissolution of hy-droxyapatite crystals of bone; inhibits osteoclast activity

Therapeutic outcome: Decreased symptoms of osteoporosis, Paget's disease

USES: Treatment and prevention of osteoporosis in postmenopausal women, treatment of osteoporosis in men, Paget's disease, treatment of corticosteroid-induced osteoporosis in postmenopausal women not receiving estrogen, or in men who are continuing corticosteroid treatment with low bone mass

CONTRAINDICATIONS:
Hypersensitivity to bisphosphonates, delayed esophageal emptying, inability to sit or stand for 30 min, hypocalcemia

Precautions: Pregnancy **C**, breastfeeding, children, CCr <35 ml/min, esophageal disease, increased esophageal cancer risk, ulcers, gastritis, poor dental health

DOSAGE AND ROUTES
Osteoporosis in postmenopausal women
Adult and geriatric: PO 10 mg daily or 70 mg qwk

Osteoporosis in men
Adult: PO 10 mg/day or 70 mg qwk

Paget's disease
Adult and geriatric: PO 40 mg daily × 6 mo, consider retreatment for relapse

Prevention of osteoporosis
Adult (postmenopausal females): PO 5 mg daily or 35 mg qwk

Corticosteroid-induced osteoporosis in postmenopausal women (not receiving estrogen)
Adult: PO 10 mg daily

Corticosteroid-induced osteoporosis in men or premenopausal women (not receiving estrogen)
Adult: PO 5 mg daily

Renal dose
Adult: PO CCr ≤35 ml/min, not recommended

Available forms: Tabs 5, 10, 35, 40, 70 mg, tabs 70 mg with 2800 IU Vit D_3, 70 mg with 5600 IU Vit D_3; oral sol 70 mg/75 ml

Implementation
- Give PO for 6 mo to be effective in Paget's disease; take with 8 oz of water 30 min before 1st food, beverage, or medication of the day
- Patient to remain upright for 30 min after dose to prevent esophageal irritation
- Store in cool environment out of direct sunlight

Tablet:
- Do not lie down for ≥30 min after dose, do not take at bedtime

Liquid:
- Use oral syringe or calibrated device; give in AM with ≥2 oz of water ≥30 min before food, beverage, or medication

---

ADVERSE EFFECTS
CNS: Headache
GI: Abdominal pain, constipation, nausea, vomiting, esophageal ulceration, acid reflux, dyspepsia, **esophageal perforation,** diarrhea, **esophageal cancer**
META: Hypophosphatemia, hypocalcemia
MS: Bone pain, **osteonecrosis of the jaw, bone fractures**
SYST: Angioedema, Stevens-Johnson syndrome, toxic epidermal necrolysis

Pharmacokinetics

Absorption	Bioavailability 60%
Distribution	Mainly to bones; protein binding 78%
Metabolism	Unknown
Excretion	Via kidneys after bound to bone
Half-life	>10 yrs

Pharmacodynamics
Unknown

INTERACTIONS
Drug classifications
Aminoglycosides, antacids, calcium supplements: decreased absorption
H_2 blockers, proton pump inhibitors (PPIs), gastric mucosal agents, NSAIDs, salicylates: adverse GI reactions

Drug/food
Caffeine, food, orange juice: decreased product absorption

Drug/lab test
Decreased: calcium, phosphate

NURSING CONSIDERATIONS
Assessment
⚠ **Assess for serious reactions: angioedema, Stevens-Johnson syndrome, toxic epidermal necrolysis, atrial fibrillation**
• Assess dental status, regular dental exams should be done; dental extractions (cover with antiinfectives) prior to procedure
• Hormonal status if a woman, prior to treatment
• Assess for **osteoporosis:** bone density testing
• For **Paget's disease:** increased skull size, bone pain, headache
• Monitor renal studies and electrolytes (calcium, potassium, magnesium, phosphorous) BUN/creatinine

• Assess for **hypercalcemia:** paresthesia, twitching, laryngospasm, Chvostek's, Trousseau's signs
• Monitor alkaline phosphatase; level of $2 \times$ upper limit of normal is indicated for Paget's disease

Patient/family education
• Teach patient to remain upright for 30 min after dose to prevent esophageal irritation; if dose is missed, skip dose, do not double doses or take later in day
• Teach patient to take in AM, only before food, other meds, to take with 6-8 oz of water (not mineral water)
• Teach patient to take calcium, vit D if instructed by provider
• Teach patient to use weight-bearing exercise to increase bone density
• Teach patient to let provider know if pregnancy is planned or suspected or if nursing
• Advise to maintain good oral hygiene

Evaluation
Positive therapeutic outcome
• Increased bone mass, absence of fractures

alfuzosin (Rx)
(al-fyoo′zoe-sin)
Uroxatral
Func. class.: Urinary tract, antispasmodic, α_1-agonist
Chem. class.: Quinazolone
Pregnancy category B

ACTION: Binds preferentially to α_{1A}-adrenoceptor subtype located mainly in the prostate, relaxing smooth muscles

Therapeutic outcome: Resolution of symptoms of benign prostatic hyperplasia

USES: Symptoms of benign prostatic hyperplasia

CONTRAINDICATIONS:
Hypersensitivity, moderate to severe hepatic impairment, not indicated for use in women or children, breastfeeding (but not used in women)

Precautions: Pregnancy **B**, geriatric, coronary artery disease, coronary insufficiency, mild hepatic disease, mild/moderate/severe renal disease, history of QT prolongation or coadministration with medications known to prolong QT interval, torsades de pointes, syncope, surgery, prostate cancer, orthostatic hypotension, ocular surgery, CAD, dysrhythmias, angina

DOSAGE AND ROUTES
Adult: PO EXT REL 10 mg daily, taken after same meal each day

Available forms: EXT REL tabs 10 mg

Implementation
• Swallow tabs whole; do not break, crush, or chew tabs
• Store in tight container in cool environment

ADVERSE EFFECTS
CNS: *Dizziness, headache,* fatigue, flushing
CV: Postural hypotension (dizziness, light-headedness, fainting) within a few hours of administration, chest pain, tachycardia, angina
GI: Nausea, abdominal pain, dyspepsia, constipation, diarrhea, liver injury, jaundice
GU: Impotence, priapism
HEMA: Thrombocytopenia
INTEG: Rash, urticaria, **angioedema,** pruritus
MISC: Body pain in general, xerostomia, rhinitis
RESP: Upper respiratory tract infection, pharyngitis, bronchitis, sinusitis

Pharmacokinetics

Absorption	Unknown
Distribution	Moderately protein bound (82%-90%)
Metabolism	Liver (by CYP3A4 enzyme)
Excretion	Urine
Half-life	10 hr

Pharmacodynamics
Unknown

INTERACTIONS
Individual drugs
Alcohol: possible increased effects of alfuzosin
Doxazosin, itraconazole, ketoconazole, prazosin, ritonavir, terazosin: do not take concurrently

Drug classifications
b-Blockers, nitrates, phosphodiesterase 5 inhibitors: increased hypotension
CYP3A4 inhibitors (ketoconazole, itraconazole, ritonavir): do not take concurrently

NURSING CONSIDERATIONS
Assessment
• Assess for prostatic hyperplasia: change in urinary patterns, baseline and throughout treatment

• Monitor CBC with differential and liver function tests; B/P and heart rate; QT prolongation
• Monitor BUN, uric acid, urodynamic studies (urinary flow rates, residual volume)
• Monitor I&O ratios, weight daily, edema; report weight gain or edema

Patient/family education
• Advise not to drive or operate machinery for 4 hr after first dose or after dosage increase

Evaluation
Positive therapeutic outcome
• Decreased symptoms of benign prostatic hyperplasia

aliskiren (Rx)
(a-lis′kir-en)
Tekturna
Func. class.: Antihypertensive
Chem. class.: Direct renin inhibitor
Pregnancy category
C (1st trimester)
D (2nd/3rd trimesters)

ACTION: Renin inhibitor that acts on the renin-angiotensin system (RAS)

Therapeutic outcome: Decrease in B/P

USES: Hypertension, alone or in combination with other antihypertensives

CONTRAINDICATIONS:
Hypersensitivity

BLACK BOX WARNING: Pregnancy **D**

Precautions: Breastfeeding, children, geriatric, angioedema, aortic/renal artery stenosis, cirrhosis, CAD, dialysis, hyper/hypokalemia, hyponatremia, hypotension, hypovolemia, renal/hepatic disease, surgery, diabetes

DOSAGE AND ROUTES
Adult: PO 150 mg/day, may increase to 300 mg/day if needed, max 300 mg/day

Available forms: Tabs 150, 300 mg

Implementation
• PO; do not use with a high-fat meal
• Give daily with a full glass of water, titrate up to achieve correct dose
• Do not discontinue abruptly; correct electrolyte/volume depletion prior to treatment
• Store in tight container at room temperature

⚠ Nurse Alert   ✴ Key NCLEX® Drug

ADVERSE EFFECTS

CNS: Headache, dizziness, **torsades de pointes, seizures**
CV: Orthostatic hypotension, hypotension
GI: *Diarrhea*
GU: Renal stones, increased uric acid
INTEG: Rash
META: Hyperkalemia
MISC: **Angioedema**, cough

Pharmacokinetics

Absorption	Poor, bioavailability 2.5%
Distribution	Steady state 7-8 days
Metabolism	Unknown
Excretion	91% unchanged in the feces
Half-life	Unknown

Pharmacodynamics

Onset	Unknown
Peak	1-3 hr
Duration	Unknown

INTERACTIONS

Individual drugs

Atorvastatin, cycloSPORINE, itraconazole, ketoconazole: increased aliskiren levels, concurrent use is not recommended
Warfarin: decreased levels of warfarin

Drug classifications

Do not use with ACE inhibitors, angiotensin II receptor antagonists, potassium-sparing diuretics, potassium supplements: increased potassium levels
Diuretics, other antihypertensives: increased hypotension
Do not use ACE inhibitors, angiotensin II receptor antagonists in diabetes mellitus

Drug/food

High-fat meal: decreased absorption

Drug/lab test

Increased: uric acid, CPK, BUN, serum creatinine, potassium
Decreased: Hct, Hgb

NURSING CONSIDERATIONS

Assessment

• Monitor renal tests: uric acid, serum creatinine, BUN may be increased; hyperkalemia may occur
• Assess for allergic reactions: angioedema may occur
• Monitor daily dependent edema in feet, legs; weight, B/P, orthostatic hypotension

• Diabetes: Identify the use of ACE inhibitors, angiotensin II receptor antagonists, do not use aliskiren

Patient/family education

> **BLACK BOX WARNING:** Teach patient to notify prescriber if pregnancy is planned or suspected; if pregnant, product will need to be discontinued (pregnancy **D** 2nd/3rd trimester, **C** 1st trimester)

• Teach patient the importance of complying with dosage schedule even if feeling better
• Instruct patient to notify if pregnancy is planned or suspected; if pregnant, product needs to be discontinued
• Teach patient how to take B/P and normal reading for age-group
• Advise patient that if dose is missed, take as soon as possible; if it is almost time for the next dose, take only that dose; do not double dose
• Instruct patient not to use OTC products, including herbs, supplements unless approved by prescriber
• Advise patient to report to prescriber immediately: dizziness, faintness, chest pain, palpitations, uneven or rapid heart beat, headache, severe diarrhea, swelling of tongue or lips, trouble breathing, difficulty swallowing, tightening of the throat
• Caution patient not to operate machinery or perform hazardous tasks if dizziness occurs
• Advise patient to rise slowly in order to avoid faintness

Evaluation

Positive therapeutic outcome
• Decrease in B/P

allopurinol (Rx)

(al-oh-pure'i-nole)
Aloprim, Zyloprim
Func. class.: Antigout drug, antihyperuricemic
Chem. class.: Xanthine enzyme inhibitor
Pregnancy category C

Do not confuse:
Zyloprim/Zovirax

ACTION: Inhibits the enzyme xanthine oxidase, reducing uric acid synthesis

Therapeutic outcome: Decreasing serum uric acid levels, decreasing joint pain

USES: Chronic gout, hyperuricemia associated with malignancies, recurrent calcium oxalate calculi, uric acid calculi

CONTRAINDICATIONS:
Hypersensitivity

Precautions: Pregnancy **C**, breastfeeding, children, renal/hepatic disease

DOSAGE AND ROUTES
Increased uric acid levels in malignancies
Adult: PO 600-800 mg/day in divided doses, for 2-3 days; start up to 1-2 days prior to chemotherapy; **IV** INF 200-400 mg/m²/day, max 600 mg/day 24-48 hr prior to chemotherapy, may be divided at 6-, 8-, 12-hr intervals
Child 6-10 yr: PO 300 mg/day, adjust dose after 48 hr
Child <6 yr: PO 150 mg/day, adjust dose after 48 hr
Child: **IV** INF 200 mg/m²/day, initially as a single dose or divided q6-12hr

Gout (mild)
Adult: PO 100 mg/day, increase qwk based on uric acid levels, max 800 mg/day, maintenance dose 100-200 mg bid-tid

Gout (moderate-severe)
Adult: PO 400-600 mg/day in a single dose or divided bid-tid, max 800 mg/day, doses >300 mg should be given in divided doses

Recurrent calculi
Adult: PO 200-300 mg/day in a single dose or divided bid-tid, max 300 mg/dose, 800 mg/day

Uric acid nephropathy prevention
Adult and child >10 yr: PO 600-800 mg daily × 2-3 days

Renal dose
Adult: PO/IV CCr 81-100 ml/min 300 mg/day; CCr 61-80 ml/min 250 mg/day; CCr 41-60 ml/min 200 mg/day; CCr 21-40 ml/min 150 mg/day; CCr 10-20 ml/min 100-200 mg/day; CCr 3-9 ml/min 100 mg/day or 100 mg every other day; CCr <3 ml/min 100 mg q24hr or longer or 100 mg every third day

Available forms: Tabs, scored, 100, 300 mg; powder for inj 500 mg/vial

Implementation
PO route
• Give with meals to prevent GI symptoms; crush and mix with food or fluids for patients with swallowing difficulties

• Increase fluid intake to 2 L/day
• Give 1-2 days before antineoplastic therapy if using for hyperuricemia associated with malignancy

Intermittent IV infusion route
• Reconstitute 30-ml vial with 25 ml of sterile water for inj; dilute to desired conc (≤6 mg/ml) with 0.9% NaCl for inj or D₅ for inj, begin inf within 10 hr

IV compatibilities: Acyclovir, aminophylline, amphotericin B lipid complex, anidulafungin, argatroban, atenolol, aztreonam, bivalirudin, bleomycin, bumetanide, buprenorphine, butorphanol, calcium gluconate, CARBOplatin, caspofungin, ceFAZolin, cefoperazone, cefoTEtan, cefTAZidime, ceftizoxime, cefTRIAXone, cefuroxime, CISplatin, cyclophosphamide, DACTINomycin, DAUNOrubicin liposome, dexamethasone, dexmedetomidine, DOCEtaxel, DOXOrubicin liposomal, enalaprilat, etoposide, famotidine, fenoldopam, filgrastim, fluconazole, fludarabine, fluorouracil, furosemide, gallium, ganciclovir, gatifloxacin, gemcitabine, gemtuzumab, granisetron, heparin, hydrocortisone phosphate, hydrocortisone succinate, HYDROmorphone, ifosfamide, linezolid, LORazepam, mannitol, mesna, methotrexate, metroNIDAZOLE, milrinone, mitoXANtrone, morphine, nesiritide, octreotide, oxytocin, PACLitaxel, pamidronate, pantoprazole, PEMEtrexed, piperacillin, piperacillin-tazobactam, plicamycin, potassium chloride, ranitidine, sodium, sulfamethoxazole-trimethoprim, teniposide, thiotepa, ticarcillin, ticarcillin clavulanate, tigecycline, tirofiban, vancomycin, vasopressin, vinBLAStine, vinCRIStine, voriconazole, zidovudine, zoledronic acid

ADVERSE EFFECTS
CNS: *Headache,* drowsiness, neuritis, paresthesia
GI: *Nausea, vomiting, anorexia, malaise,* metallic taste, cramps, peptic ulcer, diarrhea
HEMA: Agranulocytosis, thrombocytopenia, aplastic anemia, pancytopenia, leukopenia, bone marrow suppression, eosinophilia
INTEG: Dermatitis, pruritus, purpura, erythema, rash, **Stevens-Johnson syndrome**
MISC: Myopathy, arthralgia, hepatomegaly, **cholestatic jaundice, renal failure, exfoliative dermatitis**

Pharmacokinetics

Absorption	80%
Distribution	Widely distributed
Metabolism	Liver to oxypurinol
Excretion	Kidneys
Half-life	1-2 hr

Pharmacodynamics

	PO	IV
Onset	Unknown	Unknown
Peak	1½ hr	Up to 30 min
Duration	Unknown	Unknown

INTERACTIONS

Individual drugs

Ammonium chloride, potassium/sodium phosphate, vit C: increased kidney stone formation

Ampicillin, amoxicillin: increased risk of rash, avoid concurrent use

AzaTHIOprine: increased bone marrow depression

Mercaptopurine: increased bone marrow depression

Rasburicase: increased xanthine nephropathy, calculi

Theophylline: increased action of theophylline

Drug classifications

ACE inhibitors: increased hypersensitivity, toxicity

Anticoagulants (oral): increased action of oral anticoagulants

Antidiabetics (oral): increased action of antidiabetics

Antineoplastics: increased bone marrow suppression

Diuretics (thiazide): increased hypersensitivity

NURSING CONSIDERATIONS

Assessment

• Assess for **pain** including location, characteristics, onset/duration, frequency, quality, intensity or severity of pain, precipitating factors; **gout:** joint pain, swelling, may use with NSAIDs for acute gouty attacks

• Monitor uric acid levels q2wk; normal uric acid levels are 6 mg/dl or less; effect may take several wk; check I&O ratio, increase fluids to 2 L/day to prevent stone formation, toxicity

• Monitor CBC, AST, BUN, creatinine before starting treatment, monthly; check blood glucose in diabetic patients receiving oral antidiabetic agents

Patient/family education

• Tell patient to increase fluid intake to 2 L/day; to avoid taking large doses of vit C; kidney stone formation may occur; to maintain a diet enhancing urine alkalinity (e.g., milk, other dairy products); if taking for calcium oxalate stones, reduce dairy products, refined sugar, sodium, meat

• Tell patient to report skin rash, stomatitis, malaise, fever, aching; product should be discontinued

• Advise patient to avoid hazardous activities if drowsiness or dizziness occurs; response may take several days to determine

• Tell patient to avoid alcohol, caffeine; these substances increase uric acid levels and decrease allopurinol levels

• Teach patient to report side effects and adverse reactions to prescriber, including rash, itching, nausea, vomiting

Evaluation

Positive therapeutic outcome

• Decreased pain in joints
• Decreased stone formation in kidney
• Decreased uric acid level to 6 mg/dl

almotriptan (Rx)

(al-moh-trip′tan)
Axert
Func. class.: Antimigraine agent
Chem. class.: 5-HT$_1$ receptor agonist, triptan
Pregnancy category C

Do not confuse:

Axert/Antivert

ACTION: Binds selectively to the vascular 5-HT$_{1B/1D/1F}$ receptor subtype, exerts antimigraine effect; causes vasoconstriction in cranial arteries

Therapeutic outcome: Absence of migraines

USES: Acute treatment of migraine with or without aura (Adults/adolescents/children ≥12 yr)

CONTRAINDICATIONS:

Hypersensitivity, acute MI, angina, CV disease, CAD, stroke, vasospastic angina, ischemic heart disease or risk for, peripheral vascular syndrome; uncontrolled hypertension, basilar or hemiplegic migraine

Precautions: Pregnancy **C**, breastfeeding, children <18 yr, geriatric, postmenopausal women, men >40 yr, risk factors for coronary artery disease, MI, hypercholesterolemia, obesity, diabetes, impaired renal/hepatic function, sulfonamide hypersensitivity, cardiac dysrhythmias, Raynaud's disease, tobacco smoking, Wolff-Parkinson-White syndrome

DOSAGE AND ROUTES
Adult/adolescent/child ≥12 yr: PO 6.25-12.5 mg, may repeat dose after 2 hr; max 2 doses/24 hr, 25 mg/day, or 4 treatment cycles within any 30-day period

Renal/hepatic dose (CCr 10-30 ml/hr)
Adult: PO 6.25 mg initially, max 12.5 mg

Available forms: Tabs 6.25, 12.5 mg

Implementation
• Swallow tabs whole; do not break, crush, or chew tabs, without regard to food
• Provide quiet, calm environment with decreased stimulation from noise, bright light, excessive talking

ADVERSE EFFECTS
CNS: *Tingling, hot sensation, burning, feeling of pressure, tightness, numbness, dizziness, sedation,* headache, anxiety, fatigue, cold sensation, **seizures**
CV: *Flushing,* palpitations, tachycardia, **coronary artery vasospasm, MI, ventricular fibrillation, ventricular tachycardia**
EENT: Throat, mouth, nasal discomfort; vision changes
GI: Nausea, xerostomia
INTEG: Sweating
MS: *Weakness, neck stiffness,* myalgia
RESP: Chest tightness, pressure

Pharmacokinetics
Absorption	Well absorbed (~70%)
Distribution	35% protein bound
Metabolism	Liver (metabolite); metabolized by MAO-A, CYP2D6, CYP3A4
Excretion	Urine, feces
Half-life	3-4 hr

Pharmacodynamics
Onset	Unknown
Peak	1-3 hr
Duration	3-4 hr

INTERACTIONS
Individual drugs
Ergot: increased vasospastic effects, avoid concurrent use
Erythromycin, itraconazole, ketoconazole, ritonavir: increased plasma concentration of almotriptan, avoid concurrent use in renal/hepatic disease

Drug classifications
5-HT$_1$ agonists, ergot derivatives: increased vasospastic effects, avoid concurrent use
CYP2D6 inhibitors: increased almotriptan effect; do not use together
MAOIs: increased almotriptan effect; do not use together
SSRIs, SNRIs, serotonin-receptor agonists, sibutramine: increased serotonin syndrome

Drug/herb
Feverfew: avoid use
St. John's wort: increased serotonin syndrome

NURSING CONSIDERATIONS
Assessment
• Assess B/P, signs/symptoms of coronary vasospasms
• Assess for tingling, hot sensation, burning, feeling of pressure, numbness, flushing
• Assess for stress level, activity, recreation, coping mechanisms
• Assess neurologic status: LOC, blurring vision, nausea, vomiting, tingling in extremities preceding headache
• Assess for ingestion of **tyramine-containing foods** (pickled products, beer, wine, aged cheese), food additives, preservatives, colorings, artificial sweeteners, chocolate, caffeine, which may precipitate these types of headaches
• Assess for **migraine:** pain, location, aura, duration, intensity, nausea, vomiting
• Assess for **serotonin syndrome:** occurs in those taking SSRIs, SNRIs; agitation, confusion, hallucinations, diaphoresis, hypertension, diarrhea, fever, tremor, usually occurs when dose is increased

Patient/family education
• Instruct patient to use contraception while taking product, notify prescriber if pregnancy is planned or suspected, avoid breastfeeding
• Advise patient to have dark, quiet environment available
• Inform patient that product does not prevent or reduce number of migraine attacks
• Advise patient to report chest pain, drowsiness, dizziness, tingling, flushing

---

⚠ Nurse Alert   ✳ Key NCLEX® Drug

Evaluation
Positive therapeutic outcome
• Decrease in severity of migraine

TREATMENT OF OVERDOSE:
Gastric lavage followed by activated charcoal; clinical and ECG monitoring for ≥20 hr after overdose

---

alogliptin
(al'oh glip'tin)
Nesina
Func. class.: Antidiabetic
Chem. class.: Dipeptidyl peptidase-4 (DPP-4) inhibitor
Pregnancy category B

ACTION: A dipeptidyl peptidase-4 (DPP-4) inhibitor for the treatment of type 2 diabetes mellitus (monotherapy or in combination with other antidiabetic agents), potentiates the effects of the incretin hormones by inhibiting their breakdown by DPP-4

Therapeutic outcome: Decrease in polyuria, polydipsia, polyphagia; clear sensorium, absence of dizziness; improvement in A1c, daily blood glucose monitoring

USES: Type 2 diabetes mellitus (T2DM)

CONTRAINDICATIONS:
Hypersensitivity

Precautions: Pregnancy (B), breastfeeding, hepatic disease, burns, ketoacidosis, diarrhea, fever, GI obstruction, hyper/hypoglycemia, hyper/hypothyroidism, type 1 diabetes, hypercortisolism, children, ileus, malnutrition, pancreatitis, surgery, trauma, vomiting, kidney disease, adrenal insufficiency

> **BLACK BOX WARNING:** Angioedema

DOSAGE AND ROUTES
Adult: **PO** 25 mg/day; when used in combination, a lower dose of the other antidiabetic may be needed

Renal dose
Adult: **PO** CCr 30-59 ml/min: 12.5 mg/day; CCr 30 ml/min: 6.25 mg/day; intermittent hemodialysis: 6.25 mg/day; give without regard to the timing of hemodialysis

Available forms: Tab 6.25, 12.5, 25

Implementation
Give without regard to food

ADVERSE EFFECTS
CNS: Headache
GI: *Pancreatitis*
META: Hypoglycemia
RESP: Upper respiratory infection, nasopharyngitis
SYST: Rash, hypersensitivity, angioedema, **Stevens–Johnson syndrome**

Pharmacokinetics
Absorption	Unknown
Distribution	Unknown
Metabolism	Unknown
Excretion	Unchanged (urine)
Half-life	Unknown

Pharmacodynamics
Onset	Unknown
Peak	1-2 hr
Duration	Effect decreased (liver disease), increased (kidney disease)

INTERACTIONS
Drug/lab test
Increased: LFTs

NURSING CONSIDERATIONS
Assessment
• Diabetes: monitor blood glucose, glycosylated hemoglobin (A1c), LFTs, serum creatinine/BUN
• Assess for pancreatitis: can occur anytime during use
• Monitor for hypersensitivity reactions: angioedema
• Assess for Stevens-Johnson syndrome

Patient/family education
• Inform patient that diabetes is a life-long condition; product does not cure disease
• Advise patient to consume all food on diet plan, to continue other medical and lifestyle regimens
• Teach patient to carry emergency ID with prescriber, medications, and condition listed
• Teach patient to test blood glucose using a blood glucose meter

Evaluation
Positive therapeutic outcome
• Decrease in polyuria, polydipsia, polyphagia, clear sensorium, absence of dizziness, improvement in A1c, daily blood glucose monitoring

alosetron

(ah-loss'a-tron)
Lotronex
Func. class.: Antidiarrheal, anti-IBS agent; serotonin receptor antagonist
Pregnancy category B

ACTION: A potent and selective antagonist at serotonin 5-HT3 receptors; 5-HT3 receptors are extensively distributed on enteric neurons in the GI tract; antagonism at these receptors in the GI tract modulate the regulation of visceral pain, colonic transit, and GI secretions

Therapeutic outcome: Decreased irritable bowel syndrome (IBS) symptoms

USES: Severe-diarrhea-predominant IBS

CONTRAINDICATIONS: Crohn's disease, severe hepatic disease, toxic megacolon, GI adhesions/strictures/obstruction, thrombophlebitis, ulcerative colitis

> **BLACK BOX WARNING:** Ischemic colitis, severe constipation

Precautions: Pregnancy B, breastfeeding, child <18 yr

DOSAGE AND ROUTES

Adult (woman): **PO** 0.5 mg bid, may increase to 1 mg bid after 4 wk if well tolerated; discontinue if symptoms are not controlled after 4 wk

Available forms: Tab 0.5 mg

Implementation
• Give without regard to meals
• Store at room temperature, protect from light and moisture

> **BLACK BOX WARNING:** Use only after "Patient Acknowledgement Form" is signed

ADVERSE EFFECTS

GI: Constipation, abdominal pain, distention, reflux, nausea, **obstruction**, impaction, **ischemic colitis, ileus perforation, small-bowel mesenteric ischemia**

Pharmacokinetics

Absorption	Unknown
Distribution	Unknown
Metabolism	Extensively in the liver
Excretion	Unknown
Half-life	1½ hr

Pharmacodynamics

Onset	Unknown
Peak	1 hr
Duration	Unknown

INTERACTIONS

Drug classifications
CYP3A4 inhibitors, hydrALAZINE, procainamide: decreased alosetron metabolism
CYP3A4 inducers: increased alosetron metabolism

Drug/lab test
Increased: ALT

NURSING CONSIDERATIONS

Assessment

> **BLACK BOX WARNING:** Irritable bowel syndrome: Assess for constipation, diarrhea, abdominal pain, fecal incontinence; discontinue immediately if bloody diarrhea, severe constipation, rectal bleeding, or severe abdominal pain occur

> **BLACK BOX WARNING:** Only clinicians enrolled in the Lotronex prescribing program should use this product

• Geriatric women: assess for more severe side effects

Patient/family education

> **BLACK BOX WARNING:** Teach patient to report immediately, severe constipation, bloody diarrhea, rectal bleeding or worsening abdominal pain

• Instruct patient not to double doses; if a dose is missed, it should be skipped
• Advise patient that product may be taken without regard to food
• Advise patient that product does not cure disorder, but only controls symptoms
• Provide medication guide and clarify if needed, improvement in symptoms can take 1-4 wk
• Teach patient that product is used only for women with IBS

• Advise patient to report if pregnancy is planned or suspected; product should not be used during pregnancy—effects are unknown

Evaluation
Positive therapeutic outcome
• Decreasing symptoms of IBS

ALPRAZolam (Rx)
(al-pray′zoe-lam)
Apo-Alpraz 🍁, **Niravam, Xanax, Xanax XR**
Func. class.: Antianxiety/sedative/hypnotic
Chem. class.: Benzodiazepine, short/intermediate acting
Pregnancy category D
Controlled substance schedule IV

Do not confuse:
ALPRAZolam/LORazepam,
Xanax/Lanoxin/Tylox/Zantac

ACTION: Depresses subcortical levels of CNS, including limbic system, reticular formation

Therapeutic outcome: Decreased anxiety

USES: Anxiety, panic disorders with or without agoraphobia, anxiety with depressive symptoms

Unlabeled uses: Premenstrual dysphoric disorder, insomnia, PMS, alcohol withdrawal syndrome

CONTRAINDICATIONS:
Pregnancy **D**, breastfeeding, hypersensitivity to benzodiazepines, closed-angle glaucoma, psychosis, addiction

Precautions: Geriatric, debilitated, hepatic disease, obesity, severe pulmonary disease

DOSAGE AND ROUTES
Anxiety disorder
Adult: PO 0.25-0.5 mg tid, may increase q3-4days if needed, max 4 mg/day in divided doses
Geriatric: PO 0.125-0.25 mg bid; increase by 0.125 mg prn

Panic disorder
Adult: PO 0.5 mg tid, may increase up to 1 mg/day q3-4days, max 10 mg/day; EXT REL TABS (Xanax XR) give daily in AM 0.5-1 mg initially, maintenance 3-6 mg daily

Premenstrual dysphoric disorder (unlabeled)
Adult: PO 0.25 mg bid-qid, starting on day 16-18 of menses cycle, taper over 2-3 days when menses occurs, max 4 mg/day

Hepatic dose
Reduce dose

Insomnia (unlabeled)
Adult: PO 0.25-0.5 mg at bedtime

Available forms: Tabs 0.25, 0.5, 1, 2 mg; ext rel tabs (Xanax XR) 0.5, 1, 2, 3 mg; orally disintegrating tabs 0.25, 0.5, 1, 2 mg; oral sol, 1 mg/ml

Implementation
• Give with food or milk for GI symptoms; high-fat meal decreases absorption; tab may be crushed, if patient is unable to swallow medication whole, and mixed with foods or fluids; may divide total daily dose into more times/day, if anxiety occurs between doses
• Give sugarless gum, hard candy, frequent sips of water for dry mouth
• Discontinue, decrease by 0.5 mg q3days
• Place orally disintegrating tabs on tongue to dissolve and swallow, protect from moisture
• Give ext rel tab in AM

ADVERSE EFFECTS
CNS: *Dizziness, drowsiness,* confusion, headache, anxiety, tremors, stimulation, fatigue, depression, insomnia, hallucinations, memory impairment, poor coordination, **suicide**
CV: *Orthostatic hypotension,* **ECG changes, tachycardia,** hypotension
EENT: *Blurred vision,* tinnitus, mydriasis
GI: Constipation, dry mouth, nausea, vomiting, anorexia, diarrhea, weight gain/loss, increased appetite
GU: Decreased libido
INTEG: Rash, dermatitis, itching, angioedema

Pharmacokinetics
Absorption	Slow, complete
Distribution	Widely distributed; crosses placenta; crosses blood-brain barrier, protein binding 80%
Metabolism	Liver, to active metabolites
Excretion	Kidneys, breast milk
Half-life	12-15 hr

Pharmacodynamics

	PO	Oral Disintegrating
Onset	1 hr	
Peak	1-2 hr	1.5-2 hr
Duration	4-6 hr, therapeutic response 2-3 days	

INTERACTIONS

Individual drugs

Alcohol: increased CNS depression
Cigarette smoking: decreased drug level
Levodopa: decreased action of levodopa
Rifampin: decreased action of ALPRAZolam

Drug classifications

Anticonvulsants, antihistamines, opioids, sedatives/hypnotics: increased CNS depression
CYP3A4 inducers (barbiturates): decreased action of ALPRAZolam
CYP3A4 inhibitors (cimetidine, disulfiram, erythromycin, fluoxetine, isoniazid, itraconazole, ketoconazole, metoprolol, propoxyphene, propranolol, valproic acid): increased action of ALPRAZolam
Xanthines: decreased sedation

Drug/herb

Chamomile, kava, melatonin, St. John's wort, valerian: increased CNS depression

Drug/food

Grapefruit juice: increased product level, avoid concurrent use

Drug/lab test

Increased: ALT, AST, alkaline phosphatase

NURSING CONSIDERATIONS

Assessment

⚠ Assess mental status: **mood, sensorium, anxiety, affect, sleeping pattern, drowsiness, dizziness, especially geriatric; physical dependency, withdrawal symptoms: anxiety, panic attacks, agitation, seizures, headache, nausea, vomiting, muscle pain, weakness; suicidal tendencies; withdrawal seizures may occur after rapid decrease in dose or abrupt discontinuation; short duration of action makes it the product of choice in the geriatric, suicidal thoughts, behaviors**

• Monitor B/P (with patient lying, standing), pulse; if systolic B/P drops 20 mm Hg, hold product, notify prescriber

• Monitor blood studies: CBC during long-term therapy; blood dyscrasias have occurred rarely; decreased hematocrit, neutropenia may occur

• Monitor hepatic studies: AST, ALT, bilirubin, creatinine LDH, alkaline phosphatase, if on long-term treatment

• Monitor I&O; indicate renal dysfunction if on long-term treatment

⚠ Pregnancy: Assess if planned or suspected, pregnancy (D), to avoid breastfeeding

Patient/family education

• Tell patient that product may be taken with food or fluids and tabs may be crushed or swallowed whole

• Tell patient not to use for everyday stress or longer than 4 mo unless directed by prescriber; not to take more than prescribed amount; may be habit forming; not to double doses or skip doses; memory impairment is a sign of long-term use

• Tell patient to avoid OTC preparations unless approved by prescriber; alcohol and CNS depressants increase CNS depression

• Teach patient not to use during pregnancy (D), avoid breastfeeding

• Tell patient to avoid driving, activities that require alertness, since drowsiness may occur; to avoid alcohol ingestion or other psychotropic medications; to rise slowly, or fainting may occur, especially geriatric; that drowsiness may worsen at beginning of treatment

• Tell patient not to discontinue medication abruptly after long-term use; withdrawal symptoms include vomiting, cramping, tremors, seizures

Evaluation

Positive therapeutic outcome

• Decreased anxiety, restlessness, sleeplessness (short-term treatment only)

TREATMENT OF OVERDOSE:

Lavage, VS, supportive care, flumazenil

> ⚠ **HIGH ALERT**

alteplase (tissue plasminogen activator, t-PA) (Rx)
(al-ti-plaze')
Activase, Cathflo
Func. class.: Thrombolytic enzyme
Chem. class.: Tissue plasminogen activator (TPA)
Pregnancy category C

Do not confuse:
alteplase/Altace

ACTION: Produces fibrin conversion of plasminogen to plasmin; able to bind to fibrin, convert plasminogen in thrombus to plasmin, which leads to local fibrinolysis, limited systemic proteolysis

Therapeutic outcome: Lysis of thrombi in MI, pulmonary emboli (life threatening)

USES: Lysis of obstructing thrombi associated with acute MI; conditions requiring thrombolysis (e.g., PE, unclotting arteriovenous shunts, acute ischemic CVA); central venous catheter occlusion (Cathflo)

Unlabeled uses: Arterial thromboembolism, deep vein thrombosis (DVT), occlusion prophylaxis, percutaneous coronary intervention (PCI)

CONTRAINDICATIONS:
Active internal bleeding, recent CVA, severe uncontrolled hypertension, intracranial/intraspinal surgery/trauma (within 3 mo), aneurysm, brain tumor, platelets <100,000 mm³, bleeding diathesis including INR >1.7 or PT >15 sec, arteriovenous malformation, subarachnoid hemorrhage, intracranial hemorrhage, uncontrolled hypertension, seizure at onset of stroke

Precautions: Pregnancy **C**, breastfeeding, children, geriatric, neurologic deficits, mitral stenosis, recent GI/GU bleeding, diabetic retinopathy, subacute bacterial endocarditis, arrhythmias, diabetic hemorrhage retinopathy, CVA, recent major surgery, hypertension, acute pericarditis, hemostatic defects, significant hepatic disease, septic thrombophlebitis, occluded AV cannula at seriously infected site

DOSAGE AND ROUTES
Pulmonary embolism
Adult: **IV** 100 mg over 2 hr, then heparin

Acute ischemic stroke
Adult: **IV** 0.9 mg/kg, max 90 mg; give as INF over 1 hr, give 10% of dose **IV** BOL over 1st min

Myocardial infarction (standard infusion)
Adult >65 kg: **IV** a total of 100 mg, given over 3 hr; 6-10 mg given **IV** BOL over 1-2 min, then the remaining 50-54 mg over the remainder of the hr, during 2nd, 3rd hr 20 mg is given by cont **IV** INF (20 mg/hr)
Adult <65 kg: **IV** 1.25 mg/kg over 3 hr; 60% in first 1 hr (10% as a bolus), remaining 40% over next 2 hr

Myocardial infarction (accelerated infusion)
Adult >67 kg: 100 mg total dose: give 15 mg **IV** BOL, then 50 mg over 30 min, then 35 mg over 60 min
Adult <67 kg: 15 mg **IV** BOL: then 0.75 mg/kg over 30 min (max 50 mg); 0.5 mg/kg over the next 60 min (max 35 mg)

Occlusion prophylaxis (unlabeled)
Adult ≥30 kg: Max 2 mg in 2 ml; may use up to 2 doses (120 min apart)

Available forms: Powder for inj 50 mg (29 million international units/vial), 100 mg (58 million international units/vial); Cathflo Actinase: lyophilized powder for injection 2 mg

Implementation
Intermittent IV infusion route
• Give after reconstituting with provided diluent; add appropriate amount of sterile water for inj (no preservatives); 20-mg vial/20 ml or 50-mg vial/50 ml (1 mg/ml); mix by slow inversion or dilute with 0.9% NaCl, D₅W to a concentration of 0.5 mg/ml further dilution; 1.5 to <0.5 mg/ml may result in precipitation of product; use 18-G needle; flush line with 0.9% NaCl after administration; use reconstituted **IV** sol within 8 hr or discard, within 6 hr of coronary occlusion for best results
⚠ **Do not use 150 mg or more total dose; intracranial bleeding may occur**
• Give heparin therapy after thrombolytic therapy is discontinued and when thrombin time, ACT, and APTT <2 times control (about 3-4 hr), treatment can be initiated before coagulation study results, infusion should be discontinued if pretreatment is INR >1.7, PT >15 sec, or an elevated APPT is identified

• Avoid invasive procedures, inj, rect temp; apply pressure for 30 sec to minor bleeding sites; 30 min to sites of atrial puncture, followed by pressure dressing; inform prescriber if this does not attain hemostasis; apply pressure dressing
• **Cathflo Activase:** reconstitute by using 2.2 ml of sterile water provided and injecting in vial, direct flow into powder (1 mg/ml), foam will disappear after standing, swirl, do not shake, sol will be pale yellow or clear, use sol within 8 hr, instill 2 ml of reconstituted sol into occluded catheter, try to aspirate after ½ hr, if unable to remove allow 2 hrs; a second dose may be used; aspirate 5 ml of blood to remove clot and product; irrigate with normal saline
• Store powder at room temperature or refrigerate; protect from excessive light
• Avoidance of invasive procedures, inj, rectal temp
• Pressure for 30 sec to minor bleeding sites; 30 min to sites of atrial puncture followed by pressure dressing; inform prescriber if this does not attain hemostasis; apply pressure dressing

Y-site compatibilities: Eptifibatide, lidocaine, metoprolol, propranolol

Y-site incompatibilities: DOBUTamine, DOPamine, heparin, nitroglycerin

ADVERSE EFFECTS
CV: Sinus bradycardia, ventricular tachycardia, accelerated idioventricular rhythm, bradycardia, recurrent ischemic stroke, cholesterol microembolization, hypotension
EENT: Orolingual angioedema
INTEG: Urticaria, rash
SYST: GI, GU, intracranial, retroperitoneal bleeding, *surface bleeding*, anaphylaxis, fever

Pharmacokinetics

Absorption	Complete
Distribution	Unknown
Metabolism	>80% liver
Excretion	Kidneys
Half-life	35 min

Pharmacodynamics

Onset	Immediate
Peak	30-45 min
Duration	4 hr

INTERACTIONS
Individual drugs
Abciximab, clopidogrel, dipyridamole, eptifibatide, plicamycin, ticlopidine, tirofiban, valproic acid: increased bleeding
ACE inhibitors: increased orolingual angioedema
Nitroglycerin: decreased effect

Drug classifications
Anticoagulants (oral), cephalosporins (some), NSAIDs, salicylates: increased bleeding

Drug/herb
Feverfew, garlic, ginger, ginkgo, ginseng, green tea: increased risk of bleeding

Drug/lab test
Increased: PT, APTT, TT

NURSING CONSIDERATIONS
Assessment
• Treatment is not recommended in patient with acute ischemic stroke >3 hr after symptom onset, with minor neurologic deficit, or with rapidly improving symptoms
• Monitor VS q15min, B/P, pulse, respirations (including peripheral), neurologic signs, temp at least q4hr; temp >104° F (40° C) indicates internal bleeding; monitor rhythm closely; ventricular dysrhythmias may occur with hyperfusion; monitor heart, breath sounds, neurologic status, and peripheral pulses, those with severe neurologic deficit (NIHSS >22) at presentation (increased risk of hemorrhage)
⚠ Assess for bleeding during first hr of treatment and 24 hr after procedure: hematuria, hematemesis, bleeding from mucous membranes, epistaxis, ecchymosis, puncture sites; guaiac all body fluids and stools; obtain blood studies (Hct, platelets, PTT, PT, TT, APTT) before starting therapy; PT or APTT must be <2 times control before starting therapy; TT or PT q3-4hr during treatment; obtain CPK-MB to identify product effectiveness
• Assess **hypersensitivity:** fever, rash, facial swelling, dyspnea, itching, chills; mild reaction may be treated with antihistamines; report to prescriber
• **Pulmonary embolism:** monitor pulse, B/P, ABGs, rate/rhythm of respirations
• **Occlusion:** have patient exhale then hold breath when connecting/disconnecting syringe to prevent air embolism
• **Cholesterol embolism:** assess for purple toe syndrome, acute renal failure, gangrenous digits, hypertension, livedo reticularis,

pancreatitis, MI, cerebral infarction, spinal cord infarction, retinal artery occlusion, bowel infarction, rhabdomyolysis
• **Myocardial infarction:** monitor ECG; on monitor, watch for segment changes, changes in rhythm: sinus bradycardia, ventricular tachycardia, accelerated idioventricular rhythm may occur due to reperfusion, cardiac enzymes, radionuclide myocardial scanning/coronary angiography
• **Pulmonary embolism:** monitor pulse, B/P, ABGs, rate/rhythm of respirations; symptoms include dyspnea, tachypnea, chest pain, cough, hemoptysis
• **Occlusion:** have patient exhale then hold breath when connecting/disconnecting syringe to prevent air embolism

Patient/family education
• Teach patient reason for alteplase, signs and symptoms of bleeding, allergic reactions, when to notify prescriber

Evaluation
Positive therapeutic outcome
• Lysis of pulmonary thrombi
• Adequate hemodynamic state
• Absence of congestive heart failure

aluminum hydroxide (OTC)
Func. class.: Antacid, hypophosphatemic, antiulcer
Chem. class.: Aluminum product, phosphate binder
Pregnancy category C

ACTION: Neutralizes gastric acidity, binds phosphates in GI tract; these phosphates are excreted

Therapeutic outcome: Decreased acidity, healing of ulcers; decreased phosphate levels in chronic renal failure

USES: Antacid, adjunct in peptic, gastric, duodenal ulcers; hyperphosphatemia in chronic renal failure; reflux esophagitis, hyperacidity, heartburn, stress ulcer prevention in critically ill, GERD

Unlabeled uses: GI bleeding

CONTRAINDICATIONS:
Hypersensitivity to this product or aluminum products

Precautions: Pregnancy **C**, breastfeeding, geriatric, fluid restriction, decreased GI motility,

GI obstruction, dehydration, renal disease, sodium-restricted diets

DOSAGE AND ROUTES
Antacid
Adult: SUSP PO 600 mg 1 hr after meals, at bedtime; max 6 times/day

Hyperphosphatemia
Adult: PO 300-600 mg tid
Child: PO 50-150 mg/kg/day in 4-6 divided doses

GI bleeding (unlabeled)
Infant: PO 2-5 ml/dose q1-2hr
Child: PO 5-15 ml/dose q1-2hr

Available forms: SUSP 320 mg/5 ml, 600 mg/5 ml

Implementation
• 2 tsp (10 ml) neutralizes 20 mEq of acid
PO route
• Give laxatives or stool softeners if constipation occurs, especially geriatric
• Give after shaking suspension; follow with water to facilitate passage
• Tab may be chewed if patient is unable to swallow, drink 8 oz of water after chewing; or by nasogastric tube if patient unable to swallow
• Give with 8 oz of water for hyperphosphatemia unless contraindicated
• Give 1 hr before or after other medications to prevent poor absorption
• Give 15 ml 30 min after meals and at bedtime (esophagitis)
NG tube route
• May be given as prescribed q1-2hr and given by gastric tube after diluting with water (peptic ulcer)

ADVERSE EFFECTS
GI: *Constipation,* anorexia, **obstruction,** fecal impaction
META: *Hypophosphatemia,* hypercalciuria

Pharmacokinetics

Absorption	Not usually absorbed
Distribution	Widely distributed if absorbed; crosses placenta
Metabolism	Unknown
Excretion	Feces, kidneys (small amounts), breast milk
Half-life	Unknown

Pharmacodynamics

Onset	20-40 min
Peak	½ hr
Duration	1-3 hr

INTERACTIONS
Individual drugs
Allopurinol, amprenavir, delavirdine, digoxin, gabapentin, gatifloxacin, isoniazid, ketoconazole, penicillamine, phenytoin, quiNIDine, ticlopidine: decreased effect of each of these drugs

Drug classifications
Anticholinergics, cephalosporins, corticosteroids, H₂ antagonists, iron salts, phenothiazines, quinolones, tetracyclines, thyroid hormones: decreased effect of each of these drug classifications

Drug/food
High-protein meal: decreased product effect

Drug/lab test
Decreased: Phosphate Interference: Tc-99m

NURSING CONSIDERATIONS
Assessment
• Assess pain symptoms: location, duration, intensity, alleviating/precipitating factors
• Monitor phosphate levels, since product is bound in GI system; urinary pH, calcium, electrolytes; hypophosphatemia: anorexia, weakness, fatigue, bone pain, hyperreflexia
• Monitor constipation; increase bulk in diet if needed, may use stool softeners or laxatives; record amount and consistency of stools
• Monitor aluminum toxicity: severe renal disease; may also be used for hyperphosphatemia

Patient/family education
• Instruct patient to avoid phosphate-containing foods (most dairy products, eggs, fruits, carbonated beverages) during product therapy; to add cheese, corn, pasta, plums, prunes, lentils after product (hypophosphatemia)
• Instruct patient not to use for prolonged periods if serum phosphate is low or if on a low-sodium diet, shake liquid well; CHF patients should check for sodium content and use sodium-reduced products
• Instruct patient that stools may appear white or speckled; constipation may result; to report black tarry stools, which indicate gastric bleeding
• Instruct patient to check with prescriber after 2 wk of self-prescribed antacid use; may be used for 4-6 wk after symptoms subside or as prescribed
• Instruct patient to separate other medications by 2 hr
• Teach patient to notify prescriber of black tarry stools, which may indicate bleeding

Evaluation
Positive therapeutic outcome
• Absence of pain, decreased acidity
• Increased pH of gastric secretions
• Decreased phosphate levels

alvimopan (Rx)
(al-vi′moe-pan)
Entereg
Func. class.: Functional GI disorder agent
Chem. class.: Peripheral μ-opioid receptor antagonist
Pregnancy category B

ACTION: Acts within the GI tract, antagonizes opioid-induced GI dysfunction

Therapeutic outcome: Resolution of ileus

USES: Ileus, postoperative

CONTRAINDICATIONS:
Hypersensitivity

BLACK BOX WARNING: No more than 15 doses

Precautions: Pregnancy **B,** breastfeeding, renal/hepatic disease, children, GI obstruction, MI, complete GI obstruction surgery

DOSAGE AND ROUTES
Ileus, postoperative
Adult: PO 12 mg given ½-5 hr before surgery, then 12 mg bid beginning the day after surgery, max 7 days (15 doses)

Available forms: Caps 12 mg

Implementation
• Use in hospital only; therapeutic doses of opiates should not be used for >7 consecutive days
• Must register in EASE program
• Do not give >15 doses (short-term hospital only)
• Give without regard to food
• Store at room temperature

ADVERSE EFFECTS
CV: MI
GI: Dyspepsia, flatulence, constipation
GU: Urinary retention
MISC: Anemia, hypokalemia
MS: Back pain

Pharmacokinetics

Absorption	High-fat meal decreases absorption
Distribution	Protein binding 80%-94%
Metabolism	Unknown
Excretion	Kidneys (35%)
Half-life	Terminal 10-18 hr

Pharmacodynamics
Unknown

INTERACTIONS
Individual drugs
Amiodarone, bepridil, cycloSPORINE, diltiazem, itraconazole, quiNIDine, quinine, spironolactone, verapamil: increased alvimopan effect
Methylnaltrexone: duplicate therapy

Drug classifications
Opiate agonists: increased GI adverse reactions; do not give if opiate agonists were taken for ≥7 days
Opiate antagonists: duplicate therapy

NURSING CONSIDERATIONS
Assessment
• Monitor Hgb, Hct, serum potassium

Patient/family education
• Instruct the patient in the reason for the product

Evaluation
Positive therapeutic outcome
• Resolution of ileus

amantadine (Rx)
(a-man′ta-deen)
Func. class.: Antiviral, antiparkinsonian agent
Chem. class.: Tricyclic amine
Pregnancy category C

Do not confuse:
amantadine/ranitidine/rimantidine

ACTION: Prevents uncoating of nucleic acid in viral cell, preventing penetration of virus to host; causes release of dopamine from neurons

Therapeutic outcome: Resolution of infection, lessening of parkinsonism symptoms

USES: Prophylaxis or treatment of influenza type A, extrapyramidal reactions, parkinsonism, Parkinson's disease

Unlabeled uses: Neuroleptic malignant syndrome, MS-associated fatigue

CONTRAINDICATIONS:
Breastfeeding, child <1 yr, hypersensitivity, eczematic rash

Precautions: Pregnancy **C**, geriatric, epilepsy, CHF, orthostatic hypotension, psychiatric disorders, renal/hepatic disease, peripheral edema

DOSAGE AND ROUTES
Influenza type A
Adult and child >9 yr: PO 200 mg/day in single dose or divided bid
Geriatric: PO no more than 100 mg/day
Child 9-12 yr: PO 100 mg bid
Child 1-8 yr: PO 4.4-8.8 mg/kg/day divided bid-tid, max 150 mg/day

Extrapyramidal reaction/parkinsonism
Adult: PO 100 mg bid, up to 400 mg/day in EPS; give for 1 wk, then 100 mg prn up to 400 mg in parkinsonism

Renal dose
Adult: PO CCr 30-50 ml/min 200 mg first day, then 100 mg/day; CCr 15-29 ml/min 100 mg first day, then 100 mg on alternate days; CCr 15 ml/min reduce dose and interval to 200 mg q7days

MS-associated fatigue (unlabeled)
Adult: PO 200 mg daily or 100 mg bid

Neuroleptic malignant syndrome (unlabeled)
Adult: PO 100 mg bid × 3 wk

Available forms: Caps 100 mg; oral sol 50 mg/5 ml, tab 100 mg

Implementation
• **Prophylaxis:** give before exposure to influenza; continue for 10 days after contact; **treatment:** initiate within 24-48 hr after onset of symptoms, continue for 24-48 hr after symptoms disappear

- Give at least 4 hr before bedtime to prevent insomnia
- Give after meals for better absorption, to decrease GI symptoms
- Give in divided doses to prevent CNS disturbances: headache, dizziness, fatigue, drowsiness
- Store in tight, dry container
- Caps may be opened and mixed with food

ADVERSE EFFECTS

CNS: *Headache, dizziness,* drowsiness, fatigue, *anxiety,* psychosis, *depression, hallucinations,* tremors, **seizures,** confusion, *insomnia*
CV: *Orthostatic hypotension,* **CHF**
EENT: Blurred vision
GI: *Nausea, vomiting,* constipation, dry mouth, anorexia
GU: *Frequency, retention*
HEMA: **Leukopenia, agranulocytosis**
INTEG: Photosensitivity, dermatitis, livedo reticularis

Pharmacokinetics

Absorption	Unknown
Distribution	Crosses placenta
Metabolism	Not metabolized
Excretion	Urine unchanged (90%), breast milk
Half-life	11-15 hr

Pharmacodynamics

Onset	48 hr
Peak	2-4 hr
Duration	Unknown

INTERACTIONS

Individual drugs

Atropine: increased anticholinergic response
H1N1 influenza A virus vaccine: decreased effect of vaccine; avoid use 2 wk before or 48 hr after amantadine
Metoclopramide: decreased amantadine effect
Triamterene, hydrochlorothiazide: decreased excretion of amantadine

Drug classifications

Anticholinergics (other): increased anticholinergic response
CNS stimulants: increased CNS stimulation
Phenothiazines: decreased amantadine effect

Drug/lab test

Increase: BUN, creatinine, alk phos, CK, LDH, bilirubin, AST, ALT, GGT

NURSING CONSIDERATIONS

Assessment

- Mental status: may cause increased psychiatric disorders, especially in the elderly
- Assess **CHF,** confusion, mottling of skin
- Assess bowel pattern before, during treatment
- Assess skin eruptions, photosensitivity after administration of product
- Assess signs of infection
- Assess for **livedo reticularis:** mottling of the skin, usually red, edema, itching in lower extremities
- Assess for **Parkinson's disease:** gait, tremors, akinesia, rigidity, may be effective if anticholinergics have not been effective
- Assess for **toxicity:** confusion, behavioral changes, hypotension, seizures

Patient/family education

- Advise patient to change body position slowly to prevent orthostatic hypotension
- Teach about aspects of product therapy: need to report dyspnea, weight gain, dizziness, poor concentration, dysuria, complex sleep behaviors
- Advise patient to avoid hazardous activities if dizziness, blurred vision occurs
- Advise patient to take product exactly as prescribed; parkinsonian crisis may occur if product is discontinued abruptly; do not double dose; if a dose is missed, do not take within 4 hr of next dose
- Teach to avoid alcohol

Evaluation

Positive therapeutic outcome
- Absence of fever, malaise, cough, dyspnea in infection; tremors, shuffling gait in Parkinson's disease

TREATMENT OF OVERDOSE:

Withdraw product, maintain airway, administer EPINEPHrine, aminophylline, O$_2$, **IV** corticosteroids, physostigmine

ambrisentan (Rx)

(am-bri-sen'tan)
Letairis
Func. class.: Antihypertensive
Chem. class.: Vasodilator/endothelin receptor antagonist
Pregnancy category X

ACTION: Endothelin-1A receptor antagonist; endothelin-1A is vasoconstrictor

Therapeutic outcome: Decreased shortness of breath, dizziness

USES: Pulmonary arterial hypertension, alone or in combination with other antihypertensives

CONTRAINDICATIONS:
Breastfeeding, hypersensitivity

> **BLACK BOX WARNING:** Pregnancy **X**

Precautions: Children, women, geriatric, hepatitis, anemia, heart failure, jaundice, peripheral edema, hepatic disease, pulmonary edema

DOSAGE AND ROUTES
Adult: PO 5 mg/day; may increase to 10 mg if needed

Hepatic dose
Adult: Discontinue if AST/ALT >5 or if elevations are accompanied by bilirubin >2 ULN or other signs of liver dysfunction

Available forms: Tabs 5, 10 mg

Implementation
• Do not break, crush, or chew tabs
• Give daily with a full glass of water without regard to food
• Do not discontinue abruptly
• Only those facilities enrolled in the LEAP program (866-664-5327) may administer this product
• Store in tight container at room temperature

ADVERSE EFFECTS
CNS: Headache, fever, flushing, fatigue
CV: Orthostatic hypotension, hypotension, peripheral edema, palpitations
EENT: Sinusitis, rhinitis
GI: Abdominal pain, constipation, anorexia, **hepatotoxicity**
GU: Decreased sperm counts
HEMA: Anemia
INTEG: Rash, **angioedema**
RESP: Pharyngitis, dyspnea, **pulmonary edema, venoocclusive disease (VOD)**

Pharmacokinetics

Absorption	Rapid
Distribution	Protein binding 99%
Metabolism	By CYP3A4, CYP2C19, UGTa
Excretion	Unknown
Half-life	Terminal 15 hr, effective half-life 9 hr

Pharmacodynamics

Onset	Unknown
Peak	2 hr
Duration	Unknown

INTERACTIONS
Individual drugs
Cimetidine, clopidogrel, efavirenz, felbamate, FLUoxetine, modafinil, OXcarbazepine, ticlopidine: possibly increased ambrisentan
Mefloquine, niCARdipine, propafenone, quiNIDine, ranolazine, tacrolimus, testosterone: decreased ambrisentan absorption

Drug classifications
Antihypertensives (other), diuretics, MAOIs: increased hypotension
Barbiturates: need for ambrisentan dosage change
CYP3A4 inhibitors (amprenavir, aprepitant, atazanavir, clarithromycin, conivaptan, cycloSPORINE, dalfopristin, danazol, darunavir, erythromycin, estradiol, imatinib, itraconazole, ketoconazole, nefazodone, nelfinavir, propoxyphene, quinupristin, ritonavir, RU-486, saquinavir, tamoxifen, telithromycin, troleandomycin, zafirlukast), CYP2C19/ CYP3A4 (chloramphenicol, delavirdine, fluconazole, fluvoxaMINE, isoniazid, voriconazole): increased ambrisentan
CYP3A4 inducers (carBAMazepine, PHENobarbitol, phenytoin, rifampin): decreased ambrisentan

Drug/herb
Ephedra (ma huang), St. John's wort: need for ambrisentan dosage change

Drug/food
Grapefruit products: avoid use

Drug/lab test
Decreased: Hct, Hgb
Increased: LFTs

NURSING CONSIDERATIONS
Assessment
• Assess pulmonary status: improvement in breathing, ability to exercise; pulmonary edema that may indicate venoocclusive disease
• Monitor blood studies: CBC with differential; Hct, Hgb may be decreased
• Monitor liver function tests: AST, ALT, blirubin

> **BLACK BOX WARNING:** Assess pregnancy status before giving this product; pregnancy category **X**

⚠ Hepatotoxicity: assess for nausea, vomiting, pain/cramping, jaundice, anorexia, itching

Patient/family education

• Teach patient the importance of complying with dosage schedule even if feeling better
• Advise patient that if a dose is missed, take as soon as possible; if it is almost time for the next dose, take only that dose; do not double dose
• Instruct patient not to use OTC products, including herbs, supplements unless approved by prescriber
• Advise patient to report to prescriber immediately: dizziness, faintness, chest pain, palpitations, uneven or rapid heart rate, headache, edema, weight gain
• Caution patient not to operate machinery or perform hazardous tasks if dizziness occurs
• Advise patient to avoid faintness; do not get up or stand up rapidly

> **BLACK BOX WARNING:** To notify if pregnancy is planned or suspected; if pregnant, product will need to be discontinued, pregnancy test done monthly, to use two contraception methods while taking this product

• To report hepatic dysfunction: nausea/vomiting, anorexia, fatigue, jaundice, right upper quadrant abdominal pain, itching, fever, malaise
• Advise patient of importance of follow-up with labs

Evaluation

Positive therapeutic outcome
• Decrease in B/P
• Decreased shortness of breath

amifostine (Rx)
(a-mi-foss'teen)
Ethyol
Func. class.: Cytoprotective agent for CISplatin/radiation
Pregnancy category C

ACTION: Binds and detoxifies damaging metabolites of cisplatin, alkylating agents, DNA-reactive agents, and ionizing radiation by converting this product by alkaline phosphatase in tissue to an active free thiol compound

Therapeutic outcome: Decreased toxic reaction from cisplatin

USES: Used to reduce renal toxicity when CISplatin is given in ovarian cancer; reduces xerostomia (dry mouth) in radiation therapy for head, neck cancer

Unlabeled uses: To prevent or reduce cisplatin-induced neurotoxicity, cyclophosphamide-induced granulocytopenia; prevent or reduce toxicity of radiation therapy; reduce toxicity of paclitaxel, myelodysplastic syndrome (MDS)

CONTRAINDICATIONS:
Breastfeeding, hypersensitivity to mannitol, aminothiol; hypotension, dehydration

Precautions: Pregnancy **C**, children, geriatric, CV disease, hypocalcemia, MI radiation therapy, stroke, dehydration, hypotension, chemotherapy, exfoliative dermatitis

DOSAGE AND ROUTES
Reduction of renal damage with CISplatin
Adult: IV 910 mg/m² daily, within ½ hr before chemotherapy; give over 15 min; may reduce dose to 740 mg/m² if higher dose is poorly tolerated

Xerostomia prophylaxis
Adult: IV 200 mg/m² daily over 3 min as INF 15-30 min before radiation therapy

Bone marrow suppression prophylaxis, nephrotoxicity prophylaxis, neurotoxicity prophylaxis (unlabeled)
Adult: IV 100-340 mg/m²/day over 15 min prior to each dose of chemotherapy/radiation

Myelodysplastic syndrome (MDS) (unlabeled)
Adult: IV 100 mg/m² 3 ×/wk, max 300 mg/m² 3 ×/wk

Available forms: Powder for inj lyophilized 500 mg/vial

Implementation
Intermittent IV infusion route
• Give by **IV** intermittent inf after reconstituting 500 mg/9.5 ml of sterile 0.9% NaCl, further dilute with 0.9% NaCl to a concentration of 5-40 mg/ml, give at a rate over 15 min within ½ hr of chemotherapy
• Patient to be in supine position during infusion

Y-site compatibilities: Amikacin, aminophylline, amphotericin B liposome, ampicillin, ampicillin-sulbactam, aztreonam, bivalirudin, bleomycin, bumetanide, buprenorphine, butorphanol, calcium gluconate, CARBOplatin, carmustine, caspofungin, ceFAZolin, cefotaxime, cefoTEtan, cefOXitin, cefTAZidime, ceftizoxime, cefTRIAXone, cefuroxime, cimetidine, ciprofloxacin, clindamycin, cyclophosphamide, cytarabine, dacarbazine, DACTINomycin, DAPTOmycin, DAUNOrubicin, dexamethasone, dexmedetomidine, diltiazem, diphenhydrAMINE, DOBUTamine, DOCEtaxel, DOPamine, DOXOrubicin, doxycycline, droperidol, enalaprilat, epirubicin, ertapenem, etoposide, famotidine, fenoldopam, floxuridine, fluconazole, fludarabine, fluorouracil, furosemide, gallium, gentamicin, granisetron, haloperidol, heparin, hydrocortisone, HYDROmorphone, IDArubicin, ifosfamide, imipenem-cilastatin, leucovorin, levofloxacin, linezolid, LORazepam, magnesium sulfate, mannitol, mechlorethamine, meperidine, mesna, methotrexate, methylPREDNISolone, metoclopramide, metroNIDAZOLE, mezlocillin, milrinone, mitoMYcin, morphine, nalbuphine, nesiritide, netilmicin, octreotide, ondansetron, oxaliplatin, PACLitaxel, palonosetron, pantoprazole, PEMEtrexed, piperacillin, plicamycin, potassium chloride, promethazine, ranitidine, sodium bicarbonate, streptozocin, tacrolimus, teniposide, thiotepa, ticarcillin, ticarcillin/clavulanate, tigecycline, tirofiban, tobramycin, trastuzumab, trimethoprim-sulfamethoxazole, trimetrexate, vancomycin, vinBLAStine, vinCRIStine, voriconazole, zidovudine

Additive incompatibilities: Do not mix with other products or solutions

ADVERSE EFFECTS

CNS: Dizziness, somnolence, loss of consciousness, **seizures**
CV: Hypotension
EENT: Sneezing
GI: Nausea, vomiting, hiccups, diarrhea
INTEG: Flushing, feeling of warmth
MISC: Hypocalcemia, rash, chills, **anaphylaxis, toxic epidermal necrolysis, toxicoderma, Stevens-Johnson syndrome, exfoliative dermatitis, erythema multiforme**

Pharmacokinetics

Absorption	Complete
Distribution	Unknown
Metabolism	To free thiol compound
Excretion	Unknown
Half-life	5-8 min

Pharmacodynamics

Unknown

INTERACTIONS

Drug classifications
Antihypertensives: increased hypotension

Drug/lab
Decrease: calcium

NURSING CONSIDERATIONS

Assessment

• Assess for **xerostomia:** mouth lesion, dry mouth during therapy
• Assess fluid status before administration; administer antiemetic before administration to prevent severe nausea and vomiting; also, dexamethasone 20 mg **IV** and a serotonin antagonist such as ondansetron, dolasetron, or granisetron
• Monitor calcium levels before, during treatment; may cause hypocalcemia; calcium supplements may be given for hypocalcemia
• Monitor blood pressure before and q5min during infusion; antihypertensive should be discontinued 24 hr prior to infusion; if severe hypotension occurs, give **IV** 0.9% NaCl to expand fluid volume, place in modified Trendelenburg position
• **Anaphylaxis:** Assess for rash, pruritus, wheezing, laryngeal edema, discontinue; give antihistamines, EPINEPHrine depending on severity; reactions may be delayed, if severe, product should be permanently discontinued; other serious skin disorders (Stevens-Johnson syndrome, toxic epidermal necrolysis, *Toxicoderma*, erythema multiforme, exfoliative dermatitis)

Patient/family education

• Teach reason for medication and expected results
• Teach that side effects may cause severe nausea, vomiting, decreased B/P, chills, dizziness, somnolence, hiccups, sneezing

Evaluation

Positive therapeutic outcome
• Absence of renal damage

---

amikacin (Rx)

(am-i-kay′sin)
Amikin
Func. class.: Antibiotic
Chem. class.: Aminoglycoside
Pregnancy category D

Do not confuse:
Amikin/Amicar, **amikacin**/anakinra

ACTION: Interferes with protein synthesis in bacterial cell by binding to ribosomal subunit, which causes misreading of genetic code; inaccurate peptide sequence forms in protein chain, causing bacterial death

Therapeutic outcome: Bactericidal effects for the following organisms: *Pseudomonas aeruginosa, Escherichia coli, Enterobacter, Acinetobacter, Providencia, Citrobacter, Staphylococcus, Serratia, Proteus*

USES: Severe systemic infections of CNS, respiratory, GI, urinary tract, bone, skin, soft tissues caused by *Staphylococcus aureus (MSSA), Pseudomonas aeruginosa, Escherichia coli, Enterobacter, Acinetobacter, Providencia, Citrobacter, Serratia, Proteus, Klebsiella pneumoniae*

Unlabeled uses: *Mycobacterium avium* complex (intrathecal or intraventricular) in combination; aerosolization, actinomycotic mycetoma

CONTRAINDICATIONS:

Pregnancy **D**, mild to moderate infections, hypersensitivity to aminoglycosides, sulfites

Precautions: Neonates, breastfeeding, geriatric, myasthenia gravis, Parkinson's disease

> **BLACK BOX WARNING:** Hearing impairment, renal/neuromuscular disease

DOSAGE AND ROUTES
Severe systemic infections
Adult and child: IV INF 10-15 mg/kg/day in 2-3 divided doses q8-12hr in 100-200 ml D₅W over 30-60 min, not to exceed 1.5 g; **pulse dosing** (once-daily dosing) may be used with some infections; IM 10-15 mg/kg/day in divided doses q8-12hr; daily or extended internal dosing as an alternative dosing regimen
Infant: IV/IM 10 mg/kg initially, then 7.5 mg/kg q12hr

Neonate: IM/IV 10 mg/kg initially, then 7.5 mg/kg q12hr

Severe urinary tract infections
Adult: IM 10-15 mg/kg/day divided q8-12hr

Hemodialysis
Adult: IM/IV 7.5 mg/kg followed by 5 mg/kg 3 ×/wk after each dialysis session (for TIW dialysis)

Mycobacterium avian complex (unlabeled)
Adult and adolescent: IV 7.5-15 mg/kg divided q12-24hr as part of a multiple-drug regimen
Child: IV 15-30 mg/kg/day divided q12-24hr as part of a multiple-drug regimen, max 1.5 g/day

Renal dose (extended interval dosing)
Adult: IV/IM CCr 40-59 ml/min 15 mg/kg IV q36hr; CCr 20-39 ml/min 15 mg/kg IV q48hr; <20 ml/min adjust based on serum concentrations and MIC (use traditional dosing)

Traditional dosing
• Decrease dose and maintain interval or maintain dose and decrease interval

Available forms: Inj IM, IV 50, 250 mg/ml

Implementation
• Obtain C&S before administration, begin treatment before results
IM route
• Give deeply in large muscle mass, rotate inj sites
• Obtain peak 1 hr after IM, trough before next dose

Intermittent IV INF route
• **Dilute** 500 mg of product/100-200 ml of **IV** D₅W, 0.9% NaCl and **give** over ½-1 hr; dilute insufficient volume to allow inf over 1-2 hr (infants); **flush** after administration with D₅W or 0.9% NaCl; solution is clear or pale yellow; discard if precipitate or dark color develops
• In children, amount of fluid depends on ordered dose; in infants infuse over 1-2 hr
• Give in evenly spaced doses to maintain blood level

Y-site compatibilities: Acyclovir, alatrofloxacin, aldesleukin, alemtuzumab, alfentanil, amifostine, aminophylline, amiodarone, amsacrine, anidulafungin, argatroban, ascorbic acid, atracurium, atropine, aztreonam, benztropine, bivalirudin, bumetanide, buprenorphine, butorphanol, calcium chloride/gluconate, CARBOplatin, caspofungin, ceFAZolin, cefepime, cefonicid, cefotaxime, cefoTEtan, cefOXitin, cefTAZidime, ceftizoxime, cefTRIAXone, cefuroxime, chloramphenicol, chlorproMAZINE, cimetidine, cisatracurium, CISplatin, clindamycin, codeine, cyanocobalamin, cyclophosphamide, cycloSPORINE, cytarabine, DACTINomycin, DAPTOmycin, dexamethasone, dexmedetomidine, digoxin, diltiazem, diphenhydrAMINE, DOBUTamine, DOCEtaxel, DOPamine, doripenem, doxacurium, DOXOrubicin, doxycycline, enalaprilat, ePHEDrine, EPINEPHrine, epirubicin, epoetin alfa, eptifibatide, ertapenem, erythromycin, esmolol, etoposide, famotidine, fentaNYL, filgrastim, fluconazole, fludarabine, fluorouracil, foscarnet, furosemide, gemcitabine, gentamicin, glycopyrrolate, granisetron, hydrocortisone, HYDROmorphone, IDArubicin, ifosfamide, IL-2, imipenem-cilastatin, isoproterenol, ketorolac, labetalol, levofloxacin, lidocaine, linezolid, LORazepam, magnesium sulfate, mannitol, mechlorethamine, melphalan, meperidine, metaraminol, methotrexate, methoxamine, methyldopate, methylPREDNISolone, metoclopramide, metoprolol, metroNIDAZOLE, midazolam, milrinone, mitoXANtrone, morphine, multivitamins, nafcillin, nalbuphine, naloxone, niCARdipine, nitroglycerin, nitroprusside, norepinephrine, octreotide, ondansetron, oxaliplatin, oxytocin, PACLitaxel, palonosetron, pantoprazole, papaverine, PEMEtrexed, penicillin G, pentazocine, perphenazine, PHENobarbital, phenylephrine, phytonadione, piperacillin-tazobactam, potassium chloride, procainamide, prochlorperazine, promethazine, propranolol, protamine, pyridoxine, quinupristin-dalfopristin, ranitidine, remifentanil, riTUXimab, rocuronium, sargramostim, sodium acetate, sodium bicarbonate, succinylcholine, SUFentanil, tacrolimus, teniposide, theophylline, thiamine, thiotepa, ticarcillin/clavulanate, tigecycline, tirofiban, tobramycin, tolazoline, trimetaphan, urokinase, vancomycin, vasopressin, vecuronium, verapamil, vinCRIStine, vinorelbine, voriconazole, warfarin, zidovudine, zoledronic acid

ADVERSE EFFECTS
CNS: Confusion, depression, numbness, tremors, **seizures,** muscle twitching, **neurotoxicity,** dizziness, vertigo, tinnitus, **neuromuscular blockade with respiratory paralysis**
CV: Hypotension or hypertension
EENT: Ototoxicity, deafness
GI: *Nausea, vomiting, anorexia,* bilirubin
GU: Oliguria, hematuria, renal damage, azotemia, renal failure, nephrotoxicity
HEMA: Eosinophilia, **anemia**
INTEG: *Rash,* burning, urticaria, dermatitis, alopecia

Pharmacokinetics

Absorption	Well absorbed (IM), completely absorbed (**IV**)
Distribution	Widely distributed in extracellular fluids, poor in CSF; crosses placenta
Metabolism	Minimal; liver
Excretion	Mostly unchanged (79%) in kidneys, removed by hemodialysis
Half-life	2-3 hr, prolonged up to 7 hr in infants; increased in renal disease

Pharmacodynamics

	IM	IV
Onset	Rapid	Rapid
Peak	15-30 min	1-2 hr
Duration	Unknown	Unknown

INTERACTIONS
Individual drugs
Increased: masking
Acyclovir, amphotericin B, cidofovir, cycloSPORINE, vancomycin: nephrotoxicity
DimenhyDRINATE, ethacrynic acid: increased masking of ototoxicity

Drug classifications
Anesthetics, nondepolarizing neuromuscular blockers: increased neuromuscular blockade, respiratory depression

> **BLACK BOX WARNING:** Increased: Ototoxicito-IV loop diuretics

> **BLACK BOX WARNING:** Cephalosporins: inactivation of amikacin, nephrotoxicity

NSAIDs: increased serum trough and peak

Drug/lab test
Increased: BUN, creatinine, urea levels (urine)

NURSING CONSIDERATIONS
Assessment
• Assess patient for previous sensitivity reaction
• Assess patient for signs and symptoms of infection, including characteristics of wounds, sputum, urine, stool, WBC $>10,000/mm^3$, earache, temp; obtain baseline information before and during treatment
• Assess for allergic reactions: rash, urticaria, pruritus

> **BLACK BOX WARNING:** Assess renal impairment by securing urine for CCr, BUN, serum creatinine; lower dosage should be given in renal impairment; nephrotoxicity may be reversible if product is stopped at first sign

• Notify prescriber of increased BUN and creatinine, urine CCr <80 ml/min; urinalysis daily for protein, cells, casts
• Monitor blood studies: AST, ALT, CBC, Hct, bilirubin, LDH, alkaline phosphatase; Coombs' test monthly if patient is on long-term therapy
• Monitor electrolytes: potassium, sodium, chloride, magnesium monthly if patient is on long-term therapy
• Assess bowel pattern daily; if severe diarrhea occurs, product should be discontinued
• Monitor for bleeding: ecchymosis, bleeding gums, hematuria, stool guaiac daily if on long-term therapy
• Assess for **overgrowth of infection:** perineal itching, fever, malaise, redness, pain, swelling, drainage, rash, diarrhea, change in cough, sputum
• Obtain weight before treatment; calculation of dosage is usually based on ideal body weight but may be calculated on actual body weight
• Monitor VS during infusion, watch for hypotension, change in pulse
• Assess **IV** site for thrombophlebitis including pain, redness, swelling q30min; change site if needed; apply warm compresses to discontinued site

> **BLACK BOX WARNING:** Deafness by audiometric testing, ringing, roaring in ears, vertigo; assess hearing before, during, after treatment

• **Dehydration:** high specific gravity, decrease in skin turgor, dry mucous membranes, dark urine
• **Vestibular dysfunction:** nausea, vomiting, dizziness, headache; product should be discontinued if severe

Patient/family education
• Teach patient to report sore throat, bruising, bleeding, joint pain; may indicate blood dyscrasias (rare)
• Advise patient to contact prescriber if vaginal itching, loose foul-smelling stools, furry tongue occur; may indicate superinfection
• Advise patient to report hypersensitivity: rash, itching, trouble breathing, facial edema and notify prescriber

Evaluation
Positive therapeutic outcome
• Absence of signs/symptoms of infection: WBC <10,000/mm^3, temp WNL; absence of red draining wounds; absence of earache
• Reported improvement in symptoms of infection

TREATMENT OF OVERDOSE:
Withdraw product; administer EPINEPHrine, O_2, hemodialysis, exchange transfusion in the newborn; monitor serum levels of product; may give ticarcillin or carbenicillin

aMILoride (Rx)
(a-mill'oh-ride)
Midamor
Func. class.: Potassium-sparing diuretic
Chem. class.: Pyrazine
Pregnancy category B

Do not confuse:
aMILoride/amLODIPine/amiodarone

ACTION: Inhibits sodium, potassium ATPase ion exchange in the distal tubule, cortical collecting duct resulting in inhibition of sodium reabsorption and decreasing potassium secretion

Therapeutic outcome: Diuretic and antihypertensive effect while retaining potassium

USES: Edema in CHF in combination with other diuretics; for hypertension, adjunct with other diuretics to maintain potassium

Unlabeled uses: Ascites

CONTRAINDICATIONS:
Anuria, hypersensitivity, diabetic neuropathy

> **BLACK BOX WARNING:** Hyperkalemia

Precautions: Pregnancy **B,** breastfeeding, children, geriatric, dehydration, diabetes, acidosis, respiratory hyponatremia, impaired renal function

DOSAGE AND ROUTES
Adult: PO 5-10 mg daily in 1-2 divided doses; may be increased to 10-20 mg daily if needed
Infant/child (6-20 kg): PO 0.625 mg/kg/day

Renal dose
Adult: PO CCr 10-50 ml/min reduce dose by 50%; however, avoid if possible, CCr <10 ml/min contraindicated

---

Ascites (unlabeled)
Adult: PO 10 mg/day, max 40 mg

Available forms: Tabs 5 mg

Implementation
- Give in AM to avoid interference with sleep
- With food; if nausea occurs, absorption may be increased

ADVERSE EFFECTS
CNS: *Headache,* dizziness, fatigue, weakness, paresthesias, tremor, depression, anxiety, **encephalopathy**
CV: Orthostatic hypotension, dysrhythmias, angina
EENT: Blurred vision, increased intraocular pressure
ELECT: **Hyperkalemia,** dehydration, hyponatremia, hypochloremia
GI: *Nausea, diarrhea,* dry mouth, *vomiting, anorexia,* cramps, constipation, abdominal pain, jaundice
GU: *Polyuria,* dysuria, frequency, impotence
HEMA: **Aplastic anemia, neutropenia**
INTEG: *Rash, pruritus,* alopecia, urticaria
MS: *Cramps*
RESP: *Cough, dyspnea,* shortness of breath

Pharmacokinetics

Absorption	Variable (10%-50%)
Distribution	Widely distributed
Metabolism	Unchanged in urine (50%), in feces (40%)
Excretion	Renal; breast milk
Half-life	6-9 hr

Pharmacodynamics

Onset	2 hr
Peak	6-10 hr
Duration	24 hr

INTERACTIONS
Individual drugs

> **BLACK BOX WARNING:** CycloSPORINE, tacrolimus: increased hyperkalemia

Lithium: increased lithium toxicity, monitor lithium levels

Drug classifications

> **BLACK BOX WARNING:** ACE inhibitors, diuretics (potassium-sparing), potassium products, salt substitutes: increased hyperkalemia. Avoid concurrent use; if using together, monitor K level

Antihypertensives: increased action
NSAIDs: decreased effectiveness of aMILoride, avoid concurrent use

Drug/herb
Hawthorn, horse chestnut: increased aMILoride effect

Drug/food
Potassium foods: increased hyperkalemia, potassium-based salt substitutes

Drug/lab test
Interference: GTT
Increased: LFTs, BUN, potassium, sodium

NURSING CONSIDERATIONS
Assessment
- Monitor for **hyperkalemia:** *MS:* fatigue, muscle weakness; *CARDIAC:* dysrhythmias, hypotension; *NEURO:* paresthesias, confusion; *RESP:* dyspnea
- Monitor for **hypokalemia:** weakness, polyuria, polydipsia, fatigue, ECG U wave
- Assess fluid volume status: distended red veins, crackles in lung, color, quality, and specific gravity of urine, skin turgor, adequacy of pulses, moist mucous membranes, bilateral lung sounds, peripheral pitting edema; dehydration symptoms of decreasing output, thirst, hypotension, dry mouth and mucous membranes should be reported
- Monitor electrolytes: potassium, sodium, calcium, magnesium; also include BUN, ABGs, uric acid, CBC, blood glucose
- Assess B/P before, during therapy with patient lying, standing, and sitting as appropriate; orthostatic hypotension can occur rapidly

Patient/family education
- Teach patient to take medication early in the day to prevent nocturia, to avoid alcohol
- Instruct patient to take with food or milk if GI symptoms of nausea and anorexia occur
- Teach patient to maintain a weekly record of weight and notify prescriber of weight loss >5 lb
- Caution patient that this product causes an increase in potassium levels, so foods high in potassium and potassium supplements should be avoided; refer to dietitian for assistance, planning
- Caution patient not to exercise in hot weather or stand for prolonged periods since orthostatic hypotension is enhanced
- Teach patient not to use alcohol or any OTC medications without prescriber's approval; serious product reactions may occur

Adverse effects: *italics* = common; **bold** = life-threatening

• Emphasize the need to contact prescriber immediately if muscle cramps, weakness, nausea, dizziness, or numbness occurs
• Teach patient to take own B/P and pulse and record
• Advise patient that dizziness and confusion may occur; avoid driving or other hazardous activities if alertness is decreased
• Teach patient to continue taking medication even if feeling better; this product controls symptoms but does not cure the condition
• Advise patient with hypertension to continue other medical treatment (exercise, weight loss, relaxation techniques, cessation of smoking)
• Teach patient to avoid hazardous activities if dizziness occurs

Evaluation
Positive therapeutic outcome
• Prevention of hypokalemia (diuretic use)
• Decreased edema
• Decreased B/P
• Increased diuresis

TREATMENT OF OVERDOSE:
Lavage if taken orally; monitor electrolytes; administer **IV** fluids; monitor hydration, CV, renal status

---

amino acid (Rx)
(a-mee′noe)
Injection: FreAmine, HepatAmine
Solution: Aminess, Aminosyn, Branch Amin, FreAmine III, NephrAmine, Novamine, ProcalAmine, Ren Amin, Travasol, Troph Amine
Func. class.: Caloric agent
Chem. class.: Nitrogen product
Pregnancy category C

ACTION: Needed for anabolism to maintain structure; decreases catabolism, promotes healing

Therapeutic outcome: Positive nitrogen balance, decreased catabolism

USES: Hepatic encephalopathy, cirrhosis, hepatitis, nutritional support in cancer, burn, or solid organ transplant patients; to prevent nitrogen loss when adequate nutrition by mouth, gastric, or duodenal tube cannot be used; intestinal obstruction, short bowel syndrome, severe malabsorption

CONTRAINDICATIONS:
Hypersensitivity, severe electrolyte imbalances, anuria, severe liver damage, maple syrup urine disease, PKU, azotemia, genetic disease of amino acid metabolism

Precautions: Pregnancy **C**, children, renal disease, diabetes mellitus, CHF, breastfeeding, sulfite sensitivity

DOSAGE AND ROUTES
Amino acid injection
Adult: IV 80-120 g/day; 500 ml of amino acids/500 ml D$_{50}$ given over 24 hr

Amino acid solution
Adult: IV 1-1.5 g/kg/day titrated to patient's needs
Child: IV 2-3 g/kg/day titrated to patient's needs

Available forms: Inj; many strengths, types

Implementation
Continuous IV route
• Give up to 40% protein and dextrose (up to 12.5%) via peripheral vein; stronger solutions require central **IV** administration; TPN only mixed with dextrose to promote protein synthesis
• Use immediately after mixing in pharmacy under strict aseptic technique using laminar flowhood; use infusion pump, in-line filter (0.22 μm) unless mixed with fat emulsion and dextrose (3 in 1)
⚠ Use careful monitoring technique; do not speed up infusion; pulmonary edema, glucose overload will result
• Storage depends on type of solution; consult manufacturer
• Change dressing and **IV** tubing to prevent infection q24-48hr or q5-7days if transparent dressing is used

ADVERSE EFFECTS
CNS: *Dizziness, headache,* confusion, **loss of consciousness**
CV: Hypertension, **CHF, pulmonary edema**
ENDO: *Hyperglycemia, rebound hypoglycemia, electrolyte imbalances, hyperosmolar syndrome, hyperosmolar hyperglycemic nonketotic syndrome,* alkalosis, acidosis, hypophosphatemia, hyperammonemia, dehydration, hypocalcemia
GI: Nausea, vomiting, liver fat deposits, abdominal pain, jaundice
GU: Glycosuria, osmotic diuresis

INTEG: Chills, flushing, warm feeling, rash, urticaria, extravasation necrosis, phlebitis at inj site

Pharmacokinetics

Absorption	Complete bioavailability
Distribution	Widely distributed
Metabolism	Anabolism
Excretion	Kidney to urea nitrogen
Half-life	Unknown

Pharmacodynamics

Unknown

INTERACTIONS

Drug classifications

Tetracycline: decreased protein-sparing effects (inj only)

NURSING CONSIDERATIONS

Assessment

• Monitor electrolytes (potassium, sodium, calcium, chloride, magnesium), blood glucose, ammonia, phosphate, ketones; renal, liver function studies: BUN, creatinine, ALT, AST, bilirubin; urine glucose q6hr using Chemstrips, which are not affected by infusion substances; if BUN increases over 15%, therapy may need to be discontinued

• Check inj site for extravasation: redness along vein, edema at site, necrosis, pain; for a hard, tender area

• Monitor respiratory function q4hr: auscultate lung fields bilaterally for crackles; monitor respirations for quality, rate, rhythm that indicates fluid overload

• Monitor temp q4hr for increased fever, indicating infection; if infection is suspected, infusion is discontinued and tubing, bottle, catheter tip cultured; blood catheter may be obtained

⚠ **Monitor for impending hepatic coma: asterixis, confusion, fetor, lethargy**

• **Hyperammonemia:** nausea, vomiting, malaise, tremors, anorexia, seizures; increased ammonia, ketone levels may occur

Patient/family education

• Teach reason for use of amino acids as part of nutrition (TPN)

• Instruct patient to report at once to prescriber if chills, sweating are experienced

Evaluation

Positive therapeutic outcome

• Weight gain
• Decreased jaundice in liver disorders
• Increased LOC

A

aminophylline (theophylline ethylenediamine) (Rx)

(am-in-off'i-lin)
Phyllocontin
Func. class.: Bronchodilator, spasmolytic
Chem. class.: Xanthine, ethylenediamine
Pregnancy category C

ACTION: Exact mechanism unknown; relaxes smooth muscle of respiratory system by blocking phosphodiesterase, which increases cyclic AMP; increased cyclic AMP alters intracellular calcium ion movements; produces bronchodilatation, increased pulmonary blood flow, relaxation of respiratory tract

Therapeutic outcome: Increased ability to breathe

USES: Apnea in infancy for respiratory/myocardial stimulation, bronchial asthma, bronchospasm associated with chronic bronchitis, emphysema

Unlabeled uses: Methotrexate toxicity, sleep apnea, status asthmaticus

CONTRAINDICATIONS:

Hypersensitivity to xanthines, tachydysrhythmias

Precautions: Pregnancy C, breastfeeding, children, geriatric, CHF, cor pulmonale, hepatic disease, diabetes mellitus, hyperthyroidism, hypertension, seizure disorder, irritation of the rectum or lower colon, alcoholism, active peptic ulcer disease

DOSAGE AND ROUTES

Adult: PO 6 mg/kg, then 3 mg/kg q6hr × 2 doses, then 3 mg/kg q8hr maintenance, max 900 mg/day or 13 mg/kg; PO in CHF 6 mg/kg, then 2 mg/kg q8hr × 2 doses, then 1-2 mg/kg q12hr maintenance; IV 4.7 mg/kg, then 0.55 mg/kg/hr × 12 hr, then 0.36 mg/kg/hr maintenance; IV in CHF 4.7 mg/kg, then 0.39 mg/kg/hr × 12 hr; then 0.08-0.16 mg/kg/hr maintenance
Geriatric and in cor pulmonale: PO 6 mg/kg, then 2 mg/kg q6hr × 2 doses, then 2 mg/kg q8hr maintenance; IV 4.7 mg/kg, then 0.47 mg/kg/hr × 12 hr, then 0.24 mg/kg/hr maintenance
Child 9-16 yr: PO 6 mg/kg, then 3 mg/kg q4hr × 3 doses, then 3 mg/kg q6hr maintenance, max 18 mg/kg/day 12-16 yr, or 20 mg/kg/day 9-12 yr; IV 4.7 mg/kg, then 0.79 mg/kg/hr × 12 hr, then 0.63 mg/kg/hr maintenance

---

Child 6 mo-9 yr: PO 4 mg/kg q4hr × 3 doses, then 4 mg/kg q6hr maintenance, max 24 mg/kg/day; **IV** 4.7 mg/kg, then 0.95 mg/kg/hr × 12 hr, then 0.79 mg/kg/hr maintenance

Infant 6-52 wk: Dose (0.2 × age in wk) ÷ 5 × kg = 24 hr dose in mg

Neonate up to 40 wk premature postconception age: PO/IV 1 mg/kg q12hr

Neonate at birth or 40 wk postconception age: PO/IV >8 wk postnatal 1-3 mg/kg q6hr; 4-8 wk postnatal 1-2 mg/kg q8hr; up to 4 wk postnatal 1-2 mg/kg q12hr

Hepatic disease
Adult: PO 6 mg/kg, then 2 mg/kg q8hr × 2 doses, then 1-2 mg/kg q12hr maintenance; **IV** 4.7 mg/kg, then 0.39 mg/kg/hr × 12 hr, then 0.08-0.16 mg/kg/hr maintenance

Available forms: Inj 250 mg/10 ml, 500 mg/20 ml, 100 mg/100 ml in 0.45% NaCl; 200 mg/100 ml in 0.45% NaCl; rectal supp 250 mg, 500 mg; oral liq 105 mg/5 ml; tabs 100, 200 mg; cont rel tabs 225, 350 mg

Implementation
- Give around the clock to maintain blood (theophylline) levels
- If switching from **IV** to PO, give controlled-release dose at time **IV** infusion is discontinued; if giving tab (immediate release), discontinue **IV** and wait >4 hr
- If GI upset occurs, take with 8 oz of water or food
- Increase fluids to 2 L/day

PO route
- Do not break, crush, or chew enteric-coated or cont rel tabs
- Avoid giving with food

Continuous IV Infusion route
- May be diluted for **IV** inf in 100-200 ml in D_5W, $D_{10}W$, $D_{20}W$, 0.9% NaCl, 0.45% NaCl, LR
- Give loading dose over ½ hr, max rate of inf 25 mg/min, use infusion pump; after loading dose, give by cont inf
- Avoid IM inj; pain and tissue damage may occur
- Only clear sol; flush **IV** line before dose; store diluted sol for 24 hr if refrigerated

Syringe compatibilities: Heparin, metoclopramide, PENTobarbital, thiopental

Y-site compatibilities: Allopurinol, amifostine, amphotericin B sulfate complex, inamrinone, aztreonam, cefTAZidime, cimetidine, cladribine, DOXOrubicin liposome, enalaprilat, esmolol, famotidine, filgrastim, fluconazole, fludarabine, foscarnet, gallium, granisetron, heparin sodium with hydrocortisone sodium succinate, labetalol, melphalan, meropenem, netilmicin, PACLitaxel, pancuronium, piperacillin/tazobactam, potassium chloride, propofol, ranitidine, remifentanil, sargramostim, tacrolimus, teniposide, thiotepa, tolazoline, vecuronium

Y-site incompatibilities: DOBUTamine, hydrALAZINE, ondansetron

ADVERSE EFFECTS
CNS: Anxiety, restlessness, insomnia, *dizziness,* **seizures,** headache, light-headedness, muscle twitching, tremors

CV: *Palpitations, sinus tachycardia,* hypotension, flushing, **dysrhythmias,** edema

GI: *Nausea, vomiting,* diarrhea, dyspepsia, anal irritation (suppositories), epigastric pain, reflux, anorexia

GU: Urinary frequency, SIADH

INTEG: Flushing, urticaria

MISC: Hyperglycemia

RESP: Tachypnea, increased respiratory rate

Pharmacokinetics

Absorption	Well absorbed (PO), slow (PO–EXT REL), erratic (RECT)
Distribution	Widely distributed; crosses placenta
Metabolism	Liver to caffeine
Excretion	Kidneys
Half-life	3-12 hr, increased in renal disease, CHF, geriatric patients, smokers, crosses into CSF (cerebrospinal fluid)

Pharmacodynamics

	PO	PO–EXT REL	IV
Onset	15-60 min	Unknown	Immediate
Peak	1-2 hr	4-7 hr	Infusion's end
Duration	6-8 hr	8-12 hr	6-8 hr

INTERACTIONS
Individual drugs
Allopurinol (high doses), cimetidine, clarithromycin, disulfiram, erythromycin, fluvoxamine, interferon, mexiletine: decreased metabolism, increased toxicity of aminophylline

CarBAMazepine, isoniazid: increased or decreased aminophylline levels

Halothane: increased risk of dysrhythmias

⚠ Nurse Alert ❋ Key NCLEX® Drug

Ketoconazole, phenytoin, rifampin: decreased aminophylline effect

Lithium: decreased effect of lithium

Smoking: increased metabolism, decreased effect

Drug classifications

Barbiturates, β-adrenergic blockers: decreased effect of aminophylline

Benzodiazepines, β-blockers (nonselective), corticosteroids, diuretics (loop), fluoroquinolones, influenza vaccines, oral contraceptives: increased aminophylline levels

Corticosteroids, influenza vaccines: increased aminophylline toxicity

Diuretics (loop): may increase or decrease aminophylline levels

Dose-dependent reversal of neuromuscular blockade

Fluoroquinolones: decreased metabolism, increased toxicity

Sympathomimetics: increased CNS, CV adverse reactions

Tetracyclines: increased adverse reactions

Drug/herb

Cola tree, ginseng, guarana, horsetail, Siberian ginseng, tea (black, green), yerba maté: increased effects

St. John's wort: decreased effects

Drug/food

High-carbohydrate, low-protein diet: decreased elimination

Low-carbohydrate, high-protein diet, charcoal-broiled beef: increased elimination

Xanthines: increased effect

Drug/lab test

Increased: plasma free fatty acids

NURSING CONSIDERATIONS

Assessment

• Monitor theophylline blood levels (therapeutic level is 10-20 mcg/ml); toxicity may occur with small increase above 20 mcg/ml, especially geriatric; determine whether theophylline was given recently (24 hr); check for toxicity: nausea, vomiting, anxiety, restlessness, insomnia, tachycardia, dysrhythmias, seizures; notify prescriber immediately

• Monitor I&O; diuresis will occur; dehydration may result in geriatric or children in whom diuresis is great

• Monitor liver function tests: periodically, lower doses may be required in those with moderate to severe hepatic disease

• Monitor respiratory rate, rhythm, depth; auscultate lung fields bilaterally, pulmonary function tests; notify prescriber of abnormalities; check ECG for tachycardia, PVCs, PACs in patients with cardiac problems

• Monitor allergic reactions: rash, urticaria; if these occur, product should be discontinued, prescriber notified

Patient/family education

• Teach patient to take doses as prescribed, not to skip dose; to check OTC medications, current prescription medications for ephedrine, which will increase CNS stimulation; advise patient not to drink alcohol or caffeine products (tea, coffee, chocolate, colas), which will increase action

• Teach patient to avoid hazardous activities; dizziness may occur

• Teach patient if GI upset occurs, to take product with 8 oz of water or food; absorption may be decreased

• Teach patient to remain in bed 15-20 min after rect supp is inserted to prevent removal

• Instruct patient to avoid smoking because it increases metabolism; decreases blood levels and terminal half-life; dosage may need to be increased

• Teach patient to obtain blood levels of product every few months to prevent toxicity; not to change brands, since effect may not be the same

• Teach patient to increase fluids to 2 L/day to decrease viscosity of secretions

• Advise patient to report **toxicity:** nausea, vomiting, anxiety, insomnia, rapid pulse, seizures, flushing, headache, diarrhea

Evaluation

Positive therapeutic outcome

• Decreased dyspnea

• Respiratory stimulation in infants

• Clear lung fields bilaterally

⚠ HIGH ALERT

amiodarone (Rx)

(a-mee-oh′da-rone)

Cordarone, Nexterone, Pacerone

Func. class.: Antidysrhythmic (Class III)

Chem. class.: Iodinated benzofuran derivative

Pregnancy category D

Do not confuse:

amiodarone/inamrinone, Cordarone/Inocor

ACTION: Prolongs action potential duration and effective refractory period, noncompetitive α- and β-adrenergic inhibition; increases

PR and QT intervals, decreases sinus rate, decreases peripheral vascular resistance

Therapeutic outcome: Decreased amount and severity of ventricular dysrhythmias

USES: Hemodynamically unstable ventricular tachycardia, supraventricular tachycardia, ventricular fibrillation not controlled by 1st-line agents

CONTRAINDICATIONS:
Pregnancy **D**, breastfeeding, neonates, infants, severe sinus node dysfunction, hypersensitivity to this product/iodine/benzyl alcohol, cardiogenic shock

> **BLACK BOX WARNING:** 2nd-3rd degree AV block, bradycardia

Precautions: Goiter, Hashimoto's thyroiditis, electrolyte imbalances, CHF, severe respiratory disease, children, torsades de pointes

> **BLACK BOX WARNING:** Cardiac arrhythmias, pneumonitis, pulmonary fibrosis, severe hepatic disease

DOSAGE AND ROUTES
Ventricular dysrhythmias
Adult: PO loading dose 800-1600 mg/day for 1-3 wk; then 600-800 mg/day × 1 mo; maintenance 400 mg/day; **IV** loading dose (first rapid) 150 mg over the first 10 min then slow 360 mg over the next 6 hr; maintenance 540 mg given over the remaining 18 hr, decrease rate of the slow infusion to 0.5 mg/min
Child (unlabeled): PO loading dose 10-15 mg/kg/day in 1-2 divided doses for 4-14 days then 5 mg/kg/day
Child and infant: IV/INTRAOSSEOUS during CPR 5 mg/kg as a bolus (PALS guidelines)

Supraventricular tachycardia
Adult: PO 600-800 mg/day × 7 days or until desired response, then 400 mg/day × 21 days, then 200-400 mg/day maintenance
Child: PO 10 mg/kg/day (800 mg/1.72 m²/day) × 10 days or until desired response, then 5 mg/kg/day (400 mg/1.72 m²/day) × 21-28 days, then 2.5 mg/kg/day (200 mg/1.72 m²/day) (not recommended in children)

Available forms: Tabs 100, 200, 400 mg; inj 50 mg/ml

Implementation
Start with patient hospitalized and monitored

PO route
• Give reduced dosage slowly with ECG monitoring only
• Loading dose with food to decrease nausea

IV, direct route
• **Peripheral:** max 2 mg/ml for longer than 1 hr; preferred through central venous line with in-line filter; concentration >2 mg/ml should be given by central line
• **Cardiac arrest:** give 300 mg bol diluted to a total volume of 20 ml D₅W; may repeat 150 mg after 3-5 min

Intermittent IV INF route
• **Rapid loading:** add 3 ml (150 mg), 100 ml D₅W (1.5 mg/ml), give over 10 min
• **Slow loading:** add 18 ml (900 mg), 500 ml D₅W (1.8 mg/ml), give over next 6 hr

Continuous IV infusion route
• After 24 hr, dilute 50 ml to 1-6 mg/ml, give 1-6 mg/ml at 1 mg/ml for the first 6 hr, then 0.5 mg/min

Y-site compatibilities: Amikacin, bretylium, clindamycin, DOBUTamine, DOPamine, doxycycline, erythromycin, esmolol, gentamicin, insulin (regular), isoproterenol, labetalol, lidocaine, metaraminol, metroNIDAZOLE, midazolam, morphine, nitroglycerin, norepinephrine, penicillin G potassium, phentolamine, phenylephrine, potassium chloride, procainamide, tobramycin, vancomycin

Solution compatibilities: D₅W, 0.9% NaCl

ADVERSE EFFECTS
CNS: *Headache, dizziness,* involuntary movement, tremors, peripheral neuropathy, malaise, fatigue, ataxia, paresthesias, insomnia
CV: *Hypotension,* **bradycardia, sinus arrest, CHF, dysrhythmias, SA node dysfunction, AV block,** increased defibrillation energy requirement
EENT: Blurred vision, halos, photophobia, *corneal microdeposits,* dry eyes
ENDO: Hyper/hypothyroidism
GI: Nausea, vomiting, diarrhea, abdominal pain, anorexia, constipation, **hepatotoxicity**
GU: Epididymitis, ED
INTEG: Rash, photosensitivity, blue-gray skin discoloration, alopecia, spontaneous ecchymosis, **toxic epidermal necrolysis,** urticaria, **pancreatitis,** phlebitis (IV)
MISC: Flushing, abnormal taste or smell, edema, abnormal salivation, coagulation abnormalities
MS: Weakness, pain in extremities

RESP: Pulmonary fibrosis/toxicity, pulmonary inflammation, **ARDS, gasping syndrome in neonates**

Pharmacokinetics

Absorption	Slow, variable (PO) up to 65%
Distribution	Body tissues; crosses placenta
Metabolism	Liver
Excretion	Bile, kidney (minimal)
Half-life	15-100 days, increased in geriatrics

Pharmacodynamics

	PO
Onset	1-3 wk
Peak	Unknown
Duration	Up to months

INTERACTIONS
Individual drugs
CycloSPORINE, dextromethorphan, digoxin, disopyramide, flecainide, methotrexate, phenytoin, procainamide, quiNIDine, theophylline: increased blood levels, increased toxicity
Warfarin: increased bleeding

Drug classifications
Azoles, fluoroquinolones, macrolides: increased QT prolongation
β-Adrenergic blockers, calcium channel blockers: increased bradycardia
Class I antidysrhythmics: increased levels
HMG-CoA reductase inhibitors: increased myopathy
Protease inhibitors: increased amiodarone concentrations, possible serious dysrhythmias, reduce dose

Drug/herb
St. John's wort: decreased amiodarone effect

Drug/food
Grapefruit juice: toxicity

Drug/lab test
Increased: T_4, ALT, AST, GGT, alk phos, cholesterol, lipids, PT, INR
Decrease: T_3

NURSING CONSIDERATIONS
Assessment
• Monitor electrolytes: potassium, sodium, chloride
• Monitor chest x-ray, thyroid function tests
• Monitor liver function studies: AST, ALT, bilirubin, alkaline phosphatase

BLACK BOX WARNING: Monitor ECG continuously to determine product effectiveness; measure PR, QRS, QT intervals; check for PVCs, other dysrhythmias; monitor B/P continuously for hypo/hypertension; check for rebound hypertension after 1-2 hr

• Monitor for dehydration or hypovolemia, monitor PT, INR if using warfarin
• Assess for CNS symptoms: confusion, psychosis, numbness, depression, involuntary movements; if these occur, product should be discontinued
• Assess for hypothyroidism: lethargy, dizziness, constipation, enlarged thyroid gland, edema of extremities, cool, pale skin
• Monitor hyperthyroidism: restlessness, tachycardia, eyelid puffiness, weight loss, frequent urination, menstrual irregularities, dyspnea, warm, moist skin

BLACK BOX WARNING: Assess for pulmonary toxicity including ARDS, pulmonary fibrosis: dyspnea, fatigue, cough, fever, chest pain; product should be discontinued if these occur, increased at higher doses, toxicity is common

• Monitor cardiac rate, respiration: rate, rhythm, character, chest pain, ventricular tachycardia, supraventricular tachycardia or fibrillation
• Assess sight and vision before treatment and throughout therapy; microdeposits on the cornea may cause blurred vision, halos, and photophobia, to prevent corneal deposits use methylcellulose

Patient/family education
• Instruct patient to report side effects immediately to prescriber; more common at high dose NO
• Instruct patient that skin discoloration is usually reversible, but skin may turn bluish on neck, face, arms when used for long periods
• Advise patient that dark glasses may be needed for photophobia
• Instruct patient to use sunscreen and protective clothing to prevent burning associated with photosensitivity
• Instruct patient to take medication as prescribed, not to double doses, do not discontinue abruptly
• Instruct patient to complete follow-up appointment with health care provider including pulmonary function studies, chest x-ray, ophthalmic examinations

Evaluation
Positive therapeutic outcome
- Decreased ventricular tachycardia
- Decreased supraventricular tachycardia or fibrillation

TREATMENT OF OVERDOSE:
Administer O_2, artificial ventilation, ECG, DOPamine for circulatory depression, diazepam or thiopental for seizures, isoproterenol

---

amitriptyline (Rx)
(a-mee-trip'ti-leen)
Func. class.: Antidepressant—tricyclic
Chem. class.: Tertiary amine
Pregnancy category C

Do not confuse:
amitriptyline/nortriptyline/aminophylline

ACTION: Blocks reuptake of norepinephrine, serotonin into nerve endings that increase action of norepinephrine, serotonin in nerve cells

Therapeutic outcome: Decreased symptoms of depression after 2-3 wk

USES: Major depression

Unlabeled uses: Neuropathic pain, prevention of cluster/migraine headaches, fibromyalgia

CONTRAINDICATIONS:
Hypersensitivity to tricyclics, carBAMazepine; recovery phase of MI

Precautions: Pregnancy C, breastfeeding, geriatric, seizure disorders, prostatic hypertrophy, schizophrenia, psychosis, severe depression, increased intraocular pressure, closed-angle glaucoma, urinary retention, cardiac disease, renal/hepatic disease, hyperthyroidism, electroshock therapy, elective surgery

> **BLACK BOX WARNING:** Child <12 yr, suicidal patients

DOSAGE AND ROUTES
Depression
Adult/adolescent: PO 25-75 mg/day as a single dose at bedtime or in divided doses; may increase to 200 mg/day, max 300 mg/day (hospitalized)
Geriatric: PO 10-25 mg at bedtime; may be increased to 150 mg/day

Cluster/migraine headaches (unlabeled)
Adult: PO 100-300 mg/day

Pain (unlabeled)
Adult: PO 75-300 mg/day

Fibromyalgia/insomnia (unlabeled)
Adult: PO 10-50 mg nightly

Available forms: Tabs 10, 25, 50, 75, 100, 150 mg

Implementation
- Give with food or milk for GI symptoms
- Crush if patient is unable to swallow medication whole
- Give dose at bedtime if oversedation occurs during day; may take entire dose at bedtime; geriatric may not tolerate once/day dosing
- Store at room temperature; do not freeze

ADVERSE EFFECTS
CNS: *Dizziness, drowsiness,* confusion, headache, anxiety, tremors, stimulation, weakness, *insomnia,* nightmares, EPS (geriatric), increased psychiatric symptoms, **seizures, suicidal thoughts,** anxiety
CV: *Orthostatic hypotension,* **ECG changes, tachycardia, hypertension,** palpitations, dysrhythmias
EENT: *Blurred vision,* tinnitus, mydriasis, ophthalmoplegia, amblyopia
GI: *Constipation, dry mouth,* weight gain, nausea, vomiting, **paralytic ileus,** increased appetite, cramps, epigastric distress, jaundice, **hepatitis,** stomatitis
GU: *Urinary retention,* sexual dysfunction
HEMA: Agranulocytosis, thrombocytopenia, eosinophilia, leukopenia, aplastic anemia
INTEG: Rash, urticaria, sweating, pruritus, photosensitivity
RESP: Asthma exacerbation, rhinitis
SYST: Neuroleptic malignant syndrome, serotonin syndrome

Pharmacokinetics

Absorption	Well absorbed
Distribution	Widely distributed; crosses placenta
Metabolism	Liver, extensively
Excretion	Kidneys, breast milk
Half-life	10-46 hr

Pharmacodynamics

	PO
Onset	45 min
Peak	2-12 hr
Duration	Unknown

INTERACTIONS
Individual drugs
Alcohol: increased CNS depression

Amiodarone, procainamide, quiNIDine: increased QT prolongation

CarBAMazepine: increased amitriptyline levels, increased toxicity

Cimetidine, fluoxetine: increased levels, increased toxicity

CloNIDine: decreased effects

Guanethidine: decreased effects

Linezolid, methylene blue: increased serotonin syndrome, use cautiously

Drug classifications
Antidepressants, antidysrhythmics (class IC), phenothiazines: increased amitriptyline levels, toxicity

Antidysrhythmics (class IA, III), tricyclic antidepressants: increased QT prolongation

Antithyroid agents: increased risk of agranulocytosis

Barbiturates, benzodiazepines, CNS depressants, opioids, sedative/hypnotics, sympathomimetics (direct acting): increased CNS effects

MAOIs: hypertensive crisis, seizures, hyperpyretic crisis, do not use 14 days of MAOIs

Oral contraceptives: increased effects, toxicity

Sympathomimetics (indirect acting): decreased effects

Drug/herb
Chamomile, hops, kava, lavender, valerian: increased CNS depression

SAM-e, St. John's wort, yohimbe: serotonin syndrome

Drug/lab test
Increased: serum bilirubin, blood glucose, alkaline phosphatase, LFTs

Decreased: WBCs, platelets, granulocytes

NURSING CONSIDERATIONS
Assessment
• Monitor B/P (with patient lying, standing), pulse q4hr; if systolic B/P drops 20 mm Hg, hold product, notify prescriber; take VS q4hr in patients with cardiovascular disease

• Monitor blood studies: CBC, leukocytes, differential, cardiac enzymes if patient is receiving long-term therapy, thyroid function tests

• Monitor hepatic studies: AST, ALT, bilirubin

• Check weight weekly; appetite may increase with product

• Assess ECG for flattening of T wave, bundle branch block, AV block, prolongation of QTc interval, dysrhythmias in cardiac patients, avoid use immediately after MI

• Assess for EPS primarily in geriatric: rigidity, dystonia, akathisia

• Assess mental status: mood, sensorium, affect, suicidal tendencies; increase in psychiatric symptoms: depression, panic

⚠ **Assess for serotonin syndrome: may occur with other serotonergic products (hyperthermia, hypertension, rigidity, delirium)**

• Monitor urinary retention, constipation; constipation is more likely to occur in children or geriatric

• Assess for paralytic ileus, glaucoma exacerbation

• Assess for **withdrawal symptoms:** headache, nausea, vomiting, muscle pain, weakness; do not usually occur unless product was discontinued abruptly

• Identify alcohol consumption; if alcohol is consumed, hold dose until morning

• Assess for sexual dysfunction: erectile dysfunction, decreased libido; usually resolves after discontinuing product

Patient/family education
• Teach patient that therapeutic effects may take 2-3 wk

• Instruct patient to use caution in driving or other activities requiring alertness because of drowsiness, dizziness, blurred vision; to avoid rising quickly from sitting to standing, especially geriatric; management of anticholinergic effects

⚠ **Teach patient the symptoms of serotonin syndrome**

• Advise patient to avoid alcohol ingestion, other CNS depressants; overheating

• Teach patient not to discontinue medication quickly after long-term use; may cause nausea, headache, malaise

• Advise patient to wear sunscreen or large hat, since photosensitivity occurs; hyperthermia can occur

• Teach patient to increase fluids, bulk in diet if constipation, urinary retention occur, especially geriatric

• Teach patient to use gum, hard sugarless candy, or frequent sips of water for dry mouth

• Instruct patient to use contraception during treatment

⚠ **Teach patient to watch for suicidal ideation**

Adverse effects: *italics* = common; **bold** = life-threatening

Evaluation
Positive therapeutic outcome
- Decreased depression
- Absence of suicidal thoughts

TREATMENT OF OVERDOSE:
ECG monitoring, lavage, administer anticonvulsant, sodium bicarbonate

---

amLODIPine (Rx)
(am-loe'di-peen)
Norvasc
Func. class.: Antianginal, calcium channel blocker, antihypertensive
Chem. class.: Dihydropyridine
Pregnancy category C

Do not confuse:
amLODIPine/aMILoride

ACTION: Inhibits calcium ion influx across cell membrane during cardiac depolarization; produces relaxation of coronary vascular smooth muscle and peripheral vascular smooth muscle; dilates coronary vascular arteries; increases myocardial oxygen delivery in patients with vasospastic angina

Therapeutic outcome: Decreased angina pectoris, dysrhythmias, B/P

USES: Chronic stable angina pectoris, hypertension, variant angina (Prinzmetal's angina); may coadminister with other antihypertensives, antianginals

CONTRAINDICATIONS:
Hypersensitivity to this product, severe aortic stenosis, severe obstructive CAD

BLACK BOX WARNING: Hypersensitivity to dihydropyridine

Precautions: Pregnancy **C,** breastfeeding, children, geriatric, CHF, hypotension, hepatic injury, GERD

DOSAGE AND ROUTES
Coronary artery disease
Adult: PO 5-10 mg daily
Geriatric: PO 5 mg daily, may increase; max 10 mg/day

Hypertension
Adult: PO 5 mg daily initially, max 10 mg/day
Geriatric: PO 2.5 mg/day; may increase to 5 mg/day, max 10 mg/day

Hepatic dose
Adult: PO 2.5 mg/day, may increase to 10 mg/day (antihypertensive); 5 mg/day, may increase to 10 mg/day (antianginal)

Available forms: Tabs 2.5, 5, 10 mg
Implementation
- Give once a day, without regard to meals

ADVERSE EFFECTS
CNS: Headache, fatigue, dizziness, asthenia, anxiety, depression, insomnia, paresthesia, somnolence
CV: Peripheral edema, bradycardia, hypotension, palpitations, syncope, chest pain
GI: Nausea, vomiting, diarrhea, gastric upset, constipation, flatulence, anorexia, gingival hyperplasia, dyspepsia
GU: Nocturia, polyuria, sexual difficulties
INTEG: Rash, pruritus, urticaria, alopecia
MISC: Flushing, muscle cramps, cough, weight gain, tinnitus, epistaxis

Pharmacokinetics
Absorption	Well absorbed up to 90%
Distribution	Crosses placenta, protein binding 93%
Metabolism	Liver, extensively by CYP3A4
Excretion	Kidneys to metabolites (90%)
Half-life	30-50 hr; increased in geriatric, hepatic disease

Pharmacodynamics
Onset	Unknown
Peak	6-10 hr
Duration	24 hr

INTERACTIONS
Individual drugs
Alcohol, fentaNYL, quiNIDine: increased hypotension
Diltiazem: increased amLODIPine level
Lithium: increased neurotoxicity

Drug classifications
Antihypertensives, nitrates: increased hypotension
NSAIDs: decreased antihypertensive effect

Drug/food
Grapefruit juice: increased hypotension

NURSING CONSIDERATIONS
Assessment
- Assess fluid volume status: distended red veins, crackles in lung; color, quality, and specific gravity of urine, skin turgor, adequacy of

---

pulses, moist mucous membranes, bilateral lung sounds, peripheral pitting edema; dehydration symptoms of decreasing output, thirst, hypotension, dry mouth and mucous membranes should be reported

• Assess for angina: intensity, location, duration of pain

• Monitor B/P and pulse; if B/P drops, call prescriber

• Monitor ALT, AST, bilirubin daily; if these are elevated, hepatotoxicity is suspected

• Monitor platelet count: if <150,000/mm³, product is usually discontinued and another product started

• Monitor cardiac status: B/P, pulse, respiration, ECG

Patient/family education

• Advise patient to avoid hazardous activities until stabilized on product, dizziness is no longer a problem

• Instruct patient to avoid alcohol and OTC products unless directed by prescriber

• Advise patient to comply in all areas of medical regimen: diet, exercise, stress reduction, smoking cessation, product therapy; to notify prescriber of irregular heartbeat, shortness of breath, swelling of feet, face, and hands, severe dizziness, constipation, nausea, hypotension; use nitroglycerin when angina is severe

• Teach patient to use as directed even if feeling better; may be taken with other cardiovascular products (nitrates, β-blockers)

• Advise to avoid large amounts of grapefruit juice or alcohol

Evaluation

Positive therapeutic outcome

• Decreased anginal pain
• Decreased B/P
• Increased exercise tolerance

TREATMENT OF OVERDOSE:

Defibrillation, β-agonists, **IV** calcium inotropic agents, diuretics, atropine for AV block, vasopressor for hypotension

---

amoxicillin (Rx)

(a-mox-i-sill′in)

Moxatag

Func. class.: Antiinfective, antiulcer

Chem. class.: Aminopenicillin

Pregnancy category B

Do not confuse:

amoxicillin/amoxapine/Amoxil

ACTION: Interferes with cell wall replication of susceptible organisms by binding to the bacterial cell wall; the cell wall; bactericidal, lysis mediated by bacterial cell wall autolysis

Therapeutic outcome: Bactericidal effects for the following organisms: effective for gram-positive cocci *(Staphylococcus aureus, Streptococcus pyogenes, Streptococcus faecalis, Streptococcus pneumoniae)*, gram-negative cocci *(Neisseria gonorrhoeae, Neisseria meningitidis)*, gram-negative bacilli *(Haemophilus influenzae, Proteus mirabilis, Escherichia coli, Salmonella)*, in combination for *Helicobacter pylori*, gram-positive bacilli *(Corynebacterium diphtheriae, Listeria monocytogenes);* gastric ulcer, β-lactamase-negative organisms

USES: Infections of respiratory tract, skin, GI tract, GU tract, otitis media, meningitis, septicemia, sinusitis

Unlabeled uses: Lyme disease, anthrax treatment and prophylaxis, and bacterial endocarditis prophylaxis in combination with other products used for treatment of *Helicobacter pylori*

CONTRAINDICATIONS:

Hypersensitivity to penicillins

Precautions: Pregnancy **B**, breastfeeding, neonates, hypersensitivity to cephalosporins, carbapenems; severe renal disease, mononucleosis, phenylketonuria, diabetes, geriatrics, asthma, child, colitis, dialysis, eczema, pseudomembranous colitis, syphilis

DOSAGE AND ROUTES

Upper respiratory infections

Adult/adolescent and child ≥40 kg: *Mild to moderate infections:* PO 500 mg q12hr or 250 mg q8hr; *Severe infections:* 875 mg q12hr or 500 mg q8hr

Child <40 kg: *Mild to moderate infections:* 45-90 mg/kg/day in individual doses q12hr; *Severe infections:* 40 mg/kg/day divided q8hr or 45 mg/kg/day divided q12hr

Gonorrhea (not CDC approved)

Adult: PO 3 g given with 1 g probenecid as a single dose; followed by tetracycline or erythromycin

Chlamydia trachomatis

Adult: PO 500 mg/day × 1 wk

Adverse effects: italics = common; **bold** = life-threatening

Bacterial endocarditis prophylaxis
Adult: PO 2 g 1 hr prior to procedure
Child: PO 50 mg/kg/hr 1 hr prior to procedure, max 2 g

Helicobacter pylori
Adult: PO 1000 mg bid given with lansoprazole 30 mg bid, clarithromycin 500 mg bid × 2 wk; or 1000 mg bid given with omeprazole 20 mg bid, clarithromycin 500 mg bid × 2 wk; or 1000 mg tid given with lansoprazole 30 mg tid × 2 wk

Renal disease
Adult: PO CCr 10-30 ml/min 250-500 mg q12hr; CCr <10 ml/min 250-500 mg q24hr; do not use 775, 875 mg strength if CCr <30 ml/min

Available forms: Caps 250, 500 mg; chewable tabs 125, 200, 250, 400 mg; tabs 250, 500, 875 mg; ext rel tab (Moxatag) 775 mg; susp 125, 200, 250, 400 mg/5 ml

Implementation
PO route
- Identify allergies before use
- Give in even doses around the clock without regard to food; if GI upset occurs, give with food; product must be given for 10-14 days to ensure organism death and prevent superinfection; store in tight container
- The caps may be opened and contents taken with fluids
- **Suspension:** shake well before each dose, may be used alone or mixed in drinks, use immediately; susp may be stored in refrigerator for 14 days
- **Extended release:** do not crush, chew, or break; take with food

ADVERSE EFFECTS
CNS: Headache, **seizures,** agitation, confusion, dizziness, insomnia
GI: *Nausea, vomiting, diarrhea,* increased AST, ALT, abdominal pain, glossitis, colitis, **pseudomembranous colitis,** jaundice, cholestasis, **eosinophilia, thrombocytopenia, agranulocytosis**
HEMA: Anemia, increased bleeding time, **bone marrow depression, granulocytopenia, hemolytic anemia**
INTEG: *Urticaria, rash*
SYST: Anaphylaxis, respiratory distress, serum sickness, Stevens-Johnson syndrome, toxic epidermal necrolysis, exfoliative dermatitis

Pharmacokinetics

Absorption	Well absorbed (90%)
Distribution	Readily in body tissues, fluids, CSF; crosses placenta
Metabolism	Liver (30%)
Excretion	Breast milk, kidney, unchanged (70%)
Half-life	1-1.3 hr

Pharmacodynamics

Onset	½ hr
Peak	1-2 hr
Duration	Unknown

INTERACTIONS
Individual drugs
Methotrexate: increased methotrexate levels
Decreased: Hgb, WBC, platelets
Probenecid: increased amoxicillin levels, decreased renal excretion
Warfarin: increased anticoagulant effects

Drug classifications
Contraceptives (oral): decreased contraceptive effectiveness

Drug/lab test
Decreased: Hgb, WBC, platelets
Increase: AST/ALT, alk phos, LDH, eosinophils
Interference: urine glucose test (Clinitest, Benedict's reagent, cupric SO_4)

NURSING CONSIDERATIONS
Assessment
- Assess patient for previous sensitivity reaction to penicillins or other cephalosporins; cross-sensitivity between penicillin products and cephalosporins is common
- Assess patient for signs and symptoms of **infection,** including characteristics of wounds, sputum, urine, stool, WBC >10,000/mm³, earache, fever; obtain baseline information and monitor symptoms during treatment
- Obtain C&S before beginning product therapy to identify if correct treatment has been initiated
- Assess for allergic reactions during treatment: rash, urticaria, pruritus, chills, fever, joint pain; angioedema may occur a few days after therapy begins; epinephrine and resuscitation equipment should be available for **anaphylactic reactions**
- Identify urine output; if decreasing, notify prescriber (may indicate nephrotoxicity); also, increased BUN, creatinine, urinalysis, protein, blood

• Monitor blood studies: AST, ALT, CBC, Hct, bilirubin, LDH, alkaline phosphatase, Coombs' test monthly if patient is on long-term therapy
• Monitor electrolytes: potassium, sodium, chloride monthly if patient is on long-term therapy
• Assess bowel pattern daily; diarrhea, cramping, blood in stools; if severe diarrhea occurs, notify prescriber; product should be discontinued; **pseudomembranous colitis** may occur
• Monitor for bleeding: ecchymosis, bleeding gums, hematuria, stool guaiac daily if on long-term therapy
• Skin eruptions: assess after administration of penicillin to 1 wk after discontinuing product; rash is more common if allopurinol is taken concurrently
• Assess for overgrowth of infection: perineal itching, fever, malaise, redness, pain, swelling, drainage, rash, diarrhea, change in cough, sputum

Patient/family education
⚠ Teach patient to report sore throat, bruising, bleeding, joint pain; may indicate blood dyscrasias (rare)
• Advise patient to contact prescriber if vaginal itching, loose foul-smelling stools, diarrhea, sore throat, fever, fatigue, furry tongue occur; may indicate **superinfection** or **agranulocytopenia**
• Instruct patient to take all medication prescribed for the length of time ordered; not to double dose; chew form is available
• Advise patient to notify prescriber of diarrhea with blood or pus, abdominal pain, which may indicate **pseudomembranous colitis**

Evaluation
Positive therapeutic outcome
• Absence of signs/symptoms of infection (WBC <10,000/mm^3, temp WNL, absence of red draining wounds or earache)
• Prevention of endocarditis
• Resolution of ulcer symptoms

TREATMENT OF ANAPHYLAXIS:
Withdraw product, maintain airway, administer epinephrine, aminophylline, O$_2$, **IV** corticosteroids

amoxicillin/clavulanate (Rx)
(a-mox-i-sill'in)
Amoclan, Apo-Amoxi Clav ✦, Augmentin, Augmentin XR, Clavulin ✦
Func. class.: Broad-spectrum antiinfective (extended spectrum)
Chem. class.: Aminopenicillin-β-lactamase inhibitor
Pregnancy category B

Do not confuse:
Augmentin/amoxicillin

ACTION: Interferes with cell wall replication of susceptible organisms; lysis mediated by bacterial cell wall autolytic enzymes, combination increases spectrum of activity against β-lactamase resistance organisms

Therapeutic outcome: Bactericidal effects for *Actinomyces, Bacillus anthracis, Bacteroides, Bordetella pertussis, Borrelia burgdorferi, Brucella, Burkholderia pseudomallei, Clostridium perfringens, Clostridium tetani, Corynebacterium diphtheriae, Eikenella corrodens, Enterobacter, Enterococcus faecalis, Erysipelothrix rhusiopathiae, Escherichia coli, Eubacterium, Fusobacterium, Haemophilus ducreyi, Haemophilus parainfluenzae* (positive/negative beta-lactamase), *Helicobacter pylori, Klebsiella, Lactobacillus, Listeria monocytogenes, Moraxella catarrhalis, Neisseria gonorrhoeae, Neisseria meningitis, Nocardia brasiliensis, Peptococcus, Peptostreptococcus, Prevotella melaninogenica, Propionibacterium, Salmonella, Shigella, Staphylococcus aureus* (MSSA), *Staphylococcus epidermidis, Staphylococcus saprophyticus, Streptococcus agalactiae* (group B Streptococci), *Streptococcus dysgalactiae, Streptococcus pneumoniae, Streptococcus pyogenes* (group A Streptococci), *Treponema pallidum, Vibrio cholerae,* viridans streptococci

USES: Infections of lower respiratory tract, skin, GU tract; impetigo; otitis media, sinusitis, pneumonia, and endocarditis prophylaxis

CONTRAINDICATIONS:
Hypersensitivity to penicillins, severe renal disease, dialysis, jaundice

Precautions: Pregnancy **B**, breastfeeding, neonates, children, hypersensitivity to cephalosporins, GI/renal disease, asthma, colitis, diabetes, eczema, leukemia, mononucleosis, viral infections, phenylketonuria

DOSAGE AND ROUTES

Adult: PO 250-500 mg q8hr or 500-875 mg q12hr depending on severity of infection
Child ≤40 kg: PO 20-90 mg/kg/day in divided doses q8-12hr

Renal dose

Adult: PO CCr 10-30 ml/min dose q12hr; CCr <10 ml/min dose q24hr; do not use 875 mg strength if CCr <30 ml/min; Augmentin XR is contraindicated in renal disease

Available forms: Tabs 250, 500, 875 mg/125 mg clavulanate; chewable tabs 200/28.5, 400/57 mg; powder for oral susp 125, 250/28.5, 200/28.5, 400/57, 600/42.9 mg/5 ml; (XR) ext rel tabs 1000 mg amoxicillin/62.5 mg clavulanate; (ES) powder for oral susp 600 mg amoxicillin; 42.9 mg clavulanate 5 ml

Implementation

PO route

• Give in even doses around the clock; if GI upset occurs, give with food; product must be taken for 10-14 days to ensure organism death and prevent superinfection; store in tight container; cap can be opened and mixed with food or liquid; chewable tabs should be chewed
• Administer only as directed; two 250-mg tabs not equivalent to one 500-mg tab due to strength of clavulanate
• Shake susp well before each dose; may be used alone or mixed in drinks, use immediately; susp may be stored in refrigerator for 10 days

ADVERSE EFFECTS

CNS: Headache, fever, **seizures,** agitation, insomnia
GI: *Nausea, diarrhea, vomiting,* increased AST, ALT, abdominal pain, glossitis, colitis, black tongue, **pseudomembranous colitis**
GU: Oliguria, proteinuria, hematuria, *vaginitis, moniliasis,* **glomerulonephritis**
HEMA: Anemia, **bone marrow depression, granulocytopenia, leukopenia, eosinophilia,** thrombocytopenic purpura
INTEG: Rash, urticaria, dermatitis, **toxic epidermal necrolysis**
META: Hyperkalemia, hypokalemia, alkalosis, hypernatremia
SYST: Anaphylaxis, respiratory distress, serum sickness, superinfection, Stevens-Johnson syndrome, candidiasis

Absorption	Well absorbed (90%)
Distribution	Readily in body tissues, fluids, CSF; crosses placenta
Metabolism	Liver (30%)
Excretion	Breast milk; kidney, unchanged (70%), removed by hemodialysis
Half-life	1-1.3 hr

Onset	½ hr
Peak	1-2.5 hr
Duration	Unknown

INTERACTIONS

Individual drugs

Allopurinol: increased skin rash
Probenecid: increased amoxicillin levels
Warfarin: increased anticoagulant effect, monitor closely: dose adjustment may be needed

Drug classifications

Contraceptives (oral): decreased contraceptive effectiveness

Drug/food

High-fat meal: decreased absorption

Drug/lab test

Increased: AST/ALT, alk phos, LDH
Interference: urine glucose tests (Clinitest, Benedict's reagent, cupric SO_4)

NURSING CONSIDERATIONS

Assessment

• Assess patient for previous sensitivity reaction to penicillins or other cephalosporins; cross-sensitivity between penicillins and cephalosporins is common
• Assess patient for signs and symptoms of **infection,** including characteristics of wounds, sputum, urine, stool, WBC >10,000/mm³, earache, fever; obtain baseline information and during treatment
• Complete C&S before beginning product therapy to identify if correct treatment has been initiated
• Assess for **anaphylaxis:** rash, urticaria, pruritus, chills, dyspnea, laryngeal edema, fever, joint pain; angioedema may occur a few days after therapy begins; EPINEPHrine and resuscitation equipment should be available for anaphylactic reaction
• Identify urine output; if decreasing, notify prescriber (may indicate **nephrotoxicity**)

- Monitor renal studies: urinalysis, protein, blood, BUN, creatinine
- Monitor blood studies: AST, ALT, CBC, Hct, bilirubin, LDH, alkaline phosphatase, Coombs' test monthly if patient is on long-term therapy
- Monitor electrolytes: potassium, sodium, chloride monthly if patient is on long-term therapy
- Assess bowel pattern daily; diarrhea, cramping, blood in stools, report to prescriber; if severe diarrhea occurs, product should be discontinued; may indicate **pseudomembranous colitis**
- Monitor for bleeding: ecchymosis, bleeding gums, hematuria, stool guaiac daily if on long-term therapy
- Assess for **overgrowth of infection:** perineal itching, fever, malaise, redness, pain, swelling, drainage, rash, diarrhea, change in cough, sputum

Patient/family education
⚠ Teach patient to report sore throat, bruising, bleeding, joint pain; may indicate blood dyscrasias (rare)
- Advise patient to contact prescriber if vaginal itching, loose foul-smelling stools occur; may indicate **superinfection**
- Instruct patient to take all medication prescribed for the length of time prescribed
- Advise patient to notify prescriber of diarrhea with blood or pus, which may indicate **pseudomembranous colitis**

Evaluation
Positive therapeutic outcome
- Absence of signs/symptoms of infection (WBC <10,000/mm³, temp WNL)
- Reported improvement in symptoms of infection

TREATMENT OF ANAPHYLAXIS:
Withdraw product, maintain airway, administer EPINEPHrine, aminophylline, O₂, **IV** corticosteroids

amphotericin B lipid complex (ABLC)
(am-foe-ter′i-sin)
Abelcet
Func. class.: Antifungal
Chem. class.: Amphoteric polyene
Pregnancy category B ✴

ACTION: Increases cell membrane permeability in susceptible fungi by binding sterols; alters cell membrane, thereby causing leakage of cell components, cell death

Therapeutic outcome: Decreased fever, malaise, rash; negative C&S for infecting organism

USES: Indicated for the treatment of invasive fungal infections in patients who cannot tolerate or have failed conventional amphotericin B therapy; broad-spectrum activity against many fungal, yeast and mold pathogen infections, including *Aspergillus, Zygomycetes, Fusarium, Cryptococcus,* and many hard-to-treat *Candida* species; *Aspergillus fumigatus, Aspergillus, Blastomyces dermatitidis, Candida albicans, Candida guilliermondii, Candida stellatoidea, Candida tropicalis, Coccidioides immitis, Cryptococcus, Histoplasma, sporotrichosis*

Precautions: Hypersensitivity, anemia, breastfeeding, cardiac disease, children, electrolyte imbalance, geriatric, hematological/hepatic/renal disease, hypotension pregnancy (B)

DOSAGE AND ROUTES
Adult: **IV** 3-5 mg/kg/day as a single inf given at 2.5 mg/kg/hr

Available forms: Susp for inj 100 mg/20-ml vial

Implementation
- *Do not confuse four different types; these are not interchangeable: conventional amphotericin B, amphotericin B cholesteryl, amphotericin B lipid complex, amphotericin B liposome*
- May premedicate with acetaminophen, diphenhydrAMINE

IV route
- Give product only after C&S confirms organism, product needed to treat condition; make sure product is used for life-threatening infections
- Handle with aseptic technique because amphotericin B lipid complex (ABLC) has no preservatives; visually inspect parenteral products for particulate matter and discoloration before use

Filtration and dilution
- Prior to dilution, store at 36°-46° F (2°-8° C), protected from moisture and light; do not freeze; the diluted, ready-for-use admixture is stable for up to 48 hours at 36°-46° F (2°-8° C) and an additional 6 hr at room temperature; do not freeze

• Prepare the admixture for infusion by first shaking the vial until there is no evidence of yellow sediment on the bottom of the vial

• Transfer the appropriate amount of drug from the required number of vials into one or more sterile syringes using an 18-gauge needle

• Attach the provided 5-micron filter needle to the syringe; inject the syringe contents through the filter needle, into an IV bag containing the appropriate amount of D₅W injection; each filter needle may be used on the contents of no more than four 100-mg vials

• The suspension must be diluted with D₅W injection to a final concentration of 1 mg/ml; for pediatric patients and patients with cardiovascular disease, the final concentration may be 2 mg/ml; DO NOT USE SALINE SOLUTIONS OR MIX WITH OTHER DRUGS OR ELECTROLYTES

• The diluted ready-for-use admixture is stable for up to 48 hr at 36°-46° F (2°-8° C) and an additional 6 hr at room temperature; do not freeze

IV INF

• Flush IV line with D₅W injection before use or use a separate IV line; DO NOT USE AN IN-LINE FILTER

• Before infusion, shake the bag until the contents are thoroughly mixed; max rate 2.5 mg/kg/hr; if the infusion time exceeds 2 hr, mix the contents by shaking the infusion bag every 2 hr

Y-site compatibilities: Acyclovir, allopurinol, aminocaproic acid, aminophylline, amiodarone, anidulafungin, argatroban, arsenic trioxide, atracurium, azithromycin, aztreonam, bumetanide, buprenorphine, busulfan, butorphanol, CARBOplatin, carmustine, ceFAZolin, cefepime, cefotaxime, cefoTEtan, cefOXitin, cefTAZidime, ceftizoxime, cefTRIAXone, cefuroxime, chloramphenicol, chlorproMAZINE, cimetidine, cisatracurium, clindamycin, cyclophosphamide, cycloSPORINE, cytarabine, DACTINomycin dexamethasone, digoxin, diphenhydrAMINE, DOCEtaxel, doxacurium, DOXOrubicin liposomal, enalaprilat, EPINEPHrine, eptifibatide, ertapenem, etoposide, famotidine, fentaNYL, fludarabine, fluorouracil, fosphenytoin, furosemide, ganciclovir, granisetron, heparin, hydrocortisone, HYDROmorphone, ifosfamide, insulin, regular ketorolac, lepirudin, lidocaine, linezolid, LORazepam, mannitol, melphalan, meperidine, methotrexate, methylPREDNISolone, metoclopramide, mitoMYcin, mivacurium, nafcillin, nesiritide, nitroglycerin, nitroprusside, octreotide, oxaliplatin, PACLitaxel, pamidronate, pantoprazole, PEMEtrexed, pentazocine, PENTobarbital, PHENobarbital, phentolamine, piperacillin-tazobactam, procainamide, ranitidine, succinylcholine, SUFentanil, tacrolimus, telavancin, teniposide, theophylline, thiopental, thiotepa, ticarcillin, ticaracillin-clavulanate, trimethobenzamide, verapamil, vinBLAStine, vinCRIStine, zidovudine, zoledronic acid

ADVERSE EFFECTS

CNS: *Headache, fever, chills,* peripheral nerve pain, paresthesias, peripheral neuropathy, **seizures,** dizziness

CV: Bradycardia, hypotension, **cardiac arrest,** chest pain

EENT: Tinnitus, deafness, diplopia, blurred vision

GI: *Nausea, vomiting, anorexia,* diarrhea, cramps, **hemorrhagic gastroenteritis, acute liver failure**

GU: *Hypokalemia,* **azotemia, hyposthenuria, renal tubular acidosis, nephrocalcinosis, permanent renal impairment, anuria, oliguria**

HEMA: **Normochromic, normocytic anemia, thrombocytopenia, agranulocytosis, leukopenia, eosinophilia**

INTEG: *Burning, irritation,* pain, **necrosis at inj site with extravasation,** flushing, dermatitis

META: Hyponatremia, hypomagnesemia

MS: Arthralgia, myalgia, generalized pain, weakness, weight loss

RESP: Bronchospasm, dyspnea

SYST: Toxic epidermal neurolysis, exfoliative dermatitis, anaphylaxis

Pharmacokinetics

Absorption	Complete bioavailability (IV)
Distribution	Body tissues
Metabolism	Liver
Excretion	Kidneys, detectable for several weeks
Half-life	Terminal lipid complex mean 7 days

Pharmacodynamics

Onset	Immediate
Peak	2 hr
Duration	Unknown

INTERACTIONS

Individual drugs

Cidofovir: do not use concurrently

Digoxin: increased hypokalemia

Pentamidine, tacrolimus, tenofovir: increased nephrotoxicity

Drug classifications

Other nephrotoxic antibiotics (aminoglycosides, CISplatin, vancomycin, cycloSPORINE, polymyxin B), antineoplastics, salicylates): increased nephrotoxicity

Azole antifungals: decreased amphotericin B lipid complex effect; antifungals may still be used concurrently in serious resistant infections

Corticosteroids, skeletal muscle relaxants, thiazides, loop diuretics: increased hypokalemia

Drug/lab test

Increased: AST/ALT, alk phos, BUN, creatinine, LDH, bilirubin

Decreased: magnesium, potassium, Hgb, WBC, platelets

NURSING CONSIDERATIONS
Assessment

• VS every 15-30 min during first inf; note changes in pulse, B/P

• I&O ratio; watch for decreasing urinary output, change in specific gravity; discontinue product to prevent permanent damage to renal tubules

• Blood studies: CBC, potassium, sodium, calcium, magnesium every 2 wk; BUN, creatinine 2-3 ×/wk

• Weight weekly; if weight increases by more than 2 lb/wk, edema is present; renal damage should be considered

⚠ For renal toxicity: increasing BUN, serum creatinine; if BUN is .40 mg/dl or if serum creatinine is .3 mg/dl, product may be discontinued, dosage reduced

⚠ For hepatotoxicity: increasing AST, ALT, alk phos, bilirubin

⚠ For allergic reaction: dermatitis, rash; product should be discontinued, antihistamines (mild reaction) or EPINEPHrine (severe reaction) should be administered

• For hypokalemia: anorexia, drowsiness, weakness, decreased reflexes, dizziness, increased urinary output, increased thirst, paresthesias

• Infusion reactions: fever, chills, pain, swelling at site

• For ototoxicity: tinnitus (ringing, roaring in ears), vertigo, loss of hearing (rare)

Patient/family education

• Teach patient that long-term therapy may be needed to clear infection (2 wk-3 mo, depending on type of infection)

⚠ Instruct patient to notify prescriber of bleeding, bruising, or soft-tissue swelling

Evaluation
Positive therapeutic outcome

• Decreased fever, malaise, rash; negative C&S for infecting organism

---

amphotericin B liposomal (LAmB)

(am-foe-ter'i-sin)

AmBisome

Func. class.: Antifungal

Chem. class.: Amphoteric polyene

Pregnancy category B

ACTION: Increases cell membrane permeability in susceptible fungi by binding to membrane sterols; alters cell membrane, thereby causing leakage of cell components, cell death

Therapeutic outcome: Resolution of infection

USES: Empirical therapy for presumed fungal infection in febrile neutropenic patients; treatment of *Cryptococcal* Meningitis in HIV-infected patients; treatment of *Aspergillus, Candida,* and/or *Cryptococcus* infections refractory to amphotericin B deoxycholate, or in patients where renal impairment or unacceptable toxicity precludes the use of amphotericin B deoxycholate *(Aspergillus flavus, Aspergillus fumigatus, Blastomyces dermatitidis, Candida albicans, Candida krusei, Candida lusitaniae, Candida parapsilosis, Candida tropicalis, Cryptococcus neoformans)*; treatment of visceral leishmaniasis

Unlabeled uses: Coccidioidomycosis, histoplasmosis

CONTRAINDICATIONS: Hypersensitivity

Precautions: Anemia, breastfeeding, cardiac disease, children, electrolyte imbalance, geriatric, hematological/hepatic/renal disease, hypotension, pregnancy (B), severe bone marrow depression

DOSAGE AND ROUTES
Visceral leishmaniasis

Adult and child ≥1 mo: **IV** 3 mg/kg every 24 hr days 1-5, and days 14, 21 (immunocompetent), 4 mg/kg every 24 hr days 1-5, and days 10, 17, 24, 31, 38 (immunocompromised)

Cryptococcal meningitis in HIV

Adult and child ≥1 mo: **IV** 6 mg/kg/ day

Adverse effects: *italics* = common; **bold** = life-threatening

Fungal infection, empirical
Adult and child ≥1 mo: **IV** 3 mg/kg/day

Fungal infection, systemic
Adult and child ≥1 mo: **IV** 3-5 mg/kg/ day

Available forms: Powder for inj 50-mg vial

Implementation
⚠ **Do not confuse four different types; these are not interchangeable: conventional amphotericin B, amphotericin B cholesteryl, amphotericin B lipid complex, amphotericin B liposome**
• May premedicate with acetaminophen, diphenhydrAMINE

IV route
• Give only after C&S confirms organism, product needed to treat condition; make sure product is used for life-threatening infections
• Administer by IV infusion only; handle with aseptic technique as LAmB does not contain any preservatives
• Visually inspect products for particulate matter and discoloration

Reconstitution
• LAmB *must* be reconstituted using sterile water for injection (without a bacteriostatic agent); **do not reconstitute with saline or add saline to the reconstituted suspension, do not mix with other drugs;** doing so can cause a precipitate to form
• Reconstitute vials containing 50 mg of LAmB/12 ml of sterile water (4 mg/ml)
• Immediately after the addition of water, SHAKE THE VIAL VIGOROUSLY for 30 sec; the suspension should be yellow and translucent; visually inspect vial for particulate matter and continue shaking until product is completely dispersed
• Store suspension for up to 24 hours refrigerated if using sterile water for injection; do not freeze

Filtration and dilution
• Calculate the amount of reconstituted (4 mg/ml) suspension to be further diluted and withdraw this amount into a sterile syringe
• Attach the provided 5-micron filter to the syringe; inject the syringe contents through the filter, into the appropriate amount of D₅W injection; use only one filter per vial
• The suspension must be diluted with D₅W injection to a final concentration of 1-2 mg/ml before administration; for infants and small children, lower concentrations (0.2-0.5 mg/ml) may be appropriate to provide sufficient volume for infusion
• Use injection of LAmB within 6 hr of dilution with D₅W

IV INF
• Flush intravenous line with D₅W injection before infusion; if this cannot be done, then a separate IV line must be used
• An inline membrane filter may be used provided the mean pore diameter of the filter is not less than 1 micron
• Administer by IV infusion using a controlled infusion device over a period of approximately 120 min; infusion time may be reduced to approximately 60 min in patients who tolerate the infusion; if discomfort occurs during infusion, the duration of infusion may be increased

Acetaminophen and diphenhydrAMINE
• 30 min before inf to reduce fever, chills, headache
• Store protected from moisture and light; diluted solution is stable for 24 hr at room temp

Y-site compatibilities: Acyclovir, amifostine, aminophylline, anidulafungin, atropine, azithromycin, bivalirudin, bumetanide, buprenorphine, busulfan, butorphanol, CARBOplatin, carmustine, ceFAZolin, ceFOXitin, ceftizoxime, cefTRIAXone, cefuroxime, cimetidine, clindamycin, cyclophosphamide, cytarabine, DACTINomycin, DAPTOmycin, dexamethasone, dexmedetomidine, diphenhydrAMINE, doxacurium, enalaprilat, ePHEDrine, EPINEPHrine, eptifibatide, ertapenem, esmolol, etoposide, famotidine, fenoldopam, fentaNYL, fludarabine, fluorouracil, fosphenytoin, furosemide, granisetron, haloperidol, heparin, hydrocortisone, HYDROmorphone, ifosfamide, isoproterenol, ketorolac, levorphanol, lidocaine, linezolid, mesna, methotrexate, methylPREDNISolone, metoprolol, milrinone, mitoMYcin, nesiritide, nitroglycerin, nitroprusside, octreotide, oxaliplatin, oxytocin, palonosetron, pancuronium, pantoprazole, PEMEtrexed, PENTobarbital, PHENobarbital, phenylephrine, piperacillin/tazobactam, potassium chloride, procainamide, ranitidine, SUFentanil, tacrolimus, theophylline, thiopental, thiotepa, ticarcillin/clavulanate, tigecycline, trimethoprim-sulfamethoxazole, vasopressin, vinCRIStine, voriconazole, zidovudine

ADVERSE EFFECTS
CNS: *Headache, fever, chills,* peripheral nerve pain, paresthesias, peripheral neuropathy, seizures, dizziness, insomnia
CV: Bradycardia, hypotension, cardiac arrest
EENT: Tinnitus, deafness, diplopia, blurred vision
ENDO: Hyperglycemia

GI: *Nausea, vomiting, anorexia,* diarrhea, cramps, **hemorrhagic gastroenteritis, acute liver failure**
GU: *Hypokalemia,* **azotemia, hyposthenuria,** renal tubular acidosis, **nephrocalcinosis,** permanent renal impairment, anuria, oliguria
HEMA: Normochromic normocytic anemia, thrombocytopenia, agranulocytosis, leukopenia, eosinophilia, hyponatremia, hypomagnesemia
INTEG: *Burning, irritation,* pain, **necrosis at inj site with extravasation,** flushing, dermatitis, skin rash (topical route)
MS: Arthralgia, myalgia, generalized pain, weakness, weight loss
RESP: Dyspnea
SYST: Stevens–Johnson syndrome, toxic epidermal neurolysis, exfoliative dermatitis, anaphylaxis

Pharmacokinetics

Absorption	Complete bioavailability (IV)
Distribution	Body tissues
Metabolism	Liver
Excretion	Kidneys, detectable for several weeks
Half-life	Liposomal mean 4-6 days

Pharmacodynamics

Onset	Immediate
Peak	1-2 hr
Duration	Unknown

INTERACTIONS
Individual drugs
Digoxin: increased hypokalemia

Drug classifications
Other nephrotoxic antibiotics (aminoglycosides, CISplatin, vancomycin, cycloSPORINE, polymyxin B): increased nephrotoxicity
Corticosteroids, skeletal muscle relaxants, thiazides: increased hypokalemia

NURSING CONSIDERATIONS
Assessment
• VS every 15-30 min during first inf; note changes in pulse, B/P
• I&O ratio; watch for decreasing urinary output, change in specific gravity; discontinue product to prevent permanent damage to renal tubules

• Blood studies: CBC, potassium, sodium, calcium, magnesium every 2 wk, BUN, creatinine 2-3 ×/wk
• Weight weekly; if weight increases by more than 2 lb/wk, edema is present; renal damage should be considered
⚠ **For renal toxicity: increasing BUN, serum creatinine; if BUN is .40 mg/dl or if serum creatinine is .3 mg/dl, product may be discontinued, dosage reduced**
⚠ **For hepatotoxicity: increasing AST, ALT, alk phos, bilirubin, monitor LFTs**
⚠ **For allergic reaction: dermatitis, rash; product should be discontinued, antihistamines (mild reaction) or EPINEPHrine (severe reaction) administered**
⚠ **For hypokalemia: anorexia, drowsiness, weakness, decreased reflexes, dizziness, increased urinary output, increased thirst, paresthesias**
⚠ **For ototoxicity: tinnitus (ringing, roaring in ears), vertigo, loss of hearing (rare)**
⚠ **Infusion reaction: chills, fever, pain, swelling at site**

Patient/family education
• Teach patient that long-term therapy may be needed to clear infection (2 wk-3 mo, depending on type of infection)
⚠ **Instruct patient to notify prescriber of bleeding, bruising, or soft-tissue swelling**

Evaluation
Positive therapeutic outcome
• Decreased fever, malaise, rash; negative C&S for infecting organism

ampicillin (Rx)
(am-pi-sill'in)
Func. class.: Broad-spectrum antiinfective
Chem. class.: Aminopenicillin
Pregnancy category B

ACTION: Interferes with cell wall replication of susceptible organisms; the cell wall, rendered osmotically unstable, swells and bursts from osmotic pressure, lysis mediated by cell wall autolysis

Therapeutic outcome: Bactericidal effects for the following organisms: effective for gram-positive cocci (*Streptococcus aureus, Streptococcus pyogenes, Streptococcus faecalis, Streptococcus pneumoniae*), gram-negative cocci (*Neisseria meningitidis*), gram-negative bacilli *(Haemophilus influenzae, Proteus mirabilis, Salmonella, Shigella, Listeria monocytogenes)*, gram-positive bacilli

USES: Infections of respiratory tract, skin, skin structures, GI/GU tract; otitis media, meningitis, septicemia, sinusitis, and endocarditis prophylaxis

CONTRAINDICATIONS:
Hypersensitivity to penicillins, antimicrobial resistance, skin infection

Precautions: Pregnancy **B,** breastfeeding, neonates, hypersensitivity to cephalosporins, renal disease, mononucleosis

DOSAGE AND ROUTES
Renal dose
Adult and child: CCr 10-50 ml/min extend to q6-12hr; CCr <10 ml/min dose q12-16hr

Systemic infections
Adult and child ≥40 kg (88 lb): PO 250-500 mg q6hr; **IV/IM** 2-8 g daily in divided doses q4-6hr
Child <40 kg: PO 50-100 mg/kg/day in divided doses q6-8hr; **IV/IM** 50-500 mg/kg/day in divided doses q6-8hr

Bacterial meningitis
Adult/adolescent: IM/**IV** 150-200 mg/kg/day in divided doses, q3-4hr; IDSA IV 12 g divided q4hr
Infant/child: IM/**IV** 150-200 mg/kg/day in divided doses q3-4hr; IDSA dose IV 300 mg/day divided q6hr
Neonate >7 days and >2000 g: IM/**IV** 200 mg/kg/day divided q6hr; IDSA dose IV 200 mg/kg/day divided q6-8hr

Prevention of bacterial endocarditis
Adult: IM/**IV** 2 g 30 min before procedure
Child: IM/**IV** 50 mg/kg 30 min before procedure, max 2 g

GI/GU infections other than caused by *N. gonorrhoeae*
Adult and child >40 kg: PO 250-500 mg q6hr, may use larger dose for more serious infections
Child <40 kg: PO 50 mg/kg/day in divided doses q6-8hr

Available forms: Powder for inj 125, 250, 500 mg, 1, 2, 10 g; **IV** inf 500 mg, 1, 2 g; caps 250, 500 mg; powder for oral susp, 125, 250, 500 mg/5 ml

Implementation
PO route
• Give in even doses around the clock; product must be taken for 10-14 days to ensure organism death and prevent superinfection; store caps in tight container; store after reconstituting in refrigerator up to 2 wk, 1 wk room temperature
• Tabs may be crushed or caps opened and mixed with water
• Shake susp well before each dose; store for 2 wk in refrigerator or 1 wk at room temperature
IM route (painful)
• **Reconstitute** with 125 mg/0.9-1.2 ml; 250 mg/0.9-1.9 ml; 500 mg/1.2-1.8 ml; 1 g/2.4-7.4 ml; 2 g/6.8 ml
• **Give** deep in large muscle mass

IV route
• **Reconstitute** with 125 mg/0.9-1.2 ml; 250 mg/0.9-1.9 ml; 500 mg/1.2-1.8 ml; 1 g/2.4-7.4 ml; 2 g/6.8 ml
Direct IV route
• **Give** over 3-5 min in lower dosages (125-500 mg) or over 15 min in higher dosages (1-2 g)
Intermittent IV infusion route
• **Give** after diluting with 0.9% NaCl, LR, D5W, D5/0.45% NaCl; use 50 ml of sol and dilute to concentration of <30 mg/ml

Y-site compatibilities: Acyclovir, alemtuzumab, amifostine, allopurinol, argatroban, azithromycin, aztreonam, carmustine, cyclophosphamide, cytarabine, DAUNOrubicin, dexrazoxane, doxapram, DOXOrubicin liposome, enalaprilat, esmolol, etoposide phosphate, famotidine, filgrastim, fludarabine, foscarnet, gallium, gemtuzumab, granisetron, heparin, regular insulin, labetalol, lepirudin, leucovorin, liposome, magnesium sulfate, mannitol, melphalan, meperidine, milrinone, morphine, multivitamins, ofloxacin, penicillin G potassium, perphenazine, phytonadione, potassium acetate, potassium chloride, propofol, remifentanil, thiotepa, tolazoline, vecuronium, vinBLAStine, vit B with C, zoledronic acid

Y-site incompatibilities: Calcium gluconate, EPINEPHrine, fluconazole, hetastarch, HYDROmorphone, hydrALAZINE, ondansetron, sargramostim, verapamil, vinorelbine

ADVERSE EFFECTS
CNS: Lethargy, hallucinations, anxiety, depression, twitching, **coma, seizures**
GI: *Nausea, vomiting, diarrhea,* **pseudomembranous colitis,** stomatitis
GU: Oliguria, proteinuria, hematuria, *vaginitis, moniliasis,* **glomerulonephritis**

HEMA: Anemia, increased bleeding time, **bone marrow depression, granulocytope-nia, leukopenia, eosinophilia, hemolysis**
INTEG: *Rash*, urticaria, **toxic epidermal necrolysis**, erythema, multiforme
SYST: Anaphylaxis, serum sickness, Stevens-Johnson syndrome

Pharmacokinetics

Absorption	Moderate, in duodenum (35%-50%)
Distribution	Readily in body tissues, fluids, CSF; crosses placenta
Metabolism	Liver (30%)
Excretion	Breast milk; kidney un-changed (70%), removed by dialysis
Half-life	50-110 min

Pharmacodynamics

	PO	IM	IV
Onset	Rapid	Rapid	Rapid
Peak	2 hr	1 hr	Infusion's end; 1 hr
Duration	Unknown	Unknown	Unknown

INTERACTIONS

Individual drugs
Allopurinol: increased ampicillin-induced skin rash, monitor for rash
Probenecid: increased ampicillin levels, de-creased renal excretion

Drug classifications
Contraceptives (oral): decreased contraceptive effectiveness; use reliable contraception
H2 antagonists, proton pump inhibitors: de-creased ampicillin level
Oral anticoagulants: increased bleeding, moni-tor INR/PTT

Drug/lab test
Increased: eosinophil
Decreased: conjugated estrone in pregnancy, conjugated estriol, Hgb, WBC, platelets
False positive: urine glucose
Interfere: urine glucose (Clinitest, Benedict's reagent, cupric SO_4)

NURSING CONSIDERATIONS

Assessment
• Assess patient for previous sensitivity reaction to penicillins or other cephalosporins; cross-sensitivity between penicillins and cephalospo-rins is common

• Assess patient for signs and symptoms of **infection**, including characteristics of wounds, sputum, urine, stool, WBC >10,000/mm^3, earache, fever; obtain baseline information and during treatment
• Obtain C&S before beginning product therapy to identify if correct treatment has been initiated
• Assess for **allergic reactions:** rash, urticaria, pruritus, chills, fever, joint pain; an-gioedema may occur a few days after therapy be-gins; epinephrine and resuscitation equipment should be on unit for anaphylactic reaction; also, check for ampicillin rash: pruritic, red, raised; identify allergies before using
A Identify urine output, hematuria; if decreasing, notify prescriber (may indicate nephrotoxicity)
• Monitor renal studies: urinalysis, protein, blood, BUN, creatinine
• Monitor blood studies: AST, ALT, CBC, Hct, bilirubin, LDH, alkaline phosphatase, Coombs' test monthly if patient is on long-term therapy
• Monitor electrolytes: potassium, sodium, chloride monthly if patient is on long-term therapy
• Assess bowel pattern daily; if severe diarrhea occurs, product should be discontinued; may indicate pseudomembranous colitis
• Assess for **overgrowth of infection:** perineal itching, fever, malaise, redness, pain, swelling, drainage, rash, diarrhea, change in cough, sputum

Patient/family education
A Teach patient to report sore throat, bruis-ing, bleeding, joint pain; may indicate blood dyscrasias (rare)
• Advise patient to contact prescriber if vaginal itching, loose foul-smelling stools, furry tongue occur; may indicate **superinfection**
• Instruct patient to take all medication pre-scribed for the length of time ordered
• Advise patient to notify prescriber of diarrhea with blood or pus, which may indicate **pseudo-membranous colitis**
• Tab may be crushed; cap may be opened and mixed with water

Evaluation

Positive therapeutic outcome
• Absence of signs/symptoms of infection (WBC <10,000, temp WNL)
• Reported improvement in symptoms of infec-tion

**TREATMENT OF ANAPHY-
LAXIS:** Withdraw product, maintain airway, administer epinephrine, aminophylline, O₂, **IV** corticosteroids

---

ampicillin/sulbactam (Rx)
(am-pi-sill′in/sul-bak′tam)
Unasyn
Func. class.: Broad-spectrum antiinfective
Chem. class.: Aminopenicillin
Pregnancy category B (ampicillin)

ACTION: Interferes with cell wall replication of susceptible organisms; the cell wall, rendered osmotically unstable, swells and bursts from osmotic pressure; lysis due to cell wall autolytic enzymes; this combination extends the spectrum of activity and inhibits β-lactamase that may inactivate ampicillin

Therapeutic outcome: Bactericidal against *Staphylococcus aureus, Klebsiella, Bacteroides fragilis, Enterobacter, Acinetobacter calcoaceticus, Pneumococcus, Enterococcus, Streptococcus, Escherichia coli, Proteus mirabilis, Neisseria meningitidis, Neisseria gonorrhoeae, Shigella, Salmonella,* and *Haemophilus influenzae* organisms; use only with β-lactamase–producing strain of infection

USES: Skin infections, intraabdominal infections, gynecological infections, asthma, cellulitis, diabetes mellitus, diabetic foot ulcer, dialysis, diarrhea, eczema, IBS, leukemia, meningitis, nosocomial pneumonia, ulcerative colitis, *Actinobacter, Actinomyces, Bacillus anthracis, Bacteroides, Bifidobacterium, Bordetella pertussis, Borrelia burgdorferi, Brucella, Clostridium, Corynebacterium diptheriae/xerosis, Eikenella corrodens, Enterococcus faecalis, Erysipelothrix rhusiopathiae, Escherichia coli, Eubacterium, Fusobacterium, Gardnerella vaginalis, Haemophilus influenzae* (beta-lactamase negative/positive), *Helicobacter pylori, Klebsiella, Lactobacillus, Leptospira, Listeria monocytogenes, Moraxella catarrhalis, Morganella morganii, Neisseria gonorrhoeae, Pasteurella multocida, Peptococcus, Peptostreptococcus, Porphyromonas, Prevotella, Propionibacterium, Proteus mirabilis, Proteus vulgaris, Providencia rettgeri, Providencia stuartii, Salmonella, Shigella, Staphylococcus aureus* (MSSA)*/epidermidis/saprophyticus, Streptococcus agalactiae/dysgalactiae/pneumoniae/pyrogenes, Treponema pallidum,* viridans streptococci

CONTRAINDICATIONS:
Hypersensitivity to ampicillin, or sulbactam

Precautions: Pregnancy **B**, breastfeeding, neonates, hypersensitivity to cephalosporins, renal disease, mononucleosis, viral infections, syphilis

DOSAGE AND ROUTES
Adult and child >40 kg: IM/IV 1 g ampicillin and 0.5 g sulbactam to 2 g ampicillin, and 1 g sulbactam q6hr, not to exceed 4 g/day sulbactam
Child <40 kg: IV 100-200 mg/kg/day (ampicillin component) divided q6hr, max 4 g/day

Renal dose
Adult ≥40 kg: IM/IV CCr 15-29 ml/min dose q12hr; CCr 5-14 ml/min dose q24hr

Available forms: Powder for inj 1.5 g (1 g ampicillin, 0.5 g sulbactam), 3 g (2 g ampicillin, 1 g sulbactam), 15 g (10 g ampicillin, 5 g sulbactam)

Implementation
• Scratch test to assess allergy after securing order from prescriber; usually done when penicillin is only product choice
IM route
• Reconstitute by adding 3.2 ml/1.5 g or 6.4 ml/3 g; use sterile water, 0.5% or 2% lidocaine; give within 1 hr of preparation; give deep in large muscle mass, aspirate
• Do not use IM in child
• Give after C&S completed; on empty stomach

IV direct route
• Give **IV** after diluting 1.5 g/3.2 ml sterile water for inj; or 3 g/6.4 ml (250 mg ampicillin/125 mg sulbactam); allow to stand until foaming stops; give directly over 10-15 min
Intermittent IV infusion route
• Dilute further in 50 ml or more of D₅W, D₅/10.45% NaCl, 10% invert sugar in water, LR, 6% sodium lactate, isotonic NaCl; administer within 1 hr after reconstitution; give as an intermittent inf over 15-30 min

Y-site compatibilities: Alemtuzumab, amifostine, aminocaproic acid, anidulafungin, argatroban, atenolol, bivalirudin, bleomycin, CARBOplatin, carmustine, cefepime, CISplatin, codeine, cyclophosphamide, cytarabine, DAPTOmycin, DAUNOrubicin liposome, dexmedetomidine, DOCEtaxel, doxacurium, DOXOrubicin liposomal, eptifibatide, etoposide, fenoldopam, filgrastim, fludarabine, fluorouracil, foscarnet, gallium, gatifloxacin, gemcitabine, granisetron, irinotecan, levofloxacin, linezolid, methotrexate,

---

metroNIDAZOLE, octreotide, oxaliplatin, PACLi-taxel, palonosetron, pamidronate, pancuronium, pantoprazole, PEMEtrexed, remifentanil, riTUXimab, rocuronium, tacrolimus, teniposide, thiotepa, tigecycline, tirofiban, TNA, TPN, trastu-zumab, vecuronium, vinCRIStine, voriconazole, zoledronic acid

Y-site incompatibilities: IDArubicin, ondansetron, sargramostim

ADVERSE EFFECTS

CNS: Lethargy, hallucinations, anxiety, depres-sion, twitching, **coma, seizures**
GI: *Nausea, vomiting, diarrhea,* increased AST, ALT, abdominal pain, glossitis, colitis, **pseudomembranous colitis, hepatic necro-sis/failure,** black hairy tongue
GU: Oliguria, proteinuria, hematuria, *vagini-tis, moniliasis,* **glomerulonephritis,** dysuria
HEMA: Anemia, increased bleeding time, **bone marrow depression, granulocytope-nia, leukopenia, eosinophilia, hemolysis**
INTEG: Injection site reactions, rash, edema, urticaria
SYST: Anaphylaxis, serum sickness, toxic epidermal necrolysis, Stevens-Johnson syndrome, hypoalbuminemia

Pharmacokinetics

Absorption	Well absorbed (IM)
Distribution	Readily in body tissues, fluids, CSF; crosses placenta
Metabolism	Liver (10%-50%)
Excretion	Breast milk; kidney un-changed (75%)
Half-life	50-110 min (ampicillin)

Pharmacodynamics

	IM	IV
Onset	Rapid	Immediate
Peak	1 hr	Infusion's end
Duration	Unknown	Unknown

INTERACTIONS

Individual drugs

Allopurinol: ampicillin-induced skin rash, check for rash
Methotrexate: increased methotrexate level
Probenecid: increased ampicillin levels, de-creased renal excretion

Drug classifications

Oral anticoagulants: increased bleeding risk, check INR, PT

Drug/lab test

False positive: urine glucose, urine protein

NURSING CONSIDERATIONS

Assessment

• Assess patient for previous sensitivity reaction to penicillins or cephalosporins; cross-sensitivity between penicillins and cephalosporins is com-mon
• Assess patient for signs and symptoms of **infection,** including characteristics of wounds, sputum, urine, stool, WBC >10,000/mm³, earache, fever; obtain baseline information and during treatment; complete C&S before beginning product therapy to identify if correct treatment has been initiated
• Assess for **allergic reactions:** rash, urticar-ia, pruritus, chills, fever, joint pain; angioedema may occur a few days after therapy begins; epinephrine and resuscitation equipment should be on unit for anaphylactic reaction
⚠ Identify urine output; if decreasing, notify prescriber (may indicate nephrotoxicity)
• Assess renal studies: urinalysis, protein, BUN, creatinine
• Monitor blood studies: AST, ALT, CBC, Hct, bilirubin, LDH, alkaline phosphatase, Coombs' test monthly if patient is on long-term therapy
• Monitor electrolytes: potassium, sodium, chloride monthly if patient is on long-term therapy
• Assess bowel pattern daily; if severe diarrhea occurs, product should be discontinued; may indicate **pseudomembranous colitis**
• Monitor for bleeding: ecchymosis, bleeding gums, hematuria, stool guaiac daily if on long-term therapy
• Assess for superinfection: perineal itching, fever, malaise, redness, pain, swelling, drainage, rash, diarrhea, change in cough, sputum

Patient/family education

• Teach patient to report sore throat, bruising, bleeding, joint pain, persistent diarrhea; may indicate blood dyscrasias (rare) or superinfec-tion
• Advise patient to contact prescriber if vaginal itching, loose foul-smelling stools, furry tongue occur; may indicate superinfection
• Instruct patient to use another form of contra-ception other than oral contraceptives
⚠ Instruct patient to report immediately pseudomembranous colitis: fever, diarrhea with pus, blood, or mucus; may occur up to 4 wk after treatment
• Instruct patient to wear or carry emergency ID if allergic to penicillin products

Adverse effects: *italics* = common; **bold** = life-threatening

Evaluation
Positive therapeutic outcome
• Absence of signs/symptoms of infection (WBC <10,000/mm³, temp WNL, absence of red draining wounds, earache)
• Reported improvement in symptoms of infection

TREATMENT OF OVERDOSE:
Withdraw product, maintain airway, administer EPINEPHrine, aminophylline, O₂, **IV** corticosteroids for anaphylaxis

anakinra (Rx)
(an-ah-kin′rah)
Kineret
Func. class.: Antirheumatic agent (disease modifying), immunomodulator
Chem. class.: Recombinant form of human interleukin-1 receptor antagonist (IL-1Ra)
Pregnancy category B

Do not confuse:
anakinra/amikacin

ACTION: A form of human interleukin-1 receptor antagonist (IL-1Ra) produced by DNA technology; blocks activity of IL-1, resulting in decreased inflammation, cartilage degradation, bone resorption

Therapeutic outcome: Decreased pain, inflammation

USES: Reduction in signs and symptoms of moderate to severe active rheumatoid arthritis in patients 18 years of age or older who have not responded to other disease-modifying agents

CONTRAINDICATIONS:
Hypersensitivity to *Escherichia coli*–derived proteins or this product, sepsis, latex

Precautions: Pregnancy **B**, breastfeeding, children, geriatric, renal impairment, active infections, immunosuppression, neoplastic disease, asthma

DOSAGE AND ROUTES
Adult: SUBCUT 100 mg daily

Renal dose
Adult: CCr <30 ml/min; SUBCUT 100 mg every other day

Available forms: Inj, 100 mg/0.67 ml prefilled glass syringe

Implementation
• Do not use if cloudy or discolored or if particulate is present; protect from light
• Do not admix with other sol or medications, do not use filter

ADVERSE EFFECTS
CNS: Headache
CV: Cardiac arrest
EENT: Sinusitis
GI: Abdominal pain, nausea, diarrhea
HEMA: Neutropenia
INTEG: Rash, *inj site reaction,* allergic reaction
MISC: Flulike symptoms, infection
MS: *Worsening of RA, arthralgia*
RESP: *URI*

Pharmacokinetics
Absorption	Well absorbed (SUBCUT)
Distribution	Unknown
Metabolism	Unknown
Excretion	Urine
Half-life	4-6 hr

Pharmacodynamics
Onset	Unknown
Peak	3-7 hr
Duration	Unknown

INTERACTIONS
Individual drugs
Rilonacept: do not use

Drug classifications
Antibody reactions: decreased
Etanercept, TNF-blocking agents: increased risk of severe infection, do not use together
Vaccines: Avoid concurrent use; immunizations should be brought up to date before treatment

NURSING CONSIDERATIONS
Assessment
• **Rheumatoid arthritis:** assess pain, stiffness, ROM, swelling of joints during treatment
• Assess for inj site pain, swelling; usually occur after 2 inj (4-5 days)
• Assess for **infections**, stop treatment if present, do not start if patient has active infection

Patient/family education
• Teach patient about self-administration if appropriate: inj should be made in thigh, abdomen, upper arm; rotate sites at least 1 in from old site, store in refrigerator, do not freeze

---

• Advise patient to notify prescriber if pregnancy is planned or suspected, avoid breastfeeding
• Advise patient not to receive vaccines while taking this product, update vaccines before treatment

Evaluation

Positive therapeutic outcome
• Decreased inflammation, pain in joints

⚠ HIGH ALERT

anastrozole (Rx)
(an-ass-stroh′zole)
Arimidex
Func. class.: Antineoplastic
Chem. class.: Aromatase inhibitor
Pregnancy category X

ACTION: Highly selective nonsteroidal aromatase inhibitor that lowers serum estradiol concentrations; many breast cancers have strong estrogen receptors

Therapeutic outcome: Prevention of rapidly growing malignant cells

USES: Advanced breast carcinoma that has not responded to other therapy in estrogen-receptor-positive patients (usually postmenopausal); patients with advanced disease on tamoxifen, adjunct therapy in early breast cancer

CONTRAINDICATIONS:
Pregnancy **X,** hypersensitivity, breastfeeding

Precautions: Children, geriatric, cardiac/hepatic disease, premenopausal females, osteoporosis

DOSAGE AND ROUTES
Adult: PO 1 mg daily; continue for 5 yr in ERT early breast cancer who have already received 2-3 yr of tamoxifen and are switched to anastrozole

Available forms: Tabs 1 mg

Implementation
• Do not break, crush, or chew enteric products
• Give with food or fluids for GI upset; repeat dose may be needed if vomiting occurs
• Store in light-resistant container at room temperature

ADVERSE EFFECTS
CNS: Hot flashes, headache, light-headedness, depression, dizziness, confusion, insomnia, anxiety, fatigue, mood changes
CV: Chest pain, hypertension, **thrombophlebitis,** edema, **MI, CVA, cerebral infarction,** angina, *vasodilation*
GI: Nausea, vomiting, altered taste leading to anorexia, diarrhea, constipation, abdominal pain, dry mouth
GU: Vaginal bleeding, pruritus vulvae, vaginal dryness, pelvic pain, UTI
HEMA: Leukopenia
INTEG: *Rash,* **Stevens-Johnson syndrome,** anemia
MISC: Hypercholesterolemia
MS: Bone pain, myalgia, asthenia, bone loss, osteoporosis, arthralgia, fractures
RESP: Cough, sinusitis, dyspnea, **pulmonary embolism**

Pharmacokinetics

Absorption	Adequately absorbed
Distribution	Unknown
Metabolism	Liver
Excretion	Feces, urine
Half-life	50 hr

Pharmacodynamics

Onset	Unknown
Peak	4-7 hr
Duration	Unknown

INTERACTIONS
Drug/drug
• Do not use with oral contraceptives, estrogen, tamoxifen, androstenedione, DHEA

Drug/lab test
Increased: GGT, AST, ALT, alkaline phosphatase, cholesterol, LDL

NURSING CONSIDERATIONS
Assessment
• Monitor bone mineral density, cholesterol, lipid panel periodically
• Assess **serious skin reactions:** Stevens-Johnson syndrome
• Not effective in hormone receptor-negative disease, use only in post-menopausal women

Patient/family education
• Instruct patient to report any complaints, side effects to health care prescriber; if dose is missed, do not double next dose

---

• Advise patient that vaginal bleeding, pruritus, hot flashes, can occur and are reversible after discontinuing treatment
• Teach patient to take adequate calcium, vitamin D; risk of bone loss/fractures
• Inform patient that rash or lesions are temporary and may become large during beginning therapy

Evaluation
Positive therapeutic outcome
• Decreased spread of malignant cells in breast cancer

anidulafungin (Rx)
(a-nid-yoo-luh-fun′jin)
Eraxis
Func. class.: Antifungal, systemic
Chem. class.: Echinocandin
Pregnancy category C

ACTION: Inhibits fungal enzyme synthesis; causes direct damage to fungal cell wall

Therapeutic outcome: Decreased symptoms of candida infection, negative culture

USES: Esophageal candidiasis, *Aspergillosis, Candida albicans, Candida glabrata, Candida parapsilosis, Candida tropicalis*

CONTRAINDICATIONS:
Hypersensitivity to this product or other echinocandins

Precautions: Pregnancy C, breastfeeding, children, severe hepatic disease

DOSAGE AND ROUTES
Candidemia and other candidal infections
Adult: IV loading dose 200 mg on day 1, then 100 mg/day until 14 days or more since last positive culture

Esophageal candidiasis
Adult: IV loading dose 100 mg on day 1, then 50 mg/day for at least 14 days and for at least 7 days after symptoms are resolved

Available forms: Powder for injection, lyophilized 50, 100 mg

Implementation
IV route
• Visually inspect prepared infusions for particulate matter and discoloration—do not use if present; give by IV infusion only, after dilution

• **Reconstitution:** Reconstitute each 50 mg or 100 mg vial/15 ml or 30 ml of sterile water for injection, respectively (3.33 mg/ml)
• **Storage:** Reconstituted solutions are stable for ≤24 hr at room temperature
• **Dilution:** Do not use any other diluents besides dextrose 5% in water (D_5W) or sodium chloride 0.9% (NS)
• *Preparation of the 200-mg loading dose infusion:* Withdraw the contents of either four 50-mg reconstituted vials OR two 100-mg reconstituted vials and add to an IV infusion bag or bottle containing 200 ml of D_5W or NS to give a total infusion volume of 260 ml
• *Preparation of the 100-mg daily infusion:* Withdraw the contents of one 100-mg reconstituted vial OR two 50-mg reconstituted vials and add to an IV infusion bag or bottle containing 100 ml of D_5W or NS to give a total infusion volume of 130 ml
• *Preparation of a 50-mg daily infusion:* Withdraw the contents of one 50-mg reconstituted vial and add to an IV infusion bag or bottle containing 50 ml of D_5W or NS to give a total infusion volume of 65 ml
Intermittent IV INF route
• Do not mix or co-infuse with other medications
• Administer as a slow IV infusion at a rate of 1.4 ml/min or 84 ml/hr; minimum duration of infusion is 180 min for the 200-mg dose, 90 min for the 100-mg dose, and 45 min for the 50-mg dose
• Store reconstituted vials at 59°-86° F (15°-30° C) for up to 24 hr; do not freeze (dehydrated alcohol); store reconstituted vials at 36°-46° F (2°-7° C) (sterile water) for up to 24 hr; do not freeze

IV compatibilities: Acyclovir, alemtuzumab, alfentanil, allopurinol, amifostine, amikacin, aminocaproic acid, aminophylline, amiodarone hydrochloride, amphotericin B lipid complex, amphotericin B liposome, ampicillin, ampicillin sulbactam, argatroban, arsenic trioxide, atenolol, atracurium, azithromycin, aztreonam, bivalirudin, bleomycin, bumetanide, buprenorphine, busulfan, butorphanol, calcium chloride/gluconate, CARBOplatin, carmustine, caspofungin, ceFAZolin, cefepime, cefotaxime, cefoTEtan, cefOXitin, cefTAZidime, ceftizoxime, cefTRIAXone, cefuroxime, chloramphenicol, chlorproMAZINE, cimetidine, ciprofloxacin, cisatracurium, CISplatin, clindamycin, cyclophosphamide, cycloSPORINE, cytarabine, dacarbazine, DACTINomycin, DAUNOrubicin, DAUNOrubicin liposome, dexamethasone, dexmedetomidine, dexrazoxane, diazepam, digoxin, diltiazem, diphenhydrAMINE, DOBUTamine, DOCEtaxel, dolasetron, DOPamine, doripenem, doxacurium, DOXOrubicin, DOXOrubicin liposomal, doxycycline, droperidol, enalaprilat, ePHEDrine, EPINEPHrine, epirubicin, eptifibatide, erythromycin, esmolol, etoposide, etoposide phosphate, famotidine, fenoldopam, fentaNYL, fluconazole, fludarabine, fluorouracil, foscarnet, fosphenytoin, furosemide, gallium, ganciclovir, gatifloxacin, gemcitabine, gentamicin, glycopyrrolate, granisetron, haloperidol, heparin, hydrALAZINE, hydrocortisone, HYDROmorphone, hydrOXYzine, IDArubicin, ifosfamide, imipenem-cilastatin, inamrinone, insulin (regular), irinotecan, isoproterenol, ketorolac, labetalol, leucovorin, levofloxacin, lidocaine, linezolid injection, LORazepam, mannitol, mechlorethamine, melphalan, meperidine, meropenem, mesna, metaraminol, methotrexate, methyldopate, methylPREDNISolone, metoclopramide, metoprolol, metroNIDAZOLE, midazolam, milrinone, mitoMYcin, mitoXANtrone, mivacurium, morphine, moxifloxacin, mycophenolate mofetil, nafcillin, naloxone, nesiritide, niCARdipine, nitroglycerin, nitroprusside, norepinephrine, octreotide, ondansetron, oxaliplatin, oxytocin, PACLitaxel, palonosetron, pamidronate, pancuronium, pantoprazole, pentamidine, pentazocine, PENTobarbital, PHENobarbital, phentolamine, phenylephrine, piperacillin-tazobactam, polymyxin B, potassium acetate/chloride, procainamide, prochlorperazine, promethazine, propranolol, quiNIDine, quinupristin-dalfopristin, ranitidine, remifentanil, rocuronium, sodium acetate, streptozocin, succinylcholine, SUFentanil citrate, sulfamethoxazole-trimethoprim, tacrolimus, teniposide, theophylline, thiopental, thiotepa, ticarcillin, ticarcillin-clavulanate, tirofiban, tobramycin, topotecan, trimethobenzamide, vancomycin, vasopressin, vecuronium, verapamil, vinBLAStine, vinCRIStine, vinorelbine, voriconazole, zidovudine, zoledronic acid

ADVERSE EFFECTS

Candidemia/other candida infections

CNS: **Seizures,** dizziness, *headache*
CV: Deep vein thrombosis, **atrial fibrillation, right bundle branch block,** hypotension, **QT prolongation, sinus arrhythmia, thrombophlebitis superficial, ventricular extrasystoles (rare)**
GI: *Nausea; anorexia; vomiting; diarrhea; increased AST, ALT*
META: Hypokalemia

Esophageal candidiasis
CNS: *Headache*
GI: *Nausea, anorexia, vomiting, diarrhea,* **hepatic necrosis**
HEMA: **Neutropenia, thrombocytopenia, leukopenia, coagulopathy**
INTEG: *Rash,* urticaria, itching, flushing
META: Hypocalcemia, hyperglycemia, hyperkalemia, hypernatremia, hypomagnesemia (rare)
MS: *Back pain, rigors*

Pharmacokinetics

Absorption	Unknown
Distribution	Steady state after loading dose, protein binding 84%
Metabolism	Unknown
Excretion	Unknown
Half-life	Distribution 0.5-1 hr, terminal 40-50 hr

Pharmacodynamics
Unknown

INTERACTIONS
Individual drugs
CycloSPORINE: increased plasma concentrations

Drug/lab test
Increased: amylase, bilirubin, CPK, creatinine, ECG, lipase, PT
Decreased: platelets, magnesium, potassium, transferase, urea

NURSING CONSIDERATIONS
Assessment
• Assess for **infection,** clearing of cultures during treatment; obtain culture at baseline and throughout; product may be started as soon as culture is taken, those with HIV pharyngeal candidiasis may need antifungals
• **Blood dyscrasias (rare):** monitor CBC (RBC, Hct, Hgb), differential, platelet count periodically; notify prescriber of results
• Monitor hepatic studies before and during treatment: bilirubin, AST, ALT, alk phosphatase; uric acid, as needed
• Assess for **bleeding:** hematuria, heme-positive stools, bruising or petechiae, mucosa or orifices; blood dyscrasias can occur
• Assess for GI symptoms: frequency of stools, cramping, if severe diarrhea occurs, electrolytes may need to be given

Patient/family education
• Advise patient to notify prescriber if pregnancy is suspected or planned; use nonhormonal form of contraception while taking this product
• Instruct patient to avoid breastfeeding while taking this product
• Advise patient to inform prescriber of kidney or liver disease
• Advise patient to report bleeding
• Teach patient to report signs of infection: increased temp, sore throat, flulike symptoms
• Teach patient to notify prescriber of nausea, vomiting, diarrhea, jaundice, anorexia, clay-colored stools, dark urine; heptatotoxicity may occur

Evaluation
Positive therapeutic outcome
• Decreased symptoms of candidal infection, negative culture

apraclonidine ophthalmic
See Appendix B

aprepitant (Rx)
(ap-re′pi-tant)
Emend
fosaprepitant
Emend
Func. class.: Antiemetic
Chem. class:. Miscellaneous
Pregnancy category B

ACTION: Selective antagonist of human substance P/neurokinin 1 (NK_1) receptors, decreasing emetic reflex

Therapeutic outcome: Decreased nausea, vomiting during chemotherapy

USES: Prevention of nausea, vomiting associated with cancer chemotherapy (highly emetogenic/moderately emetogenic) including high-dose cisplatin; used in combination with other antiemetics; postop nausea, vomiting

CONTRAINDICATIONS:
Hypersensitivity

Precautions: Pregnancy **B**, breastfeeding, children, geriatric, hepatic disease

DOSAGE AND ROUTES
Highly emetogenic (aprepitant)
Adult: PO day 1 (1 hr prior to chemotherapy) aprepitant 125 mg with 12 mg 1st dose of aprepitant on day 1 of regimen (fosaprepitant)

Moderately emetogenic
Adult: PO day 1 dexamethasone 12 mg 125 mg aprepitant with PO, with PO ondansetron 8 mg × 2; days 2 and 3 PO 80 mg aprepitant only (aprepitant); **IV** inf 115 mg over 15 min, 30 min prior to chemotherapy as an alternative to the 1st dose of aprepitant on day 1 of regimen (fosaprepitant)

Prevention of postop nausea/vomiting
Adult: PO 40 mg within 3 hr of induction of anesthesia

Available forms: Caps 40, 80, 125 mg; powder for inj 115, 150 mg; combo pack cap 80-125 mg

Implementation
PO route
• Give PO on 3-day schedule, given with other antiemetics
• Take first dose 1 hr prior to chemotherapy
• Store at room temperature; keep in original bottles, blisters

IV route
• Only approved as a substitute for the 1st dose of aprepitant in 3-day regimen
• Reconstitution: use aseptic technique; inject 5 ml 0.9% NaCl into the vial, directing stream to wall of vial to prevent foam; swirl; do not shake
• Prepare inf bag with 110 ml 0.9% NaCl/115 mg; 145 ml/150 mg do not dilute or reconstitute with any divalent cations such as calcium, magnesium, including LR, Hartmann's sol
• Withdraw the entire volume from vial and transfer to inf bag; total volume 115 ml (1 mg/1 ml)
• Gently invert bag 2-3 times; reconstituted sol is stable for 24 hr at lower room temperature or <25° C
• Visually inspect for particulates and discoloration
• Infuse over 15 min, stable for 24 hr at room temperature

ADVERSE EFFECTS
CNS: *Headache, dizziness,* insomnia, anxiety, depression, confusion, peripheral neuropathy
CV: Bradycardia, tachycardia, DVT, hypertension, hypotension
GI: *Diarrhea; constipation;* abdominal pain; anorexia; gastritis; increased AST, ALT; *nausea;* vomiting; heartburn
GU: Increased BUN, serum creatine, proteinuria, dysuria

HEMA: Anemia, **thrombocytopenia, neutropenia**
INTEG: Pruritus, rash, urticaria
MISC: Asthenia, fatigue, dehydration, fever, hiccups, tinnitus, alopecia
SYST: Anaphylaxis

Pharmacokinetics

Absorption	Unknown
Distribution	95% protein bound
Metabolism	Liver (CYP3A4 enzymes to an active metabolite)
Excretion	Not in kidneys
Half-life	10-12 hr

Pharmacodynamics

Unknown

INTERACTIONS
Individual drugs
Paroxetine: decreased action of both products

Drug classifications
CYP2C9 substrates (phenytoin, TOLBUTamide, warfarin), oral contraceptives: decreased action
CYP3A4 inhibitors (clarithromycin, diltiazem, itraconazole, ketoconazole, nefazodone, nelfinavir, ritonavir, troleandomycin): increased aprepitant action
CYP3A4 inducers (carBAMazepine, phenytoin, rifampin): decreased aprepitant action
CYP3A4 substrates (ALPRAZolam, cisapride, dexamethasone, DOCEtaxel, etoposide, ifosfamide, imatinib, irinotecan, methylPREDNISolone, midazolam, PACLitaxel, pimozide, triazolam, vinBLAStine, vinCRIStine, vinorelbine): increased action

Drug/food
Grapefruit juice: decreased effect

NURSING CONSIDERATIONS
Assessment
• Assess for hypersensitivity reactions: pruritus, rash, urticaria, anaphylaxis
• Assess for absence of nausea, vomiting during chemotherapy
• CBC, LFTs, creatinine baseline and periodically

Patient/family education
• Teach to report diarrhea, constipation
• Advise to take only as prescribed
• Advise to report all medication to prescriber prior to taking this medication

• Instruct to use nonhormonal form of contraception while taking this agent
• Advise those on warfarin to have clotting monitored closely during 2-wk period following administration of aprepitant
• Teach to avoid breastfeeding

Evaluation
Positive therapeutic outcome
• Absence of nausea, vomiting during cancer chemotherapy

---

arformoterol (Rx)
(ar-for-moe′ter-ole)
Brovana
Func. class.: Long-acting adrenergic β$_2$-agonist, sympathomimetic, bronchodilator
Pregnancy category C

Do not confuse:
Brovana/Boniva

ACTION: Causes bronchodilation by action on β$_2$ (pulmonary) receptors by increasing levels of cyclic AMP, which relaxes smooth muscle; produces bronchodilation, CNS, and cardiac stimulation, and increased diuresis and gastric acid secretion; longer acting than isoproterenol

Therapeutic outcome: Absence of dyspnea, wheezing after 1 hr, improved airway exchange, improved ABGs

USES: Maintenance bronchospasm prevention in COPD, including chronic bronchitis, emphysema

CONTRAINDICATIONS:
Hypersensitivity to sympathomimetics, this product, or racemic formoterol; tachydysrhythmias, severe cardiac disease, heart block, children, monotherapy in asthma

Precautions: Pregnancy C, breastfeeding, cardiac disorders, hyperthyroidism, diabetes mellitus, hypertension, prostatic hypertrophy, closed-angle glaucoma, seizures, hypoglycemia

BLACK BOX WARNING: Asthma-related death

DOSAGE AND ROUTES
COPD
Adult: NEB 15 mcg, bid, AM, PM

Available forms: Inh sol 15 mcg/2 ml

Adverse effects: *italics* = common; **bold** = life-threatening

Implementation
• Must be used by nebulization
• Store in refrigerator; if stored at room temp, discard after 6 wk or if past expiration date, whichever is sooner

ADVERSE EFFECTS
CNS: *Tremors, anxiety,* insomnia, headache, dizziness, stimulation, *restlessness,* hallucinations, flushing, irritability
CV: Palpitations, **tachycardia,** hypo/hypertension, angina, **dysrhythmias, AV block, heart failure, prolonged QT supraventricular tachycardia**
EENT: Dry nose, irritation of nose and throat
GI: Heartburn, nausea, vomiting
MISC: Flushing, sweating, anorexia, bad taste/smell changes, hypokalemia, **anaphylaxis,** *hypoglycemia*
MS: Muscle cramps
RESP: Cough, wheezing, dyspnea, **bronchospasm,** dry throat

Pharmacokinetics

Absorption	Unknown
Distribution	Crosses placenta, protein binding 52%-65%
Metabolism	Direct conjugation by CYP2D6, CYP2C19, extensively
Excretion	Urine 63%, feces 11%
Half-life	Terminal (COPD) 26 hr

Pharmacodynamics

Onset	5 min
Peak	1-1½ hr
Duration	4-6 hr

INTERACTIONS
Individual drugs
Oxytoxics: increased severe hypotension
Theophylline: increased toxicity

Drug classifications
Adrenergics, MAOIs, tricyclics: increased action of arformoterol; do not use together
Class IA/III antidysrhythmics, MAOIs, tricyclics: increased QT prolongation
Nebulized bronchodilators: increased action of nebulized bronchodilators
Other β-blockers: decreased arformoterol action, asthma-related death
Potassium-losing diuretics: increased ECG changes/hypokalemia

Drug/herb
Caffeine (kola nut, green/black tea, guarana, yerba maté, coffee, chocolate): increased stimulation

NURSING CONSIDERATIONS
Assessment

> **BLACK BOX WARNING:** Assess respiratory function: vital capacity, forced expiratory volume, ABGs; lung sounds, heart rate and rhythm, B/P, sputum (baseline and peak); actively deteriorating COPD may occur; a rescue inhaler should be readily available

• Determine that patient has not received theophylline therapy or other bronchodilators before giving dose
• Assess patient's ability to self-medicate
• Assess for allergic reactions; **anaphylaxis** may occur
• Assess **paradoxical bronchospasm;** hold medication, notify prescriber if bronchospasm occurs

Patient/family education
• Teach patient to use exactly as prescribed, that death has resulted from asthma with products similar to this one, to have a rescue inhaler always
• Advise patient not to use OTC medications; excess stimulation may occur
• An opened unit-dose vial should be used immediately

Evaluation
Positive therapeutic outcome
• Absence of dyspnea, wheezing after 1 hr, improved airway exchange, improved ABGs

▲ HIGH ALERT

argatroban (Rx)
(are-ga-troe'ban)
Argatroban
Func. class.: Anticoagulant
Chem. class.: Thrombin inhibitor
Pregnancy category B

Do not confuse:
argatroban/Aggrastat

ACTION: Direct inhibitor of thrombin that is derived from L-arginine; it reversibly binds to the thrombin active site

Therapeutic outcome: Absence or decrease of thrombosis

USES: Thrombosis prophylaxis or treatment; anticoagulation prevention/treatment of thrombosis in heparin-induced thrombocytopenia (HIT); percutaneous coronary intervention (PCI) in those with a history of HIT, deep vein thrombosis, pulmonary embolism

CONTRAINDICATIONS:
Hypersensitivity, overt major bleeding

Precautions: Pregnancy **C**, breastfeeding, children, intracranial bleeding, impaired renal function, hepatic disease, severe hypertension, after lumbar puncture, spinal anesthesia, major surgery/trauma, congenital or acquired bleeding, GI ulcers

DOSAGE AND ROUTES
DVT, pulmonary embolism
Adult: CONT **IV** inf 2 mcg/kg/min; adjust dose until steady-state aPPT is 1.5-3 × initial baseline, not to exceed 100 sec, max dose 10 mcg/kg/min

Percutaneous coronary intervention (PCI) in HIT
Adult: **IV** inf 25 mcg/kg/min and a bol of 350 mcg/kg given over 3-5 min, check ACT 5-10 min after bol is completed, proceed if ACT >300 sec; if ACT <300 sec, give another 150 mcg/kg bol and increase infusion rate to 30 mcg/kg/min; recheck ACT in 5-10 min; if ACT >450 sec, decrease infusion rate to 15 mcg/kg/min; recheck ACT in 5-10 min; once ACT is therapeutic, continue for duration of procedure

Hepatic dose
Adult: Cont inf 0.5 mcg/kg/min, adjust rate based on APTT

Available forms: Inj 100 mg/ml (2.5 ml) (must dilute 100-fold), 50 mg/50 ml, 125 mg/125 ml

Implementation
• Avoid all IM inj that may cause bleeding

IV, direct route
• **For PCI:** 350 mg/kg bol, and continuous inf of 25 mcg/kg/min, check ACT 5-10 min after bolus

Intermittent IV INF route
• **Dilute** in 0.9% NaCl, D_5, LR to a final conc 1 mg/ml; **dilute** each 2.5-ml vial 100-fold by mixing with 250 ml of diluent, mix by repeated inversion of the diluent bag for 1 min; may be slightly hazy briefly
• Dosage adjustment may be made after review of aPTT, not to exceed 10 mcg/kg/min

ADVERSE EFFECTS
CNS: Fever, **intracranial bleeding,** headache
CV: Atrial fibrillation, ventricular tachycardia, coronary thrombosis, MI, myocardial ischemia, coronary occlusion, bradycardia, chest pain, hypotension
GI: Nausea, vomiting, abdominal pain, diarrhea, **GI bleeding**
GU: Hematuria, abnormal kidney function, UTI
HEMA: Hemorrhage
MISC: *Back pain,* infection
RESP: Dyspnea, coughing, hemoptysis, pulmonary edema
SYST: Sepsis

Pharmacokinetics
Absorption	Unknown
Distribution	To extracellular fluid, 54% plasma protein binding
Metabolism	Liver
Excretion	Feces
Half-life	39-51 min

Pharmacodynamics
Unknown

INTERACTIONS
Individual drugs
Clopidogrel, dipyridamole, heparin, ticlodipine, warfarin: increased bleeding risk

Drug classifications
Antiplatelets, glycoprotein IIb/IIIa antagonists (abciximab, eptifibatide, tirofiban), NSAIDs, other anticoagulants, salicylates, thrombolytics (alteplase, reteplase, tenecteplase, urokinase): increased risk of bleeding

Drug/herb
Garlic, ginger, ginkgo, horse chestnut: increased bleeding risk

NURSING CONSIDERATIONS
Assessment
• Obtain baseline aPTT before treatment; do not start treatment if aPTT ratio ≥2.5, then aPTT 4 hr after initiation of treatment and at least daily thereafter; if aPTT above target, stop inf for 2 hr, then restart at 50%, take aPTT in 4 hr; if below target, increase inf rate by 20%, take aPTT in 4 hr, do not exceed inf rate of 0.21 mg/kg/hr without checking for coagulation abnormalities
• Monitor aPTT, which should be 1.5-3 × control, draw blood for ACT q20-30min during long PCI

⚠ Assess for bleeding gums, petechiae, ecchymosis, black tarry stools, hematuria/epistaxis, B/P, vaginal bleeding, and possible hemorrhage
• Fever, skin rash, urticaria
• **Anaphylaxis:** assess for dyspnea, rash during treatment

Patient/family education
• Advise patient to use soft-bristle toothbrush to avoid bleeding gums, avoid contact sports, use electric razor, avoid IM inj
• Instruct patient to report any signs of bleeding: gums, under skin, urine, stools; trouble breathing, wheezing, skin rash

Evaluation
Positive therapeutic outcome
• Absence or decrease of thrombosis

ARIPiprazole (Rx)

(a-rip-ip-pra′zol)
Abilify, Abilify Discmelt, Abilify Maintena
Func. class.: Antipsychotic/neuroleptic
Pregnancy category C

ACTION: Exact mechanism unknown; may be mediated through both dopamine type 2 (D_2) and serotonin type 2 (5-HT_2) antagonism

Therapeutic outcome: Decreased excitement, hallucinations, delusions, paranoia, reorganization of patterns of thought, speech

USES: Schizophrenia and bipolar disorder (adults and adolescents), agitation, mania, major depressive disorder, short-term mania or mixed episodes of bipolar disorder, irritability in autism

CONTRAINDICATIONS:
Hypersensitivity, breastfeeding, seizure disorders

Precautions: Pregnancy **C**, geriatric, renal/cardiac/hepatic disease, neutropenia

> **BLACK BOX WARNING:** Children, dementia, suicidal ideation

DOSAGE AND ROUTES
Schizophrenia
Adult: PO 10-15 mg/day; if needed, dosage may be increased to 30 mg daily after 2 wk; maintenance 15 mg/day, periodically reassess; IM/EXT REL (monthly inj susp) 400 mg qmo

Adolescent 13-17 yr: 2 mg/day, may increase to 5 mg after 2 days, then 10 mg after 2 more days, max 30 mg/day

Major depressive disorder
Adult: PO 2-5 mg/day as an adjunct to other antidepressant treatment; adjust by 5 mg at ≥1 wk (range, 2-15 mg/day)

Agitation in bipolar disorder/schizophrenia
Adult: IM 9.75 mg as a single dose; may start with a lower dose, max 30 mg/day

Bipolar disorder
Adult: 15 mg/day, may increase to 30 mg/day if needed (monotherapy): adjunctive to lithium or valproate PO 10-15 mg qd, may increase to 30 mg as needed
Child ≥10 yr/adolescent: PO 2 mg, titrate to 5 mg/day after 2 days to a target of 10 mg/day after another 2 days

Irritability associated with autism
Child ≥6 yr/adolescent: PO 2 mg/day, increase to 5 mg/day after 1 wk, may increase to 10-15 mg/day if needed, dose changes should not occur more frequently than q1wk

Potential CYP2D6 inhibitor, strong CYP3A4 inhibitors
Adult: PO reduce to 50% of usual dose, increase dose when CYP2D6, CYP3A4 inhibitor is withdrawn

Combination of strong CYP3A4/CYP2D6 inhibitors
Adult: PO reduce to 25% of usual dose
Available forms: Tabs 2, 5, 10, 15, 20, 30 mg; inj 9.75 mg/1.3 ml; orally disintegrating tab 10, 15 mg; oral sol 1 mg/ml; sol for injection 1.75 mg/1.3 ml; inj susp EXT REL 300, 400 mg

Implementation
• Administer reduced dose in geriatric
• Decreased stimulus by dimming lights, avoiding loud noises
• Supervise ambulation until patient is stabilized on medication; do not involve in strenuous exercise program because fainting is possible; patient should not stand still for a long time
• Store in tight, light-resistant container
• Available as ready to use
• Oral sol can be substituted for tablet mg per mg up to 25-mg dose; patients receiving 30-mg tablets should receive 25 mg of sol
• IM route: EXT REL monthly (Abilify Maintena)
• Do not give IV or subcut

ADVERSE EFFECTS
CNS: *Drowsiness, insomnia, agitation, anxiety, headache,* **seizures, neuroleptic malignant syndrome,** *lightheadedness, akathisia, asthenia, tremor,* **stroke, suicidal ideation,** dystonia
CV: Orthostatic hypotension, **tachycardia**
EENT: Blurred vision, rhinitis
GI: Constipation, *nausea,* vomiting, jaundice, weight gain
INTEG: *Rash*
META: Hyperglycemia, dyslipidemia
MS: Musculoskeletal pain/stiffness, myalgia
RESP: *Cough*
SYST: **Death in geriatric patients with dementia**

Pharmacokinetics

Absorption	Unknown
Distribution	Protein binding, 90%
Metabolism	Liver, extensively to major active metabolism
Excretion	Unknown
Half-life	Unknown

Pharmacodynamics
Unknown

INTERACTIONS
Individual drugs
Alcohol: increased sedation
CarBAMazepine: decreased effects of ARIPiprazole
Erythromycin, FLUoxetine, ketoconazole, quiNIDine, PARoxetine: increased effects of ARIPiprazole, reduce dose
Famotidine, valproate: decreased ARIPiprazole level
Lithium: increased EPS

Drug classifications
Antipsychotics: increased EPS
CNS depressants: increased sedation
CYP3A4/CYP2D6 inhibitors: increased effects of ARIPiprazole, reduce dose
CYPA34 inducers: decreased effects of ARIPiprazole; increase dose

Drug/herb
St. John's wort: decreased ARIPiprazole effect

NURSING CONSIDERATIONS
Assessment

> **BLACK BOX WARNING:** Assess mental status before initial administration, children/young adults may exhibit suicidal thoughts/behaviors, the smallest amount of product should be given; elderly patients with dementia-related psychosis are at increased risk of death

• Check for swallowing of PO medication; check for hoarding or giving of medication to other patients
• Monitor I&O ratio; palpate bladder if urinary output is low
• Monitor bilirubin, CBC, liver function tests qmo
• Assess affect, orientation, LOC, reflexes, gait, coordination, sleep pattern disturbances
• Monitor B/P standing and lying; also pulse, respirations; take q4hr during initial treatment; establish baseline before starting treatment; report drops of 30 mm Hg; watch for ECG changes
• Assess for dizziness, faintness, palpitations, tachycardia on rising
• Assess for EPS, including akathisia (inability to sit still, no pattern to movements), tardive dyskinesia (bizarre movements of the jaw, mouth, tongue, extremities), pseudoparkinsonism (rigidity, tremors, pill rolling, shuffling gait)
⚠ Assess for neuroleptic malignant syndrome: hyperthermia, increased CPK, altered mental status, muscle rigidity
• Monitor weight, lipid profile, fasting blood glucose
• Assess skin turgor daily
• Assess for constipation, urinary retention daily; if these occur, increase bulk and water in diet

Patient/family education
• Advise patient that orthostatic hypotension may occur and to rise from sitting or lying position gradually
• Advise patient to avoid hot tubs, hot showers, tub baths; hypotension may occur
• Instruct patient to avoid abrupt withdrawal of this product; EPS may result; product should be withdrawn slowly
• Teach patient to avoid OTC preparations (cough, hayfever, cold) unless approved by prescriber, because serious product interactions may occur; avoid use with alcohol, CNS depressants; increased drowsiness may occur
• Advise patient to avoid hazardous activities if drowsy or dizzy

---

Adverse effects: *italics* = common; **bold** = life-threatening

• Explain importance of compliance with product regimen
• Advise patient, family to report impaired vision, tremors, muscle twitching, urinary retention
• Instruct patient to take extra precautions to stay cool in hot weather, that heat stroke may occur

> **BLACK BOX WARNING:** Teach patient to report suicidal thoughts/behaviors immediately

Evaluation
Positive therapeutic outcome
• Decreased emotional excitement, hallucinations, delusions, paranoia; reorganization of patterns of thought, speech

TREATMENT OF OVERDOSE:
Lavage if orally ingested; provide airway; *do not induce vomiting*

---

ascorbic acid (vitamin C) (OTC, Rx)
(as-kor'bic)
Acerda C, Apo-C ✦, Ascor L-500, Cenolate, Equaline Vitamin C, Walgreens Gold Seal, and many more
Func. class.: Vitamin C, water-soluble vitamin
Pregnancy category C

ACTION: Needed for wound healing, collagen synthesis, antioxidant, carbohydrate metabolism

Therapeutic outcome: Replacement and supplementation of vit C

USES: Vit C deficiency, scurvy, delayed wound and bone healing, chronic disease, before gastrectomy, dietary supplement

Unlabeled uses: Common cold prevention

CONTRAINDICATIONS:
Tartrazine, sulfite sensitivity; G6PD deficiency

Precautions: Pregnancy **C**, gout, diabetes, renal calculi (large doses)

DOSAGE AND ROUTES
RDA
Neonate and up to 6 mo: PO 30 mg/day
Infant: PO 40-50 mg/day
Child 1-3 yr: PO 15 mg/day
Child 4-8 yr: PO 25 mg/day

Child 9-13 yr: PO 45 mg/day
Child 14-18 yr: PO 65 mg/day (females), 75 mg/day (males)
Adult: PO 50-500 mg/day

Scurvy
Adult: PO/SUBCUT/IM/**IV** 100 mg-250 mg daily × 2 wk, then 50 mg or more daily
Child: PO/SUBCUT/IM/**IV** 100-300 mg daily × 2 wk, then 35 mg or more daily

Wound healing/chronic disease/fracture
May be given with zinc
Adult: SUBCUT/IM/**IV**/PO 200-500 mg daily for 1-2 mo
Child: SUBCUT/IM/**IV**/PO 100-200 mg added doses for 1-2 mo

Urine acidification
Adult: 4-12 g daily in divided doses
Child: 500 mg q6-8hr

Available forms: Tabs 25, 50, 100, 250, 500, 1000, 1500 mg; effervescent tabs 1000 mg; chewable tabs 100, 250, 500 mg; time-release tabs 500, 750, 1000, 1500 mg; time-release caps 500 mg; crystals 4 g/tsp; powder 4 g/tsp; liquid 35 mg/0.6 ml; sol 100 mg/ml; syr 20 mg/ml, 500 mg/5 ml; inj SUBCUT, IM, **IV** 100, 250, 500 mg/ml

Implementation
PO route
• Swallow time rel tabs or caps whole; do not break, crush, or chew
• Mix oral sol with foods or fluids
IM route
• Not to be diluted; give deep in large muscle mass

IV, direct route
• Give undiluted by *direct* **IV** 100 mg over at least 1 min, rapid inf may cause fainting
Intermittent IV infusion route
• Give by intermittent inf after diluting with D₅W, D₁₀W, 0.9% NaCl, 0.45% NaCl, LR, Ringer's sol, dextrose/saline, dextrose/Ringer's combinations; temp will increase pressure in ampules; wrap with gauze before breaking

Syringe compatibilities: Metoclopramide, aminophylline, theophylline

Syringe incompatibilities: CeFAZolin, doxapram

Y-site compatibilities: Warfarin

ADVERSE EFFECTS

CNS: Headache, insomnia, dizziness, fatigue, flushing

GI: Nausea, vomiting, diarrhea, anorexia, heartburn, cramps

GU: Polyuria, urine acidification, oxalate or urate renal stones, dysuria

HEMA: Hemolytic anemia in patients with G6PD

INTEG: Inflammation at inj site

Pharmacokinetics	
Absorption	Readily absorbed (PO)
Distribution	Widely distributed; crosses placenta
Metabolism	Oxidation
Excretion	Kidneys, inactive; breast milk
Half-life	Unknown

Pharmacodynamics
Unknown

INTERACTIONS

Drug/lab test

False positive: negative in glucose tests (Clinitest, Tes-Tape)

False negative: occult blood (large dose), urine bilirubin, leukocyte determination

NURSING CONSIDERATIONS

Assessment

• Assess nutritional status for inclusion of foods high in vit C: citrus fruits, cantaloupe, tomatoes
• Assess for vit C deficiency before, during, and after treatment; scurvy (gingivitis, bleeding gums, loose teeth); poor bone development
• Monitor I&O ratio, polyuria; in patients receiving large doses, renal stones may occur; urine pH (acidification)
• Monitor ascorbic acid levels throughout treatment if continued deficiency is suspected
• Assess inj sites for inflammation, pain, redness, thrombophlebitis if in large doses

Patient/family education

• Teach patient necessary foods to be included in diet that are rich in vit C: citrus fruits, cantaloupe, tomatoes, chili peppers (red)
• Teach patient that smoking decreases vit C levels; not to exceed prescribed dose; increases will be excreted in urine, except time release
• Teach patient not to exceed RDA recommended dose, urinary stones may occur
• Teach patient using ascorbic acid for acidification of urine to test urine pH periodically

Evaluation

Positive therapeutic outcome

• Absence of anorexia, irritability, pallor, joint pain, hyperkeratosis, petechiae, poor wound healing
• Reversal of scurvy: bleeding gums, gingivitis, loose teeth

---

asenapine (Rx)

(a-sen′a-peen)

Saphris

Func. class.: Antipsychotic, atypical

Chem. class.: Dibenzazepine

Pregnancy category C

ACTION: Unknown; may be mediated through both dopamine type 2 (D_2) and serotonin type 2 ($5\text{-}HT_{2A}$) antagonism

Therapeutic outcome: Decrease in delusions, hallucinations

USES: Bipolar 1 disorder, schizophrenia

CONTRAINDICATIONS:

Breastfeeding, hypersensitivity

Precautions: Pregnancy **C,** children, geriatric patients, cardiac/renal/hepatic disease, breast cancer, Parkinson's disease, dementia, seizure disorder, CNS depression, agranulocytosis, QT prolongation, torsades de pointes, suicidal ideation, substance abuse, diabetes mellitus

> **BLACK BOX WARNING:** Increased mortality in elderly patients with dementia-related psychosis

DOSAGE AND ROUTES

Schizophrenia

Adult: SL 5 mg bid, max 20 mg/day

Bipolar 1 disorder

Adult: SL 10 mg bid, may decrease to 5 mg bid as needed, max 20 mg/day

Available forms: SL tab 5, 10 mg

Implementation

PO route

• Give anticholinergic agent for EPS
• Avoid use with CNS depressants
• **SL tab:** remove tab, place tab under tongue; after it dissolves, swallow; advise not to chew, crush or swallow tabs, not to eat or drink for 10 min

---

Adverse effects: *italics* = common; **bold** = life-threatening

- Supervise ambulation until patient is stabilized on medication; do not involve in strenuous exercise program because fainting is possible; patient should not stand still for a long time
- Increase fluids to prevent constipation
- Store in tight, light-resistant container

ADVERSE EFFECTS

CNS: *EPS, pseudoparkinsonism, akathisia, dystonia, tardive dyskinesia, drowsiness, insomnia, agitation, anxiety, headache,* **seizures, neuroleptic malignant syndrome,** dizziness, **suicidal ideation, drowsiness, depression**
CV: Orthostatic hypotension, **sinus tachycardia, heart failure, QT prolongation, stroke, bundle branch block**
ENDO: Hyperglycemia, hyperlipidemia
GI: *Nausea,* vomiting, *constipation,* weight gain, increased appetite; oral hypoesthesia/parasthesia (SL)
HEMA: Thrombocytopenia, agranulocytosis, anemia, leukopenia
INTEG: Serious allergic reaction (anaphylaxis, angioedema)

Pharmacokinetics

Absorption	Unknown
Distribution	Protein binding 95%
Metabolism	Liver
Excretion	Unknown
Half-life	Terminal 24 hr

Pharmacodynamics

Onset	Unknown
Peak	½-1½ hr
Duration	Unknown

INTERACTIONS

Individual drugs
Alcohol: increased sedation
Chloroquine, clarithromycin, droperidol, erythromycin, haloperidol, methadone, pentamidine: increased QT prolongation
CarBAMazepine: increased asenpine excretion

Drug classifications
Other CNS depressants: increased sedation
CYP2D6 inhibitors/substrates (SSRIs), other antipsychotics: increased EPS
Class IA/III antidysrhythmics, some phenothiazines, β-agonists, local anesthetics, tricyclics: increased QT prolongation

CYP2D6 inducers (carBAMazepine, barbiturates, phenytoin, rifampin): decreased asenapine action
SSRIs: increased serotonin syndrome

Drug/herb
Kava: increased CNS depression, increased EPS
Betel palm: increased EPS

Drug/lab test
Increased: cholesterol, glucose, LFTs, lipids, prolactin levels, triglycerides
Decreased: sodium

NURSING CONSIDERATIONS

Assessment
⚠ **Assess mental status before initial administration; watch for suicidal thoughts and behaviors; dementia and death may occur in the elderly**
- Assess for affect, orientation, LOC, reflexes, gait, coordination, sleep pattern disturbances
- Monitor B/P standing and lying, pulse, respirations; take these q4hr during initial treatment; establish baseline before starting treatment; report drops of 30 mm Hg; watch for ECG changes; QT prolongation may occur
- Monitor for dizziness, faintness, palpitations, tachycardia on rising
- Assess for **EPS,** including akathisia, tardive dyskinesia (bizarre movements of the jaw, mouth, tongue, extremities), pseudoparkinsonism (rigidity, tremors, pill rolling, shuffling gait)
⚠ **Assess for neuroleptic malignant syndrome: hyperthermia, increased CPK, altered mental status, muscle rigidity**
- Assess for constipation daily; increase bulk and water in diet if needed
- Assess for weight gain, hyperglycemia, metabolic changes in diabetes

Patient/family education
- Caution patient that orthostatic hypotension may occur and to rise from sitting or lying position gradually
- Teach patient to avoid hot tubs, hot showers, tub baths; hypotension may occur
- Advise patient to avoid abrupt withdrawal of this product; EPS may result; product should be withdrawn slowly
- Advise patient to avoid OTC preparations (cough, hay fever, cold) unless approved by prescriber, serious product interactions may occur; avoid use of alcohol, increased drowsiness may occur
- Advise patient to avoid hazardous activities if drowsy or dizzy

- Advise patient about compliance with product regimen
- Advise patient that heat stroke may occur in hot weather; take extra precautions to stay cool
- Advise patient to use contraception, inform prescriber if pregnancy is planned or suspected
- Advise patient to report suicidal thoughts/behaviors immediately

Evaluation
Positive therapeutic outcome
- Therapeutic response: decrease in emotional excitement, hallucinations, delusions, paranoia; reorganization of patterns of thought, speech

TREATMENT OF OVERDOSE:
Lavage if orally ingested; provide airway; *do not induce vomiting*

aspirin (OTC)
(as'pir-in)
APC-ASA Coated Aspirin ✦, A.S.A., Ascriptin Enteric, Aspergum, Aspirin ✦, Aspir-Low, Aspirtrin ✦, Bayer Aspirin, Bayer Children's Aspirin, Bufferin, Ecotrin, Equaline, Good Sense Aspirin, Halfprin, PMS-ASA ✦, St. Joseph Children's, St. Joseph's Adult, Walgreens Aspirin Adult
Func. class.: Nonopioid analgesic
Chem. class.: Salicylate
Pregnancy category D (3rd trimester)

Do not confuse:
Ascendin/Afrin

ACTION: Blocks pain impulses in CNS, reduces inflammation by inhibition of prostaglandin synthesis; antipyretic action results from vasodilatation of peripheral vessels; decreases platelet aggregation

Therapeutic outcome: Decreased pain, inflammation, fever; absence of MI, transient ischemic attacks, thrombosis

USES: Mild to moderate pain or fever including rheumatoid arthritis, osteoarthritis, thromboembolic disorders, transient ischemic attacks, rheumatic fever, post-MI, prophylaxis of MI, ischemic stroke, angina; acute MI

Unlabeled uses: Prevention of cataracts (long-term use), prevention of pregnancy loss in women with clotting disorders

CONTRAINDICATIONS:
Pregnancy **D** (3rd trimester), breastfeeding, children <12 yr, children with flulike symptoms, hypersensitivity to salicylates, tartrazine (FDC yellow dye #5), GI bleeding, bleeding disorders, vit K deficiency, peptic ulcer, acute bronchospasm, agranulocytosis, increased intracranial pressure, intracranial bleeding, nasal polyps, urticaria

Precautions: Abrupt discontinuation, acetaminophen/NSAIDs hypersensitivity, acid/base imbalance, alcoholism, ascites, asthma, bone marrow suppression, geriatric patients, dehydration, G6PD deficiency, gout, heart failure, anemia, renal/hepatic disease, pre/postoperatively, gastritis, pregnancy **C** 1st trimester

DOSAGE AND ROUTES
Arthritis
Adult: PO 3 g/day in divided doses q4-6hr
Child >25 kg (55 lb): PO or RECT 90-130 mg/kg/day in divided doses

Kawasaki's disease (unlabeled)
Child: PO 80-100 mg/kg/day in 4 divided doses, maintenance 3-5 mg/kg/day

MI, stroke prophylaxis
Adult: PO 50-325 mg/day

Pain/fever
Adult: PO/RECT 325-650 mg q4hr prn, max 4 g/day
Child 2-11 yr: PO 10-15 mg/kg/dose q4hr, max 4 g/day

Thromboembolic disorders
Adult: PO 325-650 mg/day or bid

Transient ischemic attacks (risk)
Adult: PO 50-325 mg/day (grade 1A)

Prevention of recurrent MI
Adult: PO 75-162 mg/day

CABG
Adult: PO 325 mg/day starting 6 hr post-procedure, continue for 1 yr

PTCA
Adult: PO 325 mg 2 hr presurgery

Evolving MI with ST segment elevation (STEMI)
Adult: PO 160-325 mg nonenteric, chewed and swallowed immediately, maintenance 75-162 mg qd

Available forms: Tabs 81, 325, 500, 650, 800 mg; chewable tabs 81 mg; supp 300, 600, mg; gum 227 mg; enteric coated tabs 81, 325, 500, 975 mg; ext rel 800 mg; del rel tabs 325, 500 mg; supp 300, 600 mg

Implementation
PO route
- Do not break, crush, or chew enteric product
- Administer to patient crushed or whole; chewable tab should be chewed
- Give with food or milk to decrease gastric symptoms; separate by 2 hr of enteric product; absorption may be slowed
- Give antacids 1-2 hr after enteric products
- Give with 8 oz of water and have patient sit upright for 30 min after dose; discard tabs if vinegar-like smell is present; avoid if allergic to tartrazine
- Give ½ hr before planned exercise

Rectal route
- Place suppository in refrigerator for at least 30 min before removing wrapper

ADVERSE EFFECTS
CNS: Stimulation, drowsiness, dizziness, confusion, **seizures,** headache, flushing, hallucinations, **coma**
CV: Rapid pulse, pulmonary edema
EENT: Tinnitus, hearing loss
ENDO: Hypoglycemia, hyponatremia, hypokalemia
GI: *Nausea, vomiting,* **GI bleeding,** diarrhea, heartburn, anorexia, **hepatitis,** GI ulcer
HEMA: **Thrombocytopenia, agranulocytosis, leukopenia, neutropenia, hemolytic anemia,** increased PT, PTT, bleeding time
INTEG: *Rash,* urticaria, bruising
RESP: Wheezing, hyperpnea, **bronchospasm**
SYST: Reye's syndrome (children), anaphylaxis, laryngeal edema

Pharmacokinetics

Absorption	Well absorbed, small intestine (PO); erratic (enteric); slow (RECT)
Distribution	Rapidly, widely distributed; crosses placenta, protein binding 90%
Metabolism	Liver, extensively
Excretion	Inactive metabolites, kidney; breast milk
Half-life	15-20 min (low doses); 9 hr (high doses)

Pharmacodynamics

	PO	RECT
Onset	15-30 min	Slow
Peak	1-2 hr	4-5 hr
Duration	4-6 hr	6-7 hr

INTERACTIONS
Individual drugs
Alcohol, cefamandole, clopidogrel, eptifibatide, heparin, plicamycin, ticlopidine, tirofiban: increased risk of bleeding
Ammonium chloride, nizatidine: increased salicylate level
Insulin, methotrexate, phenytoin, valproic acid, warfarin: increased effects of each specific product
Nitroglycerin: increased hypotension
Probenecid: decreased effects of probenecid
Spironolactone, sulfinpyrazone: decreased effects

Drug classifications
ACE inhibitors: decreased antihypertensive effect
Antacids (high doses), corticosteroids, urinary alkalizers: decreased effects of aspirin
Anticoagulants, thrombolytics: increased risk of bleeding
Diuretics (loop), sulfonylamides, NSAIDs, β-blockers: decreased effect of each specific product
NSAIDs, antiinflammatories, steroids: increased gastric ulcers
Penicillins, oral hypoglycemics, sulfonamides, thrombolytic agents: increased effects of each specific product
Salicylates: decreased blood glucose levels
Urinary acidifiers: increased salicylate levels

Drug/herb
Feverfew, garlic, ginger, ginkgo, ginseng *(Panax),* horse chestnut: increased risk of bleeding

Drug/food
Foods acidifying urine may increase aspirin levels
Fish oil (omega-3-fatty acids): increased risk of bleeding

Drug/lab test
Increased: coagulation studies, liver function studies, serum uric acid, amylase, CO_2, urinary protein
Decreased: serum potassium, cholesterol
Interference: VMA, 5-HIAA, xylose tolerance test, TSH, pregnancy test

---

⚠ Nurse Alert   ✸ Key NCLEX® Drug

NURSING CONSIDERATIONS
Assessment
- Assess for **pain:** character, location, intensity, ROM before and 1 hr after administration
- Monitor liver function studies: AST, ALT, bilirubin, creatinine if patient is on long-term therapy
- Monitor renal function studies: BUN, urine creatinine if patient is on long-term therapy
- Monitor blood studies: CBC, Hct, Hgb, PT if patient is on long-term therapy
- Check I&O ratio; decreasing output may indicate renal failure (long-term therapy)
- ⚠ Assess hepatotoxicity: dark urine, clay-colored stools, yellowing of the skin and sclera, itching, abdominal pain, fever, diarrhea if patient is on long-term therapy
- Assess for **allergic reactions:** rash, urticaria; if these occur, product may have to be discontinued; in patients with asthma, nasal polyps, allergies, severe allergic reactions may occur
- Assess for **ototoxicity:** tinnitus, ringing, roaring in ears; audiometric testing needed before, after long-term therapy
- Monitor **salicylate level:** therapeutic level 150-300 mcg/ml for chronic inflammation
- Check edema in feet, ankles, legs
- Identify prior product history; there are many product interactions

Patient/family education
- Teach patient to report any symptoms of renal/hepatic toxicity, visual changes, ototoxicity, allergic reactions, bleeding (long-term therapy)
- Instruct patient to take with 8 oz of water and sit upright for 30 min after dose to facilitate product passing into the stomach; to discard tabs if vinegar-like smell is present; to avoid if allergic to tartrazine
- Instruct patient not to exceed recommended dosage; acute poisoning may result
- Advise patient to read label on other OTC products; many contain aspirin
- Inform patient that the therapeutic response takes 2 wk (arthritis)
- Teach patient to report tinnitus, confusion, diarrhea, sweating, hyperventilation
- Advise patient to avoid alcohol ingestion; GI bleeding may occur
- Advise patient with allergies, nasal polyps, asthma, that allergic reactions may develop
- Instruct patient to read labels on other OTC products; may contain salicylates
- Teach patient not to give to children or teens with flulike symptoms or chicken pox; Reye's syndrome may develop

- ⚠ Instruct patient not to use during 3rd trimester of pregnancy (D)
- Teach patient to take with a full glass of water

Evaluation
Positive therapeutic outcome
- Decreased pain
- Decreased inflammation
- Decreased fever
- Absence of MI
- Absence of transient ischemic attacks, thrombosis

TREATMENT OF OVERDOSE:
Lavage, activated charcoal; monitor electrolytes, VS

---

atazanavir (Rx)
(at-a-za-na′veer)
Reyataz
Func. class.: Antiretroviral
Chem. class.: Protease inhibitor
Pregnancy category B

ACTION: Inhibits human immunodeficiency virus (HIV-1) protease, which prevents maturation of the infectious virus

Therapeutic outcome: Decreasing symptoms of HIV

USES: HIV-1 infection in combination with other antiretroviral agents

CONTRAINDICATIONS:
Hypersensitivity

Precautions: Pregnancy **B**, breastfeeding, children, geriatric, liver disease, alcoholism, antimicrobial resistance, AV block, diabetes, dialysis, elderly, women, hemophilia, hypercholesterolemia, immune reconstitution syndrome, lactic acidosis, pancreatitis, cholelithiasis, serious rash

DOSAGE AND ROUTES
Antiretroviral-naive patients
Adult: PO 400 mg daily
Child ≥6 yr/adolescent ≤40 kg: PO 300 mg with ritonavir 100 mg qd
Child ≥6 yr/adolescent 20 to <40 kg: PO 200 mg with ritonavir 100 mg qd
Child ≥6 yr/adolescent 15 to <20 kg: PO 150 mg with ritonavir 80 mg qd

Antiretroviral-experienced patients
Adult: PO 300 mg daily and ritonavir 100 mg daily

Pregnant adult/adolescent (2nd/3rd trimester) with H₂ blocker or tenofovir: PO 400 mg with ritonavir 100 mg qd
Child ≥6 yr/adolescent ≥40 kg: PO 300 mg with ritonavir 100 mg qd
Child ≥6 yr/adolescent 20 to <40 kg: PO 200 mg with ritonavir 100 mg qd

Hepatic dose
Adult: PO (Child-Pugh B) 300 mg daily; (Child-Pugh C) do not use

Available forms: Caps 100, 150, 200, 300 mg

Implementation
• Administer with food; take 2 hr before or 1 hr after antacid or didanosine; swallow cap whole

ADVERSE EFFECTS
CNS: Headache, depression, dizziness, insomnia, peripheral neuropathy
GI: *Diarrhea, abdominal pain, nausea,* vomiting, **hepatotoxicity,** cholelithiasis
INTEG: *Rash,* **Stevens-Johnson syndrome,** *photosensitivity,* DRESS
MISC: Fatigue, fever, arthralgia, back pain, cough, lipodystrophy, pain, gynecomastia, nephrolithiasis, **lactic acidosis, hyperbilirubinemia** (pregnancy, females, obesity)

Pharmacokinetics

Absorption	Rapid, increased with food
Distribution	86% protein bound
Metabolism	Liver extensively by CYP3A4
Excretion	27% excreted unchanged in urine/feces (minimal)
Half-life	7 hr

Pharmacodynamics

Onset	Unknown
Peak	2 hr
Duration	Unknown

INTERACTIONS
Individual drugs
Chlorazepate, clarithromycin, cycloSPORINE, diazepam, irinotecan, midazolam, pimozide, sildenafil, sirolimus, tacrolimus, triazolam, warfarin: increased levels resulting in toxicity
Didanosine, efavirenz, rifampin: decreased atazanavir levels
Indinavir: increased hyperbilirubinemia
Ritonavir, teleprevir: decreased teleprevir levels when used with atazanavir and ritonavir

Drug classifications
Antacids, H₂-receptor antagonists, proton pump inhibitors, CYP3A4 inducers: decreased atazanavir levels
Antidepressants (tricyclics), antidysrhythmics, ergots, calcium channel blockers, HMG-CoA reductase inhibitors, immunosuppressants, other protease inhibitors: increased levels resulting in increased toxicity
Contraceptives (oral), estrogens: increased effects
CYP3A4 substrates, CYP3A4 inhibitors: increased atazanavir levels

Drug/herb
Red yeast rice: myopathy, rhabdomyolysis
St. John's wort: decreased atazanavir levels, avoid concurrent use

Drug/lab test
Increased: AST, ALT, total bilirubin, amylase, lipase, CK
Decreased: Hgb, neutrophils, platelets

NURSING CONSIDERATIONS
Assessment
⚠ **Immune reconstitution syndrome: when given with combination antiretroviral therapy**
⚠ **Assess for hepatic failure**
• Assess for signs of infection, anemia
• Monitor liver function studies: ALT, AST, bilirubin
• Monitor bowel pattern before, during treatment; if severe abdominal pain with bleeding occurs, product should be discontinued; monitor hydration
• If pregnant, call Antiretroviral Pregnancy Registry 800-258-4263
• Monitor viral load, CD4 count throughout treatment
⚠ **Serious rash (Stevens-Johnson syndrome, DRESS): most rashes last 1-4 wk; if serious, discontinue product**
⚠ **Immune Reconstitution syndrome: time of onset is variable**

Patient/family education
• Advise to take as prescribed with other antiretrovirals as prescribed; if dose is missed, take as soon as remembered up to 1 hr before next dose; do not double dose; do not share with others
• Teach that product must be taken daily to maintain blood levels for duration of therapy
• Teach that photosensitivity may occur; use protective clothing or stay out of the sun

• Instruct to notify prescriber if diarrhea, nausea, vomiting, rash occur; dizziness, lightheadedness; ECG may be altered
• Inform that product interacts with many products and St. John's wort; advise prescriber of all products, herbal products used
• Advise that redistribution of body fat may occur; the effect is not known
• Teach that product does not cure HIV-1 infection or prevent transmission to others, only controls symptoms
⚠ Advise that if taking sildenafil with atazanavir, there may be an increased risk of phosphodiesterase type 5 inhibitor–associated adverse events, including hypotension and prolonged penile erection; notify physician promptly of these symptoms

Evaluation
Positive therapeutic outcome
• Increasing CD4 counts; decreased viral load, resolution of symptoms of HIV-1 infection

atenolol (Rx)

(a-ten'oh-lole)
Tenormin
Func. class.: Antihypertensive
Chem. class.: β-Blocker; β₁-, β₂-blocker (high doses)
Pregnancy category D

Do not confuse:
atenolol/albuterol/Altenol,
Tenormin/thiamine/Imuran

ACTION: Competitively blocks stimulation of β-adrenergic receptor within vascular smooth muscle; produces negative chronotropic activity (decreases rate of SA node discharge, increases recovery time), slows conduction of AV node, decreases heart rate, negative inotropic activity, decreases O_2 consumption in myocardium; also decreases renin-aldosterone-angiotensin system at high doses, inhibits β₂-receptors in bronchial system at higher doses

Therapeutic outcome: Decreased B/P, heart rate, prevention of angina pectoris, MI

USES: Mild to moderate hypertension; prophylaxis of angina pectoris; suspected or known MI (**IV** use), MI prophylaxis

CONTRAINDICATIONS:
Pregnancy **D**, hypersensitivity to β-blockers, cardiogenic shock, 2nd- or 3rd-degree heart block, sinus bradycardia, cardiac failure

Precautions: Major surgery, breastfeeding, diabetes mellitus, renal disease, thyroid disease, CHF, COPD, asthma, well-compensated heart failure, dialysis, myasthenia gravis, Raynaud's disease, pulmonary edema

> **BLACK BOX WARNING:** Abrupt discontinuation

DOSAGE AND ROUTES
Adult: PO 25-50 mg daily, increasing q1-2wk to 100 mg daily; may increase to 200 mg daily for angina or up to 100 mg for hypertension
Child: PO 0.8-1 mg/kg/dose initially, range 0.8-1.5 mg/kg/day, max 2 mg/kg/day
Geriatric: PO 25 mg/day initially

Chronic stable angina
Adult: PO 50 mg q day, then 100 mg/day prn after 7 days, max 200 mg/day

Post MI, MI prophylaxis
Adult: PO 1000 mg/day, in 1-2 divided doses, may need for 1-3 yr post MI

Renal dose
Adult: PO CCr 15-35 ml/min, max 50 mg/day; CCr <15 ml/min max 25 mg/day; hemodialysis 25-50 mg after dialysis

Available forms: Tabs 25, 50, 100 mg

Implementation
PO route
• Given before meals, at bedtime; tablet may be crushed or swallowed whole; give with food to prevent GI upset; reduced dosage in renal dysfunction; take at same time each day
• Store protected from light, moisture; place in cool environment

ADVERSE EFFECTS
CNS: *Insomnia, fatigue, dizziness, mental changes,* memory loss, hallucinations, depression, lethargy, drowsiness, strange dreams, catatonia
CV: Profound hypotension, bradycardia, CHF, *cold extremities, postural hypotension, 2nd- or 3rd-degree heart block*
EENT: Sore throat, dry burning eyes, blurred vision, stuffy nose
ENDO: Increased hypoglycemic response to insulin
GI: *Nausea, diarrhea,* vomiting, **mesenteric arterial thrombosis, ischemic colitis**
GU: Impotence, decreased libido
HEMA: Agranulocytosis, thrombocytopenia, purpura

INTEG: Rash, fever, alopecia
RESP: Bronchospasm, dyspnea, wheezing, pulmonary edema

Pharmacokinetics

Absorption	50%-60% (PO)
Distribution	Crosses placenta; protein binding (5%-15%)
Metabolism	Not metabolized
Excretion	Breast milk, kidneys (50%), feces (50%—unabsorbed product)
Half-life	7 hr

Pharmacodynamics

	PO
Onset	1 hr
Peak	2-4 hr
Duration	24 hr

INTERACTIONS

Individual drugs
Digoxin, diltiazem, hydrALAZINE, methyldopa, prazosin, reserpine, verapamil: increased hypotension, bradycardia
EPHEDrine, pseudoephedrine: increased hypertension
DOPamine, insulin, theophylline: decreased effect of each of these drugs

Drug classifications
Amphetamines: increased hypertension
Anticholinergics, antihypertensives: cardiac glycosides, increased hypotension, bradycardia
Antidiabetic agents (oral) MAOIs: decreased effect of each of these drugs
Sympathomimetics (cough, cold preparations): mutual inhibition

Drug/herb
Hawthorn: increased atenolol effect
Ephedra (ma huang): decreased atenolol effect

Drug/lab test
Increased: uric acid, potassium, triglyceride, blood glucose, BUN, ANA titer

NURSING CONSIDERATIONS

Assessment
• Monitor **hypertension,** B/P during beginning treatment, periodically thereafter; pulse q4hr; note rate, rhythm, quality: apical/radial pulse before administration; notify prescriber of any significant changes (pulse <50 bpm); ECG
• Hypotension: may be caused in hemodialysis
• Hypoglycemia: may be masked in diabetes mellitus

• Check for baselines in renal, liver function tests before therapy begins
• Assess for edema in feet, legs daily; monitor I&O, daily weight; check for jugular vein distention, crackles bilaterally, dyspnea (CHF)

Patient/family education

> **BLACK BOX WARNING:** Teach patient not to discontinue product abruptly; taper over 2 wk (angina) as directed; may cause precipitate angina if stopped abruptly; take at same time each day

• Teach patient not to use OTC products containing α-adrenergic stimulants (such as nasal decongestants, OTC cold preparations); to limit alcohol, smoking; to limit sodium intake as prescribed
• Teach patient how to take pulse and B/P at home; advise when to notify prescriber
• Instruct patient to comply with weight control, dietary adjustments, modified exercise program
• Advise patient to carry/wear emergency ID for products, allergies, conditions being treated; tell patient product controls symptoms but does not cure
• Caution patient to avoid hazardous activities if dizziness, drowsiness is present
• Teach patient to report symptoms of CHF: difficult breathing, especially on exertion or when lying down, night cough, swelling of extremities or bradycardia, dizziness, confusion, depression, fever
• Teach patient to take product as prescribed, not to double doses, skip doses; take any missed doses as remembered if at least 6 hr until next dose
• Advise to change position slowly
• Advise patient that product may mask symptoms of hypoglycemia in diabetic patients
⚠ Advise patient to use contraception while taking this product, avoid breastfeeding

Evaluation
Positive therapeutic outcome
• Decreased B/P in hypertension (after 1-2 wk)
• Absence of dysrhythmias
• Absence of MI
• Decreased angina/pain
• Increased activity tolerance

TREATMENT OF OVERDOSE:
Lavage, **IV** atropine for bradycardia, **IV** theophylline for bronchospasm, digoxin, O$_2$, diuretic for cardiac failure, hemodialysis, **IV** glucose for

hyperglycemia, **IV** diazepam (or phenytoin) for seizures

atomoxetine (Rx)

(at-o-mox′eh-teen)
Strattera
Func. class.: Psychotherapeutic—miscellaneous
Pregnancy category C

ACTION: A selective norepinephrine reuptake inhibitor; may inhibit the presynaptic norepinephrine transporter; exact mechanism of action is unknown

Therapeutic outcome: Decreased hyperactivity, impulsivity, increased attention, organization, ability to complete tasks

USES: Attention deficit hyperactivity disorder

CONTRAINDICATIONS:

Hypersensitivity, closed-angle glaucoma, arteriosclerosis, cardiac disease, cardiomyopathy, heart failure, jaundice, MAOI therapy, history of pheochromocytoma

Precautions: Pregnancy **C**, breastfeeding, hypertension, hepatic disease, angioedema, bipolar disorder, dysrhythmias, CAD, hypo/hypertension

> **BLACK BOX WARNING:** Children <6 yr, suicidal ideation

DOSAGE AND ROUTES
Child ≤70 kg, <6 yr: PO 0.5 mg/kg/day, increase after 3 days to a target daily dose of 1.2 mg/kg in AM or evenly divided doses AM, late afternoon; max 1.4 mg/kg/day or 100 mg daily, whichever is less
Adult and child >70 kg: PO 40 mg daily, increase after 3 days to a target daily dose of 80 mg in AM or evenly divided doses AM, late afternoon; max 100 mg daily

Maintenance
Adolescent ≤15 yr and child ≥6 yr: PO 1.2-1.8 mg/kg/day

Initial dosage titration with strong CYP2D6 inhibitors
Adult and child >6 yr weighing >70 kg: PO 40 mg/day each AM or 2 evenly divided doses, titrate to target of 80 mg/day if symptoms do not improve after 4 wk and dose is well tolerated

Hepatic dose
Child-Pugh B: reduce dose by 50%
Child-Pugh C: reduce dose by 75%

Available forms: Caps 10, 18, 25, 40, 60, 80, 100 mg

Implementation
• Swallow whole; do not break, crush, or chew
• Give without regard to food
• Provide gum, hard candy, frequent sips of water for dry mouth

ADVERSE EFFECTS
CNS: *Insomnia,* dizziness, headache, irritability, crying, mood swings, fatigue, hypoesthesia, lethargy, paresthesia
CV: *Palpitations,* hot flushes, tachycardia, increased B/P
ENDO: Growth retardation
GI: Dyspepsia, nausea, anorexia, dry mouth, weight loss, vomiting, diarrhea, constipation, **hepatic injury**
GU: Urinary hesitancy, retention, dysmenorrhea, erectile disturbance, ejaculation failure, impotence, prostatitis, abnormal orgasm, male pelvic pain
INTEG: Exfoliative dermatitis, sweating, rash
MISC: Cough, rhinorrhea, dermatitis, ear infection

Pharmacokinetics

Absorption	Unknown
Distribution	Protein binding, 98%
Metabolism	Liver
Excretion	Kidneys
Half-life	Unknown

Pharmacodynamics
Unknown

INTERACTIONS
Individual drug
Albuterol: increased cardiovascular effects

Drug classifications
CYP2D6 inhibitors (amiodarone, cimetidine [weak], citalopram, clomiPRAMINE, delavirdine, escitalopram, FLUoxetine, gefitinib, imatinib, PARoxetine, propafenone, quiNIDine [potent], ritonavir, sertraline, thioridazine, venlafaxine): increased effects of atomoxetine
⚠ **MAOIs or within 14 days of MAOIs, vasopressors: hypertensive crisis**
Pressor agents: increased cardiovascular effects

NURSING CONSIDERATIONS
Assessment
- Monitor VS, B/P; check patients with cardiac disease more often for increased B/P
- **Hepatic injury:** may cause liver failure: monitor LFT; assess for jaundice, pruritus, flulike symptoms, upper right quadrant pain

> **BLACK BOX WARNING:** Assess mental status: mood, sensorium, affect, stimulation, insomnia, aggressiveness, suicidal ideation in children/young adults

- Assess appetite, sleep, speech patterns
- Assess for attention span, decreased hyperactivity in ADHD persons, growth rate, weight; therapy may need to be discontinued

Patient/family education
- Advise patient to avoid OTC preparations unless approved by prescriber, no tapering needed when discontinuing product
- Advise patient to avoid alcohol ingestion
- Advise patient to avoid hazardous activities until stabilized on medication
- Advise patient to get needed rest; patients will feel more tired at end of day; do not take dose late in day, insomnia may occur

> **BLACK BOX WARNING:** Advise to report suicidal ideation

- Teach patient to notify prescriber immediately if erection >4 hr

Evaluation
Positive therapeutic outcome
- Decreased hyperactivity (ADHD)

---

atorvastatin (Rx)
(a-tore′va-stat-in)
Lipitor
Func. class.: Antilipidemic
Chem. class.: HMG-CoA reductase inhibitor
Pregnancy category X

ACTION: Inhibits HMG-CoA reductase enzyme, which reduces cholesterol synthesis, high doses lead to plaque regression

Therapeutic outcome: Decreased cholesterol levels and LDLs, increased HDLs

USES: As an adjunct in primary hypercholesterolemia (types Ia, Ib), dysbetalipoproteinemia, elevated triglyceride levels; prevention of cardiovascular disease by reduction of heart risk in those with mildly elevated cholesterol

CONTRAINDICATIONS:
Pregnancy **X**, breastfeeding, hypersensitivity, active liver disease

Precautions: Past liver disease, alcoholism, severe acute infections, trauma, severe metabolic disorders, electrolyte imbalance

DOSAGE AND ROUTES
Adult: PO 10-20 mg daily, usual range 10-80 mg, dosage adjustments may be made in 2-4 wk intervals, max 80 mg/day; patients requiring >45% reduction in LDL may be started at 40 mg daily

Available forms: Tabs 10, 20, 40, 80 mg

Implementation
- Administer total daily dose at any time of day
- Store in cool environment in airtight, light-resistant container

ADVERSE EFFECTS
CNS: Headache, asthenia, **Lou Gehrig's disease (ALS)**
EENT: Lens opacities
GI: *Abdominal cramps, constipation, diarrhea, heartburn,* nausea, dyspepsia, *flatus,* **liver dysfunction, pancreatitis,** increased serum transaminase
GU: Impotence
INTEG: Rash, pruritus, alopecia, photosensitivity (rare)
MISC: Hypersensitivity
MS: Myalgia, **rhabdomyolysis,** arthralgia
RESP: Pharyngitis, sinusitis

Pharmacokinetics
Absorption	Unknown
Distribution	Unknown
Metabolism	Liver
Excretion	Bile, feces, kidneys
Half-life	14 hr

Pharmacodynamics
Unknown

INTERACTIONS
Individual drugs
Clofibrate, cycloSPORINE, erythromycin, gemfibrozil, niacin: **increased risk of rhabdomyolysis**
Colestipol: decreased action of atorvastatin
Digoxin: increased action of digoxin

Erythromycin: increased levels of atorvastatin
Warfarin: increased action of warfarin

Drug classifications
Antifungals (azole): possible rhabdomyolysis
Contraceptives (oral): increased levels

Drug/herb
St. John's wort: decreased effect

Drug/food
Grapefruit juice: possible toxicity
Oat bran may reduce effectiveness

Drug/lab test
Increased: bilirubin, alkaline phosphatase, ALT,
AST, CK
Interference: thyroid function tests

NURSING CONSIDERATIONS
Assessment
• **Hypercholesterolemia:** assess nutrition:
fat, protein, carbohydrates; nutritional analysis
should be completed by dietitian before treatment; assess for muscle pain, tenderness; obtain
CPK if these occur, product may need to be
discontinued; monitor triglycerides, cholesterol
at baseline and throughout treatment; LDL and
VLDL should be watched closely; if increased,
product should be discontinued
• Monitor bowel pattern daily; diarrhea may be
a problem
• Monitor liver function studies q1-2mo during
the first 1½ yr of treatment; AST, ALT, liver function tests may be increased
• Monitor renal studies in patients with
compromised renal system: BUN, I&O ratio,
creatinine
• Assess eyes via ophthalmic exam 1 mo after
treatment begins, annually

Patient/family education
• Inform patient that compliance is needed for
positive results to occur, not to double doses
• Teach patient that risk factors should be
decreased: high-fat diet, smoking, alcohol
consumption, absence of exercise
• Advise patient to notify prescriber if the GI
symptoms of diarrhea, abdominal or epigastric
pain, nausea, vomiting; chills, fever, sore throat;
muscle pain, weakness occur
• Advise patient that treatment will take several
years
• Advise patient that blood work and eye exam
will be necessary during treatment
• Advise not to take if pregnant (pregnancy **X**)
or breastfeeding

• Advise patient to stay out of the sun, use
protective clothing, or use sunscreen to prevent
photosensitivity (rare)

Evaluation
Positive therapeutic outcome
• Decreased cholesterol levels, serum triglycer-
ide
• Improved HDL:LDL ratio

atovaquone (Rx)
(a-toe'va-kwon)
Mepron
Func. class.: Antiprotozoal
Chem. class.: Aromatic diamide derivative;
analog of ubiquinone
Pregnancy category C

ACTION: Interferes with DNA/RNA synthesis in protozoa

Therapeutic outcome: Antiprotozoal for
Pneumocystis jiroveci only

USES: *P. jiroveci* infections in patients
intolerant of trimethoprim/sulfamethoxazole
(co-trimoxazole), prophylaxis, *Toxoplasma
gondii,* toxoplasmosis

CONTRAINDICATIONS:
Hypersensitivity or history of developing life-
threatening allergic reactions to any component
of the formulation, benzyl alcohol sensitivity

Precautions: Pregnancy **C**, breastfeeding, GI/hepatic disease, neonates, respiratory
insufficiency

DOSAGE AND ROUTES
**Acute, mild, moderate *Pneumocys-
tis jiroveci* pneumonia (PCP)**
Adult and adolescent 13-16 yr: PO 750 mg
tid with food for 21 days

***Pneumocystis jiroveci* pneumonia
prophylaxis**
Adult and adolescent: PO 1500 mg daily with
meal

Available forms: Susp 750 mg/5 ml

Implementation
• Give with food (preferably fatty); to increase
absorption of the product and higher plasma
concentrations; give tid × 3 wk
• Give oral suspension after shaken
• Take all contents of foil pouch

ADVERSE EFFECTS

CNS: *Dizziness, headache, anxiety,* insomnia, asthenia, fever
CV: Hypotension
GI: *Nausea, vomiting, diarrhea,* anorexia, increased AST and ALT, **acute pancreatitis,** constipation, abdominal pain
HEMA: Anemia, **neutropenia**
INTEG: Pruritus, urticaria, *rash*
META: Hyperkalemia, hypoglycemia, hyponatremia
OTHER: Cough, dyspnea

Pharmacokinetics

Absorption	Poor; increased when taken with fatty foods
Distribution	Unknown
Metabolism	Hepatic recycling
Excretion	Feces, unchanged (94%)
Half-life	2-3 days

Pharmacodynamics

Onset	Unknown
Peak	1-8 hr
Duration	Unknown

INTERACTIONS

Individual drugs

Rifampin, rifabutin, tetracycline: decreased effectiveness of atovaquone, avoid concurrent use
Zidovudine: increased level of zidovudine, monitor for toxicity

Drug/lab test

Increase: AST, ALT, alk phos
Decrease: glucose, neutrophils, Hgb, sodium

NURSING CONSIDERATIONS

Assessment

• Assess for **Pneumocystis jiroveci:** monitor WBC, bilateral lung sounds, sputum for C&S; these should be checked before, periodically during, after treatment; after collection of 1st sputum, therapy may begin
• Monitor for signs of **infection;** anemia; monitor bowel pattern before, during treatment
• Monitor respiratory status: rate, character, wheezing, dyspnea; ABGs, chest films
• Assess for dizziness, confusion, hallucination
• Assess for allergies before treatment, reaction of each medication; place allergies on chart; notify all people giving products

Patient/family education

• Instruct patient to take with food, preferably fatty foods, to increase plasma concentrations
• Advise patient to take product exactly as prescribed

Evaluation

Positive therapeutic outcome

• Decreased temperature
• Ability to breathe
• Three negative sputum cultures

⚠ HIGH ALERT

atropine (Rx)

(a′troe-peen)
Atreza, AtroPen, Sal-Tropine
Func. class.: Antidysrhythmic, anticholinergic parasympatholytic, antimuscarinic
Chem. class.: Belladonna alkaloid
Pregnancy category C

Do not confuse:
atropine/Akarpine

ACTION: Blocks acetylcholine at parasympathetic neuroeffector sites; increases cardiac output, heart rate by blocking vagal stimulation in heart; dries secretions by blocking vagus

Therapeutic outcome: Drying of secretions, increased heart rate, cycloplegia, mydriasis

USES: Bradycardia <40-50 bpm, bradydysrhythmia, reversal of anticholinesterase agents, insecticide poisoning, blocking cardiac vagal reflexes, decreasing secretions before surgery, antispasmodic with GU and biliary surgery, bronchodilator, AV heart block

CONTRAINDICATIONS:

Hypersensitivity to belladonna alkaloids, closed-angle glaucoma, GI obstructions, myasthenia gravis, thyrotoxicosis, ulcerative colitis, prostatic hypertrophy, tachycardia/tachydysrhythmias, asthma, acute hemorrhage, severe hepatic disease, myocardial ischemia, paralytic ileus

Precautions: Pregnancy **C,** breastfeeding, child <6 yr, geriatric, renal disease, CHF, hyperthyroidism, COPD, hypertension, intraabdominal infections, Down syndrome, spastic paralysis, gastric ulcer

---

DOSAGE AND ROUTES

Bradycardia/bradydysrhythmias

Adult: **IV** bol 0.5-1 mg given q3-5min, not to exceed 3 mg

Child: **IV** bol 0.01-0.03 mg/kg up to 0.4 mg or 0.3 mg/m²; may repeat q4-6hr, min dose 0.1 mg to avoid paradoxical reaction, max single dose 0.5 mg

Organophosphate poisoning

Adult and child: IM (AtroPen)/**IV** 1-2 mg qhr until muscarinic symptoms disappear; may need 6 mg qhr

Adult and child ≥90 lb, usually >10 yr: 2 mg IM (AtroPen)

Child 40-90 lb, usually 4-10 yr: 1 mg IM (AtroPen)

Child 15-40 lb, 6 mo-4 yr: 0.5 mg IM (AtroPen)

Infant <15 lb: IM/IV 0.05 mg/kg q5-20min

Presurgery

Adult and child >20 kg: SUBCUT/IM/ **IV** 0.4-0.6 mg 30-60 min before anesthesia

Child <20 kg: IM/SUBCUT 0.01 mg/kg up to 0.4 mg ½-1 hr preop, max 0.6 mg/dose

Available forms: Inj 0.05, 0.1, 0.4, 0.5, 0.8, 1 mg/ml; tabs 0.4 mg; inj prefilled autoinjectors (AtroPen) 0.5, 1, 2 mg

Implementation

PO route

• PO without regard to meals
• Give increased bulk, water in diet if constipation occurs (anticholinergic effect)

IM route

• Expect atropine flush 15-20 min after inj; it may occur in children and is not harmful

AtroPen

• Use no more than 3 AtroPen injections unless under the supervision of trained provider
• Use as soon as symptoms appear (tearing, wheezing, muscle fasciculations, excessive oral secretions)

IV route

• Give **IV** undiluted or diluted with 10 ml sterile water; give at a rate of 0.6 mg/min; give through Y-tube or 3-way stopcock; do not add to **IV** sol; may cause paradoxical bradycardia lasting 2 min

Y-site compatibilities: Amrinone, etomidate, famotidine, heparin, hydrocortisone sodium succinate, meropenem, nafcillin, potassium chloride, SUFentanil, vit B/C

ADVERSE EFFECTS

CNS: Headache, dizziness, involuntary movement, confusion, psychosis, anxiety, **coma,** flushing, drowsiness, insomnia, weakness, delirium (geriatric)

CV: Hypo/hypertension, paradoxical bradycardia, angina, PVCs, **tachycardia,** ectopic ventricular beats, **bradycardia**

EENT: Blurred vision, photophobia, glaucoma, eye pain, pupil dilatation, nasal congestion

GI: Dry mouth, nausea, vomiting, abdominal pain, anorexia, constipation, **paralytic ileus,** abdominal distention, altered taste

GU: Retention, hesitancy, impotence, dysuria

INTEG: Rash, urticaria, contact dermatitis, dry skin, flushing

MISC: Suppression of breastfeeding, decreased sweating, **anaphylaxis**

Pharmacokinetics

Absorption	Well absorbed (PO, SUBCUT, IM)
Distribution	Crosses blood-brain barrier, placenta
Metabolism	Liver
Excretion	Kidneys, unchanged (70%-90%); breast milk
Half-life	13-40 hr

Pharmacodynamics

	PO	IM/ SUB-CUT	IV	Ophth
Onset	½-2 hr	15 min	2-4 min	½ hr
Peak	½-1 hr	30 min	2-4 min	30-60 min
Duration	4-6 hr	4-6 hr	4-6 hr	1-2 wk

INTERACTIONS

Individual drugs

Amantadine: increased anticholinergic effects
Ketoconazole, levodopa: decreased absorption
Potassium chloride (oral): increased mucosal lesions

Drug classifications

Antacids: decreased absorption of atropine
Antidepressants (tricyclic), antiparkinson agents: increased anticholinergic effect

NURSING CONSIDERATIONS

Assessment

• Monitor I&O ratio; check for urinary retention and daily output in geriatric or postoperative patients

---

Adverse effects: *italics* = common; **bold** = life-threatening

• Monitor ECG for ectopic ventricular beats, PVC, tachycardia in cardiac patients
• Monitor for bowel sounds; check for constipation; abdominal distention and constipation may occur
• Monitor respiratory status: rate, rhythm, cyanosis, wheezing, dyspnea, engorged neck veins
• Monitor cardiac rate: rhythm, character, B/P continuously
• Monitor allergic reaction: rash, urticaria

Patient/family education
• Advise patient not to perform strenuous activity in high temperatures; heat stroke may result
• Instruct patient to take as prescribed; not to skip doses
• Instruct patient to report change in vision; blurring or loss of sight; trouble breathing; sweating; flushing, chest pain, allergic reactions, constipation, urinary retention, to use sunglasses to protect the eyes
• Caution patient not to operate machinery if drowsiness occurs
• Advise patient not to take OTC products without approval of physician
• Teach patient not to freeze or expose to light (Astropen)

Evaluation
Positive therapeutic outcome
• Decreased dysrhythmias
• Increased heart rate
• Decreased secretions, GI, GU spasms
• Bronchodilatation

TREATMENT OF OVERDOSE:
O_2, artificial ventilation, ECG; administer DO-Pamine for circulatory depression; administer diazepam or thiopental for seizure; assess need for antidysrhythmics

atropine ophthalmic
See Appendix B

axitinib
Inlyta
Func. class.: Antineoplastic, biologic response modifier, signal transduction inhibitor (STI)
Chem. class.: Tyrosine kinase inhibitor
Pregnancy category D

ACTION: Inhibits receptor tyrosine kinases including vascular endothelial growth factor receptors (VEGFR)-1, VEGFR-2, and VEGFR-3; inhibits tumor growth and phosphorylation of VEGFR-2 and VEGF-mediated endothelial cell proliferation

Therapeutic outcome: Decreased spread of malignancy

USES: Treatment of advanced renal cell cancer after failure of one prior systemic therapy

CONTRAINDICATIONS:
Pregnancy (D), breastfeeding

Precautions: Risk for or history of thromboembolic disease, recent GI bleeding, untreated brain metastasis, recent GI bleeding, GI perforation, fistula, surgery, moderate hepatic disease, uncontrolled hypertension, hyper/hypothyroidism, proteinuria, infertility, end-stage renal disease (CrCl <15 ml/min); not intended for use in adolescents, children, infants, neonates

DOSAGE AND ROUTES
Adult: PO 5 mg bid (at 12 hr intervals), may increase to 7 mg bid and then to 10 mg bid in those not receiving antihypertensives who tolerate the lower dosage for at least 2 consecutive wk with no more than grade 2 adverse reactions. Reduce to 3 mg bid if a dose reduction is needed; if further reduction is necessary, reduce to 2 mg bid
Adult receiving a strong CYP 3A4/5 inhibitor: Reduce dose by 1/2, adjust as needed

Available forms: Tab 1, 5 mg

Implementation
• Give with or without food; swallow tablet whole with a glass of water
• If patient vomits or misses a dose, an additional dose should not be taken; the next dose should be taken at the usual time
• Store at room temperature

ADVERSE EFFECTS
CNS: Dizziness, headache, reversible posterior leukoencephalopathy syndrome (RPLS), fatigue
CV: Hypertension, arterial thromboembolic events (ATE), venous thromboembolic events (VTE)
ENDO: Hypothyroidism, hyperthyroidism
GI: Lower GI bleeding/perforation/fistula. abdominal pain, constipation, diarrhea, dysgeusia, dyspepsia, dysphonia, hemorrhoids, nausea, mucosal inflammation, stomatitis, vomiting, increased ALT/AST
GU: Proteinuria
HEMA: Bleeding intracranial bleeding, anemia, polycythemia, decreased/increased

hemoglobin, lymphopenia thrombocytopenia, neutropenia

INTEG: Palmar-plantar erythrodysesthesia (hand and foot syndrome) rash, dry skin, pruritus, alopecia, erythema

MISC: Weight loss dehydration metabolic and electrolyte laboratory abnormalities included

MS: Asthenia, arthralgia, musculoskeletal pain, myalgia

RESP: Cough, dyspnea

Pharmacokinetics

Absorption	Unknown
Distribution	Protein binding >99%
Metabolism	Liver
Excretion	Unknown
Half-life	2.5-6.1 hr

Pharmacodynamics

Onset	Unknown
Peak	Unknown
Duration	Unknown

INTERACTIONS
Individual drugs

CYP3A4/5 inhibitor, strong, moderate (ketoconazole, boceprevir, chloramphenicol, conivaptan, delavirdine, fosamprenavir, imatinib, indinavir, isoniazid, itraconazole, dalfopristin; quinupristin, posaconazole, ritonavir, telithromycin, tipranavir [boosted with ritonavir], darunavir [boosted with ritonavir], aldesleukin, IL-2, amiodarone, aprepitant, fosaprepitant atazanavir, bromocriptine, clarithromycin, crizotinib, danazol, diltiazem, dronedarone, erythromycin, fluvoxaMINE, lanreotide, lapatinib, miconazole, mifepristone, nefazodone, nelfinavir, niCARdipine, octreotide, pantoprazole, saquinavir, tamoxifen, verapamil, voriconazole, grapefruit juice): increased axitinib effect

CYP3A4/5 inducers, strong/moderate (rifampin, carBAMazepine, dexamethasone, phenytoin, PHENobarbital, rifabutin, rifapentine, St. John's wort, ethanol, bexarotene, bosentan, efavirenz, etravirine, griseofulvin, metyrapone, modafinil, nafcillin, nevirapine, OXcarbazepine, vemurafenib, pioglitazone, topiramate): decreased effect of axitinib

CYP3A4/5 inhibitor and inducers (quiNINE): increased or decreased axitinib effect

Drug/lab test

Increase: creatinine, lipase, amylase, sodium, potassium, glucose

Decrease: bicarbonate, calcium, albumin, glucose, phosphate, sodium

Increase or decrease: sodium, glucose

Drug/herb

St. John's wort: decreased effect of axitinib

NURSING CONSIDERATIONS
Assessment

• Bleeding: monitor for GI bleeding or perforation; temporarily discontinue therapy if a patient develops any bleeding that requires treatment

• Surgery: discontinue ≥24 hr before surgery, may be resumed after adequate wound healing

• Hepatic/renal disease: dosage should be reduced in patients with moderate (Child-Pugh Class B) hepatic disease, monitor liver function tests (ALT, AST, bilirubin) before and periodically during therapy; monitor CCr before and during treatment

• Hypertension: B/P should be well controlled before starting treatment; monitor patients for hypertension and administer antihypertensive therapy as needed before and during therapy; dose should be reduced for persistent hypertension; therapy should be discontinued if B/P remains elevated after a dosage reduction or if there is evidence of hypertensive crisis; after discontinuation monitor B/P for hypotension in those receiving antihypertensives

• Hyper/hypothyroidism: monitor thyroid function tests before and periodically during therapy; thyroid disease should be treated with thyroid medications

• Monitor for proteinuria before and periodically during therapy; product may need to be decreased or discontinued if moderate to severe proteinuria occurs

• Pregnancy/breastfeeding: pregnancy category D; determine if the patient is pregnant or breastfeeding before using this product; may also cause infertility

Patient/family education

• Instruct patient to use contraception during treatment (pregnancy category D) or to avoid use of this product; to notify prescriber if pregnancy is planned or suspected, not to breastfeed

• Instruct patient to notify prescriber of bleeding that is severe or that requires treatment

• Teach patient that product will be discontinued ≥24 hr before surgery; may be resumed after adequate wound healing

• Teach patient that laboratory testing will be required before and periodically during product use

• Teach patient how to monitor B/P and that B/P products should be continued as directed by prescriber

Evaluation
Positive therapeutic outcome
• Decreased spread of malignancy

⚠ HIGH ALERT

azaCITIDine (Rx)
(a-za-sie-ti′deen)
Vidaza
Func. class.: Antineoplastic hormone
Chem. class.: DNA demethylation agent
Pregnancy category D

Do not confuse:
azaCITIDine/azaTHIOprine

ACTION: Cytotoxic by producing damage to double-strand DNA during DNA synthesis

Therapeutic outcome: Improved blood counts in refractor anemia

USES: Myelodysplastic syndrome (MDS)

CONTRAINDICATIONS:
Pregnancy **D**, hypersensitivity to this product or mannitol, advanced malignant hepatic tumors

Precautions: Breastfeeding, children, geriatric, renal/hepatic disease; baseline albumin <30 g/L; a man should not father a child while taking this product

DOSAGE AND ROUTES
Adult: SUBCUT 75 mg/m^2 daily × 7 days, q4wk, premedicate with antiemetic; dose may be increased to 100 mg/m^2 if no response is seen after 2 treatment cycles; minimum treatment 4 cycles

Available forms: Powder for inj, 100 mg

Implementation
• Increase patient's fluid intake to 2-3 L/day to prevent dehydration, unless contraindicated
• Assist patient with rinsing of mouth tid-qid with water, club soda; brushing of teeth bid-tid with soft brush or cotton-tipped applicator for stomatitis; use unwaxed dental floss
• Provide a nutritious diet with iron, vitamin supplement, low fiber, few dairy products
• Use cytotoxic handling procedures

SUBCUT route
• **Reconstitute** with 4 ml sterile water for inj (25 mg/ml), **inject** diluents slowly into vial, **invert** vial 2-3 times and gently rotate; sol will be cloudy, use immediately; divide doses >4 ml into two syringes; invert the contents 2-3 times and gently roll syringe between the palms for 30 sec immediately before administration; rotate inj site

IV intermittent INF route
• **Reconstitute** each vial with 4 ml sterile water for inj, **shake** well until all solids are dissolved, (10 mg/ml) withdraw sol and **inject** in 50-100 NS or LR, **infuse** over 10-40 min

ADVERSE EFFECTS
CNS: Anxiety, depression, dizziness, fatigue, headache, fever, insomnia
CV: Cardiac murmur, hypotension, tachycardia, peripheral edema, chest pain
GI: Diarrhea, nausea, vomiting, anorexia, constipation, abdominal pain, distention, tenderness, hemorrhoids, mouth hemorrhage, tongue ulceration, stomatitis, dyspepsia, **hepatotoxicity, hepatic coma**
GU: Real failure, renal tubular acidosis, dysuria, UTI
HEMA: Leukopenia, anemia, thrombocytopenia, neutropenia, ecchymosis, febrile neutropenia, petechiae
INTEG: Irritation at site, rash, sweating, pyrexia, pruritus
META: Hypokalemia
MS: Weakness, arthralgia, muscle cramps, myalgia, back pain
RESP: Cough, dyspnea, pharyngitis, **pleural effusion**

Pharmacokinetics
Absorption	Rapid
Distribution	Unknown
Metabolism	Liver
Excretion	Urine
Half-life	35-49 min

Pharmacodynamics
Onset	Unknown
Peak	½ hr
Duration	Unknown

INTERACTIONS
Drug classifications
Antineoplastics, other: increased bone marrow depression

NURSING CONSIDERATIONS
Assessment
- Assess for CNS symptoms: fever, headache, chills, dizziness
- Monitor **bone marrow suppression** with patients with baseline WBC 3 × 10⁹/L, absolute neutrophil count (ANC) = 1.5 × 10⁹/L, and platelets = 75 × 10⁹/L, adjust dose; ANC < 0.5 × 10⁹/L, platelets < 25 × 10⁹/L, give 50% dose next course; ANC 0.5-1.5 × 10⁹/L, platelets 25-50 × 10⁹/L, give 67% next course
- Assess buccal cavity q8hr for dryness, sores, or ulceration, white patches, oral pain, bleeding, dysphagia
- Assess for bruising, bleeding, blood in stools, urine, sputum, emesis; myelodysplastic syndrome (MDS), splenomegaly

Patient/family education
- Instruct patient to avoid foods with citric acid or hot or rough texture if stomatitis is present; to drink adequate fluids
- Instruct patient to report stomatitis; any bleeding, white spots, ulcerations in mouth; tell patient to examine mouth daily, report symptoms
- Instruct patient to avoid crowds, persons with known infections; not to receive immunizations
- Advise patient to use contraception during and for several months after therapy, pregnancy **D** not to breastfeed, not to father a child while receiving this product

Evaluation
Positive therapeutic outcome
- Improvement in blood counts in refractory anemia, or refractory anemia with excess blasts

---

azaTHIOprine (Rx)
(ay-za-thye'oh-preen)
Azasan, Imuran
Func. class.: Immunosuppressant
Chem. class.: Purine antagonist
Pregnancy category D

Do not confuse:
Imuran/Imferon/Elmiron/IMDUR/Enduron/Tenormin, **azaTHIOprine**/azaCITIDine

ACTION: Produces immunosuppression by inhibiting purine synthesis in cells

Therapeutic outcome: Absence of graft rejection, slowing of rheumatoid arthritis

USES: Renal transplants to prevent graft rejection, refractory rheumatoid arthritis

Unlabeled uses: Myasthenia gravis, chronic ulcerative colitis, Crohn's disease, Behçet's syndrome

CONTRAINDICATIONS:
Pregnancy **D**, breastfeeding, hypersensitivity

Precautions: Severe renal/hepatic disease, geriatric, thiopurine methyltransferase deficiency, infection

> **BLACK BOX WARNING:** Bone marrow suppression, neoplastic disease; must be used by experienced clinician

DOSAGE AND ROUTES
Renal dose
CCr 10-50 ml/min 75% of dose; CCr <10 ml/min 50% of dose

Prevention of rejection
Adult and child: IV 3-5 mg/kg/day, then maintenance (PO) of at least 1-3 mg/kg/day

Refractory rheumatoid arthritis
Adult: PO 1 mg/kg/day; may increase dosage after 2 mo by 0.5 mg/kg/day and then q4wk; not to exceed 2.5 mg/kg/day

Available forms: Tabs 50, 75, 100 mg; inj **IV** 100 mg

Implementation
PO route
- Give with meals to reduce GI upset; nausea is common

IV route
- Prepare in biological cabinet using gown, gloves, mask
Direct, IV route
- **Dilute** to 10 mg/ml with 0.9% NaCl, 0.45% NaCl, D₅W, **give** over 5 min
Intermittent IV INF route
- **Reconstitute** 100 mg/10 ml of sterile water for inj; rotate to dissolve; **further dilute** with 50 ml or more saline or glucose in saline, **give** over ½-1 hr

Y-site compatibilities: Alfentanil, atracurium, atropine, benztropine, calcium gluconate, cycloSPORINE, enalaprilat, epoetin alfa, erythromycin, fentaNYL, fluconazole, folic acid, furosemide, glycopyrrolate, heparin, insulin, mannitol, mechlorethamine, metoprolol, naloxone, nitroglycerin, oxytocin, penicillin G, potassium chloride, propranolol, protamine, SUFentanil, trimetaphan, vasopression

Solution compatibilities: D₅W, NaCl 0.9%, NaCl 0.45%

Adverse effects: *italics* = common; **bold** = life-threatening

ADVERSE EFFECTS

GI: Nausea, vomiting, stomatitis, esophagitis, **pancreatitis, hepatotoxicity, jaundice, hepatic veno-occlusive disease**
HEMA: Leukopenia, thrombocytopenia, anemia, pancytopenia, bleeding
INTEG: Rash, alopeia
MISC: Raynaud's symptoms, **serum sickness**, secondary malignancy, infection
MS: Arthralgia, muscle wasting

Pharmacokinetics

Absorption	Readily (PO)
Distribution	Crosses placenta
Metabolism	Liver to mercaptopurine
Excretion	Kidney, minimal
Half-life	3 hr

Pharmacodynamics

	PO	IV
Onset	Unknown	Unknown
Peak	4 hr	Unknown
Duration	Unknown	Unknown

INTERACTIONS

Individual drugs

Do not admix with other products
Allopurinol: increased action of azaTHIOprine
CycloSPORINE: increased myelosuppression
Sulfamethoxazole-trimethoprim: increased leukopenia
Warfarin: decreased action of warfarin

Drug classifications

ACE inhibitors: increased leukopenia
Antineoplastics: increased myelosuppression
Toxoids, vaccines: decreased immune response

Drug/lab test

Increased: liver function tests
Decreased: uric acid
Interference: CBC, diff count

NURSING CONSIDERATIONS

Assessment

• Assess symptoms of **rheumatoid arthritis:** pain in joints, stiffness, poor range of motion, mobility, inflammation before and during treatment
• Monitor **blood studies:** CBC, Hgb, WBC, platelets during treatment monthly; if leukocytes are <3000/mm^3 or platelets <100,000/mm^3, product should be discontinued or reduced; decreased Hgb level may indicate bone marrow suppression

• **Bone marrow suppression:** severe leukopenia, pancytopenia, thrombocytopenia
• Monitor liver function studies: alkaline phosphatase, AST, ALT, amylase, bilirubin; and for **hepatotoxicity:** dark urine, jaundice, itching, light-colored stools; product should be discontinued
• Monitor I&O, weight daily, report decreasing urine output, toxicity may occur
• Assess for **infection:** increased temp, WBC; sputum, urine

Patient/family education

• Teach patient to take as prescribed, do not miss doses; if dose is missed on daily regimen, skip dose; if on multiple dosing/day, take as soon as remembered
• Teach patient that therapeutic response may take 3-4 mo in rheumatoid arthritis, to continue with prescribed exercise, rest, other medications; that product is needed for life in renal transplant
• Instruct patient to report fever, rash, severe diarrhea, chills, sore throat, fatigue, since serious **infections** may occur; or clay-colored stools and cramping **(hepatotoxicity)**
• Advise patient to use contraceptive measures during treatment for 16 wk after ending therapy; product is teratogenic (pregnancy **D**)
• Advise patient to avoid vaccinations
• Tell patient to avoid crowds and persons with known infections to reduce risk of infection
• Teach patient to take with food to decrease GI intolerance
• Teach patient regarding multiple significant drug/drug interactions
• Instruct patient not to use OTC medications without approval of prescriber
• Advise patient to use soft-bristled toothbrush to prevent bleeding

Evaluation

Positive therapeutic outcome

• Absence of graft rejection
• Immunosuppression in autoimmune disorders
• Increased joint mobility without pain in rheumatoid arthritis

azelaic acid topical
See Appendix B

A

azelastine (Rx)

(ay′ze-lass-teen)
Optivar
Func. class.: Leukotriene synthesis inhibitor
Chem. class.: Phthalazinone derivative
Pregnancy category C

ACTION: Inhibits the synthesis and release of leukotrienes; antagonizes action of acetylcholine, histamine, serotonin

Therapeutic outcome: Decreased nasal stuffiness, itching, swollen eyes

USES: Seasonal allergic rhinitis

CONTRAINDICATIONS:

Hypersensitivity

Precautions: Pregnancy C

DOSAGE AND ROUTES

Adult and child ≥12 yr: NASAL 2 sprays/nostril bid

Available forms: Spray 137 mcg/actuation

Implementation

• Remove cap/safety clip from spray pump
• Prime pump if using for first time, push 4 times quickly, away from face, blow your nose, then place tip of pump into one nostril, while holding other nostril closed, tilt head forward, and spray into nostril
• Put cover/safety clip back on

ADVERSE EFFECTS

CNS: Sedation (more common with increased dosages), drowsiness
MISC: Weight increase, myalgia

Pharmacokinetics

Absorption	Unknown
Distribution	Unknown
Metabolism	Liver, extensively
Excretion	Feces
Half-life	25-42 hr

Pharmacodynamics

Onset	Unknown
Peak	4-5 hr
Duration	Unknown

INTERACTIONS

Individual drugs

Alcohol: increased CNS depression

Drug classifications

CNS depressants, opioids, sedative/hypnotics: increased CNS depression

NURSING CONSIDERATIONS

Assessment

• Assess respiratory status: rate, rhythm, increase in bronchial secretions, wheezing, chest tightness; provide fluids to 2 L/day to decrease secretion thickness

Patient/family education

• Teach patient all aspects of product uses; to notify prescriber if confusion, sedation occur; to avoid driving and other hazardous activity if drowsiness occurs; to avoid alcohol and other CNS depressants that may potentiate effect
• Caution patient not to exceed recommended dosage; dysrhythmias may occur

Evaluation

Positive therapeutic outcome
• Absence of runny or congested nose

azelastine nasal agent

See Appendix B

azelastine ophthalmic

See Appendix B

azilsartan

(ay-zil-sar′tan)
Edarbi
(Pronunciation)
Func. class.: Antihypertensive
Chem class.: Angiotensin II receptor antagonist
Pregnancy category D

ACTION: Antagonizes angiotensin II at the AT_1 receptor in tissues like vascular smooth muscle and the adrenal gland. Two angiotensin II receptors, AT_1 and AT_2, have been identified; azilsartan exhibits more than a 10,000-fold greater affinity for the AT_1 receptor than the AT_2 receptor.

Therapeutic outcome: Decreased B/P

USES: Hypertension, alone or in combination with other antihypertensives

CONTRAINDICATIONS:

BLACK BOX WARNING: Pregnancy **D** (2nd/3rd trimesters)

Adverse effects: *italics* = common; **bold** = life-threatening

Precautions: Angioedema, African descent, renal disease, renal artery stenosis, children, geriatrics, heart failure, hypovolemia, breast-feeding, pregnancy C 1st trimester

DOSAGE AND ROUTES

Adult: PO 80 mg/day, may give an initial dose of 40 mg/day in patients receiving high-dose diuretic therapy

Available forms: Tabs 40, 80 mg

Implementation
- May administer without regard to food
- Use original package to protect from light, moisture, and heat

ADVERSE EFFECTS

CNS: Dizziness, fatigue, asthenia, syncope
CV: Hypotension, orthostatic hypotension
GI: Nausea, diarrhea
HEMA: Anemia
INTEG: Angioedema
MS: Muscle cramps
RESP: Cough

Pharmacokinetics

Absorption	Absolute bioavailability (60%) not affected by food; steady state within 5 days and no accumulation in plasma occurs with once-daily dosing; hydrolyzed to the active metabolite, azilsartan, in GI tract during absorption, rapidly absorbed
Distribution	Protein binding, >99%, to serum albumin
Metabolism	Metabolized by CYP2C9
Excretion	55% eliminated (feces), 42% (urine)
Half-life	Elimination half-life 11 hr

Pharmacodynamics

Onset	Unknown
Peak	1.5-3 hr
Duration	Unknown

INTERACTIONS

Individual drugs
CycloSPORINE: in those with poor renal function, increased renal failure risk: monitor closely
Lithium: increased lithium toxicity

Sodium phosphate monobasic monohydrate, sodium phosphate dibasic anhydrous: increased phosphate nephropathy

Drug classifications
Antidiabetics: increased hypoglycemia
NSAIDs in those with poor renal function: monitor closely: Increased renal failure risk
Other antihypertensives, other angiotensin receptor antagonists, MAOIs: increased hypotensive effect

Drug/herb
Ephedra: decreased antihypertensive effect
Hawthorn: increased antihypertensive effect

NURSING CONSIDERATIONS

Assessment
- **Angioedema:** Assess for facial swelling, difficulty breathing

> **BLACK BOX WARNING:** Pregnancy **D** (2nd/3rd trimester), can cause fetal death

- Response and adverse reactions especially in renal disease
- B/P, pulse during beginning therapy and periodically thereafter; note rhythm, rate, quality; obtain electrolytes before beginning therapy

Patient/family education
- Instruct patient to comply with dosage schedule even if feeling better
- Instruct patient to notify prescriber of facial swelling; if pregnancy is planned or suspected (D 2nd/3rd trimester)
- Advise patient that diarrhea, dehydration, excessive perspiration, vomiting, may lead to fall in B/P, to consult prescriber if these occur
- Instruct patient to rise slowly from lying or sitting to minimize orthostatic hypotension; that product may cause dizziness
- Instruct patient to avoid OTC medications unless approved by prescriber; to inform all health care providers of product use
- Instruct patient to use proper technique for obtaining B/P

Evaluation
Positive therapeutic outcome
- Decreased B/P

⚠ Nurse Alert   ✱ Key NCLEX® Drug

azithromycin (Rx)
(ay-zi-thro-my'sin)
Zithromax, Zmax
Func. class.: Antiinfective
Chem. class.: Macrolide (azalide)
Pregnancy category B

Do not confuse:
azithromycin/erythromycin, **Zithromax**/Zinacef

ACTION: Binds to 50S ribosomal subunits of susceptible bacteria and suppresses protein synthesis; much greater spectrum of activity than erythromycin; more effective against gram-negative organisms

Therapeutic outcome: Bacteriostatic against the following susceptible organisms: PO, acute pharyngitis/tonsillitis (group A streptococcal); acute skin/soft tissue infections; community-acquired pneumonia

USES: Mild to moderate infections of the upper respiratory tract, in children: acute otitis media, lower respiratory tract; uncomplicated skin and skin structure infections, nongono-coccal urethritis, or cervicitis; prophylaxis of disseminated *Mycobacterium avium* complex (MAC); *Bacillus anthracis, Bacteroides bivius, Bordetella pertussis, Borrelia burgdorferi, Campylobacter jejuni,* CDC coryneform group G, *Chlamydia trachomatis, Chlamydophila pneumoniae, Clostridium perfringens, Gardnerella vaginalis, Haemophilus ducreyi/influenzae* (beta-lactamase negative/positive), *Helicobacter pylori, Klebsiella granulomatis, Legionella pneumoniae/moraxella/catarrhalis, Mycobacterium avium/intracellulare, Mycoplasma genitalium/hominis/pneumoniae, Neisseria gonorrhoeae, Peptostreptococcus, Prevotella bivia, Rickettsia tsutsugamushi, Salmonella typhi, Staphylococcus aureus* (MSSA)/*epidermidis, Streptococcus, Toxoplasma gondii, Treponema pallidum, Ureaplasma urealyticum, Vibrio cholerae,* viridans streptococci

CONTRAINDICATIONS:
Hypersensitivity to azithromycin, erythromycin, or any macrolide, hepatitis, jaundice

Precautions: Pregnancy **B**, breastfeeding, child <6 mo for otitis media, child <2 yr for pharyngitis, geriatric, renal/hepatic/cardiac disease, tonsillitis, QT prolongation, ulcerative colitis, torsades de pointes, sunlight exposure, sodium restriction, myasthenia gravis, pseudo-membranous colitis, contact lenses, hypokalemia, hypomagnesemia

DOSAGE AND ROUTES
Most infections
Adult: PO 500 mg on day 1, then 250 mg daily on days 2-5 for a total dose of 1.5 g or 500 mg a day × 3 days
Child 2-15 yr: PO 10 mg/kg on day 1, then 5 mg/kg × 4 days

Pelvic inflammatory disease
Adult: PO/**IV** 500 mg **IV** q24hr × 2 doses, then 250 mg PO q24hr × 7-10 days

Cervicitis, chlamydia, chancroid, nongonococcal urethritis, syphilis
Adult: PO 1 g single dose

Gonorrhea
Adult: PO 2 g single dose

Endocarditis prophylaxis
Adult: PO 500 mg 1 hr prior to procedure
Child: PO 15 mg/kg 1 hr prior to procedure

Community-acquired pneumonia
Adult: PO 500 mg on day 1, then 250 mg PO once daily on days 2-5
Adolescent/child, infant ≥6 mo: Susp PO 10 mg/kg on day 1, then 5 mg/kg/day on days 2-5
Adult/adolescent, child ≥34 kg: Ext Rel Susp PO 2 g as a single dose (≥1 hr before or 2 hr after a meal)
Infant ≥6 mo and child weighing 5 to <34 kg and adolescent weighing <34 kg: Ext Rel Susp PO 60 mg/kg as a single dose (≥1 hr before or 2 hr after a meal)
Adult and adolescent ≥16 yr: Initially, 500 mg **IV** infusion as a single daily dose × 2 days or more then 500 mg PO/day to complete a 7-10 day course
Adolescent <16 yr, child, infant ≥3 mo: **IV** 10 mg/kg, max 500 mg qd × 2 days, then conversion to oral therapy as soon as possible to complete a 5-day course. After **IV** loading doses have been given, oral dosage is 5 mg/kg/day, max 250 mg/dose

Disseminated MAC infections
Adult: PO 600 mg/day in combination with ethambutol 15 mg/kg/day

MAC in HIV
Adult/adolescent: PO 1.2 g qwk, alone or with rifabutin

Lower respiratory tract infections
Adult: PO 500 mg day 1, then 250 mg × 4 days
Child: PO 5-12 mg/kg/day × 5 days

Acute otitis media
Child >6 mo: PO 30 mg/kg as a single dose or 10 mg/kg daily × 3 days or 10 mg/kg as a single dose on day 1, max 500 mg/day, then 5 mg/kg on days 2-5, max 250 mg/day

Prevention of acute otitis media
Child: PO 10 mg/kg qwk × 6 mo

Bacterial conjunctivitis
Adult/adolescent/child ≥1 yr: ophth 1 drop in affected eye bid × 2 days, then 1 drop on days 2-6

Available forms: Tabs 250, 500, 600 mg; powder for inj 500 mg; powder for oral susp 1 g/packet; susp 100, 200 mg/5 ml; ophthalmic drops 1% sol

Implementation
PO route
• Provide adequate intake of fluids (2 L) during diarrhea episodes
• Give with a full glass of water; give susp 1 hr before or 2 hr after meals; tabs may be taken without regard to food; do not give with fruit juices
• Store at room temperature
• Reconstitute 1 g packet for susp with 60 ml water, mix, rinse glass with more water and have patient drink to consume all medication; packets not for pediatric use
• Do not take aluminum/magnesium-containing antacids or food simultaneously with this product

Intermittent IV infusion route
• **Reconstitute** 500 mg product/4.8 ml sterile water for inj (100 mg/ml), shake; **dilute** with ≥ 250 ml 0.9% NaCl, 0.45% NaCl, or LR to 1-2 mg/ml; diluted solution is stable for 24 hr or 7 days if refrigerated
• **Give** 1 mg/ml sol over 3 hr or 2 mg/ml sol over 1 hr, never give IM or as a bolus

Y-site compatibilities: Alemtuzumab, alfentanil, aminophylline, ampicillin, ampicillin-sulbactam, bumetanide, buprenorphine, butorphanol, calcium chloride/gluconate, carmustine, ceFAZolin, cefepime, cefoperazone, cefoTEtan, cefOXitin, ceftaroline, cefTAZidime, ceftizoxime, ceftobiprole, cimetidine, cisatracurium, cyclophosphamide, cycloSPORINE, DAUNOrubicin liposome, dexamethasone, dexrazoxane, digoxin, diltiazem, DOBUTamine, DOXOrubicin liposomal, doxycycline, enalaprilat, EPINEPHrine, esmolol, etoposide, etoposide phosphate, fluconazole, foscarnet, fosphenytoin, gallium, ganciclovir, gatifloxacin, gemcitabine, granisetron, haloperidol, heparin, hydrocortisone phosphate/succinate, HYDROmorphone, hydrOXYzine, ifosfamide, inamrinone, isoproterenol, labetalol, lepirudin, magnesium sulfate, mannitol, meropenem, mesna, methohexital, methotrexate, methylPREDNISolone, metoclopramide, metroNIDAZOLE, milrinone, minocycline, mivacurium, nalbuphine, naloxone, nitroglycerin, nitroprusside, ofloxacin, oxytocin, PACLitaxel, PENTobarbital, phenylephrine, piperacillin, potassium acetate/phosphates, procainamide, prochlorperazine, promethazine, propranolol, ranitidine, remifentanil, succinylcholine, SUFentanil, sulfamethoxazole-trimethoprim, tacrolimus, telavancin, teniposide, thiotepa, ticarcillin, trimethobenzamide, vancomycin, vecuronium, verapamil, zidovudine, zoledronic acid

ADVERSE EFFECTS
CNS: Dizziness, headache, vertigo, somnolence, fatigue
CV: Palpitations, chest pain, **QT prolongation, torsades de pointes (rare)**
EENT: Hearing loss, tinnitus, loss of smell (anosmia)
GI: *Nausea, diarrhea,* **hepatotoxicity,** abdominal pain, stomatitis, heartburn, dyspepsia, flatulence, melena, **cholestatic jaundice, pseudomembranous colitis,** tongue discoloration
GU: Vaginitis, moniliasis, nephritis
HEMA: Anemia
INTEG: Rash, urticaria, pruritus, photosensitivity, pain at injection site
SYST: Angioedema, Stevens-Johnson syndrome, toxic epidermal necrolysis

Pharmacokinetics

Absorption	Rapid (PO) up to 50%
Distribution	Widely distributed
Metabolism	Unknown, minimal metabolism
Excretion	Unchanged (bile); kidneys, minimal
Half-life	11-70 hr

Pharmacodynamics

	PO	IV
Onset	Unknown	Unknown
Peak	2-4 hr	End of infusion
Duration	24 hr	24 hr

INTERACTIONS

Individual drugs

Bromocriptine, carBAMazepine, cycloSPORINE, digoxin, disopyramide, methylPREDNISolone, nelfinavir, phenytoin, tacrolimus, theophylline, triazolam: increased effects of specific products

Ergotamine: ergot toxicity

⚠ **Amiodarone, droperidol, methadone, nilotinib, propafenone, quiNIDine: increased QT prolongation**

⚠ **Pimozide: increased dysrhythmias; fatal reaction; do not use concurrently**

Triazolam: decreased clearance of triazolam

Drug classifications

Aluminum, magnesium antacids: decreased levels of azithromycin, separate by ≥2 hr

Anticoagulants (orals): increased effect of oral anticoagulants

Drug/food

Decreased: absorption—food (suspension)

Drug/lab test

Increased: bilirubin, alkaline phosphatase, CPK, BUN, creatinine, AST, ALT, potassium, blood glucose

Decreased: blood glucose, potassium, sodium

NURSING CONSIDERATIONS

Assessment

⚠ **QT prolongation, torsades de pointes: assess for patients with serious bradycardia, ongoing pro-arrhythmic conditions, or elderly; more common in these patients**

• Assess for signs and symptoms of **infection:** drainage, fever, increased WBC >10,000/mm^3, urine culture positive, sore throat, sputum culture positive

• Monitor respiratory status: rate, character, wheezing, tightness in chest; discontinue product if these occur

• Monitor allergies before treatment, reaction of each medication; place allergies on chart, notify all people giving products; skin eruptions, itching

• Monitor I&O ratio, renal studies; report hematuria, oliguria in renal disease; check urinalysis, protein, blood

• Monitor liver studies: AST, ALT, bilirubin, LDH, alkaline phosphatase; CBC with diff

• Monitor C&S before product therapy; product may be taken as soon as culture is taken; C&S may be repeated after treatment

• Assess for **serious skin reactions:** Stevens-Johnson syndrome, toxic epidermal necrolysis, angioedema, discontinue if rash occurs

• Assess for **pseudomembranous colitis:** blood or pus in diarrhea stool, abdominal pain, fever, fatigue, anorexia; obtain CBC, serum albumin

• Assess for **superinfection:** sore throat, mouth, tongue; fever, fatigue, diarrhea, anogenital pruritus

Patient/family education

• Instruct patient to report sore throat, black furry tongue, fever, loose foul-smelling stool, vaginal itching, discharge, fatigue; may indicate **superinfection**

• Caution patient not to take aluminum/magnesium-containing antacids or food simultaneously with this product; blood levels of azithromycin will be decreased

• Instruct patient to notify prescriber of diarrhea stools, dark urine, pale stools, yellow discoloration of eyes or skin, severe abdominal pain; **cholestatic jaundice** is a severe adverse reaction

• Teach patient to take Zmax 1 hr prior to or 2 hr after a meal; shake well before use

• Teach patient to complete dosage regimen; to notify prescriber if symptoms continue

• Teach patient to use protective clothing or stay out of the sun: photosensitivity may occur

• Teach patient to notify prescriber if pregnancy is suspected

⚠ **Cardiovascular death has occurred in those with serious bradycardia or ongoing hypokalemia, hypomagnesemia; avoid use**

Evaluation

Positive therapeutic outcome

• C&S negative for infection

• WBC within 5000-10,000/mm^3

azithromycin ophthalmic

See Appendix B

baclofen (Rx)

(bak'loe-fen)
Gablofen, Lioresal
Func. class.: Skeletal muscle relaxant, central acting
Chem. class.: GABA, chlorophenyl derivative
Pregnancy category C

Do not confuse:
Lioresal/Lotensin

ACTION: Inhibits synaptic responses in CNS by stimulating GABA$_B$ receptor subtype, which decreases neurotransmitter function, decreasing frequency, severity of muscle spasms

Therapeutic outcome: Decreased spasticity of muscles

USES: Spasticity in spinal cord injury, multiple sclerosis

CONTRAINDICATIONS:
Hypersensitivity

Precautions: Pregnancy **C**, breastfeeding, geriatric, peptic ulcer, renal/hepatic disease, stroke, seizure disorder, diabetes mellitus

> **BLACK BOX WARNING:** Abrupt discontinuation

DOSAGE AND ROUTES
Adult: PO 5 mg tid × 3 days, then 10 mg tid × 3 days, then 15 mg tid × 3 days, then 20 mg tid × 3 days, then titrated to response, max 80 mg/day; IT use implantable IT inf pump; use screening trial of 3 separate bol doses if needed 24 hr apart (50 mcg/ml, 75 mcg/1.5 ml, 100 mcg/2 ml); patients who do not respond to 100 mcg should not be considered for chronic IT therapy; initial double screening dose that produced result and give over 24 hr, increase by 10%-30% q24hr only; maintenance 1200-1500 mcg/day
Child 2-7 yr: PO 10-15 mg/day divided q8hr; titrate every 3 days by 5-15 mg/day to max 40 mg/day
Child ≥8 yr: As above, max 60 mg/day
Child: IT initial test dose same as adult; for small children, initial dose of 25 mcg/dose may be used; 25-1200 mcg/day inf, titrated to response in screening phase
Geriatric: PO 5 mg bid-tid

Available forms: Tabs 10, 20 mg; IT inj 10 mg/20 ml (500 mcg/ml), 10 mg/5 ml (2000 mcg/ml); pharmacy can prepare extemporaneous liquid preparations

Implementation
PO route
• Give with meals for GI symptoms; gum, frequent sips of water for dry mouth
• Store in airtight container at room temperature

IT route
• **For screening,** dilute to a concentration of 50 mcg/ml with NaCl for inj (preservative free); give test over 1 min; watch for decreasing muscle tone, frequency of spasm; if inadequate, use two more test doses q24hr; **maintenance inf** via implantable pump of 500-2000 mcg/ml dosage because individual titration is required
• Do not give IT dose by inj, **IV, IM, SUBCUT,** epidural

ADVERSE EFFECTS
CNS: *Dizziness, weakness, fatigue, drowsiness,* headache, disorientation, insomnia, paresthesias, tremors, **seizures, coma;** life-threatening CNS depression, CNS infection (IT)
CV: Hypotension, chest pain, palpitations, edema; **cardiovascular collapse (IT)**
EENT: Nasal congestion, blurred vision, mydriasis, tinnitus
GI: *Nausea,* constipation, vomiting, increased AST, alkaline phosphatase, abdominal pain, dry mouth, anorexia
GU: Urinary frequency, hematuria
INTEG: Rash, pruritus
RESP: Dyspnea, respiratory failure (IT)

Pharmacokinetics

Absorption	Good (PO)
Distribution	Widely, crosses placenta
Metabolism	Liver, partially
Excretion	Kidney, unchanged 70%-80%
Half-life	2½-4 hr

Pharmacodynamics

	PO/IT
Onset	0.5-1 hr
Peak	4 hr
Duration	4-8 hr

INTERACTIONS
Individual drugs
Alcohol: CNS depression

Drug classifications
Antidepressants (tricyclics), barbiturates, MAOIs, opioids, sedative/hypnotics: increased CNS depression
Antihypertensives: increased hypotension

Drug/herb
Kava, valerian: increased CNS depression

Drug/lab test
Increased: AST, ALT, alkaline phosphatase, blood glucose

NURSING CONSIDERATIONS
Assessment
• **Multiple sclerosis:** spasms, spasticity, ataxia, mobility, improvement should occur
• Monitor B/P, weight, blood glucose, and hepatic function periodically
⚠ **Check for increased seizure activity in patients with epilepsy; this product decreases seizure threshold, monitor ECG**
• Check I&O ratio; check for urinary retention, frequency, hesitancy
• Allergic reactions: rash, fever, respiratory distress; severe weakness, numbness in extremities
• Assess CNS depression: dizziness, drowsiness, psychiatric symptoms
• Check dosage, as individual titration is required
• Assess for **withdrawal symptoms:** CNS depression, dizziness, drowsiness, psychiatric symptoms
• **Intrathecal:** Have emergency equipment nearby; assess test dose and titration, if there is no response, check pump and catheter for proper functioning

Patient/family education
⚠ **Advise patient not to discontinue medication quickly; hallucinations, spasticity, tachycardia will occur; product should be tapered off over 1-2 wk**
• Advise patient not to take with alcohol, other CNS depressants
• Teach patient to avoid hazardous activities if drowsiness, dizziness occurs; to rise slowly to prevent orthostatic hypotension
• Teach patient to avoid using OTC medications: cough preparations, antihistamines, unless directed by prescriber
• Teach patient to notify prescriber if nausea, headache, tinnitus, insomnia, confusion, constipation, or inadequate, painful urination continues
• May require 1-2 mo for full response

Evaluation
Positive therapeutic outcome
• Decreased pain, spasticity

TREATMENT OF OVERDOSE:
Induce emesis of conscious patient, activated charcoal, dialysis, physostigmine to reduce life-threatening CNS side effects

⚠ HIGH ALERT
basiliximab (Rx)
(bas-ih-liks'ih-mab)
Simulect
Func. class.: Immunosuppressant
Chem. class.: Murine/human monoclonal antibody (interleukin-2) receptor antagonist
Pregnancy category B

ACTION: Binds to and blocks the IL-2 receptor, which is selectively expressed on the surface of activated T-lymphocytes; impairs the immune system to antigenic challenges

Therapeutic outcome: Prevention of graft rejection

USES: Acute allograft rejection in renal transplant patients when used with cycloSPORINE and corticosteroids

CONTRAINDICATIONS:
Hypersensitivity to mannitol/murine, exposure to viral infections, breastfeeding

Precautions: Pregnancy **B**, children, geriatric, human anti-murine antibody

BLACK BOX WARNING: Infections

DOSAGE AND ROUTES
Adult/child ≥35 kg: IV 20 mg × 2 doses; first dose within 2 hr before transplant surgery; second dose given 4 days after transplantation
Child <35 kg: IV 10 mg × 2 doses; first dose within 2 hr before transplant surgery; second dose given 4 days after transplantation

Available forms: Powder for inj 10, 20 mg

Implementation

Intermittent IV INF route
• **Reconstitute** 10 mg vial/2.5 ml or 20 mg vial in 5 ml sterile water for inj; shake gently to dissolve, **dilute** reconstituted sol in 25 ml (10 mg vial) or 50 ml (20 mg vial) with 0.9% NaCl or D$_5$, gently invert bag, do not shake, **give** over ½ hr, do not admix
• Storage of reconstituted sol refrigerated for up to 24 hr or at room temp for 4 hr

ADVERSE EFFECTS

CNS: *Pyrexia, chills, tremors, headache, insomnia, weakness,* dizziness; psychiatric/behavioral changes (child)
CV: *Chest pain,* angina, **cardiac failure,** hypo/hypertension, edema
GI: *Vomiting, nausea, diarrhea,* constipation, abdominal pain, GI bleeding, gingival hyperplasia, stomatitis
INTEG: *Acne,* pruritus, impaired wound healing
META: Acidosis, hypercholesterolemia, hyperuricemia, hypo/hyperkalemia, hypocalcemia, hypophosphatemia
MISC: Infection, moniliasis, **anaphylaxis,** anemia, allergic reaction, dysuria, CMV infection, candidiasis
MS: Arthralgia, myalgia
RESP: *Dyspnea, wheezing, cough,* **pulmonary edema**

Pharmacokinetics

Absorption	Unknown
Distribution	Unknown
Metabolism	Unknown
Excretion	Unknown
Half-life	7 days (adult)
	9½ days (child)

Pharmacodynamics

Onset	Unknown
Peak	½ hr (adult)
Duration	Unknown

INTERACTIONS

Drug classifications
Immunosuppressants: increased immunosuppression

Drug/lab test
Increased: BUN, cholesterol, uric acid, creatinine, potassium, calcium, blood glucose, Hgb, Hct
Decreased: Hgb, Hct, platelets, magnesium, phosphate

NURSING CONSIDERATIONS
Assessment

> **BLACK BOX WARNING:** Assess for infection, increased temp, WBC, sputum, urine, may be fatal (bacterial, protozoal, fungal)

• Monitor blood studies: Hgb, WBC, platelets during treatment qmo; if leukocytes are <3000/mm^3, product should be discontinued
• Monitor liver function studies: alkaline phosphatase, AST, ALT, bilirubin
• Assess hepatotoxicity: dark urine, jaundice, itching, light-colored stools; product should be discontinued
⚠ Assess for anaphylaxis, hypersensitivity: dyspnea, wheezing, rash, pruritus, hypotension, tachycardia; if severe hypersensitivity reactions occur, product should not be used again

Patient/family education

> **BLACK BOX WARNING:** Instruct patient to report fever, chills, sore throat, fatigue, since serious infection may occur; avoid crowds, persons with known upper respiratory infections; use contraception during treatment

Evaluation
Positive therapeutic outcome
• Absence of graft rejection

---

beclomethasone (Rx)
(be-kloe-meth′a-sone)
QVAR
Func. class.: Synthetic glucocorticoid (long acting)
Chem. class.: Beclomethasone diester
Pregnancy category C

Do not confuse:
beclomethasone/betamethasone

ACTION: Prevents inflammation by suppression of migration of polymorphonuclear leukocytes, fibroblasts, reversal of increased capillary permeability and lysosomal stabilization; does not suppress hypothalamus and pituitary function

Therapeutic outcome: Decreased inflammation and normal immunity

USES: Seasonal, perennial allergic/vasomotor rhinitis, nasal polyps, chronic steroid-dependent asthma

---

CONTRAINDICATIONS:
Hypersensitivity, status asthmaticus (primary treatment)

Precautions: Pregnancy **C,** breastfeeding, child <12, nasal disease/surgery, nonasthmatic bronchial disease, bacterial, fungal, viral infections of mouth, throat, lungs, HPA suppression, osteoporosis, Cushing's syndrome, diabetes mellitus, measles, cataracts, corticosteroid hypersensitivity, glaucoma, herpes infection

DOSAGE AND ROUTES
Adult and child >12 yr: Oral inh 48-80 mcg bid (alone) or 40-160 mcg bid (with inhaled corticosteroids), max 320 bid
Child 5-12 yr: Oral inh 40 mcg bid, max 80 mcg bid

Available forms: Oral inh 40, 80, 250 ✚ mcg /metered spray

Implementation
Oral route
• Give PO, using a spacer device for proper dose
• Shake oral aerosol well, use spacer
• Use after cleaning aerosol top daily with warm water; dry thoroughly
• Store in cool environment; do not puncture or incinerate container

Nasal route
• Shake inhaler, invert, tilt head backward, insert nozzle into nostril, away from septum; hold other nostril closed and depress activator, inhale through nose, exhale through mouth

ADVERSE EFFECTS
CNS: *Headache;* psychiatric/behavioral changes (child)
EENT: *Candidal infection of oral cavity, hoarseness,* sore throat, dysgeusia, loss of taste/smell
ENDO: Hypothalamic-pituitary (HPA) suppression
GI: Dry mouth, dyspepsia
MISC: Angioedema, adrenal insufficiency, facial edema, Churg-Strauss syndrome (rare)
RESP: Bronchospasm, wheezing, cough

Pharmacokinetics

Absorption	Locally only
Distribution	Not distributed
Metabolism	Lungs, liver (by CYP3A)
Excretion	Feces, urine
Half-life	2.8 hr

Pharmacodynamics

	Inh	Nasal
Onset	1-4 wk	10 min
Peak	Unknown	Unknown
Duration	Unknown	Unknown

NURSING CONSIDERATIONS
Assessment
• Assess adrenal suppression: 17-KS, plasma cortisol for decreased levels, adrenal function periodically for HPA axis suppression during prolonged therapy; monitor growth and development
• Assess blood studies, neutrophils, decreased platelets; WBC with diff at baseline and q3mo; if neutrophils are <1000/mm^3, discontinue treatment
• Check nasal passages during long-term treatment for changes in mucus; check for burning, stinging; assess for glucocorticoid withdrawal: dizziness, hypotension, fatigue, muscle/joint pain; notify prescriber immediately
• Assess respiratory status: rest, rhythm, characteristics; auscultate lung bilaterally before and throughout treatment
• Assess for fungal infections in mucous membranes

Patient/family education
• Teach patient to gargle/rinse mouth after each use to prevent oral fungal infections
• Teach patient that in times of stress, systemic corticosteroids may be needed to prevent adrenal insufficiency; do not discontinue oral product abruptly, taper slowly
• Teach patient to continue using product even if mild nasal bleeding occurs; is usually transient
• Teach patient method of administration after providing written instructions from manufacturer
• Clean inhaler by wiping with dry cloth
• Teach patient the symptoms of **adrenal insufficiency:** nausea, anorexia, fatigue, dizziness, dyspnea, weakness, joint pain, depression

Evaluate
Positive therapeutic outcome
• Decrease in runny nose, improved symptoms of bronchial asthma

beclomethasone nasal agent
See Appendix B

Adverse effects: *italics* = common; **bold** = life-threatening

belatacept (Rx)

(bel-a-ta′sept)
Nulojix
Func. class.: Biologic response modifier
Chem. class.: Fusion protein
Pregnancy category C

ACTION: Activated T lymphocytes are the mediators of immunologic rejection, and this product is a selective T-cell costimulation blocker; blocks the CD28 mediated co-stimulation of T lymphocytes by binding to CD80 and CD86 on antigen-presenting cells; inhibits T lymphocyte proliferation and the production of the cytokines interleukin-2, interferon-gamma, interleukin-4, and TNF-alpha.

Therapeutic outcome: Absence of kidney transplant rejection

USES: Kidney transplant rejection prophylaxis given with basiliximab induction, mycophenolate mofetil, corticosteroids

CONTRAINDICATIONS:

Hypersensitivity

BLACK BOX WARNING: Infection, organ transplant, requires an experienced clinician, secondary malignancy, post-transplant lymphoproliferation disorder (PTLD)

Precautions: Breastfeeding, child/infant/neonate, pregnancy C, diabetes mellitus, progressive multifocal leukoencephalopathy, immunosuppression, sunlight exposure, TB

DOSAGE AND ROUTES

Adult: **IV** 10 mg/kg rounded to nearest 12.5 mg increment give over 30 min the day of transplantation (day 1) but before transplantation, on day 5 approximately 96 hours after the day 1 dose 1, at the end of wk 2, at the end of wk 4, at the end of wk 8, and at the end of wk 12; maintenance dosage is 5 mg/kg rounded to nearest 12.5 mg increment given over 30 min at the end of wk 16 and q4wk ± 3 days thereafter; doses should be calculated on actual body weight on the transplantation day unless the patient's weight varies by >10%

Available forms:
Powder for inj 250 mg

Implementation

BLACK BOX WARNING: Only providers skilled in the use of immunosuppressant and management of transplant should use these products

IV route
• Visually inspect products for particulate matter, discoloration whenever solution/ container permit, discard if present
• Calculate the number of drug vials required to provide total infusion dose
• Reconstitute each vial/10.5 ml of sterile water for injection, 0.9% sodium chloride, D₅W using the silicone-free disposable syringe provided with each vial and an 18G to 21G needle. If silicone-free disposable syringe is dropped or becomes contaminated, use a new silicone-free disposable syringe from inventory. If you need additional silicone-free disposable syringes, call 1-888-685-6549. If the powder is accidentally reconstituted using a different syringe than the one provided, the solution may develop a few translucent particles. Discard any solutions prepared using siliconized syringes.
• Using aseptic technique, inject the diluent into the vial and direct the stream of diluent to the glass wall of the vial. To minimize foaming, rotate the vial and invert with gentle swirling until the contents are dissolved. Do not shake when reconstituted (25 mg/ml), should be clear to slightly opalescent and colorless to pale yellow. Do not use if opaque particles, discoloration, or other foreign particles are present.
• Calculate the total volume of the reconstituted 25 mg/ml sol required to provide the total inf dose. Further dilute this volume with a volume of inf fluid equal to the volume of the reconstituted drug sol required to provide the prescribed dose. Use either NS or D₅W if drug was reconstituted with SWFI; use NS if drug was reconstituted with NS; use D₅W if drug was reconstituted with D₅W. With the same silicone-free disposable syringe used for reconstitution, withdraw the required amount of belatacept sol from the vial, inject it into the inf container, gently rotate the inf container to ensure mixing; final concentration in inf container should range (2-10 mg/ml). Volume of 100 ml will be appropriate for most patients and doses, but total inf volumes ranging from 50-250 ml may be used. Discard any unused drug solution remaining in the vials; after reconstitution, immediately transfer the reconstituted sol from the vial to the inf bag or bottle; complete within 24 hr.

IV INF route
- Give over 30 min, use an infusion set and a sterile, nonpyrogenic low-protein-binding filter (0.2-1.2 mm), use a separate line
- Storage: refrigerate, protect from light ≤24 hr; max 4 hr of the total 24 hr can be at room temp and room light

ADVERSE EFFECTS

CNS: **Guillain-Barré syndrome,** anxiety, dizziness, fever, insomnia, tremor
EENT: Pharyngitis, stomatitis
GI: Abdominal pain, constipation, diarrhea, nausea, vomiting
GU: **Renal tubular necrosis, renal failure,** proteinuria, urinary incontinence
HEMA: Anemia, neutropenia, leukopenia, leukoencephalopathy
INTEG: Acne, alopecia
META: Hypercholesterolemia, hyperglycemia, hyper/hypokalemia, hypocalcemia, hypophosphatemia, hypomagnesemia
MS: Arthralgia
SYST: **Secondary malignancy, post-transplant lymphoproliferation disorder (PTLD), wound dehiscence, BK-virus associated neuropathy**

Pharmacokinetics

Absorption	Unknown
Distribution	Steady-state by week 8 after transplantation and by month 6 during the maintenance phase
Metabolism	Unknown
Excretion	Unknown
Half-life	Half life range 6.1-15.1 days during receipt of 10 mg/kg IV doses; 3.1-11.9 days during receipt of 5 mg/kg IV doses

Pharmacodynamics

Onset	Unknown
Peak	Unknown
Duration	Unknown

INTERACTIONS

Individual drugs
Basiliximab induction, mycophenolate mofetil: increased effect

Drug classifications
Corticosteroids: increased belatacept effect
Vaccines: avoid concurrent use
Immunosuppressives: avoid increased dose

NURSING CONSIDERATIONS
Assessment

BLACK BOX WARNING: Transplant rejection: flu-like symptoms, decreasing urinary output, malaise; some may experience pain in area (rare; monitor BUN/Creatinine)

BLACK BOX WARNING: Infection: Monitor for fever, chills, increased WBC, wound dehiscences

BLACK BOX WARNING: Post-transplant lymphoproliferation disorder (PTLD): May lead to secondary malignancy (lymphoma) or infectious mononucleosis-like lesions; may be treated with antivirals or immunosuppressant may need to be discontinued

- Hyperlipidemia: Monitor cholesterol, triglycerides; an antilipidemic may be needed
- Store refrigerated, protected from light ≤24 hr; max 4 hr of the total 24 hr can be at room temperature and room light

Evaluation
Positive therapeutic outcome
- Absence of renal transplant rejection

Patient/family education
- Teach reason for product and expected result
- Teach to avoid exposure to sunlight, tanning beds, risk of secondary malignancy
- Teach to avoid crowds, persons with known infections
- Advise that repeated lab test will be needed
- Advise to avoid with vaccines
- Advise that immunosuppressants will be needed for life to prevent rejection; teach symptoms of rejection and to call provider immediately

belimumab (Rx)
(be-lim'ue-mab)
Benlysta
Func. class.: Monoclonal antibody
Chem. class.: Disease-modifying antirheumatic drugs (DMARDs)
Pregnancy category C

ACTION: Inhibits B lymphocyte stimulator (BLyS), which is needed for B-cell survival; normally, soluble BLyS binds to its receptors on B cells and allows B-cell survival; binds BLyS and prevents binding to its receptors on B cells

Therapeutic outcome: Decreasing symptoms of SLE: decreased fever, malaise, joint pains, myalgias, fatigue

USES: Active, autoantibody-positive, systemic lupus erythematosus (SLE) in combination with standard therapy

CONTRAINDICATIONS:
Hypersensitivity

Precautions: African descent patients, depression, children/infants, immunosuppression, infection, pregnancy C, breastfeeding, suicidal ideation, vaccination, geriatrics, secondary malignancy, cardiac disease, requires experienced clinician

DOSAGE AND ROUTES
Adult: 10 mg/kg IV over 1 hr q2wk for the first 3 doses, then q4wk

Available forms: Powder for injection 120, 400 mg

Implementation
• Use only by health care providers prepared to manage anaphylaxis should administer this product, may give premedication for prophylaxis against infusion and hypersensitivity reactions

Intermittent IV infusion route
• Visually inspect particulate matter and discoloration whenever solution and container permits
• Give as IV infusion only, do not give IV bolus or push, give over 1 hr and slow or stop if infusion reactions occur
• Do not give with any other agents in the same IV line
• Allow to stand at room temperature for 10-15 min before using
• Reconstitute with the appropriate amount of sterile water for injection (80 mg/ml); add 1.5 ml of sterile water (120 mg/vial) or 4.8 ml of sterile water (400 mg/vial)
• Direct the stream of sterile water toward the side of the vial to minimize foaming; gently swirl for 60 sec and allow to sit during reconstitution, gently swirling for 60 secs q5min until the powder is dissolved; do not shake; reconstitution is complete in 10 to 30 min
• If a mechanical reconstitution device (swirler) is used, max 500 rpm swirled for ≤30 min
• The solution should be opalescent, and colorless to pale yellow, and without particles; small air bubbles are expected; protect from sunlight

• Dilution: Only dilute in NS for injection; dilute reconstituted solution with enough normal saline to 250 ml. From a 250-ml infusion bag or bottle of normal saline, withdraw and discard a volume equal to the volume of the reconstituted solution required for dose; add the required volume of the reconstituted solution the infusion bag/bottle; gently invert to mix
• Discard any unused solution
• Storage in refrigerator or at room temp; total time from reconstitution to completion of inf max 8 hr

ADVERSE EFFECTS
CNS: Anxiety, depression, dizziness, fever, headache, insomnia, migraine, suicidal ideation
CV: Bradycardia, hypotension
GI: Diarrhea, nausea
MISC: Bronchitis, cystitis, dyspnea, leukopenia, myalgia, nasopharyngitis, pharyngitis, rash
SYST: Anaphylaxis, angioedema, antibody formation, infection, influenza, secondary malignancy

Pharmacokinetics

Absorption	Unknown
Distribution	Unknown
Metabolism	Unknown
Excretion	Unknown
Half-life	Terminal half-life 19.4 days; distribution half-life 1.75 days

Pharmacodynamics

Onset	Unknown
Peak	Unknown
Duration	Unknown

INTERACTIONS
Individual drugs
IV cyclophosphamide, biologic therapies (riTUXimab, ofatumumab): avoid concurrent use

Drug classifications
Vaccines: avoid concurrent use

NURSING CONSIDERATIONS
Assessment
• **SLE:** Monitor for decreasing fever, malaise, fatigue, joint pain, myalgias
• **Suicidal ideation:** More common in those with preexisting depression
• **Infection:** Determine if a chronic or acute infection is present, may be fatal when used with this product; do not begin therapy if any products are being used for a chronic infection;

leukopenia may occur with this product and susceptibility to infections increased
• **Anaphylaxis, infusion site reactions:** If these occur, stop infusion
• **African descent patients:** Use cautiously in these patients, may not respond to this product
• Cardiac disease: Monitor closely for cardiovascular side effects, bradycardia, hypotension
⚠ **Pregnancy: Determine if pregnant or if pregnancy is planned or suspected, if pregnant call 877-681-6269 to enroll in registry**

Patient/family education
⚠ **Teach patient to notify prescriber if pregnancy is planned or suspected, use reliable contraception during and for 4 mo after final treatment, to avoid breastfeeding**
⚠ **Advise patient to seek treatment immediately for serious hypersensitive reactions**
• Advise patient not to receive live vaccinations during treatment

Evaluation
• Decreasing symptoms of SLE: decreasing fatigue, fever, malaise

benazepril (Rx)
(ben-a′za-pril)
Lotensin
Func. class.: Antihypertensive
Chem. class.: ACE inhibitor
Pregnancy category D

Do not confuse:
benazepril/Benadryl

ACTION: Selectively suppresses renin-angiotensin-aldosterone system; inhibits ACE, preventing conversion of angiotensin I to angiotensin II

Therapeutic outcome: Decreased B/P in hypertension

USES: Hypertension, alone or in combination with thiazide diuretics

Unlabeled uses: CHF

CONTRAINDICATIONS:
Breastfeeding, children, hypersensitivity to ACE inhibitors, angioedema

> **BLACK BOX WARNING:** Pregnancy **D**

Precautions: Impaired renal/liver function, dialysis patients, hypovolemia, blood dyscrasias, CHF, COPD, asthma, geriatric, bilateral renal artery stenosis

DOSAGE AND ROUTES
Adult: PO 10 mg daily initially, then 20-40 mg/day divided bid or daily (without a diuretic); 5 mg PO daily (with a diuretic); max 80 mg daily
Geriatric: PO based on clinical response

Renal dose
Adult: PO 5 mg daily with CCr <30 ml/min; increase as needed to max of 40 mg/day

Available forms: Tabs 5, 10, 20, 40 mg

Implementation
• Store in air-tight container at 86° F (30° C) or less
• Severe hypotension may occur after 1st dose of this medication; decreased hypotension may be prevented by reducing or discontinuing diuretic therapy 3 days before beginning benazepril therapy
• Storage in tight container at 86° F (30° C) or less

ADVERSE EFFECTS
CNS: Anxiety, hypertonia, insomnia, paresthesia, headache, dizziness, fatigue
CV: Hypotension, postural hypotension, syncope, palpitations, angina
GI: Nausea, constipation, vomiting, gastritis, diarrhea, melena, **hepatotoxicity**
GU: Increased BUN, creatinine, decreased libido, impotence, urinary tract infection
HEMA: Agranulocytosis, neutropenia
INTEG: Rash, flushing, sweating
META: Hyperkalemia, hyponatremia
MISC: Angioedema, Stevens-Johnson syndrome
MS: Arthralgia, arthritis, myalgia
RESP: Cough, asthma, bronchitis, dyspnea, sinusitis

Pharmacokinetics
Absorption	<40%
Distribution	Unknown; crosses placenta
Metabolism	Liver metabolites; protein binding 97%
Excretion	Kidney, breast milk (minimal)
Half-life	10-11 hr (metabolite); increased in renal disease

Pharmacodynamics
Onset	Unknown
Peak	½-1 hr
Duration	Unknown

INTERACTIONS
Individual drugs
Alcohol: increased hypotension (large amounts)
Azathioprine: increased myelosuppression
Digoxin, lithium: increased serum levels

Drug classifications
Antihypertensives, diuretics, nitrates, phenothi-
azines: increased hypotension
Diuretics (potassium-sparing), potassium
supplements: increased hyperkalemia
NSAIDs: decreased hypotensive effects

Drug/herb
Ephedra (Ma huang): decreased antihyperten-
sive effect
Hawthorn: increased antihypertensive effect

Drug/lab test
Increased: AST, ALT, alkaline phosphatase,
bilirubin, uric acid, blood glucose
False positive: ANA titer
Positive: ANA titer

NURSING CONSIDERATIONS
Assessment
• **Hypertension:** B/P, pulse baseline and
periodically; monitor, check for orthostatic
hypotension, syncope; if changes occur, dosage
change may be required; notify prescriber of
changes; monitor compliance
• Monitor **blood dyscrasias:** neutrophils,
decreased platelets; WBC with differential at
baseline, q3mo; if neutrophils <1000/mm³,
discontinue treatment
• Monitor renal studies: protein, BUN,
creatinine; watch for increased levels that may
indicate nephrotic syndrome and renal failure;
monitor urine for protein; monitor renal symptoms: polyuria, oliguria, frequency, dysuria
• Establish baselines in renal, liver function
tests before therapy begins
• Check potassium levels throughout treatment,
although **hyperkalemia** rarely occurs; diuretic
should be discontinued 3 days prior to initiation
with benazepril; if hypertension is not controlled, a diuretic can be added; measure B/P
at peak 2-4 hr and trough (before next dose);
this product is less effective in African-American
descendants
• Assess for allergic reactions: rash, fever, pruritus, urticaria; product should be discontinued
if antihistamines fail to help; **angioedema is
more common in African-American descendants, Stevens-Johnson syndrome**

Patient/family education
• Instruct patient not to discontinue product
abruptly; advise patient to tell all persons associated with care
• Teach patient not to use OTC products
(cough, cold, allergy) unless directed by prescriber; serious side effects can occur; xanthines
such as coffee, tea, chocolate, cola can prevent
action of product
• Emphasize the importance of complying
with dosage schedule, even if feeling better;
to continue with medical regimen to decrease
B/P: exercise, cessation of smoking, decreasing
stress, diet modifications
• Emphasize the need to rise slowly to sitting or
standing position to minimize orthostatic hypotension, not to exercise in hot weather because
increased hypotension can occur
⚠ **Teach patient to notify prescriber of
mouth sores, sore throat, fever, swelling
of hands or feet, irregular heartbeat, chest
pain, coughing, shortness of breath, bruising, bleeding, swelling of face, tongue, lips,
difficulty breathing**
• Caution patient to report excessive perspiration, dehydration, vomiting, diarrhea; may lead
to fall in B/P
• Instruct patient to use caution in hot weather
• Caution patient that product may cause dizziness, fainting, light-headedness; may occur during first few days of therapy; to avoid activities
that may be hazardous
• Teach patient how to take B/P; teach normal
readings for age group; ensure patient takes
own B/P
• Instruct patient to avoid potassium-containing
products (salt substitutes)

> **BLACK BOX WARNING:** Advise patient to
> notify prescriber of pregnancy (**D**), product will
> need to be discontinued

Evaluation
Positive therapeutic outcome
• Decreased B/P in hypertension

TREATMENT OF OVERDOSE:
0.9% NaCl **IV** inf, hemodialysis

⚠ HIGH ALERT

bendamustine (Rx)

(ben-da-muss′teen)

Treanda

Func. class.: Antineoplastic alkylating agent

Chem. class.: Nitrogen mustard

Pregnancy category D

ACTION: Cross-linking DNA, which causes single strand and double strand breaks, inhibits several mitotic checkpoints, combines alkylating and antimetabolite properties

Therapeutic outcome: Improvement in blood counts and morphology

USES: Chronic lymphocytic leukemia, non-Hodgkin's lymphoma

CONTRAINDICATIONS:

Pregnancy **D**, fetal harm may occur; hypersensitivity to this product or mannitol, children, hepatic disease, renal impairment, breastfeeding

Precautions: Hyperuricemia, infusion-related reactions, myelosuppression, infection, skin reactions

DOSAGE AND ROUTES

Chronic lymphocytic leukemia

Adult: **IV** inf 100 mg/m^2 over 30 min on days 1, 2, q28days up to 6 cycles

Non-Hodgkin's lymphoma

Adult: **IV** inf 120 mg/m^2 over 60 min on days 1, 2, q21days up to 8 cycles

Renal/hepatic dose

Adult: **IV** inf CCr <40 ml/min, do not use; AST or ALT 2.5-10 × upper limit normal (ULN) or bilirubin 1.5-3 × ULN, do not use

Available forms: Powder for inj 25, 100 mg

Implementation

⚠ Give allopurinol for 1-2 wk to those at high risk for tumor lysis syndrome; usually develops in first treatment cycle

• Give blood transfusions or RBC colony-stimulating factors to counter anemia

• Give antiemetic 30-60 min before giving product to prevent vomiting

• Give all medications PO, if possible avoid IM inj if platelets are <100,000/mm^3

• Store reconstituted sol in refrigerator for 24 hr, or room temperature for 3 hr; protect from light; store vials at room temperature

Intermittent IV inf route

• Prepare in biological cabinet wearing gown, gloves, mask; avoid contact with skin; can cause burning and stain the skin brown; use cytotoxic handling procedures

• After reconstituting 100 mg product/20 ml or 25 mg/5 ml sterile water for inj (5 mg/ml), sol should be clear, colorless to pale yellow, completely dissolve in 5 min; if particulate is present, do not use

• Use within 30 min of reconstitution, withdraw the volume needed and **further dilute** in 500 ml NS or D$_{2.5\%/0.45\%}$ NS to a final conc 0.2-0.6 mg/ml; doses ≤100 mg/m^2, **give** over 30 min; doses >100 mg/m^2, **give** over 60 min

• Monitor for infusion reaction, may use antihistamines or corticosteroids in grade 1, 2 reaction; if grade 3 or 4, discontinue if needed

ADVERSE EFFECTS

CNS: Asthenia, fatigue, fever, headache, chills

CV: Hypertension, **hypertensive crisis**

GI: *Nausea, vomiting,* diarrhea, hyperbilirubinemia, constipation, stomatitis, anorexia, weight loss

GU: **Renal failure**

HEMA: **Thrombocytopenia, leukopenia, anemia, lymphocytopenia, neutropenia, secondary malignancy, toxic epidermal necrolysis, tumor lysis syndrome**

INTEG: Bulbous rash, pruritus, extravasation

META: Hyperuricemia

SYST: **Anaphylaxis,** infection, dehydration, **severe skin toxicities, tumor lysis syndrome, Stevens-Johnson syndrome**

Pharmacokinetics

Absorption	Unknown
Distribution	Protein binding 95%
Metabolism	Hydrolysis via cytochrome P450 1A2; two metabolites are produced
Excretion	90% unchanged (feces)
Half-life	40 min

Pharmacodynamics

Unknown

INTERACTIONS

Individual drugs

Aspirin: increased risk of bleeding

CloZAPine: do not use due to risk of agranulocytosis

Drug classifications
Anticoagulants, NSAIDs, platelet inhibitors, thrombolytics: increased risk of bleeding
Antineoplastics (other), radiation: increased toxicity
CYP1A2 inducers (barbiturates, carBAMazepine, rifampin): decreased bendamustine
CYP1A2 inhibitors (atazanavir, cimetidine, ciprofloxacin, enoxacin, ethyl estradiol, fluvoxaMINE, mexiletine, norfloxacin, tacrine, thiabendazole, zileuton): increased bendamustine
Myelosuppressive agents: increased myelosuppression
Vaccines (live): increased adverse reactions, decreased antibody reaction

Drug/lab test
Increased: LFTs

NURSING CONSIDERATIONS
Assessment
• **Blood dyscrasias:** assess CBC, differential, platelet count weekly; withhold product if WBC is <1000 or platelet count is <75,000; notify prescriber of results
• Monitor hepatic studies: AST, ALT, bilirubin
• Monitor renal studies: BUN, serum uric acid, urine CCr before, during therapy; I&O ratio; report fall in urine output of 30 ml/hr; electrolytes
• Assess for cold, cough, fever (may indicate beginning infection)
• Assess bleeding: hematuria, guaiac, bruising, petechiae, mucosa, orifices q8hr
• **Serious skin toxicities:** assess for toxic epidermal necrolysis, Stevens-Johnson syndrome, product should be discontinued
• **Tumor lysis syndrome:** monitor uric acid, potassium, may occur during first treatment cycle, use allopurinol in those at high risk for TLS, usually during the first 2 wk, provide adequate hydration

Patient/family education
• Teach patient to avoid crowds, persons with upper respiratory infections
• Advise patient to report immediately fever, sore throat, flulike symptoms—indicates infection
• Advise patient to report immediately allergic reaction, facial swelling, difficulty breathing, itchy rash
• Teach patient not to breastfeed until reaction is known; males should also use contraception during and for 3 mo after
⚠ Advise patient to avoid use of aspirin, ibuprofen, razors, commercial mouthwash

• Instruct patient to report signs of anemia (fatigue, irritability, shortness of breath, faintness)
• Instruct patient to report signs of infection
⚠ Teach patient to use contraception during therapy and for 3 mo after (pregnancy D)
• Advise patient to report signs of infection, myelosuppression, skin toxicities, diarrhea, nausea, vomiting

Evaluation
Positive therapeutic outcome
• Improvement in blood counts and morphology

benzocaine topical
See Appendix B

benztropine (Rx)
(benz'troe-peen)
Cogentin
Func. class.: Cholinergic blocker, antiparkinson agent
Chem. class.: Tertiary amine
Pregnancy category C

ACTION: Blockade of central acetylcholine receptors in the CNS; neurotransmitters are balanced, balances cholinergic activity

Therapeutic outcome: Decreased involuntary movements

USES: Parkinsonian symptoms, EPS associated with neuroleptic products, acute dystonia, hypersalivation

CONTRAINDICATIONS: Hypersensitivity, closed-angle glaucoma, dementia, tardive dyskinesia

Precautions: Pregnancy C, breastfeeding, children, geriatric, tachycardia, renal/hepatic disease, product abuse history, dysrhythmias, hypo/hypertension, psychosis; myasthenia gravis, GI/GU obstruction, child ≤3 yr, peptic ulcer, megacolon, prostate hypertrophy

DOSAGE AND ROUTES
Drug-induced extrapyramidal symptoms
Adult: IM/IV 1-4 mg daily/bid; give PO dose as soon as possible; PO 1-2 mg bid/tid; increase by 0.5 mg q5-6days
Child >3 yr: IM/IV 0.02-0.05 mg/kg/dose 1-2 ×/day
Geriatric: PO 0.5 mg daily-bid, increase by 0.5 mg q5-6days; max 4 mg/day

Parkinsonian symptoms
Adult: PO 1-2 mg daily, in 1-2 divided doses; increased 0.5 mg q5-6days titrated to patient response; max 6 mg daily

Acute dystonic reactions
Adult: IM/IV 1-2 mg, may increase to 1-2 mg bid (PO)

Available forms: Tabs 0.5, 1, 2 mg; inj 1 mg/ml

Implementation
PO route
• Give with or after meals to prevent GI upset; may give with fluids other than water; hard candy, frequent drinks, gum to relieve dry mouth
• Give at bedtime to avoid daytime drowsiness in patient with parkinsonism
• May be crushed and mixed with food
• Store at room temperature
IM route
• Inject deeply in muscle; use filtered needle to remove solution from ampule
• Give in large muscle mass for dystonic symptoms
IV direct route
• Give parenteral dose with patient recumbent to prevent postural hypotension; give undiluted 1 mg/1 min

Syringe compatibilities: ChlorproMAZINE, fluphenazine, metoclopramide, perphenazine, thiothixene

Y-site compatibilities: Fluconazole, tacrolimus

ADVERSE EFFECTS
CNS: Confusion; anxiety, restlessness, irritability, delusions, hallucinations, headache, sedation, depression, incoherence, dizziness, memory loss; delirium (geriatric)
CV: Palpitations, tachycardia, hypotension, bradycardia
EENT: Blurred vision, photophobia, dilated pupils, difficulty swallowing
GI: *Dryness of mouth, constipation,* nausea, vomiting, abdominal distress, **paralytic ileus**
GU: Hesitancy, retention, dysuria
INTEG: Rash, urticaria, dermatoses
MISC: Increased temperature, flushing, decreased sweating, **hyperthermia, heat stroke,** numbness of fingers

Pharmacokinetics

Absorption	Good (PO, IM), complete (**IV**)
Distribution	Unknown
Metabolism	Unknown
Excretion	Unknown
Half-life	Unknown

Pharmacodynamics

	IM/IV	PO
Onset	15 min	1 hr
Peak	Unknown	Unknown
Duration	6-10 hr	6-10 hr

INTERACTIONS
Individual drugs
Bethanechol: decreased cholinergic effects
Disopyramide, quiNIDine: increased anticholinergic effects, reduce dose

Drug classifications
Antidepressants (tricyclic), antihistamines, phenothiazines: increased anticholinergic amantadine effects
Antidiarrheals, antacids: decreased absorption

NURSING CONSIDERATIONS
Assessment
• Assess for **parkinsonism**, EPS: shuffling gait, muscle rigidity, involuntary movements, loss of balance, pill rolling, muscle spasms, drooling before and during treatment
• Paralytic ileus: assess for abdominal pain, intermittent constipation/diarrhea
• Monitor I&O ratio; retention commonly causes decreased urinary output, distention, frequency, incontinence
• Monitor for urinary hesitancy, retention; palpate bladder if retention occurs
• Monitor for constipation, cramping, pain in abdomen, abdominal distention; increase fluids, bulk, exercise if this occurs
• Assess for tolerance over long-term therapy; dosage may have to be increased or changed
• Assess for mental status: affect, mood, CNS depression, worsening of mental symptoms during early therapy
• Assess for benztropine "buzz" or "high," patients may imitate EPS

Patient/family education
• Teach patient to report urinary hesitancy/retention, dysuria

• Teach patient to use caution in hot weather; product may increase susceptibility to stroke since perspiration is decreased; patient should remain indoors
• Advise patient not to discontinue this product abruptly; to taper off over 1 wk to prevent withdrawal symptoms (insomnia, involuntary movements, anxiety, tachycardias), to take as directed, not to double doses
• Advise patient that tabs may be crushed, mixed with food; may take whole dose at bedtime if approved by prescriber
• Caution patient to avoid driving or other hazardous activities; drowsiness, dizziness may occur
• Teach patient to avoid OTC medication: cough, cold preparations with alcohol, antihistamines, antacids, or antidiarrheals within 2 hr unless directed by prescriber; increased CNS depression may occur
• Advise patient to rise from sitting or recumbent position slowly to minimize orthostatic hypotension
• Teach patient to use good oral hygiene; to use sugarless gum, hard candy, frequent sips of water to decrease dry mouth; if dry mouth continues, saliva substitutes may be prescribed
• Instruct patient that doses should not be doubled, but missed dose may be taken up to 2 hr before next dose

Evaluation
Positive therapeutic outcome
• Absence of involuntary movements (pill rolling, tremors, muscle spasms) after 2 days of treatment

betamethasone topical
See Appendix B

betamethasone (augmented) topical
See Appendix B

betaxolol ophthalmic
See Appendix B

bethanechol (Rx)
(be-than'e-kol)
Urecholine
Func. class.: Urinary tract stimulant, cholinergic
Chem. class.: Synthetic choline ester
Pregnancy category C

ACTION: Stimulates muscarinic acetylcholine receptors directly; mimics effects of parasympathetic nervous system stimulation; stimulates gastric motility, micturition; increases lower esophageal sphincter pressure

Therapeutic outcome: Absence of continued urinary retention

USES: Urinary retention (postoperative, postpartum), neurogenic atony of bladder with retention

Unlabeled uses: Ileus

CONTRAINDICATIONS:
Hypersensitivity, severe bradycardia, asthma, severe hypotension, hyperthyroidism, peptic ulcer, parkinsonism, seizure disorders, CAD, COPD, coronary occlusion, mechanical obstruction, peritonitis, recent urinary or GI surgery, GI/GU obstruction

Precautions: Pregnancy **C**, breastfeeding, child <8 yr, hypertension

DOSAGE AND ROUTES
Adult: PO 10-50 mg bid-qid
Child: PO 0.3-0.6 mg/kg/day divided in 3-4 doses/day

Ileus (unlabeled)
Adult: PO/SUBCUT 10-20 mg tid-qid; before meals (PO)

Available forms: Tabs 5, 10, 25, 50 mg

Implementation
PO route
• Give increased doses as prescribed if tolerance occurs
• To avoid nausea and vomiting, take on an empty stomach; 1 hr before or 2 hr after meals
• Store at room temperature

ADVERSE EFFECTS
CNS: Dizziness, headache, malaise
CV: Hypotension, bradycardia, reflex tachycardia, **cardiac arrest, circulatory collapse**
EENT: Miosis, increased salivation, lacrimation, blurred vision

GI: *Nausea, bloody diarrhea, belching, vomiting, cramps, fecal incontinence*
GU: Urgency
INTEG: Rash, urticaria, flushing, increased sweating
RESP: Acute asthma, dyspnea, bronchoconstriction

Pharmacokinetics

Absorption	Poor (PO)
Distribution	Does not cross blood-brain barrier
Metabolism	Unknown
Excretion	Kidneys
Half-life	Unknown

Pharmacodynamics

	PO	SUBCUT
Onset	30-90 min	5-15 min
Peak	1 hr	15-30 min
Duration	1-6 hr	2 hr

INTERACTIONS
Individual drugs
Procainamide, quiNIDine: decreased action of procainamide and quiNIDine

Drug classifications
Anticholinergics: decreased action
Anticholinesterase agents, cholinergic agonists: increased action, increased toxicity
Ganglionic blockers: increased severe hypotension

Drug/lab test
Increased: AST, lipase/amylase, bilirubin

NURSING CONSIDERATIONS
Assessment
• Assess **urinary patterns:** retention, urgency
• Monitor B/P, pulse, respirations; observe after parenteral dose for 1 hr
• Check I&O ratio; check for urinary retention or incontinence; if bladder emptying does not occur, notify prescriber; catheterization may be needed
• Assess for **toxicity:** bradycardia, hypotension, bronchospasm, headache, dizziness, seizures, sweating, cramping, respiratory depression; product should be discontinued if toxicity occurs; administer atropine

Patient/family education
• Instruct patient to take product exactly as prescribed; 1 hr before meals or 2 hr after meals; do not double doses; if dose is missed, take within 1 hr of scheduled dose

• Caution patient to make position changes slowly; orthostatic hypotension may occur
• Instruct patient to report cramping, diarrhea with blood, flushing to prescriber

Evaluation
Positive therapeutic outcome
• Absence of urinary retention
• Absence of abdominal distention

TREATMENT OF OVERDOSE:
Administer atropine 0.6-1.2 mg **IV** or IM (adult)

⚠ HIGH ALERT

bevacizumab (Rx)
(beh-va-kiz′you-mab)
Avastin
Func. class.: Antineoplastic—miscellaneous
Chem. class.: Monoclonal antibody
Pregnancy category C

Do not confuse:
Avastin/Astelin

ACTION: DNA-derived monoclonal antibody selectively binds to and inhibits activity of human vascular endothelial growth factor to reduce microvascular growth and inhibition of metastatic disease progression

Therapeutic outcome: Decreased tumor size

USES: Metastatic carcinoma of the colon or rectum in combination, renal cell carcinoma, glioblastoma, non–small cell lung cancer

Unlabeled uses: Adjunctive in breast, renal/pancreatic/neovascular/ovarian cancer, (wet) macular degeneration

CONTRAINDICATIONS:
Hypersensitivity

Precautions: Pregnancy **C,** breastfeeding, children, geriatric, CHF, blood dyscrasias, CV disease, hypertension, surgery, thromboembolic disease, hamster protein/murine hypersensitivity

BLACK BOX WARNING: GI perforation, wound dehiscence

Adverse effects: *italics* = common; **bold** = life-threatening

DOSAGE AND ROUTES
Colorectal cancer
Adult: IV INF in combination with 5-fluorouracil 5 mg/kg q14 days given over 90 min; if well tolerated, the next infusion may be given over 60 min; if 60 min infusions are well tolerated, subsequent infusions may be given over 30 min; (second-line) 5 mg/kg q2wk or 7.5 mg/kg q3wk with fluoropyrimidine and irinotecan or fluoropyramide and oxaliplatin-based agent

Non–small cell lung cancer
Adult: IV 15 mg/kg over 60-90 min with CARBOplatin and paclitaxel

Metastatic renal cell carcinoma
Adult: IV 15 mg/kg q2wk with interferon alfa 9 million units SUBCUT 3 × per wk, up to 52 wk

Available forms: Inj 25 mg/ml

Implementation
IV intermittent infusion route
• Do not give by **IV** bolus or **IV** push
• Give as **IV** inf over 90 min for first dose and 60 min thereafter, if well tolerated

> **BLACK BOX WARNING: Wound dehis-cence:** do not give for ≥28 days after surgery, make sure wounds are healed prior to use

ADVERSE EFFECTS
CNS: *Asthenia, dizziness,* **intracranial hemorrhage (malignant glioma),** headache, fatigue, confusion
CV: Deep vein thrombosis, hypo/hypertension, **hypertensive crisis,** heart failure
GI: Nausea, vomiting, anorexia, diarrhea, constipation, abdominal pain, colitis, stomatitis, **GI hemorrhage/perforation**
GU: Proteinuria, urinary frequency/urgency, **nephrotic syndrome,** ovarian failure
HEMA: **Leukopenia, neutropenia, thrombocytopenia, microangiopathic hemolytic anemia, thromboembolism, bleeding**
META: Bilirubinemia, hypokalemia
MISC: Exfoliative dermatitis, hemorrhage, non-GI fistula formation, *alopecia, impaired wound healing,* **osteonecrosis of the jaw,** antibody formation
RESP: Dyspnea, upper respiratory infection

Absorption	Unknown
Distribution	Steady state 100 days
Metabolism	Unknown
Excretion	Unknown
Half-life	20 days

Pharmacodynamics

Onset	Unknown
Peak	Unknown
Duration	Steady state 100 days

INTERACTIONS
Individual drugs
SUNItinib: avoid concurrent use; microangiopathic hemolytic anemia may occur, avoid concurrent use

NURSING CONSIDERATIONS
Assessment
• Monitor B/P q3-4wk
• Assess for symptoms of infection; may be masked by product
• Monitor **CNS reaction:** dizziness, confusion
• Assess for **CHF:** crackles, jugular vein distention, dyspnea during treatment
• Assess **GU status** (proteinuria); nephrotic syndrome may occur; monitor urinalysis for increasing protein level; products should be held if protein ≥2 g/24 hr

> **BLACK BOX WARNING: Wound dehis-cence:** hold for ≥28 days until incision is healed

⚠ **Assess for GI perforation, serious bleeding, nephrotic syndrome, hypertensive crisis; product should be discontinued permanently; for surgery, product should be discontinued temporarily**
⚠ **Reversible posterior leukoencephalopathy syndrome (RPLS): discontinue if this disorder develops**

Patient/family education
• Instruct patient to avoid hazardous tasks, since confusion, dizziness may occur
• Instruct patient to report signs of infection: sore throat, fever, diarrhea, vomiting
• Advise patient not to become pregnant while taking this product, or for several months after discontinuing treatment
• Advise patient to notify prescriber if pregnant or planning a pregnancy

---

Evaluation
Positive therapeutic outcome
• Decrease in size of tumors

> **⚠ HIGH ALERT**
>
> ## bicalutamide (Rx)
> (bi-kal-yut'ah-mide)
> **Casodex**
> *Func. class.:* Antineoplastic hormone
> *Chem. class.:* Nonsteroidal antiandrogen
> **Pregnancy category X**

Do not confuse:
Casodex/Kapidex

ACTION: Competitively inhibits the action of androgens by binding to cytosol androgen receptors in target tissue

Therapeutic outcome: Prevention of growth of malignant cells

USES: Stage D-2 metastatic prostate cancer in combination with luteinizing hormone–releasing hormone (LHRH) analog

CONTRAINDICATIONS:
Pregnancy **X,** women, hypersensitivity

Precautions: Breastfeeding, geriatric, renal/hepatic disease, diabetes mellitus

DOSAGE AND ROUTES
Adult: PO 50 mg daily with LHRH

Available forms: Tabs 50 mg

Implementation
• Give at same time each day (for both products) either AM or PM with or without food
• Give only with LHRH treatment

ADVERSE EFFECTS
CNS: Dizziness, paresthesia, insomnia, anxiety, neuropathy, headache
CV: Hot flashes, hypertension, chest pain, **CHF,** edema
GI: *Diarrhea, constipation, nausea,* vomiting, increased liver enzyme test, anorexia, dry mouth, melena, abdominal pain, **hepatitis, hepatotoxicity**
GU: Nocturia, hematuria, UTI, impotence, gynecomastia, urinary incontinence, frequency, dysuria, retention, urgency, breast tenderness, decreased libido
INTEG: Rash, sweating, dry skin, pruritus, alopecia

MISC: Infection, anemia, dyspnea, bone pain, headache, asthenia, *back pain,* flulike symptoms

Pharmacokinetics

Absorption	Well absorbed
Distribution	Unknown
Metabolism	Liver
Excretion	Urine, feces
Half-life	5.2 days

Pharmacodynamics

Onset	Unknown
Peak	31½ hr
Duration	Unknown

INTERACTIONS
Drug classifications
Anticoagulants: increased anticoagulation
CYP3A4 inhibitors (amiodarone, antiretrovirals, protease inhibitors, clarithromycin, dalfopristin, quinupristin, delavirdine, efavirenz, erythromycin, FLUoxetine, fluvoxaMINE, imatinib, mifepristone, RU-486, nefazodone, some azole antifungals): increased bicalutamide effects
CYP3A4 inducers (barbiturates, bosentan, carBAMazepine, dexamethasone, nevirapine, OXcarbazepine, phenytoins, rifabutin, rifampin, rifapentine): decreased bicalutamide effects

Drug/herb
St. John's wort: may require dosage change

Drug/food
Grapefruit juice: do not use together

Drug/lab test
Increased: AST, ALT, bilirubin, BUN, creatinine
Decreased: Hgb, WBC

NURSING CONSIDERATIONS
Assessment
• Assess for diarrhea, constipation, nausea, vomiting
• Assess for hot flashes, gynecomastia; assure patient that these are common side effects
• Monitor prostate-specific antigen (PSA) liver function tests

Patient/family education
• Teach patient to recognize and report signs of anemia, renal/hepatic toxicity
• Advise patient that hair may be lost, but loss is reversible after therapy is discontinued
• Advise patient not to use other products unless approved by prescriber
• Advise patient to use contraception

Evaluation
Positive therapeutic outcome
- Decreased tumor size, spread of malignancy

bimatoprost ophthalmic
See Appendix B

bisacodyl (Rx, OTC)
(bis-a-koe′dill)
Alophen, Correctol, Dacodyl, Dulcolax, Ex-Lax Ultra Tab, Femilax, Feminine, Femitrol, Good Sense Women's, Leader Laxative, ratio-Bisacodyl ❖, Top Care Laxative, Veracolate, Walgreens Gentle, Walgreens Women's
Func. class.: Laxative, stimulant
Chem. class.: Diphenylmethane
Pregnancy category C

ACTION: Acts directly on intestine by increasing motor activity; thought to irritate colonic intramural plexus; increases water in the colon

Therapeutic outcome: Decreased constipation

USES: Short-term treatment of constipation, bowel or rectal preparation for surgery, examination

CONTRAINDICATIONS:
Hypersensitivity, rectal fissures, abdominal pain, nausea, vomiting, appendicitis, acute surgical abdomen, ulcerated hemorrhoids, acute hepatitis, fecal impaction, intestinal/biliary tract obstruction

Precautions: Pregnancy **C,** breastfeeding

DOSAGE AND ROUTES
Adult ≥12 yr: PO 5-15 mg in PM or AM; may use up to 30 mg for bowel or rectal preparation; RECT 10 mg (single dose), 30 ml enema
Child 6-11 yr: PO 5 mg as a single dose; RECT 5 mg as a single dose

Available forms: Tabs del rel 5, 10 mg; enteric coated tabs 5 mg; supp 5, 10 mg; enema 10 mg/30 ml

Implementation
Oral route
- Swallow tabs whole; do not break, crush, or chew

- Give alone with water only for better absorption; do not take within 1 hr of antacids, milk
- Administer in AM or PM (oral dose)
Rectal route
- Lubricate before insertion, patient should retain for ½ hr
- Insert high in rectum

ADVERSE EFFECTS
CNS: Muscle weakness
GI: *Nausea, vomiting, anorexia, cramps,* diarrhea, rectal burning (supp)
META: Protein-losing enteropathy, alkalosis, hypokalemia, **tetany,** electrolyte and fluid imbalances

Pharmacokinetics
Absorption	Poor
Distribution	Unknown
Metabolism	Liver, minimally
Excretion	Kidneys
Half-life	Unknown

Pharmacodynamics
	PO	Rect
Onset	6-10 hr	15-60 min
Peak	Unknown	Unknown
Duration	Unknown	Unknown

INTERACTIONS
Drug classifications
Antacids, gastric acid pump inhibitors, H_2-blockers: increased gastric irritation

Drug/food
Increased irritation—dairy products: separate by 2 hr

Drug/lab test
Increased: sodium phosphate
Decreased: calcium, magnesium

Drug/herb
Flax, lily of the valley, pheasant's eye, senna, squill: increased laxative action

NURSING CONSIDERATIONS
Assessment
- Monitor blood, urine electrolytes if used often by patient; check I&O ratio to identify fluid loss
- Assess **GI symptoms:** cramping, rectal bleeding, nausea, vomiting; if these symptoms occur, product should be discontinued; identify cause of constipation; identify whether fluids, bulk, or exercise are missing from lifestyle
- Multiple products/routes may be used for bowel prep

Patient/family education
- Discuss with the patient that adequate fluid and bulk consumption is necessary
- Advise patient that normal bowel movements do not always occur daily
- Teach patient not to use in presence of abdominal pain, nausea, vomiting; tell patient to notify prescriber if constipation is unrelieved or if symptoms of electrolyte imbalance occur: muscle cramps, pain, weakness, dizziness, excessive thirst
- Teach patient to take with a full glass of water; do not take with dairy products
- Teach patient to identify bulk, water, constipating products, exercise in patient's life
- Instruct patient not to use laxatives for long-term therapy because bowel tone will be lost; 1 wk use is usually sufficient

Evaluation
Positive therapeutic outcome
- Decreased constipation within 3 days

bismuth subsalicylate (OTC)
(bis′meth sub-sa-li′si-late)
Bismatrol, Equaline Stomach Relief, Good Sense Stomach Relief, Kao-Tin, Leader Pink Bismuth, Maalox Total Stomach Relief, Peptic Relief, Pepto-Bismol, Pink Bismuth, Top Care Stomach Relief, Walgreens Soothe
Func. class.: Antidiarrheal/weak antacid
Chem. class.: Salicylate
Pregnancy category C

ACTION: Inhibits prostaglandin synthesis responsible for GI hypermotility, intestinal inflammation; stimulates absorption of fluid and electrolytes; binds toxins produced by *Escherichia coli*

Therapeutic outcome: Absence of loose, watery stools

USES: Diarrhea (cause undetermined); prevention of diarrhea when traveling; may be included to treat *Helicobacter pylori,* heartburn, indigestion, nausea

CONTRAINDICATIONS:
Child <3 yr; flulike symptoms; history of GI bleeding; renal disease, varicella, hypersensitivity to this product or salicylates

Precautions: Pregnancy **C**, breastfeeding, geriatric, anticoagulant therapy, gout, diabetes mellitus, immobility, bleeding disorders, previous hypersensitivity to NSAIDs, *Clostridium difficile*–associated diarrhea when used with antiinfectives for *H. pylori*

DOSAGE AND ROUTES
Antidiarrheal
Adult: PO 2 tab or 30 ml/15 ml extra/max strength q30min or 2 tabs q6min, max 4.2 g/24 hr

Antiulcer (unlabeled)
Adult: PO 524 mg q30-60min or 1048 mg q1hr, max 4.2 g/24 hr; given with metronidazole or tetracycline

Available forms: Tabs 262 mg; chewable tabs 262, mg; susp 87 mg/5 ml, 130 mg/15 ml, 262 mg/15 ml, 525 mg/15 ml

Implementation
- **Suspension:** Shake susp before use; chewable tabs should not be swallowed whole

ADVERSE EFFECTS
CNS: Confusion, twitching, **neurotoxicity (high dose)**
EENT: Hearing loss, tinnitus, metallic taste, blue gums, black tongue (chew tabs)
GI: Increased fecal impaction (high doses), dark stools, constipation, diarrhea, nausea
HEMA: Increased bleeding time

Pharmacokinetics
Absorption	Salicylate >90%
Distribution	None
Metabolism	None
Excretion	Feces (unchanged)
Half-life	Unknown

Pharmacodynamics
Onset	1 hr
Peak	2 hr
Duration	4 hr

INTERACTIONS
Individual drugs
Methotrexate: increased toxicity
Tetracycline: decreased absorption, separate by ≥2 hr

Drug classifications
Anticoagulants (oral): increased effect of anticoagulants

Antidiabetics (oral): increased effect of antidiabetics

Quinolones: decreased absorption of quinolones

Salicylates: increased risk of salicylate toxicity

Drug/lab test
Interference: radiographic studies of GI system

NURSING CONSIDERATIONS
Assessment
• **Diarrhea:** Assess bowel pattern (frequency, consistency, shape, volume, color) before product therapy, after treatment; check weight, bowel sounds; identify factors contributing to diarrhea (bacteria, diet, medications, tube feedings)

• Monitor skin turgor; dehydration may occur in severe diarrhea; monitor electrolytes (potassium, sodium, chloride) if diarrhea is severe or continues long term

Patient/family education
• Teach patient to stop use if symptoms do not improve within 2 days or become worse, or if diarrhea is accompanied by high fever

• Teach patient to increase fluids for rehydration

• Tell patient to chew or dissolve chewable tabs in mouth; do not swallow whole; shake susp before using

• Tell patient to avoid other salicylates unless directed by prescriber; not to give to children because of possibility of Reye's syndrome

• Tell patient that stools may turn gray; tongue may darken; impaction may occur in debilitated patients

Evaluation
Positive therapeutic outcome
• Decreased diarrhea or absence of diarrhea when traveling; resolution of ulcers

bisoprolol (Rx)
(bis-oh′pro-lole)

Zebeta

Func. class.: Antihypertensive

Chem. class.: β₁-Blocker (selective)

Pregnancy category C

Do not confuse:
Zebeta/Diabeta/Zetia

ACTION: Preferentially and competitively blocks stimulation of β₁-adrenergic receptor within cardiac muscle (decreases rate of SA node discharge, increases recovery time), slows conduction of AV node, decreases heart rate, which decreases O_2 consumption in myocardium; decreases renin-aldosterone-angiotensin system; inhibits β₂-receptors in bronchial and vascular smooth muscle at high doses

Therapeutic outcome: Decreased B/P, heart rate

USES: Mild to moderate hypertension

Unlabeled uses: Stable angina, stable CHF

CONTRAINDICATIONS:
Hypersensitivity to β-blockers, cardiogenic shock, heart block (2nd or 3rd degree), sinus bradycardia, CHF, cardiac failure

Precautions: Pregnancy **C**, breastfeeding, children, major surgery, diabetes mellitus, renal/hepatic/thyroid/peripheral vascular/aortic/mitral valve disease, COPD, asthma, well-compensated heart failure, myasthenia gravis

> **BLACK BOX WARNING:** Abrupt discontinuation

DOSAGE AND ROUTES
Renal/hepatic dose
Adult: PO CCr <40 ml/min 2.5 mg, titrate upward

Hypertension
Adult: PO 2.5-5 mg/day, may increase if necessary to 20 mg once daily, max 20 mg/day; reduce to 2.5 mg in bronchospastic disease

Angina (unlabeled)
Adult: PO 5-20 mg/day

Heart failure (unlabeled)
Adult: PO 1.25 mg/day × 48 hr, then 2.5 mg/day for 1st mo, then 5 mg/day, max 10 mg/day

Available forms: Tabs 5, 10 mg

Implementation
• Give daily; give with food to prevent GI upset; may be crushed

• Store protected from light, moisture; place in cool environment

ADVERSE EFFECTS
CNS: Vertigo, headache, insomnia, fatigue, dizziness, mental changes, memory loss, hallucinations, depression, lethargy, drowsiness, strange dreams, catatonia, peripheral neuropathy

CV: Ventricular dysrhythmias, **profound hypotension, bradycardia, CHF,** cold extremities, postural hypotension, **2nd- or 3rd-degree heart block**

EENT: Sore throat, dry burning eyes

ENDO: Increased hypoglycemic response to insulin

GI: Nausea, diarrhea, vomiting, **mesenteric arterial thrombosis,** ischemic colitis, flatulence, gastritis, gastric pain

GU: Impotence, decreased libido

HEMA: Agranulocytosis, thrombocytopenia, purpura, *eosinophilia*

INTEG: Rash, flushing, alopecia, pruritus, sweating

MISC: Facial swelling, weight gain, decreased exercise tolerance

MS: Joint pain, arthralgia

RESP: Bronchospasm, dyspnea, wheezing, cough, nasal stuffiness

Pharmacokinetics

Absorption	Well absorbed
Distribution	Unknown; protein binding (30%)
Metabolism	Liver, inactive metabolites
Excretion	Urine, unchanged (50%)
Half-life	9-12 hr

Pharmacodynamics

Onset	Unknown
Peak	2-4 hr
Duration	24 hr

INTERACTIONS

Individual drugs

Amiodarone, digoxin: increased bradycardia
Guanethidine, reserpine: increased hypotension

Drug classifications

ACE inhibitors, α-blockers, calcium channel blockers, diuretics: increased antihypertensive effect
Antidiabetics: increased antidiabetic effect
Calcium channel blockers: increased myocardial depression
Ergots: increased peripheral ischemia
NSAIDs, salicylates: decreased antihypertensive effects, may mask hypoglycemic symptoms

Drug/herb

Hawthorn: increased β-blocking effect
Ephedra: decreased β-blocking effect

Drug/lab test

Increased: AST, ALT, blood glucose, BUN, uric acid, potassium, lipoprotein, ANA titer
Interference: glucose/insulin tolerance tests

NURSING CONSIDERATIONS

Assessment

• **Hypertension:** Monitor B/P during beginning treatment, periodically thereafter; pulse: note rate, rhythm, quality; apical/radial pulse before administration; notify prescriber of any significant changes (pulse <50 bpm)

• Check for baselines in renal, liver function tests before therapy begins

• **CHF:** assess for edema in feet, legs daily, monitor I&O, daily weight; check for jugular vein distention, crackles, bilaterally, dyspnea (CHF)

• Monitor skin turgor, dryness of mucous membranes for hydration status, especially geriatric

Patient/family education

> **BLACK BOX WARNING:** Teach patient not to discontinue product abruptly; may cause precipitate angina if stopped abruptly; evaluate noncompliance

• Teach patient not to use OTC products containing α-adrenergic stimulants (such as nasal decongestants, cold preparations); to avoid alcohol, smoking; to limit sodium intake as prescribed

• Teach patient how to take pulse and B/P at home; advise when to notify prescriber

• Instruct patient to comply with weight control, dietary adjustments, modified exercise program

• Tell patient to carry/wear emergency ID to identify product being taken, allergies; tell patient product controls symptoms but does not cure

• Caution patient to avoid hazardous activities if dizziness, drowsiness present

• Teach patient to take product as prescribed, not to double doses, skip doses; take any missed doses as soon as remembered if at least 8 hr until next dose

• Advise patient to report bradycardia, dizziness, confusion, depression, fever, cold extremities

• Teach diabetic patient drug may mask signs of hypoglycemia or alter blood glucose levels

Evaluation

Positive therapeutic outcome

• Decreased B/P in hypertension (after 1-2 wk)

TREATMENT OF OVERDOSE:

Lavage, **IV** atropine for bradycardia, **IV** theophylline for bronchospasm, digoxin, O$_2$, diuretic for cardiac failure, hemodialysis, **IV** glucose for hypoglycemia, **IV** diazepam (or phenytoin) for seizures

⚠ HIGH ALERT

bivalirudin (Rx)

(bye-val-i-rue'din)

Angiomax

Func. class.: Anticoagulant

Chem. class.: Thrombin inhibitor

Pregnancy category B

ACTION: Direct inhibitor of thrombin that is highly specific; able to inhibit free and clot-bound thrombin

Therapeutic outcome: Anticoagulation in percutaneous transluminal coronary angioplasty (PTCA), used with aspirin; heparin-induced thrombocytopenia with thrombosis syndrome

USES: Unstable angina in patients undergoing PTCA, used with aspirin; heparin-induced thrombocytopenia; heparin-induced thrombocytopenia with thrombosis syndrome

CONTRAINDICATIONS:

Hypersensitivity, active bleeding, cerebral aneurysm, intracranial hemorrhage, recent surgery, CVA

Precautions: Pregnancy **B**, breastfeeding, children, geriatric, renal function impairment, hepatic disease, asthma, blood dyscrasias, thrombocytopenia, GI ulcers, hypertension, inflammatory bowel disease, vitamin K deficiency

DOSAGE AND ROUTES

PCI/PTCA

Adult: IV bol 0.75 mg/kg, then **IV** inf 1.75 mg/kg/hr for 4 hr; another **IV** inf may be used at 0.2 mg/kg/hr for ≤20 hr; this product is intended to be used with aspirin (325 mg daily) adjusted to body weight

HIT/HITTS

Adult: IV bol 0.75 mg/kg, then cont INF 1.75 mg/kg/hr for duration of procedure

Renal dose

Adult: IV GFR 30-59 ml/min, give 1.75 mg/kg/hr; GFR 10-29 ml/min, give 1 mg/kg/hr; dialysis-dependent patients, give 0.25 mg/kg/hr

Available forms: Inj, lyophilized 250 mg vial

Implementation

• Prior to PTCA, give with aspirin, 325 mg **IV** direct 1 mg/kg as a bolus; then intermittent infusion

Intermittent IV infusion route

• To each 250-mg vial add 5 ml of sterile water for inj, swirl until dissolved, further dilute reconstituted vial with 50 ml of D_5W or 0.9% NaCl (5 mg/ml); the dose is adjusted to body weight, run at 2.5 mg/kg/hr, do not admix before or during administration

• Give reduced dose in renal impairment

Y-site compatibilities: Abciximab, acyclovir, alfentanil, allopurinol, amifostine, amikacin, aminocaproic acid, aminophylline, amphotericin B liposome, ampicillin, ampicillin-sulbactam, anidulafungin, argatroban, arsenic trioxide, atenolol, atracurium, atropine, azithromycin, aztreonam, bleomycin, bumetanide, buprenorphine, busulfan, butorphanol, calcium chloride/gluconate, capreomycin, CARBOplatin, carmustine, ceFAZolin, cefepime, cefoperazone, cefotaxime, cefoTEtan, cefOXitin, cefTAZidime, ceftizoxime, cefTRIAXone, cefuroxime, chloramphenicol, cimetidine hydrochloride, ciprofloxacin, cisatracurium, CISplatin, clindamycin, cyclophosphamide, cycloSPORINE, cytarabine, dacarbazine, DACTINomycin, DAPTOmycin, DAUNOrubicin, DAUNOrubicin liposome, dexamethasone, dexmedetomidine, dexrazoxane, digoxin, diltiazem, diphenhydrAMINE, DOCEtaxel, dolasetron, DOPamine, DOXOrubicin, DOXOrubicin liposomal, doxycycline, droperidol, enalaprilat, ePHEDrine, EPINEPHrine, epirubicin, epoprostenol, eptifibatide, ertapenem, erythromycin, esmolol, etoposide, etoposide phosphate, famotidine, fenoldopam, fentaNYL, fluconazole, fludarabine, fluorouracil, foscarnet, fosphenytoin, furosemide, gallium, ganciclovir, gatifloxacin, gemcitabine, gentamicin, glycopyrrolate, granisetron, haloperidol, heparin, hydrALAZINE, hydrocortisone, HYDROmorphone, hydrOXYzine, IDArubicin, ifosfamide, imipenem-cilastatin, inamrinone, insulin, irinotecan, isoproterenol, ketorolac, labetalol, leucovorin, levofloxacin, lidocaine, linezolid, LORazepam, magnesium, mannitol, mechlorethamine, melphalan, meperidine, meropenem, mesna, methohexital, methotrexate, methyldopate, methylPREDNISolone, metoclopramide, metoprolol, metroNIDAZOLE, midazolam, milrinone, mitoMYcin, mitoXANtrone, mivacurium, morphine, moxifloxacin, mycophenolate, nafcillin, nalbuphine, naloxone, nesiritide, niCARdipine, nitroglycerin, nitroprusside, norepinephrine, octreotide, ofloxacin, ondansetron, oxaliplatin, oxytocin, PACLitaxel, palonosetron, pamidronate, pancuronium, PEMEtrexed, PENTobarbital, PHENobarbital, phenylephrine, piperacillin, piperacillin-tazobactam, polymyxin B, potassium acetate/chloride/phosphates, procainamide, promethazine, propranolol, ranitidine, remifentanil, rocuronium, sodium acetate/bicarbonate/phosphates, streptozocin, succinylcholine, SUFentanil, sulfamethoxazole-trimethoprim, tacrolimus, teniposide, theophylline, thiopental, thiotepa, ticarcillin, ticarcillin-clavulanate, tigecycline, tirofiban, tobramycin, topotecan, vasopressin, vecuronium, verapamil, vinBLAStine, vinCRIStine, vinorelbine, voriconazole, warfarin, zidovudine, zoledronic acid

ADVERSE EFFECTS

CNS: *Headache, insomnia, anxiety, nervousness*
CV: *Hypo/hypertension, bradycardia,* ventricular fibrillation
GI: *Nausea, vomiting, abdominal pain, dyspepsia*
HEMA: **Hemorrhage, thrombocytopenia**
MISC: Pain at inj site, pelvic pain, urinary retention, fever, **anaphylaxis**, infection
MS: *Back pain*

Pharmacokinetics

Absorption	Unknown
Distribution	No protein binding
Metabolism	Unknown
Excretion	Kidneys
Half-life	25 min

Pharmacodynamics

Onset	Unknown
Peak	Unknown
Duration	1 hr

INTERACTIONS

Individual drugs
Aspirin, treprostinil: increased risk of bleeding

Drug classifications
Anticoagulants, thrombolytics: increased risk of bleeding

Drug/herb
Agrimony, alfalfa, angelica, anise, bilberry, black haw, bogbean, buchu, cat's claw, chamomile, chondroitin, devil's claw, dong quai, evening primrose, fenugreek, feverfew, fish oils, garlic, ginger, ginkgo, ginseng, horse chestnut, Irish moss, kava, kelp, kelpware, khella, licorice, lovage, lungwort, meadowsweet, motherwort, mugwort, nettle, papaya, parsley (large amounts), pau d'arco, pineapple, poplar, prickly ash, red clover, safflower, saw palmetto, senega, skullcap, tonka bean, turmeric, wintergreen, yarrow: increased risk of bleeding
Coenzyme Q10, flax, glucomannan, goldenseal, guar gum: decreased anticoagulant effect

NURSING CONSIDERATIONS

Assessment
⚠ **Assess for fall in B/P or Hct that may indicate hemorrhage, hematoma, hemorrhage at puncture site are more common in the elderly**
• Assess for fever, skin rash, urticaria
• Assess **bleeding:** check arterial and venous sites, IM inj sites, catheters; all punctures should be minimized
• PCI use: assess for possible thrombosis, stenosis, unplanned stent, prolonged ischemia, decreased reflow

Patient/family education
• Explain reason for product and expected results
• Teach patient not to use other OTC products unless approved by prescriber
• Teach patient not to use hard-bristle toothbrush, regular razor to avoid any injury: hemorrhage may result

Evaluation
Positive therapeutic outcome
• Anticoagulation in PTCA

⚠ HIGH ALERT

bleomycin (Rx)
(blee-oh-mye'sin)
Blenoxane ✦
Func. class.: Antineoplastic, antibiotic
Chem. class.: Glycopeptide
Pregnancy category D

ACTION: Inhibits synthesis of DNA, RNA, protein; derived from *Streptomyces verticillus;* phase specific in the G_2 and M phases; a nonvesicant, sclerosing agent

Therapeutic outcome: Prevention of rapidly growing malignant cells

USES: Cancer of head, neck, penis, cervix, vulva of squamous cell origin, Hodgkin's/non-Hodgkin's disease, testicular carcinoma, as a sclerosing agent for malignant pleural effusion

CONTRAINDICATIONS:
Pregnancy **D**, breastfeeding, hypersensitivity, prior idiosyncratic reaction

---

Precautions: Renal/hepatic/respiratory disease, patients >70 yr old

> **BLACK BOX WARNING:** Idiosyncratic reaction, pulmonary fibrosis

DOSAGE AND ROUTES
Adult and child: IM/SUBCUT/IV 0.25-0.5 units/kg q1-2wk or 10-20 units/m²; then 1 unit/day or 5 units/wk; may also be given by cont INF; max total dose, 400 units in lifetime

Hodgkin's disease (test dose)
Adult and child (unlabeled): IM/IV/SUBCUT <2 units for first 2 doses followed by 24 hr observation

Malignant pleural effusion
Adult: 60 units diluted in 100 ml of 0.9% NaCl intrapleural inj given through a thoracotomy tube following drainage of excess pleural fluid and complete lung expansion, remove after 4 hr

Renal Dose
Adult/child: CCr 40-50 ml/min reduce dose by 30%; CCr 30-39 ml/min reduce dose by 40%; CCr 20-29 ml/min reduce dose by 45%; CCr 10-19 ml/min reduce dose by 55%; CCr 5-10 ml/min reduce dose by 60%

Available forms: Powder for inj 15, 30 units/vial

Implementation
• Avoid contact with skin; very irritating; wash completely to remove
• Give fluids IV or PO before chemotherapy to hydrate patient
• Give antacid before oral agent; give antiemetic 30-60 min before giving product and prn to prevent vomiting; give antibiotics for prophylaxis of infection
• Provide liquid diet: carbonated beverages, gelatin may be added if patient is not nauseated or vomiting
• Rinse mouth tid-qid with water, club soda; brush teeth bid-qid with soft brush or cotton-tipped applicators for stomatitis; use unwaxed dental floss

IM/SUBCUT route
• IM test dose in lymphoma
• Reconstitute with 1-5 ml sterile water for inj; D₅W, 0.9% NaCl, rotate inj sites

INTRAPLEURAL route
• Give 60 units/50-100 ml of 0.9% NaCl, administered by physician through thoracotomy tube

IV route
• Product should be prepared by experienced personnel using proper precautions
• Two test doses 2-5 units before initial dose in lymphoma; monitor for anaphylaxis
• Give by direct IV after reconstituting 15 units or less/5 ml or more of 0.9% NaCl; give 15 units or less/10 min through Y-tube or 3-way stopcock initial dose; monitor for anaphylaxis

Intermittent IV infusion route
• Administer after diluting 50-100 ml 0.9% NaCl, D₅W and giving at prescribed rate

Y-site compatibilities: Acyclovir, alfentanil, allopurinol, amifostine, amikacin, aminocaproic acid, aminophylline, amiodarone, ampicillin, ampicillin-sulbactam, anidulafungin, atenolol, atracurium, azithromycin, aztreonam, bivalirudin, bumetanide, buprenorphine, busulfan, butorphanol, calcium chloride/gluconate, CARBOplatin, carmustine, caspofungin, ceFAZolin, cefepime, cefotaxime, cefoTEtan, cefOXitin, cefTAZidime, ceftizoxime, cefTRIAXone, cefuroxime, chloramphenicol, chlorproMAZINE, cimetidine, ciprofloxacin, cisatracurium, CISplatin, clindamycin, codeine, cyclophosphamide, cycloSPORINE, cytarabine, dacarbazine, DACTINomycin, DAPTOmycin, DAUNOrubicin, dexamethasone, dexmedetomidine, dexrazoxane, digoxin, diltiazem, diphenhydrAMINE, DOBUTamine, DOCEtaxel, DOPamine, doxacurium, DOXOrubicin, DOXOrubicin liposomal, doxycycline, droperidol, enalaprilat, ePHEDrine, EPINEPHrine, epirubicin, ertapenem, erythromycin, esmolol, etoposide, famotidine, fenoldopam, fentaNYL, filgrastim, fluconazole, fludarabine, fluorouracil, foscarnet, fosphenytoin, furosemide, ganciclovir, gatifloxacin, gemcitabine, gentamicin, glycopyrrolate, granisetron, haloperidol, heparin, hydrALAZINE, hydrocortisone sodium succinate, HYDROmorphone, hydrOXYzine, IDArubicin, ifosfamide, imipenem-cilastatin, inamrinone, insulin (regular), irinotecan, isoproterenol, ketorolac, labetalol, leucovorin, levofloxacin, levorphanol, lidocaine, linezolid, LORazepam, magnesium sulfate, mannitol, mechlorethamine, melphalan, meperidine, meropenem, mesna, metaraminol, methohexital, methotrexate, methyldopate, methylPREDNISolone, metoclopramide, metoprolol, metroNIDAZOLE, midazolam, milrinone, minocycline, mitoMYcin, mitoXANtrone, mivacurium, morphine, nafcillin, nalbuphine, naloxone, nesiritide, niCARdipine, nitroglycerin, nitroprusside, norepinephrine, octreotide, ondansetron, oxaliplatin, palonosetron, pamidronate, pancuronium, pantoprazole, PEMEtrexed, pentamidine, pentazocine,

---

PENTobarbital, PHENobarbital, phenylephrine, piperacillin, piperacillin-tazobactam, polymyxin B, potassium chloride, potassium phosphates, procainamide, prochlorperazine, promethazine, propranolol, quiNIDine, ranitidine, remifentanil, riTUXimab, rocuronium, sargramostim, sodium acetate, sodium bicarbonate, sodium phosphates, succinylcholine, SUFentanil, sulfamethoxazole-trimethoprim, tacrolimus, teniposide, theophylline, thiopental, thiotepa, ticarcillin, ticarcillin-clavulanate, tirofiban, tobramycin, tolazoline, trastuzumab, trimethobenzamide, vancomycin, vasopressin, vecuronium, verapamil, vinBLAStine, vinCRIStine, vinorelbine, voriconazole, zidovudine

ADVERSE EFFECTS
CNS: Pain at tumor site, headache, confusion
CV: **MI, stroke**
GI: *Nausea, vomiting, anorexia, stomatitis, weight loss,* ulceration of mouth, lips
GU: Hemolytic-uremic syndrome
IDIOSYNCRATIC REACTION: Hypotension, confusion, fever, chills, wheezing
INTEG: *Rash, hyperkeratosis, nail changes, alopecia,* pruritus, acne, striae, peeling, hyperpigmentation, phlebitis
RESP: **Fibrosis, pneumonitis,** wheezing, **pulmonary toxicity**
SYST: **Anaphylaxis,** radiation recall, Raynaud's phenomenon

Pharmacokinetics

Absorption	Well absorbed (IM, SUBCUT, intrapleural, intraperitoneal)
Distribution	Widely distributed
Metabolism	Liver, 30%
Excretion	Kidneys, unchanged (50%)
Half-life	2 hr; increased in renal disease

Pharmacodynamics
Unknown

INTERACTIONS
Individual drugs
Filgrastim, sargramostim: increased toxicity
Fosphenytoin, phenytoin: decreased phenytoin levels
Radiation: increased toxicity, bone marrow suppression

Drug classifications
Anesthetics (general), antineoplastics: increased toxicity
Live virus vaccines: avoid concurrent use

Drug/lab test
Increased: uric acid

NURSING CONSIDERATIONS
Assessment
• Assess buccal cavity q8hr for dryness, sores or ulceration, white patches, oral pain, bleeding, dysphagia; obtain prescription for viscous lidocaine (Xylocaine)
⚠ **Assess symptoms indicating anaphylaxis: rash, pruritus, urticaria, purpuric skin lesions, itching, flushing, wheezing, hypotension; have emergency equipment available**

> **BLACK BOX WARNING: Pulmonary toxicity/fibrosis:** Assess pulmonary function tests; chest x-ray before, during therapy; monitor q2wk during treatment; pulmonary diffusion capacity for carbon monoxide (DL_{CO}) monthly; if <40% of pretreatment value, stop treatment; assess for dyspnea, crackles, unproductive cough, chest pain, tachypnea, fatigue, increased pulse, pallor, lethargy, more common in the elderly, radiation therapy, pulmonary disease

• Monitor CBC, differential, platelet count weekly; withhold product for WBC <4000/mm³ or platelet count <100,000/mm³; notify prescriber of results for WBC <20,000/mm³, platelets <150,000/mm³

> **BLACK BOX WARNING: Idiosyncratic reaction:** assess hypotension, mental confusion, fever, chills, wheezing

• Monitor temp (may indicate beginning of infection)
• Monitor liver function tests before, during therapy (bilirubin, AST, ALT, LDH) as needed or monthly
• Assess for bleeding: hematuria, stool guaiac, bruising or petechiae, mucosa or orifices q8hr; inflammation of mucosa, breaks in skin
• Treat pulmonary infection prior to treatment; identify dyspnea, crackles, unproductive cough, chest pain, tachypnea
• Identify effects of alopecia on body image; discuss feelings about body changes; if edema in feet, joint pain, stomach pain, shaking present, prescriber should be notified; identify inflammation of mucosa, breaks in skin

Patient/family education
• Teach patient to avoid use of products containing aspirin or ibuprofen, razors, commercial

mouthwash; bleeding may occur; to report symptoms of bleeding (hematuria, tarry stools)
• Instruct patient to report signs of anemia (fatigue, headache, irritability, faintness, shortness of breath)
• Instruct patient to report any changes in breathing or coughing even several months after treatment; to avoid crowds and persons with respiratory tract or other infections
• Inform patient that hair may be lost during treatment; a wig or hairpiece may make patient feel better; new hair may be different in color, texture
• Caution patient not to have any vaccinations without the advice of the prescriber; serious reactions can occur
• Advise patient contraception is needed during treatment and for several months after completion of therapy, pregnancy **D**

Evaluation

Positive therapeutic outcome
• Prevention of rapid division of malignant cells

---

boceprevir
(boe-se′pro-vir)
Victrelis
Func. class.: Antiviral, anti-hepatitis agents
Pregnancy category X

ACTION: Prevents hepatitis C viral (HCV) replication by blocking the activity of HCV NS3/4A serine protease. Hepatitis C virus NS3/4A serine protease is an enzyme responsible for the conversion of HCV encoded polyproteins to mature/functioning viral proteins.

Theurapeutic outcome: Resolution of hepatitis C infection

USES: Hepatitis C infection in combination with peginterferon alfa and ribavirin

CONTRAINDICATIONS:
Pregnancy (X), male partners of women who are pregnant

Precautions: Breastfeeding, anemia, neutropenia, thrombocytopenia, HIV, hepatitis B, decompensated hepatic disease, in liver or other organ transplants, neonates, infants, children, adolescents <18 years of age, hypersensitivity

DOSAGE AND ROUTES
Chronic hepatitis C infection (genotype 1) compensated liver disease (without cirrhosis, previously untreated with interferon and ribavirin therapy, null responders/partial responders/relapsers)
Adult: PO Before starting therapy, give peginterferon alfa and ribavirin 4 wk, then add boceprevir 800 mg (four 200-mg capsules) PO tid (7-9 hr). Treatment length is determined by HCV RNA concentrations at treatment wk 4, 8, 12, and 24. If the patient has undetectable HCV RNA concentrations at wk 8 and 24, discontinue all three medications at wk 28 (previously untreated); wk 36 (partial responders/relapsers). If HCV RNA is detectable at wk 8 but undetectable at wk 24, the three-drug regimen through wk 36, then give only peginterferon alfa and ribavirin through treatment wk 48. If the patient has a poor response to peginterferon alfa and ribavirin during the initial 4 wk, continue treatment with all three medications for a total of 48 wks. Discontinue the three-drug regimen if the HCV RNA concentration >100 IU/ml at treatment wk 12 or a detectable HCA RNA concentration at treatment wk 24.

Chronic hepatitis C infection (genotype 1) compensated liver disease with cirrhosis
Adult: PO Before starting therapy with boceprevir, peginterferon alfa and ribavirin must be given 4 wk; then add boceprevir 800 mg (four 200-mg capsules) PO tid (q7-9hr) to peginterferon alfa and ribavirin for an additional 44 wk (48 wk total)

Available forms: Cap 200 mg

Implementation
• Only use in combination with peginterferon alfa and ribavirin; never give as monotherapy
• Discontinue in hepatitis C virus (HCV) RNA concentrations ≥100 IU/ml at wk 12 or a confirmed detectable HCV RNA concentrations at wk 24
• Any contraindication to peginterferon alfa or ribavirin also applies to boceprevir
• Give with food

ADVERSE EFFECTS
When used in combination with peginterferon/ribavarin
CNS: *Asthenia, chills,* dizziness, *fatigue,* insomnia, irritability
GI: Diarrhea, decreased appetite, dysgeusia, nausea, vomiting, xerostomia

---

HEMA: Anemia (Hgb <10 g/dl), neutropenia, thrombocytopenia
INTEG: *Alopecia, rash,* xerosis
MISC: *Arthralgia, exertional dyspnea,* drug rash with eosinophilia and systemic symptoms (DRESS) syndrome, exfoliative dermatitis, Stevens-Johnson syndrome, toxic epidermal necrolysis

Pharmacokinetics

Absorption	Unknown
Distribution	75% protein binding
Metabolism	By the enzyme aldoketoreductase (AKR) to a ketone-reduced metabolite; undergoes oxidative metabolism by the hepatic isoenzyme CYP3A4/5 and is a substrate for the drug efflux transporter, P-glycoprotein (PGP)
Excretion	Feces (79%),urine (9%)
Half-life	3.4 hrs

Pharmacodynamics

Onset	Unknown
Peak	2 hrs
Duration	Unknown

INTERACTIONS
Individual drugs
Alfuzosin, cisapride, ezetimibe, lovastatin, niacin with simvastatin and boceprevir, oral midazolam, pimozide, sildenafil, simvastatin, tadalafil (pulmonary arterial hypertension), triazolam: Increased, life-threatening reactions of each product: do not use concurrently

Acetaminophen, alfentanil, aliskiren, almotriptan, alosetron, ALPRAZolam, aminophylline, amiodarone, amitriptyline, amLODIPine, ARIPiprazole, astemizole, atorvastatin, bepridil, boceprevir, bosentan, budesonide, bupivacaine, buprenorphine, busPIRone, carvedilol, cevimeline, chloroquine, cilostazol, cinacalcet, citalopram, clarithromycin, clomiPRAMINE, clonazePAM, clopidogrel, cloZAPine, colchicine, cyclobenzaprine, cycloSPORINE, dapsone, DAUNOrubicin, desipramine, desloratadine, dexamethasone, dexlansoprazole, dextromethorphan, diazepam, diclofenac, digoxin, diltiazem, disopyramide, disulfiram, DOCEtaxel, dolasetron, donepezil, DOXOrubicin, droperidol, dutasteride, ebastine, eletriptan, eplerenone, erlotinib, erythromycin, estazolam, eszopi-

clone, ethosuximide, etoposide, exemestane, felodipine, fentaNYL, fexofenadine, finasteride, flecainide, flunitrazepam, flurazepam, galantamine, gefitinib, glyburide, granisetron, halofantrine, haloperidol, HYDROcodone, ifosfamide, imipramine, indiplon, irinotecan, isradipine, itraconazole, ivermectin, ixabepilone, ketoconazole, lansoprazole, lidocaine, loperamide, loratadine, losartan, maraviroc, mefloquine, meloxicam, mirtazapine, mitoMYcin, montelukast, morphine, nateglinide, niCARdipine, NIFEdipine, nisoldipine, nortriptyline, omeprazole, ondansetron, oxybutynin, oxyCODONE, PACLitaxel, palonosetron, paricalcitol, plicamycin, posaconazole, prasugrel, praziquantel, propafenone, quazepam, QUEtiapine, quinacrine, quiNIDine, ramelteon, repaglinide, rifabutin, risperiDONE, ropivacaine, salmeterol, selegiline, sertraline, sibutramine, silodosin, sirolimus, sitaxsentan, solifenacin, SUFentanil, SUNItinib, systemic corticosteroids, tacrolimus, telithromycin, teniposide, terfenadine, testosterone, theophylline, tiaGABine, tinidazole, tolterodine, tolvaptan, traMADol, traZODone, vardenafil, venlafaxine, verapamil, vinBLAStine, vinCRIStine, voriconazole, warfarin, and others: increased effect, adverse reactions of each product; use cautiously; may need to reduce dose

Drosperinone: increased hyperkalemia
Ethinyl estradiol: decreased estrogen levels
Methadone: decreased effect of this product
Efavirenz, ritonavir, atazanavir, lopinavir with ritonavir: possible treatment failure

Drug classifications
Ergots (dihydroergotamine, ergotamine, ergonovine, methylergonovine): do not use concurrently

Phosphodiesterase type 5 (PDE5) inhibitors (for erectile dysfunction): increased effect, adverse reactions of each product

CYP3A4 inhibitors (phenytoin, carBAMazepine, PHENobarbital, rifampin): decreased boceprevir effect

Drug/herb
Do not use with St. John's wort

Drug/lab test
Decreased: Hgb

NURSING CONSIDERATIONS
Assessment
⚠ Pregnancy: Obtain a pregnancy test prior to, monthly during, and for 6 months after treatment is completed; those who

are not willing to practice strict contraception should not receive treatment; report any cases of prenatal ribavirin exposure to the Ribavirin Pregnancy registry at (800) 593-2214

• **Anemia:** Monitor Hgb, CBC with differential prior to, at treatment wks 2, 4, 8, and 12, and as needed. If Hgb is less than 10 g/dl, decrease ribavirin dosage; if Hgb is less than 8.5 g/dl, discontinuation of therapy is recommended; dosage should not be altered based on adverse reactions; anemia may be managed through ribavirin dose modifications; never alter the dose of boceprevir. If anemia persists despite a reduction in ribavirin dose, consider discontinuing boceprevir. If management of anemia requires permanent discontinuation of ribavirin, treatment with boceprevir MUST also be permanently discontinued. Once boceprevir has been discontinued, it must not be restarted; monitor CBC with differential at treatment wks 4, 8, 12, and at other treatment points as needed

⚠ **Serious skin disorders (DRESS, Stevens-Johnson syndrome, toxic epidermal necrolysis, exfoliative dermatitis):** These reactions may be due to combination use with peginterferon alfa, ribavirin; if serious skin reactions occur, discontinue all three products

Patient/family education
⚠ Instruct patient to use 2 forms of effective contraception (intrauterine devices and barrier methods)
• Instruct patient to take with food to increase absorption
• Instruct patient to use precautions to prevent transmission of hepatitis C
• Instruct patient to inform prescriber of all medications, herbs, supplements used

Evaluation
Positive therapeutic outcome
• Resolution of hepatitis C infection

boric acid otic
See Appendix B

⚠ **HIGH ALERT**

bortezomib (Rx)
(bor-tez'oh-mib)
Velcade
Func. class.: Antineoplastic—miscellaneous
Chem. class.: Proteasome inhibitor
Pregnancy category D

ACTION: Reversible inhibitor of chymotrypsin-like activity in mammalian cells; causes a delay in tumor growth by disrupting normal homeostatic mechanisms

Therapeutic outcome: Decreased growth and spread of malignant cells

USES: Multiple myeloma previously untreated or when at least two other treatments have failed; mantle cell lymphoma

CONTRAINDICATIONS:
Pregnancy **D**, breastfeeding, hypersensitivity to this product, boron, or mannitol

Precautions: Peripheral neuropathy, children, geriatric, renal/hepatic disease, hypotension, tumor lysis syndrome, thrombocytopenia, infection, diabetes mellitus, bone marrow suppression

DOSAGE AND ROUTES
Multiple myeloma (previously untreated)
Adult: IV bol/subcut Give for 9 6-wk cycles; cycle 1-4, 1.3 mg/m²/dose given on days 1, 4, 8, 11, then a 10-day rest period (days 12-21) and again on days 22, 25, 29, 32, then a 10-day rest period (days 33-42) given with melphalan (9 mg/m²/day on days 1-4) and predniSONE (60 mg/m²/day on days 1-4); this 6-wk cycle is considered one course; in cycles 5-9, give bortezomib 1.3 mg/m²/dose on days 1, 8, 22, 29 with melphalan (9 mg/m²/day on days 1-4) and predniSONE (60 mg/m²/day on days 1-4); this 6-wk cycle is considered one course; at least 72 hr should elapse between consecutive doses

Mantle cell lymphoma
Adult: IV bol/subcut 1.3 mg/m²/dose (days 1, 4, 8, 11) followed by 10-day rest period (days 12 to 21); max 8 cycles

Neuropathic pain
Grade 1 with pain or grade 2, reduce to 1 mg/m²; grade 2 with pain or grade 3, hold product until toxicity resolves, then start at 0.7 mg/m²

---

qwk; grade 4 hematologic toxicities, withhold use

Hepatic dose
Adult: IV bilirubin >1.5 × ULN reduce to 0.7 mg/m² in cycle 1, consider dose escalation to 1 mg/m² or further reduction to 0.5 mg/m² in next cycles based on tolerability

Available forms: Lyophilized powder for inj 3.5 mg

Implementation
IV direct
- **Reconstitute** each vial with 3.5 ml 0.9% NaCl (1 mg/ml), sol should be clear/colorless; **inject** bol over 3-5 sec
- Store unopened product at room temperature, protect from light
- Use protective clothing during handling, preparation; avoid contact with skin
- Monitor for extravasation at inj site

SC route
- Reconstitute with 1.4 ml NS (2.5 mg/ml) or 3.5 ml NS (1 mg/ml); the 1 mg/ml may be used for local inj site reaction with the 2.5 mg/ml solution; the final product should be a clear, colorless solution; if any discoloration or particulate matter is observed, do not use
- Store reconstituted at room temperature, give within 8 hr of reconstitution, store ≤8 hr in a syringe; total storage time must be ≤8 hr when exposed to normal light
- Determine the volume of reconstituted bortezomib to be administered by multiplying the desired dose in mg/m² by the patient's BSA and dividing the result by the concentration (1 mg/ml or 2.5 mg/ml); discard unused drug, as no preservative is present
- Place a sticker that indicates subcut use on the syringe

SC inj
- Inject subcutaneously in the thigh or abdomen; do not inject into a site that is tender, bruised, erythematous, or indurated; rotate injection sites; new sites should be at least 1 inch from an old site
- Use of gloves and protective clothing are recommended to prevent skin contact

ADVERSE EFFECTS
CNS: Anxiety, insomnia, dizziness, headache, peripheral neuropathy, rigors, paresthesia, fever
CV: Hypotension, edema, **CHF**
GI: Abdominal pain, constipation, diarrhea, dyspepsia, *nausea*, vomiting, anorexia
HEMA: Anemia, **neutropenia, thrombocytopenia**

MISC: Dehydration, weight loss, herpes zoster, *rash*, pruritus, blurred vision
MS: Fatigue, malaise, weakness, arthralgia, bone pain, muscle cramps, myalgia, back pain, tumor lysis syndrome
RESP: Cough, pneumonia, dyspnea, URI, ARDs, pneumonitis, interstitial pneumonia, lung infiltration

Pharmacokinetics

Absorption	Unknown
Distribution	Protein binding 83%
Metabolism	P450 enzymes (3A4, 2D6, 2C19, 2C9, 1A2)
Excretion	Unknown
Half-life	9-15 hr

Pharmacodynamics
Unknown

INTERACTIONS
Individual drugs
Amiodarone, amprenavir, chloramphenicol, CISplatin, colchicine, cycloSPORINE, dapsone, didanosine, disulfiram, DOCEtaxel, gold salts, INH, iodoquinal, isoniazid, lamiVUDine, metroNIDAZOLE, nitrofurantoin, oxaliplatin, PACLitaxel, penicillamine, phenytoin, ritonavir, stavudine, sulfaSALAzine, thalidomide, vinBLAStine, vinCRIStine, zacatabine, zidovudine, and others: increased peripheral neuropathy

Drug classifications
Anticoagulants, NSAIDs, platelet inhibitors, salicylates, thrombolytics: increased bleeding risk
Antihypertensives: increased hypotension
Antivirals, statins, HMG-CoA reductase inhibitors: increased peripheral neuropathy
Hematopoietic pregenitor cells (sargramostim, filgrastim): do not use within 24 hr of chemotherapy
Oral hypoglycemics: increased hypo/hyperglycemia
Products that induce or inhibit CYP3A4: increased toxicity or decreased efficacy
Decreased: effect of norethindrone, estradiol, combination oral contraceptives, another nonhormonal contraceptive should be used
Fatal pulmonary toxicity: assess for risk factors, or new worsening pulmonary symptoms
Tumor lysis syndrome: usually with those with a high tumor burden

Adverse effects: *italics* = common; **bold** = life-threatening

Drug/herb
St. John's wort: toxicity or decreased efficacy

NURSING CONSIDERATIONS
Assessment
• Assess hematologic status: platelets, CBC throughout treatment

Patient/family education
⚠ **Teach to use contraception while on this product, avoid breastfeeding**
• Advise diabetic to monitor blood glucose levels
• Instruct to contact prescriber if new or worsening peripheral neuropathy, severe vomiting, diarrhea
• Advise to avoid driving, operating machinery until effect is known
• Advise to avoid using other medications unless approved by prescriber

Evaluation
Positive therapeutic outcome
• Improvement of multiple myeloma symptoms

---

bosentan (Rx)
(boh-sen-tan)
Tracleer
Func. class.: Vasodilator
Chem. class.: Endothelin receptor antagonist
Pregnancy category X

ACTION: Peripheral vasodilation occurs via antagonism of the effect of endothelin on endothelium and vascular smooth muscle

Therapeutic outcome: Decreased pulmonary arterial hypertension

USES: Pulmonary arterial hypertension with WHO class III, IV symptoms

Unlabeled uses: Septic shock to improve microcirculatory blood flow

CONTRAINDICATIONS:
Hypersensitivity, CVA, CAD

Precautions: Breastfeeding, children, geriatric, mitral stenosis, impaired hepatic function

> **BLACK BOX WARNING:** Pregnancy **X**, hepatic disease

DOSAGE AND ROUTES
Adult >40 kg and child >12 yr: PO 62.5 mg bid × 4 wk, then 125 mg bid
Adult <40 kg and child >12 yr: PO 62.5 mg bid

Adults taking a protease inhibitor for ≥10 days
Adult: PO 62.5 mg qday or every other day based on tolerance

Hepatic dose
Adult: PO
• Baseline AST/ALT <3× ULN: no dosage change, monitor LFTs qmo, reduce or interrupt if elevated
• AST/ALT >3 and ≤5× ULN: repeat test; if confirmed, reduce to 62.5 mg bid or interrupt; monitor LFTs q2wk, if interrupted, restart when LFTs <3× ULN, check LFTs within 3 days
• Increase in AST/ALT >5 and ≤5× ULN: during treatment, repeat test to confirm, discontinue, monitor LFTs q2wk until LFTs <3× ULN, restart at starting dose
• AST/ALT >8× ULN: discontinue permanently

Available forms: Tabs 62.5, 125 mg

Implementation
• Store at room temperature
• Only available through the TAP program 866-228-3546

ADVERSE EFFECTS
CNS: Headache, flushing, fatigue, fever
CV: *Hypo/hypertension,* palpitations, edema of lower limbs, fluid retention
GI: Abnormal liver function, dyspepsia, **hepatotoxicity,** diarrhea
HEMA: Anemia, leukopenia, neutropenia, lymphopenia, thrombocytopenia
INTEG: Pruritus, **Stevens-Johnson syndrome, toxic epidermal necrolysis,** rash
MISC: Anaphylaxis, oligospermia, **tumor lysis syndrome**
SYST: Secondary malignancy

Pharmacokinetics	
Absorption	50% absorbed
Distribution	Protein binding >98%
Metabolism	Liver (metabolites); metabolized CYP2C9, CYP3A4, and possibly CYP2C19; steady state 3-5 days
Excretion	Biliary
Half-life	5 hr

B

Pharmacodynamics

Unknown

INTERACTIONS
Individual drugs
CycloSPORINE A, glyBURIDE: do not coadminister

CycloSPORINE A, ketoconazole: increased bosentan level

CycloSPORINE: decreased cycloSPORINE level

GlyBURIDE: glyBURIDE level decreased significantly, bosentan also decreased, increased liver function tests

Ketoconazole: increased bosentan level

Simvastatin: decreased effects

Warfarin: decreased anticoagulation

Drug classifications
Contraceptives (hormonal), statins: decreased effects

CYP2C9, CYP3A4 inhibitors: increased bosentan effects

Drug/lab test
Increased: ALT, AST

Decreased: Hgb, Hct

NURSING CONSIDERATIONS
Assessment
⚠ **Serious skin toxicities:** angioedema occurring 8-21 days after initiating therapy
- Assess B/P, pulse during treatment until stable
- Assess hepatic toxicity: AST, ALT, bilirubin; liver enzymes may increase; if ALT/AST >3 and ≤5 × ULN, decrease dose or interrupt treatment and monitor AST/ALT q2wk; if >2 × ULN, and bilirubin >2 × ULN or signs of hepatitis, hepatic disease, stop treatment; vomiting, jaundice; product should be discontinued
- Assess blood studies: Hct, Hgb after 1 mo, 3 mo, then q3mo may be decreased
- Pulmonary hypertension/CHF: fluid retention, weight gain, increased leg edema; may occur within wks

Patient/family education
- Instruct patient to report jaundice, dark urine, joint pain, fatigue, malaise, bruising, easy bleeding

BLACK BOX WARNING: Pregnancy (**X**), monitor pregnancy test monthly

- Caution patient to avoid pregnancy; to use nonhormonal form of contraception; hormonal contraceptives may not be effective
- Instruct patient to take without regard to food

Evaluation
Positive therapeutic outcome
- Decrease in pulmonary hypertension

bosutinib
(boe-sue'ti-nib)
Bosulif
Func. class.: Antineoplastic biologic response modifiers
Chem. class.: Signal transduction inhibitors (STIs), tyrosine kinase inhibitor
Pregnancy category D

ACTION: Inhibits an enzyme (bcr-abl tyrosine kinase) created in patients with chronic myeloid leukemia (CML)

USES: Treatment of CML; Philadelphia-chromosome–positive patients in blast-cell crisis

CONTRAINDICATIONS:
Pregnancy (D), hypersensitivity

Precautions: Breastfeeding, children, diarrhea, geriatric patients, hepatic disease, bone marrow suppression, infection, thrombocytopenia, neutropenia, immunosuppression

DOSAGE AND ROUTES
Adult: PO 500 mg daily with food, may increase to 600 mg/day in those who have not developed grade 3 toxicity or in patients who do not reach complete hematological response by wk 8 or complete cytogenic response (CCyR) by wk 12

Hepatic dosage
Adult: PO Any baseline hepatic impairment: Start at 200 mg/day; liver transaminase >5 × ULN hold dose until levels ≤2.5 × ULN, then resume at 400 mg/day; liver transaminase level ≥3 × ULN and bilirubin >2 × ULN and alk phos <2 × ULN, discontinue

Dosage adjustments for treatment related toxicity
Hematologic toxicity: ANC <1000 × 10^6/L or platelet count <50,000 × 10^6/L: hold dose until ANC ≥1000 × 10^6/L and platelets ≥50,000 × 10^6/L; if recovery within 2 wks, resume therapy at the same dose; if blood counts remain low after 2 wks, upon recovery, resume at 100 mg/day less than the previous dose
Diarrhea: Grade 3 or 4 diarrhea (≥7 stools/day compared with baseline): hold therapy until recovery to grade 1 toxicity or lower; resume therapy at 400 mg/day

Other nonhematologic toxicity: Significant or moderate or severe toxicity: hold therapy until toxicity resolves; resume therapy at 400 mg/day

Available forms: Tabs 100, 500 mg

Implementation
PO route
• Give with food; swallow whole
• If dose is missed, take give within 12 hr of missed dose; if >12 hr have passed, skip dose
• Follow cytotoxic handling procedures

ADVERSE EFFECTS

CNS: Headache, dizziness
GI: Nausea, vomiting, anorexia, abdominal pain, diarrhea
HEMA: Neutropenia, thrombocytopenia, bleeding
INTEG: Rash, pruritus
MS: Arthralgia, myalgia
RESP: Cough, dyspnea, pleural effusion, edema
OTHER: Elevated LFTs

Pharmacokinetics

Absorption	Unknown
Distribution	Protein binding 96%
Metabolism	CYP3A4
Half-life	22.5 hr

Pharmacodynamics

Onset	Unknown
Peak	Unknown
Duration	Unknown

INTERACTIONS

Individual drugs
Simvastatin: Increased plasma concentrations

Drug classifications
CYP3A4 inhibitors (ketoconazole, itraconazole, erythromycin, clarithromycin): increased bosutinib concentrations
Simvastatin, calcium channel blockers, ergots: increased plasma concentrations
CYP3A4 inducers (dexamethasone, phenytoin, carBAMazepine, rifampin, PHENobarbital), antacids, proton-pump inhibitors: decrease bosutinib concentrations

Drug/food
Grapefruit juice: increased bosutinib effect; avoid use while taking product

Drug/herb
St. John's wort: Decreased bosutinib concentration

NURSING CONSIDERATIONS
Assessment
• Myelosuppression: Assess for anemia, thrombocytopenia, neutropenia; obtain a CBC weekly × 1 mo, then monthly as needed
• Monitor LFTs every mo × 3 mo, then as clinically indicated

Patient/family education
• Teach patient to immediately report adverse reactions, bleeding
• Teach patient about reason for treatment, expected results
• Advise patient to use effective contraception during treatment and up to 30 days after discontinuing treatment

Evaluation
Positive therapeutic outcome
• Decrease in leukemic cells or size of tumor

⚠ HIGH ALERT

brentuximab (Rx)
(bren-tak′see-mab)
Adcetris
Func. class.: Monoclonal antibody; antineoplastic
Pregnancy category D

ACTION: The anticancer activity is due to the binding of the ADC to CD30-expressing cells, followed by the internalization and transportation of the ADC-CD30 complex to lysosomes, and the release of MMAE via selective proteolytic cleavage. MMAE binds to tubulin and disrupts the microtubule network within the cell, inducing cell cycle arrest and apoptotic death of the cells

Therapeutic outcome: Decreasing symptoms of Hodgkin's disease (increased lymph nodes, night sweats, weight loss, splenomegaly, hepatomegaly)

USES: For the treatment of Hodgkin's disease after failure of autologous stem cell transplant (ASCT) or after failure of at least 2 prior multi-agent chemotherapy regimens in patients who are not ASCT candidates; For the treatment of non-Hodgkin's lymphoma (NHL): For the treatment of systemic anaplastic large cell lymphoma (sALCL) after failure of at least one prior multi-agent chemotherapy regimen

---

CONTRAINDICATIONS:
Hypersensitivity, pregnancy D

> **BLACK BOX WARNING:** Progressive multifocal leukoencephalopathy (PML)

Precautions: Breastfeeding, children, infants, neonates, neutropenia, peripheral neuropathy, tumor lysis syndrome (TLS)

DOSAGE AND ROUTES
Adult: IV 1.8 mg/kg IV over 30 minutes every 3 weeks until a maximum of 16 cycles, disease progression, or unacceptable toxicity. For patients >100 kg, max weight used for dosage calculation should be 100 kg, which translates to no more than 180 mg/dose

Dose adjustments for toxicity due to peripheral neuropathy:
For Grade <3: No dosage adjustments are recommended; For new or worsening grade 2/3: Interrupt treatment until toxicity resolves to grade ≤1; when resuming treatment, reduce dosage to 1.2 mg/kg IV q3wk; For Grade 4: Discontinue treatment

Dose adjustments for toxicity due to neutropenia:
For neutropenia Grade <3: No dosage adjustments; For Grade 3/4 neutropenia: Interrupt treatment until toxicity resolves to baseline or grade ≤2; consider the use of growth factors (CSFs) for subsequent cycles of therapy; For Grade 4 neutropenia despite the use of growth factors: Discontinue treatment or reduce the dose to 1.2 mg/kg IV q3wk

Available forms: Powder for injection 50 mg

Implementation:
Intermittent IV infusion route
• Visually inspect for particulate matter and discoloration whenever solution and container permit
• Give only as an IV infusion, do not give as an IV push or bolus
• Use cytoxic handling procedures
• Do not mix with, or administer as an infusion with, other IV products
• Calculate the dose (mg) and the number of vials required. For patients weighing >100 kg, use 100 kg to calculate the dose; reconstitute each 50 mg vial/10.5 ml of sterile water for injection (5 mg/ml)
• Direct the stream of sterile water toward the wall of the vial and not directly at the cake or powder; gently swirl the vial to aid in dissolution, do not shake
• Discard any unused portion left in the vial
• After reconstitution, dilute immediately with ≥100 ml of 0.9% sodium chloride, 5% dextrose, or lactated ringers solution to a final concentration (0.4 mg/ml-1.8 mg/ml)
• Use the diluted solution immediately or store in refrigerator for ≤24 hrs after reconstitution; do not freeze
• Infuse over 30 min

ADVERSE EFFECTS
CNS: Headache, dizziness, *fever,* peripheral neuropathy, anxiety, chills, confusion, *fatigue,* paresthesias, insomnia, night sweats, **progressive multifocal leukoencephalopathy (PML)**
CV: Peripheral edema, supraventricular arrhythmia
GI: *Abdominal pain, nausea, vomiting,* constipation, *diarrhea,* weight loss
HEMA: Anemia, neutropenia, thrombocytopenia
INTEG: *Rash,* pruritus, alopecia, xerosis
RESP: Pneumothorax, pneumonitis, pulmonary embolism, dyspnea, *cough*
SYST: Anaphylaxis, tumor lysis syndrome, antibody formation, Stevens-Johnson syndrome

Pharmacokinetics

Absorption	Unknown
Distribution	Protein binding, 68%-82%
Metabolism	Small amount, potent inhibitors or inducers of CYP3A4, may alter action
Excretion	Unknown
Half-life	Terminal 4-6 days; three components are released: MMAE (monomethyl auristatin E), ADC, and the total antibody; the half-life of MMAE a component is 3.43-3.6 days

Pharmacodynamics

Onset	Unknown
Peak	ADC: End of infusion MME: 1-3 days
Duration	Unknown

INTERACTIONS
Individual drugs
Boceprevir, dalfopristin; delavirdine, isoniazid, indinavir, itraconazole, ketoconazole, qui-

nupristin, rifampin, ritonavir, telithromycin, tipranavir: increased brentuximab component action:

Bleomycin: increased non-infectious pulmonary toxicity; do not use together

Drug/herb
St. John's wort: increased brentuximab component action

NURSING CONSIDERATIONS
Assessment
⚠ **Tumor lysis syndrome (TLS): Assess for hyperkalemia, hyperphosphatemia, hypocalcemia; may develop renal failure may use allopurinol or rasburicase to prevent TLS; monitor serum BUN/Creatinine**
⚠ **Pregnancy: determine if pregnancy is planned or suspected, pregnancy D**
⚠ **Progressive multifocal leukoencephalopathy (PML): Assess for weakness, or paralysis, vision loss, impaired speech, and cognitive deterioration; often fatal**
• Monitor CBC and differential

Patient/family education
⚠ **Teach patient to report immediately weakness, change in vision, impaired speech**
⚠ **Advise patient to use reliable contraception, pregnancy D; avoid breastfeeding**
• Use the diluted sol immediately or store in refrigerator for ≤24 hr after reconstitution; do not freeze

Evaluation
Positive therapeutic outcome
• Decreasing symptoms of Hodgkin's disease (increased lymph nodes, night sweats, weight loss, splenomegaly, hepatomegaly)

brimonidine ophthalmic
See Appendix B

brinzolamide ophthalmic
See Appendix B

bromfenac ophthalmic
See Appendix B

bromocriptine (Rx)
(broe-moe-krip′teen)
Cycloset, Parlodel
Func. class.: Antiparkinsonian agent; DOPamine receptor agonist
Chem. class.: Ergot alkaloid derivative
Pregnancy category B

Do not confuse:
bromocriptine/benztropine/brimonidine, Parlodel/pindolol/Provera

ACTION: Inhibits prolactin release by activating postsynaptic dopamine receptors; activation of striatal dopamine receptors may be reason for improvement in Parkinson's disease

Therapeutic outcome: Decreased involuntary movements in Parkinson's disease; decreased breastfeeding; decreased hormone levels in acromegaly; absence of amenorrhea in hyperprolactinemia

USES: Parkinson's disease, amenorrhea/galactorrhea caused by hyperprolactinemia, infertility, acromegaly, pituitary adenomas, adjunct in type 2 diabetes

Unlabeled uses: Neuroleptic malignant syndrome, alcoholism, premenstrual syndrome, mastalgia, cocaine withdrawal, premenstrual breast syndromes

CONTRAINDICATIONS:
Hypersensitivity to ergot, bromocriptine; severe ischemic disease, severe peripheral vascular disease, uncontrolled hypertension, preeclampsia, migraine

Precautions: Pregnancy **B**, breastfeeding, children, hepatic/renal disease, pituitary tumors, peptic ulcer disease, sulfite hypersensitivity, pulmonary fibrosis, dementia, GI bleeding, bipolar disorder

DOSAGE AND ROUTES
Hyperprolactinemia
Adult: PO 1.25-2.5 mg with meals; may increase by 2.5 mg q3-7days; usual dosage 2.5-15 mg/day

Acromegaly
Adult: PO 1.25-2.5 mg/day × 3 days at bedtime; may increase by 1.25-2.5 mg q3-7days; usual range 20-30 mg/day; max 100 mg/day

B

Type 2 diabetes (Cycloset only)
Adult: PO (initially) 0.8 mg qd in AM within 2hr of waking, titrate by 0.8 mg/day no more than qwk to max 1.6-4.8 mg/day

Parkinson's disease
Adult: PO 1.25 mg bid with meals; may increase q2-4wk by 2.5 mg/day; not to exceed 100 mg/day, levodopa should be continued while bromocriptine is being instituted

Pituitary adenoma
Adult: PO 1.25 mg bid-tid, may increase over several weeks to 10-20 mg/day

Neuroleptic malignant syndrome (unlabeled)
Adult: PO 2.5-10 mg tid

Cocaine withdrawal (unlabeled)
Adult: PO 0.625 mg qid × 42 days

Alcoholism (unlabeled)
Adult: PO 7.5 mg/day

Mastalgia (unlabeled)
Adult: PO 2.5-7.5 bid, starting 10-14 days prior to menses, discontinue when menses begins

Available forms: Caps 5 mg; tabs 2.5 mg; Cycloset tabs 0.8 mg

Implementation
• Give with meals or milk to prevent GI symptoms; crush tab if patient has swallowing difficulty
• Give at bedtime so dizziness, orthostatic hypotension do not occur
• Store at room temperature in air-tight container

ADVERSE EFFECTS
CNS: *Headache,* depression, restlessness, anxiety, nervousness, confusion, **seizures,** hallucinations, *dizziness,* fatigue, drowsiness, abnormal involuntary movements, psychosis
CV: *Orthostatic hypotension,* decreased B/P, palpitations, extrasystole, **shock,** dysrhythmias, bradycardia, **MI**
EENT: Blurred vision, diplopia, burning eyes, nasal congestion
GI: *Nausea, vomiting, anorexia,* cramps, constipation, diarrhea, dry mouth, GI hemorrhage
GU: Frequency, retention, incontinence, diuresis
INTEG: *Rash on face, arms,* alopecia, coolness, pallor of fingers, toes, peripheral edema

Absorption	Poorly absorbed
Distribution	Unknown
Metabolism	Liver, completely
Excretion	85%-98% feces
Half-life	4 hr (initial); 50 hr (terminal)

Pharmacodynamics

Onset	½-1½ hr
Peak	1-3 hr
Duration	8-12 hr

INTERACTIONS
Individual drugs
Alcohol: increased disulfiram-like reaction
Chloramphenicol, levodopa, probenecid: increased neurologic effects
Haloperidol, loxapine, methyldopa, metoclopramide, reserpine: decreased levels of bromocriptine
Levodopa: increased neurologic effects
Metoclopramide: decreased effect of bromocriptine

Drug classifications
Antihypertensives: increased hypotension
Butyrophenones, CYP3A4 inhibitors, phenothiazines, thioxanthenes: decreased bromocriptine effect
Contraceptives (oral), estrogens, MAOIs, phenothiazines, progestins: decreased levels of bromocriptine
CYP3A4 inducers: increased bromocriptine effect
Salicylates, sulfonamides: increased neurologic effects

Drug/herb
Horehound: increased serotonin effect

Drug/lab test
Increased: growth hormone, AST, ALT, BUN, CK, uric acid, alkaline phosphatase

NURSING CONSIDERATIONS
Assessment
• Assess symptoms of **Parkinson's disease** (EPS): shuffling gait, muscle rigidity, involuntary movements, pill rolling, muscle spasms, drooling before, during treatment
• Assess for resolution of symptoms of **neuroleptic malignant syndrome:** decreased temp, seizures, sweating, pulse
• Monitor for change in size of soft tissue volume in acromegaly

• Pregnancy: may cause postpartum conception, use pregnancy testing q4wk or if menstruation does not occur
• Monitor B/P; establish baseline, compare with other readings; this product decreases B/P and causes orthostatic hypotension; patient should remain recumbent for 2-4 hr after first dose; supervise ambulation

Patient/family education
• Advise patient to change position slowly to prevent orthostatic hypotension
• Tabs may be crushed and mixed with food; bromocriptine to be taken within 2 hr of rising
• Caution patient to use contraceptives during treatment with this product; pregnancy may occur; to use methods other than oral contraceptives/subdermal implants
• Teach patient that therapeutic effect for Parkinson's disease may take 2 mo: galactorrhea, amenorrhea
• Caution patient to avoid hazardous activity if dizziness, drowsiness occurs during treatment start-up
• Advise patient to avoid alcohol and OTC medication unless approved by prescriber
• Teach patients with acromegaly to notify prescriber immediately if severe headache, nausea, vomiting, blurred vision occur; indicates change in or enlargement of tumor
• Advise patient to report symptoms of MI immediately
• Teach patient to take with food, avoid alcohol

Evaluation
Positive therapeutic outcome
• Parkinson's disease: decreased slow movements, decreased drooling
• Decreased breast engorgement with accompanied pain, tenderness
• Acromegly: decreased growth hormone levels

budesonide (Rx)
(byoo-des′oh-nide)
Entocort EC, Pulmicort, Pulmicort Flexhaler, Pulmicort Respules, Pulmicort Turbohaler, Rhinocort Aqua, Uceris
Func. class.: Glucocorticoid
Pregnancy category C

ACTION: Prevents inflammation by depression of migration of polymorphonuclear leukocytes, fibroblasts, reversal of increased capillary permeability and lysosomal stabilization; does not suppress hypothalamus and pituitary function

USES: Rhinitis; prophylaxis for asthma; Crohn's disease, ulcerative colitis

CONTRAINDICATIONS:
Hypersensitivity, status asthmaticus

Precautions: Pregnancy **C**; inhaled form pregnancy **B**; breastfeeding, children, TB, fungal, bacterial, systemic viral infections, ocular herpes simplex, nasal septal ulcers; hepatic disease (caps)

DOSAGE AND ROUTES
Rhinitis (Rhinocort Aqua)
Adult and child >6 yr: Spray/inh 256 mcg/day (2 sprays in each nostril AM, PM, or 4 sprays in each nostril AM)

Asthma
Adult and child >6 yr: INH 400-1200 mcg/day

Crohn's disease, ulcerative colitis (Uceris)
Adult: PO 9 mg daily AM × 8 wk

Laryngotracheobronchitis (croup) (unlabeled)
Infant ≥3 months-child ≤5 yr: (Pulmicort Respules INH susp) 2 mg inhaled as a single dose

Available forms: Dry powder for INH 90, 180, 200 mg/actuation (Pulmicort Flexhaler); 32 mcg/actuation (Rhinocort Aqua) nasal spray; susp for inh 0.5 mg/2 ml, 0.25 mg/2 ml; ext rel tab (Uceris) 9 mg; cap 3 mg

Implementation
PO route (Crohn's disease)
• Swallow caps whole; do not break, crush, or chew
• May repeat 8-wk course if needed; may taper to 6 mg/day for 2 wk before cessation
Oral inh route (dry powder for inh) (Pulmicort Turbuhaler)
• A new Turbuhaler should be primed before use, per the priming instructions that come with the device; while priming the Turbuhaler and loading the dose, hold in upright position; to load the dose on a primed inhaler, twist the brown grip fully to the right as far as it will go, then twist it back fully to the left; there will be the sound of a "click"
• When inhaling, the Turbuhaler may be held upright or horizontally; turn head away from the inhaler and breathe out; place the mouthpiece between the lips and inhale deeply and forcefully; remove the inhaler from the mouth and exhale normally; do not blow or exhale into the

mouthpiece; do not chew or bite on the mouthpiece; if more than one dose is required, repeat the steps
• After the last dose, rinse the mouth with water; do not swallow the water; keep inhaler clean and dry

Inh susp route for nebulization (Pulmicort Respules)
• Use via jet nebulizer connected to an air compressor with adequate airflow, and equipped with a mouthpiece or suitable face mask; do not use ultrasonic nebulizers
• See manufacturer's direction on use of nebulizer and preparation of the solution
• Gently shake the ampule in a circular motion before opening it and placing the suspension in the nebulizer reservoir; using the "blow by" technique (i.e., holding the face mask or open tube near the patient's nose and mouth) is not recommended; use inh susp separately in the nebulizer
• Store inhal susp upright at controlled room temperature and protected from light; after opening the envelope, the shelf life of the unused respules is 2 wk; return unused respules to the aluminum foil envelope to protect from light; opened respule should be used promptly

Intranasal inhalation route
• Instruct patient on proper nasal inhalation priming and use; shake inhaler well; prior to initial use, the Rhinocort Aqua container must be shaken gently and the pump must be primed by actuating 8 times; if used daily, the pump does not need to be reprimed; if not used for 2 consecutive days, reprime with 1 spray or until a fine spray appears; if not used for more than 14 days, rinse the applicator and reprime with 2 sprays or until a fine spray appears; blow nose gently, without squeezing; with head upright, spray into each nostril; sniff while squeezing the bottle quickly and firmly; after use, rinse the tip of the bottle with hot water, taking care not to suck water into the bottle, and dry with a clean tissue; replace the cap
• To avoid the spread of infection, do not use the container for more than one person
• Store at 59°-86° F (15°-30° C); keep away from heat, open flame

ADVERSE EFFECTS

CNS: *Headache,* insomnia, hypertonia, syncope, dizziness, drowsiness
CV: Chest pain, hypertension, sinus tachycardia, palpitation
EENT: *Sinusitis, pharyngitis,* rhinitis, oral candidiasis

ENDO: Adrenal insufficiency, growth suppression in children
GI: Dry mouth, dyspepsia, nausea, vomiting, abdominal pain
MISC: Ecchymosis, fever, *hypersensitivity,* flulike symptoms, epistaxis, dysuria
MS: Back pain, myalgias, fractures
RESP: Nasal irritation, cough, nasal bleeding, *respiratory infections,* **bronchospasm**

Pharmacokinetics

Absorption	39%
Distribution	In airways, protein binding 85%-90%
Metabolism	Liver
Excretion	In urine (60%), small amounts in feces, enters breast milk
Half-life	2-3.6 hr

Pharmacodynamics

Onset	Respules 2-8 days, Rhinocort Aqua 10 hr
Peak	Respules 4-6 wk, Rhinocort Aqua 2 wk
Duration	Unknown

INTERACTIONS

Individual drugs
Varicella live vaccine: avoid concurrent use in pediatric patients

Drug classifications
CYP3A inhibitors: increased budesonide effect; dose adjustment may be required

NURSING CONSIDERATIONS
Assessment
• Assess respiratory status: rate, rhythm, increase in bronchial secretions, wheezing, chest tightness; provide fluids to 2 L/day to decrease thickness of secretions; check for oral candidiasis
• For **bronchospasm**, stop treatment and give bronchodilator
• With viral infections, corticosteroid use can mask infections
• For increased intraocular pressure, discontinue use if increase occurs

Patient/family education
• Teach patient to notify prescriber of pharyngitis, nasal bleeding, oral candidiasis
• Instruct patient not to exceed recommended dosage; adrenal suppression may occur

- Teach patient to carry/wear emergency ID identifying steroid use
- Instruct patient to read and follow package directions
- Instruct patient to prevent exposure to infections, especially viral
- Advise to use good oral hygiene if using by nebulizer or inhaler
- Teach patient to avoid breastfeeding
- Teach patient that product is not a bronchodilator and is not to be used for asthma; to use regularly
- Teach how to use as described in "administer"
- Advise to notify prescriber if symptoms persist after 3 wk, that results usually take 2 wk
- Advise to notify prescriber if exposure to measles, chickenpox occurs

Evaluation
Positive therapeutic outcome
- Absence of asthma, rhinitis

budesonide nasal agent
See Appendix B

bumetanide (Rx)
(byoo-met′a-nide)
Func. class.: Loop diuretic, antihypertensive
Chem. class.: Sulfonamide derivative
Pregnancy category C

ACTION: Acts on the ascending loop of Henle in the kidney to inhibit the reabsorption of the electrolytes sodium and chloride

Therapeutic outcome: Decreased edema in lung tissue and peripherally; decreased B/P

USES: Edema in congestive heart failure, renal/hepatic disease, ascites, heart failure

CONTRAINDICATIONS:
Hypersensitivity to sulfonamides, anuria, hepatic coma

BLACK BOX WARNING: Electrolyte imbalance

Precautions: Pregnancy **C,** breastfeeding, neonates, severe renal disease, ascites, hepatic cirrhosis, blood dyscrasias, ototoxicity, hyperuricemia, hypokalemia, hyperglycemia, oliguria, hypomagnesemia, hypovolemia

BLACK BOX WARNING: Dehydration

DOSAGE AND ROUTES
Adult/adolescent: PO 0.5-2 mg daily may give 2nd or 3rd dose at 4-5 hr intervals; max 10 mg/day; may be given on alternate days or intermittently; IM/IV 0.5-1 mg; may give 2nd or 3rd dose at 2-3 hr intervals; max 10 mg/day
Child (unlabeled): PO/IM/IV 0.015-0.1 mg/kg/day or every other day, max 10 mg/day

Available forms: Tabs 0.5, 1, 2 mg; inj 0.25 mg/ml

Implementation
- Give in AM to avoid interference with sleep
- Potassium replacement if potassium level is <3.0 mg/dl whole, or use oral solutions; product may be crushed if patient is unable to swallow

PO route
- With food, if nausea occurs; absorption may be reduced; the safest dosage schedule is on alternate days

IV route
- Do not use solution that is yellow or has a precipitate or crystals

IV, direct route
- Give undiluted through Y-tube or 3-way stopcock; give 20 mg or less/min

Intermittent IV infusion route
- May be added to 0.9% NaCl, D_5W, $D_{10}W$, $D_{20}W$, invert sugar 10% in electrolyte #1, LR, sodium lactate ⅙ mol/L; use within 24 hr to ensure compatibility; give through Y-tube or 3-way stopcock; give at 4 mg/min or less; use infusion pump

Syringe compatibility: Doxapram

Y-site compatibilities: Acyclovir, alfentanil, allopurinol, amifostine, amikacin, aminocaproic acid, aminophylline, amiodarone, amoxicillin, amphotericin B lipid complex (Abelcet), amphotericin B liposome (AmBisome), anidulafungin, ascorbic acid injection, atenolol, atracurium, atropine, aztreonam, benztropine, bivalirudin, bleomycin, buprenorphine, butorphanol, calcium chloride/gluconate, CARBOplatin, caspofungin, cefamandole, ceFAZolin, cefepime, cefmetazole, cefonicid, cefoperazone, cefotaxime, cefoTEtan, cefOXitin, cefTAZidime, ceftizoxime, ceftobiprole, cefTRIAXone, cefuroxime, cephalothin, cephapirin, chloramphenicol, cimetidine, cisatracurium, CISplatin, cladribine, clarithromycin, clindamycin, codeine, cyanocobalamin, cyclophosphamide, cycloSPORINE, cytarabine, DACTINomycin, DAPTOmycin, dexamethasone, dexmedetomidine, digoxin, diltiazem, diphenhydrAMINE, DOBUTamine,

DOCEtaxel, DOPamine, doripenem, doxacurium, DOXOrubicin, doxycycline, enalaprilat, ePHEDrine, EPINEPHrine, epirubicin, epoetin alfa, eptifibatide, ertapenem, erythromycin, esmolol, etoposide, famotidine, fentaNYL, filgrastim, fluconazole, fludarabine, fluorouracil, folic acid, furosemide, gatifloxacin, gemcitabine, gentamicin, glycopyrrolate, granisetron, heparin, hydrocortisone sodium succinate, HYDROmorphone, hydrOXYzine, IDArubicin, ifosfamide, imipenem-cilastatin, indomethacin, insulin (regular), irinotecan, isoproterenol, ketorolac, labetalol, levofloxacin, lidocaine, linezolid, LORazepam, magnesium sulfate, mannitol, mechlorethamine, melphalan, meperidine, metaraminol, methotrexate, methoxamine, methyldopa, methylPREDNISolone, metoclopramide, metoprolol, metroNIDAZOLE, mezlocillin, micafungin, miconazole, milrinone, mitoXANtrone, morphine, moxalactam, multiple vitamins injection, mycophenolate, nafcillin, nalbuphine, naloxone, netilmicin, nitroglycerin, nitroprusside, norepinephrine, octreotide, ondansetron, oxacillin, oxaliplatin, oxytocin, palonosetron, pamidronate, pancuronium, pantoprazole, PEMEtrexed, penicillin G potassium/sodium, pentazocine, PENTobarbital, PHENobarbital, phenylephrine, phytonadione, piperacillin, piperacillin-tazobactam, polymyxin B, potassium chloride, procainamide, promethazine, propofol, propranolol, protamine, pyridoxine, quiNIDine, ranitidine, remifentanil, rifampin, ritodrine, riTUXimab, rocuronium, sodium acetate, sodium bicarbonate, succinylcholine, SUFentanil, tacrolimus, teniposide, theophylline, thiamine, thiotepa, ticarcillin, ticarcillin-clavulanate, tigecycline, tirofiban, TNA, tobramycin, tolazoline, TPN, traMADol, trastuzumab, trimetaphan, urokinase, vancomycin, vasopressin, vecuronium, verapamil, vinCRIStine, vinorelbine, voriconazole

ADVERSE EFFECTS

CNS: Headache, fatigue, weakness, vertigo, encephalopathy
CV: *Hypotension,* chest pain, ECG changes, **circulatory collapse,** dehydration
EENT: Loss of hearing
ELECT: *Hypokalemia, hypochloremic alkalosis, hypomagnesemia, hyperuricemia, hypocalcemia, hyponatremia*
ENDO: *Hyperglycemia*
GI: *Nausea,* diarrhea, dry mouth, vomiting, anorexia, cramps, **acute pancreatitis,** upset stomach, abdominal pain, **jaundice**
GU: *Polyuria,* **renal failure,** *glycosuria,* premature ejaculation, hypercholesterolemia

HEMA: **Thrombocytopenia, leukopenia, granulocytopenia, hemoconcentration**
INTEG: *Rash, pruritus, purpura,* **Stevens-Johnson syndrome,** sweating, photosensitivity
MS: Muscular cramps, stiffness, arthritis

Pharmacokinetics

	PO/IM
Absorption	Rapidly, completely absorbed
	PO/IM/IV
Distribution	Crosses placenta, protein binding >91%
Metabolism	Liver (30%-40%)
Excretion	Breast milk, urine (50% unchanged), feces (20%)
Half-life	1-1½ hr; 6-15 hr neonates

Pharmacodynamics

	PO	IM	IV
Onset	½-1 hr	40 min	5 min
Peak	1-2 hr	1-2 hr	½ hr
Duration	3-6 hr	4-6 hr	3-6 hr

INTERACTIONS
Individual drugs
Digoxin: increased toxicity
Indomethacin: decreased diuretic and antihypertensive effects of bumetanide
Lithium: decreased renal clearance causing increased toxicity
Metolazone: increased diuresis, electrolyte loss
Probenecid: decreased diuretic effect

Drug classifications
Aminoglycosides: increased ototoxicity
Antidiabetics: decreased antidiabetic effects
NSAIDs: decreased diuretic effect
Potassium-wasting products: increased hypokalemia

Drug/herb
Hawthorn, horse chestnut: increased diuretic effect

NURSING CONSIDERATIONS
Assessment
• Assess patient for tinnitus, hearing loss, ear pain; periodic testing of hearing is needed when high doses of this product are given by **IV** route
• Assess fluid volume status: I&O ratio and record, distended red veins, crackles in lung, color, quality and specific gravity of urine, skin turgor, adequacy of pulses, moist mucous membranes, bilateral lung sounds, peripheral pitting edema; dehydration symptoms of decreasing output, thirst, hypotension, dry mouth and mu-

Adverse effects: *italics* = common; **bold** = life-threatening

cous membranes should be reported; if urinary output decreases or azotemia occurs, product should be discontinued

- Monitor for electrolyte imbalances: potassium, sodium, calcium, magnesium; also include BUN, blood pH, ABGs, uric acid, CBC, blood glucose; severe electrolyte imbalances should be corrected before starting treatment
- Assess B/P before and during therapy with patient lying, standing, and sitting as appropriate; orthostatic hypotension can occur rapidly
- Monitor for **digoxin toxicity** (anorexia, nausea, vomiting, confusion, paresthesia, muscle cramps) in patients taking digoxin; lithium toxicity in those taking lithium

Patient/family education
- Teach patient to take the medication early in the day to prevent nocturia
- Instruct the patient to take with food or milk if GI symptoms of nausea and anorexia occur
- Teach patient to maintain weekly record of weight and notify prescriber of weight loss of >5 lb
- Caution the patient that this product causes a loss of potassium, so food rich in potassium should be added to the diet; refer to a dietitian for assistance in planning
- Caution the patient not to exercise in hot weather or stand for prolonged periods since orthostatic hypotension will be enhanced
- Teach patient not to use alcohol or any OTC medications without prescriber's approval; serious product reactions may occur
- Emphasize the need to contact prescriber immediately if muscle cramps, weakness, nausea, dizziness, or numbness occur
- Teach patient to take own B/P and pulse and record
- Caution the patient that orthostatic hypotension may occur; patient should rise slowly from sitting or reclining positions and lie down if dizziness occurs
- Teach patient to continue taking medication even if feeling better; this product controls symptoms but does not cure the condition
- Advise the patient with hypertension to continue other medical treatment (exercise, weight loss, relaxation techniques, cessation of smoking)

Evaluation
Positive therapeutic outcome
- Decreased edema
- Decreased B/P
- Increased diuresis

buprenorphine (Rx)
(byoo-pre-nor'feen)
Buprenex, Butrans, Subutex
Func. class.: Opioid analgesic, partial agonist
Chem. class.: Thebaine derivative
Pregnancy category C
Controlled substance schedule V (parenteral); schedule III (tablet)

Do not confuse:
Buprenex/Bumex

ACTION: Depresses pain impulse transmission at the spinal cord level by interacting with opioid receptors

Therapeutic outcome: Relief of pain

USES: Moderate to severe pain, opiate agonist withdrawal

Unlabeled uses: Cocaine

CONTRAINDICATIONS:
Hypersensitivity, ileus, status asthmaticus

> **BLACK BOX WARNING:** Respiratory depression

Precautions: Pregnancy **C**, breastfeeding, substance abuse/alcoholism, increased intracranial pressure, MI (acute), severe heart disease, respiratory depression, renal/hepatic/pulmonary disease, hypothyroidism, Addison's disease

> **BLACK BOX WARNING:** QT prolongation, use of heating pad, accidental exposure, potential for overdose/poisoning, substance abuse

DOSAGE AND ROUTES
Adult: IM/IV 0.3 mg q6hr prn; may repeat; reduce dosage in geriatric, may repeat after 30-60 min; EPIDURAL (unlabeled) 4 mcg/kg or 2 mcg/kg (epidural injection), remove over 48 hr; TD: each patch is worn for 7 days (moderate-severe pain); **opioid-naive patients** (those taking <30 mg oral morphine or equivalent prior to beginning treatment with TD buprenorphine), 5 mcg/hr q7days, overestimating dose can be fatal; **conversion from other opiate agonist therapy,** titrate from other opioids for up to 7 days to no more than 30 mg oral morphine or equivalent prior to beginning TD therapy, begin with 5 mcg/hr q7days; for those with daily dose of 30-80 mg oral morphine or equivalent, start

with 10 mcg/hr q7days; for those >80 mg oral morphine or equivalent start with 20 mcg/hr q7days

Child 2-12 yr: IM/IV 2-6 mcg/kg q4-6hr

Opiate dependence
Adult/adolescent ≥16 yr: SL 8 mg day 1, 16 mg day 2, then maintenance 16 mg daily

Available forms: Inj 0.3 mg/ml (1-ml vials); SL tab 2, 8 mg as base, TD system 5, 10, 20 mcg/hr (weekly)

Implementation
• Give by inj (**IM**, **IV**), only with resuscitative equipment available; give slowly to prevent rigidity

SL route
• Do not chew, dissolve under tongue or take 2 or more at same time

Transdermal route
• Apply to clean, dry, intact skin, each patch should be worn for 7 days, may use first aid tape if edge of patch is not adhering

> **BLACK BOX WARNING:** Do not apply direct heat source to patch

• Apply to upper outer arm, upper chest/back, or side of chest

IM route
• **Give** deep in large muscle mass; rotate sites of inj

IV route
• **Give IV** direct undiluted over ≥3-5 min (0.3 mg/2 min); give slowly
• With antiemetic if nausea, vomiting occur
• When pain is beginning to return; determine dosage interval by patient response; rapid injection will increase side effects

Syringe compatibilities: Glycopyrrolate, haloperidol, heparin, midazolam

Y-site compatibilities: Acyclovir, alfentanil, allopurinol, amifostine, amikacin, aminocaproic acid, amphotericin B liposome (AmBisone), anidulafungin, ascorbic acid injection, atenolol, atracurium, atropine, aztreonam, benztropine, bivalirudin, bleomycin, bumetanide, butorphanol, calcium chloride/gluconate, CARBOplatin, cefamandole, ce-FAZolin, cefepime, cefoperazone, cefotaxime, cefoTEtan, cefOXitin, cefTAZidime, ceftizoxime, cefTRIAXone, cefuroxime, chloramphenicol, chlorproMAZINE, cimetidine, cisatracurium, CISplatin, cladribine, clindamycin, cyanocobalamin, cyclophosphamide, cycloSPORINE, cytarabine, D₅W-dextrose 5%, DACTINomycin, DAPTOmycin, dexamethasone, dexmedetomi-

dine, digoxin, diltiazem, diphenhydrAMINE, DOBUTamine, DOCEtaxel, DOPamine, doxacurium, DOXOrubicin HCl, doxycycline, enalaprilat, ePHEDrine, EPINEPHrine, epirubicin, epoetin alfa, eptifibatide, ertapenem, erythromycin, esmolol, etoposide, famotidine, fenoldopam, fentaNYL, filgrastim, fluconazole, fludarabine, gatifloxacin, gemcitabine, gentamicin, glycopyrrolate, granisetron, heparin, hydrocortisone, hydrOXYzine, IDArubicin, ifosfamide, imipenem-cilastatin, inamrinone, insulin (regular), irinotecan, isoproterenol, ketorolac, labetalol, lactated Ringer's injection, levofloxacin, lidocaine, linezolid, LORazepam, magnesium sulfate, mannitol, mechlorethamine, melphalan, meperidine, metaraminol, methicillin, methotrexate, methoxamine, methyldopate, methylPREDNISolone, metoclopramide, metoprolol, metroNIDAZOLE, mezlocillin, miconazole, midazolam, milrinone, minocycline, mitoXANtrone, morphine, moxalactam, multiple vitamins injection, mycophenolate mofetil, nafcillin, nalbuphine, naloxone, nesiritide, netilmicin, nitroglycerin, nitroprusside, norepinephrine, octreotide, ondansetron, oxacillin, oxaliplatin, oxytocin, palonosetron, pamidronate, pancuronium, papaverine, PEMEtrexed, penicillin G potassium/sodium, pentamidine, pentazocine, phenylephrine, phytonadione, piperacillin, piperacillin-tazobactam, polymyxin B, potassium chloride, procainamide, prochlorperazine promethazine, propofol, propranolol, protamine, pyridoxine, quiNIDine, ranitidine, remifentanil, Ringer's injection, riTUXimab, rocuronium, sodium acetate, succinylcholine, SUFentanil, tacrolimus, teniposide, theophylline, thiamine, thiotepa, ticarcillin, ticarcillin-clavulanate, tigecycline, tirofiban, TNA (3-in-1), tobramycin, tolazoline, TPN, trastuzumab, trimetaphan, urokinase, vancomycin, vasopressin, vecuronium, verapamil, vinCRIStine, vinorelbine, voriconazole

Additive compatibilities: Atropine, bupivacaine, diphenhydrAMINE, droperidol, glycopyrrolate, haloperidol, hydrOXYzine, promethazine, scopolamine

Additive incompatibilities: Diazepam, floxacillin, furosemide, LORazepam

ADVERSE EFFECTS
CNS: *Drowsiness, dizziness, confusion, headache, sedation, euphoria,* **increased intracranial pressure,** amnesia
CV: Palpitations, bradycardia, change in B/P, tachycardia
EENT: Tinnitus, blurred vision, *miosis,* diplopia

GI: *Nausea,* vomiting, anorexia, constipation, cramps, dry mouth
GU: Dysuria, urinary retention
INTEG: *Rash,* urticaria, bruising, flushing, diaphoresis, pruritus
RESP: Respiratory depression, dyspnea, hypo/hyperventilation

Pharmacokinetics

Absorption	Well absorbed (IM)
Distribution	Crosses placenta
Metabolism	Liver, extensively by CYP3A4
Excretion	Kidneys, feces, breast milk
Half-life	2.2 hr (**IV**); 26 hr (transdermal); 37 hr (SL)

Pharmacodynamics

	IM	IV
Onset	15 min	Immediate
Peak	1 hr	5 min
Duration	6 hr (Epidural route: duration is dose-dependent)	6 hr

INTERACTIONS
Individual drugs
Alcohol: increased respiratory depression, hypotension, sedation

Drug classifications

> **BLACK BOX WARNING:** Antidysrhythmics (class IA, III): increased QT prolongation

Antihistamines, antipsychotics, CNS depressants, MAOIs, sedatives/hypnotics, skeletal muscle relaxants: increased respiratory depression, hypotension
CYP3A4 inducers (carBAMazepine, PHENobarbital, phenytoin, rifampin): decreased buprenorphine effect
CYP3A4 inhibitors (erythromycin, indinavir, ketoconazole, ritonavir, saquinavir): increased buprenorphine effect
Opioids: increased CNS depression

Drug/herb
St. John's wort: increased CNS depression

NURSING CONSIDERATIONS
Assessment
• Assess **pain characteristics:** location, intensity, type, severity before medication administration and after treatment

> **BLACK BOX WARNING:** Potential for overdose may occur from chewing, swallowing, snorting, or injecting extracted product from TD formulation

> **BLACK BOX WARNING: QT prolongation:** Assess often in those taking class Ia, III antidysrhythmics; patients with hypokalemia or cardiac instability (TD), max TD 20 mcg/hr q7 days

• Monitor VS after parenteral route; note muscle rigidity, product history, liver, kidney function tests, respiratory dysfunction: respiratory depression, character, rate, rhythm; notify prescriber if respirations are <10/min
• Monitor CNS changes: dizziness, drowsiness, hallucinations, euphoria, LOC, pupil reaction; withdrawal in opioid-dependent persons; if dependence occurs within 2 wk of discontinuing product, **withdrawal symptoms** will occur
• Monitor allergic reactions: rash, urticaria
• Monitor bowel pattern; severe constipation can occur

Patient/family education
• Instruct patient to report any symptoms of CNS changes, allergic reactions
• Caution patients to avoid CNS depressants: alcohol, sedative/hypnotics for at least 24 hr after taking this product

> **BLACK BOX WARNING:** Advise that psychologic dependence leading to substance abuse may result when used for extended periods; long-term use is not recommended

• Advise to avoid driving, other hazardous activities until reaction is known
• Discuss with patient that dizziness, drowsiness, and confusion are common; to avoid getting up without assistance; to avoid hazardous activities
• Discuss in detail all aspects of the product

Evaluation
Positive therapeutic outcome
• Relief of pain

TREATMENT OF OVERDOSE:
Naloxone 0.4 mg ampule diluted in 10 ml 0.9% NaCl, give by direct **IV** push 0.02 mg q2min (adult)

B

buPROPion (Rx)

(byoo-proe′pee-on)

Aplenzin, Budeprion SR, Buproban, Wellbutrin, Wellbutrin SR, Wellbutrin XL, Zyban

Func. class.: Antidepressant— miscellaneous, smoking deterrent

Chem. class.: Aminoketone

Pregnancy category C

Do not confuse:

buPROPion/busPIRone, **Zyban**/Diovan/Zagam

ACTION: Inhibits reuptake of DOPamine, norepinephrine, serotonin

Therapeutic outcome: Decreased symptoms of depression after 2-3 wk

USES: Depression (Wellbutrin), smoking cessation (Zyban); seasonal affective disorder

Unlabeled uses: Neuropathic pain, enhancement of weight loss, attention-deficit/ hyperactivity disorder (ADHD)

CONTRAINDICATIONS:

Hypersensitivity, head trauma, stroke, intracranial mass, eating disorders, seizure disorder

Precautions: Pregnancy **C**, breastfeeding, geriatric, renal/hepatic disease, recent MI, cranial trauma, seizure disorders

> **BLACK BOX WARNING:** Children <18 yr, suicidal thinking/behavior (young adults)

DOSAGE AND ROUTES

Depression

Adult: PO 100 mg bid initially, then increase after 3 days to 100 mg tid if needed, max 150 mg single dose; ER/SR, initially 150 mg AM, increase to 300 mg/day if initial dose is tolerated, after no less than 4 days; after several wk, titrate to 200 mg bid; Aplenzin 174 mg qAM; may increase to 348 mg qAM on day 4; may increase to 522 mg after several weeks if needed

Geriatric: PO 50-100 mg/day, may increase by 50-100 mg q3-4days

Smoking cessation (Zyban)

Adult: SR 150 mg q day × 3 days, then 150 mg bid for remainder of treatment, initiate 1-2 wk before targeted "quit day," continue for 7-12 wk; in combination with nicotine TD, 150 mg q day × 3 days, then 150 mg bid for remainder of treatment, give ≥8 hr apart, max 300 mg/ day, initiate 1-2 wk before targeted "quit day," continue for 7-12 wk, may be continued for 8-20 wk

Seasonal affective disorder

Adult: PO (Wellbutrin XL) 150 mg as a single dose in the AM, after 1 wk may be increased to 300 mg/day; (Aplenzin) 174 mg/day in AM, after 7 days may increase to 348 mg/day

Available forms: Tabs 75, 100 mg; sus rel tabs (**SR**) 150 mg; ext rel tab (XL) 100, 150, 300 mg (SR-12 hr, XL-24 hr); ext rel tab (Aplenzin) 174, 348, 522 mg

Implementation

• Give with food or milk for GI symptoms

• Give sugarless gum, hard candy, or frequent sips of water for dry mouth

• **When switching to Aplenzin from Wellbutrin, Wellbutrin SR, or XL use these equivalents: 174 buPROPion HBr = 150 mg buPROPion HCl; 348 mg buPROPion HBr = 300 mg buPROPion HCl; 522 mg buPROPion HBr = 450 mg buPROPion HCl**

• **Wellbutrin immediate rel**, separate by ≥6 hr, give in 3 divided doses; **Wellbutrin SR,** if multiple doses are used, separate by ≥8 hr; **Wellbutrin XL,** give q day in AM; Zyban SR, give in 2 divided doses ≥8 hr apart; **Aplenzin ER,** give q day in AM, a larger dose of Aplenzin is needed because these products are not equivalent

• Store at room temperature; do not freeze

ADVERSE EFFECTS

CNS: *Headache, agitation, confusion,* **seizures,** delusions, *insomnia, sedation, tremors,* dizziness, akinesia, bradykinesia, **suicidal ideation,** mania, hot flashes

CV: **Dysrhythmias,** *hypertension,* palpitations, *tachycardia,* hypotension, **complete AV block, QRS prolongation (overdose)**

EENT: *Blurred vision, auditory disturbance,* tinnitus

GI: *Nausea, vomiting, dry mouth,* anorexia, diarrhea, increased appetite, *constipation,* altered taste

GU: Impotence, frequency, retention, *menstrual irregularities,* nocturia, altered libido

INTEG: *Rash,* pruritus, *sweating,* **Stevens-Johnson syndrome**

MISC: *Weight loss or gain*

Absorption	Well absorbed; bioavailability poor
Distribution	Unknown
Metabolism	Liver extensively
Excretion	Kidneys
Half-life	14 hr, steady state 1½-5 wk

Pharmacodynamics

Onset	Up to 4 wk
Peak	Unknown
Duration	Unknown

INTERACTIONS

Individual drugs

Alcohol, levodopa, theophylline: increased risk of seizures

CarBAMazepine, cimetidine, PHENobarbital, phenytoin: decreased buPROPion effect

Cimetidine: increased buPROPion levels

Ritonavir: increased buPROPion toxicity

Tamoxifen: decreased effect of tamoxifen

Do not use within 14 days of MAOIs

Drug classifications

Antidepressants, benzodiazepines, MAOIs, phenothiazines, steroids (systemic): increased risk of seizures

CYP2D6/CYP2B6 inhibitors: increased buPROPion effect

CYP450, CYP2D6 products: decreased buPROPion effects

CYP2D6, CYP2B6 inducers: decreased buPROPion effect

MAOIs: acute toxicity

Drug/herb

Kava, valerian: increased CNS depression

Drug/lab test

Positive urine drug screen for amphetamine possible

NURSING CONSIDERATIONS

Assessment

• Monitor B/P (with patient lying, standing), pulse q4hr; if systolic B/P drops 20 mm Hg hold product, notify prescriber; take vital signs q4hr in patients with CV disease

• Assess smoking cessation progress after 7-12 wk, if progress has not been made, product should be discontinued

⚠ Assess for increased risk of seizures; if patient has used CNS depressant or CNS stimulants, dosage of buPROPion should not be exceeded

• Monitor blood studies: CBC, leukocytes, differential, cardiac enzymes if patient is receiving long-term therapy

• Monitor hepatic studies: AST, ALT, bilirubin if on long-term treatment

• Check weight weekly; appetite may increase with product

• Assess ECG for flattening of T wave, bundle branch block, AV block, dysrhythmias in cardiac patients

• Assess for EPS primarily in geriatric: rigidity, dystonia, akathisia

> **BLACK BOX WARNING:** Assess mental status: mood, sensorium, affect, suicidal tendencies; increase in psychiatric symptoms: depression, panic

• Monitor urinary retention, constipation; constipation is more likely to occur in children or geriatric

• Identify alcohol consumption; if alcohol was consumed, hold dose

Patient/family education

• Teach patient that therapeutic effects may take 2-3 wk; not to increase dose without prescriber's approval; that treatment for smoking cessation lasts 7-12 wk

• Teach patient to use caution in driving or other activities requiring alertness because of drowsiness, dizziness, blurred vision; to avoid rising quickly from sitting to standing, especially geriatric

• Teach patient to avoid alcohol ingestion; alcohol may increase risk of seizures, obtain approval for other products

• Teach patient to increase fluids, bulk in diet if constipation, urinary retention occur, especially geriatric; notify prescriber immediately if urinary retention occurs

• Teach patient to take gum, hard sugarless candy, or frequent sips of water for dry mouth

• Advise patient not to use with nicotine patches unless directed by prescriber, may increase B/P

> **BLACK BOX WARNING:** Teach patient that risk of seizures increases when dose is exceeded or if patient has seizure disorder; suicidal ideas, behavior, hostility, depression may occur in children or young adults

• Teach patient to notify prescriber if pregnancy is suspected or planned

---

Evaluation
Positive therapeutic outcome
- Decrease in depression
- Absence of suicidal thoughts
- Smoking cessation

TREATMENT OF OVERDOSE:
ECG monitoring, induce emesis, lavage, activated charcoal, administer anticonvulsant

busPIRone (Rx)
(byoo-spye'rone)
BuSpar, BuSpar Dividose, PMS-Buspirone ✤
Func. class.: Antianxiety, sedative
Chem. class.: Azaspirodecanedione
Pregnancy category B

Do not confuse:
busPIRone/buPROPion

ACTION: Acts by inhibiting the action of serotonin (5-HT) by binding to serotonin and dopamine receptors; also increases norepinephrine metabolism; has shown little potential for abuse, a good choice in substance abuse

Therapeutic outcome: Decreased anxiety

USES: Management and short-term relief of generalized anxiety disorders

CONTRAINDICATIONS:
Hypersensitivity, child <18 yr

Precautions: Pregnancy **B**, breastfeeding, geriatric, impaired renal/hepatic function

DOSAGE AND ROUTES
Adult: PO 7.5 mg tid; may increase by 5 mg/day q2-3days; max 60 mg/day

Renal/hepatic dose
Adult: PO reduce by 25%-50% in mild to moderate hepatic disease, do not use in severe hepatic disease, CCr 11-70 ml/min reduce dose by 25%-50%, CCr <10 ml/min do not use

Available forms: Tabs 5, 7.5, 10, 15, 30 mg

Implementation
- Give with food or milk for GI symptoms (avoid grapefruit juice); sugarless gum, hard candy, frequent sips of water for dry mouth
- May be crushed

ADVERSE EFFECTS
CNS: *Dizziness, headache, depression, stimulation, insomnia, nervousness, light-headedness, numbness, paresthesia, incoordination, tremors,* excitement, involuntary movements, confusion, akathisia, nightmares, hostility
CV: *Tachycardia, palpitations,* hypo/hypertension, **CVA, CHF, MI**
EENT: *Sore throat, tinnitus, blurred vision, nasal congestion,* red, itching eyes, change in taste, smell
GI: *Nausea, dry mouth, diarrhea, constipation,* flatulence, increased appetite, rectal bleeding
GU: Frequency, hesitancy, menstrual irregularity, change in libido
INTEG: *Rash,* edema, pruritus, alopecia, dry skin
MISC: *Sweating,* fatigue, weight gain, fever, **serotonin syndrome**
MS: *Pain, weakness,* muscle cramps, spasms
RESP: Hyperventilation, chest congestion, shortness of breath

Pharmacokinetics
Absorption	Rapid
Distribution	Protein binding 86%
Metabolism	Liver, extensively
Excretion	Feces
Half-life	2-3 hr

Pharmacodynamics
Onset	Unknown
Peak	40-90 min
Duration	Unknown

INTERACTIONS
Individual drugs
Alcohol: increased CNS depression; avoid use

Drug classifications
Products metabolized by CYP3A4 (erythromycin, itraconazole, nefazodone, ketoconazole, ritonavir, several other protease inhibitors): increased busPIRone levels
MAOIs, procarbazine: increased B/P, do not use together
Products induced by CYP3A4 (rifampin, phenytoin, PHENobarbital, carBAMazepine, dexamethasone): decreased busPIRone action
Psychotropics: increased CNS depression, avoid use
Selective serotonin reuptake inhibitors (SNRIs, serotonin receptor agonists): increase serotonin syndrome

---

Adverse effects: *italics* = common; **bold** = life-threatening

Drug/food
Grapefruit juice: increased peak concentration of busPIRone

NURSING CONSIDERATIONS
Assessment
• Assess anxiety reaction: inability to sleep, apprehension, dread, foreboding, or uneasiness related to unidentified source of danger
• Assess for previous product dependence or tolerance; if patient is product dependent or tolerant, amount of medication should be restricted
• Monitor B/P (lying, standing), pulse; if systolic B/P drops 20 mm Hg, hold product, notify prescriber; check I&O; may indicate renal dysfunction
• Monitor mental status: mood, sensorium, affect, sleeping patterns, drowsiness, dizziness, suicidal tendencies; withdrawal symptoms when dose is reduced or product discontinued
• Assess for CNS reaction, some reactions may be unpredictable

Patient/family education
• Teach patient that product may be taken consistently with or without food; if dose is missed take as soon as remembered; do not double doses
• Caution patient to avoid OTC preparations unless approved by the prescriber; to avoid alcohol ingestion and other psychotropic medications unless prescribed; that 1-2 wk of therapy may be required before therapeutic effects occur; to avoid large amounts of grapefruit juice
• Caution patient to avoid driving and activities requiring alertness since drowsiness may occur; until medication response is known, tell patient that drowsiness may worsen at beginning of treatment
• Instruct patient not to discontinue medication abruptly after long-term use; if dose is missed, do not double
• Advise patient to rise slowly or fainting may occur, especially in geriatric
⚠ **Serotonin syndrome: Teach patient to report immediately (fever, tremor, sweating, diarrhea, delirium)**

Evaluation
Positive therapeutic outcome
• Increased well-being
• Decreased anxiety, restlessness, sleeplessness, dread

---

busulfan (Rx)
(byoo-sul'fan)
Busulfex, Myleran
Func. class.: Antineoplastic alkylating agent
Chem. class.: Bifunctional alkylating agent
Pregnancy category D

Do not confuse:
Myleran/Leukeran

ACTION: Changes essential cellular ions to covalent bonding with resultant alkylation; this interferes with normal biological function of DNA; activity is not phase specific; action is due to myelosuppression

Therapeutic outcome: Prevention of rapid growth of malignant cells in chronic myelocytic leukemia

USES: Chronic myelocytic leukemia, bone marrow ablation, stem cell transplant preparation in CML

CONTRAINDICATIONS:
Pregnancy **D** (3rd trimester), breastfeeding, radiation, chemotherapy, blastic phase of chronic myelocytic leukemia, hypersensitivity

Precautions: Child-bearing-age men and women, leukopenia, thrombocytopenia, anemia, hepatotoxicity, renal toxicity, seizures, tumor lysis syndrome, hyperkalemia, hyperphosphatemia, hypocalcemia, hyperuricemia

BLACK BOX WARNING: Neutropenia, secondary malignancy, thrombocytopenia

DOSAGE AND ROUTES
Chronic myelocytic leukemia
Adult: PO 4-8 mg/day or 1.8-4 mg/m^2/day initially; reduce dosage if WBC levels reach 30,000-40,000/mm^3; stop if WBC ≤20,000/mm^3; maintenance 1-3 mg/day
Child: PO 0.06-0.12 mg/kg/day or 1.8-4.6 mg/m^2/day, reduce if WBC is 30,000-40,000/mm^3; discontinue if WBC ≤20,000/mm^3

Allogenic hemopoietic stem cell transplantation in chronic myelogenous leukemia
Adult: IV 0.8 mg/kg over 2 hr, q6hr × 4 days (total 16 doses); give cyclophosphamide IV 60

---

mg/kg over 1 hr/day for 2 days, starting after 16th dose of busulfan

Available forms: Tabs 2 mg; sol for inj 6 mg/ml

Implementation
• Give 1 hr before or 2 hr after meals to lessen nausea and vomiting; give at same time daily
• Increased fluid intake to 2-3 L/day to prevent urate deposits, calculus formation
• Administer antibiotics for prophylaxis of infection; may be prescribed since infection potential is high
• Store in tight container

Intermittent IV infusion route
• Prepared in biologic cabinet using gloves, gown, mask; **dilute** with 10 times volume of product with D_5W or 0.9% NaCl, (0.5 mg/ml); when withdrawing product, use needle with 5-micron filter provided, remove amount needed, remove filter and **inject** product into diluent; always add product to diluent, not vice versa; stable for 8 hr at room temperature (using D_5W) or 12 hr refrigerated; **give** by central venous catheter over 2 hr q6hr × 4 days, use infusion pump, do not admix
• Give antiemetics before **IV** route, on schedule
• In those with history of seizures give phenytoin before **IV** route, to prevent seizures (using 0.9% NaCl)

Y-site compatibilities: Acyclovir, amphotericin B lipid complex, amphotericin B liposome, anidulafungin, atenolol, bivalirudin, bleomycin, caspofungin, codeine, DAPTOmycin, dexmedetomidine, diltiazem, DOCEtaxel, ertapenem, fenoldopam, gatifloxacin, granisetron, HYDROmorphone, levofloxacin, linezolid, LORazepam, meperidine, metroNIDAZOLE, milrinone, nesiritide, octreotide acetate, ondansetron, palonosetron, pancuronium, piperacillin-tazobactam, riTUXimab, sodium acetate, tacrolimus, tigecycline, tirofiban, trastuzumab, vasopressin

ADVERSE EFFECTS
PO route
CV: *Hypotension,* **thrombosis,** *chest pain,* **tachycardia, atrial fibrillation, heart block, pericardial effusion, cardiac tamponade** (high dose with cyclophosphamide)
GI: Anorexia, constipation, dry mouth, nausea, vomiting, *diarrhea*
RESP: **Alveolar hemorrhage,** atelectasis, cough, hemoptysis, hypoxia, pleural effusion, pneumonia, sinusitis, **pulmonary fibrosis**

IV route
CNS: **Cerebral hemorrhage, coma, seizures,** *anxiety, depression, dizziness, headache,* encephalopathy, weakness, mental changes
EENT: *Pharyngitis, epistaxis, cataracts*
GI: *Diarrhea, nausea, vomiting, weight loss*
GU: Impotence, sterility, amenorrhea, gynecomastia, **renal toxicity,** hyperuremia, adrenal insufficiency–like syndrome
HEMA: **Thrombocytopenia, leukopenia, pancytopenia, severe bone marrow depression**
INTEG: Dermatitis, hyperpigmentation, alopecia
MISC: Chromosomal aberrations
RESP: **Irreversible pulmonary fibrosis,** pneumonitis

Pharmacokinetics

Absorption	Rapidly absorbed
Distribution	Unknown; crosses placenta
Metabolism	Liver, extensively
Excretion	Kidneys, breast milk
Half-life	2.5 hr

Pharmacodynamics
Unknown

INTERACTIONS
Individual drugs
Acetaminophen, itraconazole: decreased busulfan clearance
Cyclophosphamide: cardiac tamponade
Phenytoin: decreased busulfan level
Radiation: increased toxicity, bone marrow suppression
Thioguanine: hepatotoxicity

Drug classifications
Anticoagulants, salicylates: increased risk of bleeding
Antineoplastics: increased toxicity, bone marrow suppression
Live virus vaccines: decreased antibody reaction

Drug/lab test
False positive: breast, bladder, cervix, lung cytology tests

NURSING CONSIDERATIONS
Assessment
• Monitor CBC, differential, platelet count weekly; withhold product for WBC <15,000/mm³ or platelets <150,000/mm³; notify prescriber of results; institute thrombocytopenia

---

Adverse effects: *italics* = common; **bold** = life-threatening

precautions, levels to withhold product are different in children

> **BLACK BOX WARNING:** Assess bone marrow status prior to chemotherapy, bone marrow suppression may be prolonged (up to 2 mo); seizure history

• **Pulmonary fibrosis:** Monitor pulmonary function tests, chest x-ray films before, during therapy; chest film should be obtained q2wk during treatment; check for dyspnea, crackles, nonproductive cough, chest pain, tachypnea; pulmonary fibrosis may occur up to 10 yr after treatment with busulfan
• Assess for increased uric acid levels, swelling, joint pain primarily in extremities; patient should be well hydrated to prevent urate deposits
• Monitor renal function studies: BUN, serum uric acid, urine CCr before, during therapy; I&O ratio; report fall in urine output of 30 ml/hr; check for hyperuricemia
• Monitor for cold, fever, sore throat (may indicate beginning infection); identify edema in feet, joint or stomach pain, shaking; prescriber should be notified
• Assess for bleeding: hematuria, guaiac, bruising or petechiae, mucosa or orifices q8hr; no rectal temps

> **BLACK BOX WARNING:** Assess for secondary malignancy within 5-8 yr of chronic oral therapy, long-term follow-up may be required

Patient/family education
• Teach patient to avoid use of products containing aspirin or ibuprofen, razors, commercial mouthwash since bleeding may occur; to report symptoms of bleeding (hematuria, tarry stools)
• Instruct patient to report signs of anemia (fatigue, headache, irritability, faintness, shortness of breath); symptoms of **infection** (fever, sore throat, cough); jaundice; congestion; skin pigmentation; darkening of skin; sudden weakness, weight loss **(may resemble adrenal insufficiency)**
• Instruct patient to report any changes in breathing or coughing even several months after treatment; to avoid crowds and persons with respiratory tract or other infections
• Teach patient that hair loss may occur; discuss the use of wigs or hair pieces
• Caution patient not to have any vaccinations without the advice of the prescriber; serious reactions can occur

⚠ Advise patient that contraception is needed during treatment and for ≥3 months after the completion of therapy (pregnancy D); avoid breastfeeding; may cause infertility; discuss family planning before initiating therapy

Evaluation
Positive therapeutic outcome
• Decreased leukocytes to normal limits
• Absence of sweating at night
• Increased appetite, increased weight

butoconazole vaginal antifungal
See Appendix B

butorphanol (Rx)
(byoo-tor'fa-nole)
Func. class.: Mixed opiate analgesic
Chem. class.: Opioid antagonist, partial agonist
Pregnancy category C
Controlled substance schedule IV

ACTION: Depresses pain impulse transmission at the spinal cord level by interacting with opioid receptors

Therapeutic outcome: Relief of pain

USES: Moderate to severe pain, general anesthesia induction/maintenance, headache, migraine, preanesthesia

CONTRAINDICATIONS:
Hypersensitivity to this product or preservative, addiction (opioid)

Precautions: Pregnancy **C**, breastfeeding, child <18 yr, addictive personality, increased ICP, respiratory depression, renal/hepatic disease, ileus, COPD

DOSAGE AND ROUTES
Moderate to severe pain
Adult: IM 1-4 mg q3-4hr prn; **IV** 0.5-2 mg q3-4hr prn; **nasal** spray in 1 nostril; may give another dose 1-1½ hr later; may repeat if needed in q3-4hr after last dose
Geriatric: IV ½ adult dose at 2× the interval; **intranasal** if no relief in 90-120 min, may repeat with 1 spray

Severe pain
Adult: INTRANASAL 1 spray in each nostril q3-4hr

Renal/hepatic dose
Adult: INTRANASAL max 1 mg, followed by 1 mg in 90-120 min; IM/IV give 50% of dose (0.5 mg **IV**, 1 mg IM); do not repeat within 6 hr

Available forms: Inj 1, 2 mg/ml; INTRANASAL 10 mg/ml

Implementation
- Store in light-resistant container at room temperature

Nasal route
- Prime before first use, point sprayer away from face, pump activator 7 times until a fine, wide spray occurs; if not used for 48 hr, reprime by pumping 1-2 times
- If more than 1 spray is needed, use other nostril
- Do not share with others
- Nasal congestion/irritation may occur

IM route
- Give deeply in large muscle mass; rotate inj sites

Intranasal route
- Give 1 spray in nostril
- Remove clip and cover, prime before using until spray appears; pump must be reprimed q48hr; close nostril with finger and spray once quickly; have patient sniff

IV direct route
- Give **IV** undiluted at a rate of ≤2 mg/>3-5 min; titrate to patient response

Syringe compatibilities: Atropine, chlorproMAZINE, cimetidine, diphenhydrAMINE, droperidol, fentaNYL, hydrOXYzine, meperidine, methotrimeprazine, metoclopramide, midazolam, morphine, pentazocine, perphenazine, prochlorperazine, promethazine, scopolamine, thiethylperazine

Syringe incompatibilities: DimenhyDRINATE, PENTobarbital

Y-site compatibilities: Acyclovir, alfentanil, allopurinol, amifostine, amikacin, aminocaproic acid, aminophylline, amphotericin B liposome (AmBisome), anidulafungin, ascorbic acid injection, atenolol, atracurium, atropine, aztreonam, benztropine, bivalirudin, bleomycin, bumetanide, buprenorphine, calcium chloride/gluconate, CARBOplatin, caspofungin, cefamandole, ceFAZolin, cefepime, cefoperazone, cefotaxime, cefoTEtan, cefOXitin, cefTAZidime, ceftizoxime, cefTRIAXone, cefuroxime, cephalothin, chlorproMAZINE, cimetidine, cisatracurium, CISplatin, cladribine, clindamycin, cyanocobalamin, cyclophosphamide, cycloSPORINE, cytarabine, DACTINomy-cin, DAPTOmycin, dexamethasone phosphate, dexmedetomidine, digoxin, diltiazem, diphenhydrAMINE, DOBUTamine, DOCEtaxel, DOPamine, doxacurium, DOXOrubicin, DOXOrubicin liposomal, doxycycline, enalaprilat, ePHEDrine, EPINEPHrine, epirubicin, epoetin alfa, eptifibatide, ertapenem, erythromycin, esmolol, etoposide, famotidine, fenoldopam, fentaNYL, filgrastim, fluconazole, fludarabine, fluorouracil, gatifloxacin, gemcitabine, gentamicin, glycopyrrolate, granisetron, heparin, hydrocortisone, hydrOXYzine, IDArubicin, ifosfamide, imipenem-cilastatin, irinotecan, isoproterenol, ketorolac, labetalol, lactated Ringer's injection, levofloxacin, lidocaine, linezolid injection, LORazepam, magnesium, mannitol, mechlorethamine, melphalan, meperidine, metaraminol, methicillin, methotrexate, methoxamine, methyldopate, methylPREDNISolone, metoclopramide, metoprolol, metroNIDAZOLE, mezlocillin, milrinone, minocycline, mitoXANtrone, morphine, multiple vitamins injection, mycophenolate mofetil, nafcillin, nalbuphine, naloxone, nesiritide, netilmicin, niCARdipine, nitroglycerin, nitroprusside, norepinephrine, octreotide, ondansetron, oxacillin, oxaliplatin, oxytocin, palonosetron, pamidronate, pancuronium, papaverine, PEMEtrexed, penicillin G potassium/sodium, pentazocine, PHENobarbital, phenylephrine, phytonadione, piperacillin, piperacillin-tazobactam, polymyxin B, potassium chloride, procainamide, prochlorperazine, promethazine, propofol, propranolol, protamine, pyridoxine, quiNIDine, ranitidine, remifentanil, Ringer's injection, riTUXimab, rocuronium, sargramostim, sodium acetate, succinylcholine, SUFentanil, tacrolimus, teniposide, theophylline, thiamine, thiotepa, ticarcillin, ticarcillin-clavulanate, tigecycline, tirofiban, TNA, tobramycin, tolazoline, TPN, trastuzumab, urokinase, vancomycin, vasopressin, vecuronium, verapamil, vinCRIStine, vinorelbine, voriconazole

ADVERSE EFFECTS
CNS: *Drowsiness, dizziness, confusion, headache, sedation, euphoria, weakness, hallucinations,* insomnia (nasal)
CV: Palpitations, bradycardia, hypotension
EENT: Tinnitus, blurred vision, miosis, diplopia, nasal congestion, unpleasant taste
GI: *Nausea, vomiting, anorexia, constipation, cramps*
GU: Urinary retention
INTEG: Rash, urticaria, bruising, flushing, diaphoresis, pruritus
RESP: **Respiratory depression**

Pharmacokinetics

Absorption	Well absorbed (IM, nasal); complete (**IV**)
Distribution	Crosses placenta, protein binding 80%
Metabolism	Liver, extensively
Excretion	Feces (10%-15%); kidneys, unchanged (small amounts)
Half-life	2-9 hr

Pharmacodynamics

	IM	IV	Nasal
Onset	5-15 min	1 min	15 min
Peak	30-60 min	4-5 min	1-2 hr
Duration	3-4 hr	2-4 hr	4-5 hr

INTERACTIONS

Individual drugs
Alcohol: increased respiratory depression, hypotension, sedation

Drug classifications
Antipsychotics, CNS depressants, opioids, MAOIs, sedative/hypnotics, skeletal muscle relaxants: increased respiratory depression, hypotension

MAOIs: do not use 2 wk before butorphanol, fatal reaction

NURSING CONSIDERATIONS

Assessment
• Monitor VS after parenteral administration; note muscle rigidity, product history, liver, kidney function tests, respiratory dysfunction: respiratory depression, character, rate, rhythm; notify prescriber if respirations are <10/min
• Monitor CNS changes: dizziness, drowsiness, hallucinations, euphoria, LOC, pupil reaction
• Monitor allergic reactions: rash, urticaria
• Assess for withdrawal symptoms in opioid-dependent patient; pulmonary embolism, vascular occlusion, abscesses, ulcerations

Patient/family education
• Instruct patient to report any symptoms of CNS changes, allergic reactions; to avoid CNS depressants: alcohol, sedative/hypnotics for at least 24 hr after taking this product
• Discuss with patient that dizziness, drowsiness, and confusion are common; to avoid getting up without assistance, hazardous activities
• Discuss in detail all aspects of the product

Nasal route
• Teach patient to blow nose to clear both nostrils before using
• Patient should replace clip and cover after use; caution patient not to shake medication
• Teach patient how to use nasal product
• Teach patient to avoid hazardous activities

Evaluation

Positive therapeutic outcome
• Pain relief

TREATMENT OF OVERDOSE:
Narcan 0.4-2 mg **IV**, O_2, **IV** fluids, vasopressors

cabozantinib

(ka'boe-zan'ti-nib)

Cometriq

Func. class.: Antineoplastic biologic response modifiers

Chem. class.: Signal transduction inhibitor (STI)

Pregnancy category D

ACTION: Inhibits abnormal tyrosine kinase associated with growth and development of metastatic medullary thyroid cancer

USES: Treatment of progressive metastatic medullary thyroid cancer

CONTRAINDICATIONS:

Pregnancy (D), hypersensitivity

Precautions: Breastfeeding, children, geriatric patients, cardiac/renal/hepatic/dental disease, bone marrow suppression, wound dehiscence, skin disease, MI, hypertension, proteinuria, infertility, surgery, thrombocytopenia, neutropenia, immunosuppression

> **BLACK BOX WARNING** Bleeding, fistula, GI bleeding/perforations

DOSAGE AND ROUTES

Renal dosage

Adult: PO 140 mg/day until disease progression or unacceptable toxicity

• Avoid the concomitant use of strong 3A4 inhibitors or inducers if possible; temporary interruption of therapy and a dosage reduction may be necessary in patients who develop toxicity or intolerable side effects

Available forms: Tabs 60, 100, 140 mg

Implementation

• Take on an empty stomach; do not eat for 2 hr before and 1 hr after use; swallow whole; do not open or crush caps

• Do not take with grapefruit juice

• Do not take a missed dose within 12 hr of the next dose; if the next dose is in ≥12 hr, take the missed dose; if the next dose is in <12 hr, skip the missed dose and take the next dose at the scheduled time

• Store at room temperature

Dosage adjustments for treatment-related toxicity:

Grade 4 hematologic toxicity, grade 3 or higher nonhematologic toxicity, or intolerable grade 2 toxicity: Hold until resolution/improvement, then reduce the daily dosage by 40 mg (eg, 140 mg/day to 100 mg/day or 100 mg/day to 60 mg/day)

Dosage guidance in patients on strong CYP3A4 inducers/inhibitors:

Strong CYP3A4 inhibitors: Avoid use if possible; if a strong CYP3A4 inhibitor is used, reduce the daily cabozantinib dosage by 40 mg; resume the prior dosage after 2 or 3 days if the strong CYP3A4 inhibitor is discontinued

Strong CYP3A4 inducers: Avoid chronic concomitant use if possible; if a strong CYP3A4 inducer is required, increase the daily cabozantinib dosage by 40 mg, max 180 mg/day; resume the prior dosage after 2 or 3 days if the strong CYP3A4 inducer is discontinued

ADVERSE EFFECTS

CNS: Headache, dizziness

GI: Nausea, vomiting, dyspepsia, anorexia, abdominal pain, diarrhea, GI bleeding/fistula/perforation

HEMA: Neutropenia, thrombocytopenia, bleeding

INTEG: Rash

META: Hypokalemia

MISC: Fatigue, hypothyroidism, elevated liver enzymes

MS: Arthralgia, myalgia

Pharmacokinetics

Distribution	Protein binding 99%, metabolized by CYP3A4

INTERACTIONS

Individual drugs

Increase: cabozantinib concentrations—CYP3A4 inhibitors (ketoconazole, itraconazole, erythromycin, clarithromycin)

Increase: plasma concentrations of simvastatin, calcium channel blockers, ergots

Decrease: cabozantinib concentrations—CYP3A4 inducers (dexamethasone, phenytoin, carBAMazepine, rifampin, PHENobarbital)

Drug/food

Increase: cabozantinib effect—grapefruit juice; avoid use while taking product

Drug/herb

Cabozantinib concentration—St. John's wort

NURSING CONSIDERATIONS

Assessment

• Proteinuria: monitor urine protein regularly; discontinue if nephritic syndrome occurs

• GI bleeding/fistula/perforation: can be fatal

• Wound dehiscence: discontinue product 20 days before surgery

Patient/family education
• Teach patient to report adverse reactions immediately: bleeding
• Explain reason for treatment, expected results
• Teach that effect on male infertility is unknown

Evaluation
Positive therapeutic outcome
• Decrease in size, spread of tumor

---

calcitonin (rDNA) (Rx)
(kal-sih-toh′nin)
Fortical
calcitonin (salmon) (Rx)
Miacalcin
Func. class.: Parathyroid agents (calcium regulator)
Chem. class.: Polypeptide hormone
Pregnancy category C

ACTION: Decreases bone resorption, blood calcium levels; increases deposits of calcium in bones; opposes parathyroid hormone

Therapeutic outcome: Lowered calcium level, decreasing symptoms of Paget's disease

USES: Paget's disease, postmenopausal osteoporosis, hypercalcemia

CONTRAINDICATIONS:
Hypersensitivity to this product or fish

Precautions: Pregnancy **C**, breastfeeding, children, renal disease, osteogenic sarcoma, pernicious anemia

DOSAGE AND ROUTES
rDNA
Paget's disease
Adult: SUBCUT 0.5 mg/day initially; may require 0.5 mg bid × 6 mo, then decrease until symptoms reappear

Salmon
Postmenopausal osteoporosis
Adult: SUBCUT/IM 100 international units/day; nasal 200 international units (1 spray) alternating nostrils daily, activate pump before 1st dose

Paget's disease
Adult: SUBCUT/IM 100 international units daily, maintenance 50-100 international units daily or every other day, or 3 × per wk

Hypercalcemia
Adult: SUBCUT/IM 4 international units/kg q12hr, increase to 8 international units/kg q12hr if response is unsatisfactory

Available forms: Inj 200 international units/ml; nasal spray 200 international units/actuation

Implementation
• Store at <77° F (25° C); protect from light
SUBCUT route (human)
• **Give** by SUBCUT route only; rotate inj sites; use within 6 hr of reconstitution; **give** at bedtime to minimize nausea, vomiting, rotate sites
IM route (salmon)
• **Give** after test dose of 10 international units/ml, 0.1 ml intradermally; watch 15 min; **give** only with EPINEPHrine and emergency meds available
• IM inj in deep muscle mass slowly; rotate sites; preferred route if volume is >2 ml
Nasal route
• Use alternating nostrils for nasal spray; allow to warm to room temperature, prime to get full spray

ADVERSE EFFECTS
CNS: Headache, **tetany,** chills, weakness, dizziness, fever, tremors
CV: Chest pressure
EENT: Nasal congestion, eye pain
GI: Nausea, diarrhea, vomiting, anorexia, abdominal pain, salty taste, epigastric pain
GU: Diuresis, nocturia, urine sediment, frequency
INTEG: Rash, flushing, pruritus of earlobes, edema of feet, inj site reaction
MS: Swelling, tingling of hands, backache
RESP: Dyspnea
SYST: Anaphylaxis

Pharmacokinetics	
Absorption	Completely absorbed
Distribution	Unknown
Metabolism	Rapid; kidneys, tissue, blood
Excretion	Kidneys, inactive metabolite
Half-life	1 hr

Pharmacodynamics	
	SUBCUT
Onset	15 min
Peak	4 hr
Duration	8-24 hr

INTERACTIONS
Individual drugs
Lithium: decreased lithium effect

Drug classifications
Bisphosphonates (Paget's disease): decreased effect of nasal spray

NURSING CONSIDERATIONS
Assessment
• **Anaphylaxis, hypersensitivity:** inabilities to breathe, rash, fever; have emergency equipment nearby
• Assess for GI symptoms, polyuria, flushing, head swelling, tingling, headache; may indicate hypercalcemia; nervousness, irritability, twitching, seizures, spasm, paresthesia indicate hypocalcemia during beginning of treatment
• Identify nutritional status; check diet for sources of vit D (milk, some seafood), calcium (dairy products, dark green vegetables), phosphates
• Monitor BUN, creatinine, uric acid, chloride, electrolytes, urine pH, urinary calcium, magnesium, phosphate, urinalysis (calcium should be kept at 9-10 mg/dl; vit D 50-135 international units/dl), alkaline phosphatase baseline and q3-6mo; check urine sediment for casts throughout treatment; monitor urine hydroxyproline in Paget's disease, biochemical markers of bone formation/absorption, radiologic evidence of fracture; bone density (osteoporosis)
• **Toxicity (can occur rapidly):** Assess for increased product level, since toxic reactions occur rapidly; have parenteral calcium or gluconate on hand if calcium level drops too low; check for tetany (irritability, paresthesia, nervousness, muscle twitching, seizure, tetanic spasm)

Patient/family education
• Teach method of inj if patient will be responsible for self-medication
• Instruct patient to notify prescriber for hypercalcemic relapse: renal calculi, nausea, vomiting, thirst, lethargy, deep bone or flank pain
• Teach patient that warmth and flushing occur and last 1 hr
• Provide a low-calcium diet as prescribed (Paget's disease, hypercalcemia)
• Advise patients with osteoporosis to increase calcium and vit D in diet and to continue with moderate exercise to prevent continued bone loss

• Advise patients to report difficulty swallowing or change in side effects to prescriber immediately

Evaluation
Positive therapeutic outcome
• Calcium levels 9-10 mg/dl
• Decreasing symptoms of Paget's disease, including pain
• Decreased bone loss in osteoporosis

calcitriol (Rx)
(kal-si-tree´ole)
Calcijex, Rocaltrol, Vectical
Func. class.: Parathyroid agent (calcium regulator)
Chem. class.: Vitamin D hormone
Pregnancy category C

Do not confuse:
calcitriol/Calciferol

ACTION: Increases intestinal absorption of calcium, provides calcium for bones, increases renal tubular resorption of phosphate

Therapeutic outcome: Calcium at normal level

USES: Hypocalcemia in chronic renal disease, hyperparathyroidism, pseudohypoparathyroidism

CONTRAINDICATIONS: Hypersensitivity, hyperphosphatemia, hypercalcemia, vit D toxicity

Precautions: Pregnancy **C**, breastfeeding, renal calculi, CV disease

DOSAGE AND ROUTES
Hypocalcemia (stage 5 chronic kidney disease, on dialysis)
Adult and child ≥6 yr: PO 0.25 mcg/day **IV** 0.5 mcg tid, initially; may increase by 0.25 every other day q4-8wk
Child 1-5 yr: PO 0.25-2 mcg/day

Renal osteodystrophy
Adult and child ≥3 yr: PO 0.25 mcg/day, may increase to 0.5 mcg/day
Child <3 yr: PO 0.01-0.015 mcg/kg/day

Hypoparathyroidism
Adult and child ≥6 yr: PO 0.25 mcg/day, may increase q2-4wk, maintenance 0.5-2 mcg/day
Child 1-5 yr: PO 0.25-0.75 mcg daily
Child <1 yr: PO 0.04-0.08 mcg/kg/day

Available forms: Caps 0.25, 0.5 mcg; inj 1 mcg/ml, 2 mcg/ml; oral sol 1 mcg/ml; top 3 mcg/g

Implementation
PO route
• Do not break, crush, or chew caps
• Give with meals for GI symptoms
• Store protected from light, heat, moisture

IV route
• Give by direct **IV** over 1 min

ADVERSE EFFECTS
CNS: Drowsiness, headache, vertigo, fever, lethargy, hallucinations
CV: Palpitations, hypertension
EENT: Blurred vision, photophobia
GI: Nausea, diarrhea, vomiting, jaundice, anorexia, dry mouth, constipation, cramps, metallic taste
GU: Polyuria, hypercalciuria, hyperphosphatemia, hematuria, thirst
MS: Myalgia, arthralgia, decreased bone development, weakness
SYST: Anaphylaxis

Pharmacokinetics

Absorption	Well absorbed
Distribution	To liver, crosses placenta
Metabolism	Liver
Excretion	Bile
Half-life	3-6 hr, undergoes hepatic recycling, excreted in bile

Pharmacodynamics

Onset	2-6 hr
Peak	10-12 hr
Duration	Up to 5 days

INTERACTIONS
Individual drugs
Cholestyramine, mineral oil: decreased absorption of calcitriol
Phenytoin: increased vit D metabolism
Verapamil: increased dysrhythmias

Drug classifications
Antacids (magnesium): increased hypermagnesemia
Calcium supplements, diuretics (thiazide): increased hypercalcemia
Cardiac glycosides: increased dysrhythmias
Vitamin D products: increased toxicity
Vitamins (fat-soluble): decreased calcitriol absorption

Drug/food
Large amounts of high-calcium foods may cause hypercalcemia

Drug/lab test
False: increased cholesterol
Interference: alkaline phosphatase, electrolytes

NURSING CONSIDERATIONS
Assessment
• Assess GI symptoms, polyuria, flushing, head swelling, tingling, headache; may indicate hypercalcemia
• **Hypercalcemia:** dry mouth, metallic taste, polyuria, bone pain, muscle weakness, headache, fatigue, change in LOC, dysrhythmias, increased respirations, anorexia, nausea, vomiting, cramps, diarrhea, constipation; paresthesia, twitching, Chvostek's/Trousseau's sign, **hypocalcemia**
• Identify nutritional status; check diet for sources of vit D (milk, some seafood), calcium (dairy products, dark green vegetables), phosphates
• Monitor BUN, creatinine, uric acid, chloride, electrolytes, urine pH, urinary calcium, magnesium, phosphate, urinalysis (calcium should be kept at 9-10 mg/dl; vit D 50-135 international units/dl), alkaline phosphatase baseline and q3-6mo

Patient/family education
• Teach patient the symptoms of hypercalcemia (renal stones, nausea, vomiting, anorexia, lethargy, thirst, bone or flank pain) and about foods rich in calcium
• Advise patient to avoid products with sodium: cured meats, dairy products, cold cuts, olives, beets, pickles, soups, meat tenderizers in chronic renal failure
• Advise patient to avoid products with potassium: oranges, bananas, dried fruit, peas, dark green leafy vegetables, milk, melons, beans in chronic renal failure
• Advise patient to avoid OTC products containing calcium, potassium, or sodium in chronic renal failure
• Instruct patient to avoid all preparations containing vit D
• Instruct patient to monitor weight weekly; maintain fluid intake

Evaluation
Positive therapeutic outcome
• Calcium levels 9-10 mg/dl

---

calcium carbonate (Rx) (PO-OTC, Rx)

Acid Free, Alka-Mints, Amitone, Apo-Cal ✿, Calcarb, Calci-Chew, Calci-Mix, Calcite ✿, Cal-Gest, Caltrate, Equaline Calcium, Leader Calcium, Maalox Antacid, Os-Cal 500, Rolaids Extra Strength Soft-chew, Tums, Tums E-X, Walgreens Calcium

Func. class.: Antacid, calcium supplement

Chem. class.: Calcium product

calcium acetate (OTC)

(kal′see-um ass′e-tate)

Calphron, Eliphos, PhosLo

Pregnancy category C

Do not confuse:
Os-Cal/Asacol

ACTION: Neutralizes gastric acidity

Therapeutic outcome: Neutralized gastric acidity; calcium at normal levels

USES: Antacid, calcium supplement; not suitable for chronic therapy, hyperphosphatemia, hypertension in pregnancy, osteoporosis, prevention/treatment of hypocalcemia, hypoparathyroidism

CONTRAINDICATIONS:

Hypersensitivity, hypercalcemia, hyperparathyroidism, bone tumors

Precautions: Pregnancy C, breastfeeding, geriatric, fluid restriction, decreased GI motility, GI obstruction, dehydration, renal disease

DOSAGE AND ROUTES

Nutritional supplement including osteoporosis prophylaxis

Adult ≥51 yr: PO 1000-1500 mg/day elemental calcium (2500-3750 calcium carbonate)

Adult 19-50 yr: PO 1000 mg/day elemental calcium (2500 mg calcium carbonate)

Chronic hypocalcemia

Adult: PO 2-4 g/day elemental calcium (5-10 g calcium carbonate) in 3-4 divided doses

Child: PO 45-65 mg/kg/day elemental calcium (112.5-162.5 mg/kg calcium carbonate) in 4 divided doses

Neonate: PO 50-150 mg/kg/day elemental calcium (125-375 mg/kg/day in 4-6 divided doses, max 1 g/day)

Supplementation

Adolescent and child 9-18 yr: PO 1300 mg elemental calcium (3250 mg calcium carbonate)

Child 4-8 yr: PO 800 mg/day elemental calcium (2000 mg calcium carbonate)

Child 1-3 yr: PO 500 mg/day elemental calcium (1250 mg calcium carbonate)

Infant 6-12 mo: PO 270 mg/day elemental calcium based on total intake

Neonate and infant <6 mo: PO 210 mg/day elemental calcium based on total intake

Hyperphosphatemia

Adult: PO Individualized on response

Heartburn, dyspepsia, hyperacidity (OTC)

Adult: PO 1-2 tabs q2hr, max 9 tabs/24 hr (Alka-mints); chew 2-4 tab q1hr prn, max 16 tabs (Tums regular strength); chew 2-4 tab q1hr prn, max 10 tabs (Tums E-X); chew 2-3 tabs q1hr prn, max 10 tabs/24 hr (Tums Ultra); chew 2 tabs q2-3hr, max 19 tabs/24 hr (Titralac Extra Strength)

Available forms: Calcium carbonate: chewable tabs 350, 420, 450, 500, 750, 1000, 1250 mg; tabs 500, 600, 650, 667, 1000, 1250, 1500 mg; gum 300, 450 500 mg; susp 1250 mg/5 ml; caps 1250 mg; powder 6.5 g/packet; **calcium acetate:** tabs 250 mg (65 mg Ca), 667 mg (169 mg Ca), 668 mg (169 mg Ca), 1 g (250 mg Ca); caps 500 mg (125 mg Ca)

Implementation
PO route

• Administer as antacid 1 hr after meals and at bedtime

• Administer as supplement 1½ hr after meals and at bedtime

• Administer only with regular tablets or capsules; do not give with enteric-coated tablets

• Administer laxatives or stool softeners if constipation occurs

ADVERSE EFFECTS

GI: *Constipation,* anorexia, nausea, vomiting, flatulence, diarrhea, rebound hyperacidity, eructation

GU: Calculi, hypercalciuria

Absorption	⅓ absorbed by small intestines, must have adequate vit D for absorption
Distribution	Unknown
Metabolism	Unknown
Excretion	Feces, urine, crosses placenta
Half-life	Unknown

Pharmacodynamics

Onset	20 min
Peak	Unknown
Duration	20-180 min

INTERACTIONS

Individual drugs
Atenolol, etidronate, phenytoin, risedronate, ketoconazole: decreased levels of each drug
Digoxin: increased toxicity from hypercalcemia
QuiNIDine: increased quiNIDine levels

Drug classifications
Amphetamines: increased levels of amphetamines
Calcium channel blockers, fluoroquinolones, iron products, salicylates, tetracyclines: decreased levels of each specific product
Thiazide diuretics: increased hypercalcemia

Drug/lab test
False increase: chloride
False decrease: magnesium, oxylate, lipase
False positive: benzodiazepines

NURSING CONSIDERATIONS

Assessment
• Monitor Ca^+ (serum, urine); Ca^+ should be 8.5-10.5 mg/dl, urine Ca^+ should be 150 mg/day, monitor weekly
⚠ **Assess for milk-alkali syndrome: nausea, vomiting, disorientation, headache**
• Assess for constipation; increase bulk in the diet if needed
• Assess for **hypercalcemia:** headache, nausea, vomiting, confusion; hypocalcemia: paresthesia, twitching, colic, dysrhythmias, Chvostek's/Trousseau's sign
• Assess those taking digoxin for toxicity
• Assess those taking for abdominal pain, heartburn, indigestion before, after administration

Patient/family education
• Advise patient to increase fluids to 2 L unless contraindicated, to add bulk to diet for constipation; notify prescriber of constipation
• Advise patient not to switch antacids unless directed by prescriber, not to use as antacid for >2 wk without approval by prescriber
• Teach patient that therapeutic dose recommendations are figured as elemental calcium
• Advise to avoid excessive use of alcohol, caffeine, tobacco
• Teach to avoid spinach, cereals, dairy products in large amounts

Evaluation
Positive therapeutic outcome
• Absence of pain, decreased acidity
• Decreased hyperphosphatemia in renal failure (Acetate)

CALCIUM SALTS

calcium chloride (Rx)
calcium gluceptate (Rx)
calcium gluconate (Rx)
calcium lactate (PO-OTC, IV-Rx)
Func. class.: Electrolyte replacement—calcium product
Pregnancy category C

ACTION: Cation needed for maintenance of nervous, muscular, skeletal systems, enzyme reactions, normal cardiac contractility, coagulation of blood; affects secretory activity of endocrine, exocrine glands

Therapeutic outcome: Calcium at normal level, absence of increased magnesium, potassium

USES: Prevention and treatment of hypocalcemia, hypermagnesemia, hypoparathyroidism, neonatal tetany, cardiac toxicity caused by hyperkalemia, lead colic, hyperphosphatemia, vit D deficiency, osteoporosis prophylaxis, calcium antagonist toxicity (calcium channel blocker toxicity)

CONTRAINDICATIONS:
Hypercalcemia, digoxin toxicity, ventricular fibrillation, renal calculi

Precautions: Pregnancy **C**, breastfeeding, children, renal disease, respiratory disease, cor pulmonale, digitalized patient, respiratory failure, diarrhea, dehydration

---

DOSAGE AND ROUTES

Calcium chloride

Adult: **IV** 500 mg-1 g q1-3days as indicated by serum calcium levels; give at <1 ml/min; **IV** 200-800 mg injected in ventricle of heart

Calcium gluceptate

Adult: **IV** 5-20 ml; IM 2-5 ml

Calcium gluconate

Adult: PO 0.5-2 g bid-qid; **IV** 0.5-2 g at 0.5 ml/min (10% sol); max **IV** dose 3 g
Child: PO/IV 500 mg/kg/day in divided doses

Calcium lactate

Adult: PO 325 mg-1.3 g tid with meals
Child: PO 500 mg/kg/day in divided doses

Available forms: Many; check product listings

Implementation
PO route
• Give PO with or following meals to enhance absorption
• Store at room temperature
IM route
• Do not give chloride, gluconate IM
IV route
• Administer **IV** undiluted or diluted with equal amounts of 0.9% NaCl for inj to a 5% sol; give 0.5-1 ml/min
• Give through small-bore needle into large vein; if extravasation occurs, necrosis will result (**IV**); IM inj may cause severe burning, necrosis, and tissue sloughing; warm sol to body temp before administering (only gluconate/gluceptate)
• Provide seizure precautions: padded side rails, decreased stimuli (noise, light); place airway suction equipment, padded mouth gag if calcium levels are low
• Patient should remain recumbent 30 min after **IV** dose

Calcium chloride

Syringe compatibilities: Milrinone

Y-site compatibilities: DOBUTamine, EPINEPHrine, esmolol, inamrinone, morphine, paclitaxel

Additive compatibilities: Amikacin, amphotericin B, ampicillin, ascorbic acid, bretylium, cefTRIAXone, cephapirin, chloramphenicol, DOPamine, hydrocortisone, isoproterenol, lidocaine, methicillin, norepinephrine, penicillin G potassium, penicillin G sodium, PENTobarbital, PHENobarbital, verapamil, vit B/C

Calcium gluceptate

Additive compatibilities: Ascorbic acid inj, isoproterenol, lidocaine, norepinephrine, phytonadione, sodium bicarbonate

Calcium gluconate

Syringe compatibilities: Aldesleukin, allopurinol, amifostine, aztreonam, ceFAZolin, cefepime, ciprofloxacin, cladribine, DOBUTamine, enalaprilat, EPINEPHrine, famotidine, filgrastim, granisetron, heparin/hydrocortisone, labetalol, melphalan, midazolam, netilmicin, piperacillin/tazobactam, potassium chloride, prochlorperazine, propofol, sargramostim, tacrolimus, teniposide, thiotepa, tolazoline, vinorelbine, vit B/C

Additive compatibilities: Amikacin, aminophylline, ascorbic acid inj, bretylium, cephapirin, chloramphenicol, corticotropin, dimenhyDRINATE, erythromycin, furosemide, heparin, hydrocortisone, lidocaine, magnesium sulfate, methicillin, norepinephrine, penicillin G potassium, penicillin G sodium, PHENobarbital, potassium chloride, tobramycin, vancomycin, verapamil, vit B/C

ADVERSE EFFECTS
CV: *Shortened QT interval, heart block,* hypotension, bradycardia, dysrhythmias; **cardiac arrest (IV)**
GI: Vomiting, nausea, constipation
HYPERCALCEMIA: Drowsiness, lethargy, muscle weakness, headache, constipation, **coma,** anorexia, nausea, vomiting, polyuria, thirst
INTEG: Pain, burning at **IV** site, severe venous thrombosis, necrosis, extravasation

Pharmacokinetics

Absorption	Complete bioavailability (**IV**)
Distribution	Readily extracellular; crosses placenta, protein binding 40%-50%
Metabolism	Liver
Excretion	Feces (80%), kidney (20%), breast milk
Half-life	Unknown

Pharmacodynamics

	PO	IV
Onset	Unknown	Immediate
Peak	Unknown	Rapid
Duration	Unknown	½-1½ hr

INTERACTIONS
Individual drugs
Atenolol: decreased effect

Phenytoin, tetracyclines, thyroid: decreased absorption when calcium is taken PO

Verapamil: decreased effects, increased toxicity

Drug classifications
Antacids: milk-alkali syndrome (renal disease)

Digoxin glycosides: increased dysrhythmias

Diuretics (thiazide): increased hypercalcemia

Fluoroquinolones: decreased absorption of fluoroquinolones when calcium is taken PO

Iron salts: decreased absorption of iron when calcium is taken PO

Drug/herb
Lily of the valley, pheasant's eye, shark cartilage, squill: increased side effects, action

Drug/lab test
Increased: calcium

NURSING CONSIDERATIONS
Assessment
• Monitor ECG for decreased QT interval and T-wave inversion: in hypercalcemia, product should be reduced or discontinued

• Monitor calcium levels during treatment (9-10 mg/dl is normal level), urine calcium if hypercaluria occurs

• Assess cardiac status: rate, rhythm, CVP (PWP, PAWP if being monitored directly)

• Assess digitalized patients closely, an increase in calcium increases digoxin toxicity risk

• **Hypocalcemia:** muscle twitching, paresthesia, dysrhythmias, laryngospasm

Patient/family education
• Caution patient to add food high in vit D content; to add calcium-rich foods to diet: dairy products, shellfish, dark green leafy vegetables; decrease oxalate-rich and zinc-rich foods: nuts, legumes, chocolate, spinach, soy

• Advise patient to prevent injuries, avoid immobilization

Evaluation
Positive therapeutic outcome
• Decreased twitching, paresthesias, muscle spasms

• Absence of tremors, seizures, dysrhythmias, dyspnea, laryngospasm, negative Chvostek's sign, negative Trousseau's sign

---

candesartan (Rx)
(can-deh-sar′tan)

Atacand

Func. class.: Antihypertensive

Chem. class.: Angiotensin II receptor (type AT_1)

Pregnancy category
C (1st trimester),
D (2nd/3rd trimesters)

ACTION: Blocks the vasoconstrictor and aldosterone-secreting effects of angiotensin II; selectively blocks the binding of angiotensin II to the AT_1 receptor found in tissues

Therapeutic outcome: Decreased B/P

USES: Hypertension, alone or in combination; CHF NYHA Class II-IV and ejection fraction ≤40%

CONTRAINDICATIONS:
Hypersensitivity

> **BLACK BOX WARNING:** Pregnancy **D** (2nd/3rd trimesters)

Precautions: Pregnancy **C** (1st trimester), breastfeeding, children, geriatric, hypersensitivity to ACE inhibitors, volume depletion, renal/hepatic impairment, renal artery stenosis, hypotension

DOSAGE AND ROUTES
Adult: PO (single agent) 16 mg daily initially in patients who are not volume depleted, range 8-32 mg/day; with diuretic or volume depletion, 2-32 mg/day as a single dose or divided bid

Adult and child ≥6 yr and weight >50 kg: PO 8-16 mg/day or divided bid, adjust to B/P, usual range 4-32 mg/day max 30 mg/day

Child ≥6 yr and weight <50 kg: PO 4-8 mg/day or divided bid, adjust to B/P

Child ≥1 yr and <6 yr: PO 0.2 mg/kg/day in 1 dose or divided in 2 doses/day, adjust B/P, max 0.4 mg/kg/day

Heart failure
Adult: PO 4 mg/day, may be doubled ≥2 wk, target dose 32 mg/day

Renal/hepatic dose
Adult: PO ≤8 mg/day in severe renal disease/moderate hepatic disease, adjust dose as needed

Available forms: Tabs 4, 8, 16, 32 mg

Implementation
- Administer without regard to meals
- Oral liquid (compounded) shake well, do not freeze

ADVERSE EFFECTS
CNS: *Dizziness,* fatigue, headache, syncope
CV: Chest pain, peripheral edema, hypotension, palpitations
EENT: Sinusitis, rhinitis, pharyngitis
GI: *Diarrhea,* nausea, abdominal pain, vomiting
GU: **Renal failure**
MS: Arthralgia, pain
RESP: *Cough, upper respiratory infection*
SYST: **Angioedema**

Pharmacokinetics

Absorption	Well absorbed
Distribution	Bound to plasma proteins
Metabolism	Extensive
Excretion	Feces, urine, breast milk
Half-life	9 hr

Pharmacodynamics

Onset	Unknown
Peak	2 hr
Duration	24 hr

INTERACTIONS
Individual drugs
Lithium: increased lithium level
Potassium: increased hyperkalemia

Drug classifications
α-Blockers, ACE inhibitors, β-blockers, calcium channel blockers: increased hypotension
Diuretics (potassium sparing): increased hypokalemia
NSAIDs, salicylates: decreased effect

Drug/herb
Astragalus, cola tree: increased or decreased antihypertensive effect
Ephedra: decreased antihypertensive effect
Hawthorn: increased antihypertensive effect

NURSING CONSIDERATIONS
Assessment
- **Serious hypersensitivity reactions:** Assess for angioedema, anaphylaxis; facial swelling, difficulty breathing (rare)
- **Heart failure:** Assess for jugular vein distention, weight, edema, dyspnea, crackles
- Assess B/P, pulse q4hr; note rate, rhythm, quality

- Monitor electrolytes: potassium, sodium, chloride; total CO_2
- Obtain baselines in renal, liver function tests before therapy begins
- Assess blood studies: BUN, creatinine, liver function tests before treatment
- Monitor for edema in feet, legs daily
- Assess for skin turgor, dryness of mucous membranes for hydration status; for angioedema: facial swelling, dyspnea

> **BLACK BOX WARNING:** Assess for pregnancy; this product can cause fetal death when given in pregnancy (**D**), 2nd/3rd trimester

- Assess for adverse reactions, especially in renal disease

Patient/family education
- Teach patient not to take the product if breastfeeding or pregnant, or having had an allergic reaction to this product
- If a dose is missed, instruct patient to take as soon as possible, unless it is within 1 hour before next dose
- Advise patient to comply with dosage schedule, even if feeling better
- Teach patient to notify prescriber of fever, swelling of hands or feet, irregular heartbeat, chest pain
- Advise patient that excessive perspiration, dehydration, diarrhea may lead to fall in blood pressure—consult prescriber if these occur
- Inform patient that product may cause dizziness, fainting; light-headedness may occur
- Advise patient to avoid all OTC medications unless approved by prescriber; to inform all health care providers of medication use
- Caution patient to rise slowly to sitting or standing position to minimize orthostatic hypotension
- Teach proper technique for obtaining B/P and acceptable parameters

> **BLACK BOX WARNING:** Teach patient to notify prescriber immediately if pregnant (**D**) 2nd/3rd trimester, (**C**) 1st trimester, not to use if breastfeeding

Evaluation
Positive therapeutic outcome
- Decreased B/P

capecitabine (Rx)
(cap-eh-sit'ah-bean)
Xeloda
Func. class.: Antineoplastic, antimetabolite
Chem. class.: Fluoropyrimidine carbamate
Pregnancy category D

Do not confuse:
Xeloda/Xenical

ACTION: Competes with physiologic substrate of DNA synthesis, thus interfering with cell replication in the S phase of cell cycle (before mitosis); also interferes with RNA and protein synthesis; product is converted to 5-fluorouracil (5-FU)

Therapeutic outcome: Decreasing symptoms of breast cancer

USES: Monotherapy for paclitaxel-anthracycline-resistant metastatic breast, colorectal cancer when 5-FU monotherapy is preferred; treatment of patients with colorectal cancer who have undergone complete resection of their primary tumor

CONTRAINDICATIONS:
Pregnancy **D**, infants, hypersensitivity to 5-FU, severe renal impairment (CCr <30 ml/min), DPD deficiency

Precautions: Renal/hepatic disease, breast-feeding, children, geriatric

DOSAGE AND ROUTES
Metastatic breast cancer resistant to both paclitaxel and anthracycline or resistant to paclitaxel and when further anthracycline therapy is not indicated
Adult: PO 2500 mg/m^2/day divided q12hr after meal ×2 wk, repeat q3wk

Breast cancer (locally advanced/metastatic) with docetaxel, previously treated with anthracycline
Adult: PO 2500 mg/m^2/day divided q12hr after a meal on days 1-14, with docetaxel 75 mg/m^2 IV on day 1

Advanced/metastatic breast cancer (HER2 positive), who have received anthracycline, taxane, and trastuzumab
Adult: PO 2000 mg/m^2/day divided q12hr after a meal on days 1-14 with lapatinib 1250 mg/day on days 1-21, repeat q21days

Metastatic/locally advanced breast cancer, resistant to anthracycline, and a taxane or taxane resistant and when further anthracycline is contraindicated
Adult: PO 2000 mg/m^2/day divided q12hr on days 1-14 with ixabepilone 40 mg/m^2 IV over 3 hr, repeat q3wk

As an adjuvant in Dukes C colorectal cancer with a complete resection when fluoropyrimidine alone is preferred
Adult: PO 2500 mg/m^2/day divided q12hr within 30 min of a meal ×2 wk, repeat q3wk for 8 cycles

First-line in metastatic colorectal cancer when fluoropyrimidine alone is preferred
Adult: PO 2500 mg/m^2/day divided q12hr after a meal ×2 wk repeat q3wk

Renal dose
Adult: PO CCr 30-50 ml/min; decrease initial dose to 75% of usual dose; CCr < 30 ml/min contraindicated

Available forms: Tabs 150, 500 mg

Implementation
• **Dosage adjustments of capecitabine monotherapy based on the most severe toxicity OR when used in combination with ixabepilone based on nonhematologic toxicity:** *Grade 1 toxicity:* Maintain current dosage; *Grade 2 toxicity (1st appearance):* interrupt therapy until toxicity is resolved to grade 0–1; do not replace missed doses, begin the next cycle with 100% of the starting dose; *Grade 2 toxicity (2nd appearance):* interrupt therapy until toxicity is resolved to grade 0–1; do not replace missed doses, begin the next cycle with 75% of the starting dose; *Grade 2 toxicity (3rd appearance):* interrupt therapy until toxicity is resolved to grade 0–1; do not replace missed doses, begin the next cycle with 50% of the starting dose; *Grade 2 toxicity (4th appearance):* discontinue treatment permanently; *Grade 3 toxicity (1st appearance):* interrupt therapy until toxicity is resolved to grade 0-1

• Help patient to rinse mouth tid-qid with water or club soda, brush teeth bid-qid with soft brush or cotton-tipped applicators for stomatitis, use unwaxed dental floss

ADVERSE EFFECTS

CNS: Dizziness, headache, *paresthesia, fatigue,* insomnia
CV: Venous thrombosis
GI: *Nausea, vomiting, anorexia, diarrhea, stomatitis, abdominal pain, constipation, dyspepsia,* **intestinal obstruction, necrotizing enterocolitis,** hyperbilirubinemia, **hepatic failure**
HEMA: Neutropenia, lymphopenia, thrombocytopenia, anemia
INTEG: *Hand and foot syndrome,* dermatitis, nail disorder
MISC: Eye irritation, edema, myalgia, limb pain, *pyrexia,* dehydration
RESP: *Cough, dyspnea,* **pulmonary embolism**

Pharmacokinetics

Absorption	Readily absorbed, decreased with food
Distribution	Unknown
Metabolism	Liver, extensively
Excretion	Kidneys
Half-life	45 min

Pharmacodynamics

Onset	Unknown
Peak	1½ hr
Duration	Unknown

INTERACTIONS

Individual drugs
Leucovorin: increased toxicity
Phenytoin: increased phenytoin level

Drug classifications
Antacids (aluminum, magnesium): increased capecitabine

> **BLACK BOX WARNING:** Anticoagulants: increased risk of bleeding

Food/drug
Increased absorption; give within 30 min of a meal

Drug/lab test
Increased: bilirubin
Decreased: Hgb/Hct/RBC, neutrophils, platelets, WBC

NURSING CONSIDERATIONS

Assessment
• **Bone marrow suppression:** Monitor CBC, differential, platelet count weekly; withhold product if WBC <4000/mm³ or platelet count is <75,000/mm³ or RBC, Hct, Hgb is low; notify prescriber of results; frequently monitor INR in those receiving warfarin
• Assess buccal cavity q8hr for dryness, sores or ulceration, white patches, pain, bleeding, dysphagia; obtain prescription for viscous lidocaine (Xylocaine)
• Assess symptoms indicating severe allergic reaction: rash, pruritus, urticaria, purpuric skin lesions, itching, flushing; product should be discontinued
• Monitor temp q4hr (may indicate beginning of infection)
• Assess for **hand/foot syndrome:** paresthesia, tingling, painful/painless swelling, blistering, erythema with severe pain of hands/feet
• Assess for **toxicity:** severe diarrhea (multiple times/day or at night), nausea, vomiting, stomatitis
• Assess **GI symptoms:** frequency of stools, cramping; if severe diarrhea occurs, fluids/electrolytes may need to be given
• Monitor liver function tests before and during therapy (bilirubin, AST, ALT, LDH) as needed or monthly; note jaundice of skin or sclera, dark urine, clay-colored stools, itchy skin, abdominal pain, fever, diarrhea

> **BLACK BOX WARNING:** Assess for bleeding: hematuria, stool guaiac, bruising or petechiae, mucosa or orifices q8hr; inflammation of mucosa, breaks in skin, monitor INR and PT in those taking anticoagulants

Patient/family education
• Advise patient to avoid use of products containing aspirin or ibuprofen, razors, commercial mouthwash, since bleeding may occur; to report symptoms of bleeding (hematuria, tarry stools)
• Instruct patient to report signs of **anemia** (fatigue, headache, irritability, faintness, shortness of breath); **infection:** increased temp, sore throat, flulike symptoms
⚠ Advise patient not to become pregnant while taking this product; not to use while breastfeeding
• Advise patient not to double dose, if dose is missed
• Advise patient to report immediately severe diarrhea, vomiting, stomatitis, fever ≥100° F, hand/foot syndrome, anorexia

Evaluation
Positive therapeutic outcome
• Prevention of rapid division of malignant cells

captopril (Rx)
(kap'toe-pril)
Apo-Capto ✦, Capoten
Func. class.: Antihypertensive
Chem. class.: Angiotensin-converting enzyme (ACE) inhibitor
Pregnancy category D

Do not confuse:
captopril/Capitrol/carvedilol

ACTION: Selectively suppresses renin-angiotensin-aldosterone system; inhibits ACE; prevents conversion of angiotensin I to angiotensin II

Therapeutic outcome: Decreased B/P in hypertension; decreased preload, afterload in CHF

USES: Hypertension, CHF, left ventricular dysfunction (LVD) after MI, diabetic nephropathy, proteinuria

CONTRAINDICATIONS:
Breastfeeding, children, hypersensitivity, heart block, potassium-sparing diuretics, bilateral renal artery stenosis, angioedema

> **BLACK BOX WARNING:** Pregnancy **D** (2nd/3rd trimester)

Precautions: Dialysis patients, hypovolemia, leukemia, scleroderma, LE, blood dyscrasias, CHF, diabetes mellitus, renal/hepatic disease, thyroid disease, African descent, pregnancy (C) 1st trimester, collagen-vascular disease, hyperkalemia, hyponatremia

DOSAGE AND ROUTES
Hypertension
Adult: Initial dose: PO 12.5-25 mg bid-tid; may increase to 50 mg bid-tid at 1-2 wk intervals; usual range 25-150 mg bid-tid; max 450 mg/day
Child: PO 0.3-0.5 mg/kg/dose, titrate up to 6 mg/kg/day in 1-4 divided doses

Neonate: PO 0.05-0.1 mg/kg bid-tid, may increase as needed

CHF
Adult: PO 25 mg tid; may increase to 50 mg bid-tid; after 14 days may increase to 150 mg tid if needed

Diabetic nephropathy
Adult: PO 25 mg tid

Renal dose
Adult: PO CCr >50 ml/min, no change; CCr 10-50 ml/min, decrease dose by 25%; CCr <10 ml/min, decrease dose by 50%

Available forms: Tabs 12.5, 25, 50, 100 mg

Implementation
• Store in air-tight container at 86° F (30° C) or less
• Severe hypotension may occur after first dose of this medication; decreasing hypotension may be prevented by reducing or discontinuing diuretic therapy 3 days before beginning captopril therapy
• Administer 1 hr before or 2 hr after meals
• **Oral sol:** May crush tab and dissolve in water, give within ½ hr, make sure tab is completely dissolved

ADVERSE EFFECTS
CNS: Fever, chills
CV: *Hypotension,* postural hypotension, *tachycardia,* angina
GI: Loss of taste, increased liver function tests
GU: Impotence, dysuria, nocturia, proteinuria, **nephrotic syndrome, acute reversible renal failure,** polyuria, oliguria, frequency
HEMA: **Neutropenia, agranulocytosis, pancytopenia, thrombocytopenia,** anemia
INTEG: Rash, pruritus
MISC: **Angioedema,** hyperkalemia
RESP: **Bronchospasm,** *dyspnea, cough*

Pharmacokinetics

Absorption	Well absorbed
Distribution	Widely distributed; crosses placenta, excreted in breast milk (small amounts)
Metabolism	Liver (50%)
Excretion	Kidneys, unchanged (50%)
Half-life	2 hr increase in renal disease

Pharmacodynamics

Onset	¼-1 hr
Peak	1 hr
Duration	6-12 hr

INTERACTIONS
Individual drugs
Alcohol (acute ingestion): increased hypotension (large amounts)

Digoxin, lithium: increased serum levels, toxicity

Insulin: increased hypoglycemia

Drug classifications
Antacids, NSAIDs, salicylates: decreased captopril effect

Antidiabetics (oral): increased hypoglycemia

Antihypertensives, diuretics, nitrates, phenothiazines: increased hypotension

Diuretics (potassium-sparing), potassium supplements: increased toxicity, do not use

Sympathomimetics: do not use

Drug/herb
Ephedra: decreased antihypertensive effect

Hawthorn: increased antihypertensive effect

Drug/food
Food: decreased absorption of captopril

Drug/lab test
Increased: AST, ALT, alkaline phosphatase, bilirubin, uric acid, potassium

Decreased: platelets, WBC, RBC, Hgb/Hct

False positive: urine acetone, ANA titer

NURSING CONSIDERATIONS
Assessment
⚠ **Blood dyscrasias: Monitor blood studies: decreased platelets; WBC with diff baseline, periodically q3mo, if neutrophils are <1000/mm³, discontinue treatment**

• **Hypertension:** Monitor B/P, check for orthostatic hypotension, syncope; if changes occur, dosage change may be required

• Monitor renal studies: protein, BUN, creatinine; watch for increased levels that may indicate nephrotic syndrome and renal failure; monitor renal symptoms: polyuria, oliguria, frequency, dysuria, potassium

• Establish baselines in renal, liver function tests before therapy begins and check periodically; monitor for increased liver function studies; watch for increased uric acid, glucose

• Check potassium levels throughout treatment, although hyperkalemia rarely occurs

• **CHF:** Assess for edema, dyspnea, wet crackles, increased B/P, weight gain

• **Assess for allergic reactions:** rash, fever, pruritus, urticaria; product should be discontinued if antihistamines fail to help

Patient/family education
• Caution patient not to discontinue product abruptly; advise patient to tell all persons associated with care

• Teach patient not to use OTC products (cough, cold, allergy) unless directed by prescriber; serious side effects can occur; xanthines such as coffee, tea, chocolate, cola can prevent action of product

• Teach patient importance of complying with dosage schedule, even if feeling better; to continue with medical regimen to decrease B/P: exercise, smoking cessation, decreasing stress, diet modifications

• Emphasize the need to rise slowly to sitting or standing position to minimize orthostatic hypotension; not to exercise in hot weather or increased hypotension can occur

• Teach patient to notify prescriber of mouth sores, sore throat, fever, swelling of hands or feet, irregular heartbeat, chest pain, coughing, shortness of breath

• Caution patient to report excessive perspiration, dehydration, vomiting, diarrhea; may lead to fall in B/P

• Caution patient that product may cause dizziness, fainting, light-headedness; may occur during first few days of therapy; to avoid activities that may be hazardous, avoid activities that require concentration

• Teach patient how to take B/P, and teach normal readings for age-group; ensure patient takes regularly

> **BLACK BOX WARNING:** Advise patient to tell prescriber if pregnancy is suspected or planned, pregnancy **(D)**

Evaluation
Positive therapeutic outcome
• Decreased B/P in hypertension

TREATMENT OF OVERDOSE:
0.9% NaCl **IV** infusion, hemodialysis

carbachol ophthalmic
See Appendix B

carBAMazepine (Rx)
(kar-ba-maz'e-peen)
Carbatrol, Equetro, Mazepine, Novo-Carbamaz, TEGretol, TEGretol-XR
Func. class.: Anticonvulsant
Chem. class.: Iminostilbene derivative
Pregnancy category D

Do not confuse:
TEGretol/Toradol

ACTION: Exact mechanism unknown; appears to decrease polysynaptic responses and block posttetanic potentiation

Therapeutic outcome: Absence of seizures; decreased trigeminal neuralgia pain

USES: Tonic-clonic, complex-partial, mixed seizures; trigeminal neuralgia; bipolar disorder

Unlabeled uses: Neurogenic pain, psychotic behavior with dementia, diabetic neuropathy, agitation, hiccups

CONTRAINDICATIONS:
Pregnancy **D**, hypersensitivity to carBAMazepine or tricyclics

> **BLACK BOX WARNING:** Bone marrow suppression

Precautions: Glaucoma, renal/hepatic/cardiac disease, psychosis, breastfeeding, child <6 yr, alcoholism, hepatic porphyria, AV or bundle branch block

> **BLACK BOX WARNING:** Hematologic disease, agranulocytosis, leukopenia, neutropenia, thrombocytopenia, Asian patients

DOSAGE AND ROUTES
Seizures
Adult and child >12 yr: PO 200 mg bid; may be increased by 200 mg/day in weekly intervals, give in divided doses q6-8hr; maintenance 800-1200 mg/day; max 1600 mg/day (adult); max child 12-15 yr 1000 mg/day; max child >15 yr 1200 mg/day; adjustment is needed to minimum dose to control seizures; EXT REL give bid; RECT administration of oral SUSP 200 mg/10 ml or 6 mg/kg as a single dose
Child 6-12 yr: PO tabs 100 mg bid or SUSP 50 mg qid; may increase by <100 mg qwk, max 1000 mg/day, usual dose 15-30 mg/kg/day; EXT REL tabs daily-bid

Child <6 yr: PO 10-20 mg/kg/day in 2-3 divided doses or 4 divided doses (susp), may increase qwk

Trigeminal neuralgia
Adult: PO 100 mg/bid; may increase 100 mg q12hr until pain subsides; max 1200 mg/day; maintenance is 200-400 mg bid

Bipolar disorder
Adult: PO (Equetro only) (regular release) 200 mg bid, may adjust dose 3-4 days to achieve carBAMazepine level to 8-12 mcg/ml micro response; max 1600 mg/day

Agitation due to dementia (unlabeled)
Adult: PO 100 mg bid, may increase to 250-300 mg/day

Hiccups (unlabeled)
Adult: PO 200 mg tid

Available forms: Chewable tabs 100, 200 mg; oral susp 100 mg/5 ml; ext rel tabs 100, 200, 400 mg; ext rel caps (Carbatrol) 200, 300 mg

Implementation
• Do not break, crush, or chew ext rel tabs and caps; ext rel caps may be opened and beads mixed with food; chewable tabs should be chewed, not swallowed whole
• Give with food for GI symptoms
• Shake oral susp before use
• **Suspension:** Turn off N/G, internal feeding 15 min before and hold for 15 min after; mix an equal amount of water, D_5W, 0.9% NaCl when giving by NG tube, flush tube with 15-30 ml of above sol
• Store at room temperature

ADVERSE EFFECTS
CNS: *Drowsiness,* dizziness, confusion, fatigue, **paralysis,** headache, hallucinations, **worsening of seizures,** unsteadiness, speech disturbances, **suicidal ideation, neuroleptic malignant syndrome (when used with psychotropics)**
CV: Hypertension, CHF, hypotension, aggravation of CAD, dysrhythmias, **AV block**
EENT: Tinnitus, dry mouth, blurred vision, diplopia, nystagmus, conjunctivitis
ENDO: Syndrome of inappropriate antidiuretic hormone (SIADH) (geriatric)
GI: *Nausea, constipation, diarrhea,* anorexia, vomiting, abdominal pain, stomatitis, glossitis, increased liver enzymes, **hepatitis, hepatic porphyria, hypercholesterolemia, pancreatitis**

GU: Frequency, retention, albuminuria, glycosuria, impotence, increased BUN, **renal failure**
HEMA: Thrombocytopenia, leukopenia, **agranulocytosis, leukocytosis, aplastic anemia, eosinophilia,** increased pro-time, lymphadenopathy
INTEG: *Rash,* **Stevens-Johnson syndrome,** urticaria, photosensitivity, **toxic epidermal necrolysis, DRESS,** alopecia
MS: Osteoporosis
RESP: Pulmonary hypersensitivity (fever, dyspnea, pneumonitis)

Pharmacokinetics

Absorption	Slow; completely absorbed
Distribution	Widely distributed; protein binding 76%
Metabolism	Extensively, liver, metabolized by CYP3A4
Excretion	Urine, feces, breast milk
Half-life	18-65 hr, then 8-29 hr after first month

Pharmacodynamics

Onset	Slow
Peak	4-5 hr (PO), 1.5 hr (susp)
Duration	Unknown

INTERACTIONS

Individual drugs

Benzodiazepines, darunavir, delavirdine, doxycycline, felbamate, haloperidol, nefazodone, OXcarbazepine, PHENobarbital, phenytoin, primidone: decreased effect of these products
Cimetidine, clarithromycin, danzol, diltiazem, erythromycin, FLUoxetine, fluvoxaMINE, isoniazid, propoxyphene, valproic acid, verapamil, voriconazole: increased carBAMazepine levels
CISplatin, darunavir, delavirdine, DOXOrubicin, felbamate, nefazodone, OXcarbazepine, PHENobarbital, phenytoin, primidone, rifampin, theophylline: decreased carBAMazepine levels
Contraceptives (oral): decreased effect of oral contraceptives
Desmopressin, lithium, hypressin, vasopressin: increased effects of each specific product
Doxycycline: decreased effect of doxycycline
Lithium: increased CNS toxicity
Phenytoin: increased and decreased plasma levels; decreased carBAMazepine plasma levels
Thyroid hormones: decreased effect of thyroid hormones
Warfarin: decreased effect of warfarin

Drug classifications

CYP3A4 inducers: decreased carBAMazepine levels
CYP3A4 inhibitors: increased carBAMazepine levels
⚠ MAOIs: fatal reaction; do not use together
⚠ Do not use with: NNRTIs (non-nucleoside reverse-transcriptase inhibitors), nefazodone

Drug/herb

Echinacea: decreased carBAMazepine metabolism, increased levels
St. John's wort: decreased anticonvulsant action

Drug/food

Grapefruit juice: increased peak concentration of carBAMazepine

Drug/lab test

Decreased: serum calcium, sodium
Increased: cholesterol

NURSING CONSIDERATIONS
Assessment

> **BLACK BOX WARNING:** Serious skin reactions: Asian patient, obtain genetic test prior to administration

• Assess for **seizures:** character, location, duration, intensity, frequency, presence of aura
• Assess for **trigeminal neuralgia:** facial pain including location, duration, intensity, character, activity that stimulates pain
• Monitor liver function tests (AST, ALT) and urine function tests, BUN, urine protein periodically during treatments; serum calcium may be decreased and lead to osteoporosis; cholesterol periodically
• **Bone marrow depression:** Assess blood studies: RBC, Hct, Hgb, reticulocyte counts qwk for 4 wk then q3-6mo if on long-term therapy; if myelosuppression occurs, product should be discontinued
⚠ Serious skin, multi-organ hypersensitivity (Stevens-Johnson syndrome, toxic epidermal necrolysis, DRESS): May be increased in HLA-A 3101 gene and may be fatal
• Check blood levels during treatment or when changing dose; therapeutic level 4-12 mcg/ml
• Assess for **blood dyscrasias:** fever, sore throat, bruising, rash, jaundice, epistaxis (long-term treatment only)
⚠ Assess mental status: mood, sensorium, affect, behavioral changes, suicidal thoughts/behaviors

- **Toxicity:** Assess for bone marrow depression, nausea, vomiting, ataxia, diplopia, CV collapse, Stevens-Johnson syndrome

Patient/family education
- Teach patient to carry/wear emergency ID stating patient's name, products taken, condition, prescriber's name, phone number
- Caution patient to avoid driving, other activities that require alertness until stabilized on medication
- Teach patient not to discontinue medication quickly after long-term use
- Teach patient to use a nonhormonal type of contraception to prevent harm to the fetus
- Advise patient to use sunscreen to prevent burns
- Teach patient to take exactly as prescribed; do not double or omit doses
- Teach patient to report immediately chills, rash, light-colored stools, dark urine, yellowing of skin/eyes, abdominal pain, sore throat, mouth ulcers, bruising, blurred vision, dizziness, **skin rash, fever**
- Teach patient to notify if pregnancy is planned or suspected, pregnancy **(D)**, avoid breastfeeding

Evaluation
Positive therapeutic outcome
- Decreased seizure activity

TREATMENT OF OVERDOSE:
Lavage, VS

⚠ HIGH ALERT

CARBOplatin (Rx)
(kar'boe'pla-tin)
Func. class.: Antineoplastic alkylating agent
Chem. class.: Platinum coordination compound
Pregnancy category D

Do not confuse:
CARBOplatin/CISplatin

ACTION: Produces interstrand DNA cross-links and to a lesser extent DNA-protein cross-links; activity is not cell cycle phase specific

Therapeutic outcome: Prevention of rapidly growing malignant cells

USES: Initial treatment of advanced ovarian cancer in combination with other agents; palliative treatment of recurrent ovarian carcinoma after treatment with other antineoplastic agents

CONTRAINDICATIONS:
Pregnancy **D,** hypersensitivity to this product, breastfeeding, significant bleeding, aluminum products used to prepare or administer CARBOplatin

> **BLACK BOX WARNING:** Severe bone marrow depression, platinum compound hypersensitivity

Precautions: Geriatric patients, radiation therapy within 1 mo, other cancer, chemotherapy within 1 mo, renal disease, liver disease

> **BLACK BOX WARNING:** Anemia, infection

DOSAGE AND ROUTES
Dosing with the Calvert equation
Adult: The total CARBOplatin dose (in mg) for adults may be calculated using the Calvert equation: *total dose (mg/m^2) = target AUC × (GFR + 25)*
Child: Calculate CARBOplatin dose (mg/m^2) in children as follows: *total dose (mg/m^2) = target AUC × [(0.93 × GFR) + 15]*

Advanced ovarian cancer
Adult (single agent): IV INF initially 300 mg/m^2 on day 1 with cyclophosphamide, 600 mg/m^2 IV on day 1, repeat q4wk × 6 cycles; refractory tumors 360 mg/m^2 single dose, may repeat q4wk as needed; do not repeat until neutrophils are >2000 mm^3 and platelets are >100,000/mm^3

Renal dose
Adult: IV INF CCr 41-59 ml/min 250 mg/m^2, CCr 16-40 ml/min 200 mg/m^2; do not use in CCr <15 ml/min

Available forms: Lyophilized powder for inj 50, 150, 450 mg vials; aqueous sol for inj 50 mg/5 ml vial, 150 mg/15 ml vial, 450 mg/45 mg vial, 600 mg/60 ml vial

Implementation
- Antiemetic 30-60 min before giving product to prevent vomiting, and prn

IV route
- Do not use needles or IV administration sets containing aluminum; may cause precipitate or loss of potency
- Use cytotoxic handling procedures
- **Reconstitute** CARBOplatin 50, 150, or 450 mg with 5, 15, or 45 ml respectively of sterile

---

water for inj, D₅W, or NaCl (10 mg/ml); then further **dilute** with the same sol to 0.5-4 mg/ml; **give** over 15 min or more (**intermittent INF**)
• **Continuous IV INF** over 24 hr; max dose based on (GFR = 125 mg/ml)
• Store protected from light at room temperature; reconstituted sol is stable for 8 hr at room temperature

Y-site compatibilities: Acyclovir, alfentanil, allopurinol, amifostine, amikacin, aminocaproic acid, aminophylline, amiodarone, amphotericin B lipid complex, amphotericin B liposome, ampicillin, ampicillin sulbactam, anidulafungin, atenolol, atracurium, azithromycin, aztreonam, bivalirudin, bleomycin, bumetanide, buprenorphine, butorphanol, calcium chloride/gluconate, caspofungin, ceFAZolin, cefepime, cefoperazone, cefotaxime, cefoTEtan, cefOXitin, cefTAZidime, ceftizoxime, cefTRIAXone, cefuroxime, cimetidine, ciprofloxacin, cisatracurium, CISplatin, cladribine, clindamycin, codeine, cyclophosphamide, cycloSPORINE, cytarabine, DAPTOmycin, DAUNOrubicin, dexamethasone, dexmedetomidine, dexrazoxane, digoxin, diltiazem, diphenhydrAMINE, DOBUTamine, DOCEtaxel, DOPamine, doripenem, doxacurium, DOXOrubicin, DOXOrubicin liposomal, doxycycline, droperidol, enalaprilat, ePHEDrine, EPINEPHrine, epirubicin, ertapenem, erythromycin, esmolol, etoposide, famotidine, fenoldopam, fentaNYL, filgrastim, fluconazole, fludarabine, fluorouracil, foscarnet, fosphenytoin, furosemide, ganciclovir, gatifloxacin, gemcitabine, gentamicin, granisetron, haloperidol, heparin, hydrocortisone, HYDROmorphone, hydrOXYzine, IDArubicin, ifosfamide, imipenem-cilastatin, inamrinone, insulin (regular), irinotecan, isoproterenol, ketorolac, labetalol, levofloxacin, levorphanol, lidocaine, linezolid injection, LORazepam, magnesium sulfate, mannitol, melphalan, meperidine, meropenem, mesna, methohexital, methotrexate, methylPREDNISolone, metoclopramide, metoprolol, metroNIDAZOLE, micafungin, midazolam, milrinone, minocycline, mitoXANtrone, mivacurium, morphine, nafcillin, nalbuphine, naloxone, nesiritide, niCARdipine, nitroglycerin, nitroprusside, norepinephrine, octreotide, ofloxacin, ondansetron, oxaliplatin, PACLitaxel, palonosetron, pamidronate, pancuronium, pantoprazole, PEMEtrexed, pentamidine, PENTobarbital, PHENobarbital, phentolamine, piperacillin, piperacillin-tazobactam, potassium chloride, potassium phosphates, prochlorperazine, promethazine, propofol, propranolol, ranitidine, remifentanil, riTUXimab, rocuronium, sargramostim,

sodium acetate, sodium bicarbonate, sodium phosphates, succinylcholine, SUFentanil, sulfamethoxazole-trimethoprim, tacrolimus, teniposide, theophylline, thiotepa, ticarcillin, ticarcillin-clavulanate, tigecycline, tirofiban, TNA, tobramycin, topotecan, TPN, trastuzumab, trimethobenzamide, vancomycin, vasopressin, vecuronium, verapamil, vinBLAStine, vinCRIStine, vinorelbine, voriconazole, zidovudine

Solution compatibilities: D₅/0.2% NaCl, D₅/0.45% NaCl, D₅/0.9% NaCl, 0.9% NaCl, D₅W, sterile water for inj

Solution incompatibilities: Sodium bicarbonate

ADVERSE EFFECTS
CNS: **Seizures, central neurotoxicity,** peripheral neuropathy, dizziness, confusion
CV: Cardiac abnormalities (**fatal CV events**), **stroke**
EENT: Tinnitus, hearing loss, *vestibular toxicity*, visual changes
GI: Severe nausea, vomiting, diarrhea, weight loss, mucositis, anorexia, constipation, taste change
HEMA: **Thrombocytopenia, leukopenia, pancytopenia, neutropenia, anemia,** bleeding
INTEG: Alopecia, dermatitis, rash, erythema, pruritus, urticaria
META: Hypomagnesemia, hypocalcemia, hypokalemia, hyponatremia, hyperuremia
SYST: **Anaphylaxis**

Pharmacokinetics

Absorption	Complete
Distribution	Unknown
Metabolism	Liver
Excretion	Kidneys
Half-life	Initial 1-2 hr; postdistribution 2½-6 hr; increased in renal disease

Pharmacodynamics

Onset	½ hr
Peak	Unknown
Duration	4-6 hr

INTERACTIONS
Individual drugs
Amphotericin B: increased nephrotoxicity or ototoxicity
Aspirin, anticoagulants, platelet inhibitors: increased risk of bleeding
Phenytoin: decreased levels, monitor levels

Radiation: increased toxicity, bone marrow suppression

Drug classifications

Aminoglycosides: ototoxicity, increased nephrotoxicity

Antineoplastics, bone marrow–suppressing products: increased bone marrow suppression

Myelosuppressives: increased myelosuppression

NSAIDs: increased risk of bleeding

Thrombolytic agents: increased risk of bleeding

Drug/lab test

Increased: AST, BUN, alkaline phosphatase, bilirubin, creatinine

Decreased: platelets, neutrophils, WBC, RBC, Hgb/Hct, calcium, potassium, magnesium, phosphate

NURSING CONSIDERATIONS

Assessment

> **BLACK BOX WARNING:** To be used only by person experienced in the use of chemotherapeutic products, in a specialized care setting

> **BLACK BOX WARNING: Bone marrow depression:** Monitor CBC, differential, platelet count weekly; withhold product if neutrophil count is <2000/mm³ or platelet count is <100,000/mm³; notify prescriber of results, calcium, magnesium, phosphate, potassium, sodium, uric acid, CCR, bilirubin; creatinine clearance < 60 ml/min may be responsible for increased bone marrow suppression; assess frequently for infection

• Assess for **anaphylaxis:** pruritus, wheezing, tachycardia; may occur within a few minutes of use; notify physician after discontinuing products; resuscitation equipment should be available

• **Peripheral neuropathy:** may be increased in geriatrics

• Delay dental work until blood counts have returned to normal; regular toothbrushes, dental floss and toothpicks should not be used, use soft bristle toothbrush

• Monitor renal function studies: BUN, creatinine, serum uric acid, urine CCr before, during therapy; I&O ratio; report fall in urine output to <30 ml/hr

• Monitor temp q4hr (may indicate beginning of infection)

⚠ Monitor liver function tests before, during therapy (bilirubin, AST, ALT, LDH) as needed or monthly; note jaundice of skin or sclera, dark urine, clay-colored stools, itchy skin, abdominal pain, fever, diarrhea

• Assess for **bleeding:** hematuria, stool guaiac, bruising or petechiae, mucosa or orifices; inflammation of mucosa, breaks in skin; avoid all IM injections if platelets <50,000/mm³

• Identify effects of alopecia on body image; discuss feelings about body changes

Patient/family education

• Advise patient to report ringing/roaring in the ears, numbness, tingling in face, extremities, weight gain

• Teach patient to avoid use of products containing aspirin or ibuprofen, NSAIDs, alcohol, razors, commercial mouthwash, since bleeding may occur; to report symptoms of bleeding (hematuria, tarry stools)

• Instruct patient to report signs of **anemia** (fatigue, headache, irritability, faintness, shortness of breath); sore throat, bleeding, bruising, chills, back pain, blood in stools, dyspnea

• Instruct patient to report any changes in breathing or coughing even several months after treatment; to avoid crowds and persons with respiratory tract or other infections

• Advise patient that hair may be lost during treatment; a wig or hairpiece may make patient feel better; new hair may be different in color, texture

• Caution patient not to have any vaccinations without the advice of the prescriber; serious reactions can occur

• Teach patient that contraception is needed during treatment and for several months after the completion of therapy; not to breastfeed during treatment; to notify prescriber if pregnancy is planned or suspected

⚠ Teach patient that impotence or amenorrhea can occur; that this is reversible after treatment is discontinued; to notify prescriber if pregnancy is planned or suspected; pregnancy (D), that contraception should be used if patient is fertile

⚠ Teach patient not to breastfeed

• Teach patient to notify prescriber immediately of fever, fatigue, sore throat, bleeding, bruising, chills, back pain, blood in stools, dyspnea

Evaluation

Positive therapeutic outcome

• Prevention of rapid division of malignant cells

carboprost (Rx)

(kar'boe-prost)
Hemabate
Func. class.: Oxytocic, abortifacient
Chem. class.: Prostaglandin
Pregnancy category C

ACTION: Stimulates uterine contractions, causing complete abortion in approximately 16 hr

Therapeutic outcome: Loss of fetus; decreased postpartum bleeding

USES: Abortion between 13 and 20 wk gestation; postpartum hemorrhage caused by uterine atony not controlled by other methods

CONTRAINDICATIONS:

Hypersensitivity to this product or benzyl alcohol, severe renal/hepatic/cardiac/respiratory disease, PID

Precautions: Pregnancy C, asthma, anemia, jaundice, diabetes mellitus, seizure disorders, past uterine surgery

DOSAGE AND ROUTES
To induce abortion
Adult: IM 100 mcg (0.4 ml) test dose, then IM 250 mcg, then 250 mcg q1½-3½hr, may increase to 500 mcg if no response, max 12 mg total dose

Postpartum hemorrhage
Adult: IM 250 mcg, repeat at 15-90 min intervals, max total dosage 2 mg

Available forms: Inj 250 mcg/ml

Implementation
• Give only by trained personnel in a hospital that can provide emergency services
• Incomplete abortion may occur in 20% of patients
• Give antiemetics to prevent nausea/vomiting
• Give IM inj in deep muscle mass; rotate inj sites if additional doses are given
• Have crash cart available on unit
• Store in refrigerator

ADVERSE EFFECTS
CNS: *Fever, chills,* headache
GI: *Nausea, vomiting, diarrhea*

Absorption	Well absorbed (nasal)
Distribution	Widely distributed (extracellular fluid)
Metabolism	Liver, rapidly
Excretion	Kidneys
Half-life	3-9 min

Pharmacodynamics

Onset	Unknown
Peak	16 hr
Duration	Unknown

INTERACTIONS
Drug classifications
Oxytocics: increased effects

NURSING CONSIDERATIONS
Assessment
• Monitor B/P, pulse; watch for change that may indicate hemorrhage
⚠ For length, duration of contraction; notify physician of contractions lasting >1 min or absence of contractions
⚠ Assess for incomplete abortion; pregnancy must be terminated by another method; product is teratogenic

Patient/family education
• Advise patient to report increased blood loss, abdominal cramps, increased temp, or foul-smelling lochia

Evaluation
Positive therapeutic outcome
• Loss of fetus
• Control of bleeding

carfilzomib

(car-fil'zoe-mib)
Kyprolis
Func. class.: Antineoplastic biologic response modifiers
Chem. class.: Signal transduction inhibitors (STIs)
Pregnancy category D

ACTION: Antiproliferative and proapoptotic activity

USES: Multiple myeloma in those who have received 2 therapies (including bortezomib and immunomodulatory agents)

CONTRAINDICATIONS:

Pregnancy (D), hypersensitivity

Precautions: Breastfeeding, children, cardiac disease, cardiac arrest, dysrhythmias, MI, infusion-related reactions, pulmonary/hepatic disease, edema, thrombocytopenia, neutropenia, tumor lysis syndrome

DOSAGE AND ROUTES

Adult: IV 20 mg/m^2 over 2-10 min on days 1, 2, 8, 9, 15, 16, then 12 days' rest (days 17-28), then may increase to 27 mg/m^2 on days 1, 2, 8, 9, 15, 16, repeated every 28 days; refer to package insert for dosage adjustments for treatment-related toxicity

Available forms: Powder for injection 60 mg

Implementation

• Premedicate with dexamethasone 4 mg PO/IV before all carfilzomib 20-mg/m^2 doses during cycle 1 and before all carfilzomib 27-mg/m^2 doses in cycle 2; dexamethasone may be given in subsequent cycles if infusion-related reactions occur

• Hydration with 250-500 ml of NS or other IV fluids before each dose in cycle 1; additional hydration with 250-500 ml may be given after the carfilzomib infusion in cycle 1, continue hydration as needed

• Do not mix with other products

• Flush IV line with NS or D$_5$ for injection, before and after use

Reconstitution:

• Add 29 ml of sterile water for injection to the inside wall of the vial to minimize foaming (2 mg/mL); to mix, gently swirl and/or invert the vial slowly for about 1 min or until the cake or powder completely dissolves; do not shake; if foaming occurs, allow the solution to rest for 2-5 min or until foaming subsides; visually inspect for particulate and discoloration before use

IV injection route

• Give over 2-10 min; do not give as an IV bolus; the reconstituted sol may be stored in the vial/syringe at room temperature × 4 hr or ≤24 hr refrigerated

IV infusion route

• May further dilute in D$_5$W; measure and inject the correct dose from the reconstituted vial into 50 ml D$_5$W

• Administer IV over 2-10 min

• The diluted solution may be stored at room temperature × 4 hr or ≤24 hr refrigerated

ADVERSE EFFECTS

CNS: Headache, dizziness, insomnia

CV: Heart failure

GI: Nausea, vomiting, dyspepsia, anorexia, diarrhea

HEMA: Neutropenia, thrombocytopenia

META: Hyperglycemia, hypercalcemia, hypomagnesemia, hyponatremia, hypophosphatemia

MISC: Fatigue

MS: Arthralgia, myalgia

Pharmacokinetics

Absorption	Protein binding 97%

NURSING CONSIDERATIONS

Assessment

• Tumor lysis syndrome (TLS): hydrate well; assess for hyperuricemia, hyperkalemia, hyperphosphatemia, hypocalcemia, uremia

• Hematologic toxicity grade 3 and 4, neutropenia, and thrombocytopenia: platelet nadirs occur day 8 of each 28-day cycle; counts return to baseline before the start of the next cycle; monitor blood and platelet counts frequently; hold dose for grade 3 or 4 neutropenia or grade 4 thrombocytopenia, can require dosage reduction

• Serious liver toxicity: AST/ALT and bilirubin elevations and rare cases of fatal hepatic failure have occurred; monitor hepatic enzymes frequently; withhold doses until resolution or return to baseline in grade 3 or 4 AST/ALT or bilirubin elevations

• Serious cardiac toxicity: fatal cardiac arrest, CHF with decreased left ventricular function/ejection fraction, myocardial ischemia, and pulmonary edema; those with NYHA class III/IV CHF, MI within 6 mo, cardiac arrhythmias (conduction abnormalities) may be at increased risk; monitor for cardiac complications; withhold doses until resolution or return to baseline for grade 3 or 4 cardiac toxicity

• Infusion-related reactions: can occur 24 hr after dose; premedication with dexamethasone is recommended; assess for fever, chills, arthralgia, myalgia, facial flushing, facial edema, vomiting, weakness, shortness of breath, hypotension, syncope, chest tightness, angina

Patient/family education

⚠ Teach patient/family to promptly report infusion-related symptoms (fever, chills, arthralgia, myalgia, facial flushing, facial edema, vomiting, weakness, shortness of breath, hypotension, syncope, chest tightness, angina)

Evaluation
Positive therapeutic outcome
• Decreased spread of multiple myeloma

carisoprodol (Rx)
(kar-i-soe-proe′dole)
Soma
Func. class.: Skeletal muscle relaxant, central acting
Chem. class.: Meprobamate congener
Pregnancy category C
Controlled substance schedule IV

Do not confuse:
Soma/Soma compound

ACTION: Depresses CNS by blocking interneuronal activity in descending reticular formation of spinal cord, producing sedation

Therapeutic outcome: Relaxation of skeletal muscles

USES: Relieving pain, stiffness in musculo-skeletal disorders

CONTRAINDICATIONS:
Hypersensitivity to these products or carbamates, intermittent porphyria

Precautions: Pregnancy **C**, breastfeeding, geriatric, renal/hepatic disease, substance abuse, seizure disorder, CNS depression, abrupt discontinuation, Asian patients

DOSAGE AND ROUTES
Adult and child ≥16 yr: PO 250-350 mg tid and at bedtime, max 3 wk of use

Available forms: Tabs 350 mg

Implementation
• Give with meals for GI symptoms
• Have patient use gum, frequent sips of water for dry mouth
• Store in tight container at room temperature
• Use for short term (2-3 wk), potential for habituation

ADVERSE EFFECTS
CNS: *Dizziness, weakness, drowsiness,* headache, tremor, depression, insomnia, ataxia, irritability, **seizures**
CV: Postural hypotension, tachycardia
EENT: Diplopia, temporary loss of vision
GI: Nausea, vomiting, hiccups, epigastric discomfort
HEMA: Eosinophilia
INTEG: Rash, pruritus, fever, facial flushing, **erythema multiforme**
RESP: Asthmatic attack
SYST: **Angioedema, anaphylaxis**

Pharmacokinetics
Absorption	Well absorbed
Distribution	Crosses placenta
Metabolism	Liver, extensively, substrate of CYP2C19
Excretion	Kidney, unchanged; breast milk
Half-life	8 hr

Pharmacodynamics
Onset	½ hr
Peak	4 hr
Duration	4-6 hr

INTERACTIONS
Individual drugs
Alcohol: increased CNS depression
Meprobamate: do not use together

Drug classifications
Antidepressants (tricyclic), barbiturates, opioids, sedative/hypnotics: increased CNS depression
CYP2C19 inhibitors (FLUoxetine, fluvoxaMINE, isoniazid, modafinil): increased carisoprodol effect
CYP2C19 inducers (rifampin): decreased carisoprodol effect

Drug/herb
Kava, valerian: increased CNS depression
St. John's wort: increased metabolism of carisoprodol

Drug/lab test
Increased: eosinophils
Decreased: RBC, WBC, platelets

NURSING CONSIDERATIONS
Assessment
• **Pain:** Monitor ROM, atrophy, stiffness, and pain in muscles; assess throughout treatment
• Monitor **ECG in seizure patients;** poor seizure control has occurred with patients taking this product
• Assess for **idiosyncratic reaction** within a few min or 1 hr of administration (disorientation, restlessness, weakness, euphoria, blurred vision); patient should be reassured that reaction is temporary, withhold and notify prescriber
• Check for **allergic reactions:** rash, fever

• **CNS depression:** Assess for dizziness, drowsiness, psychiatric symptoms, abuse potential
• **Abrupt discontinuation:** withdrawal reactions do occur but may be mild; dependence may occur

Patient/family education
• Caution patient not to take with alcohol, other CNS depressants
• Advise patient to avoid altering activities while taking this product, to avoid rapid position changes, postural hypotension occurs
• Caution patient to avoid hazardous activities if drowsiness or dizziness occurs
• Caution patient to avoid using OTC medication such as cough preparations, antihistamines, unless directed by prescriber
• Teach patient to report **allergic reactions** immediately: rash, swelling of tongue/lips, hives, dyspnea
• Advise patient to take with food for GI symptoms

Evaluation
Positive therapeutic outcome
• Decreased pain, spasticity

TREATMENT OF OVERDOSE:
Activated charcoal, lavage, dialysis

⚠ HIGH ALERT

carmustine (Rx)
(kar-mus'teen)
BiCNU, Gliadel
Func. class.: Antineoplastic alkylating agent
Chem. class.: Nitrosourea
Pregnancy category D

ACTION: Alkylates DNA, RNA; inhibits enzymes that allow synthesis of amino acids in proteins; also responsible for cross-linking DNA strands; activity is not cell cycle phase specific

Therapeutic outcome: Prevention of rapidly growing malignant cells

USES: Brain tumors such as glioblastoma, medulloblastoma, astrocytoma, ependymoma, brain stem glioma, metastic brain tumors; multiple myeloma (with prednisone), non-Hodgkin's, Hodgkin's disease, other lymphomas; GI, breast, bronchogenic, and renal carcinomas; wafer, as adjunct to surgery/radiation in newly diagnosed high-grade malignant glioma patients

Unlabeled uses: Malignant melanoma

CONTRAINDICATIONS:
Pregnancy **D**, breastfeeding, hypersensitivity, leukopenia, thrombocytopenia

Precautions: Dental disease, extravasation, females, infection, leukopenia, neutropenia, secondary malignancy, thrombocytopenia

> **BLACK BOX WARNING:** Bone marrow suppression, pulmonary fibrosis

DOSAGE AND ROUTES
Brain tumors, Hodgkin's disease, malignant lymphoma, multiple myeloma
Adult: IV 75-100 mg/m^2 over 1-2 hr × 2 days or 150-200 mg/m^2 × 1 dose q6-8wk or 40 mg/m^2/day × 5 days q6wk or 150-200 mg/m^2 q6wk
Child (unlabeled): IV 200-250 mg/m^2 as a single dose q4-6wk
Adult: Intracavitary up to 8 wafers inserted into resection cavity

Available forms: Powder for inj 100 mg; wafer 7.7 mg intracavitary

Implementation
• RBC colony-stimulating factors to counter anemia may be required
• Give fluids **IV** or PO before chemotherapy to hydrate patient
• Provide antiemetic, serotonin antagonists, dexamethasone prn: nausea, vomiting can begin 2 hr after a dose and last ≤6 hr and may be severe; antibiotics for prophylaxis of infection
• Give all medications PO, if possible; avoid IM inj if platelets are <100,000/mm^3

> **BLACK BOX WARNING:** Carmustine should not be given until platelets >100,000/mm^3 and WBC >4000/mm^2

Wafer route
• Foil pouches may be kept at room temperature for 6 hr, if unopened
• If wafers are broken into several pieces, do not use

Intermittent IV infusion route
• Do not use with PVC IV tubing, do not admix
• Administer after **diluting** 100 mg/3 ml ethyl alcohol (provided); then **further dilute** 27 ml sterile water for inj; **then dilute** with 100-500 ml 0.9% NaCl or D$_5$W; **give** over 1 hr or more; use only glass containers; reduce rate if discomfort is felt
• Flush **IV** line after carmustine with 10 ml 0.9% NaCl to prevent irritation at site

---

• Store reconstituted sol in refrigerator for 24 hr or room temperature for 8 hr

Y-site compatibilities: Amifostine, amphotericin B lipid complex, amphotericin B liposome, anidulafungin, aztreonam, bivalirudin, bleomycin, caspofungin, cefepime, codeine, DAPTOmycin, dexmedetomidine, DOCEtaxel, ertapenem, etoposide, fenoldopam, filgrastim, fludarabine, gemcitabine, granisetron, levofloxacin, melphalan, meperidine, mitoXANtrone, nesiritide, octreotide, ondansetron, PACLitaxel, palonsetron, pamidronate, pantoprazole, PEMEtrexed, piperacillin-tazobactam, riTUXimab, sargramostim, sodium acetate, tacrolimus, teniposide, thiotepa, tigecycline, tirofiban, trastuzumab, vinCRIStine, vinorelbine, voriconazole

ADVERSE EFFECTS

GI: *Nausea, vomiting, anorexia, stomatitis,* **hepatotoxicity**
GU: *Azotemia,* **renal failure**
HEMA: **Thrombocytopenia, leukopenia, myelosuppression, anemia**
INTEG: Pain, burning, hyperpigmentation at inj site, alopecia
RESP: **Fibrosis, pulmonary infiltrate**
SYST: **Secondary malignant neoplastic disease**

Pharmacokinetics

Absorption	Completely absorbed
Distribution	Readily penetrates CSF
Metabolism	Liver, rapid
Excretion	Kidneys, breast milk
Half-life	Unknown

Pharmacodynamics

Unknown

INTERACTIONS

Individual drugs

Aspirin: increased risk of bleeding
Cimetidine, radiation: increased toxicity
Digoxin: decreased effects of digoxin
Phenytoin: decreased effects of phenytoin

Drug classifications

Anticoagulants: increased risk of bleeding
Antineoplastics: increased toxicity
Live vaccines: increased adverse reactions; decreased antibody reaction
Myelosuppressive agents: increased myelosuppression

Drug/lab test

Increased: bilirubin, prolactin, uric acid, LFTs
Decreased: platelets, WBC, neutrophils, Hct

NURSING CONSIDERATIONS

Assessment

• Assess buccal cavity q8hr for dryness, sores or ulceration, white patches, pain, bleeding, dysphagia; obtain prescription for viscous lidocaine (Xylocaine)
• Assess symptoms indicating severe allergic reaction: rash, pruritus, urticaria, purpuric skin lesions, itching, flushing; product should be discontinued

> **BLACK BOX WARNING: Bone marrow depression:** Monitor CBC, differential, platelet count weekly; withhold product if WBC <4000/mm³ or platelet count is <100,000/ mm³; notify prescriber of results

• Monitor renal function studies: BUN, creatinine, urine CCr before and during therapy; I&O ratio; report fall in urine output to <30 ml/ hr, may use allopurinol for hyperuricemia with increased fluids
• Monitor temp q4hr (may indicate beginning of infection)
• Monitor liver function tests before, during therapy (bilirubin, AST, ALT, LDH), monitor regularly, hepatotoxicity occurs rarely; note yellowing of skin or sclera, dark urine, clay-colored stools, itchy skin, abdominal pain, fever, diarrhea; hepatotoxicity can be serious and fatal
• Assess for **bleeding:** hematuria, stool guaiac, bruising or petechiae, mucosa or orifices q8hr; inflammation of mucosa, breaks in skin

> **BLACK BOX WARNING:** Only to be used by an experienced clinician in use of cancer, immune suppression

> **BLACK BOX WARNING: Pulmonary fibrosis/ infiltrate:** Monitor pulmonary function tests, chest x-ray films before, during therapy; chest film should be obtained q2wk during treatment; monitor for dyspnea, cough, pulmonary fibrosis; infiltrate occurs after high doses or several low-dose courses (>1400 mg/m² cumulative dose), may occur months or years after treatment

• Identify effects of alopecia on body image; discuss feelings about body changes

Patient/family education

• Teach patient to avoid use of products containing aspirin or ibuprofen, razors, commercial mouthwash, since bleeding may occur; to report symptoms of bleeding (hematuria, tarry stools)

• Advise patient to avoid foods with citric acid, hot flavor, or rough texture if stomatitis is present

BLACK BOX WARNING: Instruct patient to report signs of anemia (fatigue, headache, irritability, faintness, shortness of breath); avoid smoking

• Advise patient that hair may be lost during treatment; a wig or hairpiece may make patient feel better; new hair may be different in color, texture
• Caution patient not to have any vaccinations without the advice of the prescriber; serious reactions can occur
⚠ Advise patient that contraception is needed during treatment and for several months after completion of therapy; product has teratogenic properties

Evaluation
Positive therapeutic outcome
• Prevention of rapid division of malignant cells

carteolol ophthalmic
See Appendix B

carvedilol (Rx)
(kar-veh'dee-lol)
Coreg, Coreg CR
Func. class.: Antihypertensive α/β-blocker
Pregnancy category C

Do not confuse:
carvedilol/Captopril/Carteolol

ACTION: A mixture of nonselective β-blocking and α-blocking activity; decreases cardiac output, exercise-induced tachycardia, reflex orthostatic tachycardia; causes reduction in peripheral vascular resistance and vasodilatation

Therapeutic outcome: Decreased B/P in hypertension

USES: Essential hypertension alone or in combination with other antihypertensives, CHF, LV dysfunction following MI, cardiomyopathy

CONTRAINDICATIONS:
Hypersensitivity, asthma, class IV decompensated cardiac failure, 2nd- or 3rd-degree heart block, cardiogenic shock, severe bradycardia, pulmonary edema, severe hepatic disease

Precautions: Pregnancy C, breastfeeding, children, geriatric, cardiac failure, hepatic injury, peripheral vascular disease, anesthesia, major surgery, diabetes mellitus, thyrotoxicosis, emphysema, chronic bronchitis, renal disease

BLACK BOX WARNING: Abrupt discontinuation

DOSAGE AND ROUTES
Essential hypertension
Adult: PO 6.25 mg bid × 7-14 days if tolerated well, then increase to 12.5 mg bid × 7-14 days if tolerated well, may be increased if needed to 25 mg bid, max 50 mg daily; ext rel cap 20 mg/day, may increase after 7-14 days to 40 mg/day, max 80 mg/day

Congestive heart failure
Adult: PO 3.125 mg bid × 2 wk; if well tolerated, give 6.25 mg bid × 2 wk, then double q2wk to max dose 25 mg bid <85 kg or 80 mg bid >85 kg; ext rel cap (Coreg CR) 10 mg/day × 2 wk, increase to 20, 40, 80 mg/day over successive intervals of 2 wk

Postmyocardial infarction
Adult: PO 6.25 mg bid with food ×3-10 days, a lower starting dose may be used if indicated, titrate upward as tolerated, may increase to 12.5 mg bid, then titrate to 25 mg bid; PO ext rel 20 mg/day with food, a lower starting dose of 10 mg/day and titrate upwards after 3-10 days, increase to 40 mg/day as required

Available forms: Tabs 3.125, 6.25, 12.5, 25 mg; ext rel cap 10, 20, 40, 80 mg

Implementation
• Give with food in morning; tablets may be crushed or swallowed whole, give with food to decrease orthostatic hypotension; do not break, crush, or chew ext rel cap; decreased anginal pain
• Administer reduced dosage in renal dysfunction

BLACK BOX WARNING: Do not discontinue prior to surgery

ADVERSE EFFECTS
CNS: *Dizziness,* somnolence, insomnia, ataxia, hyperesthesia, paresthesia, vertigo, depression, *fatigue,* weakness, headache
CV: *Bradycardia, postural hypotension,* dependent edema, *peripheral edema,* **AV block, extrasystoles,** hypo/hypertension, palpitations, peripheral ischemia, **CHF, pulmonary edema**
GI: *Diarrhea,* abdominal pain, increased alkaline phosphatase, increased ALT/AST
GU: Decreased libido, *impotence,* UTI

INTEG: Rash, Stevens-Johnson syndrome
MISC: Injury, back pain, viral infection, hypertriglyceridemia, **thrombocytopenia,** *hyperglycemia,* abnormal weight gain, aplastic anemia
RESP: Rhinitis, pharyngitis, dyspnea, **bronchospasm,** cough, **lung edema**

Pharmacokinetics

Absorption	Readily and extensively absorbed
Distribution	>98% protein binding
Metabolism	Extensively liver
Excretion	Via bile into feces
Half-life	Terminal half-life 7-10 hr, increased in the geriatric, hepatic disease

Pharmacodynamics

Unknown

INTERACTIONS
Individual drugs
Alcohol (acute ingestion), cimetidine: increased toxicity
Clonidine: decreased heart rate, B/P
Digoxin: increased concentrations of digoxin
Reserpine, levodopa: increased hypotension, bradycardia
Rifampin: decreased levels of carvedilol

Drug classifications
Antihypertensives, nitrates: increased toxicity
Antidiabetic agents: increased hypoglycemia
Calcium channel blockers: increased conduction disturbance
CYP2D6 inhibitors (FLUoxetine, quiNIDine): increased digoxin
MAOIs: increased bradycardia, hypotension
NSAIDs, thyroid hormones: decreased levels of carvedilol

Drug/herb
Ephedra: decreased antihypertensive effect
Hawthorn: increased antihypertensive effect

Drug/lab test
Increased: blood glucose, potassium, triglycerides, uric acid, bilirubin, cholesterol, creatinine
Decreased: sodium, HDL

NURSING CONSIDERATIONS
Assessment
• Monitor I&O, weight daily
• **Hypertension:** Monitor B/P during beginning treatment and periodically thereafter; pulse q4hr, note rate, rhythm, quality

• Monitor apical/radial pulse before administration; notify prescriber of significant changes, pulse <50 bpm hold product, notify prescriber
• **CHF:** Assess for edema in feet and legs daily, fluid overload: dyspnea, weight gain, jugular vein distention, fatigue, crackles

Patient/family education
• Teach patient not to break, crush, or chew ext rel cap
• Instruct patient to comply with dosage schedule even if feeling better, that improvement may take several weeks
• Teach patient to rise slowly to sitting or standing position to minimize orthostatic hypotension
• Encourage patient to report bradycardia, dizziness, confusion, depression, fever, weight gain, shortness of breath, cold extremities, rash, sore throat, bleeding, bruising
• Teach patient to take pulse at home; advise when to notify prescriber

> **BLACK BOX WARNING:** Encourage patient not to discontinue product abruptly, taper over 1-2 wk, life-threatening dysrhythmias may occur

• Advise patient to avoid hazardous activities until stabilized on medication; dizziness may occur
• Teach patient that product may mask hypoglycemia
• Advise patient to avoid all OTC medications unless approved by prescriber
• Advise patient to carry/wear emergency ID with product name, prescriber at all times
• Advise patient to inform all health care providers of products, supplements taken
• Teach patient to report if pregnancy is planned or suspected, pregnancy (C), avoid breastfeeding

Evaluation
Positive therapeutic outcome
• Decreased B/P
• Decreased symptoms of CHF or angina

cefaclor
See cephalosporins—2nd generation

cefadroxil
ceFAZolin
See cephalosporins—1st generation

cefdinir
cefditoren pivoxil
cefepime
cefotaxime
See cephalosporins—3rd generation

cefoTEtan
cefOXitin
See cephalosporins—2nd generation

cefpodoxime
See cephalosporins—3rd generation

cefprozil
See cephalosporins—2nd generation

ceftaroline (Rx)
(sef-tar'oh-leen)
Teflaro
Func. class.: Cephalosporin
Pregnancy category B

ACTION: Inhibits cell wall synthesis through binding to essential penicillin-binding protein (PBP)

Therapeutic outcome: Negative C&S, resolution of symptoms of infection

USES: Acute bacterial skin/skin structure infections (ABSSI), bacterial community acquired pneumonia

CONTRAINDICATIONS:
Cephalosporin hypersensitivity

Precautions: Antimicrobial resistance, breastfeeding, carbapenem/penicillin hypersensitivity, child/infant/neonate, coagulopathy, colitis, dialysis, diarrhea, geriatrics, GI disease, hypoprothrombinemia, IBS, pregnancy **B**, pseudomembranous colitis, renal disease, ulcerative colitis, viral infection, vitamin K deficiency

DOSAGE AND ROUTES
Adult: IV 600 mg q12hr × 5-14 days (skin/skin structure infections), × 5-7 days (bacterial community acquired pneumonia)

Renal dose
Adult: IV CCr >30-≤50 ml/min 400 mg q12hr; CCr ≥15-≤30 ml/min 300 mg q12hr, CCr <15 ml/min 200 mg q12hr

Available forms: Powder for injection 400 mg, 600 mg

Implementation
- Obtain C&S before use
- Visually inspect for particulate matter or discoloration if solution or container permit
- **Reconstitute:** add 20 mg of sterile water to 400 or 600 mg vial (20 ml/ml for 400 mg), (30 mg/ml for 600 mg), mix gently until dissolved: **Dilute:** in 250 ml of 0.9% NaCl, 0.45% NaCl, LR, D5, D2.5, give over 1 hr, do not admix, use within 6 hrs at room temperature or 24 hr refrigerated
- Store reconstituted solution in the refrigerator

ADVERSE EFFECTS
CNS: Dizziness, **seizures**
CV: Bradycardia, palpitations, **phlebitis**
ENDO: Hyperkalemia, hypokalemia
GI: Diarrhea, nausea, vomiting, constipation, abdominal pain, **pseudomembranous colitis (rare)**, elevated hepatic enzymes
HEMA: Thrombocytopenia, neutropenia, anemia, eosinophilia
INTEG: Rash, **anaphylaxis**

Pharmacokinetics
Absorption	Unknown
Distribution	Unknown
Metabolism	Not hepatically metabolized
Excretion	In urine 88%, feces 6%
Half-life	2.66 hr

Pharmacodynamics
Unknown

INTERACTIONS
Drug classifications
Anticoagulants: increased prothrombin time risk

Drug/lab test
Increased: LFTs
Decreased: potassium, eosinophils, platelets

NURSING CONSIDERATIONS
Assessment
- **Assess for infection:** vital signs, sputum, WBC prior to and during therapy
- **Assess for hypersensitivity:** prior to use, obtain a history of hypersensitivity reactions to cephalosporins, carbapenems, penicillins; cross sensitivity may occur
- **Assess for anaphylaxis (rare):** rash, pruritus, laryngeal edema, dyspnea, wheezing; discontinue and notify health care provider immediately, keep emergency equipment nearby
- **Monitor for pseudomembranous colitis:** diarrhea, abdominal pain, fever, bloody

stools; report immediately if these occur, may occur several weeks after terminating therapy

Patient/family education
• Explain reason for treatment and expected result
⚠ Instruct patient to report immediately **rash, itching, difficulty breathing, bloody diarrhea, fever, abdominal pain**

Evaluation
Positive therapeutic outcome
• Negative C&S, resolution of symptoms of infection

---

cefTAZidime
ceftibuten
ceftizoxime
cefTRIAXone
See cephalosporins—3rd generation

cefuroxime
See cephalosporins—2nd generation

⚠ HIGH ALERT

celecoxib (Rx)
(cel-eh-cox'ib)
CeleBREX
Func. class.: Nonsteroidal antiinflammatory, antirheumatic
Chem. class.: COX-2 inhibitor
Pregnancy category C (1st/2nd trimesters), D (3rd trimester)

Do not confuse:
CeleBREX/CeleXA/Cerebra/Cerebyx

ACTION: Inhibits prostaglandin synthesis by selectively inhibiting cyclooxygenase 2 (COX-2), an enzyme needed for biosynthesis

Therapeutic outcome: Decreased pain, inflammation

USES: Acute, chronic rheumatoid arthritis, osteoarthritis, acute pain, primary dysmenorrhea, ankylosing spondylitis, juvenile rheumatoid arthritis (JRA)

Unlabeled uses: Colorectal adenoma prophylaxis

CONTRAINDICATIONS:
Pregnancy **D** (3rd trimester), hypersensitivity to salicylates, iodides, other NSAIDs, sulfonamides

BLACK BOX WARNING: CABG

Precautions: Pregnancy **C** (1st/2nd trimester), breastfeeding, children <18 yr, geriatric, renal/hepatic disease, hypertension, severe dehydration, bleeding, GI, cardiac disorders, PVD, asthma

BLACK BOX WARNING: GI bleeding/perforation, peptic ulcer disease, MI, stroke

DOSAGE AND ROUTES
Do not exceed recommended dose, deaths have occurred

Acute pain/primary dysmenorrhea
Adult: PO 400 mg initially, then 200 mg if needed on first day, then 200 mg bid prn on subsequent days, if needed; start with ½ dose in poor CYP2C9 metabolizers
Geriatric: PO use lowest possible dose

Osteoarthritis
Adult: PO 200 mg/day as a single dose or 100 mg bid; start with ½ dose in poor CYP2C9 metabolizers

Rheumatoid arthritis
Adult: PO 100-200 mg bid; start with ½ dose in poor CYP2C9 metabolizers

Ankylosing spondylitis
Adult: PO 200 mg daily or in divided dose (bid); start with ½ dose in poor CYP2C9 metabolizers

Juvenile rheumatoid arthritis (JRA)
Adolescent and child ≥2 yr (>25 kg): PO 100 mg bid; start with ½ dose in poor CYP2C9 metabolizers
Child ≥2 yr (10-25 kg): PO 50 mg bid; start with ½ dose in poor CYP2C9 metabolizers

Colorectal adenoma prophylaxis (unlabeled)
Adult: PO 200-400 mg bid for up to 3 yr

Hepatic dose (Child-Pugh class II)
Adult: PO reduce dose by 50%

Available forms: Caps 50, 100, 200, 400 mg

Implementation
• Do not break, crush, chew, or dissolve caps; caps may be opened and mixed with applesauce, ingest immediately with water
• Administer with food or milk to decrease gastric symptoms
• Do not increase dose

ADVERSE EFFECTS
CNS: *Fatigue, anxiety, depression, nervousness, paresthesia,* dizziness, insomnia, headache
CV: Stroke, MI, tachycardia, CHF, angina, palpitations, dysrhythmias, hypertension, fluid retention
EENT: Tinnitus, hearing loss, blurred vision, glaucoma, cataract, conjunctivitis, eye pain
GI: *Nausea, anorexia, vomiting, constipation, dry mouth,* diverticulitis, gastritis, gastroenteritis, hemorrhoids, hiatal hernia, stomatitis, **GI bleeding/ulceration**
GU: Nephrotoxicity: dysuria, hematuria, azotemia, cystitis, UTI, renal papillary necrosis
HEMA: Blood dyscrasias, epistaxis, anemia
INTEG: Purpura, rash, pruritus, sweating, erythema, petechiae, photosensitivity, alopecia, bruising, hot flashes, **serious sometimes fatal Stevens-Johnson syndrome, toxic epidermal necrolysis**
RESP: Pharyngitis, shortness of breath, pneumonia, coughing

Pharmacokinetics

Absorption	Well absorbed (PO)
Distribution	Crosses placenta, protein binding ~97%
Metabolism	Liver by CYP2C9
Excretion	Feces/kidneys, small amount
Half-life	11 hr

Pharmacodynamics

Onset	Unknown
Peak	3 hr
Duration	Unknown

INTERACTIONS
Individual drugs
Aspirin: decreased effectiveness; increased adverse reactions
Fluconazole: increased celecoxib level
Furosemide, cidofovir: decreased effect of each drug
Lithium: increased toxicity
Warfarin: increased anticoagulant effects

Drug classifications
ACE inhibitors: may decrease effects of ACE inhibitors
Anticoagulants, antiplatelets, SSRIs, salicylates, thrombolytics: increased risk of bleeding
Antineoplastics: increased risk of hematologic toxicity
Bisphosphonates: increased toxicity
Glucocorticoids, NSAIDs: increased adverse reactions
Thiazide diuretics: decreased effectiveness of diuretics

Drug/herb
Feverfew: decreased effect of feverfew
Garlic, ginger, ginkgo: increased bleeding risk

Drug/lab test
Increased: ALT, AST, BUN, cholesterol, glucose, potassium, sodium
Decreased: glucose, sodium, WBC, platelets

NURSING CONSIDERATIONS
Assessment
• Assess for **pain** of rheumatoid arthritis, osteoarthritis; check ROM, inflammation of joints, characteristics of pain

> **BLACK BOX WARNING:** Assess for cardiac disease that may be worse after taking this product; MI, stroke, do not use in coronary artery bypass graft (CABG)

• Monitor CBC during therapy; watch for decreasing platelets; if low, therapy may need to be discontinued, restarted after hematologic recovery; LFTs, serum creatinine BUN, stool guaiac

> **BLACK BOX WARNING:** Assess for blood dyscrasias (thrombocytopenia): bruising, fatigue, bleeding, poor healing

• Assess for **GI toxicity:** black, tarry stools; abdominal pain
⚠ **Assess for serious skin disorders: Stevens-Johnson syndrome, toxic epidermal necrolysis; may be fatal**

Patient/family education

> **BLACK BOX WARNING:** Do not exceed recommended dose; notify prescriber, immediately of chest pain, skin eruptions, stop product

• Teach patient that product must be continued for prescribed time to be effective; to avoid other NSAIDs, sulfonamides

C

> **BLACK BOX WARNING:** Caution patient to report bleeding, bruising, fatigue, malaise, since blood abnormalities do occur; to report GI symptoms: black tarry stools, cramping

• Teach patient to take with a full glass of water to enhance absorption
• Teach patient to check with prescriber to determine when product should be discontinued before surgery; advise patient to notify prescriber if pregnancy is planned or suspected
• Advise patient to report possible respiratory infection: fever, shortness of breath, coughing, painful swallowing
⚠ Teach patient to report if pregnancy is planned or suspected, pregnancy (C) prior to 3 wk, (D) after 30 wk

Evaluation
Positive therapeutic outcome
• Decreased pain in arthritic conditions
• Decreased inflammation in arthritic conditions
• Decreased number of polyps (FAP)

cephalexin
See cephalosporins—1st generation

CEPHALOSPORINS— 1ST GENERATION
cefadroxil (Rx)
(sef-a-drox′ill)
Apo-Cefadroxil ✦
ceFAZolin (Rx)
(sef-a′zoe-lin)
cephalexin (Rx)
(sef-a-lex′in)
Keflex, Panixine
Pregnancy category B

Do not confuse:
cephalexin/cefaclor

ACTION: Inhibits bacterial cell wall synthesis, rendering cell wall osmotically unstable, leading to cell death by binding to cell wall membrane, lysis mediated by cell wall autolytic enzymes

cefadroxil

Therapeutic outcome: Bactericidal effects for the following: gram-negative bacilli *Escherichia coli, Proteus mirabilis, Klebsiella pneumoniae* (UTI only); gram-positive organisms *Streptococcus pneumoniae, Strepto-*

coccus pyogenes, Staphylococcus aureus/ epidermidis

USES: Upper, lower respiratory tract, urinary tract, skin infections; otitis media; tonsillitis, UTI

ceFAZolin

Therapeutic outcome: Bactericidal effects for the following: gram-negative organisms *Haemophilus influenzae, Escherichia coli, Proteus mirabilis, Klebsiella*; gram-positive organisms *Staphylococcus aureus*

USES: Upper, lower respiratory tract, urinary tract, skin infections; bone, joint, biliary, genital infections; endocarditis, surgical prophylaxis, septicemia; *Streptococcus*

cephalexin

Therapeutic outcome: Bactericidal effects for the following: gram-negative organisms *Haemophilus influenzae, Escherichia coli, Proteus mirabilis, Klebsiella pneumoniae*; gram-positive organisms *Streptococcus pneumoniae, Streptococcus pyogenes, Streptococcus agalactiae, Staphylococcus aureus*

USES: Upper, lower respiratory tract, urinary tract, skin, bone infections; otitis media

CONTRAINDICATIONS:
Hypersensitivity to cephalosporins, infants <1 mo

Precautions: Pregnancy **B**, breastfeeding, hypersensitivity to penicillins, renal disease

DOSAGE AND ROUTES
cefadroxil
Adult: PO 1-2 g daily or divided q12hr, give a loading dose of 1 g initially
Child: PO 30 mg/kg/day in divided doses bid, max 2 g/day

Renal dose
Adult: PO CCr 25-50 ml/min, 1 g, then 500 mg q12hr; CCr 10-24 ml/min, 1 g, then 500 mg q24hr; CCr <10 ml/min, 1 g, then 500 mg q36hr

Available forms: Caps 500 mg; tabs 1 g; oral susp 125, 250, 500 mg/5 ml

ceFAZolin
Life-threatening infections
Adult: IM/**IV** 1-2 g q6-8hr, max 12 g/day
Child >1 mo: IM/**IV** 75-100 mg/kg/day in 3-4 divided doses, max 6 g/day

Mild/moderate infections
Adult: IM/IV 250 mg-1 g q8hr, max 12 g/day
Child >1 mo: IM/IV 25-50 mg/kg in 3-4 equal doses, max 6 g/day or 2 g as a single dose

Renal dose
Adult: IM/IV following loading dose CCr 35-54 ml/min dose q8hr; CCr 10-34 ml/min 50% of dose q12hr; CCr <10 ml/min 50% of dose q18-24hr
Child: IM/IV CCr >70 ml/min, no dosage adjustment; CCr 40-70 ml/min following loading dose, reduce dose to 7.5-30 mg/kg q12hr; CCr 20-39 ml/min, give 3.125-12.5 mg/kg after loading dose q12hr; CCr 5-19 ml/min, 2.5-10 mg/kg after loading dose q24hr

Available forms: Inj 500 mg, 1, 5, 10, 20 g; infusion 500 mg, 1 g/50 ml, 50 mg/500 ml vial

cephalexin

Moderate infections
Adult: PO 250-500 mg q6hr, max 4 g/day
Child: PO 25-100 mg/kg/day in 4 equal doses, max 4 g/day

Moderate skin infections
Adult: PO 500 mg q12hr

Endocarditis prophylaxis
2 g 1 hr before procedure

Severe infections
Adult: PO 500 mg-1 g q6hr, max 4 g
Child: PO 50-100 mg/kg/day in 4 equal doses, max 4 g/day

Renal dose
Adult: PO CCr 10-40 ml/min 250-500 mg, then 250-500 mg q8-12hr; CCr <10 mg/min 250-500 mg, then 250-500 mg q12-24hr

Available forms: Caps 250, 500 mg; tabs 250, 500 mg, 1 g; oral susp 125, 250 mg/5 ml

cefadroxil

Implementation
• Give in even doses around the clock; if GI upset occurs, give with food; product must be given for 10-14 days to ensure organism death and prevent superinfection
• Shake susp, refrigerate, discard after 2 wk

ceFAZolin

Implementation
IM route
• Reconstitute 250-500 mg of product with 2 ml sterile or bacteriostatic water for inj, or 0.9% NaCl; reconstitute 1 g of product with 2.5 ml; give deep in large muscle mass, massage

IV route
• Check for irritation, extravasation, phlebitis daily, change site q72hr
• For direct IV dilute in 2 ml/50 mg or 2.5 ml/1 g of sterile water for inj; give over 5 min
• For intermittent inf dilute reconstituted sol (500 mg or 1 g) in 50-100 ml D5W, D10W, D5/0.25% NaCl, D5/0.45% NaCl, D5/0.9% NaCl, D5/LR, or LR, 0.9% NaCl; give over 30-60 min; may be refrigerated up to 96 hr or stored 24 hr at room temperature

Syringe compatibilities: Heparin, Salbutamol, vit B complex

Syringe incompatibilities: Ascorbic acid inj, cimetidine, lidocaine, vit B/C

Y-site compatibilities: Acyclovir, alfentanil, allopurinol, alprostadil, amifostine, amikacin, aminocaproic acid, aminophylline, amphotericin B liposome, anidulafungin, ascorbic acid injection, atenolol, atracurium, atropine, aztreonam, benztropine, bivalirudin, bleomycin, bumetanide, buprenorphine, butorphanol, calcium gluconate, CARBOplatin, cefamandole, cefmetazole, cefonicid, cefoperazone, cefoTEtan, cefOXitin, cefpirome, cefTAZidime, ceftizoxime, cefTRIAXone, cefuroxime, cephalothin, cephapirin, chloramphenicol, cimetidine, CISplatin, clindamycin, codeine, cyanocobalamin, cyclophosphamide, cycloSPORINE, cytarabine, DACTINomycin, DAPTOmycin, dexamethasone, dexmedetomidine, digoxin, diltiazem, DOCEtaxel, doxacurium, doxapram, DOXOrubicin liposomal, enalaprilat, ePHEDrine, EPINEPHrine, epirubicin, epoetin alfa, eptifibatide, esmolol, etoposide, fenoldopam, fentaNYL, filgrastim, fluconazole, fludarabine, fluorouracil, folic acid (as sodium salt), foscarnet, furosemide, gallium, gatifloxacin, gemcitabine, gentamicin, glycopyrrolate, granisetron, heparin, hydrocortisone, hydrOXYzine, IDArubicin, ifosfamide, imipenem-cilastatin, indomethacin, insulin (regular), irinotecan, isoproterenol, ketorolac, lidocaine, linezolid, LORazepam, LR's injection, mannitol, mechlorethamine, melphalan, meperidine, metaraminol, methicillin, methotrexate, methoxamine, methyldopate, methylPREDNISolone, metoclopramide, metoprolol, metroNIDAZOLE, mezlocillin, miconazole, midazolam, milrinone, morphine, moxalactam, multiple vitamins injection, nafcillin, nalbuphine, naloxone, nesiritide, niCARdipine, nitroglycerin, nitroprusside, norepinephrine, octreotide, ondansetron, oxacillin, oxaliplatin, oxytocin, PACLitaxel, palonosetron, pamidronate, pancuronium, pantoprazole, penicillin G potassium/sodium, peritoneal dialysis solution, perphenazine, PHENobarbital, phenylephrine, phytonadione, piperacillin, Plasma-Lyte M in dextrose 5%, polymyxin B, potassium chloride, procainamide, propofol, propranolol, ranitidine, remifentanil, Ringer's injection, ritodrine, riTUXimab, sargramostim, sodium acetate, sodium bicarbonate, succinylcholine, SUFentanil, tacrolimus, teniposide, tenoxicam, theophylline, thiamine, thiotepa, ticarcillin, ticarcillin-clavulanate, tigecycline, tirofiban, TNA, tolazoline, trastuzumab, trimetaphan, urokinase, vasopressin, vecuronium, verapamil, vinCRIStine, vitamin B complex with C, voriconazole, warfarin, zoledronic acid

Y-site incompatibilities: Amiodarone, hetastarch, HYDROmorphone, IDArubicin, vinorelbine tartrate

cephalexin

Implementation
• Do not break, crush, or chew caps
• Give in even doses around the clock; if GI upset occurs, give with food; product must be taken for 10-14 days to ensure organism death and prevent superinfection
• Shake susp, refrigerate, discard after 2 wk, use calibrated oral syringe, spoon or measuring cup

ADVERSE EFFECTS
CNS: Headache, dizziness, weakness, paresthesia, fever, chills, **seizures** (high doses)
GI: Nausea, vomiting, *diarrhea, anorexia,* pain, glossitis, bleeding; increased AST, ALT, bilirubin, LDH, alkaline phosphatase; abdominal pain, **pseudomembranous colitis**
GU: Proteinuria, vaginitis, pruritus, candidiasis, increased BUN, **nephrotoxicity, renal failure**
HEMA: Leukopenia, thrombocytopenia, agranulocytosis, anemia, neutropenia, lymphocytosis, eosinophilia, pancytopenia, hemolytic anemia
INTEG: Rash, urticaria, dermatitis
MS: Arthralgia, arthritis
RESP: Dyspnea
SYST: Anaphylaxis, serum sickness, superinfection, **Stevens-Johnson syndrome**

cefadroxil

Pharmacokinetics

Absorption	Well absorbed
Distribution	Widely distributed; crosses placenta
Metabolism	Not metabolized
Excretion	Unchanged by kidneys; enters breast milk
Half-life	1½-2 hr

Pharmacodynamics

	PO
Onset	Rapid
Peak	1½-2 hr
Duration	12-24 hr

ceFAZolin

Pharmacokinetics

Absorption	Well absorbed
Distribution	Widely distributed; crosses placenta
Metabolism	Not metabolized
Excretion	Unchanged by kidneys; enters breast milk
Half-life	1½-2½ hr

Pharmacodynamics

	IM	IV
Onset	Rapid	10 min
Peak	1-2 hr	Infusion's end
Duration	6-12 hr	Unknown

cephalexin

Pharmacokinetics

Absorption	Well absorbed
Distribution	Widely distributed; crosses placenta
Metabolism	Not metabolized
Excretion	Kidneys, unchanged; enters breast milk
Half-life	½-1 hr; increased in renal disease

Pharmacodynamics

Onset	15-30 min
Peak	1 hr
Duration	6-12 hr

INTERACTIONS
Individual drugs
Probenecid: increased toxicity

Drug classifications
Aminoglycosides, diuretics (loop): increased toxicity

Anticoagulants: increased protime; use cautiously

Oral contraceptives: decreased effectiveness possible; use another form of contraception

Drug/lab test
Increased: AST, ALT, alkaline phosphatase, LDH, BUN, creatinine, bilirubin

False positive: urinary protein, direct Coombs' test, urine glucose

Interference: cross-matching

NURSING CONSIDERATIONS
Assessment
• Assess patient for previous sensitivity reaction to penicillins or other cephalosporins; cross-sensitivity between penicillins and cephalosporins is common

• Assess patient for signs and symptoms of **infection** including characteristics of wounds, sputum, urine, stool, WBC $>10,000/mm^3$, earache, fever; obtain baseline information and during treatment

• Obtain C&S before beginning product therapy to identify if correct treatment has been initiated

• Assess for **anaphylaxis**: rash, urticaria, pruritus, chills, fever, joint pain; angioedema may occur a few days after therapy begins; epinephrine and resuscitation equipment should be available for anaphylactic reaction

• Identify urine output; if decreasing, notify prescriber (may indicate **nephrotoxicity**); also check for increased BUN, creatinine

• Monitor blood studies: AST, ALT, CBC, Hct, bilirubin, LDH, alkaline phosphatase, Coombs' test monthly if patient is on long-term therapy

• Monitor electrolytes: potassium, sodium, chloride monthly if patient is on long-term therapy

• Assess bowel pattern daily; if severe diarrhea occurs, product should be discontinued; may indicate **pseudomembranous colitis**

• Monitor for bleeding: ecchymosis, bleeding gums, hematuria, stool guaiac daily if on long-term therapy

• Assess for **superinfection**: perineal itching, fever, malaise, redness, pain, swelling, drainage, rash, diarrhea, change in cough, sputum

Patient/family education
• Teach patient to report sore throat, bruising, bleeding, joint pain; may indicate **blood dyscrasias** (rare)

• Advise patient to contact prescriber if vaginal itching, loose foul-smelling stools, furry tongue occur; may indicate superinfection

• Instruct patient to take all medication prescribed for the length of time ordered

• Advise patient to notify prescriber of diarrhea with blood, pus, mucus, which may indicate **pseudomembranous colitis**

Evaluation
Positive therapeutic outcome
• Absence of signs/symptoms of infection (WBC $<10,000/mm^3$, temp WNL, absence of red draining wounds, earache)

• Reported improvement in symptoms of infection

• Negative C&S

TREATMENT OF ANAPHYLAXIS: EPINEPHrine, antihistamines, resuscitate if needed

CEPHALOSPORINS— 2ND GENERATION
cefaclor (Rx)
(sef'a-klor)
Ceclor, Raniclor
cefoTEtan (Rx)
(sef'oh-tee-tan)
Cefotan
cefOXitin (Rx)
(se-fox'i-tin)
Mefoxin
cefprozil (Rx)
(sef-proe'zill)
Cefzil
cefuroxime (Rx)
(sef-yoor-ox'eem)
Ceftin, Cefuroxime, Zinacef
Func. class.: Antiinfective
Chem. class.: Cephalosporin (2nd generation)
Pregnancy category B

Do not confuse:
cefaclor/cephalexin, Cefotan/Ceftin, cefprozil/ceFAZolin/cefuroxime, Cefzil/Ceftin

ACTION: Inhibits bacterial cell wall synthesis, rendering cell wall osmotically unstable, leading to cell death by binding to cell wall membrane

cefaclor

Therapeutic outcome: Bactericidal effects for the following: gram-negative bacilli *Haemophilus influenzae, Escherichia coli, Proteus mirabilis, Klebsiella;* gram-positive organisms *Streptococcus pneumoniae, Streptococcus pyogenes, Staphylococcus aureus*

USES: Upper and lower respiratory tract, urinary tract, skin infections; otitis media; bone, joint infections

cefoTEtan

Therapeutic outcome: Bactericidal effects for the following: gram-negative organisms *Citrobacter, Haemophilus influenzae, Escherichia coli, Enterobacter aerogenes, Proteus mirabilis, Klebsiella, Salmonella, Shigella, Acinetobacter, Bacteroides fragilis, Neisseria, Serratia;* gram-positive organisms *Streptococcus pneumoniae, Streptococcus pyogenes, Staphylococcus aureus*

USES: Serious upper or lower respiratory tract, urinary tract, gynecologic, skin, bone, joint, gonococcal, intraabdominal infections

cefOXitin

Therapeutic outcome: Bactericidal effects for the following: gram-negative bacilli *Bacteroides fragilis, Haemophilus influenzae, Escherichia coli, Proteus, Klebsiella, Neisseria gonorrhoeae;* gram-positive organisms *Streptococcus pneumoniae, Streptococcus pyogenes, Staphylococcus aureus;* anaerobes including *Clostridium*

USES: Lower respiratory tract, urinary tract, skin, bone, gynecologic, gonococcal infections; septicemia, peritonitis

cefprozil

Therapeutic outcome: Bactericidal effects for the following: gram-negative bacilli *Haemophilus influenzae, Escherichia coli;* gram-positive organisms *Streptococcus pneumoniae, Streptococcus pyogenes, Staphylococcus aureus*

USES: Pharyngitis/tonsillitis, otitis media, secondary bacterial infection of acute bronchitis, and acute bacterial exacerbation of chronic bronchitis and uncomplicated skin and skin structure infections; acute sinusitis

cefuroxime

Therapeutic outcome: Bactericidal effects for the following: gram-negative bacilli *Haemophilus influenzae, Escherichia coli, Neisseria, Proteus mirabilis, Klebsiella;* gram-positive organisms: *Streptococcus pneumoniae, Streptococcus pyogenes, Staphylococcus aureus*

USES: Serious lower respiratory tract, urinary tract, skin, bone, joint, gonococcal infections; septicemia, meningitis

CONTRAINDICATIONS:
Hypersensitivity to cephalosporins or related antibiotics, seizures

Precautions: Pregnancy **B,** breastfeeding, children, renal/GI disease, diabetes mellitus, coagulopathy

DOSAGE AND ROUTES
cefaclor

Adult: PO 250-500 mg q8hr, max 4 g/day; EXT REL 375 mg q12hr; max 1.5 mg/day (cap, oral susp); 1 g/day (EXT REL)
Child >1 mo: PO 20-40 mg/kg daily in divided doses q8hr, or total daily dose may be divided and given q12hr, max 1 g/day

Available forms: Caps 250, 500 mg; oral susp 125, 187, 250, 375 mg/5 ml; EXT REL tab 500 mg

cefoTEtan
Adult: IV/IM 1-2 g q12hr × 5-10 days

Perioperative prophylaxis
Adult: IV 1-2 g ½-1 hr before surgery

Renal dose
Adult: IM/IV CCr 30-50 ml/min 1-2 g, then 1-2 g q8-12hr; CCr 10-29 ml/min 1-2 g, then 1-2 g q12-24hr; CCr 5-9 ml/min 1-2 g, then 0.5-1 g q12-24hr; CCr <5 ml/min 1-2 g, then 0.5-1 g q24-48hr

Available forms: Inj 1, 2, 10 g

cefOXitin
Adult: IM/IV 1-2 g q6-8hr

Uncomplicated gonorrhea (outpatient)
Adult/adolescent/child ≥45 kg: IM 2 g as single dose with 1 g PO probenecid at same time

Renal dose
Adult: IM/IV after loading dose CCr 30-50 ml/min 1-2 g q8-12hr; CCr 10-29 ml/min 1-2 g q12-24hr; CCr <10 ml/min 0.5-1 g q12-24hr

Severe infections
Adult: IM/IV 2 g q4hr
Child ≥3 mo: IM/IV 80-160 mg/kg/day divided q4-6hr; max 12 g/day

Available forms: Powder for inj 1, 2, 10 g

cefprozil

Renal dose
CCr <30 ml/min 50% of dose

Upper respiratory infections
Adult: PO 500 mg q24hr × 10 days

Otitis media
Child 6 mo-12 yr: PO 15 mg/kg q12hr × 10 days

Lower respiratory infections
Adult: PO 500 mg q12hr × 10 days

Skin/skin structure infections
Adult: PO 250-500 mg q12hr × 10 days

Available forms: Tabs 250, 500 mg; susp 125, 250 mg/5 ml

cefuroxime
Oral tablets and suspension are not bio-equivalent

Lower respiratory tract infections (mild-moderate)/uncomplicated skin/skin structure infections
Adult/adolescent: PO 250-500 mg q12hr × 5-10 days; IV/IM 750 mg q8hr
Child (unlabeled): PO 125 mg q12hr; 750 mg IV or IM q8hr
Adolescent/child/infant ≥3 mo: IV/IM 50-100 mg/kg/day divided q6-8hr (not to exceed adult dose)

Serious lower respiratory tract infections/serious skin/skin structure infections
Adult: IV/IM 0.75-1.5 g q8hr; life-threatening infections or infections caused by less-susceptible organisms, IV 1.5 g q6hr
Adolescent/child/infant ≥3 mo: IV/IM 50-150 mg/kg/day divided q6-8hr; max 6 g/day

Impetigo
Child: PO (tab unlabeled) 250 mg PO q12hr
Child/infant ≥3 mo: (PO-Susp) 30 mg/kg/day divided into two doses; max 1000 mg/day

Urinary tract infection (UTI)
Adult/adolescent: PO 250 mg q12hr × 7-10 days; IV/IM 0.75-1.5 g q8hr (general) or 0.75 g q8hr (uncomplicated)
Adolescent/child/infant ≥3 mo: IV/IM 50-100 mg/kg/day in divided doses q6-8hr (max adult dose)

Bone and joint infections
Adult: IV/IM 1.5 g q8hr; for life-threatening infections or infections caused by less-susceptible organisms, 1.5 g IV q6hr
Adolescent/child/infant ≥3 mo: IV/IM 150 mg/kg/day in divided doses q8hr; max 6 g/day

Upper respiratory tract infections (e.g., pharyngitis, tonsillitis)
Adult/adolescent: PO (tabs) 250 mg q12hr × 10 days
Child/infant ≥3 mo: PO (susp) 20 mg/kg/day divided into 2 doses × 10 days, max 500 mg/day

Acute bacterial maxillary sinusitis
Adult/adolescent: PO (tabs) 250 mg bid × 10 days
Child (who can swallow tablets whole): PO (tabs) 250 mg bid × 10 days
Child/infant ≥3 mo: PO (susp) 15 mg/kg bid × 10 days, max 1000 mg/day

Early Lyme disease
Adult/adolescent: PO (tabs) 500 mg q12hr × 20 days
Child (unlabeled): PO (susp) 30 mg/kg/day in 2 divided doses (max 1000 mg/day) or 1000 mg/day × 14-21 days

Acute otitis media
Child (who can swallow whole tablets): PO (tabs) 250 mg bid × 10 days
Child/infant ≥3 mo: PO (susp) 30 mg/kg/day divided into 2 doses × 10 day, max 1000 mg/day

Septicemia
Adult: IV/IM 1.5-3 g q8hr, max 9 g/day
Adolescent/child/infant ≥3 mo: IV/IM 200-240 mg/kg/day divided doses q6-8hr, max 9 g/day

Renal dose
Adult: CCr 10-20 ml/min: IV/IM 0.75-1.5 g, then 750 mg q12hr; CrCl <10 ml/min: IV/IM 0.75-1.5 g, then 750 mg q24hr
Child: The frequency of dosing should be modified consistent with the recommendations for adults

Available forms: Tabs 125, 250, 500 mg: inj 150, 750 mg, 1.5, 7.5 g; inj 750 mg; 1.5 g powder, susp 125, 250 mg/5 ml

Implementation
cefaclor
• Do not break, crush, chew, or cut EXT REL tabs
• Give in even doses around the clock; if GI upset occurs, give with food; product must be

given for 10-14 days to ensure organism death and prevent superinfection
• Shake susp, refrigerate, discard after 2 wk
• Swallow EXT REL whole

cefoTEtan
IM route
• Reconstitute 1 g/2 ml or 2 g/3 ml of sterile or bacteriostatic water for inj; may be diluted with 0.5% of 1% lidocaine to prevent pain; give deep in large muscle mass, massage

IV route
• May be stored 96 hr refrigerated or 24 hr at room temperature
• Check for irritation, extravasation, phlebitis daily; change site q72hr
• For direct **IV** dilute in 1 g/10 ml or more and give over 5 min
• For intermittent inf further dilute in 50-100 ml of 0.9% NaCl or D₅W; give over 3-5 min; discontinue primary line while running intermittent inf

Y-site compatibilities: Allopurinol, amifostine, aztreonam, diltiazem, famotidine, filgrastim, fluconazole, fludarabine, heparin, regular insulin, melphalan, meperidine, morphine, PACLitaxel, sargramostim, tacrolimus, teniposide, theophylline, thiotepa

cefOXitin
IM route
• Reconstitute 1 g/2 ml of sterile water for inj; may be diluted with 0.5% or 1% lidocaine to prevent pain; give deep in large muscle mass, massage

IV route
• Check for irritation, extravasation, phlebitis daily; change site q72hr
• For direct **IV**, dilute 1 g/10 ml or 2 g/20 ml of sterile water for inj; shake, let stand until clear; give over 3-5 min
• For intermittent inf further dilute with 50-100 ml of D₅W, D₁₀W, D₅/0.25% NaCl, D₅/0.45% NaCl, D₅/0.9% NaCl, 0.9% NaCl D₅/LR, D₅/0.02%, sodium bicarbonate, Ringer's, or LR; give over 15-30 min; may store 96 hr refrigerated or 24 hr room temperature
• For cont inf dilute in 500-1000 ml; give over prescribed rate

Syringe compatibilities: Heparin, insulin

Y-site compatibilities: Acyclovir, amifostine, aztreonam, cyclophosphamide, diltiazem, famotidine, fluconazole, foscarnet,

HYDROmorphone, magnesium sulfate, meperidine, morphine, ondansetron, perphenazine, temiposide, thiotepa

Y-site incompatibilities: Hetastarch

cefprozil
IM route
• Reconstitute with 1 g/2 ml or 2 g/3 ml of sterile or bacteriostatic water for inj; may be diluted with 0.5% or 1% lidocaine to prevent pain; give deep in large muscle mass, massage

IV route
• Check for irritation, extravasation, phlebitis daily; change site q72hr
• For direct **IV**, dilute 1 g/10 ml or more and give over 5 min
• For intermittent inf further dilute with 50-100 ml of 0.9% NaCl or D₅W; give over 3-5 min; discontinue primary line while running intermittent inf

Syringe incompatibilities: Doxapram

Y-site compatibilities: Famotidine, fluconazole, fludarabine, regular insulin, meperidine, morphine, sargramostim

Additive incompatibilities: Aminoglycosides, tetracyclines, heparin

cefuroxime
• Give for 10-14 days to ensure organism death, prevent superinfection
• Give with food if needed for GI symptoms
• Five after C&S obtained

ADVERSE EFFECTS
CNS: Dizziness, headache, fatigue, paresthesia, fever, chills, confusion
GI: *Diarrhea,* nausea, vomiting, anorexia, dysgeusia, glossitis, bleeding; increased AST, ALT, bilirubin, LDH, alkaline phosphatase; abdominal pain, loose stools, flatulence, heartburn, stomach cramps, colitis, jaundice, **pseudomembranous colitis**
GU: Vaginitis, pruritus, candidiasis, increased BUN, **nephrotoxicity, renal failure,** pyuria, dysuria, reversible interstitial nephritis
HEMA: Leukopenia, thrombocytopenia, **agranulocytosis,** anemia, **neutropenia, lymphocytosis, eosinophilia, pancytopenia, hemolytic anemia, leukocytosis, granulocytopenia**
INTEG: Rash, urticaria, dermatitis, **Stevens-Johnson syndrome**
RESP: Dyspnea
SYST: Anaphylaxis, **serum sickness,** superinfection

cefaclor

Pharmacokinetics

Absorption	Well absorbed
Distribution	Widely distributed; crosses placenta
Metabolism	Not metabolized
Excretion	Unchanged by kidneys (60%-80%); enters breast milk
Half-life	36-54 min; increased in renal disease

Pharmacodynamics

Onset	15 min
Peak	½-1 hr
Duration	Unknown

cefoTEtan

Pharmacokinetics

Absorption	Well absorbed (IM)
Distribution	Widely distributed; crosses placenta
Metabolism	Not metabolized
Excretion	Kidneys, unchanged; enters breast milk
Half-life	5 hr; increased in renal disease

Pharmacodynamics

	IM	IV
Onset	Rapid	Immediate
Peak	1-3 hr	Infusion's end
Duration	Unknown	Unknown

cefOXitin

Pharmacokinetics

Absorption	Well absorbed (IM)
Distribution	Widely distributed; crosses placenta
Metabolism	Not metabolized
Excretion	Kidneys, unchanged; enters breast milk
Half-life	½-1 hr; increased in renal disease

Pharmacodynamics

	IM	IV
Onset	Rapid	Immediate
Peak	½ hr	Infusion's end
Duration	Unknown	Unknown

cefprozil

Pharmacokinetics

Absorption	Well absorbed
Distribution	Widely distributed; crosses placenta
Metabolism	Not metabolized
Excretion	Kidneys (60%), unchanged; enters breast milk
Half-life	1.3 hr (normal renal function); 2 hr (hepatic disease); 5¼-6 hr (end-stage renal disease)

Pharmacodynamics

Unknown

INTERACTIONS

Individual drugs

Antacids: decreased absorption of cephalosporins

Furosemide: increased effect/toxicity

Plicamycin, valproic acid: increased bleeding

Probenecid: decreased excretion of product and increased blood levels/toxicity

Drug classifications

Aminoglycosides: increased effect/toxicity

Anticoagulants, antiplatelets, NSAIDs, thrombolytics: increased bleeding (cefotetan)

H_2-blockers: decreased effects of cephalosporins

Oral contraceptives: decreased effectiveness possible; use additional form of contraception

Drug/lab test

False: increased creatinine (serum urine), urinary 17-KS

False positive: urinary protein, direct Coombs' test, urine glucose (Clinitest)

Interference: cross-matching

NURSING CONSIDERATIONS

Assessment

• Assess patient for previous sensitivity reaction to penicillins or other cephalosporins; cross-sensitivity between penicillins and cephalosporins is common

• Assess patient for signs and symptoms of **infection** including characteristics of wounds, sputum, urine, stool, WBC >10,000/mm^3, earache, fever; obtain baseline information and during treatment

• Obtain C&S before beginning product therapy to identify if correct treatment has been initiated

• Assess for **anaphylaxis**: rash, urticaria, pruritus, dyspnea, chills, fever, joint pain; angioedema may occur a few days after therapy begins; epinephrine and resuscitation equipment should be available for anaphylactic reaction
• Identify urine output; if decreasing, notify prescriber (may indicate **nephrotoxicity**); also check for increased BUN, creatinine
• Monitor blood studies: AST, ALT, CBC, Hct, bilirubin, LDH, alkaline phosphatase, Coombs' test monthly if patient is on long-term therapy
• Monitor electrolytes: potassium, sodium, chloride monthly if patient is on long-term therapy
• Assess bowel pattern daily; if severe diarrhea occurs, product should be discontinued; may indicate **pseudomembranous colitis**
• Monitor for bleeding: ecchymosis, bleeding gums, hematuria, stool guaiac daily if on long-term therapy
• Assess for **overgrowth of infection**: perineal itching, fever, malaise, redness, pain, swelling, drainage, rash, diarrhea, change in cough, sputum

Patient/family education
• Teach patient to report sore throat, bruising, bleeding, joint pain; may indicate **blood dyscrasias** (rare); **symptoms of hypersensitivity**
• Advise patient to contact prescriber if vaginal itching, loose foul-smelling stools, furry tongue occur; may indicate **superinfection**
• Instruct patient to take all medication prescribed for the length of time ordered; to use yogurt or buttermilk to maintain intestinal flora, decrease diarrhea
• Advise patient to notify prescriber of diarrhea with blood or pus, which may indicate **pseudomembranous colitis**

Evaluation
Positive therapeutic outcome
• Absence of signs/symptoms of infection (WBC $<10,000/mm^3$, temp WNL, absence of red draining wounds, earache)
• Reported improvement in symptoms of infection
• Negative C&S

TREATMENT OF ANAPHYLAXIS: EPINEPHrine, antihistamines, resuscitate if needed

CEPHALOSPORINS— 3RD/4TH GENERATION
cefdinir (Rx)
(sef'dih-ner)
Omnicef
cefditoren pivoxil (Rx)
(sef-dit'oh-ren pih-vox'il)
Spectracef
(4th generation) cefepime (Rx)
(sef'e-peem)
Maxipime
cefixime (Rx)
(sef-iks'ime)
Cefixime, Suprax
cefotaxime (Rx)
(sef-oh-taks'eem)
Claforan
cefpodoxime (Rx)
(sef-poe-docks'eem)
Vantin
cefTAZidime (Rx)
(sef'tay-zi-deem)
Ceptaz, Fortaz, Tazicef, Tazidime
ceftibuten (Rx)
(sef-ti-byoo'tin)
Cedax
ceftizoxime (Rx)
(sef-ti-zox'eem)
Cefizox
cefTRIAXone (Rx)
(sef-try-ax'one)
Rocephin

Func. class.: Broad-spectrum antibiotic
Chem. class.: Cephalosporin (3rd generation)
Pregnancy category B

Do not confuse:
cefTAZidime/ceftizoxime, **Vantin**/Ventolin

ACTION: Inhibits bacterial cell wall synthesis, rendering cell wall osmotically unstable, leading to cell death

cefdinir

Therapeutic outcome: Bactericidal effects for the following: *Citrobacter diversus, Escherichia coli, Haemophilus influenzae, Haemophilus parainfluenzae, Klebsiella pneu-*

moniae, Moraxella catarrhalis, Proteus mirabilis, Staphylococcus aureus, Staphylococcus epidermidis, Streptococcus agalactiae (group B), *Streptococcus pneumoniae, Streptococcus pyogenes,* viridans streptococci alpha

USES: Uncomplicated skin and skin structure infections, community-acquired pneumonia, acute exacerbations of chronic bronchitis, acute maxillary sinusitis, pharyngitis, tonsillitis, otitis media

cefditoren pivoxil

Therapeutic outcome: Bactericidal effects for the following organisms: *Haemophilus influenzae, Haemophilus parainfluenzae, Streptococcus pneumoniae, Moraxella catarrhalis, Streptococcus pyogenes, Staphylococcus aureus*

USES: Acute bacterial exacerbation of chronic bronchitis, pharyngitis/tonsillitis; uncomplicated skin, skin structure infections, community-acquired pneumonia, viridans streptococci

cefepime

Therapeutic outcome: Bactericidal effects for the following: *Acinetobacter calcoaceticus, Acinetobacter lwoffii, Aeromonas hydrophila, Citrobacter diversus, Citrobacter freundii, Enterobacter, Escherichia coli, Gardnerella vaginalis, Hafnia alvei, Klebsiella, Moraxella catarrhalis, Morganella morganii, Neisseria gonorrhoeae, Neisseria meningitidis, Proteus, Providencia rettgeri, Providencia stuartii, Pseudomonas aeruginosa, Salmonella, Serratia liquefaciens, Serratia marcescens, Shigella, Staphylococcus epidermidis, Staphylococcus saprophyticus, Streptococcus agalactiae, Streptococcus bovis,* viridans streptococci, *Yersinia enterocolitica*

USES: Lower respiratory tract, urinary tract, skin, bone, febrile neutropenia, intraabdominal infection

cefixime

Therapeutic outcome: Bactericidal effects for the following organisms: *Escherichia coli, Proteus mirabilis, Streptococcus pyogenes, Haemophilus influenzae, Moraxella catarrhalis, Streptococcus pneumoniae*

USES: Uncomplicated UTI, pharyngitis/tonsillitis, otitis media, acute bronchitis, exacerbations of chronic bronchitis, uncomplicated gonorrhea

cefotaxime

Therapeutic outcome: Bactericidal effects for the following: *Haemophilus influenzae, Haemophilus parainfluenzae, Escherichia coli, Enterococcus faecalis, Neisseria gonorrhoeae, Neisseria meningitidis, Proteus mirabilis, Klebsiella, Citrobacter, Serratia, Salmonella, Shigella Pseudomonas;* grampositive organisms *Streptococcus pneumoniae, Streptococcus pyogenes, Staphylococcus aureus*

USES: Lower serious respiratory tract, urinary tract, skin, bone, gonococcal infections; bacteremia, septicemia, meningitis, skin, skin structure infections, CNS infections, perioperative prophylaxis, intraabdominal infections, PID, UTI, ventriculitis

cefpodoxime

Therapeutic outcome: Bactericidal effects for the following: *Neisseria gonorrhoeae, Haemophilus influenzae, Escherichia coli, Proteus mirabilis, Klebsiella;* gram-positive organisms *Streptococcus pneumoniae, Streptococcus pyogenes, Staphylococcus aureus*

USES: Upper and lower respiratory tract, urinary tract, skin infections; otitis media, STDs

cefTAZidime

Therapeutic outcome: Bactericidal effects for the following: *Haemophilus influenzae, Escherichia coli, Enterobacter aerogenes, Proteus mirabilis, Klebsiella, Citrobacter, Enterobacter, Salmonella, Serratia, Pseudomonas aeruginosa, Shigella, Acinetobacter, Bacteroides fragilis, Neisseria; Streptococcus pneumoniae, Streptococcus pyogenes, Staphylococcus aureus*

USES: Serious upper or lower respiratory tract, urinary tract, skin, gynecologic, bone, joint, intraabdominal infections; septicemia, meningitis, febrile neutropenia

ceftibuten

Therapeutic outcome: Bactericidal effects for the following: *Haemophilus influenzae, Escherichia coli; Streptococcus pneumoniae, Streptococcus pyogenes, Staphylococcus aureus*

USES: Pharyngitis, tonsilitis, otitis media, secondary bacterial infection of acute bronchitis

---

C

ceftizoxime

Therapeutic outcome: Bactericidal effects for the following: *Bacteroides, Haemophilus influenzae, Escherichia coli, Enterobacter aerogenes, Proteus mirabilis, Klebsiella, Enterobacter; Streptococcus pneumoniae, Streptococcus pyogenes, Staphylococcus aureus, Neisseria gonorrhoeae*

USES: Serious lower respiratory tract, urinary tract, skin, intraabdominal infections; septicemia, meningitis; bone, joint infections, PID

cefTRIAXone

Therapeutic outcome: Bactericidal effects on the following: gram-negative organisms *Haemophilus influenzae, Escherichia coli, Enterobacter aerogenes, Proteus mirabilis, Klebsiella, Citrobacter, Enterobacter, Salmonella, Shigella, Acinetobacter, Bacteroides fragilis, Neisseria, Serratia;* gram-positive organisms *Streptococcus pneumoniae, Streptococcus pyogenes, Staphylococcus aureus*

USES: Serious lower respiratory tract, urinary tract, skin, gonococcal, intraabdominal infections; septicemia, meningitis; bone, joint infections, otitis media, PID

CONTRAINDICATIONS:
Hypersensitivity to cephalosporins, infants <1 mo

Precautions: Pregnancy **B,** breastfeeding, children, hypersensitivity to penicillins, renal/GI disease, geriatrics, pseudomembranous colitis, viral infection, vit K deficiencies

DOSAGE AND ROUTES

cefdinir

Uncomplicated skin and skin structure infections/community-acquired pneumonia
Adult and child ≥13 yr: PO 300 mg q12hr × 10 days
Child 6 mo-12 yr: PO 7 mg/kg q12hr or 14 mg/kg q24hr × 10 days

Acute exacerbations of chronic bronchitis/acute maxillary sinusitis
Adult and child ≥13 yr: PO 300 mg q12hr or 600 mg q24hr × 10 days

Pharyngitis/tonsillitis
Adult and child ≥13 yr: PO 300 mg q12hr or 600 mg q24hr × 5-10 days
Child 6 mo-12 yr: PO 7 mg/kg q12hr × 5-10 days or 14 mg/kg q24hr × 5-10 days

Renal dose
(CCr <30 ml/min)
Adult: 300 mg/day
Child: 7 mg/kg/day

Available forms: Caps 300 mg, oral susp 125 mg/5 ml, 250 mg/5 ml

cefditoren pivoxil
Adult: PO 200-400 mg bid × 10 days

Renal dose
Adult: PO CCr 30-49 ml/min, max 200 mg bid; CCr <30 ml/min, max 200 mg daily

Available forms: Tabs 200 mg

cefepime

Febrile neutropenia
Adult/adolescent >16 yr/child ≥40 kg: IV 2 g q3hr × 7 days or until neutropenia resolves
Infant ≥2 mo/child/adolescent ≤16 yr and weighing up to 40 kg: IV 50 mg/kg/dose q8hr × 7-10 days or until resolution

Urinary tract infections (mild to moderate)
Adult: IV/IM 0.5-1 g q12hr × 7-10 days

Urinary tract infections (severe)
Adult/adolescent >16 yr/child ≥40 kg: IV 2 g q12hr × 10 days

Pneumonia (moderate to severe)
Adult: IV 1-2 g q12hr × 10 days

Available forms: Powder for inj 500 mg, 1, 2 g; 1 g/50 ml, 2 g/100 ml

cefixime

Mild to moderate pharyngitis, tonsillitis, bronchitis
Adult/adolescent/child >45 kg: PO 400 mg/day divided q12-24hr
Child ≤45 kg and infant ≥6 mo: PO 8 mg/kg/day divided q12-24hr

Uncomplicated urinary tract infection (UTI)
Adult/adolescent/child >45 kg: PO 400 mg/day divided q12-24hr
Child ≤45 kg and infant ≥6 mo: PO 8 mg/kg/day divided q12-24hr max: 400 mg/day × 7-14 days is recommended by the American Academy of Pediatrics (AAP) for the treatment of initial UTI in febrile infants and young children 2-24 mo
Infant 2-5 mo (unlabeled): PO 8 mg/kg/day × 7-14 days is recommended by the American Academy of Pediatrics (AAP) for the treatment of initial UTI in febrile infants and young children

Mild to moderate otitis media
Adult/adolescent/child >45 kg: PO 400 mg/day divided q12-24hr
Child ≤45 kg: PO 8 mg/kg/day divided q12-24hr, max: 400 mg/day
Infant ≥6 mo: PO 8 mg/kg/day divided q12-24hr

Gonorrhea of uncomplicated cervicitis, or urethritis due to *N. gonorrhoeae*
Adult/adolescent: PO As alternative therapy, 400 mg as a single dose with a regimen effective against uncomplicated genital *C. trachomatis* infection (e.g., azithromycin as a single dose or doxycycline for 7 days) if chlamydial infection is not ruled out. The CDC states that cefixime is only acceptable if IM cefTRIAXone is not an option due to rising cefixime MICs for gonorrhea. If cefixime is used, test-of-cure should be done at the infected site 1 wk after treatment. Cefixime is not recommended for infections of the pharynx.
Child ≥45 kg: PO 400 mg as a single dose with a regimen effective against uncomplicated genital *C. trachomatis* infection (e.g., azithromycin as a single dose or doxycycline for 7 days) if chlamydial infection is not ruled out. Cefixime is not recommended for infections of the pharynx. Cefixime is an alternative to cefTRIAXone per the American Academy of Pediatrics (AAP).

Renal dose
CCr 21-59 ml/min give 65% of dose; CCr <20 ml/min give 50% of dose

Available forms: Tabs 400 mg; powder for oral susp 100 mg/5 ml; cap 400 mg

cefotaxime
Adult/adolescent/child ≥50 kg: IV/IM (uncomplicated infections) 1 g q12hr, (moderate-severe infections) 1-2 g q8hr, (severe infections) 2 g q6-8hr, (life-threatening infections) 2 g q4hr, max 12 g/day
Adolescent/child <50 kg and infant: IV/IM 50-180 mg/kg/day divided q6-8hr, max 2 g/dose, (severe infections 200-225 mg/kg/day divided q4-6hr max 12 hr)
Neonate >7 days: IV/IM 50 mg/kg/dose q8-12hr

Available forms: Powder for inj 500 mg, 1, 2, 10 g; 1, 2 g premixed frozen

cefpodoxime
Pneumonia
Adult >13 yr: PO 200 mg q12hr for 14 days

Uncomplicated gonorrhea
Adult >12 yr: PO 200 mg single dose

Skin and skin structure
Adult >13 yr: PO 400 mg q12hr for 7-14 days

Pharyngitis and tonsillitis
Adult >13 yr: PO 100 mg q12hr for 5-10 days
Child 5 mo-12 yr: PO 5 mg/kg q12hr (max 100 mg/dose or 200 mg/day) × 5-10 days

Uncomplicated UTI
Adult >13 yr: PO 100 mg q12hr for 7 days; dosing interval increased in presence of severe renal impairment

Acute otitis media
Child 5 mo-12 yr: PO 5 mg/kg q12hr for 10 days

Available forms: Tabs 100, 200 mg; granules for susp 50, 100 mg/5 ml

cefTAZidime
Adult: IV/IM 1-2 g q8-12hr × 5-10 days
Child: IV 30-50 mg/kg q8hr, max 6 g/day
Neonate: IV 30-50 mg/kg q12hr

Renal dose
Adult: IV CCr 31-50 ml/min 1 g q12hr; CCr 16-30 ml/min 1 g q24hr; CCr 6-15 ml/min 1 g loading dose, then 0.5 mg q24hr; CCr <5 ml/min 1 g loading dose, then 0.5 g q48hr

Available forms: Inj 250, 500 mg, 1, 2, 6 g

ceftibuten
Adult: PO 400 mg daily × 10 days
Child 6 mo-12 yr: PO 9 mg/kg daily × 10 days

Renal dose
Adult: PO CCr 30-49 ml/min 200 mg q24hr; CCr 5-29 ml/min 100 mg q24hr

Available forms: Caps 400 mg; susp 90, 180 mg/5 ml

ceftizoxime
Adult: IM/IV 1-2 g q8-12hr, may give up to 4 g q8hr in life-threatening infections
Child >6 mo: IM/IV 50 mg/kg q6-8hr

Renal dose
Adult: IM/IV CCr 50-79 ml/min 500-1500 mg q8hr; CCr 5-49 ml/min 250-1000 mg q12hr

PID
Adult: IV 2 g q8hr, may increase to 4 g q8hr in severe infections

Available forms: Premixed 1 g, 2 g/50 ml

C

cefTRIAXone
Adult: **IM/IV** 1-2 g daily, max 4 g q12-24hr
Child: **IM/IV** 50-75 mg/kg/day in equal doses q12-24hr

Uncomplicated gonorrhea
Adult: 250 mg IM as single dose
Reduce dosage in severe renal impairment (CCr <10 ml/min)

Available forms: Inj 250, 500 mg, 1, 2, 10 g

Implementation
cefdinir
PO route
• Give oral susp after adding 39 ml water to the 60 ml bottle; 65 ml water to the 12.0 ml bottle; discard unused portion after 10 days, give without regard to food, do not give within 2 hr of antacids, iron supplements

cefditoren pivoxil
• Give for 10 days to ensure organism death, prevent superinfection
• Give with food if needed, do not give with antacids
• Give after C&S is completed

cefepime

IV route
• Check for irritation, extravasation, phlebitis daily; change site q72hr
• For **intermittent inf** dilute with 50-100 ml of D_5W, give over 30 min

Solution compatibilities: 0.9% NaCl, D_5, 0.5, 1.0% lidocaine, bacteriostatic water for inj with parabens/benzyl alcohol

cefixime
• Give for 10-14 days to ensure organism death, prevent superinfection

cefotaxime

IV route
• **Dilute** 1 g/10 ml D_5W, NS, sterile water for inj and **give** over 3-5 min by Y-tube or 3-way stopcock; may be **diluted further** with 50-100 ml of 0.9% NaCl or D_5W; **run** over ½-1 hr; discontinue primary inf during administration; or may be diluted in larger volume of sol and given as a cont inf
• Give for 10-14 days to ensure organism death, prevent superinfection
• Thaw frozen container at room temperature or refrigeration, do not force thaw by immersion or microwave; visually inspect container for leaks

Syringe compatibilities: Heparin, oflaxacin

Y-site compatibilities: Acyclovir, alfentanil, alprostadil, amifostine, amikacin, aminocaproic acid, aminophylline, anidulafungin, ascorbic acid injection, atenolol, atracurium, atropine, aztreonam, benztropine, bivalirudin, bleomycin, bumetanide, buprenorphine, butorphanol, caffeine, calcium chloride/gluconate, CARBOplatin, cefamandole, cefmetazole, cefonicid, cefoperazone, cefoTEtan, cefOXitin, cefTAZidime (L-arginine), cefTRIAXone sodium, cefuroxime, cimetidine, CISplatin, clindamycin, codeine, cyanocobalamin, cyclophosphamide, cycloSPORINE, cytarabine, DACTINomycin, DAPTOmycin, dexamethasone, dexmedetomidine, digoxin, diltiazem, DOCEtaxel, DOPamine, doxacurium, doxycycline, enalaprilat, ePHEDrine, EPINEPHrine, epirubicin, epoetin alfa, eptifibatide, erythromycin, esmolol, etoposide, famotidine, fenoldopam, fentaNYL, fludarabine, fluorouracil, folic acid, furosemide, gatifloxacin, gentamicin, glycopyrrolate, granisetron, heparin, hydrocortisone, HYDROmorphone, ifosfamide, imipenem-cilastatin, insulin (regular), isoproterenol, ketorolac, lidocaine, linezolid, LORazepam, LR, magnesium sulfate, mannitol, mechlorethamine, melphalan, meperidine, metaraminol, methicillin, methotrexate, methoxamine, methyldopate, metoclopramide, metoprolol, metroNIDAZOLE, mezlocillin, miconazole, midazolam, milrinone, minocycline, mitoXANtrone, morphine, moxalactam, multiple vitamins, mycophenolate, nafcillin, nalbuphine, naloxone, nesiritide, netilmicin, nitroglycerin, nitroprusside, norepinephrine, normal saline, octreotide, ofloxacin, ondansetron, ornidazole, oxacillin, oxaliplatin, oxytocin, PACLitaxel, palonosetron, pamidronate, pancuronium, pantoprazole, papaverine, pefloxacin, PEMEtrexed, penicillin G potassium/sodium, pentamidine, pentazocine, PENTobarbital, peritoneal dialysis solution, perphenazine, PHENobarbital, phenylephrine, phenytoin, phytonadione, piperacillin, polymyxin B, potassium chloride, procainamide, prochlorperazine, promethazine, propofol, propranolol, protamine, quiNIDine, quinupristin, ranitidine, remifentanil, Ringer's injection, ritodrine, riTUXimab, rocuronium, sargramostim, sodium acetate/bicarbonate, sodium fusidate, sodium lactate, succinylcholine, SUFentanil, sulfamethoxazole-trimethoprim, tacrolimus, teniposide, theophylline, thiamine, thiotepa, ticarcillin, ticarcillin-clavulanate, tigecycline, tirofiban, TNA, tobramycin, tolazoline, TPN, trastuzumab, trimetaphan, urokinase, vancomycin, vasopressin, vecuronium, verapamil, vinorelbine, voriconazole

cefpodoxime
PO route
- Do not break, crush, or chew tabs due to taste
- Give for 10-14 days to ensure organism death, prevent superinfection
- With food for better absorption, do not give within 2 hr of antacids, H_2 receptor antagonists
- Shake susp well, refrigerate, discard after 2 wk

cefTAZidime
IM route
- **Fortaz, Tazidime vials:** Reconstitute 500 mg or 1 g with 1.5 or 3 ml, respectively, of sterile or bacteriostatic water for injection, or 0.5%-1% lidocaine (approx. 280 mg/ml)
- **Tazicef vials:** Reconstitute 1 g/3 ml sterile water for injection (approx. 280 mg/ml)
- **Ceptaz vials:** Reconstitute 1 g/3 ml sterile or bacteriostatic water for injection or 0.5%-1% lidocaine (approx. 250 mg/ml)
- Withdraw the dose, making sure the needle remains in the vial; ensure that no CO_2 bubbles are present; inject deeply in large muscle mass; aspirate prior to injection

IV route
- If possible, visually inspect for particulate matter and discoloration
- **Fortaz, Tazicef, Tazidime packs:** Reconstitute 1 or 2 g/100 ml sterile water for injection or other compatible **IV** sol (10 or 20 mg/ml, respectively). Reconstitution is done in two stages. First, inject 10 ml of the diluents into the pack and shake well to dissolve and become clear; CO_2 pressure inside the container will occur; insert a vent needle to release the pressure; add remaining diluents and remove vent needle
- **Fortaz, Tazicef, Tazidime vials:** Reconstitute 500 mg, 1 g, 2 g with 5, 10, 10 ml, respectively, of sterile water for injection or other compatible **IV** sol (100, 95-100, or 170-180 mg/ml, respectively; shake well to dissolve
- **Fortaz, Tazidime-ADD-Vantage vials** (for **IV** only): Reconstitute 1 or 2 g with NS, ½ NS, D_5W in either 50 or 100 ml flexible diluents container; to release CO_2 pressure, insert a vent needle after dissolving; remove vent before using
- **Ceptaz packs:** Reconstitute 1 or 2 g/100 ml sterile water for injection or compatible **IV** sol (10 or 20 mg/ml, respectively). Reconstitution is done in two stages. First, inject 10 ml of the diluent into the pack and shake well to dissolve; add the remaining diluents; insert as vent needle before giving

- **Ceptaz vials:** Reconstitute 1 or 2 g/10 ml of sterile water for injection or compatible **IV** sol (90-95, or 170-180 mg/ml, respectively)
- **Ceptaz ADD-Vantage vials** (for **IV** infusion only): Reconstitute 1 or 2 g with NS, ½ NS, or D_5W in either 50 or 100 ml diluent container as appropriate

Direct intermittent IV infusion route
- **Vials:** Withdraw the correct dose, making sure the needle opening remains in the solution; make sure there are no CO_2 bubbles in the syringe before injection; inject directly over 3-5 min or slowly into the tubing of a free-flowing compatible IV solution

Intermittent IV infusion route
- **Vials:** Withdraw the correct dose, making sure the needle opening remains in the solution; make sure there are no CO_2 bubbles in the syringe before injection; infusion packs and ADD-Vantage systems are ready for infusion after reconstitution; infuse over 15-30 min

ceftibuten
- Administer for 10 days to ensure organism death, prevent superinfection
- Administer after C&S
- Administer on empty stomach

ceftizoxime
IM route
- Reconstitute 250 mg/0.9 ml, 500 mg/1.8 ml, 1 g/3.6 ml, 2 g/7.2 ml; may be diluted with 0.5% or 1% lidocaine to prevent pain; give deep in large muscle mass, massage

IV route
- Check for irritation, extravasation, phlebitis daily; change site q72hr
- For intermittent inf reconstitute 250 mg/2.4 ml, 500 mg/4.8 ml, 1 g/9.6 mg/2 g/19.2 ml sterile water for inj, D_5W, or 0.9% NaCl; do not use sol with benzyl alcohol for neonates; may be further diluted in 50-100 ml of D_5W, $D_{10}W$, 0.9% NaCl, or LR; give over 30-60 min
- May store 96 hr refrigerated, 24 hr room temperature

Y-site compatibilities: Acyclovir, allopurinol, amifostine, aztreonam, enalaprilat, esmolol, famotidine, fludarabine, foscarnet, HYDROmorphone, labetalol, melphalan, meperidine, morphine, ondansetron, sargramostim, teniposide, thiotepa, vinorelbine

Additive compatibilities: Clindamycin, metroNIDAZOLE

Additive incompatibilities: Aminoglycosides

cefTRIAXone
• Give IM inj deep in large muscle mass
• Give for 10-14 days to ensure organism death, prevent superinfection

IV route
• Give **IV** after diluting 250 mg/2.4 ml of 500 mg/4.8 ml, 1 g/9.6 ml, 2 g/19.2 ml D$_5$W, water for inj, 0.9% NaCl; may be further diluted with 50-100 ml of 0.9% NaCl, D$_5$W, D$_{10}$W, shake; run over ½-1 hr
• Do not mix with calcium salts

Y-site compatibilities: Acyclovir, allopurinol, aztreonam, cisatracurium, diltiazem, DOXOrubicin liposome, fludarabine, foscarnet, heparin, melphalan, meperidine, methotrexate, morphine, PACLitaxel, remifentanil, sargramostim, tacrolimus, teniposide, theophylline, vinorelbine, warfarin, zidovudine

Additive compatibilities: Amino acids or sodium bicarbonate, metroNIDAZOLE

ADVERSE EFFECTS
CNS: Headache, dizziness, weakness, paresthesia, fever, chills, **seizures,** dyskinesia (cefdinir)
CV: Heart failure, syncope (cefdinir)
EENT: *Oral candidiasis*
GI: *Nausea, vomiting, diarrhea, anorexia,* pain, glossitis, **bleeding;** increased AST, ALT, bilirubin, LDH, alkaline phosphatase; abdominal pain, **pseudomembranous colitis,** cholestasis (cefotaxime)
GU: Proteinuria, vaginitis, pruritus, *candidiasis,* increased BUN, **nephrotoxicity, renal failure**
HEMA: Leukopenia, thrombocytopenia, agranulocytosis, anemia, **neutropenia, lymphocytosis, eosinophilia, pancytopenia, hemolytic anemia**
INTEG: Rash, urticaria, dermatitis
MS: Arthralgia (cefditoren)
RESP: Dyspnea
SYST: Anaphylaxis, serum sickness, Stevens-Johnson syndrome, toxic epidermal necrolysis

cefdinir

Pharmacokinetics

Absorption	Well absorbed
Distribution	Widely distributed; crosses placenta
Metabolism	Not metabolized
Excretion	Kidneys, unchanged; enters breast milk
Half-life	1.7 hr

Pharmacodynamics
Unknown

cefditoren pivoxil

Pharmacokinetics

Absorption	Well absorbed after it is broken down (prodrug)
Distribution	Widely
Metabolism	Unknown
Excretion	Unknown
Half-life	100 mins

Pharmacodynamics

Onset	Rapid
Peak	0.5-3 hr
Duration	12 hrs

cefepime

Pharmacokinetics

Absorption	Well absorbed (IM)
Distribution	Widely distributed; crosses placenta
Metabolism	Not metabolized
Excretion	Kidneys, unchanged; enters breast milk
Half-life	2 hr; increased in renal disease

Pharmacodynamics

	IM	IV
Onset	Rapid	Immediate
Peak	79 min	Infusion's end
Duration	Unknown	Unknown

cefixime

Pharmacokinetics

Absorption	Unknown
Distribution	Protein binding 65%-70%
Metabolism	Unknown
Excretion	Urine, bile
Half-life	3-4 hr

Pharmacodynamics

Onset	Unknown
Peak	2-6 hr
Duration	Unknown

cefotaxime

Pharmacokinetics

Absorption	Widely distributed
Distribution	Breast milk, small amounts
Metabolism	Liver, active metabolites
Excretion	40%-65% unchanged, kidney
Half-life	1 hr

Pharmacodynamics

	IV	IM
Onset	5 min	30 min
Peak	Unknown	Unknown
Duration	Unknown	Unknown

cefpodoxime

Pharmacokinetics

Absorption	Well absorbed
Distribution	Widely distributed; crosses placenta, protein binding 13%-38%
Metabolism	Not metabolized
Excretion	Kidneys, unchanged; enters breast milk
Half-life	1-1.5 hr, increased in renal disease

Pharmacodynamics

Unknown

cefTAZidime

Pharmacokinetics

Absorption	Well absorbed (IM)
Distribution	Widely distributed; crosses placenta
Metabolism	Not metabolized
Excretion	Kidneys, unchanged; enters breast milk
Half-life	1-2 hr; increased in renal disease

Pharmacodynamics

	IM	IV
Onset	Rapid	Immediate
Peak	1.5-2 hr	Infusion's end

ceftibuten

Pharmacokinetics

Absorption	Well absorbed
Distribution	Widely distributed; crosses placenta
Metabolism	Not metabolized
Excretion	Kidneys, unchanged; enters breast milk
Half-life	1-1½ hr; increased in renal disease

Pharmacodynamics

Unknown

ceftizoxime

Pharmacokinetics

Absorption	Well absorbed (IM)
Distribution	Widely distributed; crosses placenta, protein binding 30%
Metabolism	Not metabolized
Excretion	Kidneys, unchanged; enters breast milk
Half-life	1½-2 hr; increased in renal disease

Pharmacodynamics

	IM	IV
Onset	Rapid	Immediate
Peak	1 hr	Infusion's end

cefTRIAXone

Pharmacokinetics

Absorption	Well absorbed
Distribution	Widely distributed; crosses placenta; enters CSF, protein binding 58%-96%
Metabolism	Liver
Excretion	Kidneys, partly
Half-life	6-9 hr

Pharmacodynamics

	IM	IV
Onset	Rapid	Immediate
Peak	1.5-4 hr	30 min

INTERACTIONS

Individual drugs

Many products should not be used with calcium salts (mixed or administered) or H_2 blockers antacids (PO)

CycloSPORINE: increased cycloSPORINE levels
Furosemide, probenecid: increased toxicity
Iron: decreased absorption of cefdinir
Plicamycin, valproic acid: increased bleeding

Drug classifications
Aminoglycosides: increased toxicity
Anticoagulants, NSAIDs, thrombolytics: increased bleeding

Drug/food
Iron-rich cereal, infants' formula: decreased absorption

Drug/lab test
Increased: ALT, AST, alkaline phosphatase, LDH, bilirubin, BUN, creatinine
False increase: creatinine (serum urine), urinary 17-KS
False positive: urinary protein, direct Coombs' test, urine glucose
Interference: cross-matching

NURSING CONSIDERATIONS
Assessment
• Assess patient for previous sensitivity reaction to penicillins or other cephalosporins; cross-sensitivity between penicillins and cephalosporins is common
• Assess patient for signs and symptoms of **infection** including characteristics of wounds, sputum, urine, stool, WBC >10,000/mm^3, fever; obtain baseline information and during treatment
• Obtain C&S before beginning product therapy to identify if correct treatment has been initiated
• Assess for **anaphylaxis:** rash, urticaria, pruritus, chills, fever, joint pain; angioedema may occur a few days after therapy begins; epinephrine and resuscitation equipment should be available for anaphylactic reaction
• Identify urine output; if decreasing, notify prescriber (may indicate **nephrotoxicity**); also check for increased BUN, creatinine
• Monitor blood studies: AST, ALT, CBC, Hct, bilirubin, LDH, alkaline phosphatase, Coombs' test monthly if patient is on long-term therapy
• Monitor electrolytes: potassium, sodium, chloride monthly if patient is on long-term therapy
• Assess bowel pattern daily; if severe diarrhea occurs, product should be discontinued; may indicate **pseudomembranous colitis**
• Monitor for **bleeding:** ecchymosis, bleeding gums, hematuria, stool guaiac daily if on long-term therapy

• Assess for **overgrowth of infection:**
perineal itching, fever, malaise, redness, pain, swelling, drainage, rash, diarrhea, change in cough, sputum
• Monitor heart rate during direct IV infusion (cefotaxime)

Patient/family education
• Teach patient to report sore throat, bruising, bleeding, joint pain; may indicate blood dyscrasias (rare)
• Advise patient to contact prescriber if vaginal itching, loose foul-smelling stools, furry tongue occur; may indicate superinfection
• Advise patient to notify prescriber of diarrhea with blood or pus, may indicate pseudomembranous colitis
• Cefditoren can be taken with oral contraceptives

Evaluation
Positive therapeutic outcome
• Absence of signs/symptoms of infection (WBC <10,000/mm^3, temp WNL, absence of red draining wounds, earache)
• Reported improvement in symptoms of infection
• Negative C&S

TREATMENT OF ANAPHY-LAXIS: EPINEPHrine, antihistamines, resuscitate if needed

cephradine
See cephalosporins—1st generation

certolizumab pegol (Rx)
(ser'tue-liz'oo-mab) (pegh'ol)
Cimzia
Func. class.: Biologic response modifier
Chem. class.: Anti-TNF (tissue necrosis factor) agent
Pregnancy category B

ACTION: Monoclonal antibody that neutralizes the activity of tumor necrosis factor-α (TNF-α) found in Crohn's disease; decreased infiltration of inflammatory cells

Therapeutic outcome: Absence of fever, mucus in stools

USES: Crohn's disease (moderate-severe) that has not responded to conventional therapy, rheumatoid arthritis (moderate-severe)

Adverse effects: *italics* = common; **bold** = life-threatening

CONTRAINDICATIONS:
Influenza, **IV** administration, sepsis, hypersensitivity

> **BLACK BOX WARNING:** Infection, neoplastic disease

Precautions: Pregnancy **B**, breastfeeding, children, geriatric patients, AIDS, coagulopathy, diabetes, fungal infection, heart failure, hepatitis, human anti-chimeric antibody, immunosuppression, leukopenia, MS, cancer, neurologic disease, surgery, thrombocytopenia, TB, vaccinations, renal disease

DOSAGE AND ROUTES
Crohn's disease (moderate-severe)
Adult: SUBCUT 400 mg given as 2 inj at wk 0, 2, 4; if clinical response occurs, give 400 mg q4wk

Rheumatoid arthritis (moderate-severe)
Adult: SUBCUT 400 mg q2wk × 3 doses, then 200 mg q2wk; given with methotrexate

Available forms: Powder for inj 400 mg kit

Implementation
• Store in refrigerator; do not freeze
SUBCUT route
• Give by SUBCUT only
• Allow reconstitution to warm to room temp; add 1 ml sterile water for inj to each vial; two vials will be needed for Crohn's disease
• Gently swirl; do not shake; full reconstitution may take up to 30 min; reconstituted product may remain at room temp for up to 2 hr or refrigerated up to 24 hr
• Warm to room temperature if reconstituted product has been refrigerated
• Use 2 syringes and 2 20-G needles
• Withdraw reconstituted sol from each vial into separate syringes; each will contain 200 mg; switch 20-G to 23-G needle; inject into 2 separate sites in abdomen or thigh

ADVERSE EFFECTS
CNS: *Dizziness*, syncope, peripheral neuropathy, fever, **seizures, demyelinating disease of CNS**
CV: Hypotension, **heart failure, MI, cardiac dysrhythmia**
EENT: Optic neuritis, retinal hemorrhage, uveitis
GI: Increased LFTs, **hepatitis, bowel obstruction**

GU: UTI, renal disease
HEMA: Anemia, aplastic anemia, pancytopenia, thrombocytopenia
INTEG: *Rash, urticaria,* **angioedema**
RESP: Dyspnea, URI
SYST: Anaphylaxis, malignancies, serum sickness, bleeding, antibody formation, infection, lupus-like symptoms, lymphadenopathy, arthralgia, **suicidal ideation**

Pharmacokinetics
Absorption	Unknown
Distribution	Unknown
Metabolism	Unknown
Excretion	Unknown
Half-life	Terminal 14 days

Pharmacodynamics
Onset	Unknown
Peak	54-171 hr
Duration	Unknown

INTERACTIONS
Individual drugs
Abatacept, adalimumab, anakinra, etanercept, infliximab, do not use concurrently, rilonacept: increased possible infections
Adalimumab, etanercept, infliximab: increased possible malignancies

Drug classifications
Immunosuppressive agents: increased possible infections, do not use concurrently
Live vaccines, toxoids: do not administer concurrently

NURSING CONSIDERATIONS
Assessment
• Monitor antibody test (ANA), hepatitis B serology, CBC
• Assess for rheumatoid arthritis, ROM, pain
• Assess GI symptoms: nausea, vomiting, abdominal pain, hepatitis, increased LFTs
• Monitor periodic blood counts (CBC)
• Assess CV status: B/P, pulse, chest pain
⚠ Assess for allergic reaction, anaphylaxis: rash, dermatitis, urticaria, dyspnea, hypotension, fever, chills; discontinue if severe, administer epinephrine, corticosteroids, antihistamines; assess for allergies to murine proteins before starting therapy

> **BLACK BOX WARNING:** Assess **infections:** discontinue if infection occurs; do not administer to patients with active infections

BLACK BOX WARNING: Identify TB, risk for HBV before beginning treatment; a TB test should be obtained; if present, TB should be treated prior to receiving infliximab

Patient/family education
• Instruct patient not to breastfeed while taking this product

BLACK BOX WARNING: Advise patient to notify prescriber of GI symptoms, hypersensitivity reactions, infections, fluid retention, redness, pain, swelling at injection site

BLACK BOX WARNING: Caution patient not to operate machinery, drive if dizziness, vertigo occur

Evaluation
Positive therapeutic outcome
• Absence of fever, mucus in stools

cetirizine (Rx)
(se-tear'i-zeen)
All Day Allergy, All Day Allergy Children's, GNP All Day Allergy, GNP Children's All Day Allergy, Good Sense All Day Allergy, Good Sense Children's All Day Allergy, Publix Allergy Children's, Reactine ✦, Top Care Children's All Day Allergy, ZyrTEC, ZyrTEC Children's
Func. class.: Antihistamine, peripherally selective (2nd generation)
Chem. class.: Piperazine, H_1 histamine antagonist
Pregnancy category B

Do not confuse:
ZyrTEC/Xanax/Zantac

ACTION: Acts on blood vessels, GI, respiratory system by competing with histamine for H_1-receptor site; decreases allergic response by blocking pharmacologic effects of histamine; minimal anticholinergic/sedative action

Therapeutic outcome: Absence of allergy symptoms, rhinitis, and chronic idiopathic urticaria

USES: Rhinitis, allergy symptoms, and chronic idiopathic urticaria

CONTRAINDICATIONS:
Hypersensitivity to this product or hydrOXYzine, breastfeeding, newborn or premature infants, severe hepatic disease

Precautions: Pregnancy **B**, children, geriatric, respiratory disease, closed-angle glaucoma, prostatic hypertrophy, bladder neck obstruction, asthma

DOSAGE AND ROUTES
Perennial/seasonal allergic rhinitis or idiopathic urticaria
Adult and child ≥6 yr: PO 5-10 mg daily
Child 2-5 yr: PO 2.5 mg daily, may increase to 5 mg daily or 2.5 mg bid
Child 1-2 yr: PO 2.5 mg daily, may increase to 2.5 mg q12hr
Child 6-11 mo: PO 2.5 mg daily
Geriatric: PO 5 mg daily, may increase to 10 mg/day

Self-treatment of hay fever/other respiratory allergies
Adult/adolescent/child ≥6 yr: PO 10 mg/day, oral SOL 5-10 mg/day

Renal dose
Adult: PO CCr 11-31 ml/min 5 mg daily

Hemodialysis
Adult: PO 5 mg/day

Hepatic dose
Adult: PO 5 mg daily

Available forms: Tabs 5, 10 mg; syr 5 mg/5 ml; prefilled spoons 1 mg/ml; oral sol 5 mg/5 ml; liquid filled cap 10 mg; chew tab 5, 10 mg

Implementation
• Give without regard to meals
• Store in tight, light-resistant container
• **Caps:** swallow whole, do not break, cut, chew, crush
• **Chew tabs:** chew before swallowing, may use without or with water
• **Oral liquid:** use calibrated measuring device

ADVERSE EFFECTS
CNS: *Headache,* stimulation, *drowsiness,* sedation, *fatigue,* confusion, blurred vision, tinnitus, restlessness, tremors, parodoxical excitation in children or geriatric
GI: *Dry mouth,* increased liver function tests, constipation
INTEG: Rash, eczema, photosensitivity, urticaria
RESP: *Thickening of bronchial secretions;* dry nose, throat

Pharmacokinetics

Absorption	Well absorbed, rapid
Distribution	Protein binding 93%
Metabolism	Liver
Excretion	Kidneys
Half-life	8.3 hr, decreased in children, increased in renal/hepatic disease

Pharmacodynamics

Onset	½ hr
Peak	1-2 hr
Duration	24 hr

INTERACTIONS

Individual drugs
Alcohol: increased CNS depression
Ritonavir: increased cetirizine effect

Drug classifications
CNS depressants, opioids, sedative/hypnotics: increased CNS depression
MAOIs: increased anticholinergic effect

Drug/food
Prolongs absorption by 1.7 hr

Drug/lab test
False negative: skin allergy tests (discontinue antihistamine 3 days before testing)

NURSING CONSIDERATIONS

Assessment
• Assess respiratory status: rate, rhythm; increase in bronchial secretions, wheezing, chest tightness; provide fluids to 2 L/day to decrease secretion thickness
• Assess for **allergy symptoms:** pruritus, urticaria, watering eyes, baseline, during treatment

Patient/family education
• Teach all aspects of product uses; to notify prescriber if confusion, sedation, hypotension occur; to avoid driving or other hazardous activity if drowsiness occurs; to avoid alcohol or other CNS depressants that may potentiate effect
• Instruct patient to take without regard to meals
• Instruct patient not to exceed recommended dose; dysrhythmias may occur
• Advise patient to avoid using if breastfeeding
• Advise patient to avoid exposure to sunlight; burns may occur
• Advise patient to use sugarless gum, candy, frequent sips of water to minimize dry mouth
• Advise patient to avoid alcohol, OTC antihistamines, other CNS depressants

Evaluation
Positive therapeutic outcome
• Absence of runny or congested nose, rashes

TREATMENT OF OVERDOSE:
Lavage, diazepam, vasopressors, phenytoin IV

cetrorelix (Rx)
(set-roe-ree′lix)
Cetrotide
Func. class.: Gonadotropin-releasing
Chem. class.: Synthetic decapeptide
Pregnancy category X

ACTION: Inhibitor of pituitary gonadotropin secretion; initially increases LH and FSH, induces a rapid suppression of gonadotropin secretion

Therapeutic outcome: Pregnancy

USES: For inhibition of premature LH surges in women undergoing controlled ovarian hyperstimulation

CONTRAINDICATIONS:
Pregnancy **X,** breastfeeding, hypersensitivity, latex allergy, renal disease

Precautions: Geriatric

DOSAGE AND ROUTES

Single-dose regimen
Adult: SUBCUT 3 mg when serum estradiol level is at appropriate stimulation response, usually on stimulation day 7; if hCG has not been given within 4 days after inj of 3 mg cetrorelix, give 0.25 mg daily until day of hCG administration

Multiple-dose regimen
Adult: SUBCUT 0.25 mg is given on stimulation day 5 (either morning or evening) or 6 (morning) and continued daily until day hCG is given

Available forms: Inj 0.25, 3 mg

Implementation
SUBCUT route
• Give SUBCUT using abdomen, 1 inch away from navel, or upper thigh; swab inj area with disinfectant, clean a 2-in circle and allow to dry, pinch up area between thumb and finger, insert needle at 45-90 degrees to surface; if blood is drawn into the syringe, reposition needle without removing it; rotate inj sites
• Do not administer if patient is pregnant
• Protect from light

ADVERSE EFFECTS

CNS: Headache
CV: Edema
ENDO: Ovarian hyperstimulation syndrome, abdominal pain (gyn)
GI: Nausea, vomiting, diarrhea
INTEG: Pain on inj; local site reactions, bruising, pruritus
OTHER: Rapid weight gain
RESP: Shortness of breath
SYST: Fetal death, anaphylaxis

Pharmacokinetics

Absorption	Unknown
Distribution	Protein binding 86%
Metabolism	Liver to metabolites
Excretion	Feces/urine
Half-life	Depends on dosage

Pharmacodynamics

Unknown

NURSING CONSIDERATIONS

Assessment

• Assess for suspected pregnancy; product should not be used, pregnancy X
• Assess for **latex allergy;** product should not be used
• Monitor ALT, AST, GGT, alkaline phosphatase, serum progesterone, LH; ovarian ultrasound days 7-14
• Assess for **anaphylaxis** during first infusion

Patient/family education

• Instruct to report abdominal pain, vaginal bleeding, nausea, vomiting, diarrhea, shortness of breath, peripheral edema
• Teach self-administration technique if needed

Evaluation

Positive therapeutic outcome
• Pregnancy

---

cetuximab (Rx)

(se-tux'i-mab)
Erbitux
Func. class.: Antineoplastic—miscellaneous, monoclonal antibody
Chem. class.: Epidermal growth factor receptor inhibitor
Pregnancy category C

ACTION: Not fully understood; binds to epidermal growth factor receptors (EGFRs); inhibits phosphorylation and activation of receptor-associated kinase resulting in inhibition of cell growth

Therapeutic outcome: Decrease in tumor size

USES: Alone or in combination with irinotecan for EGFR expressing metastatic colorectal carcinoma, head/neck cancer

CONTRAINDICATIONS:

Hypersensitivity to this product or murine proteins

Precautions: Pregnancy **C**, breastfeeding, child, geriatric, CV/renal/hepatic disease, ocular, pulmonary disorders

> **BLACK BOX WARNING:** Arrhythmias, CAD, platinum-based therapy infusion-related reactions, radiation, cardiac, respiratory arrest

DOSAGE AND ROUTES

Adult: IV INF 400 mg/m^2 loading dose given over 120 min, max INF rate 5 ml/min, weekly maintenance dose (all other infusions) is 250 mg/m^2 given over 60 min, max INF rate 5 ml/min (10 mg/min); premedicate with an H$_1$ antagonist (diphenhydrAMINE 50 mg **IV**); dosage adjustments are made for INF reactions or dermatologic toxicity; other protocols are used

Available forms: Sol for inj 100 mg/50 ml, 200 mg/100 ml

Implementation

Intermittent infusion route
• Administer by **IV** infusion only, do not give by **IV** push or bolus
• Do not shake or dilute
• Do not dilute with other products
• **Infusion pump:** draw up volume of a vial using appropriate syringe/needle (a vented spike or other appropriate transfer device); fill Erbitux into sterile evacuated container/bag, repeat until calculated volume has been put into the container. Use a new needle for each vial; give through in-line filter (low protein binding 0.22-micrometer); affix inf line and prime before starting inf, max rate 5 ml/min; flush line at end of inf with 0.9% NaCl
• **Syringe pump:** Draw up volume of a vial using appropriate syringe/needle (a vented spike); place syringe into syringe driver of a syringe pump and set rate; use an in-line filter 0.22 micrometer (low protein binding); connect inf line and start inf after priming; repeat until calculated volume has been given

---

Adverse effects: *italics* = common; **bold** = life-threatening

• Use a new needle and filter for each vial, max 5 ml/min rate; use 0.9% NaCl to flush line after inf
• Do not piggyback to patient inf line
• Observe patient for adverse reactions for 1hr after inf

> **BLACK BOX WARNING:** Inf reactions: if mild (grade 1 or 2) reduce all doses by 50%; if severe (grade 3 or 4) permanently discontinue

• Store refrigerated 36°-46° F, discard unused portions

ADVERSE EFFECTS

CNS: *Headache, insomnia, depression,* aseptic meningitis
CV: Cardiac arrest
GI: *Nausea, diarrhea, vomiting, anorexia, mouth ulceration, dehydration, constipation, abdominal pain*
HEMA: Leukepenia, anemia
INTEG: Rash, pruritus, acne, dry skin, toxic epidermal necrolysis, angioedema, *blepharitis, cheilitis, cellulitis, cysts, alopecia, skin/nail disorder,* acute infusion reactions, other skin toxicities
MISC: *Conjunctivitis, asthma, malaise, fever,* renal failure, hypomagnesemia
MS: *Back pain*
RESP: Interstitial lung disease, *cough,* dyspnea, pulmonary embolus, *peripheral edema,* respiratory arrest
SYST: Anaphylaxis, sepsis, infection

Pharmacokinetics

Absorption	Unknown
Distribution	Unknown
Metabolism	Unknown
Excretion	Unknown
Half-life	114 hrs

Pharmacodynamics

Onset	Unknown
Peak	168-235 g/ml, trough 41-85 g/ml
Duration	Steady state by 3rd weekly infusion

INTERACTIONS
Drug/lab test
Increase: LFTs

NURSING CONSIDERATIONS
Assessment

> **BLACK BOX WARNING:** Monitor pulmonary changes: lung sounds, cough, dyspnea; interstitial lung disease may occur, may be fatal; discontinue therapy if confirmed

• Cardiac arrest: monitor electrolytes; in those undergoing radiation therapy, electrolytes may be decreased
⚠ Assess for toxic epidermal necrosis, angioedema, anaphylaxis
• Assess GI symptoms: frequency of stools, dehydration, abdominal pain, stomatitis
• Obtain **K-RAS mutation** in metastatic colorectal carcinoma; if K-RAS mutation in codon 12 or 13 is detected, then patient should not receive anti-EGFR antibody therapy

Patient/family education

> **BLACK BOX WARNING:** Instruct patient to report adverse reactions immediately: SOB, severe abdominal pain, skin eruptions

• Explain reason for treatment, expected results

> **BLACK BOX WARNING:** Instruct patient to use contraception during treatment

• Advise patient to wear sunscreen and hat to limit sun exposure; sun exposure can exacerbate any skin reactions

Evaluation
Positive therapeutic outcome
• Decrease growth, spread of EGFR expressing metastatic colorectal carcinoma

charcoal, activated (OTC)
Actidose-Aqua, Actidose with Sorbitol, Charcoal Plus, Charcoal Plus DS, Charcocaps, EZ Char
Func. class.: Antiflatulent/antidote
Pregnancy category D

Do not confuse:
Actidose/Actos

ACTION: Binds poisons, toxins, irritants; increases adsorption in GI tract; inactivates toxins and binds until excreted

Therapeutic outcome: Prevention of toxicity and death resulting from absorption of products

---

USES: Poisoning, overdose

Unlabeled uses: Diarrhea, flatulence

CONTRAINDICATIONS:
Pregnancy **D**, hypersensitivity to this product, unconsciousness, semiconsciousness, poisoning of cyanide, mineral acids, alkalis, gag reflex, depression, ethanol intoxication, intestinal obstruction, absent bowel sounds

Precautions: Pregnancy **(C)**, hypersensitivity to quiNIDine, quiNINE

DOSAGE AND ROUTES
Poisoning
Children should not get more than 1 dose of products with sorbitol
• Tabs/caps should not be used in poisonings
Adult/adolescents: PO (activated charcoal aqueous susp) 5-10 × estimated weight of drug/chemical ingested or 50-100 g dose, may repeat q4-6hr as needed; (activated charcoal with sorbitol susp) 50 g as a single dose, do not use multiple dosing
Child: PO (activated charcoal aqueous susp) 1-2 g/kg/dose or 25-50 g dose, may repeat as needed q4-6hr
Infant: PO (activated charcoal aqueous susp) 1 g/kg/dose, may repeat as needed q4-6hr

Available forms: Powder 15, 25✚, 30, 40, 120, 125, 240 g/container; oral susp 12.5 g/60 ml, 15 g/72 ml, 15 g/120 ml, 25 g/120 ml, 30 g/120 ml, 50 g/240 ml; ✚15 g/120 ml, 25 g/125 ml, 50 g/225 ml, 50 g/250 ml

Implementation
• Use stool softener or laxative to lessen constipation unless sorbitol has been given
• Give after inducing vomiting unless vomiting is contraindicated (i.e., cyanide or alkalis); mix with 8 oz of water or fruit juice to form thick syrup; do not use dairy products to mix charcoal; repeat dose if vomiting occurs soon after dose
• Space at least 2 hr before or after other products, or absorption will be decreased; use a laxative to promote elimination; constipation occurs often
• If patient unable to swallow, dilute to a less thick sol; keep container tightly closed to prevent absorption of gases
⚠ **Give through a nasogastric tube if patient is unable to swallow**

ADVERSE EFFECTS
GI: *Nausea, black stools,* vomiting, constipation, diarrhea, abdominal pain
OTHER: Pulmonary aspiration

Pharmacokinetics
Absorption	None
Distribution	None
Metabolism	None
Excretion	Feces (unchanged)
Half-life	Unknown

Pharmacodynamics
Onset	1 min
Peak	Unknown
Duration	4-12 hr

INTERACTIONS
Individual drugs
Acetylcysteine: inactivation
Acarbose, acetaminophen, aspirin, barbiturates, carBAMazepine, digoxin, furosemide, ipecac, methotrexate, phenothiazine, phenytoin: decreased effects

NURSING CONSIDERATIONS
Assessment
• Assess neurologic status including LOC, pupil reactivity, cough reflex, gag reflex, and swallowing ability before administration; do not give if neurologic status is impaired; aspiration may occur unless a protected airway is present
• Assess toxin, poison ingested, time of ingestion, and amount
• Monitor respiration, pulse, B/P to determine charcoal effectiveness if taken for barbiturate/opioid poisoning, serum
• Not used for all types of overdose

Patient/family education
• Tell patient stools will be black
• Teach patient about overdose/poison prevention and about keeping poison control chart available
• Teach patient to drink 8 glasses of water/day to prevent constipation

Evaluation
Positive therapeutic outcome
• Alert, PERL (poisoning)
• Absence of distention
• Absence of odor in wounds

Adverse effects: *italics* = common; **bold** = life-threatening

chlordiazePOXIDE (Rx)
(klor-dye-az-e-pox′ide)
Librium
Func. class.: Antianxiety
Chem. class.: Benzodiazepine, long-acting
Pregnancy category D
Controlled substance schedule IV

Do not confuse:
Librium/Librax

ACTION: Potentiates the actions of GABA, an inhibitory neurotransmitter, especially in the limbic system, reticular formation, which depresses the CNS

Therapeutic outcome: Decreased anxiety, successful alcohol withdrawal, relaxation

USES: Short-term management of anxiety, acute alcohol withdrawal, preoperative relaxation

CONTRAINDICATIONS:
Pregnancy **D**, breastfeeding, child <6 yr, hypersensitivity to benzodiazepines, closed-angle glaucoma, psychosis

Precautions: Geriatric, debilitated, renal/hepatic disease, suicidal ideation, abrupt discontinuation

DOSAGE AND ROUTES
Mild anxiety
Adult: PO 5-10 mg tid-qid
Geriatric: PO 5 mg bid initially, increase as needed
Child >6 yr: PO 5 mg bid-qid, max 10 mg bid-tid

Severe anxiety
Adult: PO 20-25 mg tid-qid

Preoperatively
Adult: PO 5-10 mg tid-qid on day before surgery

Alcohol withdrawal
Adult: PO 50-100 mg q4-6hr prn, max 300 mg/day

Renal disease
Adult: PO CCr <10 ml/min give 50% dose

Available forms: Caps 5, 25 mg

Implementation
PO route
• Give with food or milk for GI symptoms; do not open capsules; provide sugarless gum, hard candy, frequent sips of water for dry mouth

ADVERSE EFFECTS
CNS: *Dizziness, drowsiness,* confusion, headache, anxiety, tremors, stimulation, fatigue, depression, insomnia, hallucinations
CV: *Orthostatic hypotension,* **ECG changes, tachycardia,** hypotension, edema
EENT: *Blurred vision,* tinnitus, mydriasis
GI: Constipation, dry mouth, nausea, vomiting, anorexia, diarrhea
GU: Irregular periods, decreased libido
HEMA: Agranulocytosis
INTEG: Rash, dermatitis, itching

Pharmacokinetics

Absorption	Well absorbed (PO); slow, erratic (IM)
Distribution	Widely distributed; crosses placenta, blood-brain barrier
Metabolism	Liver extensively
Excretion	Kidneys, breast milk
Half-life	5-30 hr (increased in geriatric)

Pharmacodynamics

	PO	IM	IV
Onset	30 min	15-30 min	1-5 min
Peak	Within 2 hr	Unknown	Unknown
Duration	4-6 hr	Unknown	Up to 1 hr

INTERACTIONS
Individual drugs
Alcohol: increased CNS depression
Cimetidine, disulfiram, FLUoxetine, isoniazid, ketoconazole, metoprolol, propranolol, valproic acid: increased action of chlordiazePOXIDE
Levodopa: decreased action of levodopa

Drug classifications
CNS depressants: increased CNS depression
Contraceptives (oral): increased effect of chlordiazePOXIDE
CYP3A4 inhibitors (barbiturates, protease inhibitors, rifamycins): decreased effect of chlordiazePOXIDE

Drug/lab test
Increased: LFTs
False increase: 17-OHCS
False positive: pregnancy test (some methods)

NURSING CONSIDERATIONS
Assessment
• Assess **anxiety reaction:** inability to sleep, apprehension, dread, foreboding, or uneasiness related to unidentified source of danger
• Assess for previous **product dependence** or tolerance; if product dependent or tolerant, amount of medication should be restricted
• Monitor B/P (with patient lying, standing), pulse; if systolic B/P drops 20 mm Hg, hold product, notify prescriber
• Monitor blood studies: CBC during long-term therapy; **blood dyscrasias** have occurred rarely
• Monitor hepatic studies: AST, ALT, bilirubin, creatinine, LDH, alkaline phosphatase during long-term therapy
⚠ **Monitor mental status: mood, sensorium, affect, sleeping patterns, drowsiness, dizziness, suicidal tendencies, paradoxical reactions such as excitement, stimulation, acute rage**
⚠ **Assess for pregnancy, product should not be used during pregnancy D**

Patient/family education
• Instruct patient that product may be taken with food; if dose is missed take as soon as remembered; do not double doses
• Tell patient to avoid OTC preparations unless approved by prescriber; to avoid alcohol ingestion or other psychotropic medications unless directed by a prescriber
• Caution patient to avoid driving and activities requiring alertness, since drowsiness may occur; until medication response is known, tell patient that drowsiness may worsen at beginning of treatment
⚠ **Instruct patient not to discontinue medication abruptly after long-term use; product should be tapered over 1 wk**
• Caution patient to rise slowly or fainting may occur, especially in geriatric
⚠ **Advise patient that product should be avoided during pregnancy**
⚠ **Advise patient to report immediately suicidal thoughts/behaviors**

Evaluation
Positive therapeutic outcome
• Increased well being
• Decreased anxiety, restlessness, sleeplessness, dread
• Successful alcohol withdrawal

TREATMENT OF OVERDOSE:
Lavage, VS, supportive care

chloroquine (Rx)
(klor'oh-kwin)
Aralen
Func. class.: Antimalarial
Chem. class.: Synthetic 4-aminoquinoline derivative
Pregnancy category C

ACTION: Inhibits parasite replications, transcription of DNA to RNA by forming complexes with DNA of parasite

Therapeutic outcome: Decreased symptoms of malaria, amebiasis

USES: Malaria caused by *Plasmodium vivax, Plasmodium malariae, Plasmodium ovale, Plasmodium falciparum* (some strains), amebiasis

CONTRAINDICATIONS:
Hypersensitivity, retinal field changes

Precautions: Pregnancy **C**, breastfeeding, children, blood dyscrasias, severe GI disease, neurologic disease, alcoholism, hepatic disease, G6PD deficiency, psoriasis, eczema, seizures, preexisting auditory damage, infection, torsades de pointes

> **BLACK BOX WARNING:** Infection

DOSAGE AND ROUTES
Acute malaria attacks
Adult: **PO** 1000 mg (600 mg base), then 500 mg (300 mg base) in 6-8 hr, then 500 mg (300 mg base) q day × 2 days for a total of 2.5 g (1.5 g base) in 3 days
Adult/adolescent of low body weight, child/infant: **PO** 16.5 mg (10 mg base)/kg, max 600 mg base, then 8.3 mg (5 mg base)/kg max 300 mg base, 6 hr after 1st dose, then 8.3 mg (5 mg base)/kg, max 300 mg base 24 hr after 1st dose, then 8.3 mg (5 mg base)/kg max 300 mg base 36 hr after 1st dose

Adverse effects: *italics* = common; **bold** = life-threatening

Malaria prophylaxis (in areas with chloroquine–sensitive *P. falciparum*)
Adult: **PO** 500 mg (300 mg base) q wk on same day of each wk, starting 2 wk before travel and 8 wk after leaving

Extraintestinal amebiais
Adult: **PO** 1 g (600 mg base) q day × 2 days, then 500 mg (300 mg base) for ≥2-3 wk
Child (unlabeled): **PO** 16.6 mg (10 mg base)/ kg (max 300 mg base) q day × 2-3wk

Available forms: Tabs 250 mg (150 mg base), 500 mg (300 mg base) phosphate

Implementation
PO route
- Give with meals to decrease GI symptoms; better to take on empty stomach 1 hr before or 2 hr after meals
- Give antiemetic if vomiting occurs
- Give after C&S is completed; monthly to detect resistance

IM route
- Give IM after aspirating to prevent inj into bloodstream
- Store in tight, light-resistant container at room temp; keep inj in cool environment

Additive compatibility: Promethazine

ADVERSE EFFECTS
CNS: Headache, stimulation, fatigue, **seizure,** psychosis, hallucinations, insomnia
CV: Hypotension, **heart block, asystole with syncope,** ECG changes, cardiomyopathy
EENT: *Blurred vision, corneal changes, retinal changes, difficulty focusing,* tinnitus, vertigo, deafness, photophobia, corneal edema
GI: *Nausea, vomiting, anorexia,* diarrhea, cramps
HEMA: **Thrombocytopenia, agranulocytosis, hemolytic anemia, leukopenia**
INTEG: Pruritus, pigmentary changes, skin eruptions, lichen planus–like eruptions, eczema, **exfoliative dermatitis**

Pharmacokinetics

Absorption	Well absorbed
Distribution	Widely
Metabolism	Liver
Excretion	Kidneys, feces
Half-life	3-5 days

Pharmacodynamics

	PO	IM
Onset	Rapid	Rapid
Peak	1-3 hr	30 min
Duration	6-8 hr	Unknown

INTERACTIONS
Individual drugs
Ampicillin, rabies vaccine (ID): decreased effects
Cimetidine: decreased oral clearance, metabolism
Kaolin: decreased absorption
Magnesium: decreased action of chloroquine

Drug classifications
CYP2D6 inhibitors (amiodarone, chlorpheniramine, FLUoxetine, haloperidol, ritonavir, PARoxetine, terbinafine, ticlopidine), CYP3A4 inhibitors (clarithromycin, diltiazem, doxycycline, erythromycin, itraconazole, ketoconazole, verapamil): increased effects
Antacids (aluminum): decreased absorption
Class IA, III antidysrhythmics: increased QT prolongation, torsades de pointes

Drug/lab test
Decreased: Hgb, platelets, WBC

NURSING CONSIDERATIONS
Assessment

> **BLACK BOX WARNING:** Assess for **infection:** resistance is common, not to be used for *P. falciparum* acquired in areas of resistance or where prophylaxis has failed

- Monitor **ECG,** baseline and periodically during therapy; watch for depression of T waves, widening of QRS complex
- Assess for **allergic reactions:** pruritus, rash, urticaria
- Assess for **ototoxicity:** tinnitus, vertigo, change in hearing; audiometric testing should be done before, after treatment
- Assess for **blood dyscrasias:** malaise, fever, bruising, bleeding (rare)
- Assess mental status often: affect, mood, behavioral changes; psychosis may occur
- Assess for **toxicity:** blurring vision, difficulty focusing, headache, dizziness, decreased knee and ankle reflexes, product should be discontinued immediately

Patient/family education
- Advise patient that compliance with dosage schedule, duration is necessary

---

- Instruct patient that scheduled appointments must be kept or relapse may occur
- Caution patient to avoid alcohol while taking product
- Instruct diabetic to use blood glucose monitor to obtain correct result
- Teach patient to report weakness, fatigue, loss of appetite, nausea, vomiting, yellowing of skin or eyes, tingling/numbness of hands/feet
- Advise patient that urine may turn rust brown color
- Instruct patient to use sunglasses in bright sunlight to prevent photophobia

⚠ Keep away from pets, children; overdose is fatal

Evaluation
Positive therapeutic outcome
- Decreased symptoms of malaria

TREATMENT OF OVERDOSE:
Induce vomiting, gastric lavage, administer barbiturate (ultrashort-acting), vasopressor; tracheostomy may be necessary

chlorpheniramine (OTC, Rx)
(klor-fen-ir′a-meen)
AHIST, Aller-Chlor, Allergy, Chlor-Pheniton, Chlor-Trimeton, Diabetic Tussin Allergy Relief, ED-Chlor-Tann, Equaline Allergy, Equate Chlortabs Allergy, Good Sense Allergy, Leader Allergy, P-Tann, Tana Hist-PD, Teldrin, Top Care Allergy, Wal-finate Allergy
Func. class.: Antihistamine (1st generation, nonselective)
Chem. class.: Alkylamine, H_1-receptor antagonist
Pregnancy category B

Do not confuse:
Teldrin/Tedral

ACTION: Acts on blood vessels, GI, respiratory system by competing with histamine for H_1-receptor site; decreases allergic response by blocking histamine

Therapeutic outcome: Absence of allergy symptoms and rhinitis

USES: Allergy symptoms, rhinitis, conjunctivitis (allergic)

CONTRAINDICATIONS:
Newborns/neonates

Precautions: Pregnancy **B**, breastfeeding, geriatric, increased intraocular pressure, renal/cardiac disease, hypertension, bronchial asthma, seizure disorder, hyperthyroidism, prostatic hypertrophy, GI obstruction, peptic ulcer disease, emphysema, hypersensitivity to H_1-receptor antagonists, lower respiratory tract disease, stenosed peptic ulcers, bladder neck obstruction, closed-angle glaucoma, children

DOSAGE AND ROUTES
Adult/child ≥12 yr: PO 4 mg tid-qid, max 24 mg/day; EXT REL 8-12 mg bid-tid, max 24 mg/day
Child 6-12 yr: PO 2 mg q4-6hr, max 12 mg/day; EXT REL 8 mg at bedtime or daily; EXT REL not recommended for child <6 yr

Available forms: Chewable tabs 2 mg; tabs 4, 8, 12 mg; ext rel tabs 8, 12 mg; ext rel caps 8, 12 mg; syr 1, 2, 2.5 mg/5 ml

Implementation
PO route
- Swallow time rel tabs and caps whole
- Do not break, crush, chew, or open time rel tabs
- Chewable tabs should be chewed and not swallowed whole
- Avoid use in children ≤6 yr
- May give without regard to meals
- Store in tight container at room temp

IM/SUBCUT route
- Use only 20 and 100 mg/ml strengths; does not need to be reconstituted or diluted

Syrup
- Use dosing utensil to measure correct dose

IV route
Give undiluted by direct **IV** (10 mg/ml strength only); administer 10 mg over 1 min or more

Additive incompatibilities: Calcium chloride, kanamycin, norepinephrine, pentobarbital

ADVERSE EFFECTS
CNS: *Dizziness, drowsiness,* poor coordination, fatigue, anxiety, euphoria, confusion, paresthesia, neuritis
EENT: Blurred vision, dilated pupils, tinnitus, nasal stuffiness, dry nose, throat, mouth
GI: Nausea, anorexia, diarrhea
GU: *Retention,* dysuria, frequency
HEMA: Thrombocytopenia, agranulocytosis, hemolytic anemia

INTEG: Photosensitivity
RESP: Increased thick secretions, wheezing, chest tightness

Pharmacokinetics

Absorption	Well absorbed (PO, SUBCUT, IM, **IV**)
Distribution	Widely distributed; crosses blood-brain barrier
Metabolism	Liver, mostly
Excretion	Kidneys, metabolite; breast milk (minimal)
Half-life	12-15 hr

Pharmacodynamics

	PO	PO-ER	SUB-CUT	IM	IV
Onset	15-30 min	Unknown	Unknown	Unknown	Unknown
Peak	1-2 hr	Unknown	Unknown	Unknown	Unknown
Duration	4-12 hr	8-24 hr	4-12 hr	4-12 hr	4-12 hr

INTERACTIONS

Individual drugs
Alcohol: increased CNS depression
Atropine, haloperidol, quiNIDine: increased anticholinergic reactions

Drug classifications
Barbiturates, CNS depressants, opiates, sedative/hypnotics, tricyclics: increased CNS depression
MAOIs: increased effect of chlorpheniramine
Phenothiazines: increased anticholinergic reactions

Drug/lab test
False negative: skin allergy tests (discontinue antihistamines 3 days before testing)

NURSING CONSIDERATIONS

Assessment
• Assess respiratory status: rate, rhythm, increase in bronchial secretions, wheezing, chest tightness; provide fluids to 2 L/day to decrease secretion thickness
• Monitor I&O ratio: be alert for urinary retention, frequency, dysuria, especially geriatric; product should be discontinued if these occur
• **IV** administration may result in rapid drop in B/P, sweating, dizziness, especially in geriatric

Patient/family education
• Teach all aspects of product use; to notify prescriber if confusion, sedation, hypotension, or difficulty voiding occurs; to avoid driving and other hazardous activity if drowsiness occurs; to avoid alcohol and other CNS depressants that may potentiate effect
• Teach patient not to exceed recommended dosage; dysrhythmias may occur
• Advise patient hard candy, gum, frequent rinsing of mouth may be used for dryness

Evaluation
Positive therapeutic outcome
• Absence of running or congested nose, rashes, conjunctivitis

TREATMENT OF OVERDOSE:
Administer lavage, diazepam, vasopressors, phenytoin IV

chlorproMAZINE (Rx)
(klor-proe'ma-zeen)
Func. class.: Antipsychotic/neuroleptic/antiemetic
Chem. class.: Phenothiazine, aliphatic
Pregnancy category C

Do not confuse:
chlorproMAZINE/chlorothiazide/chlorproPAMIDE/chlorthalidone/prochlorperazine

ACTION: Depresses cerebral cortex, hypothalamus, limbic system, which control activity, aggression; blocks neurotransmission produced by dopamine at synapse; exhibits a strong α-adrenergic, anticholinergic blocking action; mechanism for antipsychotic effects is unclear

Therapeutic outcome: Decreased signs and symptoms of psychosis; control of nausea, vomiting, intractable hiccups, decreased anxiety preoperatively

USES: Psychotic disorders, Tourette's syndrome, mania, schizophrenia, anxiety, intractable hiccups (adults), nausea, vomiting, preoperative relaxation, acute intermittent porphyria, behavioral problems in children, nonpsychotic patients with dementia

Unlabeled uses: Vascular headache

CONTRAINDICATIONS:
Hypersensitivity, circulatory collapse, liver damage, cerebral arteriosclerosis, coronary disease,

---

severe hypo/hypertension, blood dyscrasias, coma, child <6 mo, brain damage, bone marrow depression, alcohol and barbiturate withdrawal, closed-angle glaucoma

Precautions: Pregnancy **C,** breastfeeding, geriatric, seizure disorders, hypertension, hepatic/cardiac disease, prostate enlargement, pulmonary/Parkinson's disease

> **BLACK BOX WARNING:** Dementia; increased mortality in elderly patients with dementia-related psychosis

DOSAGE AND ROUTES
Psychosis
Adult: PO 10-50 mg q1-4hr initially, then increase up to 2 g/day if necessary; IM 10-50 mg q1-4hr, usual dose 300-800 mg/day
Geriatric: PO 10-25 mg daily-bid, increased by 10-25 mg/day q4-7day, max 800 mg/day
Child >6 mo: PO 0.55 mg/kg q4-6hr; IM 0.5 mg/kg q6-8hr

Nausea and vomiting
Adult: PO 10-25 mg q4-6hr prn; IM 25-50 mg q3hr prn; max 400 mg/day; **IV** 25-50 mg daily-qid
Child ≥6 mo: PO 0.55 mg/kg q4-6hr; IM q6-8hr; IM ≤5 yr or ≤22.7 kg 40 mg; max IM 5-10 yr or 22.7-45.5 kg 75 mg

Intractable hiccups/acute intermittent porphyria
Adult: PO 25-50 mg tid-qid; IM 25-50 mg (used only if PO dose does not work); **IV** 25-50 mg in 500-1000 ml saline (only for severe hiccups)

Available forms: Tabs 10, 25, 50, 100; inj 25 mg/ml

Implementation
PO route
• Periodically attempt dosage reduction in patients with behavioral problems
• Give with full glass of water, milk; or give with food to decrease GI upset
• Store in tight, light-resistant container, oral sol in amber bottle
IM route
• Store in tight, light-resistant container
• Use gloves to prepare product; if product touches skin, wash with soap and water to prevent contact dermatitis
• Inject in deep muscle mass; do not give SUBCUT; may be diluted with 0.9% NaCl, 2% procaine as prescribed; do not administer sol with a precipitate

• Remain lying down after IM inj for at least 30 min
Rectal route
• Give after placing in refrigerator for 30 min if too soft to insert; this route is used for nausea, vomiting, hiccups
• Avoid skin contact with injection solution; may cause contact dermatitis

Direct IV
• Give by direct **IV** by diluting with 0.9% NaCl to a concentration of 1 mg/1 ml; administer at a rate of 1 mg/2 min, never give undiluted
• Give by intermittent IV infusion diluting 50 mg/500-1000 ml of D_5W, $D_{10}W$, 0.9% NaCl, 0.45% NaCl, LR, Ringer's over ½ hr or combinations (used for intractable hiccups)

Syringe compatibilities: Atropine, benztropine, butorphanol, diphenhydrAMINE, doxapram, droperidol, fentaNYL, glycopyrrolate, HYDROmorphone, hydrOXYzine, meperidine, metoclopramide, midazolam, morphine, pentazocine, perphenazine, prochlorperazine, promazine, promethazine, scopolamine

Syringe incompatibilities: Cimetidine, dimenhyDRINATE, heparin, PENTobarbital, thiopental

Y-site compatibilities: Alfentanil, amikacin, amphotericin B lipid complex, amsacrine, anidulafungin, ascorbic acid injection, atenolol, atracurium, atropine, benztropine, bleomycin sulfate, buprenorphine, butorphanol, calcium chloride/gluconate, caspofungin, cimetidine, cisatracurium, CISplatin, cladribine, codeine, cyanocobalamin, cyclophosphamide, cycloSPORINE, cytarabine, DACTINomycin, DAPTOmycin, dexmedetomidine, digoxin, diltiazem, diphenhydrAMINE, DOBUTamine, DOCEtaxel, DOPamine, doxacurium, DOXOrubicin, DOXOrubicin liposomal, doxycycline, enalaprilat, ePHEDrine, EPINEPHrine, epirubicin, erythromycin, esmolol, etoposide, famotidine, fenoldopam, fentaNYL, filgrastim, fluconazole, gatifloxacin, gemcitabine, gentamicin, glycopyrrolate, granisetron, hydrocortisone, HYDROmorphone, hydrOXYzine, IDArubicin, ifosfamide, isoproterenol, labetalol, levofloxacin, lidocaine, LORazepam, LR, magnesium sulfate, mannitol, mechlorethamine, meperidine, methicillin, methoxamine, methyldopa, methylPREDNISolone, metoclopramide, metoprolol, metroNIDAZOLE, miconazole, midazolam, milrinone, minocycline, mitoXANTrone, morphine, multiple vitamins injection, mycophenolate mofetil, nafcillin, nalbuphine, naloxone, netilmicin, nitroglycerin, norepinephrine, octreotide, ondansetron, oxacillin, oxaliplatin, palonosetron, pamidronate, pancuronium, papaverine, penicillin G potassium, pentamidine, pentazocine, phytonadione, polymyxin B, potassium chloride, procainamide, prochlorperazine, promethazine, propofol, propranolol, protamine sulfate, pyridoxine, quiNIDine, quinupristin-dalfopristin, ranitidine, Ringer's injection, ritodrine, riTUXimab, rocuronium, sodium acetate, succinylcholine, SUFentanil, tacrolimus, teniposide, theophylline, thiamine, thiotepa, tirofiban, TNA, tolazoline, TPN, trimetaphan, vancomycin, vasopressin, vecuronium, verapamil, vinCRIStine, vinorelbine, vitamin B complex with C, voriconazole, zoledronic acid

ADVERSE EFFECTS

CNS: Neuroleptic malignant syndrome, dizziness, *extrapyramidal symptoms: pseudoparkinsonism, akathisia, dystonia, tardive dyskinesia,* seizures, *headache*

CV: *Orthostatic hypotension,* hypertension, cardiac arrest, ECG changes, tachycardia

EENT: Blurred vision, glaucoma, dry eyes

ENDO: SIADH

GI: *Dry mouth, nausea, vomiting, anorexia, constipation,* diarrhea, cholestatic jaundice, weight gain

GU: Urinary retention, enuresis, impotence, amenorrhea, gynecomastia, breast engorgement

HEMA: Anemia, leukopenia, leukocytosis, agranulocytosis

INTEG: *Rash,* photosensitivity, dermatitis

RESP: Laryngospasm, dyspnea, respiratory depression

SYST: Death in geriatric patients with dementia

Pharmacokinetics

Absorption	Variable (PO); well absorbed (IM)
Distribution	Widely distributed; crosses placenta
Metabolism	Liver, GI mucosa extensively
Excretion	Kidneys
Half-life	30 hr

Pharmacodynamics

	PO	RECT	IM	IV
Onset	½-1 hr	12 hr	Unknown	Rapid
Peak	Unknown	Unknown	Unknown	Unknown
Duration	4-6 hr*	3-4 hr	4-8 hr	Unknown

*Duration PO ext rel is 10-12 hr.

INTERACTIONS

Individual drugs

Alcohol: increased effects of both products, oversedation

Aluminum hydroxide, magnesium hydroxide: decreased absorption

Bromocriptine, levodopa: decreased antiparkinsonian activity

EPINEPHrine: increased toxicity

Lithium: decreased chlorproMAZINE levels

Valproic acid: increased valproic acid level

Warfarin: decreased anticoagulant effect

Drug classifications

Antacids: decreased absorption

Anticholinergics, antidepressants, antiparkinsonian agents: increased anticholinergic effects

Anticonvulsants: decreased seizure threshold

Antidepressants, antihistamines, barbiturate anesthetics, opioids, sedative/hypnotics: increased CNS depression

Antithyroid agents: increased agranulocytosis

Barbiturates: decreased serum chlorproMAZINE

β-Adrenergic blockers: increased effect of both products

Drug/lab test

Increased: liver function tests

Decreased: WBC, platelets, Hgb/Hct

False positive: pregnancy tests, PKU

False negative: urinary steroids, 17-OHCS

NURSING CONSIDERATIONS

Assessment

• Assess mental status: orientation, mood, behavior, presence of hallucinations, and type before initial administration and monthly; this product should significantly reduce psychotic behavior

• Assess any potentially reversible cause of behavior problems in geriatric before, during therapy

• Check for swallowing of PO medication; check for hoarding or giving of medication to other patients

• Monitor I&O ratio; palpate bladder if low urinary output occurs, especially in geriatric; urinalysis recommended before, during prolonged therapy

• Monitor bilirubin, CBC, liver function studies, ocular exam; agranulocytosis, glaucoma, cholestatic jaundice may occur

• Assess respirations q4hr during initial treatment; establish baseline before starting treatment; report drops of 30 mm Hg; obtain baseline ECG, Q wave, and T wave changes

---

⚠ Nurse Alert ✦ Key NCLEX® Drug

- Check for dizziness, faintness, palpitations, tachycardia on rising; severe orthostatic hypotension is common
⚠ **Identify for neuroleptic malignant syndrome: hyperpyrexia, muscle rigidity, increased CPK, altered mental status; product should be discontinued**
- Assess for **EPS** including akathisia (inability to sit still, no pattern to movements), tardive dyskinesia (bizarre movements of the jaw, mouth, tongue, extremities), pseudoparkinsonism (rigidity, tremors, pill rolling, shuffling gate); an antiparkinsonian product should be prescribed
- Assess for constipation, urinary retention daily; if these occur, increase bulk, water in diet

Patient/family education
- Teach patient to use good oral hygiene; frequent rinsing of mouth, sugarless gum, candy, or ice chips for dry mouth
- Caution patient to avoid hazardous activities until product response is determined; dizziness, blurred vision may occur
- Inform patient that orthostatic hypotension occurs often and to rise from sitting or lying position gradually, to remain lying down after IM inj for at least 30 min; tell patient to avoid hot tubs, hot showers, tub baths, since hypotension may occur; tell patient that in hot weather heat stroke may occur; take extra precautions to stay cool
- Advise patient to avoid abrupt withdrawal of this product, or extrapyramidal symptoms may result; product should be withdrawn slowly
- Teach patient to avoid OTC preparations (cough, hay fever, cold) unless approved by prescriber, since serious product interactions may occur; avoid use with alcohol, CNS depressants, since increased drowsiness may occur
- Caution patient to use sunscreen and sunglasses to prevent burns
- Teach patient about extrapyramidal symptoms and necessity of meticulous oral hygiene, since oral candidiasis may occur
- Instruct patient to take antacids 2 hr before or after taking this product
- Instruct patient to report sore throat, malaise, fever, bleeding, mouth sores; if these occur, CBC should be drawn and product discontinued
- Teach that urine may turn pink or reddish-brown
- Teach patient to use contraceptive measures

Evaluation
Positive therapeutic outcome
- Decrease in emotional excitement, hallucinations, delusions, paranoia

- Reorganization of patterns of thought, speech
- Increase in target behaviors

TREATMENT OF OVERDOSE:
Lavage if orally ingested; provide airway, *do not induce vomiting or use epinephrine*

cholecalciferol
See vitamin D

cholestyramine (Rx)
(koe-less-tear'a-meen)
Prevalite, Questran, Questran Light
Func. class.: Antilipemic
Chem. class.: Bile acid sequestrant
Pregnancy category C

Do not confuse:
Questran/Quarzan

ACTION: Adsorbs, combines with bile acids to form an insoluble complex that is excreted through feces; loss of bile acids lowers LDL, cholesterol levels

Therapeutic outcome: Decreasing cholesterol levels and low-density lipoproteins, decreased pruritus

USES: Primary hypercholesterolemia (especially type IIa/IIb hyperlipoproteinemia), pruritus associated with biliary obstruction

Unlabeled uses: Diarrhea caused by excess bile acid

CONTRAINDICATIONS:
Hypersensitivity; complete biliary obstruction; hyperlipidemia III, IV, V

Precautions: Pregnancy **C,** breastfeeding, children, PKU

DOSAGE AND ROUTES
Adult: PO 4 g daily-bid, max 24 g/day
Child: PO 240 mg/kg/day in 3 divided doses; administer with food or drink, max 8 g/day, titrated up over several weeks to decrease GI effects

Available forms: Powder for susp 4 g/ cholestyramine/packet or scoop; tab 1 g

Implementation
- Give product daily-bid, at bedtime; give all other medications 1 hr before cholestyramine or 4-6 hr after cholestyramine to avoid poor absorption; do not take dry; mix product with

applesauce or stir into beverage (2-6 oz); let stand for 2 min; do not mix with carbonated beverages; avoid inhaling powder, avoid GI tube administration, take with food
• Provide supplemental doses of vit A, D, E, K if levels are low
• Doses are expressed in anhydrous cholestyramine resin; amount of resin varies with each product

ADVERSE EFFECTS

CNS: Headache, dizziness, drowsiness, vertigo, tinnitus, anxiety
GI: *Constipation, abdominal pain, nausea,* fecal impaction, hemorrhoids, flatulence, vomiting, steatorrhea, peptic ulcer
HEMA: **Bleeding,** increased pro-time
INTEG: Rash, irritation of perianal area, tongue, skin
META: Decreased vit A, D, K, red cell folate content, **hyperchloremic acidosis**
MS: Muscle, joint pain

Pharmacokinetics

Absorption	Not absorbed
Distribution	Not distributed
Metabolism	Not metabolized; LDL lowered in 4-7 days, serum cholesterol lowered in 1 mo
Excretion	Binds with bile acids, feces
Half-life	Unknown

Pharmacodynamics

Onset	24-48 hr
Peak	1-3 wk
Duration	2-4 wk

INTERACTIONS

Individual drugs
Acetaminophen, amiodarone, clofibrate, gemfibrozil, glipiZIDE, iron, oral vancomycin, penicillin G, propranolol, thyroid hormones, warfarin: decreased absorption of each specific product

Drug classifications
Cardiac glycosides, corticosteroids, tetracyclines, thiazides, vit A, D, E, K: decreased absorption

Drug/lab test
Increased: AST, ALT, alkaline phosphatase
Decreased: Na, K

NURSING CONSIDERATIONS

Assessment
• Assess nutrition: fat, protein, carbohydrates, nutritional analysis should be completed by dietitian
• Assess skin integrity after patient has been receiving product; itching, pruritus often occur from bile deposits on skin
• Monitor cardiac glycoside level if both products are being administered; cardiac glycoside levels will be decreased, may need to adjust dose of cardiac glycoside, if this product is increased or decreased
• **Hypercholesterolemia:** Monitor for signs of vit A, D, E, K deficiency; fasting LDL, HDL, total cholesterol, triglyceride levels, electrolytes if on extended therapy, diet history
• Monitor bowel pattern daily; increase bulk, water in diet if constipation develops
• **Pruritus:** Assess for itching

Patient/family education
⚠ Teach patient symptoms of hypoprothrombinemia: bleeding mucous membranes, dark tarry stools, hematuria, petechiae; report immediately
• Teach patient to take with food, never use dry
• Teach patient importance of compliance
• Teach patient that risk factors should be decreased: high-fat diet, smoking, alcohol consumption, absence of exercise
• Have patient mix product with 6 oz of milk, water, fruit juice; do not mix with carbonated beverages; rinse glass to make sure all medication is taken or may mix product in applesauce; allow to stand for 2 min before mixing

Evaluation
Positive therapeutic outcome
• Decreased cholesterol level (hyperlipidemia)
• Decreased diarrhea, pruritus (excess bile acids)

---

cidofovir (Rx)
(si-doh-foh'veer)
Vistide
Func. class.: Antiviral
Chem. class.: Nucleotide analog
Pregnancy category C

ACTION: Suppresses cytomegalovirus (CMV) replication by selective inhibition of viral DNA synthesis

Therapeutic outcome: Decreased symptoms of CMV

USES: CMV retinitis in patients with HIV, used with probenecid

CONTRAINDICATIONS:
Hypersensitivity to this product or probenecid; sulfa products, direct intraocular injection

> **BLACK BOX WARNING:** Proteinuria, renal disease/failure

Precautions: Pregnancy **C**, breastfeeding, children <6 mo, geriatric, preexisting cytopenias, renal function impairment, platelet count <25,000/mm^3

> **BLACK BOX WARNING:** Neutropenia, infertility, secondary malignancy

DOSAGE AND ROUTES
Adult: IV 5 mg/kg qwk × 2 wk; then 3 mg/kg q2wk, give with probenecid

Renal dose
Adult: IV CCr ≤55 ml/min, do not use; SCr increase of 0.3-0.4 mg/dl above baseline, decrease dose to 3 mg/kg; SCr increase of ≥0.5 mg/dl above baseline or ≥2+ proteinuria, discontinue

Available forms: Inj 75 mg/ml

Implementation
• Allow to warm to room temperature
• If product comes in contact with skin, wash with soap and water immediately
• If zidovudine is used, reduce dose to 50% in cidofovir treatment days

Intermittent IV infusion route
• **Dilute** in 100 ml 0.9% NaCl sol before administration; probenecid must be given PO 2 g 3 hr before the cidofovir INF and 1 g at 2 and 8 hr after ending the cidofovir INF; **give** 1 L of 0.9% NaCl sol IV with each INF of cidofovir, **give** saline INF over 1-2 hr period immediately before cidofovir INF; patient should be given a second L if the patient can tolerate the fluid load (second L given at time of cidofovir or immediately afterward and should be given over a 1-3 hr period)

> **BLACK BOX WARNING:** Use cytotoxic handling procedures

• **Administer** after diluting in 100 ml of 0.9% NaCl
• **Give** slowly; do not give by BOL IV, IV, SUBCUT inj

• **Use** diluted sol within 24 hr, do not refrigerate or freeze; do not use sol with particulate matter or discoloration
• Do not admix

ADVERSE EFFECTS
CNS: *Fever, chills,* **coma,** confusion, abnormal thought, *dizziness,* bizarre dreams, *headache,* psychosis, tremors, somnolence, paresthesia, *amnesia, anxiety, insomnia,* **seizures**
CV: **Dysrhythmias,** hypo/hypertension
EENT: Retinal detachment in CMV retinitis
GI: Abnormal liver function tests, *nausea, vomiting, anorexia, diarrhea,* abdominal pain, **hemorrhage**
GU: **Hematuria,** increased creatinine, BUN, **nephrotoxicity**
HEMA: **Granulocytopenia, thrombocytopenia, irreversible neutropenia, anemia, eosinophilia**
INTEG: *Rash, alopecia, pruritus, acne,* urticaria, pain at inj site, phlebitis
RESP: Dyspnea

Pharmacokinetics
Absorption	Unknown
Distribution	Unknown
Metabolism	Unknown
Excretion	Unknown
Half-life	Terminal 2.6 hr

Pharmacodynamics
Unknown

INTERACTIONS
Individual drugs

> **BLACK BOX WARNING:** Amphotericin B, foscarnet, pentamidine **IV:** increased nephrotoxicity; wait 7 days after use to begin cidofovir

Drug classifications
Aminoglycosides, NSAIDs, salicylates: increased nephrotoxicity; wait 7 days after use to begin cidofovir

NURSING CONSIDERATIONS
Assessment
• Obtain culture before treatment is initiated; cultures of blood, urine, and throat may all be taken; CMV is not confirmed by this method; the diagnosis is made by an ophthalmic exam

BLACK BOX WARNING: Monitor renal, liver function, increased hematopoietic studies and BUN; serum creatinine, AST, ALT, creatinine, CCr, A-G ratio, baseline and drip treatment, blood counts should be done q2wk; watch for decreasing granulocytes, Hgb; if low, therapy may have to be discontinued and restarted after hematologic recovery; blood transfusions may be required, renal failure/Fanconi syndrome can also occur

- Assess for GI symptoms: severe nausea, vomiting, diarrhea; severe symptoms may necessitate discontinuing product
- Assess electrolytes and minerals: calcium, phosphorous, magnesium, sodium, potassium; watch closely for tetany during first administration
- Assess for symptoms of **blood dyscrasias** (anemia, granulocytopenia); bruising, fatigue, bleeding, poor healing; assess for leukopenia, neutropenia, thrombocytopenia: WBCs, platelets q2day during 2 ×/day dosing and qwk thereafter; check for leukopenias, with daily WBC count in patients with prior leukopenia, with other nucleoside analogs, or for whom leukopenia counts are <1000 cells/mm^3 at start of treatment
- Assess allergic reactions: flushing, rash, urticaria, pruritus
- Monitor serum creatinine or CCr at least q2wk; give only to those with creatinine levels ≤1.5 mg/dl, CCr >55 ml/min, urine protein <100 mg/dl

Patient/family education

BLACK BOX WARNING: Advise to notify prescriber if sore throat, swollen lymph nodes, malaise, fever occur; may indicate other infections

- Advise to report perioral tingling, numbness in extremities, and paresthesias; report rash immediately
- ⚠ Teach that serious product interactions may occur if OTC products are ingested; check first with prescriber
- Teach that product is not a cure, but will control symptoms
- Advise that regular ophthalmic exams, renal studies must be continued
- Advise that major toxicities may necessitate discontinuing product
- ⚠ Advise to use contraception during treatment and that infertility may occur; men should use barrier contraception for 90 days after treatment

Evaluation
Positive therapeutic outcome
- Decreased symptoms of CMV

TREATMENT OF OVERDOSE:
Discontinue product; use hemodialysis, and increase hydration

cilastatin
See imipenem/cilastatin

cilostazol (Rx)
(sih-los′tah-zol)
Pletal
Func. class.: Platelet aggregation inhibitor
Chem. class.: Quinolinone derivative
Pregnancy category C

Do not confuse:
Pletal/Plendil

ACTION: Multifactorial effects (antithrombotic, antiplatelet vasodilation)

Therapeutic outcome: Increased walking distance

USES: Intermittent claudication associated with PVD

CONTRAINDICATIONS:
Hypersensitivity, acute MI, active bleeding conditions, hemostatic conditions

BLACK BOX WARNING: CHF

Precautions: Pregnancy **C,** breastfeeding, children, geriatric, past liver disease, renal/cardiac disease, increased bleeding risk, low platelet count, platelet dysfunction, smoking

DOSAGE AND ROUTES
Adult: PO 100 mg bid taken ≥30 min before or 2 hr after breakfast and dinner or 50 mg bid, if using products that inhibit CYP3A4 and CYP2C19; 12 wk of treatment may be needed for beneficial effect

Available forms: Tabs 50, 100 mg

Implementation
- Give bid ≥1 hr before or 2 hr after meals with a full glass of water; do not give with grapefruit juice

ADVERSE EFFECTS

CNS: *Dizziness, headache*
CV: *Palpitations, tachycardia,* **nodal dysrhythmia,** postural hypotension
EENT: Blindness, diplopia, ear pain, tinnitus, retinal hemorrhage
GI: *Nausea, vomiting, diarrhea, GI discomfort,* colitis, cholelithiasis, ulcer, esophagitis, gastritis, anorexia, *flatulence, dyspepsia*
GU: Cystitis, frequency, vaginitis, **vaginal hemorrhage,** hematuria
HEMA: Bleeding (epistaxis, hematuria, retinal hemorrhage, GI bleeding), thrombocytopenia, anemia, polycythemia; **aplastic anemia**
INTEG: *Rash,* urticaria, dry skin, **Stevens-Johnson syndrome**
MISC: *Back pain,* headache, *infection, myalgia, peripheral edema,* chills, fever, malaise, diabetes mellitus
RESP: *Cough, pharyngitis, rhinitis,* asthma, pneumonia

Pharmacokinetics

Absorption	Unknown
Distribution	95%-98% protein binding
Metabolism	Hepatic extensively by CYP450 enzymes (active metabolite)
Excretion	Urine (74%), feces (20%)
Half-life	11-13 hr

Pharmacodynamics

Unknown

INTERACTIONS

Individual drugs

Abciximab, eptifibatide, ticlopidine, tirofiban: increased bleeding tendencies
Clarithromycin, diltiazem, erythromycin, omeprazole, verapamil: increased cilostazol levels
Fluconazole, FLUoxetine, fluvoxaMINE, gemfibrozil, isoniazid, itraconazole, ketoconazole, omeprazole, voriconazole: may increase cilostazol levels; exercise caution when coadministering and reduce dose to 50 mg bid

Drug classifications

Anticoagulants, NSAIDs, thrombolytics: may increase bleeding tendencies
CYP3A4 inducers: decreased cilostazol
Protease inhibitors, CYP3A4 inhibitors, CYP2C19 inhibitors: increased cilostazol levels

Drug/food

Grapefruit juice: do not use; toxicity may occur
High-fat meals: increased cilostazol action; avoid giving with food

Drug/herb

Feverfew, garlic, ginger, ginkgo biloba: decreased cilostazol action

NURSING CONSIDERATIONS

Assessment

> **BLACK BOX WARNING:** Assess for underlying CV disease since CV risk is great; for severe headache, signs of toxicity

- Assess for CV lesions with repeated oral administration
- Assess for CHF
- Monitor blood studies: CBC, Hct, Hgb, pro-time if patient is on long-term therapy; thrombocytopenia, neutropenia may occur

Patient/family education

- Teach patient to avoid hazardous activities until effect is known
- Advise patient to report any unusual bleeding to prescriber
- Caution patient to report side effects such as diarrhea, skin rashes, subcutaneous bleeding
- Teach patient that effects may take 2-4 wk, treatment of up to 12 wk may be required for necessary effect
- Teach patients with CHF about potential risks
- Advise patient to take ≥1 hr before or 2 hr after meals
- Advise patient that reading patient package insert is necessary
- Advise patient to discontinue tobacco use, not to drink grapefruit juice
- Advise that there are many drug and herb interactions; obtain approval by prescriber before use

Evaluation

Positive therapeutic outcome
- Increased walking distance and duration
- Decreased pain

cimetidine (OTC, Rx)
(sye-met'i-deen)
Acid Reducer, Equaline Acid Reducer, Good Sense Heartburn Relief, Nu-Cimet ✤, Tagamet, Tagamet HB
Func. class.: H₂-receptor antagonist
Chem. class.: Imidazole derivative
Pregnancy category B

ACTION: Inhibits histamine at H₂-receptor site in the gastric parietal cells, which inhibits gastric acid secretion

Therapeutic outcome: Healing of duodenal or gastric ulcers; prevention of duodenal ulcers; decreases symptoms of gastroesophageal reflux disease (GERD) and Zollinger-Ellison syndrome

USES: Short-term treatment of duodenal and gastric ulcers and maintenance; management of GERD, Zollinger-Ellison syndrome; prevention of upper GI bleeding; prevent, relieve heartburn, acid indigestion, upper GI bleeding

Unlabeled uses: Prevention of aspiration pneumonitis, stress ulcers

CONTRAINDICATIONS:
Hypersensitivity

Precautions: Pregnancy **B,** breastfeeding, child <16 yr, geriatric, organic brain syndrome, renal/hepatic disease

DOSAGE AND ROUTES
Treatment of active ulcers
Adult/adolescent ≥16 yr: PO 300 mg qid with meals, at bedtime × 8 wk or 400 mg bid, 800 mg at bedtime; after 8 wk give at bedtime dose only; **IV BOL** 300 mg/20 ml 0.9% NaCl over 1-2 min q6hr; **IV INF** 300 mg/50 ml in D₅W over 15-20 min; IM 300 mg q6hr, max 2400 mg **Child:** PO 20-40 mg/kg/day; IM/**IV** 5-10 mg/kg q6-8hr

Prophylaxis of duodenal ulcer
Adult and child >16 yr: 400 mg at bedtime or 300 mg bid

GERD
Adult: PO 800-1600 mg/day in divided doses × ≤12 wk

Hypersecretory conditions (Zollinger-Ellison syndrome)
Adult: PO/IM/IV 300-600 mg q6hr; may increase to 12 g/day if needed; OTC use up to 200 mg daily or bid, max 2 ×/wk

Upper GI bleeding prophylaxis
Adult: IV 50 mg/hr; lowered in renal disease

Heartburn
Adult/child ≥12 yr: PO 200 mg Tagamet HB up to bid, may use prior to eating, max 400 mg/day, max daily use up to 2 wk

Renal dose
Adult: PO/IV CCr <30 ml/min 300 mg q12hr

Available forms: Tabs 100, 200, 300, 400, 800 mg; liquid 200, 300 mg/5 ml; inj 300 mg/2 ml, 300 mg/50 ml 0.9% NaCl

Implementation
PO route
• Give with meals for lengthened product effect; antacids 1 hr before or 1 hr after cimetidine
IM route
• May give undiluted
• Give at end of dialysis
• Inject deeply into large muscle mass, aspirate

IV route
• Give by **direct IV** after diluting 300 mg/20 ml of 0.9% NaCl for inj; give over ≥5 min
• Give **intermittent IV** by diluting 300 mg/50 ml of D₅W; run over ≥30 min
• Give by **cont inf** after using total daily dose (900 mg) diluted in 100-1000 ml D₅W given over 24 hr
• Store diluted sol at room temperature up to 48 hr

Y-site incompatibilities: Amsacrine

Y-site compatibilities: Acyclovir, alfentanil, amifostine, amikacin, aminocaproic acid, aminophylline, amphotericin B lipid complex/liposome, anakinra, anidulafungin, ascorbic acid injection, atenolol, atracurium, atropine, aztreonam, benztropine, bivalirudin, bleomycin, bumetanide, buprenorphine, butorphanol, calcium chloride/gluconate, CARBOplatin, caspofungin, cefamandole, ceFAZolin, cefmetazole, cefonicid, cefotaxime, cefoTEtan, cefOXitin, cefTAZidime, ceftizoxime, cefTRIAXone, cefuroxime, cephalothin, cephapirin, chlorproMAZINE, cisatracurium, CISplatin, cladribine, clarithromycin, clindamycin, codeine, cyanocobalamin, cyclophosphamide, cycloSPORINE, cytarabine, DACTINomycin, DAPTOmycin, dexamethasone, dexmedetomidine, digoxin, diltiazem, diphenhydrAMINE, DOBUTamine, DOCEtaxel, DOPamine, doripenem, doxacurium, doxapram, DOXOrubicin, DOXOrubicin liposome, enalaprilat, ePHEDrine, EPINEPHrine, epirubicin, epoetin alfa, eptifibatide, ertapenem, erythromycin, esmolol, etoposide, famotidine, fenoldopam, fentaNYL, filgrastim, fluconazole, fludarabine, fluorouracil, folic acid, foscarnet, gallium, gatifloxacin, gemcitabine, gentamicin, glycopyrrolate, granisetron, heparin, hydrocortisone, HYDROmorphone, hydrOXYzine, IDArubicin, ifosfamide, imipenem-cilastatin, irinotecan, isoproterenol, ketorolac, labetalol, levofloxacin, lidocaine, linezolid, LORazepan, LR, magnesium sulfate, mannitol, mechlorethamine, melphalan, meperidine, metaraminol, meropenem, methicillin, methotrexate, methoxamine, methyldopate, methylPREDNISolone, metoclopramide, metoprolol, metroNIDAZOLE, mezlocillin, miconazole, midazolam, milrinone, minocycline, mitoXANtrone, morphine, moxalactam, multiple vitamins injection, mycophenolate, nafcillin, nalbuphine, naloxone, nesiritide, netilmicin, niCARdipine, nitroglycerin, nitroprusside, norepinephrine, octreotide, ondansetron, oxacillin, oxaliplatin, oxytocin, PACLitaxel, palonosetron, pamidronate, pancuronium, pantoprazole, papaverine, PEMEtrexed, penicillin G sodium/potassium, pentamidine, pentazocine, phenylephrine, phytonadione, piperacillin, piperacillin/ tazobactam, polymyxin B, potassium chloride, procainamide, prochlorperazine, promethazine, propofol, propranolol, protamine, pyridoxine, quiNIDine, quinupristin-dalfopristin, ranitidine, remifentanil, Ringer's ritodrine, riTUXimab, rocuronium, sargramostim, sodium acetate/bicarbonate, succinylcholine, SUFentanil, tacrolimus, teniposide, theophylline, thiamine, thiotepa, ticarcillin, ticarcillin-clavulanate, tigecycline, tirofiban, TNA, tobramycin, tolazoline, topotecan, TPN, trastuzumab, trimetaphan, urokinase, vancomycin, vasopressin, vecuronium, verapamil, vinCRIStine, vinorelbine, voriconazole, zidovudine, zoledronic acid

ADVERSE EFFECTS

CNS: *Confusion, headache,* depression, dizziness, anxiety, weakness, psychosis, tremors, **seizures**

CV: Bradycardia, tachycardia, **dysrhythmias**

GI: *Diarrhea,* abdominal cramps, **paralytic ileus,** *jaundice*

GU: Gynecomastia, galactorrhea, impotence, increase in BUN, creatinine

HEMA: Agranulocytosis, thrombocytopenia, neutropenia, aplastic anemia, increase in pro-time

INTEG: Urticaria, rash, alopecia, sweating, flushing, **exfoliative dermatitis**

RESP: Pneumonia

Pharmacokinetics

Absorption	Well absorbed (PO, IM); completely absorbed (**IV**)
Distribution	Widely distributed; crosses placenta
Metabolism	Liver (30%)
Excretion	Kidneys, unchanged (70%); breast milk
Half-life	1½-2 hr; increased in renal disease

Pharmacodynamics

	PO	IM/IV
Onset	½ hr	10 min
Peak	45-90 min	½ hr
Duration	4-5 hr	4-5 hr

INTERACTIONS

Individual drugs

CarBAMazepine, chloroquine, lidocaine, metronidazole, moricizine, phenytoin, quiNIDine, quiNINE, valproic acid, warfarin: increased toxicity (CYP450 pathway)

Carmustine: increased bone marrow suppression

Itraconazole: decreased absorption of itraconazole

Ketoconazole: decreased absorption of ketoconazole

Sucralfate: decreased cimetidine absorption

Drug classifications

Antacids: decreased absorption of cimetidine

Antidepressants (tricyclic), benzodiazepines, β-adrenergic blockers, calcium channel blockers, phenytoins, sulfonylureas, theophyllines: increased toxicity (CYP450 pathway)

Drug/lab test

Increased: alkaline phosphatase, AST, creatinine, prolactin

False positive: Hemoccult, Gastroccult tests

False negative: TB skin tests

NURSING CONSIDERATIONS

Assessment

• **Ulcer symptoms:** Assess patient with ulcers or suspected ulcers: epigastric or abdominal pain, hematemesis, occult blood in stools, blood in gastric aspirate before and/or throughout treatment

Patient/family education

• Advise patient that any gynecomastia or impotence that develops is reversible after treatment is discontinued

- Caution patient to avoid driving, other hazardous activities until stabilized on this medication; drowsiness or dizziness may occur
- Advise patient to avoid black pepper, caffeine, alcohol, harsh spices, extremes in temperature of food; tell patient to avoid OTC preparations: aspirin, cough, cold preparations; condition may worsen
- Advise patient that smoking decreases the effectiveness of the product; smoking cessation should be considered
- Teach patient that product must be continued for prescribed time to be effective and taken exactly as prescribed; doses are not to be doubled; to take missed dose when remembered up to 1 hr before next dose
- Instruct patient to report bruising, fatigue, malaise; blood dyscrasias may occur

⚠ **Have patient report to prescriber immediately any diarrhea, black tarry stools, sore throat, dizziness, confusion, or delirium**

Evaluation

Positive therapeutic outcome
- Decreased pain in abdomen
- Healing of ulcers
- Absence of gastroesophageal reflux
- Gastric pH of ≥5

cinacalcet (Rx)

(sin-a-kal′set)
Sensipar
Func. class.: Calcium receptor agonist
Chem. class.: Polypeptide hormone
Pregnancy category C

ACTION: Directly lowers PTH levels by increasing sensitivity of calcium sensing receptors to extracellular calcium

Therapeutic outcome: Decreased symptoms of hypercalcemia

USES: Hypercalcemia in parathyroid carcinoma, secondary hyperparathyroidism in chronic kidney disease on dialysis, primary hyperparathyroidism

CONTRAINDICATIONS:

Hypersensitivity, hypocalcemia

Precautions: Pregnancy C, breastfeeding, children, seizure disorders, hepatic disease

DOSAGE AND ROUTES

Parathyroid carcinoma
Adult: PO 30 mg bid, titrate q2-4wk, with sequential doses of 30 mg bid, 60 mg bid, 90 mg bid, 90 mg tid-qid to normalize calcium levels

Secondary hyperparathyroidism
Adult: PO 30 mg daily, titrate no more frequently than 2-4 wks with sequential doses of 30, 60, 90, 120, 180 mg daily

Available forms: Tabs 30, 60, 90 mg

Implementation
- Swallow tabs whole; do not break, crush, chew, or divide tabs
- Can be used alone or in combination with vit D sterols and/or phosphate binders
- Take with food or shortly after meal

Secondary hyperthyroidism
- Titrate q2-4wk to target iPTH consistent with National Kidney Foundation—Kidney Disease Outcomes Quality Initiative (NKF-K/DOQI) for chronic kidney disease patient on dialysis of 150-300 pg/ml; if iPTH drops below 150-300 pg/ml, reduce dose of cinacalcet and/or vit D sterols or discontinue treatment
- Store at <77° F (25° C)

ADVERSE EFFECTS

CNS: Dizziness, asthenia, **seizures,** tetany, hallucinations, depression
CV: Hypertension, dysrhythmia exacerbation
GI: Nausea, diarrhea, vomiting, anorexia
MISC: Access infection, noncardiac chest pain, hypocalcemia
MS: Myalgia

Pharmacokinetics

Absorption	93%-97% bound to plasma
Distribution	Unknown
Metabolism	Proteins metabolized by CYP3A4, 2D6, 1A2
Excretion	Renal (80% renal, 15% feces)
Half-life	30-40 hr

Pharmacodynamics

Unknown

INTERACTIONS

Individual drugs
Flecainide, thioridazine, vinBLAStine: increased levels of CYP2D6 inhibitors; adjustments may be necessary

Drug classifications
Products metabolized by CYP3A4 inhibitors
(erythromycin, itraconazole, ketoconazole):
increased cinacalcet levels
Tricyclics: increased levels of CYP2D6 inhibitors)

Drug/food
High-fat meal: increased action

NURSING CONSIDERATIONS

Assessment
• Assess for **hypocalcemia:** cramping, seizures, tetany, myalgia, paresthesia
• Monitor calcium, phosphorous within 1
wk and iPTH 1-4 wk after initiation or dosage
adjustment when maintenance is established;
measure calcium, phosphorus monthly; iPTH
q1-3mo, target range 150-300 pg/ml for iPTH
level; biochemical markers of bone formation/
resorption, radiologic evidence of fracture; if
calcium <8.4 mg/dl, do not start therapy
• **Renal disease (without dialysis):** These
patients should not receive treatment with this
product, high risk of hypocalcemia

Patient/family education
• Instruct patient to take with food or shortly
after a meal, to take tabs whole
• Instruct patient to immediately report cramping, seizures, muscle pain, tingling, tetany

Evaluation
Positive therapeutic outcome
• Calcium levels 9-10 mg/dl, decreasing symptoms of hypercalcemia

---

ciprofloxacin (Rx)
(sip-ro-floks'a-sin)
Cipro, Cipro XR
Func. class.: Antiinfectives, broad-
spectrum
Chem. class.: Fluoroquinolone
Pregnancy category C

Do not confuse:
ciprofloxacin/cephalexin

ACTION: Interferes with conversion of intermediate DNA fragments into high-molecular-
weight DNA in bacteria; DNA gyrase inhibitor

Therapeutic outcome: Bactericidal action against the following: gram-positive organisms *Staphylococcus epidermidis,* methicillin-
resistant strains of *Staphylococcus aureus;*
gram-negative organisms *Escherichia coli,*
Klebsiella species, *Enterobacter, Salmonella,
Proteus vulgaris, Pseudomonas aeruginosa,
Serratia, Campylobacter jejuni*

USES: Adult urinary tract infections (including complicated); chronic bacterial prostatitis;
acute sinusitis; infectious diarrhea; typhoid
fever; complicated intraabdominal infections;
nosocomial pneumonia; exposure to inhalation
anthrax

CONTRAINDICATIONS:
Hypersensitivity to quinolones

Precautions: Pregnancy **C,** breastfeeding, children, geriatric, renal disease, seizure
disorder, stroke, CV disease, hepatic disease, QT
prolongation, hypokalemia

> **BLACK BOX WARNING:** Tendon pain/rupture,
> tendonitis, myasthenia gravis

DOSAGE AND ROUTES
Uncomplicated urinary tract infec-
tions
Adult: PO 250 mg q12hr × 3 days or XL 500
mg q24hr × 3 days

Complicated/severe urinary tract
infections
Adult: PO 500 mg q12hr or XL 1000 mg q24hr
× 7-14 days; **IV** 400 mg q12hr

Respiratory, bone, skin, joint infec-
tions (mild-moderate)
Adult: PO 500-750 mg q12hr × 7-14 days; **IV**
400 mg q12hr

Nosocomial pneumonia
Adult: **IV** 400 mg q8hr × 10-14 days

Intraabdominal infections, compli-
cated
Adult: PO 500 mg q12hr × 7-14 days, **IV**
400 mg q12hr × 7-14 days, usually given with
metroNIDAZOLE

Acute sinusitis, mild/moderate
Adult: PO 500 mg q12hr × 10 days; **IV** 400
mg q12hr × 10 days

Inhalational anthrax (postexpo-
sure)
Adult: PO 500 mg q12hr × 60 days; **IV** 400
mg q12hr × 60 days
Child: PO 15 mg/kg/dose q12hr × 60 days,
max 500 mg/dose; **IV,** 10 mg/kg q12hr, max
400 mg/dose

Infectious diarrhea
Adult: PO 500-750 mg q12hr × 5-7 days

Chronic bacterial prostatitis
Adult: PO 500 mg q12hr × 28 days; **IV** 400 mg q12hr × 28 days

Pyelonephritis, acute uncomplicated/UTI
Adult: PO 250 mg q12hr; 500 mg q12hr (severe) × 7-14 days, q4-6wk

Renal dose
Adult: PO CCr 30-50 ml/min PO 250-500 mg q12hr; CCr 5-29 ml/min PO 250-500 mg q18hr; **IV** 200-400 mg q18-24hr

Available forms: Tabs 100, 250, 500, 750 mg; ext rel tabs (XR) 500, 1000 mg; powder for oral susp 5%, 10%; inj 200 mg/20 ml, 400 mg/40 ml, 200 mg/100 ml D_5, 400 mg/200 ml D_5; oral susp 250, 500 mg/5 ml

Implementation
PO route
- Obtain C&S before use
- Give around the clock to maintain proper blood levels
- Administer 6 hr before or 2 hr after antacids, zinc, iron, calcium; use adequate fluids to prevent crystalluria
- Do not give oral sup by GI tube
- Limit intake of alkaline soda, products with milk, dairy products, alkaline antacids, sodium bicarbonate

IV route
- Check for irritation, extravasation, phlebitis daily
- For **intermittent inf,** dilute to 1-2 mg/ml of D_5W, 0.9% NaCl; give over 60 min; it will remain stable under refrigeration for 2 wk, diluted vials can be stored for 14 days at room temperature or in refrigerator, do not freeze

Y-site incompatibilities: Heparin, mezlocillin

ADVERSE EFFECTS
CNS: *Headache,* dizziness, fatigue, insomnia, depression, *restlessness,* **seizures,** confusion, hallucinations
GI: *Nausea,* increased ALT, AST, flatulence, heartburn, *vomiting, diarrhea,* oral candidiasis, dysphagia, **pseudomembranous colitis,** dry mouth, **abdominal pain, pancreatitis**
GU: Crystalluria, interstitial neuritis
HEMA: Bone marrow depression, agranulocytosis, eosinophilia

INTEG: *Rash,* pruritus, urticaria, photosensitivity, flushing, fever, chills, **toxic epidermal necrolysis,** injection site reactions
MISC: Anaphylaxis, Stevens-Johnson syndrome, visual impairment, **QT prolongation, pseudotumor cerebri**
MS: Tremor, arthralgia, tendon rupture

Pharmacokinetics
Absorption	Well absorbed (75%) (PO)
Distribution	Widely distributed
Metabolism	Liver (15%)
Excretion	Kidneys (40%-50%)
Half-life	1-2 hr; increased in renal disease

Pharmacodynamics
	PO	IV
Onset	Rapid	Immediate
Peak	1-2 hr	Infusion's end

INTERACTIONS
Individual drugs
Alfuzosin, arsenic trioxide, astemizole, chloroquine, cloZAPine, cyclobenzaprine, dasatinib, dolasetron, droperidol, flecainide, haloperidol, lapatinib, levomethadyl, methadone, octreotide, ondansetron, paliperidone, palonosetron, pentamidine, probucol, propafenone, ranolazine, risperiDONE, sertindole, SUNItinib, tacrolimus, terfenadine, vardenafil, vorinostat, ziprasidone: increased QT prolongation; less likely than other quinolones
CYP1A2 inhibitors: increased levels of CYP1A2 inhibitors
Calcium, enteral feeding, iron, sucralfate, zinc sulfate: decreased ciprofloxacin absorption
CycloSPORINE: increased nephrotoxicity
Probenecid: increased blood levels of ciprofloxacin, increased toxicity
Theophylline: increased theophylline levels, monitor blood levels, reduce dose
Warfarin: increased warfarin effect, monitor blood levels

Drug classifications
Antacids (containing magnesium, aluminum), iron salts: decreased absorption of ciprofloxacin
β-agonists, class IA/III antidysrhythmics, halogenated anesthetics, local anesthetics, macrolides, phenothiazines, tetracyclines, tricyclics: increased QT prolongation

BLACK BOX WARNING: Corticosteroids: increased tendonitis, tendon rupture

Drug/food
Dairy products, food: decreased absorption

Drug/lab test
Increased: AST, ALT, bilirubin, BUN, creatinine, alkaline phosphatase, LDH, glucose, proteinuria, albuminuria
Decreased: WBC, glucose

NURSING CONSIDERATIONS
Assessment
• Assess patient for previous sensitivity reaction
• Assess patient for signs and symptoms of **infection** including characteristics of wounds, sputum, urine, stool, WBC >10,000/mm³, fever; obtain baseline information before, during treatment
• Obtain C&S before beginning product therapy to identify if correct treatment has been initiated
• Assess for **anaphylaxis:** rash, urticaria, dyspnea, pruritus, chills, fever, joint pain; may occur a few days after therapy begins; epinephrine and resuscitation equipment should be available for anaphylactic reaction
• Identify urine output; if decreasing, notify prescriber (may indicate nephrotoxicity); also check for increased BUN, creatinine
• Monitor blood studies: AST, ALT, CBC, Hct, bilirubin, LDH, alkaline phosphatase, Coombs' test monthly if patient is on long-term therapy
• Monitor electrolytes: potassium, sodium, chloride monthly if patient is on long-term therapy

BLACK BOX WARNING: Myasthenia gravis: avoid use in these patients, increases muscle weakness

⚠ **QT prolongation: monitor for changes in QTc if taking other products that increase QT**
• Assess for **CNS symptoms:** headache, dizziness, fatigue, insomnia, depression, seizures
• Monitor for bleeding: ecchymosis, bleeding gums, hematuria, stool guaiac daily if on long-term therapy
• Assess for **overgrowth of infection:** perineal itching, fever, malaise, redness, pain, swelling, drainage, rash, diarrhea, change in cough, sputum

BLACK BOX WARNING: Assess for tendon pain, especially in children

BLACK BOX WARNING: Tendonitis, tendon rupture: discontinue at first sign of tendon pain, inflammation; increased in those >60 yr, those taking corticosteroids, organ transplant recipients

⚠ **Pseudomotor cerebri: may occur at excessive doses**

Patient/family education
• Teach patient to report sore throat, bruising, bleeding, joint pain; may indicate blood dyscrasias (rare)
• Teach patient to contact prescriber if adverse reaction occurs or if inflammation or pain in tendon occurs before, 6 hr after
• Instruct patient to take all medication prescribed for the length of time ordered; product must be taken around the clock to maintain blood levels; do not give medication to others

BLACK BOX WARNING: Teach patient to report tendon pain, chest pain, palpitations

• Advise patient to rinse mouth frequently, use sugarless candy or gum for dry mouth, to drink fluids to prevent crystals in urine
⚠ **Teach patient to notify prescriber if rash occurs, discontinue product**
• Teach patient to notify prescriber if pregnancy is planned or suspected, **(C)** do not breastfeed

Evaluation
Positive therapeutic outcome
• Absence of signs/symptoms of infection (WBC <10,000/mm³, temp WNL, absence of red draining wounds)
• Reported improvement in symptoms of infection
• Ext rel and regular release are not interchangeable
• Do not add or stop products without prescriber's approval
• Use calibrated measuring device for suspension

ciprofloxacin ophthalmic
See Appendix B

cisatracurium (Rx)

(sis-a-tra-cyoor'ee-um)

Nimbex

Func. class.: Neuromuscular blocker (nondepolarizing)

Pregnancy category B

ACTION: Inhibits transmission of nerve impulses by binding with cholinergic receptor sites, antagonizing action of acetylcholine

Therapeutic outcome: Paralysis of body for administration of anesthesia

USES: Facilitation of endotracheal intubation, skeletal muscle relaxation during mechanical ventilation surgery, or general anesthesia

CONTRAINDICATIONS:

Hypersensitivity

Precautions: Pregnancy **B**, breastfeeding, children <2 yr, electrolyte imbalances, dehydration, cardiac/neuromuscular/respiratory disease

DOSAGE AND ROUTES

Adult: IV 0.15 and 0.2 mg/kg depending on desired time to intubate and length of surgery: use peripheral nerve stimulation to evaluate dosage

Child 2-12 yr: IV 0.1 mg/kg over 5-10 sec with halothane or opioid anesthesia

Available forms: Inj 2, 10 mg/ml

Implementation

IV route

• Use nerve stimulator by anesthesiologist to determine neuromuscular blockade

• Give anticholinesterase to reverse neuromuscular blockade

• Give by slow **IV** only by qualified person; do not administer IM

• Store in light-resistant area

• Reassure if communication is difficult during recovery from neuromuscular blockage

ADVERSE EFFECTS

CV: Bradycardia, tachycardia; increased, decreased B/P

EENT: Increased secretions

INTEG: Rash, flushing, pruritus, urticaria

RESP: Prolonged apnea, bronchospasm, cyanosis, respiratory depression

Pharmacokinetics

Unknown

Pharmacodynamics

Onset	1-3 min
Peak	2-5 min
Duration	30-40 min

INTERACTIONS

Individual drugs

CarBAMazepine, phenytoin: decreased duration of neuromuscular blockade

Isoflurane, lithium: increased neuromuscular blockade

Succinylcholine: decreased neuromuscular blockade

Drug classifications

Aminoglycosides, antibiotics (polymix), β-adrenergic blockers, opioids: increased neuromuscular blockade

NURSING CONSIDERATIONS

Assessment

• Assess for electrolyte imbalances (K, Mg), may lead to increased action of this product

• Assess vital signs (B/P, pulse, respirations, airway) until fully recovered; rate, depth, pattern of respirations; strength of handgrip

• Assess I&O ratio; check for urinary retention, frequency, hesitancy

• Assess recovery: decreased paralysis of face, diaphragm, legs, arms, rest of body

• Assess allergic reactions: rash, fever, respiratory distress, pruritus; product should be discontinued

Evaluation

Positive therapeutic outcome

• Paralysis of jaw, eyelid, head, neck, rest of body

TREATMENT OF OVERDOSE:

Edrophonium or neostigmine, atropine, monitor VS; mechanical ventilation

---

⚠ HIGH ALERT

CISplatin (Rx)

(sis′pla-tin)
Func. class.: Antineoplastic alkylating agent
Chem. class.: Inorganic heavy metal
Pregnancy category D

Do not confuse:
CISplatin/CARBOplatin

ACTION: Alkylates DNA, RNA; inhibits enzymes that allow synthesis of amino acids in proteins; activity is not cell cycle phase specific

Therapeutic outcome: Prevention of rapidly growing malignant cells

USES: Advanced bladder cancer; adjunctive in metastatic testicular cancer and metastatic ovarian cancer; osteosarcoma; soft tissue sarcomas; head, neck, esophageal, prostatic, lung, and cervical cancer; lymphoma

CONTRAINDICATIONS:
Pregnancy **D**, breastfeeding

BLACK BOX WARNING: Bone marrow suppression, platinum compound hypersensitivity, renal disease/failure, preexisting hearing impairment

Precautions: Geriatric patients, vaccination

DOSAGE AND ROUTES
Dosage protocols may vary

Metastatic testicular cancer
Adult: **IV** 20 mg/m² daily × 5 days, repeat q3wk for 2 cycles or more, depending on response

Advanced bladder cancer
Adult: **IV** 50-70 mg/m² q3-4wk

Metastatic ovarian cancer
Adult: **IV** 100 mg/m² q4wk or 75-100 mg/m² q3wk with cyclophosphamide therapy

Available forms: Inj 0.5 mg/ml ♣, 1 mg/ml

Implementation
• Hydrate patient with 0.9% NaCl over 8-12 hr before treatment
• Give all medications PO, if possible; avoid IM inj when platelets <100,000/mm³
• Give EPINEPHrine, antihistamines, corticosteroids for hypersensitivity reaction; antiemetic 30-60 min before giving product to prevent vomiting, and prn; allopurinol or sodium bicarbonate to maintain uric acid level, alkalinization of urine; antibiotics for prophylaxis of infection; diuretic (furosemide 40 mg **IV**) or mannitol after infusion
• Prepare in biological cabinet using gown, gloves, mask; do not allow product to come in contact with skin; use soap and water if contact occurs

Intermittent IV infusion route
• Give after **diluting** 10 mg/10 ml or 50 mg/50 ml sterile water for inj; **withdraw** prescribed dose, **dilute** ½ dose with 1000 ml D₅ 0.2 NaCl or D₅ 0.45 NaCl with 37.5 g mannitol; **IV** inf is **given** over 3-4 hr; use a 0.45 μm filter; total dose 2000 ml over 6-8 hr; check site for irritation, phlebitis; do not use equipment containing aluminum

Continuous IV infusion route
• Give over 24 hr × 5 days

Syringe compatibilities: Bleomycin, cyclophosphamide, doxapram, droperidol, fluorouracil, furosemide, heparin, leucovorin, methotrexate, metoclopramide, vinBLAStine, vinCRIStine

Y-site compatibilities: Acyclovir, alfentanil, allopurinol, amikacin, aminophylline, amiodarone, ampicillin, ampicillin-sulbactam, anidulafungin, atenolol, atracurium, azithromycin, aztreonam, bivalirudin, bleomycin, bumetanide, buprenorphine, butorphanol, calcium chloride/gluconate, carmustine, caspofungin, ceFAZolin, cefoperazone, cefotaxime, cefoTEtan, cefOXitin, cefTAZidime, ceftizoxime, cefTRIAXone, cefuroxime, chlorproMAZINE, cimetidine, ciprofloxacin, cisatracurium, cladribine, clindamycin, codeine, cyclophosphamide, cycloSPORINE, cytarabine, DACTINomycin, DAPTOmycin, DAUNOrubicin, dexamethasone, dexmedetomidine, dexrazoxane, digoxin, diltiazem, diphenhydrAMINE, DOBUTamine, DOCEtaxel, DOPamine, doripenem, doxacurium, DOXOrubicin, DOXOrubicin liposomal, doxycycline, droperidol, enalaprilat, ePHEDrine, EPINEPHrine, epirubicin, ertapenem, erythromycin, esmolol, etoposide, famotidine, fenoldopam, fentaNYL, filgrastim, fluconazole, fludarabine, fluorouracil, foscarnet, fosphenytoin, furosemide, ganciclovir, gatifloxacin, gemcitabine, gentamicin, glycopyrrolate, granisetron, haloperidol, heparin, hydrocortisone, HYDROmorphone, IDArubicin, ifosfamide, imipenem-cilastatin, inamrinone, indomethacin, irinotecan, isoproterenol, ketorolac, labetalol, leucovorin, levofloxacin,

Adverse effects: *italics* = common; **bold** = life-threatening

levorphanol, lidocaine, linezolid, LORazepam, magnesium sulfate, mannitol, melphalan, meperidine, meropenem, methohexital, methotrexate, methylPREDNISolone, metoclopramide, metoprolol, metroNIDAZOLE, midazolam, milrinone, minocycline, mitoMYcin, mitoXANtrone, mivacurium, nafcillin, naloxone, nesiritide, niCARdipine, nitroglycerin, nitroprusside, norepinephrine, octreotide, ofloxacin, ondansetron, oxaliplatin, PACLitaxel, palonosetron, pamidronate, pancuronium, PEMEtrexed, pentamidine, pentazocine, PENTobarbital, PHENobarbital, phenylephrine, phenytoin, piperacillin, polymyxin B, potassium chloride/phosphates, procainamide, prochlorperazine, promethazine, propofol, propranolol, quiNIDine, quinupristin-dalfopristin, ranitidine, remifentanil, riTUXimab, sargramostim, sodium acetate/bicarbonate/phosphates, succinylcholine, SUFentanil, sulfamethoxazole-trimethoprim, tacrolimus, teniposide, theophylline, thiopental, ticarcillin, ticarcillin-clavulanate, tigecycline, tirofiban, TNA, tobramycin, topotecan, trastuzumab, vancomycin, vasopressin, vecuronium, verapamil, vinBLAStine, vinCRIStine, vinorelbine, voriconazole, zidovudine, zoledronic acid

Additive compatibilities: CARBOplatin, cyclophosphamide, floxuridine, hydrOXYzine, ifosfamide, leucovorin, magnesium sulfate, mannitol, ondansetron, potassium chloride

Additive incompatibilities: Fluorouracil, mesna, thiotepa

Solution compatibilities: D_5/0.225% NaCl, D_5/0.45% NaCl, D_5/0.9% NaCl, D_5/0.45% NaCl with mannitol 1.875%, D_5/0.33% NaCl with mannitol 1.875%, D_5/0.33% NaCl with KCl 20 mEq and mannitol 1.875%, 0.9% NaCl, 0.45% NaCl, 0.3% NaCl, 0.225% NaCl, water

Solution incompatibilities: Sodium bicarbonate 5%, 0.1% NaCl, water

ADVERSE EFFECTS

CNS: Seizures, *peripheral neuropathy*
CV: Cardiac abnormalities
EENT: *Tinnitus, hearing loss, vestibular toxicity,* blurred vision, altered color perception
GI: *Severe nausea, vomiting, diarrhea, weight loss*
GU: Renal tubular damage, *renal insufficiency,* impotence, sterility, amenorrhea, gynecomastia, hyperuremia
HEMA: Thrombocytopenia, leukopenia, pancytopenia
INTEG: *Alopecia,* dermatitis

META: *Hypomagnesemia,* hypocalcemia, hypokalemia, hypophosphatemia
RESP: Fibrosis
SYST: Anaphylaxis

Pharmacokinetics

Absorption	Complete
Distribution	Widely distributed, accumulates in body tissues for several months
Metabolism	Liver
Excretion	Kidneys
Half-life	30-100 hr

Pharmacodynamics

Unknown

INTERACTIONS

Individual drugs

Alcohol, aspirin: increased risk of bleeding
Bumetanide, ethacrynic acid, furosemide: ototoxicity
Phenytoin: decreased phenytoin effect

Drug classifications

Aminoglycosides, diuretics (loop), salicylates: increased nephrotoxicity
Myelosuppressive agents, radiation: increased myelosuppression
NSAIDs: increased risk of bleeding
Vaccines, live virus: decreased antibody response

Drug/lab test

Increased: uric acid, BUN, creatinine
Decreased: CCr, calcium, phosphate, potassium, magnesium
Positive: Coombs' test

NURSING CONSIDERATIONS

Assessment

> **BLACK BOX WARNING:** Monitor for **bone marrow depression:** CBC, differential, platelet count weekly; withhold product if WBC count is <4000/mm³ or platelet count is <100,000/mm³; notify prescriber of results if WBC <20,000/mm³, platelets <150,000/mm³

> **BLACK BOX WARNING:** Monitor **renal toxicity:** BUN, creatinine, serum uric acid, urine CCr before, during therapy; I&O ratio; report fall in urine output to <30 ml/hr; dose should not be given if BUN <25 mg/dl; creatinine <1.5 mg/dl

---

• Assess for **anaphylaxis:** wheezing, tachycardia, facial swelling, fainting; discontinue product and report to prescriber; resuscitation equipment should be nearby, may occur within minutes; often EPINEPHrine, corticosteroids, antihistamines may alleviate symptoms

• Monitor temp q4hr (may indicate beginning of infection)

• Monitor liver function tests before, during therapy (bilirubin, AST, ALT, LDH) as needed or monthly; note yellowing of skin or sclera, dark urine, clay-colored stools, itchy skin, abdominal pain, fever, diarrhea

• Assess for increased uric acid levels, swelling, joint pain primarily in extremities; patient should be well hydrated to prevent urate deposits

• Assess for **bleeding:** hematuria, stool guaiac, bruising or petechiae, mucosa or orifices q8hr; note inflammation of mucosa, breaks in skin

• Identify dyspnea, crackles, nonproductive cough, chest pain, tachypnea

> **BLACK BOX WARNING: Ototoxicity:** more common in genetic variants TPMT 3B and 3C in children; use audiometric testing baseline and before each dose

• Identify effects of alopecia on body image; discuss feelings about body changes

• Identify edema in feet, joint pain, stomach pain, shaking; prescriber should be notified

Patient/family education

⚠ Teach patient to avoid use of products containing aspirin or ibuprofen, NSAIDs, alcohol (may cause GI bleeding), razors, commercial mouthwash; to report symptoms of bleeding (hematuria, tarry stools, bruising, petechiae)

• Advise patient to report numbness, tingling in face or extremities, poor hearing or joint pain, swelling

⚠ Instruct patient to report signs of anemia (fatigue, headache, irritability, faintness, shortness of breath)

• Instruct patient to report any changes in breathing or coughing even several months after treatment; to avoid crowds and persons with respiratory tract or other infections

• Advise patient that hair may be lost during treatment; a wig or hairpiece may make patient feel better; new hair may be different in color, texture

• Tell patient not to have any vaccinations without the advice of the prescriber; serious reactions can occur

⚠ Caution patient contraception is needed during treatment and for 4 months after the completion of therapy, pregnancy D

> **BLACK BOX WARNING: Ototoxicity:** teach patient to report loss of hearing, ringing or roaring in the ears

Evaluation
Positive therapeutic outcome
• Prevention of rapid division of malignant cells

citalopram (Rx)
(sigh-tal′oh-pram)
CeleXA
Func. class.: Antidepressant
Chem. class.: Selective serotonin reuptake inhibitor (SSRI)
Pregnancy category C

Do not confuse:
CeleXA/CeleBREX/Cerebyx/Cerebra/Zyprexa

ACTION: Inhibits CNS neuron uptake of serotonin but not of norepinephrine; weak inhibitor of CYP450 enzyme system, making it more appealing than other products

Therapeutic outcome: Decreased symptoms of depression after 2-3 wk

USES: Major depressive disorder

Unlabeled uses: Premenstrual disorders, panic disorder, social phobia, obsessive-compulsive disorder in adolescents, anxiety, hot flashes, menopause, adjunct in schizophrenia, PTSD

CONTRAINDICATIONS: Hypersensitivity

Precautions: Pregnancy C, breastfeeding, geriatric, renal/hepatic disease, seizure disorder, hypersensitivity to escitalopram, bradycardia, recent MI

> **BLACK BOX WARNING:** Children, suicidal ideation

DOSAGE AND ROUTES
Depression
Adult: PO 20 mg daily AM or PM, may increase if needed to 40 mg/day after 1 wk; maintenance: after 6-8 wk of initial treatment, continue for 24 wk (32 wk total), reevaluate long-term usefulness (max 60 mg/day)

Hepatic dose/geriatric
Adult: PO 20 mg/day, may increase to 40 mg/day if no response

Panic disorder (unlabeled)
Adult: PO 20-60 mg/day

Premenstrual dysphoria, social phobia
Adult: PO 10-30 mg/day used intermittently in premenstrual dysphoria

Available forms: Tabs 10, 20, 40 mg; oral SOL 10 mg/5 ml

Implementation
- Give with food or milk for GI symptoms
- Give dosage at bedtime if oversedation occurs during day
- Leave orally disintegrating tabs on tongue and allow to dissolve before swallowing
- Store at room temperature; do not freeze

⚠ **Do not give within 14 days of MAOIs**

ADVERSE EFFECTS
CNS: *Headache, nervousness, insomnia, drowsiness, anxiety, tremor, dizziness, fatigue, sedation, poor concentration, abnormal dreams, agitation,* **seizures,** apathy, euphoria, hallucinations, delusions, psychosis, **suicidal attempts, malignant neuroleptic-like syndrome reactions**

CV: *Hot flashes, palpitations,* angina pectoris, **hemorrhage,** hypertension, tachycardia, 1st-degree AV block, bradycardia, **MI,** thrombophlebitis, QT prolongation, orthostatic hypotension, torsades de pointes

EENT: Vision changes, ear/eye pain, photophobia, tinnitus

GI: *Nausea, diarrhea, dry mouth, anorexia, dyspepsia, constipation, cramps, vomiting, taste changes, flatulence, decreased appetite*

GU: *Dysmenorrhea, decreased libido, urinary frequency, urinary tract infection,* amenorrhea, cystitis, impotence, urine retention

INTEG: *Sweating, rash, pruritus,* acne, alopecia, urticaria, photosensitivity

MS: *Pain,* arthritis, twitching

RESP: *Infection, pharyngitis, nasal congestion, sinus headache, sinusitis, cough, dyspnea, bronchitis,* asthma, hyperventilation, pneumonia

SYST: *Asthenia, viral infection, fever, allergy, chills,* hyponatremia (geriatric patients), **serotonin syndrome,** neonatal abstinence syndrome

Pharmacokinetics
Absorption	Well absorbed
Distribution	Unknown
Metabolism	Liver, by CYP1A2, CYP2D6
Excretion	Kidneys, steady state 28-35 days
Half-life	Unknown

Pharmacodynamics
Unknown

INTERACTIONS
Individual drugs
Alcohol: increased CNS depression

CarBAMazepine, cloNIDine: decreased citalopram levels

Lithium, tramadol, traZODone: increased serotonin syndrome

Pimoside, ziprasidone: increased QTc interval; do not use together

Drug classifications
Anticoagulants, antiplatelets, NSAIDs, salicylates, thrombolytics: increased risk of bleeding

Antidepressants (tricyclics): increased effect, use cautiously

Antifungals (azole), macrolides: increased citalopram levels

β-Adrenergic blockers: increased plasma levels of β-blockers

Barbiturates, benzodiazepines, CNS depressants, sedatives/hypnotics: increased CNS depression

MAOIs: hypertensive crisis, seizures, fatal reactions; do not use together

Quinolones: increased QTc interval; do not use together

Serotonin receptor agonists, SNRIs, SSRIs: increased serotonin syndrome

Drug/herb
SAM-e, St. John's wort: serotonin syndrome; do not use with citalopram; fatal reaction may occur

Yohimbe: increased CNS stimulation

Drug/lab test
Increased: serum bilirubin, blood glucose, alkaline phosphatase

Decreased: VMA, 5-HIAA

False increase: increased urinary catecholamines

NURSING CONSIDERATIONS
Assessment
- Monitor B/P (lying, standing), pulse q4hr; if systolic B/P drops 20 mm Hg, hold product

and notify prescriber; take vital signs q4hr in patients with cardiovascular disease
• Monitor blood studies: CBC, leukocytes, differential, cardiac enzymes if patient is receiving long-term therapy; check platelets; bleeding can occur
• Monitor hepatic studies: AST, ALT, bilirubin
• Check weight qwk; appetite may increase with product
⚠ Assess ECG for flattening of T wave, bundle branch block, AV block, dysrhythmias in cardiac patients, torsades de pointes, QT prolongation (effect is dose dependent)
• Assess EPS primarily in geriatric: rigidity, dystonia, akathisia

BLACK BOX WARNING: Assess mental status: mood, sensorium, affect, suicidal tendencies; increase in psychiatric symptoms: depression, panic

• Monitor urinary retention, constipation; constipation is more likely to occur in children or geriatric
• Assess for **serotonin syndrome:** increased heart rate, sweating, dilated pupils, tremors, twitching, hyperthermia, agitation
• Identify patient's alcohol consumption; if alcohol is consumed, hold dose until AM

Patient/family education
• Teach patient that therapeutic effects may take 4-6 wk, not to discontinue abruptly
• Instruct patient to use caution in driving or other activities requiring alertness because of drowsiness, dizziness, blurred vision; to avoid rising quickly from sitting to standing, especially geriatric patients

BLACK BOX WARNING: Advise that suicidal ideas, behavior may occur in children or young adults

• Caution patient to avoid alcohol ingestion, other CNS depressants
• Instruct patient to increase fluids, bulk in diet if constipation, urinary retention occur, especially geriatric
• Advise patient to take gum, hard sugarless candy, or frequent sips of water for dry mouth
• Teach patient how to use orally disintegrating tabs
• Teach patient to report **serotonin syndrome:** sweating, dilated pupils, tremors, twitching, extreme heat, agitation

Evaluation
Positive therapeutic outcome
• Decrease in depression
• Absence of suicidal thoughts

clarithromycin (Rx)
(clare-i-thro-mye'sin)
Biaxin, Biaxin Filmtab, Biaxin XL
Func. class.: Antiinfective
Chem. class.: Macrolide
Pregnancy category C

ACTION: Binds to 50S ribosomal subunits of susceptible bacteria and suppresses protein synthesis

Therapeutic outcome: Bactericidal action against the following: *Streptococcus pneumoniae, Streptococcus pyogenes, Mycoplasma pneumoniae, Corynebacterium diphtheriae, Bordetella pertussis, Listeria monocytogenes, Haemophilus influenzae, Staphylococcus aureus, Mycobacterium avium (MAC), Legionella pneumophila, Moxarella catarrhalis, Neisseria gonorrhoeae,* complex infections in AIDS patients, *Helicobacter pylori* in combination with omeprazole, *Helicobacter parainfluenzae*

USES: Mild to moderate infections of the upper respiratory tract, lower respiratory tract; uncomplicated skin and skin structure infections

CONTRAINDICATIONS:
Hypersensitivity to this product or other macrolides, torsades de pointes, QT prolongation

Precautions: Pregnancy C, breastfeeding, geriatric, renal/hepatic disease, QT prolongation

DOSAGE AND ROUTES
Acute exacerbation of chronic bronchitis
Adult: PO 250-500 mg q12hr × 7-14 days or 1000 mg/day × 7 days (XL)

Pharyngitis/tonsillitis
Adult: PO 250 mg q12hr × 10 days

Community-acquired pneumonia
Adult: PO 250 mg q12hr × 7-14 days or 1000 mg/day × 7 days (XL)

Endocarditis prophylaxis
Adult: PO 500 mg 1 hr before procedure

Adverse effects: *italics* = common; **bold** = life-threatening

MAC prophylaxis/treatment
Adult: PO 500 mg bid, will require an additional antiinfective for active infection

H. pylori infection
Adult: PO 500 mg/bid plus omeprazole 2 × 20 mg qAM (days 1-14), then omeprazole 20 mg qAM (days 15-28)

Acute maxillary sinusitis
Adult: PO 500 mg q12hr × 14 days

Most infections
Child: PO 7.5 mg/kg q12hr × 10 days, max 500 mg/dose for MAC

Renal dose
Adult: PO CCr 30-60 ml/min; decrease dose by 50% if using with ritonavir; CCr <30 ml/min reduce dose by 50%

Available forms: Tabs 250, 500 mg; oral susp 125, 250 mg/5 ml; ext rel tab (XL) 500 mg

Implementation
• Do not break, crush, or chew ext rel tab
• Ensure adequate fluid intake (2 L) during diarrhea episodes
• Give q12hr to maintain serum level
• Store at room temperature
• **Susp:** Shake well, store at room temperature, discard after 2 wk

ADVERSE EFFECTS
CV: Ventricular dysrhythmias, QT prolongation
GI: Nausea, vomiting, diarrhea, **hepatotoxicity,** abdominal pain, stomatitis, heartburn, anorexia, abnormal taste, **pseudomembranous colitis, tooth/tongue discoloration, pancreatitis**
GU: Vaginitis, moniliasis, interstitial nephritis, azotemia
HEMA: Leukopenia, thrombocytopenia, increased INR
INTEG: Rash, urticaria, pruritus, **Stevens-Johnson syndrome, toxic epidermal necrolysis**
MISC: Headache, hearing loss

Pharmacokinetics

Absorption	50%
Distribution	Widely distributed
Metabolism	Liver
Excretion	Kidneys, unchanged (20%-30%)
Half-life	4-6 hr

Pharmacodynamics

Onset	Unknown
Peak	2 hr
Duration	Unknown

INTERACTIONS
Individual drugs
ALPRAZolam, busPIRone, carBAMazepine, cyclo-SPORINE, digoxin, disopyramide, felodipine, fluconazole, omeprazole, tacrolimus, theophylline: increased levels, increased toxicity
CarBAMazepine: increased toxicity, from increased levels of carBAMazepine, increased oral anticoagulants effect
Cisapride, pimozide: increased effect, increased dysrhythmias
Digoxin: increased blood levels of digoxin, increased digoxin effects, increased oral anticoagulants effect
Midazolam, tacrolimus: increased effects
Rifabutin, rifampin, nevirapine, etravirine, benzodiazepine: decreased levels
Theophylline: increased toxicity from increased levels of theophylline, increased oral anticoagulant effect
Zidovudine: increased or decreased action

Drug classifications
All products metabolized by CYP3A enzyme system: increased action, risk of toxicity
Antidiabetics: increased toxicity
Calcium channel blockers, benzodiazepines: increased effects
Class IA, III antidysrhythmics or other products that prolong QT: increased QT prolongation
Ergots: increased levels, increased toxicity
HMG-CoA reductase inhibitors: increased levels
Oral anticoagulants: increased effects of oral anticoagulants

Drug/food
Do not use with grapefruit juice

Drug/lab test
Increased: 17-OHCS/17-KS, AST, ALT, BUN, creatinine, LDH, total bilirubin
Decreased: folate assay, WBC

NURSING CONSIDERATIONS
Assessment
• Assess patient for signs and symptoms of **infection** including characteristics of wounds, sputum, urine, stool, WBC >10,000/mm^3, earache, fever; obtain baseline information before, during treatment; obtain C&S before beginning product therapy to identify if correct treatment

has been initiated, product may be given as soon as culture is taken, repeat after treatment

• Bleeding: check INR if anticoagulants are taken
• Monitor blood studies: AST, ALT, CBC, Hct, bilirubin, LDH, alkaline phosphatase, Coombs' test monthly if patient is on long-term therapy
• Assess bowel pattern daily; if severe diarrhea occurs, product should be discontinued and prescriber should be notified of all products used
• Assess for overgrowth of infection: perineal itching, fever, malaise, redness, pain, swelling, drainage, rash, diarrhea, change in cough, sputum
⚠ **Assess for QT prolongation, ventricular dysrhythmias: monitor ECG, cardiac status in those with cardiac abnormalities**
⚠ **Assess for serious skin reaction: Stevens-Johnson syndrome, toxic epidermal necrolysis, product should be discontinued immediately**

Patient/family education
• Advise patient to contact physician if vaginal itching, loose foul-smelling stools, furry tongue occur; may indicate superinfection
• Instruct patient to take all medication prescribed for the length of time ordered
• Advise prescriber if pregnancy is planned or suspected
• Teach patient to notify prescriber of diarrhea, dark urine, pale stools, yellowing of eyes/skin, severe abdominal pain

Evaluation
Positive therapeutic outcome
• Absence of signs/symptoms of infection: WBC <10,000/mm³, temp WNL, absence of red draining wounds
• Reported improvement in symptoms of infection

---

clavulanate
See amoxicillin/clavulanate, ticarcillin/clavulanate

---

clevidipine (Rx)
(klev-id'i-peen)
Cleviprex
Func. class.: Calcium channel blocker (L-type)
Chem. class.: Dihydropyridine
Pregnancy category C

ACTION: L-type calcium channels mediate the influx of calcium during depolarization in arterial smooth muscle; reduces mean arterial B/P by decreasing systemic vascular resistance

Therapeutic outcome: Decreased B/P

USES: Treatment of hypertension when oral therapy is not feasible

CONTRAINDICATIONS:
Hypersensitivity to this product, eggs, or soya lecithin; defective lipid metabolism; severe aortic stenosis; pancreatitis

Precautions: Pregnancy **C**, breastfeeding, children <18 yr, heart failure, hyperlipidemia, hypertension, labor, phenochromocytoma

DOSAGE AND ROUTES
Adult: CONT **IV** 1-2 mg/hr; dose may be doubled q90sec initially; as B/P reaches goal, adjust dose less frequently (5-10 min) with smaller increases in dose; most patients require 4-6 mg/hr, max 32 mg/hr; no more than 1000 ml should be infused per 24 hr period due to lipid load restrictions

Available forms: Single dose vial 50, 100 ml (0.5 mg/ml), intravenous emulsion

Implementation
Intermittent IV infusion route
• Do not give through same line as other medications, do not dilute
• Gently invert several times before use; do not use if discolored or if particulate matter is present
• Give through central or peripheral line at 1-2 mg/hr, use infusion device
• Store vials in refrigerator, do not freeze; leave vials in carton until use; product is photosensitive but protection from light during administration is not required

ADVERSE EFFECTS
CNS: Headache
CV: Hypotension, **MI, sinus tachycardia,** syncope, **reflex tachycardia, atrial fibrillation**
GI: Nausea, vomiting
GU: Renal failure

Pharmacokinetics

Absorption	Unknown
Distribution	Protein binding >99%
Metabolism	By esterases in blood, extravascular tissues
Excretion	Urine 63%-74%, feces 7%-22%
Half-life	Initially 1 min; terminal 15 min; increased in hepatic disease

Adverse effects: *italics* = common; **bold** = life-threatening

Pharmacodynamics

Onset	2-4 min
Peak	6-12 hr
Duration	Unknown

NURSING CONSIDERATIONS
Assessment
• Assess cardiac status: B/P, pulse, respiration, ECG; some patients have developed severe angina, acute MI after calcium channel blockers if obstructive CAD is severe; if not transitioned to other antihypertensive therapies following clevidipine infusion, patients should be monitored ≥8 hr for rebound hypertension; monitor for rebound hypertension following drug stoppage
• **Renal failure:** Monitor I&O ratio, weight daily; peripheral edema, dyspnea, jugular vein distention, crackles (perioperative hypertensive patients)

Patient/family education
⚠ Instruct patient to notify prescriber immediately if neurological symptoms, visual changes, or symptoms of CHF occur
• Instruct patient to continue follow-up for hypertension
• Teach patient to notify prescriber if pregnancy is planned or suspected or if breastfeeding

Evaluation
Positive therapeutic outcome
• Decreased B/P

---

clindamycin HCl (Rx)
(klin-dah-my′sin)
Cleocin HCl
clindamycin palmitate (Rx)
Cleocin Pediatric
clindamycin phosphate (Rx)
Cleocin Phosphate
Func. class.: Antiinfective—miscellaneous
Chem. class.: Lincomycin derivative
Pregnancy category B

ACTION: Binds to 50S subunit of bacterial ribosomes; suppresses protein synthesis

Therapeutic outcome: Absence of infection

USES: Infections caused by staphylococci, streptococci, *Rickettsia, Fusobacterium, Actinomyces, Peptococcus, Bacteroides, Pneumocystis jiroveci*

CONTRAINDICATIONS:
Hypersensitivity to this product or lincomycin, tartrazine dye, ulcerative colitis/enteritis

> **BLACK BOX WARNING:** Pseudomembranous colitis

Precautions: Pregnancy **B**, breastfeeding, geriatric, renal/liver/GI disease, asthma, allergy

> **BLACK BOX WARNING:** Diarrhea

DOSAGE AND ROUTES
Adult: PO 150-450 mg q6hr, max 1.8 g/day; IM/**IV** 1.2-2.7 g/day in 2-4 divided doses q6-12hr, max 2700 mg/day
Child >1 mo: PO 8-25 mg/kg/day in divided doses q6-8hr; IM/**IV** 20-40 mg/kg/day in divided doses q6-8hr in 3-4 equal doses
Neonate: 15-20 mg/kg/day divided q6-8hr

PID
Adult: **IV** 900 mg q8hr plus gentamicin

Bacterial endocarditis prophylaxis
Adult: 600 mg 1 hr before procedure

P. jiroveci pneumonia (unlabeled)
Adult: PO 1200-1800 mg/day in divided doses with 15-30 mg primaquine/day × 21 days

Acne vulgaris
Adult/adolescent: Top (gel, lotion, sol), apply a thin film to affected areas bid for up to 12 wk
Adult/adolescent/child ≥2 yr: Top (foam), apply to affected areas daily; if no improvement in 8 wk, discontinue

Bacterial vaginosis, nonpregnant
Adult/adolescent female: Intravaginal 1 applicator full (100 mg clindamycin/5 g cream) at bedtime × 7 days

Available forms: Phosphate: inj 150, 300, 600 mg base/4 ml; 900 mg base/ml; inj inf in D$_5$ 300, 600, 900 mg; top pledget/foam/gel/lotion/solution/1%; Vag cream 2%; Vag suppository 100 mg; **HCl:** caps 75, 150, 300 mg; **palmitate:** oral sol 75 mg/5 ml

Implementation
• Obtain C&S before use
PO route
• Do not break, crush, or chew caps
• Give with 8 oz of water; give with meals for GI symptoms
• Shake liquids well
• Do not refrigerate oral preparations; stable at room temperature for 2 wk

---

⚠ Nurse Alert   ✴ Key NCLEX® Drug

Oral sol
• Do not refrigerate reconstituted product, store at room temperature ≤2 wk
• Reconstitute granules with most of 75 ml of water, shake well, add remaining water, shake well (75 mg/5 ml)

IM route
• If more than 600 mg must be given, divide into 2 inj
• Give deeply in large muscle mass; rotate sites

IV route
• Visually inspect parenteral products for particulate matter and discoloration prior to use
• **Vials:** Dilute 300 and 600 mg doses with 50 ml of a compatible diluent. Dilute 900 mg doses with 50-100 ml of a compatible diluent. Dilute 1200 mg doses with 100 ml of a compatible diluent, final concentration max 18 mg/ml
• **ADD-Vantage vials:** Dilute 600 and 900 mg ADD-Vantage containers with 50 or 100 mg, respectively, of NS or D_5W
• **Storage:** When diluted in D_5W, NS, or LR, solutions with concentrations of 6, 9, or 12 mg/ml are stable for 16 days at room temperature or 32 days under refrigeration when stored in glass bottles or minibags. When diluted in D_5W, solutions with a concentration of 18 mg/ml are stable for 16 days at room temperature

Intermittent IV infusion
• Infuse over at least 10-60 min, infusion rates max 30 mg/min and ≤1.2 g should be infused in a 1 hr period
• Infuse 300 mg doses over 10 min; 600 mg doses over 20 min, 900 mg doses over 30 min, and 1200 mg doses over 40 min

Continuous IV infusion
• Give first dose rapidly, and then follow with continuous infusion; rate is based on desired serum clindamycin levels
• To maintain serum concentrations above 4 mcg/ml, use a rapid infusion rate of 10 mg/min for 30 min and a maintenance rate of 0.75 mg/min; to maintain serum concentrations above 5 mcg/ml, use a rapid infusion rate of 15 mg/min for 30 min and a maintenance rate of 1 mg/min; to maintain serum concentrations above 5 mcg/ml, use a rapid infusion rate of 20 mg/min for 30 min and a maintenance rate of 1.25 mg/min

Syringe compatibilities: Amikacin, aztreonam, gentamicin, heparin

Syringe incompatibilities: Tobramycin

Y-site compatibilities: Acyclovir, alfentanil, amifostine, amikacin, aminocaproic acid, aminophylline, amiodarone, amphotericin B cholesteryl, amphotericin B lipid complex, amsacrine, anakinra, anidulafungin, ascorbic acid injection, atenolol, atracurium, atropine, aztreonam, benztropine, bivalirudin, bleomycin, bumetanide, buprenorphine, butorphanol, calcium chloride/gluconate, CARBOplatin, cefamandole, ceFAZolin, cefmetazole, cefonicid, cefoperazone, cefotaxime, cefoTEtan, cefOXitin, cefpirome, cefTAZidime, ceftizoxime, ceftobiprole, cefuroxime, cephalothin, cephapirin, chloramphenicol, cimetidine, cisatracurium, CISplatin, codeine, cyanocobalamin, cyclophosphamide, cycloSPORINE, cytarabine, DACTINomycin, DAPTOmycin, dexamethasone, dexmedetomidine, digoxin, diltiazem, diphenhydrAMINE, DOCEtaxel, DOPamine, doxacurium, DOXOrubicin, DOXOrubicin liposomal, doxycycline, enalaprilat, ePHEDrine, EPINEPHrine, epirubicin, epoetin alfa, eptifibatide, esmolol, etoposide, famotidine, fenoldopam, fentaNYL, fludarabine, fluorouracil, folic acid, foscarnet, furosemide, gatifloxacin, gemcitabine, gemtuzumab, gentamicin, glycopyrrolate, granisetron, heparin, hydrocortisone, HYDROmorphone, ifosfamide, imipenemcilastatin, indomethacin, insulin (regular), irinotecan, isoproterenol, ketorolac, levofloxacin, lidocaine, linezolid, LORazepam, LR, magnesium sulfate, mannitol, mechlorethamine, melphalan, meperidine, metaraminol, methicillin, methotrexate, methoxamine, methyldopate, methylPREDNISolone, metoclopramide, metoprolol, metroNIDAZOLE, mezlocillin, miconazole, milrinone, morphine, moxalactam, multiple vitamins injection, nafcillin, nalbuphine, naloxone, nesiritide, netilmicin, niCARdipine, nitroglycerin, nitroprusside, norepinephrine, octreotide, ondansetron, oxacillin, oxaliplatin, oxytocin, PACLitaxel, palonosetron, pamidronate, pancuronium, pantoprazole, PEMEtrexed, penicillin G potassium/sodium, pentazocine, perphenazine, PHENobarbital, phenylephrine, phytonadione, piperacillin, piperacillin-tazobactam, potassium chloride, procainamide, propofol, propranolol, protamine, pyridoxine, ranitidine, remifentanil, Ringer's, ritodrine, riTUXimab, rocuronium, sargramostim, sodium acetate/bicarbonate, succinylcholine, SUFentanil, tacrolimus, teniposide, theophylline, thiamine, thiotepa, ticarcillin, ticarcillin-clavulanate, tigecycline, tirofiban, TNA, tobramycin, tolazoline, TPN, trimetaphan, urokinase, vancomycin, vasopressin, vecuronium, verapamil, vinCRIStine, vinorelbine, vitamin B complex/C, voriconazole, zidovudine, zoledronic acid

Y-site incompatibilities: IDArubicin

Adverse effects: *italics* = common; **bold** = life-threatening

ADVERSE EFFECTS

GI: *Nausea, vomiting, abdominal pain, diarrhea,* **pseudomembranous colitis,** *anorexia, weight loss,* increased AST, ALT, bilirubin, alkaline phosphatase, jaundice
GU: *Vaginitis,* urinary frequency
INTEG: Rash, urticaria, pruritus, erythema, pain, abscess at inj site
SYST: Stevens-Johnson syndrome, exfoliative dermatitis

Pharmacokinetics

Absorption	Well absorbed (PO, IM), minimal (TOP)
Distribution	Widely distributed; crosses placenta
Metabolism	Liver, extensively
Excretion	Kidneys, breast milk
Half-life	2½ hr

Pharmacodynamics

	PO	IM	IV
Onset	Rapid	Rapid	Rapid
Peak	½-1 hr	1½ hr	Infusion's end

INTERACTIONS

Individual drugs

Erythromycin, chloramphenicol: decreased action of clindamycin
Kaolin: decreased absorption

Drug/lab test

Increased: alkaline phosphatase, bilirubin, CPK, AST, ALT

NURSING CONSIDERATIONS

Assessment

• Assess any patient with compromised renal system; product is excreted slowly in poor renal system function; toxicity may occur rapidly
• Assess patient for signs and symptoms of infection including characteristics of wounds, sputum, urine, stool, WBC >10,000/mm^3, fever; obtain baseline information before, during treatment; complete C&S testing before beginning product therapy; this will identify if correct treatment has been initiated, give product as soon as culture is taken
• Assess for allergic reactions: rash, urticaria, pruritus, chills, fever, joint pain; may occur a few days after therapy begins; epinephrine and resuscitation equipment should be available in case of an anaphylactic reaction
• Identify urine output; if decreasing, notify prescriber (may indicate nephrotoxicity); also look for increased BUN and creatinine levels

• Monitor blood studies: AST, ALT, CBC, Hct, bilirubin, LDH, alkaline phosphatase, Coombs' test monthly if patient is on long-term therapy
• Monitor electrolytes: potassium, sodium, chloride monthly if patient is on long-term therapy

> **BLACK BOX WARNING:** Assess bowel pattern daily; if severe diarrhea occurs, product should be discontinued; may indicate **pseudomembranous colitis**

• Monitor for bleeding: ecchymosis, bleeding gums, hematuria, stool guaiac daily if on long-term therapy, may occur several weeks after therapy is terminated
• Assess for overgrowth of infection: perineal itching, fever, malaise, redness, pain, swelling, drainage, rash, diarrhea, change in cough, sputum
⚠ Assess for serious skin infections: Stevens-Johnson syndrome, exfoliative dermatitis

Patient/family education

• Tell patient to take oral product with full glass of water; may take with food if GI symptoms occur; antiperistaltic products may worsen diarrhea
• Teach patient aspects of product therapy: need to complete entire course of medication to ensure organism death (10-14 days); culture may be taken after medication course has been completed
• Advise patient to report sore throat, fever, fatigue; may indicate **superinfection**
• Advise patient that product must be taken at equal intervals around clock to maintain blood levels

> **BLACK BOX WARNING:** Teach patient to report diarrhea with pus, mucus

Evaluation

Positive therapeutic outcome
• Decreased temp, negative C&S

TREATMENT OF HYPERSENSITIVITY: Withdraw product; maintain airway; administer EPINEPHrine, aminophylline, O_2, **IV** corticosteroids

clindamycin topical
See Appendix B

clobetasol topical
See Appendix B

---

clomiPHENE (Rx)
(kloe'mi-feen)
Clomid, Serophene
Func. class.: Ovulation stimulant
Chem. class.: Nonsteroidal antiestrogenic
Pregnancy category X

Do not confuse:
clomiPHENE/clomiPRAMINE,
Serophene/Sarafem

ACTION: Increases LH, FSH release from the pituitary, which increases maturation of ovarian follicle, ovulation, development of corpus luteum

Therapeutic outcome: Pregnancy

USES: Female infertility (ovulatory failure)

CONTRAINDICATIONS:
Pregnancy **X**, hypersensitivity, hepatic disease, undiagnosed uterine bleeding, uncontrolled thyroid or adrenal dysfunction, intracranial lesion, ovarian cysts, endometrial carcinoma

Precautions: Hypertension, depression, seizures, diabetes mellitus, abnormal ovarian enlargement, ovarian hyperstimulation

DOSAGE AND ROUTES
Adult: PO 50-100 mg daily $\times$ 5 days or 50 mg daily beginning on day 5 of the menstrual cycle, may increase to 100 mg/day $\times$ 5 days with next cycle; may be repeated until conception occurs or 3 (max 6) cycles of therapy have been completed

Available forms: Tabs 50 mg

Implementation
• Give after discontinuing estrogen therapy
• Give at same time daily to maintain product level; begin on 5th day of menstrual cycle
• Avoid heat, moisture, light, store at room temperature
• Give without regard to food

ADVERSE EFFECTS
CNS: *Headache, depression,* restlessness, anxiety, nervousness, fatigue, insomnia, dizziness, flushing
CV: Vasomotor flushing, phlebitis, **deep vein thrombosis**
EENT: Blurred vision, diplopia, photophobia
GI: *Nausea, vomiting, constipation,* abdominal pain, bloating

GU: Polyuria, frequency of urination, **birth defects, spontaneous abortions,** multiple ovulation, breast pain, oliguria, abnormal uterine bleeding, ovarian cyst, hypertrophy of ovary
INTEG: *Rash, dermatitis,* urticaria, alopecia

Pharmacokinetics

Absorption	Well distributed
Distribution	Unknown
Metabolism	Liver, extensively
Excretion	Feces
Half-life	5 days

Pharmacodynamics
Unknown

NURSING CONSIDERATIONS
Assessment
• Determine liver function tests before therapy: AST, ALT, alkaline phosphatase
• Monitor serum progesterone, urinary excretion of pregnanediol to identify occurrence of ovulation
• Pelvic exam should be done to determine ovary size, condition of cervix
• Endometrial biopsy may be done in women over 35 to rule out endometrial carcinoma

Patient/family education
• Advise patient that multiple births are common after product is taken
• Instruct patient to notify prescriber immediately if low abdominal pain occurs; may indicate ovarian cyst, cyst rupture
⚠ **Advise patient to notify prescriber of photophobia, blurred vision, diplopia, abnormal bleeding**
• Teach patient if dose is missed, double at next time; if more than one dose is missed, call prescriber
• Instruct patient that response usually occurs 4-10 days after last day of treatment
• Teach patient method for taking, recording basal body temp to determine whether ovulation has occurred; if ovulation can be determined (there is a slight decrease in temp, then a sharp increase for ovulation), to attempt coitus 3 days before and every other day until after ovulation
⚠ **Teach patient if pregnancy (X) is suspected, to notify prescriber immediately**

Evaluation
Positive therapeutic outcome
• Fertility

clomiPRAMINE (Rx)
(klom-ip′ra-meen)
Anafranil
Func. class.: Tricyclic antidepressant
Chem. class.: Tertiary amine
Pregnancy category C

Do not confuse:
clomiPRAMINE/clomiPHENE/desipramine/
Norpramin

ACTION: Potentiates serotonin and nor-epinephrine uptake; moderate anticholinergic effect

Therapeutic outcome: Decreased signs and symptoms of obsessive-compulsive disorder, decreased depression

USES: Obsessive-compulsive disorder

Unlabeled uses: Dysphoria, anxiety, agoraphobia and other phobias

CONTRAINDICATIONS:
Hypersensitivity to this product, carBAMazepine, tricyclics, immediately after MI

Precautions: Pregnancy **C**, breastfeeding, geriatric, seizures, cardiac disease, glaucoma, prostatic hypertrophy, urinary retention

> **BLACK BOX WARNING:** Suicidal ideation, children

DOSAGE AND ROUTES
Obsessive-compulsive disorder
Adult: PO 25 mg at bedtime; increase gradually over 4 wk to a dosage of 75-250 mg/day in divided doses
Child 10-18 yr: PO 25 mg/day gradually increased max over 2 wk 3 mg/kg/day or 200 mg/day, whichever is smaller

Available forms: Caps 25, 50, 75 mg

Implementation
• Do not break, crush, or chew caps
• Give without regard to food; during initial dosing and titration, give with meals
• Store in tight container, at room temperature; do not freeze

ADVERSE EFFECTS
CNS: *Dizziness, tremors, mania,* **seizures,** aggressiveness, drowsiness, headache, EPS, **neuroleptic malignant syndrome,** insomnia, agitation, anxiety, impaired memory

CV: Hypotension, tachycardia, **cardiac arrest,** hypertension, palpitations
EENT: Blurred vision, altered taste, tinnitus, increased intraocular pressure
ENDO: Galactorrhea, hyperprolactinemia
GI: *Constipation, dry mouth, nausea, dyspepsia,* weight gain, **hepatic toxicity**
GU: *Delayed ejaculation, anorgasmia,* retention, decreased libido
HEMA: Agranulocytosis, neutropenia, pancytopenia
INTEG: Diaphoresis, photosensitivity, abnormal skin odor, flushing, rash, pruritus
META: Hyponatremia
RESP: Pharyngitis, rhinitis, bronchospasm
SYST: Suicide in children/adolescents

Pharmacokinetics
Absorption	Well absorbed
Distribution	Widely distributed
Metabolism	Liver, extensively
Excretion	Kidneys, breast milk
Half-life	19-37 hr; steady state 1-2 wk

Pharmacodynamics
Onset	≥2 wk
Peak	2-6 hr
Duration	Unknown

INTERACTIONS
Individual drugs
Alcohol: increased CNS depression
CarBAMazepine: decreased clomiPRAMINE action
Cimetidine, FLUoxetine, fluvoxaMINE, sertraline: increased clomiPRAMINE level; do not use together
CloNIDine, EPINEPHrine, norepinephrine: severe hypertension; avoid use
CloNIDine, haloperidol, levodopa: decreased effect of these products
Phenytoin: decreased clomiPRAMINE action

Drug classifications
Barbiturates: decreased clomiPRAMINE levels
CNS depressants, general anesthetics: increased effects; do not use together
CYP1A2, CYP2D6: increased clomiPRAMINE level
MAOIs: hypertensive crisis, seizures; do not use together
SSRIs, SNRIs: increased serotonin syndrome
Other tricyclics, phenothiazines, quinolones: QT prolongation

Skeletal muscle relaxants, opiates: decreased action of these products

Drug/herb

SAM-e, St. John's wort: serotonin syndrome, do not use together

Drug/lab test

Increased: prolactin, TBG, AST, ALT, blood glucose

Decreased: serum thyroid hormone (T_3, T_4)

NURSING CONSIDERATIONS

Assessment

• Monitor B/P (with patient lying, standing), pulse q4hr; if systolic B/P drops 20 mm Hg hold product, notify prescriber; take VS q4hr in patients with cardiovascular disease

• Monitor blood studies: CBC, leukocytes, differential, cardiac enzymes if patient is receiving long-term therapy and signs of blood dyscrasias

⚠ Serotonin syndrome: hyperpyrexia, rigidity, irregular pulse, diaphoresis

⚠ Monitor hepatic studies: AST, ALT, bilirubin

⚠ Check weight weekly; appetite may increase with product

⚠ Assess ECG for flattening of T wave, QTc prolongation bundle branch block, AV block, dysrhythmias in cardiac patients, may lead to cardiac collapse

• Assess for EPS primarily in geriatric: rigidity, dystonia, akathisia

> **BLACK BOX WARNING:** Assess mental status: mood, sensorium, affect, suicidal tendencies; increase in psychiatric symptoms: depression, panic, frequency of obsessive-compulsive behaviors

• Monitor urinary retention, constipation; constipation is more likely to occur in children or geriatric

• Assess for **withdrawal symptoms:** headache, nausea, vomiting, muscle pain, weakness; do not usually occur unless product was discontinued abruptly

• Identify alcohol consumption; if alcohol is consumed, hold dose until morning

Patient/family education

• Teach patient that therapeutic effects may take 4-6 wk

• Teach patient to use caution in driving or other activities requiring alertness because of drowsiness, dizziness, blurred vision; to avoid rising quickly from sitting to standing, especially geriatric

• Teach patient to avoid alcohol ingestion, other CNS depressants

• Teach patient not to discontinue medication quickly after long-term use: may cause nausea, headache, malaise

• Teach patient to wear sunscreen or large hat, since photosensitivity occurs

• Teach patient to increase fluids, bulk in diet if constipation, urinary retention occur, especially geriatric

⚠ Serotonin syndrome: teach patient to report immediately sweating, diarrhea, twitching

⚠ Abrupt discontinuation: do not stop abruptly

• Teach patient to take gum, hard sugarless candy, or frequent sips of water for dry mouth

• Advise patient to notify prescriber if pregnancy is planned or suspected

> **BLACK BOX WARNING:** Teach patient that suicidal ideas, behavior may occur in children/young adults, report immediately

Evaluation

Positive therapeutic outcome

• Decrease in depression

• Absence of suicidal thoughts

TREATMENT OF OVERDOSE:

ECG monitoring, induce emesis, lavage, activated charcoal, administer anticonvulsant

clonazePAM (Rx)

(kloe-na'zi-pam)

KlonoPIN

Func. class.: Anticonvulsant

Chem. class.: Benzodiazepine derivative

Pregnancy category D

Controlled substance schedule IV

Do not confuse:

clonazePAM/LORazepam/clorazepate/cloNIDine, KlonoPIN/cloNIDine

ACTION: Inhibits spike, wave formation in absence seizures (petit mal), decreases amplitude, frequency, duration, spread of discharge in minor motor seizures

Therapeutic outcome: Decreased frequency, severity of seizures

USES: Absence, atypical absence, akinetic, myoclonic seizures, Lennox-Gastaut syndrome, panic disorder

CONTRAINDICATIONS:

Pregnancy **D**, hypersensitivity to benzodiaz-epines, acute closed-angle glaucoma, psychosis, severe liver disease

Precautions: Open-angle glaucoma, chronic respiratory disease, renal/hepatic disease, breastfeeding, geriatric

DOSAGE AND ROUTES

Lennox-Gastaut syndrome/atypical absence seizures/akinetic and myoclonic seizures

Adult: PO max 1.5 mg/day in 3 divided doses; may be increased 0.5-1 mg q3day until desired response; max 20 mg/day

Child <10 yr or <30 kg: PO 0.01-0.03 mg/kg/day in divided doses q8hr, max 0.05 mg/kg/day; may be increased 0.25-0.5 mg q3day until desired response; max 0.1-0.2 mg/kg/day

Geriatric: PO 0.25 daily-bid initially, increase by 0.25 daily q7-14day as needed

Panic disorder

Adult: PO 0.25 mg bid, increase to 1 mg/day after 3 days, max 4 mg/day

Available forms: Tabs 0.5, 1, 2 mg; **orally disintegrating tabs** 0.125, 0.25, 0.5, 1, 2 mg

Implementation

PO route

• Give on empty stomach for best absorption

Rectal route

• IV sol may be used rectally, 1 ml syringe inserted 3 cm into rectum

• Oral susp may be used rectally (1 mg/ml of product with 1 ml of water), use plastic tube (volume 2.2-3.3 ml)

• Store at room temperature

ADVERSE EFFECTS

CNS: *Drowsiness,* dizziness, confusion, behavioral changes, tremors, insomnia, headache, **suicidal tendencies,** slurred speech, anterograde amnesia

CV: Palpitations, bradycardia, tachycardia

EENT: *Increased salivation, nystagmus, diplopia,* abnormal eye movements

GI: *Nausea, constipation,* polyphagia, anorexia, xerostomia, diarrhea, gastritis, sore gums

GU: Dysuria, enuresis, nocturia, retention, libido changes

HEMA: Thrombocytopenia, leukocytosis, eosinophilia

INTEG: Rash, alopecia, hirsutism

RESP: **Respiratory depression,** dyspnea, congestion

Pharmacokinetics

Absorption	Well absorbed
Distribution	Crosses blood-brain barrier, placenta
Metabolism	Liver, protein binding 85%
Excretion	Kidneys
Half-life	18-50 hr

Pharmacodynamics

Onset	½-1 hr
Peak	1-2 hr
Duration	6-12 hr

INTERACTIONS

Individual drugs

Alcohol: increased CNS depression
CarBAMazepine: decreased clonazePAM effect
Cimetidine, clarithromycin, diltiazem, erythromycin, FLUoxetine: increased clonazePAM effect
PHENobarbitol: decreased clonazePAM effect
Phenytoin: decreased clonazePAM levels

Drug classifications

Anticonvulsants, antidepressants, barbiturates, general anesthetics, opiates, sedative/hypnotics: increased CNS depression
Azoles, oral contraceptives: increased clonazePAM effect
CYP3A4 inducers: decreased clonazePAM effect

Drug/herb

Ginkgo, melatonin: increased clonazePAM effect
Ginseng, St. John's wort: decreased clonazePAM effect
Kava, chamomile, valerian: increased sedative effect

Drug/lab test

Increased: AST, alkaline phosphatase
Decreased: platelets, WBC

NURSING CONSIDERATIONS

Assessment

• Assess for **blood dyscrasias:** fever, sore throat, bruising, rash, jaundice, epistaxis (long-term treatment only)

• Assess **seizures:** duration, type, intensity, with or without aura

⚠ **Assess mental status: mood, sensorium, affect, memory (long, short), especially geriatric; behavioral changes, suicidal thoughts/behaviors**

• Assess seizure activity including type, location, duration, and character; provide seizure precaution

• Assess renal studies: urinalysis, BUN, urine creatinine

• Monitor blood studies: RBCs, Hct, Hgb, reticulocyte counts weekly for 4 wk, then monthly
• Monitor hepatic studies: ALT, AST, bilirubin, creatinine
⚠ **Abrupt discontinuation: do not discontinue abruptly, seizures may increase**
• Assess for signs of physical withdrawal if medication suddenly discontinued
• Assess eye problems: need for ophthalmic examinations before, during, after treatment (slit lamp, fundoscopy, tonometry)
• Assess allergic reaction: red raised rash; if this occurs, product should be discontinued
• Monitor for **toxicity:** bone marrow depression, nausea, vomiting, ataxia, diplopia, cardiovascular collapse; monitor drug levels during initial treatment (therapeutic 20-80 ng/ml)

Patient/family education
• Teach patient to carry/wear emergency ID card stating patient's name, products taken, condition, physician's name, phone number
• Caution patient to avoid driving, other activities that require alertness
• Caution patient to avoid alcohol ingestion or CNS depressants; increased sedation may occur
⚠ **Teach patient not to discontinue medication quickly after long-term use; taper off over several weeks**
⚠ **Teach patient to notify prescriber of yellowing skin/eyes, pale stools, bleeding, fever, extreme fatigue, sore throat, suicidal thoughts/behaviors**
⚠ **Teach patient to notify prescriber immediately if suicidal thoughts, behaviors occur**

Evaluation
Positive therapeutic outcome
• Decreased seizure activity

TREATMENT OF OVERDOSE:
Lavage, activated charcoal, VS, flumazenil, monitor electrolytes

---

cloNIDine (Rx)
(klon′i-deen)
Catapres, Catapres-TTS, Duraclon, Kapvay, Nexiclon
Func. class.: Antihypertensive, centrally acting analgesic
Chem. class.: Centrally acting α-adrenergic agonist
Pregnancy category C

Do not confuse:
cloNIDine/KlonoPIN/clonazePAM,
Catapres/Cataflam/catarase

ACTION: Inhibits sympathetic vasomotor center in CNS, which reduces impulses in sympathetic nervous system; B/P, pulse rate, cardiac output decreased; prevents pain signal transmission in CNS by α-adrenergic receptor stimulation of the spinal cord

Therapeutic outcome: Decreased B/P in hypertension

USES: Mild to moderate hypertension, used alone or in combination; severe pain in cancer patients (epidural), attention-deficit/hyperactivity disorder (ADHD)

Unlabeled uses: Opioid withdrawal, prevention of vascular headaches, treatment of menopausal symptoms, dysmenorrhea, attention-deficit/hyperactivity disorder (ADHD), autism, cycloSPORINE nephrotoxicity prophylaxis, diabetic neuropathy, ethanol/nicotine/opiate agonist withdrawal, Tourette's syndrome, hypertensive emergency, neonatal abstinence syndrome, scleroderma renal crisis

CONTRAINDICATIONS:
Hypersensitivity; (epidural) bleeding disorders, anticoagulants

Precautions: Pregnancy C, breastfeeding, child <12 yr (transdermal), geriatric, MI (recent), diabetes mellitus, chronic renal failure, Raynaud's disease, thyroid disease, depression, COPD, asthma, noncompliant patients

> **BLACK BOX WARNING:** Labor

DOSAGE AND ROUTES
Hypertension
Adult: PO/TD 0.1 mg bid, then increase by 0.1-0.2 mg/day at weekly intervals, until desired response; range 0.2-0.6 mg/day in divided doses
Geriatric: PO 0.1 mg at bedtime, may increase gradually
Child: PO 5-10 mcg/kg/day in divided doses q8-12hr, max 0.9 mg/day

Opioid withdrawal (unlabeled)
Adult: PO 0.3-1.2 mg/day; may decrease by 50% × 3 days, then decrease by 0.1-0.2 mg/day or discontinue

Severe pain
Adult: CONT EPIDURAL INF 30 mcg/hr
Child: CONT EPIDURAL INF 0.5 mcg/kg/hr, then titrate to response

Menopausal symptoms (unlabeled)
Adult: TD 0.1 mg patch q1wk; PO 0.05-0.4 mg daily

ADHD/tic disorders in children/autism (unlabeled)
Adolescent/child ≥6 yr: PO 0.05 mg/kg/day in 3-4 divided doses; may increase by 0.1 mg/day qwk up to 0.4 mg/day; EXT REL (Kapvay): 0.1 mg at bedtime, increase dose by 0.1 mg/day up to 0.4 mg/day

Tourette's syndrome (unlabeled)
Adult: PO 0.15-0.2 mg/day

Available forms: Tabs 0.025 ✿, 0.1, 0.2, 0.3 mg; transdermal sys 2.5, 5, 7.5 mg delivering 0.1, 0.2, 0.3 mg/24 hr, respectively; inj 100, 500 mcg/ml, ext rel tab 0.1 mg (Kapvay), 0.17 mg (Nexiclon)

Implementation
PO route
- Give last dose at bedtime
- Do not crush, cut, chew, or break ER tabs; Kapvay is not interchangeable with other products

Transdermal route
- Apply patch weekly; remove old patch and wash off residue; apply to site without hair; best absorption over chest or upper arm; rotate sites with each application; clean site before application; apply firmly, especially around edges, may secure with adhesive tape if loose; fold sticky sides together and discard
- Should be removed before MRI
- Store patches in cool environment, tabs in tight container

ADVERSE EFFECTS
CNS: *Drowsiness, sedation, headache, fatigue,* nightmares, insomnia, mental changes, anxiety, depression, hallucinations, delirium, syncope, dizziness
CV: *Orthostatic hypotension, palpitations,* **CHF,** ECG abnormalities, sinus tachycardia
EENT: Taste change, parotid pain
ENDO: Hyperglycemia
GI: *Nausea, vomiting, malaise,* constipation, *dry mouth*
GU: Impotence, dysuria, *nocturia,* gynecomastia
INTEG: *Rash,* alopecia, facial pallor, pruritus, hives, edema, burning papules, excoriation (TD patches)
MISC: *Withdrawal symptoms*
MS: Muscle, joint pain, leg cramps

Pharmacokinetics

Absorption	Well absorbed (PO, TD)
Distribution	Widely distributed; crosses blood-brain barrier
Metabolism	Liver, extensively
Excretion	Kidneys, unchanged (45%)
Half-life	12-21 hr

Pharmacodynamics

	PO	TD
Onset	½-1 hr	3 days
Peak	2-4 hr	Unknown
Duration	8-12 hr	8 hr (after removal)

INTERACTIONS
Individual drugs
Alcohol: increased CNS depression
Levodopa: decreased levodopa effect
Prazosin: decreased hypotensive effects
Verapamil, diltiazem: AV block

Drug classifications
Amphetamines, appetite suppressants, MAOIs, tricyclics: decreased hypotensive effects
Anesthetics, opiates, sedatives/hypnotics: increased CNS depression
Antidepressants (tricyclic), β-adrenergic blockers: life-threatening increase in B/P
Diuretics, nitrates: increased hypotensive effects

Drug/herb
Aconite: increased toxicity, death
Ephedra, ginseng: decreased antihypertensive effect
Hawthorn: increased antihypertensive effect

Drug/lab test
Increased: blood glucose
Decreased: VMA, urinary catecholamines, aldosterone

NURSING CONSIDERATIONS
Assessment
- Assess **cancer pain:** location, intensity, character, alleviating, aggravation factors, baseline and frequency
- Perform blood studies: neutrophils, decreased platelets
- Perform renal studies: protein, BUN, creatinine; watch for increased levels that may indicate nephrotic syndrome: polyuria, oliguria, frequency
- Monitor baselines for renal/liver function tests before therapy begins; check potassium levels, although hyperkalemia rarely occurs

C

• Monitor B/P, pulse if the product is being used for **hypertension;** notify prescriber of changes

• Assess for **opiate withdrawal** (unlabeled) in patients receiving the product for opioid withdrawal, including fever, diarrhea, nausea, vomiting, cramps, insomnia, shivering, dilated pupils, weakness

• Check for edema in feet, legs daily; monitor I&O; check for decreasing output

• Assess **allergic reaction:** rash, fever, pruritus, urticaria; product should be discontinued if antihistamines fail to help

• ADHD: monitor B/P, pulse, palpitations, syncope

• Assess for symptoms of **CHF:** edema; dyspnea, wet crackles, B/P, weight gain, report significant changes, more common in the elderly

Patient/family education

⚠ **Instruct patient not to discontinue product abruptly, or withdrawal symptoms may occur: anxiety, increased B/P, headache, insomnia, increased pulse, tremors, nausea, sweating**

• Caution patient not to use OTC (cough, cold, or allergy), alcohol or CNS depressant products unless directed by prescriber

• Teach patient to comply with dosage schedule even if feeling better; product controls symptoms, does not cure

• Caution patient to change position slowly, to rise slowly to sitting or standing position to minimize orthostatic hypotension, especially geriatric

• Instruct patient to notify physician of mouth sores, sore throat, fever, swelling of hands or feet, irregular heartbeat, chest pain, signs of **angioedema,** increased weight

• Teach patient about excessive perspiration, dehydration, vomiting; diarrhea may lead to fall in B/P; consult prescriber if these occur

• Tell patient that product may cause dizziness, fainting; light-headedness may occur during first few days of therapy; use hard candy, saliva product, or frequent rinsing of mouth for dry mouth

• **Transdermal:** teach patient how to use patch; that patch comes in two parts: product patch and overlay to keep patch in place; not to trim or cut patch

• Advise patient that compliance is necessary; not to skip or stop product unless directed by prescriber

• Teach patient that product may cause skin rash or impaired perspiration

• Teach patient that response may take 2-3 days if product is given TD; instruct on administration of patch; return demonstration

• Teach patient to avoid hazardous activities, since product may cause drowsiness, dizziness

• Teach patient to administer 1 hr before meals

Evaluation

Positive therapeutic outcome

• Decrease in B/P in hypertension

• Decrease in withdrawal symptoms

• Decrease in pain

• Decrease in vascular headaches

• Decrease in dysmenorrhea

• Decrease in menopausal symptoms

TREATMENT OF OVERDOSE:

Supportive treatment; administer tolazoline, atropine, DOPamine prn

---

clopidogrel (Rx)

(klo-pid′oh-grel)

Plavix

Func. class.: Platelet aggregation inhibitor

Chem. class.: Thienopyridine derivative

Pregnancy category B

Do not confuse:

Plavix/Paxil/Elavil

ACTION: Inhibits first and second phases of ADP-induced effects in platelet aggregation

Therapeutic outcome: Decreased possibility of stroke, MI by decreasing platelet aggregation

USES: Reducing the risk of stroke, MI, vascular death, peripheral arterial disease in high-risk patients, acute coronary syndrome, transient ischemic attack (TIA), unstable angina

CONTRAINDICATIONS:

Hypersensitivity, active bleeding

Precautions: Pregnancy **B,** breastfeeding, children, past liver disease, increased bleeding risk, neutropenia, agranulocytosis, renal disease, Asian/Black/Caucasian patients

BLACK BOX WARNING: CYP2C19 allele (poor metabolizers)

Adverse effects: *italics* = common; **bold** = life-threatening

DOSAGE AND ROUTES
Recent MI, stroke, peripheral arterial disease, TIA
Adult: PO 75 mg daily with aspirin

Acute coronary syndrome
Adult: PO loading dose 300 mg then 75 mg daily with aspirin

Available forms: Tabs 75, 300 mg

Implementation
• Give with food to decrease gastric symptoms
• Product should be discontinued 5 days before elective surgery if an antiplatelet action is not desired

ADVERSE EFFECTS
CNS: Headache, dizziness, depression, syncope, hyperesthesia, neuralgia, confusion, hallucinations
CV: Edema, hypertension, chest pain
GI: Nausea, vomiting, diarrhea, GI discomfort, **GI bleeding, pancreatitis,** hepatic failure
GU: Glomerulonephritis
HEMA: *Epistaxis,* purpura, **bleeding (major/minor from any site), neutropenia, aplastic anemia, agranulocytosis, thrombotic thrombocytopenic purpura**
INTEG: Rash, pruritus
MISC: UTI, hypercholesterolemia, chest pain, fatigue, **intracranial hemorrhage, toxic epidermal necrolysis, Stevens-Johnson syndrome,** flu-like syndrome, **anaphylaxis**
MS: Arthralgia, back pain
RESP: Upper respiratory tract infection, dyspnea, rhinitis, bronchitis, cough, **bronchospasm**

Pharmacokinetics
Absorption	Rapidly absorbed
Distribution	Unknown
Metabolism	Liver, extensively, protein binding 95%
Excretion	Kidneys, unchanged product
Half-life	6 hr

Pharmacodynamics
Onset	Unknown
Peak	1-3 hr
Duration	Unknown

INTERACTIONS
Individual drugs
Abciximab, aspirin, eptifibatide, rifampin, ticlopidine, tirofiban, treprostinil: increased bleeding tendencies
Fluvastatin, phenytoin, tamoxifen, TOLBUTamide, torsemide, warfarin: increased action of each specific product

Drug classifications
Anticoagulants, NSAIDs, SSRIs, thrombolytics: increased bleeding tendencies
CYP3A4 inhibitors/substrates (atorvastatin, cerivistatin, esomeprazole, omeprazole, simvistatin): decreased effects

> **BLACK BOX WARNING:** CYP2C19 inhibitors: avoid use

NSAIDs: increased action of some NSAIDs
Proton pump inhibitors (PPIs): decreased clopidogrel effect

Drug/herb
Bilberry, saw palmetto: decreased clopidogrel effect
Feverfew, fish oil, garlic, ginger, ginkgo biloba, green tea, horse chestnut, omega-3 fatty acids: increased clopidogrel effect

Drug/lab test
Increased: AST, ALT, bilirubin, uric acid, total cholesterol, nonprotein nitrogen (NPN)

NURSING CONSIDERATIONS
Assessment

> **BLACK BOX WARNING:** CYP2C19 allele (poor metabolizers): Consider using another antiplatelet product, higher CV reaction occurs after acute coronary syndrome or PCI, tests are available to determine CYP2C19 allele

• Assess for symptoms of stroke, MI during treatment
• Assess for thrombotic/thrombocytic purpura; fever, thrombocytopenia, neurolytic anemia
• Monitor liver function tests: AST, ALT, bilirubin, creatinine if patient is on long-term therapy (4 mo or more)
• Monitor blood studies: CBC, Hct, Hgb, protime, cholesterol if patient is on long-term therapy; thrombocytopenia, neutropenia may occur

Patient/family education
• Advise patient that blood work will be necessary during treatment

• Advise patient to report any unusual bleeding to prescriber, that it may take longer to stop bleeding
• Teach patient to take without regard to food
• Caution patient to report diarrhea, skin rashes, subcutaneous bleeding, chills, fever, sore throat
• Teach patient to tell all health care providers that clopidogrel is being used; may be held for 5 days before surgery

Evaluation
Positive therapeutic outcome
• Absence of stroke

---

clotrimazole topical
See Appendix B

clotrimazole vaginal antifungal
See Appendix B

cloZAPine (Rx)
(kloz′a-peen)
Clozaril, Fazaclo, Versacloz
Func. class.: Antipsychotic
Chem. class.: Tricyclic dibenzodiazepine derivative
Pregnancy category B

Do not confuse:
Clozaril/Clinoril/Colazal

ACTION: Interferes with dopamine receptor binding with lack of EPS and tardive dyskinesia; also acts as an adrenergic, cholinergic, histaminergic, serotoninergic antagonist

Therapeutic outcome: Decreased psychotic behavior

USES: Management of psychotic symptoms in schizophrenic patients for whom other antipsychotics have failed, recurrent suicidal behavior; orally disintegrating tabs are not used for recurrent suicidal behavior

Unlabeled uses: Agitation, bipolar disorder, dementia, psychosis in Parkinson's disease

CONTRAINDICATIONS:
Hypersensitivity, severe granulocytopenia (WBC <3500/mm[3] before therapy), coma

---

BLACK BOX WARNING: Myeloproliferative disorders, severe CNS depression, agranulocytosis, leukopenia, neutropenia, seizure disorders

Precautions: Pregnancy **B**, breastfeeding, children <16 yr, geriatric, renal/hepatic/cardiac/CV/pulmonary disease, seizures, prostatic enlargement, closed-angle glaucoma, stroke

BLACK BOX WARNING: Bone marrow suppression, hypotension, myocarditis, orthostatic hypotension, seizures, elderly patients with dementia-related psychosis

DOSAGE AND ROUTES
Schizophrenia
Adult: PO 12.5 mg daily or bid; may increase by 25-50 mg/day; normal range 300-450 mg/day 1-2 ×/wk; do not increase dosage more than 2 times/wk; dose > 500 mg requires 3 divided doses; max 900 mg/day; use lowest dosage to control symptoms; if dose is to be discontinued, taper over 1-2 wk
Adolescent, child ≥9 yr (unlabeled): PO 6.25-12.5 mg initially slowly titrate

Dementia with multiple behavioral disturbances (unlabeled)
Geriatric: PO 12.5 mg qd at bedtime, may increase by 12.5 mg every other day; max 50 mg/day

Available forms: Tabs 25, 50, 100, 200 mg; orally disintegrating tabs 25, 100 mg; Fazaclo 12.5, 25, 100, 150, 200 mg; oral suspension 50 mg/ml

Implementation
• Decrease dosage in geriatric since metabolism is slowed
• Give with full glass of water, milk; or give with food to decrease GI upset
• Store in tight, light-resistant container; oral sol in amber bottle
• Patient-specific registration is required before administration; if WBC <3500 cells/mm[3] or ANC <2000 cells/mm[2], therapy should not be started, pharmacist may only dispense the 7, 14, 28 day supply upon receipt of lab report that is appropriate
• **Orally disintegrating tab:** do not push through foil, leave in foil blister until ready to take, peel back foil, place tab in mouth, allow to dissolve, swallow; water is not needed

---

Adverse effects: *italics* = common; **bold** = life-threatening

ADVERSE EFFECTS

CNS: *Sedation, salivation, dizziness, head-ache, tremors, sleep problems, akinesia, fever,* **seizures,** *sweating, akathisia, confusion, fatigue, insomnia, depression, slurred speech, anxiety,* **neuroleptic malignant syndrome,** agitation, dystonia, obsessive-compulsive symptoms

CV: *Tachycardia, hypo/hypertension,* chest pain, ECG changes, orthostatic hypotension

EENT: Blurred vision

GI: *Drooling or excessive salivation, constipation, nausea, abdominal discomfort, vomiting, diarrhea,* anorexia, weight gain, dry mouth, heartburn, dyspepsia, gastroesophageal reflux

GU: *Urinary abnormalities,* incontinence, ejaculation dysfunction, frequency, urgency, retention, dysuria

HEMA: **Leukopenia, neutropenia, agranulocytosis, eosinophilia**

MS: Weakness; pain in back, neck, legs; spasm; rigidity

RESP: Dyspnea, nasal congestion, lower respiratory tract infection

OTHER: Diaphoresis

SYST: **Death in geriatric patients with dementia,** aggravation of diabetes mellitus

Pharmacokinetics

Absorption	Well absorbed
Distribution	Widely distributed; crosses blood-brain barrier, placenta; 95% protein binding
Metabolism	Liver, CYP1A2, 2D6, 3A4
Excretion	Kidneys (50%), feces (30%) (metabolites)
Half-life	8-12 hr

Pharmacodynamics

Onset	Unknown
Peak	Unknown
Duration	8-12 hr

INTERACTIONS

Individual drugs

Alcohol: increased CNS depression

Caffeine, citalopram, erythromycin, FLUoxetine, fluvoxaMINE, ketoconazole, risperiDONE, ritonavir, sertraline: increased cloZAPine levels

CarBAMazepine, omeprazole, PHENobarbital, rifampin: decreased cloZAPine level

Digoxin: increased plasma concentration of digoxin

Warfarin: increased plasma concentrations

Drug classifications

Benzodiazepines: increased hypotension, respiratory, cardiac arrest, collapse

β-blockers, class IA/III antidysrhythmics, and other drugs that increase QT: increased QT prolongation

CNS depressants, psychoactives: increased CNS depression

CYP1A2 inducers: decreased cloZAPine levels

CYP1A2 inhibitors, CYP3A4 inhibitors: increased cloZAPine level

Highly protein-bound products: increased plasma concentrations

Drug/food

Caffeine: increased cloZAPine levels

Drug/lab test

Increased: liver function tests, cardiac enzymes, cholesterol, blood glucose, bilirubin, PBI, cholinesterase, ^{131}I, Hct/Hgb, erythrocyte sedimentation rate

Decreased: WBC

False positive: pregnancy tests, PKU

False negative: urinary steroids, 17-OHCS

NURSING CONSIDERATIONS

Assessment

• Assess for **myocarditis** if suspected, discontinue; myocarditis usually occurs during first month of treatment

> **BLACK BOX WARNING:** Assess for **seizures;** usually occurs with higher doses (>600 mg/day) or dosage change >100 mg/day; do not use in uncontrolled seizure disorder; use cautiously in those with a predisposition to seizures

• Assess mental status: orientation, mood, behavior, presence of hallucinations, and type before initial administration and monthly; this product should significantly reduce psychotic behavior

• Check for swallowing of PO medication; check for hoarding or giving of medication to other patients

• Monitor I&O ratio; palpate bladder if low urinary output occurs, especially in geriatric; urinalysis recommended before, during prolonged therapy

BLACK BOX WARNING: Bone marrow depression: Monitor bilirubin, CBC, liver function test monthly; discontinue treatment if WBC <3000/mm³ or if ANC <1500/mm³; test qwk; may resume when normal; if WBC <2000/mm³ or ANC <1000/mm³, discontinue; **if agranulocytosis develops, never restart product**

• Assess affect, orientation, LOC, reflexes, gait, coordination, sleep pattern disturbances

BLACK BOX WARNING: Hypotension: Monitor B/P with patient sitting, standing, and lying; take pulse and respirations q4hr during initial treatment; establish baseline before starting treatment; report drops of 30 mm Hg

• Check for dizziness, faintness, palpitations, tachycardia on rising
• Assess for **neuroleptic malignant syndrome:** hyperpyrexia, muscle rigidity, increased CPK, altered mental status; product should be discontinued
• Assess for **EPS** including akathisia (inability to sit still, no pattern to movements), tardive dyskinesia (bizarre movements of the jaw, mouth, tongue, extremities), pseudoparkinsonism (rigidity, tremors, pill rolling, shuffling gate)
• Assess for constipation, urinary retention daily; if these occur, increase bulk, water in diet

Patient/family education
• Teach patient to use good oral hygiene; frequent rinsing of mouth, sugarless gum for dry mouth
• Caution patient to avoid hazardous activities until product response is determined
• Inform patient that orthostatic hypotension occurs often and to rise from sitting or lying position gradually
• Caution patient to avoid hot tubs, hot showers, tub baths, since hypotension may occur
• Teach patient to avoid OTC preparations (cough, hay fever, cold) unless approved by prescriber, since serious product interactions may occur; avoid use with alcohol, CNS depressants; increased drowsiness may occur
• Teach patient about EPS and necessity of meticulous oral hygiene, since oral candidiasis may occur
• Teach patient to report sore throat, malaise, fever, bleeding, mouth sores; if these occur, CBC should be performed and product discontinued
• Advise patient that in hot weather, heat stroke may occur; take extra precautions to stay cool

BLACK BOX WARNING: Teach patient symptoms of agranulocytosis and need for blood test qwk for 6 mo, then q2wk; report flulike symptoms

Evaluation
Positive therapeutic outcome
• Decrease in emotional excitement, hallucinations, delusions, paranoia
• Reorganization of patterns of thought, speech

TREATMENT OF ANAPHYLAXIS: Withdraw product, maintain airway; if diabetic, check blood glucose levels

codeine (Rx)
(koe′deen)
Func. class.: Opiate, phenanthrene derivative
Pregnancy category C
Controlled substance schedule II, III, IV, V (depends on content)

Do not confuse:
codeine/Lodine/Iodine/Cardene

ACTION: Depresses pain impulse transmission at the spinal cord level by interacting with opioid receptors; decreases cough reflex, GI motility

Therapeutic outcome: Pain relief, decreased cough, decreased diarrhea depending on route

USES: Moderate to severe pain

Unlabeled uses: Diarrhea, nonproductive cough

CONTRAINDICATIONS:
Hypersensitivity to opiates, respiratory depression, increased intracranial pressure, seizure disorders, severe respiratory disorders, breastfeeding

BLACK BOX WARNING: Children (tonsillectomy/adenoidectomy)

Precautions: Pregnancy **C**, geriatric, cardiac dysrhythmias, prostatic hypertrophy, bowel impacton

DOSAGE AND ROUTES
Pain
Adult: PO IM/SUBCUT 15-60 mg q4hr prn
Child: PO 6-17 yr 3 mg/kg/day in divided doses q4hr prn

Cough
Adult: PO 10-20 mg q4-6hr, max 120 mg/day

Renal dose
Adult: PO CCr 10-50 ml/min 75% of dose; CCr <10 ml/min 50% of dose

Diarrhea (unlabeled)
Adult: PO 30 mg; may repeat qid prn

Available forms: Tabs 15, 30, 60 mg; oral sol 30 mg/5 ml; inj 15, 30 mg/ml, 30 mg/5 ml sol

Implementation
• Give with antiemetic if nausea, vomiting occur
• Administer when pain is beginning to return, determine dosage interval by patient response; continuous dosing of medication is more effective given prn; explain analgesic effect
• Medication should be slowly withdrawn after long-term use to prevent withdrawal symptoms
• Store in light-resistant container at room temp
PO route
• May be given with food or milk to lessen GI upset
IM/SUBCUT route
• Do not give if cloudy, or a precipitate has formed

ADVERSE EFFECTS
CNS: *Drowsiness, sedation,* dizziness, agitation, dependency, lethargy, restlessness, euphoria, **seizures,** hallucinations, headache, confusion
CV: Bradycardia, palpitations, orthostatic hypotension, tachycardia, **circulatory collapse**
GI: *Nausea, vomiting, anorexia, constipation,* dry mouth
GU: Urinary retention
INTEG: Flushing, rash, urticaria, pruritus
RESP: Respiratory depression, respiratory paralysis, dyspnea
SYST: Anaphylaxis

Pharmacokinetics
Absorption	Bioavailability 60%-90%
Distribution	Widely distributed; crosses placenta, protein binding 7%
Metabolism	Liver, extensively by CYP3A4 to morphine; altered in ethnic groups
Excretion	Kidneys (up to 15%), breast milk
Half-life	3-4 hr

Pharmacodynamics
	PO	IM	SUBCUT
Onset	30-60 min	30-60 min	15-30 min
Peak	1-2 hr	30-60 min	Unknown
Duration	4 hr	4 hr	4 hr

INTERACTIONS
Individual drugs
Alcohol: increased CNS depression

Drug classifications
Antipsychotics, CYP2D6, sedative, hypnotics, opiates, skeletal muscle relaxants: increased CNS depression
MAOIs: increased toxicity; use cautiously

Drug/lab test
Increased: amylase, lipase

NURSING CONSIDERATIONS
Assessment
• Assess **pain:** intensity, type, alleviating factors, type, location, need for pain medication, tolerance, use pain scoring
• Assess GI function: nausea, vomiting, constipation
• Assess **cough:** type, duration, ability to raise secretion for productive cough; do not use to suppress a productive cough
• Monitor VS after parenteral route; note muscle rigidity, product history, renal/hepatic function tests, respiratory dysfunction: respiratory depression, character, rate, rhythm; notify prescriber if respirations are <10/min
• Monitor CNS changes: dizziness, drowsiness, hallucinations, euphoria, LOC, pupil reaction

> **BLACK BOX WARNING:** Child (tonsillectomy/adenoidectomy): deaths have occurred, use is contraindicated

• Monitor allergic reactions: rash, urticaria

C

• Respiratory dysfunction: respiratory depression, character, rate, rhythm; notify prescriber if respirations are <10/min, shallow

Patient/family education
• Teach patient to report any symptoms of CNS changes, allergic reactions; to avoid CNS depressants: alcohol, sedative/hypnotics for at least 24 hr after taking this product
• Discuss with patient that dizziness, drowsiness, and confusion are common
• Advise patient to avoid getting up without assistance
• Discuss in detail with patient all aspects of the product
• Advise patient not to breastfeed
• Teach patient that physical dependency may result after extended periods
• Advise patient to use sugarless gum, rinse mouth after, for dry mouth

Evaluation
Positive therapeutic outcome
• Decreased pain
• Decreased cough
• Decreased diarrhea

TREATMENT OF OVERDOSE:
Naloxone 0.4 ampule diluted in 10 ml 0.9% NaCl and given by direct **IV** push 0.02 mg q2min (adult)

colchicine (Rx)
(kol'chih-seen)
Colcrys
Func. class.: Antigout agent
Chem. class.: Colchicum autumnale alkaloid
Pregnancy category C

ACTION: Inhibits microtubule formation of lactic acid in leukocytes, which decreases phagocytosis and inflammation in joints

Therapeutic outcome: Decreased pain, inflammation of joints

USES: Gout, gouty arthritis (prevention, treatment); to arrest progression of neurologic disability in multiple sclerosis

Unlabeled uses: Hepatic cirrhosis, familial Mediterranean fever, pericarditis, amyloidosis, Behçet's syndrome, biliary cirrhosis, dermatitis herpetiformis, idiopathic thrombocytopenic purpura, Paget's disease, pseudogout, pulmonary fibrosis

CONTRAINDICATIONS:
Pregnancy **D** (injectable), hypersensitivity; serious GI disorders, severe renal/hepatic/cardiac disorders

Precautions: Pregnancy **C** (**PO**), breastfeeding, children, geriatric, blood dyscrasias, hepatic disease

DOSAGE AND ROUTES
Gout prevention
Adult: PO 0.6-1.8 mg daily depending on severity

Gout treatment
Adult: 1.2 mg initially, then 0.6 mg 1 hr later (1.8 mg); those on strong CYP3A4 inhibitor (past 14 days) 0.6 mg initially, then 0.3 mg 1 hr later

Renal dose
Adult: PO CCr <30 ml/min for acute gout, do not repeat course for 2 wk; familial Mediterranean fever 0.3 mg daily, increase cautiously

Mediterranean fever (unlabeled)
Adult: PO (on no interacting products): 1.2-2.4 mg/day in 1-2 divided doses; strong CYP3A4 inhibitor/increase cautiously; P-glycoprotein inhibitors within 14 days: max 0.6 mg/day in 1-2 divided doses; moderate CYP3A4 inhibitors with 14 day max 1.2 mg/day in 1-2 divided doses
Adolescent: PO 1.2-2.4 mg/day in 1-2 divided doses, titrate by 0.3 mg/day
Child 6-12 yr: PO 0.9-1.8 mg/day in 1-2 divided doses
Child 4-6 yr: PO 0.3-1.8 mg/day in 1-2 divided doses

Available forms: Tabs 0.5, 0.6, 1 mg ✤

Implementation
PO route
• Give without regard to food
• Cumulative doses ≤4 mg, renal patients ≤2 mg, when reached, administer only for 3 wks

ADVERSE EFFECTS
GI: *Nausea, vomiting, anorexia, malaise,* metallic taste, cramps, peptic ulcer, diarrhea
GU: Hematuria, **oliguria, renal damage**
HEMA: Agranulocytosis, thrombocytopenia, aplastic anemia, pancytopenia
INTEG: Chills, dermatitis, pruritus, purpura, erythema
MISC: Myopathy, alopecia, reversible azoospermia, peripheral neuritis

Pharmacokinetics

Absorption	Well absorbed
Distribution	WBCs
Metabolism	Deacetylates in liver
Excretion	Feces (metabolites/active product)
Half-life	4.4 hr

Pharmacodynamics

	PO
Onset	Unknown
Peak	½-2 hr
Duration	Unknown

INTERACTIONS
Individual drugs
CycloSPORINE, radiation: increased bone marrow depression

Ethanol: increased GI effects

Vitamin B$_{12}$: decreased action of vit B$_{12}$; may cause reversible malabsorption

Drug classifications
Bone marrow depressants: increased bone marrow depression

Moderate/strong CYP3A4 inhibitors, reduce dose: increased colchicine level/toxicity

NSAIDs: increased GI effects

Drug/food
Grapefruit juice: increased colchicine level

Drug/lab test
Increased: alkaline phosphatase, AST

Decreased: platelets, WBC, granulocytes

False positive: urine Hgb

Interference: urinary 17-hydroxycorticosteroids

NURSING CONSIDERATIONS
Assessment
• Assess pain and mobility of joints, uric acid levels returning to normal

• Monitor I&O ratio; observe for decrease in urinary output; CBC, platelets, reticulocytes before, during therapy (q3mo); may cause aplastic anemia, agranulocytosis, decreased platelets

• Assess for **toxicity:** weakness, abdominal pain, nausea, vomiting, diarrhea, product should be discontinued, report symptoms immediately

Patient/family education
• Caution patient to avoid alcohol, OTC preparations that contain alcohol

• Instruct patient to report any pain, redness, or hard area, usually in legs; rash, sore throat, fever, bleeding, bruising, weakness, numbness, tingling, nausea, vomiting, abdominal pain

• Teach patient importance of complying with medical regimen (diet, weight loss, product therapy); bone marrow depression may occur

• Advise patient to tell all providers of product use, surgery may increase possibility of acute gout symptoms

Evaluation
Positive therapeutic outcome
• Decreased stone formation on x-ray
• Decreased pain in kidney region
• Absence of hematuria
• Decreased pain in joints

TREATMENT OF OVERDOSE:
Discontinue medication, may need opioids to treat diarrhea

colesevelam (Rx)
(coal-see-vel′am)

Welchol

Func. class.: Antilipemic

Chem. class.: Bile acid sequestrant

Pregnancy category B

ACTION: Adsorbs, combines with bile acids to form insoluble complex that is excreted through feces; loss of bile acids lowers cholesterol levels

Therapeutic outcome: Decreasing LDL cholesterol

USES: Elevated LDL cholesterol, alone or in combination with HMG-CoA reductase inhibitor; type 2 diabetes (adjunct)

CONTRAINDICATIONS:
Hypersensitivity, bowel disease, primary biliary cirrhosis, triglycerides >300 mg/dl, bowel obstruction, pancreatitis, biliary obstruction; dysphagia, fat-soluble vitamin deficiency

Precautions: Pregnancy **B,** breastfeeding, children

DOSAGE AND ROUTES
Monotherapy
Adult: PO 3 625 mg tabs bid with meals or 6 tabs daily with a meal; may increase to 7 tabs if needed

Combination therapy
Adult: PO 3 tabs bid with meals or 6 tabs daily with a meal given with an HMG-CoA reductase inhibitor

Type 2 diabetes, adjunct (to improve glycemic control)

Adult and geriatric: PO approx 3.8 g (6 tabs)/day or approx 1.9 g (3 tabs) bid

Heterozygous familial hypercholesterolemia

Females (postmenarchal and >10 yr) and males ≥10 yr: PO 1.875 g packet bid or 3.75 g packet q day dissolved in 4-8 oz of water with a meal

Available forms: Tabs 625 mg, powder for oral susp 3.75 g/packet

Implementation

• Give product daily, bid with meals; give all other medications 4 hr before colesevelam to avoid poor absorption; take with liquid
• Give supplemental doses of vit A, D, K if levels are low

Powder for oral susp

• Empty contents of packet into a cup/glass; add ½-1 cup (4-8 oz) of water, fruit juice, or diet soda; stir well before drinking

ADVERSE EFFECTS

GI: *Constipation, abdominal pain, nausea,* fecal impaction, hemorrhoids, flatulence, vomiting, GI obstruction
MISC: Hypertriglycerides, hypoglycemia
MS: Muscle, joint pain

Pharmacokinetics

Absorption	Unknown
Distribution	Unknown
Metabolism	Unknown
Excretion	Feces
Half-life	Unknown

Pharmacodynamics

LDL decreased in 4-7 days

INTERACTIONS

Individual drugs

Digoxin, diltiazem, gemfibrozil, glyBURide, fluoroquinolones, iron, mycophenolate, penicillin G, phenytoin, propanolol, warfarin: decreased absorption of each specific product
Thyroid hormones: decreased absorption of thyroid

Drug classifications

Corticosteroids: decreased corticosteroid action
Oral contraceptives: decreased action of oral contraceptives
Tetracyclines: decreased absorption of tetracyclines
Thiazides: decreased absorption of thiazides
Vitamins (fat-soluble): decreased absorption of fat-soluble vitamins

Drug/lab test

Increased: liver function tests

NURSING CONSIDERATIONS

Assessment

• Assess cardiac glycoside level if both products are being administered
• Assess for signs of vit A, D, K deficiency
• Monitor fasting LDL, HDL, total cholesterol, triglyceride levels, electrolytes if on extended therapy
• Monitor bowel pattern daily; increase bulk, H_2O in diet for constipation

Patient/family education

• Teach the importance of compliance; toxicity may result if doses missed, timing of dose 4 hr after other meds
• Teach that risk factors should be decreased: high-fat diet, smoking, alcohol consumption, absence of exercise

Evaluation

Positive therapeutic outcome

• Decreased cholesterol level (hyperlipidemia); diarrhea, pruritus (excess bile acids), collagenase *Clostridium histolyticum*

conivaptan (Rx)

(kon-ih-vap′tan)
Vaprisol
Func. class.: Vasopressin receptor antagonist
Pregnancy category C

ACTION: Dual arginine vasopressin (AVP) antagonist with affinity for V_{1A}, V_2 receptors; level of AVP in circulating blood is critical for regulation of water, electrolyte balance and is usually elevated in euvolemic/hypervolemic hyponatremia

Therapeutic outcome: Correct serum sodium levels

USES: Euvolemia hyponatremia in those hospitalized, not indicated for CHF, hypervolemia, hyponatremia

CONTRAINDICATIONS:

Hypersensitivity, hypovolemia

Adverse effects: *italics* = common; **bold** = life-threatening

Precautions: Pregnancy **C**, breastfeeding, orthostatic/renal disease, heart failure, rapid correction of serum sodium

DOSAGE AND ROUTES
Adult: **IV** INF loading dose 20 mg given over 30 min, then CONT **IV** over 24 hr; after 1 day, give for an additional 1-3 days as a CONT INF of 20 mg/day total, can be titrated up to 40 mg/day if serum sodium is not rising at the desired rate; max time 4 days

Hepatic/renal dose
Adult: **IV** Child-Pugh A-C or CCr 30-60 ml/min: Give **IV** loading dose over 10 min, then cont **IV** INF 10 mg over 24 hr × 2-4 days

Available forms: 5 mg/ml (20 mg/4 ml) in single-use ampule; 20 mg/100 ml in D$_5$W for injection

Implementation
IV route
• Withdraw 4 ml (20 mg) of conivaptan, add to 100 ml D$_5$W, gently invert several times to mix, give over 30 min; in large vein, change site q24hr to minimize vascular irritation
Continuous IV infusion route
• Withdraw 4 ml (20 mg) of conivaptan, add to 250 ml D$_5$W, gently invert several times to mix, give over 24 hr; or 40 mg in 250 ml D$_5$W, gently invert several times to mix, give over 24 hr

ADVERSE EFFECTS
CNS: Headache, confusion, insomnia
CV: **Atrial fibrillation,** hypo/hypertension, orthostatic hypotension, phlebitis
GI: Nausea, vomiting, constipation, dry mouth
GU: Hematuria, polyuria, UTI, pollakiuria
HEMA: Anemia
INTEG: Erythemia, inj site reaction
META: Dehydration, hypo/hyperglycemia, hypokalemia, hypomagnesia, hyponatremia
MISC: Oral candidiasis, pain, peripheral edema, pneumonia

Pharmacokinetics

Absorption	Unknown
Distribution	Protein binding 99%
Metabolism	By CYP3A4
Excretion	Unknown
Half-life	Terminal 5 hr

Pharmacodynamics
Unknown

INTERACTIONS
Drug classifications
CYP3A4 substrates (alfuzosin, ARIPiprazole, bexarolene, bortezomib, bosentan, bupivacaine, buprenorphine, carBAMazepine, cevimeline, cilostazol, cinacalcet, clopidogrel, colchicine, cyclobenzaprine, dapsone, darifenacin, disopyramide, DOCEtaxel, donepezil, DOXOrubicin, dutasteride, eletriptan, eplerenone, ergots, erlotinib, eszopiclone, ethinyl estradiol, ethosuximide, etoposide, fentaNYL, galantamine, gefitinib, halofantrine, ifosfamide, irinotecan, levobupivacaine, levomethadyl, lidocaine, loperamide, loratadine, mefloquine, methadone, modafinil, PACLitaxel, pimozide, praziquantel, quiNIDine, quiNINE, ramelteon, reboxetine, repaglinide, rifabutin, sibutramine, sildenafil, sirolimus, SUFentanil, SUNItinib, tacrolimus, tamoxifen, teniposide, testosterone, tiaGABine, tinidazole, trimetrexate, vardenafil, vinca alkaloids, ziprasidone, zolpidem, zonisamide): increased effects, do not use concurrently

NURSING CONSIDERATIONS
Assessment
⚠ Monitor renal/hepatic function
⚠ Assess frequent sodium volume status; overly rapid correction of sodium concentration (>12 mEq/L per 24 hr) may result in osmotic demyelination syndrome
• Assess neurologic status: confusion, headache
• Assess CV status: atrial fibrillation, hyper/hypotension, orthostatic hypotension; monitor B/P, pulse
• Monitor other electrolytes (magnesium and potassium)

Patient/family education
• Advise patient to report neurologic changes: headache, insomnia, confusion
• Teach patient administration procedure and expected result
• Advise patient to report inj site pain, redness, swelling

Evaluation
Positive therapeutic outcome
• Correction of serum sodium levels

CONTRACEPTIVES, HORMONAL

MONOPHASIC, ORAL
ethinyl estradiol/ desogestrel (Rx)
Apri, Cesia, Desogen, Kariva, Mircette, Ortho-Cept, Reclipsen, Solia, Velivet
ethinyl estradiol/ drospirenone (Rx)
Ocella, Yasmin, Yaz 28
ethinyl estradiol/ ethynodiol (Rx)
Kelnor 1/35, Zovia 1/35, Zovia 1/50
ethinyl estradiol/ levonorgestrel (Rx)
Alesse, Aviane-28, Enpresse, Jolessa, Lessina, Levlen, Levlite, Levora, Lutera, Nordette, Portia, Quasense, Seasonique, Sronyx
ethinyl estradiol/ norethindrone (Rx)
Brevicon, Genora 0.5/35, Genora 1/35, Junel 21 1/20, Junel 21 1.5/20, Loestrin 21 1.5/30, Loestrin 21 1/20, Microgestin, Modicon, Necon 0.5/35, N.E.E 1/35, Nelova 0.5/35E, Nelova 1/35E, Norcept-E 1/35, Norethin 1/35E, Norinyl 1+35, Norlestrin 1/50, Norlestrin 2.5/50, Nortrel 1/35, Nortrel 7/7/7
ethinyl estradiol/ norgestimate (Rx)
MonoNessa, Ortho-Cyclen, Previfem, Sprintec, Tri-Sprintec
ethinyl estradiol/norgestrel (Rx)
Cryselle, Lo/Ovral, Low-Ogestrel, Ogestrel, Ovral
mestranol/norethindrone (Rx)
Genora 1/50, Nelova 1/50m, Norethin 1/50m, Norinyl 1+50, Ortho-Novum 1/50

BIPHASIC, ORAL
ethinyl estradiol/ norethindrone (Rx)
Nelova 10/11, Ortho-Novum 10/11

TRIPHASIC, ORAL
ethinyl estradiol/ desogestrel (Rx)
Cyclessa

ethinyl estradiol/ norethindrone (Rx)
Necor 7/7/7, Nortrel 7/7/7, Ortho-Novum 7/7/7, Tri-Norinyl
ethinyl estradiol/ norgestimate (Rx)
Ortho Tri-Cyclen, Ortho Tri-Cyclen Lo
ethinyl estradiol/ levonorgestrel (Rx)
Enpresse, Tri-Levlen, Triphasil

EXTENDED CYCLE, ORAL
ethinyl estradiol/ levonorgestrel (Rx)
Seasonale

PROGESTIN, ORAL
norethindrone (Rx)
Errin, Ortho Micronor, Camila, Jolivette, Nor-Q D

PROGRESSIVE ESTROGEN, ORAL
ethinyl estradiol/ norethindrone acetate (Rx)
Estrostep, Estrostep Fe

EMERGENCY
levonorgestrel/ethinyl estradiol (Rx)
Preven
levonorgestrel (Rx)
Plan B
medroxyprogesterone (Rx)
Depo-Provera

INTRAUTERINE
levonorgestrel (Rx)
Mirena

IMPLANT
etonogestrel (Rx)
Implanon

VAGINAL RING
ethinyl estradiol/etonogestrel (Rx)
Nuva Ring

TRANSDERMAL
ethinyl estradiol/norelgestromin (Rx)
Ortho Evra

ACTION: Prevents ovulation by contraceptives suppressing FSH, LH; *monophasic:*

Adverse effects: *italics* = common; **bold** = life-threatening

estrogen/progestin (fixed dose) used during a 21-day cycle; ovulation is inhibited by suppression of FSH and LH; thickness of cervical mucus and endometrial lining prevents pregnancy; *biphasic:* ovulation is inhibited by suppression of FSH and LH; alteration of cervical mucus, endometrial lining prevents pregnancy; *triphasic:* ovulation is inhibited by suppression of FSH and LH; change of cervical mucus, endometrial lining prevents pregnancy; variable doses of estrogen/progestin combinations may be similar to natural hormonal fluctuations; *extended cycle:* estrogen/progestin continuous for 84 days, off for 7 days, result 4 menstrual periods/yr; *progressive estrogen:* constant progestin with 3 progressive doses of estrogen; *progestin-only pill, implant, intrauterine:* change of cervical mucus and endometrial lining prevents pregnancy; ovulation may be suppressed

Therapeutic outcome: Prevention of pregnancy, decreased severity of endometriosis, hypermenorrhea

USES: To prevent pregnancy, regulation of menstrual cycle, treatment of acne in women >14 yr that other treatment has failed, emergency contraception; *injection:* inhibits gonadotropin secretion, ovulation, follicular maturation; *emergency:* inhibits ovulation and fertilization, decreases transport of sperm and egg from fallopian tube to uterus; *vaginal ring, transdermal:* inhibits ovulation, prevents sperm entry into uterus; *antiacne:* may decrease sex hormone binding globulin, results in decreased testosterone

CONTRAINDICATIONS:

Pregnancy **X,** breastfeeding, women 40 yr and over, reproductive cancer, thrombophlebitis, MI, hepatic tumors, hepatic disease, CAD, CVA, breast cancer, jaundice, stroke, vaginal bleeding

Precautions: Depression, hypertension, renal disease, seizure disorders, lupus erythematosus, rheumatic disease, migraine headache, amenorrhea, irregular menses, gallbladder disease, diabetes mellitus, heavy smoking, acute mononucleosis, sickle cell disease

> **BLACK BOX WARNING:** Tobacco smoking

DOSAGE AND ROUTES

Monophasic
Adult: PO take first tab on Sunday after start of menses × 21 days; skip 7 days; then repeat cycle; start on 1st day of menses × 21 days; skip 7 days, then repeat cycle; may contain 7 placebo tabs, where 1 tab is taken daily

Biphasic
Adult: PO Take 10 days of small progestin, then large progestin; estrogen is the same during cycle; skip 7 days, then repeat cycle; may contain 7 placebo tabs, where 1 tab is taken daily

Triphasic
Adult: PO estrogen dose remains constant, progestin changes throughout 21 day cycle, some products contain 28 tabs per month

Extended cycle
Adult: PO start taking on first day of menses; continue for 84 days of active tab, then 7 days of placebo; repeat cycle

Progestin
Adult: PO start on 1st day of menses, then daily and continuously

Progressive estrogen
Adult: PO progestin dose remains constant, estrogen increases q7days throughout 21-day cycle, may include 7 placebo tabs for 28-day cycle

Emergency
Adult and adolescent: Give within 72 hr of intercourse, repeat 12 hr later; Plan B 1 tab, then 1 tab 12 hr later; Preven 2 tab, then 2 tab 12 hr later; Ovral (unlabeled) 2 white tabs; Lo/Ovral (unlabeled) 4 white tabs; Levlen (unlabeled), Nordette (unlabeled) 4 orange tabs; Triphasil (unlabeled), Tri-Levlen (unlabeled) 4 yellow tabs

Injectable
Adult: IM (Depo-Provera) 150 mg within 5 days of start of menses, or within 5 days postpartum (must not be breastfeeding); if breastfeeding, give 6 wk postpartum, repeat q3mo

Intrauterine
Adult: To be inserted using the levonorgestrel-releasing intrauterine system (LRIS) by those trained in procedure; inserted into uterine cavity within 7 days of the onset of menstruation; use should not exceed 5 years per implant

Vaginal ring
Adult: VAG insert 1 ring on or prior to day 5 of cycle, leave in place 3 wk; remove for 1 wk, then repeat

Transdermal
Adult: Transdermal apply patch within 7 days of menses, change weekly × 3 wk; no patch wk 4, repeat cycle

Implant
Adult: Subdermal in inner side of upper arm on days 1-5 of menses, replace q3yr

Acne
Adult: PO (Ortho Tri-Cyclen) take daily × 21 days, off 7 days

Implementation
PO route
• If GI symptoms occur, medication may be taken with food; take at same time each day
Implant route
• Inject 6 cap subdermally
• Implant is effective for 5 yr, should be removed after that
IM route
• Administer inj deep in large muscle mass after shaking susp well; ensure pregnancy has not occurred if inj are 2 wk or more apart

ADVERSE EFFECTS
CNS: Depression, fatigue, dizziness, nervousness, anxiety, headache
CV: Increased B/P, **cerebral hemorrhage, thrombosis, pulmonary embolism,** fluid retention, edema, MI
EENT: Optic neuritis, retinal thrombosis, cataracts
ENDO: Decreased glucose tolerance, increased TBG, PBI, T_4, T_3, temporary infertility
GI: *Nausea,* vomiting, cramps, diarrhea, bloating, constipation, change in appetite, **cholestatic jaundice,** weight change
GU: Breakthrough bleeding, amenorrhea, spotting, dysmenorrhea, galactorrhea, endocervical hyperplasia, vaginitis, cystitis-like syndrome, breast change
HEMA: Increased fibrinogen, clotting factor
INTEG: *Chloasma, melasma,* acne, rash, urticaria, erythema, pruritus, hirsutism, alopecia, photosensitivity

Pharmacokinetics	
Absorption	Unknown
Distribution	Unknown
Metabolism	Unknown
Excretion	Breast milk
Half-life	Unknown

Pharmacodynamics
Unknown

INTERACTIONS
Individual drugs
Griseofulvin, rifampin: decreased effectiveness of oral contraceptive

Drug classifications
Analgesics, antibiotics, anticonvulsants, antihistamines: decreased action of oral contraceptives
Anticoagulants (oral): decreased action of oral anticoagulants

Drug/herb
Black cohosh: altered action
Saw palmetto, St. John's wort: decreased oral contraceptive effect

Drug/food
Grapefruit juice: increased peak level

Drug/lab test
Increased: pro-time; clotting factors VII, VIII, IX, X; TBG, PBI, T_4, platelet aggregation, BSP, triglycerides, bilirubin, AST, ALT
Decreased: T_3, antithrombin III, folate, metyrapone test, GTT, 17-OHCS

NURSING CONSIDERATIONS
Assessment
• Assess for reproductive changes: change in breasts, tumors, positive Pap smear; product should be discontinued if changes occur
• Monitor glucose, thyroid function, liver function tests, B/P

Patient/family education
• Teach patient about detection of clots using Homans' sign; teach monitoring technique for heat, redness, pain, swelling
• Teach patient to use sunscreen or to avoid sunlight; photosensitivity can occur
• Teach patient to take at same time each day to ensure equal product level; to take another tab as soon as possible if one is missed
• Teach patient that after product is discontinued, pregnancy may not occur for several mo
• Instruct patient to report GI symptoms that occur after 4 mo
⚠ Advise patient to use another birth control method during first 3 wk of oral contraceptive use
⚠ Teach patient to report abdominal pain, change in vision, shortness of breath, change in menstrual flow, spotting, breakthrough bleeding, breast lumps, swelling, headache, severe leg pain, mental changes; that continuing medical care is needed: Pap smear and gynecologic exam q6mo

> **BLACK BOX WARNING:** Teach patient not to smoke, increased risk of CV side effects

• Teach patient to notify physicians and dentist of oral contraceptive use

---

Adverse effects: *italics* = common; **bold** = life-threatening

Evaluation

Positive therapeutic outcome
- Absence of pregnancy
- Decreased severity of endometriosis
- Decreased severity of hypermenorrhea

cotrimoxazole

See trimethoprim/sulfamethoxazole

⚠ HIGH ALERT

crizotinib

(kriz-oh′ti-nib)

XALKORI

Func. class.: Antineoplastic; biologic response modifiers

Pregnancy category D

ACTION: An inhibitor of receptor tyrosine kinases (anaplastic lymphoma kinase (ALK), hepatocyte growth factor receptor (HGFR, c-Met), recepteur d'origine nantais (RON).

Therapeutic outcome: Decreased spread of malignancy

USES: Locally advanced or metastatic non–small-cell lung cancer (NSCLC) that is anaplastic lymphoma kinase (ALK)-positive as detected by an FDA-approved test

CONTRAINDICATIONS:

Pregnancy D, breastfeeding, hypersensitivity

Precautions: Pneumonitis, severe hepatic disease, congenital long QT syndrome, neonates, infants, children, adolescents, severe renal impairment, end-stage renal disease, vision disorders

DOSAGE AND ROUTES

Adult: PO 250 mg bid; continue as long as is beneficial

Dose adjustments for hematologic toxicities

For Grade 1-2: No dosage adjustment needed

For Grade 3: Interrupt treatment until toxicity resolves to grade ≤2, then, continue with the same dosage schedule. In case of recurrence after a grade 4 event with dose reduction, interrupt treatment until toxicity resolves to grade ≤2; when resuming treatment, reduce dosage to 250 mg PO daily

For Grade 4: Interrupt treatment until toxicity resolves to grade ≤2; when resuming treatment, reduce dosage to 200 mg PO bid. In case

of grade 4 recurrence, permanently discontinue treatment

Dose adjustment for hepatic laboratory abnormalities

For Grade 1: No dosage adjustment necessary:

For Grade 2 ALT/AST elevations with grade ≤1 total bilirubin elevations: No dosage adjustment necessary

For Grade 3-4 ALT/AST elevations with grade ≤1 total bilirubin elevations: Interrupt treatment until toxicity resolves to grade ≤1 or baseline; when resuming treatment, reduce dosage to 200 mg PO bid; in case of recurrence, interrupt treatment until toxicity resolves to grade ≤1, and when resuming treatment, reduce dosage to 250 mg PO daily; permanently discontinue treatment in case of further recurrence

For Grade 2-4 ALT/AST elevations with concurrent Grade 2-4 total bilirubin elevations (in the absence of cholestasis or hemolysis): Permanently discontinue treatment

Dose adjustment for pneumonitis not attributable to NSCLC progression, other pulmonary disease, infection, or radiation effect

For any grade pneumonitis: Permanently discontinue

Dose adjustment for QTc prolongation:

For Grade 1–2 QTc prolongation: No dosage adjustment necessary

For Grade 3 QTc prolongation: Interrupt treatment until toxicity resolves to grade ≤1; when resuming treatment, reduce dosage to 200 mg PO bid; in case of recurrence, interrupt treatment until toxicity resolves to grade ≤1 and when resuming treatment, reduce dosage to 250 mg PO daily; permanently discontinue in case of further recurrence

For Grade 4 QTc prolongation: Permanently discontinue

Available forms: Caps 200, 250 mg

Implementation

- May be taken orally with or without food
- Have the patient swallow capsule whole; do not crush or chew
- If a dose is missed, it can be taken up to 6 hr before the next dose is due to maintain the twice daily regimen. Do not take both doses at the same time
- Store capsules at room temperature

ADVERSE EFFECTS

CNS: Dizziness, balance disorder, presyncope, neuropathy (motor and sensory), burning sen-

---

sation, dysesthesia, hyperesthesia, hypoesthesia, neuralgia, paresthesias, peripheral neuropathy (motor and sensory), headache, insomnia

CV: QT prolongation, **disseminated intravascular coagulation (DIC), septic shock,** bradycardia

EENT: *Diplopia, photopsia,* photophobia, *blurred vision,* visual field defect, *vitreous floaters,* visual brightness, *reduced visual acuity,* esophageal disorders, dyspepsia

GI: *Nausea, diarrhea, vomiting, constipation,* decreased appetite, dysgeusia, abdominal pain, abdominal discomfort/pain, stomatitis, oral ulceration, elevated hepatic enzymes, hyperbilirubinemia, glossodynia, glossitis, cheilitis, mucosal inflammation, oropharyngeal pain/discomfort, oral pain, esophageal disorder, dysphagia, epigastric discomfort/pain, burning, esophagitis, **esophageal obstruction**/pain/ spasm, **esophageal ulceration,** gastroesophageal reflux, odynophagia, and reflux esophagitis

HEMA: Grade 3/4 neutropenia, thrombocytopenia, lymphopenia

MISC: Fatigue, fever, *edema,* localized/ peripheral edema, chest pain (unspecified), chest discomfort, musculoskeletal chest pain, arthralgia, back pain, rash

RESP: Severe, life-threatening pneumonitis, pneumonia, hypoxia, acute respiratory distress syndrome (ARDS), dyspnea, empyema, **pulmonary hemorrhage, pulmonary embolism,** upper respiratory tract infection (nasopharyngitis, pharyngitis, rhinitis), cough

Pharmacokinetics

Absorption	43%
Distribution	Steady state 15 days, protein binding 91%, distribution tissue, plasma
Metabolism	By 3YPA4/5, oxidation to metabolites
Excretion	63% feces, unchanged 53%; 22% urine, unchanged 2, 3%
Half-life	Terminal 42 hr

Pharmacodynamics

Onset	Unknown
Peak	4-6 hr
Duration	Unknown

INTERACTIONS
Drug classifications

CYP2B6 substrates (prasugrel, selegiline, cyclophosphamide): increased action of these products

β-agonists, Class IA antiarrhythmics (disopyramide, procainamide, quiNIDine), Class III antiarrhythmics (amiodarone, dofetilide, ibutilide, sotalol), halogenated anesthetics, local anesthetics, tricyclic antidepressants: increased QT prolongation, torsades de pointes

CYP3A4 inhibitors (ketoconazole, atazanavir, indinavir, itraconazole, nefazodone, nelfinavir, ritonavir, voriconazole, boceprevir, delavirdine, isoniazid, dalfopristin, quinupristin, tipranavir): increased crizotinib

CYP3A4 inducers (rifampin, carBAMazepine, PHENobarbital, phenytoin, rifabutin); antacids, H2-blockers, proton pump inhibitors (PPIs): decreased crizotinib

CYP3A4 substrates (alfentanil, cycloSPORINE, ergotamine, dihydroergotamine fentaNYL, sirolimus, colchicine): avoid concurrent use

Individual drugs

Abarelix, alfuzosin, amoxapine, apomorphine, arsenic trioxide, asenapine, chloroquine, ciprofloxacin, citalopram, clarithromycin, cloZAPine, cyclobenzaprine, dasatinib, dolasetron, dronedarone, droperidol, eribulin, erythromycin, ezogabine, flecainide, fluconazole, gatifloxacin, gemifloxacin, grepafloxacin, halofantrine, haloperidol, iloperidone, indacaterol, lapatinib, levofloxacin, levomethadyl, lopinavir/ritonavir, magnesium sulfate, maprotiline, mefloquine, methadone, moxifloxacin, nilotinib, norfloxacin, octreotide, ofloxacin, OLANZapine, ondansetron, paliperidone, palonosetron, pentamidine, certain phenothiazines (chlorpromazine, mesoridazine, thioridazine, fluPHENAZine, perphenazine, prochlorperazine, trifluoperazine), pimozide, posaconazole, potassium sulfate, probucol, propafenone, QUEtiapine, quiNIDine, ranolazine, rilpivirine, risperidone, saquinavir, sodium, sparfloxacin, SUNItinib, tacrolimus, telavancin, telithromycin, tetrabenazine, troleandomycin, vardenafil, vemurafenib, venlafaxine, vorinostat, ziprasidone: increased QT prolongation, torsades de pointes

Midazolam: increased midazolam action

Drug/herb
Do not use with St. John's wort

Drug/food
Do not use with grapefruit juice

NURSING CONSIDERATIONS
Assessment
⚠ Severe, life-threatening, or fatal treatment-related pneumonitis: All cases occurred within 2 months of treatment initiation; monitor for pulmonary symptoms that may indicate pneumonitis and other causes of pneumonitis should be excluded; permanently discontinue in patients with treatment-related pneumonitis

⚠ Hepatic disease: Liver function test (LFT) abnormalities, altered bilirubin levels, may occur during treatment; monitor LFTs and bilirubin levels prior to treatment, then monthly; more frequent testing is needed in those presenting with grade 2 or greater toxicities; Laboratory alterations should be managed with dose reduction, treatment interruption, or discontinuation

⚠ QT prolongation: has been reported with the use of crizotinib; crizotinib should be avoided in these patients. Monitor ECG and electrolytes in those with CHF, bradycardia, electrolyte imbalance (hypokalemia, hypo-magnesemia), or in those who are taking concomitant medications known to prolong the QT interval; treatment interruption, dosage adjustment, or treatment discontinuation may be needed in those who develop QT prolongation

• **Vision disorders:** Generally started within 2 weeks of the start of therapy; ophthalmologic evaluation should be considered, particularly if patients experience photopsia or new/ increased vitreous floaters; caution should be used when driving or operating machinery by patients who experience vision disorders

• **Pregnancy/breastfeeding:** Identify if pregnancy is planned or suspected; pregnancy category D, avoid breastfeeding

• CBC with differential; BUN/creatinine

Patient/family education
• Missed doses can be taken up to 6 hr before the next dose is due to maintain the twice daily regimen

• Teach patient to use reliable contraception; both women and men of childbearing age should use adequate contraceptive methods during therapy and for at least 90 days after completing treatment; pregnancy D

• Teach patient to report immediately shortness of breath, cough, fatigue, visual changes

• Teach patient not to take with grapefruit juice

• Teach patient to avoid activities requiring mental alertness until effects are known

• Teach patient to report signs of QT prolongation (abnormal heartbeats, dizziness, syncope)

• Teach patient to swallow caps whole and avoid contact with broken cap

Evaluation
Positive therapeutic outcome
• Decreased spread of malignancy

cyclobenzaprine (Rx)
(sye-kloe-ben′za-preen)
Amrix, Fexmid, Flexeril
Func. class.: Skeletal muscle relaxant, central acting
Chem. class.: Tricyclic amine salt
Pregnancy category B

Do not confuse:
cyclobenzaprine/cyproheptadine

ACTION: Reduction of tonic muscle activity at the brain stem; may be related to antidepressant effects

Therapeutic outcome: Relaxation of skeletal muscle

USES: Adjunct for relief of muscle spasm and pain in musculoskeletal conditions

Unlabeled uses: Fibromyalgia

CONTRAINDICATIONS:
Acute recovery phase of MI, dysrhythmias, heart block, CHF, hypersensitivity, child <12 yr, intermittent porphyria, thyroid disease

Precautions: Pregnancy **B**, breastfeeding, geriatric, renal/hepatic disease, addictive personality, **Class IA/III antidysrhythmics, and other products that increase QT interval**

DOSAGE AND ROUTES
Musculoskeletal disorders
Adult/adolescent ≥15 yr: PO 5 mg tid × 1 wk, max 30 mg/day × 3 wk
Adult: EXT REL 15 mg q day, max 30 mg q day × 3 wk
Geriatric: PO 5 mg tid

Hepatic dose
Adult (mild hepatic disease): PO 5 mg, titrate slowly

Fibromyalgia (unlabeled)
Adult: PO 10 mg at bedtime, titrated up

Available forms: Tabs 5, 10 mg; ext rel tab 15, 30 mg

Implementation
• Give without regard to meals, give with food for GI symptoms
• Store in airtight container at room temperature

ADVERSE EFFECTS
CNS: *Dizziness, weakness, drowsiness,* headache, tremor, depression, insomnia, confusion, paresthesia, nervousness
CV: Postural hypotension, tachycardia, **dysrhythmias**
EENT: Diplopia, temporary loss of vision
GI: *Nausea,* vomiting, hiccups, dry mouth, constipation, hepatitis
GU: Urinary retention, frequency, change in libido
INTEG: Rash, pruritus, fever, facial flushing, sweating

Pharmacokinetics

Distribution	Well
Metabolism	Liver, partially
Excretion	Kidney (unchanged)
Half-life	1-3 days

Pharmacodynamics

Onset	1 hr
Peak	3-8 hr
Duration	12-24 hr

INTERACTIONS
Individual drugs
Alcohol: increased CNS depression
TraMADol: do not use within 14 days

Drug classifications
Antidepressants (tricyclic), barbiturates, opiates, sedative/hypnotics: increased CNS depression
MAOIs: do not use within 14 days
Serotonin syndrome—SSRIs, SNRIs: increased action of these products

Drug/herb
Kava: increased CNS depression

NURSING CONSIDERATIONS
Assessment
⚠ Serotonin syndrome: if using with SSRIs, SNRIs, monitor closely; if syndrome occurs, discontinue both products immediately
• Assess pain periodically: location, duration, mobility, stiffness, baseline

• Monitor ECG in epileptic patients; poor seizure control has occurred in patients taking this product
• Check for allergic reactions: rash, fever, respiratory distress
• Check for severe weakness, numbness, in extremities
• Assess for CNS depression: dizziness, drowsiness, psychiatric symptoms

Patient/family education
⚠ Teach patient not to discontinue medication quickly; insomnia, nausea, headache, spasticity, tachycardia will occur; product should be tapered off over 1-2 wk
• Caution patient not to take with alcohol, other CNS depressants
• Advise to avoid altering activities while taking this product
• Caution patient to avoid hazardous activities if drowsiness/dizziness occurs
• Caution patient to avoid using OTC medication: cough preparations, antihistamines, unless directed by prescriber
• Teach patient to use gum, frequent sips of water for dry mouth

Evaluation
Positive therapeutic outcome
• Decreased pain, spasticity; muscle spasms of acute, painful musculoskeletal conditions are generally short term; long-term therapy is seldom warranted

TREATMENT OF OVERDOSE:
Empty stomach with emesis, gastric lavage, then administer activated charcoal; use anticonvulsants if indicated; monitor cardiac function

cyclopentolate ophthalmic
See Appendix B

⚠ HIGH ALERT
cyclophosphamide (Rx)
(sye-kloe-foss'fa-mide)
Cytoxan, Procytox ✦
Func. class.: Antineoplastic alkylating agent
Chem. class.: Nitrogen mustard
Pregnancy category D

Do not confuse:
cyclophosphamide/cycloSPORINE,
Cytoxan/Cytosar/Cytotec/Cytarabine

ACTION: Alkylates DNA; responsible for cross-linking DNA strands; activity is not cell cycle phase specific

Therapeutic outcome: Prevention of rapidly growing malignant cells

USES: Hodgkin's disease, lymphomas, leukemia, multiple myeloma, neuroblastoma, retinoblastoma, Ewing's sarcoma, cancer of female reproductive tract, breast, lung, prostate; disseminated neuroblastoma, nephrotic syndrome

CONTRAINDICATIONS:
Pregnancy **D**, hypersensitivity, prostatic hypertrophy, bladder neck obstruction

Precautions: Radiation therapy, cardiac disease, anemia, dysrhythmias, child, dental disease/work, dialysis, geriatrics, heart failure, hematuria, infections, leukopenia QT prolongation, secondary malignancy surgery, tumor lysis syndrome, vaccinations, breastfeeding, severely depressed bone marrow function

DOSAGE AND ROUTES
Acute lymphocytic leukemia (ALL) (induction therapy)
Adult: PO initially 1-5 mg/kg over 2-5 days; maintenance 1-5 mg/kg; **IV** 300-1500 mg/m^2 (total dose)
Child: PO 60-250 mg/m^2 in divided doses × 6 or more days; maintenance; **IV** 10-15 mg/kg q7-10 days or 30 mg/kg q3-4wk; dose should be reduced by half when bone marrow suppression occurs

Neuroblastoma
Child and infant: PO 150 mg/m^2/day, days 1-7 with DOXOrubicin (**IV** 35 mg/m^2 on day 5) q21days × 5 cycles
Child: **IV** 70 mg/kg/day with hydration on days 1 and 2 with DOXOrubicin and vinCRIStine q21days for courses 1, 2, 4, 6, alternating with CISplatin and etoposide q21days for courses 3, 5, 7

Breast cancer
Adult: PO 100-200 mg/m^2/day or 2 mg/kg/day × 4-14 days; **IV** 500-1000 mg/m^2 on day 1 in combination with fluorouracil and methotrexate or DOXOrubicin, or DOXOrubicin alone; also cyclophosphamide 600 mg/m^2, may be given dose-dense on day 1 of q14day with DOXOrubicin (60 mg/m^2) with growth factor support

Operable node-positive breast cancer
IV (TAC regimen) Adult: 500 mg/m^2 with DOXOrubicin (50 mg/m^2 **IV**) then docetaxel (75 mg/m^2) **IV** given 1 hr later × 6 cycles q3wk

Nephrotic syndrome
Adult: PO 2-3 mg/kg/day for up to 12 wk when corticosteroids are unsuccessful

Available forms: Inj **IV** 100, 200, 500 mg, 1, 2 g; tabs 25, 50 mg

Implementation
• Give fluids **IV** or PO before chemotherapy to hydrate patient
• Give antacid before oral agent, after PM meals, before bedtime; antiemetic 30-60 min before giving product to prevent vomiting and prn; antibiotics for prophylaxis of infection
• Give top or syst analgesics for pain; give in AM so product can be eliminated before bedtime
• Use cytotoxic handling procedures
PO route
• To be taken on empty stomach; do not crush, break, chew tab, wash hands immediately if in contact with tab
• May be taken as a single dose or divided doses
• Take in AM or afternoon, avoid evening

Direct IV
• Reconstitute with NS only
• Store in tight container at room temperature
Intermittent IV infusion route
• Use cytotoxic handling procedures
• Give **IV** after diluting 100 mg/5 ml of sterile or bacteriostatic water; shake; let stand until clear; may be further diluted in up to 250 ml D$_5$ 0.9% NaCl, 0.45% NaCl, LR, D$_5$NS; SWI, 0.45% NaCl Ringer's; give 100 mg or less/min through 3-way stopcock of glucose or saline inf
• Use 21-, 23-, or 25-G needle; check site for irritation, phlebitis

Syringe compatibilities: Bleomycin, CISplatin, doxapram, DOXOrubicin, droperidol, fluorouracil, furosemide, heparin, leucovorin, methotrexate, metoclopramide, mitoMYcin, mitoXANtrone, vinBLAStine, vinCRIStine

Y-site compatibilities: Amifostine, amikacin, ampicillin, azlocillin, aztreonam, bleomycin, cefamandole, ceFAZolin, cefepime, cefoperazone, cefotaxime, cefOXitin, cefuroxime, cephalothin, cephapirin, chloramphenicol, chlorproMAZINE, cimetidine, CISplatin, cladribine, clindamycin, dexamethasone, diphenhydrAMINE, DOXOrubicin, doxycycline, droperidol, erythromycin, famotidine, filgrastim, fludarabine, fluorouracil, furosemide, gallium, ganciclovir, gentamicin, granisetron, heparin, HYDROmorphone, IDArubicin, kanamycin, leucovorin, LORazepam, melphalan, methotrexate, methylPREDNISolone, metoclopramide, metroNIDAZOLE, mezlocillin, minocycline, mitoMYcin, moxalactam, nafcillin, ondansetron, oxacillin, PACLitaxel, penicillin G potassium, piperacillin, piperacillin/tazobactam, prochlorperazine, promethazine, propofol, ranitidine, sargramostim, sodium bicarbonate, teniposide, tetracycline, thiotepa, ticarcillin, ticarcillin-clavulanate, tobramycin, trimethoprim-sulfamethoxazole, vancomycin, vinBLAStine, vinCRIStine, vinorelbine

Solution compatibilities: Amino acids 4.25%/D_{25}, D_5/0.9% NaCl, D_5W, 0.9% NaCl

ADVERSE EFFECTS

CNS: Headache, dizziness
CV: Cardiotoxicity (high doses), myocardial fibrosis, congestive heart failure, pericarditis
ENDO: Syndrome of inappropriate antidiuretic hormone (SIADH), gonadal suppression
GI: *Nausea, vomiting, diarrhea, weight loss,* colitis, **hepatotoxicity**
GU: Hemorrhagic cystitis, hematuria, neoplasms, amenorrhea, azoospermia, sterility, ovarian fibrosis, **renal tubular fibrosis**
HEMA: Thrombocytopenia, leukopenia, pancytopenia, myelosuppression
INTEG: *Alopecia,* dermatitis
META: Hyperuricemia
MISC: Secondary neoplasms, **anaphylaxis**
RESP: Pulmonary fibrosis, interstitial pneumonia

Pharmacokinetics

Absorption	Well absorbed (PO)
Distribution	Widely distributed; crosses placenta, blood-brain barrier (50%)
Metabolism	Liver to active product
Excretion	Kidneys, unchanged (30%)
Half-life	4-6½ hr

Pharmacodynamics

Unknown

INTERACTIONS

Individual drugs

Allopurinol: increased bone marrow suppression
Chloramphenicol: decreased cyclophosphamide effect

Digoxin: decreased digoxin levels
Insulin: increased hypoglycemia
Succinylcholine: increased neuromuscular blockade
Warfarin: increased warfarin action

Drug classifications

Diuretics (thiazides): increased bone marrow suppression
Barbiturates: increased toxicity of cyclophosphamide
Corticosteroids: decreased cyclophosphamide effect
Live virus vaccines: decreased antibody reaction

Drug/herb

St. John's wort: increased toxicity

Drug/lab test

Increased: uric acid
Decreased: pseudocholinesterase
False positive: Pap smear
False negative: PPD, mumps trichophytin, *Candida, Trichophyton,* Pap smear

NURSING CONSIDERATIONS

Assessment

🅐 **Assess symptoms indicating severe allergic reaction: rash, pruritus, urticaria, purpuric skin lesions, itching, flushing**
• Assess for tachypnea, ECG changes, dyspnea, edema, fatigue
🅐 **Bone marrow suppression: Monitor CBC, differential, platelet count weekly; withhold product if WBC count is <2500/mm³ or platelet count is <75,000/mm³; notify prescriber of results**
🅐 **Assess for hemorrhagic cystitis: renal function studies including BUN, creatinine, serum uric acid, urine CCr before, during therapy; I&O ratio; report fall in urine output to <30 ml/hr**
🅐 **Monitor temp q4hr (elevated temp may indicate beginning of infection)**
🅐 **Hepatotoxicity: Monitor liver function tests before, during therapy (bilirubin, AST, ALT, LDH) as needed or monthly; note jaundice of skin or sclera, dark urine, clay-colored stools, itchy skin, abdominal pain, fever, diarrhea**
🅐 **Assess for bleeding: hematuria, stool guaiac, bruising or petechiae, mucosa or orifices q8hr**
• Identify dyspnea, crackles, unproductive cough, chest pain, tachypnea
• Identify effects of alopecia on body image; discuss feelings about body changes

Patient/family education
• Teach patient to avoid use of products containing aspirin or ibuprofen, razors, commercial mouthwash, since bleeding may occur; to report symptoms of bleeding (hematuria, tarry stools, bruising)
• Instruct patient to report signs of anemia (fatigue, headache, irritability, faintness, shortness of breath)
• Teach patient to report any changes in breathing or coughing even several months after treatment
• Advise patient that hair may be lost during treatment; a wig or hairpiece may make patient feel better; new hair may be different in color, texture
• Advise patient on proper handling and disposal of chemotherapy drugs
• Teach patient not to have any vaccinations without the advice of the prescriber; serious reactions can occur
⚠ Advise patient contraception is needed during treatment and for several months after the completion of therapy
⚠ Teach patient to take adequate fluids to eliminate product

Evaluation
Positive therapeutic outcome
• Prevention of rapid division of malignant cells
• Increased appetite, increased weight

---

cycloSPORINE (Rx)
(sye-kloe-spor'een)
CycloSPORINE, modified Gengraf, Neoral, Pulminiq, SandIMMUNE
Func. class.: Immunosuppressant
Chem. class.: Fungus-derived peptide
Pregnancy category C

Do not confuse:
cycloSPORINE/CycloSERINE/cyclophosphamide, **SandIMMUNE**/SandoSTATIN

ACTION: Produces immunosuppression by inhibiting T lymphocytes

Therapeutic outcome: Absence of transplant rejection

USES: Organ transplants (liver, kidney, heart) to prevent rejection, rheumatoid arthritis, psoriasis

Unlabeled uses: Recalcitrant ulcerative colitis, aplastic anemia, Crohn's disease, GVHD, thrombocytopenia purpura, lupus, nephritis, myasthenia gravis, psoriatic arthritis

CONTRAINDICATIONS:
Hypersensitivity to polyxyethylated castor oil (inj only), psoriasis or rheumatoid arthrits in renal disease (Neoral/Gengraf), Gengraf/Neoral used with PUVA/UVB; methotrexate, coal tar, breastfeeding, ocular infections

> **BLACK BOX WARNING:** Neoplastic disease, sunlight (UV) exposure, renal disease/failure, uncontrolled, malignant hypertension; radiation in psoriasis

Precautions: Pregnancy **C**, geriatric, severe renal/hepatic disease

DOSAGE AND ROUTES
Prevention of transplant rejection (unmodified)
Adult and child: PO 15 mg/kg several hr before surgery, daily for 2 wk, reduce dosage by 2.5 mg/kg/wk to 5-10 mg/kg/day; **IV** 5-6 mg/kg several hr before surgery, daily, switch to PO form as soon as possible

Prevention of transplant rejection (modified)
Adult and child: PO 4-12 mg/kg/day divided q12hr, depends on organ transplanted

Rheumatoid arthritis (Neoral/Gengraf)
Adult: PO 2.5 mg/kg/day divided bid, may increase 0.5-0.75 mg/kg/day after 8-12 wk, max 4 mg/kg/day

Psoriasis (Neoral/Gengraf)
Adult: PO 2.5 mg/kg/day divided bid × 4 wk, then increase by 0.5 mg/kg/day q2wk, max 4 mg/kg/day

Idiopathic thrombocytopenia purpura (unlabeled)
Adult: PO 1.25-2.5 mg/kg bid

Severe aplastic anemia (unlabeled)
Adult and child: PO 12 mg/kg/day or 15 mg/kg/day (child) with antithymocyte globulin (ATG)

Available forms: Oral sol (Neoral) 100 mg/ml; soft gel cap 25, 50, 100 mg; inj 50 mg/ml; inh sol 300 mg/4.8 ml

---

Implementation
PO route
- Do not break, crush, or chew caps
- Use pipette provided to draw up oral sol; may mix with milk or juice, wipe pipette, do not wash (Neoral)
- Give for several days before transplant surgery with corticosteroids
- Microemulsion products (Neoral) and other products are not interchangeable
- Give with meals for GI upset or place product in chocolate milk (SandIMMUNE)
- Give with oral antifungal for *Candida* infections

Intermittent IV infusion route
- Give **IV** after diluting each 50 mg/20-100 ml of 0.9% NaCl or D$_5$W; run over 2-6 hr; use an inf pump, glass inf bottles only

Continuous IV infusion route
- May run over 24 hr
- **For Sandimmune parenteral:** give 1/3 of PO dose, initial dose 4-12 hr prior to transplantation as a single **IV** dose 5-6 mg/kg/day, continue the single daily dose until PO can be used

Additive compatibilities: Ciprofloxacin

Y-site compatibilities: Abciximab,
alatrofloxacin, alfentanil, amikacin, aminocaproic acid, aminophylline, amphotericin B lipid complex, anidulafungin, argatroban, ascorbic acid injection, atenolol, atracurium, atropine, azaTHIOprine, aztreonam, benztropine, bivalirudin, bleomycin, bretylium, bumetanide, buprenorphine, butorphanol, calcium chloride/gluconate, CARBOplatin, carmustine, caspofungin, cefamandole, ceFAZolin, cefmetazole, cefonicid, cefoperazone, cefotaxime, cefoTEtan, cefOXitin, ceftaroline, cefTAZidime, ceftizoxime, ceftobiprole, cefTRIAXone, cefuroxime, cephalothin, cephapirin, chloramphenicol, chlorproMAZINE, cimetidine, ciprofloxacin, CISplatin, clindamycin, codeine, cyanocobalamin, cyclophosphamide, cytarabine, DACTINomycin, DAPTOmycin, DAUNOrubicin, dexamethasone, dexmedetomidine, digoxin, diltiazem, diphenhydrAMINE, DOBUTamine, DOCEtaxel, DOPamine, doripenem, doxacurium, DOXOrubicin, doxycycline, enalaprilat, ePHEDrine, EPINEPHrine, epirubicin, epoetin alfa, eptifibatide, ertapenem, erythromycin, esmolol, etoposide, famotidine, fenoldopam, fentaNYL, fluconazole, fludarabine, fluorouracil, folic acid, furosemide, gallium, ganciclovir, gatifloxacin, gemcitabine, gentamicin, glycopyrrolate, granisetron, heparin, hydrocortisone, HYDROmorphone, hydrOXYzine, ifosfamide, imipenem-cilastatin, indomethacin, irinotecan, isoproterenol, ketorolac, labetalol, lansoprazole, levofloxacin, lidocaine, linezolid, LORazepam, mannitol, mechlorethamine, meperidine, meropenem, methicillin, methotrexate, methoxamine, methyldopate, methylPREDNISolone, metoclopramide, metoprolol, metroNIDAZOLE, mezlocillin, micafungin, miconazole, midazolam, milrinone, minocycline, mitoXANtrone, morphine, moxalactam, multiple vitamins injection, nafcillin, naloxone, nesiritide, netilmicin, nitroglycerin, nitroprusside, norepinephrine, octreotide, ondansetron, oxacillin, oxaliplatin, oxytocin, paclitaxel, palonosetron, pamidronate, pancuronium, pantoprazole, papaverine, PEMEtrexed, penicillin G potassium/sodium, pentamidine, pentazocine, phentolamine, phenylephrine, phytonadione, piperacillin, piperacillin-tazobactam, polymyxin B, potassium acetate/chloride, procainamide, prochlorperazine, promethazine, propofol, propranolol, protamine, pyridoxine, quiNIDine, quinupristin-dalfopristin, ranitidine, ritodrine, sargramostim, sodium acetate/bicarbonate, succinylcholine, SUFentanil, tacrolimus, teniposide, theophylline, thiamine, thiotepa, ticarcillin, ticarcillin-clavulanate, tigecycline, tirofiban, tobramycin, trimetaphan, urokinase, vancomycin, vasopressin, vecuronium, verapamil, vinCRIStine, vinorelbine, zoledronic acid

Solution compatibilities: D$_5$W, NaCl 0.9%

ADVERSE EFFECTS
CNS: *Tremors, headache,* **seizures,** confusion, **encephalopathy**
GI: Nausea, vomiting, diarrhea, *oral candida, gum hyperplasia,* **hepatotoxicity,** pancreatitis
GU: **Albuminuria, hematuria, proteinuria, renal failure, hemolytic uremic syndrome, nephrotoxicity**
INTEG: Rash, acne, *hirsutism,* pruritus
META: Hyperkalemia, hypomagnesemia, hyperlipidemia, hyperuricemia
MISC: *Infection, hypertension*

Pharmacokinetics

Absorption	Poorly absorbed (PO)
Distribution	Crosses placenta
Metabolism	Liver to mercaptopurine
Excretion	Kidney, minimal
Half-life	Biphasic 1.2 hr, 25 hr

Adverse effects: *italics* = common; **bold** = life-threatening

Pharmacodynamics

	PO
Onset	Unknown
Peak	4 hr
Duration	Unknown

INTERACTIONS
Individual drugs

Allopurinol, amiodarone, amphotericin B, bromocriptine, carvedilol, cimetidine, colchicine, foscarnet, imipenem-cilastatin, melphalan, metoclopramide: increased action, cycloSPORINE toxicity

Digoxin: increased digoxin level

Etoposide: increased etoposide level

Methotrexate: increased methotrexate level

Nafcillin, orlistat, PHENobarbital, phenytoin, terbinafine, ticlodipine, trimethoprim/sulfamethoxazole: decreased cycloSPORINE action

Sirolimus: increased sirolimus level

Tacrolimus: increased tacrolimus level

Drug classifications:

Androgens, antifungals (azole), β-blockers, calcium channel blockers, contraceptives (oral), corticosteroids, fluoroquinolones, macrolides, NSAIDs, selective serotonin reuptake inhibitors: increased cycloSPORINE levels, toxicity

Anticonvulsants, rifamycins: decreased cycloSPORINE levels

HMG-CoA reductase inhibitors, diuretics (potassium-sparing): increased effects of each product

Live virus vaccines: decreased antibody reaction

Drug/food

Grapefruit juice, food: increased slowed metabolism of product

NURSING CONSIDERATIONS
Assessment

• **Encephalopathy:** Assess for impaired cognition, seizures, vision changes including blindness, loss of motor function, movement disorders, psychiatric changes; dosage reduction or discontinuation may be needed in severe cases

• Monitor renal studies: BUN, creatinine at least monthly during treatment, 3 mo after treatment

• Monitor liver function studies: alkaline phosphatase, AST, ALT, bilirubin

• Monitor product blood levels during treatment

• Assess for **hepatotoxicity:** dark urine, jaundice, itching, light-colored stools; product should be discontinued

• Assess for **nephrotoxicity:** 6 wk postop, CyA trough level >200 ng/ml, intracapsular pressure <40 mm Hg, rise in creatinine 0.15 mg/dl/day

Patient/family education

• Advise patient to report fever, rash, severe diarrhea, chills, sore throat, fatigue, since serious infections may occur; also to report clay-colored stools, cramping (may indicate hepatotoxicity); tremors, bleeding gums, increased B/P

> **BLACK BOX WARNING:** Advise patient to limit UV exposure

• Caution patient to use contraceptive measures during treatment and for 12 wk after ending therapy; product is teratogenic, to notify prescriber if pregnancy is planned or suspected

• Caution patient to avoid crowds and persons with known infections to reduce risk of infection

• Teach patient to take at the same time of day, every day; do not skip or double a missed dose; not to use with grapefruit juice or receive vaccines; there are many drug interactions, do not add or discontinue products without prescriber approval

• Teach patient that treatment is lifelong to prevent rejection; to identify signs of rejection

• Advise patient to report severe diarrhea as drug loss may result

• **Nephrotoxicity:** Teach patient to notify prescriber of increased B/P, tremors of the hands, change in gums, increased hair on body/face

• Advise patient to continue with lab work and follow-up appointment

• Teach patient types of products are not interchangeable

• Teach patient not to wash syringe/container with water; a variation in dose may result

Evaluation
Positive therapeutic outcome

• Absence of graft rejection

A HIGH ALERT

cytarabine (Rx)
(sye-tare'a-been)
Ara-C, Cytosar ✦, Cytosar-U

cytarabine liposomal (Rx)
Depo Cyt
Func. class.: Antineoplastic, antimetabolite
Chem. class.: Pyrimidine nucleoside
Pregnancy category D

Do not confuse:
Cytosar ✦/Cytovene/Cytoxan

ACTION: Competes with physiologic substrate of DNA synthesis, thus interfering with cell replication in the S phase of the cell cycle (before mitosis)

Therapeutic outcome: Prevention of rapidly growing malignant cells

USES: Acute myelocytic leukemia, acute lymphocytic leukemia, chronic myelocytic leukemia, lymphomatous meningitis (IT/intraventricular)

Unlabeled uses: Hodgkin's/non-Hodgkin's lymphoma

CONTRAINDICATIONS:
Pregnancy **D**, hypersensitivity

Precautions: Renal/hepatic disease, breastfeeding, children, tumor lysis syndrome, infection, hyperkalemia, hyperphosphatemia, hyperuricemia, hypocalcemia

> **BLACK BOX WARNING:** Bone marrow suppression

DOSAGE AND ROUTES
Acute myelogenous leukemia (AML)
Adult: cont **IV** infusion 100 mg/m^2/day × 7 days q2wk as a single agent or 2-3 divided doses × 5-10 days until remission used in combination; maintenance 70-200 mg/m^2/day × 2-5 days qmo; **SUBCUT** maintenance 100 mg/m^2/day × 5 days q28days

Meningeal leukemia
Adult and child: Intrathecal 5-70 mg/m^2 variable daily × 4 days to q2-7day

Carcinomatous meningitis (liposoma)
Adult: Intrathecal 50 mg over 1-5 min q14days, during induction and consolidation wk 1, 3, 5, 7, 9, give another 50 mg wk 13; maintenance 50 mg q28days on wk 17, 21, 25, 29 use with dexamethasone 4 mg PO/IV × 5 days on each day of cytarabine

Renal dose
Adult CCr ≤60 ml/min, serum creatinine 1.5-1.9 mg/dl or increase of 0.5-1.2 mg/dl from baseline: during treatment reduce to 1 g/m^2/dose; **serum creatinine ≥2 mg/dl or change from baseline serum creatinine was 1.2 mg/dl** reduce to 100 mg/m^2/day

Available forms: Powder for inj 100, 500 mg, 1, 2 g; sus rel (Depo Cyt) liposomal for intrathecal use 10 mg/ml

Implementation
• Avoid contact with skin; very irritating; wash completely to remove
• Give fluids **IV** or PO before chemotherapy to hydrate patient
• Give antiemetic 30-60 min before giving product to prevent vomiting, and prn; antibiotics for prophylaxis of infection
• Increase fluids to 3 L/day
• Give top or syst analgesics for pain
• Give in AM so product can be eliminated before bedtime
• Use cytotoxic handling precautions

IM/SUBCUT route
• **Reconstitute** 100 mg/5 ml or 500 mg/10 ml with bacteriostatic water for inj with benzyl alcohol 0.9%; do not use sol with precipitate; stable for 48 hr

Intrathecal route
• **Liposomal: withdraw** product immediately before use; **use** within 4 hr, do not save unused portions or use in-line filter; **give** directly into CSF by intraventricular reservoir or by direct inj into lumbar site
• **Give** slowly over 1-5 min; follow with lumbar puncture; instruct patient to lie flat; **give** dexamethasone 4 mg bid PO or **IV** × 5 days beginning on day of liposomal inj

Direct IV route
• **Dilute** 100 mg/5 ml of sterile water for inj, **give** over 1-3 min through a free-flowing IV

Intermittent IV infusion route
• May be further diluted in 50-100 ml NS or D$_5$W and **give** over 30 min-24 hr, depending on dose

Continuous IV infusion route
• May be given as continuous IV infusion

Syringe compatibilities: Metoclopramide

Y-site compatibilities: Acyclovir, alfentanil, amifostine, amikacin, aminocaproic acid, aminophylline, amphotericin B lipid complex, amphotericin B liposome, ampicillin, ampicillin-sulbactam, amsacrine, anidulafungin, atenolol, atracurium, azithromycin, aztreonam, bivalirudin, bleomycin, bumetanide, buprenorphine, butorphanol, calcium chloride/gluconate, CARBOplatin, ceFAZolin, cefepime, cefoperazone, cefotaxime, cefoTEtan, cefOXitin, cefTAZidime, ceftizoxime, cefTRIAXone, cefuroxime, chlorproMAZINE, cimetidine, ciprofloxacin, cisatracurium, CISplatin, cladribine, clindamycin, codeine, cyclophosphamide, cycloSPORINE, DAUNOrubicin, dexamethasone, dexmedetomidine, dexrazoxane, digoxin, diltiazem, diphenhydrAMINE, DOBUTamine, DOCEtaxel, dolasetron, DOPamine, doxacurium, DOXOrubicin, DOXOrubicin liposomal, doxycycline, droperidol, enalaprilat, ePHEDrine, EPINEPHrine, ertapenem, erythromycin, esmolol, etoposide, famotidine, fenoldopam, fentaNYL, filgrastim, fluconazole, fludarabine, foscarnet, fosphenytoin, furosemide, gatifloxacin, gemcitabine, gemtuzumab, gentamicin, granisetron, haloperidol, heparin, hydrocortisone, HYDROmorphone, hydrOXYzine, IDArubicin, ifosfamide, imipenem-cilastatin, inamrinone, insulin (regular), irinotecan, isoproterenol, ketorolac, labetalol, leucovorin, levofloxacin, levorphanol, lidocaine, linezolid, LORazepam, magnesium sulfate, mannitol, melphalan, meperidine, meropenem, mesna, methohexital, methotrexate, methylPREDNISolone, metoclopramide, metoprolol, metroNIDAZOLE, midazolam, milrinone, minocycline, mitoXANtrone, mivacurium, morphine, nalbuphine, naloxone, nesiritide, niCARdipine, nitroglycerin, nitroprusside, norepinephrine, octreotide, ofloxacin, ondansetron, oxaliplatin, PACLitaxel, palonosetron, pamidronate, pancuronium, pantoprazole, PEMEtrexed, pentamidine, PENTobarbital, PHENobarbital, phenylephrine, piperacillin, piperacillin-tazobactam, potassium chloride/phosphates, procainamide, prochlorperazine, promethazine, propofol, propranolol, quinupristin-dalfopristin, ranitidine, rapacuronium, remifentanil, riTUXimab, rocuronium, sargramostim, sodium acetate/bicarbonate/phosphates, succinylcholine, SUFentanil, sulfamethoxazole-trimethoprim, tacrolimus, teniposide, theophylline, thiopental, thiotepa, ticarcillin, ticarcillin-clavulanate, tigecycline, tirofiban, TNA, tobramycin, trastuzumab, trimethobenzamide, vancomycin, vasopressin, vecuronium, verapamil, vinCRIStine, vinorelbine, voriconazole, zidovudine, zoledronic acid

Additive compatibilities: Corticotropin, DAUNOrubicin with etoposide, etoposide, hydrOXYzine, lincomycin, mitoXANtrone, potassium chloride, prednisoLONE, ondansetron, sodium bicarbonate, vinCRIStine

Additive incompatibilities: Carbenicillin, fluorouracil, heparin, regular insulin, nafcillin, oxacillin, penicillin G sodium

Solution compatibilities: Amino acids, 4.25%/D$_{25}$, D$_5$/LR, D$_5$/0.2% NaCl, D$_5$/0.9% NaCl, D$_{10}$/0.9% NaCl, D$_5$W, invert glucose 10% in electrolyte #1, Ringer's LR, 0.9% NaCl, sodium lactate 1/6 mol/L, TPN #57

ADVERSE EFFECTS
CNS: Neuritis, dizziness, headache, cerebellar syndrome, personality changes, ataxia, mechanical dysphasia, **coma; chemical arachnoiditis** (IT)
CV: Chest pain, **cardiopathy**
EENT: Sore throat, conjunctivitis
GI: *Nausea, vomiting, anorexia, diarrhea, stomatitis,* **hepatotoxicity,** abdominal pain, hematemesis, **GI hemorrhage**
GU: Urinary retention, **renal failure, hyperuricemia**
HEMA: **Thrombophlebitis, bleeding, thrombocytopenia, leukopenia, myelosuppression, anemia**
INTEG: *Rash, fever,* freckling, cellulitis
META: Hyperuricemia
MISC: Cytarabine syndrome—fever, myalgia, bone pain, chest pain, rash, conjunctivitis, malaise (6-12 hr after administration)
RESP: **Pneumonia,** dyspnea, **pulmonary edema** (high doses)
SYST: **Anaphylaxis, tumor lysis syndrome**

Pharmacokinetics
Absorption	Complete
Distribution	Widely distributed; crosses blood-brain barrier, placenta
Metabolism	Liver, extensively
Excretion	Kidneys
Half-life	Distribution 10 min; elimination 1-3 hr; IT 100-236 hr

Pharmacodynamics
Unknown

INTERACTIONS
Individual drugs
Digoxin oral: decreased digoxin effects
Filgrastim, G-CSF, GM-CSF, sargramostim: do not use within 24 hr
Flucytosine, methotrexate: increased toxicity, immunosuppression
Gentamicin: decreased effects
Radiation: increased toxicity, bone marrow suppression

Drug classifications
Anticoagulants, NSAIDs, platelet inhibitors, salicylates, thrombolytics: increased bleeding risk
Immunosuppressants, antineoplastics: increased toxicity, bone marrow suppression
Live virus vaccines: do not use together

NURSING CONSIDERATIONS
Assessment
• Assess buccal cavity q8hr for dryness, sores or ulceration, white patches, pain, bleeding, dysphagia; obtain prescription for viscous lidocaine (Xylocaine)
• Assess symptoms indicating **anaphylaxis:** rash, pruritus, urticaria, purpuric skin lesions, itching, flushing; resuscitation equipment should be nearby
⚠ **Assess for chemical arachnoiditis (IT): headache, nausea, vomiting, fever; neck rigidity/pain, meningism, CSF pleocytosis; may be decreased by dexamethasone**
• Assess tachypnea, dyspnea, edema, fatigue; identify dyspnea, crackles, unproductive cough, chest pain, tachypnea; pulmonary edema may be fatal (rare)
⚠ **Assess for cytarabine syndrome 6-12 hr after infusion: fever, myalgia, bone pain, chest pain, rash, conjunctivitis, malaise; corticosteroid may be ordered**
• **Bone marrow suppression:** Monitor CBC, differential, platelet count weekly; withhold product if WBC count is <1000/mm³ or platelet count is <50,000/mm³
• Assess for increased uric acid levels, swelling, joint pain primarily in extremities; patient should be well hydrated to prevent urate deposits
• Monitor renal function studies: BUN, creatinine, serum uric acid, urine CCr before and during therapy; I&O ratio; report fall in urine output to <30 ml/hr
• Monitor temp q4hr (may indicate beginning of infection)

⚠ **Hepatotoxicity: Monitor liver function tests before and during therapy (bilirubin, AST, ALT, LDH) as needed or monthly; note yellowing of skin or sclera, dark urine, clay-colored stools, pruritus, abdominal pain, fever, diarrhea; an antispasmodic may be used for GI symptoms**
• Assess for bleeding: hematuria, stool guaiac, bruising or petechiae, mucosa or orifices q8hr; identify inflammation of mucosa, breaks in skin

Patient/family education
• Advise patient that contraceptive measures are recommended during and 4 mo after therapy
• Teach patient to avoid use of products containing aspirin or ibuprofen, NSAIDs, razors, commercial mouthwash, since bleeding may occur; to report symptoms of bleeding (hematuria, tarry stools)
• Advise that fever, headache, nausea, vomiting are likely to occur but to continue using dexamethasone with IT administration
• Provide liquid diet: carbonated beverages; gelatin may be added if patient is not nauseated or vomiting
• Provide rinsing of mouth tid-qid with water, club soda; brushing of teeth bid-qid with soft brush or cotton-tipped applicators for stomatitis; use unwaxed dental floss
• Advise patient to report signs of anemia (fatigue, headache, irritability, faintness, shortness of breath)
• Advise patient to avoid foods with citric acid, hot flavor, or rough texture if stomatitis is present, to use sponge brush and rinse with water after each meal; to report stomatitis: any bleeding, white spots, ulcerations in mouth; tell patient to examine mouth daily, report any symptoms
• Instruct patient to report any changes in breathing or coughing even several months after treatment; to avoid crowds and persons with respiratory tract or other infections; neurotoxicity
• Caution patient not to have any vaccinations without the advice of the prescriber; serious reactions can occur
• Advise patient to take 3 L/day fluids to prevent renal damage

Evaluation
Positive therapeutic outcome
• Prevention of rapid division of malignant cells

Adverse effects: *italics* = common; **bold** = life-threatening

dabigatran (Rx)
(da-bye-gat'ran)
Pradaxa
Func. class.: Anticoagulant-thrombin inhibitor
Pregnancy category C

ACTION: Direct thrombin inhibitor that inhibits both free and clot-bound thrombin, prevents thrombin-induced platelet aggregation and thrombus formation by preventing conversion of fibrinogen to fibrin

Therapeutic outcome: Decreased thrombus formation/extension, absence of emboli, post-thrombotic effects

USES: Stroke/systemic embolism prophylaxis with non-valvular atrial fibrillation

CONTRAINDICATIONS:
Hypersensitivity, bleeding

Precautions: Abrupt discontinuation, anticoagulant therapy, breastfeeding, pregnancy **C,** children, geriatrics, labor, obstetric delivery, renal disease, surgery

> **BLACK BOX WARNING:** Abrupt discontinuation

DOSAGE AND ROUTES
Stroke prophylaxis
Adult: PO 150 mg bid

For conversion from an alternative anticoagulant to dabigatran
• When converting from warfarin to dabigatran, discontinue warfarin and initiate dabigatran therapy when the INR is <2.0. When converting from a parenteral anticoagulant to dabigatran, initiate dabigatran 0-2 hr before the time of the next scheduled anticoagulant dose or at the time of discontinuation of a continuously administered anticoagulant (e.g., intravenous unfractionated heparin)

For conversion from dabigatran to warfarin
Adult: CCr >50 ml/min start warfarin 3 days before discontinuing dabigatran; CCr 31-50 ml/min start warfarin 2 days before discontinuing dabigatran; CCr 15-30 ml/min start warfarin 1 day before discontinuing dabigatran

For conversion from dabigatran to parenteral anticoagulants
Adult: PO discontinue dabigatran, start parenteral anticoagulant 12 hr (CCR ≥30 ml/min), 24 hr (CCR <30 ml/min) after the last dabigatran dose

Renal dose
Adult: PO CCr 15-30 ml/min 75 mg bid

Deep vein thrombus (DVT)/pulmonary embolism prophylaxis (unlabeled)
Adult: PO 220 mg or 150 mg/day × 28-35 days, starting with ½ dose 1-4 hr after surgery

Available forms: Cap 75, 150 mg

Implementation
• Do not crush break, chew, or empty contents of capsule
• Take without regard to food
• Store in original package until time of use at room temperature, discard after 30 days, protect from moisture

ADVERSE EFFECTS
CV: Myocardial infarction
CNS: Intracranial bleeding
GI: Abdominal pain, dyspepsia, peptic ulcer, esophagitis, GERD, gastritis, **GI bleeding**
HEMA: Bleeding (any site)
INTEG: Rash, pruritus
SYST: Anaphylaxis (rare)

Pharmacokinetics

Absorption	Protein binding 35%
Distribution	Unknown
Metabolism	Unknown
Excretion	Unknown
Half-life	12-17 hr (extended in renal disease)

Pharmacodynamics

Onset	Unknown
Peak	1 hr; high-fat meal delays peak
Duration	Unknown

INTERACTIONS
Individual drugs
Amiodarone, clopidogrel, ketoconazole, quiNIDine, verapamil: increased bleeding risk
Rifampin: decreased dabigatran effect

Drug classifications
Anticoagulants, thrombolytics: increased bleeding risk

Drug/herb
St. John's wort: decreased dabigatran effect

NURSING CONSIDERATIONS
Assessment
• **Assess for bleeding:** blood in urine or emesis, dark tarry stools, lower back pain. Caution with arterial/venous punctures, catheters, NG tubes. Monitor vital signs frequently. The elderly are more prone to serious bleeding
• **Assess for thrombosis/MI/emboli:** swelling, pain, redness, difficulty breathing, chest pain, tachypnea, cough, coughing up blood, cyanosis
• **Assess for post-thrombotic syndrome:** pain, heaviness, itching/tingling, swelling, varicose veins, brownish/reddish skin discoloration, ulcers; ambulation, compression stockings and adequate anticoagulation can prevent this syndrome
• Monitor serum creatinine

Patient/family education
• Explain the purpose and expected results of this product
• Instruct patient to report if bleeding is present

Evaluation
Positive therapeutic outcome
• Decreased thrombus formation/extension, absence of emboli, post-thrombotic effects
• If dose is missed take as soon as remembered if on the same day, do not administer if <6 hr before next dose

---

⚠ HIGH ALERT

dacarbazine (Rx)
(da-kar'ba-zeen)
dacarbazine, DTIC ✤, DTIC-Dome
Func. class.: Antineoplastic—miscellaneous agent
Chem. class.: Imidazole
Pregnancy category C

ACTION: Alkylates DNA, RNA; inhibits RNA, DNA synthesis; also responsible for breakage, cross-linking DNA strands; activity is not cell cycle phase specific

Therapeutic outcome: Prevention of rapidly growing malignant cells

USES: Hodgkin's disease, malignant melanoma

Unlabeled uses: Malignant pheochromocytoma in combination with cyclophosphamide and vinCRIStine, metastatic soft tissue sarcoma in combination with other agents, carcinoma meningitis, neuroblastoma

CONTRAINDICATIONS:
Hypersensitivity, breastfeeding
Precautions: Renal disease

> **BLACK BOX WARNING:** Pregnancy **C** (1st trimester), radiation therapy, hepatic disease, bone marrow suppression, secondary malignancy

DOSAGE AND ROUTES
Metastatic malignant melanoma
Adult: IV 2-4.5 mg/kg daily × 10 days or 100-250 mg/m² daily × 5 days; repeat q3wk depending on response

Hodgkin's disease
Adult: IV 150 mg/m² daily × 5 days with other agents, repeat q4wk or 375 mg/m² on days 1 and 15 when given in combination, repeat q28day

Osteogenic sarcoma (unlabeled)
Adult and child: IV 250 mg/m²/day as a cont INF × 4 days q28day

Soft tissue sarcoma (unlabeled)
Adult and child: IV 250-300 mg/m²/day as a cont INF × 3 days q21-28day

Carcinoma meningitis (unlabeled)
Adult: Intrathecal 5-30 mg in a fixed dose 2-3 × wk until disease controlled

Available forms: Powder for inj 10, 100, 200 mg

Implementation
• Give fluids **IV** or PO before chemotherapy to hydrate patient
• Give antiemetic 30-60 min before giving product to prevent vomiting, and prn; antibiotics for prophylaxis of infection
• Provide liquid diet: carbonated beverages; gelatin may be added if patient is not nauseated or vomiting
Direct IV route
• After diluting 100 mg/9.9 ml or 200 mg/19.7 ml of sterile water for inj (10 mg/ml), give by direct **IV** over 1 min through Y-tube or 3-way stopcock
Intermittent IV infusion route
• May be further diluted in 50-250 ml of D₅W or normal saline for inj and given over 30 min

---

- Watch for extravasation; stop infusion, apply ice to area
- Store in light-resistant container in a dry area

Y-site compatibilities: Amifostine, aztreonam, filgrastim, fludarabine, granisetron, melphalan, ondansetron, PACLitaxel, sargramostim, teniposide, thiotepa, vinorelbine

ADVERSE EFFECTS

CNS: Facial paresthesia, flushing, fever, malaise, confusion, headache, **seizures, cerebral hemorrhage,** blurred vision (high doses)
GI: *Nausea, anorexia, vomiting,* **hepatotoxicity** (rare)
HEMA: **Thrombocytopenia, leukopenia,** anemia
INTEG: *Alopecia,* dermatitis, pain at inj site, photosensitivity, severe sun reactions (high doses)
MISC: Flulike symptoms, malaise, fever, myalgia, hypotension
SYST: Anaphylaxis

Pharmacokinetics

Absorption	Complete bioavailability (**IV**)
Distribution	Widely distributed; concentrates in liver
Metabolism	Liver (50%, 5% protein bound)
Excretion	Kidneys, unchanged (50%)
Half-life	Initial 35 min, terminal 5 hr

Pharmacodynamics

Unknown

INTERACTIONS

Individual drugs

PHENobarbital, phenytoin: increased metabolism; decreased dacarbazine effect
Radiation: bone marrow suppression, toxicity

Drug classifications

Aminoglycosides: increased nephrotoxicity
Anticoagulants, salicylates: increased risk of bleeding
Antineoplastics, bone marrow–suppressing products: increased toxicity, bone marrow suppression
Diuretics, loop: increased ototoxicity
Live virus vaccines: increased adverse reactions; decreased antibody reaction

NURSING CONSIDERATIONS

Assessment

- **Assess symptoms indicating severe allergic reaction:** rash, pruritus, urticaria, purpuric skin lesions, itching, flushing; product should be discontinued

> **BLACK BOX WARNING: Assess for bone marrow suppression:** Monitor CBC, differential, platelet count weekly; withhold product if WBC is <4000/mm^3 or platelet count is <75,000/mm^3

- Monitor renal function tests: BUN, creatinine, urine CCr before, during therapy; I&O ratio; report fall in urine output to <30 ml/hr
- Monitor temp q4hr (may indicate beginning of infection)

> **BLACK BOX WARNING: Assess for hepatic disease:** Monitor liver function tests before, during therapy (bilirubin, AST, ALT, LDH) as needed or monthly; note jaundice of skin or sclera, dark urine, clay-colored stools, itchy skin, abdominal pain, fever, diarrhea; hepatotoxicity can be serious and fatal

- Assess for bleeding: hematuria, stool guaiac, bruising or petechiae, mucosa or orifices q8hr; check for inflammation of mucosa, breaks in skin
- Identify effects of alopecia on body image; discuss feelings about body changes

> **BLACK BOX WARNING: Secondary malignancy:** Assess for secondary malignancy that may occur with this product

Patient/family education

- Teach patient to avoid use of products containing aspirin or ibuprofen, razors, commercial mouthwash, since bleeding may occur; to report symptoms of bleeding (hematuria, tarry stools)
- ⚠ **Instruct patient to report signs of anemia (fatigue, headache, irritability, faintness, shortness of breath)**
- Advise patient that hair may be lost during treatment; a wig or hairpiece may make patient feel better; new hair may be different in color, texture
- ⚠ **Pregnancy: Teach patient to notify prescriber if pregnancy is planned or suspected pregnancy (D)**
- Caution patient not to have any vaccinations without the advice of prescriber; serious reactions can occur

> **BLACK BOX WARNING:** Advise patient contraception is needed during treatment and for several months after the completion of therapy; product has teratogenic properties

⚠ Teach patient to report signs of infection: fever, sore throat, flulike symptoms

Evaluation
Positive therapeutic outcome
• Prevention of rapid division of malignant cells

dalfampridine (Rx)
(dal-fam′pri-deen)
Ampyra
Func. class.: Neurological agent—MS
Chem. class.: Broad-spectrum potassium channel blocker
Pregnancy category C

ACTION: Mechanism of action is not fully understood, a broad-spectrum potassium channel blocker inhibits potassium channels and increased action potential conduction in demyelinated axons

Therapeutic outcome: Ability to walk at improved speed in MS

USES: For improved walking in patients with multiple sclerosis

CONTRAINDICATIONS:
Renal failure (CCr <50 ml/min), seizures

Precautions: Pregnancy **C**, breastfeeding, renal disease, elderly

DOSAGE AND ROUTES
Adult: PO 10 mg q12hr

Renal dose
Adult: PO CCr 51-80 ml/min no dosage adjustment needed, but seizure risk is unknown; CCr ≤50 ml/min, do not use

Available forms: Ext rel tab 10 mg

Implementation
• Do not break, crush, or chew; give without regard to meals
• Do not give closer together than q12hr, seizures may occur
• Do not double doses, if a dose is missed, skip it

ADVERSE EFFECTS
CNS: *Seizures,* paresthesias, headache, dizziness, asthenia, insomnia
GI: Nausea, constipation, dyspepsia
GU: Urinary tract infection
MS: Back pain

Pharmacokinetics
Absorption	Bioavailability 96%
Distribution	Largely unbound to plasma proteins
Metabolism	Unknown
Excretion	96% is recovered in the urine
Half-life	Unknown

Pharmacodynamics
Onset	Unknown
Peak	3-4 hr (fasting), longer if taken with food
Duration	Unknown

INTERACTIONS
Individual drugs
Fampridine: do not use together

Drug classifications
4-aminopyridine (4-AP)-containing products: do not use together

NURSING CONSIDERATIONS
Assessment
• **Multiple sclerosis:** assess walking, including speed
• **Assess for seizures:** more common in those with previous seizure disorder

Patient/family education
• Advise patient to notify prescriber if pregnancy is planned or suspected, do not breastfeed
• Teach patient about expected results, side effects including seizures

Evaluation
Positive therapeutic outcome
• Ability to walk at improved speed in MS

⚠ HIGH ALERT
dalteparin (Rx)
(dahl′ta-pear-in)
Fragmin
Func. class.: Anticoagulant
Chem. class.: Low-molecular-weight heparin
Pregnancy category B

ACTION: Inhibits factor Xa/IIa (thrombin), resulting in anticoagulation

Therapeutic outcome: Absence of deep vein thrombosis

USES: Unstable angina/non-Q-wave MI; prevention/treatment of deep vein thrombosis in abdominal surgery, hip replacement patients or those with restricted mobility during acute illness; pulmonary embolism

Unlabeled uses: Antiphospholipid antibody, arterial thromboembolism (after heart valve surgery), cerebral thromboembolism, acute MI

CONTRAINDICATIONS:

Hypersensitivity to this product, heparin, pork products; active major bleeding, hemophilia, leukemia with bleeding, thrombocytopenic purpura, cerebrovascular hemorrhage, cerebral aneurysm, those undergoing regional anesthesia for unstable angina, non–Q-wave MI, dalteparin-induced thrombocytopenia

Precautions: Hypersensitivity to benzyl alcohol, pregnancy **B**, recent childbirth, breastfeeding, child, geriatric, hepatic disease, severe renal/cardiac disease, blood dyscrasias, bacterial endocarditis, acute nephritis, peptic ulcer disease, pericarditis, pericardial effusion, recent lumbar puncture, vasculitis, other diseases where bleeding is possible, uncontrolled hypertension; recent brain, spine, eye surgery; congenital or acquired disorders, hemorrhagic stroke, history of HIT

> **BLACK BOX WARNING:** Epidural anesthesia, lumbar puncture

DOSAGE AND ROUTES
Deep vein thrombosis/pulmonary embolism
Adult: SUBCUT 200 international units/kg/day during 1st month (max single dose 18,000 international units), then 150 IU/kg/day in month 2-6 (max single dose 18,000 international units), use prefilled syringe that is closest to calculated dose; if platelets are 50,000-100,000/mm³ reduce dose by 2500 international units until platelets ≥100,000/mm³; if platelets <50,000/mm³ discontinue until >50,000/mm³

Hip replacement surgery/DVT prophylaxis
Adult: SUBCUT 2500 international units 2 hr before surgery and 2nd dose in the evening the day of surgery (4-8 hr postop), then 5000 international units SUBCUT 1st postop day and daily 5-10 days

Unstable angina/non-Q-wave MI
Adult: SUBCUT 120 international units/kg q12hr × 5-8 days; max 10,000 international units q12hr × 5-8 days with concurrent aspirin, continue until stable

Deep vein thrombosis, prophylaxis for abdominal surgery
Adult: SUBCUT 2500 international units 1-2 hr prior to abdominal surgery and repeat daily × 5-10 days; in high-risk patients 5000 international units should be used

Renal dose
Adult: SUBCUT cancer patient with CCr <30 ml/min, monitor antifactor Xa in extended

Available forms: Prefilled syringes, 2500, 5000 international units/0.2 ml; 7500 international units/0.3 ml, 10,000, 15,000, 18,000 international units/ml

Implementation
SUBCUT route
- Cannot be used interchangeably unit for unit with unfractionated heparin or other LMWHs
- Do not give IM or **IV** product route; approved in SUBCUT only; do not mix with other inj or sol
- Give by SUBCUT only; have patient sit or lie down; SUBCUT inj may be 2 in from umbilicus in a U-shape, upper outer side of thigh, around navel, or upper outer quadrangle of the buttocks; rotate inj sites
- Change inj site daily, use at same time of day

ADVERSE EFFECTS
CNS: Intracranial bleeding
HEMA: Thrombocytopenia
INTEG: Alopecia, pruritus, superficial wound infection, skin necrosis, injection site reaction
SYST: Hypersensitivity, **hemorrhage, anaphylaxis** possible, **hematoma**

Pharmacokinetics
Absorption	87%
Distribution	Unknown
Metabolism	Liver
Excretion	Kidney
Half-life	3-5 hr elimination

Pharmacodynamics
Onset	Unknown
Peak	2-4 hr
Duration	Unknown

INTERACTIONS
Individual drugs
Aspirin: increased bleeding risk

Drug classifications

Anticoagulants, NSAIDs, platelet inhibitors, salicylates, thrombolytics: increased risk of bleeding

Drug/herb

Feverfew, garlic, ginger, ginkgo, horse chestnut: increased bleeding risk

NURSING CONSIDERATIONS

Assessment

• Assess for bleeding (Hct, occult blood in stools) during treatment since bleeding can occur

⚠ **Assess for bleeding gums, petechiae, ecchymosis, black tarry stools, hematuria, epistaxis, decrease in Hct, B/P; may indicate bleeding, possible hemorrhage; notify prescriber immediately; product should be discontinued**

• **Assess for hypersensitivity:** fever, skin rash, urticaria; notify prescriber immediately

• Assess for needed dosage change q1-2wk; dosage may need to be decreased if bleeding occurs

> **BLACK BOX WARNING:** Epidural anesthesia: Assess for neurologic impairment frequently when neuraxial anesthesia has been used, spinal/epidural hematomas can occur, with paralysis

Patient/family education

• Advise patient to avoid OTC preparations that contain aspirin, other anticoagulants; serious product interaction may occur

• Advise patient to use soft-bristle toothbrush to avoid bleeding gums, avoid contact sports, use electric razor, avoid IM inj

• Instruct patient to report any signs of bleeding: gums, under skin, urine, stools; unusual bruising

Evaluation

Positive therapeutic outcome

• Absence of deep vein thrombosis

TREATMENT OF OVERDOSE:

Protamine sulfate 1% given **IV**; 1 mg protamine/100 anti-Xa international units of dalteparin given

---

dantrolene (Rx)

(dan'troe-leen)

Dantrium, Revonto

Func. class.: Skeletal muscle relaxant, direct acting

Chem. class.: Hydantoin

Pregnancy category C

D

Do not confuse:

Dantrium/danazol

ACTION: Interferes with intracellular release from the sarcoplasmic reticulum of calcium necessary to initiate contraction; slows catabolism in malignant hyperthermia

Therapeutic outcome: Decreased muscle spasticity; absence of malignant hyperthermia

USES: Spasticity in multiple sclerosis, stroke, spinal cord injury, cerebral palsy, prevention and treatment of malignant hyperthermia

Unlabeled uses: Neuroleptic malignant syndrome

CONTRAINDICATIONS:

Hypersensitivity, compromised pulmonary function, active hepatic disease, impaired myocardial function

> **BLACK BOX WARNING:** Active hepatic disease

Precautions: Pregnancy **C**, breastfeeding, geriatric, peptic ulcer disease, renal/cardiac/hepatic, stroke, seizure disorder, diabetes mellitus, ALS, COPD, MS, mannitol/gelatin hypersensitivity, labor, lactase deficiency, extravasation

> **BLACK BOX WARNING:** Females >35 yr, with MS or taking estrogens

DOSAGE AND ROUTES

Spasticity

Adult: PO 25 mg/day; may increase to 25-100 mg bid-qid, max 400 mg/day

Child: PO 0.5 mg/kg/day given in divided doses bid; may increase gradually; max 400 mg daily

Malignant hyperthermia

Adult and child: **IV** 1 mg/kg; may repeat to total dose of 10 mg/kg; PO 4-8 mg/kg/day in 4 divided doses × 3 days to prevent further

---

Adverse effects: *italics* = common; **bold** = life-threatening

hyperthermia; postcrisis follow-up 4-8 mg/kg/day for 1-3 days

Prevention of malignant hyperthermia
Adult and child: PO 4-8 mg/kg/day in 3-4 divided doses × 1-2 days before procedures; give last dose 4 hr preoperatively; **IV** 2.5 mg/kg prior to anesthesia

Neuroleptic malignant syndrome (unlabeled)
Adult: PO 100-300 mg/day in divided doses, **IV** 1.25-1.5 mg/kg

Available forms: Caps 25, 50, 100 mg; powder for inj 20 mg/vial

Implementation
PO route
• Do not crush or chew caps; caps may be opened and mixed with juice and swallowed; drink immediately after mixing
• Give with meals for GI symptoms
• Store in airtight container at room temperature

IV route
• Administer **IV** after diluting 20 mg/60 ml sterile water for inj without bacteriostatic agent (333 mcg/ml); shake until clear; give by rapid **IV** push through Y-tube or 3-way stopcock; follow by prescribed doses immediately; may also give by intermittent inf over 1 hr before anesthesia; assess site for extravasation, phlebitis
• Protect diluted sol from light; use reconstituted sol within 6 hr
• Considered incompatible in sol or syringe, compatibility unknown

ADVERSE EFFECTS
CNS: *Dizziness, weakness, fatigue, drowsiness,* headache, disorientation, insomnia, paresthesias, tremors, **seizures**
CV: Hypotension, chest pain, palpitations
EENT: Nasal congestion, blurred vision, mydriasis
GI: **Hepatic injury,** *nausea,* constipation, vomiting, increased AST and alkaline phosphatase, abdominal pain, dry mouth, anorexia, hepatitis, dyspepsia
GU: Urinary frequency, nocturia, impotence, crystalluria, **hepatitis**
HEMA: **Eosinophilia, aplastic anemia, leukopenia, thrombocytopenia/lymphoma**
INTEG: Rash, pruritus, photosensitivity, extravasation (tissue necrosis)
RESP: Pleural effusion, **pulmonary edema**

Pharmacokinetics

Absorption	PO (30%-35%), poor
Distribution	Unknown
Metabolism	Liver, extensively
Excretion	Kidney
Half-life	9 hr

Pharmacodynamics

	PO	IV
Onset	Unknown	Immediate
Peak	5 hr	5 hr
Duration	Dose related	Dose related

INTERACTIONS
• Considered incompatible in sol or syringe; compatibility unknown

Individual drugs
Alcohol: increased CNS depression
Verapamil: increased dysrhythmias

Drug classifications
Antidepressants (tricyclic), antihistamines, barbiturates, opiates, sedative/hypnotics: increased CNS depression
Estrogens, hepatotoxic agents: increased hepatotoxicity

NURSING CONSIDERATIONS
Assessment
• Monitor I&O ratio; check for urinary retention, frequency, hesitancy, especially geriatric
• **Seizures:** Monitor ECG in epileptic patients; poor seizure control has occurred with patients taking this product; assess for increased seizure activity in epilepsy patient

> **BLACK BOX WARNING: Active hepatic disease:** Monitor hepatic function by frequent determination of AST, ALT, bilirubin, alkaline phosphatase, GGTP; renal function studies; CBC

• Assess for allergic reactions: rash, fever, respiratory distress
• Monitor for severe weakness, numbness in extremities
• Assess for CNS depression: dizziness, drowsiness, psychiatric symptoms

> **BLACK BOX WARNING: Assess for signs of hepatotoxicity:** Jaundice, yellow sclera, pain in abdomen, nausea, fever; product should be discontinued if these signs and symptoms occur

---

Patient/family education
- Caution patient not to discontinue product quickly, hallucinations, spasticity, tachycardia will occur; product should be tapered over 1-2 wk; notify prescriber of abdominal pain, jaundiced sclera, clay-colored stools, change in color of urine, rash, itching
- Caution patient not to take with alcohol, other CNS depressants; severe CNS depression can occur; avoid using OTC medication (cough preparations, antihistamines, alcohol, other CNS depressants), unless directed by prescriber
- Tell patient that if improvement does not occur within 6 wk, prescriber may discontinue
- Caution patient to avoid hazardous activities if drowsiness, dizziness, blurred vision occurs; wait several days to identify patient response to medication
- Teach patient to use sunscreen, protective clothing for photosensitivity
- Instruct patient to take medication as prescribed; do not double doses; take missed dose within 1 hr of scheduled time

Evaluation
Positive therapeutic outcome
- Decreased pain, spasticity
- Absence or decreased symptoms of malignant hyperthermia

TREATMENT OF OVERDOSE:
Activated charcoal, supportive care

---

dapiprazole ophthalmic
See Appendix B

DAPTOmycin (Rx)
(dap′toe-mye-sin)
Cubicin
Func. class.: Antiinfective—miscellaneous
Chem. class.: Lipopeptides
Pregnancy category B

ACTION: New class of antiinfective; binds to the bacterial membrane and results in a rapid depolarization of the membrane potential, leading to inhibition of DNA, RNA, and protein synthesis

Therapeutic outcome: Absence of infections

USES: Complicated skin, skin structure infections caused by *Staphylococcus aureus,* including methicillin-resistant strains, *Streptococcus pyogenes, S. agalactiae, S. dysgalactiae* (vancomycin-susceptible strains only), *Streptococcus pyogenes* (group A beta hemolytic), *Staphylococcus aureus, Staphylococcus epidermidis* (MRSA, MSSA), bone, joint infection, infectious arthritis, orthopedic device-related infection, osteomyelitis

CONTRAINDICATIONS:
Hypersensitivity

Precautions: Pregnancy **B**, breastfeeding, children, geriatrics, GI/renal disease, myopathy, ulcerative/pseudomembranous colitis, rhabdomyolysis, eosinophilic pneumonia

DOSAGE AND ROUTES
Adult: IV INF 4-6 mg/kg over ½ hr diluted in 0.9% NaCl, give q24hr × 7-14 days
Adolescent/child/infant ≥5 mo (unlabeled): IV 4-6 mg/kg/day

Staphylococcus aureus bacteremia, including right-sided infective endocarditis
Adult: IV INF 6 mg/kg/day × 2-6 wk, up to 8-10 mg/kg/day, treatment failures should use another agent

Renal dose
Adult: IV CCr <30 ml/min; hemodialysis, CAPD 4 mg/kg q48hr

Available forms: Lyophilized powder for inj 500 mg

Implementation
Intermittent IV infusion route
- Give after reconstitution with 10 ml 0.9% NaCl (500 mg/10 ml), further dilution is needed with 0.9% NaCl; infuse over ½ hr
Direct IV route
- Give reconstituted sol (50 mg/ml) by direct IV inj over 2 min

Y-site compatibilities: Alfentanil, amifostine, amikacin, aminocaproic acid, aminophylline, amiodarone, amphotericin B liposome, ampicillin, ampicillin-sulbactam, argatroban, arsenic trioxide, atenolol, atracurium, azithromycin, aztreonam, bivalirudin, bleomycin, bumetanide, buprenorphine, busulfan, butorphanol, calcium chloride/gluconate, CARBOplatin, carmustine, caspofungin, ceFAZolin, cefepime, cefotaxime, cefoTEtan, cefOXitin, cefTAZidime, ceftizoxime, cefTRIAXone, cefuroxime, chloramphenicol, chlorproMAZINE, cimetidine, ciprofloxacin, cisatracurium, CISplatin, clindamycin, cyclophosphamide, cycloSPORINE, dacarbazine, DACTINomycin, DAUNOrubicin, dexamethasone, dexmedetomidine, dexrazoxane, diazepam, digoxin, diltiazem, diphenhydrAMINE, DOBUTamine, DOCEtaxel, DOPamine, doripenem, doxacurium, DOXOrubicin, DOXOrubicin liposomal, doxycycline, droperidol, enalaprilat, ePHEDrine, EPINEPHrine, epirubicin, eptifibatide, ertapenem, erythromycin, esmolol, etoposide, famotidine, fenoldopam, fentaNYL, fluconazole, fludarabine, fluorouracil, foscarnet, fosphenytoin, furosemide, ganciclovir, gentamicin, glycopyrrolate, granisetron, haloperidol, heparin, hydrALAZINE, hydrocortisone, HYDROmorphone, hydrOXYzine, IDArubicin, ifosfamide, inamrinone, insulin (regular), irinotecan, isoproterenol, ketorolac, labetalol, lepuridin, leucovorin, levofloxacin, lidocaine, linezolid, LORazepam, magnesium sulfate, mannitol, mechlorethamine, melphalan, meperidine, meropenem, mesna, metaraminol, methyldopate, methylPREDNISolone, metoclopramide, metoprolol, midazolam, milrinone, mitoXANtrone, mivacurium, morphine, moxifloxacin, mycophenolate mofetil, nafcillin, nalbuphine, naloxone, niCARdipine, nitroprusside, norepinephrine, octreotide, ondansetron, oxaliplatin, oxytocin, PACLitaxel, palonosetron, pamidronate, pancuronium, PEMEtrexed, pentamidine, PHENobarbital, phenylephrine, piperacillin-tazobactam, polymyxin B, potassium acetate/chloride/phosphates, procainamide, prochlorperazine, promethazine, propranolol, quinupristin-dalfopristin, ranitidine, rocuronium, sodium acetate/bicarbonate/citrate/phosphates, succinylcholine, sulfamethoxazole-trimethoprim, tacrolimus, teniposide, theophylline, thiotepa, ticarcillin, ticarcillin-clavulanate, tigecycline, tirofiban, tobramycin, topotecan, trimethobenzamide, vasopressin, vecuronium, verapamil, vinBLAStine, vinCRIStine, vinorelbine, voriconazole, zidovudine, zoledronic acid

Solution compatibilities: 0.9% NaCl, LR

ADVERSE EFFECTS

CNS: Headache, insomnia, dizziness, confusion, anxiety, fatigue, fever
CV: Hypo/hypertension, **heart failure,** chest pain
GI: Nausea, constipation, diarrhea, vomiting, dyspepsia, **pseudomembranous colitis,** abdominal pain, stomatitis, xerostomia, anorexia
GU: Nephrotoxicity: increased BUN
HEMA: Leukocytosis, anemia, thrombocytopenia
INTEG: Rash, pruritus
META: Electrolyte imbalances
MISC: Fungal infections, UTI, anemia, hypoglycemia

MS: Muscle pain or weakness, arthralgia, pain, **rhabdomyolysis,** myopathy
RESP: Cough, **eosinophilic pneumonia,** dyspnea
SYST: Anaphylaxis, DRESS, Stevens-Johnson syndrome

Pharmacokinetics

Absorption	Unknown
Distribution	Protein binding 92%
Metabolism	Unknown
Excretion	Breast milk
Half-life	Unknown

Pharmacodynamics
Unknown

INTERACTIONS

Drug classifications
HMG-CoA reductase inhibitors: myopathy

Drug/lab test
Increased: CPK, AST, ALT, BUN, creatinine, albumin, LDH
Increased/decreased: glucose
Decreased: alk phos, magnesium, phosphate, bicarbonate

NURSING CONSIDERATIONS

Assessment
• Assess signs of infection, C&S, product may be given as soon as culture is taken
⚠ **Rhabdomyolysis: check for myopathy CPK >1000 U/L (5×ULN), discontinue product**
⚠ **Nephrotoxicity: Monitor any patient with compromised renal system: BUN, creatinine; toxicity may occur**
⚠ **Monitor I&O ratio: report hematuria, oliguria; nephrotoxicity may occur**
• **Eosinophilic pneumonia:** Assess for dyspnea, fever, cough, shortness of breath, if left untreated can lead to respiratory failure and death
• Monitor blood tests: CBC
• Monitor C&S, product may be given as soon as culture is taken
• Monitor B/P during administration; hypo/hypertension may occur
• Identify allergies before treatment, reaction of each medication

Patient/family education
• Teach all aspects of product therapy
• Advise patient to report sore throat, fever, fatigue; could indicate **superinfection; shortness of breath;** diarrhea; muscle weakness, pain
• Instruct patient to avoid breastfeeding

⚠ Nurse Alert ⬛ Key NCLEX® Drug

Evaluation

⚠ **Myopathy:** Assess for muscle pain, weakness; CPK >10× ULN; symptoms resolve after 3 days and CPK returns to normal within 7-10 days after stopping product

⚠ **Pseudomembranous colitis:** Assess for diarrhea with mucus, pus: product should be discontinued; if moderate to severe, provide fluids, electrolytes, protein supplements, and an antibacterial

Positive therapeutic outcome
• Negative culture

---

darbepoetin (Rx)

(dar′bee-poh′-eh-tin)
Aranesp
Func. class.: Hematopoietic agent
Chem. class.: Recombinant human erythropoietin
Pregnancy category C

ACTION: Stimulates erythropoiesis by the same mechanism as endogenous erythropoietin; in response to hypoxia, erythropoietin is produced in the kidney and released into the bloodstream, where it interacts with progenitor stem cells to increase red cell production

Therapeutic outcome: Decreased anemia with increased RBCs

USES: Anemia associated with chronic renal failure in patients on and not on dialysis and anemic in nonmyeloid malignancies receiving coadministered chemotherapy

CONTRAINDICATIONS:

Hypersensitivity to mammalian cell–derived products, human albumin, polysorbate 80; uncontrolled hypertension, red cell aplasia

Precautions: Pregnancy C, breastfeeding, children, seizure disorder, porphyria, hypertension, sickle cell disease, vit B₁₂, folate deficiency, chronic renal failure, dialysis, latex hypersensitivity, CABG, angina, anemia

BLACK BOX WARNING: Hgb >12 g/dl, neoplastic disease

DOSAGE AND ROUTES

Correction of anemia in chronic renal failure
Adult: SUBCUT/**IV** 0.45 mcg/kg as a single inj, titrate max target Hgb of 12 g/dl

Chemotherapy treatment
Adult: SUBCUT 2.5 mcg/kg/wk or 500 mcg q3wk

Epoetin alfa to darbepoetin conversion
Adult: SUBCUT/**IV** (epoetin alfa <2500 units/wk) 6.25 mcg/wk; (epoetin alfa 2500-4999 units/wk) 12.5 mcg/wk; (epoetin alfa 5000-10,999 units/wk) 25 mcg/wk; (epoetin alfa 11,000-17,999 units/wk) 40 mcg/wk; (epoetin alfa 18,000-33,999 units/wk) 60 mcg/wk; (epoetin alfa 34,000-89,999 units/wk) 100 mcg/wk; (epoetin alfa >90,000 units/wk) 200 mcg/wk

Available forms: Sol for inj 25, 40, 60, 100, 150, 200, 300, 500 mcg/ml

Implementation

IV/SUBCUT route
• Do not shake, do not dilute, do not mix with other products or solutions
• Check for discoloration, particulate matter; do not use if present; discard unused portion; do not pool unused portion
• Store refrigerated, do not freeze, protect from light

ADVERSE EFFECTS

CNS: **Seizures**, sweating, headache, dizziness, **stroke**
CV: *Hypo/hypertension,* **cardiac arrest,** *angina pectoris,* **thrombosis, CHF, acute MI,** dysrhythmias, chest pain, transient ischemic attacks, edema
GI: *Diarrhea, vomiting, nausea, abdominal pain, constipation*
HEMA: Red cell aplasia
MISC: *Infection, fatigue, fever,* **death,** *fluid overload,* **vascular access hemorrhage,** dehydration, sepsis
MS: *Bone pain, myalgia, limb pain, back pain*
RESP: *Upper respiratory infection, dyspnea, cough, bronchitis,* **pulmonary embolism**
SYST: Allergic reactions, **anaphylaxis**

Pharmacokinetics

Absorption	Slow, rate-limiting (SUBCUT)
Distribution	Vascular space
Metabolism	Metabolized in body (**IV**), extent unknown
Excretion	Unknown
Half-life	49 hr

Adverse effects: *italics* = common; **bold** = life-threatening

Pharmacodynamics

Onset	Onset of increased reticulocyte count 1-6 wk
Peak	34 hr
Duration	Unknown

INTERACTIONS
Individual drugs
⚠ Do not use epoetin alfa with this product

Drug classifications
Androgens: increased darbepoetin alfa effect

Drug/lab test
Increased: WBC, platelets
Decreased: bleeding time

NURSING CONSIDERATIONS
Assessment
• **Assess for serious allergic reactions:** rash, urticaria; if anaphylaxis occurs, stop product, administer emergency treatment (rare)

> **BLACK BOX WARNING:** Assess blood studies: ferritin, transferrin monthly; transferrin sat ≥20%, ferritin ≥100 ng/ml; Hgb 2 ×/wk until stabilized in target range (30%-33%), then at regular intervals; those with endogenous erythropoietin levels of <500 units/L respond to this agent, if there is lack of response, obtain folic acid, iron, B$_{12}$ levels

• Assess renal studies: urinalysis, protein, blood, BUN, creatinine
• Assess B/P, Hct; check for rising B/P as Hct rises; antihypertensives may be needed
⚠ Assess CV status: hypertension may occur rapidly, leading to hypertensive encephalopathy; Hgb >12 g/dl may lead to death
• Assess I&O ratio; report drop in output to <50 ml/hr
• Assess for **seizures** if Hgb is increased within 2 wk by 4 points
• Assess CNS symptoms: cold sensation, sweating, pain in long bones
• Assess **dialysis patients** for thrill, bruit of shunts; monitor for circulation impairment

> **BLACK BOX WARNING:** Neoplastic disease: breast, non-small cell lung, head and neck, lymphoid or cervical cancers, increased tumor progression, use lowest dose to avoid RBC transfusion

Patient/family education
• Caution patient to avoid driving or hazardous activity during beginning of treatment
• Advise patient to monitor B/P, Hgb
• Advise patient to take iron supplements, vit B$_{12}$, folic acid as directed
• Advise patient to report side effects to prescriber, to comply with treatment regimen
• Teach patient that menses may return, use contraception
• Teach home administration and review information for patients and caregivers if home administration is deemed appropriate

Evaluation
Positive therapeutic outcome
• Increased reticulocyte count, Hgb/Hct
• Increased appetite
• Enhanced sense of well-being

TREATMENT OF OVERDOSE:
If polycythemia occurs, discontinue product temporarily; perform phlebotomy if clinically indicated

darifenacin
(da-ree-fen'ah-sin)
Enablex
Func. class.: Antispasmodic/GU anticholinergic
Pregnancy category C

ACTION: Bladder smooth muscle relaxation by decreasing the action of muscarinic receptors, thereby relieving overactive bladder

Therapeutic outcome: Decreasing urgency, frequency of urination

USES: Urge incontinence, frequency, urgency in overactive bladder

CONTRAINDICATIONS:
Hypersensitivity, urinary retention, narrow-angle glaucoma (uncontrolled)
   Concurrent use of solid dosage forms of potassium chloride (the passage of potassium chloride tablets through the GI tract may be delayed); potassium chloride liquid is suitable alternative

Precautions: Severe hepatic disease (Child-Pugh C), GI/GU obstruction, controlled narrow-angle glaucoma, ulcerative colitis, myasthenia gravis, moderate hepatic disease (Child-Pugh B), elderly patients

DOSAGE AND ROUTES
Adult: PO 7.5 mg/day, initially, may increase to 15 mg/day after 14 days if needed

---

Those taking a potent CYP3A4 inhibitor
Adult: PO Max 7.5 mg/day

Hepatic dose
Adult: PO (Child-Pugh B) max 7.5 mg

Available forms: Tabs, EXT REL 7.5, 15 mg

Implementation
PO route
- Give without regard to meals
- Do not crush, break, chew EXT REL tabs
- Store at room temperature

ADVERSE EFFECTS
CNS: Dizziness, headache
EENT: Blurred vision, drying eyes, sinusitis, rhinitis
GI: Constipation, dry mouth, abdominal pain, nausea, vomiting, dyspepsia
GU: UTI, urine retention, vaginitis
INTEG: Rash, pruritus, skin drying
MISC: Bronchitis, flulike symptoms
MS: Back pain

Pharmacokinetics

Absorption	Unknown
Distribution	Unknown
Excretion	Unknown
Metabolism	Extensively in the liver
Half-life	12-19 hr

Pharmacodynamics

Onset	Unknown
Peak	7 hr
Duration	Unknown

INTERACTIONS
Drug classifications
Anticholinergics: increased anticholinergic effect
CYP3A4 inhibitors: increased darifenacin levels
Drugs metabolized by CYP2D6: increased levels of these products

NURSING CONSIDERATIONS
Assessment
- Urinary function: Assess for urgency, frequency, retention in bladder outflow obstruction
- Constipation, may add bulk in the diet

Patient/family education
- Instruct patient to advise prescriber if pregnancy (**C**) is planned or suspected; avoid breastfeeding

- Teach patient about anticholinergic symptoms (dry mouth, constipation, dry eyes, heat prostration), not to become overheated
- Teach patient to avoid hazardous activities until reaction is known, dizziness, blurred vision may occur

Evaluation
Positive therapeutic outcome
- Decreasing urgency, frequency of urination

darunavir (Rx)
(dar-ue′na-vir)
Prezista
Func. class.: Antiretroviral
Chem. class.: Protease inhibitor
Pregnancy category B

ACTION: Inhibits human immunodeficiency virus (HIV-1) protease; this prevents maturation of virus

Therapeutic outcome: Decreased viral load, increase in CD4 counts

USES: HIV-1 in combination with ritonavir and other antiretrovirals

CONTRAINDICATIONS:
Hypersensitivity

Precautions: Pregnancy **B**, breastfeeding, children, renal/hepatic disease, history of renal stones, diabetes, hypercholesterolemia, sulfonamide hypersensitivity, antimicrobial resistance, bleeding, elderly, immune reconstitution syndrome, pancreatitis

DOSAGE AND ROUTES
Treatment-naive patients
Adult: PO 800 mg with ritonavir 100 mg qd

Treatment-experienced patients
Adult: PO 600 mg with ritonavir 100 mg qd; 800 qd with ritonavir 100 mg with food (without darunavir resistance)
Child ≥3 yr/adolescent ≥40 kg: PO 800 mg/dose qd with ritonavir 100 mg/dose qd (no darunavir); resistance-associated substitutions
Child ≥6 yr/adolescent ≥30 kg, <40 kg: PO 450 mg bid with ritonavir 60 mg bid
Child ≥6 yr/adolescent ≥20 kg, <30 kg: PO 375 mg bid with ritonavir 50 mg bid
Child 3 to <6 yr (14 to <15 kg): PO 280 mg (with ritonavir 48 mg) bid with food
Child 3 to <6 yr (13 to <14 kg): PO 260 mg (with ritonavir 40 mg) bid with food

Child 3 to <6 yr (12 to <13 kg): PO 240 mg (with ritonavir 40 mg) bid with food
Child 3 to <6 yr (11 to <12 kg): PO 220 mg (with ritonavir 32 mg) bid with food
Child 3 to <6 yr (10 to <11 kg): PO 200 mg (with ritonavir 32 mg) bid with food

Available forms: Tabs 75, 150, 400, 600 mg

Implementation

- Give with food and ritonavir
- Tab should be swallowed whole

ADVERSE EFFECTS

CNS: *Headache, insomnia,* dizziness, somnolence
GI: *Diarrhea, abdominal pain, nausea, vomiting,* anorexia, dry mouth, **hepatitis, hepatotoxicity**
GU: Nephrolithiasis
INTEG: Rash, angioedema, **Stevens-Johnson syndrome,** toxic epidermal necrolysis, exanthematous pustulosis
MS: Pain
OTHER: Asthenia, **insulin-resistant hyperglycemia,** hyperlipidemia, **ketoacidosis,** lipodystrophy

Pharmacokinetics

Absorption	Unknown
Distribution	Protein binding 95%
Metabolism	By CYP3A4
Excretion	Feces 79.5%, urine 13.9%
Half-life	Terminal 15 hr

Pharmacodynamics

Onset	Unknown
Peak	2.5-4 hr
Duration	Unknown

INTERACTIONS

Individual drugs

Artemether/lumefantrine: increased side effects (CYP3A4 substrate)
Atorvastatin, lovastatin, simvastatin: increased myopathy
CarBAMazepine, efavirenz, fluconazole, fosphenytoin, nevirapine, PHENobarbital, phenytoin: decreased darunavir levels
Clarithromycin, zidovudine: increased levels of both products
Delavirdine, itraconazole, ketoconazole: increased darunavir levels
Telaprevir, rilpivirine: increased levels of these products; monitor for adverse reactions
Isoniazid: increased levels of isoniazid

⚠ Midazolam, pimozide, rifampin, triazolam: life-threatening dysrhythmias
Tenofovir: avoid concurrent use; decreased levels of both products

Drug classifications

⚠ Ergots: life-threatening dysrhythmias; do not use concurrently
Oral contraceptives: increased levels of oral contraceptives
Rifamycins: decreased darunavir levels

Drug/herb

Red yeast rice: increased myopathy, rhabdomyolysis
St. John's wort: decreased darunavir levels; avoid concurrent use

Drug/food

Darunavir: increased absorption

Drug/lab test

Increased: LFTs, bilirubin, uric acid
Decreased: WBC, neutrophils, platelets

NURSING CONSIDERATIONS

Assessment

- Assess for complaints of lower back, flank pain; indicates kidney stones
- Assess for signs of infection, anemia, the presence of other STDs
- **Serious skin reaction:** angioedema, Stevens-Johnson syndrome, toxic epidermal necrolysis; discontinue immediately, notify prescriber
- **Hepatotoxicity:** Monitor liver function tests: ALT, AST, bilirubin, amylase; all may be elevated in those with underlying liver disease, product should be discontinued in those with increased LFTs
- Monitor viral load, CD4 during treatment; viral load should be decreasing, CD4 increasing
- Assess bowel pattern before, during treatment; if severe abdominal pain with bleeding occurs, product should be discontinued; monitor hydration
- **Hyperlipidemia:** Cholesterol, triglycerides, LDL may be elevated, monitor serum cholesterol, lipid panel throughout treatment

Patient/family education

- Teach patient to use nonhormonal birth control, do not breastfeed
- Instruct patient to take as prescribed; if dose is missed, take as soon as remembered up to 1 hr before next dose; do not double dose
- Advise patient that product must be taken at same time of day to maintain blood levels for duration of therapy

▲ Advise patient that hyperglycemia may occur; watch for increased thirst, weight loss, hunger; dry, itchy skin; notify prescriber
• Teach patient to increase fluids to prevent kidney stones; if stone formation occurs, treatment may need to be interrupted
• Teach patient that product does not cure AIDS, only controls symptoms; do not donate blood, do not share, notify all health care providers of use, do not use with any other products without prescriber's approval

Evaluation
Positive therapeutic outcome
• Decreased viral load, increased CD4 counts

dasatinib (Rx)
(da-si′ti-nib)
Sprycel
Func. class.: Miscellaneous antineoplastic
Chem. class.: Protein-tyrosine kinase inhibitor
Pregnancy category D

ACTION: Inhibits a tyrosine kinase enzyme, thereby reducing cell growth in leukemia

Therapeutic outcome: Decrease in number of leukemic cells or size of tumor

USES: Treatment of accelerated, chronic blast phase CML or acute lymphoblastic leukemia (ALL); chronic phase CML with resistance or intolerance to prior therapy; Philadelphia chromosome–positive CML in chronic phase

CONTRAINDICATIONS:
Pregnancy **D**, hypersensitivity

Precautions: Breastfeeding, children, geriatric, QT prolongation, infection, thrombocytopenia, accidental exposure, edema, infertility, lactase deficiency, neutropenia, anemia, autoimmune disease with immune reconstitution syndrome

DOSAGE AND ROUTES
Accelerated or myeloid/lymphoid blast phase CML with resistance/intolerance to prior therapy
Adult: PO 140 mg daily, titrated up to 180 mg bid in those resistant to therapy

Chronic phase CML with resistance/intolerance to prior therapy
Adult: PO 100 mg daily either AM or PM

Dosage reduction for those taking a strong CYP3A4 inhibitor
Adult: 20 mg daily

Available forms: Tabs 20, 50, 70, 80, 100 mg

Implementation
• Do not break, crush, or chew tab
• Give after meal and with large glass of water
• Give nutritious diet with iron, vitamin supplement
• Store at 25° C (77° F)

ADVERSE EFFECTS
CNS: CNS hemorrhage, headache, dizziness, insomnia, neuropathy, asthenia
CV: Dsyrhythmias, chest pain, **CHF, pericardial effusion,** congestive cardiomyopathy; decreased injection fraction, QT prolongation
GI: *Nausea,* **vomiting,** *anorexia, abdominal pain,* constipation, diarrhea, GI bleeding, muscositis, stomatitis
HEMA: Neutropenia, thrombocytopenia, bleeding
INTEG: *Rash, pruritus,* alopecia
META: Fluid retention, edema, hypocalcemia, hypophosphatemia
MISC: Increased/decreased weight
MS: Pain, arthralgia, myalgia
RESP: Cough, dyspnea, pulmonary edema/hypertension, pneumonia, URI, **pleural effusion**

Pharmacokinetics

Absorption	Unknown
Distribution	Protein binding 96%
Metabolism	By CYP3A4
Excretion	Feces 85%, urine 4%
Half-life	Terminal 1.3-5 hr

Pharmacodynamics

Onset	0.5-6 hr
Peak	Unknown
Duration	Unknown

INTERACTIONS
Individual drugs
Clarithromycin, erythromycin, itraconazole, ketoconazole, nefazodone, telithromycin: increased dasatinib concentrations
Simvastatin: increased concentrations of this product

Drug classifications
Class IA/III antidysrhythmics and other products that increase QT prolongation: increased QT prolongation

Adverse effects: *italics* = common; **bold** = life-threatening

CYP3A4 inducers (dexamethasone, phenytoin, carBAMazepine, rifampin, PHENobarbital), H₂ blockers (famotidine), proton pump inhibitors (omeprazole): decreased dasatinib concentrations

HMG-CoA reductase inhibitors (rare): increased myopathy, rhabdomyolysis

CYP3A4 substrates (alfentanil, cycloSPORINE, ergots, fentaNYL, pimozide, quiNIDine, sirolimus, tacrolimus): altered action

Protease inhibitors: increased dasatinib concentrations

Drug/herb
St. John's wort: decreased dasatinib concentration

Drug/food
Grapefruit: do not use

NURSING CONSIDERATIONS
Assessment
• **Myelosuppression:** Monitor ANC and platelets; in chronic phase if ANC is $<1 \times 10^9$/L and/or platelets $<50 \times 10^9$/L, stop until ANC $>1.5 \times 10^9$/L and platelets $>75 \times 10^9$/L; in accelerated phase/blast crisis if ANC $<0.5 \times 10^9$/L and/or platelets $<10 \times 10^9$/L, determine whether cytopenia is related to biopsy/aspirate, if not, reduce dose by 200 mg, if cytopenia continues, reduce dose by another 100 mg; if cytopenia continues for 4 wk, stop product until ANC $\geq 1 \times 10^9$/L, monitor CBC qwk $\times$ 8 wk, then qmo
• Assess for hepatotoxicity: monitor liver function tests before treatment and qmo; if liver transaminases $>5 \times$ IULN, withhold until transaminase levels return to $<2.5 \times$ IULN
• **Monitor for signs of fluid retention, edema:** weigh, monitor lung sounds, assess for edema, some fluid retention is dose dependent, may result in CHF, congestive cardiomyopathy, decreased injection fraction
⚠ **QT prolongation: more common in those with hypokalemia, hypomagnesemia, congenital long QT syndrome, those taking products that prolong QT, correct electrolyte imbalances before use**

Patient/family education
• Instruct patient to report adverse reactions immediately: SOB, swelling of extremities, bleeding, bruising
• Teach patient reason for treatment, expected result
• Teach patient to use contraception, pregnancy **D,** avoid breastfeeding; **men should use condoms**

• Teach patient to take at same time of day, not to crush or chew, not to use grapefruit juice

Evaluation
Positive therapeutic outcome
• Decrease in number of leukemic cells

⚠ HIGH ALERT

DAUNOrubicin (Rx)
(daw-noe-roo'bi-sin)
Cerubidine
DAUNOrubicin citrate liposome (Rx)
DaunoXome
Func. class.: Antineoplastic, antibiotic
Chem. class.: Anthracycline glycoside
Pregnancy category D

Do not confuse:
DAUNOrubicin/DOXOrubicin

ACTION: Inhibits DNA synthesis, primarily; derived from *Streptomyces coeruleorubidus;* replication is decreased by binding to DNA, which causes strand splitting; cell cycle specific (S phase); a vesicant

Therapeutic outcome: Prevention of rapidly growing malignant cells; immunosuppression

USES: Acute lymphocytic leukemia (ALL), acute myelogenous leukemia (AML); liposomal Kaposi's sarcoma

CONTRAINDICATIONS:
Pregnancy **D,** breastfeeding, hypersensitivity, systemic infections, cardiac disease, bone marrow depression

BLACK BOX WARNING: IM/Subcut use

Precautions: Renal/hepatic disease, gout, tumor lysis syndrome, MI, infection, thrombocytopenia

BLACK BOX WARNING: Bone marrow suppression, cardiac disease, extravasation, renal failure, hepatic disease, requires a specialized care setting and an experienced clinician

DOSAGE AND ROUTES
Use decreased dose for those >60 yr

DAUNOrubicin

In combination
Adult: IV 45-60 mg/m²/day × 3 days, then 2 days of subsequent courses in combination, max 400-600 mg/m² total cumulative dose
Child: IV 25-60 mg/m² depending on cycle (AML); ≤2 yr or <0.5 m²: 1 mg/kg on day 1 weekly in combination with vinCRIStine and predniSONE, base dose on body weight, not surface area (ALL); >2 yr or 0.5 m²: 25 mg/m² day 1 q wk in combination with vinCRIStine and predniSONE (ALL)

DAUNOrubicin citrate liposome
Adult: IV 40 mg/m² q2wk (Kaposi's sarcoma); 100 mg/m² q3wk (multiple myeloma, unlabeled); IV 100-140 mg/m² q3wk (non-Hodgkin's lymphoma, unlabeled; metastatic breast cancer, unlabeled; IV escalating doses of 75, 100, 125, 135, 150 mg/m²/day × 3 days (AML, unlabeled)

Renal dose
Adult: IV serum Cr >3 mg/dl reduce dose by 50%

Hepatic dose
Adult: IV serum bilirubin 1.2-3 mg/dl reduce dose by 50%; bilirubin >3 mg/dl reduce dose by 75%; bilirubin >5 mg/dl omit dose

Available forms: Inj 20 mg powder/vial, sol for inj 5 mg/ml (DaunoXome); liposome: dispersion for inj 2 mg/ml

Implementation
• Avoid contact with skin; very irritating; wash completely to remove
• Give fluids IV or PO before chemotherapy to hydrate patient; give antiemetic 30-60 min before giving product to prevent vomiting, and prn; antibiotics for prophylaxis of infection
• Provide liquid diet: carbonated beverages; gelatin may be added if patient is not nauseated or vomiting

> **BLACK BOX WARNING:** To be used in a care setting with emergency equipment available

> **BLACK BOX WARNING:** To be used by a clinician knowledgeable in cytotoxic therapy

• Help patient rinse mouth tid-qid with water, club soda, brush teeth bid-qid with soft brush or cotton-tipped applicators for stomatitis, use unwaxed dental floss
• Product should be prepared by experienced personnel using proper precautions
• Do not give by IM/SUBCUT inj

Cerubidine

IV route
• Give after diluting 20 mg/4 ml sterile water for inj (5 mg/ml); rotate; further dilute in 10-15 ml 0.9% NaCl; give over 3-5 min by direct IV through Y-tube or 3-way stopcock of inf of D₅W or 0.9% NaCl
Intermittent IV infusion route
• Dilute further in 50-100 ml 0.9% NaCl, LR, D₅W; give over 15 min (50 ml), 30 min (100 ml)

Y-site compatibilities: Amifostine, anidulafungin, atenolol, bivalirudin, bleomycin, CARBOplatin, caspofungin, CISplatin, codeine, cyclophosphamide, cytarabine, DACTINomycin, DAPTOmycin, dexmedetomidine, etoposide, fenoldopam, filgrastim, gemcitabine, gemtuzumab, granisetron, melphalan, meperidine, methotrexate, nesiritide, octreotide, ondansetron, oxaliplatin, PACLitaxel, palonosetron, quinupristin-dalfopristin, riTUXimab, sodium acetate/bicarbonate, teniposide, thiotepa, tigecycline, trastuzumab, vinCRIStine, vinorelbine, voriconazole, zoledronic acid

Y-site incompatibilities: Fludarabine

Solution compatibilities: D₅.₃/0.3% NaCl, D₅W, Normosol-R, Ringer's, 0.9% NaCl

DaunoXome

IV route
• Dilute with D₅W (1 mg/ml), give over 60 min, do not use in-line filter, reconstituted sol may be stored ≤6 hr refrigerated; do not admix

ADVERSE EFFECTS
DAUNOrubicin
CNS: Fever, chills
CV: CHF, pericarditis, myocarditis, peripheral edema, fatal myocarditis, left ventricular failure, QT prolongation, ST-T wave changes, QRS voltage changes, tachycardia, SVT, PVCs
GI: *Nausea, vomiting, anorexia, mucositis,* **hepatotoxicity**
GU: Impotence, sterility, amenorrhea, gynecomastia
HEMA: Thrombocytopenia, leukopenia, anemia
INTEG: *Rash, extravasation,* dermatitis, reversible alopecia, cellulitis, thrombophlebitis at inj site
MISC: Anaphylaxis, tumor lysis syndrome

DAUNOrubicin citrate liposome
CNS: Fatigue, headache, depression, insomnia, dizziness, malaise, neuropathy
CV: Chest pain, edema

GI: Abdominal pain, nausea, vomiting, *diarrhea*, constipation, stomatitis
INTEG: *Alopecia*, sweating, *pruritus*
MISC: *Allergic reactions, chest pain, fever,* edema, flulike symptoms
MS: *Rigors*, arthralgia, back pain
RESP: *Cough, dyspnea, rhinitis, sinusitis*

Pharmacokinetics

Absorption	Complete
Distribution	Widely distributed; crosses placenta
Metabolism	Liver, extensively
Excretion	Biliary (40%-50%)
Half-life	18½ hr, liposome 55½ hr

Pharmacodynamics

Unknown

INTERACTIONS

Arsenic trioxide, chloroquine, clarithromycin, dasatinib, dolasetron, droperidol, erythromycin, flecainide, halofantrine, haloperidol, levomethadyl, methadone, ondansetron, palonosetron, pentamidine, propafenone, risperidone, sparfloxacin, vorinstat, ziprasidone: increase QT prolongation, torsades de pointes

Individual drugs

Cyclophosphamide, radiation: increased toxicity

Drug classifications

Antineoplastics: increased toxicity
Class IA/III antidysrhythmics, some phenothiazines, tricyclic antidepressants (high doses): increased QT prolongation, torsades de pointes
Live virus vaccines: decreased antibody reaction
NSAIDs, salicylates: increased risk of bleeding, anticoagulants, platelet inhibitors, thrombolytics
Hematopoietic progenitor cells: given within 24 hr: decreased DAUNOrubicin given within 24 hr

Drug/lab test

Increased: uric acid

NURSING CONSIDERATIONS

Assessment

• Assess buccal cavity q8hr for dryness, sores or ulceration, white patches, pain, bleeding, dysphagia; obtain prescription for viscous lidocaine (Xylocaine)
• Assess symptoms indicating severe allergic reaction: rash, pruritus, urticaria, purpuric skin lesions, itching, flushing; product should be discontinued

> **BLACK BOX WARNING: Cardiac toxicity:** assess chest x-ray, echocardiography, radionuclide angiography, MUGA, ECG; watch for ST-T wave changes, low QRS and T, QT prolongation possible, dysrhythmias (sinus tachycardia, heart block, PVCs); watch for CHF (jugular vein distention, weight gain, edema, crackles), may occur after 2-6 mo of treatment, cumulative dose (400-550 mg/m²), 450 mg/m² if used in combination with radiation, cyclophosphamide

> **BLACK BOX WARNING:** Monitor CBC, **bone marrow suppression,** differential, platelet count weekly, leukocyte nadir within 2 wk after administration, recovery within 3 wk; do not administer if absolute granulocyte count is <750/mm³ (liposome)

• Assess for increased uric acid levels, swelling, joint pain primarily in extremities; patient should be well hydrated to prevent urate deposits
• **Acute renal failure, uric acid nephropathy:** Monitor renal function tests: BUN, creatinine, serum uric acid, urine CCr baseline and before each dose; I&O ratio; report fall in urine output to <30 ml/hr, provide aggressive alkalinization of the urine as use of allopurinol can prevent urate nephropathy
• Monitor temp q4hr (may indicate beginning of infection)
• **Hepatotoxicity:** Monitor liver function tests baseline and before each dose (bilirubin, AST, ALT, LDH) as needed or monthly; note jaundice of skin or sclera, dark urine, clay-colored stools, itchy skin, abdominal pain, fever, diarrhea; hepatotoxicity can be severe
• Assess for bleeding: hematuria, stool guaiac, bruising or petechiae, mucosa or orifices q8hr; check for inflammation of mucosa, breaks in skin
• Identify effects of alopecia on body image; discuss feelings about body changes
⚠ **Tumor lysis syndrome: hyperkalemia, hyperphosphatemia, hyperuricemia, hypocalcemia**

> **BLACK BOX WARNING: Extravasation:** swelling, pain, decreased blood return, if extravasation occurs stop infusion, remove tubing, attempt to aspirate the drug prior to removing the needle, elevate area, treat with ice

---

Patient/family education
• Teach patient to avoid use of products containing aspirin or ibuprofen, razors, commercial mouthwash, since bleeding may occur; to report symptoms of bleeding (hematuria, tarry stools)
• Instruct patient to report signs of **anemia** (fatigue, headache, irritability, faintness, shortness of breath); signs of **infection;** bleeding, bruising, shortness of breath, swelling, change in heart rate; to avoid crowds, those with known infections
• Advise patient that hair may be lost during treatment; a wig or hairpiece may make patient feel better; new hair may be different in color, texture
• Caution patient not to have any vaccinations without the advice of the prescriber; serious reactions can occur
⚠ **Advise patient that contraception is needed during treatment and for 4 mo after the completion of therapy, pregnancy D**
• Advise patient to avoid alcohol, aspirin, NSAIDs
• Inform patient that urine and other body fluids may be red-orange for 48 hr
• Teach patient to avoid crowds, those with known infections

Evaluation
Positive therapeutic outcome
• Prevention of rapid division of malignant cells

---

delavirdine (Rx)
(de-la-veer′deen)
Rescriptor
Func. class.: Antiretroviral
Chem. class.: Nonnucleoside reverse transcriptase inhibitor (NNRTI)
Pregnancy category C

ACTION: Binds directly to reverse transcriptase and blocks RNA, DNA-dependent polymerase activities causing a disruption of the enzyme's site

Therapeutic outcome: Improvement of HIV-1 infection

USES: HIV-1 in combination with at least 2 other antiretrovirals

CONTRAINDICATIONS:
Hypersensitivity

Precautions: Pregnancy **C,** breastfeeding, children, hepatic disease, exfoliative dermatitis,

hepatitis, immune reconstitution syndrome, achlorhydria, antimicrobial resistance

DOSAGE AND ROUTES
Adult and child ≥16 yr: PO 400 mg tid; max 1200 mg/day

Available forms: Tabs 100, 200 mg

Implementation
• Add 4 tabs/3-4 oz of water, let stand, stir, swallow, rinse glass, swallow; use only 100 mg tabs for dispersion
• Do not give within 1 hr of antacids or didanosine
• Take in equal intervals around the clock
• Always use as combination therapy; this product is not recommended for initial treatment; due to inferior, virologic effect, it is no longer listed as part of any preferred regimens

ADVERSE EFFECTS
CNS: Headache, fatigue, anxiety, insomnia, fever
GI: Diarrhea, anorexia, abdominal pain, nausea, vomiting, dyspepsia, **hepatotoxicity**
GU: Nephrotoxicity
HEMA: Neutropenia, leukopenia, thrombocytopenia, anemia, granulocytopenia
INTEG: Rash, pruritis
MISC: Cough
MS: Pain, myalgia
SYST: Stevens-Johnson syndrome, immune reconstitution syndrome (combination therapy)

Pharmacokinetics
Absorption	Well
Distribution	98% protein bound
Metabolism	Liver, extensively by CYP3A4
Excretion	Kidneys, feces
Half-life	2-11 hr

Pharmacodynamics
Onset	Unknown
Peak	1 hr
Duration	8 hr

INTERACTIONS
Individual drugs
Alprazolam, amprenavir, atorvastatin, clarithromycin, dapsone, felodipine, indinavir, lovastatin, midazolam, NIFEdipine, saquinavir, simvastatin: increased level of each specific product

---

Adverse effects: *italics* = common; **bold** = life-threatening

Alprazolam, astemizole, cisapride, midazolam, pimozide, sildenafil, terfenadine,
triazolam: life-threatening reactions; do
not combine

Clarithromycin, quiNIDine, warfarin: increased
level of both products

Didanosine: decreased delavirdine levels,
decreased action of didanosine

FLUoxetine, ketoconazole: increased level of
delavirdine

Drug classifications

Amphetamines, antidysrhythmics, benzodiazepines, calcium channel blockers, ergots,
sedative/hypnotics, opiates: increased serious
life-threatening adverse reaction

Antacids, anticonvulsants, protease inhibitors,
rifamycins: decreased delavirdine levels

Contraceptives (oral): decreased action of oral
contraceptives

CYP3A4, 2D6 inhibitors: increased levels

Ergots: increased levels of ergots

Drug/herb

St. John's wort: decreased delavirdine level

NURSING CONSIDERATIONS

Assessment

• Assess CBC, blood chemistry, plasma HIV
RNA, absolute $CD4^+/CD8^+/$cell counts/%,
serum β_2 microglobulin, serum ICD+24 antigen
levels

• Assess signs of infection, anemia

• Assess liver function tests: ALT, AST; renal
studies

• Assess C&S before product therapy; product
may be taken as soon as culture is taken; repeat
C&S after treatment; determine the presence of
other STDs

• Assess bowel pattern before, during treatment; if severe abdominal pain with bleeding occurs, product should be discontinued; monitor
hydration

• Assess allergies before treatment, reaction to
each medication; place allergies on chart

• Assess plasma delavirdine concentrations
(trough 10 mcm)

• HIV: Obtain hepatitis B virus (HBV) screening
to ensure proper treatment, if co-infected, a fully
suppressive antiretroviral regimen with produc-
tions against both

• **Serious skin reactions: Stevens-Johnson
syndrome;** any rash may occur within 1-3 wk
of beginning treatment; if rash is not severe,
manage with diphenhydrAMINE, hydrOXYzine,
topical corticosteroids

• Immune reconstitution syndrome: When
treated with combination therapy; development
of opportunistic infections (*Mycobacterium
avium* complex [MAC]), cytomegalovirus
(CMV), *Pneumocystis jiroveci* pneumonia
(PCP), or TB

• **Delavirdine toxicity:** severe nausea, vomiting, maculopapular rash

Patient/family education

• Advise patient to take as prescribed; if dose is
missed, take as soon as remembered up to 1 hr
before next dose; do not double dose

• Advise patient that product must be taken in
equal intervals around the clock to maintain
blood levels for duration of therapy

• Advise patient that tabs may be dissolved;
drink right away, rinse cup with water, and drink
that to get all medication

• Instruct patient to make sure health care provider knows of all the medications being taken

• Advise patient that if severe rash, mouth
sores, swelling, aching muscles/joints, or eye
redness occur, stop taking and notify health care
provider

• Advise patient not to breastfeed if taking this
product

• Teach patient that this product is not a cure,
only controls symptoms

Evaluation

Positive therapeutic outcome

• Increased $CD4^+$ cell count

• Decreased viral load

• Improvement in symptoms of HIV

demecarium ophthalmic
See Appendix B

denosumab (Rx)
(den-oh'sue-mab)
Prolia, Xgeva
Func. class.: Bone resorption inhibitor
Chem. class.: Monoclonal antibody, bone
resorption
Pregnancy category C

ACTION: Neutralizes activity of receptor
activator nuclear factor kappa-B ligand (RANKL)
by binding to it and blocking its interaction with
cell surface receptors, use of a RANKL inhibitor
may reduce bone turnover and decrease tumor
burden

Therapeutic outcome: Increased/main-
tained bone density

USES: Osteoporosis in postmenopausal
women or men at high risk for fractures, who

are receiving androgen deprivation therapy for prostate cancer, and women receiving aromastase inhibitor therapy for breast cancer; prevention of skeletal-related events in bone metastases from solid tumors; giant cell tumor of bone (Xgeva); increase bone mass

CONTRAINDICATIONS:
Hypersensitivity, hypocalcemia

Precautions: Anemia, breastfeeding, child/infant/neonate, coagulopathy, diabetes mellitus, dialysis, eczema, hypoparathyroidism, immunosuppression, latex hypersensitivity, malabsorption syndrome, neonates, neoplastic disease, pancreatitis, parathyroid disease, pregnancy **C**, dental/renal/thyroid disease, TB, Vitamin D deficiency

DOSAGE AND ROUTES
Postmenopausal osteoporosis
Adult female: Subcut 60 mg q6mo with 1000 mg calcium and 400 international units vitamin D, max 60 mg q6mo

Bone metastases from solid tumors
Adult: SUBCUT 120 mg q4wk, max 120 mg q4wk; administer with calcium and vitamin D as necessary to prevent hypocalcemia

Giant cell tumor of bone (Xgeva)
Adult: SUBCUT 120 mg q4wk, then 2 more doses on days 8 and 15 of 1st month only; use calcium, vitamin D as needed

Prevention of skeletal-related events in bone metastases from solid tumors (Xgeva)
Adult: SUBCUT: 120 mg q4wk

Available forms: Solution for injection 60 mg/ml (Prolia); 120 mg/1.7 ml (Xgeva)

Implementation
SUBCUT route
• Give acetaminophen before and for 72 hr after to decrease pain
• Do not use if particulate matter or discoloration is present; solution is clear and colorless to slightly yellow with small white/opalescent particles, remove from refrigerator and allow to warm to room temperature (15-30 min)
• **Use of prefilled syringe with needle safety guard:** Leave green guard in original position until after administration, remove and discard needle cap immediately before injection, give by SUBCUT injection in upper arm, thigh, or abdomen; after injection, point needle away from people and slide green guard over needle

• **Use of single-use vials:** Use 27G needle, give in upper arm/thigh, or abdomen, do not re-insert needle in vial, discard supplies as appropriate
• Avoid direct sunlight/heat, do not freeze, use within 14 days after removal from refrigerator, store unopened containers in refrigerator

ADVERSE EFFECTS
CNS: Chills, fever, flushing, headache, vertigo, neuropathic pain
CV: Angina, **atrial fibrillation**
GI: Abdominal pain, constipation, *diarrhea*, flatulence, GERD, *vomiting, nausea*
GU: Cystitis, lactation suppression
HEMA: **Anemia, neutropenia**
INTEG: Atopic dermatitis, pruritus
META: Hypercholesterolemia, hypocalcemia, hypophosphatemia
MS: Back/bone pain, MS pain, myalgia, **osteonecrosis of the jaw**
RESP: Cough, *dyspnea*
SYST: **Infection, secondary malignancy**

Pharmacokinetics
Absorption	Bioavailability 62%
Distribution	Unknown
Metabolism	Unknown
Excretion	Unknown
Half-life	25.4 days

Pharmacodynamics
Onset	Unknown
Peak	Maximum serum concentration 3-21 days
Duration	Steady state 6 months

INTERACTIONS
Drug classifications
Immunosuppressives, corticosteroids: possible increased infection
Antineoplastics, corticosteroids: possible increased osteonecrosis of the jaw

NURSING CONSIDERATIONS
Assessment
• **Assess for acute acute-phase reaction:** fever, myalgia, headache, flulike symptoms, for 72 hr after injection, usually resolves after 72 hr
• Monitor blood tests: serum calcium/creatinine/BUN/magnesium/phosphate
⚠ **Assess for hypocalcemia (may be fatal):** paresthesia, twitching, laryngospasm, Chvostek's/Trousseau's signs; preexisting hypocalcemia prior to treatment; patient with

Adverse effects: *italics* = common; **bold** = life-threatening

vitamin D deficiency may require higher doses of vitamin D
- **Assess for hypercalcemia:** nausea, vomiting, anorexia, weakness, thirst, constipation, dysrhythmias
- **Monitor dental status:** correct dental complications prior to product use, good oral hygiene should be maintained; if dental work is to be performed, antiinfectives should be given to prevent osteonecrosis of the jaw
- **Assess for infection:** Do not start treatment in those with active infections, infections should be resolved first

Patient/family education
- Advise patient to report hypercalcemic relapse: nausea, vomiting, bone pain, thirst
- Teach patient to continue with dietary recommendations including additional calcium and vitamin D
- Advise patient to avoid use in pregnancy and breastfeeding, notify prescriber if pregnancy is planned or suspected
- Instruct patient to use acetaminophen prior to and for 72 hrs after injection to lessen bone pain
- Explain the purpose of this product and expected results
- Advise patient to avoid OTC, Rx, or herbs and supplements unless approved by prescriber
- Teach patient to use regular exercise, stop smoking, and avoid alcohol to maintain bone health
- Advise patient to inform all health care providers of product use, avoid dental procedures/surgery if possible, practice good oral hygiene
- Teach patient that lab tests and follow-up exams will be required

Evaluation
Positive therapeutic outcome
- Increased/maintained bone density

---

desipramine (Rx)
(dess-ip′ra-meen)
Norpramin
Func. class.: Antidepressant, tricyclic
Chem. class.: Dibenzazepine, secondary amine
Pregnancy category C

ACTION: Blocks reuptake of norepinephrine, serotonin into nerve endings, increasing action of norepinephrine, serotonin in nerve cells

Therapeutic outcome: Decreased depression

USES: Depression

Unlabeled uses: Chronic pain, ADHD, bulimia, diabetic neuropathy, panic disorder, social phobia

CONTRAINDICATIONS:
Hypersensitivity to tricyclics, carBAMazepine; closed-angle glaucoma, acute MI, MAOIs

Precautions: Pregnancy **C,** breastfeeding, geriatric, severe depression, increased intraocular pressure, seizure disorder, CV disease, urinary retention, cardiac dysrhythmias, cardiac conduction disturbances, family history of sudden death, prostatic hypertrophy, thyroid disease

> **BLACK BOX WARNING:** Suicidal patients, children <18 yr

DOSAGE AND ROUTES
Major depression
Adult: PO 50-75 mg/day in 1-4 divided doses; titrate by 25-50 mg qwk up to 300 mg/day in single or divided doses (inpatient), 200 mg/day (outpatient)
Geriatric: PO 25 mg/day at bedtime, titrate qwk; may increase to 150 mg/day
Child >12 yr: PO 25-50 mg/day in divided doses, max 150 mg/day
Child 6-12 yr: PO 1-3 mg/kg/day in divided doses, give >3 mg/kg/day with close medical monitoring; max 5 mg/kg/day

Available forms: Tabs 10, 25, 50, 75, 100, 150 mg

Implementation
- Increase fluids, bulk in diet for constipation, especially in geriatric
- Take with food or milk for GI symptoms
- Crush if patient is unable to swallow medication whole
- Give dosage at bedtime if oversedation occurs during day; may take entire dose at bedtime; geriatric may not tolerate once a day dosing
- Store at room temperature
- Provide assistance with ambulation during beginning of therapy for drowsiness/dizziness
- Provide safety measures, primarily in the geriatric
- Check to see that PO medication is swallowed

ADVERSE EFFECTS

CNS: *Dizziness, drowsiness,* confusion, headache, anxiety, tremors, stimulation, weakness, insomnia, nightmares, EPS (geriatric), increased psychiatric symptoms, paresthesia, suicidal ideation, impaired memory, **seizures, serotonin syndrome**

CV: *Orthostatic hypo/hypertension,* ECG changes, *tachycardia, palpitations*

EENT: *Blurred vision,* tinnitus, mydriasis, ophthalmoplegia

ENDO: SIADH

GI: *Diarrhea, dry mouth,* nausea, vomiting, **paralytic ileus,** increased appetite, cramps, epigastric distress, jaundice, **hepatitis,** stomatitis, constipation, weight gain

GU: *Retention,* **acute renal failure**

HEMA: Agranulocytosis, thrombocytopenia, eosinophilia, leukopenia

INTEG: Rash, urticaria, sweating, pruritus, photosensitivity

Pharmacokinetics

Absorption	Well
Distribution	Widely, protein binding 92%
Metabolism	Extensively, liver
Excretion	Unknown
Half-life	12-24 hr

Pharmacodynamics

Unknown

INTERACTIONS

Individual drugs

Alcohol: increased CNS depression

Cimetidine, diltiazem, fluvoxaMINE, FLUoxetine, PARoxetine, sertraline, verapamil: increased desipramine level

CloNIDine: increased life-threatening B/P elevations, do not use concurrently

EPINEPHrine, norepinephrine: increased hypertension

Gatifloxacin, levofloxacin, moxifloxacin, sparfloxacin, SUNItinib, vorinostat, ziprasidone: **increased serotonin syndrome, neuroleptic malignant syndrome**

Drug classifications

Barbiturates, opioids, CNS depressants: increased CNS depression

MAOIs: increased hyperpyrexia, seizures, excitation; do not use within 14 days of MAOIs

SSRIs, SNRIs, serotonin-receptor agonists, other tricyclic antidepressants: increased serotonin syndrome, neuroleptic malignant syndrome

Class IA/III dysrhythmics, tricyclic antidepressants: increased QT interval

Drug/herb

Kava, valerian: increased CNS depression

St. John's wort: may increase serotonin syndrome; avoid concurrent use

Drug/lab test

Increase: serum bilirubin, blood glucose, alkaline phosphatase

Decreased: sodium

NURSING CONSIDERATIONS

Assessment

• Monitor B/P (lying, standing), pulse q4hr; if systolic B/P drops 20 mm Hg, hold product, notify prescriber; take vital signs q4hr in patients with CV disease

• Monitor blood studies: CBC, leukocytes, differential, cardiac enzymes if patient is receiving long-term therapy

• Monitor hepatic studies: AST, ALT, bilirubin

• Check weight qwk; appetite may increase with this product

• Monitor **ECG** for flattening T wave, bundle branch block, AV block, dysrhythmias in cardiac patients

• Assess for **EPS** primarily in geriatric: rigidity, dystonia, akathisia

• Assess for **seizure activity** in those with a history of seizures

> **BLACK BOX WARNING:** Assess mental status: mood, sensorium, affect, **suicidal tendencies,** increase in psychiatric symptoms: depression, panic; this product is not indicated for children

• Assess for urinary retention, constipation; constipation most likely in children

• Assess for **withdrawal symptoms:** headache, nausea, vomiting, muscle pain, weakness; not usual unless product is discontinued abruptly

• Assess for alcohol consumption; if consumed, hold dose until morning

Patient/family education

• Advise patient that therapeutic effects may take 2-3 wk

> **BLACK BOX WARNING:** Teach patient that suicidal thoughts and behavior may occur, notify prescriber immediately

---

- Advise patient to use caution in driving, other activities requiring alertness because of drowsiness, dizziness, blurred vision
- Teach patient to avoid alcohol ingestion, other CNS depressants
- Teach patient not to discontinue medication quickly after long-term use; may cause nausea, headache, malaise
- Teach patient to wear sunscreen or large hat, since photosensitivity occurs

Evaluation
Positive therapeutic outcome
- Decreased depression

TREATMENT OF OVERDOSE:
ECG monitoring; induce emesis; lavage, activated charcoal; administer anticonvulsant

---

RARELY USED

desirudin
(deh-sihr′uh-din)
Iprivask
Func. class.: Anticoagulant; thrombin inhibitor
Pregnancy category C

ACTION: Selectively inhibits free and clot-bound thrombin, prevents activation of clotting factors

Therapeutic outcome: Decreased occurrence of deep vein thrombosis (DVT) in hip-replacement surgery

USES: Prevents DVT in hip-replacement surgery

CONTRAINDICATIONS:
Hypersensitivity to this product, mannitol (diluent), hirudins, active bleeding, coagulation disorders

Precautions: Renal disease (CCr <60 ml/min), hepatic disease, GI/respiratory bleeding ≤3 mo, severe uncontrolled hypertension, spinal/epidural anesthesia, bacterial endocarditis

DOSAGE AND ROUTES
Adult: Subcut 15 mg q12hr × 9-12 days; give first dose 5-15 min prior to surgery if a regional block is used

Renal dose
Adult: Subcut CCr 31-60 ml/min 5 mg q12hr; CCr <31 ml/min 1.7 mg q12hr

Available forms: Inj 15 mg and 0.6 mannitol diluent

Implementation
- Visually inspect particulate matter and discoloration prior to use, do not use solutions that are cloudy or contain particles
- Do not use IM

Subcut route
- Do not mix with other injections, solvents, or parenteral fluids

Reconstitution for subcut use
- Reconstitute each vial with 0.5 ml of provided diluent, shake gently until the drug is fully reconstituted; the injection should be clear, colorless; once reconstituted, each 0.5 ml contains 15.75 mg desirudin; use immediately; however, it remains stable ≤ 24 hrs at room temperature and protected from light. Discard any unused solution

Subcut inj
- Have patient sit or lie down; using a syringe with a 26 or 27 G needle which is approximately 0.5-inch in length, withdraw the entire reconstituted solution into the syringe; inject total volume subcut; alternate between the left and right anterolateral and left and right posterolateral thigh or abdominal wall; insert whole length of the needle in a skin fold held between the thumb and forefinger; the skin fold should be held throughout the injection; to minimize bruising, do not rub the site

ADVERSE EFFECTS
CV: Thrombosis, thrombophlebitis, hypotension
CNS: Dizziness, fever
EENT: Nosebleeding
GI: Hematemesis, nausea, vomiting
HEMA: Hemorrhage, anemia
GU: Hematuria
MISC: Anaphylaxis, impaired healing edema

Pharmacokinetics

Absorption	Unknown
Distribution	Unknown
Metabolism	Unknown
Excretion	Unknown
Half-life	2 hr

Pharmacodynamics

Onset	½ hr
Peak	1-1½ hr
Duration	Unknown

INTERACTIONS
Drug classifications
Other anticoagulants, glycoprotein IIb/IIIa antagonists, NSAIDs, salicylates, thrombolytics, corticosteroids: increased bleeding risk

Drug/lab test
Decreased: Hct/Hgb

NURSING CONSIDERATIONS
Assessment
Bleeding:
• Assess for bleeding gums, black tarry stools, hematuria, epistaxis, decreased Hct/Hgb, guiac-positive stools, bleeding from hip replacement site, notify prescriber if any of these occurs
• Observe for thrombosis, ecchymosis
• Monitor aPTT q day in those with bleeding risk, aPTT should not be $>$ 2 times control

> **BLACK BOX WARNING:** Assess epidural/spinal anesthesia sites for hematomas, may result in irreversible paralysis

Patient/family education
• Teach patient to report any signs of bleeding
• Teach patient to use a soft-bristle toothbrush to avoid bleeding gums, to use an electric razor

Evaluation
Positive therapeutic outcome
• Decreased occurrence of DVT in hip replacement surgery

---

desloratadine (Rx)
(des-lor-at'ah-deen)
Clarinex, Clarinex RediTabs
Func. class.: Antihistamine, 2nd generation
Chem. class.: Selective histamine (H_1) receptor antagonist
Pregnancy category C

ACTION: Binds to peripheral histamine receptors, providing antihistamine action without sedation

Therapeutic outcome: Decreased nasal stuffiness, itching, swollen eyes

USES: Seasonal/perennial allergic rhinitis, chronic idiopathic urticaria

CONTRAINDICATIONS:
Hypersensitivity, infants/neonates

Precautions: Pregnancy C, bronchial asthma, renal/hepatic impairment, child, breastfeeding

DOSAGE AND ROUTES
Adult and child ≥12 yr: PO 5 mg daily
Child 6-11 yr: PO 2.5 mg daily
Child 1-5 yr: PO 1.25 mg daily
Child 6-11 mo: PO 1 mg daily (urticaria only)

Renal/hepatic dose
Adult: PO 5 mg every other day

Available forms: Tabs 5 mg; orally disintegrating (Reditabs) 2.5, 5 mg; syr 0.5 mg/ml

Implementation
• May administer without regard to meals
• Store in airtight container at room temperature

ADVERSE EFFECTS
CNS: Sedation (more common with increased dosages), headache, psychomotor hyperactivity, **seizures,** fatigue
GI: Hepatitis, nausea, dry mouth
MISC: Flulike symptoms

Pharmacokinetics

Absorption	Unknown
Distribution	Bound to plasma proteins (82%-87%)
Metabolism	Liver (active metabolites)
Excretion	Urine, feces (metabolites)
Half-life	8½-28 hr

Pharmacodynamics

Onset	1 hr, relief in 1 day
Peak	1½ hr
Duration	24 hr

INTERACTIONS
Drug/drug
Alcohol: increased CNS depression (rare)
Etravirine, nilotinib: increased desloratadine effect

Drug classification
Anxiolytics, antipsychotics, H_1 blockers, opiates, sedative/hypnotics, tricyclics, antidepressants: increased CNS depression (rare)

NURSING CONSIDERATIONS
Assessment
• Assess for **allergy:** hives, rash, rhinitis; monitor respiratory status; stop product 4 days before antigen skin test

---

Patient/family education
• Advise patient to avoid driving, other hazardous activities if drowsiness occurs; to observe caution until product's effects are known
• Advise patient that product may cause photosensitivity; use sunscreen or stay out of the sun to prevent burns
• Instruct patient not to exceed max dose
• Caution patient to avoid use of other CNS depressants
• Teach not to remove Reditabs from blister until ready to use; to place Reditab directly on tongue; may take with or without water

Evaluation
Positive therapeutic outcome
• Absence of running or congested nose, other allergy symptoms

desmopressin (Rx)
(des-moe-press'in)
DDAVP, Minirin, Octostim ✦, Stimate
Func. class.: Pituitary hormone
Chem. class.: Synthetic antidiuretic hormone
Pregnancy category B

ACTION: Promotes reabsorption of water by action on renal tubular epithelium in the kidney; causes smooth muscle constriction and increase in plasma factor VIII levels, which increases platelet aggregation resulting in vasopressor effect; similar to vasopressin

Therapeutic outcome: Prevention of nocturnal enuresis, decreased bleeding in hemophilia A, von Willebrand's disease type 1, control and stabilization of water in diabetes insipidus

USES: Hemophilia A, von Willebrand's disease type 1, nonnephrogenic diabetes insipidus, symptoms of polyuria/polydipsia caused by pituitary dysfunction, nocturnal enuresis

CONTRAINDICATIONS:
Hypersensitivity, nephrogenic diabetes insipidus, severe renal disease

Precautions: Pregnancy **B**, breastfeeding, CAD, hypertension, cystic fibrosis, thrombus

DOSAGE AND ROUTES
Primary nocturnal enuresis
Adult and child ≥6 yr: INTRANASAL 0.2 mg (half in each nostril) at bedtime, may increase to 40 mcg; PO 0.2 mg at bedtime, may be increased to max 0.6 mg at bedtime

Diabetes insipidus
Adult: Intranasal 0.1-0.4 ml daily in divided doses (1-4 sprays with pump); SUBCUT/**IV** 0.5-1 ml daily in divided doses
Child 3 mo-12 yr: INTRANASAL 0.05-0.3 ml daily in divided doses

Hemophilia/von Willebrand's disease
Adult and child >3 mo: IV 0.3 mcg/kg in NaCl over 15-30 min; may repeat if needed

Antihemorrhagic
Adult and child >3 mo: IV 0.3 mcg/kg
Adult and child <50 kg: Intranasal 1 spray in one nostril
Adult and child >50 kg: 1 spray each nostril
Adult: SUBCUT/IV 0.3-0.4 mg/kg as a single injection

Available forms: Inj 4, 15 mcg/ml, Rhinal Tube delivery 2.5 mg/vial (0.1 mg/ml); tabs 0.1, 0.2 mg; nasal spray pump 10 mcg/spray (0.1 mg/ml); nasal sol 1.5 mg/ml (150 mcg/dose)

Implementation
PO route
• Store at room temperature
• Draw medication into tube, insert tube into nostril to instill product and blow on other end to deliver sol into nasal cavity; rinse after use
• Store in refrigerator or cool environment

IV, direct route
• Give undiluted over 1 min in diabetes insipidus
Intermittent IV infusion route
• Give single dose diluted in 50 ml of 0.9% NaCl (adult and child >10 kg); a single dose/10 ml as an **IV** inf over 15-30 min in von Willebrand's disease or hemophilia A
• Store in refrigerator

ADVERSE EFFECTS
CNS: Drowsiness, headache, lethargy, flushing, **seizures**
CV: Increased B/P, palpitations, tachycardia
EENT: Nasal irritation, congestion, rhinitis
GI: Nausea, heartburn, cramps
GU: *Vulval pain*
META: Hyponatremia, hyponatremia-induced seizures
SYST: Anaphylaxis (IV)

Pharmacokinetics

Absorption	Nasal (up to 20%)
Distribution	Unknown
Metabolism	Unknown
Excretion	Unknown; breast milk
Half-life	8 min (initial), 76 min (terminal)

Pharmacodynamics

	PO	Intra-nasal	SUBCUT/IV
Onset	1 hr	1 hr	Rapid
Peak	4-7 hr	1-4 hr	15-30 min
Duration	Unknown	8-20 hr	3 hr

INTERACTIONS

Individual drugs

Alcohol, demeclocycline, EPHINEPHrine (large doses), heparin, lithium: decreased antidiuretic action

CarBAMazepine, chlorpropamide, clofibrate: increased antidiuretic action

Drug classifications

Pressor products: increased pressor effect

NURSING CONSIDERATIONS

Assessment

• Monitor I&O ratio, urine osmolality, specific gravity, weight daily; check for edema in extremities; if water retention is severe, diuretic may be prescribed; check pulse, B/P when giving product **IV** or SUBCUT

• Assess for **water intoxication:** lethargy, behavioral changes, disorientation, neuromuscular excitability, dehydration, poor skin turgor, severe thirst, dry skin, tachycardia

• Assess intranasal use: nausea, congestion, cramps, headache; usually decreased with decreased dosage

• Monitor for enuresis during treatment **(nocturnal enuresis)**

• Assess for allergic reaction, including anaphylaxis **(IV route)**

• Assess for nasal mucosa changes: congestion, edema, discharge, scarring (nasal route)

• Monitor urine volume osmolality and plasma osmolality (diabetes insipidus)

• Monitor factor VIII coagulant activity before using for hemostasis

Patient/family education

• Use demonstration, return demonstration to teach technique for nasal instillation

• Teach patient to notify prescriber of dyspnea, vomiting, cramping, drowsiness, headache, nasal congestion

• Caution patient to avoid OTC products (cough, hay fever), since these preparations may contain epinephrine and decrease product response; do not use with alcohol

• Advise patient to carry/wear emergency ID or other identification specifying disease and medication used

• Advise patient if dose is missed, take when remembered, up to 1 hr before next dose; do not double doses; avoid fluids from 1 hr to up to 8 hr after PO dose

• Teach patient to report upper respiratory infection, nasal congestion

Evaluation

Positive therapeutic outcome

• Absence of severe thirst

• Decreased urine output, osmolality

• Absence of bleeding (hemophilia)

desonide topical
See Appendix B

desoximetasone topical
See Appendix B

desoxyephedrine nasal agent
See Appendix B

desoxyribonuclease
See fibrinolysin/desoxyribonuclease

desvenlafaxine (Rx)
Pristiq
Func. class.: Antidepressant, serotonin-receptor norepinephrine reuptake inhibitor (SNRI)
Pregnancy category C

ACTION: May work by blocking the central presynaptic reuptake of 5-HT and NE, resulting in an increased sustained level of these neurotransmitters.

Therapeutic outcome: Decreased depression, increased sense of well-being and renewed interest in activities

USES: Major depressive disorder

Unlabeled uses: Vasomotor symptoms (hot flashes) associated with menopause

CONTRAINDICATIONS:

Hypersensitivity to this product or venlafaxine, MAOI therapy

Precautions: CNS depression, abrupt discontinuation, hypertension, hepatic/renal disease, hyponatremia, geriatric patients, pregnancy C, labor and delivery, breastfeeding, angina, bleeding, cardiac dysrhythmias, MI, stroke, mania, hypovolemia, dehydration, increased intraocular pressure

> **BLACK BOX WARNING:** Children, suicidal ideation

DOSAGE AND ROUTES

Adult: **PO** Initially, 50 mg daily; max 400 mg/day with adjustments as needed; spray: apply sparingly to area bid, rub gently (plaque psoriasis only)

Vasospastic effects of menopause (unlabeled)
Adult: **PO** 100-150 mg/day

Available forms: Ext rel tabs 50, 100 mg

ADVERSE EFFECTS

CNS: *Dizziness,* drowsiness, *headache,* tremor, paresthesias, asthenia, **suicidal thoughts and behaviors, seizures,** chills, yawning, hot flashes, flushing, *irritability, insomnia, anxiety, abnormal dreams, fatigue*
CV: Palpitations, sinus tachycardia, increased blood pressure, orthostatic hypotension
EENT: Blurred vision, mydriasis, tinnitus, bruxism
GI: *Nausea,* xerostomia, *diarrhea,* constipation, vomiting, anorexia, weight loss, dysgeusia, hypercholesterolemia, hypertriglyceridemia
GU: Urinary retention/hesitancy, orgasm dysfunction, decreased libido, impotence, proteinuria
HEMA: Impaired platelet aggregation
INTEG: Photosensitivity, hyperhidrosis, diaphoresis
SYST: Serotonin syndrome, neuroleptic malignant syndrome-like symptoms, toxic epidermal necrolysis, rash, Stevens-Johnson syndrome, erythema multiforme, angioedema; neonatal abstinence syndrome (fetal exposure)

Pharmacokinetics

Absorption	Unknown
Distribution	Protein binding 30%; enters breast milk
Metabolism	Liver, 55%
Excretion	Urine, unchanged, 45%
Half-life	Elimination 11 hr, increased in hepatic/renal disease

Pharmacodynamics

Onset	Unknown
Peak	7.5 hr
Duration	24 hr

INTERACTIONS
Individual drugs
Dexfenfluramine, dexmethylphenidate, dextromethorphan, fenfluramine, linezolid, lithium, nefazodone, meperidine, methylphenidate, mirtazapine, pentazocine, phentermine, promethazine, sibutramine, SUMAtriptan, traZODone, tryptophan: do not administer concurrently; increased serotonin syndrome, neuroleptic malignant syndrome-like reactions
Zolpidem: increased hallucinations, delusions, disorientation

Drug classifications
Anticoagulants, NSAIDs, platelet inhibitors, salicylates, thrombolytics: increased bleeding risk
Alcohol, antihistamines, opioids, sedatives/hypnotics: increased CNS depression
Ergots, MAOIs, serotonin receptor agonists (almotriptan, eletriptan, frovatriptan, methylene blue IV, naratriptan, rizatriptan, sumatriptan, zolmitriptan), SSRIs, other SNRIs, TCAs, tricyclics: do not administer concurrently; increased serotonin syndrome, neuroleptic malignant syndrome-like reactions

Drug/herb
Kava, valerian: increased desvenlafaxine action

Drug/lab test
Increased: sodium, cholesterol, triglycerides
False positive: amphetamine, phencyclidine

NURSING CONSIDERATIONS
Assessment

> **BLACK BOX WARNING: Suicidal thoughts/ behaviors:** Assess mental status and mood, identify suicidal ideation

• **Serotonin syndrome, neuroleptic malignant syndrome-like symptoms:** Assess for nausea/vomiting, sedation, dizziness, diaphoresis (sweating), facial flush, hallucinations, mental status changes, myoclonia, restlessness, shivering, elevated blood pressure, hyperthermia, muscle rigidity, autonomic instability, and mental status changes; if serotonin syndrome occurs discontinue desvenlafaxine, and any other serotonergic agents
• Monitor B/P baseline and periodically during treatment, lipid levels, signs of glaucoma
• Assess appetite and nutritional intake, weight loss is common, change diet as need to support weight

Patient/family education
• Teach patient to take as directed, not to double or skip doses; if a dose is missed, take as soon as remembered unless close to next dose, do not discontinue abruptly, decreased gradually

> **BLACK BOX WARNING:** Advise patient to report immediately suicidal thoughts or behaviors, have family members look for symptoms of suicidal ideation

• Inform patient not to operate machinery or engage in hazardous activities until reaction ins known, may cause dizziness, drowsiness
• Teach patient to avoid all others products unless approval by prescriber
• Teach patient to report if pregnancy is planned or suspected, pregnancy C, or if breastfeeding
⚠ Teach patient to report immediately allergic reactions including, **rash, hives, difficulty breathing, or swelling of face, lips**
• Advise patient that continuing follow-up exams will be needed

Evaluation
Positive therapeutic outcome
• Decreased depression, increased sense of well-being and renewed interest in activities

dexamethasone (Rx)
(dex-ah-meth′ah-sone)
Baycadvor, Decadron, Dexasone ✽, Dex Pak, Maxidex ✽, Zena-Pak
dexamethasone sodium phosphate (Rx)
Func. class.: Corticosteroid, synthetic
Chem. class.: Glucocorticoid, long-acting
Pregnancy category C

D

Do not confuse:
Decadron/Percodan

ACTION: Decreases inflammation by suppressing migration of polymorphonuclear leukocytes, fibroblasts, reversing increased capillary permeability and lysosomal stabilization, suppresses normal immune response, no mineralocorticoid effects

USES: Inflammation, allergies, neoplasms, cerebral edema, septic shock, collagen disorders, dexamethasone suppression test for Cushing syndrome, adrenocortical insufficiency, TB, meningitis, acute exacerbations of MS

CONTRAINDICATIONS:
Psychosis, hypersensitivity to corticosteroids, sulfites, or benzyl alcohol, idiopathic thrombocytopenia, acute glomerulonephritis, amebiasis, fungal infections, nonasthmatic bronchial disease, child <2 yr, AIDS, TB, glaucoma, ocular infection

Precautions: Pregnancy **C,** breastfeeding, diabetes mellitus, osteoporosis, seizure disorders, ulcerative colitis, CHF, myasthenia gravis, renal disease, peptic ulcer, esophagitis, recent MI, hypertension, TB, active hepatitis, psychosis, sulfite hypersensitivity, thromboembolic disorders, abrupt discontinuation, coagulopathy, ulcerative colitis, seizure disorders

DOSAGE AND ROUTES
Inflammation
Adult: PO 0.75-9 mg/day, in divided doses q6-12hr; or phosphate IM 0.5-9 mg/day divided q6-12hr
Child: PO 0.024-0.34 mg/kg/day in divided doses q6-12hr

Shock
Adult: IV (phosphate) single dose 1-6 mg/kg or **IV** 40 mg q2-6hr as needed up to 72 hr

Adverse effects: *italics* = common; **bold** = life-threatening

Cerebral edema
Adult: IV (phosphate) 10 mg, then 4-6 mg IM q6hr × 2-4 days, then taper over 1 wk
Child: PO/IM/**IV** loading dose 1-2 mg/kg, then 1-1.5 mg/kg/day, max 16 mg/day divided q4-6hr for 2-4 days, then taper down qwk

Adrenocortical insufficiency
Adult: PO 0.75-9 mg/day in divided doses
Child: PO 0.03-0.3 mg/kg/day divided in 2-4 doses

Suppression test
Adult: PO 1 mg at 11 PM or 0.5 mg q6hr × 48 hr

Available forms: Dexamethasone: tabs 0.5, 0.75, 1, 1.5, 2, 4, 6 mg; elix 0.5 mg/5 ml; oral sol 0.5 mg/5 ml, 1 mg/ml; **sodium phosphate** 4, 10 mg/ml; ophth implant 0.7 mg; ophth susp drops/sol 0.1%

Implementation
PO route
• Give with food or milk to decrease GI symptoms
• Provide assistance with ambulation in patient with bone tissue disease to prevent fractures
IM route
• IM inj deep in large muscle mass; rotate sites; avoid deltoid; use 21-G needle
• In one dose in AM to prevent adrenal suppression; avoid SUBCUT administration, may damage tissue

Direct IV route (sodium phosphate)
• IV undiluted direct over 1 min or less
• Titrated dose; use lowest effective dose
Intermittent IV infusion route
• Diluted with 0.9% NaCl or D₅W and give as an IV inf at prescribed rate

Dexamethasone sodium phosphate

Syringe compatibilities: Acetaminophen, caffeine, dimenhydrAMINE, furosemide, granisetron, hyaluronidase, ketamine, metoclopramide, octreotide, oxyCODONE, palonosetron, ranitidine, salbutamol, SUFentanil, traMADol

Y-site compatibilities: Acetaminophen, acyclovir, alfentanil, allopurinol, amifostine, amikacin, aminocaproic acid, aminophylline, amphotericin B cholesteryl, amphotericin B lipid complex, amphotericin B liposome, amsacrine, anidulafungin, argatroban, ascorbic acid injection, atenolol, atracurium, atropine, aztreonam, benztropine, bivalirudin, bleomycin, bumetanide, buprenorphine, butorphanol, CARBOplatin, carmustine, cefamandole, ceFAZolin, cefepime, cefonicid, cefoperazone, cefoTEtan, cefOXitin, cefpirome, ceftaroline, cefTAZidime, ceftizoxime, ceftobiprole, cefTRIAXone, chloramphenicol, cimetidine, cisatracurium, CISplatin, cladribine, clindamycin, codeine, cyanocobalamin, cyclophosphamide, cycloSPORINE, cytarabine, DACTINomycin, DAPTOmycin, DAUNOrubicin liposome, dexmedetomidine, digoxin, diltiazem, DOCEtaxel, DOPamine, doripenem, doxacurium, DOXOrubicin, DOXOrubicin liposomal, enalaprilat, ePHEDrine, EPINEPHrine, epoetin alfa, eptifibatide, ertapenem, etoposide, etoposide phosphate, famotidine, fentaNYL, filgrastim, fluconazole, fludarabine, fluorouracil, folic acid, fosaprepitant, foscarnet, furosemide, ganciclovir, gatifloxacin, gemcitabine, glycopyrrolate, granisetron, heparin, hydrocortisone, HYDROmorphone, ifosfamide, imipenem-cilastatin, indomethacin, insulin (regular), irinotecan, isoproterenol, ketorolac, lansoprazole, leucovorin, levofloxacin, lidocaine, linezolid, liposome, LORazepam, LR, mannitol, mechlorethamine, melphalan, meropenem, metaraminol, methadone, methyldopate, methylPREDNISolone, metoclopramide, metoprolol, metroNIDAZOLE, mezlocillin, milrinone, morphine, multiple vitamins injection, nafcillin, nalbuphine, naloxone, nitroglycerin, nitroprusside, norepinephrine, octreotide, ondansetron, oxacillin, oxaliplatin, oxyCODONE, oxytocin, PACLitaxel, palonosetron, pamidronate, pancuronium, PEMEtrexed, penicillin G potassium/sodium, PENTobarbital, PHENobarbital, phenylephrine, phytonadione, piperacillin, piperacillin-tazobactam, potassium chloride, procainamide, propofol, propranolol, pyridoxine, ranitidine, remifentanil, Ringer's, ritodrine, riTUXimab, sargramostim, sodium acetate/bicarbonate, succinylcholine, SUFentanil, tacrolimus, telavancin, teniposide, theophylline, thiamine, thiotepa, ticarcillin, ticarcillin-clavulanate, tigecycline, tirofiban, TNA, tolazoline, topotecan, trastuzumab, trimetaphan, urokinase, vancomycin, vasopressin, vecuronium, verapamil, vinCRIStine, vinorelbine, vitamin B complex/C, voriconazole, zidovudine, zoledronic acid

ADVERSE EFFECTS
CNS: *Depression, flushing, sweating,* headache, mood changes, euphoria, psychosis, **seizures,** insomnia, **pseudotumor cerebri**
CV: *Hypertension,* **circulatory collapse, thromboembolism, heart failure, dysrhythmias,** tachycardia, edema, cardiomyopathy
EENT: Fungal infections, increased intraocular pressure, blurred vision, cataracts, glaucoma

---

ENDO: Hypothalmic-pituitary-adrenal axis suppression, hyperglycemia, sodium, fluid retention
GI: *Diarrhea, nausea, abdominal distention,* **GI hemorrhage,** *increased appetite,* **pancreatitis**
HEMA: **Thrombocytopenia,** transient leukocytosis, **thromboembolism**
INTEG: Acne, poor wound healing, ecchymosis, petechiae, hirsutism, **angioedema**
META: Hypokalemia
MS: Fractures, osteoporosis, weakness, arthralgia, myopathy

Pharmacokinetics

Absorption	Unknown
Distribution	Unknown
Metabolism	Liver
Excretion	Kidneys
Half-life	1-2 days

Pharmacodynamics

	PO	IM
Onset	1 hr	Unknown
Peak	1-2 hr	8 hr
Duration	2½ days	6 days-3 wk

INTERACTIONS
Individual drugs
Alcohol, amphotericin B, cycloSPORINE, digoxin, indomethacin: increased side effects
Ambemonium, isoniazid, neostigmine, sometrem: decreased effects of each specific product
Bosentan, carBAMazepine, cholestyramine, colestipol, ePHEDrine, ethotoin, phenytoin, rifampin, theophylline: decreased action of dexamethasone
CycloSPORINE, tacrolimus: increased effect of each drug
Ketoconazole, NSAIDs: increased action of dexamethasone

Drug classifications
Antacids, barbiturates: decreased action of dexamethasone
Antibiotics (macrolide), contraceptives (hormonal), estrogens, salicylates: increased action of dexamethasone
Anticholinesterases, anticoagulants, anticonvulsants, antidiabetics, salicylates, toxoids/vaccines: decreased effects of each specific product
Antidiabetics: increased effect of these products

Diuretics, NSAIDs, salicylates: increased side effects
Quinolones: increased risk of tendinitis, tendon rupture
Thiazide diuretics: decreased potassium levels

Drug/lab test
Increased: cholesterol, Na, blood glucose, uric acid, Ca, urine glucose
Decreased: Ca, potassium, T_4, T_3, thyroid ^{131}I uptake test, urine 17-OHCS, 17-KS, PBI
False negative: skin allergy tests

NURSING CONSIDERATIONS
Assessment
• Monitor K, blood, urine glucose while on long-term therapy; hypokalemia and hyperglycemia
• Monitor weight daily; notify prescriber of weekly gain >5 lb
• Monitor B/P, pulse; notify prescriber of chest pain
• Monitor I&O ratio; be alert for decreasing urinary output, increasing edema
• Monitor plasma cortisol levels during long-term therapy (normal: 138-635 nmol/L when assessed at 8 AM), prolonged use can cause **cushingoid symptoms** (buffalo hump, moon face, increased B/P)
• **Assess infection:** fever, WBC even after withdrawal of medication; product masks infection
• **Assess potassium depletion:** paresthesias, fatigue, nausea, vomiting, depression, polyuria, dysrhythmias, weakness
• Assess edema, hypertension, cardiac symptoms
• Assess mental status: affect, mood, behavioral changes, aggression
⚠ **Abrupt withdrawal: acute adrenal insufficiency and death may occur following abrupt discontinuation of systemic therapy; withdraw gradually**

Patient/family education
• Advise that emergency ID as corticosteroid user should be carried or worn
• Teach to notify prescriber if therapeutic response decreases; dosage adjustment may be needed
• Teach not to discontinue abruptly or **adrenal crisis** can result
• Teach to avoid OTC products: salicylates, alcohol in cough products, cold preparations unless directed by prescriber
• Instruct patient to contact prescriber if surgery, trauma, stress occurs, dosage may need to be adjusted

• Teach patient all aspects of product use, including cushingoid symptoms
• Instruct patient to notify prescriber of infection
• Teach patient to take with food or milk
• Teach patient that bruising may occur easily
• Teach patient that if on long-term therapy, a high-protein diet may be needed
• Teach symptoms of adrenal insufficiency: nausea, anorexia, fatigue, dizziness, dyspnea, weakness, joint pain
• Advise patient to avoid exposure to chickenpox or measles, persons with infections

Evaluation
Positive therapeutic outcome
Decreased inflammation

dexamethasone ophthalmic
See Appendix B

dexamethasone topical
See Appendix B

dexlansoprazole (Rx)
(dex-lan-so-prey′zole)
Dexilant
Func. class.: Anti-ulcer–proton pump inhibitor
Chem. class.: Benzimidazole
Pregnancy category B

ACTION: Suppresses gastric secretion by inhibiting hydrogen/potassium ATPase enzyme system in gastric parietal cell; characterized as gastric acid pump inhibitor, since it blocks final step of acid production

Therapeutic outcome: Reduction in gastric pain, swelling, fullness

USES: Gastroesophageal reflux disease (GERD), severe erosive esophagitis, heartburn

CONTRAINDICATIONS:
Hypersensitivity

Precautions: Pregnancy **B**, breastfeeding, children, proton-pump hypersensitivity, gastric cancer, hepatic disease, vit B_{12} deficiency

DOSAGE AND ROUTES
Erosive esophagitis
Adult: PO 60 mg qd for up to 8 wk; maintenance: PO 30 mg qd for up to 6 mo

GERD
Adult: PO: 30 mg qd × 4 wk

Hepatic disease
Adult: PO (Child-Pugh B): max 30 mg/day

Available forms: Del rel caps 30, 60 mg

Implementation
• Swallow del rel cap whole; do not break, crush, chew; caps may be opened and contents sprinkled on food, use immediately; do not chew contents of caps, give without regard to food

ADVERSE EFFECTS
CNS: Headache, dizziness, confusion, agitation, amnesia, depression, **anxiety, seizures,** insomnia
CV: Chest pain, angina, bradycardia, palpitations, **CVA,** hypertension, **MI**
EENT: Tinnitus
GI: Diarrhea, abdominal pain, vomiting, nausea, constipation, flatulence, colitis, dysgeusia
HEMA: Anemia, **neutropenia, thrombocytopenia, pernicious anemia, thrombosis**
INTEG: Rash, urticaria, pruritus
META: Gout
MS: Arthralgia, myalgia
RESP: Upper respiratory infections, cough, epistaxis, dyspnea
SYST: Anaphylaxis, Stevens-Johnson syndrome, toxic epidermal necrolysis, exfoliative dermatitis, pneumonia

Pharmacokinetics
Absorption	57%-64%
Distribution	Protein binding 97%
Metabolism	Liver extensively
Excretion	Urine, feces; clearance decreased in geriatric, renal/hepatic disease
Half-life	Plasma 1-2 hr, 4-5 hr

Pharmacodynamics
Unknown

INTERACTIONS
Individual drugs
Ampicillin, calcium carbonate, delavirdine, iron, itraconazole, ketoconazole: decreased absorption of each specific product

Drug classifications
CYP2C19, CYP3A4 (fluvoxamine, voriconazole): increased dexlansoprazole effect
Sucralfate: delayed absorption of dexlansoprazole

Drug/lab test
Increased: LFTs, bilirubin, creatinine, glucose, lipids
Decreased: platelets, magnesium

NURSING CONSIDERATIONS
Assessment
• Assess GI system: bowel sounds q8hr, abdomen for pain, swelling, anorexia; monitor serum magnesium
⚠ **Anaphylaxis, serious skin disorders requiring emergency intervention (rare)**
⚠ **Hepatotoxicity: Hepatitis, jaundice, monitor liver enzymes (AST, ALT, alkaline phosphatase) during treatment if hepatic adverse reactions occur (rare)**
• **Hypomagnesemia:** Usually 3 months to 1 yr after beginning therapy; monitor magnesium level, assess for irregular heart beats, muscle spasms; in children fatigue, upset stomach, dizziness; magnesium supplement may be used

Patient/family education
• Instruct patient to report severe diarrhea; product may have to be discontinued
• Inform diabetic patient that hypoglycemia may occur
• Encourage patient to avoid hazardous activities; dizziness may occur
• Tell patient to avoid alcohol, salicylates, ibuprofen; may cause GI irritation
• Teach patient to report allergic reactions, symptoms of low magnesium levels
⚠ **Teach patient to notify prescriber if pregnancy is planned or suspected, not to breastfeed**
• Advise patient to swallow cap whole, not to chew, crush

Evaluation
Positive therapeutic outcome
• Absence of gastric pain, swelling, fullness

---

dexmethylphenidate (Rx)
(dex′meth-ul-fen′ih-dayt)
Focalin, Focalin XR
Func. class.: Central nervous system (CNS) stimulant, psychostimulant
Pregnancy category C
Controlled substance schedule II

Do not confuse:
dexmethylphenidate/methylphenidate

ACTION: Increases release of norepinephrine and dopamine into the extraneuronal space, also blocks reuptake of norepinephrine and dopamine into the presynaptic neuron; mode of action in treating attention-deficit-hyperactivity disorder (ADHD) is unknown

Therapeutic outcome: Increased alertness, decreased fatigue, ability to stay awake (narcolepsy), increased attention span, decreased hyperactivity (ADHD)

USE: ADHD

CONTRAINDICATIONS:
Hypersensitivity to methylphenidate, anxiety, history of Tourette's syndrome; children <6 yr, glaucoma, concurrent treatment with MAOIs or within 14 days of discontinuing treatment with MAOIs, breastfeeding, tics, psychosis

Precautions: Pregnancy C, hypertension, depression, seizures, CV disorders, alcoholism

> **BLACK BOX WARNING:** Substance abuse

DOSAGE AND ROUTES
Adult: PO EXT REL 10 mg/day, may adjust to 20 mg/day in 10 mg increments
Child >6 yr: PO 2.5 mg bid with doses at least 4 hr apart, gradually increase to a max of 20 mg/day (10 mg bid); for those taking methylphenidate, use ½ of methylphenidate dose initially, then increase as needed to max 20 mg/day; EXT REL 5 mg/day, may adjust to 20 mg/day in 5 mg increments

Available forms: Tabs 2.5, 5, 10 mg; ext rel caps (Focalin XR) 5, 10, 15, 20, 25, 30, 35, 40 mg

Implementation
• Do not break, crush, or chew ext rel caps
• Twice daily at least 4 hr apart; ext rel once a day
• Without regard to meals
• Med guide should be provided by dispenser

ADVERSE EFFECTS
CNS: Dizziness, headache, drowsiness, nervousness, insomnia, **toxic psychosis, neuroleptic malignant syndrome (rare),** Tourette's syndrome
CV: Palpitations, B/P changes, angina, **dysrhythmias, tachycardia, MI, stroke**
GI: *Nausea, anorexia,* abnormal liver function, **hepatic coma,** *abdominal pain*
HEMA: Leukopenia, anemia, **thrombocytopenic purpura**

INTEG: **Exfoliative dermatitis,** urticaria, rash, erythema multiforme
MISC: *Fever,* arthralgia, scalp hair loss

Pharmacokinetics

Absorption	Readily absorbed
Distribution	Unknown
Metabolism	Liver
Excretion	Kidneys
Half-life	2.2 hr

Pharmacodynamics

	PO	EXT REL
Onset	½-1 hr	Unknown
Peak	1-1½ hr	4 hr
Duration	4 hr	8 hr

INTERACTIONS
Drug classifications
Anticoagulants (coumarin), anticonvulsants, selective serotonin reuptake inhibitors, tricyclics: increased effects
Antihypertensives: decreased effects
Decongestants, vasoconstrictors: increased sympathomimetic effect
MAOIs: hypertensive crisis if coadministered or given within 14 days
Vasopressors: hypertensive crisis

Drug/herb
Melatonin: increased synergistic effect

NURSING CONSIDERATIONS
Assessment

> **BLACK BOX WARNING:** Assess for previous or current substance abuse; psychotic episodes may occur, especially with parental abuse

• Assess VS, B/P; may reverse antihypertensives; check patients with cardiac disease more often for increased B/P
• Assess CBC, differential, platelet counts during long-term therapy, urinalysis; in diabetes: blood/urine glucose; insulin changes may have to be made, since eating will decrease
• Assess height, growth rate q3mo in children; growth rate may be decreased
• Assess mental status: mood, sensorium, affect, stimulation, insomnia, aggressiveness
⚠ **Assess withdrawal symptoms: headache, nausea, vomiting, muscle pain, weakness**
• Assess appetite, sleep, speech patterns
• Assess for attention span, decreased hyperactivity in persons with ADHD

Patient/family education
• Advise patient to decrease caffeine consumption (coffee, tea, cola, chocolate); may increase irritability, stimulation
• Advise patient to avoid OTC preparations unless approved by prescriber
• Caution patient to taper off product over several wk to avoid depression, increased sleeping, lethargy
• Caution patient to avoid alcohol ingestion
• Caution patient to avoid hazardous activities until stabilized on medication
• Advise patient to get needed rest; patients will feel more tired at end of day
• Notify all health providers including school nurse of medication and schedule
• Discuss information instructions provided in patient information section
• Teach patient to notify prescriber if pregnancy is planned or suspected, avoid breastfeeding

Evaluation
Positive therapeutic outcome
• Decreased hyperactivity or ability to stay awake

TREATMENT OF OVERDOSE:
Administer fluids; hemodialysis or peritoneal dialysis; antihypertensive for increased B/P; administer short-acting barbiturate before lavage

---

dextroamphetamine (Rx)
(dex-troe-am-fet′a-meen)
Dexedrine, ProCentra
Func. class.: Cerebral stimulant
Chem. class.: Amphetamine
Pregnancy category C
Controlled substance schedule II

ACTION: Increases release of norepinephrine, dopamine in cerebral cortex to reticular activating system

Therapeutic outcome: Increased alertness, decreased fatigue, ability to stay awake (narcolepsy); increased attention span, decreased hyperactivity (ADHD)

USES: Narcolepsy, attention-deficit disorder with hyperactivity

Unlabeled use: Obesity

CONTRAINDICATIONS:
Hypersensitivity to sympathomimetic amines, hyperthyroidism, hypertension, glaucoma, severe

---

arteriosclerosis, drug abuse, anxiety, anorexia nervosa, tartrazine dye hypersensitivity

> **BLACK BOX WARNING:** Symptomatic CV disease, substance abuse

Precautions: Pregnancy **C,** breastfeeding, child <3 yr, Gilles de la Tourette's disorder, depression, cardiomyopathy, bipolar disorder, abrupt discontinuation, acute MI; benzyl alcohol, salicylate hypersensitivity; hypercortisolism, obesity, psychosis, seizure disorder

DOSAGE AND ROUTES
Narcolepsy
Adult: PO 5 mg bid, titrate daily dose by no more than 10 mg/wk, max 60 mg/day
Child 6-12 yr: PO 5 mg daily increasing by no more than 5 mg/day at weekly intervals

ADHD
Adult: PO 5-60 mg/day in divided doses
Child 6-12 yr: PO 5 mg daily-bid increasing by 5 mg/day at weekly intervals
Child 3-5 yr: PO 2.5 mg daily increasing by 2.5 mg/day at weekly intervals (max 40 mg/day)

Available forms: Tabs 5, 10 mg, oral sol 5 mg/5 ml

Implementation
• Give at least 6 hr before bedtime to avoid sleeplessness; titrate to patient's response; lowest dosage should be used to control symptoms
• Give gum, hard candy, frequent sips of water for dry mouth at beginning of treatment; these symptoms tend to lessen with time
• Store all forms at room temperature

ADVERSE EFFECTS
CNS: *Hyperactivity, insomnia, restlessness, talkativeness,* dizziness, headache, chills, stimulation, dysphoria, irritability, aggressiveness, tremor, dependence, addiction
CV: *Palpitations,* **tachycardia,** hypertension, decrease in heart rate, **dysrhythmias**
GI: *Anorexia,* dry mouth, diarrhea, constipation, weight loss, metallic taste
GU: Impotence, change in libido
INTEG: Urticaria

Absorption	Well absorbed
Distribution	Widely distributed; crosses placenta
Metabolism	Liver
Excretion	Kidneys, pH dependent: increased pH, increased reabsorption
Half-life	10-30 hr; increased when urine is alkaline

Pharmacodynamics

Onset	½ hr; ext rel 1 hr
Peak	1-3 hr; ext rel 2 hr
Duration	4-10 hr; ext rel 8 hr

INTERACTIONS
Individual drugs
AcetaZOLAMIDE, sodium bicarbonate: increased effect of dextroamphetamine
Ammonium chloride, ascorbic acid, guanethidine: decreased effect of dextroamphetamine
Haloperidol: increased CNS effect
Phenytoin: decreased absorption of phenytoin

Drug classifications
Adrenergic blockers: decreased adrenergic blocking effect
Antacids: increased effect of dextroamphetamine
Antidepressants (tricyclic), phenothiazines: increased CNS effect
Antidiabetics: decreased antidiabetic effect
Antihistamines: decreased antihistamine effect
Antihypertensives: decreased antihypertensive effect
Barbiturates: decreased absorption of barbiturate
MAOIs: hypertensive crisis if used within 14 days
SSRIs, SNRIs, serotonin-receptor agonists: do not use concurrently: increased serotonin syndrome, neuroleptic malignant syndrome

Drug/herb
Eucalyptus: decreased stimulant effect
St. John's wort: increased serotonin syndrome

Drug/food
Caffeine (cola, coffee, tea [green/black]): increased amine effect

Drug/lab test
Increase: plasma corticosteroids, urinary steroids

NURSING CONSIDERATIONS
Assessment

> **BLACK BOX WARNING: Cardiac disease:**
> monitor VS, B/P, since this product may reverse
> antihypertensives; check patients with cardiac
> disease more often for increased B/P

• Monitor CBC, urinalysis; for diabetic patients
monitor blood, urine glucose; insulin changes
may be required, since eating will decrease
• Monitor height and weight q3mo since growth
rate in children may be decreased; appetite is
suppressed so weight loss is common during the
first few months of treatment
• Monitor mental status: mood, sensorium,
affect, stimulation, insomnia; aggressiveness may
occur; depression with crying spells may occur
after product has worn off
• Assess for **physical dependency;** should
not be used for extended time except in ADHD;
dosage should be decreased gradually to prevent
withdrawal symptoms
• Assess for **narcoleptic symptoms** before
medication and after; ability to stay awake
should increase significantly
• In children or adults with ADHD, monitor for
improved organizational skills, attention span,
attending to tasks, impulse control, socialization, and ability to get along better with others
• Assess for **withdrawal symptoms:** headache, nausea, vomiting, muscle pain, weakness;
product tolerance develops after long-term use;
dosage should not be increased if tolerance
develops; this medication has a high abuse
potential

Patient/family education
• Advise patient to decrease caffeine consumption (coffee, tea, cola, chocolate), which may increase irritability and stimulation; to avoid OTC
preparations unless approved by prescriber; to
avoid alcohol ingestion; these may cause serious
drug interactions
• Advise patient to take before meals (obesity)
• Caution patient to taper off product over several weeks, or depression, increased sleeping,
lethargy may occur
• Caution patient to avoid hazardous activities
until patient is stabilized on medication
• Instruct patient not to double doses if medication is missed; prescriber may suggest product
holidays (ADHD) during the school year to
assess progress and determine continued need
for product
• Instruct patient/family to notify prescriber if
significant side effects occur: tremors, insomnia,
palpitations, restlessness, product changes may
be needed
• Inform patient that if dry mouth occurs, to
use frequent sips of water, sugarless gum, hard
candy during beginning therapy; dry mouth
lessens with continued treatment
• Advise patient to get needed rest; patients will
feel more tired at end of day; to give last dose at
least 6 hr before bedtime to avoid insomnia

Evaluation
Positive therapeutic outcome
• Decreased activity in ADHD
• Absence of sleeping during day in narcolepsy

TREATMENT OF OVERDOSE:
Administer fluids, hemodialysis, peritoneal
dialysis, antihypertensives for increased B/P;
ammonium chloride for increased excretion

---

dextromethorphan (OTC)
(dex-troe-meth-or′fan)
**Balminil ✚, Benlyn ✚, Buckley's
DM, Buckley's Mixture, Delsym 12-
Hour, ElixSure Cough, Koffex, Robafen
Cough Gels, Robitussin, Robitussin
Cough with Honey, Robitussin Long-
Acting Cough, Scot-Tussin Diabetes
CF, Silphen-DM, Top Care Day Time
Cough, Top Care Tussin Cough
Suppressant Long Acting, Triaminic
Long-Acting Cough, Tylenol Children's
Simply Cough, Vicks DayQuil Cough,
Vicks Formula 44 Cough Relief,
Wal-Tussin**
Func. class.: Antitussive, nonopioid
Chem. class.: Levorphanol derivative
Pregnancy category C

ACTION: Depresses cough center in medulla by direct effect related to levorphanol
Therapeutic outcome: Absence of cough

USES: Nonproductive cough carried by
minor respiratory tract infections or irritants
that might be inhaled

CONTRAINDICATIONS:
Hypersensitivity

Precautions: Pregnancy **C,** fever, hepatic
disease, asthma/emphysema, chronic cough

DOSAGE AND ROUTES

Adult and child ≥12 yr: PO 10-20 mg q4hr, or 30 mg q6-8hr, max 120 mg/day; SUS REL LIQUID 60 mg q12hr, max 120 mg/day

Child 6-12 yr: PO 5-10 mg q4hr; SUS REL LIQUID 30 mg bid, max 60 mg/day; LOZENGE 5-10 mg q1-4hr, max 60 mg/day

Child 2-5 yr: 2.5-5 mg q4hr or 7.5 mg q6-8hr, max 30 mg/day; ext rel not recommended

Available forms: Liquid 7.5, 15 mg/5 ml; syr 15 mg/15 ml, 10 mg/5 ml; 15 mg/5 ml, 30 mg/15 ml; caps 15 mg; gel caps 15 mg; EXT REL SUSP 30 mg/5 ml

Implementation

• Give **chew tabs:** chew well; **syrup:** use calibrated measuring device; **ext rel susp:** shake well, use calibrated measuring device
• Administer decreased dosage to geriatric patients; their metabolism may be slowed; do not provide water within 30 min of administration because it dilutes product
• Shake susp before administration

ADVERSE EFFECTS

CNS: *Dizziness,* sedation, confusion, ataxia, fatigue
GI: *Nausea*

Pharmacokinetics	
Absorption	Rapid (PO); slow (SUS REL)
Distribution	Unknown
Metabolism	Liver
Excretion	Kidneys
Half-life	Terminal 11 hr

Pharmacodynamics		
	PO	PO-sus
Onset	15-30 min	Unknown
Peak	Unknown	Unknown
Duration	3-6 hr	12 hr

INTERACTIONS

Individual drugs

Alcohol: increased CNS depression
Amiodarone, quiNIDine, sibutramine: increased adverse reactions
Furazolidone, linezolid, procarbazine: increased hypotension, hyperpyrexia; do not give within 2 wk (MAOI activity)

Drug classifications

Antihistamines, antidepressants, opiates, sedative-hypnotics: increased CNS depression

MAOIs: increased hypotension, hyperpyrexia, do not give within 2 wk of MAOIs
Serotonin receptor agonists, SSRIs: increased serotonin syndrome

NURSING CONSIDERATIONS

Assessment

• Assess **cough:** type, frequency, character including sputum; provide adequate hydration to 2 L/day to decrease viscosity of secretions

Patient/family education

• Caution patient to avoid driving or other hazardous activities until stabilized on this medication; may cause drowsiness, dizziness in some individuals
• Advise patient to avoid smoking, smoke-filled rooms, perfumes, dust, environmental pollutants, cleaners, which increase cough; may use gum, hard candy to prevent dry mouth
• Advise patient to avoid alcohol or other CNS depressants while taking this medication; drowsiness will be increased
• Caution patient that any cough lasting over a few days should be assessed by prescriber

Evaluation

Positive therapeutic outcome
• Absence of dry, irritating cough

dextrose (D-glucose) (Rx)

Func. class.: Caloric agent

ACTION: Needed for adequate utilization of amino acids; decreases protein, nitrogen loss; prevents ketosis

Therapeutic outcome: Provides calories, prevents severe hypoglycemia

USES: Increases intake of calories; increases fluids in patients unable to take adequate fluids, calories orally; acute hypoglycemia

CONTRAINDICATIONS:

Hyperglycemia, delirium tremens, hemorrhage (cranial/spinal), CHF, anuria, allergy to corn products, concentrated products

Precautions: Renal/ liver/cardiac disease, diabetes mellitus, carbohydrate intolerance

DOSAGE AND ROUTES

Hypoglycemia

Adult: PO/IV 10-25 mg per mg/dose (20-50 ml of a 50% sol), may need subsequent continuous IV infusion of 10% dextrose

Acute symptomatic hypoglycemia (infants/neonates)

Neonate/infant: IV 250-500 mg/kg/dose (25% sol)

Available forms: Inj IV 2.5%, 5%, 10%, 20%, 25%, 30%, 38.5%, 40%, 50%, 60%, 70%; oral gel 40%; chewable tabs 5 g

Implementation

PO route

⚠ **Do not use concentrated solutions IM/IV; 25%, 50% may be used IV**

• Oral glucose preparations (gel, chewable tabs) are to be used for conscious patients only; serum blood glucose should be monitored after first oral dose; if glucose has not increased by 20 mg/100 ml in 20-30 min, dose should be repeated and serum glucose checked again
• To reduce contamination all IV sets should be replaced ≤24 hr

IV route

• Give only protein (4%) and dextrose (up to 12.5%) via peripheral vein; stronger sol requires central **IV** administration
• May be given undiluted via prepared sol; give 10% sol (5 ml/15 sec), 20% sol (1000 ml/3 hr or more), 50% sol (500 ml/30-60 min); too rapid **IV** administration may cause fluid overload and hyperglycemia
⚠ **Never discontinue hypertonic products abruptly**

ADVERSE EFFECTS

CNS: Confusion, **loss of consciousness,** dizziness
CV: Hypertension, **CHF, pulmonary edema, intracranial hemorrhage**
ENDO: Hyperglycemia, rebound hypoglycemia, hyperosmolar syndrome, hyperglycemic nonketolytic syndrome, aluminum toxicity, hypokalemia, hypomagnesium
GI: Nausea
GU: *Glycosuria, osmotic diuresis*
INTEG: Chills, flushing, warm feeling, rash, urticaria, extravasation necrosis
RESP: Pulmonary edema

Pharmacokinetics

Absorption	Well absorbed (PO); completely absorbed (**IV**)
Distribution	Widely distributed
Metabolism	Unknown
Excretion	Unknown
Half-life	Unknown

Pharmacodynamics

	PO	IV
Onset	Rapid	Immediate
Peak	Rapid	Immediate
Duration	Rapid	Immediate

INTERACTIONS

Drug classifications

Corticosteroids: increased fluid retention/electrolyte excretion

Drug/lab test

Increased: glucose

NURSING CONSIDERATIONS

Assessment

• Assess I&O, skin turgor, edema, electrolytes (potassium, sodium, calcium, chloride, magnesium), blood glucose, ammonia, phosphate
• Monitor inj site for extravasation: redness along vein, edema at site, necrosis, pain, hard tender area; site should be changed immediately
• Monitor temp for increased fever, indicating infection; if infection suspected, inf is discontinued and tubing, bottle, catheter tip cultured
• Monitor glucose level, I&O, weight, fluid overload
• Assess nutritional status: calorie count by dietitian; GI system function

Patient/family education

• Teach patient reason for dextrose infusion
• Provide literature and information on when and how to use oral products for hypoglycemia
• Review hypo/hyperglycemia symptoms
• Review blood glucose monitoring procedure

Evaluation

Positive therapeutic outcome

• Increased weight
• Blood glucose level at normal limits for patient
• Adequate hydration

diazepam (Rx)

(dye-az′e-pam)
Diastat, Diazemuls ✦, Valium

Func. class.: Antianxiety, anticonvulsant, skeletal muscle relaxant, central acting
Chem. class.: Benzodiazepine, long-acting
Pregnancy category D
Controlled substance schedule IV

Do not confuse:

diazepam/Ditropan/LORazepam

ACTION: Potentiates the actions of GABA, especially in limbic system, reticular formation; enhances presympathetic inhibition, inhibits spinal polysynaptic afferent paths

Therapeutic outcome: Decreased anxiety, restlessness, insomnia

USES: Anxiety, acute alcohol withdrawal, adjunct in seizure disorders; preoperative skeletal muscle relaxation; rectally for acute repetitive seizures

CONTRAINDICATIONS:
Pregnancy **D**, hypersensitivity to benzodiazepines, closed-angle glaucoma, coma, myasthenia gravis, ethanol intoxication, hepatic disease, sleep apnea

Precautions: Breastfeeding, geriatric, debilitated, addiction, child <6 mo, asthma, renal disease, bipolar disorder, COPD, CNS depression, labor, Parkinson's disease, neutropenia, psychosis, seizures, substance abuse, smoking

DOSAGE AND ROUTES
Anxiety/convulsive disorders
Adult: PO 2-10 mg bid-qid; IM/IV 2-10 mg q3-4hr
Geriatric: PO 1-2 mg daily-bid, increase slowly as needed
Child >6 mo: IM/IV 0.04-0.3 mg/kg/dose q2-4hr, max 0.6 mg/kg in an 8-hr period

Precardioversion
Adult: IV 5-15 mg 5-10 min precardioversion

Preendoscopy
Adult: IV 2.5-20 mg, IM 5-10 mg ½ hr preendoscopy

Muscle relaxation
Adult: PO 2-10 mg tid-qid or EXT REL 15-30 mg daily; IM/IV 5-10 mg repeat in 2-4 hr
Geriatric: PO 2-5 mg bid-qid; IM/IV 2-5 mg, may repeat in 2-4 hr

Tetanic muscle spasms
Child >5 yr: IM/IV 5-10 mg q3-4hr prn
Infant >30 days: IM/IV 1-2 mg q3-4hr prn

Status epilepticus
Adult: IM/IV 5-10 mg, 2 mg/min, may repeat q10-15min; max 30 mg; may repeat in 2-4 hr if seizures reappear
Child >5 yr: IV 1 mg slowly; IM 1 mg q2-5min
Child 1 mo-5 yr: IV 0.2-0.5 mg slowly; IM 0.2-0.5 mg slowly q2-5min up to 5 mg; may repeat in 2-4 hr prn

Seizures other than status epilepticus
Adult: RECT 0.2 mg/kg, may repeat 4-12 hr later
Child 6-11 yr: RECT 0.3 mg/kg, may repeat 4-12 hr later
Child 2-5 yr: RECT 0.5 mg/kg, may repeat 4-12 hr later

Alcohol withdrawal
Adult: IV 10 mg initially, then 5-10 mg q3-4hr prn

Available forms: Tabs 2, 5, 10 mg; inj 5 mg/ml; oral sol 5 mg/5 ml; rectal 2.5 (pediatric), 10, 20 mg, twin packs; ext rel cap 15 mg

Implementation
PO route
• Give with food or milk for GI symptoms
• Crush tab if patient is unable to swallow medication whole
• Reduce opioid dosage by one third if given concomitantly with diazepam
• Check to see if PO medication has been swallowed
• **Concentrate:** use calibrated dropper only; mix with water, juice, pudding, applesauce; consume immediately
Rectal route
• Do not use more than 5 ×/mo or for an episode q5day (Diastat)

Direct IV route
• Administer **IV** into large vein; do not dilute or mix with any other product; give **IV** 5 mg or less/min or total dose over 3 min or more (children, infants); cont inf is not recommended; inject closest vein insertion as possible; **do not dilute or mix with other products**
• Check **IV** site for thrombosis or phlebitis, which may occur rapidly

Sterile emulsion for injection route
• Use **IV** only, within 6 hr, flush line after use and after 6 hr

ADVERSE EFFECTS
CNS: *Dizziness, drowsiness,* confusion, headache, anxiety, tremors, stimulation, fatigue, depression, insomnia, hallucinations, ataxia, fatigue
CV: *Orthostatic hypotension,* **ECG changes, tachycardia,** hypotension
EENT: *Blurred vision,* tinnitus, mydriasis, nystagmus
GI: Constipation, dry mouth, nausea, vomiting, anorexia, diarrhea
HEMA: **Neutropenia**

INTEG: Rash, dermatitis, itching
RESP: Respiratory depression

Pharmacokinetics

Absorption	Rapid (PO); erratic (IM)
Distribution	Widely distributed; crosses blood-brain barrier, placenta; protein binding 99%
Metabolism	Liver, extensively, CYP2C19, CYP3A4
Excretion	Kidneys, breast milk
Half-life	20-80 hr

Pharmacodynamics

	PO	IM	IV
Onset	½ hr	15 min	Immediate
Peak	1-2 hr	½-1½ hr	15 min
Duration	2-3 hr	1-1½ hr	15 min-1 hr

INTERACTIONS

Individual drugs
Alcohol: increased CNS depression

Amiodarone, cimetidine, clarithromycin, dalfopristin, delavirdine, diltiazem, disulfiram, efavirenz, erythromycin, fluconazole, fluvoxaMINE, imatinib, itraconazole, ketoconazole, IV miconazole, nefazodone, niCARdipine, quinupristin, ranolazine, troleandomycin, valproic acid, verapamil, voriconazole, zafirlukast, zileuton: increased diazepam effect

Cimetidine, valproic acid: increased toxicity

CYP3A4 inducers (carBAMazepine, ethetoin, fosphenytoin, phenytoins, rifampin), smoking: decreased diazepam effect

Disulfiram, isoniazid, propranolol, valproic acid: decreased metabolism of diazepam

Drug classifications
Barbiturates, CNS depressants, CYP3A4 inhibitors, SSRIs: increased toxicity

CNS depressants: increased CNS depression

CYP3A4 inducers (barbiturates): decreased diazepam effect

Oral contraceptives: decreased metabolism of diazepam

Drug/lab test
Increased: AST/ALT, serum bilirubin

NURSING CONSIDERATIONS

Assessment
• **Assess degree of anxiety;** what precipitates anxiety and whether product controls symptoms; other signs of anxiety: dilated pupils, inability to sleep, restlessness, inability to focus

• **Assess for alcohol withdrawal symptoms,** including hallucinations (visual, auditory), delirium, irritability, agitation, fine to coarse tremors

• Monitor B/P (with patient lying, standing), pulse, respiratory rate; if systolic B/P drops 20 mm Hg, hold product, notify prescriber; monitor respirations q5-15min if given **IV**

• Monitor blood studies: CBC during long-term therapy; blood dyscrasias have occurred (rarely); hepatic studies: ALT, AST

• **Monitor for seizure control:** type, duration, and intensity of seizures; what precipitates seizures

• Monitor hepatic studies: AST, ALT, bilirubin, creatinine, LDH, alkaline phosphatase

• Assess mental status: mood, sensorium, affect, sleeping pattern, drowsiness, dizziness, **suicidal tendencies,** and ability of product to control these symptoms; check for tolerance, **withdrawal symptoms:** headache, nausea, vomiting, muscle pain, weakness after long-term use

• Assess for muscle spasms, pain relief

Patient/family education
• Advise patient that product may be taken with food; that product is not to be used for everyday stress or used longer than 4 mo unless directed by prescriber; take no more than prescribed amount; may be habit forming

• Caution patient to avoid OTC preparations unless approved by a prescriber; to avoid alcohol, other psychotropic medications unless prescribed; that smoking may decrease diazepam effect by increasing diazepam metabolism; **not to discontinue medication abruptly after long-term use, gradually taper**

• Inform patient to avoid driving, activities that require alertness; drowsiness may occur; to rise slowly or fainting may occur, especially in geriatric

• Advise patient not to become pregnant while using this product

• Inform patient that drowsiness may worsen at beginning of treatment

⚠ Teach patient to notify prescriber if pregnancy is planned or suspected (D), avoid breastfeeding

Evaluation

Positive therapeutic outcome
• Decreased anxiety, restlessness, insomnia

TREATMENT OF OVERDOSE:
Lavage, VS, supportive care, flumazenil

⚠ Nurse Alert　　　★ Key NCLEX® Drug

dibucaine topical
See Appendix B

diclofenac ophthalmic
See Appendix B

diclofenac epolamine (Rx)
(dye-kloe′fen-ak)
Flector
diclofenac potassium (Rx)
Cambia, Cataflam, Voltaren Rapide ♣, Zipsor
diclofenac sodium (Rx)
Apo-Diclo ♣, Novo-Difenac ♣, Nu-Diclo ♣, Pennsaid, Sandoz Diclofenac ♣, Solaraze Topical Gel, Voltram Topical Gel, Voltaren, Voltaren XR
Func. class.: Nonsteroidal antiinflammatory drug (NSAID), nonopioid analgesic
Chem. class.: Phenylacetic acid
Pregnancy category C

Do not confuse:
Cataflam/Catapres

ACTION: Inhibits COX-1, COX-2 by blocking arachidonate, resulting in analgesic, antiinflammatory, antipyretic effects

Therapeutic outcome: Decreased pain, inflammation

USES: Acute, chronic rheumatoid arthritis, osteoarthritis, ankylosing spondylitis, analgesia, primary dysmenorrhea; patch: mild to moderate pain

CONTRAINDICATIONS:
Hypersensitivity to aspirin, iodides, other NSAIDs, bovine protein; asthma, serious CV disease; eczema, exfoliative dermatitis, skin abrasions (gel patch)

> **BLACK BOX WARNING:** Treatment of perioperative pain in CABG surgery

Precautions: Breastfeeding, children, bleeding disorders, GI/cardiac disorders, hypersensitivity to other antiinflammatory agents, CCr <30 ml/min, accidental exposure, acute bronchospasm, hypersensitivity to benzyl alcohol; pregnancy (C) (tabs, del rel tab, ext rel tab, top gel) (Voltaren); pregnancy (B) (top gel) (Solaraze);

top patch, top sol, cap, powder for oral solution (pregnancy C <30 wk, D >30 wk)

> **BLACK BOX WARNING:** GI bleeding, MI, stroke

DOSAGE AND ROUTES
Osteoarthritis
Adult: PO (Cataflam) 50 mg bid-tid, max 150 mg/day; DEL REL (Voltaren) 50 mg bid-tid or 75 mg bid, max 150 mg/day; EXT REL (Voltaren-XR) 100 mg daily, max 150 mg/day; TOP gel 1% (Voltaren gel) 4 g for each lower extremity qid, max 16 g/day; 2 g for each upper extremity qid, max 8 g/day; TOP SOL (Pennsaid) apply 40 drops to each affected knee qid, apply 10 drops at a time, spread over entire knee

Rheumatoid arthritis
Adult: PO (Cataflam) 50 mg tid-qid, max 200 mg/day; DEL REL (Voltaren) 50 mg tid-qid or 75 mg bid, max 200 mg/day; EXT REL (Voltaren-XR) 100 mg qd, may increase to 200 mg/day, max 200 mg/day

Ankylosing spondylitis
Adult: PO DEL REL (Voltaren) 25 mg qid and 25 mg at bedtime, max 125 mg/day

Acute migraine with/without aura
Adult: PO (powder for oral SOL) (Cambia) 50 mg as a single dose; mix contents of packet in 1-2 oz water

Mild to moderate pain
Adult: PO (Zipsor) 25 mg qid

Dysmenorrhea or nonrheumatic inflammatory conditions
Adult: PO (Cataflam) 50 mg tid or 100 mg initially, then 50 mg tid, max 200 mg 1st day, then 150 mg/day, immediate release only

Pain of strains/sprains
Adult: TOP patch (Flector) apply patch to area bid

Actinic keratosis
Adult: TOP gel (Solaraze) apply to area bid

Renal dose
Avoid use of top gel, patch, sol, potassium oral tab in advanced renal disease

Available forms: Epolamine: topical patch 1.3%; **potassium:** tabs 50 mg tabs liquid filled 25 mg; **sodium:** del rel tabs (enteric-coated) 25, 50, 75, 100 mg; Pennsaid: top sol 1.5%; oral powder for sol 50 mg; ext rel 100 mg; topical gel 1%, 3%

Implementation
PO route
- Do not break, crush, chew, or dissolve enteric-coated or ext rel tabs
- Administer with food or milk to decrease gastric symptoms
- Remain upright for ½ hr
- Store at room temperature

Topical route (patch) (Flector)
- Wash hands before handling patch
- Remove and release liner before administering
- Use only on normal, intact skin
- Remove before bath, shower, swimming, do not use heat or occlusive dressings
- Discard removed patch in trash away from children, pets
- Store at room temperature

Topical route (gel)
- Apply to intact skin, do not use heat or occlusive dressings
- Use only for osteoarthritis: mild-moderate pain
- Store at room temperature, avoid heat, do not freeze

Ophthalmic route
- Administer with patient recumbent or tilting head back; pull down on lower lid; when conjunctival sac is exposed, instill 1 drop; wait a few minutes before instilling other drops

ADVERSE EFFECTS
CNS: *Dizziness, headache,* drowsiness, fatigue, tremors, confusion, insomnia, anxiety, depression, nervousness, paresthesia, muscle weakness
CV: CHF, tachycardia, peripheral edema, palpitations, dysrhythmias, hypo/hypertension, fluid retention, **MI, stroke**
EENT: Tinnitus, hearing loss, blurred vision, **laryngeal edema**
GI: Nausea, anorexia, vomiting, diarrhea, **jaundice, cholestatic hepatitis,** constipation, flatulence, cramps, dry mouth, peptic ulcer, **GI bleeding, hepatotoxicity,** hematemesis
GU: Nephrotoxicity: dysuria, hematuria, oliguria, azotemia, cystitis, **UTI**
HEMA: Blood dyscrasias, epistaxis, anemia
INTEG: Purpura, rash, pruritus, sweating, erythema, petechiae, photosensitivity, alopecia
META: Hyperglycemia, hypoglycemia
RESP: Dyspnea, **bronchospasm**
SYST: Anaphylaxis, Stevens-Johnson syndrome

Pharmacokinetics

Absorption	Well absorbed (PO, ophth)
Distribution	Crosses placenta; 99% bound to plasma proteins
Metabolism	Liver (50%)
Excretion	Breast milk
Half-life	1-2 hr, patch 12 hr

Pharmacodynamics

	PO	Ophth	TOP (Patch)
Onset	Unknown	Unknown	Unknown
Peak	2-3 hr	Unknown	12 hr
Duration	Unknown	Unknown	Unknown

INTERACTIONS
Individual drugs
Aspirin: increased GI side effects
Cidofovir, cycloSPORINE, digoxin, lithium, methotrexate, phenytoin: increased toxicity

Drug classifications
ACE inhibitors, β-blockers, diuretics: decreased antihypertensive effect
Anticoagulants, NSAIDs, platelet inhibitors, salicylates, SSRIs, thrombolytics: increased risk of bleeding
Antidiabetic agents: increased need for dosage adjustment
Diuretics: decreased effect of these products
Diuretics (potassium-sparing): hyperkalemia
NSAIDs, bisphosphonates, corticosteroids: increased GI side effects

Drug/herb
Garlic, ginger, ginkgo: monitor for bleeding; increased bleeding risk

NURSING CONSIDERATIONS
Assessment

> **BLACK BOX WARNING: CABG:** do not use oral, top, gel, patch in perioperative pain in CABG surgery for 10-14 days

> **BLACK BOX WARNING: Stroke/MI:** may increase CHF and hypertension, increased CV thrombotic events that may be fatal; those with CV disease may be at greater risk

- **Assess for pain of rheumatoid arthritis, osteoarthritis, ankylosing spondylitis;** check ROM, inflammation of joints, characteristics of pain

• Assess ophthalmic patients for pain, inflammation, redness, swelling
• Assess for asthma, aspirin hypersensitivity, nasal polyps; may develop hypersensitivity
• Monitor liver function tests (may be elevated) and uric acid (may be decreased in serum, increased in urine) periodically; also BUN, creatinine, electrolytes (may be elevated)
⚠ Monitor for blood dyscrasias (thrombocytopenia): bruising, fatigue, bleeding, poor healing; monitor blood counts during therapy; watch for decreasing platelets; if low, therapy may need to be discontinued, restarted after hematologic recovery; stool guaiac

Patient/family education
• Teach patient that product must be continued for prescribed time to be effective; to avoid aspirin, NSAIDs, acetaminophen, or other OTC medications unless approved by prescriber, alcoholic beverages; to contact prescriber before surgery regarding when to discontinue this product
• Caution patient to report bleeding, bruising, fatigue, malaise, since **blood dyscrasias** do occur
• Advise patient to report **hepatotoxicity:** flulike symptoms, nausea, vomiting, jaundice, pruritus, lethargy
• Instruct patient to use sunscreen to prevent photosensitivity
• Teach patient to avoid use in 3rd trimester of pregnancy
• Instruct patient to use caution when driving; drowsiness, dizziness may occur
• Teach patient to take with a full glass of water to enhance absorption; remain upright for ½ hr; if dose is missed, take as soon as remembered within 2 hr if taking 1-2 ×/day; do not double doses
• Advise to notify all providers that product is being used
⚠ Teach patient to notify prescriber if pregnancy is planned or suspected (C, tabs) (C <30 wk, D >30 wk caps, topical patch/ solution, powder for oral solution)

Evaluation
Positive therapeutic outcome
• Decreased pain in arthritic conditions
• Decreased inflammation in arthritic conditions
• Decreased ocular irritation

RARELY USED
dicyclomine
(dye-sye′kloe-meen)
Bentyl, Bentylol ✤, Formulex ✤, Lomine ✤
Func. class.: Gastrointestinal anticholinergic

USES: Treatment of peptic ulcer disease in combination with other products; infant colic, urinary incontinence, IBS

CONTRAINDICATIONS:
Hypersensitivity to anticholinergics, closed-angle glaucoma, GI obstructions, myasthenia gravis, paralytic ileus, GI atony, toxic megacolon, dementia

DOSAGE AND ROUTES
Adult: PO 10-20 mg tid-qid; IM 20 mg q4-6hr, max 160/day
Child >2 yr: PO 10 mg tid-qid
Child 6 mo-2 yr: PO 5 mg tid-qid

didanosine (Rx)
(dye-dan′oh-seen)
ddI, Pediatric Videx, Videx EC
Func. class.: Antiretroviral
Chem. class.: Synthetic purine nucleoside reverse transcriptase inhibitor (NRTI)
Pregnancy category B

ACTION: Nucleoside analog incorporating into cellular DNA by viral reverse transcriptase, thereby terminating the cellular DNA chain and preventing viral replication

Therapeutic outcome: Antiviral against the retroviruses, primarily HIV-1

USES: HIV-1 infection in combination with at least 2 other antiretrovirals

CONTRAINDICATIONS:
Hypersensitivity, lactic acidosis, pancreatitis, phenylketonuria

Precautions: Pregnancy **B**, breastfeeding, children, renal disease, sodium-restricted diets, elevated amylase, preexistent peripheral neuropathy, hyperuricemia, gout, CHF, noncirrhotic portal hypertension

BLACK BOX WARNING: Hepatic disease, lactic acidosis, pancreatitis

---

DOSAGE AND ROUTES
Ext rel cap
Adult/adolescent/child ≥6 yr and ≥60 kg: PO ext rel cap 400 mg daily; if used with tenofovir, reduce to 250 mg daily

Adult/adolescent/child ≥6 yr and 25 kg to <60 kg: PO ext rel cap 250 mg daily; if used with tenofovir, reduce to 200 mg daily

Adolescent 20 kg to <25 kg: PO ext rel cap 200 mg daily

Oral dosage (powder for oral solution)
Adult ≥60 kg: PO 200 mg bid or 400 mg daily; if used with tenofovir, reduce to 250 mg daily

Adult <60 kg: PO 125 mg bid or 250 mg daily; if used with tenofovir, reduce to 200 mg daily

Adolescent/child/infant >8 mo: PO 120 mg/m^2 q12hr, max adult dosing

Infant ≤8 mo/neonate ≥2 wk: PO 100 mg/m^2 q12hr

Renal dose
Adult: PO CrCl ≥60 ml/min: no change

Adult/adolescent ≥60 kg: PO CCr 30-59 ml/min: reduce oral solution to 100 mg q12hr or 200 mg q24hr, reduce ext rel capsules to 200 mg daily; CCr 10-29 ml/min: reduce oral solution to 150 mg q24hr, reduce ext rel capsules to 125 mg q24hr; CCr <10 ml/min: reduce oral solution to 100 mg q24hr, reduce ext rel capsules to 125 mg q24hr

Adult/adolescent <60 kg: PO CCr 30-59 ml/min: reduce oral solution to 75 mg q12hr or to 150 mg q24hr, reduce ext rel capsules to 125 mg daily; CCr 10-29 ml/min: reduce oral solution to 100 mg q24hr, reduce ext rel capsules to 125 mg daily; CCr <10 ml/min: reduce oral solution to 75 mg q24hr, ext rel capsules are not recommended

Intermittent hemodialysis/continuous ambulatory peritoneal dialysis
≥60 kg, give 100 mg oral solution or 125 mg ext rel capsules q24hr; <60 kg, give 75 mg oral solution q24hr, ext rel capsules are not recommended

Available forms: Powder for oral sol 10 mg/ml; del rel caps 125, 200, 250, 400 mg

Implementation
• Give on empty stomach 1 hr before or 2 hr after meals q12hr; food decreases effectiveness of product; adjust dose in renal impairment
• Pediatric powder for oral sol should be prepared in the pharmacy; shake before using
• Packets for oral sol must be mixed with ½ glass of water, not fruit juice; stir until dissolved; drink immediately
• Store caps, tabs in tightly closed bottle at room temperature; store oral sol after dissolving at room temperature ≤4 hr
• Do not take dapsone at same time as ddI

ADVERSE EFFECTS
CNS: Peripheral neuropathy, seizures, confusion, *anxiety,* hypertonia, abnormal thinking, asthenia, *insomnia, CNS depression,* pain, dizziness, chills, fever

CV: Hypertension, vasodilatation, dysrhythmia, syncope, CHF, palpitations

EENT: Ear pain, otitis, photophobia, visual impairment, retinal depigmentation, optic neuritis

GI: Pancreatitis, *diarrhea, nausea,* vomiting, *abdominal pain,* constipation, stomatitis, dyspepsia, liver abnormalities, flatulence, taste perversion, dry mouth, oral thrush, melena, increased ALT, AST, alkaline phosphatase, amylase, hepatic failure, noncirrhotic portal hypertension

GU: Increased bilirubin, uric acid

HEMA: Leukopenia, granulocytopenia, thrombocytopenia, anemia

INTEG: *Rash, pruritus,* alopecia, ecchymosis, hemorrhage, petechiae, sweating

MS: Myalgia, arthritis, myopathy, muscular atrophy

RESP: Cough, pneumonia, dyspnea, asthma, epistaxis, hypoventilation, sinusitis

SYST: Lactic acidosis, anaphylaxis

Pharmacokinetics
Absorption	Rapidly absorbed (up to 40%)
Distribution	Unknown
Metabolism	Not metabolized
Excretion	Kidneys (55%), feces
Half-life	0.8-1.6 hr, shorter in children

Pharmacodynamics
Onset	Unknown
Peak	Up to 1 hr, del rel 2 hr
Duration	Unknown

INTERACTIONS
Individual drugs
Allopurinol, tenofovir: increased didanosine level

Dapsone, ketoconazole: decreased absorption of each specific product

Gatifloxacin, gemifloxacin, grepafloxacin, levofloxacin, lomefloxacin, moxifloxacin, norfloxacin, sparfloxacin, trovafloxa-

cin: Do not use didanosine with these products (PO)
Itraconazole: decreased concentrations
Methadone: decreased didanosine level
Stavudine: increased pancreatitis risk

Drug classifications
Aluminum, antacids, magnesium: increased side effects
Antiretrovirals, other: decreased concentration
Fluoroquinolones, tetracyclines: decreased concentrations of each specific product

Drug/food
Do not use with acidic juices
Decreased: absorption 50%, do not use with food

NURSING CONSIDERATIONS
Assessment

> **BLACK BOX WARNING: Pancreatitis:** do not use in those with symptoms of pancreatitis (may be dose-related) or advanced HIV, alcoholism, history of pancreatitis

• **Assess for peripheral neuropathy:** tingling or pain in hands and feet, distal numbness; onset usually occurs 2-6 mo after beginning treatment; if these occur during therapy, product may be decreased or discontinued
• **Assess for pancreatitis:** abdominal pain, nausea, vomiting, elevated liver enzymes; product should be discontinued since condition can be fatal
• Assess children by dilated retinal examination q6mo to rule out retinal depigmentation
• Monitor CBC, differential, platelet count monthly, viral load, CD4$^+$ count; notify prescriber of results
• Monitor renal function studies: BUN, serum uric acid, urine CCr before, during therapy; these may be elevated throughout treatment

> **BLACK BOX WARNING:** Lactic acidosis, severe hepatomegaly, pancreatitis: assess for abdominal pain, nausea, vomiting, elevated hepatic enzymes; product should be discontinued because condition can be fatal

• Monitor temp; may indicate beginning of infection
• Monitor liver function tests before, during therapy (bilirubin, AST, ALT, amylase, alkaline phosphatase) as needed or monthly

Patient/family education
• Advise patient to take on empty stomach; not to mix powder with fruit juice; to drink powder immediately after mixing; to use exactly as prescribed
• Instruct patient to report signs of **infection:** increased temp, sore throat, flulike symptoms; to avoid crowds and those with known infections
• Instruct patient to report signs of **anemia:** fatigue, headache, faintness, shortness of breath, irritability
• Advise patient to report numbness/tingling in extremities
• Instruct patient to report **bleeding;** avoid use of razors and commercial mouthwash
• Advise patient that hair may be lost during therapy; a wig or hairpiece may make patient feel better
• Caution patient to avoid OTC products and other medications without approval of prescriber; to avoid alcohol
• Teach patient not to have any sexual contact without use of a condom; needles should not be shared; blood from infected individual should not come in contact with another's mucous membranes

Evaluation
Positive therapeutic outcome
• Absence of opportunistic infection, symptoms of HIV

---

difenoxin with atropine
See diphenoxylate with atropine

⚠ HIGH ALERT

digoxin (Rx)
(di-jox′in)
Apo-Digoxin ✦, Lanoxin
Func. class.: Inotropic antidysrhythmic, cardiac glycoside
Chem. class.: Digitalis preparation
Pregnancy category C

Do not confuse:
Lanoxin/Lasix/Lonox/Lomotil/Xanax/Levoxine

ACTION: Inhibits sodium-potassium ATPase, which makes more calcium available for contractile proteins, resulting in increased cardiac output; increases force of contraction (positive inotropic effect); decreases heart rate (negative chronotropic effect); decreases AV conduction speed

Therapeutic outcome: Decreased edema, pulse, respiration, crackles

USES: Rapid digitalization in acute and chronic CHF, atrial fibrillation, atrial flutter, atrial tachycardia; cardiogenic shock, paroxysmal atrial tachycardia

CONTRAINDICATIONS:
Hypersensitivity to digoxin, ventricular fibrillation, ventricular tachycardia, **carotid sinus syndrome, 2nd- or 3rd-degree heart block**

Precautions: Pregnancy **C,** breastfeeding, geriatric, renal disease, acute MI, AV block, severe respiratory disease, hypothyroidism, sinus nodal disease, hypokalemia, electrolyte disturbances, hypertension, cor pulmonale, Wolff-Parkinson-White syndrome

DOSAGE AND ROUTES
Loading dose: IV
Adult: IV 400-600 mcg as a single dose, effect in 5-30 min, max effect 1-4 hr, give subsequent doses of 100-300 mcg q6-8hr
Adolescent/child >10 yr: IV 8-12 mcg/kg, divided into 3 or more doses, with the first dose equaling approximately half of the total, give subsequent doses q4-8hr
Child 5-10 yr: IV 15-30 mcg/kg divided into 3 or more doses, with the first dose equaling approximately half of the total, give subsequent doses q4-8hr
Child 2-4 yr: IV 25-35 mcg/kg, divided into 3 or more doses, with the first dose equaling approximately half of the total, give subsequent doses q4-8hr
Child <2 yr/infant: IV 30-50 mcg/kg, divided into 3 or more doses, with the first dose equaling approximately half of the total, give subsequent doses q4-8hr
Full-term neonate: IV 20-30 mcg/kg, divided into 3 or more doses, with the first dose equaling approximately half of the total, give subsequent doses q4-8hr
Premature neonate: IV 15-25 mcg/kg, divided into 3 or more doses, with the first dose equaling approximately half of the total, give subsequent doses q4-8hr

Loading dose: oral dosage (tablets)
Tablets are 60%-80% bioavailable; oral elixir should be used to obtain the appropriate dose in infants, young pediatric patients, or patients with very low body weight
Adult/adolescent/child >10 yr: PO Total dose of 10-15 mcg/kg, in 3 divided doses, give half of the total loading dose initially, then one-fourth the loading dose q4-8hr × 2 doses
Child 5-10 yr: PO Total dose of 20-45 mcg/kg, in 3 divided doses, give half of the total loading dose initially, then one fourth of the loading dose q4-8hr × 2 doses

Loading dose: oral dosage (elixir)
Elixir is approximately 70%-85% bioavailable
Adult/adolescent/child >10 yr: PO Total dose of 10-15 mcg/kg, give half of the total loading dose initially, then additional fractions of the planned total dose at 4-8 hr
Child 5-10 yr: PO Total dose of 20-35 mcg/kg, give half of the total loading dose initially, then additional fractions of the planned total dose at 4-8 hr
Child 2-4 yr: PO Total dose of 30-45 mcg/kg, give half of the total loading dose initially, then additional fractions of the planned total dose at 4-8 hr
Infant/child <2 yr: PO Total dose of 35-60 mcg/kg, give half of the total loading dose initially then additional fractions of the planned total dose at 4-8 hr
Full-term neonate: PO Total dose of 25-35 mcg/kg, give half of the total loading dose initially, then additional fractions of the planned total dose at 4-8 hr
Premature neonate: PO Total dose of 20-30 mcg/kg, give half of the total loading dose initially, then additional fractions of the planned total dose at 4-8 hr

Maintenance dose: IV
Adult: IV 125-350 mcg/day, depending on CrCl, daily; usual daily maintenance dose for the CHF in adult based on corrected CrCl (ml/min per 70 kg) and lean body weight (LBW) are listed below
- LBW 50-59 kg
  CrCl ≥100 ml/min: 175 mcg IV daily
  CrCl 70-99 ml/min: 150 mcg IV daily
  CrCl 60-69 ml/min: 125 mcg IV daily
- LBW 60-69 kg
  CrCl ≥90 ml/min: 200 mcg IV daily
  CrCl 70-89 ml/min: 175 mcg IV daily
  CrCl 60-69 ml/min: 150 mcg IV daily
- LBW 70-79 kg
  CrCl ≥100 ml/min: 250 mcg IV daily
  CrCl 90-99 ml/min: 225 mcg IV daily
  CrCl 70-89 ml/min: 200 mcg IV daily
  CrCl 60-69 ml/min: 175 mcg IV daily
- LBW 80-89 kg
  CrCl ≥100 ml/min: 275 mcg IV daily
  CrCl 80-99 ml/min: 250 mcg IV daily
  CrCl 70-79 ml/min: 225 mcg IV daily
  CrCl 60-69 ml/min: 200 mcg IV daily
- LBW 90-99 kg
  CrCl ≥90 ml/min: 300 mcg IV daily
  CrCl 80-89 ml/min: 275 mcg IV daily

CrCl 70-79 ml/min: 250 mcg IV daily
CrCl 60-69 ml/min: 225 mcg IV daily
• LBW ≥100 kg
CrCl ≥100 ml/min: 350 mcg IV daily
CrCl 90-99 ml/min: 325 mcg IV daily
CrCl 80-89 ml/min: 300 mcg IV daily
CrCl 70-79 ml/min: 275 mcg IV daily
CrCl 60-69 ml/min: 250 mcg IV daily
Child >10 yr: 25%-35% of the IV digitalizing dose IV daily
Child 5-10 yr: 25%-35% of the IV digitalizing IV in 2 daily doses
Child 2-4 yr: 25%-35% of the IV digitalizing dose IV in 2 daily doses
Child <2 yr/infant: 25%-35% of the IV digitalizing dose IV in 2 daily doses
Full-term neonate: 25%-35% of the IV digitalizing dose in 2 daily doses
Preterm neonate: 20%-30% of the IV digitalizing dose in 2 daily doses

Maintenance dose: oral dosage (tablets)

Adult/adolescent/child >10 yr: PO 3.4-5.1 mcg/kg/day
• LBW 40-49 kg
CrCl ≥70 ml/min: 187.5 mcg PO daily
CrCl ≥60-69 ml/min: 125 mcg PO daily
• LBW 50-59 kg
CrCl ≥90 ml/min: 250 mcg PO daily
CrCl 60-89 ml/min: 187.5 mcg PO daily
• LBW 60-69 kg
CrCl ≥100 ml/min: 312.5 mcg PO daily
CrCl 60-99 ml/min: 250 mcg PO daily
• LBW 70-79 kg
CrCl ≥80 ml/min: 312.5 mcg PO daily
CrCl 60-79 ml/min: 250 mcg PO daily
• LBW 80-89 kg
CrCl ≥90 ml/min: 375 mcg PO daily
CrCl 60-89 ml/min: 312.5 mcg PO daily
• LBW 90-99 kg
CrCl ≥90 ml/min: 437.5 mcg PO daily
CrCl 70-89 ml/min: 375 mcg PO daily
CrCl 60-69 ml/min: 312.5 mcg PO daily
• LBW ≥100 kg
CrCl ≥100 ml/min: 500 mcg PO daily
CrCl 80-99 ml/min: 437.5 mcg PO daily
CrCl 60-79 ml/min: 375 mcg PO daily
Child 5-10 yr: PO 6.4-12.9 mcg/kg/day PO in 2 divided doses is the recommended starting maintenance dose

Maintenance dose: oral dosage (elixir)

Adult/adolescent/child >10 yr: PO 3-4.5 mcg/kg/day daily
• LBW 40-49 kg
CrCl ≥100 ml/min: 170 mcg PO daily

CrCl 90-99 ml/min: 160 mcg PO daily
CrCl 80-89 ml/min: 150 mcg PO daily
CrCl 70-79 ml/min: 140 mcg PO daily
CrCl 60-69 ml/min: 130 mcg PO daily
• LBW 50-59 kg
CrCl ≥100 ml/min: 213 mcg PO daily
CrCl 90-99 ml/min: 200 mcg PO daily
CrCl 80-89 ml/min: 188 mcg PO daily
CrCl 70-79 ml/min: 175 mcg PO daily
CrCl 60-69 ml/min: 163 mcg PO daily
• LBW 60-69 kg
CrCl ≥100 ml/min: 255 mcg PO daily
CrCl 90-99 ml/min: 240 mcg PO daily
CrCl 80-89 ml/min: 225 mcg PO daily
CrCl 70-79 ml/min: 210 mcg PO daily
CrCl 60-69 ml/min: 195 mcg PO daily
• LBW 70-79 kg
CrCl ≥100 ml/min: 298 mcg PO daily
CrCl 90-99 ml/min: 280 mcg PO daily
CrCl 80-89 ml/min: 263 mcg PO daily
CrCl 70-79 ml/min: 245 mcg PO daily
CrCl 60-69 ml/min: 228 mcg PO daily
• LBW 80-89 kg
CrCl ≥100 ml/min: 340 mcg PO daily
CrCl 90-99 ml/min: 320 mcg PO daily
CrCl 80-89 ml/min: 300 mcg PO daily
CrCl 70-79 ml/min: 280 mcg PO daily
CrCl 60-69 ml/min: 260 mcg PO daily
• LBW 90-99 kg
CrCl ≥100 ml/min: 383 mcg PO daily
CrCl 90-99 ml/min: 360 mcg PO daily
CrCl 80-89 ml/min: 338 mcg PO daily
CrCl 70-79 ml/min: 315 mcg PO daily
CrCl 60-69 ml/min: 293 mcg PO daily
• LBW ≥100 kg
CrCl ≥100 ml/min: 425 mcg PO daily
CrCl 90-99 ml/min: 400 mcg PO daily
CrCl 80-89 ml/min: 375 mcg PO daily
CrCl 70-79 ml/min: 350 mcg PO daily
CrCl 60-69 ml/min: 325 mcg PO daily
Child 5-10 yr: PO 5.6-11.3 mcg/kg/day in 2 divided doses
Child 2-4 yr: PO 9.4-13.1 mcg/kg/day in 2 divided doses
Child <2 yr/infant: PO 11.3-18.8 mcg/kg/day in 2 divided doses
Full-term neonate: PO 7.5-11.3 mcg/kg/day in 2 divided doses
Preterm neonate: PO 4.7-7.8 mcg/kg/day in 2 divided doses

Renal dose
IV route
• CrCl 50-59 ml/min
LBW 50-59 kg: 125 mcg IV once daily
LBW 60-69 kg: 150 mcg IV once daily
LBW 70-79 kg: 175 mcg IV once daily

LBW 80-89 kg: 200 mcg IV once daily
LBW 90-99 kg: 225 mcg IV once daily
LBW ≥100 kg: 250 mcg IV once daily
• CrCl 40-49 ml/min
LBW 50-59 kg: 100 mcg IV once daily
LBW 60-69 kg: 125 mcg IV once daily
LBW 70-79 kg: 150 mcg IV once daily
LBW 80-89 kg: 175 mcg IV once daily
LBW 90-99 kg: 200 mcg IV once daily
LBW ≥100 kg: 225 mcg IV once daily
• CrCl 30-39 ml/min
LBW 50-59 kg: 100 mcg IV once daily
LBW 60-69 kg: 125 mcg IV once daily
LBW 70-89 kg: 150 mcg IV once daily
LBW 90-99 kg: 175 mcg IV once daily
LBW ≥100 kg: 200 mcg IV once daily
• CrCl 20-29 ml/min
LBW 50-69 kg: 100 mcg IV once daily
LBW 70-79 kg: 125 mcg IV once daily
LBW 80-99 kg: 150 mcg IV once daily
LBW ≥100 kg: 175 mcg IV once daily
• CrCl 10-19 ml/min
LBW 50-59 kg: 75 mcg IV once daily
LBW 60-79 kg: 100 mcg IV once daily
LBW 80-89 kg: 125 mcg IV once daily
LBW ≥90 kg: 150 mcg IV once daily
• CrCl <10 ml/min
LBW 50-69 kg: 75 mcg IV once daily
LBW 70-89 kg: 100 mcg IV once daily
LBW 90-99 kg: 125 mcg IV once daily
LBW ≥100 kg: 150 mcg IV once daily

Oral dosage (tablets)
• CrCl 40-59 ml/min
LBW 50-69 kg: 187.5 mcg PO once daily
• CrCl 50-59 ml/min
LBW 70-89 kg: 250 mcg PO once daily
LBW ≥90 kg: 312.5 mcg PO once daily
• CrCl 30-39 ml/min
LBW 50-59 kg: 125 mcg PO once daily
LBW 60-79 kg: 187.5 mcg PO once daily
LBW 80-99 kg: 250 mcg PO once daily
LBW ≥100 kg: 312.5 mcg PO once daily
• CrCl 20-29 ml/min
LBW 50-69 kg: 125 mcg PO once daily
LBW 70-89 kg: 187.5 mcg PO once daily
LBW ≥90 kg: 250 mcg PO once daily
• CrCl <20 ml/min
LBW 50-69 kg: 125 mcg PO once daily
LBW 70-99 kg: 187.5 mcg PO once daily
LBW ≥100 kg: 250 mcg PO once daily

Oral dosage (elixir)
• CrCl 50-59 ml/min
LBW 50-59 kg: 150 mcg PO once daily
LBW 60-69 kg: 180 mcg PO once daily
LBW 70-79 kg: 210 mcg PO once daily
LBW 80-89 kg: 240 mcg PO once daily

LBW 90-99 kg: 270 mcg PO once daily
LBW ≥100 kg: 300 mcg PO once daily
• CrCl 40-49 ml/min
LBW 50-59 kg: 138 mcg PO once daily
LBW 60-69 kg: 165 mcg PO once daily
LBW 70-79 kg: 193 mcg PO once daily
LBW 80-89 kg: 220 mcg PO once daily
LBW 90-99 kg: 248 mcg PO once daily
LBW ≥100 kg: 275 mcg PO once daily
• CrCl 30-39 ml/min
LBW 50-59 kg: 125 mcg PO once daily
LBW 60-69 kg: 150 mcg PO once daily
LBW 70-79 kg: 175 mcg PO once daily
LBW 80-89 kg: 200 mcg PO once daily
LBW 90-99 kg: 225 mcg PO once daily
LBW ≥100 kg: 250 mcg PO once daily
• CrCl 20-29 ml/min
LBW 50-59 kg: 113 mcg PO once daily
LBW 60-69 kg: 135 mcg PO once daily
LBW 70-79 kg: 158 mcg PO once daily
LBW 80-89 kg: 180 mcg PO once daily
LBW 90-99 kg: 203 mcg PO once daily
LBW ≥100 kg: 225 mcg PO once daily
• CrCl <20 ml/min
LBW 50-59 kg: 100 mcg PO once daily
LBW 60-69 kg: 120 mcg PO once daily
LBW 70-79 kg: 140 mcg PO once daily
LBW 80-89 kg: 160 mcg PO once daily
LBW 90-99 kg: 180 mcg PO once daily
LBW ≥100 kg: 200 mcg PO once daily

The daily maintenance dose can also be estimated using the patient's CrCl and loading dose (LD) according to the method of Jelliffe and Brooker daily % loss = $14 + $ CrCl/5

Available forms: Caps 0.05, 0.1, 0.2 mg; elix 0.05 mg/ml; tabs 0.125, 0.25, 0.5 mg; inj 0.5 ✦, 0.25 mg/ml; pediatric inj 0.1 mg/ml

Implementation
• Do not give at same time as antacids or other products that decrease absorption
PO route
• **Bioavailability varies between different oral dosage forms of digoxin and between different brands of the same dosage form. Changing from one preparation to another may require dosage adjustments.**
• All dosage forms may be administered without regard to meals.
• Tab may be crushed and administered with food or fluids
• Pediatric elixir should be administered using a calibrated measuring device
Injectable routes
• IV is preferred over IM, as it is less painful
• PO should replace parenteral therapy as soon as possible

- Visually inspect parenteral products for particulate matter and discoloration prior to use

IV route
- May be given undiluted or each 1 ml may be diluted in 4 ml of sterile water for injection, NS, D₅W, or LR; diluent volumes less than 4 ml will cause precipitation; use diluted solutions immediately
- Inject over at least 5 min via Y-site or 3-way stopcock; in patients with pulmonary edema, administer over 10-15 min to avoid inadvertent overdosage, do not flush the syringe following administration

IM route
- Do not administer more than 2 ml at any one IM injection site
- Inject deeply into gluteal muscle, then massage area

Syringe compatibilities: Heparin, milrinone

Syringe incompatibility: Doxapram

Y-site compatibilities: Amrinone, cefmetazole, ciprofloxacin, cisatracurium, diltiazem, famotidine, meperidine, meropenem, midazolam, milrinone, morphine, potassium chloride, propofol, remifentanil, tacrolimus, vit B/C

Y-site incompatibilities: Fluconazole, foscarnet

Additive compatibilities: Bretylium, cimetidine, floxacillin, furosemide, lidocaine, ranitidine, verapamil

Additive incompatibility: DOBUTamine

ADVERSE EFFECTS
CNS: *Headache,* drowsiness, apathy, confusion, disorientation, fatigue, depression, hallucinations
CV: Dysrhythmias, hypotension, bradycardia, **AV block**
EENT: Blurred vision, yellow-green halos, photophobia, diplopia
GI: Nausea, vomiting, anorexia, abdominal pain, diarrhea

Pharmacokinetics
Absorption	Unknown
Distribution	Widely distributed; 20%-25% protein bound
Metabolism	Liver, small amount; also intestinal bacteria
Excretion	Urine
Half-life	1½ days

Pharmacodynamics
	PO	IV
Onset	½-1½ hr	5-30 min
Peak	2-6 hr	1-5 hr
Duration	After steady state	6-8 days

INTERACTIONS
Individual drugs
AMILoride, cholestyramine, colestipol, metoclopramide, thyroid hormones: decreased digoxin levels
Amiodarone, diltiazem, indomethacin, NIFEdipine, propantheline, quiNIDine, verapamil: increased digoxin levels
Amphotericin B, carbenicillin, ticarcillin: increased hypokalemia, increased toxicity
Azole antifungals, macrolides, tetracyclines: increased toxicity
Calcium IV: increased hypercalcemia, hypomagnesemia, digoxin toxicity
Kaolin/pectin: decreased absorption

Drug classifications
Antacids: decreased digoxin absorption
Anticholinergics: increased digoxin blood levels
Antidysrhythmics, β-adrenergic blockers: increased bradycardia
Diuretics (thiazide) corticosteroids: increased hypokalemia, hypercalcemia, hypomagnesemia, digoxin toxicity
Sympathomimetics: increased cardiac dysrhythmia risk

Drug/herb
St. John's wort: decreased product effect

Drug/food
Flaxseed, psyllium: decreased digoxin absorption

Drug/lab test
Increased: CPK

NURSING CONSIDERATIONS
Assessment
- Assess and document apical pulse for 1 min before giving product; if pulse <60 in adult or <90 in an infant or is significantly different, take again in 1 hr; if <60 in adult, call prescriber; note rate, rhythm, character
- Monitor electrolytes: potassium, sodium, chloride, magnesium, calcium; renal function studies: BUN, creatinine; other blood studies: ALT, AST, bilirubin, Hct, Hgb, product levels (therapeutic level 0.5-2 ng/ml) before initiating treatment and periodically thereafter

    Adverse effects: *italics* = common; **bold** = life-threatening

• Monitor resolution of atrial dysrhythmias by ECG; if tachydysrhythmia develops, hold product; delay cardioversion while product levels are determined
• **Monitor ECG continuously** during parenteral loading doses and for patients with suspected toxicity; provide hemodynamic monitoring for patients with heart failure or administer multiple cardiac products

Patient/family education
• Advise patient not to stop abruptly; teach all aspects of product
• Caution patient to avoid OTC medications including cough, cold, allergy preparations, antacids, since many adverse product interactions may occur; do not take antacid at same time
• Instruct patient to notify prescriber of any loss of appetite, lower stomach pain, diarrhea, weakness, drowsiness, headache, blurred or yellow-green vision, rash, depression; teach toxic symptoms of this product and when to notify prescriber
• Advise patient to maintain a sodium-restricted diet as ordered; to take potassium supplements as ordered to prevent toxicity
• Instruct patient to report shortness of breath, difficulty breathing, weight gain, edema, persistent cough
• Teach patient purpose of product is to regulate the heart's functioning
• Teach patient as outpatient to check and record pulse for 1 min before taking dose; if there is a change of >15 bpm from usual pulse, prescriber should be notified
• Teach patient to take medication at the same time each day, take missed doses within 12 hr; do not double doses; notify prescriber if doses are missed for 2 days or more; how to monitor heart rate
• Teach patient toxic symptoms and when to notify prescriber
• Advise patient to carry/wear emergency ID describing dosage and reason for digoxin
• Advise patient to use one brand consistently

Evaluation
Positive therapeutic outcome
• Decreased weight, edema, pulse, respiration, crackles
• Increased urine output
• Serum digoxin level 0.5-2 ng/ml

TREATMENT OF OVERDOSE:
Discontinue product, administer potassium, monitor ECG, administer an adrenergic blocking agent, digoxin immune FAB

digoxin immune FAB (ovine) (Rx)
(di-jox'in)
DigiFab
Func. class.: Antidote, digoxin specific
Pregnancy category C

ACTION: Antibody fragments bind to free digoxin or to reverse toxicity by not allowing digoxin or digitoxin to bind to sites of action

Therapeutic outcome: Correction of digoxin toxicity

USES: Reversal of life-threatening digoxin or digitoxin toxicity, including severe bradycardia, ventricular tachycardia/fibrillation, severe hypertension

CONTRAINDICATIONS:
Mild digoxin toxicity, hypersensitivity to this product, papain, or ovine protein

Precautions: Pregnancy **C**, breastfeeding, children, geriatric, cardiac/renal disease, hypocalcemia, heart failure, allergy to ovine proteins

DOSAGE AND ROUTES
1 (38 mg) vial binds 0.5 mg digoxin, 1 (40 mg) DigiFab binds 0.5 mg digoxin

Digoxin toxicity (known amount) (tabs, oral sol, IM)
Adult and child: **IV** dose (mg) = dose ingested (mg) × 0.8/1000 × 38 or 40 mg vial

Toxicity (known amount) (cap, IV)
Adult and child: **IV** dose = dose ingested (mg)/0.5 × 38 or 40 mg vial

Toxicity (known amount) by serum digoxin concentrations (SDCs)
Adult and child: **IV** SDC (nanograms/ml) × kg of weight/100 × 38 or 40 mg vial

Digoxin toxicity (unknown amount)
Adult and child >20 kg: **IV** 228 mg (6 vials)
Infant and child <20 kg: **IV** 38 mg (1 vial)

Acute ingestion
Adult: **IV** 10 vials (380 mg)

Life-threatening ingestion
Adult: **IV** 20 vials (760 mg)

Skin test
Adult: ID 9.5 mcg

Available forms: Inj 38 mg/vial (binds 0.5 mg of digoxin), 40 mg/vial (binds 0.5 mg digoxin)

Implementation
- Test doses have proved to be ineffective in the general population; only use test dose in those with known allergies or those previously treated with digoxin immune FAB
- **For test dose** dilute 0.1 ml or reconstituted product (9.5 mg/ml) in 9.9 ml sterile isotonic saline, inj 0.1 ml (1:100 dilution) ID and observe for wheal with erythema; read in 20 min
- **For scratch test,** place 1 drop of sol on skin and make a scratch through the drop with a sterile needle; read in 20 min
- Give after diluting 40 mg/4 ml of sterile water (10 mg/ml), mix gently; may be further diluted with 0.9% NaCl; sol should be clear, colorless
- Give by BOL if cardiac arrest is imminent or IV over 30 min using a 0.22-μm filter
- Store reconstituted sol for up to 4 hr in refrigerator; do not freeze DigiFab

ADVERSE EFFECTS
CV: **CHF,** *ventricular rate increase,* **atrial fibrillation,** *low cardiac output,* hypotension
INTEG: *Hypersensitivity,* allergic reactions, facial swelling, redness, phlebitis
META: *Hypokalemia*
MISC: **Anaphylaxis** (rare)
RESP: **Impaired respiratory function, rapid respiratory rate**

Pharmacokinetics
Absorption	Complete
Distribution	Widely distributed into plasma, interstitial fluids
Metabolism	Unknown
Excretion	Kidneys
Half-life	Biphasic (14-20 hr); increased in renal disease

Pharmacodynamics
Onset	30 min (variable)
Peak	Unknown
Duration	Unknown

INTERACTIONS
Individual drugs
Considered incompatible with all products in syringe or sol

Drug/lab test
Interference: immunoassay (digoxin)

NURSING CONSIDERATIONS
Assessment
- **Assess for CHF:** dyspnea, crackles, peripheral edema, B/P, volume overload

- **Assess for hypokalemia:** ST depression, flat T waves, presence of U wave, ventricular dysrhythmias
- Obtain information on previous allergies: previous exposure to sheep (ovine) proteins; scratch test may be performed before use of this product; hypersensitive reactions are more common in persons with previous exposure
- Monitor VS before, during, after infusion
- Monitor heart rate, B/P q10min during inf and after completion until stabilized; hemodynamic monitoring is used for unstable or hypotensive patients; check potassium levels until toxicity is resolved
- Assess for oxygen or perfusion deficit: hypotension, chest pain, dizziness, loss of consciousness
- Assess respiratory status: auscultate lung fields for bibasilar crackles in patients with advanced CHF, B/P, volume overload

Patient/family education
- Teach that purpose of medication is to bind excess digoxin and reduce high blood levels
- Instruct patients to report fever, chills, itching, sweating, dyspnea, delayed hypersensitivity
- Advise other prescribers that this medication has been used previously

Evaluation
Positive therapeutic outcome
- Correction of digoxin toxicity
- Digoxin blood level 0.5-2 ng/ml
- Digitoxin blood level 9-25 ng/ml

dihydroergotamine
See ergotamine

dihydrotachysterol (Rx)
(dye-hye-droh-tak-iss′ter-ole)
DHT Intensol ✦, Hytakerol
Func. class.: Parathyroid agent (calcium regulator)
Chem. class.: Vitamin D analog
Pregnancy category C

ACTION: Increases intestinal absorption of calcium, increases renal tubular absorption of phosphorus; is able to regulate calcium levels by regulation of calcitonin, parathyroid hormone

Therapeutic outcome: Prevention of continued calcium loss in bones

USES: Hypoparathyroidism, pseudohypoparathyroidism, postoperative tetany

Adverse effects: *italics* = common; **bold** = life-threatening

CONTRAINDICATIONS:

Hypersensitivity, renal disease, hyperphosphatemia, hypercalcemia, hypervitaminosis D

Precautions: Pregnancy **C**, breastfeeding, renal calculi, CV disease

DOSAGE AND ROUTES

Hypoparathyroidism/pseudohypoparathyroidism

Adult: PO 0.75-2.5 mg daily × 4 days, maintenance 0.2-1 mg daily regulated by serum calcium levels

Neonate: PO 0.05-0.1 mg/day

Child/infant: PO 1-5 mg qd × 4 days then 0.5-1.5 mg qd

Rickets (vit D resistant)

Child: PO 0.25-1 mg/day

Available forms: Tabs 0.125, 0.2, 0.4 mg; caps 0.125 mg; oral sol 0.2, 0.25 mg/5 ml, 0.2 mg/ml ✿ (Intensol)

Implementation

• Do not break, crush, or chew caps
• May be increased q4wk depending on blood level; give with meals for GI symptoms
• Store in tight, light-resistant containers at room temperature
• Restrict sodium, potassium if required
• Restriction of fluids may be required for chronic renal failure

ADVERSE EFFECTS

CNS: Drowsiness, headache, vertigo, fever, lethargy, depression
CV: Dysrhythmias, hypertension
EENT: Tinnitus
GI: Nausea, diarrhea, vomiting, jaundice, anorexia, dry mouth, constipation, cramps, metallic taste, thirst
GU: Polyuria, hypercalciuria, hyperphosphatemia, **hematuria,** nocturia, renal calculi
MS: Myalgia, arthralgia, decreased bone development, weakness, ataxia

Pharmacokinetics

Absorption	Well absorbed from small intestine
Distribution	Liver, fat
Metabolism	Liver
Excretion	Feces (inactive, active metabolites)
Half-life	Unknown

Pharmacodynamics

Onset	2 wk
Peak	2 wk
Duration	2-9 wk

INTERACTIONS

Individual drugs

Cholestyramine, colestipol, mineral oil: decreased absorption of dihydrotachysterol
Phenytoin: decreased effect of dihydrotachysterol
Verapamil: increased dysrhythmias

Drug classifications

Barbiturates, corticosteroids: decreased effect of dihydrotachysterol
Calcium supplements, diuretics (thiazide): increased hypercalcemia
Cardiac glycosides: increased dysrhythmias

Drug/lab test

False increase: cholesterol

NURSING CONSIDERATIONS

Assessment

• Monitor BUN, urinary calcium, AST, ALT, cholesterol, alkaline phosphatase, creatinine, uric acid, chloride, magnesium, electrolytes, urine pH, phosphate; may increase calcium; should be kept at 9-10 mg/dl; keep vit D at 50-135 international units/dl, phosphate at 70 mg/dl; these tests should be checked before and throughout treatment
• Monitor for increased blood level, since toxic reaction may occur rapidly
• Monitor for dry mouth, metallic taste, polyuria, bone pain, muscle weakness, headache, fatigue, tinnitus, change in LOC, irregular pulse, dysrhythmias, increased respirations, anorexia, nausea, vomiting, cramps, diarrhea, constipation; may indicate hypercalcemia; if these occur, discontinue product, give laxatives, low-calcium diet
• Monitor renal status: decreased urinary output (oliguria, anuria), edema in extremities, weight gain >5 lb, periorbital edema
• Assess nutritional status; check diet for sources of vit D (milk, some seafood), calcium (dairy products, dark green vegetables); phosphates (dairy products) must be avoided

Patient/family education

• Teach symptoms of hypercalcemia and when to report symptoms to prescriber
• Teach patient about foods rich in calcium, vit D; provide list of calcium-rich foods; renal failure patients are given a renal diet

---

- Caution patient not to double doses, take exactly as prescribed

Evaluation
Positive therapeutic outcome
- Prevention of bone deficiencies
- Calcium, phosphorus at normal levels

⚠ HIGH ALERT

diltiazem (Rx)
(dil-tye′a-zem)
Cardizem, Cardizem CD, Cardizem LA, Cartia XT, Dilacor-XR, Dilt-CD, Diltia XR, Diltia XT, Diltzac, Taztia XT, Tiamate, Tiazac
Func. class.: Calcium channel blocker, antianginal, antiarrhythmic class IV, antihypertensive
Chem. class.: Benzothiazepine
Pregnancy category C

Do not confuse:
Cardizem/Cardene

ACTION: Inhibits calcium ion influx across cell membrane during cardiac depolarization, produces relaxation of coronary vascular smooth muscle, dilates coronary arteries, slows SA/AV node conduction times, dilates peripheral arteries

Therapeutic outcome: Decreased angina pectoris, dysrhythmias, B/P

USES
Oral: Angina pectoris due to hypertension, coronary artery spasm

Parenteral: Atrial fibrillation, flutter; paroxysmal supraventricular tachycardia

CONTRAINDICATIONS:
Sick sinus syndrome, 2nd- or 3rd-degree heart block, hypotension less than 90 mm Hg systolic, acute MI, pulmonary congestion, cardiogenic shock

Precautions: Pregnancy **C**, breastfeeding, children, CHF, aortic stenosis, bradycardia, GERD, hepatic disease, hiatal hernia, ventricular dysfunction, elderly

DOSAGE AND ROUTES
Hypertension
Adult: PO 60-120 mg bid (SUS REL) (Cardizem SR), max 540 mg/day, or 120-240 mg (EXT REL) daily

Prinzmetal's or variant angina, chronic stable angina
Adult: PO 30 mg qid, increasing dose gradually to 180-360 mg/day in divided doses or (SR) 60-120 mg bid; may increase to 240-360 mg/day or 120 or 180 mg EXT REL (LA, CD, XT, XR products) PO daily

Atrial fibrillation, flutter, paroxysmal supraventricular tachycardia
Adult: IV 0.25 mg/kg as BOL over 2 min initially, then 0.35 mg/kg may be given after 15 min; if no response, may give CONT INF 5-15 mg/hr for up to 24 hr

Available forms: Tabs 30, 60, 90, 120 mg; ext rel tab 120, 180, 240, 300, 360, 420 mg; ext rel caps 60, 90, 120, 180, 240, 300, 360, 420 mg; inj 5 mg/ml (5, 10 ml)

Implementation
PO route
- Store at room temperature
- **Cardizem LA ext rel tab 24 hr:** give daily, either AM or PM, without regard to meals
- **Dilacor XR/Diltia XT ext rel cap 24 hr** give daily, take on empty stomach, swallow whole, do not cut, crush, chew, open
- **Tiazac, Tiztia XT:** give daily without regard to meals
- **Conventional regular-rel tab:** give before meals and at bedtime
- **Cardizem CD or equivalent (Cartia XT) generic ext rel cap 24 hr:** give daily, without regard to meals
- Give with meals for GI symptoms; may crush and sprinkle (reg tab) on applesauce
Oral suspension (unlabeled)
- Grind 16, 90 mg diltiazem reg rel tab into fine powder
- In separate container, mix 60 ml Ora-Sweet and 60 ml Ora-Plus
- Add small amount of sol to powder to form paste, add geometric amounts of base to achieve desired vol, place in amber container

Direct IV route
- Give direct **IV** undiluted over 2 min
Continuous IV infusion route
- **Dilute** 125 mg/100 ml (1.25 mg/ml) or 250 mg/250 ml (1 mg/ml) or 250 mg/500 ml (0.5 mg/ml) of D_5W, 0.9% NaCl, D_5/0.45% NaCl; give

10 mg/hr; may increase by 5 mg/hr to 15 mg/hr; may continue inf up to 24 hr

Y-site compatibilities: Albumin, amikacin, amphotericin B, aztreonam, bretylium, bumetanide, ceFAZolin, cefotaxime, cefoTEtan, cefOXitin, cefTAZidime, cefTRIAXone, cefuroxime, cimetidine, ciprofloxacin, clindamycin, digoxin, DOBUTamine, DOPamine, doxycycline, EPINEPHrine, erythromycin, esmolol, fentaNYL, fluconazole, gentamicin, hetastarch, HYDROmorphone, imipenem-cilastatin, labetalol, lidocaine, LORazepam, meperidine, metoclopramide, metroNIDAZOLE, midazolam, milrinone, morphine, multivitamins, niCARDipine, nitroglycerin, norepinephrine, oxacillin, penicillin G potassium, pentamidine, piperacillin, potassium chloride, potassium phosphates, ranitidine, sodium nitroprusside, theophylline, ticarcillin, ticarcillin/clavulanate, tobramycin, trimethoprim-sulfamethoxazole, vancomycin, vecuronium

ADVERSE EFFECTS

CNS: *Headache, fatigue, drowsiness,* dizziness, depression, weakness, insomnia, tremor, paresthesia
CV: Dysrhythmia, *edema,* **CHF,** bradycardia, hypotension, palpitations, **heart block**
GI: *Nausea,* vomiting, diarrhea, gastric upset, *constipation,* increased LFTs
GU: Nocturia, polyuria, **acute renal failure**
INTEG: *Rash,* pruritus at inj site, flushing, photosensitivity, burning
RESP: Rhinitis, dyspnea, pharyngitis

Pharmacokinetics

Absorption	Well absorbed
Distribution	Not known
Metabolism	Liver, extensively
Excretion	Metabolites (96%)
Half-life	3½-9 hr

Pharmacodynamics

	PO	PO–sus rel	IV
Onset	½ hr	Unknown	Unknown
Peak	2-3 hr	Unknown	Unknown
Duration	6-8 hr	12 hr	Unknown

INTERACTIONS

Individual drugs

CarBAMazepine, lithium, lovastatin, methyl-PREDNISolone: increased effects of each specific product
Cimetidine: increased effects of diltiazem
CycloSPORINE: increased cycloSPORINE effect
Digoxin: increased digoxin effect
Theophylline: increased effect, toxicity

Drug classifications

Anesthetics: increased effects of anesthetics
β-Adrenergic blockers: increased bradycardia, CHF, increased β-blocker effect
Benzodiazepines: increased effect of benzodiazepines
HMG-CoA reductase inhibitors: increased effects

NURSING CONSIDERATIONS

Assessment

• **CHF:** monitor for dyspnea, weight gain, edema, jugular vein distention, rales; monitor I&O ratios daily, weight
• **Angina:** location, duration, alleviating factors, activity when pain starts
• **Dysrhythmias:** monitor B/P and pulse, respiration, ECG and intervals (PR, QRS, QT); PCWP, CVP often during infusion; if B/P drops 30 mm Hg, stop infusion and call prescriber

Patient/family education

• Caution patient to avoid hazardous activities until stabilized on product and dizziness is no longer a problem
• Instruct patient to limit caffeine consumption; to avoid grapefruit juice; to avoid alcohol and OTC products unless directed by prescriber
⚠ Tell patient to comply in all areas of medical regimen; diet, exercise, stress reduction, product therapy; to notify prescriber of irregular heartbeat, shortness of breath, swelling of feet and hands, pronounced dizziness, constipation, nausea, hypotension
• Teach patient to use as directed even if feeling better; may be taken with other cardiovascular products (nitrates, β-blockers); how to take pulse, B/P before taking product; to change position slowly
• Teach patient not to discontinue abruptly

Evaluation

Positive therapeutic outcome
• Decreased anginal pain
• Decreased B/P
• Absence of dysrhythmias

TREATMENT OF OVERDOSE:

Atropine for AV block, vasopressor for hypotension

dimenhyDRINATE (OTC, Rx)

(dye-men-hye′dri-nate)

**Apo-DimenhyDRINATE ✦,
Dramamine, Driminate, Travol Motion
Sickness, TripTone, Wal-Dram**

Func. class.: Antiemetic, antihistamine, anticholinergic

Chem. class.: H1-receptor antagonist, ethanolamine derivative

Do not confuse:
dimenhyDRINATE/diphenhydrAMINE

ACTION: Competes with histamine for H1 receptors in GI tract, blood vessels, respiratory tract; central anticholinergic activity, which results in decreased vestibular stimulation and blockade of chemoreceptor trigger zone

Therapeutic outcome: Absence of nausea, vomiting, or vertigo

USES: Motion sickness, nausea, vomiting, vertigo

Unlabeled uses: Hyperemesis gravidarum, Ménière's syndrome

CONTRAINDICATIONS:
Hypersensitivity, infants, neonates, tartrazine dye hypersensitivity

Precautions: Pregnancy (B), breastfeeding, children, geriatric patients, cardiac dysrhythmias, asthma, prostatic hypertrophy, bladder-neck obstruction, closed-angle glaucoma, stenosing peptic ulcer, pyloroduodenal obstruction

DOSAGE AND ROUTES
Adult: PO 50-100 mg q4hr; IM/IV 50 mg q4hr as needed (Canada only)

Child 6-12 yr: PO 25-50 mg q6-8hr prn, max 150 mg/day

Child 2-5 yr: PO 12.5-25 mg q6-8hr, max 75 mg/day

Available forms: Tabs 50 mg; inj 50 mg/ ml; elixir 15 mg/5 ml; chew tabs 50 mg

Implementation
• Give IM inj in large muscle mass; aspirate to avoid IV administration (Canada only)
• Tablets may be swallowed whole, chewed, or allowed to dissolve

IV route (Canada only)
• After diluting 50 mg/10 ml of NaCl inj, give 50 mg over 2 min

ADVERSE EFFECTS
CNS: Drowsiness, restlessness, headache, dizziness, insomnia, confusion, nervousness, tingling, vertigo
CV: Hypertension, hypotension, palpitation
EENT: Dry mouth, blurred vision, diplopia, nasal congestion, photosensitivity, xerostomia
GI: Nausea, anorexia, vomiting, constipation
INTEG: Rash, urticaria, fever, chills, flushing
MISC: Anaphylaxis

Pharmacokinetics
Absorption	Unknown
Distribution	May cross placenta, enter breast milk
Metabolism	Liver
Excretion	Kidneys
Half-life	Unknown

Pharmacodynamics
Onset	PO 15-30 min
Peak	PO 2 hr
Duration	PO 4-6 hr

INTERACTIONS
Individual drugs
Alcohol: increased effects

Drug classifications
Anticholinergics, tricyclics, MAOIs, opiates, sedative/hypnotics, other CNS depressants: increased effects

Drug/lab test
False negative: allergy skin testing

NURSING CONSIDERATIONS
Assessment
• Monitor VS, B/P; check patients with cardiac disease more often
• Assess for signs of toxicity of other products or masking of symptoms of disease: brain tumor, intestinal obstruction
• Observe for drowsiness, dizziness

Patient/family education
• Advise patient to avoid hazardous activities, activities requiring alertness because dizziness may occur; to request assistance with ambulation
• Advise to avoid alcohol, other CNS depressants

Evaluation
Positive therapeutic outcome
• Absence of nausea, vomiting, or vertigo

Adverse effects: *italics* = common; **bold** = life-threatening

dinoprostone (Rx)

(dye-noe-prost'one)
Cervidil, Prepidil, Prostin E-Z
Func. class.: Oxytocic, abortifacient
Chem. class.: Prostaglandin E_2
Pregnancy category C

Do not confuse:
Prepidil/bepridil

ACTION: Stimulates uterine contractions similar to labor by myometrium stimulation, causing abortion; acts within 30 hr for complete abortion

Therapeutic outcome: Beginning of labor, fetal expulsion

USES: Abortion during 2nd trimester, benign hydatidiform mole, expulsion of uterine contents in fetal deaths to 28 wk, missed abortion, cervical effacement and dilatation in term pregnancy when they have not occurred spontaneously

CONTRAINDICATIONS:

Hypersensitivity, C-section, surgery, fetal distress, multiparity, vaginal bleeding, cephalopelvic disproportion

Precautions: Pregnancy **C**, renal/hepatic/cardiac disease, asthma, anemia, jaundice, diabetes mellitus, seizure disorders, hypertension, glaucoma, uterine fibrosis, cervical stenosis, pelvic surgery, PID, respiratory disease

> **BLACK BOX WARNING:** Requires a specialized setting and an experienced clinician

DOSAGE AND ROUTES

Abortifacient/2nd trimester/missed abortion/benign hydatidiform mole/intrauterine fetal death
Adult: VAG SUPP 20 mg; repeat q3-5hr until abortion occurs; max dose 240 mg

Cervical ripening
Adult: GEL 0.5 mg vag gel placed in cervical canal, may repeat after 6 hr, max 1.5 mg/24 hr; vag insert 10 mg high in vagina, remove at onset of active labor or within 12 hr

Available forms: Vag supp 20 mg; gel 0.5 mg/3 g (prefilled syringe); vag insert 10 mg

Implementation
Suppository route
• Warm supp by running warm water over package; insert high in vagina, wear gloves to prevent absorption; have patient recumbent for at least 10 min
Gel route
• Do not allow to come in contact with skin; use soap and water to wash after use
• Gel should be at room temperature
• Place patient in dorsal or lithotomy position to insert gel into cervical canal; remove catheter; discard all items after use; keep supine 15-30 min

ADVERSE EFFECTS
CNS: *Headache,* dizziness, chills, fever, flushing
CV: Hypotension, **dysrhythmias,** DIC
EENT: Blurred vision
GI: *Nausea, vomiting, diarrhea*
GU: Vaginitis, vaginal pain, vulvitis, vaginismus
INTEG: Rash, skin color changes
MS: *Leg cramps, joint swelling,* weakness
SYST: **Anaphylactoid syndrome of pregnancy**
Insert: Uterine hyperstimulation, fever, nausea, vomiting, diarrhea, abdominal pain
Gel: Uterine contractile abnormality, GI side effects, back pain, fever
Fetal: Bradycardia (i.e., deceleration)
Suppository: Uterine rupture, anaphylaxis

Pharmacokinetics
Absorption	Rapidly absorbed
Distribution	Unknown
Metabolism	Enzymes
Excretion	Kidneys
Half-life	Unknown

Pharmacodynamics
	Gel	Supp
Onset	Rapid	10 min
Peak	30-45 min	Unknown
Duration	Unknown	2-3 hr

INTERACTIONS
Individual drugs
Alcohol: decreased oxytoxic effect

Drug classifications
Other oxytocics: increased effect

NURSING CONSIDERATIONS
Assessment

> **BLACK BOX WARNING:** Specialized setting, specialized clinician: use only with emergency equipment nearby, by a clinician experienced with use in pregnancy termination; complete abortion should result within 17 hr (insert)

- **Cervical ripening:** assess dilatation and effacement of the cervix, uterine contractions, fetal heart tones; watch for contractions lasting over 1 min, hypertonus, fetal distress; product should be slowed or discontinued
- Assess for fever that occurs approximately 30 min after supp insertion (abortion)
- Monitor for nausea, vomiting, diarrhea; these may require medication
- **Assess for hypersensitivity reaction:** dyspnea, rash, chest discomfort
- Assess respiratory rate, rhythm, depth; notify prescriber of abnormalities in pulse, B/P
- **Check vaginal discharge;** itching, irritation indicates vaginal infection

Patient/family education
- Teach patient all aspects of treatment including purpose of medication and expected results
- Tell patient that gel may produce warmth in her vagina
- Caution patient that if contractions are longer than 1 min to notify nurse or prescriber
- Advise patient to notify prescriber of cramping, pain, increased bleeding, chills, increased temp, or foul-smelling discharge; these symptoms may indicate uterine infection
- Advise patient to remain supine 10-15 min after insertion of suppository, 2 hr after insert, 15-30 min after gel

Evaluation
Positive therapeutic outcome
- Progression of labor
- Abortion

diphenhydrAMINE
(OTC, Rx)
(dye-fen-hye′dra-meen)
Allerdryl ✤, AllerMax ✤, Altaryl, Banophen, Benadryl, Benadryl Allergy, Benadryl Allergy Dye Free, Benadryl Children's Allergy, Buckley's Bedtime, Diphedryl, Diphenhist, Dytan, ElixSure Allergy, Equaline Allergy, Equaline Children's Allergy, Equate Allergy, Equate Children's Allergy, Genahist, Good Sense Children's Allergy Relief, Good Sense Diphedryl, Leader Complete Allergy, Nytol, PediaCare Children's Allergy, PediaCare Nighttime Cough, Q-Dryl Allergy, Select Brand Allergy, Siladryl, Silphen, Simply Sleep, Sleepinal, Sleep Tabs, Sominex, Top Care Allergy, Top Care Children's Allergy, Unisom ✤, Valu-Dryl, Wal-dryl Allergy, Wal-dryl Allergy Dye Free, Wal-dryl Children's Allergy, Walgreen's Sleep Aid, Walgreen's Sleep II, Wal-Som

Func. class.: Antihistamine (1st generation, nonselective), antitussive
Chem. class.: Ethanolamine derivative, H_1-receptor antagonist
Pregnancy category B

Do not confuse:
diphenhydrAMINE/dicyclomine/dimenhyDRINATE

ACTION: Acts on blood vessels, GI, respiratory system by competing with histamine for H_1-receptor site; decreases allergic response by blocking histamine

Therapeutic outcome: Absence of allergy symptoms and rhinitis, decreased dystonic symptoms, absence of motion sickness, absence of cough, ability to sleep

USES: Allergy symptoms, rhinitis, motion sickness, antiparkinsonism, nighttime sedation, infant colic, nonproductive cough, insomnia in children

CONTRAINDICATIONS:
Hypersensitivity to H_1-receptor antagonist, acute asthma attack, lower respiratory tract disease, neonates

Precautions: Pregnancy **B,** breastfeeding, children <2 yr, increased intraocular pressure, renal/cardiac disease, hypertension, bronchial asthma, seizure disorder, stenosed peptic ulcers, hyperthyroidism, prostatic hypertrophy, bladder neck obstruction

DOSAGE AND ROUTES
Adult and child >12 yr: PO 25-50 mg q4-6hr, max 300 mg/day; IM/**IV** 10-50 mg, max 300 mg/day
Child 6-12 yr: PO/IM/**IV** 5 mg/kg/day in 4 divided doses, max 300 mg/day

Nighttime sleep aid
Adult and child ≥12 yr: PO 25-50 mg at bedtime

Antitussive (syrup only)
Adult and child ≥12 yr: 25 mg q4hr, max 150 mg/24 hr
Child 6-12 yr: 12.5 mg q4hr, max 75 mg/24 hr

Renal dosage
Adult: PO CCr >50 ml/min give dose q6hr; CCr 10-50 ml/min dose q6-12hr; CCr <10 ml/min dose q12-18hr

Available forms: Caps 25, 50 mg; tabs 25, 50 mg; chew tabs 12.5 mg; elix 12.5 mg/5 ml; syr 12.5 mg/5 ml; inj 10, 50 mg/ml; orally disintegrating tabs 12.5, 25 mg

Implementation
• Avoid use in children <2 yr, death has occurred; overdose has occurred in topical gel taken orally (adult/child)
• Give 20 min before bedtime if using for sleep aid
PO route
• Give with meals if GI symptoms occur; absorption rate may be slightly decreased; cap may be opened and product mixed with food/fluids for patients with swallowing difficulties
IM route
• Give IM inj in large muscle mass; aspirate to avoid **IV** administration; rotate sites
Direct IV route
• Give **IV** undiluted ≤25 mg/min
Intermittent IV infusion route
May be diluted with 0.9% NaCl, D₅W, D₁₀W, 0.45% NaCl, D₅/0.9% NaCl, D₅/0.45% NaCl, D₅/0.25% NaCl, LR, Ringer's; give 25 mg/min or less

Syringe compatibilities: Atropine, butorphanol, chlorproMAZINE, cimetidine, cisatracurium, dimenhyDRINATE, DOXOrubicin liposome, droperidol, fentaNYL, fluphenazine,

glycopyrrolate, HYDROmorphone, hydrOXYzine, meperidine, metoclopramide, midazolam, morphine, nalbuphine, pentazocine, perphenazine, prochlorperazine, promazine, promethazine, ranitidine, remifentanil, scopolamine, SUFentanil

Syringe incompatibilities: PENTobarbital, phenytoin, thiopental

Y-site compatibilities: Abciximab, aldesleukin, alfentanil hydrochloride, amifostine, amikacin sulfate, aminocaproic acid, amphotericin B lipid complex (Abelcet), amphotericin B liposome (AmBisome), amsacrine, anidulafungin, argatroban, ascorbic acid injection, atenolol, atracurium besylate, atropine sulfate, azithromycin, benztropine mesylate, bivalirudin, bleomycin, bumetanide, buprenorphine, butorphanol, calcium chloride/gluconate, CARBOplatin, caspofungin, cefTAZidime, ceftizoxime, chlorproMAZINE, cimetidine, ciprofloxacin, cisatracurium, CISplatin, cladribine, clindamycin, codeine, cyanocobalamin, cyclophosphamide, cycloSPORINE, cytarabine, DACTINomycin, DAPTOmycin, digoxin, diltiazem, DOBUTamine, DOCEtaxel, DOPamine, doripenem, doxacurium, DOXOrubicin, DOXOrubicin liposomal, doxycycline, enalaprilat, ePHEDrine, EPINEPHrine, epirubicin, epoetin alfa, eptifibatide, ertapenem, erythromycin, esmolol, etoposide, famotidine, fenoldopam, fentaNYL, filgrastim, fluconazole, fludarabine, folic acid, gallium, gatifloxacin, gemcitabine, gemtuzumab, gentamicin, glycopyrrolate, granisetron, HYDROmorphone, hydrOXYzine, IDArubicin, ifosfamide, imipenem-cilastatin, irinotecan, isoproterenol, labetalol, levofloxacin, lidocaine, linezolid, LORazepam, LR, magnesium sulfate, mannitol, mechlorethamine, melphalan, meperidine, meropenem, metaraminol, methadone, methicillin, methotrexate, methoxamine, methyldopate, metoclopramide, metoprolol, metroNIDAZOLE, miconazole, midazolam, minocycline, mitoXANtrone, morphine, multiple vitamins injection, mycophenolate, nalbuphine, naloxone, nesiritide, netilmicin, nitroglycerin, norepinephrine, octreotide, ondansetron, oxaliplatin, oxytocin, PACLitaxel, palonosetron, pamidronate, pancuronium, papaverine, PEMEtrexed, penicillin G potassium/sodium, pentamidine, pentazocine, phenylephrine, phytonadione, piperacillin, piperacillin-tazobactam, polymyxin B, potassium chloride, procainamide, prochlorperazine, promethazine, propofol, propranolol, protamine, pyridoxine, quiNIDine, quinupristin-dalfopristin, ranitidine, remifentanil, Ringer's, ritodrine, riTUXimab, rocuronium, sargramostim, sodium acetate, succinylcholine, SUFentanil, tacrolimus,

---

teniposide, theophylline, thiamine, thiotepa, ticarcillin, ticarcillin-clavulanate, tigecycline, tirofiban, TNA, tobramycin, tolazoline, TPN, trastuzumab, trimetaphan, urokinase, vancomycin, vasopressin, vecuronium, verapamil, vinCRIStine, vinorelbine, vitamin B complex/C, voriconazole, zoledronic acid

Y-site incompatibilities: Foscarnet

ADVERSE EFFECTS

CNS: *Dizziness, drowsiness,* poor coordination, fatigue, anxiety, euphoria, confusion, paresthesia, neuritis, **seizures**
CV: Hypotension, palpitations
EENT: Blurred vision, dilated pupils, tinnitus, nasal stuffiness, dry nose, throat, mouth
GI: Nausea, anorexia, diarrhea
GU: *Retention,* dysuria, frequency
HEMA: **Thrombocytopenia, agranulocytosis, hemolytic anemia**
INTEG: Photosensitivity
MISC: **Anaphylaxis**
RESP: Increased thick secretions, wheezing, chest tightness

Pharmacokinetics

Absorption	Well absorbed (PO, IM); completely absorbed (**IV**)
Distribution	Widely distributed; crosses placenta
Metabolism	Liver (95%)
Excretion	Kidneys, breast milk
Half-life	2½-7 hr

Pharmacodynamics

	PO	IM	IV
Onset	15-60 min	30 min	Immediate
Peak	1-4 hr	1-4 hr	Unknown
Duration	4-8 hr	4-8 hr	4-8 hr

INTERACTIONS
Individual drugs
Alcohol: increased CNS depression

Drug classifications
Antidepressants (tricyclic), barbiturates, CNS depressants, opiates, sedative/hypnotics: increased CNS depression
MAOIs: increased effect of diphenhydrAMINE

Drug/lab test
False negative: skin allergy tests (discontinue antihistamines 3 days before testing)

NURSING CONSIDERATIONS
Assessment
• Assess respiratory status: rate, rhythm, increase in bronchial secretions, wheezing, chest tightness; provide fluids to 2 L/day to decrease secretion thickness
• Monitor I&O ratio: be alert for urinary retention, frequency, dysuria, especially geriatric; product should be discontinued if these occur
• Monitor CBC during long-term therapy; blood dyscrasias may occur but are rare
• If giving for dystonic reactions, assess type of involuntary movements and evaluate response to this medication
• Assess cough characteristics including type, frequency, thickness of secretions; evaluate response to this medication if using for cough
• Product should be discontinued 4 days prior to skin allergy tests

Patient/family education
• Tell patient that a false-negative result may occur with skin testing; these procedures should not be scheduled until 3 days after discontinuing use
• Caution patient to avoid hazardous activities and activities requiring alertness, since dizziness may occur; instruct patient to request assistance with ambulation
• Teach patient to use sunscreen to prevent photosensitivity
• Advise patient to avoid alcohol, other depressants; may potentiate effect; CNS depression may occur
• Teach all aspects of product uses; to notify prescriber if confusion, sedation, hypotension occur; to avoid driving and other hazardous activity if drowsiness occurs; to avoid alcohol or other CNS depressants that may potentiate effect
• Advise patient to avoid breastfeeding; **not to breastfeed (injectable)**

Evaluation
Positive therapeutic outcome
• Absence of motion sickness
• Absence of nausea, vomiting
• Ability to sleep
• Absence of cough
• Decrease in involuntary movements

TREATMENT OF OVERDOSE:
• Administer lavage, diazepam, vasopressors, phenytoin **IV**

diphenoxylate with atropine (Rx)

(dye-fen-ox′i-late)
Lomotil, Lonox
difenoxin/atropine (Rx)
(dye-fen-ox′in/a′troe-peen)
Motofen

Func. class.: Antidiarrheal
Chem. class.: Phenylpiperidine derivative, opiate agonist

Pregnancy category C
Controlled substance schedule V (diphenoxylate/atropine); IV (difenoxin/atropine (US))

Do not confuse:
Lomotil/Lamictal/Lamasil/Lanoxin/Lasix/Ludomil

ACTION: Inhibits gastric motility by acting on mucosal receptors responsible for peristalsis

Therapeutic outcome: Decreased loose stools

USES: Acute nonspecific and acute exacerbations of chronic functional diarrhea

CONTRAINDICATIONS:
Hypersensitivity, pseudomembranous colitis, child <2 yr, severe electrolyte imbalances, diarrhea associated with organisms that penetrate intestinal mucosa

Precautions: Pregnancy **C,** breastfeeding, hepatic disease, ulcerative colitis, severe hepatic disease, substance abuse, dehydration

DOSAGE AND ROUTES
diphenoxylate/atropine
Adult: PO 5 mg qid, titrated to patient response, max 8 tabs/24 hr
Child 2-12 yr: PO (liquid only) 0.3-0.4 mg/kg/day in 4 divided doses

difenoxin/atropine
Adult: PO initially 2 tabs, then 1 tab after each loose stool or q3-4hr prn, max 8 tabs/day

Available forms: diphenoxylate/atropine: tab 2.5 mg diphenoxylate/0.025 mg atropine; liq 2.5 mg diphenoxylate/0.025 mg atropine/5 ml; **difenoxin/atropine:** tabs 1 mg difenoxin/0.025 atropine

Implementation
• Give for 48 hr only; tabs may be given with food, crushed and mixed with fluids; liquid should be measured accurately

ADVERSE EFFECTS
CNS: *Dizziness, drowsiness, light-headedness, headache,* fatigue, nervousness, insomnia, confusion
EENT: Blurred vision, burning eyes
GI: *Nausea, vomiting, dry mouth, epigastric distress,* constipation, **paralytic ileus, toxic megacolon**
MISC: **Anaphylaxis, angioedema**
RESP: **Respiratory depression**

Pharmacokinetics
Absorption	Well absorbed
Distribution	Unknown
Metabolism	Liver, active metabolite
Excretion	Kidneys
Half-life	2½ hr

Pharmacodynamics
Onset	45-60 min
Peak	2 hr
Duration	3-4 hr

INTERACTIONS
Individual drugs
Alcohol: increased action of alcohol
Amantadine, amoxapine, diphenhydrAMINE, clemastine, cloZAPine, cyclobenzaprine, disopyramide, loperamide, maprotiline, olanzapine: decreased GI motility, possible toxic megacolon

Drug classifications
Anticholinergics: increased anticholinergic effect
Antimuscarinics, phenothiazines, tricyclics: decreased GI motility, possible toxic megacolon
Barbiturates: increased action of barbiturates
CNS depressants: increased action of CNS depressants
MAOIs: hypertensive crisis; do not use together
Opiates: increased action of opioids

NURSING CONSIDERATIONS
Assessment
• Monitor electrolytes (potassium, sodium, chloride) if on long-term therapy; fluid status, skin turgor
• Assess bowel pattern before, during treatment; check for rebound constipation after termination of medication; check bowel sounds

---

• Check response after 48 hr; if no response, product should be discontinued and other treatment initiated
• **Assess for abdominal distention and toxic megacolon,** which may occur in ulcerative colitis
• Assess hepatic function if on long-term therapy

Patient/family education
• Advise patient to avoid alcohol and OTC products unless directed by prescriber; may cause increased CNS depression
• Caution patient not to exceed recommended dosage; that product may be habit forming
• Advise patient that product may cause drowsiness; to avoid hazardous activities until response to product is determined
• Teach patient that dry mouth can be decreased by frequent sips of water, hard candy, sugarless gum

Evaluation
Positive therapeutic outcome
• Decreased diarrhea

---

dipivefrin ophthalmic
See Appendix B

---

dipyridamole (Rx)
(dye-peer-id′a-mole)
Persantine
Func. class.: Coronary vasodilator, antiplatelet agent
Chem. class.: Nonnitrate
Pregnancy category B

ACTION: Inhibits adenosine uptake, which produces coronary vasodilatation; increases oxygen saturation in coronary tissues, coronary blood flow; acts on small vessels with little effect on vascular resistance; may increase development of collateral circulation; decreased platelet aggregation by the inhibition of phosphodiesterases (enzymes)

Therapeutic outcome: Inhibition of platelet aggregation; absence of ischemic attacks, reinfarction

USES: Prevention of transient ischemic attacks, inhibition of platelet adhesion to prevent myocardial reinfarction, thromboembolism, with warfarin in prosthetic heart valves, prevention of coronary bypass graft occlusion with aspirin; **IV** form used to evaluate coronary

artery disease; used as alternative to exercise in thallium myocardial perfusion imaging to evaluate coronary artery disease

CONTRAINDICATIONS:
Hypersensitivity

Precautions: Pregnancy **B,** breastfeeding, hypotension, unstable angina, asthma, hepatic disease, labor

DOSAGE AND ROUTES
Inhibition of platelet adhesion
Adult: PO 75-100 mg qid in combination with aspirin or warfarin

Thallium myocardial perfusion imaging
Adult: **IV** 570 mcg/kg

Transient ischemic attacks with aspirin (unlabeled)
Adult: PO 225-400 mg/day, max 400 mg daily

Available forms: Tabs 25, 50, 75 mg; inj 10 mg/2 ml

Implementation
PO route
• Give with 8 oz of water; to improve absorption give on an empty stomach; if GI symptoms occur may give with meals
• Tabs may be crushed, mixed with food or fluids for swallowing difficulty, or swallowed whole
• Store at room temperature

Intermittent IV infusion route
• Give by **IV** after diluting to at least 1:2 ratio using D₅W, 0.45% NaCl, or 0.9% NaCl; 20-50 ml should be given; give over 4 min; do not give undiluted
• Inject thallium 201 within 5 min after product infusion
• Do not admix

ADVERSE EFFECTS
CNS: *Headache, dizziness, weakness, fainting, syncope;* **IV**: transient cerebral ischemia, weakness
CV: *Postural hypotension;* **IV**: **MI**
GI: *Nausea, vomiting,* anorexia, diarrhea
INTEG: *Rash,* flushing

Adverse effects: *italics* = common; **bold** = life-threatening

Pharmacodynamics

	PO	IV
Onset	Unknown	Unknown
Peak	1.25 hr	6 min
Duration	6 hr	½ hr
Therapeutic effect	Several mo	

INTERACTIONS

Individual drugs

Aspirin, cefamandole, cefoTEtan, cefoperazone, plicamycin, sulfinpyrazone, valproic acid: increased risk of bleeding

Digoxin: increased digoxin effect

Theophylline: prevention of coronary vasodilation

Drug classifications

Anticoagulants, NSAIDs, salicylates, thrombolytics: increased risk of bleeding

NURSING CONSIDERATIONS

Assessment

• Monitor B/P, pulse baseline and during treatment until stable; take B/P with patient lying, standing; orthostatic hypotension is common

• Assess cardiac status: chest pain, what aggravates or ameliorates condition

• If using by IV route, monitor VS before, during, and after infusion; monitor for chest pain, bronchospasm; use ECG for identifying dysrhythmias; use aminophylline up to 250 mg IV for bronchospasm and chest pain; if chest pain is unrelieved with the 250 mg dose of aminophylline, give SL dose of nitroglycerin

Patient/family education

• Teach patient that this medication is not a cure; that product may have to be taken continuously in evenly spaced doses only as directed; if a dose is missed, take one when remembered up to 4 hr; do not double doses

• Advise patient to rise slowly from sitting or lying down to prevent orthostatic hypotension

• Caution patient not to use alcohol or OTC medication unless approved by prescriber

• Caution patient to avoid hazardous activities until stabilized on medication; dizziness may occur

Evaluation

Positive therapeutic outcome

• Absence of reinfarction, ischemic attacks

TREATMENT OF OVERDOSE:

Administer **IV** phenylephrine

divalproex sodium
See valproate

DOBUTamine (Rx)
(doe-byoo'ta-meen)
DOBUTamine
Func. class.: Adrenergic direct-acting β₁-agonist, inotropic agent, cardiac stimulant
Chem. class.: Catecholamine
Pregnancy category B

Do not confuse:
DOBUTamine/DOPamine

ACTION: Causes increased contractility, increased cardiac output without marked increase in heart rate by acting on β_1-receptors in heart; minor α/β_2 effects

Therapeutic outcome: Cardiac output increased with decreased fatigue and dyspnea

USES: Cardiac decompensation due to organic heart disease or cardiac surgery

Unlabeled uses: Cardiogenic shock in children, congenital heart disease in children undergoing cardiac catherization

CONTRAINDICATIONS:

Hypersensitivity, idiopathic hypertrophic subaortic stenosis

Precautions: Pregnancy **B**, breastfeeding, children, hypertension, CAD, MI, hypovolemia, dysrhythmias, sulfite hypersensitivity, renal failure, geriatrics

DOSAGE AND ROUTES

Adult and child: IV INF 0.5-1 mcg/kg/min; titrate to 2-20 mcg/kg/min; may increase to 40 mcg/kg/min if needed

Available forms: Inj 12.5 mg/ml, 250 mg/20 ml

Implementation
Injectable administration
• Visually inspect parenteral products for particulate matter and discoloration prior to administration whenever solution and container permit

IV administration
NOTE: Infusions up to 72 hours have been given without development of tolerance. However, β-receptor desensitization may occur with prolonged infusions of any β-adrenergic agonist, including DOBUTamine, or as a consequence of sympathetic compensatory mechanisms associated with advanced congestive heart failure, resulting in alterations in DOBUTamine pharmacodynamics. Experience with intravenous DOBUTamine in controlled trials does not extend beyond 48 hours of repeated boluses and/or continuous infusions
• Must be diluted before administration
• Infuse into a large vein

Dilution
• Concentrate for injection must be diluted with at least 50 ml of a compatible IV solution (strongly alkaline [i.e., sodium bicarbonate] solutions are incompatible). A common dilution is 500 mg (40 ml) in 210 ml D_5W or NS (withdraw 40 ml from a 250 ml bag) to produce a final concentration of 2000 mcg/ml; or 1000 mg (80 ml) in 170 ml D_5W or NS (withdraw 80 ml from a 250 ml bag) to produce a final concentration of 4000 mcg/ml. Maximum concentration should not exceed 5000 mcg/ml and should be adjusted according to the fluid requirements of the patient

Infusion
• Administer diluted solution by IV infusion using a controlled infusion device
• Premixed bags of DOBUTamine in D_5W solutions may exhibit a pink color that, if present, will increase with time; this color change is due to slight oxidation of the drug, but there is no significant loss of potency.
• Do not administer DOBUTamine simultaneously with solutions containing sodium bicarbonate or strong alkaline solutions (incompatible)
• Infusion of DOBUTamine should be started at a low rate and titrated frequently to reach the optimal dosage (see Dosage); dosage titration is guided by the patient's response, including systemic blood pressure, urine flow, frequency of ectopic activity, heart rate, and (whenever possible) measurements of cardiac output, central venous pressure, and/or pulmonary capillary wedge pressure

Syringe compatibilities: Heparin, ranitidine

Syringe incompatibility: Doxapram

Y-site compatibilities: Alfentanil, alprostadil, amifostine, amikacin, aminocaproic acid, amiodarone, anidulafungin, argatroban, ascorbic acid injection, atenolol, atracurium, atropine, aztreonam, benztropine, bleomycin, bumetanide, buprenorphine, butorphanol, calcium chloride/gluconate, CARBOplatin, caspofungin, chlorproMAZINE, cimetidine, ciprofloxacin, cisatracurium, CISplatin, cladribine, clarithromycin, cloNIDine, codeine, cyanocobalamin, cyclophosphamide, cycloSPORINE, cytarabine, DACTINomycin, DAPTOmycin, dexmedetomidine, digoxin, diltiazem, diphenhydrAMINE, DOCEtaxel, DOPamine, doripenem, doxacurium, DOXOrubicin, DOXOrubicin liposomal, doxycycline, enalaprilat, ePHEDrine, EPINEPHrine, epirubicin, epoetin alfa, eptifibatide, erythromycin, esmolol, etoposide, famotidine, fenoldopam, fentaNYL, fluconazole, fludarabine, gatifloxacin, gemcitabine, gentamicin, glycopyrrolate, granisetron, HYDROmorphone, hydrOXYzine, IDArubicin, ifosfamide, irinotecan, isoproterenol, labetalol, levofloxacin, lidocaine, linezolid, LORazepam, LR, magnesium sulfate, mannitol, mechlorethamine, meperidine, meropenem, metaraminol, methoxamine, methyldopate, methylPREDNISolone, metoclopramide, metoprolol, metroNIDAZOLE, miconazole, milrinone, minocycline, mitoXANtrone, morphine, multiple vitamins injection, mycophenolate mofetil, nafcillin, nalbuphine, naloxone, netilmicin, niCARdipine, nitroglycerin, norepinephrine, octreotide, ondansetron, oxaliplatin, oxytocin, PACLitaxel, palonosetron, pamidronate, pancuronium, papaverine, pentamidine, pentazocine, phenylephrine, polymyxin B, potassium chloride, procainamide, prochlorperazine, promethazine, propofol, propranolol, protamine, pyridoxine, quiNIDine, ranitidine, remifentanil, Ringer's, ritodrine, riTUXimab, rocuronium, sodium acetate, succinylcholine, SUFentanil, tacrolimus, temocillin, teniposide, theophylline, thiamine, thiotepa, tigecycline, tirofiban, TNA, tobramycin, tolazoline, TPN, trastuzumab, trimetaphan, urokinase, vancomycin, vasopressin, vecuronium, verapamil, vinCRIStine, vinorelbine, voriconazole, zidovudine, zoledronic acid

Y-site incompatibilities: Acyclovir, alteplase, aminophylline, foscarnet, phytonadione

ADVERSE EFFECTS
CNS: *Anxiety,* headache, dizziness, fatigue
CV: Palpitations, tachycardia, hypo/hypertension, PVCs, angina
ENDO: Hypokalemia
GI: Heartburn, nausea, vomiting
MS: Muscle cramps (leg)
RESP: Dyspnea

Pharmacokinetics
Absorption	Complete
Distribution	Unknown
Metabolism	Liver
Excretion	Kidneys
Half-life	2 min

Pharmacodynamics
Onset	1-5 min
Peak	10 min
Duration	<10 min

INTERACTIONS
Individual drugs
Atomoxetine: increased pressor effect, dysrhythmias
Bretylium, oxytocin: increased dysrhythmias
Guanethidine: increased severe hypertension
Oxytocin: increased pressor effects

Drug classifications
Anesthetics (general): increased dysrhythmias
Antidepressants (tricyclic), COMT inhibitors, MAOIs, oxytocics: increased pressor response, dysrhythmias
β-Blockers: decreased action of DOBUTamine

NURSING CONSIDERATIONS
Assessment
• **Assess for hypovolemia;** if present, correct before beginning treatment with DOBUTamine; avoid use in patients with atrial fibrillation before digitalization
• **Monitor ECG for dysrhythmias, ischemia** during treatment; some patients may not need continuous ECG monitoring; also monitor PCWP, CVP, CO_2, urinary output; notify prescriber if <30 ml/hr
• **Assess for heart failure:** bibasilar crackles, S_3 gallop, dyspnea, neck vein distention in patients with cardiomyopathy or CHF
• Assess for oxygenation or perfusion deficit: decreased B/P, chest pain, dizziness, loss of consciousness
• Monitor B/P and pulse q5min during infusion; if B/P drops 30 mm Hg, stop infusion and call prescriber

• Monitor ALT, AST, bilirubin daily
• **Monitor for sulfite sensitivity,** which may be life threatening

Patient/family education
• Teach patient reason for medication and expected results, reason for all monitoring and procedures
• Advise patient to report dyspnea, headache, **IV** site discomfort, chest pain, numbness of extremities

Evaluation
Positive therapeutic outcome
• Increased cardiac output
• Decreased PCWP, adequate CVP
• Decreased dyspnea, fatigue, edema, ECG
• Increased urine output

TREATMENT OF OVERDOSE:
Discontinue product, support circulation

DOCEtaxel (Rx)
(doe-se-tax′el)
Taxotere
Func. class.: Antineoplastic, miscellaneous
Pregnancy category D

Do not confuse:
Taxotere/Taxol

ACTION: Inhibits the reorganization of the microtubule network needed for interphase and mitotic cellular functions; also causes abnormal bundles of microtubules during cell cycle and multiple esters of microtubules during mitosis

Therapeutic outcome: Prevention of rapidly growing malignant cells

USES: Locally advanced or metastatic breast cancer, non–small cell lung cancer, androgen-independent metastatic prostate cancer, post-surgery operable node-positive breast cancer, induction treatment of locally advanced squamous cell cancer of the head/neck, adjuvant treatment of breast cancer with CARBOplatin and trastuzumab, gastric adenocarcinoma

CONTRAINDICATIONS:
Pregnancy **D,** breastfeeding, hypersensitivity to this product, bilirubin exceeding upper normal limit

BLACK BOX WARNING: Hypersensitivity to other products with polysorbate 80, neutropenia (neutrophils <1500/mm³)

Precautions: Children, CV disease, pulmonary disorders, bone marrow depression, herpes zoster, pleural effusion

> **BLACK BOX WARNING:** Edema, hepatic disease, lung cancer, taxane hypersensitivity

DOSAGE AND ROUTES
• Other regimens are used

Locally advanced or metastatic breast cancer after failure of other chemotherapy
Adult: IV 60-100 mg/m^2 given over 1 hr q3wk; if neutrophil count is <500/mm^3 for >1 wk, reduce dose by 25%

Operable node-positive breast cancer; adjuvant postsurgery treatment of operable node-positive breast cancer
Adult: IV (TAC regimen) 75 mg/m^2 1 hr after DOXOrubicin 50 mg/m^2 and cyclophosphamide 500 mg/m^2 q3wk for 6 cycles

Adjuvant treatment of operable stage I-III invasive breast cancer in combination with cyclophosphamide
Adult: IV (TAC) regimen DOCEtaxel 75 mg/m^2 with cyclophosphamide 600 mg/m^2 q21day × 4 cycles

Locally advanced or metastatic non–small cell lung cancer after failure of CISplatin chemotherapy
Adult: IV 75 mg/m^2 over 1 hr q3wk; if neutrophil count is <500/mm^3 for >1 wk, reduce dose to 55 mg/m^2; if patient develops grade 3 peripheral neuropathy, stop product

Unresectable, locally advanced or metastatic non–small cell lung cancer previously treated with chemotherapy
Adult: IV 75 mg/m^2 over 1 hr, then CISplatin 75 mg/m^2 **IV** given over 30-60 min q3wk; reduce dose to 65 mg/m^2 in those with hematologic or nonhematologic toxicities

Androgen-independent metastatic prostate cancer
Adult: IV 75 mg/m^2 given over 1 hr q3wk, with 5 mg predniSONE PO bid continuously; give dexamethasone 8 mg PO at 12 hr, 3 hr, and 1 hr prior to DOCEtaxel; if neutrophil count is <500 cells/mm^3 for more than 1 wk or other toxicities occur, reduce dose to 60 mg/m^2

Squamous cell cancer of head/neck
Adult: IV 75 mg/m^2 over 1 hr, then CISplatin 100 mg/m^2 over 1 hr on day 1, then 5-FU 1000 mg/m^2/day CONT INF × 5 days, repeat cycle q3wk

Gastric adenocarcinoma
Adult: IV 75 mg/m^2 q3wk, given with CISplatin, fluorouracil

Available forms: Inj 20 mg/0.5 ml, 20 mg/ml, 80 mg/2 ml, 80 mg/4 ml

Implementation
• Give top or systemic analgesics for pain to lessen effects of stomatitis
• Give liquid diet: carbonated beverages; gelatin may be added if patient is not nauseated or vomiting
⚠ Confirm that dexamethasone was given 12 hr and 6 hr before inf begins
• Store prepared sol up to 27 hr in refrigerator

Intermittent IV infusion route
• Use gloves and cytotoxic handling precautions
• Use non-PVC bag and use non-DEHP tubing
• Allow vials to warm to room temperature, withdraw all diluent and inject in vial of docetaxel, rotate gently to mix, allow to stand to decrease foaming, then withdraw the required amount (10 mg/ml) and inject in 250 ml of 0.9% NaCl or D$_5$W, mix gently, give over 1 hr

Y-site compatibilities: Acyclovir, alfentanil, allopurinol, amifostine, amikacin, aminocaproic acid, aminophylline, amiodarone, amphotericin B lipid complex, ampicillin, ampicillin-sulbactam, anidulafungin, atenolol, atracurium, azithromycin, aztreonam, bivalirudin, bleomycin, bumetanide, buprenorphine, busulfan, butorphanol, calcium chloride/gluconate, CARBOplatin, carmustine, caspofungin, ceFAZolin, cefepime, cefonicid, cefoperazone, cefotaxime, cefoTEtan, cefOXitin, cefTAZidime, ceftizoxime, cefTRIAXone, cefuroxime, cephapirin, chloramphenicol, chlorproMAZINE, cimetidine, ciprofloxacin, cisatracurium, CISplatin, clindamycin, codeine, cyclophosphamide, cycloSPORINE, cytarabine, dacarbazine, DACTINomycin, DAPTOmycin, dexamethasone, dexmedetomidine, dexrazoxane, diazepam, digoxin, diltiazem, diphenhydrAMINE, DOBUTamine, DOPamine, doripenem, doxacurium, DOXOrubicin HCl, doxycycline, droperidol, enalaprilat, ePHEDrine, EPINEPHrine, epirubicin, ertapenem, erythromycin, esmolol, etoposide, famotidine, fenoldopam, fentaNYL, fluconazole, fludarabine, fluorouracil, foscarnet, fosphenytoin, furosemide, ganciclovir, gatifloxacin, gemcitabine, gentamicin, glycopyrrolate, granisetron, haloperidol, heparin, hydrALAZINE, hydrocortisone, HYDROmorphone, hydrOXYzine, ifosfamide, imipenem-cilastatin, inamrinone, insulin (regular), irinotecan, isoproterenol, ketorolac, labetalol, leucovorin, levofloxacin, levorphanol, lidocaine, linezolid, LORazepam, LR, magnesium sulfate, mannitol, meperidine, meropenem, mesna, methotrexate, methyldopate, metoclopramide, metoprolol, metroNIDAZOLE, midazolam, milrinone, minocycline, mitoXANtrone, mivacurium, morphine, nafcillin, naloxone, nesiritide, netilmicin, niCARdipine, nitroglycerin, nitroprusside, norepinephrine, octreotide, ofloxacin, ondansetron, oxaliplatin, palonosetron, pamidronate, pancuronium, pantoprazole, PEMEtrexed, pentamidine, pentazocine, PENTobarbital, PHENobarbital, phenylephrine, piperacillin, piperacillintazobactam, polymyxin B, potassium chloride/phosphates, procainamide, prochlorperazine, promethazine, propranolol, quiNIDine, quinupristin-dalfopristin, ranitidine, remifentanil, riTUXimab, rocuronium, sodium acetate/bicarbonate/phosphates, succinylcholine, SUFentanil, sulfamethoxazole-trimethoprim, tacrolimus, teniposide, theophylline, thiopental, thiotepa, ticarcillin, ticarcillin-clavulanate, tigecycline, tirofiban, tobramycin, tolazoline, trastuzumab, trimethobenzamide, vancomycin, vasopressin, vecuronium, verapamil, vinCRIStine, vinorelbine, voriconazole, zidovudine, zoledronic acid

ADVERSE EFFECTS
CNS: Seizures
CV: *Hypotension, fluid retention, peripheral edema,* flushing, MI, **sinus tachycardia**
GI: *Nausea, vomiting, diarrhea,* **hepatotoxicity,** stomatitis, colitis
HEMA: **Neutropenia, leukopenia, thrombocytopenia, anemia,** bleeding, infections, **myelosuppression**
INTEG: *Alopecia,* nail pain, rash, skin eruptions
MISC: Amenorrhea, fever of unknown origin, **secondary malignancy, Stevens-Johnson syndrome,** epiphora
MS: *Arthralgia, myalgia,* back pain, weakness
NEURO: *Peripheral neuropathy*
RESP: Dyspnea, **pulmonary edema, fibrosis, embolism**
SYST: **Hypersensitivity reactions,** AML, **death**

Pharmacokinetics

Absorption	Completely absorbed
Distribution	Unknown
Metabolism	Liver, extensively
Excretion	Fecal
Half-life	11.1 hr

Pharmacodynamics

Onset	Rapid
Peak	Unknown
Duration	Unknown

INTERACTIONS
Individual drugs
Anastrozole (high doses), aprepitant, clarithromycin, conivaptan, delavirdine, efavirenz (induces or inhibits), erythromycin, fluconazole, FLUoxetine, fluvoxaMINE, fosaprepitant, imatinib, itraconazole, ketoconazole, mibefradil, nefazodone, voriconazole, and others: increased CYP3A inhibition

Bosentan, carBAMazepine, nevirapine, phenytoin, fosphenytoin, rifabutin, rifampin, rifapentine, troglitazone: increased CYP3A induction

CycloSPORINE, erythromycin, ketoconazole, troleandomycin: altered metabolism of DOCEtaxel

Drug classifications
Antineoplastics, radiation: increased myelosuppression
Barbiturates: increased CYP3A induction
Live virus vaccines: decreased immune response

NURSING CONSIDERATIONS
Assessment
• **Assess CNS changes:** confusion, paresthesias, peripheral neuropathy, dysethenia, pain, weakness: if severe, product should be discontinued
• Check buccal cavity q8hr for dryness, sores or ulceration, white patches, oral pain, bleeding, dysphagia; obtain prescription for viscous lidocaine (Xylocaine) to use in mouth

> **BLACK BOX WARNING: Taxane: assess symptoms indicating severe allergic reaction, anaphylaxis:** rash, pruritus, urticaria, purpuric skin lesions, itching, flushing

> **BLACK BOX WARNING:** Monitor CBC, differential, platelet count weekly; withhold product if WBC is <1500/mm³ or platelet count is <100,000/mm³, notify prescriber of results

BLACK BOX WARNING: Use of DOCEtaxel, polysorbate 80 hypersensitivity are contraindicated

BLACK BOX WARNING: Edema: oral corticosteroids should be given as premedication; assess for fluid retention

BLACK BOX WARNING: Lung cancer: increased mortality in those with increased LFTs and a history of platinum-based products

• Monitor renal function tests: BUN, creatinine, serum uric acid, urine CCr before, during therapy; check I&O ratio; report fall in urine output to <30 ml/hr
• Monitor temp (may indicate beginning of infection)

BLACK BOX WARNING: Hepatic disease: Monitor liver function tests before, during therapy (bilirubin, AST, ALT, LDH) as needed or monthly; check for jaundice of skin and sclera, dark urine, clay-colored stools, itchy skin, abdominal pain, fever, diarrhea

BLACK BOX WARNING: Assess for bone marrow depression/bleeding: hematuria, stool guaiac, bruising or petechiae, mucosa or orifices q8hr; check for inflammation of mucosa, breaks in skin

• Assess effects of alopecia on body image; discuss feelings about body changes

Patient/family education
⚠ Inform patient that nonhormonal contraceptive measures are recommended during therapy and >4 mo after; teratogenic effects are possible, pregnancy D
• Teach patient to avoid use of products containing aspirin or ibuprofen, razors, commercial mouthwash, since bleeding may occur; to report symptoms of bleeding (hematuria, tarry stools)
• Instruct patient to report signs of **anemia** (fatigue, headache, irritability, faintness, shortness of breath) and CNS reactions (confusion, psychosis, nightmares, seizures, severe headaches)
• Instruct patient to report signs of **infection:** fever, sore throat, flulike symptoms
• Inform patient that hair may be lost during treatment; a wig or hairpiece may make patient feel better; new hair may be different in color and texture
• Inform patient that receiving vaccinations during therapy may cause serious reactions

• Instruct patient to rinse mouth tid-qid with water, club soda; brush teeth bid-qid with soft brush or cotton-tipped applicators for stomatitis; use unwaxed dental floss

Evaluation
Positive therapeutic outcome
• Prevention of rapid division of malignant cells

docosanol topical
See Appendix B

docusate calcium (OTC)
(dok′yoo-sate cal′see-um)
Kao-Tin, Stool Softener DC, Sur-Q-Lax, Walgreen's Stool Softener
docusate sodium (OTC)
Colace, Correctol, Diocto, Doc-Q-Lace, Docu DOK, Doculace, Enemeez, Equaline Stool Softener, Good Sense Stool Softener, Leader Stool Softener, Phillip's Stool Softener, Regulex ✦, Select Brand Docusate Sodium, Selex ✦, Silace, Soflax ✦, Top Care Stool Softener, Walgreen's Stool Softener
Func. class.: Laxative, emollient
Chem. class.: Anionic surfactant
Pregnancy category C

ACTION: Increases water, fat penetration in intestine; allows for easier passage of stool

Therapeutic outcome: Passage of softened stool, absence of constipation

USES: Prevent hard, dry stools, prevent constipation, soften fecal impaction (rectal route)

CONTRAINDICATIONS:
Hypersensitivity, obstruction, fecal impaction, nausea/vomiting

Precautions: Pregnancy **C**, breastfeeding

DOSAGE AND ROUTES
Adult: PO 50-300 mg/day (docusate sodium) or 240 mg (docusate calcium) prn enema 4 ml (docusate sodium)
Child >12 yr: Enema 2 ml (docusate sodium)
Child 6-12 yr: PO 40-150 mg/day (docusate sodium) in divided doses
Child 3-6 yr: PO 20-60 mg/day (docusate sodium) in divided doses
Child <3 yr: PO 10-40 mg/day (docusate sodium) in divided doses

Available forms: Docusate calcium: caps 240 mg; **docusate sodium:** caps 50, 100, 250 mg; tabs 100 mg; syr 20 mg/5 ml, 50 mg/15 ml, 100 mg/30 ml, 150 mg/15 ml; oral sol 10, 50 mg/ml; enema 283 mg/3.9 g cap

Implementation
PO route
• Dilute oral sol in juice or other fluid to disguise taste
• Give tabs or caps with 8 oz of liquid; give on empty stomach for increased absorption, results
• Store in cool environment; do not freeze

ADVERSE EFFECTS
EENT: Bitter taste, throat irritation
GI: Nausea, anorexia, cramps, diarrhea
INTEG: Rash

Pharmacokinetics

Absorption	Minimal (PO)
Distribution	Unknown
Metabolism	Not metabolized
Excretion	Bile
Half-life	Unknown

Pharmacodynamics

	PO	RECT
Onset	24-72 hr	4-6 hr
Peak	Unknown	Unknown
Duration	Unknown	Unknown

INTERACTIONS
Individual drugs
Mineral oil: toxicity

Drug/herb
Flax, senna: increased laxative action

NURSING CONSIDERATIONS
Assessment
• Assess cramping, rectal bleeding, nausea, vomiting; if these symptoms occur, product should be discontinued; identify cause of constipation; identify fluids, bulk, or exercise is missing from lifestyle

Patient/family education
• Discuss with patient that adequate fluid consumption is as necessary as bulk, exercise for adequate bowel function
• Teach patient that normal bowel movements do not always occur daily
• Advise patient not to use in presence of abdominal pain, nausea, vomiting; tell patient to notify prescriber if unrelieved constipation or if symptoms of electrolyte imbalance occur:

muscle cramps, pain, weakness, dizziness, excessive thirst
• Advise patient that product may take up to 3 days to soften stools
• Instruct patient to take oral preparation with a full glass of water and increase fluid intake unless on fluid restrictions
• Caution patients with heart disease to avoid using the Valsalva maneuver to expedite evacuation

Evaluation
Positive therapeutic outcome
• Decreased constipation within 3 days

---

dofetilide
(doff-ee-till′-lide)
Tikosyn
Func. class.: Antidysrhythmic (Class III)
Pregnancy category C

ACTION: Blocks cardiac ion channel carrying the rapid component of delayed potassium current, no effect on sodium channels

Therapeutic outcome: Absence of atrial fibrillation

USES: Atrial fibrillation, flutter, maintenance of normal sinus rhythm

CONTRAINDICATIONS:
Hypersensitivity, digoxin toxicity, aortic stenosis, pulmonary hypertension, children, severe renal disease

> **BLACK BOX WARNING:** QT prolongation, torsades de pointes, renal failure

Precautions: Pregnancy C, breastfeeding, AV block, bradycardia, electrolyte imbalance

> **BLACK BOX WARNING:** Renal disease, arrhythmias, ventricular arrhythmias/tachycardia

DOSAGE AND ROUTES
Conversion of atrial fibrillation/ atrial flutter to normal sinus rhythm; or, maintenance therapy with highly symptomatic atrial fibrillation/atrial flutter of ≥1 wk duration
Adult: PO Individualize dosage based on renal function and QTc in a monitored facility. Refer to the step-by-step procedure for determining the initial dose of dofetilide

---

Maintenance therapy of atrial fibrillation/atrial flutter after hospital discharge

Adult: PO continue dosage at discharge as from initial dosage titration. Individualize dosage based on renal function and QTc, which should be re-evaluated q3mo or as medically warranted; if the QTc >500 milliseconds (550 msec in patients with ventricular conduction abnormalities) at any time, discontinue; carefully monitor until QTc returns to baseline; if renal function deteriorates, adjust the dose as described in the dosage guidelines for patients with renal impairment

Discontinuation of dofetilide before use of interacting drugs

Adult: PO discontinue dofetilide for ≥2 days before starting a potentially interacting drug

Renal dose

Adult: PO initial dose for CCr >60 mg/ml 500 mcg bid; CCr 40-60 mg/min 250 mcg bid; CCr 20-39 mg/min 125 mcg bid; CCr <20 mg/min do not use

Available forms: Caps 125, 250, 500 mcg

Implementation

Step 1: Assess cardiac conduction: Before first dose, the QTc interval must be determined using an average of 5-10 beats; if the QTc interval is >440 msec (or >500 msec in ventricular conduction abnormalities), do not use. If baseline heart rate is <60 bpm, then the QT interval should be used

Step 2: Assess renal function: Before first dose, determine renal function using the Cockroft-Gault equation, use actual body weight to calculate creatinine clearance

Step 3: Adjust starting dose according to renal function: Refer to the Renal dose section (above) to determine the appropriate initial dose

Step 4: ECG monitoring: Begin continuous ECG monitoring starting with the first dose

Step 5: Dose adjustments: Approximately 2-3 hr after the first dose, determine the QTc interval. If the QTc interval has increased by >15% (compared with baseline), or, if the QTc interval is >500 msec (>550 msec in patients with ventricular conduction abnormalities), the initial dosage should be reduced by half as follows:

• Decrease an initial dose of 500 mcg bid to 250 mcg bid
• Decrease an initial dose of 250 mcg bid to 125 mcg bid
• Decrease an initial dose of 125 mcg bid to 125 mcg daily

Step 6: Reassess QTc interval: Reassess the QTc interval 2-3 hr after each subsequent dose; if, the QTc interval lengthens to >500 msec (or >550 msec in patients with ventricular conduction abnormalities), **discontinue**

Step 7: ECG Monitoring: Monitor continuous ECG for a minimum of 3 days or for 12 hr after conversion to normal sinus rhythm, whichever is greater

ADVERSE EFFECTS

CNS: *Syncope, dizziness,* headache, **stroke**
CV: *Hypotension, postural hypotension, bradycardia,* angina, PVCs, substernal pressure, precipitation of angina, transient hypertension, **QT prolongation, torsades de pointes, ventricular dysrhythmias,** chest pain
GI: *Nausea, vomiting,* severe diarrhea, anorexia
MISC: Angioedema
RESP: Dyspnea, respiratory infections

Pharmacokinetics	
Absorption	>90%
Distribution	Steady state 2-3 days
Metabolism	Not metabolized
Excretion	Kidneys 80%
Half-life	10 hr

Pharmacodynamics
Unknown

INTERACTIONS

Individual drugs

AMILoride, entecavir, lamiVUDine, memantine, metFORMIN, procainamide, triamterene, trospium: increased toxicity

Arsenic trioxide, chloroquine, ciprofloxacin, clarithromycin, droperidol, erythromycin, halofantrine, haloperidol, levomethadyl, methadone, pentamidine, ziprasidone: increased QT prolongation, torsades de pointes

Cimetidine, hydrochlorothiazide, ketoconazole, megestrol, metFORMIN, prochlorperazine, triamterene, trimethoprim/sulfamethoxazole, verapamil: do not use together

Drug classifications

Antiretroviral protease inhibitors: increased dofetilide levels

Class IA/III antidysrhythmics, some phenothiazines: increased QT prolongation, torsades de pointes

Diuretics, potassium depletion: increased hypokalemia

Adverse effects: *italics* = common; **bold** = life-threatening

Drug/food
• Do not use with grapefruit juice

NURSING CONSIDERATIONS
Assessment

> **BLACK BOX WARNING: Severe renal impairment:** CCr <20 ml/min: do not use for mild to moderate renal disease, monitor BUN/creatinine; adjust dose based on creatinine clearance

⚠ AF patients should receive anticoagulation prior to cardioversion

Patient/family education
• Instruct patient to notify prescriber if fast heartbeats with fainting or dizziness occur
• Instruct patient to notify all prescribers of all medications and supplements taken
• Teach patient that if a dose is missed, do not double, take next dose at usual time

Evaluation
Positive therapeutic outcome
• Increased control in atrial fibrillation

dolasetron (Rx)
(do-la′se-tron)
Anzemet
Func. class.: Antiemetic
Chem. class.: 5-HT receptor antagonist
Pregnancy category B

ACTION: Prevents nausea, vomiting by blocking serotonin peripherally, centrally, and in the small intestine

Therapeutic outcome: Control of nausea, vomiting

USES: Prevention of nausea, vomiting associated with cancer chemotherapy and prevention of postoperative nausea, vomiting

Unlabeled uses: Radiotherapy-induced nausea/vomiting

CONTRAINDICATIONS:
Hypersensitivity

Precautions: Pregnancy **B,** breastfeeding, children, geriatric, hypokalemia, electrolyte imbalances, granisetron, ondansetron, palonosetron hypersensitivity, QT prolongation

DOSAGE AND ROUTES
Prevention of nausea/vomiting associated with cancer chemotherapy
Adult and child 2-16 yr: IV 1.8 mg/kg as a single dose ½ hr before chemotherapy, max 40 mcg/kg
Adult: PO 100 mg 1 hr before chemotherapy
Child 2-16 yr: PO 1.8 mg/kg 1 hr before chemotherapy, max 100 mg

Prevention of postoperative nausea/vomiting
Adult: IV 12.5 mg as a single dose 15 min before cessation of anesthesia; PO 100 mg 2 hr before surgery (prevention only)
Child 2-16 yr: IV 0.35 mg/kg as a single dose 15 min before cessation of anesthesia; PO 1.2 mg/kg within 2 hr before surgery (prevention only)

Available forms: Tabs 50, 100 mg; inj 20 mg/ml (12.5 mg/0.625 ml)

Implementation
PO route
• Do not mix product for oral administration in juice until immediately before administration; apple or apple-grape diluted can be kept for 2 hr at room temperature
• Store at room temp 48 hr after dilution

Intermittent IV infusion route
• Administer by inj 100 mg/30 sec or less or diluted in 50 ml of compatible sol; give over 15 sec
• Store at room temperature for 24 hr after dilution
• Do not admix

ADVERSE EFFECTS
CNS: *Headache,* dizziness, fatigue, drowsiness
CV: Dysrhythmias, ECG changes, hypo/hypertension, tachycardia, bradycardia, **QT prolongation, torsades de pointes, ventricular tachycardia/fibrillation, cardiac arrest (IV)**
GI: *Diarrhea,* constipation, increased AST, ALT, abdominal pain, anorexia
GU: Urinary retention, oliguria
MISC: Rash, **bronchospasm**

Pharmacokinetics

Absorption	Completely absorbed
Distribution	Unknown
Metabolism	Liver, extensively
Excretion	Kidneys
Half-life	Unknown

Pharmacodynamics
Unknown

INTERACTIONS
Individual drugs
Arsenic trioxide, chloroquine, clarithromycin, droperidol, erythromycin, halofantrine, haloperidol, levomethadyl, methadone, pentamidine, ziprasidone: increased QT prolongation; occurs at higher dose of dolasetron

Cimetidine: increased dolasetron levels

Rifampin: decreased dolasetron levels

Drug classifications
Antidysrhythmics: increased dysrhythmias

Class IA/III antidysrhythmics, some phenothiazines, loop diuretics, thiazide: increased QT prolongation

NURSING CONSIDERATIONS
Assessment
• **QT prolongation** and QRS, PR prolongation: do not use in those with congenital long QT syndrome, hypokalemia, hypomagnesemia, complete heart block (unless a pacemaker is in place); correct electrolytes before use; monitor ECG in the elderly, renal cardiac disease

• Assess for absence of nausea, vomiting during chemotherapy

• **Assess for hypersensitivity reaction:** rash, bronchospasm

• Assess for cardiac conduction conditions; electrolyte imbalances or dysrhythmias

Patient/family education
• Instruct patient to report diarrhea, constipation, rash, or changes in respirations; may cause headache; use analgesic

• Teach patient reason for medication and expected results

Evaluation
Positive therapeutic outcome
• Absence of nausea, vomiting during cancer chemotherapy

---

donepezil (Rx)
(don-ep-ee′zill)
Aricept, Aricept ODT
Func. class.: Anti-Alzheimer's agent
Chem. class.: Reversible cholinesterase inhibitor
Pregnancy category C

ACTION: Elevates acetylcholine concentrations (cerebral cortex) by slowing degradation of acetylcholine released in cholinergic neurons; does not alter underlying dementia

Therapeutic outcome: Decreased symptoms of Alzheimer's disease

USES: Treatment of mild to severe dementia in Alzheimer's disease

Unlabeled uses: Subcortical vascular dementia, dementia with Lewy bodies

CONTRAINDICATIONS:
Hypersensitivity to this product or piperidine derivatives

Precautions: Pregnancy **C**, breastfeeding, children, sick sinus syndrome, history of ulcers, GI bleeding, hepatic disease, bladder obstruction, asthma, seizures, COPD, abrupt disconinuation, AV block, GI obstruction, Parkinson's disease, surgery

DOSAGE AND ROUTES
Adult: PO 5 mg/day at bedtime; may increase to 10 mg/day after 4-6 wk, may increase to 23 mg/day after 3 mo of 10 mg/day

Available forms: Tabs 5, 10, 23 mg; oral sol 1 mg/ml; orally disintegrating tabs 5, 10 mg (Aricept ODT)

Implementation
PO route
• Give between meals; may be given with meals for GI symptoms

• Administer dosage adjusted to response no more than q4-6wk, oral dosage forms are interchangeable

• Provide assistance with ambulation during beginning therapy; dizziness, ataxia may occur

• Oral sol: measure with calibrated oral syringe or other calibrated device

• Orally disintegrating tabs: allow to dissolve on tongue before swallowing

ADVERSE EFFECTS
CNS: Dizziness, insomnia, somnolence, headache, fatigue, abnormal dreams, syncope, **seizures,** drowsiness, agitation, depression, confusion, fever, hallucinations

CV: **Atrial fibrillation,** hypo/hypertension, **sinus bradycardia, AV block**

GI: *Nausea, vomiting,* anorexia, *diarrhea,* abdominal pain, weight loss, **GI bleeding**

GU: Frequency, UTI, incontinence

INTEG: Rash, flushing, diaphoresis, bruising

META: Hyperlipidemia

MS: Cramps, arthritis, arthralgia, back pain
RESP: Rhinitis, URI, cough, pharyngitis

Pharmacokinetics

Absorption	Well
Distribution	Unknown
Metabolism	Liver to metabolites
Excretion	Unknown
Half-life	10 hr (single dose)

Pharmacodynamics
Unknown

INTERACTIONS
Individual drugs
CarBAMazepine, dexamethasone, PHENobarbital, phenytoin, rifampin: decreased donepezil effect

Succinylcholine: synergistic effects

Drug classification
Anticholinergics: decreased activity
Cholinergic agonists, cholinesterase inhibitors: synergistic effects
NSAIDs: increased GI intolerance
CYP2D6, CYP3A4 inducers: decreased donepezil effects
CYP2D6, CYP3A4 inhibitors: increased donepezil effects

Drug/herb
St. John's wort: decreased donepezil effect

NURSING CONSIDERATIONS
Assessment
• Monitor B/P, heart rate: hypo/hypertension
• Assess mental status: affect, mood, behavioral changes, depression, complete suicide assessment
• Assess GI status: nausea, vomiting, anorexia, diarrhea
• Assess GU status: urinary frequency, incontinence

Patient/family education
• Advise patient to report side effects: twitching, nausea, vomiting, sweating, dizziness; indicates overdose
• Advise patient to use product exactly as prescribed
• Advise patient to notify prescriber of nausea, vomiting, diarrhea (dose increase or beginning treatment), or rash
• Advise patient not to increase or abruptly decrease dosage, serious consequences may result
• Instruct patient that product is not a cure

Evaluation
Positive therapeutic outcome
• Decrease in confusion; improved mood

⚠ HIGH ALERT

DOPamine (Rx)
(doe'pa-meen)
Func. class.: Agonist, vasopressor, inotropic agent
Chem. class.: Catecholamine
Pregnancy category C

Do not confuse:
DOPamine/DOBUTamine

ACTION: Causes increased cardiac output; acts on β_1- and α-receptors, causing vasoconstriction in blood vessels; when low doses are administered, causes renal and mesenteric vasodilatation; β_1 stimulation produces inotropic effects with increased cardiac output

Therapeutic outcome: Increased B/P, cardiac output

USES: Shock; to increase perfusion; hypotension, cardiogenic/septic shock

CONTRAINDICATIONS:
Hypersensitivity, ventricular fibrillation, tachydysrhythmias, pheochromocytoma, hypovolemia

Precautions: Pregnancy **C**, breastfeeding, geriatric, arterial embolism, peripheral vascular disease, sulfite hypersensitivity, acute MI

> **BLACK BOX WARNING:** Extravasation

DOSAGE AND ROUTES
Shock
Adult: IV INF 2-5 mcg/kg/min, titrate upward 5-10 mcg/kg/min, max 50 mcg/kg/min; titrate to patient's response
Child: IV 1-5 mcg/kg/min initially; usual dosage range 2-20 mcg/kg/min

COPD
Adult: IV 4 mcg/kg/min

CHF
Adult: IV 3-10 mcg/kg/min

Available forms: Inj 40, 80, 160 mg/ml; conc for **IV** inf 0.8, 1.6, 3.2 mg/ml in 250, 500 ml D$_5$W

⚠ Nurse Alert   ⭐ Key NCLEX® Drug

D

Implementation
- Store reconstituted sol for up to 24 hr if refrigerated
- Do not use discolored sol; protect from light

Continuous infusion route
- Dilute 200-400 mg/250-500 ml of D$_5$W, 0.9% NaCl, D$_5$/LR, D$_5$/0.45% NaCl, D$_5$/0.9% NaCl, LR; do not use discolored sol; sol is stable for 24 hr; give 0.5-5 mcg/kg/min; may increase by 1-4 mcg/kg/min q15-30min until desired patient response; use infusion pump

BLACK BOX WARNING: Extravasation: if extravasation occurs, stop infusion, may inject area with phentolamine 10 mg/15 ml NS

Y-site compatibilities: Alfentanil, alprostadil, amifostine, amikacin, aminocaproic acid, aminophylline, amiodarone, anidulafungin, argatroban, ascorbic acid injection, atenolol, atracurium, atropine, aztreonam, benztropine, bivalirudin, bleomycin, bumetanide, buprenorphine, butorphanol, calcium chloride/gluconate, CARBOplatin, caspofungin, cefamandole, cefmetazole, cefonicid, cefotaxime, cefoTEtan, cefOXitin, cefpirome, cefTAZidime, ceftizoxime, cefTRIAXone, cefuroxime, chlorproMAZINE, cimetidine, ciprofloxacin, cisatracurium, CISplatin, cladribine, clarithromycin, clindamycin, cloNIDine, codeine, cyanocobalamin, cyclophosphamide, cycloSPORINE, cytarabine, DACTINomycin, DAPTOmycin, dexamethasone, dexmedetomidine, digoxin, diltiazem, diphenhydrAMINE, DOBUTamine, DOCEtaxel, doripenem, doxacurium, DOXOrubicin, DOXOrubicin liposomal, doxycycline, droperidol, enalaprilat, ePHEDrine, EPINEPHrine, epirubicin, epoetin alfa, eptifibatide, ertapenem, erythromycin, esmolol, etoposide, famotidine, fenoldopam, fentaNYL, fluconazole, fludarabine, fluorouracil, folic acid, foscarnet, gatifloxacin, gemcitabine, gemtuzumab, gentamicin, glycopyrrolate, granisetron, heparin, hydrocortisone, HYDROmorphone, hydrOXYzine, IDArubicin, ifosfamide, imipenem-cilastatin, irinotecan, isoproterenol, ketorolac, labetalol, levofloxacin, lidocaine, linezolid, LORazepam, LR, magnesium sulfate, mannitol, mechlorethamine, meperidine, metaraminol, methicillin, methoxamine, methyldopate, methylPREDNISolone, metoclopramide, metoprolol, metroNIDAZOLE, mezlocillin, micafungin, miconazole, midazolam, milrinone, minocycline, mitoXANtrone, morphine, moxalactam, multiple vitamins injection, mycophenolate, nafcillin, nalbuphine, naloxone, netilmicin, niCARdipine, nitroglycerin, nitroprusside, nor-epinephrine, octreotide, ondansetron, oxacillin, oxaliplatin, oxytocin, PACLitaxel, palonosetron, pamidronate, pancuronium, pantoprazole, papaverine, PEMEtrexed, penicillin G potassium/sodium, pentamidine, pentazocine, PENTobarbital, PHENobarbital, phenylephrine, phytonadione, piperacillin, piperacillin-tazobactam, polymyxin B, potassium chloride, procainamide, prochlorperazine, promethazine, propofol, propranolol, protamine, pyridoxine, quiNIDine, ranitidine, remifentanil, Ringer's, ritodrine, riTUXimab, rocuronium, sargramostim, sodium acetate, succinylcholine, SUFentanil, tacrolimus, temocillin, teniposide, theophylline, thiamine, thiotepa, ticarcillin, ticarcillin-clavulanate, tigecycline, tirofiban, TNA, tobramycin, tolazoline, TPN, trastuzumab, trimetaphan, urokinase, vancomycin, vasopressin, vecuronium, verapamil, vinCRIStine, vinorelbine, vitamin B complex/C, voriconazole, warfarin, zidovudine, zoledronic acid

ADVERSE EFFECTS
CNS: *Headache,* anxiety
CV: *Palpitations,* **tachycardia,** *hypertension,* **ectopic beats,** *angina,* **wide QRS complex,** peripheral vasoconstriction, hypotension
GI: *Nausea, vomiting, diarrhea*
INTEG: Necrosis, tissue sloughing with extravasation, **gangrene**
RESP: Dyspnea

Pharmacokinetics

Absorption	Complete
Distribution	Widely
Metabolism	Liver
Excretion	Kidney, plasma
Half-life	2 min

Pharmacodynamics

Onset	2-5 min
Peak	Unknown
Duration	<10 min

INTERACTIONS
Individual drugs
Phenytoin: bradycardia, hypotension

Drug classifications
α-Adrenergic blockers, β-adrenergic blockers: decreased action of DOPamine
Anesthetics (general): increased dysrhythmias
Antidepressants (tricyclic): increased pressor response
Ergots: severe hypertension

Adverse effects: *italics* = common; **bold** = life-threatening

MAOIs: increased hypertension (severe), do not use within 2 wk; increased pressor effect; hypertensive crisis may result

Oxytocics: increased B/P

Drug/lab test

Increased: urinary catecholamine, serum glucose

NURSING CONSIDERATIONS

Assessment

• Monitor ECG for dysrhythmias, ischemia during treatment; some patients may not need continuous ECG monitoring; also monitor PCWP, CVP, CO_2, urinary output; notify prescriber if <30 ml/hr

• **Assess for heart failure:** bibasilar crackles, S_3 gallop, dyspnea, neck vein distention in patients with cardiomyopathy or CHF

• **Assess for oxygenation or perfusion deficit:** decreased B/P, chest pain, dizziness, loss of consciousness

• Monitor B/P and pulse q5min during inf; if B/P drops 30 mm Hg, stop inf and call prescriber

• Check for extravasation: if this occurs, administer phentolamine mixed with 0.9% NaCl

Patient/family education

• Teach patient reason for medication, expected results, reason for all monitoring and procedures

• Advise patient to report all side effects

Evaluation

Positive therapeutic outcome

• Increased cardiac output

TREATMENT OF OVERDOSE:

Discontinue product, support circulation; give a short-acting α-blocker

doripenem (Rx)

(dore-i-pen′em)

Doribax

Func. class.: Antiinfective, miscellaneous

Chem. class.: Carbapenem

Pregnancy category B

ACTION: Bactericidal, interferes with cell wall replication of susceptible organisms; osmotically unstable cell wall swells, bursts from osmotic pressure

Therapeutic outcome: Negative C&S; decreasing symptoms and signs of infection

USES: Serious infections caused by *Acinetobacter baumannii, Bacteroides caccae, Bacteroides fragilis, Bacteroides thetaiotaomicron, Bacteroides uniformis, Bacteroides vulgatus, Citrobacter freundii, Escherichia coli, Klebsiella pneumoniae, Peptostreptococcus micros, Proteus mirabilis, Pseudomonas aeruginosa, Serratia marcescens, Staphylococcus aureus, Streptococcus contellatus, Streptococcus intermedius;* complicated UTIs, pyelonephritis, complicated intraabdominal infections

CONTRAINDICATIONS:

Hypersensitivity to carbapenems (meropenem, doripenem, imipenem), penicillin, β-lactam; viral infection

Precautions: Pregnancy **B**, breastfeeding, geriatric, renal disease, seizure disorder, pseudomembranous colitis, nebulizer or inhalation use, hypersensitivity to cephalosporins, children/adolescents

DOSAGE AND ROUTES

Adult: IV 500 mg every 8 hr × 5-14 days; if improvement occurs after 3 days, switch to an appropriate oral product

Renal dose

Adult: IV CCr 30-50 ml/min 250 mg over 1 hr q8hr; CCr >10 to <30 ml/min 250 mg over 1 hr q12hr; CCr ≤10 ml/min no data

Available forms: Powder for inj 500 mg

Implementation

IV route

• Visually inspect parenteral products for particulate matter and discoloration before use, diluted range in color from clear, colorless solutions to solutions that are clear and slightly yellow

• **Reconstitution:** No bacteriostatic preservative is present; observe aseptic technique while preparing the infusion

• **500-mg dose using the 500 mg vial:** Constitute the vial with 10 ml of sterile water for injection or sodium chloride 0.9% (normal saline). Gently shake (50 mg/ml); THE CONSTITUTED SUSPENSION IS NOT FOR DIRECT INJECTION; FURTHER DILUTION IS REQUIRED. Using a syringe with a 21-G needle, withdraw the suspension and add it to an infusion bag containing 100 ml of NS or D_5W; gently shake until clear: final (4.5 mg/ml)

• **250-mg dose using the 500 mg vial:** Constitute the vial with 10 ml of sterile water for injection or sodium chloride 0.9% (normal saline). Gently shake (50 mg/ml); THE CONSTITUTED SUSPENSION IS NOT FOR DIRECT INJECTION; FURTHER DILUTION IS REQUIRED. Using a syringe with a 21-G needle, withdraw the suspension and add it to an infusion bag containing 100 ml of normal saline or D_5W; gently shake until clear; remove 55 ml of this solution and discard. The remaining infusion solution contains 250 mg (4.5 mg/ml)

• **250-mg dose using the 250 mg vial:** Constitute the vial with 10 ml of sterile water for injection or sodium chloride 0.9% (normal saline). Gently shake (25 mg/ml); THE CONSTITUTED SUSPENSION IS NOT FOR DIRECT INJECTION; FURTHER DILUTION IS REQUIRED. Using a syringe with a 21-G needle, withdraw the suspension and add it to an infusion bag containing 50 or 100 ml of normal saline or D_5W; gently shake until clear; final concentration 4.2 mg/ml (50 ml infusion bag) or 2.3 mg/ml (100 ml infusion bag)

• **Storage:** Constituted suspensions may be held in vial for up to 1 hr prior to transfer and dilution in the infusion bag. Including storage and infusion time, diluted infusion solutions are stable for up to 12 hr (NS) or 4 hr (D_5W) at controlled room temperature; diluted infusion solutions are stable for up to 72 hr (NS) or 24 hr (D_5W) refrigerated, do not freeze constituted solutions.

• If Baxter Minibag Plus infusion bags are to be used, consult the instructions provided by the infusion bag manufacturer
Intermittent IV infusion route

• Do not mix with or physically add to solutions containing other drugs, infuse over 1 hr

Solution compatibilities: D_5W, 0.9% NaCl, sterile water for inj

Y-site compatibilities: Acyclovir, amikacin, aminophylline, amiodarone, anidulafungin, atropine, azithromycin, bumetanide, calcium gluconate, CARBOplatin, caspofungin, ceftaroline, ceftobiprole, cimetidine, ciprofloxacin, CISplatin, cyclophosphamide, cycloSPORINE, DAPTOmycin, dexamethasone, digoxin, diltiazem, diphenhydrAMINE, DOBUTamine, DOCEtaxel, DOPamine, DOXOrubicin, enalaprilat, esmolol, esomeprazole, etoposide, famotidine, fentaNYL, fluconazole, fluorouracil, foscarnet, furosemide, gemcitabine, gentamicin, granisetron, heparin, hydrocortisone, HYDROmorphone, ifosfamide, insulin (regular), labetalol, levofloxacin, linezolid, LORazepam, magnesium sulfate, mannitol, meperidine, methotrexate, methylPREDNISolone, metoclopramide, metroNIDAZOLE,

micafungin, midazolam, milrinone, morphine, moxifloxacin, norepinephrine, ondansetron, PACLitaxel, pantoprazole, PHENobarbital, phenylephrine, potassium chloride, ranitidine, sodium bicarbonate/phosphates, tacrolimus, telavancin, tigecycline, tobramycin, vancomycin, voriconazole, zidovudine

ADVERSE EFFECTS
CNS: *Seizures,* headache
GI: *Diarrhea, nausea,* vomiting, **pseudomembranous colitis, hepatitis**
GU: **Renal impairments/failure**
HEMA: **Neutropenia, leukopenia, anemia**
INTEG: *Rash,* urticaria, phlebitis, erythema at inj site, **Stevens-Johnson syndrome, toxic epidermal necrolysis,** pruritus
RESP: **Pneumonitis (inhalation)**
SYST: **Anaphylaxis, Stevens-Johnson syndrome, toxic epidermal necrolysis**

Pharmacokinetics

Absorption	Unknown
Distribution	To most body fluids/tissue
Metabolism	Unknown
Excretion	Mainly unchanged in urine, 70% recovered in 48 hr
Half-life	1 hr, extended in renal disease

Pharmacodynamics
Unknown

INTERACTIONS
Individual drugs
Probenecid: increased doripenem plasma levels
Divalproex sodium, valproic acid: decreased effects

Drug/lab test
Increased: AST, ALT, LDH, BUN, alkaline phosphatase, bilirubin, creatinine
False positive: direct Coombs' test

NURSING CONSIDERATIONS
Assessment
• Assess sensitivity to carbapenem antibiotics, penicillins, cephalosporins, other beta lactams
• Monitor renal disease: lower dose may be required
• Monitor bowel pattern daily; if severe diarrhea occurs, product should be discontinued; may indicate pseudomembranous colitis
• **Monitor for infection:** temp, sputum, characteristics of wound, before, during, and after treatment

⚠ Monitor for allergic reactions, anaphylaxis: **rash, urticaria, pruritus;** may occur few days after therapy begins
• **Monitor overgrowth of infection:** perineal itching, fever, malaise, redness, pain, swelling, drainage, rash, diarrhea, change in cough, sputum

Patient/family education
• Instruct patient to report severe diarrhea; may indicate pseudomembranous colitis
• Instruct patient to report sore throat, bruising, bleeding, joint pain; may indicate blood dyscrasias (rare)
• Instruct patient to report overgrowth of infection: black, furry tongue; vaginal itching; foul-smelling stools
• Advise patient to avoid breastfeeding; product is excreted in breast milk

Evaluation
Positive therapeutic outcome
• Negative C&S
• Absence of symptoms and signs of infection

TREATMENT OF HYPERSENSITIVITY: EPINEPHrine, antihistamines; resuscitate if needed (anaphylaxis)

dorzolamide ophthalmic
See Appendix B

doxazosin (Rx)
(dox-ay′zoe-sin)
Cardura, Cardura XL
Func. class.: Peripheral α-adrenergic blocker, antihypertensive
Chem. class.: Quinazoline
Pregnancy category C

Do not confuse:
Cardura/Coumadin/Cardene/Ridaura

ACTION: Peripheral blood vessels are dilated, peripheral resistance lowered; reduction in B/P results from peripheral α-adrenergic receptors being blocked

Therapeutic outcome: Decreased B/P, decreased symptoms of benign prostatic hypertrophy (BPH)

USES: Hypertension, urinary outflow obstruction, symptoms of benign prostatic hyperplasia

CONTRAINDICATIONS:
Hypersensitivity to quinazolines

Precautions: Pregnancy **C,** breastfeeding, children, hepatic disease, geriatrics

DOSAGE AND ROUTES
BPH
Adult: PO 1 mg/day at bedtime, increase in stepwise manner to 2, 4, 8 mg/day as needed at 1-2 wk intervals, max 8 mg; ext rel tab (Cardura XL) 4 mg/day with breakfast, adjust dose q3-4wk up to 8 mg/day

Hypertension
Adult: PO 1 mg/day at bedtime, increasing up to 16 mg daily if required; usual range 4-16 mg/day
Geriatric: PO 0.5 mg nightly, gradually increase

Available forms: Tabs 1, 2, 4, 8 mg; ext rel tabs 4, 8 mg

Implementation
PO route
• **Tabs** broken, crushed, or chewed; chewed tabs taste bitter; do not break, crush, chew **XL tabs**
• **Immediate release tab:** give without regard to meals; **EXT REL tabs:** give with breakfast; when switching from immediate release to EXT REL, the final evening dose of immediate release should be taken
• Store in tight container at room temperature (86° F [30° C] or less)
• May be used in combination with other antihypertensives
• May be given with food to prevent GI symptoms

ADVERSE EFFECTS
CNS: *Dizziness,* headache, drowsiness, anxiety, depression, vertigo, weakness, fatigue, asthenia, syncope
CV: Palpitations, *orthostatic hypotension,* **tachycardia,** *edema,* **dysrhythmias,** chest pain
EENT: Epistaxis, tinnitus, dry mouth, red sclera, pharyngitis, rhinitis
GI: *Nausea,* vomiting, diarrhea, constipation, abdominal pain, **hepatitis**
GU: Incontinence, polyuria, priapism, impotence

D

Pharmacokinetics

Absorption	Well absorbed
Distribution	Not known; 98% plasma protein bound
Metabolism	Liver, extensively ($<$63%)
Excretion	Kidneys
Half-life	22 hr

Pharmacodynamics

Onset	2 hr
Peak	5-6 hr
Duration	up to 24 hr

INTERACTIONS

Individual drugs
Alcohol: increased hypotensive effects
CloNIDine: decreased antihypertensive effect

Drug classifications
Other antihypertensives, nitrates, PDE-5 inhibitors: increased hypotensive effects

NURSING CONSIDERATIONS

Assessment
• **Hypertension:** monitor B/P (lying, standing) and pulse, syncope; check for edema in feet, legs daily; I&O; monitor for weight daily; notify prescriber of changes
• **BPH:** urinary pattern changes (hesitancy, dribbling, incomplete bladder emptying, dysuria, urgency, nocturia, urgency incontinence, intermittency before and during treatment)
• Assess for orthostatic hypotension; tell patient to rise slowly from sitting or lying position; assess pulse, jugular venous distention q4hr, crackles, dyspnea, orthopnea with B/P

Patient/family education
• Teach patient not to discontinue product abruptly; emphasize the importance of complying with dosage schedule, even if feeling better; if dose is missed take as soon as remembered; take at same time each day
• Teach patient not to use OTC products (cough, cold, allergy) unless directed by prescriber; also to avoid large amounts of caffeine
• Emphasize the need to rise slowly to sitting or standing position to minimize orthostatic hypotension
• Teach patient to notify prescriber of mouth sores, sore throat, fever, swelling of hands or feet, irregular heartbeat, chest pain
• Caution patient to report excessive perspiration, dehydration, vomiting, diarrhea; may lead to fall in B/P

• Caution patient that product may cause dizziness, fainting, light-headedness; may occur during 1st few days of therapy; to avoid hazardous activities
• Teach patient how to take B/P, and normal readings for age-group; to take B/P q7days
• Inform patient that fainting occasionally occurs after 1st dose; do not drive or operate machinery for 4 hr after 1st dose or after dosage increase or take 1st dose at bedtime; may take 1-2 wk in BPH

Evaluation
Positive therapeutic outcome
• Decreased B/P in hypertension
• Decreased symptoms of BPH

TREATMENT OF OVERDOSE:
Administer volume expanders or vasopressors; discontinue product; place in supine position

---

doxepin (Rx)
(dox′e-pin)
Prudoxin Cream, Silenor ✤, Zonolon Topical Cream
Func. class.: Antidepressant, tricyclic; antianxiety
Chem. class.: Dibenzoxepin, tertiary amine
Pregnancy category
B (Topical)
C (PO)

ACTION: Blocks reuptake of norepinephrine, serotonin into nerve endings, increasing action of norepinephrine, serotonin in nerve cells; has anticholinergic effects

Therapeutic outcome: Decreased symptoms of depression after 2-3 wk

USES: Major depression, anxiety, topical: lichen simplex, atopic dermatitis, eczema

Unlabeled uses: Insomnia, migraine prophylaxis; topical: pruritus

CONTRAINDICATIONS:
Hypersensitivity to tricyclics, urinary retention, closed-angle glaucoma, prostatic hypertrophy, acute recovery from MI

Precautions: Pregnancy **C** (PO), **B** (topical), breastfeeding, geriatric, seizures

BLACK BOX WARNING: Suicidal patients, children

Adverse effects: *italics* = common; **bold** = life-threatening

DOSAGE AND ROUTES

Depression/anxiety
Adult: PO 50-75 mg/day, may increase to 300 mg/day for severely ill, give in divided doses if >150 mg/day
Geriatric: PO 25-50 mg at bedtime, increase qwk by 25-50 mg to desired dose, max 150 mg/day

Pruritus
Adult: PO 10 mg at bedtime, may increase to 25 mg at bedtime; TOP apply a thin film qid ≥3 hr apart

Available forms: Caps 10, 25, 50, 75, 100, 150 mg; oral conc 10 mg/ml; cream 5%; tabs (Silenor) 3, 6 mg

Implementation
• **Oral conc** should be diluted with 120 ml of water, milk, or orange, grapefruit, tomato, prune, pineapple juice; do not mix with grape juice
• Give with food or milk for GI symptoms; do not give with carbonated beverages
• Give dose at bedtime if oversedation occurs during day; may take entire dose at bedtime; geriatric may not tolerate once/day dosing
• Store at room temperature; do not freeze
• Provide safety measures, primarily for geriatric
• Store in tight container protected from direct sunlight
• **Topical:** apply to affected area; rub slightly, do not use occlusive dressing

ADVERSE EFFECTS

CNS: *Dizziness, drowsiness,* confusion, headache, anxiety, tremors, stimulation, weakness, insomnia, nightmares, EPS (geriatric), increased psychiatric symptoms, paresthesia, **suicidal ideation**
CV: *Orthostatic hypotension, ECG changes,* **tachycardia**, *hypertension*, palpitations, **dysrhythmias**
EENT: *Blurred vision,* tinnitus, mydriasis, ophthalmoplegia, glossitis
GI: *Diarrhea, dry mouth,* nausea, vomiting, **paralytic ileus**, increased appetite, cramps, epigastric distress, jaundice, **hepatitis**, stomatitis, constipation
GU: *Retention,* **acute renal failure**
HEMA: **Agranulocytosis, thrombocytopenia, eosinophilia, leukopenia**, pancytopenia, purpuric disorder
INTEG: Rash, urticaria, sweating, pruritus, photosensitivity

Pharmacokinetics

Absorption	Well absorbed
Distribution	Widely distributed; crosses placenta
Metabolism	Liver, extensively
Excretion	Kidneys, breast milk
Half-life	8-24 hr

Pharmacodynamics
Unknown

INTERACTIONS

Individual drugs
Alcohol: increased CNS depression
Cimetidine, FLUoxetine, fluvoxaMINE, PARoxetine, sertraline: increased doxepin effect
CloNIDine: increased hypertensive crisis; do not use together
EPINEPHrine, norepinephrine: increased hypertensive action

Drug classifications
Antiarrhythmics, 1C (propafenone, flecainide), class III, quinolones: increased QT interval
Anticholinergics: increased anticholinergic effect
Barbiturates, benzodiazepines, CNS depressants, sedative/hypnotics: increased CNS depression
MAOIs: hypertensive crisis, seizures, hyperpyretic crisis
SSRIs, SNRIs, serotonin receptor agonists: increased toxicity

Drug/herb
St. John's wort: increased serotonin syndrome

Drug/lab test
Increased: serum bilirubin, blood glucose, alkaline phosphatase, LFTs

NURSING CONSIDERATIONS

Assessment
• **Assess chronic pain:** location, severity, type, alleviating/aggravating factors before and during treatment
• Monitor B/P (with patient lying, standing), pulse q4hr; if systolic B/P drops 20 mm Hg, hold product, notify prescriber; take VS q4hr in patients with CV disease
• Monitor blood studies: CBC, leukocytes, differential, cardiac enzymes if patient is receiving long-term therapy
• Monitor liver function tests: AST, ALT, bilirubin
• Check weight weekly; appetite may increase with product
• **Assess ECG** for flattening of T wave, bundle branch block, AV block, dysrhythmias in cardiac

patients; product should be discontinued gradually several days before surgery
• Assess for EPS primarily in geriatric: rigidity, dystonia, akathisia
• **Assess depression:** mood, sensorium, affect, **suicidal tendencies;** increase in psychiatric symptoms
• Monitor urinary retention, constipation; constipation is more likely to occur in children or geriatric
• **Assess for withdrawal symptoms:** headache, nausea, vomiting, muscle pain, weakness; do not usually occur unless product was discontinued abruptly
• Identify alcohol consumption; if alcohol is consumed, hold dose until AM

Patient/family education
• Tell patient that therapeutic effects of decreased depression may take 2-3 wk, antianxiety effects sooner; to use caution in driving and other activities requiring alertness because of drowsiness, dizziness, blurred vision
• Advise patient to avoid rising quickly from sitting to standing, especially geriatric
• Teach patient to avoid alcohol ingestion, other CNS depressants: may potentiate effects; not to discontinue medication quickly after long-term use: may cause nausea, headache, malaise
• Teach patient to wear sunscreen or large hat, since photosensitivity occurs
• Teach patient that clinical worsening and suicidal ideation may occur
• Teach patient to increase fluids, bulk in diet if constipation occurs, especially geriatric; to take gum, hard sugarless candy, or frequent sips of water for dry mouth
• Teach patient to report urinary retention immediately

Evaluation
Positive therapeutic outcome
• Decrease in depression
• Absence of suicidal thoughts

TREATMENT OF OVERDOSE:
ECG monitoring, induce emesis, lavage, activated charcoal, administer anticonvulsant

⚠ HIGH ALERT
DOXOrubicin
(dox-oh-roo′bi-sin)
Adriamycin
Func. class.: Antineoplastic, antibiotic
Chem. class.: Anthracycline glycoside
Pregnancy category D

Do not confuse:
DOXOrubicin/DOXOrubicin liposomal/DAUNOrubicin

ACTION: Inhibits DNA synthesis primarily; replication is decreased by binding to DNA, which causes strand splitting; active throughout entire cell cycle; a vesicant

USES: Wilms' tumor; bladder, breast, lung, ovarian, stomach, thyroid cancer; Hodgkin's/non-Hodgkin's disease; acute lymphoblastic leukemia; myeloblastic leukemia; neuroblastomas; lymphomas; soft tissue/bone sarcomas

CONTRAINDICATIONS:
Pregnancy (D) 1st trimester, breastfeeding, hypersensitivity, systemic infections, cardiac disorders, severe myelosuppression, lifetime dose of 550 mg/m^2

BLACK BOX WARNING: Hepatic disease

Precautions: Accidental exposure, cardiac disease, dental work, electrolyte imbalance, infection, hyperuricemia

BLACK BOX WARNING: Bone marrow suppression, extravasation, heart failure, secondary malignancy; requires an experienced clinician

DOSAGE AND ROUTES
Adult: IV 60-75 mg/m^2 q3wk, or may be used in combination with other antineoplastics with 40-60 mg/m^2 q21-28d, max cumulative dose 550 mg/m^2 or 450 mg/m^2 if prior DAUNOrubicin, cyclophosphamide, mediastinal XRT

Hepatic dose
Adult: IV Bilirubin 1.2-3 mg/dl, give 50% of dose; bilirubin 3.1-5 mg/dl, give 25% of dose

Renal dose
Adult: IV CCr <10 ml/min give 75% of dose

Available forms: Powder for inj 10, 20, 50 mg; inj 2 mg/ml

Implementation
IV route
• Give antiemetic 30-60 min before product to prevent vomiting
• Give allopurinol or sodium bicarbonate to maintain uric acid levels, alkalization of urine
⚠ Use cytotoxic handling procedures: inspect for particulate and discoloration before use

---

BLACK BOX WARNING: Do not give IM, subcut

BLACK BOX WARNING: If extravasation occurs, stop inf and complete via another vein, preferably in another limb

---

• Aluminum needles may be used during administration; avoid aluminum during storage
• Rapid injection can cause facial flushing or erythema along the vein
Reconstitution:
• To avoid risks with reconstitution, the commercially available injection may be used; there are still risks involved in handling the injection
• Do not use diluents containing preservatives to reconstitute powder for injection
• Reconstitute 10, 20, 50, 100 mg of DOXOrubicin with 5, 10, 25, 50 ml, respectively, of nonbacteriostatic NS injection (2 mg/ml), shake until completely dissolved; use reconstituted solution within 24 hr; do not expose to sunlight
• **IV injection:** Inject reconstituted solution over 0.3-5 min via Y-site or 3-way stopcock into a free-flowing IV inf of NS or D₅W; a butterfly needle inserted into a large vein is preferred

---

BLACK BOX WARNING: Care should be taken to avoid extravasation because the drug is extremely irritating to extravascular tissue

---

• Increased fluid intake to 2-3 L/day to prevent urate, calculi formation
• Store at room temperature for 24 hr after reconstituting

Y-site compatibilities: Alemtuzumab, alfentanil, amifostine, amikacin, anidulafungin, argatroban, aztreonam, bivalirudin, bleomycin, bumetanide, buprenorphine, butorphanol, calcium chloride/gluconate, CARBOplatin, carmustine, caspofungin, ceftizoxime, chlorproMAZINE, cimetidine, ciprofloxacin, CISplatin, cladribine, clindamycin, cyclophosphamide, cycloSPORINE, cytarabine, DACTINomycin, DAPTOmycin, dexamethasone, diltiazem, diphenhydrAMINE, DOBUTamine, DOCEtaxel, dolasetron, DOPamine, doripenem, doxycycline, droperidol, enalaprilat, ePHEDrine, EPINEPHrine, erythromycin, esmolol, etoposide, etoposide phosphate, famotidine, fenoldopam, fentaNYL, filgrastim, fluconazole, fludarabine, gemcitabine, gentamicin, granisetron, haloperidol, hydrocortisone, HYDROmorphone, ifosfamide, imipenem cilastatin, inamrinone, isoproterenol, ketorolac, labetalol, leucovorin, levorphanol, lidocaine, linezolid, LORazepam, mannitol, mechlorethamine, melphalan, meperidine, mesna, methotrexate, metoclopramide, metoprolol, metroNIDAZOLE, midazolam, milrinone, mitoMYcin, morphine, nalbuphine, naloxone, nesiritide, niCARdipine, nitroglycerin, nitroprusside, octreotide, ofloxacin, ondansetron, oxaliplatin, PACLitaxel, palonosetron, pancuronium, phenylephrine, potassium chloride, procainamide, prochlorperazine, promethazine, propranolol, quinupristin-dalfopristin, ranitidine, sargramostim, sodium acetate, tacrolimus, teniposide, theophylline, thiotepa, ticarcillin/clavulanate, tigecycline, tirofiban, tobramycin, topotecan, trastuzumab, trimethobenzamide, vancomycin, vasopressin, vecuronium, verapamil, vinBLAStine, vinCRIStine, vinorelbine, zidovudine, zoledronic acid

ADVERSE EFFECTS
CV: Increased B/P, sinus tachycardia, PVCs, chest pain, bradycardia, extrasystoles, **irreversible cardiomyopathy, acute left ventricular failure**
GI: *Nausea, vomiting,* anorexia, *mucositis,* **hepatotoxicity**
GU: Impotence, sterility, amenorrhea, gynecomastia, hyperuricemia, urine discoloration
HEMA: **Thrombocytopenia, leukopenia, anemia**
INTEG: *Rash,* necrosis at inj site, dermatitis, reversible *alopecia,* cellulitis, thrombophlebitis at inj site
SYST: Anaphylaxis

Pharmacokinetics
Absorption	Complete
Distribution	Crosses placenta
Metabolism	Liver
Excretion	Urine, bile, breast milk
Half-life	30 min, terminal 16.5 hr

Pharmacodynamics
Onset	Unknown
Peak	Unknown
Duration	Unknown

INTERACTIONS
Individual drugs
CycloSPORINE, mercaptopurine: increased toxicity

Fluconazole, posaconazole: increased life-threatening dysrhythmias: do not use together

Fosphenytoin, phenytoin: increased effect of these drugs

Hematopoietic progenitor cell: decreased antineoplastic effect; do not use 24 hr before or after treatment

PACLitaxel: decreased clearance of DOXOrubicin

PHENobarbital: decreased DOXOrubicin effect

Progesterone: increased neutropenia, thrombocytopenia

Streptozocin: increased DOXOrubicin effect

Drug classifications
Antineoplastics, radiation: increased toxicity

Calcium channel blockers: increased cardiomyopathy

Drugs that increase QT prolongation: increased effect

Live virus vaccine: decreased antibody response

Drug/lab test
Increased: uric acid

NURSING CONSIDERATIONS
Assessment:

> **BLACK BOX WARNING: Bone marrow depression:** CBC, differential, platelet count weekly; withhold or reduce dose of product if WBC is <1500/mm³ or platelet count is <50,000/mm³; notify prescriber of these results

• Renal studies: BUN, serum uric acid, urine CCr, electrolytes before, during therapy
• I&O ratio: Report fall in urine output to <30 ml/hr
• Monitor temperature: Fever might indicate beginning infection

> **BLACK BOX WARNING: Hepatotoxicity:** hepatic studies before, during therapy: bilirubin, AST, ALT, alk phos as needed or monthly; check for jaundice of skin and sclera, dark urine, clay-colored stools, itchy skin, abdominal pain, fever, diarrhea

> **BLACK BOX WARNING: Dysrhythmias:** ECG; watch for ST-T wave changes, low QRS and T, possible dysrhythmias (sinus tachycardia, heart block, PVCs), ejection fraction before treatment, signs of irreversible cardiomyopathy, can occur up to 6 mo after treatment begins

• Bleeding: hematuria, guaiac, bruising, petechiae of mucosa or orifices every 8 hr
• Effects of alopecia on body image; discuss feelings about body changes; almost total alopecia is expected
• Buccal cavity every 8 hr for dryness, sores, ulceration, white patches, oral pain, bleeding, dysphagia
• Alkalosis if severe vomiting is present

> **BLACK BOX WARNING: Extravasation:** local irritation, pain, burning at inj site; a vesicant; if extravasation occurs, stop drug, restart at another site, apply ice, elevate extremity to reduce swelling; if resolution does not occur, surgical debridement may be required

• GI symptoms: frequency of stools, cramping
• Rinsing of mouth tid-qid with water, club soda; brushing of teeth bid-tid with soft brush or cotton-tipped applicators for stomatitis; use unwaxed dental floss

Patient/family education
• Instruct patient to add 2-3 L of fluids unless contraindicated before and for 24-48 hr after to decrease possible hemorrhagic cystitis
• Instruct patient to report any complaints, side effects to nurse or prescriber
• Advise patient that hair may be lost during treatment; that wig or hairpiece might make patient feel better; that new hair might be different in color, texture
• Instruct patient to avoid foods with citric acid, hot or rough texture
• Instruct patient to report any bleeding, white spots, ulcerations in mouth to prescriber; to examine mouth daily
• Advise patient that urine, other body fluids may be red-orange for 48 hr
• Instruct patient to avoid crowds and persons with infections when granulocyte count is low
⚠ Advise patient that barrier contraceptive measures are recommended during therapy and for 4 mo after (pregnancy [D]); to avoid breastfeeding
• Instruct patient to avoid vaccinations

Evaluation
Positive therapeutic outcome
• Decreased tumor size, decreased spread of malignancy

> **⚠ HIGH ALERT**

DOXOrubicin liposomal
(dox-oh-roo'bi-sin)
Doxil, Lipodex
Func. class.: Antineoplastic, antibiotic
Chem. class.: Anthracycline glycoside
Pregnancy category D

Do not confuse:
DOXOrubicin liposomal/DOXOrubicin/
DAUNOrubicin

ACTION: Inhibits DNA synthesis primarily; replication is decreased by binding to DNA, which causes strand splitting; active throughout entire cell cycle; a vesicant

USES: AIDS-related Kaposi's sarcoma, multiple myeloma, metastatic ovarian carcinoma

CONTRAINDICATIONS:
Pregnancy (D), breastfeeding, hypersensitivity, systemic infections, cardiac disorders

> **BLACK BOX WARNING:** Cardiotoxicity, inf reactions, myelosuppression, hepatic disease

Precautions: Children, infection, leukopenia, stomatitis, thrombocytopenia

DOSAGE AND ROUTES
Max lifetime cumulative dose 550 mg/m^2; 400 mg/m^2 for those who have received other cardiotoxics or mediastinal radiation

Kaposi's sarcoma
Adult: **IV** 20 mg/m^2 q3wk

Multiple myeloma
Adult: **IV** 30 mg/m^2 IV inf on day 4 every 3 wk plus bortezomib 1.3 mg/m^2/dose IV bolus on days 1, 4, 8, 11 of each cycle; give DOXOrubicin liposomal after bortezomib receipt on day 4; administer up to 8 treatment cycles or until disease progression or unacceptable toxicity occurs

Ovarian cancer that has progressed or recurred after platinum-based chemotherapy
Adult: **IV** 50 mg/m^2 q4wk; continue treatment for as long as the patient shows benefit and does not progress; a minimum of 4 courses is recommended

Available forms: Liposomal dispersion for inj: 2 mg/ml

Implementation
• Prepared liposomal DOXOrubicin is a translucent, red liposomal dispersion; visually inspect for particulate matter and discoloration before use
• **Pegylated liposomal DOXOrubicin (Doxil) is for IV INF use only and should not be given IM/subcut, give under the supervision of a physician who is experienced in cancer chemotherapy**

> **BLACK BOX WARNING:** Care should be taken to avoid extravasation because the drug is irritating to extravascular tissue

• Premedication with antiemetics is recommended

IV route
• **Reconstitution (Doxil):** dilute the appropriate dose, not to exceed 90 mg/250 ml D$_5$W; do not mix with any other diluent, drugs, or bacteriostatic agent, use aseptic technique; product contains no preservative or bacteriostatic agent; diluted solution must be refrigerated and used within 24 hr
• **IV INF (Doxil):** do not administer as a bolus injection or an undiluted solution; rapid injection can increase the risk of an inf-related reaction
• **An acute inf reaction can occur during the first inf and is usually resolved by slowing the rate of inf; most patients can tolerate subsequent inf**
• **Rate:** infuse at an initial rate of 1 mg/min; if no inf-related action, the rate can be increased to complete the inf over 1 hr; do not filter
• **For hematologic toxicity in patients with ovarian cancer or HIV-related Kaposi's sarcoma: Grade 1 (ANC of 1500-1900/ mm^3, platelets ≥75,000/mm^3): No dose reduction; Grade 2 (ANC of 1000-1499/ mm^3, platelets ≥50,000/mm^3 and <75,000/ mm^3: Wait until ANC ≥1500 cells/mm^3 and platelets ≥75,000 cells/mm^3; redose with no dose reduction; Grade 3 (ANC of 500-999/ mm^3, platelets ≥25,000/ mm^3 and <50,000/ mm^3): Wait until ANC ≥1500 cells/mm^3 and platelets ≥75,000 cells/mm^3; redose with no dose reduction; Grade 4 (ANC <500/mm^3, platelets <25,000/mm^3): Wait until ANC ≥1500 cells/mm^3 and platelets ≥75,000 cells/mm^3; reduce dose by 25% or continue**

with full dose with colony-stimulating factor
• Give antiemetic 30-60 min before product to prevent vomiting
• Use allopurinol or sodium bicarbonate to maintain uric acid levels, alkalinization of urine
• Avoid mixing with other products
• Increase fluid intake to 2-3 L/day to prevent urate, calculi formation
• Store refrigerated for 24 hr after reconstituting

ADVERSE EFFECTS

CNS: Paresthesias, headache, depression, insomnia, fatigue, fever
CV: Chest pain, decreased B/P, **cardiomyopathy, heart failure, dysrhythmias, tachycardia**
EENT: Optic neuritis, rhinitis, pharyngitis, stomatitis
GI: *Nausea, vomiting,* anorexia, *mucositis,* **hepatotoxicity, constipation, oral candidiasis, abdominal pain**
HEMA: **Thrombocytopenia, leukopenia, anemia, neutropenia**
INTEG: *Rash,* **necrosis at inj site,** dermatitis, reversible *alopecia,* **exfoliative dermatitis, palmar-plantar erythrodysesthesia,** thrombophlebitis at inj site
RESP: Dyspnea, cough, respiratory infections

Pharmacokinetics

Absorption	Complete
Distribution	Crosses placenta
Metabolism	Liver
Excretion	Urine, bile, breast milk
Half-life	55 hr

Pharmacodynamics

Onset	Unknown
Peak	Unknown
Duration	Unknown

INTERACTIONS

Individual drugs

CycloSPORINE, mercaptopurine: increased toxicity
Fluconazole, posaconazole: increased life-threatening dysrhythmias: do not use together
Fosphenytoin, phenytoin: increased effect of these drugs
Hematopoietic progenitor cell: decreased antineoplastic effect; do not use 24 hr before or after treatment
PACLitaxel: decreased clearance of DOXOrubicin

PHENobarbital: decreased DOXOrubicin effect
Progesterone: increased neutropenia, thrombocytopenia
Streptozocin: increased DOXOrubicin effect

Drug classifications

Antineoplastics, radiation: increased toxicity
Calcium channel blockers: increased cardiomyopathy
Drugs that increase QT prolongation: increased effect
Live virus vaccine: decreased antibody response

Drug/lab test

Increased: uric acid

NURSING CONSIDERATIONS

Assessment

> **BLACK BOX WARNING: Bone marrow depression:** CBC, differential, platelet count weekly; withhold or reduce dose of product if WBC is <1500/mm³ or platelet count is <50,000/mm³; notify prescriber of these results

• Renal studies: BUN, serum uric acid, urine CCr, electrolytes before, during therapy
• I&O ratio: Report fall in urine output to <30 ml/hr
• Monitor temperature: Fever might indicate beginning infection

> **BLACK BOX WARNING: Hepatotoxicity:** hepatic studies before, during therapy: bilirubin, AST, ALT, alk phos as needed or monthly; check for jaundice of skin and sclera, dark urine, clay-colored stools, itchy skin, abdominal pain, fever, diarrhea

> **BLACK BOX WARNING: Dysrhythmias:** ECG; watch for ST-T wave changes, low QRS and T, possible dysrhythmias (sinus tachycardia, heart block, PVCs), ejection fraction before treatment, signs of irreversible cardiomyopathy, can occur up to 6 mo after treatment begins

• Bleeding: hematuria, guaiac, bruising, petechiae of mucosa or orifices every 8 hr
• Effects of alopecia on body image; discuss feelings about body changes; almost total alopecia is expected
• Inflammation of mucosa, breaks in skin
• Buccal cavity every 8 hr for dryness, sores, ulceration, white patches, oral pain, bleeding, dysphagia
• Alkalosis if severe vomiting is present

BLACK BOX WARNING: Extravasation: local irritation, pain, burning at inj site; a vesicant; if extravasation occurs, stop drug, restart at another site, apply ice, elevate extremity to reduce swelling; if resolution does not occur, surgical debridement may be required

---

• GI symptoms: frequency of stools, cramping
• Rinsing of mouth tid-qid with water, club soda; brushing of teeth bid-tid with soft brush or cotton-tipped applicators for stomatitis; use unwaxed dental floss

Patient/family education

• Instruct patient to add 2-3 L of fluids unless contraindicated before and for 24-48 hr after to decrease possible hemorrhagic cystitis
• Instruct patient to report any complaints, side effects to nurse or prescriber
• Advise patient that hair may be lost during treatment; that wig or hairpiece might make patient feel better; that new hair might be different in color, texture
• Instruct patient to avoid foods with citric acid, hot or rough texture
• Instruct patient to report any bleeding, white spots, ulcerations in mouth to prescriber; to examine mouth daily
• Advise patient that urine, other body fluids may be red-orange for 48 hr
• Instruct patient to avoid crowds and persons with infections when granulocyte count is low
⚠ Advise patient that barrier contraceptive measures are recommended during therapy and for 4 mo after (pregnancy [D]); to avoid breastfeeding
• Instruct patient to avoid vaccinations because reactions can occur; to avoid alcohol

Evaluation

Positive therapeutic outcome
• Decreased tumor size, decreased spread of malignancy

doxycycline (Rx)

(dox-i-sye′kleen)
Adoxa, Apo-Doxy ✦, Doryx, Doxy, Doxycaps, Doxycin ✦, doxycycline calcium, doxycycline hyclate, doxycycline monohydrate, Monodox, Oracea, Periostat, Vibramycin, Vibra-Tabs
Func. class.: Antiinfective
Chem. class.: Tetracycline
Pregnancy category D

Do not confuse:
doxycycline/doxepin/dicyclomine

ACTION: Inhibits protein synthesis, phosphorylation in microorganisms by binding to 30S ribosomal subunits, reversibly binding to 30S ribosomal subunits; bacteriostatic

Therapeutic outcome: Bactericidal action against the following: gram-positive pathogens: *Bacillus anthracis, Clostridium perfringens, Clostridium tetani, Listeria monocytogenes, Nocardia, Propionibacterium acnes, Actinomyces israelii;* gram-negative pathogens *Haemophilus influenzae, Legionella pneumophila, Yersinia enterocolitica, Yersinia pestis, Neisseria gonorrhoeae, Neisseria meningitidis, Mycoplasma, Chlamydia*

USES: Syphilis, gonorrhea, lymphogranuloma venereum, uncommon gram-negative or gram-positive organisms, malaria prophylaxis, *Acinetobacter, Actinomyces israelii, Bacillus anthracis, Bacteroides, Balantidium coli, Bartonella bacilliformis, Borrelia recurrentis, Brucella, Campylobacter fetus, Chlamydia psittaci, Chlamydia trachomatis, Clostridium, Entamoeba histolytica, Enterobacter aerogenes, Enterococcus, Escherichia coli, Francisella tularensis, Fusobacterium fusiforme, Haemophilus ducreyi, Haemophilus influenzae* (beta-lactamase negative), *Haemophilus influenzae* (beta-lactamase positive), *Klebsiella granulomatis, Klebsiella, Leptospira, Listeria monocytogenes, Mycoplasma pneumoniae, Neisseria gonorrhoeae, Neisseria meningitidis, Orientia tsutsugamushi, Plasmodium falciparum, Propionibacterium acnes, Rickettsia akari, Rickettsia prowazekii, Rickettsia rickettsii, Shigella, Staphylococcus aureus* (MSSA), *Streptococcus pneumoniae, Streptococcus pyogenes* (group A beta-hemolytic streptococci), *Treponema pallidum, Treponema*

⚠ Nurse Alert   ✹ Key NCLEX® Drug

pertenue, Ureaplasma urealyticum, Vibrio cholerae, viridans streptococci, *Yersinia pestis*

Unlabeled uses: Enterocolitis, biliary tract, intraabdominal infections; epididymitis *(Chlamydia trachomatis);* chronic prostatitis *(Ureaplasma urealyticum);* traveler's diarrhea (enterotoxigenic *Escherichia coli*); Legionnaire's disease *(Legionella pneumophila);* Lyme disease *(Borrelia burgdorferi),* Lyme disease (erythema migrans); Lyme arthritis; Lyme carditis; pleural effusion; malaria (chloroquine-resistant *Plasmodium falciparum*); pelvic inflammatory disease (PID); tubo-ovarian abscess in combination; acute dental infection, dentoalveolar infection, endodontic infection; aggressive juvenile periodontitis, plague prophylaxis *(Yersinia pestis);* tularemia prophylaxis *(Francisella tularensis);* Bancroft's filariasis (elephantiasis) *(Wuchereria bancrofti);* melioidosis due to *Burkholderia pseudomallei;* leptospirosis *(Leptospira);* infection prophylaxis for gynecologic procedures/surgical infection prophylaxis for hysterosalpingogram or chromotubation/induced abortion/dilation and evacuation; methicillin-resistant *Staphylococcus aureus* (MRSA)-associated bone and joint infections

CONTRAINDICATIONS:

Pregnancy **D**, children <8 yr, esophageal ulceration, hypersensitivity to tetracyclines

Precautions: Hepatic disease, breastfeeding, pseudomembranous colitis, ulcerative colitis, sulfite hypersensitivity, excessive sunlight

DOSAGE AND ROUTES
Most infections

Adult: PO/IV 100 mg q12hr on day 1, then 100 mg/day; **IV** 200 mg in 1-2 INF on day 1, then 100-200 mg/day

Child >8 yr (≥45 kg): PO/IV 100 mg q12hr on day 1, then 100 mg/day; severe infections 100 mg q12hr; **IV** 200 mg on day 1, then 100-200 mg/day, give 200 mg dose as 1 or 2 infusions

Child ≥8 yr, <45 kg: PO 2.2 mg/kg q12hr on day 1, then 2.2 mg/kg/day, severe infections 2.2 mg/kg q12hr; **IV** 4.4 mg/kg on day 1, then 2.2-4.4 mg/kg/day in 1-2 divided doses

Gonorrhea (uncomplicated) (patients allergic to penicillin)

Adult: PO 100 mg q12hr × 7 days, or 300 mg followed 1 hr later by another 300 mg

Malaria prophylaxis

Adult: 100 mg/day 1-2 days before travel, daily during travel, and 4 wk after return

Adolescent/child ≥8 yr <45 kg: PO 2 mg/kg/day (up to 100 mg/day) begin 1-2 days before travel, continue for 4 wk after return

Chlamydia trachomatis

Adult: PO 100 mg bid × 7 days

Syphilis

Adult: PO 100 mg bid × 14 days

Anthrax

Adult and child >8 yr and ≥45 kg: IV 100 mg q12hr, change to PO when able × 60 days

Adolescent/child ≥8 yr and <45 kg: PO 2.2 mg/kg q12hr × 60 days; **IV** 100 mg q12hr, change to PO when able × 60 days

Lyme disease

Adult: PO 100 mg bid × 14-21 days

Periodontitis

Adult: 20 mg bid after sealing and root planing for ≤9 mo; give close to meal AM or PM

Available forms: Doxycycline: cap 40 mg; **doxycycline calcium:** susp 50 mg/5 ml; **doxycycline hyclate:** cap 50, 100 mg; del rel tab 75, 100, 150 mg; del rel cap 75, 100 mg; inj 100 mg; tabs 20, 100, mg; **doxycycline monohydrate:** caps 50, 100, 150 mg; tabs 50, 75, 100 mg; oral susp 25 mg/5 ml

Implementation
PO route

• Do not break, crush, or chew caps
• Give around the clock to maintain proper blood levels; give with food to increase absorption of product; do not give within 3 hr of other agents; product reactions may occur
• Give with 8 oz of water 1 hr before bedtime to prevent ulceration
• Shake liquid preparation well before giving; use calibrated device for proper dosing
• Do not give with iron, calcium, magnesium products or antacids, which decrease absorption and form insoluble chelate
• **Del rel cap:** swallow whole or open and sprinkle on applesauce
• **Susp:** shake well, use calibrated device, may give with food/milk for GI irritation

Intermittent IV infusion route

• Check for irritation, extravasation, phlebitis daily
• Dilute each 100 mg/10 ml or 200 mg/20 ml of 0.9% NaCl, sterile water for inj; each 100 mg must be further dilute in at least 100 ml of 0.9% NaCl, D₅W, Ringer's, LR, D₅/LR; give over 1-4 hr

Adverse effects: *italics* = common; **bold** = life-threatening

- Avoid rapid use, extravasation
- Store in tight, light-resistant container at room temperature; **IV** sol stable for 12 hr at room temperature, 72 hr if refrigerated; discard if precipitate forms

Y-site compatibilities: Acyclovir, alemtuzumab, alfentanil, amifostine, amikacin, aminophylline, amiodarone, anidulafungin, ascorbic acid, atracurium, atropine, aztreonam, bivalirudin, bumetanide, buprenorphine, butorphanol, calcium chloride, calcium gluconate, CARBOplatin, caspofungin, cefonicid, cefotaxime, cefTRIAXone, chlorproMAZINE, cimetidine, cisatracurium, CISplatin, clindamycin, codeine, cyanocobalamin, cyclophosphamide, cycloSPORINE, cytarabine, DACTINomycin, DAPTOmycin, dexmedetomidine, digoxin, diltiazem, diphenhydrAMINE, DOBUTamine, DOCEtaxel, DOPamine, doxacurium, DOXOrubicin, enalapril, ePHEDrine, EPINEPHrine, epirubicin, epoetin alfa, eftifibitide, ertapenem, esmolol, etoposide, etoposide phosphate, famotidine, fenoldopam, fentaNYL, filgrastim, fluconazole, fludarabine, gemcitabine, gentamicin, glycopyrrolate, granisetron, HYDROmorphone, IDArubicin, ifosfamide, imipenem/cilastatin, insulin, isoproterenol, labetalol, levofloxacin, lidocaine, linezolid, LORazepam, magnesium sulfate, mannitol, mechlorethamine, melphalan, meperidine, metaraminol, methoxamine, methyldopate, metoclopramide, metoprolol, metroNIDAZOLE, miconazole, midazolam, milrinone, mitoXANtrone, morphine, multivitamins, nalbuphine, naloxone, nesiritide, netilmicin, nitroglycerin, nitroprusside, norepinephrine, octreotide, ondansetron, oxaliplatin, oxytocin, PACLitaxel, pancuronium, pantoprazole, papaverine, pentamidine, pentazocine, perphenazine, phentolamine, phenylephrine, phytonadione, potassium chloride, procainamide, prochlorperazine, promethazine, propofol, propranolol, protamine, pyridoxine, quinupristin/dalfopristin, ranitidine, remifentanil, ritodrine, riTUXimab, rocuronium, sargramostim, sodium acetate, streptokinase, succinylcholine, SUFentanil, tacrolimus, telavancin, teniposide, theophylline, thiamine, thiotepa, tirofiban, tobramycin, tolazoline, TPN (2 in 1), trastuzumab, trimetaphan, urokinase, vancomycin, vasopressin, vecuronium, verapamil, vinCRIStine, vinorelbine, voriconazole, zoledronic acid

Y-site incompatibilities: Allopurinol, amphotericin B colloidal, amphotericin B liposome, ampicillin, ampicillin/sulbactam, azaTHIOprine, ceFAZolin, cefoperazone, cefoTEtan, cefOXitin, ceftizoxime, cefuroxime, chloramphenicol, dantrolene, dexamethasone, diazepam, diazoxide, erythromycin, fluorouracil, folic acid, furosemide, ganciclovir, heparin, hydrocortisone, inamrinone, indomethacin, ketorolac, methotrexate, methylPREDNISolone, mezlocillin, moxalactam, nafcillin, oxacillin, palonosetron, PEMEtrexed, penicillin G, PENTobarbital, PHENobarbital, phenytoin, piperacillin/tazobactam, potassium acetate, sodium bicarbonate, trimethoprim/sulfamethoxazole

ADVERSE EFFECTS
CNS: Fever, headache
CV: Pericarditis
EENT: Dysphagia, glossitis, decreased calcification of deciduous teeth, oral candidiasis, tooth discoloration
GI: *Nausea, abdominal pain, vomiting, diarrhea,* anorexia, enterocolitis, **hepatotoxicity,** flatulence, abdominal cramps, gastric burning, stomatitis
GU: *Increased BUN*
HEMA: Eosinophilia, neutropenia, thrombocytopenia, hemolytic anemia
INTEG: Rash, urticaria, photosensitivity, increased pigmentation, **exfoliative dermatitis,** pruritus, phlebitis, injection site reaction
MS: Bone growth retardation (child <8 yr), muscle, joint pain
RESP: Cough
SYST: Stevens-Johnson syndrome, angioedema, toxic epidermal necrolysis

Pharmacokinetics

Absorption	Well absorbed
Distribution	Widely distributed, crosses placenta
Metabolism	Some hepatic recycling, 90% protein binding
Excretion	Bile, feces; kidneys unchanged (20%-40%), enters breast milk
Half-life	14-17 hr; increased in severe renal disease

Pharmacodynamics

	PO	IV
Onset	1½-4 hr	Immediate
Peak	1½-4 hr	Infusion's end

INTERACTIONS
Individual drugs
Bismuth, calcium, carBAMazepine, cimetidine, cholestyramine, colestipol, kaolin/pectin, magnesium, NaHCO$_3$, phenytoin, rifampin, sucralfate, zinc: decreased effect of doxycycline

Digoxin: increased or decreased effect of digoxin, sevelamer

Iron: forms chelates, decreased absorption

Penicillins: decreased effects of penicillins

Warfarin: increased effect of warfarin

Drug classifications
Alkali products, antacids, barbiturates: decreased effect of doxycycline

Anticoagulants (oral): increased effect of anticoagulants, methotrexate

Contraceptives (oral): decreased effect of oral contraceptive

Drug/food
Decreased: absorption with dairy products

Drug/lab test
Increased: BUN, alkaline phosphatase, bilirubin, amylase, ALT, AST, eosinophils, WBC

False increase: urinary catecholamines

NURSING CONSIDERATIONS
Assessment
• Assess patient for previous sensitivity reaction

• **Assess patient for signs and symptoms of infection** including characteristics of wounds, sputum, urine, stool, WBC >10,000/mm^3, fever; obtain baseline information before, during treatment

• Obtain C&S before beginning product therapy to identify if correct treatment has been initiated

• **Assess for allergic reactions:** rash, urticaria, pruritus, chills, fever, joint pain; angioedema may occur a few days after therapy begins

• Assess bowel pattern daily; if severe diarrhea occurs, product should be discontinued

• Monitor for bleeding: ecchymosis, bleeding gums, hematuria, stool guaiac daily if on long-term therapy; blood dyscrasias may occur

• **Assess for overgrowth of infection:** perineal itching, fever, malaise, redness, pain, swelling, drainage, rash, diarrhea, change in cough, sputum

Patient/family education
• Teach patient to report sore throat, bruising, bleeding, joint pain; may indicate blood dyscrasias (rare)

• Advise patient to contact prescriber if vaginal itching, loose foul-smelling stools, furry tongue occur; may indicate superinfection; report itching, rash, pruritus, urticaria

• Instruct patient to take all medication prescribed for the length of time ordered; product must be taken around the clock to maintain blood levels; do not give medication to others

• Advise patient to notify prescriber of diarrhea with blood or pus

• Teach patient not to use with antacids, iron products, H$_2$ blockers, sevelamer

• Advise patient to take with full glass of water, if nausea occurs take with food

Evaluation
Positive therapeutic outcome
• Absence of signs/symptoms of infection (WBC <10,000/mm^3, temp WNL, absence of red draining wounds)

• Reported improvement in symptoms of infection

⚠ HIGH ALERT

dronedarone (Rx)
(drone-da-rone)
Multaq
Func. class.: Antidysrhythmic (Class III)
Chem. class.: Iodinated benzofuran derivative
Pregnancy category X

ACTION: Prolongs action potential duration and effective refractory period, noncompetitive α- and β-adrenergic inhibition; increases PR and QT intervals, decreases sinus rate, decreases peripheral vascular resistance

Therapeutic outcome: Decreased amount and severity of ventricular dysrhythmias

USES: Atrial fibrillation, atrial flutter

CONTRAINDICATIONS:
Pregnancy **X,** breastfeeding, severe sinus node dysfunction, 2nd- or 3rd-degree AV block; bradycardia, hypersensitivity, heart failure, hepatic disease, QT prolongation

BLACK BOX WARNING: NYHA class IV heart failure or class II-III with recent decompensation requiring hospitalization, permanent atrial fibrillation (cannot restore sinus rhythm)

Precautions: Children, electrolyte imbalances, elderly, Asian patients, females, atrial fibrillation/flutter

---

DOSAGE AND ROUTES
Adult: PO 400 mg bid; discontinue class I, III antidysrhythmias or strong CYP3A4 inhibitors prior to beginning treatment; max 800 mg/day
Available forms: Tabs 400 mg

Implementation
• Start with patient hospitalized and monitored
PO route
• Give reduced dosage slowly with ECG monitoring only
• Give loading dose with food to decrease nausea

ADVERSE EFFECTS
CNS: Weakness
CV: *Bradycardia,* **heart failure, QT prolongation, torsades de pointes,** atrial flutter
ENDO: Hypo/hyperthyroidism
GI: Nausea, vomiting, diarrhea, abdominal pain, **severe hepatic injury, hepatic failure**
INTEG: Rash, photosensitivity, **angioedema**
RESP: Interstitial pneumonitis, pulmonary fibrosis

Pharmacokinetics
Absorption	Slow, variable (PO) up to 65%
Distribution	Body tissues; crosses placenta
Metabolism	Liver
Excretion	Bile, kidney (minimal)
Half-life	15-100 day

Pharmacodynamics
	PO
Onset	1-3 wk
Peak	Unknown
Duration	Up to months

INTERACTIONS
Individual drugs
CycloSPORINE, dextromethorphan, digoxin, disopyramide, flecainide, methotrexate, phenytoin, procainamide, quiNIDine, theophylline: increased blood levels, increased toxicity
Dabigatran, warfarin: increased anticoagulant effect

Drug classifications
β-Adrenergic blockers, calcium channel blockers: increased bradycardia
CYP3A4 inhibitors, CYP2D6 inhibitors: increased dronedarone levels
CYP3A, CYP2D6 inducers: decreased dronedarone levels
CYP3A, CYP2D6 substrates: increased levels

Drug/herb
St. John's wort: decreased effect
Yohimbine: increased anticoagulant effect

Drug/food
Grapefruit juice: increased dronedarone effect, avoid use

Drug/lab test
Increased: T4, LFTs, bilirubin, creatinine
Decreased: potassium, magnesium

NURSING CONSIDERATIONS
Assessment
• Monitor I&O ratio; monitor electrolytes: potassium, creatinine, magnesium
• Monitor liver function studies: AST, ALT, bilirubin, alkaline phosphatase

> **BLACK BOX WARNING:** NYHA Class IV heart failure or symptomatic heart failure with recent decomposition requiring hospitalization doubles risk of death

• Monitor **ECG** to determine product effectiveness; measure PR, QRS, QT intervals; check for PVCs, other dysrhythmias; monitor B/P continuously for hypo/hypertension; check for rebound hypertension after 1-2 hr
• Monitor serum creatine, potassium, magnesium
• Monitor for dehydration or hypovolemia
• **Assess for hypothyroidism:** lethargy, dizziness, constipation, enlarged thyroid gland, edema of extremities, cool, pale skin
• **Monitor hyperthyroidism:** restlessness, tachycardia, eyelid puffiness, weight loss, frequent urination, menstrual irregularities, dyspnea, warm, moist skin
• Monitor cardiac rate, respiration: rate, rhythm, character, chest pain, ventricular tachycardia, supraventricular tachycardia or fibrillation
• Assess sight and vision before treatment and throughout therapy; microdeposits on the cornea may cause blurred vision, halos, and photophobia

Patient/family education
• Instruct patient to report weight gain, edema, difficulty breathing immediately to prescriber
• Instruct patient to use sunscreen and protective clothing to prevent burning associated with photosensitivity
• Instruct patient to take medication as prescribed, not to double doses, avoid use with all other products without approval of prescriber, do not use grapefruit juice

---

⚠ Nurse Alert   ❋ Key NCLEX® Drug

• Instruct patient to complete follow-up appointment with health care provider, including pulmonary function studies, chest x-ray
• Teach patient to use effective contraception during treatment, pregnancy **X**, do not breastfeed

Evaluation
Positive therapeutic outcome
• Decreased dysrhythmias

TREATMENT OF OVERDOSE:
Administer O₂, artificial ventilation, ECG, DOPamine for circulatory depression, diazepam or thiopental for seizures, isoproterenol

---

⚠ HIGH ALERT

droperidol (Rx)
(droe-per′i-dole)
Func. class.: Sedative-hypnotic
Chem. class.: Butyrophenone derivative
Pregnancy category C

ACTION: Acts on CNS at subcortical levels, producing tranquilization, sleep; antiemetic; mild α-blockade

Therapeutic outcome: Maintenance of anesthesia

USES: Premedication for surgery; induction, maintenance in general anesthesia; postoperatively for nausea and vomiting

CONTRAINDICATIONS:
Hypersensitivity, breastfeeding, child <2 yr

BLACK BOX WARNING: QT prolongation, torsades de pointes

Precautions: Pregnancy **C**, geriatric, CV disease (hypotension, bradydysrhythmias), renal/hepatic disease, Parkinson's disease, pheochromocytoma, CHF, hypokalemia, hypomagnesemia, cardiac hypertrophy

DOSAGE AND ROUTES
Induction, adjunct
Adult: **IV/IM** 1.25-2.5 mg, may give additional 1.25 mg with caution
Child 2-12 yr: **IV** 0.05-0.1 mg/kg titrate to response

Premedication
Adult: **IM** 2.5 mg ½-1 hr before surgery, may give 1.25-2.5 mg additionally
Child 2-12 yr: **IM** 0.05-0.1 mg/kg

Available forms: Inj 2.5 mg/ml
Implementation
• Protect from light
IM route
• Give deeply in large muscle mass

Direct IV route
• Give undiluted; give through Y-tube or 3-way stopcock at 10 mg or less/min; titrate to patient response
Intermittent IV infusion route
• May be given by adding dose to 250 ml of LR, D₅W, 0.9% NaCl; give slowly, titrate to patient response
• Give anticholinergics (benztropine, diphenhydrAMINE) for extrapyramidal reaction
• Give only with resuscitative equipment nearby

Syringe compatibilities: Atropine, bleomycin, butorphanol, chlorproMAZINE, cimetidine, CISplatin, cyclophosphamide, dimenhyDRINATE, diphenhydrAMINE, DOXOrubicin, fentaNYL, glycopyrrolate, hydrOXYzine, meperidine, metoclopramide, midazolam, mitoMYcin, morphine, nalbuphine, pentazocine, perphenazine, prochlorperazine, promazine, promethazine, scopolamine, vinBLAStine, vinCRIStine

Syringe incompatibilities: Fluorouracil, furosemide, heparin, leucovorin, methotrexate, pentobarbital

Y-site compatibilities: Amifostine, aztreonam, bleomycin, cisatracurium, CISplatin, cladribine, cyclophosphamide, cytarabine, DOXOrubicin, DOXOrubicin liposome, famotidine, filgrastim, fluconazole, fludarabine, granisetron, hydrocortisone sodium succinate, IDArubicin, melphalan, meperidine, metoclopramide, mitoMYcin, ondansetron, PACLitaxel, potassium chloride, propofol, remifentanil, sargramostim, teniposide, thiotepa, vinBLAStine, vinCRIStine, vinorelbine, vit B/C

Y-site incompatibilities: Fluorouracil, foscarnet, furosemide, leucovorin, methotrexate, nafcillin

Additive incompatibilities: Barbiturates

ADVERSE EFFECTS
CNS: EPS: Dystonia, akathisia, flexion of arms, fine tremors; dizziness, anxiety, drowsiness, restlessness, hallucinations, depression, **seizures, neuroleptic malignant syndrome**
CV: Tachycardia, *hypotension*, **QT prolongation, torsades de pointes**

EENT: Upward rotation of eyes, oculogyric crisis
INTEG: *Chills, facial sweating, shivering*
RESP: Laryngospasm, bronchospasm

Pharmacokinetics

Absorption	Well absorbed (IM)
Distribution	Crosses blood-brain barrier, placenta
Metabolism	Liver
Excretion	Kidneys, unchanged (10%)
Half-life	2-3 hr

Pharmacodynamics

	IM/IV
Onset	3-10 min
Peak	30 min
Duration	3-6 hr

INTERACTIONS
Individual drugs
Alcohol: increased CNS depression
Lithium: increased side effects of lithium

Drug classifications
Antihistamines, antipsychotics, barbiturates, CNS depressants, opiates: increased CNS depression
Antihypertensives, nitrates: increased hypotension

> **BLACK BOX WARNING:** Class IA/III antiarrhythmics, some phenothiazines, some quinolones, tricyclics, others: increased QT prolongation

Drug/herb
Chamomile, hops, kava, valerian: increased action

NURSING CONSIDERATIONS
Assessment
⚠ **Check VS q10min during IV administration, q30min after IM dose; for increasing heart rate or decreasing B/P, notify prescriber at once; do not place patient in Trendelenburg's position, sympathetic blockade may occur, causing respiratory arrest**
• Assess extrapyramidal reactions: dystonia, akathisia, extended neck, restlessness, tremors; if these occur, an anticholinergic should be given
• If given for nausea or vomiting, monitor for significant loss of fluids, bowel sounds before, during administration

> **BLACK BOX WARNING: QT prolongation, torsades de pointes:** ECG prior to and 2-3 hr after administration for serious arrhythmias

Patient/family education
• Advise patient that orthostatic hypotension is common; to rise from lying or sitting position slowly; to avoid ambulation without assistance
• Caution patient that drowsiness, dizziness may occur; to call for assistance for ambulation

Evaluation
Positive therapeutic outcome
• Decreased anxiety
• Absence of vomiting during and after surgery

DULoxetine (Rx)
(du-lox'uh-teen)
Cymbalta
Func. class.: Antidepressant, miscellaneous
Chem. class: Serotonin, norepinephrine reuptake inhibitor (SNRI)
Pregnancy category C

ACTION: Unknown, may potentiate serotoninergic, noradrenergic activity in the CNS. In studies duloxetine is a potent inhibitor of neuronal serotonin and norepinephrine reuptake

Therapeutic outcome: Decreased depression, decreased neuropathic pain

USES: Major depressive disorder (MDD), neuropathic pain associated with diabetic neuropathy, generalized anxiety disorder, fibromyalgia, chronic low back pain, osteoarthritis pain

CONTRAINDICATIONS:
Hypersensitivity, closed-angle glaucoma, alcohol intoxication, alcoholism, hepatic disease, hepatitis, jaundice

Precautions: Pregnancy **C,** breastfeeding, geriatric, mania, hypertension, cardiac/renal/hepatic disease, seizures, increased intraocular pressure, anorexia nervosa, bleeding, dehydration, diabetes, hyponatremia, hypotension, hypovolemia, orthostatic hypotension, abrupt drug withdrawal

> **BLACK BOX WARNING:** Children, suicidal ideation

DOSAGE AND ROUTES

Depression
Adult: PO 40-60 mg/day as a single dose or 2 divided doses

Diabetic neuropathy
Adult: PO 60 mg qday

Generalized anxiety disorder
Adult: PO 60 mg/day, may start with 30 mg/day × 1 wk, then increase to 60 mg/day, maintenance 60-120 mg/day

Fibromyalgia
Adult: PO 30 mg/day × 1 wk, then 60 mg/day

Musculoskeletal pain
Adult: PO 60 mg/day or 30 mg/day × 1 wk, then 60 mg/day

Renal dose
Adult: PO Start with 20 mg, gradually increase; avoid use in severe renal disease

Available forms: Caps 20, 30, 60 mg

Implementation
• Swallow caps whole; do not break, crush, or chew; do not sprinkle on food or mix with liquid
• Give without regard to food
• Store in tight container at room temperature; do not freeze
• Provide assistance with ambulation during beginning therapy, since drowsiness, dizziness occur
• Check to see if PO medication was swallowed

ADVERSE EFFECTS

CNS: Insomnia, anxiety, dizziness, tremor, somnolence, fatigue, decreased appetite, decreased weight, agitation, diaphoresis, hallucinations, **neuroleptic malignant syndrome–like reaction,** aggression, **seizures,** headache, abnormal dreams, flushing, hot flashes, chills
CV: **Thrombophlebitis,** peripheral edema, palpitations, hypertension, **supraventricular dysrhythmia,** orthostatic hypotension
EENT: *Abnormal vision*
ENDO: Hypoglycemia, SIADH
GI: Constipation, diarrhea, dysphagia, *nausea,* vomiting, anorexia, dry mouth, colitis, gastritis, abdominal pain, **hepatic failure**
GU: Abnormal ejaculation, urinary hesitation, ejaculation delayed, erectile dysfunction, urinary frequency/retention, gyn bleeding
INTEG: Photosensitivity, bruising, sweating, **Stevens-Johnson syndrome**
MS: Gait disturbances, muscle spasm, restless legs syndrome, myalgia

SYST: Anaphylaxis, angioedema, serotonin syndrome, Stevens-Johnson syndrome

Pharmacokinetics

Absorption	Well absorbed
Distribution	90% protein binding
Metabolism	Extensively metabolized (CYP2D6, CYP1A2) in the liver to an active metabolite
Excretion	70% of product recovered in urine, 20% in feces
Half-life	12 hr

Pharmacodynamics
Unknown

INTERACTIONS

Individual drugs
Alcohol: increased ALT, bilirubin

Drug classifications
⚠ **MAOIs:** coadministration (or within 14 days of MAOIs use) is contraindicated: hyperthermia, rigidity, rapid fluctuations of VS, mental status changes, neuroleptic malignant syndrome
Anticoagulants, antiplatelets, salicylates, NSAIDs: increased bleeding risk
Opioids, antihistamines, sedative/hypnotics: increased CNS depression
CYP1A2 inhibitors (fluvoxaMINE, quinolone antiinfectives); CYP2D6 inhibitors (FLUoxetine, quiNIDine, PARoxetine): increased action of DULoxetine
CYP2D6 extensively metabolized products (flecainide, phenothiazines, propafenone, tricyclics, thioridazine): narrow therapeutic index
SSRIs serotonin receptor agonists: increased serotonin syndrome, neuroleptic malignant syndrome

Drug/herb
Kava: increased CNS depression
St. John's wort: serotonin syndrome

Drug/lab test
Increased: blood glucose

NURSING CONSIDERATIONS
Assessment

> **BLACK BOX WARNING: Depression:** Assess mental status: mood, sensorium, affect, **suicidal tendencies,** increase in psychiatric symptoms; depression, panic

• Assess B/P lying, standing; pulse q4hr; if systolic B/P drops 20 mm Hg, hold product, notify prescriber; take VS q4hr in patients with CV disease
• Monitor hepatic studies: AST, ALT, bilirubin
• Monitor weight qwk; weight loss or gain; appetite may increase; peripheral edema may occur
• Offer sugarless gum, hard candy, frequent sips of water for dry mouth
• Assess for withdrawal symptoms: headache, nausea, vomiting, muscle pain, weakness; not usual unless product is discontinued abruptly
⚠ **Assess for neuroleptic malignant syndrome–like reaction**
• **Serotonin syndrome:** assess for nausea, vomiting, dizziness, facial flushing, shivering, sweating
• **Sexual dysfunction:** ejaculation dysfunction, erectile dysfunction, decreased libido, orgasm dysfunction

Patient/family education
• Advise that product is dispensed in small amounts because of suicide potential, especially in the beginning of therapy
• Teach patient/family to use caution when driving or other activities requiring alertness because of drowsiness, dizziness, blurred vision
• Advise patient to avoid alcohol ingestion, other CNS depressants, MAOIs
• **Abrupt discontinuation:** Advise patient not to discontinue medication quickly after long-term use; may cause nausea, headache, malaise
• Advise patient to wear sunscreen or large hat, since photosensitivity may occur
• Advise patient to notify prescriber if pregnancy is planned or suspected or if breastfeeding
• Tell patient that improvement may occur in 4-8 wk; up to 12 wk (geriatric patients)

> **BLACK BOX WARNING:** Advise that clinical worsening and suicide risk may occur

Evaluation
Positive therapeutic outcome
• Decreased depression

---

dutasteride (Rx)
(doo-tass′ter-ide)
Avodart
Func. class.: Sex hormone, 5α-reductase inhibitor
Chem. class.: Synthetic 4-azasteroid compound
Pregnancy category X

ACTION: Inhibits both types 1 and 2 forms of a steroid enzyme that converts testosterone to 5 μ-dihydrotestosterone (DHT), which is responsible for the initial growth of prostatic tissue

Therapeutic outcome: Decreased symptoms of benign prostatic hyperplasia (BPH)

USES: Treatment of symptomatic BPH in men with an enlarged prostate gland, or may be used in combination with tamsulosis

Unlabeled uses: Alopecia

CONTRAINDICATIONS:
Pregnancy **X,** breastfeeding, children, women, hypersensitivity

Precautions: Hepatic disease

DOSAGE AND ROUTES
Benign prostatic hyperplasia (BPH)
Adult: PO 0.5 mg/day

Alopecia (unlabeled)
Adult: PO 0.5-2.5 mg/day

Available forms: Caps 0.5 mg

Implementation
• Swallow caps whole: do not break, crush, chew, or open
• May be given without regard to meals

ADVERSE EFFECTS
GU: Decreased libido, impotence, gynecomastia, ejaculation disorders (rare), mastalgia, teratogenesis
INTEG: Serious skin infections

Pharmacokinetics

Absorption	Absolute bioavailability ~60%
Distribution	Protein binding 99%
Metabolism	Liver (CYP3A4)
Excretion	Feces
Half-life	5 wk at steady state

Pharmacodynamics

Onset	Rapid
Peak	2-3 hr
Duration	Levels detectable 4-6 mo posttreatment

INTERACTIONS

Individual drugs
Cimetidine, ciprofloxacin, diltiazem, ketoconazole, ritonavir, verapamil: increased dutasteride concentrations

Drug classifications
Antiretroviral protease inhibitors or other CYP3A4-metabolized products: increased dutasteride concentrations

Drug/lab test
Decreased: PSA

NURSING CONSIDERATIONS

Assessment
• **Assess for decreasing symptoms in BPH:** decreasing urinary retention, frequency, urgency, nocturia
• Assess PSA levels, digital rectal exam, urinary obstruction; determine the absence of urinary cancer before starting treatment
• Assess liver function tests: ALT, AST, bilirubin; blood studies: CBC with differential, serum creatitine, serum electrolytes

Patient/family education
• Advise patient to notify prescriber if therapeutic response decreases, if edema occurs

• Caution patient not to discontinue product abruptly
• Inform patient about changes in sex characteristics
• Caution patient not to donate blood for at least 6 mo after last dose to prevent possible blood administration to pregnant woman
• Advise patient and family that caps should not be handled by pregnant women or those who may become pregnant since this product can be absorbed through the skin
• Inform patient that ejaculate volume may decrease during treatment, that product rarely interferes with sexual function
• Advise patient to read patient information leaflet before starting therapy and reread it upon prescription renewal
• Teach patient product should not be used or handled by breastfeeding women
• Advise patient to swallow whole; do not crush, chew, or open
• Teach patient that drug may increase risk for developing high-grade prostate cancer

Evaluation
Positive therapeutic outcome
• Decreased levels of DHT (5 α-dihydrotestosterone)
• Decreased urinary frequency
• Decreased urinary retention
• Decreased urinary urgency
• Decreased nocturia

Adverse effects: *italics* = common; **bold** = life-threatening

ecallantide
(ee-kal'lan-tide)
Kalbitor
Func. class.: Protein inhibitor—kallikrein inhibitor
Pregnancy category C

CONTRAINDICATIONS:
Hypersensitivity

BLACK BOX WARNING: Anaphylaxis

DOSAGE AND ROUTES
Adult/adolescent ≥16 yr: Subcut 30 mg as three 10-mg injections; give additional 30-mg dose within 24 hr if attack persists

Implementation
• Using aseptic technique, withdraw 1 ml (10 mg) using a large-bore needle. Change the needle on the syringe to a needle suitable for subcut injection (27 gauge recommended)
• Inject into the skin of the abdomen, thigh, or upper arm
• Repeat the procedure for each of the three vials (30-mg total dose). The injection site for each of the three injections may be in the same or different anatomic location (abdomen, thigh, or upper arm). There is no need for site rotation. Individual injections should be separated by at least 2 inches and away from the anatomical site of attack
• The same directions for administration apply if an additional dose is required within 24 hr. Different injection sites or the same anatomical location as used for the first dose may be used
• Visually inspect parenteral products for particulate matter and discoloration prior to administration

econazole topical
See Appendix B

ecothiophate ophthalmic
See Appendix B

efavirenz (Rx)
(ef-ah-veer'enz)
Sustiva
Func. class.: Antiretroviral
Chem. class.: Nonnucleoside reverse transcriptase inhibitor (NNRTI)
Pregnancy category D

ACTION: Binds directly to reverse transcriptase and blocks RNA polymerase and DNA polymerase, causing a disruption of the enzyme's site

Therapeutic outcome: Improvement of HIV-1 infection

USES: HIV-1 in combination with other antiretrovirals

CONTRAINDICATIONS:
Pregnancy **D**, hypersensitivity

Precautions: Liver disease, breastfeeding, children <3 yr, renal disease, myelosuppression, depression, seizures

DOSAGE AND ROUTES
Given in combination with protease inhibitor or nucleoside analog reverse transcriptase inhibitors (NRTIs)
Adult and child >40 kg: PO 600 mg/day at bedtime
Child ≥3 mo:
10-14.9 kg: PO 200 mg/day at bedtime
15-19.9 kg: PO 250 mg/day at bedtime
20-24.9 kg: PO 300 mg/day at bedtime
25-32.4 kg: PO 350 mg/day at bedtime
32.5-39.9 kg: PO 400 mg/day at bedtime
Child ≥3 mo, 5-<7.5 kg: PO 150 mg/day at bedtime
Child 3.5≤5 kg: PO 100 mg/day at bedtime

Available forms: Caps 50, 100, 200 mg; tabs 600 mg

Implementation
• Give at bedtime to decrease CNS side effects, give on empty stomach

ADVERSE EFFECTS
CNS: Headache, dizziness, fatigue, impaired cognition, insomnia, abnormal dreams, depression, anxiety, drowsiness
GI: *Diarrhea,* abdominal pain, *nausea,* hyperlipidemia, constipation, increased liver function tests
GU: Hematuria, kidney stones

INTEG: *Rash,* erythema multiforme, Stevens-Johnson syndrome, toxic epidermal necrolysis, exfoliative dermatitis

Pharmacokinetics

Absorption	Well absorbed, concentrations higher in females, Africans, Asians, Hispanics
Distribution	Highly protein bound (99%)
Metabolism	Liver
Excretion	Kidneys, feces
Half-life	Terminal 52-76 hr

Pharmacodynamics

Onset	Unknown
Peak	3-5 hr
Duration	Unknown

INTERACTIONS

Individual drugs

Alcohol: increased CNS depression

Amprenavir, clarithromycin, indinavir, itraconazole, ketoconazole, lopinavir, methadone, posaconazole, saquinavir, voriconazole: decreased level of each specific product

CarBAMazepine: decreased efavirenz levels

Cisapride, midazolam, triazolam: do not give together

Ritonavir: increased levels of both products

Drug classifications

Anticonvulsants, ergots, statins (except pravastatin, fluvastatin): increased levels of each specific product

Antidepressants, antihistamines, opioids: increased CNS depression

Benzodiazepines, ergots: do not give together

CYP3A4 inhibitors (conivaptan, ambrisentan, sorafenib): decreased efavirenz metabolism

CYP3A4 inducers (carBAMazepine, rifamycins): decreased efavirenz effect

Estrogens: increased level of both products

Oral contraceptives, non-oral contraceptives: decreased level of these products

Rifamycins: decreased efavirenz action

Drug/herb

St. John's wort: decreased efavirenz level; do not use together

Drug/food

Increased: absorption of high-fat foods

Drug/lab test

Increased: ALT

False positive: cannabinoids

NURSING CONSIDERATIONS

Assessment

⚠ **Pregnancy:** Rule out pregnancy (D) before starting treatment; a type of contraception is needed, oral/non-oral contraceptives are decreased

• **HIV:** Assess CBC, blood chemistry, plasma HIV RNA, absolute $CD4^+/CD8^+/$cell counts/%, serum β_2 microglobulin, serum ICD+24 antigen levels, cholesterol, hepatic enzymes

• **Serious skin reactions:** Stevens-Johnson syndrome, toxic epidermal necrolysis

• Assess bowel pattern before, during treatment; if severe abdominal pain with bleeding occurs, product should be discontinued; monitor hydration

• **Assess for signs of toxicity:** severe nausea/vomiting, maculopapular rash

Patient/family education

• Advise patient to take as prescribed; if dose is missed, take as soon as remembered; do not double dose; take on empty stomach with water/juice

• Instruct patient to make sure health care provider knows of all the medications being taken, supplements, herbs, OTC products

• Advise patient that if severe rash occurs, stop taking and notify health care provider

⚠ **Advise patient not to breastfeed or become pregnant (pregnancy D) if taking this product**

• Advise patient that adverse reactions (rash, dizziness, abnormal dreams, insomnia) lessen after a month

• Teach patient to avoid hazardous activities if dizziness, drowsiness occurs

• Teach patient that product does not cure disease but controls symptoms; HIV can be transmitted to others even while taking this product

• Advise patient to continue safer-sex practices

Evaluation

Positive therapeutic outcome

• Increased CD4, cell counts

• Decreased viral load

• Improvement in symptoms and progression of HIV-1 infection

eletriptan (Rx)

(el-ee-trip′tan)

Relpax

Func. class.: Antimigraine agent

Pregnancy category C

ACTION: Binds selectively to the vascular $5-HT_1$-receptor subtype, exerts antimigraine effect; causes vasoconstriction in cranial arteries

Therapeutic outcome: Decreased severity of migraine

USES: Acute treatment of migraine with or without aura

CONTRAINDICATIONS:

Uncontrolled hypertension, hypersensitivity, basilar or hemiplegic migraine, ischemic bowel disease, severe renal/hepatic disease, coronary artery vasospasm, peripheral vascular disease, heart disease, acute MI, stroke, angina, CV disease

Precautions: Pregnancy **C**, breastfeeding, children, geriatric, postmenopausal women, men >40 yr, risk factors of CAD, MI, or other cardiac disease, hypercholesterolemia, obesity, diabetes, impaired renal/hepatic function

DOSAGE AND ROUTES

Adult: **PO** 20 or 40 mg, may increase if needed, max 40 mg (single dose); may repeat in 2 hr if headache improves but returns, max 80 mg/24 hr

Available forms: Tabs 20, 40 mg

Implementation

• Swallow tabs whole; do not break, crush, or chew, take with 8 oz of water

• Provide quiet, calm environment with decreased stimulation from noise, bright light, excessive talking

ADVERSE EFFECTS

CNS: *Dizziness,* headache, anxiety, paresthesia, asthenia, somnolence, flushing, fatigue, hot/cold sensation, chills, vertigo, hypertonia, **seizures, serotonin syndrome**

CV: Chest pain, palpitations, hypertension, **MI, sinus tachycardia, stroke, ventricular fibrillation/tachycardia, atrial fibrillation, AV block, bradycardia, chest pressure syndrome, coronary vasospasm**

GI: Nausea, dry mouth, vomiting

MS: *Weakness,* back pain

RESP: Chest tightness, pressure

Pharmacokinetics

Absorption	Unknown
Distribution	Unknown
Metabolism	Liver
Excretion	Urine, feces
Half-life	Unknown

Pharmacodynamics

Onset	Of pain relief 2 hr
Peak	Unknown
Duration	Unknown

INTERACTIONS

Individual drugs

Clarithromycin, erythromycin, itraconazole, ketoconazole, nelfinavir, propanolol, ritonavir: increased plasma concentration of eletriptan

Drug classifications

CYP3A4 inhibitors: increased concentration of ergots, eletriptan

SSRIs, SNRIs, serotonin-receptor agonists: increased serotonin syndrome

NURSING CONSIDERATIONS

Assessment

• **Migraine:** pain location, character, intensity, nausea, vomiting, aura

• Monitor B/P; signs/symptoms of coronary vasospasms; geriatrics may be at higher risk

• Assess for tingling, hot sensation, burning, feeling of pressure, numbness, flushing

• Assess stress level, activity, recreation, coping mechanisms

• Assess neurologic status: LOC, blurring vision, nausea, vomiting, tingling in extremities preceding headache

• Identify ingestion of tyramine foods (pickled products, beer, wine, aged cheese), food additives, preservatives, colorings, artificial sweeteners, chocolate, caffeine, which may precipitate these types of headaches

Patient/family education

• Have patient report any side effects to prescriber

• Teach patient to use contraception while taking product

• Teach patient to have dark, quiet environment

• Teach patient that product does not prevent or reduce number of migraine attacks

Evaluation

Positive therapeutic outcome

• Decreased severity of migraine

⚠ Nurse Alert   ✦ Key NCLEX® Drug

eltrombopag
Promacta
See Appendix A, Selected New Drugs

emedastine ophthalmic
See Appendix B

emtricitabine (Rx)
(em-tri-sit'uh-bean)
Emtriva
Func. class.: Antiretroviral
Chem. class.: Nucleoside reverse transcriptase inhibitor (NRTI)
Pregnancy category B

ACTION: Synthetic nucleoside analog of cytosine; inhibits replication of HIV virus by competing with the natural substrate and then becoming incorporated into cellular DNA by viral reverse transcriptase, thereby terminating cellular DNA chain

Therapeutic outcome: Decreasing symptoms of HIV

USES: HIV-1 infection with other antiretrovirals

Unlabeled uses: HBV (hepatitis B virus) infection

CONTRAINDICATIONS:
Hypersensitivity

> **BLACK BOX WARNING:** Lactic acidosis

Precautions: Pregnancy **B**, breastfeeding, children, geriatric, renal disease

> **BLACK BOX WARNING:** Hepatic insufficiency, chronic hepatitis B virus (HBV) infection

DOSAGE AND ROUTES
Oral cap and sol are not interchangeable
Adult: PO (caps) 200 mg/day; oral SOL 240 mg (24 ml) daily
Adolescent/child >33 kg: PO (caps) 200 mg/day
Child 3 mo-17 yr: oral SOL 6 mg/kg/day, max 240 mg (24 ml)
Infant <3 mo: PO oral SOL 3 mg/kg daily, do not use caps

Renal dose
Adult: PO CCr 30-49 ml/min 200 mg q48hr, SOL 120 mg q24hr; caps CCr 15-29 ml/min 200 mg q72hr, SOL 80 mg q24hr; caps CCr <15 ml/min 200 mg q96hr, SOL 60 mg q24hr

Available forms: Caps 200 mg; oral sol 10 mg/ml; oral cap and sol are not interchangeable

Implementation
- Give without regard to meals
- Store at 25° C (77° F)
- Take at same time every day
- Oral cap and sol are not interchangeable

ADVERSE EFFECTS
CNS: Headache, abnormal dreams, depression, dizziness, insomnia, neuropathy, paresthesia, *asthenia*
GI: *Nausea, vomiting, diarrhea, anorexia, abdominal pain, dyspepsia,* **hepatomegaly with stenosis (may be fatal)**
INTEG: Rash, skin discoloration
MS: Arthralgia, myalgia
RESP: Cough
SYST: Change in body fat distribution, **lactic acidosis**

Pharmacokinetics
Absorption	Rapidly, extensively absorbed
Distribution	Protein binding <4%
Metabolism	Unknown
Excretion	Excreted unchanged in urine (86%), feces (14%)
Half-life	10 hr

Pharmacodynamics
Onset	Unknown
Peak	1-2 hr
Duration	Unknown

INTERACTIONS
Efavirenz, lamiVUDine, tenofovir: Do not use together, treatment duplication
Ribavirin: Complex interactions

Drug classifications
Interferons: Decreased emtricitabine level

NURSING CONSIDERATIONS
Assessment
- Monitor liver, renal function tests: AST, ALT, bilirubin, amylase, lipase, triglycerides periodically during treatment

BLACK BOX WARNING: Assess for lactic acidosis, severe hepatomegaly with steatosis; if lab reports confirm these conditions, discontinue treatment; more common in females, obese; monitor serum lactate levels, liver function tests

BLACK BOX WARNING: Confirm that patient is free of HBV (hepatitis B virus) before starting treatment

BLACK BOX WARNING: Hepatotoxicity: Do not use in those with risk factors such as alcoholism; discontinue if hepatotoxicity occurs

BLACK BOX WARNING: Hepatitis B and HIV coinfection (unlabeled): Perform HBV screening in any patient who has HIV to ensure appropriate treatment; avoid single-drug treatments in HBV

Patient/family education

• Teach that GI complaints resolve after 3-4 wk of treatment
• Advise patient to report planned or suspected pregnancy, not to breastfeed while taking this product
• Instruct that product must be taken at same time of day to maintain blood level
• Advise that product will control symptoms, but is not a cure for HIV; patient is still infectious, may pass HIV virus on to others
• Instruct that other products may be necessary to prevent other infections
• Advise that changes in body fat distribution may occur

BLACK BOX WARNING: Lactic acidosis: notify prescriber immediately of fatigue, muscle aches/pains, abdominal pain, difficulty breathing, nausea, vomiting, change in heart rate

BLACK BOX WARNING: Hepatotoxicity: notify prescriber of dark urine, yellowing of skin/eyes, clay-colored stools, anorexia, nausea, vomiting

⚠ Instruct patient to avoid breastfeeding to reduce postnatal HIV transmission

Evaluation

Positive therapeutic outcome
• Decrease in signs/symptoms of HIV
• Decrease viral load, increase CD4 counts

enalapril/enalaprilat (Rx)

(e-nal′a-pril/e-nal′a-pril-at)
Vasotec
Func. class.: Antihypertensive
Chem. class.: Angiotensin-converting enzyme (ACE) inhibitor
Pregnancy category D

Do not confuse:
enalapril/Eldepryl/ramipril/Anafranil

ACTION: Selectively suppresses renin-angiotensin-aldosterone system; inhibits ACE; prevents conversion of angiotensin I to angiotensin II, resulting in dilatation of arterial and venous vessels

Therapeutic outcome: Decreased B/P in hypertension; decreased preload, afterload in CHF

USES: Hypertension, CHF, left ventricular dysfunction

CONTRAINDICATIONS:
Hypersensitivity, history of angioedema

BLACK BOX WARNING: Pregnancy **D**

Precautions: Breastfeeding, renal disease, hyperkalemia, hepatic failure, dehydration, bilateral renal artery/aortic stenosis

DOSAGE AND ROUTES
Hypertension
Adult: PO 2.5-5 mg/day, may increase or decrease to desired response, range 10-40 mg/day; **IV** 0.625-1.25 mg q6hr over 5 min
Child: PO 0.08 mg/kg/day in 1-2 divided doses, max 0.58 mg/kg/day in 1-2 divided doses; **IV** 5-10 mcg/kg/dose q8-24hr

CHF
Adult: PO 2.5-20 mg/day in 2 divided doses, max 40 mg/day in divided doses

Renal dose
Adult: PO CCr <30 ml/min 2.5 mg/day, increase gradually; **IV** CCr >30 ml/min 1.25 mg q6hr; CCr <30 ml/min 0.625 mg as one-time dose, increase as per B/P

Available forms: Enalapril: tabs 2.5, 5, 10, 20 mg; enalaprilat: inj 1.25 mg/ml

Implementation
PO route
• Store in air-tight container at 86° F (30° C) or less

- Severe hypotension may occur after 1st dose of this medication; hypotension may be prevented by reducing or discontinuing diuretic therapy 3 days before beginning benazepril therapy
- Give by **IV** inf of 0.9% NaCl (as ordered) to expand fluid volume if severe hypotension occurs

Direct IV route/ intermittent IV infusion
- Give undiluted over ≥5 min; use diluent provided or 50 ml D₅W, 0.9% NaCl, 0.9% NaCl in D₅W, or LR, give over ≥5 min, sol is stable for 24 hr

Y-site compatibilities: Acyclovir, alemtuzumab, alfentanil, allopurinol, amifostine, amikacin, aminophylline, amphotericin B liposome, anidulafungin, ascorbic acid, atracurium, atropine, azaTHIOprine, aztreonam, benztropine, bivalirudin, bretylium, bumetanide, buprenorphine, butorphanol, calcium chloride/gluconate, CARBOplatin, ceFAZolin, cefonicid, cefoperazone, cefotaxime, cefoTEtan, cefOXitin, cefTAZidime, ceftizoxime, cefTRIAXone, cefuroxime, cephalothin, cephapirin, chloramphenicol, cimetidine, cisatracurium, cladribine, clindamycin, cyanocobalamin, cyclophosphamide, cycloSPORINE, cytarabine, DACTINomycin, DAPTOmycin, dexamethasone, dexmedetomidine, dextran 40, digoxin, diltiazem, diphenhydrAMINE, DOBUTamine, DOCEtaxel, DOPamine, doripenem, doxacurium, DOXOrubicin, DOXOrubicin liposome, doxycycline, ePHEDrine, EPINEPHrine, epirubicin, epoetin, ertapenem, erythromycin, esmolol, etoposide, etoposide phosphate, famotidine, fenoldopam, fentaNYL, filgrastim, fluconazole, fludarabine, fluorouracil, folic acid, furosemide, ganciclovir, gemcitabine, gentamicin, granisetron, heparin, hydrocortisone, HYDROmorphone, ifosfamide, imipenem/cilastatin, indomethacin, insulin, isoproterenol, ketorolac, labetalol, levofloxacin, lidocaine, linezolid, LORazepam, magnesium sulfate, mannitol, mechlorethamine, melphalan, meperidine, meropenem, metaraminol, methicillin, methotrexate, methoxamine, methyldopate, methylPREDNISolone, metoclopramide, metoprolol, metroNIDAZOLE, mezlocillin, miconazole, midazolam, milrinone, minocycline, mitoXANtrone, morphine, moxalactam, multiple vitamin infusion, nafcillin, nalbuphine, naloxone, netilmicin, niCARdipine, nitroglycerin, nitroprusside, norepinephrine, octreotide, ondansetron, oxacillin, oxaliplatin, oxytocin, PACLitaxel, palonosetron, papaverine, PEMEtrexed, penicillin G potassium, pentamidine, pentazocine, PENTobarbital, PHENobarbital, phentolamine, phenylephrine, phytonadione, piperacillin/tazobactam, potassium chloride/phosphate, procainamide, prochlorperazine, promethazine, propofol, propranolol, protamine, pyridoxime, quinupristin/dalfopristin, ranitidine, remifentanil, ritodrine, riTUXimab, rocuronium, sodium acetate, sodium bicarbonate, succinylcholine, SUFentanil, tacrolimus, teniposide, tetracycline, theophylline, thiamine, thiotepa, ticarcillin/clavulanate, tigecycline, tirofiban, tobramycin, tolazoline, trastuzumab, trimetaphan, urokinase, vancomycin, vasopressin, vecuronium, verapamil, vinCRIStine, vinorelbine, voriconazole

Y-site incompatibilities: Amphotericin B cholesteryl sulfate, caspofungin, cefepime, dantrolene, diazepam, diazoxide, gemtuzumab, lansoprazole, phenytoin

Additive compatibilities: DOBUTamine, DOPamine, heparin, meropenem, nitroglycerin, nitroprusside, potassium chloride

ADVERSE EFFECTS
CNS: *Insomnia, dizziness,* paresthesias, headache, fatigue, anxiety
CV: *Hypotension,* chest pain, tachycardia, **dysrhythmias,** syncope, angina, **MI,** orthostatic hypotension
EENT: *Tinnitus,* visual changes, sore throat, double vision, dry burning eyes
GI: Nausea, vomiting, colitis, cramps, diarrhea, constipation, flatulence, dry mouth, loss of taste, **hepatotoxicity**
GU: Proteinuria, **renal failure,** increased frequency of polyuria or oliguria
HEMA: Agranulocytosis, neutropenia
INTEG: Rash, purpura, alopecia, hyperhidrosis, photosensitivity
META: Hyperkalemia
RESP: Dyspnea, dry cough, crackles
SYST: Toxic epidermal necrolysis, **Stevens-Johnson syndrome, angioedema**

Pharmacokinetics

Absorption	Well absorbed (PO), complete (**IV**)
Distribution	Unknown
Metabolism	Liver (active metabolite—enalaprilat)
Excretion	Kidneys (60%—enalaprilat, 20%—enalapril)
Half-life	Enalaprilat 11 hr, increased in renal disease

Pharmacodynamics

	PO	IV
Onset	1 hr	5-15 min
Peak	4-6 hr	1-4 hr
Duration	24 hr	4-6 hr

INTERACTIONS
Individual drugs
Alcohol: increased hypotension (large amounts)
Allopurinol: increased hypersensitivity
CycloSPORINE, NSAIDs: increased potassium levels
Digoxin, lithium: increased serum levels
Rifampin: decreased effects of enalapril

Drug classifications
Antacids: decreased effects of enalapril
Diuretics, general anesthesia, nitrates, other antihypertensives, phenothiazines: increased hypotension
Diuretics (potassium-sparing), potassium supplements, salt substitutes: increased potassium levels

Drug/lab test
Increased: ALT, AST, bilirubin, alkaline phosphatase, glucose, uric acid, BUN, creatinine
False positive: ANA titer

NURSING CONSIDERATIONS
Assessment
• **Bone marrow depression (rare):** monitor blood studies: neutrophils, decreased platelets with differential baseline and q3mo; if neutrophils <1000/mm^3, discontinue treatment
• **Hypertension:** monitor B/P, orthostatic hypotension, syncope; if changes occur, dosage change may be required; obtain peak/trough levels, maintain adequate hydration
• **CHF:** monitor for increased weight, rales, jugular vein distention, edema, difficulty breathing
• Monitor electrolytes: K, Na, Cl during 1st 2 wk of therapy
• Monitor renal studies: protein, BUN, creatinine; increased levels may indicate nephrotic syndrome and renal failure
• Monitor renal symptoms: polyuria, oliguria, frequency, dysuria
• Establish baselines in renal, liver function tests before therapy begins and 1 wk into therapy, avoid activities requiring coordination
• Check potassium levels throughout treatment, although hyperkalemia rarely occurs
• Check for edema in feet, legs daily
• Assess for allergic reactions: rash, fever, pruritus, urticaria; product should be discontinued if antihistamines fail to help

Patient/family education
• Advise patient not to discontinue product abruptly; advise patient to tell all persons associated with health care that product is being taken
• Teach patient not to use OTC products (cough, cold, allergy medications) unless directed by physician, to avoid potassium, salt substitutes; serious side effects can occur; xanthines, such as coffee, tea, chocolate, cola, can prevent action of product
• Instruct patient on the importance of complying with dosage schedule, even if feeling better; to continue with medical regimen to decrease B/P: exercise, cessation of smoking, decreasing stress, diet modifications
• Emphasize the need to rise slowly to sitting or standing position to minimize orthostatic hypotension; not to exercise in hot weather, which can cause increased hypotension
• Advise patient to notify prescriber of mouth sores, sore throat, fever, swelling of hands or feet, irregular heartbeat, chest pain, coughing, shortness of breath
• Caution patient to report excessive perspiration, dehydration, vomiting, diarrhea; may lead to fall in B/P
• Caution patient that product may cause skin rash or impaired perspiration; that angioedema may occur and to discontinue if it occurs
• Caution patient that product may cause dizziness, fainting, light-headedness; may occur during 1st few days of therapy; to avoid activities that may be hazardous
• Teach patient how to take B/P, normal readings for age-group

> **BLACK BOX WARNING:** Teach patient to use contraception during treatment, pregnancy **D,** to notify prescriber if pregnancy is planned or suspected

Evaluation
Positive therapeutic outcome
• Decreased B/P in hypertension

TREATMENT OF OVERDOSE:
Lavage, **IV** atropine for bradycardia; **IV** theophylline for bronchospasm, digoxin, O$_2$; diuretic for cardiac failure, hemodialysis

---

enfuvirtide (Rx)
(en-fyoo′vir-tide)
Fuzeon
Func. class.: Antiretroviral
Chem. class.: Fusion inhibitor
Pregnancy category B

ACTION: Inhibitor of the fusion of HIV-1 with CD4+ cells

Therapeutic outcome: Decreasing symptoms of HIV

USES: Treatment of HIV-1 infection in combination with other antiretrovirals

CONTRAINDICATIONS:
Breastfeeding, hypersensitivity

Precautions: Pregnancy **B**, children <6 yr, liver disease, myelosuppression, infections

DOSAGE AND ROUTES
Adult: SUBCUT 90 mg (1 ml) bid
Child 6-16 yr and <42.6 kg: SUBCUT 2 mg/kg bid, max 90 mg bid; 11-15.5 kg 27 mg/0.3 ml bid; 15.6-20 kg 36 ml/0.4 ml bid; 20.1-24.5 kg 45 mg/0.5 ml bid; 24.6-29 kg 54 mg/0.6 ml bid; 29.1-33.5 kg 63 mg/0.7 ml bid; 33.6-38 kg 72 mg/0.8 ml bid; 38.1-42.5 kg 81 mg/0.9 ml bid

Available forms: Powder for inj, lyophilized 108 mg (90 mg/ml when reconstituted)

Implementation
• Give SUBCUT, bid; rotate sites; preferred sites are upper arm, anterior thigh, abdomen

ADVERSE EFFECTS
CNS: Anxiety, peripheral neuropathy, taste disturbance, **Guillain-Barré syndrome**, insomnia, depression
GI: Abdominal pain, anorexia, constipation, **pancreatitis**
GU: **Glomerulonephritis, renal failure**
HEMA: **Thrombocytopenia, neutropenia**
INTEG: *Inj site reactions*
MISC: Influenza, cough, conjunctivitis, lymphadenopathy, myalgias, hyperglycemia, hypersensitivity, **pneumonia**, rhinitis, fatigue

Pharmacokinetics

Pharmacokinetics	
Absorption	Well absorbed
Distribution	92% protein binding
Metabolism	Undergoes catabolism
Excretion	Unknown
Half-life	Terminal 3.8 hr

Pharmacodynamics	
Onset	Unknown
Peak	8 hrs
Duration	Unknown

NURSING CONSIDERATIONS
Assessment
• Assess for signs of infection, inj site reactions
• Monitor renal studies: BUN, creatinine, renal failure may occur
• Monitor bowel pattern before, during treatment; if severe abdominal pain or constipation occurs, notify prescriber; monitor hydration
• Assess skin eruptions, rash, urticaria, itching
• Identify allergies before treatment, reaction to each medication
• CBC, blood chemistry, plasma HIV RNA, absolute CD4/CD8 cell counts/%, serum β_2 microglobulin, serum ICD+24 antigen levels, cholesterol

Patient/family education
• Instruct to notify prescriber if pregnancy is suspected or if breastfeeding
⚠ Advise that pneumonia may occur, to contact prescriber if cough, fever occur
• Teach that hypersensitive reactions may occur: rash, pruritus; stop product, contact prescriber
• Teach that this product is not a cure for HIV-1 infection but controls symptoms; HIV-1 can still be transmitted to others
• Teach that this product is to be used in combination only with other antiretrovirals

Evaluation
Positive therapeutic outcome
• Increased CD4 cell counts; decreased viral load; slowing progression of HIV-1 infection

---

⚠ HIGH ALERT

enoxaparin (Rx)
(ee-nox′a-par-in)
Lovenox
Func. class.: Anticoagulant, antithrombotic
Chem. class.: Unfractionated porcine heparin (low-molecular-weight heparin)
Pregnancy category B

Do not confuse:
enoxaparin/enoxacin, **Lovenox**/Lotronex

ACTION: Binds to antithrombin III inactivating factors Xa/IIa resulting in higher ratio of anti-factor Xa to anti-factor IIa

---

Therapeutic outcome: Prevention of deep vein thrombosis

USES: Prevention of DVT (inpatient or outpatient), pulmonary emboli (inpatient) in hip and knee replacement, abdominal surgery at risk for thrombosis; unstable angina/non–Q-wave MI, acute MI, coronary artery thrombosis

CONTRAINDICATIONS:

Hypersensitivity to this product, heparin, or pork; hemophilia; leukemia with bleeding; thrombocytopenic purpura, heparin-induced thrombocytopenia, active major bleeding

Precautions: Pregnancy **B**, breastfeeding, children, geriatric, severe renal/hepatic disease, blood dyscrasias, severe hypertension, subacute bacterial endocarditis, acute nephritis, recent burn, spinal surgery, indwelling catheters, low weight (men <57 kg, women <45 kg), hypersensitivity to benzyl alcohol

> **BLACK BOX WARNING:** Lumbar puncture, epidural/spinal anesthesia, aneurysm, coagulopathy

DOSAGE AND ROUTES
DVT/PE prophylaxis
Adult (moderate risk—general surgery, non-surgery 40-60 yr, major surgery <40 yr with no risk factors): SUBCUT 20 mg/day
Adult (higher risk—abdominal surgery, elderly-general surgery, major surgery <40 yr with no risk factors): SUBCUT 30 mg q12hr or 40 mg/day

DVT prevention before hip/knee surgery
Adult: SUBCUT 30 mg bid given 12-24 hr postoperatively for 7-10 days until DVT risk is diminished

DVT prevention before hip replacement
Adult: SUBCUT 40 mg/day started 9-15 hr preop or 30 mg q12hr started 12-24 hr postop, continued until DVT risk is diminished or patient is adequately on anticoagulant

DVT prophylaxis before abdominal surgery
Adult: SUBCUT 40 mg/day × 7-10 days to prevent thromboembolic complications, start 24 hr before surgery

Treatment of DVT/PE
Adult: SUBCUT (outpatient without PE) 1 mg/kg q12hr or 1.5 mg/kg/day (outpatient/inpatient); warfarin should be started within 72 hr and continued ≥5 days until INR is 2-3 (usually 7 days)

Prevention of ischemic complications in unstable angina/non–Q-wave/non-ST MI with aspirin
Adult: SUBCUT/**IV** 1 mg/kg q12hr until stable with aspirin 100-325 mg/day × ≥2 days

Renal dose
Adult: SUBCUT <30 ml/min 30 mg/day (thrombosis prophylaxis)

Available forms: Prefilled syringes/inj 30 mg/0.3 ml, 40 mg/0.4 ml, 60 mg/0.6 ml, 80 mg/0.8 ml, 100 mg/1 ml, 120 mg/0.8 ml, 150 mg/ml; multidose vials 100 mg/ml (3 ml)

Implementation
• Give at same time each day to maintain steady blood levels
SUBCUT route
• Administer SUBCUT deeply; do not give IM, begin 1 hr before surgery, do not aspirate, do not expel bubble from syringe before administration; sol is clear to yellow; do not use sol with precipitate; apply gentle pressure for 1 min
• Give to recumbent patient, rotate sites (left/right anterolateral, left/right posterolateral abdominal wall)
• Leave vascular access sheath in place for 6 hr after dose, then give next dose 6 hr after sheath removed

Direct IV route
• Use multidose vial for **IV** administration; use TB syringe or other graduated syringe to measure dose; give **IV** BOL through **IV** line; flush after
• If withdrawing from multidose vial, use TB syringe for proper measurement
• Prefilled syringes (30, 40 mg) are not graduated; do not use for partial doses
• Do not mix with other products or infusion fluids
⚠ Give only this product when ordered; not interchangeable with heparin or LMWHs

ADVERSE EFFECTS
CNS: Fever, confusion
GI: Nausea
HEMA: Hemorrhage from any site, hypochromic anemia, thrombocytopenia, bleeding
INTEG: Ecchymosis, inj site hematoma
META: Hyperkalemia in renal failure
MS: Osteoporosis
SYST: Edema, peripheral edema

Pharmacokinetics

Absorption	Well absorbed (90%)
Distribution	Unknown
Metabolism	Unknown
Excretion	Kidneys
Half-life	4½ hr

Pharmacodynamics

Onset	Unknown
Peak	3-5 hr
Duration	Unknown

INTERACTIONS

Drug classifications
Anticoagulants, antiplatelets, NSAIDs, RU-486, salicylates, thrombolytics: increased bleeding

Drug/herb
Feverfew, garlic, ginger, ginkgo, horse chestnut: increased bleeding risk

Drug/lab test
Increased: AST/ALT
Decreased: platelets

NURSING CONSIDERATIONS

Assessment
• Monitor blood studies (Hct, CBC, coagulation studies, occult blood in stools), anti-Xa levels q3mo; platelet count q2-3day; thrombocytopenia may occur
• Assess patient for bleeding gums, petechiae, ecchymosis, black tarry stools, hematuria, epistaxis, decrease in B/P; indicate bleeding and possible hemorrhage; notify prescriber immediately

BLACK BOX WARNING: Assess for neuro-symptoms in patients who have received spinal anesthesia

Patient/family education
• Warn patient to avoid OTC preparations unless directed by prescriber because they could cause serious product interactions
• Instruct patient to use soft-bristled toothbrush to avoid bleeding gums; to avoid contact sports; to use electric razor; to avoid IM inj
• Advise patient to report any signs of bleeding, bruising: gums, under skin, urine, stools

Evaluation
Positive therapeutic outcome
• Absence of DVT

entacapone (Rx)

(en-ta′ka-pone)
Comtan
Func. class.: Antiparkinsonian agent
Chem. class.: COMT
Pregnancy category C

ACTION: Inhibits COMT (catechol *O*-methyltransferase) and alters the plasma pharmacokinetics of levodopa; given with levodopa/carbidopa

Therapeutic outcome: Decreased symptoms of Parkinson's disease (involuntary movements)

USES: Parkinsonism in those experiencing end of dose, decreased effect as an adjunct to levodopa/carbidopa

CONTRAINDICATIONS:
Hypersensitivity

Precautions: Pregnancy **C**, breastfeeding, children, renal/hepatic disease, affective disorders, psychosis

DOSAGE AND ROUTES
Adult: PO 200 mg given with carbidopa/levodopa, max 1600 mg/day; may allow 25% dosage reduction in levodopa therapy

Available forms: Tabs 200 mg film coated

Implementation
• Adjust dosage to patient response
• Give with meals to decrease GI upset; limit protein taken with product
• Give only after MAOIs have been discontinued for 2 wk

ADVERSE EFFECTS
CNS: *Involuntary choreiform movements, dyskinesia, hypokinesia, hyperkinesia, hand tremors, fatigue, headache, anxiety, twitching, numbness, weakness, confusion, agitation, nightmares,* psychosis, hallucinations, hypomania, severe depression, dizziness, **neuroleptic malignant syndrome**
CV: *Orthostatic hypotension*
GI: *Nausea, vomiting, anorexia, abdominal distress, dry mouth, flatulence,* gastritis, GI disorder, *diarrhea, constipation,* bitter taste
INTEG: Rash, sweating, alopecia
MISC: Dark urine and other body fluids, back pain, dyspnea, purpura, fatigue, asthenia, infection-bacterial, **rhabdomyolysis**

Absorption	Well absorbed
Distribution	Protein binding 98%
Metabolism	Liver extensively
Excretion	Kidneys, feces; breast milk
Half-life	0.5 hr initial, 2.5 hr second

Pharmacodynamics

Onset	Unknown
Peak	Unknown
Duration	≤8 hr

INTERACTIONS

Individual drugs

Ampicillin, chloramphenicol, erythromycin, probenecid, rifampin: decreased excretion of entacapone

Bitolterol, DOBUTamine, DOPamine, EPHINEPHrine, isoetharine, methyldopa, norepinephrine: increased CV reactions; avoid use

Drug classifications

MAOIs: prevent catecholamine metabolism; do not use together

Drug/herb

Kava: decreased effect
Ma huang: increased B/P

NURSING CONSIDERATIONS

Assessment

• **Assess for neuroleptic malignant syndrome:** high temp, increased CPK, rigidity, change in consciousness, usually during rapid withdrawal
• Monitor B/P, respiration during initial treatment; hypotension should be reported
• Assess mental status: affect, mood, behavioral changes, depression; complete suicide assessment
• Monitor liver function enzymes: AST, ALT, alkaline phosphatase; also check LDH, bilirubin, CBC
• **Assess for involuntary movements in parkinsonism:** akinesia, tremors, staggering gait, muscle rigidity, drooling; these symptoms should improve with therapy when given with levodopa/carbidopa
• **Rhabdomyolysis:** Assess for muscle pain, tenderness, weakness, swelling of affected muscles, may lead to decreased B/P, shock

Patient/family education

• Advise patient that hallucinations, mental changes, nausea, dyskinesia can occur

• Caution patient to change positions slowly to prevent orthostatic hypotension; not to drive or operate machinery until stabilized on medication and mental performance is not affected
• Instruct patient to use product exactly as prescribed; if dose is missed, take as soon as remembered, up to 2 hr before next dose, not to discontinue abruptly, withdraw gradually
• Inform patient that urine, sweat may darken
• Instruct patient to notify prescriber if pregnancy is suspected; if breastfeeding, product is excreted in breast milk

Evaluation

Positive therapeutic outcome
• Decreased akathisia, other involuntary movements when used with levodopa/carbidopa
• Increased mood when used with levodopa/carbidopa

entecavir (Rx)

(en-te′ka-veer)
Baraclude
Func. class.: Antiretroviral nucleoside reverse transcriptase inhibitors (NRTIs)
Chem. class.: Guanosine nucleoside analog
Pregnancy category C

ACTION: Inhibits hepatitis B virus DNA polymerase by competing with natural substrates and by causing DNA termination after its incorporation into viral DNA; causes viral DNA death

Therapeutic outcome: Improved liver function tests in chronic hepatitis B (HBV)

USES: Chronic hepatitis B (HBV)

CONTRAINDICATIONS:

Hypersensitivity

Precautions: Pregnancy **C**, breastfeeding, child, geriatric, severe renal disease

> **BLACK BOX WARNING:** Hepatic disease, hepatitis, lactic acidosis, HIV

DOSAGE AND ROUTES

Chronic hepatitis B (nucleoside treatment–naive)

Adult and adolescent ≥16 yr: PO 0.5 mg/day

Chronic hepatitis B with compensated liver disease and history of hepatitis B viremia, while receiving lamiVUDine/telbivudine or known lamiVUDine resistance mutations
Adult and adolescent ≥16 yr: PO 1 mg/day

Renal dose
Adult: PO CCr ≥50 ml/min 0.5 mg/day; CCr 30-49 ml/min 0.25 mg daily, 0.5 mg/day or 1 mg q48hr for lamiVUDine refractory patient; CCr 10-29 ml/min 0.15/day, 0.3 for lamiVUDine refractory patient; CCr <10 ml/min 0.05 mg PO/day, 0.1 mg/day or 1 mg q7days for lamiVUDine refractory patient

Available forms: Tabs, film coated 0.5, 1 mg; oral sol 0.05 mg/ml

Implementation
- After hemodialysis give by mouth on empty stomach 2 hr before or after food
- Tabs: Store at room temperature
- **Oral liquid:** Use calibrated oral dosing spoon provided, may be used interchangeably with tabs
- Store in cool environment; protect from light

ADVERSE EFFECTS
CNS: *Headache*, fatigue, dizziness, insomnia
ENDO: Hyperglycemia
GI: *Dyspepsia*, nausea, vomiting, diarrhea, elevated liver function enzymes, **hepatotoxicity with steatosis**
INTEG: Alopecia, rash
SYST: Lactic acidosis

Pharmacokinetics
Absorption	100%
Distribution	Extensively to tissues, protein binding 13%
Metabolism	Unknown
Excretion	Unchanged 62%-73% via kidneys
Half-life	Terminal 128-149 hr

Pharmacodynamics
Onset	Unknown
Peak	0.5-1.5 hr
Duration	Unknown

INTERACTIONS
Drug/food
High-fat meal: decreased absorption

Drug/lab test
Increased: ALT, AST, total bilirubin, amylase, lipase, creatinine, blood glucose, urine glucose
Decreased: platelets, albumin

NURSING CONSIDERATIONS
Assessment

> **BLACK BOX WARNING:** Assess for HIV before beginning treatment because HIV resistance may occur in patients with chronic hepatitis B infection; monitor HIV RNA

⚠ **Assess for lactic acidosis, severe hepatomegaly with stenosis: increased serum lactate, increased hepatic enzymes, palpate liver; discontinue product if these occur**
- Monitor geriatric patients more carefully; may develop renal, cardiac symptoms more rapidly
- Assess for exacerbations of hepatitis (jaundice, pruritus, fatigue) after discontinuing treatment; monitor liver function tests

Patient/family education
- Teach patient not to take with food
- Teach patient to take exactly as prescribed
- Advise patient not to stop medication without approval of prescriber
- Advise that optimal duration of treatment is unknown
- Teach patient to avoid use with other medications unless approved by prescriber
- Teach patient to notify prescriber of decreased urinary output, blood in urine

> **BLACK BOX WARNING: Teach patient symptoms of lactic acidosis:** muscle pain, severe tiredness, weakness, trouble breathing, stomach pain with nausea/vomiting, coldness in arms/legs, fast/irregular heartbeat, dizziness

> **BLACK BOX WARNING: Teach patient symptoms of hepatotoxicity:** eyes/skin turns yellow, dark urine, light bowel movements, no appetite for days, nausea, stomach pain

- Advise patient that product does not cure, but lowers the amount of HBV in body
- Teach patient that product does not stop the spreading of HBV to others by sex, sharing needles, or being exposed to blood

Evaluation
Positive therapeutic outcome
- Decreased symptoms of chronic hepatitis B, improving liver function tests

enzalutamide

(en-zal-u'ta-mide)

Xtandi

Func. class.: Antineoplastic hormone
Chem. class.: Nonsteroidal antiandrogen

Pregnancy category X

ACTION: Binds to cytosolic androgen receptors in target tissue, which competitively inhibits the action to androgens

Therapeutic outcome: Decreased tumor size, decreased spread of malignancy

USES: Metastatic castration-resistant prostate cancer in those who have received DOCEtaxel

CONTRAINDICATIONS:

Pregnancy (X), women, hypersensitivity

Precautions: Breastfeeding, brain tumor, head trauma, infertility, seizures, stroke, male-mediated teratogenicity

DOSAGE AND ROUTES

Adult: PO 160 mg (4 × 40-mg caps) daily
If a patient experiences a grade 3 or higher toxicity or an intolerable adverse effect, withhold dosing for 1 wk or until symptoms improve to grade 2 or less, then resume at the same or a reduced dosage (120 or 80 mg), if warranted
The concomitant use of strong cytochrome P450 (CYP-450) 2C8 inhibitors should be avoided if possible; if a strong CYP2C8 inhibitor must be coadministered, reduce the enzalutamide dosage to 80 mg once daily

Available forms: Tabs 40 mg

Implementation

• Give at same time each day, without regard to food
• Swallow whole

ADVERSE EFFECTS

CNS: Dizziness, paresthesias, insomnia, anxiety, headache
CV: Hot flashes, hypertension
GU: Urinary frequency
INTEG: Dry skin, pruritus
MISC: Infection, asthenia

Pharmacokinetics

Absorption	Unknown
Distribution	97%-98% protein binding
Metabolism	Unknown
Excretion	Unknown
Half-life	Terminal half-life 2.8 to 10.2 days

Pharmacodynamics

Onset	Unknown
Peak	Unknown
Duration	Unknown

INTERACTIONS

Drug classifications

Anticoagulants: Increased anticoagulation
CYP3A4 inhibitors (amiodarone, antiretrovirals, protease inhibitors, clarithromycin, dalfopristin, quinupristin, delavirdine, efavirenz, erythromycin, FLUoxetine, fluvoxaMINE, imatinib, mifepristone, RU-486, nefazodone, some azole antifungals): Increased enzalutamide effects
CYP3A4 inducers (barbiturates, bosentan, carBAMazepine, dexamethasone, nevirapine, OXcarbazepine, phenytoin, rifabutin, rifampin, rifapentine): Decreased enzalutamide effects

Drug/herb

St. John's wort: Might require dosage change

NURSING CONSIDERATIONS

Assessment

• **Male-mediated teratogenicity**: a condom and another effective birth control method should be used if patient is having sex with a woman of childbearing potential during and 3 mo after end of therapy
• **Seizures**: those with a history of seizures, underlying head trauma with loss of consciousness, TIA within 12 mo, stroke, brain tumor, or drugs lowering seizure threshold should be told about danger of loss of consciousness when engaging in activities
• Assess for hot flashes, assure patient that these are common side effects

Patient/family education

• Advise patient that infertility can occur, to use a condom and another form of birth control during and for 3 mo after end of therapy if female sex partner is of childbearing potential
• Teach patient that those with seizure disorders might experience seizures because seizure threshold is decreased

---

• Advise patient not to use other products unless approved by prescriber

Evaluation
Positive therapeutic outcome
• Decreased tumor size, decreased spread of malignancy

---

ePHEDrine nasal agent
See Appendix B

---

epinastine ophthalmic
See Appendix B

⚠ HIGH ALERT

EPINEPHrine (Rx, OTC)
(ep-i-nef'rin)
Adrenaclick, Primatene Mist, Twinject, Walgreens Bronchial Mist
EPINEPHrine HCl
Adrenalin, EpiPen, EpiPen Jr.
Func. class.: Bronchodilator, nonselective adrenergic agonist, cardiac stimulant, vasopressor
Chem. class.: Catecholamine
Pregnancy category C

Do not confuse:
EPINEPHrine/ePHEDrine

ACTION: β_1- and β_2-agonist causing increased levels of cyclic AMP producing bronchodilatation, cardiac and CNS stimulation; large doses cause vasoconstriction via α-receptors; small doses can cause vasodilation via β_2-vascular receptors

Therapeutic outcome: Vasoconstrictor, cardiac stimulator, bronchodilator, decreased aqueous humor

USES: Acute asthmatic attacks, hemostasis, bronchospasm, anaphylaxis, allergic reactions, cardiac arrest, adjunct in anesthesia, shock

CONTRAINDICATIONS:
Hypersensitivity to sympathomimetics, sulfites, closed-angle glaucoma, nonanaphylactic shock during general anesthesia

Precautions: Pregnancy C, breastfeeding, cardiac disorders, hyperthyroidism, diabetes mellitus, prostatic hypertrophy, hypertension, organic brain syndrome, local anesthesia of certain areas, labor, cardiac dilatation, coronary insufficiency, cerebral arteriosclerosis, organic heart disease

DOSAGE AND ROUTES
Anaphylaxis/severe asthma exacerbation
Adult: IM/SUBCUT 0.3-0.5 mg, may repeat q10-15min (anaphylaxis) or q20min-4 hr (asthma)

Severe allergic reactions type 1
Adult/child ≥30 kg: IM 0.3 mg (EpiPen/EpiPen 2-Pak, 1:1000)
Child <30 kg: IM 0.15 mg (EpiPen Jr/EpiPen Jr 2-Pak 1:2000)
Adult/child ≥66 lb: IM/SUBCUT 0.3 mg (0.3 ml) initially (Twinject 1.1 ml 1:1000, 1 mg/ml, containing 2 doses of 0.3 mg)
Adult/child 33-66 lb: IM/SUBCUT 0.15 mg (0.15 ml) initially, may give another 0.15 mg after 10 min (Twinject 1.1 ml 1:1000 [1 mg/ml] containing 2 doses of 0.15 mg)

Status asthmaticus
Adult/adolescent: SUBCUT 0.3-0.5 mg (0.3-0.5 ml of the 1:1000 injection) q20min ×3 doses
Child/infant: SUBCUT 0.01 mg/kg-0.5 mg q20min ×3 doses

Available forms: Nasal spray (sol) 1 mg/ml; sol for inj 1 mg/ml; 1:10,000, 1:1000; inh vapor (sol) 0.22 mg/acuation; pressurized inh (sol) 0.22 mg/actuation; sol for inj 0.15 mg/0.15 ml autoinjector, 0.3 mg/0.3 ml autoinjector, 0.15 mg/0.3 ml

Implementation
• Give subcut, IM, intraosseously, IV; suspensions are for subcut use only; do not give IV
• Visually inspect parenteral products for particulate matter and discoloration prior to use; do not use solutions that are pinkish to brownish in color or contain a precipitate
• **Avoid extravasation during parenteral administration; if extravasation occurs, infiltrate the affected area with phentolamine diluted in NS**
• Store reconstituted sol refrigerated 24 hr

Direct IV injection route
• Inject EPINEPHrine directly into a vein over 5-10 min for adults or 1-3 min for children; may be given IV push in cardiac arrest
• In neonates, may administer via the umbilical vein
• During adult cardiopulmonary resuscitation (CPR): resuscitation drugs may be given IV by bolus injection into a peripheral vein, followed by an injection of 20 ml IV fluid; elevate the

---

extremity for 10-20 sec to facilitate drug delivery to the central circulation

Continuous IV infusion route
• Dilute 1 mg EPINEPHrine in 250 or 500 ml of a compatible IV infusion solution to provide a concentration of 4 or 2 mcg/ml, respectively; give into a large vein, if possible
• More concentrated solutions (16-32 mcg/ml) may be used in fluid-restricted patients when administered through a central line

IM route
• EPINEPHrine injection should preferably be into the deltoid or anterior thigh (vastus lateralis); do not administer into the gluteal muscle
• Twinject is light-sensitive and should be stored in the carrying case provided; do not refrigerate; protect from freezing; replace if solution is discolored or contains a precipitate

Subcut route
• Inject taking care not to inject intradermally
• Massage injection site well after use to enhance absorption and to decrease local vasoconstriction; injection can cause tissue irritation

Intraosseous infusion route (unlabeled)
• During CPR, the same EPINEPHrine dosage may be given via the intraosseous route when IV access is not available

Intracardiac route
• Should be reserved for extreme emergencies. Intracardiac injection should only be performed by properly trained medical personnel

Inhalation route
• Use 2.25% sol diluted in nebulizer/respirator
• Rinse mouth after inh
• 10 gtt of a 1% sol should be placed in nebulizer
• Dilute racepinephrine 2.25% sol

Endotracheal route
• Per the ACLS or PALS guidelines, the EPINEPHrine parenteral product is administered via this route
• Endotracheal (ET) administration should only be used if access to IV or intraosseous routes is not possible
• **Adult:** Dilute dose in 5-10 ml NS or sterile distilled water; administer via ET tube; endotracheal absorption of EPINEPHrine may be improved by diluting with water instead of NS
• **Child:** After dose administration, flush the ET tube with a minimum of 5 ml NS

Y-site compatibilities: Alfentanil, amikacin, amiodarone, amphotericin B liposome, anidulafungin, ascorbic acid, atracurium, aztreonam, benztropine, bivalirudin, bleomycin, bumetanide, buprenorphine, butorphanol, calcium chloride/gluconate, CARBOplatin, ca-spofungin, ceFAZolin, cefoperazone, cefotaxime, cefoTEtan, cefOXitin, cefTAZidime, ceftizoxime, cefTRIAXone, cefuroxime, chloramphenicol, chlorproMAZINE, cimetidine, cisatracurium, CISplatin, clindamycin, cyanocobalamin, cyclophosphamide, cycloSPORINE, cytarabine, DACTINomycin, DAPTOmycin, dexamethasone, dexmedetomidine, digoxin, diltiazem, diphenhydrAMINE, DOBUTamine, DOCEtaxel, DOPamine, DOXOrubicin, doxycycline, enalaprilat, epirubicin, epoetin alfa, ertapenem, erythromycin, esmolol, etoposide, etoposide phosphate, famotidine, fenoldopam, fentaNYL, fluconazole, fludarabine, folic acid, furosemide, gemcitabine, gentamicin, glycopyrrolate, granisetron, heparin, hydrocortisone, HYDROmorphone, ifosfamide, imipenem/cilastatin, isoproterenol, ketorolac, labetalol, levofloxacin, lidocaine, linezolid, LORazepam, magnesium sulfate, mannitol, mechlorethamine, meperidine, metaraminol, methicillin, methotrexate, methoxamine, methyldopa, methylPREDNISolone, metoclopramide, metoprolol, metroNIDAZOLE, midazolam, milrinone, minocycline, mitoXANtrone, morphine, multiple vitamins, nafcillin, nalbuphine, naloxone, niCARdipine, nitroglycerin, nitroprusside, norepinephrine, octreotide, ondansetron, oxacillin, oxaliplatin, oxytocin, PACLitaxel, palonosetron, pancuronium, pantoprazole, PEMEtrexed, penicillin G potassium, pentamidine, pentazocine, phentolamine, phenylephrine, phytonadione, piperacillin-tazobactam, potassium chloride, procainamide, prochlorperazine, promethazine, propofol, propranolol, protamine, pyridoxime, quinupristin/dalfopristin, ranitidine, remifentanil, ritodrine, rocuronium, sodium acetate, streptomycin, succinylcholine, SUFentanil, tacrolimus, teniposide, theophylline, thiamine, thiotepa, ticarcillin/clavulanate, tigecycline, tirofiban, tobramycin, tolazoline, trimethaphan, urokinase, vancomycin, vasopressin, vecuronium, verapamil, vinCRIStine, vinorelbine, vitamin B complex with C, voriconazole, warfarin, zoledronic acid

Y-site incompatibilities: Acyclovir, aminophylline, azaTHIOprine, carmustine, cephapirin, dantrolene, diazepam, diazoxide, fluorouracil, ganciclovir, gemtuzumab, indomethacin, micafungin, PENTobarbital, PHENobarbital, phenytoin, sodium bicarbonate, thiopental, sulfamethoxazole/trimethoprim

ADVERSE EFFECTS
CNS: *Tremors, anxiety,* insomnia, headache, dizziness, weakness, drowsiness, confusion, hallucinations, **cerebral hemorrhage**

CV: *Palpitations, tachycardia,* hypertension, *dysrhythmias,* increased T-wave
GI: *Anorexia, nausea, vomiting*
MISC: Sweating, dry eyes
RESP: *Dyspnea*

Pharmacokinetics

Absorption	Well absorbed (PO), complete (**IV**)
Distribution	Unknown, crosses placenta
Metabolism	Liver
Excretion	Breast milk
Half-life	Unknown

Pharmacodynamics

	SUB-CUT	IM	IV	INH
Onset	3-5 min	Variable	Immediate	1 min
Peak	Unknown	Unknown	Unknown	Unknown
Duration	1-4 hr	1-4 hr	Unknown	1-4 hr

INTERACTIONS

Drug classifications
β-Adrenergic blockers: decreased hypertensive effects
Antidepressants (tricyclics): increased chance of hypertensive crisis; do not use together
MAOIs: increased chance of hypertensive crisis, do not use together
Other sympathomimetics: toxicity

NURSING CONSIDERATIONS

Assessment
• **Asthma:** Monitor respiratory function: vital capacity, forced expiratory volume, ABGs, lung sounds, heart rate, rhythm (baseline); amount, color of sputum
• Monitor **ECG** during administration continuously; if B/P increases, product should be decreased; check B/P, pulse q5min after parenteral route; CVP, PCWP, SVR; inadvertent high arterial B/P can result in angina, aortic rupture, cerebral hemorrhage
• Check inj site for tissue sloughing; if this occurs, administer phentolamine mixed with 0.9% NaCl
• **Monitor for evidence of allergic reactions, paradoxical bronchospasm:** withhold dose, notify prescriber; **sulfite sensitivity,** which may be life threatening

Patient/family education
• Tell patient not to use OTC medications; extra stimulation may occur; to use this medication before other medications and allow at least 5 min between each, to prevent overstimulation
• Teach patient that paradoxical bronchospasm may occur and to stop product immediately and notify prescriber; to limit caffeine products such as chocolate, coffee, tea, and colas
• Patient should rinse mouth after inh
• Patient should report blurred vision, irritation with ophth preparations

Evaluation
Positive therapeutic outcome
• Absence of dyspnea, wheezing
• Improved airway exchange, improved ABGs
• Decreased aqueous humor
• Stabilization of heart rate and cardiac output

TREATMENT OF OVERDOSE:
Administer a β₂-adrenergic blocker, vasodilators, α-blocker

EPINEPHrine/epinephryl borate ophthalmic
See Appendix B

EPINEPHrine nasal agent
See Appendix B

⚠ HIGH ALERT

epirubicin (Rx)
(ep-i-roo'bi-sin)
Ellence, Pharmorubicin ♣
Func. class.: Antineoplastic, antibiotic
Chem. class.: Anthracycline
Pregnancy category D

Do not confuse:
epirubicin/DOXOrubicin/DAUNOrubicin/eribulin/IDArubicin

ACTION: Inhibits DNA synthesis primarily; replication is decreased by binding to DNA, which causes strand splitting; maximum cytotoxic effects at S and G₂ phases; a vesicant

Therapeutic outcome: Prevention of rapidly growing malignant cells

USES: Breast cancer as an adjuvant therapy, with axillary node involvement, after resection

Unlabeled uses: Used in combination for treatment of advanced forms of cancer

---

Adverse effects: *italics* = common; **bold** = life-threatening

CONTRAINDICATIONS:

Pregnancy **D**, breastfeeding, hypersensitivity to this product, anthracyclines, anthracenediones, baseline neutrophil count <1500 cell/mm³, severe myocardial insufficiency, recent MI, heart failure, cardiomyopathy

> **BLACK BOX WARNING:** Severe hepatic disease, IM/subcut

Precautions: Children, geriatric, renal/hepatic/cardiac disease, previous anthracycline use, accidental exposure, angina, dental disease, herpes, hyperkalemia, hyperphosphatemia, hypertension, hyperuricemia, hypocalcemia, infection, infertility, tumor lysis syndrome, ventricular dysfunction

> **BLACK BOX WARNING:** Bone marrow suppression (severe), heart failure, extravasation, secondary malignancy, requires an experienced clinician

DOSAGE AND ROUTES

Breast cancer with axillary node involvement following resection of the primary tumor in combination with cyclophosphamide and fluorouracil

Adult: **IV** 100 mg/m² on day 1 with fluorouracil and cyclophosphamide (FEC regimen) q21 days × 6 cycles or 60 mg/m² on days 1 and 8 with oral cyclophosphamide and fluorouracil q28 days × 6 cycles

Breast cancer in combination with cyclophosphamide

Adult: **IV** 60 mg/m² day 1 with cyclophosphamide (500 mg/m² IV day 1), repeated q21 days × 8 cycles, or a higher-dose regimen of epirubicin 100 mg/m² IV day 1 with cyclophosphamide (830 mg/m² IV day 1), q21 days × 8 cycles

Dosage adjustments based upon hematologic and non-hematologic toxicities:

Nadir platelet counts <50,000/mm³, absolute neutrophil counts (ANC) <250/ mm³, neutropenic fever, or Grades 3/4 non-hematologic toxicities: Day 1 dose in subsequent cycles should be reduced by 25% of the previous dose

For patients receiving divided-dose epirubicin (i.e., day 1 and 8): Day 8 dose should be reduced by 25% of the day 1 dose if the platelet counts are 75,000-100,000/mm³ and the ANC is 1000-1499/mm³; if day 8 platelet counts are <75,000/mm³, ANC <1000/mm³, or Grade 3/4

nonhematologic toxicity has occurred, omit the day 8 dose

Hepatic dose

Adult: **IV** Bilirubin 1.2-3 mg/dl or AST 2-4 × normal upper limit, 50% of starting dose; bilirubin >3 mg/dl or AST >4 × normal upper limit, 25% of starting dose

Available forms: Inj (2 mg/ml) 10 mg/5 ml, 50 mg/25 ml, 150 mg/75 ml, 200 mg/100 ml

Implementation

- Avoid contact with skin; very irritating; wash completely to remove; give fluids **IV** or PO before chemotherapy to hydrate patient
- Give antiemetic 30-60 min before giving product to prevent vomiting and prn
- Administer prophylactic antibiotic with a fluoroquinolone or trimethoprim/sulfamethoxazole if dose of epirubicin is 120 mg/m²
- Provide liquid diet: carbonated beverages; gelatin may be added if patient is not nauseated or vomiting; monitor electrolytes

> **BLACK BOX WARNING:** To be used by a clinician experienced in giving cytotoxic products

> **BLACK BOX WARNING:** Do not use IM/subcut due to severe tissue necrosis

- **Give IV, do not give IM, subcut; a vesicant: if extravasation occurs, stop and complete via another vein, preferably in another limb; avoid infusion into veins over joints or in extremities with compromised venous or lymphatic drainage**
- Rapid injection may cause facial flushing or erythema along the vein; avoid administration time of less than 3 min
- **Product should be given to those with neutrophils ≥1500/mm³, platelet count ≥100,000/mm³, and non-hematologic toxicities recovered to ≤Grade 1**
- When refrigerated, the preservative-free, ready-to-use solution may form a gelled product; and will return to solution after 2-4 hr at room temperature
- Visually inspect for particulate matter and discoloration prior to use

IV route

- Product should be prepared by experienced personnel using proper precautions; pregnant women must not handle product
- Reconstitute 50 mg and 200 mg powder for injection vials with 25 ml and 100 ml, respectively, of sterile water for injection (2 mg/ml),

shake vigorously for up to 4 min; reconstituted solutions are stable for 24 hr when stored refrigerated and protected from light or at room temperature in normal light
• Solution can be further diluted with sterile water for injection

IV injection route
• Give doses of 100-120 mg/m² into tubing of a freely flowing 0.9% sodium chloride (NS) or D₅W IV infusion over 15-20 min; the infusion time may be decreased, proportionally, in those who require lower doses; infusion times <3 min are not recommended
• Direct injection into the vein is not recommended due to the risk of extravasation; avoid use with any solution of alkaline pH as hydrolysis will occur

IV infusion route
• Dilute dose in 0.9% sodium chloride (NS) or D₅W; infuse over 30-60 min
• Avoid use with any solution of alkaline pH as hydrolysis will occur

Y-site compatibilities: Alemtuzumab, alfentanil, amifostine, amikacin, aminocaproic acid, anidulafungin, atracurium, aztreonam, bivalirudin, bleomycin, bumetanide, buprenorphine, butorphanol, calcium chloride/gluconate, CARBOplatin, caspofungin, ceFAZolin, cefotaxime, ceftizoxime, chlorproMAZINE, cimetidine, ciprofloxacin, cisatracurium, CISplatin, clindamycin, cyclophosphamide, cycloSPORINE, DAPTOmycin, dexrazoxane, digoxin, diltiazem, diphenhydrAMINE, DOBUTamine, DOCEtaxel, dolasetron, DOPamine, doxacurium, doxycycline, droperidol, enalaprilat, ePHEDrine, EPINEPHrine, ertapenem, erythromycin, etoposide, famotidine, fenoldopam, fentaNYL, fluconazole, gatifloxacin, gemcitabine, gentamicin, granisetron, haloperidol, hydrocortisone, HYDROmorphone, hydrOXYzine, ifosfamide, imipenem-cilastatin, inamrinone, insulin (regular), isoproterenol, labetalol, levofloxacin, levorphanol, lidocaine, linezolid, LORazepam, mannitol, meperidine, mesna, methotrexate, metoclopramide, metoprolol, metroNIDAZOLE, midazolam, milrinone, minocycline, mitoMYcin, mivacurium, morphine, nalbuphine, naloxone, nesiritide, niCARdipine, nitroglycerin, nitroprusside, norepinephrine, octreotide, ofloxacin, ondansetron, oxaliplatin, PACLitaxel, palonosetron, pamidronate, pancuronium, pentamidine, pentazocine, phenylephrine, potassium chloride, procainamide, prochlorperazine, promethazine, propranolol, quinupristin-dalfopristin, ranitidine, remifentanil, rocuronium, sodium acetate, succinylcholine, SUFentanil,

tacrolimus, teniposide, theophylline, thiotepa, tigecycline, tirofiban, tobramycin, trimethobenzamide, vancomycin, vasopressin, vecuronium, verapamil, vinBLAStine, vinCRIStine, vinorelbine, voriconazole, zidovudine, zoledronic acid

Y-site incompatibilities: Acyclovir, allopurinol, aminophylline, amphotericin B colloidal, amphotericin B lipid complex, amphotericin B liposome, ampicillin, ampicillin/sulbactam, azithromycin, cefepime, cefoperazone, cefoTEtan, cefOXitin, cefTAZidime, cefTRIAXone, cefuroxime, dexamethasone, diazepam, ertapenem, fluorouracil, foscarnet, fosphenytoin, furosemide, ganciclovir, gemtuzumab, heparin, hydrocortisone, ketorolac, leucovorin, magnesium sulfate, meropenem, methohexital, methylPREDNISolone, nafcillin, pantoprazole, PEMEtrexed, PENTobarbital, PHENobarbital, phenytoin, piperacillin/tazobactam, potassium phosphates, sodium bicarbonate, sodium phosphates, thiopental, ticarcillin/clavulanate, tigecycline, sulfamethoxazole/trimethoprim

ADVERSE EFFECTS
CV: Increased B/P, **sinus tachycardia, PVCs,** chest pain, **bradycardia, extrasystole,** cardiomyopathy
GI: Nausea, vomiting, diarrhea, anorexia, mucositis
GU: *Hot flashes, amenorrhea, hyperuricemia*
HEMA: Thrombocytopenia, leukopenia, anemia, neutropenia, secondary AML
INTEG: *Rash, necrosis, pain at inj site, reversible alopecia*
MISC: Infection, febrile neutropenia, lethargy, fever, conjunctivitis, tumor lysis syndrome

Pharmacokinetics

Absorption	Complete bioavailability
Distribution	Widely distributed, crosses placenta
Metabolism	Liver, extensively
Excretion	Bile (60%)
Half-life	3 min; 2.5 hr; 33 hr

Pharmacodynamics
Unknown

INTERACTIONS
Individual drugs
Cimetidine, radiation: increased toxicity
PACLitaxel: give epirubicin before PACLitaxel if given concurrently
Trastuzumab: increased ventricular dysfunction, CHF

Drug classifications
Antineoplastics: increased toxicity
Calcium channel blockers: increased heart failure
Live virus vaccines: decreased antibody response

NURSING CONSIDERATIONS
Assessment
• **Heart failure:** monitor left ventricular ejection fraction, multigated acquisition scan or echocardiogram, ECG; watch for ST-T wave changes, low QRS and T; possible dysrhythmias (sinus tachycardia, heart block, PVCs) may occur; assess tachypnea, ECG changes, dyspnea, edema, fatigue; cardiac status: B/P, pulse, character, rhythm, rate, ABGs; identify cumulative amount of anthracycline received (lifetime)
• Assess symptoms indicating severe allergic reaction: rash, pruritus, urticaria, purpuric skin lesions, itching, flushing; product should be discontinued

> **BLACK BOX WARNING: Bone marrow depression (severe):** monitor CBC, differential, platelet count weekly; withhold product if baseline neutrophil count is <1500/mm³; notify prescriber of results if WBC <20,000/mm³, platelets <150,000/mm³; leukocyte nadir occurs 10-14 days after administration; recovery by 21st day

• Infection: treat before receiving this product in regimens >120 mg/m²; prophylactic antibiotics should be given (trimethaprim-sulfamethoxazole or a quinolone)
• Assess for increased uric acid levels, swelling, joint pain, primarily extremities; patient should be well hydrated to prevent urate deposits
• Monitor renal function studies: BUN, creatinine, serum uric acid, urine CCr before, during therapy; I&O ratio; report fall in urine output to <30 ml/hr; dosage adjustment is needed for serum creatinine >5 mg/dl

> **BLACK BOX WARNING: Severe hepatic disease:** monitor liver function tests before, during therapy (bilirubin, AST, ALT, LDH) as needed or monthly; note jaundice of skin or sclera, dark urine, clay-colored stools, itchy skin, abdominal pain, fever, diarrhea

• Assess for bleeding: hematuria, stool guaiac, bruising or petechiae, mucosa or orifices q8hr; inflammation of mucosa, breaks in skin
• Identify effects of alopecia on body image; discuss feelings about body changes

> **BLACK BOX WARNING: Extravasation (vesicant):** Assess for local irritation, pain, burning, necrosis at injection site; discontinue and start at another site

Patient/family education
• Advise patient to avoid use of products containing aspirin or NSAIDs, razors, commercial mouthwash, since bleeding may occur; to report symptoms of bleeding (hematuria, tarry stools)
• Instruct patient to report signs of anemia (fatigue, headache, irritability, faintness, shortness of breath)
• Inform patient that hair may be lost during treatment; a wig or hairpiece may make patient feel better; new hair may be different in color, texture, new hair growth occurs in ≤3 mo after treatment
• Caution patient not to have any vaccinations without the advice of the prescriber; serious reactions can occur
⚠ **Advise patient to use contraception during treatment and 4 mo afterward; pregnancy D**
• Advise patient that urine may appear red for 2 days
• Instruct patient to avoid crowds, persons with known infection
• Caution patient to avoid OTC medications, supplements unless approved by prescriber
• Teach patient to report rapid heartbeat, trouble breathing, fever, nausea, vomiting, oral sores

> **BLACK BOX WARNING:** Teach patient that irreversible myocardial damage, leukopenia, menopause may occur

Evaluation
Positive therapeutic outcome
• Prevention of rapid division of malignant cells

eplerenone (Rx)
(ep-ler-ee′known)
Inspra
Func. class.: Antihypertensive
Pregnancy category B

Do not confuse:
Inspra/Spiriva

ACTION: Binds to mineralocorticoid receptor and blocks the binding of aldosterone, a component of the renin-angiotensin-aldosterone system (RAAS)

Therapeutic outcome: Absence of hypertension

USES: Hypertension, alone or in combination with thiazide diuretics, CHF, post-MI

CONTRAINDICATIONS:
Hypersensitivity, increased serum creatinine >2 mg/dl (male) or >1.8 mg/dl (female), potassium >5.5 mEq/L, type 2 diabetes with microalbuminuria, hepatic disease, CCr <30 ml/min, CCr <50 ml/min in hypertension

Precautions: Pregnancy **B**, breastfeeding, children, geriatric, impaired renal/hepatic function, hyperkalemia

DOSAGE AND ROUTES
Adult: **PO** 50 mg/day initially, may increase to 50 mg bid after 4 wk; start dose at 25 mg/day if patient is taking CYP3A4 inhibitors

CHF/post-MI
Adult: **PO** 25 mg/day initially, may increase to 50 mg/day max

Available forms: Tabs 25, 50 mg

Implementation
• Store in tight container at 86° F (30° C) or less

ADVERSE EFFECTS
CNS: Headache, *dizziness, fatigue*
CV: Angina, **MI**
GI: Increased GGT *diarrhea,* abdominal pain, increased ALT
GU: Gynecomastia, mastodynia (males), abnormal vaginal bleeding
META: *Hyperkalemia,* hyponatremia, hypercholesteremia, hypertriglyceridemia, increased uric acid
RESP: *Cough*

Pharmacokinetics	
Absorption	Unknown
Distribution	Protein binding 50%
Metabolism	Liver (CYP3A4 inhibitor)
Excretion	Urine, feces
Half-life	4-6 hr

Pharmacodynamics	
Onset	Unknown
Peak	1½ hr
Duration	Unknown

INTERACTIONS
Individual drugs
Clarithromycin, imatinib, nelfinavir, nefazodone, ritonavir, troleandomycin: do not use concurrently
Erythromycin, fluconazole, verapamil: reduce dose of eplerenone; increased eplerenone levels
Itraconazole, ketoconazole, saquinavir, verapamil: increased levels of eplerenone; reduce dose of eplerenone
Lithium: increased serum lithium levels

Drug classifications
ACE inhibitors, angiotensin II antagonists, diuretics (potassium-sparing), NSAIDs, potassium supplements: increased hyperkalemia
CYP3A4 inhibitors: increased levels of eplerenone; reduce dose of eplerenone
NSAIDs: decreased antihypertensive effect

Drug/herb
Decreased antihypertensive effect: ephedra

Drug/food
Grapefruit, grapefruit juice: increased product level by 25%
• Do not use salt substitutes with potassium

Drug/lab test
Increased: BUN, creatinine, potassium, cholesterol, lipids, uric acid
Decreased: sodium

NURSING CONSIDERATIONS
Assessment
• **Hypertension:** monitor B/P at peak/trough level of product, orthostatic hypotension, syncope when used with diuretic
• Monitor renal studies: protein, BUN, creatinine; increased liver function tests; uric acid may be increased
• Monitor potassium levels, hyperkalemia may occur

Patient/family education
• Advise patient not to discontinue product abruptly
• Advise patient not to use OTC products (cough, cold, allergy) unless directed by prescriber; do not use salt substitutes containing potassium without consulting prescriber
• Teach patient the importance of complying with dosage schedule, even if feeling better
• Teach patient that product may cause dizziness, fainting, light-headedness; may occur during first few days of therapy
• Teach patient how to take B/P, normal readings for age-group

Adverse effects: *italics* = common; **bold** = life-threatening

- Teach patient to avoid activities that require coordination

Evaluation
Positive therapeutic outcome
- Decrease in B/P

---

epoetin alfa (Rx)
(ee-poe′e-tin)
Epogen, Eprex ✦, Procrit
Func. class.: Antianemic, biologic modifier, hormone
Chem. class.: Amino acid polypeptide
Pregnancy category C

ACTION: Erythropoietin is one factor controlling rate of red cell production; product is developed by recombinant DNA technology

Therapeutic outcome: Decreased anemia with increased RBCs

USES: Anemia caused by reduced endogenous erythropoietin production, primarily end-stage renal disease; to correct hemostatic defect in uremia; anemia caused by AZT (zidovudine) treatment in HIV-positive patients; anemia caused by chemotherapy; reduction of allogeneic blood transfusion in surgery patients

Unlabeled uses: Anemia in premature preterm infants

CONTRAINDICATIONS:
Hypersensitivity to mammalian cell–derived products or human albumin; uncontrolled hypertension

Precautions: Pregnancy **C**, breastfeeding, children <1 mo, seizure disorder, porphyria, CV disease, hemodialysis, latex allergy, hypertension, history of CABG; multidose preserved formulation contains benzyl alcohol and should not be used in premature infants

---

BLACK BOX WARNING: Hgb >12 g/dl, surgery, neoplastic disease

DOSAGE AND ROUTES
Anemia due to chronic kidney disease including dialysis-dependent and dialysis-independent patients to decrease the need for red blood cell transfusion
Adult/adolescent ≥17 yr: Subcut/IV, initially, 50-100 units/kg IV/SC 3×/wk; for patients on dialysis, administer IV and initiate treatment when hemoglobin (Hgb) is <10 g/dl. If Hgb approaches or exceeds 11 g/dl, reduce or interrupt the dose. For patients not on dialysis, consider initiating treatment only when Hgb is <10 g/dl and the rate of Hgb decline indicates the likelihood of requiring a RBC transfusion and reducing the risk of alloimmunization and/or other RBC transfusion-related risks is a goal. If Hgb is >10 g/dl, reduce or interrupt the dose, and use the lowest dose sufficient to reduce the need for RBC transfusions. If the Hgb rises >1 g/dl in any 2-wk period, reduce dose by 25% or more as needed to reduce rapid responses. In contrast, if Hgb has not increased >1 g/dl after 4 wk of therapy, increase the dose by 25%. For patients who do not respond adequately over a 12-wk escalation period, increasing the dose further is unlikely to improve response and may increase risks. Use the lowest dose that will maintain a Hgb concentration sufficient to reduce the need for RBC transfusions. Evaluate other causes of anemia, and discontinue if responsiveness does not improve
Adolescent ≤16 yr/child/infant: Subcut/IV 50 units/kg 3×/wk initially; for dosage adjustments, see adult dosage

Zidovudine-induced anemia in HIV-infected patients with circulating endogenous erythropoietin concentrations ≤500 mUnits/ml who are receiving a dose of zidovudine ≤4200 mg/wk
Adult: Subcut/IV initially, 100 units/kg 3×/wk. If Hgb does not increase after 8 wk, increase by 50-100 units/kg at 4 to 8 wk intervals until Hgb is at a concentration to avoid RBC transfusions or a dose of 300 units/kg is reached. If the Hgb >12 g/dl, withhold, once Hgb <11 g/dl resume at a dose 25% below the previous dose

Anemia in patients with nonmyeloid malignancies where the anemia is due to the effect of concomitantly administered chemotherapy and at least 2 additional months of chemotherapy is planned
Adult: Subcut 150 units/kg three times weekly or 40,000 units once weekly only when the hemoglobin is <10 g/dl and only until the chemotherapy course is completed. Adjust the dose to maintain the lowest Hgb concentration sufficient to avoid RBC transfusions. If no rise in Hgb ≥1 g/dl after 4 wk of therapy and Hgb is <10 g/dl, the dosage may be increased to 300 units/kg subcut three times weekly or 60,000 units once wkly. Discontinue if after 8 wk of therapy there is no response as measured by

---

Hgb concentrations or if transfusions are still required. Reduce the dose by approximately 25% if Hgb increases by more than 1 g/dl in any 2-week period or if Hgb reaches a concentration needed to avoid RBC infusion. If Hgb is increasing and exceeds a concentration necessary to avoid blood transfusions, hold therapy and reinstitute at a dose that is 25% lower when the Hgb reaches a concentration where transfusions may be needed

Adolescent/child ≥5 yr: IV 600 units/kg qwk only when the hemoglobin is <10 g/dl and only until the chemotherapy course is completed. Adjust the dose to maintain the lowest Hgb concentration sufficient to avoid RBC transfusions. If no rise in Hgb ≤1 g/dl after 4 wk of therapy and Hgb is <10 g/dl, the dosage may be increased to 900 units/kg (up to 60,000 units) IV weekly. Discontinue after 8 wk there is no response as measured by Hgb concentrations or if transfusions are still required. Reduce the dose by approximately 25% if Hgb increases by more than 1 g/dl in any 2-wk period or if Hgb reaches a concentration needed to avoid RBC infusion. If the Hgb is increasing and exceeds a concentration necessary to avoid blood transfusions, hold therapy and reinstitute at a dose that is 25% lower when the Hgb reaches a concentration where transfusions may be needed

To reduce the need for allogenic blood transfusions in anemic patients (hemoglobin >10 and ≤13 g/dl) scheduled to undergo elective, noncardiac, nonvascular surgery
Adult: Subcut 300 units/kg/day × 10 days before surgery, on the day of surgery, and for 4 days after surgery (14 days total) or 600 units/kg once weekly, 21, 14, and 7 days before surgery plus one dose on the day of surgery

Available forms: Inj 2000, 3000, 4000, 10,000, 20,000, 40,000 units/ml

Implementation
SUBCUT route
• Before injecting, preservative-free, single-dose formulation may be admixed by using 0.9% NaCl, USP, with benzyl alcohol 0.9% at a 1:1 ratio to reduce injection site discomfort

Direct IV route
• Administer by direct route at end of dialysis by venous line, do not shake vial
• If Hct increases by 4% in 2 wk, decrease dose by 25 units/kg; increase dose if Hct does not increase by 5-6 points after 8 wk of therapy; suggested target Hct range 30%-36%

• Give additional heparin to lower chance of clots

Solution compatibilities: Do not dilute or administer with other solutions

ADVERSE EFFECTS
CNS: **Seizures,** coldness, sweating, headache
CV: *Hypertension,* **hypertensive encephalopathy, CHF,** edema, **DVT**
INTEG: Pruritus, rash, inj site reaction
MISC: Iron deficiency
MS: Bone pain
RESP: Cough

Pharmacokinetics

Absorption	Well absorbed (SUBCUT), completely absorbed (**IV**)
Distribution	Increased RBC count 2-6 wk
Metabolism	Unknown
Excretion	Unknown
Half-life	5-14 hr

Pharmacodynamics

	SUBCUT/IV
Onset	Unknown
Peak	Immediate
Duration	Unknown

INTERACTIONS
Drug classifications
Anticoagulants: need for increased heparin during hemodialysis

NURSING CONSIDERATIONS
Assessment
• Monitor renal studies: urinalysis, protein, blood, BUN, creatinine; I&O; report drop in output to <50 ml/hr

> **BLACK BOX WARNING:** Monitor blood studies: ferritin, transferrin monthly, transferrin sat ≥20%; ferritin ≥100 ng/ml; Hct 2 ×/wk until stabilized in target range (30%-36%), then at regular intervals; those with endogenous erythropoietin levels of <500 units/L respond to this agent; check for symptoms of anemia: fatigue, pallor, dyspnea; monitor Hct 2 ×/wk in chronic renal failure; cancer patients and those being treated with zidovudine should be monitored weekly, then periodically after stabilization; death may occur in Hgb >12 g/dl

• Assess for CNS symptoms: coldness, sweating, pain in long bones

• Assess CV status: B/P before, during treatment; hypertension may occur rapidly, leading to hypertension encephalopathy; antihypertensives may be needed
• Assess patient during hemodialysis for bruits, thrills, or shunts; product prevents severe anemia in chronic renal failure; clotting may need to be treated with increased anticoagulant
• **Seizures:** place on seizure precautions; assess for seizures if Hct is increased within 2 wk by 4 points, increased B/P, more common in chronic renal failure in the first 90 days of treatment
• Monitor serum iron, ferritin, transferrin levels; iron therapy may be needed to prevent recurring anemia
• Monitor B/P, check for rising B/P as Hct rises
• Monitor blood studies: BUN, creatinine, uric acid, platelets, WBC, phosphorus, potassium, bleeding time; Hct, Hgb, RBCs, reticulocytes should be checked in chronic renal failure
• For hypersensitivity reactions: Skin rashes, urticaria (rare), antibody development does not occur
⚠ For pure cell aplasia (PRCA) in absence of other causes, evaluate by testing serum for recombinant erythropoietin antibodies; any loss of response to epoetin should be evaluated

Patient/family education
• Teach patient how to take B/P
• Advise patients to take iron supplements, vit B_{12}, folic acid as directed
• Teach patient to avoid driving or hazardous activity during treatment
• Teach patients with renal disease to include high-iron and low-potassium foods in their diets (meat, dark green leafy vegetables, eggs, enriched breads)
• Teach patient the reason for treatment, expected results
• Advise patient to use contraception

Evaluation
Positive therapeutic outcome
• Increased appetite
• Enhanced sense of well-being
• Increase in reticulocyte count in 2-6 wk, Hgb, Hct

eprosartan (Rx)
(ep-roh-sar′tan)
Teveten
Func. class.: Antihypertensive
Chem. class.: Angiotensin II receptor antagonist (Subtype AT_1)
Pregnancy category C (1st trimester), D (2nd/3rd trimesters)

ACTION: Blocks the vasoconstrictor and aldosterone-secreting effects of angiotensin II; selectively blocks the binding of angiotensin II to the AT_1 receptor found in tissues

Therapeutic outcome: Decreased B/P

USES: Hypertension, alone or in combination with other antihypertensives

CONTRAINDICATIONS:
Hypersensitivity

> **BLACK BOX WARNING:** Pregnancy **D**

Precautions: Breastfeeding, children, geriatric, hypersensitivity to ACE inhibitors, renal/hepatic disease, angioedema, hyperkalemia

DOSAGE AND ROUTES
Adult: PO 600 mg/day; dose may be divided and given bid, with total daily doses ranging from 400-800 mg, max 900 mg/day

Renal dose
Adult: PO CCr ≤30 ml/min, max 600 mg/day

Available forms: Tabs 400, 600 mg

Implementation
• May be given without regard to meals

ADVERSE EFFECTS
CNS: *Dizziness*, depression, *fatigue*, headache
CV: Chest pain, palpitations
EENT: Sinusitis
GI: *Diarrhea, dyspepsia, abdominal pain*
GU: UTI
HEMA: Neutropenia
INTEG: Pruritus, **angioedema**
META: Hypertriglyceridemia
MS: *Myalgia*, arthralgia, **rhabdomyolysis**
RESP: *Cough, upper respiratory infection*, rhinitis, pharyngitis, viral infection
SYST: Anaphylaxis

Pharmacokinetics

Absorption	Absolute bioavailability ~13%; food delays absorption
Distribution	Protein binding 98%
Metabolism	Moderate renal impairment increases product levels by 30%, hepatic impairment increases levels by 40%
Excretion	Urine, feces
Half-life	5-9 hr

Pharmacodynamics

Onset	Unknown
Peak	1-2 hr
Duration	Unknown

INTERACTIONS

Drug classifications

ACE inhibitors, angiotensin II receptor antagonists, potassium sparing diuretics, potassium supplements: increased hyperkalemia

NSAIDs, salicylates: decreased antihypertensive effect

Other antihypertensives: increased antihypertensive effect

Drug/lab test

Increased: ALT, AST, alkaline phosphatase, potassium

Decreased: Hgb

NURSING CONSIDERATIONS

Assessment

• Assess B/P with position changes, pulse q4hr; note rate, rhythm, quality
• Assess electrolytes: K, Na, Cl
• Assess baselines in renal, liver function tests before therapy begins
• Assess for edema in feet, legs daily
• Assess skin turgor, dryness of mucous membranes for hydration status

Patient/family education

• Advise patient to comply with dosage schedule, even if feeling better
• Advise patient to notify prescriber of fever, swelling of hands or feet, chest pain
• Inform patient that excessive perspiration, dehydration, diarrhea may lead to fall in blood pressure; consult prescriber if these occur, maintain adequate hydration
• Inform patient that product may cause dizziness; advise to avoid hazardous activities until effect is known, to rise slowly from sitting position

> **BLACK BOX WARNING:** Advise patient not to take this medication if pregnant or breastfeeding, or if allergic reaction to this product has occurred

• Advise patient to take missed dose as soon as possible, unless within 1 hr of next dose

Evaluation

Positive therapeutic outcome
• Decreased B/P

> **⚠ HIGH ALERT**
>
> ## eptifibatide (Rx)
> (ep-tih-fib′ah-tide)
> **Integrilin**
> *Func. class.:* Antiplatelet agent
> *Chem. class.:* Glycoprotein IIb/IIIa inhibitor
> **Pregnancy category B**

ACTION: Platelet glycoprotein antagonist; reversibly prevents fibrinogen, von Willebrand factor from binding to the glycoprotein IIb/IIIa receptor, inhibiting platelet aggregation

Therapeutic outcome: Decreased platelets

USES: Acute coronary syndrome, including those undergoing percutaneous coronary intervention (PCI)

CONTRAINDICATIONS:

Hypersensitivity, active internal bleeding, recent history of bleeding, stroke within 30 days or any hemorrhagic stroke, major surgery with severe trauma, severe hypertension, history of intracranial bleeding, current or planned use of another parenteral GPIIb/IIIa inhibitor, dependence on renal dialysis, coagulopathy, AV malformation, aneurysm

Precautions: Pregnancy **B**, breastfeeding, children, geriatric, bleeding, renal function impairment

DOSAGE AND ROUTES

Acute coronary syndrome

Adult: IV BOL 180 mcg/kg as soon as diagnosed, max 22.6 mg; then IV CONT INF 2 mcg/kg/min until discharge or coronary artery bypass graft (CABG) up to 72 hr, max 15 mg/hr

PCI in patients without acute coronary syndrome

Adult: IV BOL 180 mcg/kg given immediately before PCI; then 2 mcg/kg/min × 18 hr by

---

CONT IV INF and a 2nd 180 mcg/kg BOL, 10 min after 1st BOL; continue INF for up to 18-24 hr at a rate of 1 mcg/kg/min

Renal dose
Adult: IV BOL CCr <50 ml/min 2-4 mg/dl same loading dose, then ½ usual INF dose; CCr <10 ml/min contraindicated

Available forms: Sol for inj 2 mg/ml (10 ml), 0.75 mg/ml (100 ml)

Implementation
• Aspirin and heparin may be given with this product; check for bleeding
• Discontinue heparin before removing femoral artery sheath after PCI
• Do not give discolored solutions, those with particulates; discard unused amount
• Discontinue product prior to CABG
• All medications PO if possible; avoid IM inj, all catheters

Direct IV route
• After withdrawing the BOL dose from 10-ml vial, give **IV** push over 1-2 min
• Do not use discolored sol or sol with particulate

Continuous IV infusion route
• Follow BOL dose with cont inf using infusion pump, give product undiluted directly from the 100-ml vial, spike the 100-ml vial with a vented infusion set; use caution when centering the spike on the circle of the stopper top

Y-site compatibilities: Alfentanil, alteplase, amikacin, aminophylline, amphotericin B lipid complex, amphotericin B liposome, ampicillin, ampicillin-sulbactam, anidulafungin, argatroban, atenolol, atracurium, atropine, azithromycin, aztreonam, bivalirudin, bumetanide, buprenorphine, butorphanol, calcium chloride/gluconate, ceFAZolin, cefepime, cefoperazone, cefotaxime, cefoTEtan, cefOXitin, cefTAZidime, ceftizoxime, cefTRIAXone, cefuroxime, cimetidine, ciprofloxacin, cisatracurium, clindamycin, cycloSPORINE, DAPTOmycin, dexamethasone, D₅/NaCl 0.9%, diazepam, diltiazem, diphenhydrAMINE, DOBUTamine, dolasetron, DOPamine, doxycycline, droperidol, enalaprilat, ePHEDrine, EPINEPHrine, ertapenem, erythromycin, esmolol, famotidine, fentaNYL, fluconazole, fosphenytoin, ganciclovir, gatifloxacin, gentamicin, granisetron, haloperidol, heparin, hydrocortisone, HYDROmorphone, hydrOXYzine, imipenem-cilastatin, inamrinone, isoproterenol, ketorolac, labetalol, leucovorin, levofloxacin, levorphanol, lidocaine, linezolid, LORazepam, magnesium sulfate, mannitol, meperidine, meropenem, methylPREDNISolone, metoclopramide, metoprolol, metroNIDAZOLE, micafungin, midazolam, milrinone, minocycline, mivacurium, morphine, nalbuphine, naloxone, niCARdipine, nitroglycerin, nitroprusside, NS, octreotide, ofloxacin, ondansetron, oxytocin, palonosetron, pancuronium, PEMEtrexed, PENTobarbital, PHENobarbital, phenylephrine, piperacillin, piperacillin-tazobactam, potassium chloride/phosphates, procainamide, prochlorperazine, promethazine, propranolol, ranitidine, remifentanil, rocuronium, sodium bicarbonate/phosphates, succinylcholine, SUFentanil, sulfamethoxazole-trimethoprim, teniposide, theophylline, ticarcillin, ticarcillin-clavulanate, tigecycline, tirofiban, tobramycin, trimethobenzamide, vancomycin, vecuronium, verapamil, zidovudine, zoledronic acid

Solution compatibilities: 0.9% NaCl, D₅/0.9% NaCl
• Discontinue product before CABG
• Give all medications PO if possible, avoid IM inj and catheters

ADVERSE EFFECTS
CV: Stroke, hypotension
GU: Hematuria
HEMA: Thrombocytopenia
SYST: Major/minor bleeding from any site, anaphylaxis

Pharmacokinetics

Absorption	Unknown
Distribution	Protein binding 25%
Metabolism	Limited
Excretion	Kidneys
Half-life	1.5-2 hr

Pharmacodynamics

Onset	Within 1 hr

INTERACTIONS
Individual drugs
Abciximab, aspirin, clopidogrel, dipyridamole, heparin, ticlopidine, valproate: increased bleeding

Drug classifications
Anticoagulants, NSAIDs, SSRIs, SNRIs, thrombolytics: increased bleeding
Platelet receptor inhibitors IIb, IIIa: do not give together

Drug/herb
Feverfew, garlic, ginger, ginkgo, ginseng

NURSING CONSIDERATIONS

Assessment

- **Thrombocytopenia:** Monitor platelets, Hgb, Hct, creatinine, APTT baseline, INR, within 6 hr of loading dose and daily thereafter; patients undergoing PCI should have ACT monitored; maintain APTT 50-70 sec unless PCI is to be performed; during PCI, ACT should be 200-300 sec; if platelets drop $<$100,000/mm^3, obtain additional platelet counts; if thrombocytopenia is confirmed, discontinue product; also draw Hct, Hgb, serum creatinine
- **Assess for bleeding:** gums, bruising, ecchymosis, petechiae; from GI, GU tract, cardiac catheter sites, IM inj sites

Patient/family education

- Teach patient to report bruising, bleeding, chest pain immediately
- Inform patient of reason for medication and expected results

Evaluation

Positive therapeutic outcome

- Decreased platelets

ergocalciferol

See vitamin D

eribulin (Rx)

(er′i-bue′lin)

Halaven

Func. class.: Antineoplastics, nontaxane

Pregnancy category D

Do not confuse:

eribulin/epirubicin/erlotinib

ACTION: Potent antimitotic agent, different from taxes, vinca alkaloids, epothilones; blocks cell progression in G$_2$-M phase, inhibits the growth phase of microtubules and sequesters tubules, leading to disruption of mitotic spindles and apoptotic cell death

Therapeutic outcome: Decreased spread and size of tumor

USES: Metastatic breast cancer patients who have received at least 2 chemotherapy regimens

CONTRAINDICATIONS:

Hypersensitivity, pregnancy **D**

Precautions: Bradycardia, breastfeeding, children, electrolyte imbalances, heart failure, hepatic disease, hypokalemia, hypomagnesemia, infants, infertility, neonates, neutropenia, peripheral neuropathy, QT prolongation, renal disease

DOSAGE AND ROUTES

Adult: IV 1.4 mg/m^2 over 2-5 min on days 1 and 8, repeat q21days

Recommendations for dose delay

- *For ANC $<$1000/mm^3, platelets $<$75,000/ mm^3, or grade 3 or 4 non-hematologic toxicities:* Do not administer; the day 8 dose may be delayed a maximum of 1 wk
- *For the day 8 dose, if toxicities do not resolve to $\leq$grade 2 by day 15:* Omit the dose
- *For the day 8 dose, if toxicities resolve or improve to $\leq$grade 2 by day 15:* Administer eribulin at a reduced dose (see below) and initiate the next cycle no sooner than 2 wk later

Dosage adjustments for hematologic toxicity

- *ANC $<$500/mm^3 for $>$7 days or ANC $<$1000/mm^3 with fever or infection:* Permanently reduce dosage to 1.1 mg/m^2
- *Platelets $<$25,000/mm^3 or $<$50,000/mm^3 requiring transfusion:* Permanently reduce dosage to 1.1 mg/m^2
- *If day 8 of previous cycle omitted or delayed:* Permanently reduce dosage to 1.1 mg/m^2
- *While receiving 1.1 mg/m^2, if recurrence of hematologic event occurs, or if day 8 of previous cycle omitted or delayed:* Permanently reduce dosage to 0.7 mg/m^2
- *While receiving 0.7 mg/m^2, if recurrence of hematologic event occurs, or if day 8 of previous cycle omitted or delayed:* Discontinue

Dose adjustments of eribulin for non-hematologic toxicity during treatment

- *Any grade 3 or 4 non-hematologic toxicity:* Permanently reduce dosage to 1.1 mg/m^2
- *If day 8 of previous cycle omitted or delayed:* Permanently reduce dosage to 1.1 mg/m^2
- *While receiving 1.1 mg/m^2, if recurrence of grade 3 or 4 non-hematologic toxicity occurs, or if day 8 of previous cycle omitted or delayed:* Permanently reduce dosage to 0.7 mg/m^2
- *While receiving 0.7 mg/m^2, if recurrence of grade 3 or 4 non-hematologic toxicity occurs, or if day 8 of previous cycle omitted or delayed:* Discontinue

Available forms: Solution for injection
1 mg/2 ml

Implementation

IV direct, intermittent route
• Visually inspect for particulate matter or
discoloration as solution and container permit;
withdraw required amount (0.5 mg/ml) from
single-use vial, give undiluted over 2-5 min or
diluted in 100 ml 0.9% NaCl and give as intermittent infusion, do not give through line with
dextrose or any other product
• Store at room temperature for 4 hr or 24 hr
refrigerated

ADVERSE EFFECTS

CNS: Depression, dizziness, *fatigue*, fever,
headache, insomnia, *peripheral neuropathy*
CV: QT prolongation, peripheral edema
GI: Abdominal pain, anorexia, constipation, di-
arrhea, dyspepsia, nausea, vomiting, weight loss
HEMA: Anemia, neutropenia, thrombocy-
topenia
INTEG: *Alopecia*, rash, stomatitis
META: Hypokalemia
MS: Arthralgia, myalgia, bone/back pain
RESP: Cough, dyspnea
SYST: Infection

Pharmacokinetics

Absorption	Protein binding, 49%-65%
Distribution	Unknown
Metabolism	Inhibits CYP3A4
Excretion	Feces 82%, urine 9%
Half-life	40 hr, increased levels in renal/hepatic disease

Pharmacodynamics

Unknown

INTERACTIONS

Individual drugs
**Arsenic trioxide, astemizole, bepridil, chlo-
roquine, cisapride, clarithromycin, dextromethorphan, dronedarone, droperidol,
erythromycin, halofantrine, haloperidol,
levomethadyl, methadone, pentamidine,
pimozide, posaconazole, probucol,
propafenone, quiNIDine, saquinavir,
sparfloxacin, terfenadine, troleandomycin, and ziprasidone; also to a lesser
degree abarelix, alfuzosin, amoxapine,
apomorphine, artemether; lumefantrine, asenapine, ofloxacin, cloZAPine,
cyclobenzaprine, dasatinib, dolasetron,
flecainide, gatifloxacin, gemifloxacin,**
**iloperidone, lapatinib, levofloxacin,
lopinavir; ritonavir, magnesium sulfate;
potassium sulfate; sodium sulfate, maprotiline, mefloquine, moxifloxacin, nilotinib,
norfloxacin, octreotide, ciprofloxacin,
OLANZapine, ondansetron, paliperidone,
palonosetron, QUEtiapine, ranolazine,
risperidone, sertindole, SUNItinib,
tacrolimus, telavancin, telithromycin,
tetrabenazine, venlafaxine, vardenafil,
vorinostat: increased QT prolongation**

Drug classifications
**Certain phenothiazines (chlorproMAZINE,
mesoridazine, thioridazine), class IA
antiarrhythmics (disopyramide, procainamide, quiNIDine), class III antiarrhythmics (amiodarone, bretylium, dofetilide,
ibutilide, sotalol), also to a lesser degree,
beta-agonists, halogenated anesthetics,
local anesthetics, some phenothiazines
(fluPHENAZine, perphenazine, prochlorperazine, trifluoperazine), tricyclic antidepressants: increased QT prolongation**

NURSING CONSIDERATIONS

Assessment

• Peripheral neuropathy: assess for pain, numbness in extremities
• Infection: assess for increased temperature,
sore throat, flulike symptoms
• **QT prolongation:** assess for drug interactions that may occur; monitor ECG, heart rate
• **Bone marrow depression:** CBC and differential, serum creatinine/bun/electrolytes,
liver function tests, baseline and periodically,
increased AST/ALT $>3 \times$ ULN or total bilirubin
$>1.5 \times$ ULN are at a greater chance of grade 4
or febrile neutropenia

Patient/family education

• Infection: teach patient to notify prescriber
of increased temperature, sore throat, fatigue,
flu-like symptoms
• QT prolongation: teach patient to report extra
heartbeats
• Peripheral neuropathy: teach patient to report
tingling, pain in extremities
• Teach patient reason for product and expected results
• Advise patient to report side effects to health
care provider
• Advise patient to avoid other medications,
supplements unless approved by provider, serious drug interactions may occur
• Discuss hair loss and use of wig or hairpiece

A Advise patient to notify prescriber if pregnancy is planned or suspected (pregnancy D), avoid breastfeeding

Evaluation
Positive therapeutic outcome
• Decreasing tumor spread and size

erlotinib (Rx)
(er-loe′tye-nib)
Tarceva
Func. class.: Misc. antineoplastic
Chem. class.: Epidermal growth factor receptor inhibitor
Pregnancy category D

ACTION: Not fully understood. Inhibits intracellular phosphorylation of cell surface receptors associated with epidermal growth factor receptors.

Therapeutic outcome: Decrease in tumor size

USES: Non–small cell lung cancer (NSCLC) including EGFR exon 19 deletions or exon 21 substitution mutations, pancreatic cancer

Unlabeled uses: Squamous cell, head and neck cancer

CONTRAINDICATIONS:
Pregnancy **D**, breastfeeding

Precautions: Renal, hepatic; ocular, pulmonary disorders; children; geriatric, bradycardia, heart failure, hypokalemia, infertility, QT prolongation

DOSAGE AND ROUTES
CYP3A4 inducers concurrently (such as rifampin or phenytoin)
Dosage increase is advised

CYP3A4 inhibitors (atazanavir, clarithromycin, indinavir, itraconazole, ketoconazole, telithromycin, ritonavir, saquinavir, troleandomycin, nelfinavir)
Dosage reduction may be needed.

Hepatic dose
Adult: PO interrupt if total bilirubin >3 times ULN and/or transaminases >5 times ULN

Non–small cell lung cancer (NSCLC)
Adult: PO 150 mg/day

Pancreatic cancer
Adult: PO 100 mg/day in combination with gemcitabine 1000 mg/m^2 cycle 1, days 1, 8, 15, 22, 29, 36, 43 of an 8-wk cycle; cycle 2 and subsequent cycles, days 1, 8, 15 of a 4-wk cycle

Available forms: Tabs 25, 100, 150 mg

Implementation
• Administer 1 hr before or 2 hr after food

ADVERSE EFFECTS
CNS: CVA, *anxiety, depression, headache, rigors*
CV: MI/ischemia
EENT: *Ocular changes, conjunctivitis, eye pain*
GI: *Nausea, diarrhea, vomiting, anorexia, mouth ulceration,* **hepatic failure, GI perforation**
GU: Renal impairment/failure
HEMA: DVT
INTEG: *Rash,* Stevens-Johnson–like skin reactions, toxic epidermal necrolysis
MISC: *Fatigue, infection*
RESP: Interstitial lung disease, *cough, dyspnea,* ARDS, pulmonary fibrosis
SYST: Hepatorenal syndrome

Pharmacokinetics
Absorption	Slowly absorbed
Distribution	Unknown
Metabolism	Metabolized by CYP3A4
Excretion	Feces (86%), urine (<4%)
Half-life	36 hr

Pharmacodynamics
Onset	Unknown
Peak	3-7 hr
Duration	Unknown

INTERACTIONS
Individual drugs
Metoprolol, warfarin: increased plasma concentrations
Smoking: decreased erlotinib level, dose may need to be increased

Drug classifications
CYP3A4 inducers (phenytoin, rifampin, carBAMazepine, phenobarbital), proton-pump inhibitors: decreased erlotinib levels
CYP3A4 inhibitors (clarithromycin, erythromycin, itraconazole, ketoconazole, telithromycin): increased erlotinib concentrations
HMG-CoA reductase inhibitors: increased myopathy

Drug/herb

St. John's wort: decreased erlotinib levels

Drug/food

Grapefruit juice: increased effect of erlotinib

NURSING CONSIDERATIONS

Assessment

⚠ Serious skin toxicities: toxic epidermal necrolysis, Stevens-Johnson syndrome

⚠ Assess for MI/ischemia, CVA in pancreatic cancer

⚠ Assess for pulmonary changes: lung sounds, cough, dyspnea; interstitial lung disease may occur, may be fatal; discontinue therapy if confirmed

• **Assess for ocular changes:** eye irritation, corneal erosion/ulcer, aberrant eyelash growth

• Assess for GI symptoms: frequency of stools; if diarrhea is poorly tolerated, therapy may be discontinued for up to 14 days; monitor for dehydration, fluid status during period of vomiting and diarrhea

• Monitor blood studies: INR, LFTs, PT

• **Hepatic failure:** interrupt dosing if severe changes to liver function occur (total bilirubin >3× ULN and/or transaminases >5× ULN for normal pretreatment LFTs)

⚠ GI perforation/bleeding: some cases have been fatal

Patient/family education

⚠ Teach patient to report adverse reactions immediately: SOB, severe abdominal pain, persistent diarrhea or vomiting, ocular changes, skin eruptions

• Explain reason for treatment, expected results

⚠ Advise patient to use contraception during treatment; pregnancy D, avoid breastfeeding

• Instruct patient to avoid use with other products, herbs, or supplements unless approved by provider

• Instruct patient to avoid smoking; decreases effect of this product

Evaluation

Positive therapeutic outcome

• Decrease non–small cell lung cancer cells

ertapenem (Rx)

(er-tah-pen'em)

Invanz

Func. class.: Antiinfective, miscellaneous

Chem. class.: Carbapenem

Pregnancy category B

Do not confuse:

Invanz/Aninza

ACTION: Interferes with cell wall replication of susceptible organisms

Therapeutic outcome: Bactericidal action against the following organisms: *Bacteroides fragilis, Bacteroides distasonis, Bacteroides ovatus, Bacteroides thetaiotaomicron, Bacteroides uniformis; Clostridium clostridioforme, Escherichia coli, Eubacterium lentum, Haemophilus influenzae* (β lactamase–negative), *Klebsiella pneumoniae, Moraxella catarrhalis, Peptostreptococcus* sp., *Porphyromonas asaccharolytica, Prevotella bivia, Staphylococcus aureus* (methicillin-susceptible); *Streptococcus agalactiae, Streptococcus pneumoniae* (penicillin-susceptible), *Streptococcus pyogenes*

USES: Bacteremia, *Bacteroides distasonis, Bacteroides fragilis, Bacteroides ovatus, Bacteroides thetaiotaomicron, Bacteroides uniformis, Bacteroides vulgatus, Citrobacter freundii, Citrobacter koseri, Clostridium clostridioforme, Clostridium perfringens,* community-acquired pneumonia, diabetic foot ulcer, endomyometritis, *Enterobacter aerogenes, Enterobacter cloacae, Escherichia coli, Eubacterium lentum, Fusobacterium, Haemophilus influenzae* (beta-lactamase negative), *Haemophilus influenzae* (beta-lactamase positive), *Haemophilus parainfluenzae,* intraabdominal infections, *Klebsiella oxytoca, Klebsiella pneumoniae, Moraxella catarrhalis, Morganella morganii, Peptostreptococcus, Porphyromonas asaccharolytica, Prevotella bivia, Proteus mirabilis, Proteus vulgaris, Providencia rettgeri, Providencia stuartii, Serratia marcescens,* skin infections, *Staphylococcus aureus* (MSSA), *Staphylococcus epidermidis, Streptococcus agalactiae* (group B streptococci), *Streptococcus pneumoniae, Streptococcus pyogenes* (group A beta-hemolytic streptococci), surgical infection prophylaxis, urinary tract infections

CONTRAINDICATIONS:

Hypersensitivity to this product or its components, to amide-type local anesthetics (IM only); anaphylactic reactions to β-lactams

Precautions: Pregnancy **B**, breastfeeding, children, geriatric, renal/hepatic/GI disease, seizures

DOSAGE AND ROUTES

Complicated intraabdominal infections
Adult: IM/IV 1 g/day × 5-14 days
Child 3 mo-12 yr: IM/IV 15 mg/kg bid (max 1 g/day) × 5-14 days

Complicated skin/skin structure infections
Adult/adolescent: IM/IV 1 g/day × 7-14 days
Child 3 mo-12 yr: IM/IV 15 mg/kg bid × 7-14 days

Community-acquired pneumonia
Adult/adolescent: IM/IV 1 g/day × 10-14 days
Child 3 mo-12 yr: IM/IV 15 mg/kg bid × 10-14 days, max 1 g/day

Complicated UTI
Adult/adolescent: IM/IV 1 g/day × 10-14 days
Child 3 mo-12 yr: IM/IV 15 mg/kg bid × 10-14 days

Acute pelvic infections
Adult/adolescent: IM/IV 1 g/day × 3-10 days
Child 3 mo-12 yr: IM/IV 15 mg/kg bid × 3-10 days

Surgical infection prophylaxis
Adult: IV 1 g as a single dose 1 hr prior to surgical incision

Renal dose
Adult: IM/IV CCr ≤30 ml/min, 500 mg/day

Available forms: Powder, lyophilized, 1 g

Implementation

IV route
• Visually inspect for particulate matter and discoloration before use: may be colorless to pale yellow; do not mix with other products; dextrose solutions are not compatible
• 1 g vial: For each gram reconstitute with 10 ml of either NS injection, sterile water for injection, or bacteriostatic water for injection to 100 mg/ml, shake
• 1 g dose: immediately transfer contents of the reconstituted vial to 50 ml of NS injection; for a dose <1 g (pediatric patients 3 mo to 12 yr): from the reconstituted vial, immediately withdraw a volume equal to 15 mg/kg of body weight (max 1 g/day) and dilute in NS injection to a concentration of 20 mg/ml or less

IV infusion route
• Complete the infusion within 6 hr of reconstitution, infuse over 30 min; do not co-infuse with other medications
• The reconstituted IV solution may be stored at room temperature if used within 6 hr, or stored under refrigeration for 24 hr and used within 4 hr after removal from refrigeration; do not freeze

IM route
• Reconstitute the 1 g vial of ertapenem with 3.2 ml of 1% lidocaine HCl injection (without EPINEPHrine) (280 mg/ml), agitate well to form a solution; the IM reconstituted formulation is not for IV use
• IM administration may be used as an alternative to IV administration in the treatment of infections where IM therapy is appropriate; only given via IM injection × 7 days
• For a 1 g dose: immediately withdraw the contents of the vial and inject deeply into a large muscle, aspirate prior to injection to avoid injection into a blood vessel
• For a dose <1 g (i.e., for pediatric patients 3 mo to 12 yr): immediately withdraw a volume equal to 15 mg/kg (max 1 g/day) and inject deeply into a large muscle, aspirate prior to injection to avoid injection into a blood vessel; use the reconstituted IM solution within 1 hour after preparation

Y-site compatibilities: Acyclovir, alfentanil, amifostine, amikacin, aminocaproic acid, aminophylline, amphotericin B lipid complex, amphotericin B liposome, argatroban, arsenic trioxide, atenolol, atracurium, azithromycin, aztreonam, bivalirudin, bleomycin, bumetanide, buprenorphine, busulfan, butorphanol, calcium chloride/gluconate, CARBOplatin, carmustine, chloramphenicol, cimetidine, ciprofloxacin, cisatracurium, CISplatin, cyclophosphamide, cycloSPORINE, cytarabine, dacarbazine, DACTINomycin, DAPTOmycin, dexamethasone, dexmedetomidine, dexrazoxane, digoxin, diltiazem, diphenhydrAMINE, DOCEtaxel, dolasetron, DOPamine, doxacurium, doxycycline, enalaprilat, ePHEDrine, EPINEPHrine, eptifibatide, erythromycin, esmolol, etoposide, etoposide phosphate, famotidine, fenoldopam, fluconazole, fludarabine, fluorouracil, foscarnet, fosphenytoin, furosemide, ganciclovir, gatifloxacin, gemcitabine, gemtuzumab, gentamicin, glycopyrrolate, granisetron, haloperidol, heparin, hydrocortisone, HYDROmorphone, ifosfamide, inamrinone, insulin (regular), irinotecan, isoproterenol, ketorolac, labetalol, lepirudin, leucovorin, levofloxacin, lidocaine, linezolid, LORazepam, magnesium sulfate, mannitol, mechlorethamine, melphalan, meperidine, mesna, metaraminol, methotrexate, methyldopate, methylPREDNISolone, metoclopramide, metroNIDAZOLE, milrinone, mitoMYcin, mivacurium, morphine, moxifloxacin, nalbuphine, naloxone, nesiritide, nitroglycerin, nitroprusside, norepinephrine, octreotide, oxaliplatin, oxytocin, PACLitaxel, pamidronate, pancuronium, pantoprazole, PEMEtrexed, PENTobarbital, PHENobarbital, phentolamine, phenylephrine, polymyxin B, potassium acetate/chloride/phosphates, procainamide, propranolol, ranitidine, remifentanil, rocuronium, sodium acetate/bicarbonate/phosphates, streptozocin, succinylcholine, SUFentanil, sulfamethoxazole-trimethoprim, tacrolimus, telavancin, teniposide, theophylline, thiotepa, tigecycline, tirofiban, tobramycin, trimethobenzamide, vancomycin, vasopressin, vecuronium, vinBLAStine, vinCRIStine, vinorelbine, voriconazole, zidovudine, zoledronic acid

ADVERSE EFFECTS

CNS: Insomnia, **seizures,** dizziness, *headache,* agitation, confusion, somnolence, disorientation, edema, hypotension
CV: Tachycardia, **seizures**
GI: *Diarrhea, nausea, vomiting,* **pseudomembranous colitis,** cholelithiasis, jaundice, abdominal pain
GU: *Vaginitis,* dysuria
INTEG: *Rash,* urticaria, *pruritus,* pain at inj site, *infused vein complication, phlebitis/thrombophlebitis,* erythema at inj site, dermatitis
RESP: Dyspnea, cough, pharyngitis, crackles, respiratory distress
SYST: Anaphylaxis, angioedema

Pharmacokinetics

Absorption	Almost completely absorbed (IM); completely absorbed (**IV**)
Distribution	85%-95% plasma protein bound
Metabolism	Liver (IM, **IV**)
Excretion	Urine (80%), feces (10%), breast milk (IM, **IV**)
Half-life	4 hr (**IV**)

Pharmacodynamics

	IM	IV
Onset	Unknown	Immediate
Peak	2.3 hr	Dose-dependent
Duration	Unknown	Unknown

INTERACTIONS
Individual drugs
Probenecid: increased ertapenem plasma levels; do not coadminister
Valproic acid: decreased effect of valproic acid

Drug/lab test
Increased: hepatic enzymes

NURSING CONSIDERATIONS
Assessment
• Assess for renal disease: lower dose may be required
• **Pseudomembranous colitis:** Assess bowel pattern daily; if severe diarrhea occurs, product should be discontinued
• **Assess for infection:** temp, sputum, characteristics of wound before, during, after treatment
⚠ **Assess for allergic reactions, anaphylaxis: rash, urticaria, pruritus may occur a few days after therapy begins; assess for sensitivity to carbapenem antibiotics, other β-lactam antibiotics, penicillins**
• Assess for overgrowth of infection: perineal itching, fever, malaise, redness, pain, swelling, drainage, rash, diarrhea, change in cough or sputum

Patient/family education
⚠ **Advise patient to report severe diarrhea; may indicate pseudomembranous colitis**
⚠ **Advise patient to report overgrowth of infection: black, furry tongue, vaginal itching, foul-smelling stools**
• Caution patient to avoid breastfeeding; product is excreted in breast milk

Evaluation
Positive therapeutic outcome
• Negative C&S, absence of signs and symptoms of infection

TREATMENT OF OVERDOSE:
Administer EPINEPHrine, antihistamines; resuscitate if needed (anaphylaxis)

⚠ Nurse Alert　　　　★ Key NCLEX® Drug

erythromycin base (Rx)
(eh-rith-roh-my′sin)
Apo Erythro ✦, Ery-Tab, Novo-Rythro Encap ✦, PCE

erythromycin ethylsuccinate (Rx)
Apo-Erythro-ES ✦, EES, Ery Ped, Novo-Rythro ✦

erythromycin lactobionate (Rx)
Erythrocin

erythromycin stearate (Rx)
Apo-Erythro-S ✦, Erythrocin, My-E, Novo-Rythro ✦

Func. class.: Antiinfective
Chem. class.: Macrolide
Pregnancy category B

Do not confuse:
erythromycin/azithromycin

ACTION: Binds to 50S ribosomal subunits of susceptible bacteria and suppresses protein synthesis

Therapeutic outcome: Bactericidal action against the following organisms: *Neisseria gonorrhoeae, Streptococcus pneumoniae, Mycoplasma pneumoniae, Corynebacterium diphtheriae, Bordetella pertussis, Borrelia burgdorferi, Listeria monocytogenes, Treponema pallidum;* streptococci, staphylocci; gram-negative pathogens: *Neisseria, Haemophilus influenzae* (when used with sulfonamides), *Legionella pneumophila, Chlamydia trachomatis*

USES: Mild to moderate respiratory tract, skin, soft tissue infections, Legionnaire's disease, syphilis

CONTRAINDICATIONS:
Hypersensitivity, preexisting liver disease (estolate)

Precautions: Pregnancy **B**, breastfeeding, geriatric, hepatic/GI disease, QT prolongation, seizure disorder, myasthenia gravis

DOSAGE AND ROUTES
Acne vulgaris
Adult: PO 250 mg qid

Mild to moderately severe upper respiratory tract infections (otitis media, sinusitis) or lower respiratory tract infections (pneumonia, bronchitis) caused by susceptible organisms
Adult: PO 250-500 mg (of base, estolate or stearate) q6hr or 400-800 mg (ethylsuccinate) q6hr; IV 15-20 mg/kg/day in divided doses q4-6 hr, max 4 g/day
Adolescent/child/infant: PO 20-50 mg/kg/day divided q6hr, max adult doses; IV 15-20 mg/kg/day in divided doses q4-6hr, or as a continuous infusion, max dose 4 g/day
Neonate >7 days, weighing ≥1200 g: PO 30 mg/kg/day in divided doses q8hr
Neonate >7 days, weighing <1200 g: PO 20 mg/kg/day in divided doses q12hr
Neonate ≤7 days: PO 20 mg/kg/day PO in divided doses q12hr

Pneumonia caused by *Chlamydia trachomatis* in infants and neonates
Infant/neonate: PO; the CDC recommends 50 mg/kg/day in four divided doses × 14 days (erythromycin base or ethylsuccinate)

Mycoplasma infection such as *Mycoplasma pneumoniae* pneumonia
Adult: PO 250-500 mg tid
Adult/adolescent/child/infant: IV 15-20 mg/kg/day, given in divided doses q4-6hr, or as a continuous infusion, maximum dose 4 g/day; replace by oral dosage as soon as possible

Legionnaire's disease (caused by *Legionella pneumophila*)
Adult: PO/IV 0.5-1 g q6hr × 21 days

Treatment of group A beta-hemolytic streptococcal (GAS) pharyngitis (primary rheumatic fever prophylaxis)
Adult: PO 250-500 mg (base, estolate, or stearate) q6hr or 400-800 mg (ethylsuccinate) q6hr × 10 days
Adolescent/child/infant: PO 20-50 mg/kg/day, divided q6hr × 10 days, max adult dose

Secondary prevention of rheumatic fever (prevention of recurrent attacks of rheumatic fever)
Adult/adolescent/child: PO 250 mg bid in patients allergic to penicillin and sulfADIAZINE for 10 yr or age 40 yr, whichever is longer, secondary prophylaxis (American Heart Association)

Adverse effects: italics = common; **bold** = life-threatening

Listeriosis

Adult: PO 250-500 mg (base, estolate or stearate) q6hr or 400-800 mg (ethylsuccinate) q6hr
Adolescent/child/infant: PO 20-50 mg/kg/day PO, divided q6hr, max adult doses

Cervicitis caused by *Chlamydia trachomatis*

Adult/adolescent: PO; the CDC recommends erythromycin base 500 mg qid or erythromycin ethylsuccinate 800 mg qid × 7 days as alternatives to first-line agents doxycycline or azithromycin
Pregnant female: As alternatives to first-line agents azithromycin or amoxicillin, the CDC recommends PO base 500 mg qid × 7 days, base 250 mg qid × 14 days, ethylsuccinate 800 mg qid × 7 days, ethylsuccinate PO 400 mg qid × 14 days
Child ≤45 kg: The CDC recommends base or ethylsuccinate PO 50 mg/kg/day in 4 doses × 14 days

Proctitis caused by *Chlamydia trachomatis*

Adult/adolescent: PO base 500 mg qid

Chlamydial conjunctivitis caused by *Chlamydia trachomatis* including trachoma and inclusion conjunctivitis

Pregnant and lactating woman/child <8 yr: PO 250-500 mg qid × 10-14 days

Infant pneumonia caused by *Chlamydia trachomatis*

Infant/neonate: PO (base or ethylsuccinate); the CDC recommends 50 mg/kg/day 4 divided doses × 14 days

Nongonococcal urethritis (NGU) caused by *Chlamydia trachomatis* or *Ureaplasma urealyticum*

Adult/adolescent: PO; the CDC recommends 500 mg (base) qid or 800 mg (ethylsuccinate) qid × 7 days as alternatives to first-line agents doxycycline or azithromycin
Pregnant female: PO; the CDC recommends base 500 mg qid × 7 days
Child <45 kg: PO; the CDC recommends base 50 mg/kg/day in 4 divided doses × 10-14 days, second course of therapy may be required

Ophthalmia neonatorum caused by *Chlamydia trachomatis*

Neonate: PO (erythromycin base or ethylsuccinate); the CDC recommends 50 mg/kg/day in qid × 14 days, may be repeated if condition returns

Lymphogranuloma venereum caused by *Chlamydia trachomatis*

Adult: PO (base); the CDC recommends 500 mg qid × 21 days as an alternative to doxycycline

Adjunctive treatment of diphtheria to prevent establishment of carrier state and to eradicate *Corynebacterium diphtheriae* in carriers

Adult: PO 500 mg q6hr × 10 days

Intestinal amebiasis (unable to take metroNIDAZOLE)

Adult: PO 250 mg q6hr × 10-14 days
Adolescent/child: PO 30-50 mg/kg/day, divided q6hr × 10-14 days, max adult dose

Acute pelvic inflammatory disease (PID) caused by *Neisseria gonorrhoeae*

Adult: IV 500 mg IV (lactobionate) q6hr × 3 days, then PO 250 mg (base, estolate, stearate) or PO 400 mg (ethylsuccinate) q6hr × 7 days

Pertussis (whooping cough) caused by *Bordetella pertussis* or for post-exposure pertussis prophylaxis

Adult: PO 500 mg PO qid (2 g total) × 14 days
Adolescent/child/infant: PO 40-50 mg/kg/day (max 2 g/day) in 4 divided doses × 14 days

Primary or secondary syphilis (caused by *Treponema pallidum*) in penicillin-allergic, nonpregnant patients

Adult: PO (CDC) 500 mg qid × 14 days as an alternative therapy

Surgical infection prophylaxis as a bowel preparation in combination with neomycin

Adult: It is generally recommended that if surgery is scheduled for 8 AM, 1 g erythromycin PO with neomycin sulfate PO should be given at 1 PM, 2 PM, and 11 PM on the day before surgery

Impetigo/burn wound infection (unlabeled)

Adult: PO 250-500 mg q6hr (base, estolate, stearate) or 400-800 mg (ethylsuccinate) q6hr
Adolescent/child/infant: PO 20-50 mg/day divided q6hr

Available forms: Base: enteric-coated tab 250, 333, 500 mg; film-coated tab 250, 500 mg; enteric-coated caps, 250, 333 mg; stearate: film-coated tabs, 250 mg, granules for oral susp: 200, 400 mg/5 ml powder for inj 500 mg, 1 g (lactobionate); 1 g (as glucepate)

Implementation
- Store at room temp; store susp in refrigerator
- Adequate intake of fluids (2 L) during diarrhea episodes

PO route
- Give around the clock on an empty stomach, at least 1 hr before or 2 hr after meals; may be taken with food if GI upset occurs; do not take with juices; take dose with a full glass of water: use calibrated measuring device for drops or susp; shake well
- Store susp in refrigerator
- Do not crush or chew enteric-coated tab

IV route
- Add 10 ml of sterile water for inj without preservatives to 250- or 500-mg vials and 20 ml to 1-g vial; sol is stable for 1 wk after reconstitution if refrigerated

Intermittent IV infusion route
- Dilute further in 100-250 ml of 0.9% NaCl or D₅W
- Give over 20-60 min to avoid phlebitis; assess for pain along vein; slow inf if pain occurs; apply ice to site and notify prescriber if unable to relieve pain

Continuous infusion route
- May also be administered as an inf in a dilution of 1 g/L of 0.9% NaCl, D₅W, over 4 hr

Erythromycin lactobionate

Y-site compatibilities: Acyclovir, alfentanil, amikacin, aminocaproic acid, aminophylline, amiodarone, anidulafungin, argatroban, atenolol, atosiban, atracurium, atropine, azaTHIOprine, benztropine, bivalirudin, bleomycin, bumetanide, buprenorphine, butorphanol, calcium chloride/gluconate, CARBOplatin, caspofungin, cefotaxime, cefTAZidime, cefTRIAXone, cefuroxime, chlorproMAZINE, cimetidine, CISplatin, cyanocobalamin, cyclophosphamide, cycloSPORINE, cytarabine, DACTINomycin, DAPTOmycin, dexmedetomidine, digoxin, diltiazem, diphenhydrAMINE, DOBUTamine, DOCEtaxel, DOPamine, doxacurium, doxapram, DOXOrubicin, enalaprilat, ePHEDrine, EPINEPHrine, epirubicin, epoetin alfa, eptifibatide, ertapenem, esmolol, etoposide, famotidine, fenoldopam, fentaNYL, fluconazole, fludarabine, fluorouracil, folic acid, foscarnet, gatifloxacin, gemcitabine, gentamicin, glycopyrrolate, granisetron, hydrocortisone, HYDROmorphone, hydrOXYzine, IDArubicin, ifosfamide, imipenem-cilastatin, insulin (regular), irinotecan, isoproterenol, labetalol, levofloxacin, lidocaine, LORazepam, LR, mannitol, mechlorethamine, meperidine, methicillin, methotrexate, methoxamine, methyl-dopate, methylPREDNISolone, metoclopramide, metroNIDAZOLE, miconazole, midazolam, milrinone, mitoXANtrone, morphine, multiple vitamins injection, mycophenolate nafcillin, nalbuphine, naloxone, nesiritide, netilmicin, niCARdipine, nitroglycerin, norepinephrine, octreotide, ondansetron, oxacillin, oxaliplatin, oxytocin, PACLitaxel, palonosetron, pamidronate, pancuronium, papaverine, pentamidine, pentazocine, perphenazine, phenylephrine, phytonadione, piperacillin, piperacillin-tazobactam, polymyxin B, procainamide, prochlorperazine, promethazine, propranolol, protamine, pyridoxine, quiNIDine, ranitidine, Ringer's, ritodrine, sodium acetate/bicarbonate, succinylcholine, SUFentanil, tacrolimus, temocillin, teniposide, theophylline, thiamine, thiotepa, tigecycline, tirofiban, TNA, tobramycin, tolazoline, TPN, trimetaphan, urokinase, vancomycin, vasopressin, vecuronium, verapamil, vinCRIStine, vinorelbine, vitamin B complex/C, voriconazole, zidovudine, zoledronic acid

ADVERSE EFFECTS
CNS: Seizures
CV: Dysrhythmias, QT prolongation
EENT: Hearing loss, tinnitus
GI: *Nausea, vomiting, diarrhea,* **hepatotoxicity,** abdominal pain, stomatitis, heartburn, anorexia, pruritus ani, **pseudomembranous colitis,** *esophagitis,* **hepatotoxicity**
GU: *Vaginitis, moniliasis*
INTEG: Rash, urticaria, pruritus, thrombophlebitis (**IV** site)
SYST: Anaphylaxis

Pharmacokinetics

Absorption	Well absorbed (PO)
Distribution	Widely distributed; minimally distributed (CSF); crosses placenta
Metabolism	Liver, partially
Excretion	Bile, unchanged; kidneys (minimal), unchanged
Half-life	1-3 hr

Pharmacodynamics

	PO	IV
Onset	1 hr	Rapid
Peak	1-4 hr	Infusion's end
Duration	Unknown	Unknown

INTERACTIONS
Individual drugs
Alfentanil, ALPRAZolam, bromocriptine, busPIRone, carBAMazepine, cilostazol,

---

clindamycin, cloZAPine, cycloSPORINE, diazepam, digoxin, disopyramide, felodipine, methylPREDNISolone, midazolam, quiNIDine, rifabutin, sildenafil, tacrolimus, tadalafil, theophylline, triazolam, vardenafil, vinBLAStine, warfarin: increased toxicity, increased action

Diltiazem, itraconazole, ketoconazole, nefazodone, pimozide, verapamil: increased serious dysrhythmias, do not use together

Drug classifications
Ergots: increased action, toxicity

HMG-CoA reductase inhibitors: increased action, toxicity

Products that increase QT prolongation: increased QT

Protease inhibitors: serious dysrhythmias

Drug/lab test
Increased: AST/ALT

Decreased: folate assay

False increase: 17-OHCS/17-KS

NURSING CONSIDERATIONS
Assessment
• Assess patient for previous sensitivity reaction

• **Assess patient for signs and symptoms of infection** including characteristics of wounds, sputum, urine, stool, WBC >10,000/mm³, earache, fever; obtain baseline information before, during treatment

• Obtain C&S test results before beginning product therapy to identify if correct treatment has been initiated

• Assess for allergic reactions: rash, urticaria may occur a few days after therapy begins

• Identify urine output; if decreasing, notify prescriber (may indicate nephrotoxicity); also monitor increases in BUN, creatinine

• Monitor blood studies: AST, ALT, CBC, Hct, bilirubin, LDH, alkaline phosphatase, Coombs' test monthly if patient is on long-term therapy

• Monitor electrolytes: potassium, sodium, chloride monthly if patient is on long-term therapy

• **Assess for overgrowth of infection:** perineal itching, fever, malaise, redness, pain, swelling, drainage, rash, diarrhea, change in cough, sputum

• **Pseudomembranous colitis:** assess for diarrhea with blood, mucus, abdominal pain, fever, product should be discontinued immediately

• **Anaphylaxis:** assess for generalized hives, itching, flushing, swelling of lips/tongue/throat, wheezing; have emergency equipment nearby

• **QT prolongation:** may occur (**IV** >15 mg/min), those with electrolyte imbalances, congenital QT prolongation, and the elderly are at greater risk; correct electrolyte imbalances prior to treatment; monitor ECG

Patient/family education
• Teach patient to report sore throat, bruising, bleeding, joint pain; may indicate blood dyscrasias (rare)

• Advise patient to contact prescriber if vaginal itching, loose foul-smelling stools, furry tongue occur; may indicate superinfection

• Instruct patient to take all medication prescribed for the length of time ordered

• Teach patient to avoid use with other products unless approved by prescriber

Evaluation
Positive therapeutic outcome
• Absence of signs/symptoms of infection (WBC <10,000/mm³, temp WNL, absence of red, draining wounds, earache)

• Reported improvement in symptoms of infection

TREATMENT OF OVERDOSE:
Withdraw product, maintain airway, administer EPINEPHrine, aminophylline, O₂, **IV** corticosteroids

erythromycin ophthalmic
See Appendix B

erythromycin topical
See Appendix B

escitalopram (Rx)
(es-sit-tal′oh-pram)
Lexapro
Func. class.: Antidepressant, selective serotonin reuptake inhibitor
Pregnancy category C

ACTION: Inhibits CNS neuron uptake of serotonin but not of norepinephrine

Therapeutic outcome: Decreased symptoms of depression

USES: General anxiety disorder; major depressive disorder in adults/adolescents

Unlabeled uses: Panic disorder, social phobia, autism

CONTRAINDICATIONS:
Hypersensitivity to this product or citalopram

Precautions: Pregnancy **C**, breastfeeding, geriatric, renal/hepatic disease, history of seizures

> **BLACK BOX WARNING:** Children ≤12 yr/ adolescents, suicidal ideation

DOSAGE AND ROUTES

Adult: PO 10 mg/day in AM or PM; after 1 wk if no clinical improvement is noted, dosage may be increased to 20 mg/day PM; maintenance 10-20 mg/day; reassess to determine need for treatment

Geriatric/hepatic dose: PO 10 mg/day

Available forms: Tabs 5, 10, 20 mg; oral sol 5 mg (as base)/5 ml (contains sorbitol)

Implementation

- Give with food or milk for GI symptoms; give with full glass of water
- Give crushed if patient is unable to swallow medication whole
- Give dose at bedtime if oversedation occurs during the day
- Give gum, hard candy, frequent sips of water for dry mouth
- Oral sol: measure with calibrated device
- Store at room temperature; do not freeze
- Provide assistance with ambulation during therapy, because drowsiness, dizziness occur
- Provide safety measures primarily in geriatric
- Check to see if PO medication swallowed

ADVERSE EFFECTS

CNS: *Headache, nervousness, insomnia,* **suicidal ideation,** *drowsiness, anxiety, tremor, dizziness, fatigue, sedation, poor concentration, abnormal dreams, agitation,* **seizures,** apathy, euphoria, hallucinations, delusions, psychosis, **neuroleptic malignant syndrome–like reactions,** ataxia

CV: *Hot flashes, palpitations,* angina pectoris, **hemorrhage,** hypertension, **tachycardia,** 1st-degree AV block, **bradycardia, MI, thrombophlebitis,** postural hypotension

EENT: Visual changes, ear/eye pain, photophobia, tinnitus, pupil dilation

GI: *Nausea, diarrhea, dry mouth, anorexia, dyspepsia, constipation, cramps, vomiting, taste changes, flatulence, decreased appetite,* **hepatitis**

GU: *Dysmenorrhea, decreased libido, urinary frequency, UTI, amenorrhea,* cystitis, impotence, urine retention, ejaculation disorder

INTEG: *Sweating, rash, pruritus,* acne, alopecia, urticaria, photosensitivity, bruising

MS: *Pain,* arthritis, twitching, osteopenia

RESP: *Infection, pharyngitis, nasal congestion, sinus headache, sinusitis, cough, dyspnea, bronchitis,* asthma, hyperventilation, pneumonia

SYST: *Asthenia, viral infection, fever, allergy, chills,* **serotonin syndrome, neonatal abstinence syndrome, Stevens-Johnson syndrome**

Pharmacokinetics

Absorption	Unknown
Distribution	Unknown
Metabolism	Liver
Excretion	Urine
Half-life	Unknown

Pharmacodynamics

Unknown

INTERACTIONS

Individual drugs

Alcohol: increased CNS depression

Amantadine, bromocriptine, busPIRone, lithium, traMADol, tryptophan: increased serotonin syndrome

BusPIRone: increased symptoms of OCD

CarBAMazepine, lithium, phenytoin, warfarin: increased levels or toxicity of each specific product

Cyproheptadine: decreased escitalopram effect

Diazepam: increased half-life of diazepam

Haloperidol: increased effect of haloperidol

Drug classifications

Antidepressants, opioids, sedatives: increased CNS depression

Antidysrhythmics, antipsychotics: increased levels, toxicity

Highly protein-bound products: increased side effects of escitalopram

MAOIs: do not use with or 14 days before escitalopram

NSAIDs, salicylates, anticoagulants, SSRIs, platelet inhibitors: increased bleeding risk

Phenothiazines: increased levels of phenothiazines

SSRIs, SNRIs, serotonin-receptor agonists, amphetamines: increased serotonin syndrome

Tricyclics: increased levels of tricyclics

Drug/herb

Kava: increased CNS effect

St. John's wort: do not use together, serotonin syndrome may occur

Drug/food

Grapefruit juice: increased escitalopram effect

Drug/lab test

Increased: serum bilirubin, blood glucose, alkaline phosphatase

Decreased: VMA, 5-HIAA

False increase: urinary catecholamines

NURSING CONSIDERATIONS
Assessment

> **BLACK BOX WARNING:** Assess mental status: mood, sensorium, affect, **suicidal tenden-cies,** increase in psychiatric symptoms, depression, panic, not approved for use in children

* Assess appetite in bulimia nervosa, weight daily, increase nutritious foods in diet, watch for bingeing and vomiting
⚠ **Assess allergic reactions: itching, rash, urticaria; product should be discontinued; may need to give antihistamine**
* Monitor B/P (lying/standing), pulse q4hr; if systolic B/P drops 20 mm Hg, hold product, notify prescriber; take VS q4hr in patients with cardiovascular disease
* Monitor blood studies: CBC, leukocytes, differential, cardiac enzymes if patient is receiving long-term therapy; check platelets; bleeding can occur
⚠ **Serotonin syndrome: Assess for nausea, vomiting, sedation, dizziness, sweating, facial flushing, mental changes, shivering, increased B/P: discontinue, notify prescriber**
* Monitor liver function tests: AST, ALT, bilirubin, creatinine; thyroid function studies
* Monitor weight qwk; appetite may decrease with product
⚠ **Monitor ECG for flattening of T wave, bundle branch, AV block, dysrhythmias in cardiac patients**
* Monitor alcohol consumption; if alcohol is consumed, hold dose until AM

Patient/family education

* Teach patient that therapeutic effect may take 1-4 wk, may have increased anxiety for first 5-7 days
* Advise patient to use caution in driving, other activities requiring alertness because of drowsiness, dizziness, blurred vision
* Advise patient to use sunscreen to prevent photosensitivity
* Advise patient to avoid alcohol ingestion, other CNS depressants
* Advise patient to notify prescriber if pregnant or plan to become pregnant or breastfeed

* Advise patient to change positions slowly; orthostatic hypotension may occur
* Teach patient to avoid all OTC products unless approved by prescriber
* Teach patient to report immediately signs of urinary retention

> **BLACK BOX WARNING:** Teach patient that clinical worsening and suicide risk may occur

* Teach patient using MedGuide provided
* Teach patient about drug interactions

Evaluation

Positive therapeutic outcome
* Decreased depression

TREATMENT OF OVERDOSE:
Activated charcoal, supportive care

esmolol (Rx)
(ez'moe-lole)
Brevibloc
Func. class.: β-Adrenergic blocker (anti-dysrhythmic II)
Pregnancy category C

Do not confuse:
esmolol/Osmitrol, **Brevibloc**/Brevital

ACTION: Competitively blocks stimulation of β_1-adrenergic receptors in the myocardium; produces negative chronotropic, inotropic activity (decreases rate of SA node discharge, increases recovery time), slows conduction of AV node, decreases heart rate, decreases O_2 consumption in myocardium; also decreases renin-aldosterone-angiotensin system at high doses; inhibits β_2-receptors in bronchial system at higher doses

Therapeutic outcome: Decreased supraventricular tachycardia

USES: Supraventricular tachycardias, non-compensatory sinus tachycardia, hypertensive crisis, intraoperative and postoperative tachycardia and hypertension, atrial fibrillation/flutter

Unlabeled uses: Hypertensive crisis/urgency, unstable angina

CONTRAINDICATIONS:
Heart block (2nd- or 3rd-degree), cardiogenic shock, CHF, cardiac failure, hypersensitivity, severe bradycardia

Precautions: Pregnancy **C**, breastfeeding, geriatric patients, hypotension, peripheral vascu-

---
⚠ Nurse Alert   ✳ Key NCLEX® Drug

lar disease, diabetes, hypoglycemia, thyrotoxicosis, renal disease, atrial fibrillation, bronchospasms, hyperthyroidism, myasthenia gravis

> **BLACK BOX WARNING:** Abrupt discontinuation

DOSAGE AND ROUTES
Atrial fibrillation/flutter
Adult: **IV** Loading dose 500 mcg/kg/min over 1 min; maintenance 50 mcg/kg/min for 4 min; if no response in 5 min, give 2nd loading dose; then increase INF to 100 mcg/kg/min for 4 min; if no response, repeat loading dose, then increase maintenance INF by 50 mcg/kg/min (max of 200 mcg/kg/min); titrate to patient response
Child: **IV** A total loading dose of 600 mcg/kg over 2 min, maintenance **IV** INF 200 mcg/kg/min, titrate upward by 50-100 mcg/kg/min q5-10min until B/P, heart rate reduced by >10%

Perioperative hypertension/tachycardia
Adult: **IV** immediate control 80 mg (bolus) over 30 seconds, then 150 mcg/kg/min, adjust to response, max 300 mcg/kg/min

Hypertensive emergency (unlabeled)
Adult: **IV** 250-500 mcg/kg over 1 min, then **IV** INF 50-100 mcg/kg/min × 4 min

Available forms: Inj 10 mg, 250 mg/ml

Implementation
IV route
• Check that correct concentration is being given
• The 10 mg/ml inj solution needs no dilution and may be used as an **IV** loading dose using handheld syringe
Continuous IV infusion route
• Ready-to-use bags premixed isotonic sol of 10 mg/ml and 20 mg/ml are available in 100, 250 ml bags; use controlled device, a central line is preferred, rate is based on patient's weight
• Store at room temperature for 24 hr; sol should be clear

Y-site compatibilities: Amikacin, aminophylline, ampicillin, amiodarone, atracurium, butorphanol, calcium chloride, ceFAZolin, cefmetazole, cefoperazone, cefTAZidime, ceftizoxime, chloramphenicol, cimetidine, cisatracurium, clindamycin, diltiazem, DOPamine, enalaprilat, erythromycin, famotidine, fentaNYL, gentamicin, heparin, hydrocortisone, regular insulin, labetalol, magnesium sulfate, methyldopate, metroNIDAZOLE, midazolam,

morphine, nafcillin, nitroglycerin, norepinephrine, nitroprusside, pancuronium, penicillin G potassium, phenytoin, piperacillin, polymyxin B, potassium chloride, potassium phosphate, propofol, ranitidine, remifentanil, streptomycin, tacrolimus, tobramycin, trimethoprim/sulfamethoxazole, vancomycin, vecuronium, voriconazole, zoledronic acid

Y-site incompatibilities: Furosemide

ADVERSE EFFECTS
CNS: Confusion, light-headedness, paresthesia, somnolence, fever, dizziness, fatigue, headache, depression, anxiety, **seizures**
CV: Hypotension, bradycardia, chest pain, peripheral ischemia, shortness of breath, CHF, conduction disturbances 1st-, 2nd-, 3rd-degree heart block
GI: *Nausea*, vomiting, anorexia, gastric pain, flatulence, constipation, heartburn, bloating
GU: Urinary retention, impotence, dysuria
INTEG: *Induration, inflammation at inj site*, discoloration, edema, erythema, burning, pallor, flushing, rash, pruritus, dry skin, alopecia
RESP: **Bronchospasm,** dyspnea, cough, wheezing, nasal stuffiness, **pulmonary edema**

Pharmacokinetics	
Absorption	Complete
Distribution	Unknown
Metabolism	Liver
Excretion	Kidneys
Half-life	9 min

Pharmacodynamics	
Onset	Rapid
Peak	Unknown
Duration	1-2 min

INTERACTIONS
Individual drugs
Amphetamine, ePHEDrine, EPINEPHrine, norepinephrine, phenylephrine, pseudoephedrine: increased α-adrenergic stimulation
Digoxin: increased digoxin levels
Thyroid hormones: decreased effect of esmolol, decreased action of thyroid hormone

Drug classifications
MAOIs, solatol: avoid use
General anesthetics: increased antihypertensive effect

Drug/herb
Ephedra, hawthorn: decreased antihypertensive effect

Adverse effects: *italics* = common; **bold** = life-threatening

Drug/lab test
Interference: glucose/insulin tolerance test

NURSING CONSIDERATIONS
Assessment
• **Dysrhythmias:** Monitor B/P during beginning treatment, periodically thereafter; pulse q4hr; note rate, rhythm, quality; apical/radial pulse before administration; notify prescriber of any significant changes (pulse <50 bpm); if severe, slow or stop infusion
• Check for baselines in renal, liver function tests before therapy begins
• **CHF:** Assess for edema in feet, legs daily; monitor I&O, daily weight; check for jugular vein distention, crackles bilaterally, dyspnea
• **Bronchospasm:** Assess breath sounds and respiratory patterns

Patient/family education
• Teach patient need for medication and expected results
• Caution patient to rise slowly to prevent orthostatic hypotension
• Advise patient to notify if pain, swelling occurs at **IV** site

Evaluation
Positive therapeutic outcome
• Absence of dysrhythmias

TREATMENT OF OVERDOSE:
Defibrillation, vasopressor for hypotension

---

esomeprazole (Rx)
(es′oh-mep′rah-zohl)
NexIUM
Func. class.: Anti-ulcer, proton pump inhibitor
Chem. class.: Benzimidazole
Pregnancy category B

Do not confuse:
NexIUM/NexAVAR

ACTION: Suppresses gastric secretion by inhibiting hydrogen/potassium ATPase enzyme system in the gastric parietal cell; characterized as gastric acid pump inhibitor, since it blocks final step of acid production

Therapeutic outcome: Absence of duodenal ulcers; decreased gastroesophageal reflux

USES: Gastroesophageal reflux disease (GERD), adult/child/infant; severe erosive esophagitis; treatment of active duodenal ulcers in combination with antiinfectives for *Helicobacter pylori* infection; long-term use in hypersecretory conditions

CONTRAINDICATIONS:
Hypersensitivity to proton-pump inhibitors (PPIs)

Precautions: Pregnancy **B**, breastfeeding, children, geriatric

DOSAGE AND ROUTES
Active duodenal ulcers associated with *H. pylori*
Adult: PO 40 mg/day × 10 days in combination with clarithromycin 500 mg bid × 10 days and amoxicillin 1000 mg bid × 10 days

Hepatic dose
Adult: PO/**IV** max 20 mg/day (severe hepatic disease)

GERD/erosive gastritis
Adult: PO 20 or 40 mg/day × 4-8 wk; no adjustment needed in renal, liver failure, geriatric; **IV** 20 or 40 mg/day up to 10 days
Child and adolescent 12-17 yr: PO 20 or 40 mg/day 1 hr before meals up to 8 wk
Child 1-11 yr and ≥20 kg: PO 10 mg/day 1 hr before meals for up to 8 wk
Infant ≥1 mo: **IV** 0.5 mg/kg over 10-30 min
Infant 1-11 mo (>7.5-12 kg): PO 10 mg daily up to 6 wk
Infant 1-11 mo (5-7.5 kg): PO 5 mg daily up to 6 wk
Infant 1-11 mo (3-5 kg): PO 2.5 mg daily up to 6 wk

Available forms: Del rel caps 20, 40 mg; powder for **IV** inj 20, 40 mg/vial; del rel powder for oral susp 20, 40 mg

Implementation
PO route
• Swallow caps whole; do not crush or chew; cap may be opened and sprinkled over Tbsp of applesauce
• Same time daily, 1 hr before meal
• **Oral susp (del rel):** empty contents of packet into container with 1 Tbsp of water, let stand 2-3 min to thicken, restir, give within 30 min of mixing; any residual product should be flushed with more water, taken immediately
• **NG tube (del rel oral susp):** add 15 ml water to contents of packet in syringe, shake, leave 2-3 min to thicken, shake, inject through NG tube within 30 min

IV, direct route
• Reconstitute each vial with 5 ml 0.9% NaCl, D_5W, LR; give over 3 min

---

Intermittent IV INF route
• Dilute reconstituted sol to 50 ml, give over 30 min, do not admix, flush line with D₅W, 0.9% NaCl, LR after inf

Solution compatibilities: D₅W, LR, 0.9% NaCl

ADVERSE EFFECTS
CNS: *Headache, dizziness*
GI: *Diarrhea, flatulence,* abdominal pain, constipation, dry mouth, **hepatic failure, hepatitis,** microscopic colitis
INTEG: *Rash,* dry skin
MISC: **Heart failure**
RESP: *Cough,* pneumonia
SYST: Stevens-Johnson syndrome, toxic epidermal necrolysis, exfoliative dermatitis

Pharmacokinetics

Absorption	Unknown
Distribution	97% plasma protein bound
Metabolism	Liver (metabolites)
Excretion	Urine (metabolites), feces (metabolites); in geriatric, elimination rate decreased, bioavailability increased
Half-life	1-1½ hr

Pharmacodynamics

Onset	Unknown
Peak	1½ hr
Duration	Unknown

INTERACTIONS
Individual drugs
Calcium carbonate, clopidogrel, dapsone, indinavir, iron, itraconazole, ketoconazole, vitamin B₁₂: decreased effect
Diazepam, digoxin, penicillins, saquinavir: increased effect, toxicity

Drug/lab test
Interference: sodium, Hgb, WBC, platelets, magnesium

NURSING CONSIDERATIONS
Assessment
• Assess GI system: bowel sounds q8hr, abdomen for pain, swelling, anorexia
• **Hepatic failure, hepatitis:** monitor AST, ALT, alkaline phosphatase during treatment
• **Serious skin disorders: Stevens-Johnson syndrome,** toxic epidermal necrolysis, exfoliative dermatitis

Patient/family education
• Instruct patient to report severe diarrhea; product may have to be discontinued, rash
• Advise diabetic patients that hypoglycemia may occur
• Advise patient to avoid hazardous activities; dizziness may occur
• Advise patient to avoid alcohol, salicylates, ibuprofen; may cause GI irritation
• Teach patient to take ≥1 hr prior to meal; not to crush, chew delayed-release product
• Teach patient if cap cannot be swallowed whole contents may be mixed with a tablespoon of applesauce

Evaluation
Positive therapeutic outcome
• Absence of epigastric pain, swelling, fullness

---

estradiol (Rx)
(ess-tra-dye′ole)
Estrace
estradiol cypionate (Rx)
Depo-Estradiol
estradiol topical emulsion (Rx)
Estrasorb
estradiol valerate (Rx)
Delestrogen
estradiol transdermal system (Rx)
Alora, Climara, Estraderm, Menostar, Vivelle
estradiol vaginal tablet (Rx)
Vagifem Dot
estradiol vaginal ring (Rx)
Estring, Femring
estradiol gel (Rx)
Divigel, Elestrin, Estrogel
estradiol spray (Rx)
Evamist
Func. class.: Estrogen, progestin
Chem. class.: Nonsteroidal synthetic estrogen
Pregnancy category X

ACTION: Needed for adequate functioning of female reproductive system; affects release of pituitary gonadatropins, inhibits ovulation, promotes adequate calcium use in bone structure

---

Therapeutic outcome: Decreased tumor size in prostatic cancer; increased estrogen levels in menopause, female hypogonadism

USES: Vasomotor symptoms associated with menopause, inoperable breast cancer (selected cases), prostatic cancer, atrophic vaginitis, kraurosis vulvae, hypogonadism, primary ovarian failure, prevention of osteoporosis, castration

CONTRAINDICATIONS:

Pregnancy **X**, breastfeeding, reproductive cancer, genital bleeding (abnormal, undiagnosed), protein C, S, antithrombin deficiency

> **BLACK BOX WARNING:** Breast/endometrial cancer, thromboembolic disorders, MI, stroke

Precautions: Hypertension, asthma, blood dyscrasias, gallbladder disease, CHF, diabetes mellitus, bone disease, depression, migraine headache, seizure disorders, renal/hepatic disease, family history of cancer of breast or reproductive tract, history of smoking, uterine fibroids, vaginal irritation/infection, accidental exposure of topical products to children/pets, history of angioedema

> **BLACK BOX WARNING:** Cardiac disease, dementia

DOSAGE AND ROUTES

Hormone replacement/menopause symptoms

Adult: TD 1 patch delivering 0.025, 0.0375, 0.05, 0.075, or 0.1 mg/day 2×/wk (Alora, Estraderm, Vivelle-Dot); 1 patch delivering 0.025, 0.0375, 0.05, 0.06, 0.075, or 0.1 mg/day replace q7 days (Climara); 1 patch delivering 0.025 mg/day replace q7 days, may increase to 2 patches after 4-6 wk; **GEL** apply entire unit dose packet to 5- × 7-inch area of upper thigh/day, alternate thighs; **SPRAY** (Evamist) 1 spray to inner surface of forearm/day in AM

Menopause/hypogonadism/ castration/ovarian failure

Adult: PO 1-2 mg/day 3 wk on, 1 wk off or 5 days on, 2 days off; IM 1-5 mg q3-4wk (cypionate), 1-5 mg q3-4wk; 10-20 mg q4wk (valerate); TOP Estraderm 0.05 mg/24 hr applied 2 ×/wk, Climara 0.05 mg/hr applied 1 ×/wk in a cyclic regimen; women with hysterectomy may use continuously

Prostatic cancer

Adult: IM 30 mg q1-2wk (valerate); PO 1-2 mg tid (oral estradiol)

Breast cancer (palliative treatment)

Adult: PO 10 mg tid × 3 mo or longer

Atropic vaginitis/kraurosis vulvae

Adult: VAG cream 2-4 g/day × 1-2 wk, then 1 g 1-3 ×/wk cycled; VAG tab 1/day × 2 wk, maintenance 1 tab 2 ×/wk; VAG ring inserted and left in place continuously for 3 mo

Vasomotor symptoms

Adult: TOP after cleaning and drying skin on left thigh, calf, rub in contents of pouch using both hands until completely absorbed; wash hands

Available forms: Estradiol: tabs 0.5, 1, 2 mg; **valerate:** inj 10, 20, 40 mg/ml; **transdermal** 0.025, 0.0375, 0.05, 0.06, 0.075, 0.1 mg/24-hr release rate; **vag cream** 100 mcg/g; **vag ring** 2 mg/90 days; **vag tab** 10 mcg; **topical emulsion:** 2.5 mg; **gel** 0.1% (Divigel); **spray** (Evamist) 1.53 mg/acuation

Implementation
PO route
- Give titrated dose, use lowest effective dose
- Give with food or milk to decrease GI symptoms

IM route
- Administer deeply in large muscle mass; product is painful
- Rotate syringe to mix oil and medication

Transdermal route
- May contain aluminum or other metals in backing of patch, can overheat in MRI scan and burn patients
- Apply to area free of hair to ensure adhesion on trunk of body 2 ×/wk; press firmly and hold in place for 10 sec to ensure good contact; do not apply to breasts
- Start transdermal dose 7 days before last PO dose if routes are to be changed

Topical route spray (Evamist)
- Use daily; spray to inner upper arm; may increase to 2-3 ×/day based on response; let dry for 2 min, **avoid secondary exposure to children, pets, caregivers**

Vaginal route
- Place cream in applicator by attaching tube to applicator; squeeze cream into tube to mark; insert with patient reclining
- Use a new applicator daily

ADVERSE EFFECTS

CNS: Dizziness, headache, migraine, depression, **seizures**

CV: Hypertension, thrombophlebitis, edema, **thromboembolism, stroke, pulmonary embolism, MI,** chest pain

EENT: Contact lens intolerance, increased myopia, astigmatism, throat swelling, eyelid edema

GI: *Nausea,* vomiting, diarrhea, anorexia, pancreatitis, cramps, constipation, increased appetite, increased weight, **cholestatic jaundice, hepatic adenoma**

GU: Amenorrhea, cervical erosion, breakthrough bleeding, dysmenorrhea, vaginal candidiasis, breast changes, *gynecomastia, testicular atrophy, impotence;* **increased risk of breast, endometrial cancer,** changes in libido; **toxic shock, vaginal wall ulceration/ erosion (vag ring)**

INTEG: Rash, urticaria, acne, hirsutism, alopecia, oily skin, seborrhea, purpura, erythema, pruritus, melasma; site irritation (transdermal)

META: Folic acid deficiency, hypercalcemia, hyperglycemia

Pharmacokinetics

Absorption	Well absorbed
Distribution	Widely distributed, crosses placenta
Metabolism	Unknown
Excretion	Unknown
Half-life	Unknown

Pharmacodynamics

	PO	IM	IV
Onset	Rapid	Slow	Rapid
Peak	Unknown	Unknown	Unknown
Duration	Unknown	Unknown	Unknown

INTERACTIONS

Individual drugs

Calcium, phenylbutazone, rifampin: decreased estradiol action

CycloSPORINE, dantrolene: increased toxicity

Tamoxifen: decreased tamoxifen action

Drug classifications

Anticoagulants: decreased action of anticoagulants

Anticonvulsants, barbiturates: decreased estradiol action

Corticosteroids: increased action of corticosteroids

Hypoglycemics (oral): decreased action of hypoglycemics

Drug/herb

Black cohosh, DHEA: altered estrogen effect

Saw palmetto, St. John's wort: decreased estrogen effect

Drug/food

Grapefruit juice: increased estrogen level

Drug/lab test

Increased: BSP retention test; PBI; T_4; serum sodium; platelet aggregation; thyroxine-binding globulin (TBS); prothrombin; factors VII, VIII, IX, X; triglycerides

Decreased: serum folate, serum triglyceride, T_3 resin uptake test, glucose tolerance test, antithrombin III, pregnanediol, metyrapone test

False positive: LE prep, ANA titer

NURSING CONSIDERATIONS

Assessment

> **BLACK BOX WARNING:** Assess for previous breast/endometrial cancer, thromboembolic disorders, MI, stroke, dementia

- Monitor blood glucose in patient with diabetes; hyperglycemia may occur
- Monitor B/P q4hr; watch for increase caused by water and sodium retention
- Monitor I&O ratio; be alert for decreasing urinary output and increasing edema; monitor weight daily; notify prescriber if weekly weight gain is >5 lb; if increased, diuretic may be ordered
- Obtain liver function tests baseline, periodically, including AST, ALT, bilirubin, alkaline phosphatase, periodic folic acid level
- Assess edema, hypertension, cardiac symptoms, jaundice
- Assess mental status: affect, mood, behavioral changes, aggression; depression may occur, product may need to be discontinued
- Assess female patient for intact uterus; if so, progesterone should be added to estrogen therapy to decrease risk of endometrial cancer

Patient/family education

- Tell patient to take exactly as prescribed; do not double doses
- ⚠ Advise patient that increased weight gain and symptoms of fluid retention should be reported to prescriber: edema of feet, ankles, sacral area; abnormal vaginal bleeding; breast lumps; hepatic disease (dark urine, clay-colored stools, jaundice of skin, sclera, pruritus); to report dermal rash with transdermal patch
- ⚠ Caution patient that thromboembolic symptoms should be reported: tenderness

in legs, chest pain, dyspnea, headaches, blurred vision
• Inform patient to use sunscreen and protective clothing because sunburns may occur
• Advise patient to stop smoking; smokers have a greater chance of thromboembolic disorder
• Tell patient to use nonhormonal birth control and to notify prescriber if pregnancy is suspected
• Teach patient to avoid grapefruit or grapefruit juice (PO)

Evaluation
Positive therapeutic outcome
• Reversal of menopausal symptoms
• Decrease in tumor size in prostatic or breast cancer
• Decrease in itching, inflammation of vagina
• Absence of symptoms of osteoporosis

---

estrogens, conjugated (Rx)
Cenestin, Premarin
estrogens, conjugated synthetic B (Rx)
Enjuvia
Pregnancy category X

Do not confuse:
Premarin/Provera

ACTION: Needed for adequate functioning of female reproductive system; affects release of pituitary gonadotropins; inhibits ovulation; promotes adequate calcium use in bone structures

Therapeutic outcome: Decreased tumor size in prostatic cancer; increased estrogen levels in menopause, female hypogonadism

USES: Symptoms associated with menopause, inoperable breast cancer, prostatic cancer, abnormal uterine bleeding, hypogonadism, primary ovarian failure, prevention of osteoporosis, castration, atrophic vaginitis

CONTRAINDICATIONS:
Pregnancy **X,** breastfeeding, thromboembolic disorders, reproductive cancer, genital bleeding (abnormal, undiagnosed), hypersensitivity, MI, stroke, phlebitis

BLACK BOX WARNING: Endometrial breast cancer, thromboembolic diseases

Precautions: Hypertension, asthma, blood dyscrasias, gallbladder disease, CHF, diabetes mellitus, bone disease, depression, migraine headache, seizure disorders, renal/hepatic disease, family history of cancer of breast or reproductive tract, history of smoking, dementia, hypothyroidism, obesity, SLE

DOSAGE AND ROUTES
Estrogens, conjugated
Menopause
Adult: PO 0.3-1.25 mg/day 3 wk on, 1 wk off
Prevention of osteoporosis
Adult: PO 0.3 mg/day or in a cycle
Atrophic vaginitis
Adult: VAG cream 0.5 g/day × 21 days, off 7 days, repeat
Prostatic cancer
Adult: PO 1.25-2.5 mg tid
Advanced inoperable breast cancer
Adult: PO 10 mg tid × 3 mo or longer
Abnormal uterine bleeding
Adult: IV/IM 25 mg, repeat in 6-12 hr
Castration/primary ovarian failure
Adult: PO 1.25 mg/day 3 wk on, 1 wk off
Hypogonadism
Adult: PO 2.5-7.5 mg/day × 20 days/mo

Estrogens, conjugated synthetic B
Menopause
Adult: PO 0.625 mg/day initially, may increase based on response

Available forms: Tabs 0.3, 0.45, 0.625, 0.9, 1.25, 2.5 mg; inj 25 mg/vial; vag cream 0.625 mg/g; synthetic B: tabs 0.625, 1.25 mg

Implementation
PO route
• Give titrated dose, use lowest effective dose
• Give in 1 dose in AM for prostatic cancer, vaginitis, hypogonadism
• Give with food or milk to decrease GI symptoms
IM route
• Reconstitute after withdrawing at least 5 ml of air from container and inject sterile diluent on vial side, rotate to dissolve
• Give IM inj deeply in large muscle
Vaginal route
• Place cream in applicator by attaching tube to applicator, squeeze cream into tube to mark, insert with patient recumbent
• Applicator should be washed after each use

IV, direct route
• Reconstitute as for IM, inject into distal port of running **IV** line of D₅W, 0.9% NaCl, LR, at a rate of 5 mg/min or less

Y-site compatibilities: Heparin/hydrocortisone, potassium chloride, vit B/C

ADVERSE EFFECTS
CNS: Dizziness, headache, migraine, depression, **seizures,** mood disturbances
CV: Hypertension, thrombophlebitis, edema, **thromboembolism, stroke, pulmonary embolism, MI,** chest pain
EENT: Contact lens intolerance, increased myopia, astigmatism
GI: *Nausea,* vomiting, diarrhea, anorexia, pancreatitis, cramps, constipation, increased appetite, **cholestatic jaundice, hepatic adenoma,** weight gain/loss
GU: Amenorrhea, cervical erosion, breakthrough bleeding, dysmenorrhea, vaginal candidiasis, breast changes, *gynecomastia, testicular atrophy, impotence,* **increased risk of breast, endometrial cancer,** libido changes
INTEG: Rash, urticaria, acne, hirsutism, alopecia, oily skin, seborrhea, purpura, melasma
META: Folic acid deficiency, hypercalcemia, hyperglycemia

Pharmacokinetics

Absorption	Well absorbed (PO), completely absorbed (**IV**)
Distribution	Widely distributed, crosses placenta
Metabolism	Liver, exclusively; hepatic recirculation
Excretion	Kidney
Half-life	Unknown

Pharmacodynamics

	PO	IM	IV
Onset	Rapid	Slow	Immediate
Peak	Unknown	Unknown	Unknown
Duration	Unknown	Unknown	Unknown

INTERACTIONS
Individual drugs
CycloSPORINE, dantrolene: increased toxicity
Phenylbutazone, rifampin: decreased action of estrogens
Tamoxifen, thyroid: decreased tamoxifen action

Drug classifications
Anticoagulants: decreased action of anticoagulants

Anticonvulsants, barbiturates: decreased action of estrogens
Corticosteroids: increased action of corticosteroids
Oral hypoglycemics: decreased action of hypoglycemics

Drug/food
Grapefruit juice: increased estrogen level

Drug/lab test
Increased: BSP retention test; PBI, T₄; serum sodium; platelet aggregation; thyroxine-binding globulin (TBG); prothrombin; factors VII, VIII, IX, X; triglycerides
Decreased: serum folate, serum triglyceride, T₃ resin uptake test, glucose tolerance test, antithrombin III, pregnanediol, metyrapone test
False positive: LE prep, ANA titer

NURSING CONSIDERATIONS
Assessment

> **BLACK BOX WARNING:** Breast, endometrial cancer: estrogens should not be used in known, suspected, or history of these disorders

> **BLACK BOX WARNING:** Stroke, thromboembolic disease of MI: should not be used in these conditions or known protein C deficiency, protein S deficiency or antithrombin in deficiency

• Monitor blood glucose in patient with diabetes; hyperglycemia may occur
• Monitor B/P q4hr; watch for increase caused by water and sodium retention
• Monitor I&O ratio; be alert for decreasing urinary output and increasing edema; monitor weight daily; notify prescriber if weekly weight gain is >5 lb; if increased, diuretic may be ordered
• Obtain liver function tests, including AST, ALT, bilirubin, alkaline phosphatase
• Assess edema, hypertension, cardiac symptoms, jaundice
• Assess mental status: affect, mood, behavioral changes, aggression; depression may occur; product may need to be discontinued
• Assess female patient for intact uterus; if so, progesterone should be added to estrogen therapy to decrease risk of endometrial cancer; abnormal uterine bleeding, breast exam

Patient/family education
• Caution patient to take exactly as prescribed and not to double doses

BLACK BOX WARNING: Advise patient that increased weight gain and symptoms of fluid retention should be reported to prescriber: edema of feet, ankles, sacral area; abnormal vaginal bleeding; breast lumps; hepatic disease (dark urine, clay-colored stools, jaundice of skin, sclera, pruritus)

⚠ Caution patient that thromboembolic symptoms should be reported: pain, redness, tenderness in legs; chest pain, dyspnea, headaches, blurred vision
• Inform patient that sunburns may occur and to use sunscreen and protective clothing
• Advise patient to stop smoking; smokers have a greater chance of thromboembolic disorder
• Tell patient to use nonhormonal birth control and to notify prescriber if pregnancy is suspected
• Tell patient that vasomotor symptoms improve in 2 wk, max relief 8 wk

Evaluation

Positive therapeutic outcome
• Reversal of menopause symptoms
• Decrease in tumor size in prostatic, breast cancer
• Decrease in itching, inflammation of vagina
• Absence of symptoms of osteoporosis

RARELY USED

estropipate
(ess-troe-pip′ate)
Func. class.: Estrogen

USES: Primary ovarian failure, menopausal symptoms, prevention of osteoporosis, vaginal atrophy

CONTRAINDICATIONS:
Hypersensitivity, coagulation disorders, breast and reproductive cancers, undiagnosed genital bleeding

BLACK BOX WARNING: Pregnancy (X)

DOSAGE AND ROUTES
Vaginal atrophy/vulval atrophy/menopausal symptoms
Adult (women): PO 0.75-6 mg/day, 1 wk on 1 wk off, may be used continuously in menopausal symptoms

Primary ovarian failure
Adult (women): PO 1.5-9 mg/day for 3 wk, then off for 8-10 days; if bleeding does not occur, repeat cycle

Osteoporosis prevention
Adult (women): PO 0.75 mg/day 25 days, 6 days off, repeat as needed

eszopiclone (Rx)
(es-zop′i-klone)
Lunesta
Func. class.: Sedative-hypnotic, non-benzodiazepine
Chem. class.: Cyclopyrrolone
Pregnancy category C
Controlled substance schedule IV

ACTION: Interacts with GABA receptors

Therapeutic outcome: Ability to sleep and stay asleep throughout the night

USES: Insomnia

CONTRAINDICATIONS:
Hypersensitivity

Precautions: Pregnancy **C**, breastfeeding, children, geriatric, severe hepatic disease, abrupt discontinuation, COPD, depression, labor, sleep apnea, substance abuse, suicidal ideation, ethanol intoxication

DOSAGE AND ROUTES
Adult: PO 2 mg immediately before bed, may increase to 3 mg if needed

Hepatic dose/CYP3A4 inhibitors
Adult: PO 1 mg immediately before bed in severe hepatic disease

Available forms: Tabs 1, 2, 3 mg

Implementation
• Do not break, crush, or chew tab
• For short-term use only
• Give immediately before bedtime
• Avoid use with a high-fat meal
• Provide assistance with ambulation, nightlight, call bell within reach
• Check to see product is swallowed

ADVERSE EFFECTS
CNS: Worsening depression, hallucinations, headache, daytime drowsiness, **suicidal thoughts/actions,** migraine, restlessness, anxiety, sleep driving, sleep walking
CV: Peripheral edema, chest pain

GI: Dry mouth, bitter taste (dysgeusia)
GU: Gynecomastia, dysmenorrhea
INTEG: Rash, **angioedema**

Pharmacokinetics

Absorption	Unknown
Distribution	Unknown
Metabolism	Extensively in the liver by CYP3A4, CYP2E1; protein binding 52%-59%
Excretion	Via kidneys
Half-life	6 hr, geriatric 9 hr

Pharmacodynamics

Onset	Rapid
Peak	1 hr
Duration	6 hr

INTERACTIONS
Drug classifications
CNS depressants: increased CNS depression
CYP3A4 inhibitors (clarithromycin, itraconazole, ketoconazole, nefazodone, nelfinavir, ritonavir, troleandomycin): increased toxicity due to decreased eszopiclone elimination

Drug/food
High-fat meal: decreased product action

NURSING CONSIDERATIONS
Assessment
• **Anaphylaxis, angioedema:** monitor during first dose
• **Assess sleep pattern:** ability to go to sleep, stay asleep; early morning awakenings; conservative methods used
• Monitor for abuse of this or other products

Patient/family education
• Caution patient that daytime drowsiness may occur; not to engage in hazardous activities until effect is known, memory problems may occur
• Advise patient that all other medications and supplements should be avoided unless approved by prescriber
• Advise patient to notify prescriber if pregnancy is suspected or planned
• Discuss alternative methods to improve sleep: reading, quiet environment, warm bath, milk
• Teach patient to avoid use after a high-fat meal
• Teach patient to swallow tab whole
• Teach patient not to stop drug abruptly, tolerance may occur

Evaluation
Positive therapeutic outcome
• Ability to sleep and stay asleep throughout the night

---

etanercept (Rx)
(eh-tan′er-sept)
Enbrel
Func. class.: Antirheumatic agent
(disease-modifying) (DMARDs)
Chem. class.: Anti-TNF agent
Pregnancy category B

ACTION: Binds to tumor necrosis factor (TNF), which decreases inflammation and immune response

Therapeutic outcome: Decreased pain, inflammation

USES: Acute, chronic rheumatoid arthritis that has not responded to other disease-modifying agents; polyarticular course juvenile rheumatoid arthritis (JRA), ankylosing spondylitis, plaque psoriasis, psoriatic arthritis

Unlabeled uses: Crohn's disease

CONTRAINDICATIONS:
Sepsis

Precautions: Pregnancy **B**, breastfeeding, children <4 yr, geriatric, malignancies, CHF, seizures, multiple sclerosis, latex hypersensitivity

BLACK BOX WARNING: Infection, lymphoma, neoplastic disease

DOSAGE AND ROUTES
Rheumatoid/psoriatic arthritis, ankylosing spondylitis
Adult: SUBCUT 50 mg qwk or 25 mg 2×/wk, 3-4 days apart
Child 2-17 yr: SUBCUT 0.8 mg/kg/wk, max 50 mg/wk

Plaque psoriasis
Adult: SUBCUT 50 mg 2 ×/wk × 3 mo
Adolescent and child 4-17 yr (unlabeled): SUBCUT 0.8 mg/kg/wk, max 50 mg/wk

Juvenile rheumatoid arthritis (JRA)
Adolescent and child 2-17 yr: SUBCUT 0.8 mg/kg/wk, max 50 mg/wk

Available forms: Powder for inj 25 mg; inj 50 mg/ml; auto injector, single use

---

Implementation
• If appropriate, may be administered by the patient or a caregiver after thorough instruction of proper injection preparation and administration. Assess the patient's or caregiver's ability to inject subcut and observe the first injection
• Administration of one 50 mg/ml prefilled syringe or autoinjector provides a dose equivalent to two, 25 mg prefilled syringes or two, 25 mg vials of lyophilized when vials are reconstituted and administered as recommended
• The needle cap on the prefilled syringe and on the SureClick autoinjector contain dry natural rubber (latex) and should not be handled by persons sensitive to this product

Inj route
• Visually inspect parenteral products for particulate matter and discoloration prior to use, solution should be clear and colorless, although small white particles in solution may be noted in the autoinjector or prefilled syringe

Subcut route
• Injection sites include front of the thigh; abdomen except the 2 inches around the navel; or outer area of the upper arm. Rotate injection sites. Do not administer where skin is tender, bruised, red, or hard. Also, do not inject directly into any raised, thick, red, or scaly skin patches or lesions related to psoriasis

Reconstitution and administration of the vial
• Do not mix or transfer the contents of one vial into another vial. Also, do not filter reconstituted product during preparation or administration. Do not add other medications to solutions containing etanercept. ONLY use the supplied diluent
• A vial adaptor is supplied for use when reconstituting the powder; however, the adaptor should not be used if multiple doses are going to be withdrawn from the vial. To reconstitute using the vial adaptor, slide the plunger into the flange end of the syringe. Attach the plunger to the gray rubber stopper in the syringe by turning the plunger clockwise until a slight resistance is felt. Remove the twist-off cap from the prefilled diluent syringe by turning counterclockwise. Once the twist-off cap is removed, twist the vial adapter onto the syringe clockwise until a slight resistance is felt. Place the vial adapter over the top of the vial being careful not to bump or touch the plunger; the plastic spike inside the vial adapter should puncture the gray stopper. Push the plunger down until all the liquid from the syringe is in the vial and gently swirl to dissolve the powder. After the diluent is added, some foaming may occur. Do not

shake. Generally, dissolution takes less than 10 min; the solution should be clear and colorless. Each reconstituted vial contains 25 mg/ml of etanercept. Turn the vial upside down and slowly pull the plunger down to the unit markings on the side of the syringe that correspond with the needed dose. Gently tap the syringe to make any air bubbles rise to the top of the syringe, and slowly push the plunger up to remove them. Remove the syringe from the vial adapter by turning the syringe counterclockwise and attach the 27 gauge needle
• If the vial will be used for multiple doses, use a 25-gauge needle for reconstituting and withdrawing the solution. Insert the 25 gauge needle or the vial adapter straight into the center of the gray stopper. A "pop" will be felt. Inject the diluent very slowly. After the diluent is added, some foaming may occur. Do not shake. Swirl contents gently during dissolution. Generally, dissolution takes less than 10 minutes; the solution should be clear and colorless. Write the mixing date on the supplied sticker and attach to the vial. Each reconstituted vial contains 25 mg/ml of etanercept. Withdraw the correct dose of the solution into the syringe; remove any air bubbles. Remove the 25-gauge needle from the syringe. Attach a 27-gauge needle
• Hold the barrel of the syringe with one hand and pull the needle cover straight off. Hold the syringe in one hand like a pencil and use the other hand to gently pinch a fold of skin at the cleaned injection site. Insert the needle at a 45° angle to the skin. Let go of the skin, and hold the syringe near its base to stabilize it. Push the plunger to inject all of the solution at a slow, steady rate. Withdraw the needle at the same angle as insertion. Do NOT rub the site
• Use as soon as possible after reconstitution. Place reconstituted vials for multiple doses in the refrigerator at 2-8° C (36°-46° F) within 4 hr of reconstitution and may be stored up to 14 days. DO NOT FREEZE

Use of the SureClick autoinjector
• Allow to reach room temperature, do not shake. Immediately before use, remove the needle shield by pulling it straight off
• Stretch the skin under and around the prefilled autoinjector, place the open end against the injection site at a 90° angle. Without pushing the purple button on top, push the autoinjector firmly against the skin to unlock. Press the purple button on top once and release the button. Listen for the first click. Wait for the second click or wait 15 seconds, and remove the autoinjector from injection site. Do NOT rub the site

---

• Look at the inspection window. If it is not purple, call 1-888-436-2735; do not try to reuse the autoinjector

Use of the prefilled syringe

• **Single-use:** allow to come to room temperature, do not shake. Immediately before use, remove the needle shield by pulling it straight off; do not twist off or recap. Check to see if the amount of liquid in the prefilled syringe falls between the two purple fill level indicator lines on the syringe. Hold the prefilled syringe with the covered needle pointing down. If bubbles are seen in the syringe, very gently tap the prefilled syringe to allow any bubbles to rise to the top of the syringe. Turn the syringe so that the purple horizontal lines on the barrel are directly facing you. Do not use if the syringe does not have the right amount of liquid

• Hold the barrel of the prefilled syringe with one hand and pull the needle cover straight off. Holding the syringe with the needle pointing up, check the syringe for air bubbles. If there are bubbles, gently tap until the air bubbles rise to the top of the syringe. Slowly push the plunger up to force the air bubbles out of the syringe

• Hold the syringe in one hand like a pencil and use the other hand to gently pinch a fold of skin at the cleaned injection site. Insert the needle at a 45° angle to the skin. Let go of the skin, and hold the syringe near its base to stabilize it. Push the plunger to inject all of the solution at a slow, steady rate. Withdraw the needle at the same angle as insertion. Do NOT rub the site

ADVERSE EFFECTS

CNS: Headache, asthenia, dizziness, **seizures**
CV: Heart failure
GI: Abdominal pain, dyspepsia, vomiting, **hepatitis**
HEMA: Pancytopenia, **anemia, thrombocytopenia, leukopenia, neutropenia**
INTEG: Rash, *inj site reaction*, keratoderma blenorrhagicum
RESP: Pharyngitis, rhinitis, *cough, URI,* non-URI sinusitis
SYST: Serious infections, sepsis, death, malignancies, Stevens-Johnson syndrome

Absorption	Rapidly absorbed (60%)
Distribution	Unknown
Metabolism	Unknown
Excretion	Unknown
Half-life	115 hr

Unknown

INTERACTIONS

Individual drugs

Anakinra, cyclophosphamide, rilonacept: avoid use

SulfaSALAzine: increased neutropenia

Drug classifications

Immunizations: should be brought up to date before treatment

Immunizations, live vaccines: do not give concurrently

Drug/lab test

Increased: LFTs

NURSING CONSIDERATIONS

Assessment

• **Rheumatoid arthritis:** assess for pain; check ROM, inflammation of joints, characteristics of pain

• Assess inj site for pain, swelling; usually occurs after 2 inj (4-5 days)

> **BLACK BOX WARNING: Infection:** patients using immunosuppressives, corticosteroids, methotrexate are at greater risk, assess for fever

> **BLACK BOX WARNING: Hypersensitivity: to this product, latex needle cap, benzyl alcohol; usual reaction to this product lasts 3-5 days**

Patient/family education

• Teach patient that product must be continued for prescribed time to be effective; to avoid aspirin, alcoholic beverages

• Instruct patient to use caution when driving; dizziness may occur

• Teach patient about self-administration, if appropriate: inj should be made in thigh, abdomen, upper arm; rotate sites at least 1 in from old site

Evaluation

Positive therapeutic outcome

• Decreased pain in arthritic conditions
• Decreased inflammation in arthritic conditions

ethambutol (Rx)

(e-tham'byoo-tole)

Etibi ✦, **Myambutol**

Func. class.: Antitubercular

Chem. class.: Diisopropylethylene diamide derivative

Pregnancy category B

Do not confuse:

ethambutol/Ethmozine

ACTION: Inhibits RNA synthesis, decreases tubercle bacilli replication

Therapeutic outcome: Resolution of TB infection

USES: Pulmonary TB, as an adjunct, other mycobacterial infections

CONTRAINDICATIONS:

Hypersensitivity, optic neuritis, child <13 yr

Precautions: Pregnancy **B**, breastfeeding, renal disease, diabetic retinopathy, cataracts, ocular defects, hepatic and hematopoietic disorders

DOSAGE AND ROUTES

Adult and child >13 yr: PO 15-25 mg/kg/day as a single dose or 50 mg/kg 2 ×/wk or 25-30 mg/kg 3 ×/wk

Renal dose

Adult: PO CCr 10-50 ml/min dose q24-36hr; CCr <10 ml/min dose q48hr

Retreatment

Adult: PO 25 mg/kg/day as single dose × 2 mo with at least 1 other product, then decrease to 15 mg/kg/day as single dose, max 2.5 g/day

Child: PO 15 mg/kg/day

Available forms: Tabs 100, 400 mg

Implementation

• Give with meals to decrease GI symptoms, at same time each day to maintain blood level

• Give 2 hr before antacids

• Give antiemetic if vomiting occurs

ADVERSE EFFECTS

CNS: *Headache, confusion,* fever, malaise, dizziness, *disorientation,* hallucinations, peripheral neuropathy

EENT: Blurred vision, optic neuritis, photophobia, decreased visual acuity

GI: *Abdominal distress, anorexia, nausea, vomiting*

INTEG: Dermatitis, pruritus, **toxic epidermal necrolysis,** erythema multiforme

META: *Elevated uric acid, acute gout,* liver function impairment

MISC: **Thrombocytopenia,** joint pain, **anaphylaxis**

Pharmacokinetics

Absorption	Rapidly absorbed
Distribution	Widely distributed, crosses blood-brain barrier, placenta
Metabolism	Liver
Excretion	Kidneys, unchanged
Half-life	3 hr, increased in liver, kidney disease

Pharmacodynamics

Onset	Rapid
Peak	2-4 hr
Duration	Unknown

INTERACTIONS

Drug classifications

Aluminum, antacids: decreased absorption, separate by 4 hr

Neurotoxic agents, other: increased neurotoxicity

NURSING CONSIDERATIONS

Assessment

• Obtain C&S tests including sputum tests before initiating treatment; monitor qmo to detect resistance

• Monitor liver function tests qwk × 2 wk, then q2mo: ALT, AST, bilirubin; renal studies: before, qmo: BUN, creatinine output, specific gravity, urinalysis, uric acid; decreased appetite, jaundice, dark urine, fatigue

• Assess patient's mental status often: affect, mood, behavioral changes; psychosis may occur with hallucinations, confusion

• Assess patient for vision disturbance that may indicate optic neuritis: blurred vision, change in color perception; may lead to blindness

⚠ Serious skin reaction: toxic epidermal necrolysis

Patient/family education

• Advise patient that compliance with dosage schedule and duration is necessary to eradicate disease; to keep scheduled appointments, including ophthalmic appointments, or relapse may occur

• Caution patient to report weakness, fatigue, loss of appetite, nausea, vomiting, yellowing of

skin or eyes, tingling/numbness of hands/feet, weight gain, or decreased urine output
• Instruct patient to report any vision changes; rash; hot, swollen, painful joints; numbness or tingling of extremities to physician
• Caution patient to inform prescriber if pregnancy is suspected

Evaluation
Positive therapeutic outcome
• Decreased symptoms of TB
• Decrease in acid-fast bacteria

etodolac (Rx)
(ee-toe-doe′lak)
Lodine, Lodine XL
Func. class.: Nonsteroidal antiinflammatory, nonopioid analgesic
Pregnancy category C

Do not confuse:
Lodine/codeine/iodine

ACTION: Inhibits COX 1,2; analgesic, antiinflammatory properties

Therapeutic outcome: Decreased pain, inflammation

USES: Mild to moderate pain, osteoarthritis

CONTRAINDICATIONS:
Hypersensitivity; patients in whom aspirin, iodides, or other NSAIDs have produced asthma, rhinitis, urticaria, nasal polyps, angioedema, bronchospasm; avoid in 2nd half of pregnancy

Precautions: Pregnancy **C**, breastfeeding, children, geriatric, bleeding, GI/cardiac/renal/hepatic disorders, bronchospasm, nasal polyps

> **BLACK BOX WARNING:** GI bleeding, perforation, MI, stroke

DOSAGE AND ROUTES
Osteoarthritis
Adult: PO 300 mg bid-tid, or 400-500 mg bid initially, then adjust to 600-1200 mg/day in divided doses; max 1200 mg/day; patients <60 kg max 20 mg/kg; ext rel 400-1000 mg/day

Analgesia
Adult: PO 200-400 mg q6-8hr; max 1200 mg/day; patients <60 kg max 20 mg/kg

Available forms: Caps 200, 300 mg; tabs 400, 500 mg; ext rel tabs 400, 600 mg

Implementation
• Do not break, crush, or chew ext rel tabs
• Administer with full glass of water to enhance absorption
• Administer with food or milk to decrease gastric symptoms; food will slow absorption slightly, will not decrease absorption

ADVERSE EFFECTS
CNS: Dizziness, headache, drowsiness, fatigue, tremors, confusion, insomnia, anxiety, depression, light-headedness, vertigo
CV: Tachycardia, peripheral edema, fluid retention, palpitations, dysrhythmias, CHF
EENT: Tinnitus, hearing loss, blurred vision, photophobia
GI: *Nausea, anorexia,* vomiting, diarrhea, jaundice, **cholestatic hepatitis,** constipation, flatulence, cramps, dry mouth, peptic ulcer, dyspepsia, **GI bleeding**
GU: **Nephrotoxicity, dysuria, hematuria, oliguria, azotemia, cystitis, UTI**
HEMA: **Blood dyscrasias**
INTEG: Erythema, urticaria, purpura, rash, pruritus, sweating, **Stevens-Johnson syndrome**
SYST: **Angioedema, anaphylaxis**

Pharmacokinetics
Absorption	Well absorbed
Distribution	Highly bound to plasma protein
Metabolism	Unknown
Excretion	Unknown
Half-life	7 hr

Pharmacodynamics
Onset	½ hr
Peak	1-2 hr
Duration	4-12 hr

INTERACTIONS
Individual drugs
Aspirin: may increase GI toxicity
Cidofovir, cycloSPORINE, digoxin, lithium, methotrexate, phenytoin: increased toxicity

Drug classifications
Antacids: delayed etodolac effect
β-Adrenergic blockers: decreased effect
Diuretics: decreased effectiveness of diuretics

Drug/herb
Arginine, gossypol: increased gastric irritation
Bearberry, bilberry: increased NSAIDs action

Bogbean, chondroitin, saw palmetto, turmeric: increased bleeding risk

St. John's wort: severe photosensitivity

NURSING CONSIDERATIONS
Assessment
• Assess pain: location, frequency, characteristics; relief after medication
• Assess for GI bleeding: black stools, hematemesis
• Assess for asthma, aspirin hypersensitivity, nasal polyps that may be hypersensitive to etodolac
• Monitor blood counts during therapy; watch for decreasing platelets; if low, therapy may need to be discontinued, then restarted after hematologic recovery; watch for blood dyscrasia (thrombocytopenia): bruising, fatigue, bleeding, poor healing

Patient/family education
• Inform patient that product must be continued for prescribed time to be effective; to avoid aspirin, alcoholic beverages, NSAIDs
• Caution patient to report bleeding, bruising, fatigue, malaise because blood dyscrasias can occur
• Instruct patient to use caution when driving; drowsiness, dizziness may occur
• Teach patient to take with a full glass of water to enhance absorption

Evaluation
Positive therapeutic outcome
• Decreased pain
• Decreased inflammation
• Increased mobility

⚠ HIGH ALERT

etoposide (Rx)
(e-toe'poe-side)
Toposar
etoposide phosphate (Rx)
Etopophos
Func. class.: Antineoplastic— miscellaneous
Chem. class.: Semisynthetic podophyllotoxin
Pregnancy category D

ACTION: Inhibits cells from entering mitosis, depresses DNA, RNA synthesis, cell cycle specific S and G_2, binds to a complex of DNA and topoisomerase II leading to DNA strand breaks

Therapeutic outcome: Prevention of rapid growth of malignant cells

USES: Leukemias, testicular cancer

Unlabeled uses: Lymphomas

CONTRAINDICATIONS:
Pregnancy **D**, breastfeeding, hypersensitivity

Precautions: Children, renal/hepatic disease, gout

> **BLACK BOX WARNING:** Bone marrow depression, infection, bleeding, requires an experienced clinician

DOSAGE AND ROUTES
Testicular cancer
Adult: IV 100 mg/m²/day on days 1, 2 in combination with methotrexate, leucovorin, actinomycin D, cyclophosphamide, and vinCRIStine (EMA-CO regimen) q2-3wk or 1-5 with bleomycin, CISplatin (BEP regimen) or 100 mg/m²/day on days 1, 3, 5, repeat q3wk or q4wk

Renal dose
Adult: IV CCr 45-60 ml/min reduce dose by 15%; CCr 30-44 ml/min reduce dose by 20%; CCr <30 ml/min reduce dose by 25%

Hepatic dose
Adult: IV/PO total bilirubin 1.5-3 mg/dl: reduce dose by 50%; total bilirubin 3-5 mg/dl: reduce dose by 75%; total bilirubin >5 mg/dl: hold

Available forms: Inj 20 mg/ml, caps 50 mg

Implementation
PO route
• Caps need to be refrigerated
• Give without regard to food
• Increase fluid intake to 2-3 L/day to prevent urate deposits, calculi formation
• Refrigerate oral product, do not freeze

IV route
• **Do not use acrylic or ABS plastic devices, may crack, leak**
Intermittent IV infusion route (etoposide)
• Use cytotoxic handling procedures
• Dilute 5 ml vial with D_5W or 0.9% NaCl (200-400 mcg/ml); give slowly over 30-60 min; do not give over <30 min, hypotension may occur
• 200 mcg/ml is stable for 96 hr; 400 mcg/ml 48 hr

• Use Luer-Lok tubing to prevent leakage; do not let sol come in contact with skin; if contact occurs, wash well with soap and water

Y-site compatibilities: Acyclovir, alfentanil, allopurinol, amifostine, amikacin, aminocaproic acid, aminophylline, amiodarone, amphotericin B colloidal, amphotericin B lipid complex, amphotericin B liposome, ampicillin, ampicillin-sulbactam, anidulafungin, atenolol, atracurium, aztreonam, bivalirudin, bleomycin, bumetanide, buprenorphine, butorphanol, calcium chloride/gluconate, CARBOplatin, caspofungin, ceFAZolin, cefoperazone, cefotaxime, cefoTEtan, cefOXitin, cefTAZidime, ceftizoxime, cefTRIAXone, cefuroxime, chloramphenicol, chlorproMAZINE, cimetidine, ciprofloxacin, cisatracurium, CISplatin, cladribine, clindamycin, codeine, cyclophosphamide, cycloSPORINE, cytarabine, DACTINomycin, DAPTOmycin, DAUNOrubicin, dexamethasone, dexmedetomidine, dexrazoxane, digoxin, diltiazem, diphenhydrAMINE, DOBUTamine, DOCEtaxel, DOPamine, doxacurium, DOXOrubicin, DOXOrubicin HCl, DOXOrubicin liposomal, doxycycline, droperidol, enalaprilat, ePHEDrine, EPINEPHrine, epirubicin, ertapenem, erythromycin, esmolol, famotidine, fenoldopam, fentaNYL, floxuridine, fluconazole, fludarabine, fluorouracil, foscarnet, fosphenytoin, furosemide, ganciclovir, gatifloxacin, gemcitabine, gentamicin, glycopyrrolate, granisetron, haloperidol, heparin, hydrALAZINE, hydrocortisone, HYDROmorphone, hydrOXYzine, ifosfamide, imipenem-cilastatin, inamrinone, insulin (regular), irinotecan, isoproterenol, ketorolac, labetalol, lansoprazole, leucovorin, levofloxacin, levorphanol, lidocaine, linezolid, LORazepam, magnesium sulfate, mannitol, mechlorethamine, melphalan, meperidine, meropenem, mesna, methohexital, methotrexate, methyldopate, methylPREDNISolone, metoclopramide, metoprolol, metroNIDAZOLE, micafungin, midazolam, milrinone, minocycline, mitoXANtrone, mivacurium, morphine, nafcillin, nalbuphine, naloxone, nesiritide, nitroglycerin, nitroprusside, norepinephrine, NS, octreotide, ofloxacin, ondansetron, oxaliplatin, PACLitaxel, palonosetron, pamidronate, pancuronium, PEMEtrexed, pentamidine, pentazocine, PENTobarbital, PHENobarbital, phenylephrine, piperacillin, piperacillin-tazobactam, polymyxin B, potassium chloride/phosphates, procainamide, prochlorperazine, promethazine, propranolol, quinupristin-dalfopristin, ranitidine, remifentanil, rocuronium, sargramostim, sodium acetate/bicarbonate/phosphates, succinylcholine, SUFentanil, sulfamethoxazole-trimethoprim,

tacrolimus, teniposide, theophylline, thiotepa, ticarcillin, ticarcillin-clavulanate, tigecycline, tirofiban, tobramycin, topotecan, trimethobenzamide, vancomycin, vasopressin, vecuronium, verapamil, vinBLAStine, vinCRIStine, vinorelbine, voriconazole, zidovudine, zoledronic acid

Y-site incompatibility: IDArubicin

Additive compatibilities: CARBOplatin, CISplatin, cytarabine, floxuridine, fluorouracil, hydrOXYzine, ifosfamide, ondansetron

Intermittent IV INF route (etoposide phosphate)
• Reconstitute each vial with 5 or 10 ml of D_5W, 0.9% NaCl for a concentration of 20 mg/ml or 10 mg/ml, respectively; may give diluted or undiluted to concentration of as little as 0.1 mg/ml, give over 5-210 min

Y-site compatibilities: Acyclovir, alfentanil, amifostine, amikacin, aminocaproic acid, aminophylline, amiodarone, ampicillin, ampicillin-sulbactam, anidulafungin, atenolol, atracurium, aztreonam, bivalirudin, bleomycin, bumetanide, buprenorphine, butorphanol, calcium acetate/chloride/gluconate, CARBOplatin, carmustine, caspofungin, ceFAZolin, cefonicid, cefoperazone, cefotaxime, cefoTEtan, cefOXitin, cefTAZidime, ceftizoxime, cefTRIAXone, cefuroxime, chloramphenicol, cimetidine, ciprofloxacin, cisatracurium, CISplatin, clindamycin, codeine, cyclophosphamide, cycloSPORINE, cytarabine, dacarbazine, DACTINomycin, DAPTOmycin, DAUNOrubicin, dexamethasone, digoxin, diltiazem, diphenhydrAMINE, DOBUTamine, DOCEtaxel, DOPamine, doripenem, doxacurium, DOXOrubicin, doxycycline, enalaprilat, ePHEDrine, EPINEPHrine, epirubicin, ertapenem, erythromycin, esmolol, famotidine, fenoldopam, fentaNYL, floxuridine, fluconazole, fludarabine, fluorouracil, foscarnet, fosphenytoin, furosemide, ganciclovir, gatifloxacin, gemcitabine, gentamicin, glycopyrrolate, granisetron, haloperidol, heparin, hydrALAZINE, hydrocortisone, HYDROmorphone, hydrOXYzine, IDArubicin, ifosfamide, inamrinone, insulin (regular), irinotecan, isoproterenol, ketorolac, labetalol, leucovorin, levofloxacin, levorphanol, lidocaine, linezolid, LORazepam, magnesium sulfate, mannitol, mechlorethamine, meperidine, meropenem, mesna, metaraminol, methotrexate, methyldopate, metoclopramide, metoprolol, metroNIDAZOLE, midazolam, milrinone, minocycline, mitoXANtrone, mivacurium, morphine, nafcillin, nalbuphine, naloxone, nesiritide, netilmicin, nitroglycerin, nitroprusside, norepinephrine, octreotide, ofloxacin, ondansetron, oxaliplatin, PACLitaxel, palonosetron, pamidronate, pancuronium, PEMEtrexed, pentamidine, pentazocine, PENTobarbital, PHENobarbital, phenylephrine, piperacillin, piperacillin-tazobactam, plicamycin, polymyxin B, potassium chloride/phosphates, procainamide, promethazine, propranolol, quiNIDine, quinupristin-dalfopristin, ranitidine, remifentanil, riTUXimab, rocuronium, sodium acetate/bicarbonate/phosphates, streptozocin, succinylcholine, SUFentanil, sulfamethoxazole-trimethoprim, tacrolimus, teniposide, theophylline, thiopental, thiotepa, ticarcillin, ticarcillin-clavulanate, tigecycline, tirofiban, tobramycin, tolazoline, trastuzumab, trimethobenzamide, vancomycin, vasopressin, vecuronium, verapamil, vinBLAStine, vinCRIStine, vinorelbine, voriconazole, zidovudine, zoledronic acid

ADVERSE EFFECTS

CNS: Headache, *fever,* peripheral neuropathy, paresthesia, confusion, chills, fever
CV: *Hypotension,* **MI,** dysrhythmia
GI: *Nausea, vomiting, anorexia,* **hepatotoxicity,** dyspepsia, diarrhea, constipation
GU: **Nephrotoxicity**
HEMA: **Thrombocytopenia, leukopenia, myelosuppression, anemia**
INTEG: *Rash, alopecia,* phlebitis at **IV** site, radiation recall, **Stevens-Johnson syndrome**
RESP: **Bronchospasm,** pleural effusion
SYST: **Anaphylaxis, secondary malignancy**

Pharmacokinetics

Absorption	Variably absorbed
Distribution	Rapidly absorbed, 97% protein binding, crosses placenta
Metabolism	Liver, some
Excretion	Kidneys, unchanged 50%; breast milk, feces
Half-life	3 hr initially, 15 hr terminally

Pharmacodynamics

Unknown

INTERACTIONS

Individual drugs

Conivaptan, cycloSPORINE, imatinib, nilotinib, etravirine, telithromycin: increased etoposide effect, toxicity
Filgrastim, sargramostim: decreased etoposide effect, separate ≥24 hr
Radiation: increased bone marrow depression

Drug classifications

Other antineoplastics, immunosuppressives: increased bone marrow depression
Anticoagulants, NSAIDs, platelet inhibitors, thrombolytics, salicylates: increased bleeding risk
Live virus vaccines: increased adverse reactions

Drug/food

Grapefruit juice: decreased etoposide (PO)

Drug/lab test

Decreased: platelets, RBC, WBC, neutrophils, Hgb, calcium, phosphate
Increased: uric acid, potassium

NURSING CONSIDERATIONS

Assessment

• Monitor B/P (baseline and q15min) during administration

> **BLACK BOX WARNING: Bone marrow suppression:** monitor CBC, differential, platelet count weekly; withhold product if WBC is <500/mm³ or platelet count is <75,000/mm³; notify prescriber of results; recovery will take 3 wk, treatment should be delayed

• **Nephrotoxicity:** monitor renal function tests: BUN, urine CCr before, during therapy; I&O ratio; report fall in urine output of 30 ml/hr; for decreased hyperuricemia
• Monitor for cold, fever, sore throat (may indicate beginning of infection); notify prescriber if these occur, treat active infection prior to treatment

> **BLACK BOX WARNING:** Assess for bleeding: hematuria, guaiac, bruising or petechiae, mucosa or orifices q8hr; no rectal temp; avoid IM inj; use pressure to venipuncture sites

⚠ **Injection site reaction: closely monitor site for infiltration**
⚠ **Assess for symptoms indicating severe allergic reactions: rash, pruritus, urticaria, itching, flushing, bronchospasm, hypotension; epinephrine and crash cart should be nearby**
⚠ **Geriatric patients: assess for increased alopecia, GI effects, infection, nephrotoxicity, myelosuppression**

Patient/family education

• Teach patient to avoid use of products containing aspirin or ibuprofen, razors, commercial mouthwash because bleeding may occur; to report symptoms of bleeding (hematuria, tarry stools)

⚠ Nurse Alert   ✴ Key NCLEX® Drug

• Instruct patient to report signs of anemia (fatigue, headache, irritability, faintness, shortness of breath)
• Teach patient to report any changes in breathing or coughing even several months after treatment
⚠ Advise patient that contraception will be necessary during treatment because teratogenesis may occur
⚠ Pregnancy: instruct patient to notify prescriber if pregnancy is planned or suspected, pregnancy (D)
• Caution patient that hair loss may occur during treatment; a wig or hairpiece may make patient feel better; new hair will be different in color, texture
• Advise patient to avoid vaccinations during treatment because serious reactions may occur

BLACK BOX WARNING: Infection: teach patient to report signs/symptoms of infection: fever, chills, sore throat; patient should avoid crowds and persons with known infections

• Teach patient to take as prescribed (PO), not to double dose
• Teach patient to report signs of infection (flu-like symptoms, fever, fatigue, sore throat)
• Teach patient to take B/P often, hypotension occurs

Evaluation

Positive therapeutic outcome
• Decreased spread of malignant, leukemic cells

etravirine (Rx)

(e-tra′veer-een)
INTELENCE
Func. class.: Antiretroviral
Chem. class.: Non-nucleoside reverse transcriptase inhibitor (NNRTI)
Pregnancy category B

ACTION: Binds directly to reverse transcriptase, blocking the RNA- and DNA-dependent DNA polymerase action, causing a disruption of the enzyme's catalytic site

Therapeutic outcome: Increased CD4 count, decrease viral load

USES: In combination with other antiretroviral agents for HIV infection in treatment-experienced patients with evidence of HIV replication despite ongoing antiretroviral therapy

CONTRAINDICATIONS:

Hypersensitivity, breastfeeding

Precautions: Pregnancy **B**, impaired hepatic function, children, antimicrobial resistance, geriatric patients, hepatitis, hypercholesterolemia, hypertriglycerides, immune reconstitution syndrome

DOSAGES AND ROUTES

Adult: PO 200 mg bid after a meal, max 400 mg/day; not established in treatment-naïve patients

Available forms: Tabs 100, 200 mg

Implementation
• Give in combination with other antiretrovirals with food
• Store in cool environment; protect from light

ADVERSE EFFECTS

CNS: *Headache, insomnia,* amnesia, anxiety, confusion, fatigue, nightmares, peripheral neuropathy, **seizures, stroke,** tremor
CV: Atrial fibrillation, hypertension, MI
EENT: Blurred vision
GI: *Nausea, vomiting, diarrhea, anorexia,* abdominal pain, increased AST/ALT, constipation, flatulence, gastritis, GERD, **hematemesis, hepatitis,** hepatomegaly, **pancreatitis**
GU: Renal failure
HEMA: Hemolytic anemia, neutropenia, thrombocytopenia, anemia
INTEG: *Rash,* erythema multiforme, **angioedema, Stevens-Johnson syndrome**
MS: Rhabdomyolysis
OTHER: Diabetes mellitus, gynecomastia, hyperamylasemia, hypercholesterolemia, hyperglycemia, hyperlipidemia
RESP: Dyspnea, **bronchospasm**
SYST: DRESS

Pharmacokinetics

Absorption	Unknown
Distribution	Plasma protein binding 99.9%
Metabolism	By CYP3A4, 2C9, 2C19
Excretion	Feces
Half-life	21-61 hr

Pharmacodynamics

Unknown

INTERACTIONS

Individual drugs
Atazanavir, carBAMazepine, delavirdine, fosamprenavir, fosphenytoin, phenytoin, PHENobar-

bital, rifapentine, rifampin, tipranavir: do not use concurrently

CycloSPORINE, sirolimus, tacrolimus: altered effect

CYP3A4 inducers: amiodarone, atazanavir, clarithromycin, flecainide, fosamprenavir, lidocaine, mexiletine, propafenone, quiNIDine, sildenafil, tadalafil, vardenafil: decreased levels

CYP3A4 inhibitors: fluconazole, itraconazole, ketoconazole, lopinavir, posaconazole, ritonavir, voriconazole: increased etravirine levels

Darunavir, dexamethasone, disopyramide, efavirenz, nevirapine, ritonavir, tipranavir: decreased etravirine levels

Diazepam, rifampin, voriconazole, warfarin: increased levels

Methadone: increased withdrawal symptoms

Drug classifications
HMG-CoA reductase inhibitors: increased myopathy, rhabdomyolysis

Drug/herb
St. John's wort: decreased etravirine

NURSING CONSIDERATIONS
Assessment
• **Assess symptoms of HIV and for possible infections;** increased temp

⚠ **Monitor for fatal hypersensitivity reactions: fever, rash, nausea, vomiting, fatigue, cough, dyspnea, diarrhea, abdominal discomfort; treatment should be discontinued and not restarted; incidence of rash may be worse in women**

• **Assess blood dyscrasias** (anemia, granulocytopenia): bruising, fatigue, bleeding, poor healing

• **Renal failure:** monitor renal studies: BUN, serum uric acid, CCr before, during therapy; these may be elevated throughout treatment

• Monitor hepatic studies before, during therapy: bilirubin, AST, ALT, amylase, alk phos, creatine phosphokinase, creatinine, qmo

• **HIV:** monitor blood counts q2wk; monitor viral load and CD4 counts during treatment; watch for decreasing granulocytes, Hgb; if low, therapy may have to be discontinued and restarted after hematologic recovery; blood transfusions may be required; cholesterol/lipid profile

Patient/family education
• Inform patient that product is not a cure but will control symptoms; patient is still infective, may pass AIDS virus on to others

⚠ **Instruct patient to notify prescriber of sore throat, swollen lymph nodes, malaise,** fever; other infections may occur; to stop product and notify prescriber immediately if skin rash, fever, cough, shortness of breath, GI symptoms occur; advise all health care providers that allergic reaction has occurred with etravirine

• Advise patient that follow-up visits must be continued since serious toxicity may occur; blood counts must be done

⚠ **Instruct patient to use contraception during treatment; still able to transmit disease**

• Give patient Medication Guide and Warning Card, discuss points on guide

• Inform patient that other products may be necessary to prevent other infections

• Advise patient to take medication following a meal

Evaluation
Positive therapeutic outcome
• Increased CD4 count, decreased viral load

---

everolimus (Rx)
(e-ve-ro'li-mus)
Afinitor, Afinitor Disperz, Zortress
Func. class.: Antineoplastic (miscellaneous)
Chem. class.: Immunosuppressant, macrolide
Pregnancy category D

Do not confuse:
everolimus/sirolimus/tacrolimus/temsirolimus

ACTION: Proliferation signal inhibitor that inhibits mammalian target of rapamycin (mTOR); this pathway is dysregulated in cancer

USES: Renal cell cancer in those with failed treatment with suritinib or sorafenib or SUNItinib, kidney transplant rejection prophylaxis with cycloSPORINE, subependymal giant cell astrocytoma, progressive pancreatic neuroendocrine tumor (PNET) with unresectable locally advanced metastatic disease, renal angiomyolipoma, tuberous sclerosis complex, breast cancer hormone receptor positive/HER-2 negative

Therapeutic outcome: Decreasing tumor size, decreasing spread of malignancy

CONTRAINDICATIONS:
Breastfeeding; hypersensitivity to this product, Rapamune, and torisel; pregnancy **D**

Precautions: Children, renal/hepatic disease, diabetes mellitus, infection, hyperlipidemia, plural effusion

> **BLACK BOX WARNING:** Immunosuppression, infection, renal artery thrombosis, renal impairment, renal vein thrombosis

DOSAGE AND ROUTES

Kidney transplant rejection prophylaxis (Zortress)
Adult: PO 0.75 mg q12hr with cycloSPORINE in combination with basiliximab corticosteroids, reduced doses of cycloSPORINE

Advanced renal cancer (Afinitor)
Adult: PO 10 mg qd as long as clinically beneficial; with strong CYP3A4 inducers 10 mg qd, may increase by 5-mg increments to 20 mg qd

Progressive neuroendocrine tumor (PNET) (Afinitor only)
Adult: PO 10 mg/day, reduce dose to 5 mg/day if intolerable adverse reactions occur

Subependymal giant cell astrocytoma (SEGA) (Afinitor only)
Adult/adolescent/child ≥3 yr: PO BSA ≥2.2 m² give 7.5 mg/day; BSA 1.3-21 m² give 5 mg/day; BSA 0.5-1.2 m² give 2.5 mg/day, adjust q2wk, based on trough, clinical response

Hepatic dose
Adult: PO (Child-Pugh A) Afinitor 7.5 mg/day; (Child-Pugh B) Afinitor 5 mg qd; not to be used in Child-Pugh C

Available forms: Tabs 0.25, 0.5, 0.75, 2.5 (Zortress); 2.5, 5, 7.5, 10 mg (Afinitor)

Implementation
• Swallow tabs whole with a full glass of water; do not chew, crush, or break
• Afinitor: take at same time of day, consistently with or without food; if unable to swallow, disperse in 30 ml of water
• Zortress: must take consistently with or without food, give at same time of day q12h with cycloSPORINE
• Follow procedure for proper handling of antineoplastics
• Give all medications PO if possible, avoiding IM inj; bleeding may occur
• Store protected from light, at room temperature

Afinitor adjustments for toxicity
Noninfectious pneumonitis
Grade 1, asymptomatic with radiographic findings only: No dose change
Grade 2, symptomatic but no interference with activities of daily living (ADL): Consider withholding therapy; resume Afinitor at a lower dose when symptoms improve to ≤ grade 1; discontinue Afinitor if symptoms do not improve within 4 wk
Grade 3, symptomatic and interfering with ADL and oxygen therapy indicated: Hold therapy; consider resuming Afinitor at a lower dose when symptoms improve to ≤ grade 1; consider discontinuing Afinitor if grade 3 toxicity recurs
Grade 4, life-threatening and ventilator support indicated: Discontinue therapy

Stomatitis
Grade 1, minimum symptoms and normal diet: No dose adjustment required
Grade 2, symptomatic but can eat and swallow modified diet: Hold therapy until symptoms improve to ≤ grade 1 and resume Afinitor at the same dose; if grade 2 toxicity recurs, hold therapy and resume Afinitor at a lower dose when symptoms improve to ≤ grade 1
Grade 3, symptomatic and unable to adequately eat or hydrate orally: Hold therapy; resume Afinitor at a lower dose when symptoms improve to ≤ grade 1
Grade 4, symptomatic and life-threatening: Discontinue therapy

Other nonhematologic toxicity (excluding metabolic events)
Grade 1: No dose adjustment required if toxicity is tolerable
Grade 2: No dose adjustment required if toxicity is tolerable; if toxicity is intolerable, hold therapy until symptoms improve to ≤ grade 1 and resume Afinitor at the same dose; if grade 2 toxicity recurs, hold therapy and resume Afinitor at a lower dose when symptoms improve to ≤ grade 1
Grade 3: Hold therapy; consider resuming Afinitor at a lower dose when symptoms improve to ≤ grade 1; if grade 3 toxicity recurs, consider discontinuing therapy
Grade 4: Discontinue Afinitor therapy

Metabolic events (hyperglycemia, dyslipidemia)
Grade 1 or 2: No dose adjustment required
Grade 3: Temporarily withhold therapy; resume Afinitor at a lower dose
Grade 4: Discontinue Afinitor therapy

ADVERSE EFFECTS

CNS: *Headache, insomnia, paresthesia, chills,* fever, seizure, personality changes, dizziness
CV: *Hypertension, CHF, peripheral edema*
EENT: Blurred vision, photophobia
GI: Nausea, vomiting, diarrhea, constipation, stomatitis
GU: Renal failure
HEMA: Anemia, leukopenia, thrombocytopenia
INTEG: *Rash, acne*
META: Hyperglycemia, increased creatinine, *hyperlipemia,* hypophosphatemia, weight loss
RESP: **Pleural effusion,** *dyspnea,* noninfectious pneumonitis

Pharmacokinetics

Absorption	Rapid
Distribution	Protein binding 74%
Metabolism	Extensively by CYP3A4
Excretion	Feces 80%, urine 5%
Half-life	30 hr, reduced by high-fat meal

Pharmacodynamics

Onset	Unknown
Peak	1-2 hr
Duration	Unknown

INTERACTIONS

Individual drugs
Cimetidine, cycloSPORINE, danazol, erythromycin: increased everolimus effect
CarBAMazepine, PHENobarbital, phenytoin, rifamycin, rifapentine: decreased blood levels of everolimus

Drug classifications
Antifungals, calcium channel blockers, CYP3A4 inhibitors (strong, moderate), HIV-protease inhibitors: increased everolimus effect
Immunosuppressants: increased nephrotoxicity
Vaccines: decreased effect of these products

Drug/herb
St. John's wort: may decrease the effect of everolimus

Drug/food
Alters bioavailability; use consistently with or without food; do not use with grapefruit juice

Drug/lab test
Increased: bilirubin, calcium, cholesterol, glucose, potassium, lipids, phosphate, triglycerides, uric acid

Decreased: calcium, glucose, potassium, magnesium, phosphate

NURSING CONSIDERATIONS

Assessment
• Monitor lipid profile: cholesterol, triglycerides, a lipid-lowering agent may be needed; blood glucose

> **BLACK BOX WARNING:** Monitor **immunosuppression:** Hgb, WBC, platelets during treatment qmo; if leukocytes <3000/mm^3 or platelets <100,000/mm^3, product should be discontinued or reduced; decreased hemoglobin level may indicate bone marrow suppression

• Monitor hepatic studies: alk phos, AST, ALT, amylase, bilirubin, and for hepatotoxicity: dark urine, jaundice, itching, light-colored stools; product should be discontinued

> **BLACK BOX WARNING: Infection:** bacterial/fungal infections can occur and are more common with combination immunosuppression therapy

> **BLACK BOX WARNING: Renal artery/vein thrombosis (Zortress):** may result in graft loss within 30 days after transplantation

Patient/family education

> **BLACK BOX WARNING:** Advise to report fever, rash, severe diarrhea, chills, sore throat, fatigue; serious infections may occur; clay-colored stools, cramping (hepatotoxicity)

• Advise to avoid crowds, persons with known infections to reduce risk of infection
⚠ **Teach to use contraception before, during, and 12 wk after product has been discontinued, avoid breastfeeding**
⚠ **Teach to notify prescriber if pregnancy is planned or suspected; pregnancy (D)**
• Advise not to use with grapefruit juice
• Inform to avoid live virus vaccines
• Advise to take up to 6 hr after normally scheduled time if dose is missed
• Advise that product may decrease male/female fertility
• Teach that drinking alcohol is not recommended
• Teach patient to take consistently with or without food
• Teach patient to report visual changes, weight gain, edema, shortness of breath

Evaluation
Positive therapeutic outcome
• Decreasing size of tumor, decreasing spread of malignancy

exemestane (Rx)
(x-ee-mes'tane)
Aromasin
Func. class.: Antineoplastic
Chem. class.: Aromatase inhibitor
Pregnancy category D

Do not confuse:
exemestane/ezetimibe/estramustine

ACTION: Lowers serum estradiol concentrations; many breast cancers have strong estrogen receptors

Therapeutic outcome: Prevention of rapidly growing malignant cells

USES: Advanced breast carcinoma that has not responded to other therapy in estrogen receptor–positive patients (postmenopausal)

CONTRAINDICATIONS:
Pregnancy **X**, breastfeeding, hypersensitivity, premenopausal women

Precautions: Children, geriatric, renal/hepatic disease

DOSAGE AND ROUTES
Adult: PO 25 mg/day after meals; may need 50 mg/day if taken with a potent CYP3A4 inhibitor

Available forms: Tabs 25 mg

Implementation
• Give after food or fluids for GI upset
• Store in light-resistant container at room temperature

ADVERSE EFFECTS
CNS: Headache, fatigue, depression, insomnia, anxiety, hot flashes, diaphoresis, dizziness
CV: Hypertension, edema
GI: Nausea, vomiting, increased appetite, diarrhea, constipation, abdominal pain
HEMA: *Lymphopenia*
MS: Fracture, bone loss
RESP: Cough, dyspnea

Absorption	Rapidly absorbed
Distribution	Unknown
Metabolism	Liver
Excretion	Feces, urine
Half-life	24 hr

Unknown

INTERACTIONS
Drug classifications
CYP3A4 inducers, estrogens: decreased exemestane action

NURSING CONSIDERATIONS
Assessment
• Assess B/P; hypertension may occur
• Bone mineral density, x-ray of thoracic or lumbar spine if bone changes are suspected

Patient/family education
• Instruct patient to report any complaints, side effects to prescriber; if dose is missed, do not double next dose
• Advise patient that hot flashes can occur and are reversible after discontinuing treatment
• Inform patient about who should be told about therapy
• Advise patient to use reliable contraception, pregnancy **X**, do not breastfeed

Evaluation
Positive therapeutic outcome
• Decreased spread of malignant cells in breast cancer

exenatide (Rx)
(ex-en'a-tide)
Bydureon, Byetta
Func. class.: Antidiabetic
Chem. class.: Incretin mimetic
Pregnancy category C

ACTION: Binds and activates known human GLP-1 receptor, mimics natural physiology for self-regulating glycemic control

Therapeutic outcome: Decreased polyuria, polydipsia, polyphagia; improved Hgb A1c

USES: Type 2 diabetes mellitus given in combination with metformin, sulfonylurea, or a thiazolidinedione, insulin glargine

CONTRAINDICATIONS:
Hypersensitivity

> **BLACK BOX WARNING:** Medullary thyroid carcinoma, multiple endocrine neoplasia syndrome type 2 (MEN-2), thyroid cancer

Precautions: Pregnancy **C,** geriatric, severe renal/hepatic/GI disease, vitamin D deficiency

DOSAGE AND ROUTES
Adult: SUBCUT 5 mcg bid 1 hr before morning and evening meal; may increase to 10 mcg bid after 1 mo of therapy; ext rel subcut (Bydureon) 2 mg q7 days; ext rel inj 2 mg q7 days

Available forms: Inj 5, 10 mcg pen; ext rel powder for susp for inj 2 mg

Implementation
• Store in refrigerator; unopened pen may be stored at room temperature after opening for up to 30 days
Subcut route (regular release—Byetta)
• Give SUBCUT only, do not give **IV/IM**
• Pen needles must be purchased separately and be compatible
• Prime prior to use
• Inject into thigh, abdomen, upper arm
Subcut route (extended release—Bydureon)
• Give 1× wk; the dose can be given at any time of day, without regard to meals
• Available as a single dose tray containing a vial of 2 mg, a prefilled syringe delivering 0.65 ml diluent, a vial connector, and two custom needles (23G, 5/16″) specific to this delivery system (one is a spare needle); do not substitute needles or any other components
• Inject immediately after the white/off-white powder is suspended in the diluent and transferred to the syringe
• Inject subcutaneously into the thigh, abdomen, or upper arm; rotate sites to prevent lipodystrophy
• Give 1 hr before meals, approximately 6 hr apart; if patient is NPO, may need to hold dose to prevent hypoglycemia
• Store in refrigerator; unopened pen may be stored at room temperature after opening for up to 30 days
• If added to insulin glargine, insulin detemir, a dosage reduction in these products may be required

ADVERSE EFFECTS
CNS: *Headache, dizziness,* jittery feeling, restlessness, weakness
ENDO: **Hypoglycemia,** thyroid hyperplasia

GI: Nausea, vomiting, diarrhea, dyspepsia, anorexia, gastroesophageal reflux, weight loss, **pancreatitis**
SYST: Angioedema, anaphylaxis, inj site reactions

Pharmacokinetics
Absorption	Unknown
Distribution	Unknown
Metabolism	Unknown
Excretion	Glomerular filtration
Half-life	Unknown

Pharmacodynamics
Onset	Unknown
Peak	Immediate release: 2.1 hr; ext rel: 2 wk
Duration	Unknown

INTERACTIONS
Individual drugs
Acetaminophen: may decrease the effect of acetaminophen
Acetaminophen (elixir), digoxin, lovastatin: decreased action of these products
Alcohol, disopyramide: increased hypoglycemia
Dextrothyroxine, niacin, triamterene: decreased hypoglycemia efficacy
Erythromycin, metoclopramide: do not use with exenatide

Drug classifications
ACE inhibitors, anabolic steroids, androgens, fibric acid derivatives, sulfonylureas: increased hypoglycemia
Corticosteroids, phenothiazines: increased hyperglycemia
Estrogens, MAOIs, oral contraceptives, progestins, thiazide diuretics: decreased hypoglycemia

NURSING CONSIDERATIONS
Assessment
• Monitor fasting blood, glucose, A1c levels, postprandial glucose during treatment to determine diabetes control
• **Pancreatitis:** severe abdominal pain, with/without vomiting; product should be discontinued
• Assess for hypo/hyperglycemic reaction that can occur soon after meals; for severe hypoglycemia give **IV** D₅W, then **IV** dextrose solution
⚠ **Anaphylaxis, angioedema: product should be discontinued immediately**
• Assess for nausea, diarrhea, vomiting, ability to tolerate product, may cause dehydration

---

⚠ Nurse Alert   ✦ Key NCLEX® Drug

Patient/family education
- Teach patient symptoms of hypo/hyperglycemia, what to do about each; to have glucagon emergency kit available; to carry a glucose source (candy, sugar cube) to treat hypoglycemia
- Advise patient that product must be continued on daily or weekly basis (ext rel); explain consequences of discontinuing product abruptly
- Teach patient that diabetes is a lifelong illness; product will not cure disease
- Advise patient to carry emergency ID with prescriber and medications
- Advise patient to continue weight control, dietary restrictions, exercise, hygiene
- Inform patient that regular blood glucose monitoring and A1c testing is needed
- Advise patient to notify prescriber if pregnant or intend to become pregnant
- Advise patient to read "Information for the Patient" and "Pen User Manual"; provide education on self-injection
- **A Pancreatitis: if severe abdominal pain with or without vomiting occurs, seek medical attention immediately**
- Review injection procedure, to store product in refrigerator, room temperature after first use, discard 30 days after first use, do not freeze, protect from light (Byetta)

Evaluation
Positive therapeutic outcome
- Decrease in polyuria, polydipsia, polyphagia, clear sensorium; improved A1c, weight; absence of dizziness, stable gait

ezetimibe (Rx)
(ehz-eh-tim′bee)
Ezetrol ✦, Zetia
Func. class.: Antilipemic
Pregnancy category C

ACTION: Inhibits absorption of cholesterol by the small intestine

Therapeutic outcome: Decreased cholesterol levels

USES: Hypercholesterolemia, homozygous familial hypercholesterolemia (HoFH), homozygous sitosterolemia

CONTRAINDICATIONS:
Hypersensitivity, severe hepatic disease

Precautions: Pregnancy **C**, breastfeeding, children, hepatic disease

DOSAGE AND ROUTES
Adult: PO 10 mg/day; may be given with HMG-CoA reductase inhibitor at same time; may be given with bile acid sequestrant; give ezetimibe 2 hr before or 4 hr after the bile acid sequestrant

Available forms: Tabs 10 mg

Implementation
- Give without regard to meals

ADVERSE EFFECTS
CNS: Fatigue, dizziness, headache
GI: Diarrhea, abdominal pain
MISC: Chest pain
MS: *Myalgias, arthralgias,* back pain, myopathy, **rhabdomyolysis**
RESP: Pharyngitis, sinusitis, cough, URI

Pharmacokinetics

Absorption	Unknown
Distribution	Unknown
Metabolism	Small intestine, liver
Excretion	Urine (11%), feces (78%)
Half-life	Unknown

Pharmacodynamics
Unknown

INTERACTIONS
Individual drugs
Cholestyramine: decreased ezetimibe action
CycloSPORINE: increased action of ezetimibe

Drug classifications
Antacids: decreased action of ezetimibe
Fibric acid derivatives: increased ezetimibe action

Drug/lab test
Increase: LFTs

NURSING CONSIDERATIONS
Assessment
- **Hypercholesterolemia:** obtain diet history; monitor fat content, lipid levels (triglycerides, LDL, HDL, total cholesterol), LFTs baseline and periodically during treatment
- **Myopathy/rhabdomyolysis:** monitor for increased CPK; myalgia, muscle cramps, musculoskeletal pain, lethargy, fatigue, fever; more common when combined with statins

Patient/family education
- Teach patient that compliance is needed
- Advise that risk factors should be decreased: high-fat diet, smoking, alcohol consumption, absence of exercise

• Advise patient to notify prescriber if pregnancy is suspected or planned or if breastfeeding
• Advise patient to notify prescriber if unexplained weakness, or muscle pain is present
• Teach patient to notify prescriber of dietary/herbal supplements

Evaluation

Positive therapeutic outcome
• Decreased cholesterol

---

ezogabine (Rx)
(e-zog'a-been)
Potiga
Func. class.: Anticonvulsant

ACTION: The exact mechanism of anticonvulsant effects is not fully known. However, studies indicate that the drug enhances transmembrane potassium currents, which may stabilize the resting membrane potential and reduce brain excitability. May also augment GABA-mediated currents

USES: Partial seizures, migraines

CONTRAINDICATIONS:
Hypersensitivity

Precautions: Suicidal ideation/behavior, prostatic hypertrophy, dementia, psychotic disorders, QT prolongation, congestive heart failure, ventricular hypertrophy, hypokalemia, hypomagnesemia, abrupt discontinuation, renal impairment, hepatic disease, geriatrics, pregnancy category C, breastfeeding, neonates, infants, children, adolescents

DOSAGE AND ROUTES
Adult/geriatric patient ≤65 yr: PO Initially, 100 mg tid; increase by ≤50 mg tid per day at weekly intervals depending on response, up to a maintenance dose of 200-400 mg tid depending on response; max is 400 mg tid (1200 mg/day).
Geriatric patient >65 yr: PO Initially, 50 mg tid; increase by ≤50 mg tid per day at weekly intervals depending on response; max 250 mg tid (750 mg/day).

Available forms: Film-coated tabs 50, 200, 300, 400 mg

Implementation
• Tabs should be swallowed whole without regard to meals
• Give in 3 equally divided doses

ADVERSE EFFECTS
CNS: Dizziness, drowsiness, memory impairment, tremor, vertigo, abnormal coordination, disturbance in attention, gait disturbance, aphasia, dysarthria, balance disorder, paresthesias, amnesia, dysphagia, myoclonia, hypokinesia, confusion, anxiety, hallucinations, **suicidal thoughts/behaviors,** fatigue, asthenia, malaise, euphoria
EENT: *Diplopia, blurred vision,* retinal pigment change
GI: *Nausea, constipation, dyspepsia , xerostomia, constipation, weight gain, appetite stimulation*
GU: *Urinary retention, hydronephrosis, dysuria, urinary hesitation, hematuria, chromaturia*
HEMA: **Thrombocytopenia,** leukopenia, neutropenia
INTEG: Rash, alopecia, blue skin discoloration
MISC: *Influenza, dyspnea,* **QT prolongation**
MS: Muscle spasms, weakness

Pharmacokinetics

Absorption	Rapid, 60%
Distribution	Extensively in the body, 80% protein binding
Metabolism	Extensive (glucuronidation, acetylation), metabolite (N-glucuronides)
Excretion	Renal 36% (exogabine), 18% (NAMR), 24% (N-glucuronides); fecal 14%
Half-life	Elimination 7 hr, metabolite 11 hr

Pharmacodynamics

Onset	Unknown
Peak	0.5-2 hr, increased by high-fat food
Duration	Unknown

INTERACTIONS
Individual drugs
Amantadine: increased urinary retention
Arsenic trioxide, chloroquine, chlorproMA-ZINE, clarithromycin, dextromethorphan; dronedarone, droperidol, erythromycin, grepafloxacin, halofantrine, levomethadyl, mesoridazine, methadone, pentamidine, pimozide, posaconazole, probucol, propafenone, quiNIDine, saquinavir, sparfloxacin, terfenadine, thioridazine, troleandomycin, ziprasidone: increased QT prolongation

---

Buprenorphine, butorphanol, dronabinol, ethanol, mirtazapine, nabilone, nalbuphine, opiate agonists, pentazocine, pregabalin, traMADol, traZODone, ethanol: increased CNS depression

CarBAMazepine: decreased effect of ezogabine

Digoxin: increased effect of each product

Phenytoin: decreased effect of each product

Drug classifications

Antimuscarinics, H1-blockers: increased urinary retention

Class IA antiarrhythmics (disopyramide, procainamide, quiNIDine), Class III antiarrhythmics (amiodarone, dofetilide, ibutilide, sotalol): **increased QT prolongation**

Anxiolytics, hypnotics, opiate agonists, sedatives, skeletal muscle relaxants: increased CNS depression

NURSING CONSIDERATIONS

Assessment

• **Seizures:** Assess for type, duration, location, activity, presence of aura

• **QT prolongation**: Monitor in those with known QT prolongation, congestive heart failure, ventricular hypertrophy, hypokalemia, hypomagnesemia, and in patients receiving medications known to cause QT prolongation. QT prolongation can occur within 3 hrs of dose

• **Abrupt withdrawal:** Withdraw gradually to minimize increased seizure frequency

• **Suicidal thoughts/behaviors**: Assess for any unusual changes in moods or behaviors, including emotional lability or emerging or worsening depression and suicidal ideation

Patient/family education

• Instruct patient to avoid driving or operating machinery, or performing other tasks that require mental alertness until reaction is known

• Instruct patient to avoid concurrent use of alcohol

• Instruct patient to avoid abruptly discontinuing this medication

• **Suicidal thought/behaviors:** Advise patient to notify prescriber immediately for suicidal thought/behaviors

> **⚠ HIGH ALERT**
>
> ## factor IX complex (human)
> **Alpha Nine SD, Bebulin VH, BeneFIX, Mononine, Profilnine SD**
> *Func. class.:* Hemostatic
> *Chem. class.:* Factors II, VII, IX, X
> **Pregnancy category C**

ACTION: Causes an increase in blood levels of clotting factors II, VII, IX, X; factor IX (human) has IX activity only

Therapeutic outcome: Replacement of factors II, VII, IX, X

USES: Hemophilia B (Christmas disease), factor IX deficiency, anticoagulant reversal, control of bleeding in patients with factor VIII inhibitors; reversal of overdose of anticoagulants in emergencies

CONTRAINDICATIONS:
Hypersensitivity to mouse/hamster protein, DIC, mild factor IX deficiency

Precautions: Pregnancy **C**, neonates, infants, elective surgery, hepatic disease

DOSAGE AND ROUTES
Bleeding in hemophilia A and inhibitors of factor VIII (Proplex T, Konyne 80)
Adult and child: 75 units/kg, repeat in 12 hr

Factor IX complex (human) bleeding in hemophilia B
Adult and child: **IV** Establish 25% of normal factor IX activity or 60-75 units/kg then 10-20 units/kg/day × 1-2 wk

Prophylaxis of bleeding in hemophilia B
Adult and child: **IV** 10-20 units/kg 1-2 ×/wk

Reversal of oral anticoagulant
Adult and child: 15 units/kg

Factor VII deficiency (use Proplex T only)
Adult and child: **IV** 0.5 units/kg × body weight (kg) × desired factor IX increase (in % of normal); repeat q4-6hr if needed

Factor IX (human) minor to moderate hemorrhage
Use only Alpha Nine, Alpha Nine SD
Adult and child: **IV** Dose to increase plasma factor IX level to 20%-30% in one dose

Serious hemorrhage
Adult and child: **IV** Dose to increase plasma factor IX level to 30%-50% given as daily INF

Minor hemorrhage (Mononine only)
Adult and child: **IV** dose to increase plasma factor IX level to 15%-25% (20-30 units/kg), may repeat in 24 hr if needed

Major hemorrhage
Adult and child: **IV** dose to increase plasma factor IX level to 25%-50% (75 units/kg) q18-30hr for up to 10 days

Available forms: Inj (number of units noted on label)

Implementation
IV route
- Give hepatitis B vaccine before administration
- Give **IV** after warming to room temperature 3 ml/min or less, with plastic syringe only; do not admix
- Give after dilution with provided diluent, 50 or 25 units/ml; max 10 ml/min; decrease rate if fever, headache, flushing, tingling occur
- Give after crossmatch is completed if patient has blood type A, B, AB, to determine incompatibility with factor
- Store reconstituted sol for 3 hr at room temperature or for 2 yr with refrigeration (powder); check expiration date
- Incompatible with protein products

BeneFIX
- Allow vials of concentrate/diluent to warm to room temperature
- After removing flip-top cap from vial, wipe top of vial with alcohol swab; let dry
- Peel back cover from vial adapter package; do not remove
- Place vial adapter over vial; press firmly until it snaps; attach plunger rod to diluent syringe and break plastic tip cap from diluent syringe
- Lift the package away from the adapter and connect diluent syringe; depress plunger; swirl contents

ADVERSE EFFECTS
CNS: *Headache, dizziness,* malaise, paresthesia, *lethargy, chills, fever, flushing*
CV: *Hypotension,* tachycardia, **MI, venous thrombosis, pulmonary embolism**
GI: Nausea, vomiting, abdominal cramps, jaundice, **viral hepatitis**
HEMA: Thrombosis, hemolysis, AIDS, DIC
INTEG: Rash, flushing, *urticaria,* injection-site reactions
RESP: Bronchospasm

Pharmacokinetics

Absorption	40% (PO), complete (**IV**)
Distribution	Unknown
Metabolism	Rapidly cleared from plasma, liver 30%
Excretion	Kidneys—70% unchanged
Half-life	24 hr

Pharmacodynamics

Unknown

INTERACTIONS
Individual drugs
Aminocaproic acid: increased risk of thrombosis; do not use together

Warfarin: decreased effect of warfarin

Drug classifications
Incompatible with protein products

NURSING CONSIDERATIONS
Assesment
• Monitor blood studies (coagulation factor assays by % normal: 5% prevents spontaneous hemorrhage, 30%-50% for surgery, 80%-100% for severe hemorrhage); check for bleeding q15-30min, immobilize and apply ice to affected joints

• Monitor for increased B/P, pulse

• Monitor I&O; if urine becomes orange or red, notify prescriber

• **Assess for allergic or pyrogenic reaction:** fever, chills, rash, itching; slow inf rate if not severe

⚠ **Assess for DIC: bleeding, ecchymosis, hypersensitivity, changes in coagulation tests**

Patient/family education
• Advise patient to report any signs of bleeding: gums, under skin, urine, stools, emesis; calf pain, joint pain, yellowing of eyes/skin

• Caution patient about risk of viral hepatitis, AIDS; that immunization for hepatitis B may be given first; to be tested q2-3mo for HIV, even though the risk is low

• Tell patient to carry/wear emergency ID identifying disease and treatment; avoid salicylates, NSAIDs; inform other health professionals about condition

Evaluation
Positive therapeutic outcome
• Prevention of hemorrhage

famciclovir (Rx)
(fam-sye-klo′vir)

Famvir

Func. class.: Antiviral

Chem. class.: Guanosine nucleoside

Pregnancy category B

ACTION: Inhibits DNA polymerase and viral DNA synthesis by conversion of this guanosine nucleoside to penciclovir

Therapeutic outcome: Decreasing size and number of lesions

USES: Treatment of acute herpes zoster (shingles), genital herpes, recurrent mucocutaneous herpes simplex virus (HSV) in HIV patients, initial episodes of herpes genitalis, herpes labialis in the immunocompromised

CONTRAINDICATIONS:
Hypersensitivity to this product, penciclovir, acyclovir, ganciclovir, valacyclovir, or valganciclovir

Precautions: Pregnancy **B,** breastfeeding, renal disease

DOSAGE AND ROUTES
Herpes zoster
Adult: PO 500 mg q8hr × 7 days

Renal dose
Adult: PO CCr ≥ 60 ml/min 500 mg q8hr; 40-59 ml/min 500 mg q12hr; 20-39 ml/min 500 mg q24hr; CCr <20 ml/min 250 mg q24hr

Recurrent HSV
Adult: PO 125 mg q12hr × 5 days

Renal dose
Adult: PO CCr <39 ml/min 125 mg q24hr × 5 days

Suppression of recurrent HSV
Adult: PO 250 mg q12hr up to 1 yr

Renal dose
Adult: PO CCr 20-39 ml/min 125 mg q12hr × 5 days; CCr <20 ml/min 125 mg q24hr × 5 days

Genital herpes/herpes labialis (recurrent)
Adult: PO 125 mg bid × 5 days or 1000 mg bid for 1 day; begin treatment at first sign of recurrence; immunocompetent herpes labialis: 1500 mg as a single dose

F

Suppression of recurrent genital herpes
Adult: PO 250 mg bid for up to a year

Herpes genitalis initial episodes
Adult: PO 250 mg tid × 7-10 days

Available forms: Tabs 125, 250, 500 mg

Implementation
• Give with or without meals; absorption does not appear to be lowered when taken with food
• Give within 72 hr of the appearance of rash in herpes zoster

ADVERSE EFFECTS
CNS: *Headache, fatigue, dizziness,* paresthesia, somnolence, fever
GI: Nausea, vomiting, diarrhea, constipation, abdominal pain, anorexia
GU: Decreased sperm count
INTEG: *Pruritus*
MS: Back pain, arthralgia
RESP: Pharyngitis, sinusitis

Pharmacokinetics
Absorption	Well absorbed, 77%
Distribution	Protein binding 20%
Metabolism	Intestinal tissue, blood, liver
Excretion	Breast milk, kidney, bile
Half-life	Terminal 2-3 hr

Pharmacodynamics
Onset	Unknown
Peak	1 hr
Duration	8 hr

INTERACTIONS
Individual drugs
Cimetidine: decreased metabolism
Digoxin, probenecid, theophylline: decreased renal excretion

NURSING CONSIDERATIONS
Assessment
• **Herpes zoster:** assess number and distribution of lesions; also burning, itching, or pain (early symptoms of herpes infection); neuralgia during, after treatment
• **Acute renal failure:** usually in high doses or in those >65 yr; monitor renal function tests: urine CCr, BUN before, during treatment if patient has decreased renal function; dosage may need to be lowered
• Monitor bowel pattern before, during treatment; diarrhea may occur

• Assess for posttherapeutic neuralgia during and after treatment

Patient/family education
• Teach patient how to recognize signs of beginning of infection
• Teach patient how to prevent the spread of infection to others
• Teach patient reason for medication and expected results
• Advise patient that this medication does not prevent spread of disease to others, that condoms should be used
• Advise women with genital herpes to have yearly Pap smears; cervical cancer is more likely

Evaluation
Positive therapeutic outcome
• Decreased size and spread of lesions
• Prevention of recurrence (genital herpes)
• Decreased time for healing

famotidine (Rx, OTC)
(fa-moe'ti-deen)
Pepcid, Pepcid AC
Func. class.: H₂-histamine receptor antagonist, antiulcer agent
Pregnancy category B

ACTION: Inhibits histamine at H₂-receptor site in gastric parietal cells, which inhibits gastric acid secretion while pepsin remains at a stable level

Therapeutic outcome: Healing of duodenal ulcers or gastric ulcers; prevention of duodenal ulcers; decreases symptoms of gastroesophageal reflux disease or Zollinger-Ellison syndrome, heartburn

USES: Short-term treatment of active duodenal ulcer, maintenance therapy for duodenal ulcer, Zollinger-Ellison syndrome, multiple endocrine adenomas, gastric ulcers, heartburn, gastroesophageal reflux disease

Unlabeled uses: GI disorders in those taking NSAIDs, urticaria, prevention of stress ulcers, aspiration pneumonitis, inactivation of oral pancreatic enzymes in pancreatic disorders, prevention of paclitaxel hypersensitivity reactions

CONTRAINDICATIONS:
Hypersensitivity

Precautions: Pregnancy **B**, breastfeeding, children <12 yr, geriatric, severe renal/hepatic disease

DOSAGE AND ROUTES

Active ulcer
Adult: PO 40 mg/day at bedtime × 4-8 wk, then 20 mg/day at bedtime if needed (maintenance); **IV** 20 mg q12hr if unable to take PO
Child 1-16 yr: PO 0.5 mg/kg/day at bedtime or divided bid, max 40 mg/day

Hypersecretory conditions
Adult: PO 20 mg q6hr; may give 160 mg q6hr if needed; **IV** 20 mg q12hr if unable to take PO

Heartburn relief/prevention
Adult: PO 10 mg with water, 15 min-1 hr before eating

Renal dose
Adult: PO CCr <50 ml/min; give 50% of dose or extend interval to q36-48hr

Available forms: Tabs 10, 20, 40 mg; powder for oral susp 40 mg/5 ml; inj 10 mg/ml, 20 mg/50 ml 0.9% NaCl; orally disintegrating tabs (RPD) 20, 40 mg; chew tabs 10 mg; gel cap 10 mg

Implementation
PO route
- Give antacids 1 hr before or 2 hr after famotidine; may be given with foods or liquid
- Administer oral susp after shaking well; discard unused sol after 1 mo
- Store in cool environment (oral)

Direct IV route
- Give **IV** direct after diluting 2 ml of product (10 mg/ml) in 0.9% NaCl to total volume of 5-10 ml; inject over 2 min to prevent hypotension
Intermittent IV infusion route
- Administer after diluting 20 mg of product in 100 ml of LR, 0.9% NaCl, D_5W, $D_{10}W$; run over 15-30 min
Continuous IV infusion route
- **Adults:** Dilute 40 mg/250 ml D_5W or NS, infuse over 24 hr, run at 11 ml/hr, use infusion device
- Store in cool environment (oral); **IV** sol is stable for 48 hr at room temperature; do not use discolored sol

Y-site compatibilities: Acyclovir, allopurinol, amifostine, aminophylline, amphotericin, ampicillin, ampicillin/sulbactam, inamrinone, amsacrine, atropine, aztreonam, bretylium, calcium gluconate, ceFAZolin, cefoperazone, cefotaxime, cefoTEtan, cefOXitin, cefTAZidime, ceftizoxime, cefTRIAXone, cefuroxime, cephalothin, cephapirin, chlorproMAZINE, CISplatin, cladribine, cyclophosphamide, cytarabine, dexamethasone, dextran 40, digoxin, diphenhydrAMINE, DOBUTamine, DOPa-mine, DOXOrubicin, droperidol, enalaprilat, EPINEPHrine, erythromycin lactobionate, esmolol, filgrastim, fluconazole, fludarabine, folic acid, gentamicin, granisetron, haloperidol, heparin, hydrocortisone, HYDROmorphone, hydrOXYzine, imipenem/cilastatin, regular insulin, isoproterenol, labetalol, lidocaine, LORazepam, magnesium sulfate, melphalan, meperidine, methotrexate, methylPREDNISolone, metoclopramide, mezlocillin, midazolam, morphine, nafcillin, nitroglycerin, nitroprusside, norepinephrine, ondansetron, oxacillin, PACLitaxel, perphenazine, phenylephrine, phenytoin, phytonadione, piperacillin, potassium chloride, potassium phosphate, procainamide, propofol, sargramostim, sodium bicarbonate, teniposide, theophylline, thiamine, thiotepa, ticarcillin, ticarcillin-clavulanate, verapamil, vinorelbine

ADVERSE EFFECTS
CNS: *Headache, dizziness,* paresthesia, depression, anxiety, somnolence, insomnia, fever, **seizures in renal disease**
CV: **Dysrhythmias,** QT prolongation (impaired renal functioning)
EENT: Taste change, tinnitus, orbital edema
GI: *Constipation,* nausea, vomiting, anorexia, cramps, abnormal liver enzymes, diarrhea
HEMA: **Thrombocytopenia, aplastic anemia**
INTEG: Rash, **toxic epidermal necrolysis, Stevens-Johnson syndrome**
MS: Myalgia, arthralgia
RESP: **Pneumonia**

Pharmacokinetics
Absorption	50% absorbed (PO)
Distribution	Plasma, protein binding (15%-20%)
Metabolism	Liver (30% active metabolizing)
Excretion	Kidneys (70%)
Half-life	2½-3½ hr

Pharmacodynamics
	PO	IV
Onset	30-60 min	Immediate
Peak	1-3 hr	½-3 hr
Duration	6-12 hr	8-15 hr

INTERACTIONS
Individual drugs
Cefditoren, cefpodoxime, itraconazole, ketoconazole: decreased absorption of each specific product

---

Adverse effects: *italics* = common; **bold** = life-threatening

Atazanivir, delavirdine: decreased effects of each specific product

Drug classifications
Antacids: decreased absorption of famotidine

NURSING CONSIDERATIONS
Assessment
• **Assess patient with ulcers or suspected ulcers:** epigastric, abdominal pain, hematemesis, occult blood in stools, blood in gastric aspirate before treatment; throughout treatment, monitor gastric pH (maintain at pH 5)
• Monitor I&O ratio, BUN, creatinine, CBC with differential monthly

Patient/family education
• Caution patient to avoid driving, other hazardous activities until stabilized on this medication; dizziness may occur
• Advise patient to avoid black pepper, caffeine, alcohol, harsh spices, extremes in temperature of food; tell patient to avoid OTC preparations: aspirin, cough/cold preparations; condition may worsen
• Advise patient to avoid taking OTC and prescription preparations of this product concurrently
• Tell patient that smoking decreases the effectiveness of the product; that smoking cessation should be considered
• Instruct patient that product must be continued for prescribed time to be effective and taken exactly as prescribed; doses are not to be doubled; take missed dose when remembered up to 1 hr before next dose
• Tell patient to report diarrhea, black tarry stools, sore throat, rash, dizziness, confusion, or delirium to prescriber immediately

Evaluation
Positive therapeutic outcome
• Decreased pain in abdomen
• Healing of ulcers

---

fat emulsions (Rx)
(fat ee-mul'shuns)
Intralipid 10%, Intralipid 20%, Liposyn II 10%, Liposyn II 20%, Liposyn III 10%, Liposyn III 20%, Soyacal 20%
Func. class.: Caloric
Chem. class.: Fatty acid, long chain
Pregnancy category C

ACTION: Needed for energy, heat production; consists of neutral triglycerides, primarily unsaturated fatty acids

Therapeutic outcome: Increased available calories and fatty acids

USES: Increase calorie intake, prevent fatty acid deficiency

CONTRAINDICATIONS:
Hypersensitivity to this product, eggs, soybeans, or legumes; hyperlipemia; lipid necrosis; acute pancreatitis accompanied by hyperlipemia; hyperbilirubinemia of the newborn; renal insufficiency; hepatic damage

Precautions: Pregnancy **C**, term newborns, severe liver disease, diabetes mellitus, thrombocytopenia, gastric ulcers, sepsis

> **BLACK BOX WARNING:** Preterm infants

DOSAGE AND ROUTES
Deficiency
Adult and child: IV 8%-10% of required calorie intake (intralipid)

Adjunct to TPN
Adult: IV 1 ml/min over 15-30 min (10%) or 0.5 ml/min over 15-30 min (20%); may increase to 500 ml over 4-8 hr if no adverse reactions occur; max 2.5 g/kg
Child: IV 0.1 ml/min over 10-15 min (10%) or 0.05 ml/ min over 10-15 min (20%); may increase to 1 g/kg over 4 hr if no adverse reactions occur; max 4 g/kg

Prevention of deficiency
Adult: IV 500 ml 2 ×/wk (10%), given 1 ml/min for 30 min, max 500 ml over 6 hr
Child: IV 5-10 ml/kg/day (10%), given 0.1 ml/min for 30 min, max 100 ml/hr

Available forms: Inj 10% (50, 100, 200, 250, 500 ml), 20% (50, 100, 200, 250, 500 ml)

Implementation
Intermittent IV infusion route
• Administer using infusion pump at prescribed rate; do not use in-line filter sized for lipid emulsion; clogging will occur
• Do not use mixed sol if separated or oily looking; discard unused sol
• Change **IV** tubing at each inf: infection may occur with old tubing
• Give by intermittent inf at a rate of 10% sol (1 ml/min); 20% sol (0.5 ml/min) initially for 15-30 min; may be increased to 10% sol (120 ml/hr) or 20% sol (62.5 ml/hr) if no adverse reactions occur; max 500 ml during the first day; children should be given 10% (0.1 mg/ ml) or 20% (0.05 ml/min) initially for 15-30 min,

---

may be increased 1 g/kg/4 hr, max 10% (100 ml/hr) or 20% (50 ml/hr)

ADVERSE EFFECTS
CNS: Dizziness, headache, drowsiness, **focal seizures**
CV: Shock
GI: Nausea, vomiting, **hepatomegaly**
HEMA: Hyperlipemia, hypercoagulation, thrombocytopenia, leukopenia, leukocytosis
RESP: Dyspnea, **fat in lung tissue**

Pharmacokinetics

Absorption	Completely absorbed
Distribution	Intravascular space
Metabolism	Conversion to triglycerides, then to free fatty acids
Excretion	Unknown
Half-life	Unknown

Pharmacodynamics
Unknown

NURSING CONSIDERATIONS
Assessment
• Monitor triglycerides, free fatty acid levels, platelet counts daily to prevent fat overload, thrombocytopenia
• Monitor liver function tests: AST, ALT, Hct, Hgb; notify prescriber if abnormal
• Assess nutritional status: calorie count by dietitian; monitor weight daily

Patient/family education
• Teach patient reason for use of lipids and expected results

Evaluation
Positive therapeutic outcome
• Increased weight
• Fatty acids at adequate levels

---

febuxostat (Rx)
(feb-ux'oh-stat)
Uloric
Func. class.: Antigout drug, antihyperuricemic
Chem. class.: Xanthine oxidase inhibitor
Pregnancy category C

ACTION: Inhibits the enzyme xanthine oxidase, reducing uric acid synthesis; more selective for xanthine oxidase than allopurinol

Therapeutic outcome: Decreased signs/symptoms of gout, hyperuricemia

USES: Chronic gout, hyperuricemia

CONTRAINDICATIONS:
Hypersensitivity

Precautions: Pregnancy **C**, breastfeeding, children, renal/hepatic/cardiac/neoplastic disease, stroke, MI, organ transplant, Lesch-Nyhan syndrome

DOSAGE AND ROUTES
Adult: PO 40 mg daily, may increase to 80 mg daily if uric acid levels are >6 mg/dl after 2 wk of therapy

Available forms: Tabs 40, 80 mg

Implementation
PO route
• Give without regard to meals or antacid; may crush and add to foods or fluids
• Give a few days before antineoplastic therapy

ADVERSE EFFECTS
CNS: Weakness, flushing
CV: MI, atrial fibrillation, atrial flutter, AV block, bradycardia, hyper/hypotension, palpitations, **sinus tachycardia, stroke,** angina
EENT: Retinopathy, cataracts, epistaxis
GI: *Nausea, vomiting, anorexia,* constipation, diarrhea, dyspepsia, hematemesis, **hepatitis,** hepatomegaly, weight gain/loss, cholecystitis, cholelithiasis, melena
GU: Renal failure, urinary urgency/frequency/incontinence, nephrolithiasis, hematuria
HEMA: Thrombocytopenia, anemia, pancytopenia, leukopenia, bone marrow suppression
INTEG: Rash
MISC: Arthralgia, gout flare

Pharmacokinetics

Absorption	Unknown
Distribution	Protein binding 99.2%
Metabolism	Unknown
Excretion	Feces, urine
Half-life	5-8 hr

Pharmacodynamics

Onset	Unknown
Peak	1-1.5 hr
Duration	Unknown

INTERACTIONS
Individual drugs
AzaTHIOprine: increased toxicity
Rasburicase: increased xanthine nephropathy, calculi

Adverse effects: *italics* = common; **bold** = life-threatening

Mercaptopurine, theophylline: increased myelo-suppression

Drug classifications

Antineoplastics: increased xanthine nephropathy, calculi

NURSING CONSIDERATIONS
Assessment
- **Hyperuricemia:** Monitor uric acid levels q2wk; uric acid levels should be 6 mg/dl or less
- Hepatic studies prior to use, then at 2, 4 mo, and then periodically; assess for fatigue, anorexia, right upper abdominal discomfort, dark urine, jaundice
- Monitor CBC, AST, BUN, creatinine before starting treatment, periodically, flares may occur during first 6 wk of treatment
- **Renal disease:** Monitor I&O ratio; increase fluids to 2 L/day to prevent stone formation and toxicity
- Assess for rash, hypersensitivity reactions; discontinue
- **Assess for gout:** joint pain, swelling; may use with NSAIDs for acute gouty attacks and gout flare (first 6 wk)

Patient/family education
- Inform patient that tabs may be crushed
- Teach patient to take as prescribed; if dose is missed, take as soon as remembered; do not double dose
- Teach patient to increase fluid intake to 2 L/day unless contraindicated
- Advise patient to avoid alcohol, caffeine; will increase uric acid levels
- Advise patient to report cardiovascular events to prescriber, immediately
- **Gout:** teach patient that flares may occur during first 6 wk of treatment

Evaluation
Positive therapeutic outcome
- Decreased pain in joints, decreased stone formation in kidneys, decreased uric acid levels

---

felodipine (Rx)
(feh-loh′dih-peen)
Plendil ✦, **Renedil** ✦
Func. class.: Calcium-channel blocker, antihypertensive, antianginal
Chem. class.: Dihydropyridine
Pregnancy category C

Do not confuse:
Plendil/Pindolol/Pletal/PriLOSEC/Prinival/Isordil

ACTION: Inhibits calcium ion influx across cell membrane, resulting in inhibition of excitation/contraction of vascular smooth muscle

Therapeutic outcome: Decreased B/P in hypertension

USES: Essential hypertension, alone or with other antihypertensives

CONTRAINDICATIONS:
Hypersensitivity to this product or dihydropyridines, sick sinus syndrome, 2nd- or 3rd-degree heart block, hypotension <90 mm Hg systolic

Precautions: Pregnancy **C**, breastfeeding, children, geriatric, CHF, hepatic injury, renal disease, coronary artery disease

DOSAGE AND ROUTES
Adult: PO 5 mg/day initially, usual range 2.5-10 mg/day; max 10 mg/day; do not adjust dosage at intervals of <2 wk
Geriatric: PO 2.5 mg/day

Hepatic dose
Adult: PO 2.5-5 mg/day, max 10 mg/day

Available forms: Ext rel tabs 2.5, 5, 10 mg

Implementation
PO route
- Do not break, crush, or chew ext rel tabs
- Give once a day with food for GI symptoms

ADVERSE EFFECTS
CNS: *Headache,* fatigue, drowsiness, dizziness, anxiety, depression, nervousness, insomnia, light-headedness, paresthesia, tinnitus, psychosis, somnolence
CV: **Dysrhythmias,** *edema,* **CHF,** hypotension, palpitations, **MI, pulmonary edema,** tachycardia, syncope, AV block, angina
GI: Nausea, vomiting, diarrhea, **gastric upset,** constipation, increased liver function studies, dry mouth
GU: Nocturia, polyuria
HEMA: Anemia
INTEG: Rash, pruritus, peripheral edema
MISC: Flushing, sexual difficulties, cough, nasal congestion, shortness of breath, wheezing, epistaxis, respiratory infection, chest pain, **Angioedema,** gingival hyperplasia

---

Pharmacokinetics

Absorption	Well absorbed
Distribution	Unknown; protein binding >99%
Metabolism	Liver, extensively
Excretion	Kidneys
Half-life	11-16 hr

Pharmacodynamics

Onset	2-3 hr
Peak	2½-5 hr
Duration	<24 hr

INTERACTIONS

Individual drugs

Alcohol, carBAMazepine, cimetidine, clarithromycin, conivaptan, cycloSPORINE, dalfopristin, delavirdine, diltiazem, erythromycin, itraconazole, ketoconazole, miconazole, phenytoin, propanolol, quiNIDine, quinupristin, zileuton: increased hypotension

Digoxin, disopyramide, phenytoin: increased bradycardia, increased CHF

Drug classifications

β-Adrenergic blockers: increased bradycardia, CHF

Nitrates: increased hypotension

NSAIDs: decreased antihypertensive effects

Drug/herb

Ginkgo, ginseng, hawthorn: increased antihypertensive effect

Ephedra, St. John's wort: decreased antihypertensive effect

Drug/food

Grapefruit juice: increased felodipine level

NURSING CONSIDERATIONS

Assessment

• **CHF:** Assess fluid volume status: I&O ratio and record; weight; skin turgor; adequacy of pulses; moist mucous membranes; bilateral lung sounds; peripheral pitting edema; dehydration symptoms of decreasing output, thirst, hypotension, dry mouth, and mucous membranes should be reported; for CHF: weight gain, crackles, dyspnea, edema, jugular venous distention

• Monitor ALT, AST, bilirubin daily if these are elevated

• Monitor cardiac status: B/P, pulse, respiration, ECG, periodically

• **Assess for anginal pain:** duration; intensity; ameliorating, aggravating factors

Patient/family education

• Caution patient to avoid hazardous activities until stabilized on product and dizziness is no longer a problem

• Instruct patient to limit caffeine consumption; to avoid alcohol and OTC products unless directed by prescriber

• Urge patient to comply in all areas of medical regimen: diet, exercise, stress reduction, product therapy; to notify prescriber of irregular heartbeat, shortness of breath, swelling of feet and hands, pronounced dizziness, constipation, nausea, hypotension

• Advise patient to use protective clothing, sunscreen to prevent photosensitivity

• Teach patient to change positions slowly to prevent orthostatic hypotension

• Advise patient to obtain correct pulse; to contact prescriber if pulse is <50 bpm

• Teach patient to use as directed even if feeling better; may be taken with other CV products (nitrates, β-blockers); that capsules may appear in stools but are insignificant

• Teach patient to practice good oral hygiene to prevent gingival hyperplasia

• Advise patient not to stop medication abruptly

• Advise patient to avoid grapefruit juice

Evaluation

Positive therapeutic outcome

• Decreased B/P

• Decreased anginal attacks

• Increase in activity tolerance

fenofibrate (Rx)

(fen-oh-fee′brate)

Antara, Apo-Fero-Micro ✦, Fenoglide, Lipidil Micro ✦, Lipidil Supracap ✦, Lipofem, Lofibra, Tricor, Triglide

Func. class.: Antilipemic

Chem. class.: Fibric acid derivative

Pregnancy category C

ACTION: Increases lipolysis and elimination of triglyceride-rich particles from plasma by activating lipoprotein lipase, resulting in triglyceride change in size and composition of LDL, leading to rapid breakdown of LDL; mobilizes triglycerides from tissue; increases excretion of neutral sterols

Therapeutic outcome: Decreasing cholesterol levels and low-density lipoproteins, decreased pruritus

USES: Hypercholesterolemia, patients with types IV, V hyperlipidemia who do not respond to other treatment and who are at risk for pancreatitis; Fredrickson type IV, V hypertriglyceridemia

CONTRAINDICATIONS:
Hypersensitivity, severe renal/hepatic disease, primary biliary cirrhosis, preexisting gallbladder disease, breastfeeding

Precautions: Pregnancy **C**, geriatric, peptic ulcer, pancreatitis, renal/hepatic disease, diabetes mellitus

DOSAGE AND ROUTES
Hypertriglyceridemia
Adult: PO (Antara) 43-130 mg/day; (Lofibra) 67-200 mg/day; (Tricor) 48-145 mg/day; (Triglide) 50-160 mg/day

Primary hypercholesterolemia/ mixed hyperlipidemia
Adult: PO (Antara) 130 mg/day; (Lofibra) 200 mg/day; (Tricor) 145 mg/day; (Triglide) 160 mg/day

Renal dose (geriatric)
Adult: PO (Tricor) CCr 30-80 ml/min 48 mg/day; CCr <30 ml/min contraindicated
Adult: PO (Triglide, Lipofem) CCr 11-49 ml/min 50 mg/day; (Antara) 43 mg/day; (Fenoglide) 40 mg/day; (Lofibra) 67 mg/day; (Antara, Lipofem, Lofibra, Triglide) CCr <30 ml/min, contraindicated

Available forms: Tabs (Fenoglide) 40, 120 mg; (Lofibra) 54, 160 mg; (Tricor) 48, 145 mg; (Triglide) 50, 160 mg; cap (Lipofen) 50, 150 mg; micronized cap (Antara) 43, 130 mg; (Lofibra micronized) 67, 134, 200 mg

Implementation
• Do not break, crush, or chew tabs
• Give with evening meal; if dose is increased, give with breakfast and evening meal (Lipofen, Lofibra); Triglide, Antara without regard to food; may increase q4-8wk
• Brands are not interchangeable; therapy should be discontinued if there is not adequate response after 2 mo
• Store in cool environment in tight, light-resistant container

ADVERSE EFFECTS
CNS: Fatigue, weakness, drowsiness, dizziness, insomnia, depression, vertigo
CV: Angina, hypertension, hypotension
GI: Nausea, vomiting, dyspepsia, increased liver enzymes, flatulence, hepatomegaly, gastritis, **pancreatitis, cholelithiasis**
GU: Dysuria, urinary frequency
HEMA: Anemia, **leukopenia, thrombosis, pulmonary embolism**
INTEG: *Rash,* urticaria, pruritus, photosensitivity
MISC: Polyphagia, weight gain, infection, flulike syndrome
MS: Myalgias, arthralgias, **myopathy, rhabdomyolysis**
RESP: Pharyngitis, bronchitis, cough

Pharmacokinetics
Absorption	Unknown
Distribution	Protein binding 99%
Metabolism	Liver
Excretion	Urine 60%, feces 25%
Half-life	20 hr

Pharmacodynamics
Onset	Unknown
Peak	6-8 hr
Duration	Unknown

INTERACTIONS
Individual drugs
CycloSPORINE: increased nephrotoxicity

Drug classifications
Anticoagulants (oral): increased effect of anticoagulants
Antidiabetics: increased effect of antidiabetics
Bile acid sequestrants: decreased absorption
HMG-CoA reductase inhibitors: do not use together, rhabdomyolysis may occur

Drug/herb
Red yeast rice: increased effects

Drug/food
Increased absorption

Drug/lab test
Increase: ALT, AST, BUN, CK, creatinine
Decrease: WBC, uric acid, Hgb

NURSING CONSIDERATIONS
Assessment
• **Hypercholesterolemia:** Monitor lipid levels (triglycerides, LDL, HDL, total cholesterol), fat content
• Liver function tests, baseline and periodically during treatment; CPK if muscle pain occurs, CBC, Hct, Hgh, pro-time with anticoagulant therapy

---

• **Assess for pancreatitis, cholelithiasis, renal failure, rhabdomyolysis** (when combined with HMG-CoA reductase inhibitors), myositis; product should be discontinued
• Assess nutrition: fat, protein, carbohydrates, nutritional analysis should be completed by dietitian

Patient/family education
• Inform patient that compliance is needed
• Instruct patient not to consume chipped or broken tabs (Triglide)
• Teach patient that risk factors—high-fat diet, smoking, alcohol consumption, absence of exercise—should be decreased
• Caution patient to notify prescriber if pregnancy is planned or suspected
• Teach patient to notify prescriber if the GI symptoms of diarrhea, abdominal or epigastric pain, nausea, or vomiting occur
• Instruct patient to report GU symptoms: dysuria, proteinuria, oliguria, decreased libido, impotence
• Advise patient to notify prescriber of muscle pain, weakness, fever, fatigue, epigastric pain

Evaluation
Positive therapeutic outcome
• Decrease in cholesterol to desired level after 8 wk

⚠ HIGH ALERT

fentaNYL (Rx)
(fen′ta-nill)
ABSTRAL, Actiq, Fentora, Onsolis, RAN-Fentanyl ✦
fentaNYL transdermal (Rx)
Duragesic
Func. class.: Opioid analgesic
Chem. class.: Synthetic phenylpiperidine derivative
fentaNYL nasal spray (Rx)
Lazanda
fentaNYL SL spray (Rx)
Subsys
Pregnancy category C
Controlled substance schedule II

Do not confuse:
fentaNYL/Sufenta

ACTION: Inhibits ascending pain pathways in CNS, increases pain threshold, alters pain perception by binding to opiate receptors

Therapeutic outcome: Relief of pain, supplement to anesthesia

USES: Controls moderate to severe pain; preoperatively, postoperatively; adjunct to general anesthetic, adjunct to regional anesthesia; **FentaNYL:** for anesthesia as premedication, conscious sedation; **Actiq:** for breakthrough cancer pain

CONTRAINDICATIONS:
Hypersensitivity to opiates, myasthenia gravis

> **BLACK BOX WARNING:** headache, migraine (Actiq), Astral, Fentora, Lazanda, Onsolis, emergency dept use (Abstral, Lazanda), outpatient surgeries (Duragesic TD), opioid-naive patients, respiratory disorders, depression

Precautions: Pregnancy C, breastfeeding, geriatric, increased ICP, seizure disorders, cardiac dysrhythmias, severe respiratory disorders

> **BLACK BOX WARNING:** Children, accidental exposure, ambient temperature increase, fever, skin abrasion (TD patch), substance abuse, surgery, requires an experienced clinician

DOSAGE AND ROUTES
FentaNYL

Anesthetic
Adult: IV 50-100 mcg/kg over 1-2 min, max 150 mcg/kg

Anesthesia supplement
Adult and child >12 yr: IM/IV 2-20 mcg/kg IV INF 0.025-0.25 mcg/kg/min

Induction and maintenance
Child 2-12 yr: IV 2-3 mcg/kg

Preoperatively
Adult and child >12 yr: IM/IV 50-100 mcg q30-60min before surgery

Postoperatively
Adult and child >12 yr: IM/IV 0.05-0.1 mg q1-2hr prn

Moderate/severe pain
Adult: IV/IM 50-100 mcg q1-2hr

Actiq
Adult: Transmucosal 200 mcg, redose if needed 15 min after completion of 1st dose, max 2 doses during titration period, max 4 doses/day

---

Adverse effects: *italics* = common; **bold** = life-threatening

Fentora

Adult: BUCCAL/SL 100 mcg placed above rear molar between upper cheek and gum, a second 100 mcg dose, if needed, may be started 30 min after first dose

Onsolis

Adult: transmucosal 200 mcg, titrate, max 1200 mcg/dose or 4 doses/day

ABSTRAL

Adult: SL 100 mcg, another dose may be taken 30 min after first, max 2 doses per episode of breakthrough pain, ≥2 hr must elapse before treating again, titrate stepwise over consecutive episodes

FentaNYL transdermal

Adult: 25 mcg/hr; may increase until pain relief occurs; apply patch to flat surface on upper torso and wear for 72 hr; apply new patch to different site for continued relief

FentaNYL nasal spray

Adult: 100 mcg (1 spray in 1 nostril), may re-treat after ≥2 hr, titrate upward to adequate analgesia, treat a max of 4 episodes q day

FentaNYL SL spray

Adult: SL 100 mcg sprayed under the tongue; titrate stepwise carefully

Available forms: Inj 0.05 mg/ml; lozenges 100, 200, 300, 400, 600, 800, 1200, 1600 mcg; lozenges on a stick 200, 400, 600, 800, 1200, 1600 mcg; buccal tab 100, 200, 400, 600, 800 mcg; oral dissolving film (Onsolis) 200, 400, 600, 800 mcg; transdermal patch 12, 25, 50, 75, 100 mcg/hr; SL tab (ABSTRAL) 100, 200, 300, 400, 600, 800 mcg; SL spray: 100, 200, 400, 600, 1200, 1600 mcg/spray

Implementation

• Store in light-resistant area at room temperature

Transmucosal route

• Remove foil just before administration; instruct patient to place between cheek and lower gum, moving it back and forth and sucking, not chewing (Actiq); place above rear molar (Fentora); place film on the inside of the cheek (Onsolis); all products not used or partially used should be flushed down the toilet; this product may be used SL

Transdermal route

• Apply patch to chest on a flat area with skin intact; for skin preparation, use clear water with no soap; clip hair, skin should be dry before applying patch; apply immediately after removing from package and press firmly in place with palm of hand; flush old patch down toilet immediately upon removal

Use pain dosing

• Dosage is titrated based on patient's report of pain; dosage is determined by calculating the previous 24-hr requirement and converting to equianalgesic morphine dose

• To convert to another opioid analgesic, remove transdermal patch and begin treatment with half the equal pain-controlling dose of the new analgesic in 12-18 hr

SL spray

• Open blister package with scissors immediately prior to use; spray contents under tongue; dispose of unit by placing it into disposable bags provided; seal bag, discard into trash container out of reach of children.

IV route

• Give by inj (IM, **IV**), only with resuscitative equipment available; give slowly to prevent rigidity

• Give **IV** undiluted by anesthesiologist or diluted with 5 ml or more sterile water or 0.9% NaCl given through Y-tube or 3-way stopcock given at 0.1 mg or less/1.2 min

• Muscular rigidity may occur with rapid IV administration

Syringe compatibilities: Alprostadil, atracurium, atropine, bupivacaine/ketamine, butorphanol, chlorproMAZINE, cimetidine, cloNIDine/lidocaine, dimenhyDRINATE, diphenhydrAMINE, droperidol, heparin, HYDROmorphone, hydrOXYzine, lidocaine, meperidine, metoclopramide, midazolam, morphine, pentazocine, perphenazine, prochlorperazine, promazine, promethazine, ranitidine, scopolamine

Syringe incompatibilities: PENTobarbital

Y-site compatibilities: Abciximab, acyclovir, alfentanil, alprostadil, amikacin, aminocaproic acid, aminophylline, amiodarone, amphotericin B cholesteryl, amphotericin B lipid complex, amphotericin B liposome, anidulafungin, argatroban, ascorbic acid injection, atenolol, atracurium, atropine, azaTHIOprine, aztreonam, benztropine, bivalirudin, bleomycin, bumetanide, buprenorphine, butorphanol, calcium chloride/gluconate, CARBOplatin, caspofungin, cefamandole, ceFAZolin, cefmetazole, cefonicid, cefoperazone, cefotaxime, cefoTEtan, cefOXitin, cefTAZidime, ceftizoxime, ceftobiprole, cefTRIAXone, cefuroxime, cephalothin, chloramphenicol, chlorproMAZINE, cimetidine, cisatracurium, CISplatin, clindamycin, cloNIDine, cyanocobalamin, cyclophosphamide, cycloSPORINE, cytarabine, DACTINomycin, DAPTOmycin, dexamethasone, dexmedetomidine, digoxin, diltiazem, diphenhydrAMINE, DOBUTamine, DOCEtaxel, DOPamine, doripenem, doxacurium, doxorubicin, doxycycline, enalaprilat, ePHEDrine, EPINEPHrine, epirubicin, epoetin alfa, eptifibatide, erythromycin, esmolol, etomidate, etoposide, famotidine, fenoldopam, fluconazole, fludarabine, fluorouracil, folic acid, furosemide, ganciclovir, gatifloxacin, gemcitabine, gentamicin, glycopyrrolate, granisetron, heparin, hydrocortisone, HYDROmorphone, hydrOXYzine, IDArubicin, ifosfamide, imipenem-cilastatin, inamrinone, insulin (regular), irinotecan, isoproterenol, ketorolac, labetalol, lansoprazole, levofloxacin, lidocaine, linezolid, LORazepam, LR, magnesium sulfate, mannitol, mechlorethamine, meperidine, metaraminol, methicillin, methotrexate, methotrimeprazine, methoxamine, methyldopa, methylPREDNISolone, metoclopramide, metoprolol, metroNIDAZOLE, mezlocillin, miconazole, midazolam, milrinone, minocycline, mitoXANtrone, mivacurium, morphine, moxalactam, multiple vitamins injection, mycophenolate, nafcillin, nalbuphine, naloxone, nesiritide, netilmicin, niCARdipine, nitroglycerin, nitroprusside, norepinephrine, octreotide, ondansetron, oxacillin, oxaliplatin, oxytocin, PACLitaxel, palonosetron, pamidronate, pancuronium, papaverine, PEMEtrexed, penicillin G potassium/sodium, pentamidine, pentazocine, PENTobarbital, PHENobarbital, phenylephrine, phytonadione, piperacillin, piperacillin-tazobactam, polymyxin B, potassium chloride, procainamide, prochlorperazine, promethazine, propofol, propranolol, protamine, pyridoxine, quiNIDine, quinupristin-dalfopristin, ranitidine, remifentanil, Ringer's, ritodrine, riTUXimab, rocuronium, sargramostim, scopolamine, sodium acetate/bicarbonate, succinylcholine, SUFentanil, tacrolimus, teniposide, theophylline, thiamine, thiopental, thiotepa, ticarcillin, ticarcillin-clavulanate, tigecycline, tirofiban, TNA, tobramycin, tolazoline, TPN, trastuzumab, trimetaphan, urokinase, vancomycin, vasopressin, vecuronium, verapamil, vinCRIStine, vinorelbine, vitamin B complex/C, voriconazole, zoledronic acid

Additive compatibilities: Bupivacaine, caffeine citrate, cloNIDine, droperidol, EPINEPHrine, ketamine, lidocaine, ziconotide

Additive incompatibilities: Methohexital, PENTobarbital, thiopental

Solution compatibilities: D$_5$W, 0.9% NaCl

ADVERSE EFFECTS
CNS: Dizziness, delirium, euphoria, sedation
CV: **Bradycardia, cardiac arrest,** hypo/hypertension
EENT: Blurred vision, miosis
GI: Nausea, vomiting, constipation
GU: Urinary retention
INTEG: Rash, diaphoresis
MS: Muscle rigidity
RESP: **Respiratory depression, arrest, laryngospasm**

Pharmacokinetics
Absorption	Well absorbed (IM), completely absorbed (**IV**)
Distribution	Unknown, crosses placenta
Metabolism	Extensively, liver; 80% bound to plasma proteins
Excretion	Kidneys, up to 25% unchanged; breast milk
Half-life	IV 2-4 hr; transdermal 13-22 hr; transmucosal 7 hr; buccal 4-12 hr

Pharmacodynamics
	IM	IV	TD
Onset	7-8 min	Rapid	6 hr
Peak	30 min	3-5 min	12-24 hr
Duration	1-2 hr	½-1 hr	72 hr

INTERACTIONS
Individual drugs
Alcohol: increased respiratory depression, hypotension, increased sedation

> **BLACK BOX WARNING:** Cimetidine, conivaptan, cycloSPORINE, fluconazole, itraconazole, ketoconazole, nefazodone, ranolazine, zafirlukast, zileuton: increased fentaNYL effect, fatal respiratory depression

Diazepam: increased CV depression
Droperidol: increased hypotension

Drug classifications
Antipsychotics, opioids, skeletal muscle relaxants: effects increased, protease inhibitors
CNS depressants, sedative/hypnotics: increased respiratory depression, hypotension
CYP3A4 inducers (carBAMazepine, PHENobarbital, phenytoin, rifampin): decreased fentaNYL effect

Drug/herb

St. John's wort, valerian: increased fentaNYL action

Echinacea: decreased effect of fentaNYL

Drug/lab test

Increased: amylase, lipase

NURSING CONSIDERATIONS

Assessment

• Monitor VS after parenteral route (B/P, pulse, respiration); note muscle rigidity; take drug history before administering product; check renal/liver function tests; assess for respiratory dysfunction: respiratory depression, character, rate, rhythm; notify prescriber if respirations are <10/min

• Monitor CNS changes: dizziness, drowsiness, hallucinations, euphoria, LOC, pupil reaction

• Monitor allergic reactions: rash, urticaria; product should be discontinued

• **Assess for pain:** intensity, location, duration, type, before and 15 min after IM route or 3-5 min after **IV** route

> **BLACK BOX WARNING: Headache, migraine:** Abstral, Actiq, Fentora, Lazanda, Onsolis are not to be used for this condition; Abstral, Lazanda is not to be used in the ED; Duragesic TD is not to be used for outpatient surgery patients

> **BLACK BOX WARNING: Apnea, respiratory arrest in opioid-naive patients:** Do not use Abstral, Actiq, Duragesic, Fentora, Lazanda, Onsolis, opioid tolerant are those using ≥60 ml/day oral morphine, ≥30 mg/day oxyCODONE PO, 8 mg/day HYDROmorphone, 25 mcg tid fentaNYL/hr

Patient/family education

• Discuss the dangers of children or pets getting the product

• Advise patient to report any symptoms of CNS changes, allergic reactions

• Instruct patient to avoid CNS depressants: alcohol, sedative-hypnotics for at least 24 hr after taking this product

• Teach patient that dizziness, drowsiness, confusion are common, and to avoid getting up without assistance

• Discuss in detail with patient all aspects of the product

• Teach patient CNS changes: physical dependence; not to use with alcohol, other CNS depressants

Transdermal route

> **BLACK BOX WARNING: Ambient temperature increase:** Discuss with patient that excessive heat may increase absorption; excessive perspiration may alter adhesiveness; do not use with heating pads, electric blankets, heat/tanning lamps, saunas, hot tubs, heated waterbeds, sunbathing

• Discuss with patient that hair may need to be clipped before applying

• Teach patient how to dispose of patch: place sticky sides together and flush in toilet

• May add first aid tape around the edges if there is a problem with adhesion

Evaluation

Positive therapeutic outcome

• Maintenance of anesthesia

• Decreased breakthrough cancer pain

• General pain relief

TREATMENT OF OVERDOSE:

Naloxone 0.2-0.8 **IV**, O_2, **IV** fluids, vasopressors

---

ferrous fumarate (Rx)

Ferretts, Ferrimin, Ferro-Sequels, Hemocyte, Palafer ✦, Walgreens Finest Iron

ferrous gluconate (Rx)

Apo-Ferrous Gluconate ✦, Ferate, Walgreens Gold Seal Ferrous Gluconate

ferrous sulfate (Rx)   ✳

Apo-Ferrous Sulfate ✦, Equaline Ferrous Sulfate, Leader Ferrous Sulfate, Slow Release Iron, Walgreens Gold Seal Ferrous Sulfate

ferrous sulfate, dried (Rx)

Slow Fe

carbonyl iron (OTC)

(kar'boh-nil)

ICAR Pediatric, Iron Chews

iron polysaccharide (OTC)

iFerex, Niferex, Nu-Iron

Func. class.: Hematinic

Chem. class.: Iron preparation

Pregnancy category B, C

ACTION: Replaces iron stores needed for red blood cell development, energy and O_2 transport, utilization; fumarate contains 33% elemental iron; gluconate, 12%; sulfate, 20%; iron, 30%; ferrous sulfate exsiccated

---

Therapeutic outcome: Prevention and correction of iron deficiency

USES: Iron deficiency anemia, prophylaxis for iron deficiency in pregnancy, nutritional supplementation

CONTRAINDICATIONS:
Sideroblastic anemia, thalassemia, hemosiderosis/hemochromatosis

Precautions: Pregnancy **B** (ferric gluconate complex), **C** (iron dextran, oral products); anemia (long-term), peptic ulcer disease, hemolytic anemia, cirrhosis, ulcerative colitis/regional enteritis, sulfite sensitivity

> **BLACK BOX WARNING:** Accidental exposure

DOSAGE AND ROUTES
Fumarate
Adult: PO 50-100 mg tid
Child: PO 3 mg/kg/day (elemental iron) tid-qid
Infant: PO 10-25 mg/day (elemental iron) in 3-4 divided doses, max 15 mg/day

Gluconate
Adult: PO 60 mg bid-qid
Child 6-12 yr: PO 3 mg/kg/day divided

Sulfate
Adult: PO 0.750-1.5 g/day in divided doses tid
Child 6-12 yr: 600 mg/day in divided doses

Pregnancy
Adult: PO 300-600 mg/day in divided doses

Iron polysaccharide
Adult: 100-200 mg tid
Child: PO 4-6 mg/kg/day in 3 divided doses (severe iron deficiency)

Available forms: Fumarate: tabs 63, 195, 200, 324, 325 mg; chewable tabs 100 mg; controlled-release tabs 300 mg; oral susp 100 mg/5 ml, 45 mg/0.6 ml; **gluconate:** tabs 300, 320, 325 mg; caps 86, 325, 435 mg; film-coated tabs 300 mg; elix 300 mg/5 ml; **sulfate:** tabs 195, 300, 325 mg; enteric-coated tabs 325 mg; ext rel tabs, time-rel caps 525 mg; dried: tabs 200 mg; ext rel tabs 160 mg; ext rel caps 160 mg; **iron polysaccharide:** tabs 50 mg; caps 150 mg; sol 100 mg/5 ml

Implementation
PO route
• Swallow all tabs whole; do not break, crush, or chew
• Give between meals for best absorption; may give with juice; do not give with antacids or milk, delay at least 1 hr; if GI symptoms occur, give after meals even if absorption is decreased; eggs, milk products, chocolate, caffeine interfere with absorption; ferrous gluconate is less GI irritating than ferrous sulfate
• Give **liquid** preparations through plastic straw to avoid discoloration of tooth enamel; dilute thoroughly
• Store in tight, light-resistant container
• Give at least 1 hr before bedtime because corrosion may occur in stomach
• Give for <6 mo for anemia
• Store at room temperature; protect from moisture

ADVERSE EFFECTS
GI: *Nausea, constipation, epigastric pain, black and red tarry stools,* vomiting, diarrhea
INTEG: Temporarily discolored tooth enamel and eyes
SYST: Hypersensitivity reactions (Ferrlecit)

Pharmacokinetics
Absorption	Up to 30%
Distribution	Bound to transferrin, crosses placenta
Metabolism	Recycled
Excretion	Feces, urine, skin, breast milk
Half-life	Unknown

Pharmacodynamics
Unknown

INTERACTIONS
Individual drugs
Chloramphenicol, vit C: increased absorption of iron products
Cholestyramine, L-thyroxine, levodopa, methyldopa, penicillamine, tetracycline, vitamin E: decreased absorption of each product

Drug classifications
Antacids, H_2 antagonists, proton pump inhibitors: decreased absorption of iron preparations
Fluoroquinolones: decreased absorption of fluoroquinolone

Drug/food
Caffeine, dairy products, eggs: decreased absorption

Drug/lab test
False positive: occult blood

NURSING CONSIDERATIONS
Assessment
• Monitor blood studies: Hct, Hgb, reticulocytes, bilirubin before treatment, at least monthly; iron studies (Fe, TIBC, ferritin)
• **Assess for toxicity:** nausea, vomiting, diarrhea (green, then tarry stools,) hematemesis, pallor, cyanosis, shock, coma
• Assess bowel elimination; if constipation occurs, increase water, bulk, activity before laxatives are required
• **Assess nutrition:** amount of iron in diet (meat, dark green leafy vegetables, dried beans, dried fruits, eggs); provide referral to dietitian if indicated
• Identify cause of iron loss or anemia, including salicylates, sulfonamides, antimalarials, quiNIDine

Patient/family education
• Advise patient that iron will make stools black or dark green; that iron poisoning may occur if increased beyond recommended level
• Advise patient to keep out of reach of children, pets
• Caution patient not to substitute one iron salt for another; elemental iron content differs (e.g., 300 mg ferrous fumarate contains about 100 mg elemental iron, whereas 300 mg ferrous gluconate contains only about 30 mg elemental iron)
• Caution patient to avoid reclining position for 15-30 min after taking product to avoid esophageal corrosion; to follow diet high in iron
• Caution patient to avoid taking iron, dairy products, calcium supplements, vit C together; they compete for absorption

Evaluation
Positive therapeutic outcome
• Decreased fatigue, weakness
• Improvement in Hct, Hgb, reticulocytes

TREATMENT OF OVERDOSE:
Induce vomiting; give eggs, milk until lavage can be done

fesoterodine (Rx)
(fess'oh-ter-oh-deen)
Toviaz
Func. class.: Overactive bladder product
Chem. class.: Muscarinic receptor antagonist
Pregnancy category C

ACTION: Relaxes smooth muscles in urinary tract by inhibiting acetylcholine at postganglionic sites

Therapeutic outcome: Absence of urinary frequency, urgency, incontinence

USES: Overactive bladder (urinary frequency, urgency), urinary incontinence

CONTRAINDICATIONS:
GI obstruction, ileus, pyloric stenosis, urinary retention, gastric retention, hypersensitivity, closed-angle glaucoma

Precautions: Pregnancy **C**, breastfeeding, children, renal/hepatic disease, urinary tract obstruction, ambient temperature increase, autonomic neuropathy, constipation, contact lenses, hazardous activity, GERD, gastroparesis, myasthenia gravis, prostatic hypertrophy, toxic megacolon, ulcerative colitis, possible cross-sensitivity with tolterodine

DOSAGE AND ROUTES
Adult and geriatric: PO EXT REL 4 mg/day, may increase to 8 mg/day based on response, max 4 mg/day in those taking potent CYP3A4 inhibitors

Renal dose
Adult: PO EXT REL CCr <30 ml/min max 4 mg/day in severe renal impairment

Available forms: Ext rel tabs 4, 8 mg

Implementation
• Do not break, crush, or chew ext rel product
• Give without regard to meals
• Store at room temperature; protect from moisture

ADVERSE EFFECTS
CV: Chest pain, angina, **QT prolongation**
EENT: Xerophthalmia
GI: *Nausea, vomiting,* abdominal pain, constipation, dry mouth
GU: Dysuria, urinary retention
INTEG: Rash, angioedema
MISC: Peripheral edema, insomnia
MS: Back pain
RESP: Cough
SYST: Infection

Pharmacokinetics	
Absorption	Rapid
Distribution	Protein binding 50%
Metabolism	Unknown
Excretion	Urine, feces
Half-life	7 hr

Pharmacodynamics
Unknown

INTERACTIONS
Drug classifications
Anticholinergics, antimuscarinics: increased anticholinergic effect
CYP3A4 inhibitors (antiretroviral protease inhibitors, azole antifungals), macrolide anti-infectives: increased action of fesoterodine
Diuretics: increased urinary frequency

Drug/herb
Caffeine, green tea, guarana: decreased fesoterodine

Drug/food
Grapefruit juice: increased fesoterodine level
Cola, coffee, tea: decreased fesoterodine level

NURSING CONSIDERATIONS
Assessment
• **Assess urinary patterns:** distention, nocturia, frequency, urgency, incontinence
• **Assess for allergic reactions:** rash, angioedema; if this occurs, product should be discontinued

Patient/family education
• Advise patient not to drink liquids before bedtime
• Instruct the patient on the importance of bladder maintenance

Evaluation
Positive therapeutic outcome
• Absence of urinary frequency, urgency, incontinence

---

fexofenadine (Rx, OTC)
(fex-oh-fin′a-deen)
Allegra, Allegra ODT, GNP Allergy Relief, Premier Value Allergy Relief
Func. class.: Histamine antagonist, 2nd generation
Chem. class.: Piperidine, peripherally selective
Pregnancy category C

Do not confuse:
Allegra/Viagra

ACTION: Acts on blood vessels, GI, respiratory system by competing with histamine for H_1-receptor site; decreases allergic response by blocking pharmacologic effects of histamine; less sedation rate than with other antihistamines

Therapeutic outcome: Absence of allergy symptoms and rhinitis

USES: Rhinitis, allergy symptoms, chronic idiopathic urticaria

CONTRAINDICATIONS:
Breastfeeding, newborn or premature infants, hypersensitivity, severe hepatic disease

Precautions: Pregnancy **C,** children, geriatric, respiratory disease, closed-angle glaucoma, prostatic hypertrophy, bladder neck obstruction, asthma

DOSAGE AND ROUTES
Adult and child >12 yr: PO Rx only 60 mg bid or 180 mg/day; PO OTC only 60 mg bid or 180 mg/day (self-treatment of allergic rhinitis)
Child 6-11 yr: PO 30 mg bid; Orally disintegrating tab 30 mg bid dissolved on tongue

Renal dose
Adult and child ≥12 yr: PO CCr <80 ml/min 60 mg/day
Child 2-11 yr: PO CCr <80 ml/min 30 mg/day
Child <2 yr: PO CCr <80 ml/min 15 mg/day

Available forms: Caps 60 mg; tabs 30, 60, 180 mg; oral susp 6 mg/ml; orally disintegrating tab 30 mg

Implementation
• Give without regard to meals; caps/tabs should not be given with or right before grapefruit, orange, or apple juice
• **Orally disintegrating tab:** allow to dissolve, swallow
• **Oral susp:** shake well, use calibrated measuring device
• Store in tight, light-resistant container

ADVERSE EFFECTS
CNS: Headache, stimulation, drowsiness, sedation, fatigue, confusion, blurred vision, tinnitus, restlessness, tremors, paradoxical excitation in children or geriatric
CV: Hypotension, palpitations, bradycardia, tachycardia, **dysrhythmias (rare)**
GI: Nausea, diarrhea, abdominal pain, vomiting, constipation
GU: Frequency, dysuria, urinary retention, impotence
HEMA: Hemolytic anemia, **thrombocytopenia, leukopenia, agranulocytosis, pancytopenia**
INTEG: Rash, eczema, photosensitivity, urticaria
RESP: Thickening of bronchial secretions; dry nose, throat

F

Adverse effects: *italics* = common; **bold** = life-threatening

Absorption	Well absorbed
Distribution	Unknown
Metabolism	Liver
Excretion	Kidneys
Half-life	Unknown

Pharmacodynamics

Onset	1 hr
Peak	2-3 hr
Duration	12-24 hr

INTERACTIONS

Drug classifications
Aluminum, antacids, magnesium: decreased fexofenadine effect

Drug/food
Apple, orange, grapefruit juice: decreased absorption

Drug/lab test
False negative: skin allergy tests (discontinue antihistamine 3 days before testing)

NURSING CONSIDERATIONS

Assessment
• **Allergy:** assess for itchy, runny, watery eyes; congested nose; before and during treatment
• Assess respiratory status: rate, rhythm, increase in bronchial secretions, wheezing, chest tightness; provide fluids to 2 L/day to decrease secretion thickness
• Monitor I&O ratio: be alert for urinary retention, frequency, dysuria, especially geriatric; product should be discontinued if these occur

Patient/family education
• Teach all aspects of product uses; to notify prescriber if confusion, sedation, hypotension occur; to avoid driving or other hazardous activity if drowsiness occurs; to avoid alcohol or other CNS depressants that may potentiate effect
• Instruct patient to take 1 hr before or 2 hr after meals to facilitate absorption
• Instruct patient not to exceed recommended dose; dysrhythmias may occur
• Teach patient that hard candy, gum, frequent rinsing of mouth may be used for dryness

Evaluation
Positive therapeutic outcome
• Absence of running or congested nose, rashes

TREATMENT OF OVERDOSE:
Administer lavage, diazepam, vasopressors, **IV** phenytoin

---

fibrinogen, concentrate, human
Ria STAP
See Appendix A, Selected New Drugs

fidaxomicin (Rx)
(fye-dax-oh-mye'sin)
Dificid
Func. class.: Antiinfective-macrolide
Pregnancy category B

ACTION: Bactericidal against *Clostridium difficile;* is a fermentation product obtained from *Dactylosporangium aurantiacum;* inhibits RNA synthesis by inhibiting transcription of bacterial RNA polymerases; may act at the early stages of transcription

Therapeutic outcome: Resolution of *C. difficile* based on stool culture

USES: Pseudomembranous colitis, *C. difficile*-associated diarrhea

CONTRAINDICATIONS:
Hypersensitivity

Precautions: Pregnancy B, breastfeeding, children

DOSAGE AND ROUTES
Adult: **PO** 200 mg bid × 10 days 1000 mg

Available forms: Tab 200 mg

Implementation:
• Give without regard to food
• Store at room temperature

ADVERSE EFFECTS
GI: Nausea, vomiting, abdominal pain, **GI bleeding**
HEMA: **Anemia, neutropenia**
INTEG: Rash, pruritus
META: **Metabolic acidosis,** hyperglycemia

Pharmacokinetics

Absorption	Minimal
Distribution	GI tract
Metabolism	P-glucoprotein
Excretion	Feces 92%; parent drug
Half-life	12 hr

Pharmacodynamics

Onset	Unknown
Peak	1 hr
Duration	1-5 hr

INTERACTIONS
Individual drugs
CycloSPORINE: Increased fidaxomicin action

Drug/lab test
Increased: glucose, LFTs, alk phos
Decreased: sodium bicarbonate

NURSING CONSIDERATIONS
Assessment
⚠ **Pseudomembraneous colitis: Assess for diarrhea, abdominal pain, fever, fatigue, anorexia, possible anemia, elevated WBC and low serum albumin; this product may be used in place of vancomycin; monitor CBC with differential, and stool culture (*C. difficile*); not to be used for systemic infection; obtain C&S prior to use; monitor glucose (diabetic patients); monitor fluid, electrolyte depletion**

Patient/family education
• Advise patient to report GI bleeding, or severe abdominal pain
• Teach patient to report if pregnancy is planned or suspected or if breastfeeding
• Teach patient to take without regard to food

Evaluation
Positive therapeutic outcome
• Resolution of *C. difficile*

---

filgrastim (Rx)
(fill-gras′stim)
G-CSF, granulocyte colony stimulator, Neupogen
Func. class.: Biological modifier
Chem. class.: Granulocyte colony-stimulating factor
Pregnancy category C

ACTION: Stimulates proliferation and differentiation of neutrophils; a glycoprotein

Therapeutic outcome: Absence of infection

USES: To decrease infection in patients receiving antineoplastics that are myelosuppressive; to increase WBC in patients with product-induced neutropenia; bone marrow depression

Unlabeled uses: Neutropenia in HIV infection, aplastic anemia, ganciclovir-induced neutropenia, zidovudine-induced neutropenia

CONTRAINDICATIONS:
Hypersensitivity to proteins of *Escherichia coli*

Precautions: Pregnancy **C**, breastfeeding, children, cardiac conditions, myeloid malignancies, radiation therapy, sepsis, sickle cell disease, chemotherapy, respiratory disease

DOSAGE AND ROUTES
After myelosuppressive chemotherapy
Adult and child: IV/SUBCUT 5 mcg/kg/day in a single dose × 14 days; may increase by 5 mcg/kg in each chemotherapy cycle

After bone marrow transplantation
Adult: IV/SUBCUT 10 mcg/kg as an INF (**IV**) over 4 or 24 hr, begin 24 hr after chemotherapy and 24 hr after bone marrow transplantation

Peripheral blood progenitor cell collection/therapy
Adult: 10 mcg/kg/day as a BOL or CONT INF × 4 days or more before leukapheresis, continue to last leukapheresis, may alter dose if WBC >100,000/mm^3

Severe neutropenia (chronic), idiopathic/cyclical
Adult: SUBCUT 5 mcg/kg daily

Available forms: Inj 300 mcg/ml, 480 mcg/1.6 ml, 480 mcg/0.8 ml, 3000 mcg/0.5 ml

Implementation
• Store in refrigerator; do not freeze; may store at room temp up to 24 hr
• Given by subcut injection, short IV infusion, continuous SC or IV infusion
• Avoid use within 24 hr before or after chemotherapy
• Do not shake commercial single-dose vials prior to withdrawing the dose. If the vial is shaken and froth or bubbles form, allow the vial to stand undisturbed for a few min until the froth or bubbles dissipate
• Prior to injection, filgrastim may be allowed to reach room temperature for a maximum of 24 hr. Any vial or syringe exposed to room temperature for more than 24 hr should be discarded
• Visually inspect for particulate matter and discoloration prior to use

IV route
• May be diluted with 5% dextrose. Do not dilute with NS; product may precipitate
• May be diluted to concentrations 5-15 mcg/ml; should be protected from absorption to plastic by the addition of albumin to a final albumin concentration of 2 mg/ml. Do not dilute filgrastim to a concentration <5 mcg/ml

---

Adverse effects: *italics* = common; **bold** = life-threatening

IV infusion
• Infuse IV over 15-30 min or as a continuous infusion over 24 hr

SUBCUT route
• May divide into 2 injections if dose is >1 ml
• Subcut injection: no dilution is necessary; inject by rapid subcut injection taking care not to inject intradermally
• Subcut continuous infusion: infuse subcut at a rate not to exceed 2 ml/hour

Y-site compatibilities: Acyclovir, allopurinol, amikacin, aminophylline, ampicillin, ampicillin/sulbactam, aztreonam, bleomycin, bumetanide, buprenorphine, butorphanol, calcium gluconate, CARBOplatin, carmustine, ceFAZolin, cefoTEtan, cefTAZidime, chlorproMAZINE, cimetidine, CISplatin, cyclophosphamide, cytarabine, dacarbazine, DAUNOrubicin, dexamethasone, diphenhydrAMINE, DOXOrubicin, doxycycline, droperidol, enalaprilat, famotidine, floxuridine, fluconazole, fludarabine, gallium, ganciclovir, granisetron, haloperidol, hydrocortisone, hydromorphone, hydrOXYzine, IDArubicin, ifosfamide, leucovorin, LORazepam, mechlorethamine, melphalan, meperidine, mesna, methotrexate, metoclopramide, miconazole, minocycline, mitoXANtrone, morphine, nalbuphine, netilmicin, ondansetron, plicamycin, potassium chloride, promethazine, ranitidine, sodium bicarbonate, streptozocin, ticarcillin, ticarcillin/clavulanate, tobramycin, trimethoprim-sulfamethoxazole, vancomycin, vinBLAStine, vinCRIStine, vinorelbine, zidovudine

ADVERSE EFFECTS
CNS: Fever, headache
GI: Nausea, vomiting, diarrhea, mucositis, anorexia
HEMA: Thrombocytopenia, excessive leukocytosis
INTEG: Alopecia, exacerbation of skin conditions, urticaria, cutaneous vasculitis
MS: Osteoporosis, skeletal pain
OTHER: Chest pain, hypotension
RESP: Acute respiratory distress syndrome, wheezing, alveolar hemorrhage

Pharmacokinetics

Absorption	Well absorbed (SUBCUT), completely absorbed (**IV**)
Distribution	Unknown
Metabolism	Unknown
Excretion	Unknown
Half-life	Unknown

Pharmacodynamics

	IV	SUBCUT
Onset	5-60 min	5-60 min
Peak	24 hr	2-8 hr
Duration	up to 1 wk	up to 1 wk

INTERACTIONS
Individual drugs
Lithium: do not use concurrently

Drug classifications
Antineoplastics: increased neutrophils, do not use together 24 hr before or after antineoplastics

Drug/lab test
Increased: uric acid, lactate dehydrogenase, alkaline phosphatase, WBC

NURSING CONSIDERATIONS
Assessment
• Monitor blood studies: CBC, platelet count before treatment and twice weekly; neutrophil counts (ANC) may be increased for 2 days after therapy, but treatment should continue until ANC >10,000/mm^3
• Assess for bone pain: frequency, intensity, duration; analgesics may be given; opiates should not be used
• Check B/P, heart rate, respiration; baseline, during treatment

Patient/family education
• Teach patient technique for self-administration: dose, side effects, disposal of containers and needles; provide instruction sheet

Evaluation
Positive therapeutic outcome
• Absence of infection

finasteride (Rx)
(fin-ass′te-ride)
Propecia, Proscar
Func. class.: Androgen hormone inhibitor, hair stimulant
Chem. class.: 5-α-Reductase inhibitor
Pregnancy category X

Do not confuse:
Proscar/ProSom/Prozac,
finasteride/furosemide

ACTION: Inhibits 5-α-reductase and reduction in dihydrotestosterone (DHT); DHT induces androgenic effects by binding to androgen receptors in the cell nuclei of the prostate gland, liver, skin; prevents development of benign prostatic hypertrophy (BPH)

Therapeutic outcome: Reduced prostate size

USES: Symptomatic BPH; male-pattern baldness (Propecia)

CONTRAINDICATIONS:
Pregnancy **X**, breastfeeding, children, women who are pregnant or may become pregnant should not handle tabs, hypersensitivity

Precautions: Large residual urinary volume, severely diminished urinary flow, liver function abnormalities

DOSAGE AND ROUTES
BPH
Adult: PO 5 mg/day × 6-12 mo

Male-pattern baldness
Adult: PO 1 mg/day for 3 mo or more for results

Available forms: Tabs (Propecia) 1 mg, (Proscar) 5 mg

Implementation
• Administer without regard to meals; give for a minimum of 6 mo; not all patients will respond
• Store at temp <86° F (30° C); protect from light; keep container tightly closed

ADVERSE EFFECTS
GU: Impotence, decreased libido, decreased volume of ejaculate, sexual dysfunction
INTEG: Rash
MISC: Breast tenderness, **secondary malignancy**

Pharmacokinetics
Absorption	63%, readily
Distribution	Plasma protein binding, crosses blood-brain barrier
Metabolism	Liver
Excretion	Kidneys, metabolites (39%); feces (57%)
Half-life	6-15 hr

Pharmacodynamics
Onset	Immediate
Peak	1-2 hr
Duration	14 days

INTERACTIONS
Drug classifications
Anticholinergics, bronchodilators (adrenergic), theophylline: decreased effect of finasteride

Drug/lab test
Decreased: PSA levels (finasteride)

NURSING CONSIDERATIONS
Assessment
• **BPH:** Assess urinary patterns, residual urinary volume, severely diminished urinary flow; PSA levels and digital rectal exam results before initiating therapy and periodically thereafter
• Monitor liver function tests before initiating treatment; extensively metabolized in liver

Patient/family education
• Advise patient that pregnant women or women who may become pregnant should not touch crushed tab or come into contact with semen of a patient taking this product; may adversely affect development of male fetus
• Inform patient that volume of ejaculate may be decreased during treatment; impotence and decreased libido may also occur and may continue after discontinuing treatment
• Inform patient that Propecia results may not occur for 3 mo
• Inform patient that Proscar results may not occur for 6-12 mo

Evaluation
Positive therapeutic outcome
• Decreased postvoiding dribbling, frequency, nocturia
• Increased urinary flow
• Regression of prostate size
• Hair growth within 3-6 mo

fingolimod (Rx)
(fin-gol'i-mod)
Gilenya
Func. class.: Biologic response modifier
Chem. class.: Sphingosine 1-phosphate receptor modulator
Pregnancy category C

ACTION: Binds with high affinity to sphingosine 1 phosphate receptors, blocks lymphocyte egress to lymph nodes, reducing the number of peripheral blood lymphocytes, may reduce lymphocyte migration into the CNS

Therapeutic outcome: Improved symptoms of multiple sclerosis and prevention of increasing disability

USES: To reduce frequency of exacerbation, to delay physical disability of relapsing forms of MS

CONTRAINDICATIONS:
Hypersensitivity

Precautions: AIDS, asthma, AV block, bradycardia, breastfeeding, dysrhythmias, cardiac disease, children, COPD, diabetes mellitus, heart failure, hepatic disease, HIV, hypertension, immunosuppression, infants, leukemia, lymphoma, neonates, pregnancy **C**, QT prolongation, respiratory insufficiency, sick sinus syndrome, syncope, uveitis

DOSAGE AND ROUTES
Adult: PO 0.5 mg/day

Hepatic dose
Adult: PO Child-Pugh C, total score >10: Closely monitor, fingolimod exposure is doubled

Available forms: Cap 0.5 mg

Implementation
PO route
• Watch patient for 6 hr after initial dose or if product is not given for >2 wk for development of bradycardia. Give without regard to food
• Store at room temperature, protect from moisture

ADVERSE EFFECTS
CNS: Asthenia, depression, fatigue, headache, dizziness, encephalopathy, migraine, paresthesias, **stroke**
CV: AV block, bradycardia, chest pain, hypertension, palpitations
EENT: Blurred vision, vision impairment, ocular pain, macular edema
GI: Abdominal pain, anorexia, diarrhea, jaundice, vomiting, weight loss
HEMA: Leukopenia, lymphopenia, neutropenia
INTEG: Alopecia, pruritus
MS: Back pain
RESP: Dyspnea, cough
SYST: Infection, influenza, **secondary malignancy**

Pharmacokinetics
Absorption	Protein binding (99.7%)
Distribution	Distributed to RBCs (86%)
Metabolism	Metabolized by CYP4F2 and CYP2D6 to a lesser extent
Excretion	Excreted in urine (81% inactive metabolites)
Half-life	Terminal half-life 6-9 days

Pharmacodynamics
Onset	Unknown
Peak	12-16 hr
Duration	Steady state 1-2 mo

INTERACTIONS
Individual drugs
Ketoconazole: increased fingolimod effect

Drug classifications
Class Ia/III antidysrhythmics: increased risk of torsades de pointes
Antineoplastics, immunosuppressants, immune modulating therapies: increased immunosuppression
Inactive vaccines, toxoids: decreased effects
Live vaccines: increased infection risk

NURSING CONSIDERATIONS
Assessment
• **Multiple sclerosis:** Assess for improving paresthesia, muscle weakness, clonus, muscle spasms, difficulty in moving, difficulty in coordination in balance, speech, swallowing, vision problems, fatigue; prevention of increasing disability
• **Monitor laboratory values:** obtain before initial dose, CBC, LFTs, serum bilirubin, ophthalmologic exam, antibodies to VZV if there is not a history of chickenpox or without vaccination, may give VZV vaccination of antibody-negative patient before giving product, postpone for 1 month after vaccination; obtain ECG for evidence of bradycardia, or AV block

Patient/family education
• Provide med guide to patient and explain use of product and expected results
• Advise patient that continuing follow-up exams and laboratory tests will be required on a regular basis
• Instruct patient to report any side effects resulting from therapy
• Teach patient to protect from moisture
• Advise patient to report chest pain, palpitations, jaundice

Evaluation
Positive therapeutic outcome
• Improved symptoms of multiple sclerosis and prevention of increasing disability

flecainide (Rx)
(flek′a-nide)
Tambocor
Func. class.: Antidysrhythmic (Class IC)
Pregnancy category C

ACTION: Decreases conduction in all parts of the heart, with greatest effect on the His-Purkinje system, which stabilizes the cardiac membrane

Therapeutic outcome: Absence of dysrhythmias

USES: Life-threatening ventricular dysrhythmias, sustained ventricular tachycardia; supraventricular tachydysrhythmias, paroxysmal atrial fibrillation/flutter associated with disabling symptoms

Unlabeled uses: Atrial fibrillation, single dose

CONTRAINDICATIONS:
Hypersensitivity, AV bundle branch block, cardiogenic shock

Precautions: Pregnancy C, breastfeeding, children, renal/hepatic disease, CHF, respiratory depression, myasthenia gravis, geriatric, electrolyte abnormalities, atrial fibrillation, sick sinus syndrome, torsades de pointes

> **BLACK BOX WARNING:** MI, cardiac arrhythmias, atrial fibrillation

DOSAGE AND ROUTES
PSVT/PAT
Adult: PO 50 mg q12hr; may increase every 4 days by 50 mg q12hr to desired response; max 300 mg/day

Life-threatening ventricular dysrhythmias
Adult: PO 100 mg q12hr, may increase by 50 mg q12hr q4days; max 400 mg/day

Renal dose
Adult: PO CCr <35 ml/min dose 100 mg daily or 50 mg bid initially

Available forms: Tabs 50, 100, 150 mg

Implementation
PO route
• Give reduced dosage slowly with ECG monitoring; do not increase dose <4 days apart
• Give with meals if GI upset occurs
• Therapeutic trough serum concentrations for adults range from 200-1000 ng/mL (average 500 ng/mL); toxicity is more common with trough serum concentrations >1000 ng/mL; usual therapeutic range in children is 200-500 ng/mL; in some cases, up to 800 ng/mL may be required
• Adjust dosage at intervals of ≥4 days (approximate plateau effects) following dosage adjustments; however, longer intervals are needed in patients with renal or hepatic impairment
• Frequent serum drug concentration monitoring is required for patients with severe renal (CrCl <35 ml/min) or hepatic disease, and may also be helpful in patients with CHF or in patients with moderate renal disease
• Monitoring of flecainide serum concentrations is strongly recommended in patients receiving amiodarone therapy

ADVERSE EFFECTS
CNS: *Headache, dizziness,* involuntary movement, confusion, psychosis, restlessness, irritability, paresthesias, ataxia, flushing, somnolence, depression, anxiety, malaise, fatigue, asthenia, tremors
CV: *Hypotension,* **bradycardia,** angina, PVCs, **heart block, cardiovascular collapse/arrest, dysrhythmias, CHF, fatal ventricular tachycardia,** palpitations, **QT prolongation, torsades de pointes**
EENT: Tinnitus, *blurred vision,* hearing loss, corneal deposits, dry eyes
GI: Nausea, vomiting, anorexia, constipation, abdominal pain, flatulence, change in taste, diarrhea
GU: Impotence, decreased libido, polyuria, urinary retention
HEMA: **Leukopenia, thrombocytopenia**
INTEG: Rash, urticaria, edema, swelling
RESP: Dyspnea, **respiratory depression**

Pharmacokinetics	
Absorption	Well absorbed
Distribution	Widely distributed
Metabolism	Liver
Excretion	30% kidneys, unchanged
Half-life	14 hr

Pharmacodynamics

Onset	Unknown
Peak	3 hr
Duration	Unknown

INTERACTIONS
Individual drugs
Amiodarone, cimetidine, ritonavir: increased level of flecainide

Digoxin: increased digoxin levels

Disopyramide, verapamil: increased CV depressant action

Propanolol: increased effects of both products

Drug classifications
Acidifying agents, alkalizing agents: increased or decreased effect

β-Adrenergic blockers: increased CV depressant action

Drug/herb
Hawthorn: do not use concurrently

Drug/lab test
Increased: CPK

NURSING CONSIDERATIONS
Assessment

> **BLACK BOX WARNING:** MI, CHF, cardiogenic shock: should not be used in these conditions

> **BLACK BOX WARNING:** Atrial fibrillation: avoid use, risk of ventricular dysrhythmias

> **BLACK BOX WARNING:** Cardiac dysrhythmias: discontinue in those with prolonged QRS >180 ms, or prolonged PR >300 ms; monitor ECG, B/P, pulse

• Monitor I&O ratio; electrolytes prior to use: potassium, sodium, chloride; check weight daily and for signs of CHF or pulmonary toxicity: dyspnea, fatigue, cough, fever, chest pain, jugular vein distention, crackles; if these occur, product should be discontinued

• Monitor liver function studies: AST, ALT, bilirubin, alkaline phosphatase

• Assess patient for CNS symptoms: confusion, psychosis, numbness, depression, involuntary movements; if these occur, product should be discontinued

• Monitor cardiac rate, respiration: rate, rhythm, character, chest pain; watch for ventricular tachycardia, supraventricular tachycardia, or fibrillation

• **Flecainide level:** Monitor level in those with CHF or renal failure, peak, trough

Patient/family education
• Instruct patient to report side effects immediately to prescriber

• Instruct patient to complete follow-up appointment with health care provider, including pulmonary function tests, chest x-ray

• Teach patient to change position slowly from lying or sitting to standing to minimize orthostatic hypotension

• Advise patient not to skip or double doses

• Advise patient to carry/wear emergency ID with disorder, medications taken

• Advise patient to avoid hazardous activities that require alertness until response is known

Evaluation
Positive therapeutic outcome
• Absence of dysrhythmias

fluconazole (Rx)
(floo-kon′a-zole)
Diflucan
Func. class.: Antifungal
Chem. class.: Triazole
Pregnancy category C

Do not confuse:
Diflucan/Diprivan

ACTION: Inhibits ergosterol biosynthesis, causes direct damage to membrane phospholipids in the cell wall of fungi

Therapeutic outcome: Fungistatic fungicidal against the following susceptible organisms: *Candida, Cryptococcus neoformans*

USES: Oropharyngeal candidiasis; chronic mucocutaneous candidiasis; systemic, vaginal, urinary candidiasis; cryptococcal meningitis; prevention of candidiasis in bone marrow transplant in those who receive chemotherapy and/or radiation therapy, cystitis, fungal prophylaxis, peritonitis, pneumonia, pyelonephritis

CONTRAINDICATIONS: Hypersensitivity to this product or azoles, pregnancy **D**

Precautions: Breastfeeding, renal/hepatic disease, torsades de pointes

DOSAGE AND ROUTES
Vulvovaginal candidiasis
Adult: PO 150 mg as a single dose

Serious fungal infections
Adult: PO/IV 50-400 mg initially, then 200 mg once daily for 4 wk
Child: 6-12 mg/kg/day

Oropharyngeal candidiasis
Adult: PO/IV 200 mg initially, then 100 mg/day for at least 2 wk
Child: PO/IV 6 mg/kg initially, then 3 mg/kg/day for ≥2 wk

Esophageal candidiasis
Adult: PO/IV 200 mg on 1st day, then 100 mg/day × ≥3 wk and for ≥2 wk after resolution of symptoms
Child: PO/IV 6 mg/kg on 1st day, then 3 mg/kg/day × ≥3 wk and for ≥2 wk after resolution of symptoms

Cryptococcal meningitis
Adult: PO/IV 400 mg on 1st day, then 200 mg/day × 10-12 wk after CSF culture negative
Child/infant/neonate >14 days: PO/IV 12 mg/kg on 1st day, then 6-12 mg/kg/day × 10-12 wk after negative CSF culture
Neonate 0-14 days: PO/IV 12 mg/kg on 1st day, then 6-12 mg/kg q72hr × 10-12 wk after negative CSF culture

Prevention of candidiasis in bone marrow transplant
Adult: PO/IV 400 mg/day; those anticipated to have neutrophils <500/mm^3, start several days prior to anticipated onset of neutropenia and continue for 7 days after rise of neutrophils >1000/mm^3

Renal dose
Adult: PO CCr <50 ml/min after loading dose, give 50% of usual dose

Available forms: Tabs 10, 40, 50, 100, 150, 200 mg; inj 2 mg/ml; powder for oral susp 50, 200 mg/ml

Implementation
• Take with food to reduce GI effects
PO route
• Add water in 2 portions, review manufacturer reconstitution instructions
• Shake oral susp before each use; use within 2 wk

Intermittent IV infusion route
• Give after diluting according to package directions; run at 200 mg/hr or less; do not use plastic containers in connections
• Do not admix
• Administer **IV** using an in-line filter, using distal veins; check for extravasation and necrosis q2hr

• Give product only after C&S confirms organism, product needed to treat condition
• Store protected from moisture and light, diluted sol is stable for 24 hr

Y-site compatibilities: Acyclovir, aldesleukin, alfentanil, allopurinol, amifostine, amikacin, aminocaproic acid, aminophylline, amiodarone, anidulafungin, ascorbic acid injection, atenolol, atracurium, atropine, azaTHIOprine, aztreonam, benztropine, bivalirudin, bleomycin, bumetanide, buprenorphine, butorphanol, calcium chloride, CARBOplatin, caspofungin, cefamandole, ceFAZolin, cefepime, cefmetazole, cefonicid, cefoperazone, cefoTEtan, cefOXitin, cefpirome, cefTAZidime, ceftizoxime, ceftobiprole, cephalothin, cephapirin, chlorproMAZINE, cimetidine, cisatracurium, CISplatin, codeine, cyanocobalamin, cyclophosphamide, cycloSPORINE, cytarabine, DACTINomycin, DAPTOmycin, dexamethasone, diltiazem, dimenhyDRINATE, diphenhydrAMINE, DOBUTamine, DOCEtaxel, DOPamine, doripenem, doxacurium, DOXOrubicin, DOXOrubicin liposomal, doxycycline, droperidol, drotrecogin alfa, enalaprilat, ePHEDrine, EPINEPHrine, epirubicin, epoetin alfa, eptifibatide, ertapenem, erythromycin, esmolol, etoposide, famotidine, fenoldopam, fentaNYL, filgrastim, fludarabine, fluorouracil, folic acid, foscarnet, gallium, ganciclovir, gatifloxacin, gemcitabine, gentamicin, glycopyrrolate, granisetron, heparin, hydrocortisone, HYDROmorphone, IDArubicin, ifosfamide, IV immune globulin, inamrinone, indomethacin, insulin (regular), irinotecan, isoproterenol, ketorolac, labetalol, lansoprazole, leucovorin, levofloxacin, lidocaine, linezolid, LORazepam, LR, magnesium sulfate, mannitol, mechlorethamine, melphalan, meperidine, meropenem, metaraminol, methicillin, methotrexate, methoxamine, methyldopate, methylPREDNISolone, metoclopramide, metoprolol, metroNIDAZOLE, mezlocillin, miconazole, midazolam, milrinone, minocycline, mitoXANtrone, morphine, moxalactam, multiple vitamins injection, mycophenolate, nafcillin, nalbuphine, naloxone, nesiritide, nitroglycerin, nitroprusside, norepinephrine, octreotide, ondansetron, oxacillin, oxaliplatin, oxytocin, PACLitaxel, palonosetron, pamidronate, pancuronium, papaverine, PEMEtrexed, penicillin G potassium/sodium, pentazocine, PENTobarbital, PHENobarbital, phenylephrine, phenytoin, phytonadione, piperacillin-tazobactam, polymyxin B, potassium chloride, procainamide, prochlorperazine, promethazine, propofol, propranolol, protamine, pyridoxine, quiNIDine, quinupristin-dalfopristin, ranitidine, remifentanil, Ringer's, ritodrine, riTUXimab, rocuronium, sargramostim, sodium acetate/bicarbonate, succinylcholine, SUFentanil, tacrolimus, temocillin, teniposide, theophylline, thiotepa, ticarcillin-clavulanate, tigecycline, tirofiban, TNA, tobramycin, tolazoline, TPN, trastuzumab, trimetaphan, urokinase, vancomycin, vasopressin, vecuronium, verapamil, vinCRIStine, vinorelbine, voriconazole, zidovudine, zoledronic acid

Y-site incompatibilities: Amphotericin B, ampicillin, calcium gluconate, cefotaxime, cefTRIAXone, cefTAZidime, cefuroxime, chloramphenicol, clindamycin, diazepam, digoxin, erythromycin lactobionate, furosemide, haloperidol, hydrOXYzine, imipenem/cilastatin, pentamidine, ticarcillin, trimethoprim/sulfamethoxazole

ADVERSE EFFECTS

CNS: *Headache,* seizures
CV: QT prolongation, torsades de pointes
GI: *Nausea, vomiting,* diarrhea, cramping, flatus, increased AST, ALT, **hepatotoxicity**
HEMA: Agranulocytosis, eosinophilia, leukopenia, neutropenia, thrombocytopenia
INTEG: Stevens-Johnson syndrome, angioedema, anaphylaxis, exfoliative dermatitis, toxic epidermal necrolysis

Pharmacokinetics

Absorption	Well absorbed (PO)
Distribution	Widely distributed (peritoneum, CSF)
Metabolism	<10%, liver
Excretion	80% kidneys (unchanged)
Half-life	30 hr, increased in renal disease

Pharmacodynamics

	PO	IV
Onset	Unknown	Immediate
Peak	2-4 hr	Infusion's end
Duration	Unknown	Unknown

INTERACTIONS

Individual drugs

Alfentanil, buprenorphine, ergot, fentaNYL, methadone, saquinavir, SUFentanil, zidovudine: increased effect of each specific drug
CycloSPORINE, phenytoin, rifabutin, sirolimus, tacrolimus, theophylline, zidovudine, zolpidem: increased plasma concentrations

Lovastatin, simvastatin: increased myopathy, rhabdomyolysis risk
Warfarin: increased anticoagulation

Drug classification

Contraceptives (oral), calcium-channel blockers: decreased effect
Oral sulfonylureas (glipiZIDE): hypoglycemia
Proton pump inhibitors: decreased fluconazole

Drug/herb

Gossypol: increased nephrotoxicity

Drug/lab test

Increased: alk phos, LFTs
Decreased: WBC, platelets

NURSING CONSIDERATIONS

Assessment

• **Assess for signs and symptoms of infection:** clearing of CSF culture during treatment, obtain C&S baseline and during treatment, product may be started as soon as culture is taken
• **Monitor for hepatotoxicity:** increased AST, ALT, alkaline phosphatase, bilirubin; discontinue product if hepatotoxicity occurs
• **Monitor for skin symptoms:** color, lesions, injection site reactions; if lesions progress, discontinue product

Patient/family education

• Caution patient that long-term therapy may be needed to clear infection; to take entire course of medication; take in equal intervals (PO)
• **Teach patient the signs and symptoms of hepatotoxicity:** nausea, vomiting, clay-colored stools, dark urine, anorexia, fatigue, jaundice, **skin rash;** prescriber should be notified immediately
• Inform patient that medication may be taken with food to reduce GI effects
• Advise patient to consider using alternative contraception if using oral contraceptives, pregnancy **D**

Evaluation

Positive therapeutic outcome
• Decreasing oral candidiasis, fever, malaise, rash
• Negative C&S for infecting organism

fludrocortisone (Rx)

(floo-droe-kor'ti-sone)
Func. class.: Synthetic corticosteroid
Pregnancy category C

ACTION: Promotes increased reabsorption of sodium and loss of potassium, water, hydrogen from distal tubules

Therapeutic outcome: Correction of adrenal insufficiency

USES: Adrenal insufficiency, salt-losing adrenogenital syndrome, Addison's disease

CONTRAINDICATIONS:
Children <2 yr, hypersensitivity, acute glomerulonephritis, amebiasis, psychosis, Cushing's syndrome, fungal infections

Precautions: CHF, hypertension, diabetes, pregnancy C, breastfeeding, children >2 yrs, osteoporosis

DOSAGE AND ROUTES
Adult: PO 100-200 mcg/day
Child: PO 50-100 mcg/day

Available forms: Tabs 100 mcg (0.1 mg)

Implementation
• Titrate to lowest dose
• Give with food or milk to decrease GI symptoms

ADVERSE EFFECTS
CV: Hypertension, circulatory collapse, thrombophlebitis, embolism, tachycardia, CHF, edema
CNS: Flushing, sweating, headache, paralysis, dizziness, seizure
ENDO: Weight gain, adrenal suppression, hyperglycemia
META: Hypokalemia
MISC: Hypersensitivity, cataracts, GI ulcers, anaphylaxis
MS: Fractures, osteoporosis, weakness

Pharmacokinetics	
Absorption	Unknown
Distribution	Unknown
Metabolism	Liver
Excretion	Urine
Half-life	18-36 hr

Pharmacodynamics	
Onset	Unknown
Peak	1.5 hr
Duration	Unknown

INTERACTIONS
Drug classifications
Barbiturates: decreased fludrocortisone action
Loop/thiazide diuretics, potassium-wasting products: increased potassium levels
Sodium-containing products: increased B/P

Drug/lab test
Increased: potassium, sodium
Decreased: HCT

NURSING CONSIDERATIONS
Assessment
• Assess weight daily, notify prescriber of weekly gain >5 lb
• Monitor I&O, be alert for decreasing output, increasing edema
• Monitor B/P, pulse, notify prescriber of chest pain
• Potassium depletion: assess for paresthesia, fatigue, nausea, vomiting, dysrhythmias, weakness, depression, polyuria
• Electrolytes: monitor sodium, potassium, chloride; hypokalemia is common

Patient/family education
• Teach patient that emergency ID as corticosteroid user should be carried
• Teach patient not to discontinue abruptly
• Instruct patient to notify health care provider of muscle cramps, weight gain, edema, nausea, infection, trauma, stress
• Advise patient to avoid exposure to disease, trauma

Evaluation
Positive therapeutic outcome
• Correction of adrenal insufficiency

flumazenil (Rx)

(flu-maz'e-nil)
Anexate ✦, Romazicon
Func. class.: Antidote: Benzodiazepine receptor antagonist
Chem. class.: Imidazobenzodiazepine derivative
Pregnancy category C

ACTION: Antagonizes the actions of benzodiazepines on the CNS, competitively inhibits the activity at the benzodiazepine receptor complex

Therapeutic outcome: Reversed benzodiazepine toxic effects

USES: Reversal of the sedative effects of benzodiazepines

CONTRAINDICATIONS:

Hypersensitivity to this product or benzodiazepines, serious tricyclic overdose, patients given benzodiazepine for control of life-threatening condition

Precautions: Pregnancy **C,** breastfeeding, children, geriatric, ambulatory patients, renal/hepatic disease, status epilepticus, head injury, labor and delivery, hypoventilation, panic disorder, drug/alcohol dependency

> **BLACK BOX WARNING:** Benzodiazepine dependence, seizures

DOSAGE AND ROUTES

Reversal of conscious sedation or in general anesthesia

Adult: IV 0.2 mg (2 ml) given over 15 sec; wait 45 sec, then give 0.2 mg (2 ml) if consciousness does not occur; may be repeated at 60-sec intervals as needed (max 3 mg/hr) or 1 mg/5 min
Child: IV 10 mcg (0.01 mg)/kg; cumulative dose of 1 mg or less

Management of suspected benzodiazepine overdose

Adult: IV 0.2 mg (2 ml) given over 30 sec; wait 30 sec, then give 0.3 mg (3 ml) over 30 sec if consciousness does not occur; further doses of 0.5 mg (5 ml) can be given over 30 sec at intervals of 1 min up to cumulative dose of 3 mg
Child: IV 10 mcg (0.01 mg/kg); cumulative dose of less than 1 mg

Available forms: Inj 0.1 mg/ml

Implementation

Direct IV route
• Give directly undiluted or diluted in 0.9% NaCl, D$_5$W, or LR; give over 15-30 sec into running **IV**
• Use large vein
• Check airway and **IV** access before administration
• Stable for 24 hr if drawn into a syringe or mixed with other solutions

ADVERSE EFFECTS

CNS: Dizziness, agitation, emotional lability, confusion, **seizures,** somnolence, panic attacks
CV: Hypertension, palpitations, cutaneous vasodilatation, **dysrhythmias,** bradycardia, tachycardia, chest pain

EENT: Abnormal vision, blurred vision, tinnitus
GI: Nausea, vomiting, hiccups
SYST: Headache, inj site pain, increased sweating, fatigue, rigors

Pharmacokinetics

Absorption	Complete
Distribution	Unknown
Metabolism	Liver
Excretion	Unknown
Half-life	41-79 min

Pharmacodynamics

Onset	1-2 min
Peak	10 min
Duration	Unknown

INTERACTIONS

Individual drugs
Zaleplon, zolpidem: antagonize action

Drug classifications
Benzodiazepines: antagonize action
Toxicity: mixed product overdosage

NURSING CONSIDERATIONS

Assessment
• Assess cardiac status using continuous monitoring
• Assess for seizures, protect patient from injury; most likely in those who usually experience withdrawal from sedatives
• Assess for GI symptoms: nausea, vomiting; place in side-lying position to prevent aspiration
• **Assess for allergic reactions:** flushing, rash, urticaria, pruritus

> **BLACK BOX WARNING: Seizures/benzodiazepine dependence:** Do not use in those who have used these products for interictal psychosis (IIP), or status epilepticus, use in ICU cautiously where there may be unrecognized benzodiazepine dependence

Patient/family education
• Caution patient that amnesia may continue
• Instruct patient to avoid any hazardous activities for 18-24 hr after discharge
• Caution patient not to take any alcohol or nonprescription products for 18-24 hr; serious reactions may occur

---

Evaluation
Positive therapeutic outcome
- Decreased sedation, respiratory depression
- Absence of toxicity

flunisolide nasal agent
See Appendix B

fluocinolone topical
See Appendix B

fluorometholone ophthalmic
See Appendix B

⚠ HIGH ALERT

fluorouracil (Rx)
(flure-oh-yoor'a-sil)
5-FU, Adrucil, Carac, Efudex
Func. class.: Antineoplastic, antimetabolite
Chem. class.: Pyrimidine antagonist
Pregnancy category X

Do not confuse:
fluorouracil/flucytosine

ACTION: Inhibits DNA, RNA synthesis; interferes with cell replication by competitively inhibiting thymidylate synthesis; cell cycle specific (S phase)

Therapeutic outcome: Prevention of rapidly growing malignant cells

USES: Systemic: cancer of breast, colon, rectum, stomach, pancreas; **Topical:** superficial basal cell carcinoma; multiple actinic keratoses

Unlabeled uses: Anal, biliary tract, cervical, head and neck, hepatocellular, and ovarian cancers

CONTRAINDICATIONS:
Pregnancy **X**, breastfeeding, hypersensitivity, poor nutritional status, serious infections

BLACK BOX WARNING: Bone marrow suppression

Precautions: Children, renal/hepatic disease, angina

BLACK BOX WARNING: GI bleeding

DOSAGE AND ROUTES
Doses vary widely, doses are based on actual body weight, unless obese, then based on lean body weight

Advanced colorectal cancer
Adult: IV bolus 300-500 mg/m^2/day × 4-5 days q28 days or 600-1500 mg/m^2 qwk or every other wk; continuous IV infusion: 300-1000 mg/m^2/day × 4-5 days q4wk or 300 mg/m^2/day indefinitely; high dose 3000-3400 mg/m^2 over 24-72 hr

Breast cancer
Adult: IV bolus 400-600 mg/m^2 on days 1 and 8 of every cycle with cyclophosphamide and methotrexate or 600 mg/m^2 on day 1 with cyclophosphamide and methotrexate q21-28 days

Pancreatic cancer
Adult: IV bolus 600 mg/m^2 on day 1, 8, 29, 36 with DOXOrubicin and mitoMYcin q8wk

Actinic/solar keratoses
Adult: TOP 1% cream/SOL 1-2 ×/day or 2%-5% SOL for hands

Superficial basal cell carcinoma
Adult: TOP 5% cream/SOL 2 ×/day × 3-12 wk

Available forms: Inj 50 mg/ml; cream 0.5%, 1%, 5%; SOL 1%, 2%, 5%

Implementation
- Avoid contact with skin (very irritating); wash completely to remove
- Give fluids **IV** or PO before chemotherapy to hydrate patient
- Give antiemetic 30-60 min before giving product to prevent vomiting, and prn for several days thereafter; antibiotics for prophylaxis of infection
- Provide liquid diet: carbonated beverages; gelatin may be added if patient is not nauseated or vomiting
- Rinse mouth tid-qid with water, club soda; brush teeth bid-qid with soft brush or cotton-tipped applicators for stomatitis; use unwaxed dental floss

Topical route
- The 1% strength is used on face, other higher strengths are used on other parts of the body
- Wear gloves when applying; may use with a loose dressing; use a plastic or wooden applicator

IV route
- Prepare in biological cabinet using gloves, gown, mask
- IV undiluted; may inject through Y-tube or 3-way stopcock; give over 1-3 min

---

Adverse effects: *italics* = common; **bold** = life-threatening

• May be diluted in 0.9% NaCl, D₅W; given as a continuous infusion in plastic containers; do not refrigerate/freeze; protect from light; discard unused portion

Y-site compatibilities: Acyclovir, alatrofloxacin, alfentanil, allopurinol, amifostine, amikacin, amphotericin B lipid complex, amphotericin B liposome, ampicillin, ampicillin-sulbactam, anidulafungin, argatroban, atenolol, atracurium, azithromycin, aztreonam, bivalirudin, bleomycin, bumetanide, butorphanol, calcium gluconate, CARBOplatin, ceFAZolin, cefepime, cefoperazone, cefotaxime, cefoTEtan, cefOXitin, cefTAZidime, ceftizoxime, cefTRIAXone, cefuroxime, cimetidine, cisatracurium, CISplatin, clindamycin, codeine, cyclophosphamide, cycloSPORINE, DAPTOmycin, dexamethasone, digoxin, DOCEtaxel, DOPamine, doripenem, DOXOrubicin liposomal, enalaprilat, ePHEDrine, ertapenem, erythromycin, esmolol, etoposide phosphate, famotidine, fenoldopam, fentaNYL, fluconazole, fludarabine, foscarnet, fosphenytoin, furosemide, ganciclovir, gatifloxacin, gemcitabine, gentamicin, granisetron, heparin, hydrocortisone, HYDROmorphone, ifosfamide, imipenem-cilastatin, inamrinone, isoproterenol, ketorolac, labetalol, leucovorin, levorphanol, lidocaine, linezolid, magnesium sulfate, mannitol, melphalan, meperidine, meropenem, mesna, methohexital, methotrexate, methylPREDNISolone, metoprolol, metroNIDAZOLE, milrinone, mitoMYcin, mitoXANtrone, morphine sulfate, nalbuphine, naloxone, nesiritide, nitroglycerin, nitroprusside, octreotide, ofloxacin, PACLitaxel, palonosetron, pamidronate, pancuronium, pantoprazole, PEMEtrexed, PENTobarbital, PHENobarbital, phenylephrine, piperacillin, piperacillin-tazobactam, potassium chloride/phosphates, procainamide, propofol, propranolol, ranitidine, remifentanil, riTUXimab, sargramostim, sodium acetate/bicarbonate/phosphates, succinylcholine, SUFentanil, sulfamethoxazole-trimethoprim, teniposide, theophylline, thiopental, thiotepa, ticarcillin, ticarcillin-clavulanate, tigecycline, tirofiban, tobramycin, trastuzumab, vasopressin, vecuronium, vinBLAStine, vinCRIStine, vitamin B complex/C, voriconazole, zidovudine, zoledronic acid

Y-site incompatibilities: Droperidol, vinorelbine

ADVERSE EFFECTS
SYSTEMIC use
CNS: Lethargy, malaise, weakness, acute cerebellar dysfunction

CV: **Myocardial ischemia,** angina
EENT: Epistaxis, light intolerance, lacrimation
GI: *Anorexia, stomatitis,* diarrhea, nausea, vomiting, **hemorrhage,** enteritis, glossitis
HEMA: Thrombocytopenia, leukopenia, myelosuppression, anemia, agranulocytosis
INTEG: *Rash,* fever, photosensitivity, **anaphylaxis**

Pharmacokinetics

Absorption	Completely bioavailable (**IV**), minimal (topical)
Distribution	Widely distributed, concentration in tumor
Metabolism	Liver, converted to active metabolite
Excretion	Lungs (60%-80%), kidneys (up to 15%)
Half-life	20 hr terminal

Pharmacodynamics
Unknown

INTERACTIONS
Individual drugs
Leucovorin: increased toxicity, bone marrow depression
MetroNIDAZOLE: increased toxicity
Phenytoin: decreased effect of phenytoin
Radiation: increased toxicity, bone marrow suppression

Drug classifications
Anticoagulants, NSAIDs, platelet inhibitors, thrombolytics: increased bleeding
Antineoplastics: increased toxicity, bone marrow depression
Live virus vaccines: decreased antibody response

Drug/lab test
Increased: AST, ALT, LDH, serum bilirubin, Hct, Hgb, WBC, platelets, 5-HIAA
Decreased: albumin

NURSING CONSIDERATIONS
Assessment
• Monitor ECG; watch for ST-T wave changes, low QRS and T, possible dysrhythmias (sinus tachycardia, heart block, PVCs)
• Assess buccal cavity q8hr for dryness, sores or ulceration, white patches, oral pain, bleeding, dysphagia; obtain prescription for viscous lidocaine (Xylocaine)
• Assess tachypnea, ECG changes, dyspnea, edema, fatigue; identify dyspnea, crackles, unproductive cough, chest pain, tachypnea

BLACK BOX WARNING: Bone marrow suppression: Monitor CBC, differential, platelet count daily (**IV**); withhold product if WBC is <4000/mm³ or platelet count is <100,000/mm³; notify prescriber of results if WBC <20,000/mm³, platelets <50,000/mm³; nadir of leukopenia within 2 wk, recovery 1 mo; if pretreatment of WBC <2000/mm³ or platelets <100,000/mm³, delay until recovery of counts above this level

• Monitor renal function studies: BUN, creatinine, serum uric acid, urine CCr before, during therapy; I&O ratio; report fall in urine output to <30 ml/hr
• Monitor temp q4hr (may indicate beginning of infection)
• Monitor liver function tests before, during therapy (bilirubin, AST, ALT, LDH) as needed or monthly; jaundice of skin, sclera, dark urine, clay-colored stools, itchy skin, abdominal pain, fever, diarrhea
• **Assess for bleeding:** hematuria, stool guaiac, bruising or petechiae, mucosa or orifices q8hr; inflammation of mucosa, breaks in skin
⚠ Assess for infection: those with current infections should be treated prior to receiving 5-FU, the dose reduced or discontinued if infection occurs

Patient/family education
⚠ Caution patient that contraceptive measures are recommended during therapy, pregnancy X
• **Bleeding:** Teach patient to avoid using aspirin, NSAIDs, or ibuprofen-containing products, razors, commercial mouthwash because bleeding may occur; to report symptoms of bleeding (hematuria, tarry stools), IM injections if counts are low
• **Instruct patient to report signs of anemia** (fatigue, headache, irritability, faintness, SOB)
• **Instruct patient to report signs of stomatitis** (bleeding, white spots, ulcerations in the mouth); tell patient to examine mouth daily, to report symptoms; viscous lidocaine (Xylocaine) may be used
• Teach patient to avoid crowds, persons with known infections
• Advise patient to avoid vaccinations during therapy, to use sunscreen or stay out of the sun to prevent burns; about hair loss; explore use of wigs or other products until hair regrowth occurs

Evaluation
Positive therapeutic outcome
• Prevention of rapid division of malignant cells

FLUoxetine (Rx)
(floo-ox′uh-teen)
PROzac, PROzac Weekly, Sarafem
Func. class.: Antidepressant, selective serotonin reuptake inhibitor
Pregnancy category C

Do not confuse:
PROzac/Proscar/PriLOSEC/Prosom, Sarafem/Serophene

ACTION: Inhibits CNS neuron uptake of serotonin but not of norepinephrine

Therapeutic outcome: Decreased symptoms of depression after 2-3 wk

USES: Major depressive disorder, obsessive-compulsive disorder (OCD), bulimia nervosa; *Sarafem:* premenstrual dysphoric disorder (PMDD), panic disorder, generalized anxiety disorder, social phobia

Unlabeled uses: Alcoholism, anorexia nervosa, borderline personality disorder, obesity, posttraumatic stress disorder

CONTRAINDICATIONS:
Hypersensitivity

Precautions: Pregnancy **C**, breastfeeding, geriatric, diabetes mellitus, narrow-angle glaucoma, cardiac malformations in infants (exposed to FLUoxetine in utero)

BLACK BOX WARNING: Children, suicidal ideation

DOSAGE AND ROUTES
Depression/OCD
Adult: PO 20 mg/day AM; after 4 wk if no clinical improvement is noted, dosage may be increased to 20 mg bid in AM, afternoon; max 80 mg/day; PO 90 mg weekly
Geriatric: PO 5-10 mg/day, increase as needed
Child 5-18 yr: PO 5-10 mg/day, max 20 mg/day

Alcoholism (unlabeled)
Adult: PO 20-80 mg/day

Anorexia nervosa (unlabeled)
Adult: PO 10 mg every other day-20 mg/day

Borderline personality disorder (unlabeled)
Adult: PO 20 mg/day, max 80 mg/day

Kleptomania (unlabeled)
Adult: PO 60-80 mg/day

Posttraumatic stress disorder (unlabeled)
Adult: PO 10-80 mg/day

Premenstrual dysphoric disorder (Sarafem)
Adult: PO 20 mg/day, may be taken daily 14 days before menses

Available forms: Caps 10, 20, 40 mg; tabs 10, 20 mg; oral sol 20 mg/5 ml; del rel caps (PROzac Weekly) 90 mg; tab 10, 15, 20 mg (Sarafem)

Implementation
• Give without regard to meals
• Give dose at bedtime if oversedation occurs during day; may take entire dose at bedtime; geriatric may not tolerate once/day dosing, crush if patient unable to swallow whole (tabs only)
• **PROzac Weekly:** Give on same day each week, swallow whole, do not crush, cut, chew
• Store at room temperature; do not freeze

ADVERSE EFFECTS

CNS: *Headache, nervousness, insomnia, drowsiness, anxiety, tremor, dizziness, fatigue, sedation, poor concentration, abnormal dreams, agitation,* **seizures,** apathy, euphoria, hallucinations, delusions, psychosis, **suicidal ideation, neuroleptic malignant syndrome–like reactions,** serotonin syndrome
CV: *Hot flashes, palpitations,* angina pectoris, **hemorrhage,** hypertension, **tachycardia, 1st-degree AV block, bradycardia, MI, thrombophlebitis,** generalized edema
EENT: Visual changes, ear/eye pain, photophobia, tinnitus, increased intraocular pressure
GI: *Nausea, diarrhea, dry mouth, anorexia, dyspepsia, constipation,* taste changes, flatulence, decreased appetite
GU: *Dysmenorrhea, decreased libido, urinary frequency, urinary tract infection,* amenorrhea, cystitis, impotence, urine retention
INTEG: *Sweating, rash, pruritus,* acne, alopecia, urticaria; **angioedema, exfoliative dermatitis, Stevens-Johnson syndrome, toxic epidermal necrolysis**
MS: *Pain,* arthritis, twitching
RESP: *Pharyngitis, cough, dyspnea, bronchitis,* asthma, hyperventilation, pneumonia

SYST: *Asthenia,* **serotonin syndrome, flulike symptoms, neonatal abstinence syndrome**

Pharmacokinetics

Absorption	Well absorbed
Distribution	Crosses blood-brain barrier
Metabolism	Liver, extensively to norfluoxetine
Excretion	Kidneys, unchanged (12%), metabolite (7%); steady state 28-35 days, protein binding 94%
Half-life	1-3 days metabolite up to 1 wk

Pharmacodynamics

Onset	Unknown
Peak	6-8 hr
Duration	Unknown

INTERACTIONS

Individual drugs
Alcohol: increased CNS depression
Antidiabetics: increased levels or toxicity
Bosentan, budesonide, carBAMazepine, darifenacin, diazepam, digoxin, donepezil, lithium, paricalcitol, phenytoin, thioridazine, vinBLAStine, warfarin: increased toxicity
Cyproheptadine: decreased FLUoxetine effect
BusPIRone, haloperidol, loxapine, selegiline, thiothixene, tryptophan: increased serotonin syndrome, do not use concurrently

Drug classifications
Anticoagulants, NSAIDs, platelet inhibitors, salicylates, thrombolytics: increased bleeding risk
Antidepressants, opioids, sedative/hypnotics: increased CNS depression
MAOIs: hypertensive crisis, seizures; do not use with or 14 days prior to fluoxetine
SSRIs, SNRIs, serotonin-receptor agonists, tricyclics: increased serotonin syndrome, do not use concurrently

Drug/herb
Hops, kava, lavender, valerian: increased CNS effect
St. John's wort, SAM-e: do not use together; increased risk of serotonin syndrome

Drug/lab test
Increased: serum bilirubin, blood glucose, alkaline phosphatase, BUN, CK

NURSING CONSIDERATIONS

Assessment

• Monitor B/P (lying, standing), pulse q4hr; if systolic B/P drops 20 mm hg, hold product and notify prescriber; take VS q4hr in patients with CV disease
• Monitor blood studies: CBC, leukocytes, differential, cardiac enzymes if patient is receiving long-term therapy; check platelets, bleeding can occur; thyroid growth rate (children)
• Monitor hepatic studies: AST, ALT, bilirubin
• Check weight qwk; appetite may increase with product
• Assess ECG for flattening of T-wave, bundle branch block, AV block, dysrhythmias in cardiac patients

> **BLACK BOX WARNING:** Assess mental status: mood, sensorium, affect, suicidal tendencies; increase in psychiatric symptoms: depression, panic; monitor for seizures; seizure potential is increased; Sarafem is not approved for children

• Monitor urinary retention, constipation; constipation is more likely to occur in children or geriatric
• Identify patient's alcohol consumption; if alcohol is consumed, hold dose until AM
• **Assess appetite in bulimia nervosa,** monitor weight daily, increase nutritious foods in diet, watch for bingeing and vomiting
• **Serious skin reactions:** angioedema, exfoliative dermatitis, **Stevens-Johnson syndrome,** toxic epidermal necrolysis
• Assess allergic reactions: itching, rash, urticaria, product should be discontinued; may need to give antihistamine

Patient/family education

• Teach patient that therapeutic effects may take 1-4 wk, not to discontinue abruptly
• Instruct patient to use caution in driving or other activities requiring alertness because of drowsiness, dizziness, blurred vision; to avoid rising quickly from sitting to standing, especially geriatric; to use sunscreen to prevent photosensitivity
• Caution patient to avoid alcohol ingestion, other CNS depressants
• Advise patient not to discontinue medication quickly after long-term use: may cause nausea, headache, malaise
• Instruct patient to increase fluids, bulk in diet if constipation, urinary retention occur, especially geriatric
• Advise patient to take gum, hard sugarless candy, or frequent sips of water for dry mouth

• Teach patient to avoid all OTC products unless approved by prescriber
• Advise patient to change positions slowly, orthostatic hypotension may occur
• Teach that suicidal thoughts, behavior may occur in young adults, children

Evaluation

Positive therapeutic outcome

• Decrease in depression
• Absence of suicidal thoughts
• Decreased symptoms of OCD

TREATMENT OF OVERDOSE:
Activated charcoal, supportive care

---

fluPHENAZine decanoate (Rx)
(floo-fen'ah-zeen)
Modecate ✤
fluPHENAZine hydrochloride (Rx)
Func. class.: Antipsychotic/neuroleptic
Chem. class.: Phenothiazine, piperazine
Pregnancy category C

ACTION: Depresses cerebral cortex, hypothalamus, limbic system, which control activity and aggression; blocks neurotransmission produced by dopamine at synapse; exhibits strong α-adrenergic and anticholinergic blocking action; mechanism for antipsychotic effects is unclear

Therapeutic outcome: Decreased signs and symptoms of psychosis

USES: Schizophrenia

Unlabeled uses: Agitation

CONTRAINDICATIONS:
Hypersensitivity, blood dyscrasias, coma, bone marrow depression, closed-angle glaucoma

Precautions: Pregnancy C, breastfeeding, children <12 yr, geriatric, seizure disorders, hypertension, hepatic/cardiac disease, abrupt discontinuation; accidental exposure, agranulocytosis, ambient temperature increase, angina, hypersensitivity to benzyl alcohol/parabens/sesame oil/tartrazine dye, QT prolongation, suicidal ideation, renal failure, Parkinson's disease, hypocalcemia, head trauma, prostatic hypertrophy, pulmonary disease, infection, ileus, chemotherapy, breast cancer

---

> **BLACK BOX WARNING:** Increased mortality in elderly patients with dementia-related psychosis

DOSAGE AND ROUTES

Decanoate

Adult and child >12 yr: IM/SUBCUT 12.5-25 mg q1-3wk, may increase slowly, max 100 mg/dose

HCl

Adult: PO 2.5-10 mg, in divided doses q6-8hr, max 40 mg/day; IM initially 1.25 mg then 2.5-10 mg in divided doses q6-8hr

Available forms: decanoate: inj 25 mg/ml; elixir 2.5 mg/5 ml; oral sol 5 mg/ml; **HCl:** tabs 1, 2.5, 5, 10 mg; inj 2.5 mg/ml

Implementation
PO route
• Give with food, milk, or a full glass of water to minimize gastric irritation
• Oral concentrate: Give using a calibrated measuring device. Dilute just before use with 120-240 ml of water, saline, milk, 7-Up, carbonated orange beverage, or the following juices: apricot, orange, pineapple, prune, tomato or V-8. Do not mix with beverages containing caffeine (coffee, cola), tannics (tea), or pectinates (apple juice) or with other liquid medications. Avoid spilling the solution on the skin and clothing
• Oral elixir: Give using a calibrated measuring device. Avoid spilling the solution on the skin and clothing

Injectable routes
• Visually inspect for particulate matter and discoloration prior to use; slight yellow to amber color does not alter potency, markedly discolored solutions should be discarded

IM route (fluPHENAZine HCl only)
• No dilution necessary, if irritation occurs, subsequent IM doses may be diluted with NS for injection or 2% procaine
• Inject slowly and deeply into the upper, outer quadrant of the gluteal muscle using a dry syringe and needle; aspirate prior to injection
• Keep patient in a recumbent position for at least 30 min following injection to minimize hypotensive effects
• Rotate the site of injection to avoid irritation or sterile abscess formation with repeat use

IM depot injection (fluPHENAZine decanoate or fluPHENAZine enanthate)
• FluPHENAZine decanoate or enanthate injections are administered via IM or subcut; do not use IV
• FluPHENAZine depot injections must be drawn up using a dry syringe and needle of at least 21-G; do not dilute
• Inject slowly and deeply into the upper outer quadrant of the gluteal muscle, aspirate
• Keep patient in a recumbent position for at least 30 min following the initial injection to minimize hypotensive effects; once dose-stabilized on depot formulation, this precaution may be modified
• Rotate the site of injection to avoid irritation or sterile abscess formation with repeat administration

Subcut injection route (fluPHENAZine decanoate or fluPHENAZine enanthate)
• FluPHENAZine decanoate or enanthate injections are administered via IM or SC injection only; do not administer intravenously
• FluPHENAZine depot injection solutions must be drawn up using a dry syringe and a needle of at least 21-G; do not dilute
• Inject subcut taking care not to inject intradermally
• Keep patient in a recumbent position for at least 30 min following the initial injection to minimize hypotensive effects. Once dose-stabilized on depot formulation, this precaution may be modified for ambulatory patients; rotate the injection sites

ADVERSE EFFECTS
CNS: *EPS, pseudoparkinsonism, akathisia, dystonia, tardive dyskinesia, drowsiness, headache,* **seizures, neuroleptic malignant syndrome,** drowsiness
CV: *Orthostatic hypotension,* hypertension, **cardiac arrest,** ECG changes, **tachycardia**
EENT: Blurred vision, glaucoma, dry eyes, nasal congestion
GI: *Dry mouth, nausea, vomiting, anorexia, constipation,* diarrhea, jaundice, weight gain, **paralytic ileus, hepatitis,** cholecystic jaundice
GU: Urinary retention, urinary frequency, enuresis, impotence, amenorrhea, gynecomastia
HEMA: Anemia, **leukopenia, leukocytosis, agranulocytosis, aplastic anemia, thrombocytopenia**
INTEG: *Rash,* photosensitivity, dermatitis, hyperpigmentation (long-term use)
RESP: **Laryngospasm,** dyspnea, **respiratory depression**

Pharmacokinetics

Absorption	Well absorbed (PO, IM)
Distribution	Widely absorbed, crosses blood-brain barrier, placenta
Metabolism	Liver, extensively, not dialyzable
Excretion	Kidneys (metabolites)
Half-life	HCl-4.7-15.3 hr, enanthate 3½-4 days, decanoate 6.8-14.3 days

Pharmacodynamics

	PO/IM	IM	IM
	HCl	Enanthate	Decanoate
Onset	1 hr	1-2 days	1-3 days
Peak	1½-2 hr	2-3 days	1-2 days
Duration	6-8 hr	1-3 wk	>4 wk

INTERACTIONS

Individual drugs

Alcohol, haloperidol, metyrosine, risperidone: increased effects of both products, oversedation

Amiodarone, ARIPiprazole, arsenic trioxide, astemizole, dasatinib, disopyramide, dofetilide, droperidol, erythromycin, flecainide, gatifloxacin, haloperidol, ibutilide, levomethadyl, lurasidone, ondansetron, paliperidone, palonosetron, pimozide, procainamide probucol, ranolazine, quiNIDine, sotalol, sparfloxacin, saquinavir, SUNItinib, vorinostat, ziprasidone: increased QT prolongation, torsades de pointes (at higher doses)

EPINEPHrine: increased toxicity

Levodopa: decreased antiparkinson activity

Lithium: decreased effects of lithium

Drug classifications

Anticholinergics: increased anticholinergic effects

Barbiturates: decreased effect of fluphenazine, oversedation

CNS depressants: oversedation

Smoking: decreased effects of fluphenazine

Drug/herb

Betel palm, kava: increased EPS

Cola tree, hops, kava, nettle, nutmeg: possible increased action

Henbane leaf: increased anticholinergic effect

Drug/lab test

Increased: liver function tests, cardiac enzymes, cholesterol, blood glucose, prolactin, bilirubin, cholinesterase

Decreased: hormones (blood and urine)

False positive: pregnancy tests, PKU, urinary steroids, 17-OHCS

NURSING CONSIDERATIONS

Assessment

• SSRIs, SNRIs, serotonin-receptor agonists: increased serotonin syndrome, malignant neuroleptic syndrome

> **BLACK BOX WARNING:** Increased mortality in elderly patients with dementia-related psychosis; not approved for this use

⚠ Serotonin syndrome, neuroleptic malignant syndrome: severe EPS, increased CPK, altered mental state, sinus tachycardia, change in B/P; sweating often occurs in young men; heat stress, physical exhaustion, dehydration, organic brain disease

• **QT prolongation, torsades de pointes:** ECG for changes

• Assess mental status: orientation, mood, behavior, presence and type of hallucinations before initial administration and monthly; this product should significantly reduce psychotic behavior

• Monitor bilirubin, CBC, liver function tests monthly; ophthalmic exams periodically

• Assess affect, orientation, LOC, reflexes, gait, coordination, sleep pattern disturbances

• Monitor B/P with patient sitting, standing, and lying down; take pulse and respirations q4hr during initial treatment; establish baseline before starting treatment; report drops of 30 mm Hg; obtain baseline ECG, Q-wave and T-wave changes

• Check for dizziness, faintness, palpitations, tachycardia on rising; severe orthostatic hypotension is common

• **Assess for EPS** including akathisia (inability to sit still, no pattern to movements), tardive dyskinesia (bizarre movements of the jaw, mouth, tongue, extremities), pseudoparkinsonism (rigidity, tremors, pill rolling, shuffling gait); an antiparkinson product should be prescribed

• Assess for constipation, urinary retention daily; if these occur, increase bulk, water in diet

Patient/family education

• Caution patient to avoid hazardous activities until product response is determined; dizziness, blurred vision may occur

• Inform patient that orthostatic hypotension occurs often and to rise from sitting or lying position gradually; tell patient to avoid hot tubs, hot showers, tub baths because hypotension may occur; tell patient that in hot weather, heat stroke may occur; extra precautions are necessary to stay cool

• Instruct patient to avoid abrupt withdrawal of this product, or EPS may result; product should be withdrawn slowly

• Advise patient that follow-up lab and ophthalmic exams are needed

• Teach patient to avoid OTC preparations (cough, hay fever, cold) unless approved by physician because serious product interactions may occur; avoid use with alcohol, CNS depressants; increased drowsiness may occur

• Instruct patient to use a sunscreen and sunglasses to prevent burns

• Teach patient about EPS and necessity of meticulous oral hygiene because oral candidiasis may occur

• Instruct patient to take antacids 2 hr before or after this product

• Advise patient to report sore throat, malaise, fever, bleeding, mouth sores; if these occur, CBC should be performed and product discontinued

Evaluation

Positive therapeutic outcome

• Decrease in emotional excitement, hallucinations, delusions, paranoia

• Reorganization of patterns of thought, speech

TREATMENT OF OVERDOSE:

Lavage if orally ingested; provide airway; *do not induce vomiting or use EPINEPHrine*

flurandrenolide topical
See Appendix B

flurbiprofen ophthalmic
See Appendix B

flutamide (Rx)
(floo′ta-mide)
Euflex ✹
Func. class.: Antineoplastic hormone
Chem. class.: Antiandrogen
Pregnancy category D

ACTION: Interferes with androgen uptake in the nucleus or androgen activity in target tissues; arrests tumor growth in androgen-sensitive tissue (i.e., prostate gland)

Therapeutic outcome: Prevention of rapidly growing malignant cells

USES: Metastatic prostatic carcinoma, stage D_2 in combination with LHRH agonistic analogs (leuprolide), B_2-C in combination with goserelin and radiation

CONTRAINDICATIONS:

Pregnancy **D**, hypersensitivity

> **BLACK BOX WARNING:** Severe hepatic disease

Precautions: G6PD deficiency, hemoglobinopathy, lactase deficiency, polycystic ovary syndrome, tobacco smoking

DOSAGE AND ROUTES

Adult: PO 250 mg q8hr for a daily dose of 750 mg

Available forms: Caps 125, 250 ✹ mg

Implementation

• Used in combination with LHRH agonist (leuprolide)

• Give without regard to food with a full glass of water

• Use cytotoxic handling procedures

ADVERSE EFFECTS

CNS: *Hot flashes,* drowsiness, confusion, depression, anxiety, paresthesia

GI: *Diarrhea, nausea, vomiting,* increased liver function studies, **hepatitis,** anorexia, **hepatotoxicity,** abdominal pain, cholestasis, **hepatic necrosis/failure**

GU: *Decreased libido, impotence, gynecomastia*

HEMA: Leukopenia, thrombocytopenia, hemolytic anemia

INTEG: Irritation at site, rash, photosensitivity

MISC: Edema, neuromuscular and pulmonary symptoms, hypertension, **secondary malignancy**

Pharmacokinetics	
Absorption	Well absorbed
Distribution	Unknown; protein binding
Metabolism	Liver
Excretion	Unknown
Half-life	6 hr

Pharmacodynamics

Onset	Unknown
Peak	2 hr
Duration	Unknown

INTERACTIONS
Individual drugs
Leuprolide: decreased flutamide action
Warfarin: increased PT

Drug/lab test
Increased: LFTs, BUN, creatinine
Decreased: WBC, platelets

NURSING CONSIDERATIONS
Assessment

> **BLACK BOX WARNING: Severe hepatic disease:** Monitor AST, ALT, alkaline phosphatase, which may be elevated; product may need to be discontinued; CBC, bilirubin, creatinine

• Identify CNS symptoms: drowsiness, confusion, depression, anxiety

Patient/family education
• Tell the patient to report side effects: decreased libido, impotence, breast enlargement, hot flashes, diarrhea, which occur when the two products are given together; **also nausea, vomiting; jaundice in eyes, skin; dark urine, clay-colored stools; hepatotoxicity may occur**
• Inform patient that this product is taken with leuprolide for medical castration; do not change dosing
⚠ Advise patient to use contraception during treatment, pregnancy D

Evaluation
Positive therapeutic outcome
• Prevention of rapid division of malignant cells

fluticasone (Rx)
(floo-tic′a-sone)
Flonase, Flovent HFA, Flovent Diskus ♣, Veramyst (nasal spray)
Func. class.: Corticosteroids, inhalation; antiasthmatic
Pregnancy category C

ACTION: Decreases inflammation by inhibiting mast cells, macrophages, and leukotrienes; antiinflammatory and vasoconstrictor properties

Therapeutic outcome: Decreased severity of asthma

USES: Prevention of chronic asthma during maintenance treatment in those requiring oral corticosteroids; nasal symptoms of seasonal/perennial and allergic/nonallergic rhinitis

CONTRAINDICATIONS:
Hypersensitivity to this product or milk protein, primary treatment in status asthmaticus, acute bronchospasm

Precautions: Pregnancy **C**, breastfeeding, active infections, glaucoma, diabetes, immunocompromised patients, Cushing syndrome

DOSAGE AND ROUTES
Prevention of chronic asthma during maintenance treatment in those requiring oral corticosteroids
Flovent HFA
Adult and child ≥12 yr: INH 88-440 mcg bid (in those previously taking bronchodilators alone); INH 88-220 mcg bid, max 440 mcg bid (in those previously taking inhaled corticosteroids); INH 440 mcg bid, max 880 mcg bid (in those previously taking oral corticosteroids)
Child 4-11 yr: INH 88 mg bid

Flovent Diskus ♣
Adult and child ≥12 yr: INH 100 mcg bid, max 500 mcg bid (in those previously taking bronchodilators alone); INH 100-250 mcg bid, max 500 mcg bid (in those previously taking inhaled corticosteroids); INH 500-1000 mcg bid, max 1000 mcg bid (in those previously taking oral corticosteroids)
Child 4-11 yr: INH initially 50 mcg bid, max 100 mcg bid (in those previously taking bronchodilators alone or inhaled corticosteroids)

Nasal symptoms of seasonal, perennial allergic, non-allergic rhinitis
Flonase
Adult: Nasal 2 sprays initially, in each nostril per day or 1 spray bid, when controlled, lower to 1 spray in each nostril per day
Adolescent/child >4 yr: Nasal 1 spray in each nostril per day, may increase to 2 sprays in each nostril per day, when controlled, lower to 1 spray in each nostril per day

Veramyst
Adult/child ≥12 yr: Nasal 2 sprays in each nostril per day
Child 2-11 yr: Nasal 1 spray in each nostril per day

Available forms: Oral inh aerosol 44, 110, 220 mcg; oral inh powder 50, 100, 250 mcg;

Adverse effects: *italics* = common; **bold** = life-threatening

nasal spray (Veramyst) 27.5 mcg/actuation, (Flonase) 50 mcg/actuation

Implementation

- Give at 1 min intervals
- Decrease dose to lowest effective dose after desired effect; decrease dose at 2- to 4-wk intervals
- Blow nose prior to use

Inhalation route: powder for oral inhalation (Flovent Diskus)

- Prior to initial use, remove the diskus foil pouch and throw away the foil pouch, the diskus will be in the closed position, fill in the "Pouch opened" and "Use by" dates in the blank lines on the label. The "Use by" date for Flovent diskus 50 mcg is 6 wk from the date the pouch is opened. The "Use by" date for diskus 100 mcg and 250 mcg is 2 months from the date pouch is opened
- Open the diskus by holding in one hand and using the thumb of the other to push the thumbgrip away as far as it will go until the mouthpiece shows and snaps into place
- Hold the diskus in a level, flat position with the mouthpiece toward the patient and slide the lever away from the patient as far as it will go until it clicks. The number on the dose counter will count down by 1; the diskus is now ready to use
- Before inhaling the dose, have patient breathe out as far as possible while holding the diskus level and away from the mouth. The patient should never breathe out into the mouthpiece
- Instruct the patient to put the mouthpiece to the lips and breathe in through the mouth quickly and deeply through the diskus. The patient should then remove the diskus from the mouth, hold breath for about 10 sec, and breathe out slowly
- After taking a dose, close the diskus by sliding the thumbgrip back as far as it will go. The diskus will click shut. The lever will automatically return to its original position
- The counter displays how many doses are left. The counter number will count down each time the patient uses the diskus. After 55 doses (23 doses from the sample pack), numbers 5 to 0 appear in red to warn that there are only a few doses left
- After use, instruct patient to rinse mouth with water and spit out the water; patient should not swallow it
- To avoid the spread of infection, do not use the inhaler for more than one person

Intranasal

- Prime before first use
- Shake well before each use
- Rinse tip after use, dry with tissue

ADVERSE EFFECTS

CNS: Fever, headache, nervousness, dizziness, fatigue, migraines, numbness in fingers
EENT: *Pharyngitis,* sinusitis, rhinitis, laryngitis, hoarseness, dry eyes, cataracts, nasal discharge, epistaxis, blurred vision
GI: Diarrhea, abdominal pain, nausea, vomiting, *oral candidiasis,* gastroenteritis
GU: UTI
INTEG: Urticaria, dermatitis
META: Hyperglycemia, growth retardation in children, cushingoid features
MISC: Influenza, **eosinophilic conditions, angioedema, Churg-Strauss syndrome,** adrenal insufficiency (high doses), bone mineral density reduction
MS: Osteoporosis, muscle soreness, joint pain, arthralgia
RESP: *Upper respiratory infection,* dyspnea, cough, bronchitis, **bronchospasm**

Pharmacokinetics

Absorption	30% aerosol, 13.5% powder
Distribution	Protein binding 91%
Metabolism	In liver after absorption in lung
Excretion	<5% in urine and feces
Half-life	7.8 hr

Pharmacodynamics

	Intranasal	INH
Onset	12 hr	24 hr
Peak	Several days	Several days
Duration	1-2 wk	1-2 wk

INTERACTIONS

Individual drugs

Amprenavir, atazanavir, darunavir, delavirdine, fosamprenavir, nelfinavir, ritonavir, saquinavir: increased fluticasone levels
Isoproterenol (asthma patients): increased cardiac toxicity
Mecasermin: decreased effects of mecasermin

Drug classifications

CYP3A4 inhibitors (ketoconazole, itraconazole): increased fluticasone levels
Growth hormones: decreased effects of growth hormones

Live vaccines: avoid concurrent use
Quinolones: increased tendinitis, tendon rupture

Drug/lab test
Increased: urine/serum glucose

NURSING CONSIDERATIONS
Assessment
• **Assess respiratory status:** lung sounds, pulmonary function tests during and several months after change from systemic to inhalation corticosteroids
• Assess for withdrawal symptoms from oral corticosteroids: depression, pain in joints, fatigue
⚠ **Monitor adrenal insufficiency: nausea, weakness, fatigue, hypotension, hypoglycemia, anorexia; may occur when changing from systemic to inhalation corticosteroids; may be life-threatening**
• Monitor growth rate in children; blood glucose, serum potassium in all patients
• Monitor adrenal function tests periodically: hypothalamic-pituitary-adrenal axis suppression in long-term treatment

Patient/family education
⚠ **Teach patient to report immediately cushingoid symptoms: no appetite, nausea, weakness, fatigue, decreased B/P**
• Advise patient to use bronchodilator first before using inhalation, if taking both
• Caution patient not to use for acute asthmatic attack; acute asthma may require oral corticosteroids
• Advise patient to avoid smoking, smoke-filled rooms, those with URIs, those not immunized against chickenpox or measles

Evaluation
Positive therapeutic outcome
• Decreased severity of asthma, COPD, allergies

---

fluticasone topical
See Appendix B

---

fluvastatin (Rx)
(flu′vah-stay-tin)
Lescol, Lescol XL
Func. class.: Antilipidemic
Chem. class.: HMG-CoA reductase inhibitor
Pregnancy category X

ACTION: Inhibits HMG-CoA reductase enzyme, which reduces cholesterol synthesis

Therapeutic outcome: Decreased cholesterol levels and LDLs, increased HDLs

USES: As an adjunct in primary hypercholesterolemia (types Ia, Ib), coronary atherosclerosis in CAD; secondary prevention of coronary events in patients with CAD; adjunct to diet to reduce LDL, total cholesterol, apo B levels in heterozygous familial hypercholesterolemia (LDL-C ≥190 mg/dl) or LDL-C >160 mg/dl with history of premature CV disease

CONTRAINDICATIONS:
Pregnancy **X**, breastfeeding, hypersensitivity, active liver disease

Precautions: Past liver disease, alcoholism, severe acute infections, trauma, hypotension, uncontrolled seizure disorders, severe metabolic disorders, electrolyte imbalance, myopathy, rhabdomyolysis

DOSAGE AND ROUTES
Adult: PO 20-40 mg/day in PM initially, usual range 20-80 mg, max 80 mg; may be given in 2 doses (40 mg AM, 40 mg PM); dosage adjustments may be made in 4-wk intervals or more

Heterozygous familial hypercholesterolemia
Adolescent ≥1 yr postmenarche (10-16 yr): PO 20 mg daily at bedtime, may increase q6wk, max 40 mg bid (cap) or 80 mg (ext rel)

Available forms: Caps 20, 40 mg; ext rel tab 80 mg

Implementation
• Give without regard to food at any time of day (tab) or in the evening (cap)
• Store at room temperature, protected from light

ADVERSE EFFECTS
CNS: Headache, dizziness, insomnia, confusion
EENT: Lens opacities
GI: *Nausea, constipation, diarrhea, abdominal pain, cramps, dyspepsia, flatus,* liver dysfunction, **pancreatitis**
HEMA: Thrombocytopenia, hemolytic anemia, leukopenia
INTEG: Rash, pruritus
MISC: Fatigue, influenza, photosensitivity
MS: Myalgia, *arthritis, arthralgia,* myositis, **rhabdomyolysis**

F

Pharmacokinetics

Absorption	Unknown
Distribution	Steady state 4-5 wk
Metabolism	Liver
Excretion	Feces, kidneys
Half-life	9 hr

Pharmacodynamics

Unknown

INTERACTIONS

Individual drugs

Alcohol, cimetidine, ranitidine, omeprazole: increased fluvastatin effect

Cholestyramine, colestipol: decreased fluvastatin effect; separate by ≥4 hr

Colchicine, cycloSPORINE, niacin: increased myopathy

Digoxin, phenytoin, warfarin: increased action

TraMADol: increased serotonin syndrome

Drug classifications

Fibric acid derivatives, protease inhibitors: increased myopathy

Drug/herb

Red yeast rice: increased adverse reactions

Gotu kola, St. John's wort: decreased effect

Drug/food

Grapefruit juice: possible increased fluvastatin toxicity

Drug/lab test

Increased: LFTs, CK

Decreased: platelets, WBC

NURSING CONSIDERATIONS

Assessment

• **Hypercholesterolemia:** Assess nutrition: fat, protein, carbohydrates; nutritional analysis should be completed by dietitian before treatment

• Assess fasting lipid profile (cholesterol, LDL, HDL, triglycerides) q4-6wk, then q3-6mo when stable

• Monitor bowel pattern daily; diarrhea may be a problem

• **Hepatotoxicity/pancreatitis:** Monitor liver function studies q1-2mo during the first 1½ yr of treatment; AST, ALT, liver function test results may be increased

• Monitor renal studies in patients with compromised renal system: BUN, I&O ratio, creatinine

• Obtain ophth exam before, 1 mo after treatment begins, annually; lens opacities may occur

• **Myopathy, rhabdomyolysis:** Assess for muscle pain, tenderness; obtain baseline CPK, if elevated or if symptoms occur, product should be discontinued

Patient/family education

• Inform patient that compliance is needed for positive results to occur, not to double doses

• Advise patient to notify prescriber if GI symptoms of diarrhea, abdominal or epigastric pain, nausea, vomiting, or if chills, fever, sore throat occur; also muscle pain, weakness, tenderness

• Advise patient that blood studies and eye exam will be necessary during treatment, that effect may take ≥4 wk

⚠ **Instruct patient to report suspected pregnancy, not to use during pregnancy (X)**

• Advise patient that previously prescribed regimen will continue, including diet, exercise, smoking cessation

• Instruct patient to notify all health care providers of products taken

• Teach patient to take without regard to meals, to take immediate release product in the evening, to separate by ≥4 hr with bile-acid product

Evaluation

Positive therapeutic outcome

• Decreased LDL, VLDL, total cholesterol levels

• Improved ratio of HDLs

folic acid (vitamin B₉) (PO, OTC; IM/IV, Ph)

(foe-lik a′sid)

Equaline Folic Acid, Folacin, Vitamin B₉, Walgreens Gold Seal Folic Acid

Func. class.: Vitamin B-complex group, water-soluble vitamin

Chem. class.: Supplement

Pregnancy category A

ACTION: Needed for erythropoiesis; increases RBC, WBC, and platelet formation in megaloblastic anemias

Therapeutic outcome: Absence of macrocytic, megaloblastic anemias

USES: Megaloblastic or macrocytic anemia caused by folic acid deficiency; liver disease; alcoholism; hemolysis; intestinal obstruction; pregnancy; to reduce risk of neural tube defect

CONTRAINDICATIONS:

Hypersensitivity

Precautions: Pregnancy **A**, anemias other than megaloblastic/macrocytic anemia, vit B$_{12}$ deficiency anemia, uncorrected pernicious anemia

DOSAGE AND ROUTES
RDA
Adult (pregnant/breastfeeding): PO 600 mcg/day
Adult and child ≥14 yr: PO 400 mcg
Child 9-13 yr: PO 300 mcg
Child 4-8 yr: PO 200 mcg
Child 1-3 yr: PO 150 mcg
Infant 6 mo-1 yr: PO 80 mcg
Neonate and infant <6 mo: PO 65 mcg

Megaloblastic/macrocytic anemia due to folic acid or nutritional deficiency
Pregnant/lactating: PO 800-1000 mcg

Therapeutic dose
Adult and child: PO/IM/SUBCUT/**IV** up to 1 mg/day

Maintenance dose
Adult and child >4 yr: PO/IM/**IV**/SUBCUT 0.4 mg/day
Child <4 yr: PO/IM/**IV**/SUBCUT up to 0.3 mg/day
Infant: PO/IM/**IV**/SUBCUT up to 0.1 mg/day
Pregnant/lactating: PO/IM/**IV**/SUBCUT 0.8-1 mg/day

Prevention of neural tube defects during pregnancy
Adult: PO 0.6 mg/day

Prevention of megaloblastic anemia during pregnancy
Adult: PO/IM/SUBCUT up to 1 mg/day during pregnancy

Tropical sprue
Adult: PO 3-15 mg/day

Available forms: Tabs 0.1, 0.4, 0.8, 1, 5 mg; inj 5, 10 mg/ml

Implementation
SUBCUT route
• Do not inject intradermally
IM route
• Inject deeply in large muscle mass, aspirate
Direct IV route
• Give **IV** directly, undiluted 5 mg or less over 1 min or more
Continuous IV route
• May be added to most **IV** sol or TPN
• Store in light-resistant container

ADVERSE EFFECTS
CNS: Confusion, depression, excitability, irritability
GI: Anorexia, nausea
INTEG: Flushing, pruritus, rash, erythema
RESP: Bronchospasm
SYST: Anaphylaxis (rare)

Pharmacokinetics
Absorption	Well absorbed
Distribution	Liver, crosses placenta
Metabolism	Liver (converted to active metabolite)
Excretion	Kidneys (unchanged)
Half-life	Unknown

Pharmacodynamics
Onset	Unknown
Peak	½-1 hr
Duration	Unknown

INTERACTIONS
Individual drugs
CarBAMazepine: increased need for folic acid
Fosphenytoin: decreased fosphenytoin levels, may increase seizures
Methotrexate, sulfaSALAzine, trimethoprim: decreased action of folic acid
Phenytoin: decreased phenytoin levels, may increase seizures

Drug classifications
Estrogens, glucocorticoids, hydantoins: increased need for folic acid
Sulfonamides: decreased action of folic acid

NURSING CONSIDERATIONS
Assessment
• **Megaloblastic anemia:** Assess patient for fatigue, dyspnea, weakness, activity intolerance (signs of megaloblastic anemia)
• Monitor Hgb, Hct, and reticulocyte count; folate levels: 6-15 mcg/ml baseline, throughout treatment
• Assess nutritional status: bran, yeast, dried beans, nuts, fruits, fresh vegetables, asparagus; if high folic acid foods are missing from the diet, a referral to a dietitian may be indicated
• Identify products currently taken: alcohol, oral contraceptives, estrogens, glucocorticoids, carBAMazepine, hydantoins, trimethoprim; these products may cause increased folic acid use by the body and contribute to deficiency if taking other neurotoxic products

Patient/family education
• Advise patient to take product exactly as prescribed; not to double doses, toxicity may occur
• Instruct patient to notify prescriber of side effects; rash or fever may indicate hypersensitivity
• Advise patient that urine may become more yellow
• Instruct patient to increase intake of foods rich in folic acid in diet as recommended by dietitian or health care provider
• Advise patient to avoid breastfeeding

Evaluation
Positive therapeutic outcome
• Absence of fatigue, weakness, dyspnea
• Absence of symptoms of megaloblastic anemia
• Increase in reticulocyte count within 5 days
• Absence of neural tube defect

⚠ HIGH ALERT

fondaparinux (Rx)
(fon-dah-pair'ih-nux)
Arixtra
Func. class.: Anticoagulant, antithrombotic
Chem. class.: Synthetic, selective factor Xa inhibitor
Pregnancy category B

Do not confuse:
Arixtra/Anti-Xa

ACTION: Inhibits factor Xa; interrupts blood coagulation and inhibits thrombin formation; does not inactivate thrombin (activated factor II) or affect platelets

Therapeutic outcome: Prevention of deep vein thrombosis

USES: Prevention/treatment of deep vein thrombosis, pulmonary emboli in hip and knee replacement, hip fracture or abdominal surgery, acute MI, unstable angina

CONTRAINDICATIONS:
Hypersensitivity to this product; hemophilia, leukemia with bleeding, peptic ulcer disease, hemorrhagic stroke, surgery, thrombocytopenic purpura, weight <50 kg, severe renal disease (CCr <30 ml/min), active major bleeding, bacterial endocarditis

Precautions: Pregnancy **B**, breastfeeding, children, geriatric, alcoholism, hepatic disease (severe), blood dyscrasias, heparin-induced thrombocytopenia, uncontrolled severe hypertension, acute nephritis, mild to moderate renal disease

> **BLACK BOX WARNING:** Spinal/epidural anesthesia, lumbar puncture

DOSAGE AND ROUTES
Deep vein thrombosis/PE
Adult <50 kg: SUBCUT 5 mg/day × 5 days or more until INR is 2-3; give warfarin within 72 hr of fondaparinux
Adult 50-100 kg: SUBCUT 7.5 mg/day × 5 days or more until INR is 2-3; give warfarin within 72 hr of fondaparinux
Adult >100 kg: SUBCUT 10 mg/day × 5 days or more until INR is 2-3; give warfarin within 72 hr of fondaparinux

Prevention of deep vein thrombosis
Adult: SUBCUT 2.5 mg/day, given 6 hr after surgery (hemostasis established); continue for 5-9 days; hip surgery up to 32 days; abdominal surgery up to 24 days

Renal disease
Adult: Do not use if CCr <30 ml/min; CCr 30-50 ml/min, use cautiously

Available forms: Inj 2.5 mg/0.5 ml, 5 mg/0.4 ml, 7.5 mg/0.6 ml, 10 mg/0.8 ml prefilled syringes

Implementation
• Do not mix with other products or solutions; cannot be used interchangeably (unit to unit) with other anticoagulants
• Give only after screening patient for bleeding disorders
• Store at 77° F (25° C); do not freeze
SUBCUT route
• Administer SUBCUT only; do not give IM
• Check for discolored sol or sol with particulate; if present, do not give
• Administer to recumbent patient, rotate inj sites (left/right anterolateral, left/right posterolateral abdominal wall), administer 6-8 hr after surgery
• Wipe surface of inj site with alcohol swab, twist plunger cap and remove, remove rigid needle guard by pulling straight off needle, do not aspirate, do not expel air bubble from surface
• Insert whole length of needle into skin fold held with thumb and forefinger
• When product is injected, a soft click may be felt or heard
• Give at same time each day to maintain steady blood levels

- Avoid all IM inj that may cause bleeding
⚠ Administer only this product when ordered; not interchangeable with heparin

ADVERSE EFFECTS
CNS: *Fever,* confusion, headache, dizziness, *insomnia*
GI: *Nausea, vomiting,* diarrhea, dyspepsia, *constipation,* increased AST, ALT
GU: UTI, urinary retention
HEMA: *Anemia,* minor bleeding, purpura, hematoma, **thrombocytopenia, major bleeding (intracranial, cerebral, retroperitoneal hemorrhage), postoperative hemorrhage, heparin-induced thrombocytopenia**
INTEG: Local reaction—*rash,* pruritus, inj site bleeding, increased wound drainage, bullous eruption
META: Hypokalemia
MISC: Hypotension, pain, *edema*

Pharmacokinetics

Absorption	Rapidly, completely absorbed
Distribution	Blood; does not bind to plasma proteins except 94% to ATIII
Excretion	Eliminated unchanged in 72 hr in normal renal function
Half-life	17-21 hr

Pharmacodynamics

Onset	Unknown
Peak	3 hr
Duration	Unknown

INTERACTIONS
Do not mix with other products or inf fluids

Individual drugs
Abciximab, clopidogrel, dipyridamole, eptifibatide, quiNIDine, tirofiban, valproic acid: increased risk of bleeding

Drug classifications
NSAIDs, salicylates: increased risk of bleeding

Drug/herb
Feverfew, garlic, ginger, ginkgo, ginseng, green tea, horse chestnut, kava: increased risk of bleeding

NURSING CONSIDERATIONS
Assessment

BLACK BOX WARNING: Monitor patients who have received epidural/spinal anesthesia or lumbar puncture for neurological impairment

- **Hemorrhage:** Assess for hemorrhage if coadministered with other products that may cause bleeding
- Assess blood studies (Hct, CBC, coagulation studies, platelets, occult blood in stools), anti-Xa; if platelets <100,000/mm³, treatment should be discontinued; renal studies: BUN, creatinine
- Assess for bleeding: gums, petechiae, ecchymosis, black tarry stools, hematuria; notify prescriber

Patient/family education
- Advise patient to use soft-bristle toothbrush to avoid bleeding gums, to use electric razor
- Advise patient to report any signs of bleeding: gums, under skin, urine, stools
- Caution patient to avoid OTC products containing aspirin, NSAIDs

Evaluation
Positive therapeutic outcome
- Absence of deep vein thrombosis

formoterol (Rx)
(for-moh′ter-ahl)
Foradil Aerolizer, Oxeze ✦, Perforomist
Func. class.: β-Adrenergic agonist
Chem. class.: Sympathomimetic catecholamine
Pregnancy category C

Do not confuse:
Foradil/Toradol

ACTION: Has β_1 and β_2 action; relaxes bronchial smooth muscle and dilates the trachea and main bronchi by increasing levels of cyclic AMP, which relaxes smooth muscles; causes increased contractility and heart rate by acting on β-receptors in the heart

Therapeutic outcome: Bronchodilation, increased heart rate and cardiac output from action on β-receptors in heart

USES: Maintenance, treatment of asthma, COPD, prevention of exercise-induced bronchospasm

CONTRAINDICATIONS:
Hypersensitivity to sympathomimetics, monotherapy for asthma, COPD, status asthmaticus

Precautions: Pregnancy **C**, geriatric, cardiac disorders, hyperthyroidism, diabetes

---

mellitus, prostatic hypertrophy, hypertension, African descendants

BLACK BOX WARNING: Asthma-related death

DOSAGE AND ROUTES
Maintenance, treatment of asthma
Adult and child ≥5 yr: INH AM and PM long-term, 1 cap (12 mcg) q12hr using aerolizer inhaler

Maintenance of COPD
Adult: INH 12 mcg q12hr

Prevention of exercise-induced bronchospasm
Adult and child ≥12 yr: INH prn 1 cap (12 mcg) at least 15 min before exercise, do not use additional doses for ≥12 hr

Available forms: INH powder in cap 12 mcg; nebulizer sol for inhalation 20 mcg/2 ml

Implementation
• Store at room temperature; protect from heat, moisture
Inhalation route
• Place cap in aerolizer inhaler; the cap is punctured; do not wash aerolizer inhaler
• Pull off cover, twist mouthpiece to open, push buttons in; make sure the four pins are visible; remove cap from blister pack, place cap in chamber; twist to close, press (a click will be heard), release; patient should exhale, place inhaler in mouth, inhale rapidly

ADVERSE EFFECTS
CNS: Tremors, *anxiety*, insomnia, headache, dizziness, stimulation
CV: Palpitations, tachycardia, hypertension, chest pain
GI: Nausea, vomiting, xerostomia
RESP: Bronchial irritation, dryness of oro-pharynx, **bronchospasms (overuse);** infection, inflammatory reactions (child)

Pharmacokinetics

Absorption	Rapid (INH)
Distribution	Plasma protein binding 61%-64% at concentrations of 0.1-100 ng/mL; 31%-38% at concentrations of 5-500 ng/mL
Metabolism	Liver, lungs, GI tract
Excretion	Urine, feces
Half-life	10 hr mean terminal elimination half-life

Pharmacodynamics

Onset	Unknown
Peak	5 min (INH)
Duration	Unknown

INTERACTIONS
Amoxapine, arsenic trioxide, chloroquine, clarithromycin, dasatinib, dolasetron, droperidol, erythromycin, halofantrine, levomethadyl, ondansetron, paliperidone, palonosetron, pentamidine, probucol, ranolazine, SUNItinib, vorinostat, pimozide, risperidone, ziprasidone: increased QT prolongation

Drug classifications
Class IA/III antidysrhythmics, pheno-thiazines, halogenated anesthetics, tricyclics, some quinolones: increase QT prolongation
β-blockers: decreased action of formoterol
MAOIs, antidepressants (tricyclics): serious dysrhythmias
Sympathomimetics, thyroid hormones, tricyclics, some quinolones: increased action of both products
Loop/thiazide diuretics: increased hypokalemia

NURSING CONSIDERATIONS
Assessment
• Assess respiratory function: B/P, pulse, lung sounds
• Assess I&O ratio; check for urinary retention, frequency, hesitancy
• Assess for paresthesias and coldness of extremities; peripheral blood flow may decrease

Patient/family education
• Review package insert with patient and inform about all aspects of product
• Teach correct use of inhaler; not to swallow caps
• Teach use of spacer device in children or geriatric
• Advise patient to avoid getting aerosol in eyes
• Instruct patient to rinse mouth after use
• Advise patient to wash inhaler in warm water and dry daily
• Advise patient to avoid smoking, smoke-filled rooms, persons with respiratory infections
• Asthma-related death, severe asthma exacerbations: if wheezing worsens and cannot be relieved during an acute asthma attack, immediate medical attention should be sought

---

⚠ Nurse Alert   ✴ Key NCLEX® Drug

Evaluation
Positive therapeutic outcome
- Absence of dyspnea, wheezing
- Improved airway exchange
- Improved ABGs

TREATMENT OF OVERDOSE:
Administer β-blocker

fosamprenavir (Rx)
(fos-am-pren′a-veer)
Lexiva, Telzin ✦
Func. class.: Antiretroviral
Chem. class.: Protease inhibitor
Pregnancy category C

ACTION: Prodrug of amprenavir; inhibits human immunodeficiency virus (HIV) protease, which prevents maturation of the infectious virus

Therapeutic outcome: Decreasing symptoms of HIV

USES: HIV-1 infection in combination with antiretrovirals

CONTRAINDICATIONS:
Hypersensitivity to protease inhibitors

Precautions: Pregnancy **C**, breastfeeding, geriatric, liver disease, hemolytic anemia, diabetes, sulfa sensitivity, autoimmune disease with immune reconstitution

DOSAGE AND ROUTES
Therapy-naïve patients
Adult: PO 1400 mg bid without ritonavir, or fosamprenavir 1400 mg/day and ritonavir 200 mg/day, or fosamprenavir 700 mg bid and ritonavir 100 mg bid
Adolescent/child/infant ≥4 wk: PO 30 mg/kg bid, max 1400 mg/dose, without ritonavir

Protease-experienced patients (PI)
Adult: PO 700 mg bid and ritonavir 100 mg bid
Adolescent/child ≥20 kg: PO 18 mg/kg bid with ritonavir 3 mg/kg bid
Adolescent/child 15 kg to <20 kg: PO 23 mg/kg bid with ritonavir 3 mg/kg bid
Adolescent/child 11 kg to <15 kg: PO 30 mg/kg bid with ritonavir 3 mg/kg bid
Adolescent/child <11 kg: PO 45 mg bid with ritonavir 7 mg bid
Infant ≥6 mo, 15 kg to <20 kg: PO susp 23 mg/kg bid with ritonavir 3 mg/kg bid
Infant ≥6 mo, 11 kg to <15 kg: PO susp 30 mg/kg bid with ritonavir 3 mg/kg bid

Infant ≥6 mo, <11 kg: PO susp 45 mg/kg bid with ritonavir 7 mg/kg bid

Combination with efavirenz
Adult: PO add another 100 mg/day of ritonavir for a total of 300 mg/day when all three products are given

Hepatic dose
Adult: PO (Child-Pugh 5-6) 700 mg bid without ritonavir (treatment-naive patients) or 700 mg bid with ritonavir 100 mg qd (treatment-naive or experienced patients); (Child-Pugh 7-9) 700 mg bid without ritonavir (treatment-naive patients) or 450 mg bid with ritonavir 100 mg qd (treatment-naive or experienced patients); (Child-Pugh 10-15) 350 mg bid without ritonavir (treatment-naive patients) or 300 mg bid with ritonavir 100 mg qd (treatment-naive or experienced patients)

Available forms: Tabs 700 mg (equivalent to 600 mg amprenavir); oral suspension 50 mg/ml

Implementation
- **Tabs:** Administer without regard to food
- **Oral susp:** *Adult:* give without food; *child:* give with food; if vomiting occurs within 30 min, readminister; shake oral susp vigorously prior to dosing, use calibrated device
- Patients receiving phosphodiesterase type 5 (PDE5) inhibitors may be at increased risk for PDE5 inhibitor adverse effects

ADVERSE EFFECTS
CNS: Headache, fatigue, depression, oral paresthesia
GI: *Nausea, diarrhea, vomiting, abdominal pain*
INTEG: Rash, pruritus
MISC: Redistribution or accumulation of body fat, hyperglycemia, **Stevens-Johnson syndrome**

Pharmacokinetics
Absorption	Unknown
Distribution	90% protein binding
Metabolism	In the liver by CYP3A4
Excretion	Excretion of unchanged product is minimal
Half-life	Unknown

Pharmacodynamics
Onset	Unknown
Peak	1½-4 hr
Duration	Unknown

Adverse effects: *italics* = common; **bold** = life-threatening

INTERACTIONS
Individual drugs
⚠ **Amiodarone, flecainide, lidocaine, midazolam, pimozide, propafenone, triazolam: serious life-threatening reactions**

CarBAMazepine, dexamethasone, efavirenz, lopinavir/ritonavir, nevirapine, phenytoin, ranitidine, saquinavir: decreased fosamprenavir levels, avoid concurrent use

ARIPiprazole, itraconazole, ketoconazole, rifabutin, sildenafil, vardenafil: increased effect

Methadone: decreased effect

Warfarin: increased effect of warfarin

Ritonavir with boceprevir or ritonavir with telaprevir not recommended: increased treatment failure

Decreased dose of maraviroc with product is used with ritonavir; do not use maraviroc with unboosted fosamprenavir

Drug classifications
Antacids: decreased fosamprenavir levels

⚠ **Barbiturates, proton-pump inhibitors, calcium channel blockers, ergots, H₂ receptor antagonists: serious life-threatening reactions**

Contraceptives (oral): decreased effect

Estrogens, H₂ receptor antagonists, oral contraceptives, proton-pump inhibitors: avoid use; may lose virologic response and possibly lead to resistance of fosamprenavir

HMG-CoA reductase inhibitors: increased toxicity

Drug/herb
Avoid use with St. John's wort, may lose virologic response and possibly lead to resistance of fosamprenavir

Drug/lab test
Increased: serum glucose, AST, ALT, triglycerides

NURSING CONSIDERATIONS
Assessment
• Assess bowel pattern before, during treatment; monitor hydration
• Assess skin eruptions, rash, urticaria, itching
• **HIV:** Monitor viral load, CD4 cell counts, plasma HIV RNA, serum cholesterol, lipid profile baseline, throughout treatment
⚠ **Stevens-Johnson syndrome: report immediately**
⚠ **Immune reconstitution syndrome: may occur with combination antiretroviral therapy; autoimmune disease may also develop, up to months after treatment starts**

Patient/family education
• Advise patient to avoid taking product with other medications unless directed by provider
• Teach patient that product does not cure, but does manage symptoms; that product does not prevent transmission of HIV to others
• Advise patient to use nonhormonal form of birth control while taking this product
• Instruct patient if dose is missed, take as soon as remembered up to 1 hr before next dose; do not double dose
• Instruct patient not to alter dose or stop therapy without talking to physician
• Advise physician if patient has a sulfa allergy
• Advise patient to report all medications, including herbal supplements, to prescriber

Evaluation
Positive therapeutic outcome
• Decreasing symptoms of HIV

---

foscarnet (Rx)
(foss-kar′net)
Foscavir
Func. class.: Antiviral
Chem. class.: Inorganic pyrophosphate organic analog
Pregnancy category C

ACTION: Antiviral activity is produced by selective inhibition at the pyrophosphate binding site on virus-specific DNA polymerases and reverse transcriptases at concentrations that do not affect cellular DNA polymerases

Therapeutic outcome: Virostatic agents against CMV retinitis

USES: Treatment of CMV, retinitis, herpes simplex virus (HSV) infections; used with ganciclovir for relapsing patients

CONTRAINDICATIONS: Hypersensitivity, CCr <0.4 ml/min/kg

Precautions: Pregnancy **C,** breastfeeding, children, geriatric, seizure disorders, severe anemia

> **BLACK BOX WARNING:** Renal disease, electrolyte/mineral imbalances

---

DOSAGE AND ROUTES

Acyclovir-resistant mucocutaneous herpes simplex virus infection (herpes labialis, herpes febrilis, herpes genitalis) in HIV-infected patients

Adult/adolescent (unlabeled): IV 40 mg/kg q8-12hr × 2-3 wk or until lesions are healed

Cytomegalovirus (CMV) encephalitis (unlabeled); cytomegalovirus (CMV) neurological disease (unlabeled) (including encephalitis) in HIV-infected patients

Adult/adolescent: IV 90 mg/kg q12hr or 60 mg/kg q8hr × 3 wk (or until symptomatic improvement) with ganciclovir 5 mg/kg IV q12hr × 2-3 wk

Encephalitis (unlabeled) caused by human herpesvirus 6 (HHV-6) in immunocompromised patients

Adult: IV 60 mg/kg q8hr or 90 mg/kg q12hr alone or in combination with ganciclovir 5 mg/kg IV q12hr

Cytomegalovirus (CMV) retinitis or disseminated disease (unlabeled) in HIV-infected patients, recurrent or relapsed cytomegalovirus (CMV) retinitis in HIV-infected patients

Adult: IV Induction with 90 mg/kg q12hr or 60 mg/kg IV q8hr for 14-21 days, depending upon the clinical response

Renal dose

Adult: HSV induction dosage equivalent to 80 mg/kg/day (40 mg/kg IV q12hr)

Adult: IV CCr >1.4 ml/min/kg: no change; CCr >1-1.4 ml/min/kg: decrease to 30 mg/kg q12hr; CCr >0.8-1 ml/min/kg: decrease to 20 mg/kg q12hr; CCr >0.6-0.8 ml/min/kg: decrease to 35 mg/kg/day; CCr >0.5-0.6 ml/min/kg: decrease to 25 mg/kg/day; CCr ≥0.4-0.5 ml/min/kg: decrease to 20 mg/kg/day; CCr <0.4 ml/min/kg: not recommended

HSV induction dosage equivalent to 120 mg/kg/day (40 mg/kg IV q8hr)

Adult: IV CCr >1.4 ml/min/kg: no change; CCr >1-1.4 ml/min/kg: decrease to 30 mg/kg q8hr; CCr >0.8-1 ml/min/kg: decrease to 35 mg/kg q12hr; CCr >0.6-0.8 ml/min/kg: decrease to 25 mg/kg q12hr; CCr >0.5-0.6 ml/min/kg: decrease to 40 mg/kg/day; CCr ≥0.4-0.5 ml/min/kg: decrease to 35 mg/kg/day; CCr <0.4 ml/min/kg: not recommended

CMV induction dosage equivalent to 180 mg/kg/day (60 mg/kg q8hr)

Adult: IV CCr >1.4 ml/min/kg: no change; CCr >1-1.4 ml/min/kg: decrease to 45 mg/kg q8hr; CCr >0.8-1 ml/min/kg: decrease to 50 mg/kg q12hr; CCr >0.6-0.8 ml/min/kg: decrease to 40 mg/kg q12hr; CCr >0.5-0.6 ml/min/kg: decrease to 60 mg/day; CCr ≥0.4-0.5 ml/min/kg: decrease to 50 mg/kg/day; CCr <0.4 ml/min/kg: not recommended

CMV induction dosage equivalent to 180 mg/kg/day (90 mg/kg IV q12hr)

Adult: IV CCr >1.4 ml/min/kg: no change; CCr >1-1.4 ml/min/kg: decrease to 70 mg/kg q12hr; CCr >0.8-1 ml/min/kg: decrease to 50 mg/kg q12hr; CCrl >0.6-0.8 ml/min/kg: decrease to 80 mg/kg/day; CCr >0.5-0.6 ml/min/kg: decrease to 60 mg/kg/day; CCr ≥0.4-0.5 ml/min/kg: decrease to 50 mg/kg/day; CCr <0.4 ml/min/kg: not recommended

Available forms: Inj 6000 mg/250 ml, 12,000 mg/500 ml (24 mg/ml)

Implementation

Intermittent IV infusion route

• Administer increased fluids before, during product administration to induce diuresis and minimize renal toxicity

• Administer via inf pump, at no more than 1 mg/kg/min; do not give by rapid or bolus IV; give by central venous line or peripheral vein; standard 24 mg/ml sol may be used without dilution if using by central line; dilute the 24 mg/ml sol to 12 mg/ml with D₅W or 0.9% NaCl if using peripheral vein

• Monitor patient closely during therapy; if tingling, numbness, paresthesias occur, stop inf and obtain lab sample for electrolytes

Y-site incompatibilities: Manufacturer recommends that product not be given with other medications in syringe or admixed

ADVERSE EFFECTS

CNS: *Fever,* dizziness, *headache,* **seizures,** *fatigue,* neuropathy, asthenia, encephalopathy, malaise, meningitis, *paresthesia,* depression, *confusion, anxiety*

CV: ECG abnormalities, 1st-degree AV block, nonspecific ST-T segment changes, cerebrovascular disorder, cardiomyopathy, **cardiac arrest,** atrial fibrillation, CHF, sinus tachycardia

GI: *Nausea, vomiting, diarrhea, anorexia,* abdominal pain, **pancreatitis**

GU: **Acute renal failure,** decreased CCr and increased serum creatinine, azotemia, diabetes mellitus
HEMA: Anemia, **granulocytopenia, leukopenia, thrombocytopenia, thrombosis,** lymphadenopathy, neutropenia
INTEG: *Rash,* sweating, pruritus, skin discoloration
RESP: *Coughing, dyspnea,* pneumonia, **pulmonary infiltration, pneumothorax, hemoptysis**
SYST: *Hypokalemia, hypocalcemia, hypomagnesemia,* hypophosphatemia

Pharmacokinetics

Absorption	Complete (**IV**)
Distribution	14%-17% plasma protein binding
Metabolism	Not metabolized
Excretion	Kidneys (79%-92%) unchanged, breast milk
Half-life	18-88 hr; increased in renal disease

Pharmacodynamics

Onset	48 hr
Peak	2 wk
Duration	Unknown

INTERACTIONS

Individual drugs
Acyclovir, cidofovir, CISplatin, penicillamine, tacrolimus, tenofovir, vancomycin, amphotericin B, cycloSPORINE, lithium: increased nephrotoxicity
Pentamidine: increased hypocalcemia

Drug classifications

> **BLACK BOX WARNING:** Aminoglycosides, gold compounds, NSAIDs: increased nephrotoxicity

NURSING CONSIDERATIONS

Assessment
• **General** culture should be done before treatment with foscarnet is begun; cultures of blood, urine, and throat may all be taken; CMV is not confirmed by this method; the diagnosis is made by an ophth exam

> **BLACK BOX WARNING: Renal tubular disorders:** Assess kidney: BUN, serum creatinine, creatinine clearance, if CCr <0.4 ml/min/kg, discontinue product

• Blood counts should be done q2wk; watch for decreasing granulocytes, Hgb; if low, therapy may have to be discontinued and restarted after hematologic recovery; blood transfusions may be required
• Assess for GI symptoms: severe nausea, vomiting, diarrhea; severe symptoms may necessitate discontinuing product
• Monitor electrolytes and minerals: calcium, phosphorous, magnesium, sodium, potassium; watch closely for tetany during first administration
⚠ Assess for symptoms of blood dyscrasias (anemia, granulocytopenia); bruising, fatigue, bleeding, poor healing
• **Assess for symptoms of allergic reactions:** flushing, rash, urticaria, pruritus
CMV retinitis
• Culture should be done prior to treatment (blood, urine, throat); a negative culture does not rule out CMV; ophthalmic exam should confirm diagnosis

Patient/family education
• Advise patient to notify prescriber if sore throat, swollen lymph nodes, malaise, fever occur; may indicate presence of other infections
• Advise patient to report perioral tingling, numbness in extremities, and paresthesias; inf should be stopped and electrolytes should be requested
• Caution patient that serious product interactions may occur if OTC products are ingested; check first with prescriber
• Inform patient that product is not a cure but will control symptoms
• Advise patient that ophth exams must be continued

Evaluation
Positive therapeutic outcome
• Improvement in CMV retinitis

---

fosinopril (Rx)

(foss-in-o′pril)
Monopril
Func. class.: Antihypertensive
Chem. class.: Angiotensin-converting enzyme (ACE) inhibitor
Pregnancy category D

Do not confuse:
Monopril/minoxidil/Accupril/Monoket

ACTION: Selectively suppresses renin-angiotensin-aldosterone system; inhibits ACE; prevents conversion of angiotensin I to angioten-

---

sin II; results in dilatation of arterial, venous vessels

Therapeutic outcome: Decreased B/P in hypertension

USES: Hypertension, alone or in combination with thiazide diuretics, systolic CHF

CONTRAINDICATIONS:
Breastfeeding, children, hypersensitivity to ACE inhibitors, history of ACE inhibitor–induced angioedema

> **BLACK BOX WARNING:** Pregnancy **D**

Precautions: Geriatric, impaired liver function, hypovolemia, blood dyscrasias, CHF, COPD, asthma, angioedema, hyperkalemia, renal artery stenosis, renal disease, aortic stenosis, autoimmune disorders, collagen vascular disease, febrile illness

DOSAGE AND ROUTES
Hypertension
Adult: PO 5-10 mg/day initially, then 20-40 mg/day divided bid or daily, max 80 mg/day

CHF
Adult: PO 10 mg/day, then up to 40 mg/day, increased over several weeks; use lower dose in those undergoing diuresis before fosinopril

Available forms: Tabs 10, 20, 40 mg

Implementation
• Store in tight container at 86° F (30° C)
• Severe hypotension may occur after 1st dose of this medication; hypotension may be prevented by reducing or discontinuing diuretic therapy 3 days before beginning benzapril therapy

ADVERSE EFFECTS
CNS: *Headache, dizziness,* fatigue, syncope
CV: *Hypotension,* orthostatic hypotension, tachycardia
GI: *Nausea,* constipation, *vomiting,* diarrhea, **hepatotoxicity, cholestatic jaundice, fulminant hepatic necrosis, hepatic failure, death**
GU: Increased BUN, creatinine, azotemia, **renal artery stenosis**
HEMA: Decreased Hct, Hgb, **eosinophilia, leukopenia, neutropenia, agranulocytosis**
META: *Hyperkalemia*
RESP: *Cough*
SYST: **Anaphylaxis, angioedema**

Pharmacokinetics
Absorption	30%
Distribution	Crosses placenta
Metabolism	Liver, converted to fosinoprilat
Excretion	50% kidneys (metabolites), 50% feces
Half-life	12 hr: fosinoprilat

Pharmacodynamics
Onset	1 hr
Peak	2-6 hr
Duration	24 hr

INTERACTIONS
Individual drugs
Alcohol (acute ingestion): increased hypotension (large amounts)
Digoxin, hydrALAZINE, lithium, prazosin: increased toxicity

Drug classifications
Adrenergic blockers, antihypertensives, diuretics, ganglionic blockers, nitrates: increased hypotension
Antacids: decreased absorption
Diuretics (potassium-sparing), sympathomimetics, NSAIDs, vasodilators: increased toxicity
Salicylates: decreased antihypertensive effect

Drug/herb
Hawthorn: increased antihypertensive effect
Ephedra: decreased antihypertensive effect

Drug/lab test
Increased: AST, ALT, alkaline phosphatase, glucose, bilirubin, uric acid
Positive: ANA titer
False positive: urine acetone

NURSING CONSIDERATIONS
Assessment
• **Hypertension:** Monitor B/P, check for orthostatic hypotension, syncope; if changes occur, dosage change may be required
⚠ **Collagen vascular disease: Monitor blood studies: neutrophils, decreased platelets; obtain WBC with differential at baseline and qmo × 6 mo, then q2-3mo × 1 yr; if neutrophils <1000/mm³, discontinue**
• Monitor renal studies: protein, BUN, creatinine; watch for increased levels that may indicate nephrotic syndrome and renal failure; monitor urine daily for protein; monitor renal symptoms: polyuria, oliguria, frequency, dysuria

Adverse effects: *italics* = common; **bold** = life-threatening

- Establish baselines in renal, liver function tests before therapy begins
- Check potassium levels throughout treatment although hyperkalemia rarely occurs
- **CHF:** Check for edema in feet, legs daily, monitor weight daily
- **Assess for allergic reactions:** rash, fever, pruritus, urticaria; product should be discontinued if antihistamines fail to help

Patient/family education

- Advise patient not to discontinue product abruptly; warn patient to tell all persons associated with his or her care
- Teach patient not to use OTC products (cough, cold, allergy) unless directed by prescriber because serious side effects can occur; xanthines such as coffee, tea, chocolate, cola can prevent action of product
- Teach patient the importance of complying with dosage schedule, even if feeling better; to continue with medical regimen to decrease B/P: exercise, smoking cessation, decreasing stress, diet modifications
- Emphasize the need to rise slowly to sitting or standing position to minimize orthostatic hypotension; not to exercise in hot weather or increased hypotension can occur
- Advise patient to notify prescriber of mouth sores, sore throat, fever, swelling of hands or feet, irregular heartbeat, chest pain, coughing, shortness of breath
- Instruct patient to report excessive perspiration, dehydration, vomiting, diarrhea; may lead to fall in B/P
- Caution patient that product may cause dizziness, fainting, light-headedness; may occur during 1st few days of therapy; to avoid activities that may be hazardous
- Teach patient how to take B/P, normal readings for age-group

> **BLACK BOX WARNING:** Advise patient to notify prescriber if pregnancy is planned or suspected, pregnancy **D**

Evaluation

Positive therapeutic outcome
- Decreased B/P in hypertension

TREATMENT OF OVERDOSE:
0.9% NaCl **IV** inf, hemodialysis

fosphenytoin (Rx)
(foss-fen′i-toy-in)
Func. class.: Anticonvulsant
Chem. class.: Hydantoin, phosphate phenytoin ester
Pregnancy category D

ACTION: Inhibits spread of seizure activity in motor cortex by altering ion transport; increases AV conduction; prodrug of phenytoin

Therapeutic outcome: Decreased seizures, absence of dysrhythmias

USES: Generalized tonic-clonic seizures, status epilepticus, partial seizures

CONTRAINDICATIONS:
Pregnancy **D**, hypersensitivity, bradycardia, SA and AV block, Stokes-Adams syndrome

Precautions: Breastfeeding, allergies, renal/hepatic disease, myocardial insufficiency, hypoalbuminemia, hypothyroidism, Asian patients positive for HLA-B 1502, abrupt discontinuation, agranulocytosis, alcoholism, carBAMazepine/barbiturate hypersensitivity, bone marrow suppression, CAD, geriatrics, hemolytic anemia, hyponatremia, methemoglobinemia, myasthenia gravis, psychosis, suicidal ideation

> **BLACK BOX WARNING:** Rapid IV infusion

DOSAGE AND ROUTES
All doses in PE (phenytoin sodium equivalent)

Status epilepticus
Adult and adolescent: **IV** 15-20 mg PE/kg

Nonemergency/maintenance dosing
Adult and adolescent >16 yr: **IM/IV** 10-20 mg PE/kg 10 mg dose; 4-6 mg PE/kg/day (maintenance); start maintenance 12 hr after loading dose; give in 2-3 divided doses

Available forms: Inj 150 mg (100 mg PE), 750 mg (500 mg PE), 50 mg/ml vials

Implementation
Injectable routes
- Give IM/IV; the dosage, concentration, and infusion rate of fosphenytoin should always be expressed, prescribed, and dispensed in phenytoin sodium equivalents (PE); exercise extreme caution when preparing and administering fosphenytoin; the concentration and dosage should be carefully confirmed; fatal overdoses have occurred in children when the per-ml

concentration of the product (50 mg PE/mL) was misinterpreted as the total amount of drug in the vial
• Visually inspect for particulate matter and discoloration prior to use

IV infusion route
• Prior to infusion, dilute in 5% dextrose or 0.9% saline solution to a concentration ranging from 1.5-25 mg PE/ml
• Because of the risk of hypotension, do not exceed recommended infusion rates. Continuous monitoring of ECG, B/P, and respiratory function is recommended, especially throughout the period when phenytoin concentrations peak (about 10-20 min after the end of the infusion)
• Loading doses should always be followed by maintenance doses of oral or parenteral phenytoin or parenteral fosphenytoin
• Adult: Infuse IV at a rate max 150 mg PE/min
• Elderly or debilitated adult: infuse IV at a max 3 mg PE/kg/min or 150 mg PE/min, whichever is less
• Child: infuse IV at a rate of 0.5-3 mg PE/kg/min, max 150 mg PE/min, whichever is less
• Infant, neonate: infuse IV at a rate max 0.5-3 mg PE/kg/min

Y-site compatibilities: Aminocaproic acid, amphotericin B lipid complex, amphotericin B liposome, anidulafungin, atenolol, bivalirudin, bleomycin, CARBOplatin, CISplatin, cyclophosphamide, cytarabine, DACTINomycin, DAPTOmycin, dexmedetomidine, diltiazem, DOCEtaxel, doxacurium, eptifibatide, ertapenem, etoposide, fludarabine, fluorouracil, gatifloxacin, gemcitabine, gemtuzumab, granisetron, ifosfamide, levofloxacin, linezolid, LORazepam, mechlorethamine, meperidine, methotrexate, metroNIDAZOLE, nesiritide, octreotide, oxaliplatin, oxytocin, PACLitaxel, palonosetron, pamidronate, pantoprazole, PEMEtrexed, PHENobarbital, piperacillin-tazobactam, rocuronium, sodium acetate, tacrolimus, teniposide, thiotepa, tigecycline, tirofiban, vinCRIStine, vinorelbine, voriconazole, zoledronic acid

Y-site incompatibilities: Caspofungin, DOXOrubicin, epirubicin, fenoldopam, IDArubicin, midazolam, mitoXANtrone, mycophenolate, quinupristin-dalfopristin

ADVERSE EFFECTS
CNS: *Drowsiness,* dizziness, insomnia, paresthesias, depression, **suicidal tendencies,** aggression, headache, confusion, paresthesia, emotional lability, syncope, cerebral edema
CV: Hypotension, hypertension, **CHF, shock, dysrhythmias**

EENT: Nystagmus, diplopia, blurred vision
GI: Nausea, vomiting, diarrhea, constipation, anorexia, weight loss, **hepatitis,** jaundice, gingival hyperplasia
HEMA: Agranulocytosis, leukopenia, aplastic anemia, thrombocytopenia, megaloblastic anemia
INTEG: Rash, lupus erythematosus, **Stevens-Johnson syndrome,** hirsutism, hypersensitivity, pruritus
RESP: Bronchospasm, cough
SYST: Hyperglycemia, hypokalemia, **toxic epidermal necrolysis (Asian patients positive for HLA-B 1502), DRESS, purple glove syndrome, anaphylaxis**

Pharmacokinetics

Absorption	Unknown
Distribution	Protein binding 99%
Metabolism	Liver: converted to phenytoin
Excretion	Kidneys
Half-life	Unknown

Pharmacodynamics
Unknown

INTERACTIONS
Individual drugs
Alcohol: decreased effects of fosphenytoin (chronic use)
Amiodarone, chloramphenicol, cimetidine: increased fosphenytoin level
CarBAMazepine, folic acid, rifampin, theophylline, tramadol: decreased effects of fosphenytoin
Delavirdine: do not use concurrently; decreased virologic response, resistance

Drug classifications
Antacids, antihistamines, antineoplastics, CYP1A2 inducers: decreased effects of fosphenytoin
Antidepressants (tricyclics), CYP1A2 inhibitors, estrogens, H₂-receptor antagonists, phenothiazines, salicylates, sulfonamides: increased fosphenytoin level

Drug/herb
Ginseng, valerian: decreased anticonvulsant effect
Ginkgo: increased anticonvulsant effect

Drug/lab test
Increased: glucose, alkaline phosphatase
Decreased: dexamethasone, metyrapone test serum, PBI, urinary steroids, potassium

NURSING CONSIDERATIONS
Assessment
• Assess drug level: target level 10-20 mcg/ml; toxic level 30-50 mcg/ml, wait at least 2 hr after dose before testing, 4 hr after IM dose
• **Assess seizure activity** including type, location, duration, and character; provide seizure precaution
• Assess renal studies: urinalysis, BUN, urine creatinine
• Monitor hepatic studies: ALT, AST, bilirubin, creatinine
• Assess allergic reaction: red raised rash; if this occurs, product should be discontinued
• **Monitor for toxicity:** bone marrow depression, nausea, vomiting, ataxia, diplopia, cardiovascular collapse, slurred speech, confusion
• Assess product level: toxic level 30-50 mcg/ml
⚠ **Assess for rash, discontinue as soon as rash develops, serious adverse reactions such as Stevens-Johnson syndrome can occur**
⚠ **Assess mental status: mood, sensorium, affect, memory (long, short), especially geriatric; suicidal thoughts/behaviors**
⚠ **Serious skin reactions: usually occurring within 28 days of treatment; if a rash develops, patient should be evaluated for DRESS**
• **Assess for blood dyscrasias:** fever, sore throat, bruising, rash, jaundice, epistaxis (long-term treatment only)
• Monitor blood studies: RBC, Hct, Hgb, reticulocyte counts weekly for 4 wk, then monthly; also check thyroid function tests, serum calcium, albumin, phosphorus, potassium

Patient/family education
• Teach patient the reason for and expected outcome of treatment
• Instruct patient not to use machinery or engage in hazardous activity; drowsiness, dizziness may occur
• Advise patient to carry/wear emergency ID identifying product used, name of prescriber
• Advise patient to notify prescriber of rash, bleeding, bruising, slurred speech, jaundice of skin or eyes, joint pain, nausea, vomiting, severe headache, **depression, suicidal ideation**
• Advise patient to keep all medical appointments, including lab work, physical assessment
• Advise patient to notify prescriber if pregnancy is planned or suspected; to use contraception with this product

Evaluation
Positive therapeutic outcome
• Decreased seizure activity

⚠ HIGH ALERT

fospropofol (Rx)
(fos-proe′poe-fol)
Lusedra
Func. class.: General anesthetic
Pregnancy category B

ACTION: Prodrug of propofol; produces dose-dependent CNS depression by activation of GABA receptor inhibition of NMDA subtype of glutamate receptors by channel-gating modulation

Therapeutic outcome: Anesthesia

USES: Induction or maintenance of anesthesia as part of balanced anesthetic technique; sedation in mechanically ventilated patients

CONTRAINDICATIONS:
Hypersensitivity to product

Precautions: Pregnancy **B**, breastfeeding, children, geriatric patients, respiratory depression, severe respiratory disorders, cardiac dysrhythmias, labor and delivery, renal disease, hyperlipidemia

DOSAGE AND ROUTES
Induction/maintenance
Adult <65 (healthy): *>90 kg,* initially 577.5 mg **IV** bolus, as needed give supplemental doses up to a max of 140 mg **IV**/dose to achieve desired level of sedation, give no more frequently than q4min; *61-89 kg,* initially 6.5 mg/kg (max 577.5 mg) **IV** bolus, as needed give supplemental doses up to 1.6 mg/kg/dose (max 140 mg/dose) **IV** to achieve desired level of sedation, give no more frequently than q4min; *≤60 kg,* initially 385 mg **IV** bolus, as needed give supplemental doses up to a max of 105 mg **IV**/dose to achieve desired level of sedation, give no more frequently than q4min
Adult <65 yr (severe systemic disease): *≥90 kg,* initially 437.5 mg **IV** bolus, as needed give supplemental doses up to a max of 105 mg **IV**/dose to achieve desired level of sedation, give no more frequently than q4min; *61-89 kg,* initially give 75% of standard dosing regimen, which is 4.875 mg/kg (max 437.5 mg) **IV** bolus, as needed give supplemental doses that are 75% of standard dosing regimen (up to 1.2 mg/kg/dose **IV,** max 105 mg/dose **IV**), give doses to achieve desired level of sedation, give no more frequently than q4min; *≤60 kg,* initially 297.5 mg **IV** bolus, as needed give supplemental doses

---

up to a max of 70 mg **IV**/dose to achieve desired level of sedation, give no more frequently than q4min

Geriatric: ≥*90 kg,* initially 437.5 mg **IV** bolus, as needed give supplemental doses up to a max 105 mg **IV**/dose to achieve desired level of sedation, give no more frequently than q4min; *61-89 kg,* initially give 75% of standard dosing regimen, which is 4.875 mg/kg (max 105 mg 1 dose) **IV** bolus, as needed give supplemental doses that are 75% of standard dosing regimen; give doses to achieve desired level of sedation; give no more frequently than q4min

Available forms: Inj 1050 mg/30 ml

Implementation

IV bolus route
- Visually inspect for particulate matter and discoloration
- Each vial is single patient/single use
- Draw from vial, discard unused portion
- Do not mix with other drugs prior to use
- Give by **IV** bolus in free-flowing peripheral **IV** line of D₅W, 5% dextrose/0.2% NaCl, 5% dextrose/0.45% NaCl D₅LR, LR, 0.45% NaCl, NS, 5% dextrose/0.45% NaCl/20 mEq KCl; do not mix with other fluids; flush line with NS before and after administration
- No filtration needed
- Give only with resuscitative equipment available
- Give only by qualified persons trained in anesthesia
- Store unopened vials at room temperature

ADVERSE EFFECTS

CNS: Involuntary movement, headache, jerking, fever, dizziness, shivering, tremor, confusion, somnolence, paresthesia, agitation, abnormal dreams, euphoria, fatigue, **increased intracranial pressure, impaired cerebral flow, seizures**

CV: *Bradycardia, hypotension,* hypertension, PVC, PAC, tachycardia, abnormal ECG, ST segment depression, **asystole, bradydysrhythmias**

EENT: Blurred vision, tinnitus, eye pain, strange taste, diplopia

GI: *Nausea, vomiting, abdominal cramping,* dry mouth, swallowing, hypersalivation, **pancreatitis**

GU: Urine retention, green urine, cloudy urine, oliguria

INTEG: *Flushing, phlebitis, hives, burning/ stinging at inj site,* rash, pain of extremities

MS: Myalgia

RESP: Apnea, *cough, hiccups,* dyspnea, hypoventilation, sneezing, wheezing, tachypnea, hypoxia, respiratory acidosis

Pharmacokinetics

Absorption	Unknown
Distribution	Rapid, 98% protein binding
Metabolism	Liver conjugated to inactive metabolites
Excretion	Urine 7%
Half-life	1-8 min; terminal 0.81-0.88 hr

Pharmacodynamics

Onset	15-30 sec
Peak	Unknown
Duration	Unknown

INTERACTIONS

Individual drugs
Alcohol: increased CNS depression

Drug classifications
- Alcohol, opioids, sedative/hypnotics, antipsychotics, skeletal muscle relaxants, inhalational anesthetics: increased CNS depression
- MAOIs: do not use within 10 days

Drug/herb
St. John's wort: increased fospropofol effect

Drug/lab test
Increased: LFTs, bilirubin

NURSING CONSIDERATIONS

Assessment
- Assess inj site: phlebitis, burning, stinging
- **Monitor ECG** for changes: PVC, PAC, ST segment changes; monitor VS
- Assess CNS changes: movement, jerking, tremors, dizziness, LOC, pupil reaction
- Assess for allergic reactions: hives
- **Assess for respiratory depression,** character, rate, rhythm; notify prescriber if respirations are <10/min, hypoxemia is detectable by pulse oximetry

Teach patient/family
- Teach patient that this medication will cause dizziness, drowsiness, sedation

Evaluation

Positive therapeutic outcome
- Induction of anesthesia

TREATMENT OF OVERDOSE:
Discontinue product; administer vasopressor agents or anticholinergics, artificial ventilation

frovatriptan (Rx)

(froh-vah-trip'tan)

Frova

Func. class.: Antimigraine agent
Chem. class.: 5-HT$_1$ receptor agonist

Pregnancy category C

ACTION: Binds selectively to the vascular 5-HT$_{1B}$, 5-HT$_{1D}$ receptor subtypes, exerts antimigraine effect; binds to benzodiazepine receptor sites, causes vasoconstriction in cranium

Therapeutic outcome: Absence of migraines

USES: Acute treatment of migraine with or without aura

CONTRAINDICATIONS:

Angina pectoris, history of MI, documented silent ischemia, Prinzmetal's angina, ischemic heart disease, concurrent ergotamine-containing preparations, uncontrolled hypertension, hypersensitivity, basilar or hemiplegic migraine; ischemic bowel disease; peripheral vascular disease, severe hepatic disease, prophylactic migraine treatment

Precautions: Pregnancy C, breastfeeding, children, geriatric, postmenopausal women, men >40 yr, risk factors for CAD, hypercholesterolemia, obesity, diabetes, impaired hepatic function, seizure disorder

DOSAGE AND ROUTES

Adult: PO 2.5 mg; a 2nd dose may be taken after ≥2 hr; max 3 tabs/day (7.5 mg)

Available forms: Tabs 2.5 mg

Implementation

• Ensure that tablets are swallowed whole
• Provide quiet, calm environment with decreased stimulation from noise, bright light, excessive talking

ADVERSE EFFECTS

CNS: *Hot sensation,* paresthesia, *dizziness,* headache, fatigue, cold sensation, insomnia, anxiety, somnolence, **seizures**
CV: *Flushing,* chest pain, palpitation
GI: Dry mouth, dyspepsia, abdominal pain, diarrhea, vomiting, nausea
MS: Skeletal pain

Absorption	Absolute bioavailability of PO dose ~20% in males, 30% in females
Distribution	Protein binding 15%; reversibly bound to blood cells at equilibrium 60%
Metabolism	Liver, by CYP1A2
Excretion	Urine (32%), feces (62%)
Half-life	25-29 hr

Onset	10 min-2 hr
Peak	2-4 hr
Duration	Unknown

INTERACTIONS

Individual drugs

Estrogen, propranolol: increased effects of frovatriptan

Drug classifications

CYP1A2 inhibitors (cimetidine, ciprofloxacin, erythromycin), oral contraceptives: increased frovatriptan levels
Selective serotonin reuptake inhibitors, other serotonin agonists (dextromethorphan, tramadol, antidepressants): increased toxicity

NURSING CONSIDERATIONS

Assessment

• **Migraine:** aura, alleviating/exacerbating factor, diet, character
• Assess for ingestion of tyramine-containing foods (pickled products, beer, wine, aged cheese), food additives, preservatives, colorings, artificial sweeteners, chocolate, caffeine, which may precipitate these types of headaches
• Assess B/P; signs/symptoms of coronary vasospasms
• Assess for stress level, activity, recreation, coping mechanisms
• Assess neurologic status: LOC, paresthesia, hot/cold sensations, dizziness, headache, fatigue

Patient/family education

• Instruct patient to report any side effects to prescriber
• Advise patient to use contraception while taking product
• Advise patient that photosensitivity may occur, to use sunscreen and wear protective clothing when outdoors
• Advise patient to have dark, quiet environment available

Evaluation
Positive therapeutic outcome
• Decrease in frequency, severity of migraine

TREATMENT OF OVERDOSE:
No specific antidote; monitor patient closely for ≥48 hr, treat any symptoms as necessary

fulvestrant (Rx)
(full-ves'trant)
Faslodex
Func. class.: Antineoplastic
Pregnancy category D

ACTION: Inhibits cell division by binding to competitive cytoplasmic estrogen receptors; resembles normal cell complex but inhibits DNA synthesis and estrogen response of target tissue

Therapeutic outcome: Decreased tumor size, spread of malignancy

USES: Advanced breast carcinoma in estrogen-receptor–positive patients (usually postmenopausal)

CONTRAINDICATIONS:
Pregnancy **D**, breastfeeding, children, hypersensitivity

Precautions: Hepatic disease, jaundice, thrombocytopenia, biliary tract disease, coagulopathy

DOSAGE AND ROUTES
Adult: IM 500 mg as two 5-ml inj on days 1, 15, 29 and q mo thereafter

Available forms: Inj 50 mg/ml

Implementation
• Give IM 5 ml as one inj in each buttock slowly
• Give antacid before oral agent; give product after evening meal, before bedtime
• Give antiemetic 30-60 min before giving product to prevent vomiting
• Provide liquid diet, if needed, including cola, Jell-O; dry toast or crackers may be added if patient is not nauseated or vomiting
• Increase fluids to 2 L/day unless contraindicated
• Store in refrigerator, protect from light

ADVERSE EFFECTS
CNS: *Headache,* depression, dizziness, insomnia, paresthesia, anxiety

GI: *Nausea, vomiting,* anorexia, constipation, diarrhea, abdominal pain, hepatitis, hepatic failure, hyperbilirubinemia
HEMA: Anemia
INTEG: *Rash,* sweating, *hot flashes,* inj site pain
MS: Bone pain, arthritis, back pain
RESP: Pharyngitis, dyspnea, cough
SYST: Angioedema

Pharmacokinetics

Absorption	Unknown
Distribution	Unknown
Metabolism	CYP3A4
Excretion	Feces 90%
Half-life	40 days

Pharmacodynamics
Unknown

INTERACTIONS
Drug classifications
Anticoagulants: do not use concurrently; increased bleeding

Drug/lab test
Increased: LFTs

NURSING CONSIDERATIONS
Assessment
• Monitor for side effects, report to prescriber
• Monitor for anticoagulant use

Patient/family education
• Advise patient to report any complaints, side effects to prescriber
• Teach patient to increase fluids to 2 L/day unless contraindicated
• Advise patient to report vaginal bleeding immediately
• Teach patient that tumor flare—increase in size of tumor, increased bone pain—may occur and will subside rapidly; may take analgesics for pain
• Teach patient to use contraception, pregnancy **D**

Evaluation
Positive therapeutic outcome
• Decreased tumor size, decreased spread of malignancy

F

furosemide (Rx)
(fur-oh'se-mide)
Lasix
Func. class.: Loop diuretic
Chem. class.: Sulfonamide derivative
Pregnancy category C

Do not confuse:
furosemide/torsemide,
Lasix/Lanoxin/Lomotil/Losec/Luvox

ACTION: Acts on the ascending loop of
Henle in the kidney, inhibiting reabsorption of
electrolytes sodium and chloride, causing excretion of sodium, calcium, magnesium, chloride,
water, and some potassium; decreases reabsorption of sodium and chloride and increases
excretion of potassium in the distal tubule of the
kidney; responsible for slight antihypertensive
effect and peripheral vasodilatation

Therapeutic outcome: Decreased
edema in lung tissue, peripherally; decreased
B/P

USES: Pulmonary edema, edema in CHF,
nephrotic syndrome, ascites, hepatic disease,
hypertension

Unlabeled uses: Hypercalcemia in
malignancy

CONTRAINDICATIONS:
Anuria, hypovolemia

Precautions: Pregnancy **C**, diabetes
mellitus, dehydration, severe renal disease, cirrhosis, ascites, hypersensitivity to sulfonamides,
breastfeeding, infants, electrolyte depletion

DOSAGE AND ROUTES
Adult: PO 20-80 mg/day in AM, may give
another dose in 6 hr, up to 600 mg/day; IM/**IV**
20-40 mg, increased by 20 mg q2hr until
desired response
Child: PO/IM/**IV** 2 mg/kg, may increase by 1-2
mg/kg/q6-8hr up to 6 mg/kg

Antihypercalcemia
Adult: IM/**IV** 80-100 mg q1-4hr or PO 120 mg/
day or divided bid
Child: IM/**IV** 25-50 mg, repeat q4hr if needed

Acute/chronic renal failure
Adult: PO 80 mg/day, increase by 80-120 mg/
day to desired response; **IV** 100-200 mg, max
600-800 mg

Available forms: Tabs 20, 40, 80 mg; oral
sol 8 mg/ml, 10 mg/ml; inj IM, **IV** 10 mg/ml

Implementation
• Give in AM to avoid interference with sleep
• Potassium replacement if potassium level is
<3.0 mg/dl; product may be crushed if patient
is unable to swallow
PO route
• With food or milk or use oral sol if nausea
occurs; absorption may be reduced slightly
IV route
• Do not use sol that is yellow, has a precipitate
or crystals
IV, direct route
• Give undiluted through Y-tube on 3-way
stopcock; give 20 mg or less/min
Intermittent IV inf route
• May be added to 0.9% NaCl, D$_5$W, use within
24 hr to ensure compatibility; give through
Y-tube or 3-way stopcock; give at 4 mg/min or
less, use inf pump

Y-site compatibilities: Acyclovir,
alfentanil, allopurinol, alprostadil, amifostine,
amikacin, aminocaproic acid, aminophylline,
amphotericin B cholesteryl/lipid complex/lipo-
some, anidulafungin, argatroban, ascorbic acid,
atenolol, atropine, azaTHIOprine, aztreonam,
bivalirudin, bleomycin, bumetanide, calcium
chloride/gluconate, CARBOplatin, cefamandole,
ceFAZolin, cefepime, cefmetazole, cefonicid,
cefoperazone, cefotaxime, cefoTEtan, cefOXitin,
cefTAZidime, ceftizoxime, ceftobiprole, cefTRI-
AXone, cefuroxime, cephalothin, cephapirin,
chloramphenicol, CISplatin, cladribine, clindamycin, cyanocobalamin, cyclophosphamide,
cycloSPORINE, cytarabine, DACTINomycin, DAP-
TOmycin, dexamethasone, dexmedetomidine,
digoxin, DOCEtaxel, doripenem, doxacurium,
DOXOrubicin liposome, enalaprilat, ePHEDrine,
EPINEPHrine, etoposide, fentaNYL, fludarabine,
fluorouracil, folic acid, foscarnet, gallium
nitrate, ganciclovir, granisetron, heparin,
hydrocortisone, HYDROmorphone, ifosfamide,
imipenem-cilastatin, indomethacin, insulin
(regular), isosorbide, kanamycin, leucovorin,
lidocaine, linezolid, LORazepam, LR, mannitol,
mechlorethamine, melphalan, meropenem,
methicillin, methotrexate, methylPREDNISolone,
metoprolol, metroNIDAZOLE, mezlocillin, micafungin, miconazole, mitoMYcin, moxalactam,
multiple vitamins injection, nafcillin, naloxone,
nitroprusside, octreotide, oxacillin, oxaliplatin,
oxytocin, PACLitaxel, palonosetron, pamidronate, pantoprazole, PEMEtrexed, penicillin G,
PENTobarbital, PHENobarbital, phytonadione,

---

piperacillin, piperacillin-tazobactam, potassium chloride, procainamide, propofol, propranolol, ranitidine, remifentanil, Ringer's, ritodrine, sargramostim, sodium acetate/bicarbonate, succinylcholine, SUFentanil, temocillin, teniposide, theophylline, thiopental, thiotepa, ticarcillin, ticarcillin-clavulanate, tigecycline, tirofiban, TNA, tobramycin, urokinase, vit B/C, voriconazole, zoledronic acid

Y-site incompatibilities: Amsacrine, bleomycin, DOXOrubicin, droperidol, esmolol, fluconazole, gentamicin, IDArubicin, metoclopramide, milrinone, netilmicin, ondansetron, quiNIDine, vinBLAStine, vinCRIStine

ADVERSE EFFECTS

CNS: Headache, fatigue, weakness, vertigo, paresthesias
CV: Orthostatic hypotension, chest pain, ECG changes, **circulatory collapse**
EENT: *Loss of hearing,* ear pain, tinnitus, blurred vision
ELECT: *Hypokalemia, hypochloremic alkalosis, hypomagnesemia, hyperuricemia, hypocalcemia, hyponatremia,* metabolic alkalosis
ENDO: *Hyperglycemia*
GI: *Nausea,* diarrhea, dry mouth, vomiting, anorexia, cramps, oral or gastric irritations, pancreatitis
GU: *Polyuria,* **renal failure,** *glycosuria,* bladder spasms
HEMA: Thrombocytopenia, agranulocytosis, leukopenia, neutropenia, anemia
INTEG: *Rash, pruritus, purpura,* **Stevens-Johnson syndrome,** sweating, photosensitivity, urticaria
MS: Cramps, stiffness
SYST: Toxic epidermal necrolysis

Pharmacokinetics

	PO
Absorption	GI tract (60%-70%)
	PO/IM/IV
Distribution	Crosses placenta
Metabolism	Liver (30%-40%)
Excretion	Breast milk, urine, feces
Half-life	½-1 hr

Pharmacodynamics

	PO	IM	IV
Onset	1 hr	½ hr	5 min
Peak	1-2 hr	Unknown	½ hr
Duration	6-8 hr	4-8 hr	2 hr

INTERACTIONS
Individual drugs
CISplatin, vancomycin: increased risk of ototoxicity
Digoxin: increased toxicity
Lithium: decreased renal clearance, causing increased toxicity
Probenecid: decreased furosemide effect

Drug classifications
Aminoglycosides: increased ototoxicity
Anticoagulants, salicylates: increased effects
Antihypertensives: increased antihypertensive effect
Nitrates: increased hypotensive action
Nondepolarizing skeletal muscle relaxants: increased toxicity

Drug/lab test
Interference: GTT
Increase: LDL

NURSING CONSIDERATIONS
Assessment
• **Ototoxicity:** Assess patient for tinnitus, hearing loss, ear pain; periodic testing of hearing is needed when high doses of this product are given by **IV** route
• **Hypokalemia:** acidic urine, reduced urine osmolality, nocturia, polyuria and polydipsia; hypotension, broad T-wave, U-wave, ectopy, tachycardia, weak pulse; muscle weakness, altered LOC, drowsiness, apathy, lethargy, confusion, depression; anorexia, nausea, cramps, constipation, distention, paralytic ileus; hypoventilation, respiratory muscle weakness
• Monitor for CV, GI, neurologic manifestations of hyponatremia: increased B/P, cold, clammy skin, hypovolemia or hypervolemia; anorexia, nausea, vomiting, diarrhea, abdominal cramps; lethargy, increased ICP, confusion, headache, seizures, coma, fatigue, tremors, hyperreflexia
• Monitor for neurologic, respiratory manifestations of hyperchloremia: weakness, lethargy, coma; deep rapid breathing
• **CHF:** Assess fluid volume status: I&O ratios and record, count or weigh diapers as appropriate, weight, distended red veins, crackles in lung, color, quality, and specific gravity of urine, skin turgor, adequacy of pulses, moist mucous membranes, bilateral lung sounds, peripheral pitting edema; dehydration symptoms of decreasing output, thirst, hypotension, dry mouth and mucous membranes should be reported
• Monitor electrolytes: potassium, sodium, chloride, magnesium; also include BUN, blood pH, ABGs, uric acid, CBC, blood glucose

---

Adverse effects: *italics* = common; **bold** = life-threatening

• **Hypertension:** Assess B/P before and during therapy lying, standing, and sitting as appropriate; orthostatic hypotension can occur rapidly

Patient/family education
• Teach patient to take the medication early in the day to prevent nocturia
• Instruct the patient to take with food or milk if GI symptoms of nausea and anorexia occur
• Teach patient to maintain a record of weight on a weekly basis and notify physician of weight loss of >5 lb
• Caution the patient that this product causes a loss of potassium, that food rich in potassium should be added to the diet; refer to a dietitian for assistance in planning
• Caution the patient to rise slowly from sitting or reclining positions, not to exercise in hot weather or stand for prolonged periods because orthostatic hypotension will be enhanced; lie down if dizziness occurs
• Advise patient to wear protective clothing and sunscreen to prevent photosensitivity

• Caution patient not to use alcohol or any OTC medications without physician's approval; serious product reactions may occur
• Emphasize the need to contact physician immediately if muscle cramps, weakness, nausea, dizziness, or numbness occurs
• Teach patient to take and record own B/P and pulse
• Advise patient to continue taking medication even if feeling better; this product controls symptoms but does not cure the condition
• Advise the patient with hypertension to continue other medical treatment (exercise, weight loss, relaxation techniques, cessation of smoking)

Evaluation
Positive therapeutic outcome
• Decreased edema
• Decreased B/P
• Lowered calcium level in malignancy
• Increased diuresis

gabapentin (Rx)

(gab'a-pen-tin)
Apo-Gabapentin ✶, **CO**
Gabapentin ✶, **Gen-Gabapentin,**
Gralise, Horizant, Neurontin, Novo-
Gabapentin ✶, **PMS-Gabapentin** ✶,
ratio-Gabapentin
Func. class.: Anticonvulsant
Pregnancy category C

Do not confuse:
Neurontin/Noroxin/Neoral

ACTION: Mechanism unknown; may increase seizure threshold; structurally similar to GABA; gabapentin binding sites in neocortex, hippocampus

Therapeutic outcome: Decreased seizure activity

USES: Adjunct treatment of partial seizures, with or without generalization in patients >12 yr; adjunct in partial seizures in children 3-12 yr, postherpetic neuralgia, primary restless leg syndrome (RLS) in adults

Unlabeled uses: Tremors in multiple sclerosis, neuropathic pain, bipolar disorder, migraine prophylaxis, diabetic neuropathy

CONTRAINDICATIONS:
Hypersensitivity to this product

Precautions: Pregnancy **C**, breastfeeding, children <3 yr, geriatric, renal disease, hemodialysis, suicidal thoughts, depression

DOSAGE AND ROUTES
Adult and child >12 yr: PO 900-1800 mg/day in 3 divided doses; may titrate by giving 300 mg on the first day, 300 mg bid on second day, 300 mg tid on third day; may increase to 1800 mg/day by adding 300 mg on subsequent days
Child 3-12 yr: PO 10-15 mg/kg/day in 3 divided doses, initially titrate dose upward over approximately 3 days; if 3-4 yr old, 40 mg/kg/day in 3 divided doses; all given in 3 divided doses

Postherpetic neuralgia
Adult: PO 300 mg on day 1, 600 mg/day divided bid on day 2, 900 mg/day divided tid, may titrate to 1800-3600 mg divided tid if needed; ext rel tab (Gralise only) 300 mg on day 1, then 600 mg on day 2, 900 mg on days 3-6, 1200 mg on days 7-10, 1500 mg on days 11-14, 1800 mg on day 15 and thereafter

Moderate to severe RLS (Horizant only)
Adult: PO ext rel tab 600 mg qd with food at about 5 PM; if dose is missed, take next day at 5 PM

Renal dose
Adult and child >12 yr: CCr 30-59 ml/min 200-700 mg bid; CCr 15-29 ml/min 200-700 mg/day; CCr ≤15 ml/min 100-300 mg/day

Available forms: Caps 100, 300, 400 mg; tabs 600, 800 mg; oral sol 250 mg/5 ml; Horizant: ext rel tab 600 mg

Implementation
• Do not break, crush, or chew caps, ext rel tabs; cap may be opened and contents put in applesauce or dissolved in juice; scored tab may be cut in half
• Give at least 2 hr apart when giving antacids; give without regard to meals
• Store at room temperature away from heat and light
• Provide assistance with ambulation during early part of treatment; dizziness occurs
• **Provide seizure precautions:** padded side rails, move objects that may harm patient
• **Oral sol:** measure with calibrated device
• **Ext release:** give with food at about 5 pm; bioavailability is increased with food; do not interchange Gralise with Horizant

ADVERSE EFFECTS
CNS: *Drowsiness, confusion,* dizziness, fatigue, anxiety, somnolence, ataxia, amnesia, abnormal thinking, unsteady gait, depression; 3-12 yr old: emotional lability, aggression, thought disorder, hyperkinesia, hostility, **seizures, suicidal ideation,** impaired cognition, euphoria
CV: Vasodilatation, peripheral edema, hypotension, hypertension
EENT: Dry mouth, blurred vision, diplopia, nystagmus, conjunctivitis; otitis media (child 3-12 yr)
GI: Constipation/diarrhea, weight gain, increased appetite, dental abnormalities, nausea, vomiting
GU: Impotence, bleeding, *UTI*
HEMA: **Leukopenia, thrombocytopenia,** decreased WBC
INTEG: Pruritus, abrasion, **Stevens-Johnson syndrome,** acne vulgaris
MS: Myalgia, back pain, gout
RESP: Rhinitis, pharyngitis, coughing, upper respiratory infection (child 3-12 yr)

G

Pharmacokinetics

Absorption	Unknown
Distribution	Unknown
Metabolism	None
Excretion	Urine unchanged
Half-life	5-7 hr, 130 hr in ESRD

Pharmacodynamics

Unknown

INTERACTIONS

Individual drugs
Alcohol: increased CNS depression
Cimetidine, sevelamer: decreased gabapentin levels
Morphine: increased gabapentin levels
HYDROcodone: decreased effect of HYDROcodone

Drug classifications
Antacids: decreased gabapentin levels
Antihistamines, sedatives, all other CNS depressants: increased CNS depression

Drug/lab test
Increased: LFTs
False positive: urinary protein using Ames N-multistix SG

NURSING CONSIDERATIONS

Assessment
• **Assess seizures:** aura, location, duration, frequency, activity at onset
• Assess renal studies: urinalysis, BUN, urine creatinine q3mo
⚠ **Assess mental status: mood, sensorium, affect, behavioral changes, suicidal thoughts/behaviors; if mental status changes, notify prescriber**
• Assess eye problems, need for ophth exam before, during, after treatment (slit lamp, fundoscopy, tonometry)

Patient/family education
• Advise patient to carry/wear emergency ID stating patient's name, products taken, condition, prescriber's name and phone number
• Advise patient to avoid driving, other activities that require alertness
• Teach patient not to discontinue medication quickly after long-term use, withdrawal-precipitated seizures may occur, not to double dose; if dose is missed, take if 2 hr or more before next dose
• Teach patient to gradually withdraw over 7 days; abrupt withdrawal may precipitate seizures

• Teach patient to use hard candy, gum, and frequent rinsing of mouth for dry mouth
• Teach patient to increase fluids, bulk in diet for constipation
• Advise patient to notify prescriber if pregnancy is planned or suspected, avoid breastfeeding

Evaluation
Positive therapeutic outcome
• Decreased seizure activity; document on patient's chart

TREATMENT OF OVERDOSE:
Lavage, VS

---

galantamine (Rx)
(gah-lan'tah-meen)
Razadyne, Razadyne ER, Reminyl ✦
Func. class.: Anti-Alzheimer's agent
Chem. class.: Cholinesterase inhibitor
Pregnancy category B

ACTION: Enhances cholinergic functioning by increasing acetylcholine

Therapeutic outcome: Decreased signs and symptoms of Alzheimer's dementia

USES: Mild to moderate dementia of Alzheimer's disease, vascular dementia, dementia with Lewy bodies

CONTRAINDICATIONS:
Hypersensitivity to this product, children, GI bleeding, jaundice, renal failure

Precautions: Pregnancy **B**, respiratory/renal/hepatic/cardiac disease, seizure disorder, peptic ulcer, asthma, bradycardia, heart block, geriatric patients, surgery, urinary tract obstruction, breastfeeding

DOSAGE AND ROUTES
Adult: PO 4 mg bid with morning and evening meals; after 4 wk or more may increase to 8 mg bid; after another 4 wk may increase to 12 mg bid; usual dose 16-24 mg/day in 2 divided doses; EXT REL 8 mg/day in AM; may increase to 16 mg/day after 4 wk, and 24 mg/day after another 4 wk

Hepatic dose
Adult: (Child-Pugh 7-9) PO max 16 mg/day
Adult: (Child-Pugh 10-15) avoid PO use

Renal dose
Adult: PO CCr 10-70 ml/min; max 16 mg/day;
CCr <9 ml/min: PO avoid use

Available forms: Tabs 4, 8, 12 mg; ext rel tabs 8, 16, 24 mg; oral sol 4 mg/ml

Implementation

• Give with meals, morning and evening, ext rel product can be opened and sprinkled on food; do not crush/chew
• Dose increase after minimum of 4 wk at prior dose; if dose is interrupted for several days, restart at lower dose, titrate to current dose
• Provide assistance with ambulation during beginning therapy
• Perform complete suicide assessment

ADVERSE EFFECTS

CNS: *Tremors, insomnia,* depression, dizziness, headache, somnolence, fatigue
CV: Bradycardia, chest pain
GI: *Nausea, vomiting, anorexia, abdominal distress, flatulence,* diarrhea
GU: Urinary incontinence, bladder outflow obstruction, hematuria
HEMA: Anemia
META: Weight decrease
MS: Asthenia
RESP: URI, rhinitis

Pharmacokinetics

Absorption	Rapidly and completely absorbed
Distribution	18% protein binding
Metabolism	Liver
Excretion	Kidneys; clearance decreased in geriatric, hepatic/renal disease, females (20% lower)
Half-life	Elimination 7 hr

Pharmacodynamics

Unknown

INTERACTIONS

Drug classifications

Cholinesterase inhibitors, cholinomimetics: synergistic effect
CYP3A4/CYP2D6 inducers (bosentan, carBAMazepine, fosphenytoin, nevirapine, OXcarbazepine, phenytoin, rifabutin, rifampin, rifapentine, troglitazone), anticholinergics: decreased galantamine effect
CYP3A4/CYP2D6 inhibitors (antiretroviral protease inhibitors, clarithromycin, conivaptan, delaviridine, diltiazem, efavirenz, erythromycin, fluconazole, fluvoxaMINE, imatinib, itraconazole, ketoconazole, nefazodone, niCARdipine, troleandomycin, verapamil,

voriconazole, zafirlukast): increased galantamine effect
NSAIDs: increased GI effects

Drug/herb

St. John's wort: decreased galantamine effect

NURSING CONSIDERATIONS

Assessment

• **Alzheimer's disease:** Assess mental status: affect, mood, behavioral changes, depression, memory, attention, confusion, cognitive functioning
• Assess liver function enzymes: AST, ALT, alkaline phosphatase, LDH, bilirubin, CBC
• Assess for severe GI effects: nausea, vomiting, anorexia, weight loss
• Assess B/P, heart rate, respiration during initial treatment

Patient/family education

• Teach patient or caregiver correct procedure for giving oral sol, using instruction sheet provided
• Instruct patient or caregiver to notify prescriber of severe GI effects
• Instruct patient or caregiver to report hypo/hypertension, slow heart rate
• Teach patient to take with food to prevent intolerance

Evaluation

Positive therapeutic outcome
• Decreased symptoms of dementia
• Increased coherence
• Improved cognitive performance (memory, orientation, attention, reasoning, language, praxis)

TREATMENT OF OVERDOSE:

Administer **IV** atropine titrated to effect at an initial dose of 0.5-1 mg, with subsequent doses based on clinical response; provide general supportive measures

ganciclovir (Rx)

(gan-sye'kloe-vir)
Cytovene, Vitrasert
Func. class.: Antiviral
Chem. class.: Synthetic nucleoside analog
Pregnancy category C

Do not confuse:

Cytovene/Cytosar

ACTION: Inhibits replication of herpes viruses in vitro; competitively inhibits human cytomegalovirus (CMV) DNA polymerase and is incorporated, resulting in termination of DNA elongation

Therapeutic outcome: Decreased proliferation of virus responsible for CMV retinitis

USES: Cytomegalovirus (CMV) retinitis in immunocompromised persons, including those with AIDS, after indirect ophthalmoscopy confirms diagnosis; prophylaxis of CMV in transplantation

Unlabeled uses: CMV pneumonia in organ transplant patients, CMV gastroenteritis in patients with irritable bowel syndrome, CMV pneumonitis

CONTRAINDICATIONS:
Hypersensitivity to acyclovir, famciclovir, penciclovir, valacyclovir, valganciclovir, or ganciclovir

> **BLACK BOX WARNING:** ANC <500/mm^3, platelet count <25,000/mm^3 (intravitreal)

Precautions: Pregnancy **C**, breastfeeding, children <6 mo, geriatric, preexisting cytopenias, renal function impairment, radiation therapy

> **BLACK BOX WARNING:** Secondary malignancy, bone marrow suppression, anemia, infertility, neutropenia

DOSAGE AND ROUTES
Induction treatment
Adult: **IV** 5 mg/kg/dose given over 1 hr q12hr × 2-3 wk

Maintenance treatment
Adult: **IV** INF 5 mg/kg/day given over 1 hr, daily × 7 days/wk; or 6 mg/kg/day × 5 days/wk; PO 1000 mg tid with food or 500 mg q3hr while awake; Intravitreal 4.5-mg implant

Prevention of CMV infection
Adult: **IV** 5 mg/kg/dose over 1 hr q12hr × 1-2 wk, then 5 mg/kg/day × 7 days/wk, then 6 mg/kg/day × 5 days/wk; PO 1000 mg tid, starting 10 days posttransplant × 14 days

Renal dose
Adult: **IV** CCr 50-69 ml/min, reduce to 2.5 mg/kg q12hr (induction), 2.5 mg/kg q24hr (maintenance); **PO** 1500 mg/day or 500 mg tid; **IV** CCr 25-49 ml/min reduce to 2.5 mg q24hr (induction); 1.25 mg/kg q24hr (maintenance); **PO** 1000 mg/day or 500 mg bid; **IV** CCr 10-24 ml/min reduce to 1.25 mg/kg q24hr (induc-

tion); 0.625 mg/kg q24hr (maintenance); **PO** 500 mg/day; **IV** CCr <10 ml/min reduce to 1.25 mg/kg 3×/wk after hemodialysis (induction); 0.625 mg/kg 3×/wk after hemodialysis (maintenance); **PO** 500 mg 3×/wk after hemodialysis

Available forms: Powder for inj 500 mg/vial, caps 250, 500 mg; implant, intravitreal 4.5 mg

Implementation
PO route
• Give with food, do not open or crush caps

IV route
• Product should be mixed under strict aseptic conditions using gloves, gown, and mask and using precautions for antineoplastics
Intermittent IV inf route
• Administer **IV** after reconstituting 500 mg/10 ml of sterile water for inj (50 mg/ml); shake; further dilute in 100 ml of D$_5$W, 0.9% NaCl, LR, Ringer's and run over 1 hr; use inf pump, in-line filter
• Do not give by BOL **IV**, IM, SUBCUT inj
• Use reconstituted sol within 12 hr, do not refrigerate or freeze; do not use sol with particulate matter or discoloration, fludarabine, sargramostim

Y-site compatibilities: Allopurinol, CISplatin, cyclophosphamide, enalaprilat, etoposide, filgrastim, fluconazole, gatifloxacin, granisetron, linezolid, melphalan, methotrexate, PACLitaxel, propofol, tacrolimus, teniposide, thiotepa

Y-site incompatibilities: Amsacrine, fludarabine, foscarnet, ondansetron, sargramostim, vinorelbine

Intravitreal implant route
• Implanted by surgeon only
• Handle carefully to prevent damage to coating

ADVERSE EFFECTS
CNS: *Fever,* chills, **coma,** *confusion,* abnormal thoughts, dizziness, bizarre dreams, *headache,* psychosis, tremors, somnolence, *paresthesia, weakness,* **seizures,** peripheral neuropathy
CV: Dysrhythmia, hypo/hypertension
EENT: Retinal detachment in CMV retinitis, cataracts, ocular hypertension, ocular pain, conjunctival scarring
GI: *Abnormal liver function tests, nausea, vomiting, anorexia, diarrhea, abdominal pain,* **hemorrhage, perforation, pancreatitis**
GU: **Hematuria,** *increased creatinine,* BUN

HEMA: Granulocytopenia, thrombocytopenia, irreversible neutropenia, anemia, eosinophilia, pancytopenia
INTEG: *Rash,* alopecia, *pruritus,* urticaria, pain at inj site, phlebitis
RESP: Dyspnea

Pharmacokinetics

Absorption	Completely absorbed, increased bioavailability with fatty foods
Distribution	Crosses blood-brain barrier, CSF
Metabolism	Not metabolized
Excretion	Kidneys (90%) unchanged, breast milk
Half-life	3 hr

Pharmacodynamics

Unknown

INTERACTIONS

Individual drugs

Adriamycin, amphotericin B, cycloSPORINE, dapsone, DOXOrubicin, flucytosine, mycophenolate, pentamidine, probenecid, tacrolimus, trimethoprim/sulfa combinations, vinBLAStine, vinCRIStine: increased ganciclovir toxicity

Didanosine: increased didanosine effect

Imipenem with cilastatin: increased risk for seizures

Probenecid: decreased renal clearance of ganciclovir

Radiation, zidovudine: severe granulocytopenia; do not give together

Tenofovir: increased effect

Drug classifications

Antineoplastics: severe granulocytopenia; do not give together

Nucleoside analogs, NSAIDs: increased toxicity

NURSING CONSIDERATIONS

Assessment

• **CMV retinitis:** Culture should be done before treatment with ganciclovir is initiated; cultures of blood, urine, and throat may all be taken; CMV is not confirmed by this method; the diagnosis is made by an ophthalmic exam

• Assess kidney, liver function; increases in hemopoietic studies: BUN, serum creatinine, AST creatinine clearance, ALT, A:G ratio, baseline, and drip treatment; blood counts should be done q2wk; watch for decreasing granulocytes, Hgb; if low, therapy may have to be discontinued

and restarted after hematologic recovery; blood transfusions may be required

• Assess for GI symptoms: severe nausea, vomiting, diarrhea; severe symptoms may necessitate discontinuing product

• Monitor electrolytes and minerals: calcium, phosphorus, magnesium, sodium, potassium; watch closely for tetany during 1st administration

• Assess for symptoms of allergic reactions: flushing, rash, urticaria, pruritus

• **Monitor for leukopenia/neutropenia/thrombocytopenia:** WBCs, platelets q2day during 2 ×/day dosing and qwk thereafter; check for leukopenia with daily WBC count in patients with prior leukopenia with other nucleoside analogs or for whom leukopenia counts are <1000 cells/mm^3 at start of treatment; bruising, fatigue, bleeding, poor healing

• Assess for seizures, dysrhythmias

Patient/family education

• Advise patient to notify prescriber if sore throat, swollen lymph nodes, malaise, fever occur; may indicate other infections

• Advise patient to report perioral tingling, numbness in extremities, and paresthesias

• Caution patient that serious product interactions may occur if OTC products are ingested; check first with prescriber

• Inform patient that product is not a cure, but will control symptoms

• Advise patient that regular blood tests, ophth exams must be continued

• Inform patient that major toxicities may necessitate discontinuing product

• **Instruct patient to use contraception during treatment and that infertility may occur; men should use barrier contraception for 90 days after treatment**

• Teach patient to take PO with food

• **Teach patient to report infection:** fever, chills, sore throat; blood dyscrasias: bruising, bleeding, petechiae

• Tell patient to avoid crowds, persons with respiratory infection

• Advise patient to use sunscreen to prevent burns

Evaluation

Positive therapeutic outcome

• Decreased symptoms of CMV infection

ganciclovir ophthalmic
See Appendix B

ganirelix (Rx)

(gan-i-rell'ex)
Orgalutran ✤
Func. class.: Gonadotropin-releasing hormone antagonist
Chem. class.: Synthetic decapeptide
Pregnancy category X

ACTION: Inhibitor of pituitary gonadotropin secretion; initially increases LH and FSH, induces a rapid suppression of gonadotropin secretion

Therapeutic outcome: Pregnancy

USES: For inhibition of premature LH surges in women undergoing controlled ovarian hyperstimulation

CONTRAINDICATIONS:

Pregnancy **X**, breastfeeding, hypersensitivity, latex allergy

DOSAGE AND ROUTES

Adult: Give FSH on day 2 or 3 of cycle, then SUBCUT 250 mcg/day during mid to late portion of follicular phase; continue until day of hCG administration

Available forms: Inj 250 mcg/0.5 ml

Implementation

• Administer SUBCUT using abdomen, around navel, or upper thigh, swab inj area with disinfectant, clean a 2-in circle and allow to dry, pinch up area between thumb and finger, insert needle at 45-90 degrees to surface; if positioned correctly, no blood will be drawn back into syringe; if blood is drawn into syringe, reposition needle without removing it, inject slowly
• Protect from light

ADVERSE EFFECTS

CNS: Headache
ENDO: Ovarian hyperstimulation syndrome, abdominal pain (gynecologic)
GI: Nausea
GU: *Spotting, breakthrough bleeding,* decreased urine, **fetal death**
INTEG: Pain on inj
SYST: Fetal death

Pharmacokinetics

Absorption	Unknown
Distribution	Unknown
Metabolism	To metabolites
Excretion	Unknown
Half-life	13-16 hr

Pharmacodynamics

Onset	Unknown
Peak	Unknown
Duration	Treatment length

NURSING CONSIDERATIONS
Assessment

• Monitor reproductive tests: serum progesterone, LH, estradiol, ovarian ultrasound, pelvic exam, baseline, during treatment
• Assess for suspected pregnancy; product should not be used (pregnancy **X**)
• Assess for latex allergy; product should not be used

Patient/family education

• Teach patient to report abdominal pain, vaginal bleeding

Evaluation
Positive therapeutic outcome
• Pregnancy

gatifloxacin ophthalmic

See Appendix B

gefitinib (Rx)

(ge-fi'tye-nib)
Iressa
Func. class.: Antineoplastic, miscellaneous
Chem. class.: Epidermal growth factor receptor inhibitor
Pregnancy category D

ACTION: Not fully understood; inhibits intracellular phosphorylation of cell surface receptors associated with epidermal growth factor receptors

Therapeutic outcome: Decreased growth and spread of malignant cells

USES: Advanced/metastatic non–small cell lung cancer (NSCLC) in those who have not responded to platinum or docetaxel products

CONTRAINDICATIONS:
Pregnancy **D**, breastfeeding, children, hypersensitivity

Precautions: Renal/hepatic/ocular/pulmonary disorders, geriatric

DOSAGE AND ROUTES
Adult: PO 250 mg/day

CYP3A4 inducers concurrently (such as rifampin or phenytoin)
Adult: PO 500 mg/day

Available forms: Tabs 250 mg

Implementation
• Give without regard to food

ADVERSE EFFECTS
EENT: Amblyopia, conjunctivitis, eye pain, corneal erosion/ulcer
GI: Nausea, diarrhea, vomiting, anorexia, **pancreatitis**, mouth ulceration, **hepatotoxicity**
INTEG: Rash, pruritus, acne, dry skin, **toxic epidermal neurolysis, angioedema**
MISC: Peripheral edema, hemorrhage
RESP: **Interstitial lung disease**, cough, dyspnea, pneumonia

Pharmacokinetics

Absorption	Slowly
Distribution	Unknown
Metabolism	Unknown
Excretion	In feces (86%), urine (<4%)
Half-life	Unknown

Pharmacodynamics

Onset	Unknown
Peak	3-7 hr
Duration	Unknown

INTERACTIONS
Individual drugs
Cimetidine, phenytoin, ranitidine, rifampin, sodium bicarbonate: decreased levels
Clarithromycin, erythromycin, itraconazole, ketoconazole: increased concentration
CloZAPine: increased bone marrow suppression
Metoprolol, warfarin: increased plasma concentration

Drug/herb
St. John's wort: decreased gefitinib levels

NURSING CONSIDERATIONS
Assessment
⚠ **Assess pulmonary changes: lung sounds, cough, dyspnea; interstitial lung disease may occur, may be fatal; discontinue therapy if confirmed**
• Assess ocular changes: eye irritation, corneal erosion/ulcer, aberrant eyelash growth
⚠ **Assess for pancreatitis: abdominal pain, levels of amylase, lipase**
⚠ **Assess for toxic epidermal necrosis, angioedema**
• Monitor GI symptoms: frequency of stools; if diarrhea is poorly tolerated, therapy may be discontinued for up to 14 days

Patient/family education
• Teach to report adverse reactions immediately: SOB, severe abdominal pain, occular changes, skin eruptions
• Advise of reason for treatment, expected results
• Advise to use contraception during treatment

Evaluation
Positive therapeutic outcome
• Decreased non–small cell lung cancer cells

---

gemcitabine (Rx)
(gem-sit'a-been)
Gemzar
Func. class.: Antineoplastic—miscellaneous
Chem. class.: Nucleoside analog
Pregnancy category D

Do not confuse:
Gemzar/Zinecard

ACTION: Exhibits antitumor activity by killing cells undergoing DNA synthesis (S phase) and blocking G_1/S-phase boundary

Therapeutic outcome: Prevention of growth of tumor

USES: Adenocarcinoma of the pancreas (nonresectable stage II, III, or metastatic stage IV); in combination with CISplatin for inoperable, advanced, or metastatic non–small cell lung cancer; advanced breast cancer in combination with PACLitaxel; with CARBOplatin for ovarian cancer, biliary tract cancer

CONTRAINDICATIONS:
Pregnancy **D**, breastfeeding, hypersensitivity

Adverse effects: *italics* = common; **bold** = life-threatening

Precautions: Children, geriatric, myelosuppression, radiation therapy, renal/hepatic disease

DOSAGE AND ROUTES
Pancreatic carcinoma (nonresectable stage II, III, IV)
Adult: IV 1000 mg/m^2 given over ½ hr qwk × 7 wk, then 1 wk rest period; subsequent cycles should be infused once qwk × 3 wk out of every 4 wk depending on hematologic toxicity

Non–small cell lung cancer
4 wk schedule
Adult: IV 1000 mg/m^2 given over ½ hr on days 1, 8, 15 of each 28-day cycle; give CISplatin **IV** 100 mg/m^2 on day 1 after gemcitabine

3 wk schedule
Adult: IV 1250 mg/m^2 given over ½ hr on days 1, 8 of each 21-day cycle; give CISplatin 100 mg/m^2 after the INF of gemcitabine on day 1

Advanced breast cancer
Adult: IV 1250 mg/m^2 over ½ hr on days 1 and 8 of a 21-day cycle; give with PACLitaxel on day 1, 175 mg/m^2 over 3 hr prior to gemcitabine

Available forms: Lyophilized powder for inj 20 mg/ml

Implementation
• Give increased fluid intake to 2-3 L/day to prevent dehydration, unless contraindicated
• Provide antiemetic agents before and after treatment

IV route
• Prepare in biological cabinet using gown, mask, gloves
• After reconstituting with 0.9% NaCl 5 ml/200 mg vial of product or 25 ml/1 g of product, shake (38 mg/ml); may be further diluted with 0.9% NaCl to concentrate as low as 0.1 mg/ml; discard unused portion, give over ½ hr, do not admix

Y-site compatibilities: Amifostine, amikacin, aminophylline, ampicillin, aztreonam, bleomycin, bumetanide, butorphanol, calcium gluconate, cefOXitin, cefTAZidime, ceftizoxime, cefTRIAXone, chlorproMAZINE, cimetidine, ciprofloxacin, CISplatin, clindamycin, cyclophosphamide, cytarabine, DACTINomycin, DAUNOrubicin, diphenhydrAMINE, DOBUTamine, DOCEtaxel, DOPamine, DOXOrubicin, droperidol, enalaprilat, etoposide, famotidine, floxuridine, fluconazole, fludarabine, fluorouracil, gentamicin, granisetron, haloperidol, heparin, hydrocortisone, HYDROmorphone, IDArubicin, ifosfamide, leucovorin, linezolid, LORazepam, mannitol, meperidine, mesna, metoclopramide, metroNIDAZOLE, minocycline, mitoXANtrone, morphine, nalbuphine, ondansetron, PACLitaxel, promethazine, ranitidine, streptozocin, teniposide, thiotepa, ticarcillin, tobramycin, topotecan, trimethoprim/sulfamethoxazole, vancomycin, vinBLAStine, vinCRIStine, vinorelbine, zidovudine, zoledronic acid

Y-site incompatibilities: Acyclovir, amphotericin B colloidal, amphotericin B lipid complex, amphotericin B liposome, cefepime, cefoperazone, cefotaxime, chloramphenicol, dantrolene, DAPTOmycin, diazepam, furosemide, ganciclovir, imipenem-cilastatin, irinotecan, ketorolac, lansoprazole, methotrexate, methylPREDNISolone, mitoMYcin, nafcillin, pantoprazole, PEMEtrexed, phenytoin, piperacillin, prochlorperazine, thiopental

ADVERSE EFFECTS
GI: Diarrhea, nausea, vomiting, anorexia, constipation, stomatitis
GU: Proteinuria, hematuria
HEMA: Leukopenia, anemia, neutropenia, thrombocytopenia
INTEG: Irritation at site, rash, alopecia
MISC: Dyspnea, fever, **hemorrhage**, infection, flulike syndrome, paresthesia, peripheral edema, myalgia, capillary leak syndrome

Pharmacokinetics	
Absorption	Unknown
Distribution	Crosses placenta
Metabolism	Unknown
Excretion	Unknown
Half-life	42-379 min

Pharmacodynamics
Unknown

INTERACTIONS
Individual drug
Alcohol: increased bleeding

Drug classifications
Anticoagulants, NSAIDs, salicylates: increased bleeding
Antineoplastics, radiation: increased myelosuppression, diarrhea
Live virus vaccines: decreased antibody response

Drug/lab test
Increased: BUN, AST, ALT, alkaline phosphatase, bilirubin, creatinine

---

NURSING CONSIDERATIONS
Assessment
• **Bone marrow depression:** monitor CBC, differential, platelet count before each dose; single agent: absolute granulocyte count >1000, and platelets >100,000, give complete dose; absolute granulocyte count 500-999, platelets 50,000-99,999, give 75%; absolute granulocyte count <500 or platelets <50,000, do not give; combination with PACLitaxel in breast cancer: absolute granulocyte count >1200 and platelets >75,000, give complete dose; absolute granulocyte count 1000-1199 or platelets 50,000-75,000, give 75%; absolute granulocyte 700-999 or platelets ≥50,000, give 50%; granulocyte count <700 or platelets <50,000, do not give; combination with CARBOplatin in ovarian cancer: absolute granulocyte count >1500 and platelet count >100,000, give complete dose; absolute granulocyte count 1000-1499 or platelets 75,000-99,999, give 75%; absolute granulocyte count <1000 or platelets <75,000, do not give
• **Assess for blood dyscrasias:** bruising, bleeding, petechiae
• Monitor I&O, nutritional intake
• Monitor renal/hepatic studies before, during treatment; may increase AST, ALT, alkaline phosphatase, bilirubin, BUN, creatinine
• Assess food preferences: list likes, dislikes
• Assess buccal cavity for dryness, sores or ulceration, white patches, oral pain, bleeding, dysphagia
• Assess GI symptoms: frequency of stools; cramping
• Assess signs of dehydration: rapid respirations, poor skin turgor, decreased urine output, dry skin, restlessness, weakness

Patient/family education
• Teach patient to rinse mouth tid-qid with water, club soda; brush teeth bid-tid with soft brush or cotton-tipped applicator for stomatitis; use unwaxed dental floss
• Advise patient to avoid foods with citric acid or hot or rough texture if stomatitis is present; to drink adequate fluids
• Advise patient to report stomatitis; any bleeding, white spots, ulcerations in mouth; tell patient to examine mouth daily, report symptoms
• Advise patient to report signs of anemia: fatigue, headache, faintness, shortness of breath, irritability; hematuria, dysuria
• Advise patient to use contraception during therapy and for 4 mo after (pregnancy **D**)
• Instruct patient to avoid use with NSAIDs, salicylates, alcohol; not to receive vaccinations during treatment

• Teach about possible hair loss and what can be done
• Advise to report flulike symptoms, swelling of feet/legs, bruising; bleeding of gums, blood in urine, stools, emesis
• Teach to avoid crowds, persons with known upper respiratory infections
• Advise patient to use electric razor

Evaluation
Positive therapeutic outcome
• Decrease in tumor size, decrease in spread of cancer, symptom relief

TREATMENT OF OVERDOSE:
Induce vomiting, provide supportive care

gemfibrozil (Rx)
(gem-fye′broe-zil)
Apo-Gemfibrozil ✤**, gemfibrozil,**
Gen-Gemfibrozil ✤**, Lopid, PMS-**
Gemfibrozil ✤
Func. class.: Antilipemic
Chem. class.: Fibric acid derivative
Pregnancy category C

Do not confuse:
Lopid/Levbid/Slo-bid

ACTION: Inhibits biosynthesis of VLDL, decreases triglycerides, increases HDLs

Therapeutic outcome: Decreased hepatic triglyceride production, VLDL; accelerates removal of cholesterol from liver

USES: Type IIb, IV, V hyperlipidemia as adjunct with diet therapy, hypertriglyceridemia

CONTRAINDICATIONS:
Severe renal/hepatic disease, preexisting gallbladder disease, primary biliary cirrhosis, hypersensitivity

Precautions: Pregnancy **C,** breastfeeding, renal disease, cholelithiasis

DOSAGE AND ROUTES
Adult: PO 1200 mg in divided doses bid 30 min before meals

Hepatic/renal dose
Avoid use

Available forms: Tabs 600 mg; caps 300 mg ✤

Implementation
• Give 30 min before AM and PM meals

Adverse effects: *italics* = common; **bold** = life-threatening

ADVERSE EFFECTS

CNS: Fatigue, vertigo, headache, paresthesia, dizziness, somnolence

GI: Nausea, vomiting, *dyspepsia, diarrhea, abdominal pain*

HEMA: Leukopenia, anemia, eosinophilia, thrombocytopenia

INTEG: Rash, urticaria, pruritus

MISC: Task perversion

MS: Myopathy, rhabdomyolysis

SYST: Angioedema, exfoliative dermatitis

Pharmacokinetics

Absorption	Well absorbed
Distribution	Unknown, plasma protein binding >95%
Metabolism	Liver, minimal
Excretion	Kidney, unchanged (70%), feces (6%)
Half-life	1½ hr

Pharmacodynamics

Onset	1-2 hr
Peak	1-2 hr
Duration	2-4 months

INTERACTIONS

Individual drugs

Do not use with repaglinide, simvastatin
CycloSPORINE: decreased cycloSPORINE effect
Repaglinide: increased hypoglycemic effect
Warfarin: increased anticoagulant properties

Drug classifications

Bile acid sequestrants: decreased effect of gemfibrozil, separate by >2 hr
HMG-CoA reductase inhibitors: increased risk of myositis, myalgia
Sulfonylureas: increased hypoglycemic effect

Drug/lab test

Increased: liver function tests, CK
Decreased: Hgb, Hct, WBC, potassium

NURSING CONSIDERATIONS

Assessment

• **Hypercholesteremia:** Assess nutrition: fat, protein, carbohydrates; nutritional analysis should be performed by dietitian before treatment is initiated; monitor triglycerides, cholesterol, lipids baseline, during treatment; LDL and VLDL should be watched closely and if increased, product should be discontinued

• Assess renal, liver function tests, CBC, blood glucose if patient is on long-term therapy; if liver function test results increase, product should be discontinued; monitor hematologic and hepatic function

• Monitor bowel pattern daily; diarrhea may be a problem

• **Myopathy, rhabdomyolysis:** Assess for muscle pain, tenderness; obtain baseline CPK; if elevated or if these occur, product should be discontinued

Patient/family education

• Inform patient that compliance is needed for positive results to occur; not to double doses; that product may be discontinued if no improvement in 3 mo

• Caution patient to decrease risk factors: high-fat diet, smoking, alcohol consumption, lack of exercise

• Advise patient to notify prescriber if GI symptoms of diarrhea, abdominal or epigastric pain, nausea, vomiting occur; or if chills, fever, sore throat occur; also occurrence of muscle cramps, abdominal cramps, severe flatulence

Evaluation

Positive therapeutic outcome

• Decreased cholesterol levels, serum triglyceride and improved ratio with HDLs

---

gemifloxacin (Rx)

(gem-ah-flox′a-sin)

Factive

Func. class.: Antiinfective

Chem. class.: Fluoroquinolone

Pregnancy category C

ACTION: Inhibits DNA gyrase, which is an enzyme involved in replication, transcription, and repair of bacterial DNA

Therapeutic outcome: Negative C&S, decreasing symptoms of infection

USES: Acute bacterial exacerbation of chronic bronchitis caused by *Streptococcus pneumoniae, Haemophilus influenzae, Haemophilus parainfluenzae, Moraxella catarrhalis;* community-acquired pneumonia caused by *Streptococcus pneumoniae* including multiproduct-resistant strains, *H. influenzae, M. catarrhalis, Mycoplasma pneumoniae, Chlamydia pneumoniae, Klebsiella pneumoniae*

CONTRAINDICATIONS:
Hypersensitivity to quinolones

Precautions: Pregnancy **C,** breastfeeding, children, geriatric, hypokalemia, hypomagnese-

---

mia, renal disease, seizure disorders, excessive exposure to sunlight, psychosis, increased intracranial pressure, history of QT interval prolongation, dysrhythmias, myasthenia gravis, torsades de pointes

> **BLACK BOX WARNING:** Tendon pain/rupture, tendinitis

DOSAGE AND ROUTES
Adult: PO 320 mg/day × 5-7 days depending on type of infection

Renal dose
Adult: PO CCr ≤40 ml/min 160 mg q24hr

Available forms: Tabs 320 mg

Implementation
• Give with or without food
• Theophylline should not be used with this product; toxicity may result
• Administer 2 hr before or 3 hr after antacids, iron, zinc, or buffered products; 2 hr before sucralfate

ADVERSE EFFECTS
CNS: *Dizziness, headache,* somnolence, depression, insomnia, nervousness, confusion, agitation, **seizures**
CV: QT prolongation, vasodilatation
EENT: Visual disturbances, retinal detachment
GI: Diarrhea, *nausea,* vomiting, anorexia, flatulence, heartburn, dry mouth; increased AST, ALT; constipation, abdominal pain, oral thrush, glossitis, stomatitis, **pseudomembranous colitis**
GU: Crystalluria (rare), vaginitis, interstitial nephritis
HEMA: **Thrombocytopenia, neutropenia, anemia, agranulocytosis, thrombotic thrombocytopenic purpura,** muscle weakness
INTEG: Rash, pruritus, urticaria, *photosensitivity*
SYST: **Anaphylaxis, Stevens-Johnson syndrome, toxic epidermal necrolysis, exfoliative dermatitis**

Pharmacokinetics

Absorption	Rapidly, bioavailability 71%
Distribution	Unknown
Metabolism	Unknown
Excretion	In urine as active product, metabolites
Half-life	4-12 hr

Pharmacodynamics

Onset	Unknown
Peak	1-2 hr
Duration	Unknown

INTERACTIONS
Individual drugs
Amoxapine, chloroquine, cloZAPine, dasatinib, dolasetron, dronedarone, droperidol, erythromycin, flecainide, haloperidol, lapatinib, maprotiline, methadone, octreotide, ondansetron, palonosetron, pentamidine, pimozide, propafenone, ranolazine, risperidone, sertindole, SUNItinib, tacrolimus, telithromycin, troleandomycin, vardenafil, vorinostat, ziprasidone: increased QT prolongation
Probenecid: may increase toxicity
Theophylline: toxicity; do not use concurrently

Drug classifications
Antacids containing aluminum, iron, magnesium, sucralfate, zinc: decreased absorption; give 2 hr before or 3 hr after meals
Antiarrhythmics (amiodarone, disopyramide, procainamide, quiNIDine, sotalol), antidepressants (tricyclics), β-blockers, halogenated/local anesthetics: may decrease effect, resulting in life-threatening dysrhythmias, QT prolongation
Drugs that increase QT prolongation: increased QT prolongation
NSAIDs: increased CNS stimulation

NURSING CONSIDERATIONS
Assessment
• Monitor renal, liver function tests: BUN, creatinine, AST, ALT, electrolytes
• Monitor I&O ratio; urine pH, <5.5 is ideal
• Assess CNS symptoms: insomnia, vertigo, headache, agitation, confusion
A Assess allergic reactions and anaphylaxis: rash, flushing, urticaria, pruritus, chills, fever, joint pain; may occur a few days after therapy begins; epinephrine and resuscitation equipment should be available for anaphylactic reaction
• **Pseudomembranous colitis:** Monitor bowel pattern daily; if severe diarrhea, fever, abdominal pain occurs, product should be discontinued
• **Assess for overgrowth of infection:** perineal itching, fever, malaise, redness, pain, swelling, drainage, rash, diarrhea, change in cough, sputum

Patient/family education
• Advise patient that fluids must be increased to 2 L/day to avoid crystallization in kidneys
• Instruct patient that if dizziness or light-headedness occurs, to ambulate, perform activities with assistance
• Instruct patient to complete full course of product therapy
• Teach patient to contact prescriber if adverse reactions occur
• Teach patient to avoid iron- or mineral-containing supplements or aluminum/magnesium antacids within 2 hr before or 3 hr after dosing
• Advise patient that photosensitivity may occur and sunscreen should be used
• Advise patient to use frequent rinsing of mouth, sugarless candy or gum for dry mouth
• Teach patient to avoid other medication unless approved by prescriber

Evaluation
Positive therapeutic outcome
• Negative C&S, absence of signs/symptoms of infection

⚠ HIGH ALERT

gemtuzumab (Rx)
(gem-tue-zue'mab)
Mylotarg
Func. class.: Antineoplastic—miscellaneous
Chem. class.: Monoclonal antibody
Pregnancy category D

ACTION: Composed of recombinant humanized IgG4κ antibody, binds to CD33 antigen that is released in myeloid cells

Therapeutic outcome: Decreasing signs/symptoms of leukemia

USES: Acute myeloid leukemia (AML) in patients with first relapse who are 60 yr or older

CONTRAINDICATIONS:
Pregnancy **D**, breastfeeding

BLACK BOX WARNING: Hypersensitivity to this product or murine protein, severe myelosuppression

Precautions: Children, severe renal disease

BLACK BOX WARNING: Hepatic disease, pulmonary disease, infusion-related reactions

DOSAGE AND ROUTES
Adult: IV 9 m/m^2 as a 2 hr INF; before giving INF, give diphenhydrAMINE 50 mg PO, acetaminophen 650-1000 mg PO 1 hr; then use acetaminophen 650-1000 mg q4hr for additional 2 doses prn

Available forms: Powder for inj, lyophilized 5 mg

Implementation
• Do not give **IV** push or bolus
• Protect from light, use biological safety hood, allow to come to room temperature
• Reconstitute each vial with 5 ml of sterile water for inj using sterile syringes, swirl each vial, check for discoloration or particulate matter, give over 2 hr, use a separate line with 1.2-micron terminal filter
• May be premedicated with methylPREDNISolone and antiemetics
• Store reconstituted sol for ≤8 hr in refrigerator

ADVERSE EFFECTS
CNS: *Dizziness,* insomnia, depression, headache
CV: Hypertension, **hemorrhage,** tachycardia, hypotension
HEMA: Prolonged neutropenia, thrombocytopenia
INTEG: *Rash,* herpes simplex, local reaction, petechiae, pruritus
GI: Anorexia, diarrhea, constipation, nausea, stomatitis, vomiting, **fatal liver toxicity**
GU: Hematuria, **vaginal hemorrhage**
META: Hypokalemia, hypomagnesemia
MISC: *Fever, myalgias, headache, chills,* peripheral edema
RESP: Cough, pneumonia, epistaxis, rhinitis, dyspnea

Pharmacokinetics
Absorption	Unknown
Distribution	Unknown
Metabolism	Unknown
Excretion	Unknown
Half-life	Biphasic; 45, 100 hr, respectively

Pharmacodynamics
Unknown

INTERACTIONS
Drug classifications
Antineoplastics, other, radiation: increased bone marrow suppression

---

NURSING CONSIDERATIONS
Assessment
- Assess for pulmonary symptoms: cough, dyspnea
- Monitor blood studies: BUN, creatinine, AST, ALT, electrolytes, bilirubin, CBC, uric acid
- Assess for symptoms of infection; chills, fever, headache may be masked by product
- Assess CNS reaction: LOC, mental status, dizziness, confusion
- Assess cardiac status: lung sounds; ECG before, during treatment, especially in those with cardiac disease
- Assess bone marrow depression: bruising, bleeding, blood in stools, urine, sputum, emesis

Patient/family education
- Advise patient to take acetaminophen for fever
- Instruct patient to avoid hazardous tasks, since confusion, dizziness may occur; avoid prolonged sunlight, use sunscreen
- Instruct patient to report signs of infection: sore throat, fever, diarrhea, vomiting
- Teach patient to avoid immunizations, crowds, people with known infections
- Caution patient that product is very toxic

Evaluation
Positive therapeutic outcome
- Improvement in blood counts

gentamicin (Rx)
(jen-ta-mye′sin)
Func. class.: Antiinfective
Chem. class.: Aminoglycoside
Pregnancy category C

ACTION: Interferes with protein synthesis in bacterial cell by binding to 30S ribosomal subunit, causing misreading of genetic code; inaccurate peptide sequence forms in protein chain, causing bacterial death

Therapeutic outcome: Bactericidal effects for the following organisms: *Pseudomonas aeruginosa, Proteus, Klebsiella, Serratia, Escherichia coli, Enterobacter, Citrobacter, Staphylococcus, Shigella, Salmonella, Acinetobacter, Bacillus anthracis*

USES: Severe systemic infections of CNS; respiratory, GI, and urinary tracts; bone; skin; soft tissues; caused by susceptible strains

CONTRAINDICATIONS:
Hypersensitivity to this or other aminoglycosides

> **BLACK BOX WARNING:** Pregnancy **D**

Precautions: Breastfeeding, geriatric, neonates, pseudomembranous colitis

> **BLACK BOX WARNING:** Renal disease, hearing deficits, myasthenia gravis, Parkinson's disease, infant botulism, neuromuscular disease, tinnitus

DOSAGE AND ROUTES
Severe systemic infections
Adult: IV INF 3-6 mg/kg/day in 3 divided doses q8hr; IM 3-5 mg/kg/day in divided doses q8hr
Child: IV/IM 2-2.5 mg/kg q8hr

Neonate and infant: IV/IM 2.5 mg/kg q8-12hr

Neonate <1 wk: 2.5 mg/kg q12hr

Renal dose
Adult: IM/IV CCr 70-100 ml/min reduce dose by multiplying maintenance dose by 0.85, give q8-12hr; CCr 50-69 ml/min reduce dose as above, give q12hr; CCr 25-49 ml/min reduce as above, give q24hr; CCr <25 ml/min reduce as above, give based on serum concentrations

Renal dose: extend interval (unlabeled)
Adult: IV CCr 40-59 ml/min, 5-7 mg/kg q36hr; CCr 20-39 ml/min, 5-7 mg/kg q48hr; CCr <20 ml/min, 5-7 mg/kg once, then base on serial levels

Available forms: Inj 10, 40, 60, 80, 100 mg/ml; premixed inj 40, 60, 70, 80, 90, 100, 120 mg/100 ml NS

Implementation
Intermittent IV infusion route
- Give inj deeply in large muscle mass; rotate sites

Topical route
- Wash hands, wear gloves, clean skin before applying

IV route
- Give in even doses around the clock; product must be given for 10-14 days to ensure organism death and prevent superinfection
- Give by intermittent inf over ½-1 hr, flush with 0.9% NaCl or D₅W after inf

Adverse effects: *italics* = common; **bold** = life-threatening

- Separate aminoglycosides and penicillins by ≥1 hr
- Store in tight container

Syringe compatibilities: Clindamycin, methicillin, penicillin G sodium

Y-site compatibilities: Amifostine, amiodarone, amsacrine, atracurium, aztreonam, cefpirome, ciprofloxacin, cyclophosphamide, cytarabine, diltiazem, enalaprilat, esmolol, famotidine, fluconazole, fludarabine, foscarnet, granisetron, hydromorphone, IL-2, insulin, labetalol, LORazepam, magnesium sulfate, melphalan, meperidine, meropenem, midazolam, morphine, multivitamins, ondansetron, PACLitaxel, pancuronium, perphenazine, sargramostim, tacrolimus, teniposide, theophylline, thiotepa, tolazine, vecuronium, vinorelbine, vit B with C, zidovudine

Y-site incompatibilities: IDArubicin, indomethacin

ADVERSE EFFECTS

CNS: Confusion, depression, numbness, tremors, **seizures,** muscle twitching, **neurotoxicity,** dizziness, vertigo, **encephalopathy, fever, headache, lethargy**

CV: Hypotension, hypertension, palpitations, edema

EENT: Ototoxicity, **deafness,** visual disturbances, tinnitus

GI: *Nausea, vomiting, anorexia,* increased ALT, AST, bilirubin, hepatomegaly, **hepatic necrosis,** splenomegaly

GU: Oliguria, hematuria, **renal damage, azotemia, renal failure, nephrotoxicity,** proteinuria

HEMA: Agranulocytosis, thrombocytopenia, leukopenia, eosinophilia, anemia

INTEG: *Rash,* burning, urticaria, dermatitis, alopecia, photosensitivity, **anaphylaxis**

MS: Twitching, myasthenia gravis–like symptoms

RESP: Apnea

Pharmacokinetics

Absorption	Well absorbed (IM)
Distribution	Distributed in extracellular fluids, poorly distributed in CSF; crosses placenta
Metabolism	Liver, minimal
Excretion	Mostly unchanged (79%) kidneys
Half-life	1-2 hr; infants 6-7 hr; increased in renal disease

Pharmacodynamics

	IM	IV
Onset	Rapid	Rapid
Peak	30-90 min	Infusion's end
Duration	Unknown	Unknown

INTERACTIONS
Individual drugs
Acyclovir, amphotericin B, cidofovir, CISplatin, cycloSPORINE, ethacrynic acid, foscarnet, furosemide, ganciclovir, mannitol, methoxyflurane, pamidronate, polymyxin, tacrolimus, vancomycin, zoledronic acid: increased ototoxicity, neurotoxicity, nephrotoxicity

Drug classifications
Aminoglycosides, cephalosporins, penicillins: increased otoxicity, neurotoxicity, nephrotoxicity

Nondepolarizing neuromuscular blockers: increased neuromuscular blockade, respiratory depression

Penicillins: Do not use at the same time as or physically mix with penicillins

Drug/lab test
Increase: LDH, AST, ALT, bilirubin, BUN, creatinine, eosinophils
Decrease: Hgb, WBC, platelets, granulocytes

NURSING CONSIDERATIONS
Assessment
- Assess patient for previous sensitivity reaction
- **Assess patient for signs and symptoms of infection** including characteristics of wounds, sputum, urine, stool, WBC >10,000/mm³, fever; obtain baseline during treatment
- **Neuromuscular disease (myasthenia gravis, Parkinson's disease, infant botulism):** Assess for paresthesias, tetany, Chvostek's/Trousseau's signs, confusion (adults) tetany, muscle weakness (infants); correct electrolyte imbalance
- Complete C&S before beginning product therapy; this will ensure that correct treatment has been initiated
- **Assess for allergic reactions:** rash, urticaria, pruritus, chills, fever, joint pain may occur a few days after therapy begins

> **BLACK BOX WARNING: Renal disease:**
> Identify urine output; if decreasing, notify prescriber (may indicate nephrotoxicity); also, increased BUN, creatinine, urine CCr <80 ml/min; monitor I&O ratio; urinalysis daily for proteinuria, cells, casts; report sudden change in urine output; assess urine pH if product is used for UTI; urine should be kept alkaline

---

⚠ Nurse Alert   ✳ Key NCLEX® Drug

• Monitor blood studies: AST, ALT, CBC, Hct, bilirubin, LDH, alkaline phosphatase, Coombs' test monthly if patient is on long-term therapy

• Monitor electrolytes: potassium, sodium, chloride, magnesium monthly if patient is on long-term therapy

• Monitor for bleeding: ecchymosis, bleeding gums, hematuria; assess stool guaiac daily if on long-term therapy

• **Assess for overgrowth of infection:** perineal itching, fever, malaise, redness, pain, swelling, drainage, rash, diarrhea, change in cough, sputum

• Obtain weight before treatment; calculation of dosage is usually based on ideal body weight but may be calculated on actual body weight

• Monitor VS during inf, watch for hypotension, change in pulse

• Assess **IV** site for thrombophlebitis including pain, redness, swelling q30min, change site if needed; apply warm compresses to discontinued site

• Obtain serum peak, measured at 30-60 min after **IV** inf or 60 min after IM inj, trough level measured just before next dose; blood level should be 2-4 times bacteriostatic level (based on traditional dosing)

> **BLACK BOX WARNING: Assess for deafness** by audiometric testing, ringing, roaring in ears, vertigo; assess hearing before, during, after treatment

• Assess for dehydration: high specific gravity, decrease in skin turgor, dry mucous membranes, dark urine

Patient/family education
• Teach patient to report sore throat, bruising, bleeding, joint pain; may indicate blood dyscrasias (rare)

• Advise patient to contact prescriber if vaginal itching, loose foul-smelling stools, furry tongue occur; may indicate superimposed infection

• Teach patient to drink adequate fluids

• Teach patient to avoid hazardous activities until reaction is known

Evaluation
Positive therapeutic outcome
• Absence of signs/symptoms of infection (WBC $<10,000/mm^3$, temp WNL, absence of red, draining wounds)

• Reported improvement in symptoms of infection

TREATMENT OF OVERDOSE:
Withdraw product, hemodialysis

gentamicin ophthalmic
See Appendix B

gentamicin topical
See Appendix B

glatiramer (Rx)
(glah-teer′a-mer)
Copaxone
Func. class.: Multiple sclerosis agent
Pregnancy category B

ACTION: Unknown; may modify the immune responses responsible for multiple sclerosis (MS)

Therapeutic outcome: Decreased symptoms of MS

USES: Reduction of the frequency of relapses in patients with relapsing-remitting MS after first clinical episode with MRI results consistent with MS

CONTRAINDICATIONS:
Hypersensitivity to this product or mannitol

Precautions: Pregnancy **B**, breastfeeding, children <18 yr, immune disorders, renal disease

DOSAGE AND ROUTES
Adult: SUBCUT 20 mg/day

Available forms: Inj premixed 20 mg/ml

Implementation
SUBCUT route
• Use a sterile syringe/needle to transfer the supplied diluent into the vial, rotate vial gently, do not shake; withdraw medication using a syringe with 27-G needle; administer SUBCUT into hip, thigh, arm; discard unused portion

• Use SUBCUT route only; do not give IM or **IV**

• Do not use sol that contains precipitate or is discolored

ADVERSE EFFECTS
CNS: Anxiety, hypertonia, tremor, vertigo, speech disorder, agitation, confusion, flushing
CV: Migraine, syncope, tachycardia, vasodilatation, chest pain, hypertension
EENT: Ear pain, blurred vision
GI: Nausea, vomiting, diarrhea, anorexia, gastroenteritis
GU: Urgency, dysmenorrhea, vaginal moniliasis
HEMA: Ecchymosis, lymphadenopathy
INTEG: Pruritus, rash, sweating, urticaria, erythema, injection site reaction

G

META: Edema, weight gain
MS: Arthralgia, back pain, neck pain, increased muscle tone
RESP: Bronchitis, dyspnea, laryngismus, rhinitis

Pharmacokinetics
Unknown

Pharmacodynamics
Unknown

NURSING CONSIDERATIONS
Assessment
• Monitor blood, renal, liver function tests before treatment
• Assess for CNS symptoms: anxiety, confusion, vertigo
• Assess GI status: diarrhea, vomiting, abdominal pain, gastroenteritis
• Assess cardiac status: tachycardia, palpitations, vasodilatation, chest pain

Patient/family education
• Give written, detailed instructions about the product; provide initial and return demonstrations on inj procedure; give information on use and disposal of product
• Advise patient that blurred vision, sweating may occur
• Advise patient that irregular menses, dysmenorrhea, or metorrhagia as well as breast pain may occur; use contraception during treatment
• Advise patient to notify prescriber if pregnancy is suspected or if nursing
• Advise patient not to change dosing or to stop taking product without advice of prescriber

Evaluation
Positive therapeutic outcome
• Decreased symptoms of multiple sclerosis

---

glimepiride (Rx)
(gly-meh′pih-ride)
Amaryl, CO Glimepiride ✦, ratio-Glimepiride ✦, Sandoz Glimepiride ✦
glipiZIDE (Rx)
(glip-i′zide)
Glucotrol, Glucotrol XL
Func. class.: Antidiabetic
Chem. class.: Sulfonylurea (2nd generation)
Pregnancy category C

Do not confuse:
glipiZIDE/glucotrol/glyBURIDE

ACTION: Causes functioning β cells in pancreas to release insulin, leading to drop in blood glucose levels; may improve insulin binding to insulin receptors or increase the number of insulin receptors with prolonged administration; may also reduce basal hepatic glucose secretion; not effective if patient lacks functioning β cells

Therapeutic outcome: Decrease in polyuria, polydipsia, polyphagia, clear sensorium, absence of dizziness, stable gait

USES: Type 2 diabetes mellitus

CONTRAINDICATIONS:
Hypersensitivity to sulfonylureas, type 1 diabetes, diabetic ketoacidosis

Precautions: Pregnancy C, geriatric, cardiac disease, severe renal/hepatic disease, G6PD deficiency

DOSAGE AND ROUTES
Glimepiride
Adult: PO 1-2 mg/day with breakfast, then increase by ≤2 mg/day at q1-2wk, max 8 mg/day
Geriatric: PO 1 mg/day, may increase if needed

Renal dose
Adult: PO 1 mg/day with breakfast, may titrate upward as needed

GlipiZIDE
Adult: PO 5 mg initially before breakfast, then increase by 2.5-5 mg after several days, to desired response; max 40 mg/day in divided doses or 15 mg/dose; (XL) PO 5 mg/day with breakfast, may increase to 10 mg/day; max 20 mg/day
Geriatric: PO 2.5 mg/day, may increase if needed

Hepatic dose
Adult: PO 2.5 mg initially, then increase to desired response; max 40 mg/day in divided doses or 15 mg/dose

Available forms: Glimepiride: tabs 1, 2, 4 mg; glipiZIDE: tabs 5, 10 mg scored; EXT REL tabs 2.5, 5, 10 mg

Implementation
• Do not break, crush, or chew ext rel tabs
• Convert from other oral hypoglycemic agents or insulin dosage of <40 units/day; change may be made without gradual dosage change
• Patients taking >40 units/day of insulin convert gradually by receiving oral hypoglycemic agents and 50% of previous insulin dosage for 3-5 days

---

⚠ Nurse Alert   ✦ Key NCLEX® Drug

- Monitor serum or urine glucose and ketones 3 ×/day during conversion
- **GlipiZIDE:** 30 min before meals (regular release); with breakfast (ext rel)
- **Glimepiride:** with breakfast; if patient is NPO, may need to hold dose to prevent hypoglycemia
- Give tab crushed and mixed with meal or fluids for patients with difficulty swallowing
- For severe hypoglycemia give **IV** D$_{50}$W, then **IV** dextrose solution
- Store in tight container in cool environment

ADVERSE EFFECTS
CNS: *Headache, weakness, dizziness, drowsiness,* tinnitus, fatigue, vertigo
ENDO: Hypoglycemia
GI: **Hepatotoxicity, cholestatic jaundice,** nausea, vomiting, diarrhea, heartburn
HEMA: **Leukopenia, thrombocytopenia, agranulocytosis, aplastic anemia,** increased AST, ALT, alkaline phosphatase, **pancytopenia, hemolytic anemia**
INTEG: Rash, allergic reactions, pruritus, urticaria, eczema, photosensitivity, erythema, allergic vasculitis

Pharmacokinetics

Absorption	Completely absorbed, GI tract
Distribution	Unknown
Metabolism	Liver
Excretion	Via kidneys
Half-life	2-4 hr; 5 hr glimepiride

Pharmacodynamics

	Glipizide	Glimepiride
Onset	1-1½ hr	
Peak	1-2 hr	2-3 hr
Duration	10-12 hr	

INTERACTIONS
Individual drugs
Charcoal, cholestyramine, diazoxide, isoniazid, rifampin: possible decreased action of glipiZIDE
Chloramphenicol, cimetidine, clarithromycin, clofibrate, fenfluramine, fluconazole, gemfibrozil, guanethidine, insulin, methyldopa, phenylbutazone, probenecid, sulfinpyrizine, voriconazole: increased hypoglycemia
Digoxin: increased action of digoxin

Drug classifications
Androgens, anticoagulants, fibric acid derivatives, H$_2$-antagonists, magnesium salts, MAOIs, NSAIDs, salicylates, sulfonamides, tricyclics, urinary acidifiers: increased hypoglycemia
β-Blockers: may mask symptoms of hypoglycemia
Diuretics (thiazide), corticosteroids, hydantoins, urinary alkalinizers: possible decreased action of glipiZIDE
Glycosides: increased action of glycosides

Drug/herb
Garlic, horse chestnut: increased antidiabetic effect
Chromium: decreased antidiabetic effect
Chromium, coenzyme Q10, fenugreek, ginseng: increased or decreased hypoglycemic effect
Green tea: decreased hypoglycemic effect

Drug/lab test
Increase: AST, ALT, LDH, BUN, creatinine

NURSING CONSIDERATIONS
Assessment
- **Assess for hypoglycemic/hyperglycemic reactions** that can occur soon after meals; hypoglycemic reactions (sweating, weakness, dizziness, anxiety, tremors, hunger); hyperglycemic reactions; A1c (baseline, q3mo) during treatment
- **Blood dyscrasias:** Monitor CBC

Patient/family education
- **Teach patient to check for symptoms of cholestatic jaundice:** dark urine, pruritus, yellow sclera; if these occur, prescriber should be notified
- Teach patient to use capillary blood glucose test
- Teach patient to report bleeding, bruising, weight gain, edema, SOB, weakness, sore throat
- Teach patient symptoms of hypo/hyperglycemia, what to do about each
- Instruct patient that product must be continued on daily basis; explain consequence of discontinuing product abruptly
- Caution patient to avoid OTC medications unless approved by a prescriber
- Teach patient that diabetes is a lifelong illness; that this product is not a cure
- Teach patient to avoid alcohol; inform about disulfiram reaction (nausea, headache, cramps, flushing, hypoglycemia)
- Instruct patient that all food included in diet plan must be eaten to prevent hypoglycemia
- Advise patient to use sunscreen or stay out of the sun to prevent burns
- Advise patient to carry/wear emergency ID and carry a glucagon emergency kit for emer-

gency purposes; also prescriber name, phone number, and medications taken
• Teach patient ext rel tab may appear in stool

Evaluation

Positive therapeutic outcome
• Decrease in polyuria, polydipsia, polyphagia; clear sensorium; absence of dizziness; stable gait
• Improved serum glucose, A1c

---

glyBURIDE (Rx)
(glye'byoor-ide)
Apo-GlyBURIDE ✦, DiaBeta ✦, Glynase PresTab, Novo-GlyBURIDE ✦, Nu-GlyBURIDE ✦, PMS-GlyBURIDE ✦, ratio-GlyBURIDE ✦, Sandoz GlyBURIDE ✦
Func. class.: Antidiabetic
Chem. class.: Sulfonylurea (2nd generation)
Pregnancy category C   ⬣

Do not confuse:
glyBURIDE/Glucotrol/glipiZIDE, **DiaBeta**/Zebeta

ACTION: Causes functioning β cells in pancreas to release insulin, leading to drop in blood glucose levels; may improve insulin binding to insulin receptors and increase number of insulin receptors with prolonged administration; may also reduce basal hepatic glucose secretion; not effective if patient lacks functioning β cells

Therapeutic outcome: Decrease in polyuria, polydipsia, polyphagia, clear sensorium, absence of dizziness, stable gait

USES: Type 2 diabetes mellitus

CONTRAINDICATIONS:
Hypersensitivity to sulfonylureas, type 1 diabetes, diabetic ketoacidosis, renal failure

Precautions: Pregnancy **C**, geriatric, cardiac/thyroid disease, severe renal/hepatic disease, severe hypoglycemic reactions, sulfonamide/sulfonylurea hypersensitivity, G6PD deficiency

DOSAGE AND ROUTES
DiaBeta
Adult: PO 1.25-5 mg initially, then increased to desired response at weekly intervals up to 20 mg/day; may be given as a single or divided dose
Geriatric: PO 1.25 mg initially, then increased to desired response; max 20 mg/day, maintenance 1.25-20 mg/day

Glynase PresTab (micronized)
Adult: PO 1.5-3 mg/day initially, may increase by 1.5 mg/wk, max 12 mg/day
Geriatric: PO 0.75-3 mg/day, may increase by 1.5 mg/wk

Available forms: Tabs (DiaBeta) 1.25, 2.5, 5 mg; tabs micronized (Glynase PresTab) 1.5, 3, 6 mg

Implementation
• Conversion from other oral hypoglycemic agents or insulin dosage of <40 units/day; change may be made without gradual dosage change
• Patients taking >40 units/day of insulin convert gradually by receiving oral hypoglycemic agents and 50% of previous insulin dosage for 3-5 days
• Monitor serum or urine glucose and ketones 3 ✕/day during conversion
• Give product 30 min before breakfast; if large dose is required, may be divided into two; give with meals to decrease GI upset and provide best absorption; if patient is NPO, may need to hold dose to avoid hypoglycemia, take at same time each day
• Give tab crushed and mixed with meal or fluids for patients with difficulty swallowing
• For severe hypoglycemia, give **IV** D$_{50}$W, then **IV** dextrose sol
• Store in tight container in cool environment

ADVERSE EFFECTS
CNS: *Headache, weakness,* paresthesia, tinnitus, fatigue, vertigo
EENT: Blurred vision
ENDO: Hypoglycemia
GI: Nausea, fullness, heartburn, **hepatoxicity, cholestatic jaundice,** vomiting, diarrhea, **hepatic failure** (rare)
HEMA: Leukopenia, thrombocytopenia, agranulocytosis, aplastic anemia, increased AST, ALT, alkaline phosphatase
INTEG: Rash, allergic reactions, pruritus, urticaria, eczema, photosensitivity, erythema
MS: Joint pains, vasculitis

Pharmacokinetics
Absorption	Completely absorbed GI tract
Distribution	99% plasma protein binding
Metabolism	Liver
Excretion	Urine, feces (metabolites), crosses placenta
Half-life	10 hr

Onset	2 hr
Peak	2-4 hr
Duration	24 hr

INTERACTIONS
Individual drugs

Bosentan: increased LFTs, avoid concurrent use

Charcoal, cholestyramine, isoniazid, rifampin thyroid, voriconazole: decreased action of glyBURIDE

Clarithromycin, chloramphenicol, fenfluramine, fluconazole, gemfibrozil, guanethidine, insulin, methyldopa, phenylbutazone, probenecid, sulfinpyrazone: increased hypoglycemia

Colesevelam: increased triglyceride levels

CycloSPORINE: increased action of cycloSPORINE

Diazoxide: both products may have action decreased

Digoxin: increased level

Drug classifications

Androgens, anticoagulants, antidepressants (tricyclics), β-blockers, H₂-antagonists, magnesium salts, MAOIs, NSAIDs, salicylates, sulfonamides, urinary acidifiers: increased hypoglycemia

β-Adrenergic blockers: increased masking of symptoms of hypoglycemia

Diuretics (thiazide), hydantoins, urinary alkalinizers, corticosteroids, phenothiazines, oral contraceptives, estrogens: decreased action of glyBURIDE

Drug/herb

Garlic, horse chestnut: increased antidiabetic effect

Green tea: decreased hypoglycemic effect

Drug/lab test

Increased: AST, ALT, LDH, BUN, creatinine

NURSING CONSIDERATIONS
Assessment

• Assess for hypo/hyperglycemic reactions that can occur soon after meals; hypoglycemic reactions (sweating, weakness, dizziness, anxiety, tremors, hunger); hyperglycemic reactions; A1c (baseline, q3mo) during treatment

• **Blood dyscrasias:** Monitor CBC, check liver function tests periodically, AST, LDH, and renal studies: BUN, creatinine during treatment

Patient/family education

• **Teach patient to check for symptoms of cholestatic jaundice:** dark urine, pruritus, yellow sclera; if these occur, prescriber should be notified

• Teach patient to use capillary blood glucose test

• **Teach patient symptoms of hypo/hyperglycemia,** what to do about each

• Instruct patient that product must be continued on daily basis; explain consequence of discontinuing product abruptly

• Teach patient to report bleeding, bruising, weight gain, edema, shortness of breath, weakness, sore throat

• Teach patient to take product in AM to prevent hypoglycemic reactions at night

• Caution patient to avoid OTC medications unless approved by a prescriber

• Teach patient that diabetes is a lifelong illness; that this product is not a cure

• Instruct patient that all food included in diet plan must be eaten to prevent hypoglycemia

• Advise patient to carry/wear emergency ID and carry a glucagon emergency kit for emergency purposes: have sugar packets available; also prescriber name, phone number, and medications

• Advise patient to use sunscreen or stay out of the sun to prevent burns

Evaluation
Positive therapeutic outcome

• Decrease in polyuria, polydipsia, polyphagia; clear sensorium; absence of dizziness; stable gait

• Improved serum glucose, A1c

---

glycopyrrolate (Rx)
(glye-koe-pye′roe-late)
Cuvposa, Robinul, Robinul-Forte
Func. class.: Cholinergic blocker, antispasmodic
Chem. class.: Quaternary ammonium compound
Pregnancy category B

ACTION: Inhibits action of acetylcholine at receptor sites in autonomic nervous system, which controls secretions, free acids in stomach

Therapeutic outcome: Decreased secretions in the respiratory tract, GI system

USES: Decreased secretions before surgery, reversal of neuromuscular blockade, peptic ulcer disease, irritable bowel syndrome, bradycardia, drooling

---

CONTRAINDICATIONS:

Children <3 yr, hypersensitivity, closed-angle glaucoma, myasthenia gravis, GI/GU obstruction, tachycardia, myocardial ischemia, hepatic disease, ulcerative colitis, toxic megacolon, prostatic hypertrophy

Precautions: Pregnancy **B**, breastfeeding, geriatric, pulmonary/renal disease, CHF, hyperthyroidism, CAD, Down syndrome, hiatal hernia, hypertension

DOSAGE AND ROUTES
Preoperatively
Adult: IM 4.4 mcg/kg ½-1 hr before surgery, max 0.1 mg
Child >2 yr (unlabeled): IM 4 mcg/kg 30-60 min before surgery
Child <2 yr (unlabeled): IM 4-9 mcg/kg

Intraoperative
Adult: **IV** 0.1 mg; may repeat 2-3 min prn
Child: IM/**IV** 4 mcg/kg q2-3min prn; max 0.1 mg/dose

Reversal of neuromuscular blockage
Adult and child: **IV** 200 mcg for each 1 mg of neostigmine or 5 mg **IV** of pyridostigmine simultaneously

GI disorders
Adult: PO 1-2 mg bid-tid; max 6 mg/day; IM/**IV** 100-200 mcg tid-qid, titrated to patient response

Antidysrhythmic
Adult: **IV** 100 mcg, may repeat q2min
Child: **IV** 4.4 mcg/kg, may repeat q2min, max 100 mcg

Secretion control
Child: PO 40-100 mcg/kg/dose tid-qid; IM/**IV** 4-10 mcg/kg/dose q3-4hr; max 0.2 mg/dose or 0.8 mg/24hr

Chronic drooling
Child/adolescent (3-16 yr): PO (oral solution) 0.02 mg/kg tid, titrate by 0.02 mg/kg/dose q5-7days, max 0.1 mg/kg/dose tid or 13-17 kg 1.5 mg/dose, 18-22 kg 2 mg, 23-27 kg 2.5 mg dose, ≥28 kg 3 mg/dose

Available forms: Tabs 1, 2 mg; inj 200 mcg 0.2 mg/ml; oral sol 1 mg/5 ml

Implementation
PO route
• Give PO with or after meals to prevent GI upset; may give with fluids other than water
IM route
• Give IM inj deeply in large muscle mass

Direct IV route
• Administer **IV** undiluted, give at a rate of 0.2 mg or less over 5-15 min through Y-tube or 3-way stopcock; do not add to **IV** sol
• Administer parenteral dose with patient recumbent to prevent postural hypotension

Syringe compatibilities: Atropine, benzquinamide, chlorproMAZINE, cimetidine, codeine, diphenhydrAMINE, droperidol, droperidol/fentaNYL, HYDROmorphone, hydrOXYzine, levorphanol, lidocaine, meperidine, meperidine/promethazine, midazolam, morphine, nalbuphine, neostigmine, oxymorphone, procaine, prochlorperazine, promazine, promethazine, pyridostigmine, ranitidine, scopolamine, triflupromazine, trimethobenzamide

Y-site compatibilities: Propofol

Solution compatibilities: D_5W, 0.9% NaCl, Ringer's D_5/0.45% NaCl

ADVERSE EFFECTS
CNS: Confusion, anxiety, restlessness, irritability, delusions, hallucinations, headache, sedation, depression, incoherence, dizziness, lethargy, flushing, weakness, **seizures**
CV: Palpitations, tachycardia, postural hypotension, paradoxical bradycardia
EENT: Blurred vision, photophobia, dilated pupils, difficulty swallowing, increased intraocular pressure, mydriasis, cycloplegia
GI: *Dryness of mouth, constipation,* nausea, vomiting, abdominal distress, paralytic ileus, altered taste perception
GU: Hesitancy, retention, impotence
INTEG: Urticaria, allergic reactions
MISC: Suppression of breastfeeding, nasal congestion, decreased sweating, **malignant hyperthermia**
SYST: Anaphylaxis

Pharmacokinetics

Absorption	Well absorbed (PO, SUBCUT, IM)
Distribution	Unknown
Metabolism	Not metabolized
Excretion	Unchanged in feces
Half-life	2 hr

Pharmacodynamics

	PO	IM	IV
Onset	Unknown	15-30 min	Immediate
Peak	1 hr	30-45 min	10-15 min
Duration	8-12 hr	2-7 hr	2-7 hr

⚠ Nurse Alert   ✳ Key NCLEX® Drug

INTERACTIONS
Individual drugs
Alcohol, amantadine: increased anticholinergic effect

Drug classifications
Antacids: decreased absorption of glycopyrrolate
Antidepressants (tricyclic), antihistamines, phenothiazines: increased anticholinergic effect
Antidiarrheals: decreased absorption of glycopyrrolate

NURSING CONSIDERATIONS
Assessment
• Monitor I&O ratio; retention commonly causes decreased urinary output; check for urinary hesitation; palpate bladder if retention occurs
• Monitor ECG for ectopic ventricular beats, PVC, tachycardia
• Monitor for bowel sounds; check for constipation; increase fluids, bulk, exercise if constipation occurs
• Assess mental status: affect, mood, CNS depression, worsening of psychiatric symptoms during early therapy

Patient/family education
• Caution patient not to operate machinery or engage in hazardous activities if drowsiness, blurred vision occurs
• Advise patient not to take OTC products, cough, cold preparations with alcohol, antihistamines without approval of prescriber
• Teach patient to avoid hot temperature: sweating is decreased, so heat stroke is possible
• Advise patient to notify prescriber of eye pain, blurred vision, light sensitivity
• Caution patient not to discontinue this product abruptly; tapering should be done over 1 wk

Evaluation
Positive therapeutic outcome
• Decreased secretions, bronchial, GI
• Decreased pain in GI disorders
• Reversal of neuromuscular blockade

golimumab (Rx)
(goal-lim'yu-mab)
Simponi, Simponi Aria
Func. class.: Antirheumatic agent (disease modifying), immunomodulator
Chem. class.: Monoclonal antibody, DMARDS, tumor necrosis factor (TNF) modifier
Pregnancy category B

ACTION: Monoclonal antibody specific for human tumor necrosis factor (TNF); elevated levels of TNF are found in patients with rheumatoid arthritis

Therapeutic outcome: Decreased pain, decreased inflammation in joints, better ROM

USES: Rheumatoid arthritis, ankylosing spondylitis, psoriatic arthritis, ulcerative colitis

CONTRAINDICATIONS:
Hypersensitivity active infections

Precautions: Pregnancy **B**, breastfeeding, children, geriatric patients, CNS demyelinating disease, Guillain-Barré syndrome, CHF, hepatitis B carriers, blood dyscrasias, surgery, MS, neurological disease, diabetes, immunosuppression

> **BLACK BOX WARNING:** Infection

DOSAGE AND ROUTES
Rheumatoid arthritis
Adult: SUBCUT 50 mg qmo; for RA give with methotrexate; IV (Simponi Aria only) 2 mg/kg over 30 min, repeat in 4 wk, then q8wk; give with methotrexate

Ulcerative colitis
Adult: SUBCUT 200 mg for 1 dose, then 100 mg in 2 wk; maintenance 100 mg q4wk starting at wk 6

Available forms: Inj 50 mg/0.5 ml prefilled syringe, SmartJect Auto Injector

Implementation
SUBCUT route
• Refrigerate; do not freeze; allow to warm to room temp before using
• Visually inspect solution for particulate or discoloration, solution should be clear to slightly opalescent and colorless to slightly yellow; there may be tiny white particles; do not shake
• *SmartJect autoinjector:* Allow to reach room temperature for 30 min prior to use, remove cap, inject within 5 min of removing cap, do not

Adverse effects: *italics* = common; **bold** = life-threatening

put cap back on, place the open end against the inj site at a 90-degree angle, without pushing button, push the injector firmly against the skin, press the button once and release, listen for the first click, wait for the second click or 15 sec, and remove the injector; do not rub site
• *Prefilled syringe:* Allow to warm to room temperature for 30 min, remove needle cover by pulling straight off, do not twist or recap, inject within 5 min of needle cover removal, hold the syringe in one hand like a pencil and use the other to pinch the skin, inject needle at a 45-degree angle, push plunger down as far as it will go, keep pressure on the plunger head and remove needle from skin, remove pressure from the plunger head, the needle guard will cover the needle, do not rub site

IV route (Simponi Aria)
• Calculate number of vials needed; do not shake; dilute total volume of product in NS to yield 100 ml for infusion, slowly add product, mix gently
• Infuse over 30 min; use infusion set with in-line, sterile, non-pyrogenic, low-protein binding filter (≤0.22 mm pore size)

ADVERSE EFFECTS
CNS: Dizziness, paresthesia, **CNS demyelinating disorder,** weakness
CV: Hypertension, **CHF**
GI: Hepatitis
HEMA: Agranulocytosis, aplastic anemia, leukopenia, polycythemia, thrombocytopenia, pancytopenia
INTEG: Psoriasis
MISC: Increased risk of cancer, antibody development to this drug, **risk of infection (TB, invasive fungal infections, other opportunistic infections); may be fatal,** inj site reactions

Pharmacokinetics

Absorption	Unknown
Distribution	Unknown
Metabolism	Unknown
Excretion	Unknown
Half-life	Terminal 2 wk

Pharmacodynamics

Unknown

INTERACTIONS
Individual drugs
Abatacept, adalimumab, anakinra, etanercept, immunosuppressants, inFLIXimab, rilonacept, riTUXimab: increased infection
Warfarin, cycloSPORINE, theophylline: dosage change may be needed

Drug classifications
Live vaccines: do not give concurrently; immunization should be brought up to date before treatment

NURSING CONSIDERATIONS
Assessment
• **Assess for pain,** stiffness, ROM, swelling of joints during treatment
• Check for inj site pain, swelling; usually occur after 2 inj (4-5 days)

> **BLACK BOX WARNING: Check for infections** (fever, flulike symptoms, dyspnea, change in urination, redness/swelling around any wounds), stop treatment if present; some serious infections including sepsis may occur, may be fatal; patients with active infections should not be started on this product

• **Blood dyscrasias:** CBC, differential before and periodically during treatment

Patient/family education
• Teach patient about self-administration if appropriate: inj should be made in thigh, abdomen, upper arm; rotate sites at least 1 inch from old site; do not inject in areas that are bruised, red, hard
• Advise patient that if medication is not taken when due, inject next dose as soon as remembered and inject next dose as scheduled

Evaluation
Positive therapeutic outcome
• Decreased inflammation, pain in joints

goserelin (Rx)
(goe′se-rel-lin)
Zoladex
Func. class.: Gonadotropin-releasing hormone, antineoplastic
Chem. class.: Synthetic decapeptide analog of LHRH
Pregnancy category D, X

ACTION: Inhibitor of pituitary gonadotropin secretion; initially increases LH and FSH, with increases in testosterone, reduction in sex steroid levels (substitute serum testosterone levels)

Therapeutic outcome: Decrease in tumor size and spread of malignant cells

USES: Advanced prostate cancer Stage B2-C (10.8 mg); endometriosis, advanced breast cancer, endometrial thinning (3.6 mg)

CONTRAINDICATIONS:

Pregnancy **D** (breast cancer), **X** (endometriosis), breastfeeding, nondiagnosed vaginal bleeding, children, 10.8 mg dose in women, hypersensitivity to LHRH, LHRH-agonist analogs

Precautions: Spinal cord decompression, renal disease, bone mineral density loss

DOSAGE AND ROUTES

Adult: SUBCUT 3.6 mg q4wk (implant) or 10.8 mg q12wk

Endometrial thinning

Adult: SUBCUT 1-2 depot inj; usually 1 depot, surgery performed at 4 wk; if 2 depots, surgery performed 2-4 wk after 2nd depot

Available forms: Depot inj 3.6, 10.8 mg

Implementation

Depot

• Give SUBCUT using implant, inserted by qualified person into upper subcutaneous tissue in abdominal wall q28days or q12wk (10.8 mg), do not attempt to remove air bubbles from syringe

ADVERSE EFFECTS

CNS: Headaches, **spinal cord compression,** anxiety, depression, dizziness, insomnia, lethargy, hot flashes, emotional lability
CV: Dysrhythmia, cerebrovascular accident, hypertension, **MI,** chest pain, **CHF; sudden cardiac death, stroke (men)**
ENDO: Gynecomastia, breast tenderness, hot flashes; hyperglycemia, diabetes (men)
GI: Nausea, vomiting, constipation, diarrhea, ulcer
GU: *Spotting, breakthrough bleeding, decreased libido,* renal insufficiency, urinary obstruction, urinary tract infection, impotence
INTEG: Rash, pain on inj, diaphoresis
MS: Osteoneuralgia
RESP: *COPD, URI*

Pharmacokinetics

Absorption	Well absorbed
Distribution	Unknown
Metabolism	Unknown
Excretion	Unknown
Half-life	4½ hr

Pharmacodynamics

Onset	Unknown
Peak	14-28 days
Duration	Treatment length

INTERACTIONS

Drug/lab test

Increased: alkaline phosphatase, estradiol, FSH, LH
Decreased: progesterone

NURSING CONSIDERATIONS

Assessment

• Reproductive studies: monitor pelvic ultrasound, pelvic exam, PSA, serum estradiol/testosterone, pregnancy test prior to therapy
• Monitor I&O ratios; palpate bladder for distention in urinary obstruction
• Cancer metastases: monitor for relief of bone pain (back pain), change in motor function
• Blood studies: monitor acid phosphatase; calcium in breast/prostate cancer, hypercalcemia may occur

Patient/family education

• Caution patient that gynecomastia and postmenopausal symptoms may occur but will decrease after treatment is discontinued; that bone pain may increase, then decrease
• Teach patient to contact prescriber for difficulty urinating, hot flashes occur during treatment
• Advise patient not to breastfeed while taking product; use effective nonhormonal contraception

Evaluation

Positive therapeutic outcome

• More normal levels of PSA, acid phosphatase, alkaline phosphatase; testosterone level of <25 mg/dl

---

granisetron (Rx)

(grane-iss′e-tron)
Granisol, Kytril, Sancuso
Func. class.: Antiemetic
Chem. class.: 5-HT$_3$ receptor antagonist
Pregnancy category B

ACTION: Prevents nausea, vomiting by blocking serotonin peripherally, centrally, and in the small intestine

Therapeutic outcome: Absence of nausea and vomiting

USES: Prevention of nausea, vomiting associated with cancer chemotherapy including high-dose CISplatin, radiation

Unlabeled uses: Acute nausea, vomiting after surgery

CONTRAINDICATIONS:
Hypersensitivity to this product or benzyl alcohol

Precautions: Pregnancy **B**, breastfeeding, children, geriatric, ondansetron/palonosetron/dolasetron hypersensitivity, cardiac dysrhythmias, cardiac/hepatic disease, electrolyte imbalances

DOSAGE AND ROUTES
Nausea, vomiting in chemotherapy
Adult and child ≥2 yr: **IV** 10 mcg/kg over 5 min, 30 min before the start of cancer chemotherapy, TD apply 1 patch (3.1 mg/24 hr) to upper arm 24-48 hr before chemotherapy; patch may be worn up to 7 days
Adult: PO 1 mg bid, give 1st dose 1 hr before chemotherapy and next dose 12 hr after 1st or 2 mg as a single dose anytime within 1 hr prior to chemotherapy

Nausea, vomiting in radiation therapy
Adult: PO 2 mg/day 1 hr prior to radiation

Available forms: Inj 1 mg/ml; tabs 1 mg, oral sol 2 mg/10 ml; patch TD 3.1 mg/24 hr

Implementation
IV route
• May give undiluted over 30 sec via Y-site
IV intermittent infusion route
• Dilute in 0.9% NaCl for inj or D_5W (20-50 ml), give over 5-15 min, ½ hr prior to chemotherapy
• Store at room temp for 24-hr dilution

Y-site compatibilities: Acyclovir, allopurinol, amifostine, amikacin, aminophylline, amphotericin B cholesteryl, ampicillin, ampicillin/sulbactam, amsacrine, aztreonam, bleomycin, bumetanide, buprenorphine, butorphanol, calcium gluconate, CARBOplatin, carmustine, ceFAZolin, cefepime, cefonicid, cefoperazone, cefotaxime, cefoTEtan, cefOXitin, cefTAZidime, ceftizoxime, cefTRIAXone, cefuroxime, chlorproMAZINE, cimetidine, ciprofloxacin, CISplatin, cladribine, clindamycin, cyclophosphamide, cytarabine, dacarbazine, DACTINomycin, DAUNOrubicin, dexamethasone, diphenhydrAMINE, DOBUTamine, DOPamine, DOXOrubicin, DOXOrubicin liposome, doxycycline, droperidol, enalaprilat, etoposide, famotidine, filgrastim, floxuridine, fluconazole, fluorouracil, fludarabine, furosemide, gallium, ganciclovir, gentamicin, haloperidol, heparin, hydrocortisone, HYDROmorphone, hydrOXYzine, IDArubicin, ifosfamide, imipenem-cilastatin, leucovorin, LORazepam, magnesium sulfate, melphalan, meperidine, mesna, methotrexate, methylPRED-NISolone, metoclopramide, metroNIDAZOLE, mezlocillin, miconazole, minocycline, mitoMYcin, mitoXANtrone, morphine, nalbuphine, netilmicin, ofloxacin, PACLitaxel, piperacillin, piperacillin/tazobactam, plicamycin, potassium chloride, prochlorperazine, promethazine, propofol, ranitidine, sargramostim, sodium bicarbonate, streptozocin, teniposide, thiotepa, ticarcillin, ticarcillin/clavulanate, tobramycin, trimethoprim/sulfamethoxazole, vancomycin, vinBLAStine, vinCRIStine, vinorelbine, zidovudine

Y-site incompatibilities: Amphotericin B coloidal, diazepam, phenytoin

Additive compatibilities: Dexamethasone, methylPREDNISolone

Solution compatibilities: D_5W, 0.9% NaCl
Transdermal route
• Apply to dry, clean, intact skin of upper, outer arm 24 hr prior to chemotherapy; firmly press on skin; keep on during chemotherapy; can bathe; avoid swimming, whirlpool; remove ≥24 hr after chemotherapy

ADVERSE EFFECTS
CNS: *Headache, asthenia,* anxiety, dizziness
CV: Hypertension, QT prolongation
GI: Diarrhea, *constipation,* increased AST, ALT, *nausea*
HEMA: Leukopenia, anemia, **thrombocytopenia**
MISC: Rash, **bronchospasm**

Pharmacokinetics
Absorption	Unknown
Distribution	Unknown
Metabolism	Liver
Excretion	Unknown
Half-life	10-12 hr

Pharmacodynamics
Unknown

INTERACTIONS
Individual drugs
Amoxapine, chloroquine, cloZAPine, dasatinib, dolasetron, dronedarone, droperidol, erythromycin, flecainide, haloperidol, lapatinib, maprotiline, methadone, octreotide, ondansetron, palonosetron, pentamidine, pimozide, propafenone, ranolazine, risperidone, sertindole, SUNItinib, tacrolimus, telithromycin, troleandomycin, vardenafil, vorinostat, ziprasidone: increased QT prolongation

Drug classifications

Antipsychotics: increased EPS
β-blockers, class I, III antidysrhythmics,
halogenated/local anesthetics, phenothiazines,
tricyclics: increased QT prolongation

NURSING CONSIDERATIONS

Assessment

• Assess patient for absence of nausea, vomiting
during chemotherapy
• **Assess patient for hypersensitive reaction:** rash, bronchospasm

Patient/family education

• Advise patient to report diarrhea, constipation, rash, or changes in respirations

Evaluation

Positive therapeutic outcome

• Absence of nausea, vomiting during cancer
chemotherapy

guaiFENesin (Rx, OTC)

(gwye-fen′e-sin)
Alfen, Altarussin, Balminil ♣,
Bidex, Diabetic Tussin, Elix Sure EX,
Equaline Non-Drowsy Tussin,
Equate Tussin Cough, Ganidin NR,
Good Sense Mucus Relief, Good
Sense Tussin Chest Congestion,
GuaiFENesin NR, Guiatuss, Humibid,
Iophen NR, Liquibid, Miltuss EX,
Mucinex, Mucinex Children's Mucus
Relief, Mucinex Junior Strength,
Naldecon Senior EX, Organ-1 NR,
Organidin NR, Q-Tussin, Robafen,
Robitussin GuaiFENesin ♣,
Scot-Tussin Expectorant, Siltussin
DAS, Siltussin SA, Top Care
Children's Mucus Relief, Top Care
Tussin Chest Congestion Solution,
Wal-Tussin Expectorant, XPect
Func. class.: Expectorant
Pregnancy category C

ACTION: Increases the volume and
reduces the viscosity of secretions in the trachea
and bronchi to facilitate secretion removal

Therapeutic outcome: Decreased cough

USES: Productive and nonproductive cough

CONTRAINDICATIONS:

Hypersensitivity, chronic persistent cough

Precautions: Pregnancy **C**, breastfeeding,
CHF, asthma, emphysema, fever

DOSAGE AND ROUTES

Adult and child ≥12 yr: PO 200-400 mg q4hr,
or EXT REL 600-1200 mg q12hr; max 2.4 g/day
Child 6-11 yr: PO 100-200 mg q4hr or EXT
REL 600 mg q12hr; max 1.2 g/day
Child 2-5 yr: PO: 50-100 mg q4hr; max 600 mg/
day, EXT REL 300 mg q12hr, max 600 mg/day

Available forms: Tabs 200, 400 mg; ext rel
tabs 600, 1200 mg; syr 100 mg/5 ml; oral sol
100 mg/5 ml; oral granules 50, 100 mg/packet

Implementation

• Store at room temperature; provide room humidification to assist with liquefying secretions
• Avoid fluids for ½ hr after administration

ADVERSE EFFECTS

CNS: Drowsiness, headache, dizziness
GI: Nausea, anorexia, vomiting, diarrhea

Pharmacokinetics

Absorption	Well absorbed
Distribution	Unknown
Metabolism	Unknown
Excretion	Unknown
Half-life	1 hr

Pharmacodynamics

	PO	PO–EXT REL
Onset	½ hr	Unknown
Peak	Unknown	Unknown
Duration	4-6 hr	12 hr

NURSING CONSIDERATIONS

Assessment

• **Assess cough:** type, frequency, character,
including characteristics of sputum; lung sounds
bilaterally; fluids should be increased to 2 L/day
to decrease secretion viscosity (thickness)

Patient/family education

• Caution patient to avoid driving, other hazardous activities if drowsiness occurs (rare)
• Advise patient to avoid smoking, smoke-filled
rooms, perfumes, dust, environmental pollutants, cleansers
• Instruct patient to notify prescriber if dry,
nonproductive cough lasts over 7 days

Evaluation

Positive therapeutic outcome

• Absence of dry cough
• Thinner, more productive cough that raises
secretions

---

halcinonide topical
See Appendix B

haloperidol (Rx)
(hal-oh-pehr′ih-dol)
haloperidol decanoate (Rx)
Haldol Decanoate
haloperidol lactate (Rx)
Haldol
Func. class.: Antipsychotic/neuroleptic
Chem. class.: Butyrophenone
Pregnancy category C

Do not confuse:
haloperidol/Halotestin, **Haldol**/Stadol

ACTION: Depresses cerebral cortex, hypothalamus, limbic system, which control activity and aggression; blocks neurotransmission produced by dopamine at synapse; exhibits strong α-adrenergic, anticholinergic blocking action; mechanism for antipsychotic effects unclear

Therapeutic outcome: Decreased signs and symptoms of psychosis

USES: Psychotic disorders, control of tics, vocal utterances in Tourette's syndrome, short-term treatment of hyperactive children showing excessive motor activity, prolonged parenteral therapy in chronic schizophrenia, organic mental syndrome with psychotic features, hiccups (short-term), emergency sedation of severely agitated or delirious patients, ADHD

Unlabeled uses: Nausea, vomiting in surgery, autism, migraine headache

CONTRAINDICATIONS:
Children <3 yr, hypersensitivity, coma, Parkinson's disease, CNS depression

Precautions: Pregnancy **C**, breastfeeding, geriatric, seizure disorders, hypertension, hepatic/cardiac/pulmonary disease, prostatic hypertrophy, hyperthyroidism, thyrotoxicosis, blood dyscrasias, brain damage, bone marrow depression, alcohol and barbiturate withdrawal states, angina, epilepsy, urinary retention, closed-angle glaucoma

BLACK BOX WARNING: Dementia; increased mortality in elderly patients with dementia-related psychosis

DOSAGE AND ROUTES
Acute psychosis
Adult: **IM/IV** (lactate) 2-10 mg, may repeat q1hr, convert to **PO** as soon as possible, **PO** should be 150% of total parenteral dose required
Child 6-12 yr: **IM/IV** (lactate) (unlabeled) 1-3 mg q4-8hr, max 0.15 mg/kg/day, switch to **PO** as soon as possible

Chronic schizophrenia
Adult: **IM** (decanoate) 50-100 mg q4wk, max 100 mg for 1st inj
Child 3-12 yr: **PO/IM** 0.05-0.15 mg/kg/day

Tourette's syndrome
Adult and adolescent: **PO** 0.5-2 mg bid-tid, increased until desired response occurs
Child 3-12 yr or weighing 15-40 kg: **PO** 0.25-0.5 mg/day in 2-3 divided doses, increase by 0.25-0.5 mg q5-7days, max 0.15 mg/kg/day

ADHD
Child 3-12 yr: **PO** 0.25-0.5 mg/day in 2-3 divided doses, may increase by 0.025-0.5 mg q5-7days; maintenance 0.01-0.03 mg/kg/day as a single dose

Autism (unlabeled)
Child: **PO** 0.04 mg/kg/day or 1-3 mg/day, max 4 mg/day

Migraine (unlabeled)
Adult: **PO/IM** (lactate) 5 mg at onset, may repeat once

Available forms: Tabs 0.5, 1, 2, 5, 10, 20 mg; **lactate:** oral sol 2 mg/ml; inj 5 mg/ml; **decanoate:** 50 mg/ml, 100 mg/ml

Implementation
PO route—oral liquid
• Give product in liquid form mixed in glass of juice or caffeine-free cola if hoarding is suspected; do not mix in caffeine drinks, tannics, pectins
• Give decreased dosage in geriatric because of slower metabolism
• Give PO with full glass of water, milk; or give with food to decrease GI upset
• Give antacids 2 hr before or after this product
• Store in tight, light-resistant container; oral sol in amber bottle
• Avoid skin contact with oral susp or sol: may cause contact dermatitis
IM route
• Inject in deep muscle mass, do not give SUBCUT; use 21-gauge 2-in needle; do not administer sol with a precipitate; give <3 ml per inj site; give slowly, may be painful

- Patient should remain lying down after IM inj for at least 30 min

IV route (lactate)
- Give undiluted for psychotic episode at 5 mg/min
- Only use lactate for IV

Intermittent IV infusion route
- Give after dilution in 30-50 ml of D₅W, run over ½ hr

Y-site compatibilities: Amifostine, amsacrine, aztreonam, cimetidine, cisatracurium, cladribine, DOBUTamine, DOPamine, DOXOrubicin liposome, famotidine, filgrastim, fludarabine, granisetron, lidocaine, LORazepam, melphalan, midazolam, nitroglycerin, norepinephrine, ondansetron, PACLitaxel, phenylephrine, propofol, remifentanil, SUFentanil, tacrolimus, teniposide, theophylline, thiotepa, vinorelbine

Y-site incompatibilities: Fluconazole, foscarnet, heparin, sargramostim

ADVERSE EFFECTS
CNS: *EPS, pseudoparkinsonism, akathisia, dystonia, tardive dyskinesia, drowsiness, headache,* **seizures, neuroleptic malignant syndrome,** confusion
CV: *Orthostatic hypotension,* hypertension, **cardiac arrest,** ECG changes, **tachycardia, QT prolongation, sudden death**
EENT: Blurred vision, glaucoma, dry eyes
GI: *Dry mouth, nausea, vomiting, anorexia, constipation,* diarrhea, jaundice, weight gain, **ileus, hepatitis**
GU: Urinary retention, urinary frequency, dysuria, enuresis, impotence, amenorrhea, gynecomastia
INTEG: *Rash,* photosensitivity, dermatitis
RESP: **Laryngospasm,** dyspnea, **respiratory depression**
SYST: **Risk of death (dementia)**

Pharmacokinetics

Absorption	Well absorbed (PO, IM); decanoate (IM) absorbed slowly
Distribution	High concentrations in liver, crosses placenta, protein binding 92%
Metabolism	Liver, extensively
Excretion	Kidneys, breast milk
Half-life	Terminal half-life 12-36 hr (metabolized)

Pharmacodynamics

	PO	IM	IM (decanoate)
Onset	Erratic	½ hr	3-9 days
Peak	2-6 hr	30-45 min	4-11 days
Duration	8-12 hr	4-8 hr	3 wk

INTERACTIONS
Individual drugs
Alcohol: increased effects of both products, oversedation
Amoxapine, chloroquine, cloZAPine, dasatinib, dolasetron, dronedarone, droperidol, erythromycin, flecainide, lapatinib, maprotiline, methadone, octreotide, ondansetron, palonosetron, pentamidine, pimozide, propafenone, ranolazine, risperidone, sertindole, SUNItinib, tacrolimus, telithromycin, troleandomycin, vardenafil, vorinostat, ziprasidone: increased QT prolongation, usually with IV use
CarBAMazepine: decreased effects of haloperidol
EPINEPHrine: increased toxicity
Levodopa: decreased effects of levodopa
Lithium: increased toxicity; decreased effects of lithium
PHENobarbital: decreased effects of haloperidol

Drug classifications
Anticholinergics: increased anticholinergic effects
Barbiturate anesthetics: oversedation
β-Adrenergic blockers: increased effects of both products
Class IA, III antidysrhythmics, halogenated/local anesthetics, phenothiazines, tricyclics, β-blockers: increased QT prolongation
CNS depressants: oversedation
SSRIs, SNRIs: increased serotonin syndrome, increased neuroleptic malignant syndrome

Drug/lab test
Increased: liver function tests

NURSING CONSIDERATIONS
Assessment

BLACK BOX WARNING: Assess for dementia, affect, orientation, LOC, reflexes, gait, coordination, sleep pattern disturbances, risk for death in dementia-related psychosis

- Assess mental status: orientation, mood, behavior, presence and type of hallucinations before initial administration and monthly; this

Adverse effects: *italics* = common; **bold** = life-threatening

product should significantly reduce psychotic behavior

• Monitor I&O ratio; palpate bladder if low urinary output occurs, especially in geriatric; urinalysis is recommended before, during prolonged therapy

• Monitor bilirubin, CBC, liver function tests monthly

• Assess affect, orientation, LOC, reflexes, gait, coordination, sleep pattern disturbances

• Monitor B/P with patient sitting, standing, and lying; take pulse and respirations q4hr during initial treatment; establish baseline before starting treatment; report drops of ≥30 mm Hg; obtain baseline ECG, Q-wave and T-wave changes

• Check for dizziness, faintness, palpitations, tachycardia on rising; severe orthostatic hypotension is common

• **Assess for neuroleptic malignant syndrome:** hyperpyrexia, muscle rigidity, increased CPK, altered mental status; product should be discontinued immediately; if seizures, hypo/hypertension, tachycardia occur, notify prescriber immediately

• **Assess for EPS** including akathisia (inability to sit still, no pattern to movements), tardive dyskinesia (bizarre movements of the jaw, mouth, tongue, extremities), pseudoparkinsonism (ragged tremors, pill rolling, shuffling gait); an antiparkinsonian product should be prescribed

• Assess for constipation and urinary retention daily; if these occur, increase bulk, water in diet

• **Abrupt discontinuation:** Do not withdraw abruptly, taper

⚠ QT prolongation: More common with IV use at high doses; monitor ECG in those with CV disease

Patient/family education

• Teach patient to use good oral hygiene; use frequent rinsing of mouth, sugarless gum for dry mouth; oral candidiasis may occur

• Advise patient to avoid hazardous activities until product response is determined and effects are known; dizziness, blurred vision are common

• Inform patient that orthostatic hypotension occurs often and to rise from sitting or lying position gradually; tell patient that in hot weather heat stroke may occur; take extra precautions to stay cool

• Instruct patient to avoid abrupt withdrawal of this product, or EPS may result; product should be withdrawn slowly

• Caution patient to avoid OTC preparations (cough, hay fever, cold) unless approved by prescriber, since serious product interactions may occur; avoid use with alcohol, CNS depressants since increased drowsiness may occur

• Tell patient to report impaired vision, jaundice, muscle twitching

Evaluation

Positive therapeutic outcome

• Decrease in emotional excitement, hallucinations, delusions, paranoia, reorganization of patterns of thought, speech; improvement in specific behaviors

TREATMENT OF OVERDOSE:

Lavage if orally ingested; provide airway; *do not induce vomiting*

⚠ HIGH ALERT

heparin (Rx)

(hep'a-rin)

Hepalean ✦, Heparin Leo ✦, Hep-Lock, Hep-Lock U/P, Monoject Prefill

Func. class.: Anticoagulant, antithrombotic

Pregnancy category C   ⬛

Do not confuse:

heparin/Hespan

ACTION: Prevents conversion of fibrinogen to fibrin and prothrombin to thrombin by enhancing inhibitory effects of antithrombin III

Therapeutic outcome: Prevention of thrombi

USES: Prevention and treatment of MI, open heart surgery, disseminated intravascular clotting syndrome, atrial fibrillation with embolization; as an anticoagulant in transfusion and dialysis procedures; to maintain patency of indwelling venipuncture devices; diagnosis, treatment of disseminated intravascular coagulation (DIC)

CONTRAINDICATIONS:

Bleeding, hypersensitivity

Precautions: Pregnancy **C,** children, geriatric, alcoholism, hyperlipidemia, diabetes, renal disease, heparin-induced thrombocytopenia (HIT), hemophilia, leukemia with bleeding, peptic ulcer disease, severe thrombocytopenic purpura, renal/hepatic disease (severe), blood dyscrasias, severe hypertension, subacute

---

⚠ Nurse Alert   ⭐ Key NCLEX® Drug

bacterial endocarditis, acute nephritis; benzyl alcohol products in neonates, infants, pregnancy, lactation

DOSAGE AND ROUTES

Deep vein thrombosis/pulmonary embolism

Adult: **IV BOL** 80 international units/kg, then maintenance **IV INF** 18 international units/kg/hr; if aPTT <35 (1.2×normal), increase **IV INF** rate by 4 international units/kg/hr and rebolus with 80 international units/kg; if aPTT 35-45 (1.2-1.5 × normal), increase **IV INF** by 2 international units/kg/hr and rebolus with 40 international units/kg; if aPTT 46-70 (1.5-2.3 × normal), maintain **IV INF;** if aPTT 71-90 (2.3-3 × normal), decrease **IV INF** by 2 international units/kg/hr; if aPTT >90 (>3 × normal), hold **IV INF** for 1 hr, then decrease rate 3 international units/kg/hr

Child/infant/neonate: **IV** loading dose 75 international units/kg

Child >1 yr: 20 international units/kg/hr, **infant, neonate <1 yr:** 28 international units/kg/hr as initial maintenance dose

Thrombosis prophylaxis (open heart/CV surgery)

Adult: **IV** ≥150 international units/kg, procedures <60 min up to 300 international units/kg, procedures >60 min up to 400 international units/kg, based on ACT

Thrombosis prophylaxis (PCI, not receiving abciximab)

Adult: **IV BOL** weight-adjusted with 60-100 international units/kg, maintain ACT within 250-300 sec (HemoTec) or 300-350 sec (Hemochron)

Child/infant/neonate: **IV BOL** 100-150 international units/kg

Prophylaxis for DVT/PE

Adult: **SUBCUT** 5000 units q8-12hr

IV catheter occlusion prophylaxis

Adult and child: **IV** 10-100 units/ml
Infant <10 kg: **IV** 10 units/ml

Available forms: Sol for inj 10, 100, 1000, 2000, 5000, 7500, 10,000, 20,000, 40,000 units/ml; premixed 1000 units/500 ml, 2000 units/1000 ml, 12,500 units/250 ml, 25,000 units/250 ml, 25,000 units/500 ml; lock flush preparations 10 units/ml

Implementation

• Heparin and low-molecular-weight heparins are not interchangeable

• Give at same time each day to maintain steady blood levels
• Cannot be used interchangeably (unit for unit) with LMWHs or heparinoids
• Store at room temperature

SUBCUT route
• Give SUBCUT with at least 25-G ⅜-in needle; do not massage area or aspirate fluid when giving SUBCUT inj; give in abdomen between pelvic bones, rotate sites; leave in for 10 sec; apply gentle pressure for 1 min
• Changing needles is not recommended

Heparin lock route
• **Do not mistake heparin sodium injection 10,000 units/ml and Hep-Lock U/P 10 units/ml; they have similar blue labeling; deaths in pediatric patients have occurred when heparin sodium injection vials were confused with heparin flush vials**
• Inject 10-100 units/0.5-1 ml after each inf or q8-12hr

Direct IV route
• Give loading dose undiluted over ≥1 min; use before continuous infusion

Continuous IV infusion route
• Dilute 25,000 units/250-500 ml 0.9% NaCl or D₅W (50-100 units/ml); some solutions are premixed and ready for use
• When product is added to inf sol for cont **IV**, invert container at least 6 × to ensure adequate mixing

Y-site compatibilities: Acyclovir, aldesleukin, allopurinol, amifostine, aminophylline, ampicillin, ampicillin/sulbactam, atracurium, atropine, aztreonam, betamethasone, bleomycin, calcium gluconate, ceFAZolin, cefoTEtan, cefTAZidime, cefTRIAXone, cephalothin, cephapirin, chlordiazepoxide, chlorproMAZINE, cimetidine, CISplatin, cladribine, clindamycin, conjugated estrogens, cyanocobalamin, cyclophosphamide, cytarabine, dexamethasone, digoxin, diphenhydrAMINE, DOPamine, DOXOrubicin liposome, edrophonium, enalaprilat, EPINEPHrine, erythromycin, esmolol, ethacrynate, famotidine, fentaNYL, fluconazole, fludarabine, fluorouracil, foscarnet, furosemide, gallium, granisetron, hydrALAZINE, hydrocortisone, HYDROmorphone, regular insulin, isoproterenol, kanamycin, leucovorin, lidocaine, LORazepam, magnesium sulfate, melphalan, menadiol sodium, meperidine, meropenem, methicillin, methotrexate, methoxamine, methyldopa, methylergonovine, metoclopramide, metroNIDAZOLE, midazolam, milrinone, minocycline, mitoMYcin, morphine, nafcillin, neostigmine, nitroglycerin, nitroprusside, norepinephrine, ondansetron, oxacillin, oxytocin, PACLitaxel, pancuronium, penicillin G potassium, pentazocine, phytonadione, piperacillin, piperacillin/tazobactam, propofol, potassium chloride, prednisoLONE, procainamide, prochlorperazine, propofol, propranolol, pyridostigmine, ranitidine, remifentanil, sargramostim, scopolamine, sodium bicarbonate, streptokinase, succinylcholine, tacrolimus, teniposide, theophylline, thiopental, thiotepa, ticarcillin, ticarcillin/clavulanate, trimethobenzamide, vecuronium, vinBLAStine, vinorelbine, warfarin, zidovudine

Y-site incompatibilities: Alteplase, ciprofloxacin, dacarbazine, diazepam, DOBUTamine, DOXOrubicin, ergotamine, gentamicin, haloperidol, IDArubicin, methotrimeprazine, phenytoin, promethazine, tobramycin, triflupromazine

Additive compatibilities: Aminophylline, amphotericin, ascorbic acid, bleomycin, calcium gluconate, cefepime, cephapirin, chloramphenicol, clindamycin, colistimethate, dimenhyDRINATE, doxacillin, DOPamine, enalaprilat, erythromycin, esmolol, floxacillin, fluconazole, flumazenil, furosemide, hydrocortisone, isoproterenol, lidocaine, lincomycin, magnesium sulfate, meropenem, methyldopate, methylPREDNISolone, metroNIDAZOLE/sodium bicarbonate, nafcillin, norepinephrine, octreotide, penicillin G, potassium chloride, prednisoLONE, promazine, ranitidine, sodium bicarbonate, verapamil, vit B complex, vit B complex with C

Additive incompatibilities: Amikacin, erythromycin lactobionate, gentamicin, kanamycin, meperidine, methadone, morphine, polymyxin B, streptomycin

ADVERSE EFFECTS

CNS: *Fever,* chills, headache
GU: Hematuria
HEMA: **Hemorrhage, thrombocytopenia, anemia, HIT**
INTEG: *Rash,* dermatitis, urticaria, pruritus, delayed transient alopecia, hematoma, cutaneous necrosis (SUBCUT), injection site reactions
META: Hyperlipidemia
SYST: Anaphylaxis

Pharmacokinetics

Absorption	Well absorbed (SUBCUT)
Distribution	Unknown
Metabolism	Partially in kidney, liver
Excretion	Lymph, spleen, in urine (<50% unchanged)
Half-life	1½ hr

Pharmacodynamics

	SUBCUT	IV
Onset	½-1 hr	5 min
Peak	2 hr	10 min
Duration	8-12 hr	2-6 hr

INTERACTIONS

Individual drugs
Dextran, dipyridole, ticlopidine, clopidogrel, presgrel: increased action of heparin
Digoxin: decreased action of heparin
Nicotine: decreased action of heparin

Drug classifications
Anticoagulants (oral), cephalosporins, NSAIDs, penicillins, platelet inhibitors, salicylates, antineoplastics, SSRIs, SNRIs: increased action of heparin
Antihistamines, tetracyclines, cardiac glycosides: decreased action of heparin, nitroglycerin
Corticosteroids: decreased action of corticosteroids

Drug/herb
Feverfew, garlic, ginger, ginkgo, green tea, horse chestnut: increased bleeding risk

Drug/lab test
Increased: ALT, AST, INR, pro-time, PTT, potassium
Decreased: platelets

NURSING CONSIDERATIONS

Assessment
• Assess for blood studies (Hct, occult blood in stools) q3mo if patient is on long-term therapy
• Monitor PPT, which should be 1½-2 × control, PTT; often done daily, APTT, ACT
• Monitor platelet count q2-3day; thrombocytopenia may occur on fourth day of treatment and resolve, or continue to eighth day of treatment
⚠ Bleeding, hemorrhage: Assess for bleeding gums, petechiae, ecchymosis, black tarry stools, hematuria, epistaxis, decrease in Hct, B/P; notify prescriber immediately; HIT may occur after product discontinuation
• **Monitor for hypersensitivity:** fever, skin rash, urticaria; notify prescriber immediately

Patient/family education
• Advise patient to avoid OTC preparations that may cause serious product interactions unless directed by prescriber; may contain aspirin or other anticoagulants
• Tell patient that product may be withheld during active bleeding (menstruation), depending on condition
• Caution patient to use soft-bristle toothbrush to avoid bleeding gums; avoid contact sports; use electric razor; avoid IM inj
• Instruct patient to carry/wear emergency ID or other identification identifying product taken and condition treated
• Advise patient to report any signs of bleeding: gums, under skin, urine, stools; or unusual bruising even after discontinuing product

Evaluation
Positive therapeutic outcome
• Decrease of DVT
• PTT of 1.5-2.5 × control
• Free-flowing **IV**

TREATMENT OF OVERDOSE:
Withdraw product, give protamine sulfate 1 mg protamine/100 units heparin

hepatitis B immune globulin (HBIG) (Rx)
(hep-a-tite'iss)
HepaGam B, Hyper HEP B S/D, Nabi-HB
Func. class.: Immune globulin
Pregnancy category C

ACTION: Provides passive immunity to hepatitis B

Therapeutic outcome: Passive immunity to hepatitis B

USES: Prevention of hepatitis B virus in exposed patients, including passive immunity in neonates born to HBsAg-positive mothers, prevention of hepatitis B recurrence after liver transplant in HBsAg-positive patients

CONTRAINDICATIONS:
Hypersensitivity to immune globulins, coagulation disorders

Precautions: Pregnancy **C**, breastfeeding, children, geriatric, hemophilia, active infection, IgA deficiency

DOSAGE AND ROUTES
Hepatitis B exposure in those at high risk
Adult and child: IM 0.06 ml/kg (usual 3-5 ml) within 7 days of exposure; repeat 28 days after exposure, if patient wishes not to receive the hepatitis B vaccine

Prevention of hepatitis B infection recurrence after liver transplant
Adult: IV (HepaGam B only) 20,000 international units concurrent with grafting transplanted liver, then 20,000 international units/day on days 1-7, then 20,000 international units q2wk starting on day 14, then 20,000 international units qmo, starting on month 4

Neonates born to hepatitis B surface antigen–positive mothers: IM 0.5 ml within 12 hr of birth

Available forms: Inj 1-, 4-, 5-ml vials; neonatal syringe 0.5 ml; HepaGam B sol for inj 312 units/ml; Hyper HEP B S/D 217 units/ml

Implementation
IM route
• After rotating vial, do not shake
• Only with EPINEPHrine 1:1000 on unit to treat laryngospasm
• In deltoid for better absorption (adult)

IV route (Hepa Gam B only)
• Calculate volume needed for each 20,000 international units dose by using measured potency of each lot, HBIG potency is stamped on label
• Promptly use after vial is entered, discard unused product
• Give at 2 ml/min through separate IV line, use inf pump, decrease to 1 ml/min, if infusion-related event occurs, patient becomes uncomfortable
• **Do not use HyperHEP B BS/D or Nabi-HB IV**

ADVERSE EFFECTS
CNS: Headache, dizziness, fever
GI: Nausea, vomiting
INTEG: Soreness at inj site, urticaria, erythema, swelling
SYST: Induration, **anaphylaxis, angioedema**

Pharmacokinetics

Absorption	Slowly absorbed
Distribution	Unknown
Metabolism	Unknown
Excretion	Unknown
Half-life	3 wk

Adverse effects: *italics* = common; **bold** = life-threatening

Pharmacodynamics

Onset	1-7 days
Peak	3-10 days
Duration	2-6 mo

INTERACTIONS
Drug classifications
MMR, rotavirus vaccines, varicella: do not use within 3 mo of hepatitis B immune globulin

NURSING CONSIDERATIONS
Assessment
• Assess for history of allergies, skin conditions (eczema, psoriasis, dermatitis), reactions to vaccinations
• Assess for skin reactions: rash, induration, urticaria
• Assess for sneezing, pruritus, angioedema, dysphagia, vomiting, abdominal pain
⚠ **Assess for anaphylaxis: inability to breathe, bronchospasm, hypotension, wheezing, diaphoresis, fever, flushing; epinephrine and emergency equipment should be available**
• Can be used with hepatitis B vaccine in cases of direct contact

Patient/family education
• Teach patient purpose of product and expected results
• Give patient a list of adverse reactions that need to be reported immediately: wheezing, vomiting, sneezing, abdominal pain, sweating, tightness in chest
• Advise patient that pain, rash, swelling at inj site can be expected
• Give patient written record of immunization

Evaluation
Positive therapeutic outcome
• Prevention of hepatitis B

homatropine ophthalmic
See Appendix B

hydrALAZINE (Rx)
(hye-dral′a-zeen)
Apresoline
Func. class.: Antihypertensive, direct-acting peripheral vasodilator
Chem. class.: Phthalazine
Pregnancy category C

Do not confuse:
hydrALAZINE/hydrOXYzine,
Apresoline/allopurinol

ACTION: Vasodilates arterioles in smooth muscle by direct relaxation; reduces B/P with reflex increases in heart rate, stroke volume, cardiac output

Therapeutic outcome: Decreased B/P in hypertension, decreased afterload in CHF

USES: Essential hypertension, hypertensive emergency/urgency

Unlabeled uses: CHF, preeclampsia

CONTRAINDICATIONS:
Hypersensitivity to hydrALAZINEs, mitral valvular rheumatic heart disease, CAD

Precautions: Pregnancy **C**, breastfeeding, geriatric, CVA, advanced renal disease, liver disease, SLE, dissecting aortic aneurysm

DOSAGE AND ROUTES
Hypertension
Adult: PO 10 mg qid 2-4 days, then 25 mg qid for rest of 1st wk, then 50 mg qid individualized to desired response; max 300 mg/day
Child: PO 0.75-1 mg/kg/day in 2-4 divided doses; max 25 mg/dose, increase over 3-4 wk to max 7.5 mg/kg/day or 200 mg, whichever is less

Hypertensive crisis
Adult: IV BOL 10-20 mg q4-6hr; administer PO as soon as possible; IM 10-50 mg q4-6hr
Child: IV BOL 0.1-0.6 mg/kg q4hr; IM 0.1-0.6 mg/kg q4-6hr, max 1.7-3.5 mg/kg/day

CHF
Adult: PO 10-25 mg bid, max 75 mg tid

Available forms: Inj 20 mg/ml; tabs 10, 25, 50, 100 mg

Implementation
PO route
• Give with meals to enhance absorption
• Store protected from light and heat
IM route
• Do not admix; switch to PO as soon as possible

Direct IV route
• Give by **IV** undiluted through Y-tube or 3-way stopcock, give each 10 mg over 1 min or more
• Administer with patient in recumbent position; keep in that position for 1 hr after administration

Y-site compatibilities: Heparin, hydrocortisone, potassium chloride, verapamil, vit B/C

Y-site incompatibilities: Aminophylline, ampicillin, diazoxide, furosemide, PACLitaxel

---

⚠ Nurse Alert   ✳ Key NCLEX® Drug

ADVERSE EFFECTS

CNS: *Headache, tremors, dizziness, anxiety,* peripheral neuritis, depression, fever, chills

CV: *Palpitations, reflex tachycardia, angina,* **shock,** rebound hypertension, orthostatic hypotension

GI: *Nausea, vomiting, anorexia, diarrhea,* constipation, paralytic ileus, **hepatotoxicity**

GU: Urinary retention, glomerulonephritis, hematuria

HEMA: **Leukopenia, agranulocytosis,** anemia, **thrombocytopenia**

INTEG: Rash, pruritus, urticaria

MISC: Nasal congestion, muscle cramps, *lupuslike symptoms,* flushing, edema, dyspnea

Pharmacokinetics

Absorption	Rapidly absorbed (PO); well absorbed (IM); completely absorbed (**IV**)
Distribution	Widely distributed; crosses placenta
Metabolism	GI mucosa, liver extensively
Excretion	Kidneys, urine (12%-14%)
Half-life	2-8 hr

Pharmacodynamics

	PO	IM	IV
Onset	½ hr	10-30 min	5-20 min
Peak	1-2 hr	1 hr	10-80 min
Duration	6-12 hr	Up to 12 hr	Up to 12 hr

INTERACTIONS

Individual drugs

Alcohol, levodopa: increased hypotension
Indomethacin: decreased effects of hydrALAZINE

Drug classifications

β-Adrenergic blockers: increased effects
MAOIs: severe hypotension
Other antihypertensives, thiazide diuretics: increased hypotension
Sympathomimetics (EPINEPHrine, norepinephrine): increased tachycardia, angina
NSAIDs, estrogens: decreased hydrALAZINE effects

NURSING CONSIDERATIONS

Assessment

• Assess cardiac status: B/P q5min for 2 hr, then qhr for 2 hr, then q4hr; pulse, jugular venous distention q4hr

• Monitor electrolytes, blood studies: potassium, sodium, chloride, carbon dioxide, CBC, serum glucose; LE prep, ANA titer before starting treatment

• Monitor weight daily, I&O; check for edema in feet, legs daily; check skin turgor, dryness of mucous membranes for hydration status

• Assess for crackles, dyspnea, orthopnea; peripheral edema, fatigue, weight gain, jugular vein distention (CHF)

• For fever, joint pain, rash, sore throat (lupuslike symptoms), notify prescriber

Patient/family education

• Teach patient to take with food to increase bioavailability (PO)

• Teach patient to avoid OTC preparations unless directed by prescriber

• Advise patient to notify prescriber if chest pain, severe fatigue, fever, muscle or joint pain occur

• Advise patient to rise slowly to prevent orthostatic hypertension

• Advise patient to notify prescriber if pregnancy is suspected

Evaluation

Positive therapeutic outcome
• Decreased B/P in hypertension

TREATMENT OF OVERDOSE:

Administer vasopressors, volume expanders for shock; if PO, lavage or give activated charcoal, digitalization

---

hydrochlorothiazide (Rx)

(hye-droe-klor-oh-thye′a-zide)
Apo-Hydrol ✦**, Ezide, Neo-Codema** ✦
Func. class.: Diuretic, antihypertensive
Chem. class.: Thiazide, sulfonamide derivative
Pregnancy category B

ACTION: Acts on the distal tubule in the kidney, increasing excretion of sodium, water, chloride, and potassium

Therapeutic outcome: Decreased B/P, decreased edema in lung tissues peripherally

USES: Edema, hypertension, diuresis, CHF; edema in corticosteroid, estrogen, NSAID therapy; idiopathic lower extremity edema therapy

CONTRAINDICATIONS:
Hypersensitivity to thiazides or sulfonamides, anuria, renal decompensation, pregnancy (D) preeclampsia

Precautions: Pregnancy **B,** breastfeeding, hypokalemia, renal/hepatic disease, gout, COPD, lupus erythematosus, diabetes mellitus, hyperlipidemia, CCr <30 ml/min, hypomagnesemia

DOSAGE AND ROUTES
Hypertension
Adult/adolescent: PO 12.5-25 mg/day, may increase to 50 mg/day in 1-2 divided doses
Child >6 mo: PO 1-2 mg/kg/day in divided doses; max 37.5 mg/day for 6 mo-2 yr; max 100 mg/day for 2-12 yr
Child <6 mo: PO up to 2-3.3 mg/kg/day in divided doses

Renal dose
Adult: PO CCr <30 ml/min, do not use, not effective

Available forms: Tabs 12.5, 25, 50 mg; caps 12.5 mg

Implementation
PO route
• Give in AM to avoid interference with sleep
• Provide potassium replacement if potassium level is ≤3.0 mg/dl; give whole tab or use oral sol lightly; product may be crushed if patient is unable to swallow
• Administer with food; if nausea occurs, absorption may be increased

ADVERSE EFFECTS
CNS: Drowsiness, paresthesia, depression, headache, *dizziness, fatigue, weakness,* fever
CV: Irregular pulse, *orthostatic hypotension,* palpitations, volume depletion, allergic myocarditis
EENT: Blurred vision
ELECT: *Hypokalemia,* hypercalcemia, hyponatremia, hypochloremia, hypomagnesemia
GI: *Nausea, vomiting, anorexia,* constipation, diarrhea, cramps, **pancreatitis,** GI irritation, **hepatitis**
GU: *Frequency,* polyuria, **uremia,** glucosuria, hyperuricemia, jaundice
HEMA: **Aplastic anemia, hemolytic anemia, leukopenia, agranulocytosis, thrombocytopenia, neutropenia**
INTEG: *Rash,* urticaria, purpura, photosensitivity, alopecia, erythema multiforme
META: *Hyperglycemia, hyperuricemia,* **renal failure,** increased creatinine, BUN
SYST: **Stevens-Johnson syndrome**

Absorption	Variable
Distribution	Extracellular spaces; crosses placenta
Metabolism	Excreted unchanged in urine
Excretion	Breast milk
Half-life	6-15 hr

Onset	2 hr
Peak	4 hr
Duration	6-12 hr

INTERACTIONS
Individual drugs
Amphotericin B: increased hypokalemia
Cholestyramine, colestipol: decreased absorption of hydrochlorothiazide
Diazoxide: increased hyperglycemia, hyperuricemia, hypotension
Lithium: increased toxicity

Drug classifications
Antidiabetics: decreased effect of antidiabetic agent
Cardiac glycosides, nondepolarizing skeletal muscle relaxants: increased toxicity
Diuretics (loop): increased effects of diuretic
Glucocorticoids: increased hypokalemia
NSAIDs: increased risk of renal failure

Drug/food
Licorice: increased severe hypokalemia

Drug/lab test
Increased: parathyroid test, uric acid, calcium, glucose, cholesterol, triglycerides
Decreased: potassium, sodium, Hgb, WBC, platelets

NURSING CONSIDERATIONS
Assessment
• Monitor glucose in urine if patient is diabetic
• Assess improvement in CVP q8hr
• Check for rashes, temp elevation daily
• Assess for confusion, especially in geriatric patients; take safety precautions if needed
• Monitor for acidic urine, reduced urine, osmolality, nocturia; hypotension, broad T-wave, U-wave, ectopy, tachycardia, weak pulse; muscle weakness, altered LOC, drowsiness, apathy, lethargy, confusion, depression; anorexia, nausea, cramps, constipation, distention, paralytic ileus; hypoventilation, respiratory muscle weakness
• Assess fluid volume status: I&O ratios, record, count, or weigh diapers as appropriate; weight;

distended red veins; crackles in lungs; color, quality, and specific gravity of urine; skin turgor; adequacy of pulses; moist mucous membranes; bilateral lung sounds; peripheral pitting edema; assess for dehydration: symptoms of decreasing output, thirst, hypotension; dry mouth and mucous membranes should be reported

• Monitor electrolytes: potassium, sodium, calcium, magnesium; also include BUN, blood pH, ABGs, uric acid, CBC, blood glucose, renal function

• Assess B/P before, during therapy with patient lying, standing, and sitting as appropriate; orthostatic hypotension can occur rapidly

Patient/family education

• Teach patient to take the medication early in the day to prevent nocturia

• Instruct patient to take with food or milk if GI symptoms of nausea and anorexia occur

• Teach patient to maintain a weekly record of weight and notify prescriber of weight loss >5 lb

• Caution patient that this product causes a loss of potassium and that food rich in potassium should be added to the diet; refer to a dietitian for assistance in planning

• Caution patient to rise slowly from sitting or reclining positions, not to exercise in hot weather or stand for prolonged periods since orthostatic hypotension will be enhanced; lie down if dizziness occurs

• Teach patient not to use alcohol or any OTC medications without prescriber's approval; serious product reactions may occur

• Emphasize the need to contact prescriber immediately if muscle cramps, weakness, nausea, dizziness, or numbness occurs

• Teach patient to take own B/P and pulse and record findings

• Teach patient to continue taking medication even if feeling better; this product controls symptoms but does not cure the condition

• Advise patient with hypertension to continue other medical treatment (exercise, weight loss, relaxation techniques, cessation of smoking)

Evaluation

Positive therapeutic outcome

• Decreased edema

• Decreased B/P

• Increased diuresis

TREATMENT OF OVERDOSE:

Lavage if taken orally, monitor electrolytes, administer dextrose in saline, monitor hydration, CV, renal status

HYDROcodone (Rx)
(hye-droe-koe'done)
Hycodan ✤, Tussigon
HYDROcodone/acetaminophen (Rx)
Co-Gesic, Dolorex Forte, Duocet, Hycet, Hydrocet, Hydrogesic, Liquicet, Lorcet, Lortab, Margesic H, Maxidone, NorCo, Panlor, Polygesic, Stagesic, T-Gesic, Vanacet, Vicodin, Vicodin ES, Vicodin HP, Xodol, Zamicet, Zydone
HYDROcodone/ibuprofen (Rx)
Ibudone, Reprexain, Vicoprofen
Func. class.: Antitussive opioid analgesic/ nonopioid analgesic

Pregnancy category C
Controlled substance schedule III

Do not confuse:
HYDROcodone/hydrocortisone,
Hycodan/Vicodin

ACTION: Acts directly on cough center in medulla to suppress cough; binds to opiate receptors in the CNS to reduce pain

Therapeutic outcome: Pain relief, decreased cough, decreased diarrhea

USES: Hyperactive and nonproductive cough, mild to moderate pain

CONTRAINDICATIONS:
Acne rosacea/vulgaris, Cushing's, measles, perioral dermatitis, varicella, abrupt discontinuation, hypersensitivity to this product or benzyl

Precautions: Pregnancy **C**, breastfeeding, neonates, addictive personality, increased ICP, MI (acute), severe heart disease, respiratory depression, renal/hepatic disease, bowel impaction, urinary retention, viral infection, ulcerative colitis, seizures, sulfite hypersensitivity, psychosis, hypertension, hyperthyroidism

DOSAGES AND ROUTES
Analgesic
Adult: PO 2.5-10 mg q3-6hr prn, max 60 mg/day

Antitussive
Adult: PO 5 mg q4-6hr prn, max 30 mg/24 hr

Adverse effects: *italics* = common; **bold** = life-threatening

Available forms: HYDROcodone: bulk powder; **HYDROcodone/acetaminophen:** 5 mg HYDROcodone/500 mg acetaminophen (Co-Gesic, Lorcet, Lortab 5/500, Stagesic, Vicodin); 7.5 mg HYDROcodone/400 mg acetaminophen (Zydone), 7.5 mg HYDROcodone/500 mg acetaminophen (Lortab 7.5/500), 7.5 mg HYDROcodone/750 mg acetaminophen (Vicodin ES), 5 mg HYDROcodone/325 acetaminophen, 10 mg HYDROcodone/325 acetaminophen (Norco), 10 mg HYDROcodone/500 mg acetaminophen (Lortab 10/500), 10 mg HYDROcodone/650 mg acetaminophen (Lorcet 10/650, Vicodin HP), 10 mg HYDROcodone/660 acetaminophen (Vicodin HP); caps 5 mg HYDROcodone/500 mg acetaminophen (Stagesic, Zydone); **HYDROcodone/ibuprofen:** tabs 7.5 mg HYDROcodone/200 mg ibuprofen (Vico-profen)

Implementation

• Do not break, crush, or chew tabs; only scored tabs may be broken
• Give with antiemetic if nausea, vomiting occur
• Give when pain is beginning to return; determine dosage interval by patient response; continuous dosing of medication is more effective than given prn
• Medication should be slowly withdrawn after long-term use to prevent withdrawal symptoms
• Max 4 g acetaminophen with combination product
• Store in light-resistant container at room temperature
• May be given with food or milk to lessen GI upset

ADVERSE EFFECTS

CNS: *Drowsiness,* dizziness, light-headedness, confusion, headache, sedation, euphoria, dysphoria, weakness, hallucinations, disorientation, mood changes, dependence, **seizures**
CV: Palpitations, tachycardia, bradycardia, change in B/P, **circulatory depression,** syncope, **cardiac arrest (child)**
EENT: Tinnitus, blurred vision, miosis, diplopia
GI: *Nausea, vomiting, anorexia, constipation,* cramps, dry mouth, ulcers
GU: Increased urinary output, dysuria, urinary retention
INTEG: Rash, urticaria, flushing, pruritus
RESP: Respiratory depression, pulmonary edema, bronchopneumonia, **respiratory arrest (child)**

Pharmacokinetics

Absorption	Well absorbed
Distribution	Unknown; crosses placenta
Metabolism	Liver, extensively
Excretion	Kidneys
Half-life	3½-4½ hr

Pharmacodynamics

	PO (analgesic)	PO (antitussive)
Onset	10-20 min	Unknown
Peak	30-60 min	Unknown
Duration	4-6 hr	4-6 hr

INTERACTIONS

Individual drugs
Alcohol: increased CNS depression

Drug classifications
Antidepressants (tricyclics), CNS depressants, general anesthetics, opioids, phenothiazines, sedative/hypnotics, skeletal muscle relaxants: increased CNS depression
MAOIs: increased severe reactions

Drug/herb
Lavender, valerian: increased CNS depression

Drug/lab test
Increased: amylase, lipase

NURSING CONSIDERATIONS

Assessment
• **Assess pain:** intensity, type, location, duration, precipitating factor before and 1 hr after giving product, titrate upward by 25%; assess need for pain medication, physical dependency
• Monitor VS after parenteral route; note muscle rigidity; product history; liver; renal function tests; cough; and respiratory dysfunction: respiratory depression, character, rate, rhythm; notify prescriber if respirations are <10/min
• **Monitor CNS changes:** dizziness, drowsiness, hallucinations, euphoria, LOC, pupil reaction
• Monitor allergic reactions: rash, urticaria
• Obtain history of ulcers if using ibuprofen combination product
• **Bowel status:** constipation; provide fluids, fiber in diet, may need stimulant laxative

Patient/family education
• Instruct patient to report any symptoms of CNS changes, allergic reactions; to avoid CNS depressants: alcohol, sedative/hypnotics for at least 24 hr after taking this product

---

⚠ Nurse Alert   ✳ Key NCLEX® Drug

• Teach patient that dizziness, drowsiness, and confusion are common and to avoid getting up without assistance, driving, or other hazardous activities

• Discuss in detail all aspects of the product

Evaluation
Positive therapeutic outcome
• Decreased pain
• Decreased cough

TREATMENT OF OVERDOSE:
Naloxone HCl (Narcan) 0.2-0.8 **IV**, O_2, **IV** fluids, vasopressors

---

hydrocortisone (Rx)
(hy-droh-kor'tih-sone)
Cortef, Colocort, Cortena
hydrocortisone acetate (Rx)
Anucort, Anusol, Cortifoam, Hemril, Protocort, Rectasol
hydrocortisone sodium succinate (Rx)
A-hydroCort, Solu-Cortef
Func. class.: Short-acting glucocorticoid
Chem. class.: Natural nonfluorinated, group IV potency (valerate), group VI potency (acetate and plain)
Pregnancy category C

Do not confuse:
hydrocortisone/HYDROcodone

ACTION: Decreases inflammation by suppressing migration of polymorphonuclear leukocytes and fibroblasts and reversing increased capillary permeability and lysosomal stabilization (systemic); antipruritic, antiinflammatory (topical)

Therapeutic outcome: Decreased inflammation

USES: Severe inflammation, septic shock, adrenal insufficiency, ulcerative colitis, collagen disorders, asthma, COPD, Hodgkin disease, SLE, Stevens-Johnson syndrome, ulcerative colitis, TB

CONTRAINDICATIONS:
Hypersensitivity, fungal infections

Precautions: Pregnancy **C**, breastfeeding, diabetes mellitus, glaucoma, osteoporosis, seizure disorders, ulcerative colitis, CHF, myas-thenia gravis, renal disease, esophagitis, peptic ulcer, metastatic carcinoma, septic shock, Cushing syndrome, hepatic disease, hypothyroidism, coagulopathy, thromboembolism, children <2 yr, psychosis, idiopathic thrombocytopenia (IM), acute glomerulonephritis, amebiasis, nonasthmatic bronchial disease, AIDS, TB, recent MI (associated with left-ventricular rupture)

DOSAGE AND ROUTES
Adrenal insufficiency/inflammation
Adult: PO 20-240 mg daily in divided doses; IM/IV 100-500 mg (succinate), may repeat q2-6hr, then 50-100 mg IM as needed

Shock prevention
Adult: IM/IV 50 mg/kg repeated q4hr; repeat q24hr as needed (succinate)
Child: IM/IV 0.16-1 mg/kg or 6-30 mg/m² given daily or bid (succinate)

Colitis
Adult: PO 20-240 mg (base)/day in 2-4 divided doses; enema 100 mg nightly for 21 days
Child: PO 2-8 mg (base)/kg/day or 60-240 mg (base)/m²/day in 3-4 divided doses

Topical route
Adult and child >2 yr: Apply to affected area daily-qid

Available forms: Hydrocortisone: enema 100 mg/60 ml; tabs 5, 10, 20 mg; **acetate:** rectal aerosol foam: 10%; **cypionate:** tabs 5, 10, 20 mg; **succinate:** inj 100, 250, 500, 1000 mg vial

Implementation
PO route
• Give with food or milk to decrease GI symptoms
Rectal route
• Use applicator provided
• Clean applicator after each use
• Retain for 1 hr if possible
Topical route
• Apply only to affected areas; do not get in eyes
• Cleanse and dry area before applying medication, then cover with occlusive dressing (only if prescribed); seal to normal skin; change q12hr; systemic absorption may occur; use only on dermatoses; do not use on weeping, denuded, or infected area
• Use for a few days after area has cleared
• Store at room temperature
Nasal route
• Patient should clear nasal passages before administration; use decongestant if needed; shake inhaler, invert, tilt head backward, insert

H

---

nozzle into nostril, away from septum; hold other nostril closed and depress activator, inhale through nose, exhale through mouth

IM route
• Give deeply in large muscle mass; rotate sites; avoid deltoid; use 21-gauge needle

IV route
• **Succinate:** IV in mix-o-vial or reconstitute 250 mg or less/2 ml bacteriostatic water for injection, mix gently; give direct IV over 1 min or more; may be further diluted in 100, 250, 500, or 1000 ml of D_5W, D_5/0.9% NaCl, 0.9% NaCl given over ordered rate

Sodium succinate preparations

Y-site compatibilities: Acyclovir, allopurinol, amifostine, ampicillin, amphotericin B cholesteryl, inamrinone, amsacrine, atracurium, atropine, aztreonam, betamethasone, calcium gluconate, cefepime, cefmetazole, cephalothin, cephapirin, chlordiazePOXIDE, chlorproMAZINE, cisatracurium, cladribine, cyanocobalamin, cytarabine, dexamethasone, digoxin, diphenhydrAMINE, DOPamine, DOXOrubicin liposome, droperidol, edrophonium, enalaprilat, EPINEPHrine, esmolol, conjugated estrogens, ethacrynate, famotidine, fentaNYL, fentaNYL/droperidol, filgrastim, fludarabine, fluorouracil, foscarnet, furosemide, gallium, granisetron, heparin, hydrALAZINE, regular insulin, isoproterenol, kanamycin, lidocaine, LORazepam, magnesium sulfate, melphalan, menadiol, meperidine, methicillin, methoxamine, methylergonovine, minocycline, morphine, neostigmine, norepinephrine, ondansetron, oxacillin, oxytocin, PACLitaxel, pancuronium, penicillin G potassium, pentazocine, phytonadione, piperacillin/tazobactam, prednisoLONE, procainamide, prochlorperazine, propofol, propranolol, pyridostigmine, remifentanil, scopolamine, sodium bicarbonate, succinylcholine, tacrolimus, teniposide, theophylline, thiotepa, trimethaphan, trimethobenzamide, vecuronium, vinorelbine

Y-site incompatibilities: Diazepam, ergotamine tartrate, IDArubicin, phenytoin, sargramostim

ADVERSE EFFECTS

CNS: Depression, flushing, sweating, headache, mood changes, **pseudotumor cerebri,** euphoria, insomnia, **seizures**
CV: Hypertension, **circulatory collapse, thrombophlebitis, embolism,** tachycardia, edema, heart failure

EENT: Fungal infections, increased intraocular pressure, blurred vision, cataracts, glaucoma
GI: Diarrhea, nausea, abdominal distention, **GI hemorrhage,** increased appetite, **pancreatitis,** vomiting
HEMA: Thrombocytopenia
INTEG: Acne, poor wound healing, ecchymosis, petechiae
MISC: Adrenal insufficiency (after stress/withdrawal)
MS: Fractures, osteoporosis, weakness

Pharmacokinetics

Absorption	Well absorbed (PO); systemic (topical)
Distribution	Crosses placenta
Metabolism	Liver, extensively
Excretion	Kidney
Half-life	3-5 hr, adrenal suppression 3-4 days

Pharmacodynamics

	PO	IM	IV	TOPICAL
Onset	1-2 hr	20 min	Rapid	Min to hr
Peak	1 hr	4-8 hr	1-2 hr	Hr to days
Duration	1½ days	1½ days	1½ days	Hr to days

INTERACTIONS

Individual drugs

Alcohol, amphotericin B, cycloSPORINE, digoxin: increased side effects
Bosentan, carBAMazepine, cholestyramine, colestipol, ePHEDrine, phenytoin, rifampin, theophylline: decreased action of hydrocortisone

Drug classifications

Acetaminophen, NSAIDs, salicylates: increased risk of GI bleeding
Anticoagulants, calcium supplements, toxoids, vaccines: decreased action of each specific drug
Anticonvulsants: decreased effects of anticonvulsant
Antidiabetics: decreased effects of antidiabetics
Barbiturates: decreased action of hydrocortisone
Diuretics: increased side effects
Live virus vaccines/toxoids: increased neurologic reactions

Drug/herb

Ephedra: decreased hydrocortisone levels

Drug/lab test

Increased: cholesterol, sodium, blood glucose, uric acid, calcium, urine glucose

Decreased: calcium, potassium, T_4, T_3, thyroid ^{131}I uptake test, urine 17-OHCS, 17-KS

False negative: skin allergy tests

NURSING CONSIDERATIONS

Assessment

• **Adrenal insufficiency (cushingoid symptoms):** nausea, anorexia, shortness of breath, moon face, fatigue, dizziness, weakness, joint pain before and during treatment; monitor plasma cortisol levels during long-term therapy (normal level is 138-635 nmol/L when obtained at 8 AM); check adrenal function periodically for hypothalamic-pituitary-adrenal axis suppression

• Monitor potassium, blood glucose, urine glucose while patient is on long-term therapy; hypokalemia and hyperglycemia may occur

• Monitor I&O ratio; be alert for decreasing urinary output and increasing edema; weigh daily; notify prescriber of weekly gain >5 lb or edema, hypertension, cardiac symptoms

• **Assess for infection:** increased temp, WBC even after withdrawal of medication; product masks infection symptoms; if fever develops, product should be discontinued

• Check for potassium depletion: paresthesias, fatigue, nausea, vomiting, depression, polyuria, dysrhythmias, weakness

• Assess mental status: affect, mood, behavioral changes, aggression

• Check nasal passages during long-term treatment for changes in mucus (nasal)

• Assess for systemic absorption: increased temp, inflammation, irritation (topical)

• GI effects: nausea, vomiting, anorexia or appetite stimulation, diarrhea, constipation, abdominal pain, hiccups, gastritis, pancreatitis, GI bleeding/perforation with long-term treatment

Patient/family education

• Teach patient all aspects of product use, including cushingoid symptoms

• Advise patient to carry/wear emergency ID as corticosteroid user; not to discontinue abruptly; adrenal crisis can result

• Instruct patient to notify prescriber if therapeutic response decreases; dosage adjustment may be needed

• Instruct patient to notify prescriber of signs of infection

• Teach patient that product can mask infections and cause hyperglycemia (diabetic)

• Teach patient to avoid live-virus vaccines if using steroids long term

• Caution patient to avoid OTC products unless directed by prescriber: salicylates, alcohol in cough products, cold preparations

• **Teach patient symptoms of adrenal insufficiency:** nausea, anorexia, fatigue, dizziness, dyspnea, weakness, joint pain; and when to notify prescriber

• Advise patient that long-term therapy may be needed to resolve infection (1-2 mo depending on type of infection)

• Teach patient to report immediately abdominal pain, black tarry stools, as GI bleeding/perforation can occur

• Advise patient not to discontinue abruptly or adrenal crisis can result; product should be tapered

Nasal route

• Instruct patient to clear nasal passages if sneezing attack occurs, then repeat dose; to continue using product even if mild nasal bleeding occurs; bleeding is usually transient

• Teach method of instillation after providing written instruction from manufacturer on instillation

Evaluation

Positive therapeutic outcome

• Decrease in runny nose (nasal)

• Decreased inflammation

• Absence of severe itching, patches on skin, flaking (top)

• Decreased GI symptoms

---

hydrocortisone topical
See Appendix B

⚠ HIGH ALERT

HYDROmorphone (Rx)

(hye-droe-mor′fone)

Dilaudid, Dilaudid-HP, Exalgo, Hydromorph Contin ✚

Func. class.: Antitussive, opioid analgesic agonist

Chem. class.: Phenanthrene derivative, guaifenesin

Pregnancy category C

Controlled substance schedule II

Do not confuse:

HYDROmorphone/meperidine/morphine, Dilaudid/Demerol

ACTION: Inhibits ascending pain pathways in CNS, increases pain threshold, alters pain perception

---

Therapeutic outcome: Decreased cough, decreased pain

USES: As an antitussive to suppress cough; moderate to severe pain

CONTRAINDICATIONS:
Hypersensitivity to this product, sulfite, COPD, cor pulmonale, emphysema, GI obstruction, ileus, increased intracranial pressure, obstetric delivery, status asthmaticus

> **BLACK BOX WARNING:** Respiratory depression, opioid-naive patients, substance abuse, accidental exposure, potential for overdose/poisoning

Precautions: Pregnancy **C,** breastfeeding, children <18 yr, increased ICP, addictive personality, renal/hepatic disease, MI (acute), abrupt discontinuation, adrenal insufficiency, angina, asthma, biliary tract disease, bladder obstruction, hypothyroidism, hypovolemia, hypoxemia, IBD, IV use, labor, latex hypersensitivity, myxedema, seizure disorders, sleep apnea

DOSAGE AND ROUTES
Analgesic
Adult: PO (oral solution) 2.5-10 mg q3-6hr or (tabs) 2-4 mg q4-6hr; ext rel (Exalgo): Convert to ext rel by giving total daily dose of immediate release in one daily dose, titrate if needed ext rel q3-4days until adequate pain relief; use 25%-50% increase for each titration step, if more than 2 doses of rescue medication is needed in 24 hr consider titration; **IV** 0.2-1 mg q2-3hr; give over 2-3 min; **IM/SUBCUT** 1-2 mg q4-6hr prn, may be increased (opioid-naive patients may require lower dose); **RECT** 3 mg q6-8hr prn
Geriatric: PO 1-2 mg q4-6hr

Available forms: Powder of injection 250 mg; inj 1, 2, 4, 10 mg/ml; tabs 2, 4, 8 mg; oral sol 5 mg/5 ml; supp 3 mg, ext rel tab 8, 12, 16, 32 mg

Implementation
• Give with antiemetic if nausea, vomiting occur
• Give when pain is beginning to return; determine dosage interval by patient response; continuous dosing of medication is more effective given prn; explain analgesic effect
• Withdraw medication slowly after long-term use to prevent withdrawal symptoms
• Store in light-resistant container at room temperature

PO route
• May be given with food or milk to lessen GI upset

Extended release

> **BLACK BOX WARNING:** Do not use extended-release products in opioid-naive patients

• **Converting from oral opioids;** conversion ratios are approximate; initiate ext rel tabs at 50% of calculated total daily equivalent dose of ext rel, give q24hr; max increase q2-3days, consider titration increases of 25%-50% in each step
• **Converting from transdermal patch (fentaNYL)** initiate ext rel tabs 18 hr after removal of patch; for each 25 mcg/hr dose of transdermal fentaNYL the dose is 12 mg q24hr, start dose at 50% of calculated HYDROmorphone ext rel dose q24hr; titrate no more often than q3-4days, consider dose increases of 25%-50% with each step; if more than 2 rescue doses are required in 24 hr, consider titration
SUBCUT route
• Do not give if sol is cloudy or a precipitate has formed; rotate inj sites
• Use short 30-G needle, make sure not to inject intradermally
Direct IV route
• Give after diluting with 5 ml or more of sterile water or 0.9% NaCl for inj
• Give slowly at 2 mg over 3-5 min or less through Y-connector or 3-way stopcock
IV infusion route
• Dilute each 0.1-1 mg/ml in 0.9% NaCl, deliver by opioid syringe infusion; may be diluted in D₅W, D₅/NaCl, 0.45% NaCl or 0.9% NaCl for larger amounts and through an infusion pump

Syringe compatibilities: Atropine, bupivacaine, cefTAZidime, chlorproMAZINE, cimetidine, diphenhydrAMINE, fentaNYL, glycopyrrolate, haloperidol, hydrOXYzine, LORazepam, midazolam, pentazocaine, PENTobarbital, prochlorperazine, promethazine, ranitidine, scopolamine, thiethylperazine, trimethobenzamide

Y-site compatibilities: Acyclovir, allopurinol, amifostine, amikacin, amsacrine, aztreonam, cefamandole, cefepime, cefoperazone, cefotaxime, cefOXitin, cefTAZidime, ceftizoxime, cefuroxime, chloramphenicol, CISplatin, cladribine, clindamycin, cyclophosphamide, cytarabine, diltiazem, DOBUTamine, DOPamine, DOXOrubicin, doxycycline, EPINEPHrine, erythromycin lactobionate, famotidine, fentaNYL, filgrastim, fludarabine, foscarnet, furosemide, gentamicin, granisetron, heparin, kanamycin, labetalol, LORazepam, magnesium sulfate, melphalan, methotrexate, metroNIDAZOLE, midazolam, milrinone, morphine, nafcillin, niCARdipine, nitroglycerin, norepinephrine, ondansetron, oxacillin, PACLitaxel, penicillin G potassium, piperacillin, piperacillin/tazobactam, propofol, ranitidine, teniposide, thiotepa, ticarcillin, tobramycin, trimethoprim/sulfamethoxazole, vancomycin, vecuronium, vinorelbine

Y-site incompatibilities: Ampicillin, diazepam, minocycline, PHENobarbital, phenytoin, sargramostim

Additive compatibilities: Bupivacaine, cloNIDine, fluorouracil, heparin, midazolam, ondansetron, potassium chloride, promethazine, verapamil, ziconotide

Additive incompatibilities: Sodium bicarbonate, thiopental

Solution compatibilities: D_5W, D_5/0.45% NaCl, D_5/0.9% NaCl, D_5/LR, D_5/Ringer's, 0.45% NaCl, 0.9% NaCl, Ringer's, LR

ADVERSE EFFECTS
CNS: Dizziness, drowsiness, *sedation, confusion,* headache, euphoria, mood changes, **seizures**
CV: *Hypotension, bradycardia,* palpitations, change in B/P, tachycardia, peripheral vasodilatation
EENT: Miosis, diplopia, blurred vision, tinnitus
GI: *Nausea, constipation, vomiting, anorexia,* dry mouth, cramps, paralytic ileus
GU: Increased urinary output, dysuria, urinary retention
INTEG: Urticaria, rash, flushing, bruising, diaphoresis, pruritus
RESP: **Respiratory depression,** dyspnea

Pharmacokinetics
Absorption	Well absorbed (PO), complete (**IV**)
Distribution	Unknown; crosses placenta
Metabolism	Liver, extensively
Excretion	Kidneys
Half-life	Varied

Pharmacodynamics
	PO/IM/SUBCUT	IV	RECT
Onset	15-30 min	10-15 min	15-30 min
Peak	30-60 min	15-30 min	30-90 min
Duration	4-5 hr	2-3 hr	4-5 hr

INTERACTIONS
Individual drugs
Alcohol: increased respiratory depression, hypotension, sedation

Drug classifications
Antipsychotics, opiates, sedative/hypnotics, skeletal muscle relaxants: increased effects
MAOIs: increased severe reactions
Opiate antagonists: decreased HYDROmorphone effects

Drug/herb
Chamomile, hops, kava, lavender, St. John's wort, valerian: increased action

Drug/lab test
Increased: amylase

NURSING CONSIDERATIONS
Assessment
• **Assess pain control,** sedation by scoring on 0-10 scale; around-the-clock dosing is best for pain control
• Monitor VS after parenteral route; note muscle rigidity; product history

BLACK BOX WARNING: Respiratory dysfunction; respiratory depression; monitor character, rate, rhythm; notify prescriber if respirations are <10/min

• Monitor CNS changes: dizziness, drowsiness, hallucinations, euphoria, LOC, pupil reaction
• Monitor allergic reactions: rash, urticaria; bowel function, constipation

Patient/family education
• Instruct patient to report any symptoms of CNS changes, allergic reactions; to avoid CNS depressants: alcohol, sedative-hypnotics for at least 24 hr after taking this product
• Advise patient that dizziness, drowsiness, and confusion are common and to avoid getting up without assistance, driving, or other hazardous activities
• Discuss in detail all aspects of the product

Evaluation
Positive therapeutic outcome
- Decreased pain
- Decreased cough

TREATMENT OF OVERDOSE:
Naloxone HCl (Narcan) 0.2-0.8 **IV**, O$_2$, **IV** fluids, vasopressors

---

hydroxychloroquine (Rx)
(hye-drox-ee-klor'oh-kwin)
Apo-Hydroxyquine ✤, Plaquenil
Func. class.: Antimalarial, antirheumatic (DMARDs)
Chem. class.: 4-Aminoquinoline derivative
Pregnancy category C

ACTION: Impairs complement-dependent antigen-antibody reactions

Therapeutic outcome: Resolution of infection

USES: Malaria caused by *Plasmodium vivax, P. malariae, P. ovale, P. falciparum* (some strains); LE, rheumatoid arthritis

CONTRAINDICATIONS:
Hypersensitivity to this product or chloroquine, retinal field changes

> **BLACK BOX WARNING:** Children (long-term), ocular disease

Precautions: Pregnancy **C**, breastfeeding, blood dyscrasias, severe GI disease, neurologic disease, alcoholism, hepatic disease, G6PD deficiency, psoriasis, eczema

DOSAGE AND ROUTES
Malaria
Adult: PO **suppression or prevention** 400 mg qwk, begin 1-2 wk before travel, continue 4 wk after returning; **treatment** 800 mg, then 400 mg after 6-8 hr, then 400 mg/day on 2nd and 3rd day, total dose 2 g
Child: PO **suppression or prevention** 6.4 mg/kg (5 mg/kg base) qwk, begin 1-2 wk before travel, continue 4 wk after returning; **treatment** 10 mg/kg, 6.4 mg/kg (5 mg/kg base), at 6, 24, 48 hr after 1st dose

Lupus erythematosus
Adult: PO 400 mg (310 mg base) daily-bid; length depends on patient response; **maintenance** 200-400 mg/day

Rheumatoid arthritis
Adult: PO 400-600 mg/day for 4-12 wk; then 200-300 mg/day after good response

Available forms: Tabs 200 mg

Implementation
PO route
- Give before or after meals with milk, at same time each day to maintain product level
- Tabs may be crushed and mixed with food, fluids
- Malaria prophylaxis should be started 2 wk prior to exposure and 4-6 wk after leaving exposure area
- Store in tight, light-resistant container at room temperature; keep inj in cool environment

ADVERSE EFFECTS
CNS: Headache, stimulation, fatigue, irritability, **seizures**, bad dreams, dizziness, confusion, psychosis, decreased reflexes
CV: Hypotension, heart block, **asystole with syncope**
EENT: *Blurred vision, corneal changes, retinal changes, difficulty focusing,* tinnitus, vertigo, deafness, photophobia, corneal edema
GI: *Nausea, vomiting, anorexia,* diarrhea, cramps
HEMA: **Thrombocytopenia, agranulocytosis, leukopenia, aplastic anemia**
INTEG: Pruritus, pigmentation changes, skin eruptions, lichen planus–like eruptions, eczema, **exfoliative dermatitis**, alopecia, **Stevens-Johnson syndrome**, photosensitivity

Pharmacokinetics
Absorption	Well absorbed
Distribution	Widely distributed, crosses placenta
Metabolism	Liver
Excretion	Urine/feces
Half-life	3-5 day

Pharmacodynamics
Onset	Rapid
Peak	1-2 hr
Duration	Days-weeks

INTERACTIONS
Individual products
Magnesium, aluminum products: decreased malarial action
Digoxin: increased levels
Methotrexate: decreased levels
Rabies vaccine: increased antibody titer

Drug classifications
Live-virus vaccines, botulinum toxoids: decreased effects

NURSING CONSIDERATIONS
Assessment
• **Assess for lupus erythematosus, malaria symptoms** before treatment and daily
• **Assess for rheumatoid arthritis:** pain, swelling, ROM, temp of joints, for decreased reflexes: knee, ankle
• Assess ophthalmic exam baseline, q6mo if long-term treatment or product dosage >150 mg/day
• Assess hepatic studies qwk: AST, ALT, bilirubin
• **Blood dyscrasias:** Assess blood studies: CBC, platelets; WBC, RBC, platelets may be decreased; if severe, product should be discontinued; malaise, fever, bruising, bleeding (rare)
• Assess for decreased reflexes: knee, ankle
• Assess ECG during therapy
• Assess for depression of T-waves, widening of QRS complex
• **Assess allergic reactions:** pruritus, rash, urticaria
• **Assess for ototoxicity** (tinnitus, vertigo, change in hearing); audiometric testing should be done before, after treatment
⚠ **Assess for toxicity: blurring vision, difficulty focusing, headache, dizziness, knee, ankle reflexes; product should be discontinued immediately**

Patient/family education
• Teach patient to use sunglasses in bright sunlight to decrease photophobia
• Teach patient that urine may turn rust or brown
• Teach patient to report hearing, vision problems; fever, fatigue, bruising, bleeding, which may indicate blood dyscrasias

Evaluation
Positive therapeutic outcome
• Decreased symptoms of malaria, LE, rheumatoid arthritis

TREATMENT OF OVERDOSE:
Induce vomiting; gastric lavage; administer barbiturate (ultra–short-acting), vasopressor, ammonium chloride; tracheostomy may be necessary

hydroxyurea (Rx)
(hye-drox-ee-yoo-ree'ah)
Droxia, Hydrea
Func. class.: Antineoplastic, antimetabolite
Chem. class.: Synthetic urea analog
Pregnancy category D

Do not confuse:
hydroxyurea/hydrOXYzine

ACTION: Acts by inhibiting DNA synthesis without interfering with RNA or protein synthesis; incorporates thymidine into DNA, causing direct damage to DNA strands; cell cycle specific (S phase)

Therapeutic outcome: Prevention of rapidly growing malignant cells

USES: Melanoma, chronic myelogenous leukemia, recurrent or metastatic ovarian cancer, squamous cell carcinoma of the head and neck, sickle cell anemia

CONTRAINDICATIONS:
Pregnancy **D**, breastfeeding, hypersensitivity, leukopenia (<2500/mm³), thrombocytopenia (<100,000/mm³), anemia (severe), bone marrow suppression, dental disease, geriatrics, HIV, hyperkalemia, hyperphosphatemia, hyperuricemia, hypocalcemia, infection, infertility, IM injection, tumor lysis syndrome, vaccinations

> **BLACK BOX WARNING:** Requires an experienced clinician, secondary malignancy

Precautions: Renal disease (severe)

DOSAGE AND ROUTES
Ovarian cancer, malignant melanoma
Adult: PO 80 mg/kg as a single dose q3day or 20-30 mg/kg as a single dose daily

Ovarian cancer in combination with radiation
Adult: PO 80 mg/kg as a single dose q3day; should be started 7 days before irradiation

Sickle cell anemia
Adult: PO 15 mg/kg/day, may increase by 5 mg/kg/day q12wk; max 35 mg/kg/day

Renal disease
Adult: CCr <59 ml/min use 50% of dose

Available forms: Caps 200, 300, 400, 500 mg

Implementation

• Do not crush or chew caps; for difficulty swallowing, caps may be opened and contents mixed with water

• Avoid contact with skin, very irritating; wash completely to remove

• Give fluids **IV** or PO before chemotherapy to hydrate patient

• Give antiemetic 30-60 min before giving product and prn to prevent vomiting; antibiotics for prophylaxis of infection

• Provide liquid diet: carbonated beverages; gelatin may be added if patient is not nauseated or vomiting

ADVERSE EFFECTS

CNS: Headache, confusion, hallucinations, dizziness, **seizures**

CV: Angina, ischemia

GI: Nausea, vomiting, anorexia, diarrhea, stomatitis, constipation, **hepatotoxicity**, pancreatitis

GU: Increased BUN, uric acid, creatinine, temporary renal function impairment

HEMA: Leukopenia, anemia, thrombocytopenia, megaloblastic erythropoiesis

INTEG: *Rash*, urticaria, pruritus, dry skin, facial erythema

MISC: Fever, chills, malaise, secondary cancers, **tumor lysis syndrome**

META: Hyperphosphatemia, hyperuricemia, hypocalcemia

RESP: Pulmonary fibrosis, diffuse pulmonary infiltrates

Pharmacokinetics

Absorption	Well absorbed
Distribution	Crosses blood-brain barrier
Metabolism	Liver (50%)
Excretion	Kidneys, unchanged (50%), eliminated as CO_2
Half-life	Terminal 3.5-4.5 hr

Pharmacodynamics

Onset	Unknown
Peak	1-4 hr
Duration	Unknown

INTERACTIONS

Individual drugs

Didanosine, stavudine: increased pancreatitis/hepatotoxicity

Probenecid, sulfinpyrazone: increased uric acid levels

Radiation: increased toxicity

Drug classifications

Anticoagulants, NSAIDs, thrombolytics, salicylates, platelet inhibitors: increased bleeding

Antineoplastics: increased toxicity

Hematopoietic progenitor cells (sargramostim, filgrastim): do not use within 24 hr before or after antineoplastic

Live-virus vaccines: do not use together

Drug/lab test

Increased: BUN, creatinine, LFTs, uric acid

Decreased: Hgb, WBC, platelets

NURSING CONSIDERATIONS

Assessment

• Assess buccal cavity q8hr for dryness, sores or ulceration, white patches, oral pain, bleeding, dysphagia; obtain prescription for viscous lidocaine (Xylocaine)

• Assess symptoms indicating severe allergic reaction: rash, pruritus, urticaria, purpuric skin lesions, itching, flushing

• **Bone marrow suppression:** Determine the hemoglobin concentration, total leukocyte count, and platelet count at least once a week during entire course; if the WBC ≤2500/mm³ or platelets ≤100,000/mm³, interrupt Hydrea until the values rise significantly toward normal concentrations. If severe anemia occurs, manage it without interrupting Hydrea receipt. For Droxia, monitor blood counts q2wk and interrupt drug receipt if neutrophils <2000/mm³, platelets <80,000/mm³, hemoglobin <4.5 g/dl, or if reticulocytes <80,000/mm³ when the hemoglobin concentration is <9 g/dl. After recovery, Droxia may be resumed at a lower dose; Droxia therapy requires an experienced clinician knowledgeable in the use of this medication for the treatment of sickle cell anemia

⚠ Assess for increased uric acid levels, swelling, joint pain primarily in extremities; patient should be well hydrated to prevent urate deposits

⚠ Monitor renal function studies: BUN, creatinine, serum uric acid, urine CCr before, during therapy; I&O ratio; report fall in urine output to <30 ml/hr

⚠ Monitor temp (may indicate beginning of infection)

⚠ Monitor liver function tests before, during therapy (bilirubin, AST, ALT, LDH) as needed or monthly

---

⚠ Cutaneous vasculitic toxicity and gangrene: more common in those receiving interferon
⚠ Assess for bleeding: hematuria, stool guaiac, bruising or petechiae, mucosa or orifices q8hr
⚠ Assess for tumor lysis syndrome: hyperkalemia, hyperphosphatemia, hyperuricemia, hypocalcemia, uric acid nephropathy, acute renal failure; metabolic acidosis can occur, aggressive alkalinization of urine and allopurinol can prevent this
⚠ Severe allergic reaction: assess for rash, urticaria, itching, flushing
⚠ Neurotoxicity: assess for headaches, hallucinations, seizures, dizziness
⚠ Pulmonary reactions: assess for pulmonary fibrosis, fever, dyspnea, diffuse pulmonary infiltrates

Patient/family education
⚠ Teach patient to notify prescriber if pregnancy is planned or suspected, pregnancy (D)
• Teach patient to avoid use of products containing aspirin or ibuprofen, razors, commercial mouthwash, since bleeding may occur; instruct patient to report symptoms of bleeding (hematuria, tarry stools)
• Teach patient to rinse mouth tid-qid with water, club soda; brush teeth bid-qid with soft brush or cotton-tipped applicators for stomatitis; use unwaxed dental floss
• Instruct patient to report signs of anemia (fatigue, headache, irritability, faintness, shortness of breath)
• Advise patient to report any changes in breathing or coughing even several mo after treatment; to avoid crowds and persons with respiratory tract or other infections
• Caution patient not to have any vaccinations without the advice of the prescriber; serious reactions can occur
⚠ Advise patient to notify prescriber of fever, chills, sore throat, nausea, vomiting, anorexia, diarrhea, bleeding, bruising; may indicate blood dyscrasias; mental status change

Evaluation
Positive therapeutic outcome
• Prevention of rapid division of malignant cells

hydrOXYzine (Rx)
(hye-drox´i-zeen)
Vistaril
Func. class.: Antianxiety, sedative, hypnotic, antihistamine, antiemetic
Chem. class.: Piperazine derivative
Pregnancy category C

Do not confuse:
hydrOXYzine/hydrALAZINE, **Vistaril**/Versed

ACTION: Depresses subcortical levels of CNS, including limbic system, reticular formation; anticholinergic, antiemetic, antihistaminic responses; competes with H_1-receptor sites

Therapeutic outcome: Absence of allergy symptoms, rhinitis, pruritus, absence of nausea/vomiting, sedation, absence of anxiety

USES: Anxiety preoperatively; postoperatively to prevent nausea, vomiting; to potentiate opioid analgesics; sedation; pruritus; prevention of alcohol withdrawal

CONTRAINDICATIONS: Pregnancy (1st trimester), breastfeeding, acute asthma, hypersensitivity to this product or cetirizine

Precautions: Pregnancy C (2nd/3rd trimesters), geriatric, debilitated patients, renal/hepatic disease, closed-angle glaucoma, COPD, prostatic hypertrophy, asthma

DOSAGE AND ROUTES
Anxiety
Adult: PO 25-100 mg tid-qid, max 600 mg/day; IM 50-100 mg q4-6hr
Geriatric: PO max 50 mg/day
Child >6 yr: PO 50-100 mg/day in divided doses
Child <6 yr: PO 50 mg/day in divided doses

Alcohol withdrawal
Adult: IM 50-100 mg, then q4-6hr

Preoperatively/postoperatively (nausea/vomiting)
Adult: IM 25-100 mg q4-6hr
Child: IM 0.5-1.1 mg/kg as a single dose

Pruritus
Adult: PO 25 mg tid-qid; IM 50-100 mg, then q4-6hr prn, switch to PO as soon as feasible
Child ≥6 yr: PO 50-100 mg/day in divided doses; IM 0.5-1 mg/kg/dose q4-6hr prn, use PO when possible
Child <6 yr: PO 50 mg/day in divided doses

Renal dose
Adult: PO CCr <50 ml/min reduce dose by 50%

Available forms: Tabs 10, 25, 50 mg; caps 25, 50, 100 mg; oral sol 10 mg/5 ml; oral susp 25 mg/5 ml; inj 25, 50 mg/ml

Implementation
PO route
- Give without regard to meals
- May crush tab if patient is unable to swallow whole
- Caps may be opened and product mixed with food/fluids for patients with swallowing difficulties
- Shake oral susp before giving

IM route
- Give IM inj in large muscle mass; aspirate to prevent **IV** administration; use Z-track method; severe necrosis can result with improper technique; never give **IV/SUBCUT**

Syringe compatibilities: Atropine, atropine/meperidine, benzquinamide, bupivacaine, butorphanol, chlorproMAZINE, cimetidine, codeine, diphenhydrAMINE, doxapram, droperidol, fentaNYL, fluPHENAZine, glycopyrrolate, HYDROmorphone, lidocaine, meperidine, meperidine/atropine, methotrimeprazine, metoclopramide, midazolam, morphine, nalbuphine, oxymorphone, pentazocine, perphenazine, procaine, prochlorperazine, promazine, promethazine, remifentanil, scopolamine, SUFentanil, thiothixene

Syringe incompatibilities: Aminophylline, chloramphenicol, dimenhyDRINATE, heparin, penicillin G potassium, PENTobarbital, PHENobarbital, phenytoin

Additive compatibilities: CISplatin, cyclophosphamide, cytarabine, dimenhyDRINATE, etoposide, lidocaine, mesna, methotrexate, nafcillin

ADVERSE EFFECTS
CNS: *Dizziness, drowsiness,* confusion, headache, tremors, fatigue, depression, **seizures**
CV: Hypotension
GI: Dry mouth, nausea, diarrhea, increased appetite, weight gain

Pharmacokinetics
Absorption	Well absorbed
Distribution	Not known
Metabolism	Liver, completely
Excretion	Feces, urine, bile
Half-life	3 hr

Pharmacodynamics
	PO/IM
Onset	15-60 min
Peak	2-4 hr
Duration	4-6 hr

INTERACTIONS
Individual drugs
Alcohol: increased CNS depression
Atropine, disopyramide, haloperidol, quiNIDine: increased anticholinergic reactions

Drug classifications
Analgesics, barbiturates, CNS depressants, opiates, sedative/hypnotics: increased CNS depression
Antidepressants, antihistamines, MAOIs, phenothiazines: increased anticholinergic reactions

Drug/lab test
False negative: skin allergy testing
False increase: 17-hydroxycorticosteroids

NURSING CONSIDERATIONS
Assessment
- Anticholinergic effects: dry mouth, dizziness, confusion, hypotension, increased sedation; monitor B/P
- Assess respiratory status: rate, rhythm, increase in bronchial secretions, wheezing, chest tightness; provide fluids to 2 L/day to decrease secretion thickness
- Monitor I&O ratio: be alert for urinary retention, frequency, dysuria, especially in geriatric; product should be discontinued if these occur
- Observe for drowsiness, dizziness
- Assess cough characteristics including type, frequency, thickness of secretions; evaluate response to this medication if using for cough

Patient/family education
- Caution patient to avoid hazardous activities and activities requiring alertness, since dizziness may occur; instruct patient to request assistance with ambulation
- Advise patient to avoid alcohol, other CNS depressants including cough, cold preparations; CNS depression may occur
- Teach all aspects of product use; to notify prescriber if confusion, sedation, hypotension occur; to avoid driving and other hazardous activity if drowsiness occurs
- Caution patient not to exceed recommended dosage; dysrhythmias may occur
- Tell patient hard candy, gum, frequent rinsing of mouth may be used for dryness

---

Evaluation
Positive therapeutic outcome
- Absence of nausea, vomiting
- Decreased anxiety

TREATMENT OF OVERDOSE:
Lavage if orally ingested, VS, supportive care, **IV** norepinephrine for hypotension

Hylan G-F 20
Synvisc, Synvisc One
See Appendix A, Selected New Drugs

hyoscyamine (Rx)
(hye-oh-sye′a-meen)
Anaspaz, Colidrops, Colytrol Pediatric, Cystospaz-M, ED-SPAZ, HydroMax-DT, HydroMax-FT, HydroMax-SR, HyoMax, HyoMax SL, Hyosyne, Levsin SL, Medispax, NuLev, Oscimin, Spasdel, Symax
Func. class.: Anticholinergic/antispasmodics
Chem. class.: Belladonna alkaloid
Pregnancy category C

ACTION: Inhibits muscarinic actions of acetylcholine at postganglionic parasympathetic neuroeffector sites, reduces rigidity, tremors, hyperhidrosis of parkinsonism

Therapeutic outcome: Absence of peptic ulcer after treatment

USES: Treatment of peptic ulcer disease in combination with other products; other GI disorders, other spastic disorders, IBS, urinary incontinence

CONTRAINDICATIONS:
Hypersensitivity to anticholinergics, closed-angle glaucoma, GI obstruction, myasthenia gravis, paralytic ileus, GI atony, toxic megacolon, prostatic hypertrophy, urinary tract obstruction

Precautions: Pregnancy **C**, geriatric, hyperthyroidism, CAD, dysrhythmias, CHF, ulcerative colitis, hypertension, hiatal hernia, renal/hepatic disease, urinary retention

DOSAGE AND ROUTES
Adult/adolescent/child ≥12 yr: PO/SL 0.125-0.25 mg q4hr; ext rel 0.375-0.75 mg q12hr
Adult: IM/SUBCUT/**IV** 0.25-0.5 mg single dose or 2-4×/day q6hr

Geriatric: Max 1.5 mg/day in divided doses or max 4 biphasic tabs
Child 2-12 yr: PO SL 0.0625-0.125 q4hr

Available forms: Tabs 0.125, 0.15 mg; ext rel caps 0.375 mg; time rel tabs 0.375 ml; sol 0.125 mg/ml; elix 0.125 mg/ml; inj 0.5 mg/ml, SL tab 0.125 mg, tab biphasic 0.125, 0.375 mg; orally disintegrating tab 0.125 mg

Implementation
PO route
- Do not break, crush, or chew time rel caps
- Give ½ hour before meals for better absorption
- Give decreased dose to geriatric patients; metabolism may be slowed
- Store in tight container protected from light

IV route
- Use undiluted, inject slowly

ADVERSE EFFECTS
CNS: *Confusion, stimulation in geriatric,* headache, insomnia, dizziness, drowsiness, anxiety, weakness, hallucination
CV: *Palpitations,* tachycardia
EENT: *Blurred vision,* photophobia, mydriasis, cycloplegia, increased ocular tension
GI: *Dry mouth, constipation, paralytic ileus,* heartburn, nausea, vomiting, dysphagia, absence of taste
GU: *Urinary hesitancy, retention,* impotence
INTEG: Urticaria, rash, pruritus, anhidrosis, fever, allergic reactions

Pharmacokinetics
Absorption	Well
Distribution	Cross blood-brain barrier, placenta
Metabolism	Liver
Excretion	Urine
Half-life	3½ hr

Pharmacodynamics
	PO	IM/IV/SUBCUT
Onset	30 min	2-3 min
Peak	Unknown	Unknown
Duration	4-6 hr	4-6 hr

INTERACTIONS
Individual drugs
Amantadine: increased anticholinergic effect
Ketoconazole, levodopa: decreased effects

Adverse effects: *italics* = common; **bold** = life-threatening

Drug classifications

Antacids: decreased hyoscyamine effect
Antidepressants (tricyclics), antihistamines, H_1, MAOIs: increased anticholinergic effect
Phenothiazines: decreased effect of phenothiazines

NURSING CONSIDERATIONS

Assessment

• Monitor VS, cardiac status: checking for dysrhythmias, increased rate, palpitations
• Monitor I/O ratio; check for urinary retention or hesitancy
• Monitor GI complaints: pain, bleeding (frank or occult), nausea, vomiting, anorexia

Patient/family education

• Teach patient to avoid driving, other hazardous activities until stabilized on medication
• Teach patient to avoid alcohol or other CNS depressants; will enhance sedating properties of this product
• Teach patient to avoid hot environments; heat stroke may occur; product suppresses perspiration
• Teach patient to use sunglasses when outside to prevent photophobia; may cause blurred vision
• Teach patient to use gum, hard candy, frequent rinsing of mouth for dryness of oral cavity
• Teach patient to increase fluids, bulk, exercise to decrease constipation

Evaluation

Positive therapeutic outcome
• Absence of epigastric pain, bleeding, nausea, vomiting

ibandronate (Rx)

(eye-ban'dro-nate)

Boniva

Func. class.: Bone-resorption inhibitor, electrolyte modifier

Chem. class.: Bisphosphonate

Pregnancy category C

ACTION: Inhibits bone resorption, apparently without inhibiting bone formation and mineralization; absorbs calcium phosphate crystals in bone and may directly block dissolution of hydroxyapatite crystals of bone; more potent than other products

Therapeutic outcome: Increased bone mineral density

USES: Osteoporosis and prophylaxis

Unlabeled uses: Hypercalcemia, osteolytic metastases, Paget's disease

CONTRAINDICATIONS:

Achalasia, esophageal stricture, hypocalcemia, intraarterial administration, renal failure, hypersensitivity to bisphosphonates

Precautions: Pregnancy **C**, breastfeeding, children, geriatric, anemia, chemotherapy, coagulopathy, dental disease, diabetes mellitus, dysphagia, GI/renal disease, GERD, hypertension, infection, multiple myeloma, phosphate hypersensitivity, vitamin D deficiency

DOSAGE AND ROUTES

Postmenopausal osteoporosis

Adult: PO 2.5 mg/day or 150 mg qmo; **IV** BOL 3 mg q3mo

Prophylaxis

Adult: PO 2.5 mg/day or 150 mg qmo

Paget's disease (unlabeled)

Adult: IV 2 mg as a single dose

Osteolytic metastases (unlabeled)

Adult: IV 6 mg over 1 hr × 3 days, repeat q4wk

Hypercalcemia (unlabeled)

Adult: IV INF 2 mg over 2 hr

Renal dose

Adult: PO CCr <30 ml/min, avoid use

Available forms: Tabs 2.5, 150 mg; sol for inj 3 mg/ml

Implementation

PO route

• Give early AM with a glass of water; if qmo, give on same day of each month

• Store at room temperature

Direct IV route

• Use single-dose prefilled syringe; discard unused portion; give over 15-30 sec

• Store at room temperature

• Do not use if discolored or if sol contains particulates

ADVERSE EFFECTS

CNS: Fever, insomnia, dizziness, headache

CV: Hypertension, **atrial fibrillation**

EENT: Ocular pain/inflammation, uveitis

GI: Constipation, nausea, vomiting, diarrhea, dyspepsia

INTEG: Rash, inj site reaction

META: *Hypomagnesemia, hypophosphatemia, hypocalcemia,* hypercholesterolemia

MS: Bone pain, myalgia, osteonecrosis of the jaw

Pharmacokinetics

Absorption	Poor
Distribution	Taken up primarily by bones, 86%-99% protein binding
Metabolism	Unknown
Excretion	Primarily by kidneys
Half-life	5-60 hr

Pharmacodynamics

Onset	Unknown
Peak	0.5-2 hr
Duration	Up to 1 mo

INTERACTIONS

Individual drugs

Calcium, vitamin D, iron, aluminum, magnesium salts: decreased ibandronate effect, separate by 1 hr

CycloSPORINE, tacrolimus: possible increased neurotoxicity

Drug classifications

Aminoglycosides, NSAIDs, radiopaque contrast agents: possible increased neurotoxicity

Loop diuretics: increased hypocalcemia

Drug/food

• Do not take with food, calcium

Drug/lab test

Increased: cholesterol

Decreased: alk phos, magnesium, calcium, phosphate

NURSING CONSIDERATIONS
Assessment
• **Osteoporosis:** before and during treatment; monitor DEXA scan for bone mineral density, correct electrolyte imbalances (calcium, magnesium, phosphate) before starting therapy
• Assess for blood studies: electrolytes, Ca, P, Mg; creatinine/BUN
• Assess for atrial fibrillation
• **Assess dental health;** before dental extraction, give antiinfectives; **osteonecrosis of the jaw may occur**
• Assess for bone pain; use analgesics; may begin within 24 hr, or even years after treatment, pain usually subsides after treatment is discontinued

Patient/family education
• **Teach patient to report hypercalcemic relapse:** nausea, vomiting, bone pain, thirst; unusual muscle twitching, muscle spasms, severe diarrhea, constipation
• Advise patient to continue with dietary recommendations, including calcium and vit D
• Instruct patient to obtain an analgesic from provider for bone pain
• Advise patient that if nausea/vomiting occur, small, frequent meals may help
• Teach patient to report vision symptoms: blurred vision, edema, inflammation; report to prescriber
• Teach to report if pregnancy is planned or suspected or if planning to breastfeed, pregnancy (C)
• Encourage to exercise regularly, to stop smoking, and decrease alcohol
• Advise to take in AM at least 60 min before other meds, food, beverages, to take monthly dose on same day
• Teach to sit upright ≥60 min after PO dose

Evaluation
Positive therapeutic outcome
• Increased bone mineral density

ibritumomab (Rx)
(ee-brit-u-moe'mab)
Zevalin
Func. class.: Radiopharmaceutical
Pregnancy category D

ACTION: High affinity for indium-111, yttrium-90; induces CD20⁺ B-cell lines

Therapeutic outcome: Decrease in tumor size, spread of malignancy

USES: Non-Hodgkin's lymphoma, B-cell NHL

CONTRAINDICATIONS:
Pregnancy **D**, hypersensitivity to murine proteins, prior murine antibody exposure

> **BLACK BOX WARNING:** Hypersensitivity to this agent, neutropenia, thrombocytopenia

Precautions: Breastfeeding, children, geriatric, cardiac conditions, immunizations after therapy

> **BLACK BOX WARNING:** Altered biodistribution, infusion-related reaction

DOSAGE AND ROUTES
Adult:
Step 1: IV RiTUXimab 250 mg/m² given first; premedicate with acetaminophen 650 mg and diphenhydrAMINE 50 mg
Adult (baseline platelets ≥150,000/mm³)
Step 2: 7-9 days after step 1, give a second dose of riTUXimab 250 mg/m² IV; within 4 hr of completing the riTUXimab infusion, give Y-90 ibritumomab tiuxetan 0.4 mCi/kg (14.8 MBq/kg) **IV** over 10 min; the dose given should be within 10% of the actual prescribed dose of Y-90 ibritumomab tiuxetan, the total dose given max 32 mCi (1184 MBq) regardless of the patient's weight
Adult (baseline platelets 100,000-149,000/mm³)
Step 2: 7-9 days after step 1, give a second dose of riTUXimab 250 mg/m² IV; within 4 hr of completing the riTUXimab infusion, give Y-90 ibritumomab tiuxetan 0.3 mCi/kg (11.1 MBq/kg) **IV** over 10 min; the dose given should be within 10% of the actual prescribed dose of Y-90 ibritumomab tiuxetan; the total dose given max 32 mCi (1184 MBq) regardless of the patient's weight
Adult (baseline platelets <100,000/mm³)
Do not use

Available forms: Inj 3.2 mg/2 ml

Implementation
• Do not use as BOL or **IV** direct
• Provide increased fluid intake to 2-3 L/day to prevent dehydration, unless contraindicated
• Keep emergency equipment nearby with EPINEPHrine, antihistamines, corticosteroids

IV infusion route
• See manufacturer's product labeling for preparation

⚠ Nurse Alert   ✦ Key NCLEX® Drug

ADVERSE EFFECTS
CV: Cardiac dysrhythmias
GI: *Nausea, vomiting, anorexia,* abdominal pain, diarrhea
GU: Renal failure
HEMA: Leukopenia, neutropenia, thrombocytopenia, anemia
INTEG: *Irritation at site, rash,* fatal mucocutaneous infections (rare)
OTHER: Fever, chills, asthenia, headache, angioedema, hypotension, myalgia, bronchospasm, hemorrhage, infections, cough, dyspnea, dizziness, anxiety
SYST: Stevens-Johnson syndrome, secondary malignancies (AML, MDS), fatal infections

Pharmacokinetics

Absorption	Unknown
Distribution	Unknown
Metabolism	Unknown
Excretion	Unknown
Half-life	30 hr

Pharmacodynamics

Unknown

NURSING CONSIDERATIONS
Assessment
• Assess for infection, murine antibody titers

> **BLACK BOX WARNING: Assess for signs of fatal infusion reaction:** hypoxia, pulmonary infiltrates, ARDS, MI, ventricular fibrillation, cardiogenic shock; most fatal infusion reactions occur with first infusion; potentially fatal

• Assess biodistribution: first image 2-24 hr, second image 48-72 hr, third image 90-120 hr (optimal)
• **Assess for signs of severe mucocutaneous reactions:** Stevens-Johnson syndrome, lichenoid dermatitis, toxic epidermal lysis; occur 1-13 wk after product was given
⚠ Assess for tumor lysis syndrome: acute renal failure requiring hemodialysis, hyperkalemia, hypocalcemia, hyperuricemia, hyperphosphatemia

> **BLACK BOX WARNING: Bone marrow depression:** Monitor CBC, differential, platelet count weekly; withhold product if WBC is <3500/mm^3 or platelet count <150,000/mm^3; notify prescriber of these results

• Monitor GI symptoms: frequency of stools
• Assess for signs of dehydration: rapid respirations, poor skin turgor, decreased urine output, dry skin, restlessness, weakness

Patient/family education
• Teach patient radiation safety precautions, disposal of body fluids
• Teach patient symptoms of infection
• Teach patient decreased blood count precautions
• Advise patient to report adverse reactions
• Advise patient to use contraception during and for 12 mo after therapy, pregnancy **D**
• Teach patient neutropenia and bleeding precautions

Evaluation
Positive therapeutic outcome
• Improvement in blood counts
• Decreased evidence of disease

---

ibuprofen (OTC, Rx)
(eye-byoo-proe′fen)
Advil, Advil Children's, Advil Infant's Concentrated, Advil Junior Strength, Apo-Ibuprofen ✦, Caldolor, ElixSure IB, Genpril, Ibren, IBU, Infants Leader Ibu-drops, Midol Cramps and Body Aches Formula, Motrin ✦, Motrin IB, Motrin Infant's, Motrin Junior Strength, Pamprin IB ✦, Samson-8 Select Brand, Top Care Infant, Wal-Profen
ibuprofen lysine (Rx)
NeoProfen

ACTION: Inhibits COX-1, COX-2 by blocking arachidonate; analgesic, antiinflammatory, antipyretic

Therapeutic outcome: Decreased pain, inflammation, fever

USES: Rheumatoid arthritis, osteoarthritis, primary dysmenorrhea, dental pain, musculoskeletal disorders, fever, migraine, patent ductus arteriosus

CONTRAINDICATIONS:
Avoid IV after 30 wk of pregnancy (**D**), hypersensitivity to this product, NSAIDs, salicylates, asthma, severe renal/hepatic disease

---

> **BLACK BOX WARNING:** Perioperative pain in CABG

Precautions: Pregnancy (**C**) (1st and 2nd trimester), breastfeeding, children, geriatric, bleeding disorders, GI disorders, cardiac disorders, hypersensitivity to other antiinflammatory agents, CHF, CCr <25 ml/min

> **BLACK BOX WARNING:** GI bleeding, MI, stroke

DOSAGE AND ROUTES
Self-treatment of minor aches/pain
Adult/adolescent: PO (OTC product) 200 mg q4-6hr, may increase to 400 mg q4-6hr; max 1200 mg/day

Analgesia
Adult: PO 200-400 mg q4-6hr; max 3.2 g/day; OTC use max 1200 mg/day
Child: PO 4-10 mg/kg/dose q6-8hr

Moderate to severe pain (hospitalized patients) (Caldolor)
Adult: IV 400-800 mg q6hr as an adjunct to opiate agonist therapy

Dysmenorrhea
Adult: PO 400 mg q4hr; max 1200 mg/day

Antipyretic
Child 6 mo-12 yr: PO 5 mg/kg (temp <102.5° F or 39.2° C), 10 mg/kg (temp >102.5° F), may repeat q6-8hr; max 40 mg/kg/day

Antiinflammatory
Adult: PO 400-800 mg tid-qid; max 3.2 g/day
Child: PO 30-40 mg/kg/day in 3-4 divided doses; max 50 mg/kg/day

Patent ductus arteriosus (PDA) (Neoprofen)
Premature neonate ≤32 wk gestation who weighs 500-1500 g: IV 10 mg/kg initially, then if needed, 2 doses 5 mg/kg at 24 hr intervals; if oliguria occurs, hold dose

Available forms: Tabs 100, 200, 300, 400, 600, 800 mg; liqui-gel caps 200 mg; oral susp 100 mg/5 ml; liquid 100 mg/5 ml; chew tabs 50, 100 mg; drops 50 mg/1.25 ml; inj 10 mg/ml (NeoProfen); inj (Caldolor) 100 mg/ml

Implementation
PO route
• Administer to patient crushed or whole; 800-mg tab may be dissolved in water

• Give with food or milk to decrease gastric symptoms; give 2 hr before or 30 min after meals; absorption may be slowed
• Shake susp well before use
• Store at room temperature
• **Do not use in pregnancy after 30 wk gestation**

IV route
• Must be well hydrated prior to administration
• Dilute to ≤4 mg/ml (0.9% NaCl, LR, D$_5$); infuse over ≥30 min
• Discard unused portion
Intermittent IV infusion route
• Visually inspect for particulate
• Ibuprofen lysine: dilute with dextrose or saline to appropriate volume (10 mg/ml of ibuprofen is recommended) given within 30 min of preparation: give via port that is nearest insertion site; give over 15 min
• Check for extravasation; do not give in same line with TPN, interrupt TPN for 15 min before and after product administration

ADVERSE EFFECTS
CNS: *Headache,* dizziness, drowsiness, fatigue, tremors, confusion, insomnia, anxiety, depression
CV: Tachycardia, peripheral edema, palpitations, dysrhythmias, **CV thrombotic events, MI, stroke**
EENT: Tinnitus, hearing loss, blurred vision
GI: *Nausea, anorexia,* vomiting, diarrhea, jaundice, **hepatitis,** constipation, flatulence, cramps, dry mouth, peptic ulcer, **GI bleeding, ulceration, necrotizing enterocolitis, GI perforation**
GU: **Nephrotoxicity,** dysuria, hematuria, oliguria, azotemia
HEMA: **Blood dyscrasias,** increased bleeding time
INTEG: Purpura, rash, pruritus, sweating, urticaria, **necrotizing fasciitis,** photosensitivity, photophobia
META: Hyperkalemia, hyperuricemia, hypoglycemia, hyponatremia
SYST: **Anaphylaxis, Stevens-Johnson syndrome**

Pharmacokinetics

Absorption	Well absorbed
Distribution	Not known; crosses placenta
Metabolism	Liver, extensively
Excretion	Kidneys, unchanged (10%)
Half-life	1.8-2 hr

Pharmacodynamics

Onset	½ hr
Peak	1-2 hr
Duration	4-6 hr

INTERACTIONS
Individual drugs
Alcohol, aspirin: increased GI reactions

Aspirin: decreased ibuprofen action

CycloSPORINE, lithium, methotrexate: increased toxicity

Furosemide: decreased effect of furosemide

Radiation: increased risk of blood dyscrasias

Valproic acid, warfarin: increased risk of bleeding

Drug classifications
Anticoagulants, antiplatelet agents, salicylates, thrombolytics: increased risk of bleeding

Anticoagulants (oral): increased toxicity

Antidiabetics (oral): increased hypoglycemia

Antihypertensives: decreased effect of antihypertensives

Antineoplastics: increased risk of blood dyscrasias

Corticosteroids, NSAIDs: increased GI reactions

Diuretics: decreased effectiveness of diuretics (thiazides)

Drug/herb
Feverfew, garlic, ginger, ginkgo, ginseng *(Panax):* increased risk of bleeding

Drug/lab test
Increased: BUN, creatinine, LFTs

Decreased: Hgb/Hct, blood glucose, WBC, platelets

NURSING CONSIDERATIONS
Assessment
• **Assess for infection;** may mask symptoms

• **Assess pain:** location, duration, type, intensity before dose, 1 hr after

• Assess musculoskeletal status: ROM before dose, 1 hr after

• Monitor liver function tests: AST, ALT, bilirubin, creatinine if patient is on long-term therapy, monitor electrolytes as needed

> **BLACK BOX WARNING:** Perioperative pain in CABG: MI and stroke can result for 10-14 days, can be fatal

• **Nephrotoxicity:** Monitor renal function tests: BUN, urine creatinine if patient is on long-term therapy

• Assess cardiac status: edema (peripheral), tachycardia, palpitations; monitor B/P, pulse for character, quality, rhythm

• Monitor blood studies: CBC, Hct, Hgb, protime if patient is on long-term therapy

• Check I&O ratio; decreasing output may indicate renal failure if patient is on long-term therapy

• Assess for history of peptic ulcer disorder; asthma, aspirin, hypersensitivity, check closely for hypersensitivity reactions

> **BLACK BOX WARNING:** GI bleeding/perforation: chronic use can cause gastritis with or without bleeding; in those with a prior history of peptic ulcer disease or GI bleeding, initiate treatment at lower dose; geriatrics are at greater risk, as are those who consume >3 alcohol drinks/day

• **Assess for allergic reactions:** rash, urticaria; if these occur, product may have to be discontinued

• Assess for vision changes: blurring, halos; may indicate corneal, retinal damage

• Identify prior product history; there are many product interactions

• Identify fever: length of time in evidence and related symptoms

Patient/family education
• Teach patient to use sunscreen, sunglasses, and protective clothing to prevent photosensitivity, photophobia

• Advise patient to read label on other OTC products

• Inform patient that the therapeutic response takes 1 mo (arthritis)

• Caution patient to avoid alcohol ingestion, salicylates, NSAIDs; GI bleeding may occur

• Advise patient with allergies that allergic reactions may develop

• Advise patient to use sunscreen to prevent photosensitivity

• Advise patient to report use of this product to all health care providers

• **Nephrotoxicity:** advise to report change in urinary pattern, weight increase, edema, increased pain in joints, fever, blood in urine; monitor fluid status, BUN, creatinine

⚠ **Pregnancy: notify prescriber if pregnancy (C) is planned or suspected; avoid during 3rd trimester; pregnancy (D) IV after 30 wk**

Evaluation
Positive therapeutic outcome
• Decreased pain
• Decreased inflammation

- Decreased fever
- Increased mobility

TREATMENT OF OVERDOSE:
Lavage, activated charcoal, induce diuresis

⚠ HIGH ALERT

ibutilide (Rx)
(eye-byoo′te-lide)
Corvert
Func. class.: Antidysrhythmic (Class III)
Chem. class.: Methane sulfonamide
Pregnancy category C

ACTION: Prolongs duration of action potential and effective refractory period

USES: For rapid conversion of atrial fibrillation/flutter occurring within 1 wk of coronary artery bypass or valve surgery

CONTRAINDICATIONS:
Hypersensitivity

Precautions: Pregnancy **C**, breastfeeding, children <18 yr; geriatric, sinus node dysfunction, 2nd- or 3rd-degree AV block, electrolyte imbalances, bradycardia, renal/hepatic disease, CHF

BLACK BOX WARNING: QT prolongation, torsades de pointes, ventricular arrhythmias, ventricular tachycardia, cardiac dysrhythmias

DOSAGE AND ROUTES
Atrial fibrillation/flutter
Adult: IV INF (≥60 kg) 1 vial (1 mg) given over 10 min, may repeat same dose in 10 min; IV INF (<60 kg) 0.01 mg/kg given over 10 min, may repeat same dose in 10 min

Available forms: Inj 1 mg/10 ml

Implementation
IV route
- Give reduced dosage slowly with ECG monitoring only
- Give undiluted or diluted in 50 ml of 0.9% NaCl or D₅W (0.017 mg/ml), give over 10 min
- Solution is stable for 48 hr refrigerated or 24 hr at room temperature
- Do not admix with other solution, products
- **Ice compress after stopping inf for extravasation; remove tubing and attempt to aspirate product, elevate affected areas**

- Stop infusion as soon as arrhythmia is stopped
- Do not use if discolored or if particulate is present

ADVERSE EFFECTS
CNS: *Headache*
CV: *Hypotension, bradycardia,* **sinus arrest, CHF, dysrhythmias,** hypertension, extrasystoles, ventricular tachycardia, bundle branch block, AV block, palpitations, supraventricular extrasystoles, syncope, **prolonged QT interval, torsades de pointes**
GI: Nausea

Pharmacokinetics

Absorption	Unknown
Distribution	Unknown
Metabolism	Liver
Excretion	Kidney
Half-life	6 hr

Pharmacodynamics
Unknown

INTERACTIONS
Individual drugs
Digoxin: masking of cardiotoxicity

Drug classifications
Antidepressants (tricyclics/tetracyclics): prodysrhythmia
Antihistamines, H₂-receptor antagonists, antidepressants, tetracyclines, tricyclics, phenothiazines: increased prodysrhythmia
Class Ia antidysrhythmics (disopyramide, quiNIDine, procainamide), class III agents (amiodarone, sotalol): do not use within 5 hr of ibutilide

Drug/herb
Do not use with hawthorn
Ginger: increased antiarrhythmic action

NURSING CONSIDERATIONS
Assessment

BLACK BOX WARNING: ECG continuously for >4 hr to determine product effectiveness; measure PR, QRS, QT intervals, check for PVCs, other dysrhythmias; discontinue if atrial fibrillation/flutter ceases; continue until QT interval corrected for heart rate (QTc) returns to baseline; if used ≥2 days, anticoagulation must be adequate

- Monitor I&O ratio; monitor electrolytes: potassium, sodium, chloride

---

- Monitor liver function tests: AST, ALT, bilirubin, alkaline phosphatase
- Monitor ECG continuously to determine product effectiveness; measure PR, QRS, QT intervals; check for PVCs, other dysrhythmias; monitor B/P continuously for hypo/hypertension; check for rebound hypertension after 1-2 hr; discontinue product when atrial fibrillation/flutter ceases
- Monitor for dehydration or hypovolemia
- Assess for CNS symptoms: confusion, psychosis, numbness, depression, involuntary movements; if these occur product should be discontinued
- Monitor cardiac rate, respiration; rate, rhythm, character, chest pain, ventricular tachycardia, supraventricular tachycardia or fibrillation

Patient/family education
- Instruct patient to report side effects immediately to prescriber

Evaluation
Positive therapeutic outcome
- Decrease in atrial fibrillation/flutter

---

icosapent
(eye-koe'sa-pent)
Vascepa
Func. class.: Antilipidemic
Chem. class.: Omega-3 fatty acid ethyl-ester
Pregnancy category C

ACTION: Inhibits hepatic very-low-density lipoprotein (VLDL) and triglyceride synthesis; enhances clearance of triglycerides from circulating VLDL particles

Therapeutic outcome: Decrease in triglycerides

USES: As adjunct to diet in adults with severe hypertriglyceridemia (500 mg/dl)

CONTRAINDICATIONS:
Hypersensitivity to icosapent ethyl

Precautions: Hepatic disease, bleeding, breastfeeding, children, fish/shellfish hypersensitivity, thrombolytic/anticoagulation therapy, pregnancy (C)

DOSAGE AND ROUTES
Adult: PO 2 g bid

Available forms: Soft gel cap 1 g

Implementation
- Give with food, swallow whole
- Store at room temperature

ADVERSE EFFECTS
HEMA: Ecchymosis, epistaxis
MS: Arthralgia

Pharmacokinetics
Absorption	Unknown
Distribution	Protein binding 99%
Metabolism	Unknown
Excretion	Unknown
Half-life	89 hr

Pharmacodynamics
Onset	Unknown
Peak	5 hr
Duration	Unknown

INTERACTIONS
Drug classifications
Anticoagulants, platelet inhibitors, thrombolytics: increased effects of these agents

Drug/lab test
Increased: bleeding time

NURSING CONSIDERATIONS
Assessment
- **Hypertriglyceridemia:** Obtain diet history including fat, cholesterol in diet; cholesterol, triglyceride levels periodically during treatment
- **Liver disease:** Monitor LFTs baseline, periodically in those with liver disease
- **Bleeding:** Monitor ecchymosis, epistaxis, bleeding time; use cautiously in anticoagulant/thrombolytic therapy
- **Fish/shellfish hypersensitivity:** Identify fish hypersensitivity, use cautiously

Patient/family education
- Teach patient that blood work may be necessary during treatment
- Advise patient to report bleeding if anticoagulants or thrombolytics are used
- Advise patient not to break, crush, open, or dissolve caps
- Inform patient that previously prescribed regimen will continue: low-cholesterol diet, exercise program, smoking cessation

Evaluation
Positive therapeutic outcome
- Decrease in triglycerides

⚠ HIGH ALERT

IDArubicin (Rx)

(eye-da-roo′bi-sin)

Idamycin PFS

Func. class.: Antineoplastic, antibiotic
Chem. class.: Anthracycline glycoside

Pregnancy category D

Do not confuse:
IDArubicin/DOXOrubicin/DAUNOrubicin/
epirubicin, **Idamycin**/Adriamycin

ACTION: Not cell cycle specific; topo-isomerase II inhibitor, a vesicant; intercalculat-ing between DNA base pairs, causing shape change, low free radicals

Therapeutic outcome: Prevention of rapidly growing malignant cells

USES: Used in combination with other antineoplastics for acute myelocytic leukemia in adults

Unlabeled uses: Breast cancer, liquid tumors

CONTRAINDICATIONS:

Pregnancy **D,** breastfeeding, hypersensitivity

> **BLACK BOX WARNING:** Myelosuppression, bilirubin >5 mg/dl

Precautions: Children, gout, bone marrow depression, preexisting CV disease

> **BLACK BOX WARNING:** Renal/hepatic disease, heart failure

DOSAGE AND ROUTES

Adult: **IV** 8-12 mg/m²/day × 3 days in combi-nation with cytarabine (induction)

Renal/hepatic dose

Adult: **IV** if bilirubin is 2.5-5 mg/dl, give 50% of dose; if bilirubin >5 mg/dl, do not use; if CCr >2.5 mg/dl, reduce dose

Available forms: Inj 1 mg/ml

Implementation

• Store at room temp for 3 days after reconsti-tuting or for 7 days refrigerated

IV route

• Avoid contact with skin; very irritating; wash completely to remove

• Administer antiemetic 30-60 min before giving product and prn to prevent vomiting; ad-minister antibiotics for prophylaxis of infection

Intermittent IV infusion route

• Product should be prepared by experienced personnel using proper precautions (biological cabinet, wearing gown, gloves, mask)

• Do not give IM/subcut

• Give after reconstituting 5-mg vial with 5 ml of 0.9% NaCl (1 mg/1 ml); give over 10-15 min through Y-tube or 3-way stopcock of inf of D_5 or 0.9% NaCl; discard unused portion

• Apply ice compress after stopping infusion (extravasation)

Y-site compatibilities: Amifostine, amikacin, aztreonam, cimetidine, cladribine, cyclophosphamide, cytarabine, diphenhy-drAMINE, droperidol, erythromycin, filgrastim, granisetron, imipenem/cilastatin, magnesium sulfate, mannitol, melphalan, metoclopromide, potassium chloride, ranitidine, sargramostim, thiotepa, vinorelbine

Y-site incompatibilities: Acyclovir, ampicillin/sulbactam, ceFAZolin, cefTAZidime, clindamycin, dexamethasone, etoposide, furosemide, gentamicin, hydrocortisone, LORaz-epam, meperidine, methotrexate, mezlocillin, sargramostim, sodium bicarbonate, vancomycin, vinCRIStine

ADVERSE EFFECTS

CNS: Fever, chills, headache, **seizures**
CV: **Dysrhythmias, CHF, pericarditis, myocarditis,** peripheral edema, angina, **MI, myocardial toxicity**
GI: Nausea, vomiting, abdominal pain, mucosi-tis, diarrhea, **hepatotoxicity**
GU: **Nephrotoxicity,** red urine
HEMA: **Thrombocytopenia, leukopenia, anemia**
INTEG: Rash, **extravasation,** dermatitis, reversible alopecia, urticaria, thrombophlebitis, tissue necrosis at inj site, radiation recall
SYST: **Infection,** tumor lysis syndrome

Pharmacokinetics

Absorption	Complete bioavailability
Distribution	Rapidly distributed, protein binding 97%
Metabolism	Liver, extensively
Excretion	Bile
Half-life	22 hr

Pharmacodynamics

Unknown

INTERACTIONS

Individual drugs

Cyclophosphamide: increased cardiotoxicity

Radiation: increased toxicity

Trastuzumab: increased CHF, ventricular
dysfunction

Drug classifications

Anticoagulants, salicylates, NSAIDs, thrombolytics: increased bleeding risk, avoid concurrent
use

Antineoplastics: increased toxicity

**Class IA/III, some phenothiazines, other
products that increase QT prolongation:
increased ECG changes (QT prolongation,
changes in QRS voltage)**

Corticosteroids: decreased IDArubicin effect

Live virus vaccines: decreased antibody response

Drug/lab test

Increased: uric acid, phosphate, potassium

Decreased: calcium, platelets, neutrophils

NURSING CONSIDERATIONS

Assessment

• **Assess for tumor lysis syndrome:** hyperkalemia, hyperphosphatemia, hyperuricemia,
hypocalcemia

• **Assess symptoms indicating severe allergic reaction:** rash, pruritus, urticaria, purpuric
skin lesions, itching, flushing; product should be
discontinued

• Assess for tachypnea, dyspnea, edema, fatigue

> **BLACK BOX WARNING: Assess for cardiac
> toxicity:** CHF, dysrhythmias, cardiomyopathy;
> cardiac studies should be done before and
> periodically during treatment; ECG, chest x-ray,
> MUGA

> **BLACK BOX WARNING:** Monitor CBC,
> differential, platelet count weekly; severe
> myelosuppression can occur

• Monitor renal function studies: BUN, uric
acid, urine CCr, electrolytes, before, during
therapy

• Monitor temp (may indicate beginning of
infection)

> **BLACK BOX WARNING:** Monitor liver function
> tests before, during therapy (bilirubin, AST,
> ALT, LDH) as needed or monthly; note jaundice
> of skin and sclera, dark urine, clay-colored
> stools, itchy skin, abdominal pain, fever, diar-
> rhea; hepatotoxicity can be severe

• Assess for bleeding: hematuria, stool guaiac,
bruising or petechiae, mucosa or orifices, assess
for inflammation of mucosa, breaks in skin

• Identify effects of alopecia on body image;
discuss feelings about body changes

> **BLACK BOX WARNING:** Assess for local irrita-
> tion, pain, burning at injection site, extravasa-
> tion, a vesicant

Patient/family education

• Teach patient to avoid use of products containing aspirin or ibuprofen, razors, commercial
mouthwash, since bleeding may occur; to report
symptoms of bleeding (hematuria, tarry stools)

• Instruct patient to report signs of anemia (fatigue, headache, irritability, faintness, shortness
of breath)

• Advise patient that hair may be lost during
treatment; a wig or hairpiece may make patient
feel better; new hair may be different in color,
texture

• Teach patient to rinse mouth tid-qid with
water, club soda; brush teeth bid-qid with soft
brush or cotton-tipped applicators for stomatitis; use unwaxed dental floss

• Tell patient not to have any vaccinations
without the advice of the prescriber; serious
reactions can occur

⚠ **Teach patient to report if pregnancy is
planned or suspected, pregnancy (D)**

⚠ **Advise patient that contraception is
needed during treatment and for several mo
after the completion of therapy**

⚠ **Teach patient to report signs of CHF,
cardiac toxicity, beginning infection**

• Advise patient to avoid crowds, those with
upper respiratory illness

• Advise that all body fluids change color

Evaluation

Positive therapeutic outcome

• Prevention of rapid division of malignant cells

⚠ HIGH ALERT

ifosfamide (Rx)
(i-foss′fa-mide)
Ifex
Func. class.: Antineoplastic alkylating agent
Chem. class.: Nitrogen mustard
Pregnancy category D

Do not confuse:
ifosfamide/cyclophosphamide

ACTION: Alkylates DNA, RNA; inhibits enzymes that allow synthesis of amino acids in proteins; also responsible for cross-linking DNA strands; activity is not cell cycle stage specific

Therapeutic outcome: Prevention of rapidly growing malignant cells

USES: Testicular cancer

Unlabeled uses: Soft-tissue sarcoma, Ewing's sarcoma, non-Hodgkin's lymphoma, lung/pancreatic cancer, sarcoma, bladder, breast, cervical, thymic cancer, desmoid tumor, Ewing sarcoma, rhabdomyosarcoma

CONTRAINDICATIONS:
Pregnancy **D**, hypersensitivity

> **BLACK BOX WARNING:** Bone marrow suppression

Precautions: Renal/hepatic disease, breastfeeding, children, accidental exposure, dehydration, dental disease, infection, IM injection, ocular exposure, varicella

> **BLACK BOX WARNING:** Coma, hemorrhagic cystitis

DOSAGE AND ROUTES
Adult: **IV** 1.2-2 g/m²/day × 5 days; repeat course q3wk; give with mesna, epirubicin, ondansetron alpha

Renal dose
Adult: **IV** CCr 31-60 ml/min give 75% of dose; CCr 10-30 ml/min give 50% of dose; CCr <10 ml/min, do not give

Available forms: Inj 1, 3 g vials

Implementation
• Administer antiemetic 30-60 min before product to prevent vomiting

• Visually inspect parenteral products for particulate matter and discoloration prior to use
• Store powder at room temperature

IV route
• Give as an intermittent infusion or continuous infusion
• Well hydrate with at least 2 L/day of oral or IV fluids should be given to prevent bladder toxicity
• Must be given in combination with mesna to prevent hemorrhagic cystitis
• Close hematologic monitoring is recommended. WBC count, platelet count, and hemoglobin should be obtained prior to each use and periodically thereafter
• A urinalysis should be performed prior to each dose to monitor for hematuria

Reconstitution and further dilution
• Reconstitute 1 or 3 g with 20 or 60 ml, respectively, of sterile water for injection or bacteriostatic water for injection containing parabens or benzyl alcohol to give IV solutions containing 50 mg/ml
• Solutions may be diluted further to achieve concentrations of 0.6-20 mg/ml in the following solutions: 5% dextrose for injection, 0.9% sodium chloride for injection, lactated Ringer's injection, or sterile water for injection
• Infuse slowly over at least 30 min
• Diluted and reconstituted solutions refrigerated and used within 24 hours

Y-site compatibilities: Allopurinol, amifostine, aztreonam, filgrastim, fludarabine, gallium, granisetron, melphalan, ondansetron, PACLitaxel, piperacillin/tazobactam, propofol, sargramostim, teniposide, thiotepa, vinorelbine

Additive compatibilities: CARBOplatin, CISplatin, etoposide, fluorouracil, mesna

ADVERSE EFFECTS
CNS: Facial paresthesia, fever, malaise, somnolence, confusion, depression, hallucinations, dizziness, disorientation, **seizures, coma,** cranial nerve dysfunction, **encephalopathy**
GI: Nausea, vomiting, anorexia, **hepatotoxicity,** stomatitis, constipation, diarrhea, dyslipidemia, hyperglycemia
GU: **Hematuria, nephrotoxicity, hemorrhagic cystitis,** dysuria, urinary frequency, retrograde ejaculation
HEMA: **Thrombocytopenia, leukopenia, anemia**
INTEG: Dermatitis, alopecia, pain at inj site, hyperpigmentation
META: Metabolic acidosis

Pharmacokinetics

Absorption	Complete bioavailability
Distribution	Saturation at high dosages
Metabolism	Liver
Excretion	Breast milk
Half-life	15 hr, depends on dose

Pharmacodynamics

Unknown

INTERACTIONS
Individual drugs
Allopurinol: increased toxicity
Radiation: increased bone marrow suppression

Drug classifications
Anticoagulants, NSAIDs, salicylates, thrombolytics: increased bleeding risk
Antineoplastics: increased bone marrow suppression
CYP3A4 inducers, barbiturates: increased toxicity
CYP3A4 inhibitors: decreased ifosfamide effect
Live virus vaccines: decreased antibody response
Do not use within 24 hr of hematopoietic progenitor cells

NURSING CONSIDERATIONS
Assessment
⚠ Monitor CBC, differential, platelet count weekly; withhold product if WBC is <2000 or platelet count is <50,000; notify prescriber of results if WBC <10,000/mm³, platelets <100,000/mm³, severe myelosuppression
• Monitor renal function studies: BUN, serum uric acid, urine CCr before, during therapy; I&O ratio; report fall in urine output of 30 ml/hr
• Monitor for cold, fever, sore throat (may indicate beginning of infection); identify edema in feet and joints, stomach pain, shaking; prescriber should be notified
• Assess for bleeding: hematuria, guaiac, bruising or petechiae, mucosa or orifices; no rect temp

BLACK BOX WARNING: I&O ratio; monitor for hematuria; hemorrhagic cystitis can occur; increase fluids to 3 L/day; urinalysis prior to each dose; do not give at night

• Monitor liver function tests before, during therapy (ALT, AST, LDH); jaundice of skin, sclera, dark urine, clay-colored stools, itching, abdominal pain, fever, diarrhea that may indicate liver involvement

Patient/family education
• Teach patient to avoid use of products containing aspirin or NSAIDs, razors, commercial mouthwash, since bleeding may occur; to report symptoms of bleeding (hematuria, tarry stools)
• Instruct patient to report signs of anemia (fatigue, headache, irritability, faintness, shortness of breath)
• Advise patient to report any changes in breathing or coughing even several mo after treatment; to avoid crowds and persons with respiratory tract or other infections
• Teach patient that hair loss is common; discuss the use of wigs or hairpieces; that hair may be a different texture when regrowth occurs
• Caution patient not to have any vaccinations without the advice of the prescriber; serious reactions can occur
• Teach patient to notify prescriber if pregnancy is planned or suspected, pregnancy (D)
• Advise patient that contraception is needed during treatment and for several mo after completion of therapy
• Advise patient to report confusion, hallucinations, extreme drowsiness, numbness, tingling; avoid use of alcohol for ≥4 months after treatment
• Teach patient to avoid driving, hazardous activities until reaction is known
• Instruct patient to drink extra fluids in order to urinate often to prevent hemorrhagic cystitis

Evaluation
Positive therapeutic outcome
• Prevention of rapid division of malignant cells
• Absence of swelling at night
• Increased appetite, increased weight

iloperidone (Rx)
(ill-o-pehr′ih-dohn)
Fanapt
Func. class.: Antipsychotic
Chem. class.: Benzisoxazole derivative
Pregnancy category C

ACTION: Unknown; may be mediated through both dopamine type 2 (D₂) and serotonin type 2 (5-HT₂) antagonism; high receptor binding affinity for norepinephrine (alpha 1)

Therapeutic outcome: Decreased signs/symptoms of schizophrenia

USES: Schizophrenia
Unlabeled uses: Agitation

CONTRAINDICATIONS:
Breastfeeding, hypersensitivity

Precautions: Pregnancy **C**, children, geriatric patients, renal/hepatic disease, breast cancer, Parkinson's disease, dementia with Lewy bodies, seizure disorder, QT prolongation, bundle branch block, acute MI, ambient temperature increase, AV block, stroke, substance abuse, suicidal ideation, tardive dyskinesia, torsades de pointes, blood dyscrasias, dysphagia

> **BLACK BOX WARNING:** Increased mortality in elderly patients with dementia-related psychosis

DOSAGE AND ROUTES
Adult: PO 1 mg bid, day 1; 2 mg bid, day 2, 4 mg bid, day 3; 6 mg bid, day 4; 8 mg bid, day 5; 10 mg bid, day 6; 12 mg bid, day 7; max 24 mg/day in two divided doses; reduce dose by 50% in poor metabolizer of CYP2D6 or when used with strong CYP2D6/CYP3A4 inhibitors

Available forms: Tabs 1, 2, 4, 6, 8, 10, 12 mg; titration pack

Implementation
- Give reduced dose in geriatric patients
- Give anticholinergic agent on order from prescriber, to be used for EPS
- Avoid use with CNS depressants
- Provide decreased stimulus by dimming lights, avoiding loud noises
- Provide supervised ambulation until patient is stabilized on medication; do not involve in strenuous exercise program because fainting is possible; patient should not stand still for a long time
- Give increased fluids to prevent constipation
- Provide sips of water, candy, gum for dry mouth
- Store in tight, light-resistant container (PO); store unopened vials in refrigerator; protect from light; do not freeze

ADVERSE EFFECTS
CNS: *EPS, pseudoparkinsonism, akathisia, dystonia, tardive dyskinesia; drowsiness,* **seizures, neuroleptic malignant syndrome,** dizziness, delirium, depression, paranoia, fatigue, hostility, lethargy, restlessness, vertigo, tremor, drowsiness
CV: Orthostatic hypotension, **heart failure, AV block, QT prolongation,** tachycardia
EENT: Blurred vision, cataracts, nystagmus, tinnitus

GI: *Nausea,* vomiting, *anorexia, constipation,* jaundice, weight gain/loss, abdominal pain, stomatitis, xerostomia
GU: Hyperprolactinemia, urinary retention/incontinence, testicular pain, **renal failure**
MISC: Renal artery occlusion
HEMA: Agranulocytosis, leukopenia, neutropenia

Pharmacokinetics
Absorption	Unknown
Distribution	Unknown
Metabolism	Extensively, liver (major metabolite) CYP2D6, CYP3A4
Excretion	Urine
Half-life	Terminal 18 hr extensive metabolizers; 33 hr poor metabolizers

Pharmacodynamics
Onset	Unknown
Peak	2-4 hr
Duration	Unknown

INTERACTIONS
Individual drugs
Alcohol: increased sedation
Chloroquine, clarithromycin, droperidol, erythromycin, haloperidol, methadone, pentamidine: increased QT prolongation

Drug classifications
CYP2D6, CYP3A4 inducers (carBAMazepine, barbiturates, phenytoins, rifampin): decreased iloperidone action
CYP2D6, CYP3A4 inhibitors (delavirdine, indinavir, itraconazole, dalfopristin, ritonavir, tipranavir): increased iloperidone effect, decreased clearance, reduce dose
Class IA/ III antidysrhythmics, some phenothiazines, β-agonists, local anesthetics, tricyclics: increased QT prolongation
Other CNS depressants: increased sedation
SSRIs, SNRIs, serotonin-agonists: increased serotonin syndrome, neuroleptic malignant syndrome

Drug/lab test
Increased: prolactin levels, cholesterol, glucose, lipids, triglycerides
Decreased: potassium

NURSING CONSIDERATIONS
Assessment
- Assess mental status before initial administration

- Monitor I&O ratio; palpate bladder if urinary output is low
- Monitor bilirubin, CBC, hepatic studies qmo
- Monitor glucose, hyperglycemia may occur
- Monitor urinalysis before, during prolonged therapy, monitor potassium, magnesium and lipid panel
- Assess affect, orientation, LOC, reflexes, gait, coordination, sleep pattern disturbances
- Monitor B/P standing and lying; also pulse, respirations; take these q4hr during initial treatment; establish baseline before starting treatment; report drops of 30 mm Hg; watch for ECG changes; QT prolongation may occur
- Assess for dizziness, faintness, palpitations, tachycardia on rising
- **Assess for EPS,** including akathisia, tardive dyskinesia (bizarre movements of the jaw, mouth, tongue, extremities), pseudoparkinsonism (rigidity, tremors, pill rolling, shuffling gait)

> **BLACK BOX WARNING:** Assess for serious reactions in the geriatric patient: fatal pneumonia, heart failure, sudden death, not to be used in the elderly with dementia

- **Assess for neuroleptic malignant syndrome:** hyperthermia, increased CPK, altered mental status, muscle rigidity
- Assess for constipation, urinary retention daily; if these occur, increase bulk and water in diet
- Monitor weight gain, hyperglycemia, metabolic changes in diabetes

Patient/family education
- Teach that orthostatic hypotension may occur and to rise from sitting or lying position gradually
- Advise to avoid hot tubs, hot showers, tub baths; hypotension may occur
- Teach to avoid abrupt withdrawal of this product; EPS may result; product should be withdrawn slowly; to review symptoms of neuroleptic malignant syndrome
- Teach to avoid OTC preparations (cough, hay fever, cold) unless approved by prescriber; serious product interactions may occur; avoid use of alcohol; increased drowsiness may occur
- Advise to avoid hazardous activities if drowsy or dizzy
- Teach compliance with product regimen
- Teach to report impaired vision, tremors, muscle twitching
- Teach that heat stroke may occur in hot weather; take extra precautions to stay cool
- Advise to use contraception; inform prescriber if pregnancy is planned or suspected

Evaluation
Positive therapeutic outcome
- Decrease in emotional excitement, hallucinations, delusions, paranoia; reorganization of patterns of thought, speech

TREATMENT OF OVERDOSE:
Lavage if orally ingested; provide airway; *do not induce vomiting*

---

imatinib (Rx)
(im-ah-tin′ib)
Gleevec
Func. class.: Antineoplastic—miscellaneous
Chem. class.: Protein-tyrosine kinase inhibitor
Pregnancy category D

ACTION: Inhibits Bcr-Abl tyrosine kinase created in chronic myeloid leukemia (CML), also inhibits tyrosine kinases including EGF, FGF, PDGF, SCF, VEGF, NGF

Therapeutic outcome: Decreased tumor size, prevention of spread of cancer

USES: Treatment of chronic myeloid leukemia (CML), Philadelphia chromosome positive in blast cell crisis or chronic failure after treatment failure with interferon alfa; gastrointestinal stromal tumors (GIST), positive for C-KIT; chronic eosinophilic leukemia, acute lymphocytic leukemia, dermatofibrosarcoma protuberans, myelodysplastic syndrome, systemic mastocytosis

CONTRAINDICATIONS:
Pregnancy **D,** hypersensitivity

Precautions: Breastfeeding, children, geriatric, cardiac/renal/hepatic/dental disease, GI bleeding, bone marrow suppression, infection, thrombocytopenia, neutropenia, immunosuppression

DOSAGE AND ROUTES
Treatment of Philadelphia chromosome positive (Ph+) chronic myelogenous leukemia (CML) chronic phase as initial therapy
Adult: PO 400 mg/day, continue as long as is beneficial; may increase to 600 mg/day in the absence of severe adverse reactions and severe non-leukemia–related neutropenia or thrombocytopenia

---

Adverse effects: *italics* = common; **bold** = life-threatening

Adolescent/child >2 yr: PO 340 mg/m²/day, max 600 mg/day; daily dose may be given as a single dose or split into 2 doses given once in the morning and once in the evening

Adult patients with Ph+ CML in chronic phase after failure of interferon-alfa therapy
Adult: PO 400 mg/day; continue as long as is beneficial; may increase to 600 mg/day

Pediatric patients with Ph+ CML in chronic phase whose disease has recurred after hematopoietic stem cell transplant or who are resistant to interferon-alfa therapy
Adolescent/child >3 yr: PO 260 mg/m²/day; may be given as single daily dose or may be divided and given once in the morning and once in the evening; may increase to 340 mg/m²/day

Adult patients with Ph+ CML in accelerated phase or blast crisis
Adult: PO 600 mg/day, continue as long as is beneficial, may increase to 800 mg/day (400 mg bid)

Adult patients with resistant or relapsed Ph+ acute lymphocytic leukemia (ALL)
Adult: PO 600 mg/day, continue as long as is beneficial

Adult patients with *Kit* (CD117) positive unresectable and/or metastatic GIST
Adult: PO 400-600 mg/day, may increase to 400 mg bid

Adjuvant treatment of *Kit* (CD117) positive GIST after complete gross resection
Adult: PO 400 mg/day

Hypereosinophilic syndrome (HES) and/or chronic eosinophilic leukemia (CEL) who have the FIPL1L1-PDGFR alpha fusion kinase (mutational analysis or FISH demonstration of CHIC2 allele deletion) and for patients with HES and/or CEL who are FIPL1L1-PDGFR alpha fusion kinase negative or unknown
Adult: PO 400 mg/day in those who are FIPL1L-PDGFR alpha fusion kinase negative or unknown; for HES/CEL patients with demonstrated FIP1L1-PDGFR alpha fusion kinase, 100 mg/day, may increase to 400 mg

Myelodysplastic syndrome (MDS)/myeloproliferative disease (MPD) associated with the PDGFR (platelet-derived growth factor receptor) gene rearrangements
Adult: PO 400 mg/day

Aggressive systemic mastocytosis (ASM) without D816V c-Kit mutation or with c-Kit mutation status unknown
Adult: PO 400 mg/day in those without the FIP1L1-PDGFR alpha c-Kit mutation. If c-Kit status is unknown or not available, give 400 mg/day

Unresectable, recurrent, and/or metastatic dermatofibrosarcoma protuberans (DFSP)
Adult: PO 400 mg bid (800 mg/day)

Hepatic dose
Adult: PO total bilirubin 1.5-3 × ULN and any AST, decrease initial dose to 400 mg/day; total bilirubin >3 × ULN and any AST, decrease initial dose to 300 mg/day

Renal dose
Adult: PO CCr 40-59 ml/min, max 600 mg/day; CCr 20-39 ml/min decrease initial dose by 50%, max 400 mg/day; CCr <20 ml/min use with caution 100 mg/day

Available forms: Tabs 100, 400 mg

Implementation
PO route
• Give with meal and large glass of water to decrease GI symptoms, doses of 800 mg should be given 400 mg bid
• Tab may be dispersed in a glass of water or apple juice, use 50 ml of liquid for 100 mg tab, 200 ml/400 mg
• Store at 25° C (77° F)
• Continue as long as is beneficial

ADVERSE EFFECTS
CNS: **CNS hemorrhage,** headache, dizziness, insomnia, **subdural hematoma**
CV: **Hemorrhage, heart failure,** cardiac tamponade, hypereosinophilia, cardiac toxicity
EENT: Blurred vision, conjunctivitis
GI: *Nausea,* **hepatotoxicity,** *vomiting, dyspepsia,* **GI hemorrhage,** *anorexia,* abdominal pain, GI perforation, diarrhea
HEMA: **Neutropenia, thrombocytopenia, bleeding**
INTEG: *Rash, pruritus,* alopecia, photosensitivity

META: Edema, fluid retention, hypokalemia
MISC: Fatigue, epistaxis, pyrexia, night sweats, increased weight, flulike symptoms, hypothyroidism
MS: Cramps, pain, arthralgia, myalgia
RESP: Cough, dyspnea, nasopharyngitis, pneumonia, URI, pleural effusion, edema

Pharmacokinetics

Absorption	Well absorbed; bound to plasma protein (98%)
Distribution	Unknown
Metabolism	Liver (metabolites)
Excretion	Feces, primarily (metabolites)
Half-life	18-40 hr

Pharmacodynamics

Onset	Unknown
Peak	2-4 hr
Duration	24 hr (imatinib), 40 hr (metabolite)

INTERACTIONS
Individual drugs
Acetaminophen: increased hepatotoxicity
Simvastatin: increased plasma concentrations
Warfarin: increased plasma concentration of warfarin; avoid coadministration; use low-molecular-weight anticoagulants instead

Drug classifications
Calcium channel blockers, ergots: increased plasma concentrations
CYP3A4 inducers (carBAMazepine, dexamethasone, PHENobarbital, phenytoin, rifampin): decreased imatinib concentrations
CYP3A4 inhibitors (clarithromycin, erythromycin, ketoconazole, itraconazole): increased imatinib concentrations

Drug/herb
St. John's wort: decreased imatinib concentration

Drug/lab test
Increased: bilirubin, amylase, LFTs
Decreased: albumin, calcium, potassium, sodium, phosphate, platelets, neutrophils, leukocytes, lymphocytes

NURSING CONSIDERATIONS
Assessment
• **Bone marrow suppression:** Assess ANC and platelets; in chronic phase if ANC <1 × 10^9/L and/or platelets <50 × 10^9/L, stop until ANC >1.5 × 10^9/L and platelets >75 × 10^9/L; in accelerated phase/blast crisis if ANC <0.5 × 10^9/L and/or platelets <10 × 10^9/L, determine whether cytopenia is related to biopsy/aspirate; if not, reduce dose by 200 mg; if cytopenia continues, reduce dose by another 100 mg; if cytopenia continues for 4 wk, stop product until ANC ≥1 × 10^9/L

⚠ **Assess for hepatotoxicity:** monitor liver function tests before treatment, qmo if line transaminases are >5 × IULN, withhold imatinib until transaminase levels return to <2.5 × IULN

⚠ **Renal toxicity:** monitor bilirubin, if >3 × IULN, withhold imatinib until bilirubin levels return to <1.5 × IULN

• Assess GI symptoms: frequency of stools
• Assess signs of fluid retention, edema: weigh, monitor lung sounds, 50-ml fluid retention is dose dependent

⚠ **Monitor CBC for first month, biweekly next month, and periodically thereafter; neutropenia (2-3 wk), thrombocytopenia (3-4 wk) and anemia may occur, may need dosage decrease or discontinuation**

Patient/family education
• Instruct patient to report adverse reactions immediately: shortness of breath, swelling of extremities, bleeding
• Teach patient reason for treatment, expected result
• Instruct patient to eat a nutritious diet with iron, vit supplement, low fiber, few dairy products
• Teach patient not to stop or change dose; to avoid hazardous activities until response is known, dizziness may occur
• Teach patient to take with food and water; for those unable to swallow tabs, to mix in liquid (30 ml for 100 mg or 200 ml for 400 mg); after dissolved, stir and consume
• Advise patient to avoid OTC products unless approved by prescriber

⚠ **Teach patient to notify prescriber if pregnancy is planned or suspected, pregnancy (D), do not breastfeed**

Evaluation
Positive therapeutic outcome
• Decrease in leukemic cells, size of tumors

imipenem/cilastatin (Rx)

(i-me-pen'em sye-la-stat'in)
Primaxin IM, Primaxin IV
Func. class.: Antiinfective, miscellaneous penicillin
Chem. class.: Carbapenem
Pregnancy category C

Do not confuse:
imipenem/Omnipen, **Primaxin**/Premarin

ACTION: Interferes with cell wall replication of susceptible organisms; osmotically unstable cell wall swells and bursts from osmotic pressure; addition of cilastatin prevents renal inactivation that occurs with high urinary concentrations of imipenem

Therapeutic outcome: Bactericidal action against the following: *Streptococcus pneumoniae,* group A β-hemolytic streptococci, *Staphylococcus aureus,* enterococcus; gram-negative organisms: *Klebsiella, Proteus, Escherichia coli, Acinetobacter, Serratia, Pseudomonas aeruginosa; Salmonella, Shigella, Haemophilus influenzae, Listeria* spp.

USES: Serious infections caused by gram-positive or gram-negative organisms

CONTRAINDICATIONS:
Hypersensitivity, IM hypersensitivity to local anesthetics of the amide type, or carbapenems, AV block, shock (IM)

Precautions: Pregnancy **C,** breastfeeding, children, geriatric, hypersensitivity to cephalosporins, penicillins, seizure disorders, renal disease, head trauma, pseudomembranous colitis, ulcerative colitis, diabetes mellitus

DOSAGE AND ROUTES
Intraabdominal infections, gynecologic infections, lower respiratory tract infections, skin and skin structure infections, bone and joint infections, septicemia, endocarditis, febrile neutropenia (unlabeled), and polymicrobial infections for fully susceptible organisms including gram-positive/gram-negative aerobes and anaerobes
Adult ≥70 kg: IV 250 mg q6hr (mild infections); 500 mg q6-8hr (moderate infections); 500 mg q6hr (severe life-threatening infections)
Adult 60-<70 kg: IV 250 mg q8hr (mild infections); 250 mg q6hr (moderate or severe life-threatening infections)
Adult 50-<60 kg: IV 125 mg q6hr (mild infections) 250 mg q6hr (moderate or severe life-threatening infections)
Adult 40-<50 kg: IV 125 mg q6hr (mild infections); 250 mg q6-8hr (moderate infections); 250 mg q6hr (severe life-threatening infections)
Adult 30-<40 kg: IV 125 mg q8hr (mild infections); 125 mg q6hr or 250 mg q8hr (moderate infections); 250 mg q8hr (severe life-threatening infections)
Adolescent/child/infant ≥3 mo: IV 15-25 mg/kg q6hr
Infant 1-3 mo weighing ≥1500 g: IV 25 mg/kg q6hr
Neonate 1-4 wk weighing ≥1500 g: IV 25 mg/kg q8hr
Neonate <7 days weighing ≥1500 g: IV 25 mg/kg q12hr

Moderately susceptible organisms, primarily some strains of *P. aeruginosa*
Adult ≥70 kg: IV 500 mg q6hr (mild infections); 500 mg q6hr or 1 g q8hr (moderate infections); 1 g q6-8hr (life-threatening infections)
Adult 60-≤70 kg: IV 500 mg q8hr (mild infections); 500 mg q8hr or 750 mg q8hr (moderate infections); 0.75-1 g q8hr (life-threatening infections)
Adult 50-≤60 kg: IV 250 mg q6hr (mild infections); 250-500 mg q6hr (moderate infections); 500 mg q6hr or 750 mg q8hr (life-threatening infections)
Adult 40-≤50 kg: IV 250 mg q6hr (mild infections); 250 mg q6hr or 500 mg q8hr (moderate infections); 500 mg q6-8hr (life-threatening infections)
Adult 30-≤40 kg: IV 250 mg q8hr (mild infections); 250 mg q6-8hr; 250 mg q6hr or 500 mg q8hr (life-threatening infections)
Adolescent/child/infant >3 mo: IV 15-25 mg/kg q6hr
Infant 1-3 mo weighing ≥1500 g: IV 25 mg/kg q6hr
Neonate 1-4 wk weighing ≥1500 g: IV 25 mg/kg q8hr
Neonate <7 days weighing ≥1500 g: IV 25 mg/kg q12hr

Mild to moderate lower respiratory tract, skin and skin structure, or gynecologic infections
Adult/adolescent/child ≥12 yr: IM 500 or 750 mg q12hr, max 1.5 g/day

Mild to moderate intraabdominal infections, including acute gangrenous or perforated appendicitis and appendicitis with peritonitis

Adult/adolescent/child ≥12 yr: IM 750 mg q12hr, max 1.5 g/day

Community-acquired pneumonia (CAP) in ICU patients with risk factors for *Pseudomonas* infection

Imipenem; cilastatin in combination with ciprofloxacin or an aminoglycoside plus a respiratory fluoroquinolone or an advanced macrolide

Adult ≥70 kg: IV 500 mg q6-8hr
Adult 60-≤70 kg: IV 250 mg q6hr
Adult 50-≤60 kg: IV 250 mg q6hr
Adult 40-≤50 kg: IV 250 mg q6-8hr
Adult 30-≤40 kg: IV 125 mg q6hr or 250 mg q8hr

Empiric treatment of aspiration pneumonia

Adult: IV 500-1000 mg q6hr × 10 days

Renal dose

Adult ≥70 kg (reduce normal dose of 1 g/day to): IV CCr 41-70 ml/min 250 mg q8hr; CCr 6-40 ml/min 250 mg q12hr; **(reduce normal dose of 1.5 g/day to):** CCr 41-70 ml/min 250 mg q6hr; CCr 21-40 ml/min 250 mg q8hr; CCr 6-20 ml/min 250 mg q12hr; **(reduce normal dose of 2 g/day to):** CCr 41-70 ml/min 500 mg q8hr; CCr 21-40 ml/min 250 mg q6hr; CCr 6-20 250 mg q12hr

Available forms: Powder for sol inj 250, 500; powder for susp 500 mg

Implementation
IM route
- Reconstitute 500 mg/2 ml lidocaine without epiNEPHrine; shake well, withdraw and administer entire vial; give inj deep in large muscle mass, aspirate, product for IM is not for IV use

Intermittent IV infusion route
- Reconstitute each 250 or 500 mg/10 ml of compatible diluent; shake well; transfer the resulting susp to ≥100 ml of compatible diluent; add 10 ml to each previously reconstituted vial and shake to ensure all medication is used; transfer the remaining contents of the vial to the inf container; do not administer susp by direct inj
- Give each 250- or 500-mg dose over 20-30 min, and each 1-g dose over 40-60 min; administer over 15-20 min for pediatric patients; do not administer direct **IV**; do not admix with other antibiotics

Y-site compatibilities: Acyclovir, alfentanil, amifostine, amikacin, aminocaproic acid, andulafungin, argatroban, ascorbic acid, atenolol, atracurium, atropine, benztropine, bivalirudin, bleomycin, bumetanide, buprenorphine, butorphanol, CARBOplatin, carmustine, caspofungin, cefamandole, ceFAZolin, cefoperazone, cefotaxime, cefoTEtan, cefOXitin, cefTAZidime, ceftizone, cefuroxime, chloramphenicol, cimetidine, CISplatin, clindamycin, codeine, cyanocobalamin, cyclophosphamide, cycloSPORINE, cytarabine, DACTINomycin, dexamethasone, dexrazoxane, digoxin, diltiazem, diphenhydrAMINE, DOCEtaxel, dolasetron, DOPamine, doxacurium, DOXOrubicin, DOXOrubicin liposomal, doxycycline, enalaprilat, famotidine, fludarabine, foscarnet, granisetron, IDArubicin, regular insulin, melphalan, methotrexate, ondansetron, propofol, tacrolimus, teniposide, thiotepa, vinorelbine, zidovudine

Y-site incompatibilities: Fluconazole, meperidine, sargramostim

ADVERSE EFFECTS
CNS: Fever, somnolence, **seizures,** confusion, dizziness, weakness, myoclonus, drowsiness
CV: Hypotension, palpitations, tachycardia
GI: *Diarrhea, nausea, vomiting,* **pseudomembranous colitis, hepatitis,** glossitis, gastroenteritis, abdominal pain, jaundice
GU: Renal toxicity/failure
HEMA: **Agranulocytosis, eosinophilia, neutropenia,** decreased Hgb, Hct
INTEG: Rash, urticaria, pruritus, pain at inj site, phlebitis, erythema at inj site, erythema multiforme
MISC: Hearing loss, tinnitus, electrolyte abnormalities
RESP: Chest discomfort, dyspnea, hyperventilation
SYST: **Anaphylaxis, Stevens-Johnson syndrome, toxic epidermal necrolysis, angioedema**

Pharmacokinetics

Absorption	Complete bioavailability (IV)
Distribution	Widely distributed; crosses placenta
Metabolism	Liver
Excretion	Kidneys, unchanged (70%-80%); breast milk
Half-life	1 hr; increased in renal disease

Adverse effects: *italics* = common; **bold** = life-threatening

Pharmacodynamics

	IM	IV
Onset	Unknown	Rapid
Peak	Unknown	20 min-1 hr

INTERACTIONS
Individual drugs
Aminophylline, cycloSPORINE, ganciclovir, theophylline: increased risk of seizures
Probenecid: increased imipenem plasma levels
Valproic acid: decreased effect of valproic acid

Drug classifications
β-Lactam antibiotics: increased antagonistic effect

Drug/lab test
Increased: AST, ALT, LDH, BUN, alkaline phosphatase, bilirubin, creatinine, potassium, chloride
Decreased: sodium
False positive: direct Coombs' test

NURSING CONSIDERATIONS
Assessment
• Assess patient for previous penicillin sensitivity reaction or sensitivity to other β-lactams, may have sensitivity to this product
• **Assess patient for signs and symptoms of infection,** including characteristics of wounds, sputum, urine, stool, WBC >10,000/mm³, fever; obtain baseline information before, during treatment
• Complete C&S tests before beginning product therapy to identify if correct treatment has been initiated
• **Assess for allergic reactions, anaphylaxis:** rash, urticaria, pruritus, chills, wheezing, laryngeal edema, fever, joint pain; angioedema may occur a few days after therapy begins; epiNEPHrine, resuscitation equipment should be available for anaphylactic reaction
• Identify urine output; if decreasing, notify prescriber (may indicate nephrotoxicity); also check for increased BUN, creatinine, electrolytes
• Monitor blood studies: AST, ALT, CBC, Hct, bilirubin, LDH, alkaline phosphatase, Coombs' test monthly if patient is on long-term therapy
• Monitor electrolytes: potassium, sodium, chloride monthly if patient is on long-term therapy
• Assess bowel pattern daily; if severe diarrhea occurs, product should be discontinued; may indicate pseudomembranous colitis
• **Monitor for bleeding:** ecchymosis, bleeding gums, hematuria, stool guaiac daily if patient is on long-term therapy

• Assess for overgrowth of infection: perineal itching, fever, malaise, redness, pain, swelling, drainage, rash, diarrhea, change in cough, sputum

Patient/family education
• Advise patient to report sore throat, bruising, bleeding, joint pain; may indicate blood dyscrasias (rare)
• Advise patient to contact prescriber if vaginal itching, loose foul-smelling stools, furry tongue occur; may indicate superinfection
• Advise patient to notify prescriber of diarrhea with blood or pus; may indicate pseudomembranous colitis
⚠ Instruct patient to report seizures immediately

Evaluation
Positive therapeutic outcome
• Absence of signs/symptoms of infection (WBC <10,000/mm³, temp WNL, absence of red, draining wounds)
• Reported improvement in symptoms of infection

TREATMENT OF ANAPHYLAXIS: EPINEPHrine, antihistamines, resuscitate if needed

imipramine (Rx)
(im-ip′ra-meen)
Tofranil, Tofranil PM
Func. class.: Antidepressant, tricyclic
Chem. class.: Dibenzazepine, tertiary amine
Pregnancy category D

Do not confuse:
imipramine/desipramine

ACTION: Blocks reuptake of norepinephrine and serotonin into nerve endings, increasing action of norepinephrine and serotonin in nerve cells; has anticholinergic effects

Therapeutic outcome: Decreased symptoms of depression after 2-3 wk; decreased bedwetting in children

USES: Depression, enuresis in children

Unlabeled uses: Chronic pain, migraine headaches, cluster headaches as adjunct, incontinence

---

⚠ Nurse Alert   ✴ Key NCLEX® Drug

CONTRAINDICATIONS:
Pregnancy **D**, hypersensitivity to this product or carBAMazepine; acute MI

Precautions: Suicidal patients, severe depression, increased intraocular pressure, closed-angle glaucoma, urinary retention, cardiac/hepatic disease, hyperthyroidism, electroshock therapy, elective surgery, breastfeeding, geriatric, seizure disorders, prostatic hypertrophy, MI, hypersensitivity to tricyclics, AV block, bundle-branch block, ileus, QT prolongation

BLACK BOX WARNING: Children other than for enuresis; suicidal ideation

DOSAGE AND ROUTES
Depression
Adult: PO 75-100 mg/day in divided doses; may increase by 25-50 mg up to 200 mg, 200 mg/day (outpatients), 300 mg/day (inpatients); may give daily dose at bedtime
Geriatric: PO 25-50 mg at bedtime, may increase to 100 mg/day in divided doses
Child ≥6 yr (unlabeled): PO 1.5 mg/kg/day in divided doses; max 2.5 mg/kg/day

Enuresis
Child 6-12 yr: PO 10-25 mg at bedtime, max 50 mg

Available forms: Tabs 10, 25, 50 mg; caps 75, 100, 125, 150 mg

Implementation
PO route
• Do not break, crush, or chew caps
• Give with food or milk
• Store in tight container at room temp; do not freeze

ADVERSE EFFECTS
CNS: *Dizziness, drowsiness,* confusion, headache, anxiety, tremors, stimulation, weakness, insomnia, nightmares, EPS (geriatric), increased psychiatric symptoms, paresthesia, **seizures,** ataxia
CV: *Orthostatic hypotension, ECG changes, tachycardia,* hypertension, palpitations, **dysrhythmias**
EENT: Blurred vision, tinnitus, mydriasis
ENDO: Hyperglycemia, hypothyroidism/hyperthyroidism, goiter, SIADH
GI: *Diarrhea, dry mouth,* nausea, vomiting, **paralytic ileus,** increased appetite, cramps, epigastric distress, jaundice, **hepatitis,** stomatitis, constipation, taste change, weight gain

GU: *Retention,* **acute renal failure,** impotence, decreased libido
HEMA: **Agranulocytosis, thrombocytopenia, eosinophilia, leukopenia**
INTEG: Rash, urticaria, sweating, pruritus, photosensitivity, hyperpigmentation (rare)

Pharmacokinetics
Absorption	Well absorbed
Distribution	Widely distributed; crosses placenta
Metabolism	Liver, extensively
Excretion	Kidneys, breast milk
Half-life	6-20 hr

Pharmacodynamics
	PO
Onset	1 hr
Peak	Unknown
Duration	Unknown

INTERACTIONS
Individual drugs
Alcohol: increased effects
CloNIDine: hyperpyretic crisis, seizures, hypertensive episode
CloNIDine, guanethidine: decreased effects
Gatifloxacin, levofloxacin, moxifloxacin, ziprasidone: increased QT interval

Drug classifications
MAOIs: hyperpyretic crisis, hypertensive episode, seizures
SSRIs, SNRIs, serotonin-receptor agonists: increased serotonin syndrome, increased neuroleptic malignant syndrome; avoid concurrent use
Sympathomimetics (direct acting [EPINEPHrine]), barbiturates, benzodiazepines, CNS depressants: increased effects
Sympathomimetics (indirect acting [ePHEDrine]): decreased effects
Tricyclic antidepressants, class IA/III antidysrhythmics: increased QT interval

Drug/herb
St. John's wort: serotonin syndrome

Drug/lab test
Increased: serum bilirubin, blood glucose, alkaline phosphatase, LFTs
Decreased: VMA, 5-HIAA, urinary catecholamines

NURSING CONSIDERATIONS
Assessment
• Monitor B/P (with patient lying, standing), pulse q4hr; if systolic B/P drops 20 mm Hg, hold product, notify prescriber; take vital signs q4hr in patients with CV disease
• Monitor blood studies: CBC, leukocytes, differential, cardiac enzymes if patient is receiving long-term therapy
• Monitor hepatic studies: AST, ALT, bilirubin
• Check weight weekly; appetite may increase with product
• **QT prolongation:** Assess ECG for flattening of T wave, bundle branch block, AV block, dysrhythmias in cardiac patients
• Assess for EPS primarily in geriatric: rigidity, dystonia, akathisia
• Assess mental status: mood, sensorium, affect, suicidal tendencies; increase in psychiatric symptoms: depression, panic
• Monitor urinary retention, constipation; constipation is more likely to occur in children or geriatric
⚠ **Assess for withdrawal symptoms: headache, nausea, vomiting, muscle pain, weakness, diarrhea, insomnia, restlessness; do not usually occur unless product was discontinued abruptly**
• Identify alcohol consumption; if alcohol is consumed, hold dose until AM

Patient/family education
• Teach patient that therapeutic effects may take 2-3 wk
• Teach patient to use caution in driving and other activities requiring alertness because of drowsiness, dizziness, blurred vision; to avoid rising quickly from sitting position, especially geriatric; orthostatic hypotension may occur
• Teach patient to avoid alcohol ingestion, other CNS depressants during treatment
• Teach patient not to discontinue medication quickly after long-term use: may cause nausea, headache, malaise
• Teach patient to wear sunscreen or large hat, since photosensitivity occurs
• Teach patient to increase fluids, bulk in diet if constipation, urinary retention occur, especially geriatric
• Teach patient to take gum, hard sugarless candy, frequent sips of water for dry mouth

Evaluation
Positive therapeutic outcome
• Decreased depression
• Absence of suicidal thoughts

• Decreased enuresis in children
• Decreased pain

TREATMENT OF OVERDOSE:
ECG monitoring, lavage, activated charcoal, administer anticonvulsant

---

immune globulin IM (IMIg, IgIM) (Rx)
Bay Gam 15%, Flebogamma 5%, Flebogamma DIF 5%, Gamunex 10%, Privigen 10%, Vivaglobin 10%

immune globulin IV (IGIV, IVIG) (Rx)
Bay Gam 15%, Carimune DF, Flebogamma 5%, Flebogamma 10% DIF, Gammaked, Gammaplex, Gammar-P IV, Gammagard S/D, Gamunex, Iveegram EN, Polygam S/D, Privigen, Vivaglobin

immune globulin SC (SCIG, IGSC) (Rx)
Bay Gam 15%, Flebogamma 5%, Flebogamma DIF 5%, Gammagard Liquid 10%, Gammaked, Gammaplex, Gamunex 10%, Hizentra, Privigen 10%, Vivaglobin

Func. class.: Immune serum
Chem. class.: IgG
Pregnancy category C

Do not confuse:
Iveegam/Invega

ACTION: Provides passive immunity to hepatitis A, measles, varicella, rubella, immune globulin deficiency; contains γ-globulin antibodies (IgG)

Therapeutic outcome: Absence of infection

USES: Immunodeficiency syndrome, B-cell chronic lymphocytic leukemia, Kawasaki's syndrome, bone marrow transplantation, pediatric HIV infection, agammaglobulinemia, hepatitis A, B exposure, measles exposure, measles vaccine complications, purpura, rubella exposure, chickenpox exposure, chronic inflammatory demyelinating polyneuropathy, multifocal motor neuropathy

Unlabeled uses: IV posttransfusion purpura, Guillain-Barré syndrome

---

CONTRAINDICATIONS:

Coagulopathy, hemophilia, IgA deficiency, thrombocytopenia

Precautions: Pregnancy **C**, breastfeeding, children, agammaglobulinemia, bleeding, hypogammaglobulinemia, infection, IV, viral infection

DOSAGE AND ROUTES

Immune globulin IM (IMIg, IgIM)

Hepatitis A prophylaxis

Adult, geriatric, adolescent, child, infant (unlabeled): IM 0.02 ml/kg for those who have not received Hepatitis A vaccine and have been exposed in the last 2 wk

Measles prophylaxis (exposed in last 6 days)

Adult: IM 0.25 ml/kg (immunocompetent)
Child (unlabeled): IM 0.5 ml/kg as a single dose, max 15 ml (immunocompromised)

Varicella prophylaxis

Adult: IM 0.6-1.2 ml/kg as soon as possible and if varicella-zoster immune globulin is not available

Rubella prophylaxis in exposed/ susceptible who will not consider a therapeutic abortion

Adult: Pregnant women IM 0.55 ml/kg

Immunoglobulin deficiency

Adult: 1.32 ml/kg, then 0.66 ml/kg (at least 100 mg/kg) q3-4wk

Immune globulin IV (IVIG, IGIV)

Primary immunodeficiency
Gammagard S/D

Adult/adolescent/child: IV 300-600 mg/kg q3-4wk

Polygam S/D

Adult/adolescent/child: IV 100 mg/kg qmo; initially 200-400 mg/kg may be used

Gammar-P IV

Adult: IV 200-400 mg/kg q3-4wk
Adolescent/child: IV 200 mg/kg q3-4wk

Gamunex

Adult/adolescent/child: IV INF 300-600 mg/ kg (3-6 ml/kg) q3-4wk; initial infusion rate 1 mg/kg/min (max 8 mg/kg/min)

Iveegam EN

Adult/adolescent/child: IV 200 mg/kg qmo; max 800 mg/kg qmo

Panglobulin NF/Carimune NF

Adult/adolescent/child: IV 200 mg/kg qmo

Gammagard Liquid/Flebogamma 5%

Adult/adolescent/child: IV 300-600 mg/kg q3-4wk

Privigen

Adult/adolescent/child ≥3 yr: IV 200-800 mg q3-4wk

Idiopathic thrombocytopenic purpura (ITP)
Panglobulin NF/Carimune NF

Adult/child: IV 400 mg/kg qd × 2-5 days; in acute ITP of childhood, only 2 of the 5 days are needed if initial platelets are 30,000-50,000 mcl after 2 doses

Gammagard S/D/Polygam S/D

Adult/adolescent/child: IV 1000 mg/kg as a single dose; may give on alternate days for up to 3 doses

Gamunex

Adult/adolescent/child: IV INF total dose of 2000 mg/kg, divided as 1000 mg/kg (10 ml/ kg) given on 2 consecutive days; initial rate is 1 mg/kg/min (max 8 mg/kg/min), if after 1st dose adequate platelets are observed after 24 hr, may withhold 2nd dose

Privigen

Adult/adolescent ≥15 yr: 1 g/kg/day × 2 days

Kawasaki disease
Iveegam EN

Child: IV 400 mg/kg qd × 4 consecutive days or a single dose of 2000 mg/kg over 10 hr; give with aspirin 100 mg/kg/day through 14th day of illness, then 3-5 mg/kg each day thereafter for 5 wk

Gammagard S/D/Polygam S/D

Infant/child: IV 1000 mg/kg (single dose) or 400 mg/kg/day × 4 days beginning within 7 days of fever onset, with aspirin 80-100 mg/kg/ day × 4 divided doses

Immune globulin SC (SCIG/IgSC)

Adult/child >2 yr: SC infusion 100-200 mg/ kg qwk; **Vivaglobin** brand of SGIG 160 mg IgG/ ml, SC inj; max 15 ml for injection, given at max of 20 ml/hr

Hizentra

Adult/child: 1.53 × previous IGIV dose in g divided by number of wk between IGIV dose; multiply dose in g × 5 for dose in ml, adjust by 1.3 trough before last IGIV treatment, give by subcut infusion qwk

Available forms: IM (Bay Gam) inj 2, 10 ml vial; **IV** (Gamimune N) 5%, 10% sol; powder for inj (Carimune NF) 1-, 3-, 6-, 12-g vials; (Gammagard S/D) 50 mg protein/ml in 2.5-, 5-, 10-g vials; (Gammar-P IV) 1-, 2.5-, 5-, 10-g vials; (Iveegam) 500 mg, 1-, 2.5-, 5-g vials; (Panglobulin) 6-, 12-g vials; (Polygam S/D) 2.5-, 5-, 10-g vials; sol for inj (Gamunex) 1-, 2.5-, 5-, 10-, 20-g vials; human sol for inj: Flebogamma 5%, 10% DIF; subcut inj 10%, 16%, 20% single use

Implementation
IM route
• Give IM (IGIM) inj in deltoid or anterolateral thigh in adults or anterolateral thigh in young children; if large amounts are given, several injections may be needed
• Do not give the IM preparation **IV**, SUBCUT, or intradermally
• Sol should be transparent and clear or slightly colored
• Store at 36°-46° F (2°-8° C)

IV route
• Warm to room temperature before administration (diluent, powder for inj)
• A transfer device is provided by manufacturer; this product should not be agitated or shaken
• Do not give the **IV** preparation SUBCUT, IM, or intradermally
• Check for adverse reaction during inf; stop inf if adverse reactions occur

Y-site compatibilities: Fluconazole, sargramostim

Gamimune N: Dilute **IV** with D$_5$; give 0.01 ml/kg/min; may increase to 0.02-0.04 ml/kg/min if no adverse reactions occur; may increase to 0.08 ml/kg/hr; sol should be refrigerated; do not freeze

Gammagard S/D: Reconstitute with sterile water for inj (50 mg protein/ml); give within 2 hr of reconstitution; give 0.5 ml/kg/hr; may increase to 4 ml/kg/hr if no adverse reactions occur; use inf set provided

Gammar-P IV: Give 0.01 ml/kg/min (50 mg/ml sol) over 15-30 min; may increase to 0.02 ml/kg/min; if adverse reactions are not present, may increase to 0.03-0.06 ml/kg/min; do not freeze; store at room temperature

Iveegam (5%): Give 1-2 ml/min; refrigerate, do not freeze

ADVERSE EFFECTS
CNS: Headache, fatigue, malaise
GI: Abdominal pain
HEMA: Thromboembolism (Vivaglobin)
INTEG: Pain at inj site, rash, pruritus, chills
MS: Arthralgia, chest pain
SYST: Lymphadenopathy, **anaphylaxis**

Pharmacokinetics

Absorption	Well absorbed (IM); completely absorbed (**IV**)
Distribution	Rapidly
Metabolism	Liver, catabolism
Excretion	Kidneys
Half-life	3-4 wk

Pharmacodynamics

	IM	IV
Onset	Unknown	Rapid
Peak	Unknown	Unknown
Duration	Unknown	Unknown

INTERACTIONS
Drug classifications
Live virus vaccines: do not give within 3 mo

Drug/lab test
Interference: glucose testing system

NURSING CONSIDERATIONS
Assessment
• Assess for exposure date: this product should be given within 6 days of measles, 1 wk of hepatitis B, 14 days of hepatitis A; if the date of exposure is outside these limits, immune globulin will not be effective
• Monitor blood studies in leukemia, idiopathic thrombocytopenic purpura: WBCs (leukemia), platelets
• Identify the number of inj of this product patient has received; multiple inj may lead to sensitization (diaphoresis, fever, chills, malaise)
• Assess for anaphylaxis in patient receiving **IV** immune globulin: diaphoresis, flushing, nausea, vomiting, wheezing, difficulty breathing, hypotension, chest tightness, fever, weakness, sneezing, abdominal pain; VS should be monitored during inf and 1 hr after beginning inf; emergency equipment should be available with epinephrine and antihistamines to treat anaphylaxis

Patient/family education
• Advise patient that passive immunity is temporary; explain reason for and expected results of this product
• Advise patient that pain and tenderness may occur at inj site

Evaluation
Positive therapeutic outcome
- Prevention of infection
- Increased platelets

TREATMENT OF ANAPHY-
LAXIS: EPINEPHrine, diphenhydrAMINE, O_2, vasopressors, corticosteroids

indacaterol
(in-da-kat′er-ol)
Arcapta Neohaler
Func. class.: β₂-agonist, long-acting
Pregnancy category C

ACTION: An agonist at β₂-receptors. These receptors are present in large numbers in the lungs and are located on bronchiolar smooth muscle. Stimulation of β₂-receptors in the lung causes relaxation of bronchial smooth muscle, which produces bronchodilation and an increase in bronchial airflow. These effects may be mediated, in part, by increased activity of adenyl cyclase, an intracellular enzyme responsible for the formation of cyclic-3′,5′-adenosine monophosphate (cAMP); has >24 times greater agonist activity at β₂-receptors (primarily in the lung) than at β₁-receptors (primarily in the heart)

USES: Bronchitis, chronic obstructive pulmonary disease (COPD), emphysema

CONTRAINDICATIONS:
Acute bronchospasm, acute asthma attack, status asthmaticus, acute respiratory insufficiency, monotherapy of asthma

Precautions: Cardiac arrhythmias, congenital long QT syndrome, diabetes mellitus, hypertension, hyperthyroidism (thyrotoxicosis, thyroid disease), hypokalemia, ischemic cardiac disease (coronary artery disease), milk protein hypersensitivity, pheochromocytoma, QT prolongation, seizure disorder, severe hepatic disease, tachycardia, torsades de pointes history, unusual responsiveness to other sympathomimetic amines; not indicated for neonates, infants, children, or adolescents under the age of 18 years, pregnancy C, breastfeeding

> **BLACK BOX WARNING:** Asthma-related deaths

DOSAGE AND ROUTES
Adult: INH 75 mcg (contents of 1 capsule) inhaled once daily; administer at the same time every day, max 1 dose in 24 hours

Available forms:
Powder for inhalation: 75 mcg

Implementation
Inhalation route
- For oral inhalation use only; *not* to swallow the capsules; always use the Neohaler inhaler; this inhaler should not be used with any other products; do *not* use with a spacer
- To administer, use dry hands to remove a capsule from the blister pack immediately before use and place into the capsule chamber of the Neohaler inhaler; click the inhaler closed; do not place capsule into the mouthpiece; then, holding upright, depress buttons fully one time to pierce capsule; a click will be heard; have patient breathe out fully away from inhaler; place inhaler in the mouth with lips closed around the mouthpiece and buttons positioned to the left and right (not up and down), then breathe deeply, rapidly, steadily in through the inhaler. A whirring sound should be heard; if no sound is heard, check the chamber—capsule may be stuck. Gently tap the base of the device to loosen capsule if necessary. After inhalation, the patient should hold breath as long as comfortable while removing inhaler from the mouth; check the chamber to see if any powder remains in the capsule; repeat inhalation steps until no powder remains. Most patients can empty the capsule in one or two inhalations. After administration, open the chamber and discard the empty capsule
- The gelatin capsule might break into very small pieces, which can pass through the inhaler screen and reach the mouth. Accidental inhalation or ingestion of these pieces is harmless; piercing the capsule more than once increases the risk of shattering capsule; do not wash inhaler; keep it dry. A clean, dry, lint-free cloth may be used to wipe out the inhaler
- Use the new inhaler provided with each new prescription
- To avoid the spread of infection, do not share the inhaler

ADVERSE EFFECTS
CNS: Headache, tremor
CV: **Sinus tachycardia,** hypertension, **QT prolongation and ST-T wave changes, prolonged QTc (an increase of >60 ms from baseline), nonsustained ventricular tachy-**

cardia, supraventricular tachycardia (SVT) episodes, intermittent ectopic atrial rhythm
ENDO: Hyperglycemia
GI: Nausea, dry mouth (xerostomia)
META: Hypokalemia
MS: Muscle cramps/spasm, musculoskeletal pain
RESP: Paradoxical bronchospasm, cough, dyspnea, sputum purulence or volume, wheezing, nasopharyngitis, pneumonia, sinusitis and upper respiratory tract infection

Pharmacokinetics

Absorption	Unknown
Distribution	Steady state 12-15 days protein binding 94%-96%
Metabolism	By CYP3A4, CYP1A1, CYP2D6, UTG1A1
Excretion	Renal 2%-6%, fecally >90%
Half-life	Terminal 45.5-126 hrs

Pharmacodynamics

Onset	5 min
Peak	15 min
Duration	Unknown

INTERACTIONS

Individual drugs

Amoxapine, some antipsychotics (phenothiazines, pimozide, haloperidol risperidone, sertindole ziprasidone), arsenic trioxide, astemizole, bepridil, cisapride, citalopram, chloroquine, clarithromycin, dasatinib, dolasetron, dronedarone, droperidol, erythromycin, flecainide, halofantrine, levomethadyl, maprotiline, methadone, ondansetron, paliperidone, palonosetron, pentamidine, probucol, propafenone, some quinolones (ofloxacin, gatifloxacin, gemifloxacin, grepafloxacin, levofloxacin, moxifloxacin, sparfloxacin), ranolazine, sunitinib, terfenadine, thioridazine, troleandomycin, vorinostat, tetrabenazine: increased QT prolongation

Aminophylline, theophylline: increased hypokalemia

Furazolidone, procarbazine, rasagiline: increased cardiovascular reactions

Drug classifications

Class IA/III antiarrhythmics, halogenated anesthetics, tricyclic antidepressants: increased QT prolongation

Corticosteroids: increased hypokalemia
MAOIs: increased cardiovascular reactions

NURSING CONSIDERATIONS

Assessment

> **BLACK BOX WARNING:** Asthma-related death; not to be used in asthma

• **COPD, emphysema, bronchospasm:** Monitor pulmonary function tests
⚠ **QT prolongation: Monitor ECG, ejection fraction for QT prolongation**
• **Paradoxical bronchospasm: If paradoxical bronchospasm occurs, discontinue this medication immediately, use a short-acting beta-agonist for rescue therapy, as appropriate**

Patient/Family Education

• Teach patient/family to report dyspnea, wheezing, bronchospasm
• Teach patient/family not to use with other products unless approved by prescriber; there are many interactions

> **BLACK BOX WARNING:** Not to use for asthma

indapamide (Rx)

(in-dap'a-mide)
Lozide ✦
Func. class.: Diuretic, thiazide-like, antihypertensive
Chem. class.: Thiazide-like sulfonamide derivative
Pregnancy category D

ACTION: Acts on proximal section of distal renal tubule by inhibiting reabsorption of sodium, may act by direct vasodilatation caused by blocking of calcium channels

Therapeutic outcome: Decreased B/P; decreased edema in lung tissues, peripherally

USES: Edema of CHF, hypertension, diuresis

CONTRAINDICATIONS: Hypersensitivity to this product or sulfonamides, anuria, hepatic coma

Precautions: Breastfeeding, hypokalemia, severe renal disease, hepatic disease, ascites, dehydration, CCr <30 ml/min (not effective), diabetes mellitus, gout, pregnancy (**B**), cardiac dysrhythmias

DOSAGE AND ROUTES
Edema
Adult: PO 2.5 mg/day in AM; may be increased to 5 mg/day if needed after 1 wk

Antihypertensive
Adult: PO 1.25-5 mg/day; may increase to 5 mg/day over 8 wk

Available forms: Tabs 1.25, 2.5 mg

Implementation
- Give in AM to avoid interference with sleep
- Provide potassium replacement if potassium level is <3.0 mg/dl; give whole
- Give with food and milk if nausea occurs, absorption may be increased

ADVERSE EFFECTS
CNS: Depression, *headache, dizziness, fatigue, weakness, nervousness, agitation,* extremity numbness
CV: Orthostatic hypotension, palpitations, volume depletion, PVCs, dysrhythmias, vaculitis
EENT: Blurred vision, nasal congestion, increased intraocular pressure
ELECT: *Hypokalemia, hypercalcemia, hyponatremia, hypochloremic alkalosis, hypomagnesemia,* hyperuricemia, hyperglycemia
GI: *Nausea,* vomiting, anorexia, constipation, diarrhea, cramps, abdominal pain, dry mouth, hypercholesterolemia
GU: *Frequency, polyuria, nocturia,* impotence
HEMA: **Agranulocytosis,** anemia
INTEG: Rash, *pruritus,* **Stevens-Johnson syndrome**
MS: Cramps

Pharmacokinetics
Absorption	Well absorbed
Distribution	Widely distributed
Metabolism	Liver, 7%
Excretion	Unchanged (urine)
Half-life	14-18 hr

Pharmacodynamics
Onset	1-2 hr
Peak	2 hr
Duration	Up to 36 hr

INTERACTIONS
Individual drugs
Amphotericin B: decreased potassium
Cholestyramine, colestipol: decreased absorption
Diazoxide: hyperglycemia
Digoxin, lithium: increased toxicity
Indomethacin: decreased hypotensive effect

Drug classifications
Anticoagulants, antidiabetics, antigout agents: decreased effects
Diuretics (other), steroids: decreased potassium
Muscle relaxants, steroids: increased toxicity
NSAIDs: decreased hypotensive effects

Drug/food
Licorice: increased severe hypokalemia

Drug/herb
Hawthorn: increased antihypertensive effect

Drug/lab test
Increased: calcium, parathyroid test, glucose, uric acid

NURSING CONSIDERATIONS
Assessment
- Check for rashes, temp elevation daily
- Monitor patients that receive cardiac glycosides for increased hypokalemia, toxicity
- Monitor for hypokalemia: acidic or reduced urine, osmolality, nocturia; hypotension, broad T-wave, U-wave, ectopy, tachycardia, weak pulse; muscle weakness, altered LOC, drowsiness, apathy, lethargy, confusion, depression; anorexia, nausea, cramps, constipation, distention, paralytic ileus; hypoventilation, respiratory muscle weakness
- Monitor for hypomagnesemia: agitation, muscle twitching, paresthesias, hyperactive reflexes, positive Babinski reflex, dysphagia, nystagmus, seizures, tetany; nausea, vomiting, diarrhea, anorexia, abdominal distention; ectopy, tachycardia, broad, flat- or inverted T-waves, depressed ST segment, prolonged QT interval, decreased cardiac output, hypotension
- Monitor for hyponatremia: increased B/P, cold, clammy skin, hypo/hypervolemia; anorexia, nausea, vomiting, diarrhea, abdominal cramps; lethargy, increased ICP, confusion, headache, seizures, coma, fatigue, tremors, hyperreflexia
- Monitor for manifestations of hyperchloremia: weakness, lethargy, coma, deep rapid breathing
- Assess fluid volume status: I&O ratios and record, weight, distended red veins, crackles in lung, color, quality and specific gravity of urine, skin turgor, adequacy of pulses, moist mucous membranes, bilateral lung sounds, peripheral pitting edema; dehydration symptoms of decreasing output, thirst, hypotension, dry mouth and mucous membranes should be reported

- Monitor electrolytes: potassium, sodium, calcium, magnesium; also include BUN, blood pH, ABGs, uric acid, CBC, blood glucose
- Assess B/P before, during therapy with patient lying, standing, and sitting as appropriate; orthostatic hypotension can occur rapidly

Patient/family education
- Teach patient to take the medication early in the day to prevent nocturia, to avoid alcohol
- Instruct the patient to take with food or milk if GI symptoms of nausea and anorexia occur
- Teach patient to maintain weekly record of weight and notify prescriber of weight loss >5 lb
- Caution the patient that this product causes a loss of potassium, so food rich in potassium should be added to the diet; refer to a dietitian for assistance in planning
- Caution the patient to rise slowly from sitting or reclining positions, not to exercise in hot weather or stand for prolonged periods, since orthostatic hypotension will be enhanced; lie down if dizziness occurs
- Teach patient not to use alcohol or any OTC medications without prescriber's approval; serious product reactions may occur
- Emphasize the need to contact prescriber immediately if muscle cramps, weakness, nausea, dizziness, or numbness occur
- Teach patient to take own B/P and pulse and record findings
- Instruct patient to continue taking medication even if feeling better; this product controls symptoms but does not cure the condition
- Advise the patient with hypertension to continue other medical treatment (exercise, weight loss, relaxation techniques, cessation of smoking)
- Do not stop product abruptly

Evaluation
Positive therapeutic outcome
- Decreased edema
- Decreased B/P
- Increased diuresis

TREATMENT OF OVERDOSE:
Lavage, monitor electrolytes, administer **IV** fluids, monitor hydration, CV, renal status

indinavir (Rx)
(en-den´a-veer)
Crixivan
Func. class.: Antiretroviral
Chem. class.: Protease inhibitor
Pregnancy category C

Do not confuse:
indinavir/Denavir

ACTION: Inhibits HIV-1 protease; this prevents maturation of the infectious virus

Therapeutic outcome: Decreased signs/symptoms of HIV-1 infection

USES: HIV-1 in combination with at least 2 other antiretrovirals

Unlabeled uses: Prevention of HIV-1 after exposure

CONTRAINDICATIONS:
Hypersensitivity, breastfeeding

Precautions: Pregnancy **C,** children, renal/hepatic disease, history of renal stones, diabetes, hypercholesterolemia, hemophilia, autoimmune disease, immune reconstitution syndrome

DOSAGE AND ROUTES
Adult: PO 800 mg q8hr; 400 mg bid with ritonavir 400 mg bid; or 800 mg bid with ritonavir 100-200 mg bid; decrease dose to 600 mg bid when given with lopinavir, ritonavir

Hepatic dose
Adult: PO 600 mg q8hr

Available forms: Caps 200, 400 mg

Implementation
- Do not break, crush, or chew caps
- Give with water 1 hr before or 2 hr after meals; may be given with other liquids or small meal; do not give with high-fat, high-protein meals
- Give in equal intervals around the clock
- Dosage adjustment will need to be considered when given with efavirenz
- Give water to 1.5 L/day minimum, to prevent nephrolithiasis

ADVERSE EFFECTS
CNS: *Headache, insomnia,* dizziness, somnolence
GI: *Diarrhea, abdominal pain, nausea, vomiting,* anorexia, dry mouth
GU: Nephrolithiasis

INTEG: Rash
MISC: Asthenia, **insulin-resistant hyperglycemia,** hyperlipidemia, **ketoacidosis,** lipodystrophy
MS: Pain

Pharmacokinetics

Absorption	Unknown
Distribution	Unknown
Metabolism	60% protein binding; liver
Excretion	<20% unchanged, urine; 83% feces
Half-life	Terminal 2 hr

Pharmacodynamics

Unknown

INTERACTIONS

Individual drugs

Amiodarone, alfuzosin, pimozide: life-threatening dysrhythmias
Clarithromycin, zidovudine: increased levels of both products
Isoniazid: increased isoniazid level
Midazolam, rifampin, triazolam: increased life-threatening dysrhythmias

Drug classifications

Anticonvulsants: decreased effect of both products
CYP3A4 inducers (barbiturates, carBAMazepine, efavirenz, fluconazole, modafinil, nevirapine, nonnucleoside reverse transcriptase inhibitors, phenytoin, rifamycins): decreased indinavir levels
CYP3A4 inhibitors (aprepitant, azole antifungals, delavirdine, itraconazole, ketoconazole, nefazodone, protease inhibitors, verapamil); phosphotriesterases: increased indinavir levels
CYP3A4 substrates (azole antifungals, benzodiazepines, calcium channel blockers, immunosuppressants, macrolides, sildenafil, SSRIs, statins, tadalafil, vardenafil): decreased effect of these substrates
Ergots: increased life-threatening dysrhythmias
Oral contraceptives: increased levels of oral contraceptives
Statins (atorvastatin, lovastatin, simvastatin): increased myopathy

Drug/herb

St. John's wort: decreased indinavir level, avoid use

Drug/food

High fat, high protein, grapefruit juice: decreased absorption

Drug/lab test

Increased: AST, ALT, amylase, total bilirubin

NURSING CONSIDERATIONS

Assessment

• Assess for lower back, flank pain: indicates kidney stones
• Monitor signs of infection, anemia
• Monitor liver studies: ALT, AST; total bilirubin, amylase; all may be elevated
• Determine the presence of other STDs
• Assess bowel pattern before, during treatment; if severe abdominal pain with bleeding occurs, product should be discontinued; monitor hydration
• Assess skin eruptions: rash, urticaria, itching
• Assess allergies before treatment, reaction to each medication; place allergies on chart
• Monitor viral load CD4 during treatment

Patient/family education

• Advise to take as prescribed; if dose is missed, take as soon as remembered up to 1 hr before next dose; do not double dose
• Advise that product must be taken in equal intervals around the clock to maintain blood levels for duration of therapy
• Instruct patient to increase fluids to prevent kidney stones; if stone formation occurs, treatment may need to be interrupted
• Inform patient that product does not cure AIDS, controls symptoms only; not to donate blood
• Advise patient that hyperglycemia may occur; watch for symptoms (thirst, hunger, dry, itchy skin); notify prescriber

Evaluation

Positive therapeutic outcome
• Decreased signs/symptoms of infection, HIV

---

indomethacin (Rx)

(in-doe-meth′a-sin)
Indocin, Nu-Indo ✦
Func. class.: NSAID (nonsteroidal antiinflammatory), antirheumatic
Chem. class.: Acetic acid derivative
Pregnancy category B (1st trimester), D (2nd/3rd trimesters)

Do not confuse:

Indocin/Endocet, **minocin**/Vicodin

ACTION: Inhibits prostaglandin synthesis by decreasing enzyme needed for biosynthesis; analgesic, antiinflammatory, antipyretic

---

Adverse effects: *italics* = common; **bold** = life-threatening

Therapeutic outcome: Decreased pain, inflammation; closure of patent ductus arteriosus (premature infants)

USES: Rheumatoid arthritis, ankylosing spondylitis, osteoarthritis, bursitis, tendinitis, acute gouty arthritis; closure of patent ductus arteriosus in premature infants (**IV**)

CONTRAINDICATIONS:
Pregnancy **D** (3rd trimester) hypersensitivity, asthma, aortic coarctation, bleeding, salicylate/NSAID hypersensitivity, GI bleeding

> **BLACK BOX WARNING:** Perioperative pain in CABG

Precautions: Pregnancy **B** (1st trimester), breastfeeding, children, bleeding disorders, GI disorders, cardiac disorders, asthma, diabetes, acute bronchospasm, ulcerative colitis, seizures, Parkinson's disease, renal/hepatic disease, depression, neonates

> **BLACK BOX WARNING:** Stroke, GI bleeding, MI

DOSAGE AND ROUTES
Arthritis/antiinflammatory
Adult: PO 25-50 mg bid-tid, max 200 mg/day; SUS REL 75 mg daily; may increase to 75 mg bid

Acute gouty arthritis
Adult: PO 50 mg tid; use only for acute attack, then reduce dosage

Patent ductus arteriosus
Longer or repeated treatment courses may be necessary for very premature infants
Infant <2 days: IV 0.2 mg/kg, then 0.1 mg/kg × 2 doses at 12, 24 hr
Infant 2-7 days: IV 0.2 mg/kg, then 0.2 mg/kg × 2 doses at 12, 24 hr
Infant >7 days: IV 0.2 mg/kg, then 0.25 mg/kg × 2 doses at 12, 24 hr

Available forms: Caps 25, 50 mg; sus rel caps 75 mg; oral susp 5 mg/ ml; inj 1-mg vials; supp 50 mg

Implementation
PO route
• Swallow sus rel cap whole; do not break, crush, or chew sus rel cap
• Give with food or milk to decrease gastric symptoms and prevent ulceration
• Shake susp; do not mix with other liquids

Rectal route
• Have patient retain rect supp for 1 hr after insertion
• Store at room temperature

IV route
• Give after diluting 1 mg with 1 or 2 ml saline or sterile water for inj without preservative; give 1 or 0.5 mg/ml, respectively, do not dilute further; give over 5-35 sec to avoid dramatic shift in cerebral blood flow; avoid extravasation

Y-site compatibilities: Furosemide, insulin (regular), potassium chloride, sodium bicarbonate, sodium nitroprusside

ADVERSE EFFECTS
CNS: Dizziness, drowsiness, fatigue, confusion, insomnia, anxiety, depression, *headache*
CV: Tachycardia, peripheral edema, palpitations, dysrhythmias, hypertension, **CV thrombotic events, MI, stroke**
EENT: Tinnitus, hearing loss, blurred vision
GI: *Nausea,* anorexia, *vomiting,* diarrhea, jaundice, **cholestatic hepatitis,** *constipation,* flatulence, cramps, dry mouth, peptic ulcer, **ulceration, perforation, GI bleeding**
GU: Nephrotoxicity **(dysuria, hematuria, oliguria, azotemia)**
HEMA: **Blood dyscrasias,** prolonged bleeding
INTEG: Purpura, rash, pruritus, sweating

Pharmacokinetics

Absorption	Well absorbed (PO); erratic (RECT); complete (**IV**)
Distribution	Crosses blood-brain barrier; placenta, 99% plasma protein binding
Metabolism	Liver, extensively
Excretion	Breast milk; urine 60%, feces 33%
Half-life	1 hr first pass, 2.6-11.2 hr second pass

Pharmacodynamics

	PO	PO–ext rel	IV
Onset	30 min	½ hr	2 day
Peak	2 hr	Unknown	Unknown
Duration	4-6 hr	4-6 hr	Unknown

INTERACTIONS
Individual drugs
Abciximab, aspirin, clopidogrel, eptifibatide, plicamycin, ticlodipine, tirofiban: increased bleeding risk

Cidofovir, cycloSPORINE, lithium, methotrexate, probenecid: increased toxicity

Digoxin, penicillamine, phenyton: increased effect of each specific product

Drug classifications
Aminoglycosides: increased effects of aminoglycosides

Anticoagulants, SNRIs, SSRIs, thrombolytics: increased risk of bleeding

Antihypertensives: decreased effect of antihypertensives

Diuretics (potassium sparing): increased hyperkalemia

NURSING CONSIDERATIONS
Assessment
• Assess for patent ductus arteriosus: respiratory rate, character, heart sounds
• Assess for joint pain (duration, intensity, ROM), baseline and during treatment
• Assess for confusion, mood changes, hallucinations, especially in geriatric
• Assess renal, liver, blood studies: BUN, creatinine, AST, ALT, Hgb before treatment, periodically thereafter; if renal function decreases, do not give subsequent doses

> **BLACK BOX WARNING:** Assess for cardiac disease, CV, thrombotic events (MI, stroke) prior to administration, not to be used for perioperative pain in CABG surgery

> **BLACK BOX WARNING:** GI bleeding/perforation: chronic use can lead to GI bleeding: use cautiously in those with a history of active GI disease

> **BLACK BOX WARNING:** MI, stroke: risk may be greater with longer-term use and in those with CV risk factors

Patient/family education
• Advise patient to report change in vision, blurring, rash, tinnitus, black stools
• Tell patient not to use for any other condition than prescribed
• Advise patient to avoid use with OTC medications for pain unless approved by prescriber, to report use to all providers

• Advise patient to avoid hazardous activities, since dizziness or drowsiness can occur
• Instruct patient to use sunscreen to prevent photosensitivity

Evaluation
Positive therapeutic outcome
• Decreased stiffness
• Increased joint mobility
• Decreased pain

---

inFLIXimab (Rx)
(in-fliks′ih-mab)
Remicade
Func. class.: Monoclonal antibody
Chem. class.: Tumor necrosis factor modifiers
Pregnancy category B

Do not confuse:
inFLIXimab/riTUXimab, **Remicade**/Renacidin

ACTION: Monoclonal antibody that neutralizes the activity of tumor necrosis factor α (TNFα) that has been found in Crohn's disease; decreased infiltration of inflammatory cells

Therapeutic outcome: Decreased cramping and blood in stools

USES: Crohn's disease, fistulizing, moderate to severe; rheumatoid arthritis given with methotrexate, plaque psoriasis, ankylosing spondylitis, ulcerative colitis, psoriatic arthritis, psoriasis

Unlabeled uses: Behçet's syndrome, uveitis, juvenile arthritis

CONTRAINDICATIONS:
Hypersensitivity to murines, moderate to severe CHF (NYHA class III/IV)

Precautions: Pregnancy **B**, breastfeeding, children, geriatric, COPD, hepatotoxicity, hematologic abnormalities, hepatitis B, Guillain-Barré syndrome, seizures, multiple sclerosis

> **BLACK BOX WARNING:** Infection, neoplastic disease, TB

DOSAGE AND ROUTES
Crohn's disease (moderate to severe/fistulizing)
Adult/adolescent/child ≥6 yr: **IV** INF 5 mg/kg initially, then repeat dose 2, 6 wk, q8wk thereafter, may increase to 10 mg/kg if needed (adults)

Adverse effects: *italics* = common; **bold** = life-threatening

Rheumatoid arthritis

Adult: IV 3 mg/kg initially, and 2, 6 wk and q8wk thereafter, max 10 mg/kg/dose

Available forms: Powder for inj 100 mg

Implementation

Intermittent IV infusion route

• Administer immediately after reconstitution; reconstitute each vial with 10 ml of sterile water for inj, further dilute total dose/250 ml of 0.9% NaCl inj to a total conc of between 0.4 and 4 mg/ml; use 21-G or smaller needle for reconstitution, direct sterile water at glass wall of vial, gently swirl, do not shake, may foam; allow to stand for 5 min, give within 3 hr

• Give over ≥2 hr, use polyethylene-lined inf with in-line, sterile, low-protein-bind filter

• Do not admix

• Provide refrigerated storage, do not freeze

ADVERSE EFFECTS

CNS: *Headache, dizziness, depression, vertigo, fatigue, anxiety, fever,* **seizures,** *chills, flulike symptoms,* demyelinating disease
CV: Chest pain, hypo/hypertension, tachycardia, **CHF, acute coronary syndrome**
GI: *Nausea, vomiting, abdominal pain, stomatitis, constipation, dyspepsia, flatulence*
GU: Dysuria, frequency
HEMA: Anemia, leukopenia, thrombocytopenia, pancytopenia
INTEG: *Rash, dermatitis, urticaria,* dry skin, sweating, flushing, hematoma, pruritus, keratoderma blennorrhagicum
MS: Myalgia, back pain, arthralgia
RESP: URI, pharyngitis, bronchitis, cough, dyspnea, sinusitis
SYST: Anaphylaxis, fatal infections, sepsis, malignancies, immunogenicity, Stevens-Johnson syndrome, toxic epidermal necrolysis

Pharmacokinetics

Absorption	Unknown
Distribution	Vascular compartment
Metabolism	Unknown
Excretion	Unknown
Half-life	9½ days

Pharmacodynamics

Unknown

INTERACTIONS

Drug classifications

Live virus vaccines: do not administer live vaccines concurrently

TNF blockers (abatacept, anakinra, golimumab, rilonacept): increased infections, neutropenia; avoid concurrent use

NURSING CONSIDERATIONS

Assessment

• Assess GI symptoms: nausea, vomiting, abdominal pain

• Take periodic blood counts: CBC

• Assess CV status: B/P, pulse, chest pain

⚠ Assess for allergic reaction, anaphylaxis: rash, dermatitis, urticaria, fever, chills, dyspnea, hypotension; discontinue if severe; administer epinephrine, corticosteroids, antihistamines; assess for allergy to murine proteins before starting therapy

BLACK BOX WARNING: Fatal infections: discontinue if infection occurs, do not administer to patients with active infections; identify TB before beginning treatment, a TB test should be obtained; if present, TB should be treated before giving infliximab; exercise caution when switching one DMARD to another

• Report suspected adverse reactions to the FDA (1-800-FDA-1088)

BLACK BOX WARNING: Assess for neoplastic disease in those <18 yr, including heptosplenic T-cell lymphoma, usually occurs in those with inflammatory bowel disease

Patient/family education

• Instruct patient to report infusion reaction immediately

• Instruct patient to notify prescriber immediately if infection occurs

• Advise patient not to breastfeed while taking this product

• Advise patient to notify prescriber of GI symptoms, hypersensitivity reactions

• Advise patient not to operate machinery or drive if dizziness, vertigo occurs

• Teach patient to avoid live virus vaccinations, bring up to date prior to use

Evaluation

Positive therapeutic outcome

• Absence of blood in stool

• Reported improvement in comfort

• Weight gain

🅐 HIGH ALERT

INSULINS

RAPID ACTING

insulin glulisine (Rx)
Apidra, Apidra SoloStar
insulin aspart (Rx)
Novolog, Novolog Flexpen, Novolog PenFill, NovoMix 30 ✦, NovoRapid ✦
insulin lispro (Rx)
Humalog

SHORT ACTING

insulin, regular (OTC)
Humulin R ✦, Novolin R, ReliOn R
insulin, regular concentrated (Rx)
Humulin RU-500

INTERMEDIATE ACTING

insulin, isophane suspension (NPH) (OTC)
Humulin N, Novolin ge NPH ✦, Novolin N, Novolin N Prefilled, ReliOn N

LONG ACTING

insulin detemir (Rx)
Levemir
insulin glargine (Rx)
Lantus

MIXTURES

insulin, isophane suspension and regular insulin (Rx)
Humulin 70/30, Humalin 30/70 ✦, Novolin 70/30, Novolin 70/30 Prefilled, ReliOn 70/30
isophane insulin suspension (NPH) and insulin mixtures (Rx)
Humulin 50/50
insulin lispro mixture (Rx)
Humalog KwikPen Mix 50/50, Humalog Mix 25 ✦, Humalog Mix 50 ✦, Humalog Mix 75/25, Humalog Mix 50/50

insulin aspart mixture (Rx)
Novolog 70/30, Novolog Mix Flexpen Prefilled Syringe 70/30
Func. class.: Antidiabetic, pancreatic hormone
Chem. class.: Modified structures of endogenous human insulin
Pregnancy category B, C

Do not confuse:
Lantus/lente

ACTION: Decreases blood glucose; by transport of glucose into cells and the conversion of glucose to glycogen, indirectly increases blood pyruvate and lactate, decreases phosphate and potassium; insulin may be human (processed by recombinant DNA technologies)

Therapeutic outcome: Decreased blood glucose levels in diabetes mellitus

USES: Type 1 diabetes mellitus, type 2 diabetes mellitus, gestational diabetes, insulin lispro may be used in combination with sulfonylureas in children >3 yr

CONTRAINDICATIONS:
Hypersensitivity to protamine; creosol (aspart)

Precautions: Pregnancy **B** (lispro, detemir, aspart, regular), **C** (all others)

DOSAGE AND ROUTES
Insulin glulisine
Adult/adolescent/child ≥4 yr: SUBCUT dosage individualized, give within 15 min before or 20 min after starting a meal
Adult: IV dilute to 1 unit/ml in INF systems with 0.9% NaCl, using PVC Viaflex INF bags and PVC tubing, use dedicated line

Insulin aspart
Adult/adolescent/child ≥6 yr: Intermittent SUBCUT total daily dose is given as 2-4 inj/day just prior to beginning of a meal; in general, 50%-70% of total daily insulin may be given as insulin aspart, the remainder should be intermediate or long-acting insulin; CONTINUOUS SUBCUT used with external insulin pump via cont SUBCUT insulin INF (CSII), the insulin dose should be based on the insulin dose from the previous regimen

Insulin lispro
Adult/adolescent/child ≥3 yr: SUBCUT 15 min before meals; **continuous subcut infusion (external insulin pump)** the total daily dose should be based on the insulin dose in previous regimen, 50% of total dose can be given as meal-related boluses and the remainder as basal infusion

Human regular
Adult: SUBCUT ½-1 hr before meals

Insulin, isophane suspension
Adult: SUBCUT dosage individualized by blood, urine glucose; usual dose 7-26 units; may increase by 2-10 units/day if needed

Insulin detemir
Adult/adolescent/child ≥2 yr: SUBCUT 1 or 2 times/day; if 1 time, give with evening meal

Insulin glargine
Adult and child ≥6 yr: SUBCUT 10 international units/day, range 2-100 international units/day

Regular insulin (ketoacidosis)
Adult: IV 5-10 units, then 5-10 units/hr until desired response, then switch to SUBCUT dose; IV/INF 2-12 units (50 units/500 ml of normal saline)
Child: IV 0.1 units/kg

Replacement
Adult and child: SUBCUT 0.5-1 units/kg/day qid given 30 min before meals
Adolescent: SUBCUT 0.8-1.2 mg/kg/day; this dosage is used during rapid growth

Available forms: NPH inj 100 units/ml; **regular** inj 100 units/ml, cartridges 100 units/ml; **insulin analog** inj 100 units/ml; **isophane insulin** inj 100 units/ml, cartridges 100 units/ml; **insulin lispro** 100 units/ml, 1.5-ml cartridges; insulin lispro Humalog Pen sol for inj 100 units/ml; **insulin glulisine** inj 100 units/ml; **insulin glargine** inj 100 units/ml; **insulin detemir** inj 100 units/ml in 10 vials, 3-ml cartridges; **insulin aspart** inj 100 mg/ml (Flexpen, PenFill)

Implementation
• Store at room temperature for <1 mo (some insulins); keep away from heat and sunlight; refrigerate all other supply; NPH, premixed insulins are cloudy; regular, rapid-acting analogs, long-acting analogs are clear; do not freeze—**IV** route, regular only

SUBCUT route
• Give after warming to room temperature by rotating in palms to prevent injecting cold insulin; use only insulin syringes with markings or syringe matching units/ml; rotate inj sites within one area: abdomen, upper back, thighs, upper arm, buttocks; keep record of sites
• Give increased dosages if tolerance occurs
• Premixed insulins and NPH are cloudy suspensions
• Regular human insulin, rapid-acting analogs, and long-acting analogs are clear; do not use if cloudy, thick, or discolored

CONT SUBCUT route (insulin infusion CSII)
• Do not mix with other insulins when using a pump
• Insulin lispro 3 ml cartridges are to be used in Disetronic H-TRON plus V100 pump using Disetronic rapid inf sets; the inf set and the cartridge adapter should be changed q3day; replace 3 ml cartridge q6days

IV route (insulin glulisine only)
• Dilute to 1 international unit/ml in infusion systems with 0.9% NaCl using PVC viaflex inf bags and PVC tubing; use dedicated line; do not admix

IV route (regular only)
⚠ When regular insulin is administered IV, monitor glucose, potassium often to prevent fatal hypoglycemia, hypokalemia
• IV direct, undiluted via vein, Y-site, 3-way stopcock; give at 50 units/min or less
• Give by cont inf after diluting with IV sol and run at prescribed rate; use IV inf pump for correct dosing; give reduced dose at serum glucose level of 250 mg/100 ml

Additive compatibilities: Bretylium, cimetidine, lidocaine, meropenem, ranitidine, verapamil

Additive incompatibilities: Aminophylline, amobarbital, chlorothiazide, cytarabine, DOBUTamine, PENTobarbital, PHENobarbital, phenytoin, secobarbital, sodium bicarbonate, thiopental

Y-site compatibilities: Amiodarone, ampicillin, ampicillin/sulbactam, aztreonam, ceFAZolin, cefoTEtan, DOBUTamine, esmolol, famotidine, gentamicin, heparin, heparin/hydrocortisone, imipenem/cilastatin, indomethacin, magnesium sulfate, meperidine, meropenem, midazolam, morphine, nitroglycerin, oxytocin, PENTobarbital, potassium chloride, propofol, ritodrine, sodium bicarbonate, sodium nitro-

prusside, tacrolimus, terbutaline, ticarcillin,
ticarcillin/clavulanate, tobramycin, vancomycin,
vit B/C

Y-site incompatibilities: Nafcillin

ADVERSE EFFECTS
EENT: Blurred vision, dry mouth
INTEG: Flushing, rash, urticaria, warmth, *lipodystrophy,* lipohypertrophy, swelling, redness
META: *Hypoglycemia,* rebound hyperglycemia (Somogyi effect 12-72 hr or longer)
MISC: Peripheral edema
SYST: Anaphylaxis

Pharmacokinetics

Absorption	Rapidly absorbed (SUBCUT)
Distribution	Widely distributed
Metabolism	Liver, muscle, kidney
Excretion	Kidneys
Half-life	Regular 3-5 min; NPH 10 min

INTERACTIONS
Individual drugs
Alcohol: increased hypoglycemia
DOBUTamine: increased insulin need
EPINEPHrine: decreased hypoglycemia
Fenfluramine, guanethedine, phenylbutazone, sulfinpyrazone, tetracycline: decreased insulin need

Drug classifications
Anabolic steroids, β-adrenergic blockers, hypoglycemics (oral), salicylates: increased hypoglycemia
Contraceptives (oral), corticosteroids, diuretics (thiazide), thyroid hormones: decreased hypoglycemia
Estrogens: increased insulin need
MAOIs: decreased insulin need

Drug/lab test
Increased: VMA
Decreased: potassium, calcium
Interference: liver, thyroid function tests

Pharmacodynamics

Rapid acting	
Insulin glulisine	Onset 15-30 min, peak ½-1½ hr, duration 3-4 hr
Insulin aspart	Onset 10-20 min, peak 1-3 hr, duration 3-5 hr
Insulin lispro	Onset 15-30 min, peak ½-1½ hr, duration 3-4 hr
Short acting	
Insulin regular	Onset 30 min, peak 2.5-5 hr, duration up to 6 hr
Intermediate acting	
Insulin, isophane suspension (NPH)	Onset 1.5-4 hr, peak 4-12 hr, duration up to 24 hr
Long acting	
Insulin detemir	Onset 0.8-2 hr, peak unknown, duration up to 24 hr (concentration dependent)
Insulin glargine	Onset 1.5 hr, no peak identified, duration ≥ 24 hr
Mixtures	
Insulin, isophane suspension and regular insulin (70/30)	Onset 10-20 hr, peak 2.4 hr, duration up to 24 hr
Isophane insulin suspension (NPH) and insulin mixtures (50/50)	Onset ½-1 hr, peak dual, duration 10-16 hr

NURSING CONSIDERATIONS
Assessment
• Fasting blood glucose, also Hgb A1c may be tested to identify treatment effectiveness q3mo
• Urine ketones during illness; insulin requirements may increase during stress, illness, surgery
• For hypoglycemic reaction that can occur during peak time (sweating, weakness, dizziness, chills, confusion, headache, nausea, rapid weak pulse, fatigue, tachycardia, memory lapses, slurred speech, staggering gait, anxiety, tremors, hunger)
• For hyperglycemia: acetone breath, polyuria, fatigue, polydipsia, flushed, dry skin, lethargy

Patient/family education
• Advise patient that blurred vision occurs; not to change corrective lens until vision is stabilized 1-2 mo
• Advise patient to keep insulin, equipment available at all times; carry a glucagon kit, candy, or lump sugar to treat hypoglycemia
• Inform patient that product does not cure diabetes but controls symptoms
• Advise patient to carry emergency ID as diabetic
• Instruct patient to recognize hypoglycemia reaction: headache, tremors, fatigue, weakness
• Instruct patient to recognize hyperglycemia reaction: frequent urination, thirst, fatigue, hunger
• Teach patient the dosage, route, mixing instructions, any diet restrictions, disease process
• Teach patient the symptoms of ketoacidosis: nausea, thirst, polyuria, dry mouth, decreased B/P, dry, flushed skin, acetone breath, drowsiness, Kussmaul respirations
• Advise patient that a plan is necessary for diet, exercise; all food on diet should be eaten; exercise routine should not vary
• Teach patient about blood glucose testing; make sure patient is able to determine glucose level
• Advise patient to avoid OTC products unless directed by prescriber

Evaluation
Positive therapeutic outcome
• Decrease in polyuria, polydipsia, polyphagia; clear sensorium; absence of dizziness; stable gait
• Blood glucose level under control

TREATMENT OF OVERDOSE:
Glucose 25 g **IV,** via dextrose 50% sol, 50 ml, or glucagon 1 mg

interferon alfacon-1 (Rx)
(in-ter-feer'on al'fa-kon)
Infergen
Func. class.: Recombinant type 1 interferon
Pregnancy category C

ACTION: Induces biologic responses and has antiviral, antiproliferative, and immunomodulatory effects

Therapeutic outcome: Decreased signs/symptoms of hepatitis C

USES: Chronic hepatitis C infections in those 18 yr and older with compensated liver disease who have anti-HCV antibodies or HCV RNA, may use in combination with ribavirin

Unlabeled uses: Hairy cell leukemia when used with G-CSF

CONTRAINDICATIONS:
Hypersensitivity to α-interferons, or products from *Escherichia coli,* uncompensated hepatic disease, autoimmune hepatitis

Precautions: Pregnancy **C,** breastfeeding, children <18 yr, thyroid disorders, myelosuppression, hepatic disease, alcoholism, geriatric patients, seizure disorder, hepatitis

> **BLACK BOX WARNING:** Cardiac disease, autoimmune disorder, infection, depression

DOSAGE AND ROUTES
Adult: Monotherapy: SUBCUT 9 mcg as a single inj 3 ×/wk × 24 wk; leave at least 48 hr between injections; those who did not respond or relapsed after discontinuation, give 15 mcg 3×/wk × 48 wk; **combination:** subcut 15 mcg/day with ribavirin 1000 mg/day PO (<75 kg), 1200 mg/day PO (≥75 kg) give in 2 divided doses for up to 48 wks, use stepwise dose reduction in the interferon dose from 15 mcg to 9 mcg to 6 mcg for serious adverse reactions

Available forms: Inj 9 mcg/0.3 ml, 15 mcg/0.5 ml

Implementation
• Do not shake vial; use 1 dose per vial; discard unused portion; use proper inj sites; rotate sites, discard unused product

---

ADVERSE EFFECTS

CNS: Headache, fatigue, fever, rigors, insomnia, dizziness, agitation, nervousness, anxiety, lability, abnormal thinking, depression

CV: Hypertension, palpitation, tachycardia

EENT: Tinnitus, earache, conjunctivitis, eye pain

GI: Abdominal pain, nausea, diarrhea, anorexia, dyspepsia, vomiting, constipation, flatulence, hemorrhoids, decreased salivation

GU: Dysmenorrhea, vaginitis, menstrual disorders

HEMA: Granulocytopenia, thrombocytopenia, leukopenia, ecchymosis, **aplastic anemia**

INTEG: Alopecia, pruritus, rash, erythema, dry skin

MISC: Anaphylaxis, angioedema, flulike illness

MS: Back, limb, neck, skeletal pain, rigors

RESP: Pharyngitis, upper respiratory infection, cough, sinusitis, rhinitis, respiratory tract congestion, epistaxis, dyspnea, bronchitis

Pharmacokinetics	
Unknown	

Pharmacodynamics	
Onset	Unknown
Peak	24-36 hr
Duration	Unknown

INTERACTIONS

Individual drugs

Eflornithine (systemic): increased hearing loss, consider serial audiograms

Drug classifications

NRTIs: increased effect, use together cautiously

NURSING CONSIDERATIONS

Assessment

⚠ **Pregnancy: determine if patient is pregnant before use with ribavirin, pregnancy (X) when used with ribavirin**

• Assess CBC, liver function tests, ECG, platelet counts, heme concentration, ANC, serum creatinine concentration, albumin, bilirubin, TSH, T_4

> **BLACK BOX WARNING: Hemolytic anemia:** ribavirin may be used with this product and cause hemolytic anemia, cardiac symptoms

• Assess for myelosuppression, low dose if neutrophil count is $<500 \times 10\text{-}6/L$ or if platelets are $<50 \times 10\text{-}9/L$, monitor for infection

• Assess for hypersensitivity; discontinue immediately if hypersensitivity occurs

Patient/family education

• Provide patient or family member with written, detailed instructions about the product

• Caution patient to use contraception during treatment

⚠ **Teach patient to report if pregnancy is planned or suspected; pregnancy (C), when combined with ribavirin pregnancy (X)**

• Teach patient to use OTC analgesics to decrease flulike symptoms

• If patient will be self-administering injection, teach all aspects of product use, administration, disposal; provide med guide

Evaluation

Positive therapeutic outcome

• Decreased hepatitis C signs/symptoms

---

interferon beta-1a (Rx)

(in-ter-feer′on)

Avonex, Rebif

interferon beta-1b (Rx)

Betaseron, Extavia

Func. class.: Multiple sclerosis agent, immune modifier

Chem. class.: Interferon, *Escherichia coli* derivative

Pregnancy category C

ACTION: Antiviral, immunoregulatory; action not clearly understood; biologic response-modifying properties mediated through specific receptors on cells, inducing expression of interferon-induced gene products

Therapeutic outcome: Decreased symptoms of multiple sclerosis

USES: Ambulatory patients with relapsing or remitting multiple sclerosis

Unlabeled uses: May be useful in treatment of AIDS, AIDS-related Kaposi's sarcoma, malignant melanoma, metastatic renal cell carcinoma, cutaneous T-cell lymphoma, acute non-A/non-B hepatitis

CONTRAINDICATIONS:

Hypersensitivity to natural or recombinant interferon-beta or human albumin, hamster protein, rotavirus vaccine

Precautions: Pregnancy **C**, breastfeeding, children <18 yr, chronic progressive multiple sclerosis, depression, mental disorders, seizure disorders, latex allergy, autoimmune disorders, bone marrow suppression, hepatotoxicity, cardiac disease, alcoholism, chickenpox, herpes zoster

DOSAGE AND ROUTES

Interferon beta-1a

Remitting-relapsing multiple sclerosis

Adult: IM (Avonex) 30 mcg qwk; SUBCUT (Rebif) 22 or 44 mcg 3 ×/wk with each dose 48 hr apart, titrate to full dose over 4-wk period

Interferon beta-1b

Relapsing/remitting multiple sclerosis

Adult: SUBCUT 0.0625 mg every other day for wk 1 and 2; then 0.125 mg every other day for wk 3 and 4; then 0.1875 mg every other day for wk 5 and 6; then 0.25 mg every other day thereafter; higher doses should not be used

Available forms: Beta-1a (Avonex): 33 mcg (6.6 million international units/vial) (auto-injector pen); (Rebif) 22 mcg, 44 mcg/0.5 ml; beta-1b: powder for inj 0.3 mg (9.6 m international units)

Implementation

• Reconstitute 0.3 mg (9.6 million international units)/1.2 ml of supplied diluent (0.2 mg or 8 million international units concentration); rotate vial gently, do not shake; withdraw 1 ml using a syringe with 27-G needle; administer SUBCUT only into hip, thigh, arm; discard unused portion

Interferon beta-1a

• Reconstitute with 1.1 ml of diluent, swirl, give within 6 hr
• Store in refrigerator; do not freeze
• Visually inspect parenteral products for particulate matter and discoloration prior to use

IM route
• Premedication with acetaminophen or ibuprofen and give at bedtime to lessen flulike symptoms
• Interferon beta-1a (Avonex) 30 mcg is equivalent to 6 million IU
• If a dose is missed, give it as soon as possible; continue the regular schedule but do not give 2 injections within 2 days of each other; all products are for single-use only. Do not re-use needles, syringes, prefilled syringes, or autoinjectors
• Injection sites should be rotated to minimize the likelihood of injection site reactions
• Do not inject into an area of the body where skin is irritated, reddened, bruised, infected, or scarred

• The injection site should be checked after 2 hours for redness, edema, or tenderness
• The manufacturer of Avonex offers free training on IM use for patients and health care partners. Contact MS ActiveSource for more information (800-456-2255)

Reconstitution and administration of Avonex lyophilized powder for IM route
• Use appropriate aseptic technique for preparation of solution
• Sites for injection include the thigh or upper arm
• Slowly add 1.1 ml sterile water for injection, USP, preservative-free (supplied by manufacturer) to the vial. Rapid addition of the diluent may cause foaming, making it difficult to withdraw the solution
• Gently swirl the vial to aid in dissolution; do not shake. Final concentration should be 30 mcg/ml (6 million IU/ml)
• The reconstituted solution should be clear to slightly yellow without particles. Discard if the reconstituted product contains particulate matter or is discolored
• Withdraw 1 ml of reconstituted solution into a syringe. Attach the sterile needle and inject IM
• A 25 gauge, 1″ needle may be substituted for the 23 gauge, 1¼″ needle provided by the manufacturer, if needed
• *Storage:* Use within 6 hours of reconstitution; store reconstituted solution refrigerated; do NOT freeze. Discard any unused solution; both drug and diluent vials are single-use only

Administration of Avonex prefilled syringe
• Patients may self-inject only if provider determines that it is appropriate, and with medical follow-up, and after proper training in IM injection technique
• The first injection should be performed under the supervision of an appropriately qualified person
• If self-injecting, rotate between thighs. With help from another person, may rotate between thighs and upper arms
• Wash hands prior to handling the Dose Pack
• Remove prefilled syringe from the refrigerator to warm to room temperature (usually 30 min before use). Do not use external heat sources such as hot water to warm the syringe
• Hold the syringe so the cap is facing down and the 0.5 mL mark is at eye level. Be sure the amount of liquid in the syringe is the same or very close to the 0.5 mL mark. If the correct amount of liquid is not in the syringe, do not use it and call the pharmacist

---

• Hold syringe upright so that the rubber cap faces up. Remove the cap by bending it at a 90 degree angle until it snaps free

• Attach the needle by pressing it onto the syringe and turning it clockwise until it locks in place. Be careful not to push the plunger while attaching the needle

• Use the alcohol wipe to clean the skin at the injection site you choose. Then, pull the protective cover straight off the needle; do not twist the cover off

• Inject intramuscularly at a 90 degree angle into the thigh or upper arm as directed by the provider

• Use gauze pad to apply pressure for a few seconds after the injection

• Dispose of used needles and syringes in a puncture-resistant container and discard appropriately

• Instruct patients to contact the health care provider if a skin reaction occurs that does not resolve in a few days

• A 25 gauge, 1″ needle for intramuscular injection may be substituted for the 23 gauge, 1¼″ needle provided by the manufacturer, if deemed appropriate by the physician

• Refer to the Patient Medication Guide for detailed instructions for preparing and giving a dose

• *Storage:* Store refrigerated, if refrigeration is unavailable, may store at 77 degrees F or less for up to 7 days; after removal from refrigerator, do not store product above 25 degrees C. If the product has been exposed to conditions other than recommended, discard the product. Do not expose to high temperatures. Do not freeze. Protect from light

Administration of Avonex prefilled autoinjector

• Patients may self-inject only if their provider determines that it is appropriate, and with medical follow-up, and after proper training in IM technique

• The first injection should be performed under the supervision of provider

• Remove one Administration Dose Pack from the refrigerator to warm to room temperature (about 30 min before use). Do not use external heat sources such as hot water to warm the syringe Dose Pack

• Wash hands prior to handling Dose Pack contents

• Ensure tamper-evident cap has not been removed or is loose. Then grasp the cap and bend it at a 90-degree angle until it snaps off. Pull off the sterile foil from the needle cover

• Hold the Avonex pen with the glass syringe tip pointing up. Press the needle onto the glass syringe tip. Gently turn the needle clockwise until firmly attached. Do not remove plastic cover from the needle

• Hold Pen with one hand and using other hand, hold onto the injector shield (grooved area) tightly and quickly pull up on the injector shield until the injector shield covers the needle all the way. The plastic needle cover will pop off after the injector shield has been fully extended

• When the injector shield is extended the right way, there will be a small blue rectangular area next to the oval medication display window. Check the display window and make sure the Avonex is clear and colorless

• Do not use the injection if the liquid is colored, cloudy, or has lumps or particles. Air bubbles will not affect your dose

• Do not push down on the injector shield and the blue activation button at the same time until you are ready to give injection

• Avonex pen should be injected into the upper, outer thigh

• Use the alcohol wipe to clean the skin at the injection site you choose and allow it to dry prior to injection

• Hold Pen at 90-degree angle to the injection site. Firmly push the body of the pen down against the thigh to release the safety lock. Safety lock is released when blue rectangle area above the oval medication display window is gone. Push down on blue activation button with thumb and count to 10. You will hear a click if the injection is given the right way

• After counting to 10, pull the pen straight out of the skin. Use gauze pad to apply pressure for a few seconds

• The circular display window on the pen will be yellow if you have received the full dose

• Cover exposed needle with pen cover. Do not hold the pen cover with your hands while inserting the needle

• Dispose of used needles and syringes in a puncture-resistant container and discard appropriately

• Instruct patients to contact the health care provider if a skin reaction occurs that does not resolve in a few days

• Refer to the Patient Medication Guide for detailed instructions for preparing and giving a dose

• *Storage:* Store at 36°-46° F (2°-8° C). If refrigeration is unavailable, may store at 77° F (25° C) or less for up to 7 days. After removal from refrigerator, do not store product above 77° F (25° C). If the product has been exposed to conditions other than recommended, discard the product and do not use. Do not expose to high temperatures. Do not freeze. Protect from light

Subcutaneous administration

• Give at the same time (preferably late in the afternoon or evening) on the same days of the week at least 48 hr apart

• Do not give on two consecutive days. If a dose is missed, administer the dose as soon as possible then skip the following day. Return to the regular schedule the following week

• Premedication with acetaminophen or ibuprofen may lessen the severity of flulike symptoms

• Interferon beta-1a (Rebif) 44 mcg is equivalent to 12 million IU

• Rotate injection sites. Appropriate injection sites include thigh, outer surface of upper arm, stomach, or buttocks. Do not inject into an area where the skin is irritated, reddened, bruised, or infected

• A "Starter Pack" containing a lower dose of Rebif syringes is available for the initial titration period. Patients and/or caregivers should be trained and understand appropriate preparation and administration

• The manufacturer offers complimentary services including injection training and reimbursement support. Contact MS LifeLines at 877-44-REBIF

Injection (Rebif)

• Interferon beta-1a (Rebif) is available in a prefilled syringe with a 29-gauge needle

• Inject subcutaneously into the outer surface of the upper arm, abdomen, thigh, or buttock. Do not inject the area near the navel or waistline. Take care not to inject intradermally

• Discard any unused solution. Prefilled syringes do not contain preservatives and are single-use only

Interferon beta-1b

• Reconstitute by injecting diluent provided (1.2 ml) into vial, swirl (8 milli-international units/ml), use 27-G needle for inj

• Give acetaminophen for fever, headache; use SUBCUT route only; do not give IM or **IV**

• Store reconstituted sol in refrigerator; do not freeze; do not use sol that contains precipitate or is discolored

Subcut route

• The manufacturers of Betaseron and of Extavia offer materials to assist with training on subcut use: call 1-800-788-1467 (Betaseron), 1-888-669-6682 (Extavia)

• Premedication with acetaminophen or ibuprofen and use of product at bedtime may lessen the severity of flulike symptoms

• Visually inspect parenteral products for particulate matter and discoloration prior to use. Do not use if particulate matter is present

Reconstitution

• Add 1.2 ml of 0.54% sodium chloride injection (supplied by the manufacturer) to the vial by using the vial adapter to attach the prefilled syringe that contains the diluent. Keep the plunger depressed, and gently swirl; do not shake. If you take your thumb off the plunger, the solution may come back into the syringe before the product is fully reconstituted. If foaming occurs, allow the vial to sit until the foam settles; final concentration (250 mcg interferon beta-1b/ml, which corresponds to 8 million International Units/ml)

• If not used immediately, store in the refrigerator for up to 3 hr; do not freeze; discard any unused portion after 3 hr

Injection

• Withdraw the desired amount of the reconstituted solution into the syringe by turning the vial and syringe to get the vial on top. Pull the plunger back to get the desired amount of product; turn the syringe to point the needle upward, and tap the syringe and release any air bubbles. Twist the vial adapter to remove it and the vial

• Choose an injection site on the upper, back arms; abdomen; buttocks; or front thighs. Do not inject within 2 in of the navel or in a site where the skin is red, bruised, infected, broken, painful, uneven, or scabbed; rotate injection sites to minimize injection site reactions such as necrosis or localized infection

• Inject subcutaneously. Take care not to inject intradermally

ADVERSE EFFECTS

CNS: *Headache, fever, pain, chills, mental changes,* depression, hypertonia, **suicide attempts, seizures**

CV: *Migraine, palpitations, hypertension,* tachycardia, peripheral vascular disorders

EENT: Conjunctivitis, blurred vision

GI: *Diarrhea, constipation, vomiting, abdominal pain*

GU: *Dysmenorrhea, irregular menses, metrorrhagia,* cystitis, breast pain

HEMA: Decreased lymphocytes, ANC, **WBC,** *lymphadenopathy,* anemia

INTEG: *Sweating,* inj site reaction

MS: *Myalgia,* **myasthenia**

RESP: *Sinusitis,* dyspnea

Pharmacokinetics

Absorption	50% is absorbed
Distribution	Unknown
Metabolism	Unknown
Excretion	Unknown
Half-life	8 min-4½ hr (beta-1b), 8.6 hr (beta-1a)

Pharmacodynamics

	Beta-1a	Beta-1b
Onset	Up to 12 hr	Rapid
Peak	48 hr	2-8 hr
Duration	4 days	Unknown

INTERACTIONS

Individual drugs
Zidovudine: decreased clearance

Drug classifications
Antiretrovirals (NNRTIs, NRTIs, protease inhibitors): increased hepatic damage
Antineoplastics: increased myelosuppression

Drug/herb
Astragalus, echinacea, melatonin: change in immunomodulation

Drug/lab test
Increased: liver function tests
Interference: vaccines, toxoids; avoid concurrent use

NURSING CONSIDERATIONS

Assessment
• Monitor blood, renal, liver function tests: CBC, differential, platelet counts, BUN, creatinine, ALT, urinalysis; if neutrophil count is <750/mm³, or if AST, ALT is 10 × greater than ULN, or if bilirubin is 5 × greater than ULN, discontinue product; when neutrophil count exceeds 750/mm³ and liver function or renal studies return to normal, treatment may resume at 50% original dosage
• Assess for CNS symptoms: headache, fatigue, depression; if depression occurs and is severe, product should be discontinued
• Assess for multiple sclerosis symptoms
• Assess mental status: depression, depersonalization, suicidal thoughts, insomnia
• Monitor GI status: diarrhea or constipation, vomiting, abdominal pain
• Monitor cardiac status: increased B/P, tachycardia

Patient/family education
• Provide patient or family member with written, detailed instructions about the product; provide initial and return demonstrations on inj procedure; give information on use and disposal of product
• Inform patient that blurred vision, sweating may occur
• Advise female patients that irregular menses, dysmenorrhea, or metrorrhagia as well as breast pain may occur; use contraception during treatment; product may cause spontaneous abortion
• Teach patient to use sunscreen to prevent photosensitivity
• Instruct patient to notify prescriber if pregnancy is suspected
• Teach patient inj technique and care of equipment
• Instruct patient to notify prescriber of increased temp, chills, muscle soreness, fatigue

Evaluation
Positive therapeutic outcome
• Decreased symptoms of multiple sclerosis

interferon gamma-1b (Rx)
(in-ter-feer′on)
Actimmune
Func. class.: Biologic response modifier
Chem. class.: Lymphokine, interleukin type
Pregnancy category C

ACTION: Species-specific protein synthesized in response to viruses; potent phagocyte-activating effects; capable of mediating the killing of *Staphylococcus aureus, Toxoplasma gondii, Leishmania donovani, Listeria monocytogenes, Mycobacterium avium-intracellulare;* enhances oxidative metabolism of macrophages; enhances antibody-dependent cellular cytotoxicity

Therapeutic outcome: Decreased signs/symptoms of infection (serious) in chronic granulomatous disease

USES: Serious infections associated with chronic granulomatous disease, osteopetrosis

Unlabeled uses: Osteoporosis, *Mycobacterium avium* complex (MAC), ovarian cancer, pulmonary fibrosis

CONTRAINDICATIONS:
Hypersensitivity to interferon γ, *Escherichia coli*–derived products

Precautions: Pregnancy **C**, breastfeeding, children <1 yr, cardiac disease, seizure/CNS disorders, myelosuppression

DOSAGE AND ROUTES

Adult: SUBCUT 50 mcg/m^2 (1.5 million units/m^2) for patient with a surface area of >0.5 m^2; 1.5 mcg/kg/dose for patient with a surface area of <0.5/m^2; give on Monday, Wednesday, Friday for 3 ×/wk dosing

Available forms: Inj 100 mcg (2 million units)/single-dose vial

Implementation

• Give at bedtime to minimize adverse reactions; administer acetaminophen for fever, headache; use 50% of the dosage prescribed if severe reactions occur or discontinue treatment until reactions subside

• Give in right or left deltoid and anterior thigh; warm to room temperature before use; do not leave at room temperature >12 hr (unopened vial); does not contain preservatives

• Store in refrigerator upon receipt; do not freeze; do not shake

ADVERSE EFFECTS

CNS: *Headache, fatigue,* depression, fever, chills
GI: *Nausea, anorexia,* abdominal pain, weight loss, diarrhea, vomiting, colitis
HEMA: **Leukopenia, thrombocytopenia,** neutropenia
INTEG: Rash, pain at inj site, **Stevens-Johnson syndrome**
MS: Myalgia, arthralgia

Pharmacokinetics

Absorption	Slowly absorbed 89%
Distribution	Unknown
Metabolism	Unknown
Excretion	Unknown
Half-life	5.9 hr

Pharmacodynamics

Onset	Unknown
Peak	7 hr
Duration	Unknown

INTERACTIONS

Individual drugs

Aminophylline, theophylline: increased levels

Drug classifications

Myelosuppressive agents: increased myelosuppression

Protease inhibitors, nucleoside reverse transcriptase inhibitors (NRTIs), nonnucleoside reverse transcriptase inhibitors (NNRTIs): increased liver toxicity

NURSING CONSIDERATIONS

Assessment

• Monitor blood, renal, hepatic studies: CBC with differential, platelet count, BUN, creatinine, ALT, urinalysis before, q3mo during treatment

• Assess for infection: headache, fever, chills, fatigue; these are common adverse reactions

• Monitor CNS symptoms: headache, fatigue, depression

Patient/family education

• Provide patient or family member with written, detailed instructions about the product; provide initial and return demonstrations on inj procedure; give information on use and disposal of product

• Caution patient to use contraception during treatment

Evaluation

Positive therapeutic outcome

• Decreased serious infections

• Improvement in existing infections and inflammatory conditions

ipilimumab

(ip-i-lim'ue-mab)
Yervoy
Func. class.: Antineoplastic; biologic response modifier
Pregnancy category C

ACTION: A recombinant, human monoclonal antibody that binds to the cytotoxic T-lymphocyte-associated antigen 4 (CTLA-4); action is indirect, possibly through T-cell mediated antitumor immune responses

Therapeutic outcome: Decreased spread of malignant cells

USES: Treatment of unresectable or metastatic malignant melanoma

CONTRAINDICATIONS:

Hypersensitivity

Precautions: Pregnancy, breastfeeding, Crohn's disease, hepatitis, immunosuppression, inflammatory bowel disease, iritis, ocular disease, organ transplant, pancreatitis, renal disease, rheumatoid arthritis, sarcoidosis, systemic lupus erythematosus, thyroid disease, ulcerative colitis, uveitis

DOSAGE AND ROUTES

Adult and geriatric: IV 3 mg/kg over 90 min q3wk × 4 doses. Permanently discontinue if the full treatment course is not completed within 16 wk from first dose or for severe or life-threatening adverse reactions; withhold a dose for any moderate endocrine or immune-mediated adverse reactions; if the moderate adverse reaction completely or partially resolves (Grade 0-1) and if the patient is receiving less than 7.5 mg predniSONE or equivalent per day, resume at a dose of 3 mg/kg IV every 3 wk until all 4 planned doses or 16 wk from first dose, whichever occurs earlier; if moderate adverse reactions are persistent or if the corticosteroid dose cannot be reduced to 7.5 mg predniSONE or equivalent per day, permanently discontinue

Available forms: Solution for inj 50 mg/10 ml, 200 mg/40 ml

Implementation
Intermittent IV infusion route
• Visually inspect parenteral products for particulate matter and discoloration before using whenever solution and container permit; solution may have a pale yellow color and have translucent-to-white, amorphous particles; discard the vial if the solution is cloudy, if there is pronounced discoloration, or if particulate matter is present

• Allow vials to stand at room temperature for 5 min before infusion preparation; withdraw the required volume and transfer into an IV bag. Discard partially used vials or empty vials; dilute with 0.9% sodium chloride injection, or 5% dextrose injection, to a final concentration (1-2 mg/ml); mix diluted solution by gentle inversion; do not admix

• Give infusion over 90 min through an IV line with a low-protein binding in-line filter, do not give with other products; after each infusion, flush the line with 0.9% sodium chloride Injection, or 0.5% dextrose injection

• Store once diluted, store for no more than 24 hr refrigerated or at room temperature

ADVERSE EFFECTS
CNS: Severe and fatal immune-mediated neuropathies, fatigue, fever, headache
EENT: Episcleritis, iritis, Uveitis
ENDO: Severe and fatal immune-mediated endocrinopathies
GI: Severe and fatal immune-mediated enterocolitis, hepatitis; pancreatitis, abdominal pain, colitis, constipation, decreased appetite, diarrhea, nausea, vomiting
INTEG: Severe and fatal immune-mediated dermatitis, pruritus, rash, urticaria

MISC: Anemia, cough, dyspnea, eosino-philia, nephritis
SYST: Antibody formation, **Stevens-Johnson syndrome, toxic epidermal necrolysis**

> **BLACK BOX WARNING:** Adrenal insuf-ficiency, diarrhea, Gullain-Barré syndrome, hepatic disease, myasthenia gravis, hyper-hypothyroidism, hypopituitarism, peripheral neuropathy, serious rash

Pharmacokinetics
Absorption	Unknown
Distribution	Steady state (end of 3rd dose)
Metabolism	Unknown
Excretion	Unknown
Half-life	Terminal 14.7 days

Pharmacodynamics
Onset	Unknown
Peak	Unknown
Duration	Unknown

NURSING CONSIDERATIONS
Assessment
• **Serious skin disorders: Stevens-Johnson syndrome, toxic epidermal necrolysis: permanently discontinue in these or rash complicated by full thickness dermal ulceration or necrotic, bullous, or hemor-rhagic manifestations like bullous rash; give systemic corticosteroids at a dose of 1-2 mg/kg/day of predniSONE or equivalent; when dermatitis is controlled, taper corti-costeroids over a period of at least 1 month. Withhold in those with moderate to severe reactions;** for mild to moderate dermatitis (localized rash and pruritus), give topical or systemic corticosteroids

• **Hepatotoxicity:** Monitor liver function tests baseline and before each dose; rule out infectious or malignant causes and increase the frequency of liver function test monitoring until resolution; permanently discontinue in those with Grade 3-5 give systemic corticosteroids at a dose of 1-2 mg/kg/day of prednisone or equivalent

• **Neuropathy:** Monitor for motor or sensory neuropathy (unilateral or bilateral weakness, sensory alterations, or paresthesias) before each dose; permanently discontinue if severe neuropathy (interfering with daily activities) such as Guillain-Barré-like syndromes occur

- **Endocrinopathy:** Monitor thyroid function tests at baseline and before each dose; monitor hypophysitis, adrenal insufficiency, adrenal crisis, hyperthyroidism, hypothyroidism (fatigue, headache, mental status changes, abdominal pain, unusual bowel habits, hypotension, or nonspecific symptoms that may resemble other causes)

Patient/family education
⚠️ Instruct patient/family to report immediately allergic reaction, skin rash, severe abdominal pain, yellowing of skin, eyes; tingling of extremities, change in bowel habits
⚠️ Discuss reason for treatment and expected results

Evaluation
Positive therapeutic outcome
- Decreasing spread of malignant melanoma

ipratropium (Rx)
(i-pra-troe'pee-um)
Atrovent HFA
Func. class.: Anticholinergic, bronchodilator
Chem. class.: Synthetic quaternary ammonium compound
Pregnancy category B

Do not confuse:
Atrovent/Alupent

ACTION: Inhibits interaction of acetylcholine at receptor sites on the bronchial smooth muscle, resulting in decreased cyclic guanosine monophosphate (cyclic GMP) and bronchodilatation

Therapeutic outcome: Bronchodilatation

USES: COPD; rhinorrhea (nasal spray)

CONTRAINDICATIONS:
Hypersensitivity to this product, atropine, bromide, soybean, or peanut products

Precautions: Pregnancy **B**, breastfeeding, children <12 yr, angioedema, heart failure, surgery, acute bronchospasm, closed-angle glaucoma, prostatic hypertrophy, bladder neck obstruction, urinary retention

DOSAGE AND ROUTES
Bronchospasm in chronic bronchitis/emphysema
Adult: INH 2 sprays (17 mcg/spray) 3-4×/day, max 12 INH/24 hr, SOL 500 mcg (1 unit dose) given 3-4×/day by nebulizer; nasal spray: 2 sprays (42 mcg/spray) 3-4×/day
Child 5-12 yr: NASAL 2 sprays in each nostril 3×/day

Rhinorrhea perennial rhinitis
Adult/child ≥6 yr: INTRANASAL 2 sprays (43 mcg)/nostril bid or tid
Child 5-12 yr: INTRANASAL 2 sprays (0.03%) in each nostril 3×/day

Available forms: Aerosol 17 mcg/actuation; nasal spray 0.03%, 0.06%; sol for inh 0.0125% ♣, 0.02%

Implementation
- Give after shaking container; have patient exhale, place mouthpiece in mouth, inhale slowly, hold breath, remove, exhale slowly; allow at least 1 min between inhalations
- Give this medication before other medications and allow at least 5 min between each
Nebulizer route
- Use solution in nebulizer with a mouthpiece rather than a face mask
Intranasal route
- Prime pump, initially requires 7 actuations of the pump, priming again is not necessary if used regularly; tilt head backward after dose
- Store in light-resistant container; do not expose to temperature over 86° F (30° C)

ADVERSE EFFECTS
CNS: *Anxiety, dizziness, headache,* nervousness
CV: Palpitations
EENT: Dry mouth, blurred vision, nasal congestion
GI: *Nausea, vomiting, cramps*
INTEG: Rash
RESP: *Cough, worsening of symptoms,* bronchospasm

Pharmacokinetics
Absorption	Minimal
Distribution	Does not cross blood-brain barrier
Metabolism	Liver, minimal
Excretion	Unknown
Half-life	2 hr

Pharmacodynamics

Onset	5-15 min
Peak	1-1½ hr
Duration	3-6 hr

INTERACTIONS
Individual drugs
Disopyramide: increased anticholinergic action

Drug classifications
Antihistamines, phenothiazines: increased anticholinergic action
Bronchodilators (other): increased toxicity

Drug/herb
Belladonna: increased anticholinergic effect
Green tea (large amounts), guarana: increased bronchodilator effect

NURSING CONSIDERATIONS
Assessment
• Monitor respiratory function: vital capacity, FEV, ABGs, lung sounds, heart rate, rhythm (baseline, during treatment); if severe bronchospasm is present, a more rapid medication is required
• Monitor for evidence of allergic reactions, paradoxical bronchospasm; withhold dose and notify prescriber; identify if patient is allergic to belladonna products or atropine; allergy to this product may occur

Patient/family education
• Advise patient not to use OTC medications unless approved by prescriber; extra stimulation may occur; to use this medication before other medications and allow at least 5 min between each to prevent overstimulation
• Teach patient that compliance is necessary with number of inhalations/24 hr, or overdose may occur
• Instruct geriatric patients to use spacer device
• Teach patient the proper use of the inhaler; review package insert with patient; to avoid getting aerosol in eyes: blurring may result; to wash inhaler in warm water daily and dry; to avoid smoking, smoke-filled rooms, persons with respiratory tract infections
• Teach patient if paradoxical bronchospasm occurs to stop product immediately and notify prescriber; to limit caffeine products such as chocolate, coffee, tea, and colas
• Instruct patient on administration of dose, not to use more than prescribed; serious side effects may occur; if dose is missed, take when remembered; space other doses on new time schedule; do not double doses

• Instruct patient to "prime" the inhaler before using for the first time by releasing 2 test sprays into the air, away from the face
• Teach patient that each inhaler has 200 actuations or sprays

Evaluation
Positive therapeutic outcome
• Absence of dyspnea, wheezing after 1 hr
• Improved airway exchange
• Improved ABGs

---

irbesartan (Rx)
(er-be-sar′tan)
Avapro
Func. class.: Antihypertensive
Chem. class.: Angiotensin II receptor (type AT₁)
Pregnancy category C (1st trimester), D (2nd/3rd trimesters)

Do not confuse:
Avapro/Anaprox

ACTION: Blocks the vasoconstrictor and aldosterone-secreting effects of angiotensin II; selectively blocks the binding of angiotensin II to the AT_1 receptor found in tissues

Therapeutic outcome: Decreased B/P

USES: Hypertension, alone or in combination, nephropathy in patients with type 2 diabetes mellitus; proteinuria

Unlabeled uses: Heart failure

CONTRAINDICATIONS:
Hypersensitivity

> **BLACK BOX WARNING:** Pregnancy **D** (2nd/3rd trimesters)

Precautions: Pregnancy **C** (1st trimester), breastfeeding, children <6 yr, geriatric, renal/hepatic disease, renal artery stenosis, hypersensitivity to ACE inhibitors, African descent, angioedema

DOSAGE AND ROUTES
Hypertension
Adult: PO 150 mg/day; may be increased to 300 mg/day; volume-depleted patients: start with 75 mg/day

Nephropathy in patients with type 2 diabetes mellitus

Adult: PO maintenance dose 300 mg/day, start 75 mg/day

Available forms: Tabs 75, 150, 300 mg

Implementation
• Administer without regard to meals
• May be used with other antihypertensives, diuretic

ADVERSE EFFECTS

CNS: Dizziness, anxiety, *headache, fatigue,* syncope
CV: Hypotension
GI: *Diarrhea, dyspepsia,* hepatitis, cholestasis
HEMA: **Thrombocytopenia**
MISC: Edema, chest pain, rash, tachycardia, UTI, **angioedema,** hyperkalemia
RESP: *Cough, upper respiratory infection,* rhinitis, pharyngitis, sinus disorder

Pharmacokinetics	
Absorption	Well absorbed
Distribution	Bound to plasma proteins (90%)
Metabolism	Liver (minimal) by CYP2C9
Excretion	Feces, urine
Half-life	11-15 hr

Pharmacodynamics
Unknown

INTERACTIONS

Drug classifications
CYP2C9 inhibitors (amiodarone, delavirdine, fluconazole, FLUoxetine, fluvastatin, fluvoxaMINE, imatinib, sulfonamides, sulfinpyrazone, voriconazole, zafirlukast): increased irbesartan level
Diuretics (potassium sparing), ACE inhibitors, potassium salt substitutes: increased hyperkalemia
NSAIDs: decreased antihypertensive effect

Drug/herb
Astragalus, cola tree: increased or decreased antihypertensive effect
Black cohosh, goldenseal, hawthorn, kelp: increased antihypertensive effect
Guarana, khat, licorice, yohimbe: decreased antihypertensive effect

NURSING CONSIDERATIONS

Assessment
• Hypotension: For severe hypotension, place in supine position and give IV infusion of NS; drug may be continued after B/P is restored
• Assess B/P, pulse q4hr; note rate, rhythm, quality
• Monitor electrolytes: potassium, sodium, chloride
• Obtain baselines for renal, liver function tests before therapy begins
• Monitor for edema in feet, legs daily
• Assess for skin turgor, dryness of mucous membranes for hydration status

Patient/family education
• Advise patient to comply with dosage schedule, even if feeling better
• Inform patient that product may cause dizziness, fainting, light-headedness
• Caution patient to rise slowly to sitting or standing position to minimize orthostatic hypotension

> **BLACK BOX WARNING:** Advise patient to notify prescriber if pregnancy is suspected; pregnancy (D) 2nd/3rd trimester, (C) 1st trimester

• Teach patient not to stop product abruptly
• Teach patient to take without regard to food

Evaluation
Positive therapeutic outcome
• Decreased B/P

⚠ HIGH ALERT

irinotecan (Rx)
(ear-een-oh-tee′kan)
Camptosar
Func. class.: Antineoplastic hormone
Chem. class.: Topoisomerase inhibitor
Pregnancy category D

ACTION: Cytotoxic by producing damage to single-strand DNA during DNA synthesis, binds to topoisomerase I

Therapeutic outcome: Prevention in growth of tumor

USES: Metastatic carcinoma of colon or rectum, or 1st-line treatment in combination with fluorouracil (5-FU) and leucovorin for metastatic carcinoma of colon or rectum

---

CONTRAINDICATIONS:

Pregnancy **D**, hypersensitivity

Precautions: Breastfeeding, children, geriatric, irradiation, hepatic disease

> **BLACK BOX WARNING:** Myelosuppression, diarrhea

DOSAGE AND ROUTES

First-line treatment of colorectal cancer in combination with 5-fluorouracil: IV dosage (with bolus 5-FU/leucovorin)

Adult: IV 125 mg/m² over 90 min followed by leucovorin (20 mg/m² IV bolus) and then 5-FU (500 mg/m² IV bolus) on days 1, 8, 15, and 22; the next course begins on day 43 or when toxicity has recovered to NCI grade 1 or less

Intravenous dosage (with infusional 5-FU/leucovorin)

Adult: IV 180 mg/m² over 90 min followed by leucovorin (200 mg/m² IV over 2 hr) then 5-FU bolus and continuous infusion (400 mg/m² IV bolus, then 600 mg/m² IV infusion over 22 hr); give days 1, 15, and 29, while leucovorin and 5-FU are given on days 1, 2, 15, 16, 29, and 30; the next course begins on day 43 or when toxicity has recovered to NCI grade 1 or less

Single-agent treatment of metastatic colorectal cancer that has recurred or progressed after 5-fluorouracil-based therapy

IV route (weekly dosage schedule)
Adult: IV 125 mg/m² over 90 min qwk × 4 wk, q6wk

IV route (q3wk dosage schedule)
Adult: IV 350 mg/m² over 90 min, q3wk

Available forms: Inj 20 mg/ml

Implementation

• Use cytotoxic handling precautions

IV route
• Premedicate with antiemetic, dexamethasone 10 mg plus another antiemetic agent, such as a 5-HT₃ blocker, given at least 30 min before use
• Prior to beginning a course of therapy, the granulocyte count should be ≥1500, the platelet count ≥100,000 and treatment-related diarrhea should be fully resolved

Dilution
• Dilute appropriate dose in D₅W (preferred) or NS injection to a final concentration of 0.12-2.8 mg/ml

• Store up to 24 hr at room temperature and room lighting; because of possible microbial contamination during preparation, an admixture prepared with D₅W or NS should be used within 6 hr; solutions prepared with D₅W, refrigerated and protected from light, can be stored for up to 48 hr; avoid refrigeration if prepared with NS
Intravenous infusion
• Infuse intravenously over 90 min

ADVERSE EFFECTS

CNS: Fever, headache, chills, dizziness
CV: Vasodilatation, edema, **thromboembolism**
GI: Severe diarrhea, *nausea, vomiting,* anorexia, constipation, cramps, flatus, stomatitis, dyspepsia, **hepatotoxicity**
HEMA: Leukopenia, anemia, **neutropenia**
INTEG: Irritation at site, rash, sweating, alopecia
MISC: Asthenia, weight loss, back pain
RESP: Dyspnea, increased cough, rhinitis

Pharmacokinetics

Absorption	Complete
Distribution	Widely, 30%-68% bound to plasma proteins, increased risk of toxicity in those homozygous for UGT1A128
Metabolism	Unknown
Excretion	Urine/bile
Half-life	6-12 hr

Pharmacodynamics

Unknown

INTERACTIONS

Individual products

CarBAMazepine, PHENobarbital, phenytoin: decreased irinotecan levels
Dexamethasone: increased lymphocytopenia, hyperglycemia
Fluorouracil: increased toxicity
Prochlorperazine: increased akathisia
Radiation: increased myelosuppression, diarrhea

Drug classifications

Anticoagulants, NSAIDs: increased bleeding risk
Antineoplastics: increased myelosuppression, diarrhea
CYP3A4 inhibitors (ketoconazole): increased irinotecan levels
CYP3A4 inducers (phenytoin, carBAMazepine, PENTobarbital): decreased irinotecan levels
Diuretics: increased dehydration

Drug/herb
St. John's wort: decreased product level; avoid concurrent use

Drug/lab test
Increased: ALK phos, AST, LFTs, bilirubin
Decreased: platelets, WBC, neutrophils, Hgb/Hct

NURSING CONSIDERATIONS
Assessment
• Assess for CNS symptoms: fever, headache, chills, dizziness

> **BLACK BOX WARNING:** Assess CBC, differential, platelet count weekly; use colony-stimulating factor if WBC is <2000/mm³, platelet count is <100,000/mm³, Hgb ≤9 g/dl, neutrophils ≤1000/mm³; notify prescriber of these results, product should be discontinued and colony-stimulating factor given

• Assess buccal cavity for dryness, sores or ulceration, white patches, oral pain, bleeding, dysphagia

> **BLACK BOX WARNING:** Assess GI symptoms: frequency of stools; cramping; severe life-threatening diarrhea may occur with fluid and electrolyte imbalances; treat diarrhea within 24 hr of use with 0.25-1 mg atropine IV; treat diarrhea >24 hr of use with loperamide; diarrhea >24 hr (late diarrhea) can be fatal

• Assess early diarrhea and other cholinergic symptoms, treat with atropine; late diarrhea can be life threatening, must be treated promptly with loperimide
• Assess signs of dehydration: rapid respirations, poor skin turgor, decreased urine output; dry skin, restlessness, weakness
• Assess for bone marrow depression: bruising, bleeding, blood in stools, urine, sputum, emesis

Patient/family education
• Advise patient to avoid foods with citric acid or hot or rough texture if stomatitis is present; to drink adequate fluids
• Advise patient to report stomatitis; any bleeding, white spots, ulcerations in mouth; tell patient to examine mouth daily, report symptoms
• Advise patient to report signs of anemia: fatigue, headache, faintness, shortness of breath, irritability, infection, rash
• Advise patient to use contraception during therapy; **to report if pregnancy is planned or suspected, pregnancy (D)**
• Advise patient to avoid vaccinations while taking this product

• Instruct patient to report diarrhea that occurs 24 hr after administration; severe dehydration can occur rapidly
• Teach patient to avoid salicylates, NSAIDs, alcohol; bleeding may occur; to avoid all of these products unless approved by prescriber

Evaluation
Positive therapeutic outcome
• Decrease in tumor size, decrease in spread of cancer

iron, carbonyl
See ferrous fumarate

iron dextran (Rx)
DexFerrum, InFed
Func. class.: Hematinic
Chem. class.: Ferric hydroxide complex with dextran
Pregnancy category C

Do not confuse:
Imferon/Imuran/Roferon-A/Interferon

ACTION: Iron is carried by transferrin to the bone marrow, where it is incorporated into hemoglobin

Therapeutic outcome: Prevention and resolution of iron-deficiency anemia

USES: Iron-deficiency anemia

CONTRAINDICATIONS:

> **BLACK BOX WARNING:** Hypersensitivity

Precautions: Pregnancy **C**, breastfeeding, infants <4 mo, children, acute renal disease, asthma, rheumatoid arthritis (**IV**), all anemias excluding iron-deficiency anemia, hepatic/cardiac/renal disease, neonates, ankylosing spondylitis, lupus, hypotension

DOSAGE AND ROUTES
Adult and child: IM 0.5 ml as a test dose by Z-track, then no more than the following total dose including test dose per day:
Adult/adolescent/child >15 kg: IM 100 mg/day
Child 10-15 kg: IM 100 mg/kg
Child/infant >4 mo (5-9.9 kg): IM 50 mg/day
Infant >4 mo (<5 kg): IM 25 mg/day

Total dose (in ml):

$$[0.0442 \times (\text{desired Hb} - \text{observed Hb}) \times \text{LBW}] + (0.26 \times \text{LBW})$$

(LBW = lean body weight in kg)

Available forms: Inj IM/IV 50 mg/ml (2 ml, 10 ml vials)

Implementation
IM route
• Discontinue oral iron before parenteral; give only after test dose of 25 mg by preferred route; wait at least 1 hr before giving remaining portion
• Give IM inj deep in large muscle mass; use Z-track method and 19-G, 20-G 2-, 3-inch needle; ensure needle is long enough to place product deep in muscle; change needles after withdrawing medication and injecting to prevent skin and tissue staining

IV route
• Give IV after flushing tubing with 10 ml of 0.9% NaCl; give undiluted; give 1 ml (50 mg) or less over 1 min or more; flush line after use with 10 ml of 0.9% NaCl; patient should remain recumbent for 30-60 min to prevent orthostatic hypotension
• IV inj requires single-dose vial without preservative; verify on label IV use is approved
• Give by cont inf after diluting in 50-250 ml of 0.9% NaCl for inf; administer over 4-5 hr
• Give only with epinephrine available in case of anaphylactic reaction during dose
• Store at room temperature in cool environment

ADVERSE EFFECTS
CNS: Headache, paresthesia, dizziness, shivering, weakness, **seizures**
CV: Chest pain, **shock,** hypotension, tachycardia
GI: *Nausea,* vomiting, metallic taste, abdominal pain
HEMA: Leukocytosis
INTEG: Rash, pruritus, urticaria, fever, sweating, chills, brown skin discoloration, pain at inj site, necrosis, sterile abscesses, phlebitis
MISC: Anaphylaxis
RESP: Dyspnea

Absorption	Well absorbed; lymphatics over wk or mo
Distribution	Crosses placenta
Metabolism	Slow; blood loss, desquamation
Excretion	Breast milk, feces, urine, bile
Half-life	6 hr

Unknown

INTERACTIONS
Individual drugs
Chloramphenicol: decreased reticulocyte response
Oral iron: do not use together, increased toxicity

Drug/lab test
False increase: serum bilirubin
False decrease: serum calcium
False positive: ^{99m}Tc diphosphate bone scan, iron test (large doses >2 ml)

NURSING CONSIDERATIONS
Assessment
• Observe for 1 hr after test dose
• Monitor blood studies: Hct, Hgb, reticulocytes, transferrin, plasma iron concentrations, ferritin, total iron-binding bilirubin before treatment, at least monthly

> **BLACK BOX WARNING:** Assess for allergic reaction and anaphylaxis; rash, pruritus, fever, chills, wheezing; notify prescriber immediately, keep emergency equipment available

• Assess cardiac status: anginal pain, hypotension, tachycardia
• Assess for nutrition: amount of iron in diet (meat, dark green leafy vegetables, dried fruits, eggs); cause of iron loss or anemia, including salicylates, sulfonamides
• Monitor pulse, B/P during IV administration
• Assess for toxicity: nausea, vomiting, diarrhea, fever, abdominal pain (early symptoms); cyanotic lips, nailbeds, seizures, CV collapse (late symptoms)

Patient/family education
• Caution patient that iron poisoning may occur if increased beyond recommended level; to not take oral iron preparation or vitamins containing iron unless approved by prescriber
• Advise patient that delayed reaction may occur 1-2 days after administration and last 3-4

Adverse effects: *italics* = common; **bold** = life-threatening

days (**IV**) or 3-7 days (**IM**); report fever, chills, malaise, muscle/joint aches, nausea, vomiting, backache

- Advise patient to avoid breastfeeding
- Advise patient that stools may become dark

Evaluation
Positive therapeutic outcome
- Increased serum iron levels, Hct, Hgb

TREATMENT OF OVERDOSE:
Discontinue product, treat allergic reaction, give diphenhydrAMINE or EPINEPHrine as needed for anaphylaxis; give iron-chelating product in acute poisoning

---

iron polysaccharide
See ferrous fumarate

iron sucrose (Rx)
Venofer
Func. class.: Hematinic
Chem. class.: Ferric hydroxide complex with dextran
Pregnancy category B

ACTION: Iron is carried by transferrin to the bone marrow, where it is incorporated into hemoglobin

Therapeutic outcome: Improved signs/symptoms of iron deficiency anemia; iron levels improved

USES: Iron deficiency anemia

Unlabeled uses: Dystrophic epidermolysis bullosa (DEB)

CONTRAINDICATIONS:
Hypersensitivity, all anemias excluding iron deficiency anemia, iron overload

Precautions: Pregnancy **B**, breastfeeding (**IV**), children, geriatric, abdominal pain, anaphylactic shock, arthralgia, chest pain, cough, diarrhea, dizziness, dyspnea, edema, increased LFTs, fever, headache, heart failure, hyper/hypotension, infection, MS pain, nausea/vomiting, seizures, weakness

DOSAGE AND ROUTES
Adult: **IV** 5 ml (100 mg of elemental iron) given during dialysis, most will need 1000 mg of elemental iron over 10 sequential dialysis sessions

Available forms: Inj 20 mg/ml

Implementation
⚠ Give only with epinephrine, solu-medrol in case of anaphylactic reaction during dose
- Do not use if particulate is present, or if sol is discolored

IV route
- Give directly in dialysis line by slow inj or inf; give by slow inj at 1 ml/min (5 min/vial); inf dilute each vial exclusively in a maximum of 100 ml of 0.9% NaCl, give at rate of 100 mg of iron/15 min, discard unused portions
- Store at room temperature in cool environment, do not freeze
- Do not use with other IV products

ADVERSE EFFECTS
CNS: Headache, dizziness
CV: Chest pain, hypo/hypertension, hypervolemia, **heart failure**
GI: *Nausea, vomiting, abdominal pain*
INTEG: Rash, pruritus, urticaria, fever, sweating, chills
MISC: **Anaphylaxis,** hyperglycemia
RESP: Dyspnea, pneumonia, cough

Pharmacokinetics

Absorption	Unknown
Distribution	Unknown
Metabolism	Unknown
Excretion	Urine
Half-life	6 hr

Pharmacodynamics
Unknown

INTERACTIONS
Individual drugs
Chloramphenicol: decreased iron sucrose
Dimercaprol, iron (oral): increased toxicity; do not use together

Drug/lab test
Increased: glucose

NURSING CONSIDERATIONS
Assessment
- Monitor blood studies: Hct, Hgb, reticulocytes, transferrin, plasma iron concentrations, ferritin, total iron binding, bilirubin before treatment, at least monthly
- Assess for allergy: anaphylaxis, rash, pruritus, fever, chills, wheezing; notify prescriber immediately, keep emergency equipment available
- Assess cardiac status: hypotension, hypertension, hypervolemia

---

• Assess for toxicity: nausea, vomiting, diarrhea, fever, abdominal pain (early symptoms), cyanotic-looking lips and nailbeds, seizures, CV collapse (late symptoms)

Patient/family education
• Teach patient that iron poisoning may occur if increased beyond recommended level; not to take oral iron preparations
• Teach patient to report itching, rash, chest pain, headache, vertigo, nausea, vomiting, abdominal pain, joint/muscle pain, numbness, tingling

Evaluation
Positive therapeutic outcome
• Increased serum iron levels, Hct, Hgb

TREATMENT OF OVERDOSE:
Discontinue product, treat allergic reaction, give diphenhydrAMINE or epinephrine as needed, give iron-chelating product in acute poisoning

isoflurophate ophthalmic
See Appendix B

isoniazid (Rx)
(eye-soe-nye′a-zid)
Isotamine ✦
Func. class.: Antitubercular
Chem. class.: Isonicotinic acid hydrazide
Pregnancy category C

ACTION: Bactericidal interference with lipid, nucleic acid biosynthesis

Therapeutic outcome: Resolution of TB infection

USES: Treatment, prevention of TB

CONTRAINDICATIONS:
Hypersensitivity

> **BLACK BOX WARNING:** Acute liver disease

Precautions: Pregnancy **C,** diabetic retinopathy, cataracts, ocular defects, renal disease, **IV** drug users, people >35 yr, postpartum period, HIV, neuropathy

> **BLACK BOX WARNING:** Female (African descent, Hispanic), alcoholism

DOSAGE AND ROUTES
Treatment
Adult/adolescent with or without HIV: PO/IM 5 mg/kg/day up to 300 mg/day or 15 mg/kg 2-3 ×/week, max 900 mg 2-3 ×/wk
Child and infant HIV positive: PO/IM 10-15 mg/kg/day; max 300 mg/day

Available forms: Tabs 100, 300 mg; inj 100 mg/ml

Implementation
• Give antiemetic for vomiting
• Provide a list of foods to avoid while taking this product
PO route
• Give with meals to decrease GI symptoms; absorption is better when taken on empty stomach, 1 hr before or 2 hr after meals
IM route
• Give inj deep in large muscle mass, massage; rotate inj sites, warm inj to room temperature to dissolve crystals

ADVERSE EFFECTS
Hypersensitivity: Fever, skin eruptions, lymphadenopathy, vasculitis
CNS: *Peripheral neuropathy, dizziness,* memory impairment, **toxic encephalopathy, seizures,** psychosis, slurred speech
EENT: Blurred vision, optic neuritis
GI: *Nausea, vomiting,* epigastric distress, **jaundice, fatal hepatitis**
HEMA: Agranulocytosis, hemolytic anemia, aplastic anemia, thrombocytopenia, eosinophilia, methemoglobinemia
MISC: Dyspnea, vit B$_6$ deficiency, pellagra, hyperglycemia, metabolic acidosis, gynecomastia, rheumatic syndrome, systemic lupus erythematosus–like syndrome

Pharmacokinetics
Absorption	Well absorbed
Distribution	Widely
Metabolism	Liver
Excretion	Kidneys
Half-life	1-4 hr

Pharmacodynamics
	PO	IM
Onset	Rapid	Rapid
Peak	1-2 hr	45-60 min
Duration	6-8 hr	6-8 hr

INTERACTIONS
Individual drugs
Alcohol, carBAMazepine, cycloSERINE, ethionamide, meperidine, phenytoin, rifampin, warfarin: increased toxicity

BCG vaccine, ketoconazole: decreased effectiveness

Drug classifications
Antacids, aluminum: decreased absorption

Benzodiazepines: increased toxicity

SSRIs, SNRIs: increased serotonin syndrome

Drug/food
Tyramine foods: increased toxicity

Drug/lab test
Increased: LFTs, bilirubin, glucose

Decreased: platelets, granulocytes

NURSING CONSIDERATIONS
Assessment
• Obtain C&S tests, including sputum tests, before treatment; monitor every mo to detect resistance

> **BLACK BOX WARNING:** Monitor liver function tests weekly; obtain baseline in all patients, those >35 yr and all women should be monitored periodically; monitor ALT, AST, bilirubin; increased results may indicate hepatitis; renal studies during treatment, monthly: BUN, creatinine, output, specific gravity, urinalysis, uric acid; those with fast acetylation (genetic) may metabolize product more than 5 times faster (Black, Asian, and some Caucasians are at greater risk); fatal hepatitis is a greater risk in Blacks/Hispanics after birth

• Assess mental status often: affect, mood, behavioral changes; psychosis may occur with hallucinations, confusion

• Assess hepatic status: decreased appetite, jaundice, dark urine, fatigue

• Assess for visual disturbance that may indicate optic neuritis: blurred vision, change in color perception; may lead to blindness

Patient/family education
• Instruct patient that compliance with dosage schedule for duration is necessary; not to skip or double doses; that scheduled appointments must be kept or relapse may occur

• Caution patient to avoid alcohol while taking product or hepatotoxicity may result; to avoid ingestion of aged cheeses, fish or hypertensive crisis may result; give patient written directions on which foods to avoid while taking this medication

• Tell patient to report peripheral neuritis: weakness, tingling/numbness of hands/feet, fatigue; hepatotoxicity: loss of appetite, nausea, vomiting, jaundice of skin or eyes

> **BLACK BOX WARNING: Fatal hepatitis:** teach patient to notify prescriber immediately of yellow skin/eyes, dark urine, loss of appetite

Evaluation
Positive therapeutic outcome
• Decreased symptoms of TB
• Culture negative for TB

TREATMENT OF OVERDOSE:
Pyridoxine

---

isosorbide dinitrate (Rx)
(eye-soe-sor'bide)
Apo-ISDN ✦, Dilatrate-SR, Isochren, IsoDitrate, Isordil
isosorbide mononitrate (Rx)
Apo-ISMN ✦, Imdur
Func. class.: Antianginal, vasodilator
Chem. class.: Nitrate
Pregnancy category C

Do not confuse:
Imdur/Imuran/Inderal/K-Dur

ACTION: Relaxation of vascular smooth muscle, which leads to decreased preload, afterload, thus decreasing left ventricular end-diastolic pressure, and systemic vascular resistance and reducing cardiac O_2 demand

Therapeutic outcome: Relief and prevention of angina pectoris

USES: Treatment, prevention of chronic stable angina pectoris

CONTRAINDICATIONS:
Hypersensitivity to this product or nitrates, severe anemia, closed-angle glaucoma

Precautions: Pregnancy **C**, breastfeeding, children, orthostatic hypotension, MI, CHF, severe renal/hepatic disease, increased ICP, cerebral hemorrhage, acute MI, geriatrics, GI disease, syncope

---

DOSAGE AND ROUTES
Dinitrate
Adult: PO 5-20 mg bid-tid, initially, maintenance 10-40 mg bid-tid; SL buccal tab 2.5-5 mg; may repeat q5-10min × 3 doses; ext rel 40-80 mg q8-12hr, max 160 mg/day

Mononitrate
Adult: PO (Monoket) 10-20 mg bid, 7 hr apart; (Imdur) initiate at 30-60 mg/day as a single dose, increase q3day as needed; may increase to 120 mg/day; max 240 mg/day

Available forms: Dinitrate: sus rel caps 40 mg; SR tabs 40 mg; tabs 5, 10, 20, 30, 40 mg; SL tabs 2.5, 5 mg; chew tabs 5, 10 mg; mononitrate: tabs (Monoket) 10, 20 mg; ext rel tabs (Imdur) 30, 60, 120 mg

Implementation
PO route
- Swallow sus rel cap and ext rel tab whole; do not break, crush, or chew
- Do not swallow SL tab; tab should be dissolved under tongue
- Chew tab should be chewed thoroughly
- Give 1 hr before or 2 hr after meals with 8 oz of water

SL route
- Hold SL tab under tongue until dissolved (a few min); do not take anything PO when SL tab is in place

ADVERSE EFFECTS
CNS: *Vascular headache, flushing, dizziness,* weakness
CV: *Orthostatic hypotension,* tachycardia, **collapse,** syncope
GI: Nausea, vomiting
INTEG: Pallor, sweating, rash
MISC: Twitching, hemolytic anemia, **methemoglobinemia,** tolerance, xerostomia

Pharmacokinetics

Absorption	Well absorbed
Distribution	Unknown
Metabolism	Liver
Excretion	Urine, metabolites
Half-life	Dinitrate 1 hr, mononitrate 5 hr

Pharmacodynamics

	Sus rel	SL	PO
Onset	Up to 4 hr	2-5 min	15-30 min
Peak	Unknown	Unknown	Unknown
Duration	5 hr	2 hr	5-6 hr

INTERACTIONS
Individual drugs
Alcohol: increased hypotension
Rosiglitazone: increased myocardial ischemia; avoid concurrent use
⚠ **Sildenafil, tadalafil, vardenafil: fatal hypotension, do not use together**

Drug classifications
Antihypertensives, β-adrenergic blockers, calcium channel blockers, diuretics, phenothiazines: increased hypotension
Sympathomimetics: increased heart rate, B/P

NURSING CONSIDERATIONS
Assessment
- **Assess for pain:** duration, time started, activity being performed, character, intensity
⚠ **Methemoglobinemia (rare): assess for cyanosis of lips, nausea/vomiting, coma, shock; usually caused by high dose of product, but may occur with normal dosing**
- Monitor for orthostatic B/P, pulse at baseline, during treatment and periodically thereafter

Patient/family education
- Teach patient that tolerance may occur if taken over long periods; to prevent, allow intervals of 12-14 hr/day without product
- Advise patient to treat headache with OTC analgesics
- Instruct patient to not skip or double doses; if dose is missed take when remembered if 2 hr before next dose (dinitrate), 6 hr before next dose (sus rel), or 8 hr before next dose (mononitrate)
- Caution patient to avoid alcohol and OTC medications unless approved by prescriber
- Inform patient that product may be taken before stressful activity: exercise, sexual activity
- Advise patient that SL tab may sting mucous membranes
- Caution patient to avoid driving and hazardous activities if dizziness occurs
- Advise patient to comply with complete medical regimen
- Caution patient to make position changes slowly to prevent orthostatic hypotension

---

⚠ Teach patient not to use with sildenafil, tadalafil, vardenafil with nitrates; may cause serious drop in B/P

⚠ Teach patient not to discontinue abruptly; may cause heart attack

⚠ Teach patient to use at beginning of angina symptoms, may repeat every 15 min; if no relief seek medical attention immediately

Evaluation

Positive therapeutic outcome
- Decrease in, prevention of anginal pain

---

itraconazole (Rx)

(it-tra-kon′a-zol)

Onmel, Sporanox

Func. class.: Antifungal (systemic)
Chem. class.: Triazole derivative

Pregnancy category C

ACTION: Alters cell membranes and inhibits several fungal enzymes

Therapeutic outcome: Fungistatic against *Histoplasma capsulatum, Blastomyces dermatitis, Cryptococcus neoformans, Aspergillus fumigatus, Candida*

USES: Histoplasmosis, blastomycosis (pulmonary and extrapulmonary), aspergillosis onychomycosis of toenail/fingernail

Unlabeled uses: Dermatomycosis, chromoblastomycosis, coccidioidomycosis, pityriasis versicolor, sebopsoriasis, vaginal candidiasis, cryptococcal, subcutaneous mycoses, dimorphic infections, fungal keratitis, alternariosis, zygomycosis

CONTRAINDICATIONS:

Hypersensitivity, fungal meningitis, onychomycosis, or dermatomycosis in cardiac dysfunction; in pregnant women (pregnancy **C**)

> **BLACK BOX WARNING:** Heart failure, ventricular dysfunction, coadministration with other drugs

Precautions: Pregnancy **C**, breastfeeding, children, cardiac/renal/hepatic disease, achlorhydria or hypochlorhydria (product-induced), dialysis, hearing loss, cystic fibrosis neuropathy

DOSAGE AND ROUTES

Dose varies with type of infection
Adult: PO 200 mg/day with food; may increase to 400 mg/day if needed; life-threatening infections may require a loading dose of 200 mg tid × 3 days
Child: PO 2-10 mg/kg/day

Available forms: Caps 100 mg; oral sol 10 mg/ml; tab 200 mg

Implementation
PO route
- Swallow caps whole; do not break, crush, or chew
- Give caps after full meal to ensure absorption
- Give with food or milk to prevent nausea and vomiting
- Take 2 hr before administration of other products that increase gastric pH
- Store in tight container at room temperature; do not freeze
- *Oral sol and caps are not interchangeable on a mg/mg basis*
- **Oral sol:** patient should swish in mouth vigorously

ADVERSE EFFECTS

CNS: Headache, dizziness, insomnia, somnolence, depression
CV: Hypertension, CHF
GI: Nausea, vomiting, anorexia, diarrhea, cramps, *abdominal pain,* flatulence, **GI bleeding, hepatotoxicity**
GU: Gynecomastia, impotence, decreased libido
INTEG: Pruritus, fever, rash, **toxic epidermal necrolysis, Stevens-Johnson syndrome**
MISC: Edema, fatigue, malaise, hypokalemia, tinnitus, **rhabdomyolysis**
RESP: Rhinitis, sinusitis, upper respiratory infection, pulmonary edema

Pharmacokinetics

Absorption	Variable
Distribution	Tissue, plasma, CSF, 99.8% protein bound
Metabolism	Liver, extensively, inhibits CYP4503A enzyme
Excretion	Feces, breast milk
Half-life	IV 35.4 hr; terminal 29.4 hr; PO 64 hr; pediatric 35.8 hr

Pharmacodynamics

Onset	Unknown
Peak	4 hr
Duration	Unknown

INTERACTIONS
Individual drugs
BusPIRone: increased busPIRone levels, toxicity

Busulfan, clarithromycin, cycloSPORINE, atorvastatin, carBAMazepine, disopyramide, QUEtiapine, diazepam, digoxin, felodipine, fentaNYL, indinavir, isradipine, niCARdipine, NIFEdipine, nimoldipine, phenytoin, ritonavir, saquinavir, tacrolimus, warfarin: increased toxicity

CarBAMazepine, isoniazid: decreased itraconazole action

Didanosine: decreased antifungal action

Dofetilide, **dronedarone,** levomethadyl, pimozide, quiNIDine: life-threatening CV reaction

ALPRAZolam, clorazepate, clorazepine, diazepam, estazolam, flurazepam, midazolam (oral), triazolam: increased sedation

QuiNIDine: increased tinnitus, hearing loss, increased toxicity

Rifamycins: decreased action of itraconazole

Drug classifications
Antacids, H$_2$-receptor antagonists: decreased action of itraconazole

Calcium channel blockers: increased edema

Contraceptives (oral): decreased effect

Proton pump inhibitors: decreased itraconazole action

Hepatotoxic products: hepatotoxicity

Oral hypoglycemics: increased effects of oral hypoglycemics

Drug/food
Increased: absorption

Drug/lab test
Increased: LFTs

NURSING CONSIDERATIONS
Assessment
• Assess for infection: WBC, sputum baseline, periodically, may start treatment before obtaining results

⚠ **Monitor for hepatotoxicity: increasing AST, ALT, alkaline phosphatase, bilirubin**

• Monitor for allergic reaction: dermatitis, rash; product should be discontinued, antihistamines (mild reaction) or epinephrine (severe reaction) administered; check inj site for thrombophlebitis

• Monitor for hypokalemia, check potassium level: anorexia, drowsiness, weakness, decreased reflexes, dizziness, increased urinary output, increased thirst, paresthesias; if these occur, product should be decreased or discontinued and potassium administered

Patient/family education
• Advise patient that long-term therapy may be needed to clear infection (1 wk-6 mo depending on type of infection)

• Teach patient side effects and when to notify prescriber

• Instruct patient to avoid hazardous activities if dizziness occurs

• Instruct patient to take 2 hr before administration of other products that increase gastric pH (antacids, H$_2$-blockers, omeprazole, sucralfate, anticholinergics)

• Teach patient importance of compliance with product regimen

• Instruct patient to notify prescriber of GI symptoms, signs of liver dysfunction (fatigue, jaundice, nausea, anorexia, vomiting, dark urine, pale stools)

Evaluation
Positive therapeutic outcome
• Decreased fever, malaise, rash
• Negative C&S for infectious organism

RARELY USED
ivacaftor
(eye′va-kaf′tor)
Kalydeco
Func. class.: Respiratory agent
Pregnancy category B

USES: Cystic fibrosis in those with G551D mutation in the *CFTR* gene

DOSAGE AND ROUTES
Renal dose
Adult/adolescent/child ≥6 yr: PO 150 mg every 12 hr with fat-containing food

ixabepilone (Rx)
(ix-ab-ep′i-lone)
Ixempra
Func. class.: Antineoplastic—miscellaneous
Chem. class.: Epothilone
Pregnancy category D

ACTION: Microtubule stabilizing agent; microtubules are needed for cell division

Therapeutic outcome: Decreased tumor size, decreased spread of malignancy

USES: Breast cancer

CONTRAINDICATIONS:

Pregnancy **D**, hypersensitivity to products with polyoxyethylated castor oil, breastfeeding, neutropenia $<1500/mm^3$, thrombocytopenia $<100,000/mm^3$

BLACK BOX WARNING: Hepatic disease

Precautions: Children, geriatric, alcoholism, bone marrow suppression, cardiac dysrhythmias, cardiac/renal disease, diabetes mellitus, peripheral neuropathy, ventricular dysfunction

DOSAGE AND ROUTES

Breast cancer, metastatic or locally advanced given with capecitabine, and resistant to anthracycline, taxane

Adult: IV INF 40 mg/m^2 over 3 hr q3wk plus capecitabine PO 2000 mg/m^2/day in 2 divided doses on days 1-14 q21day; in those with BSA >2.2 m^2, dose should be calculated for a BSA of 2.2 m^2

Breast cancer, metastatic or locally advanced resistant/refractory to anthracyclines, taxanes, capecitabine

Adult: IV INF 40 mg/m^2 over 3 hr q3wk; in those with BSA >2.2 m^2, dose should be calculated for a BSA of 2.2 m^2

Dosage reduction in those taking a strong CYP3A4 inhibitor

Adult: IV INF 20 mg/m^2 over 3 hr q3wk

Available forms: Powder for inj 15, 45 mg

Implementation
• Premedicate with histamine antagonists 1 hr prior to use, prevents hypersensitivity
• Give antiemetic 30-60 min before giving product and prn

IV route
• Let kit stand at room temperature for 30 min; to reconstitute, withdraw supplied diluent (8 ml for 15 mg vials, 23.5 ml for 45 mg vials); slowly inject solution into vial; gently swirl and invert to mix, final conc 2 mg/ml; further dilute in LR in DEHP-free bags; final conc should be 0.2-0.6 mg/ml; after added, mix by manual rotation
• Diluted sol is stable for 6 hr at room temperature; inf must be completed within 6 hr
• Use in-line filter 0.2-1.2 mcm
• Give over 3 hr

ADVERSE EFFECTS

CNS: *Peripheral neuropathy,* chills, fatigue, fever, flushing, headache, insomnia, impaired cognition, asthenia
CV: Bradycardia, *hypotension,* abnormal ECG, angina, atrial flutter, cardiomyopathy, chest pain, edema, MI, vasculitis
GI: *Nausea, vomiting, diarrhea,* abdominal pain, anorexia, colitis, constipation, gastritis, jaundice, GERD, **hepatic failure,** trismus
GU: Renal failure
HEMA: Neutropenia, thrombocytopenia, anemia, infections, coagulopathy
INTEG: *Alopecia,* rash, hot flashes
META: Hypokalemia, metabolic acidosis
MS: *Arthralgia, myalgia*
RESP: Bronchospasm, cough, dyspnea
SYST: *Hypersensitivity reactions,* anaphylaxis, dehydration, **radiation recall reaction**

Pharmacokinetics

Absorption	Unknown
Distribution	Unknown
Metabolism	Liver by CYP3A4
Excretion	Feces 65%, urine 21%
Half-life	Terminal 52 hr

Pharmacodynamics

Unknown

INTERACTIONS

Drug classifications
CYP3A4 inducers (aminoglutethimide, barbiturates, bexarotene, bosentan, carBAMazepine, dexamethasone, efavirenz, griseofulvin, modafinil, nafcillin, nevirapine, OXcarbazepine, phenytoin, rifamycin, topiramate): decreased ixabepilone levels
CYP3A4 inhibitors (amiodarone, amprenavir, aprepitant, atazanavir, chloramphenicol, clarithromycin, conivaptan, cycloSPORINE, danazol, darunavir, dalforpristan, delavirdine, diltiazem, erythromycin, estradiol, fluconazole, fluvoxaMINE, fosamprenavir, imatinib, indinavir, isoniazid, itraconazole, ketoconazole, lopinavir, miconazole, nefazodone, nelfinavir, propoxyphene, ritonavir, RU-486, saquinavir, tamoxifen, telithromycin, troleandomycin, verapamil, voriconazole, zafirlukast): increased ixabepilone level

Drug/herb
St. John's wort: avoid use

Drug/food
Grapefruit products: avoid use

Drug/lab test

Increased: LFTs, bilirubin

Decreased: platelets, neutrophils, RBC, potassium

NURSING CONSIDERATIONS
Assessment

• Monitor CBC, differential, platelet count prior to therapy, qwk; withhold product if WBC is <1500/mm³ or platelet count is <100,000/mm³, notify prescriber

• Monitor temp q4hr (may indicate beginning infection)

> **BLACK BOX WARNING:** Monitor liver function tests before, during therapy (bilirubin, AST, ALT, LDH) prn or qmo; check for jaundiced skin and sclera, dark urine, clay-colored stools, itchy skin, abdominal pain, fever, diarrhea

• Monitor VS during 1st hr of inf; check IV site for signs of infiltration

• **Cardiac ischemia:** Monitor cardiac function in those with cardiac function that is impaired; chest pain, ECG changes may occur

⚠ **Assess for hypersensitive reactions, anaphylaxis including hypotension, dyspnea, angioedema, generalized urticaria;** discontinue inf immediately; keep emergency equipment available

• Assess effects of alopecia on body image; discuss feelings about body changes

Patient/family education

• Teach patient to report signs of infection: fever, sore throat, flulike symptoms

• Teach patient to report signs of anemia: fatigue, headache, faintness, shortness of breath

• Teach patient to report any complaints or side effects to nurse or prescriber

• Caution patient that hair may be lost during treatment; a wig or hairpiece may make patient feel better; new hair may be different in color, texture

• Advise patient that pain in muscles and joints 2-5 days after inf is common

• Advise patient to use nonhormonal type of contraception

• Instruct patient to avoid receiving vaccinations while on this product

Evaluation
Positive therapeutic outcome

• Decreased tumor size, decreased spread of malignancy

ketoconazole (Rx)

(kee-toe-koe′na-zole)

Func. class.: Antifungal

Chem. class.: Imidazole derivative

Pregnancy category C

ACTION: Alters cell membrane and inhibits several fungal enzymes leading to cell death

Therapeutic outcome: Fungistatic/fungicidal against susceptible organisms: *Blastomycoses, Candida, Coccidioides, Cryptococcus, Histoplasma;* topical route: tinea cruris, tinea corporis, tinea versicolor, *Pityrosporum ovale*

USES: Systemic candidiasis, chronic mucocandidiasis, oral thrush, candiduria, coccidioidomycosis, histoplasmosis, chromomycosis, paracoccidioidomycosis, blastomycosis, tinea cruris, tinea corporis, tinea versicolor, *Pityrosporum ovale*

Unlabeled uses: Cushing's syndrome, advanced prostatic cancer

CONTRAINDICATIONS:

Breastfeeding, hypersensitivity, fungal meningitis

> **BLACK BOX WARNING:** Coadministration with other drugs; ergot derivatives, cisapride, or triazolam may cause fatal cardiac arrhythmias due to inhibition of CYP3A4 enzyme system

Precautions: Pregnancy **C**, children <2 yr, renal disease, achlorhydria (product induced)

> **BLACK BOX WARNING:** Hepatic disease

DOSAGE AND ROUTES

Adult: PO 200-400 mg once/day for 1-2 wk (candidiasis), 6 wk (other infections); 400 mg tid (prostate cancer, unlabeled)

Child >2 yr: 3.3-6.6 mg/kg/day as single daily dose

Available forms: Tabs 200 mg; oral susp ✿ 100 mg/5 ml topical (see Appendix B)

Implementation

PO route

• Give in the presence of acid products only; do not use alkaline products, proton pump inhibitors, H$_2$-antagonists, or antacids within 2 hr of product; may give coffee, tea, acidic fruit juices, cola; give with food to decrease GI symptoms; dissolve tab/4 ml of aqueous sol 0.2 N HCl, use straw to avoid contact, rinse with water afterward and swallow

• Give with HCl if achlorhydria is present

• Store in tight container at room temperature

Topical route

• Use enough medication to cover fungally infected and surrounding area; rub in; do not use occlusive dressing; do not get in eyes

Shampoo

• Hair should be wet; apply shampoo, lather, rub gently into scalp and hair for 1 min; rinse; reapply × 3 min; continue treatment 2 ×/wk for 1 mo, no more than once q3day

• Store in tight container at room temp

ADVERSE EFFECTS

CNS: Headache, dizziness, somnolence

GI: Nausea, vomiting, anorexia, diarrhea, abdominal pain, **hepatotoxicity**

GU: Gynecomastia, impotence

HEMA: **Thrombocytopenia, leukopenia, hemolytic anemia**

INTEG: Pruritus, fever, chills, photophobia, rash, dermatitis, purpura, urticaria

SYST: **Anaphylaxis**

Pharmacokinetics

Absorption	pH dependent; decreased pH, increased absorption
Distribution	Widely distributed; crosses placenta
Metabolism	Liver, partially
Excretion	Feces, bile, breast milk
Half-life	Biphasic: 2 hr, 8 hr

Pharmacodynamics

Onset	Unknown
Peak	1-3 hr
Duration	Unknown

INTERACTIONS

Individual drugs

Alcohol: increased hepatotoxicity

Alfentanil, ALPRAZolam, amprenavir, ARIPiprazole, atorvastatin, carBAMazepine, cerivastatin, clarithromycin, cyclophosphamide, cycloSPORINE, donepezil, eletriptan, erythromycin, fentaNYL, ifosfamide, indinavir, lovastatin, midazolam, nelfinavir, nisoldipine, quiNIDine, ritonavir, saquinavir, sildenafil, simvastatin, SUFentanil, tamoxifen, triazolam, vinBLAStine, vinCRIStine, zolpidem: increased toxicity, inhibition of CYP3A4 pathway

---

ChlordiazePOXIDE, clonazePAM, clorazepate, diazepam, estazolam, flurazepam,
prazepam, quazepam: increased effect of
CNS depression; avoid concurrent use
ddI, isoniazid, phenytoin, rifampin: decreased
effect of ketoconazole
Paclitaxel: inhibited metabolism
Theophylline: decreased effectiveness
Warfarin: increased effects of warfarin

Drug classifications
**Antacids, anticholinergics, gastric acid
pump inhibitors, H₂-receptor agonists:
decreased ketoconazole action**
Anticoagulants (oral): increased effects of oral
anticoagulants
**Calcium channel blockers, corticosteroids,
vinca alkaloids: increased effect, toxicity**
Hepatotoxic agents: increased hepatotoxicity

Drug/lab test
Increased: alkaline phosphatase, LFTs, lipids
Decreased: Hgb, WBC, platelets

NURSING CONSIDERATIONS
Assessment
• Assess for signs and symptoms of infection:
drainage, sore throat, urinary pain, hematuria,
fever
• Obtain cultures for C&S before beginning
treatment; therapy may be started after culture is
taken

> **BLACK BOX WARNING: Monitor for
> hepatotoxicity:** increased AST, ALT, alkaline
> phosphatase, bilirubin; discontinue product
> if hepatotoxicity occurs; nausea, vomiting,
> jaundice, clay-colored stools, fatigue

• Use cautiously in those with hepatic disease
⚠ **Using with CYP3A4 inhibitors can lead to
increased product level, toxicity**

Patient/family education
• Advise patient that long-term therapy may be
needed to clear infection (1 wk-6 mo depending
on infection)
• Advise patient to avoid hazardous activities if
dizziness occurs
• Instruct patient to take 2 hr before administration of other products that increase gastric
pH (antacids, H₂-blockers, omeprazole, sucralfate, anticholinergics)
• Stress the importance of compliance with
product regimen, that testing will be done
periodically to indicate infection has been
eradicated

• Instruct patient to divide dose with meals to
decrease nausea
• Instruct patient not to use any products (OTC,
herbal) unless approved by prescriber

> **BLACK BOX WARNING:** Advise patient to
> notify prescriber of GI symptoms, signs of liver
> dysfunction (fatigue, nausea, anorexia, vomit-
> ing, dark urine, pale stools)

• Teach patient proper hygiene: hand washing,
nail care, use of concomitant topical agents if
prescribed
• Caution patient to avoid alcohol, since nausea,
vomiting, hypertension may occur
• Advise patient to use sunscreen or avoid
direct sunlight to prevent photosensitivity
• Advise patient to notify prescriber of sore
throat, fever, skin rash, which may indicate
superinfection
• Advise patient to use sunglasses to prevent
photophobia (rare)
• Teach patient to notify prescriber if pregnancy
is planned or suspected, and not to breastfeed

Evaluation
Positive therapeutic outcome
• Decreased oral candidiasis, fever, malaise,
rash
• Negative C&S for infectious organism
• Absence of dandruff, scaling

ketoconazole topical
See Appendix B

ketoprofen (OTC, Rx)
(ke-to-proe'fen)
Apo-Keto ✦
Func. class.: NSAID; nonopioid analgesic,
antirheumatic
Chem. class.: Propionic acid derivative
**Pregnancy category C (1st trimester),
D (2nd/3rd trimesters)**

ACTION: Inhibits COX-1, COX-2; analgesic,
antiinflammatory, antipyretic

Therapeutic outcome: Decreased pain,
inflammation

USES: Mild to moderate pain; osteoarthritis;
rheumatoid arthritis; dysmenorrhea; OTC relief
of minor aches, pains

CONTRAINDICATIONS:
Pregnancy **D**, 2nd/3rd trimesters; hypersensitivity to this product, NSAIDs, salicylates

K

> **BLACK BOX WARNING:** Perioperative pain in CABG

Precautions: Pregnancy (**C**) (1st trimester), breastfeeding, children, geriatric, bleeding/GI/cardiac disorders, hypersensitivity to other antiinflammatory agents, asthma, severe renal/hepatic disease, ulcer disease

> **BLACK BOX WARNING:** GI bleeding, MI, stroke

DOSAGE AND ROUTES
Antiinflammatory
Adult: PO 50 mg qid or 75 mg tid, max 300 mg/day or ext rel 200 mg/day

Analgesic
Adult: PO 25-50 mg q6-8hr, max 300 mg/day

Available forms: Caps 50, 75 mg; ext rel caps 200 mg

Implementation
- Store at room temperature
- Give with antacids, milk, or food for GI upset
- Swallow whole; do not break, crush, chew, or open ext rel cap
- Give with 8 oz of water and sit upright for 30 min after dose to prevent ulceration
- Give with food or milk to decrease gastric symptoms; give 30 min before or 2 hr after meals; absorption may be slowed

ADVERSE EFFECTS
CNS: Dizziness, drowsiness, fatigue, confusion, insomnia, depression, headache
CV: Tachycardia, peripheral edema, palpitations, dysrhythmias, hypertension, **CV thrombotic events, MI, stroke**
EENT: Tinnitus, hearing loss, blurred vision
GI: *Nausea, anorexia, vomiting, diarrhea,* jaundice, **hepatitis,** constipation, flatulence, cramps, dry mouth, peptic ulcer, **GI bleeding**
GU: **Nephrotoxicity: dysuria, hematuria, oliguria, azotemia**
HEMA: **Blood dyscrasias**
INTEG: Purpura, rash, pruritus, sweating
SYST: Anaphylaxis

Pharmacokinetics

Absorption	Well absorbed
Distribution	Not known
Metabolism	Liver
Excretion	Kidneys
Half-life	2-4 hr; 5.4 hr (ext rel)

Pharmacodynamics

Onset	Unknown
Peak	1.2 hr; 6.8 hr (ext rel)
Duration	Unknown

INTERACTIONS
Individual drugs
Alcohol, cidofovir: increased adverse GI reactions, toxicity
Aspirin: increased ketoprofen levels, increased adverse GI reactions
Clopidogrel, eptifibatide, ticlopidine, tirofiban: increased risk of bleeding
CycloSPORINE, lithium, methotrexate, phenytoin: increased ketoprofen levels, increased toxicity
Insulin: increased hypoglycemia
Probenecid: increased ketoconazole levels

Drug classifications
Anticoagulants, thrombolytics: increased risk of bleeding
Antihypertensives: decreased effect of antihypertensives
Antineoplastics: increased hematologic toxicity
Corticosteroids: increased adverse GI reactions
Diuretics: decreased effectiveness of diuretics
NSAIDs: increased adverse GI reactions
Sulfonylureas: increased hypoglycemia

Drug/herb
Feverfew, garlic, ginger, ginkgo, ginseng *(Panax):* increased risk of bleeding

Drug/lab test
Increased: bleeding time, BUN, alkaline phosphatase, AST, ALT, creatinine, LDH

NURSING CONSIDERATIONS
Assessment
- **Assess for pain:** type, location, intensity; ROM before and 1-2 hr after treatment
- Monitor renal, liver function tests: AST, ALT, bilirubin, creatinine, BUN, urine creatinine, CBC Hct, Hgb, pro-time if patient is on long-term therapy
- Check I&O ratio; decreasing output may indicate renal failure (long-term therapy)
- **Assess hepatotoxicity:** dark urine, clay-colored stools, jaundice of skin and sclera, itching, abdominal pain, fever, diarrhea if patient is on long-term therapy
- Assess for allergic reactions: rash, urticaria; if these occur, product may have to be discontinued

- Assess for ototoxicity: tinnitus, ringing, roaring in ears; audiometric testing needed before, after long-term therapy
- Assess for vision changes: blurring, halos; may indicate corneal, retinal damage
- Check edema in feet, ankles, legs
- Identify prior product history; there are many product interactions

> **BLACK BOX WARNING:** Assess for CV thrombotic events: MI, stroke

> **BLACK BOX WARNING:** For GI bleeding: blood in sputum, emesis, stools

Patient/family education
- Teach patient to report any symptoms of hepatotoxicity, renal toxicity, vision changes, ototoxicity, allergic reactions, bleeding (long-term therapy)
- Advise patient to take with 8 oz of water and sit upright for 30 min after dose to prevent ulceration, not to crush or chew ext rel products
- Caution patient not to exceed recommended dosage, acute poisoning may result; to take as prescribed; do not double dose
- Advise patient to read label on other OTC products; many contain other antiinflammatories
- Advise patient to use sunscreen, protective clothing to prevent photosensitivity
- Inform patient that the therapeutic response takes 2 wk (arthritis)
- Teach patient to report tinnitus, confusion, diarrhea, sweating, hyperventilation, blurred vision, fever, joint aches
- Caution patient to avoid alcohol ingestion; GI bleeding may occur
- Teach patient to report use to all providers
- Teach patient to report planned or suspected pregnancy, D (2nd/3rd trimester)/C (1st trimester); avoid breastfeeding

Evaluation
Positive therapeutic outcome
- Decreased pain
- Decreased inflammation
- Increased mobility
- Decreased fever

ketorolac (systemic, nasal) (Rx)
(kee′toe-role-ak)
Acular, Sprix, Toradol ✦
Func. class.: Nonsteroidal antiinflammatory (NSAID), nonopioid analgesic
Chem. class.: Acetic acid
Pregnancy category C; D (third trimester)

ACTION: Inhibits prostaglandin synthesis by decreasing an enzyme needed for biosynthesis; analgesic, antiinflammatory, antipyretic effects

Therapeutic outcome: Decreased pain, inflammation, ocular itching

USES: Mild to moderate pain (short term); decreased ocular itching in seasonal allergic conjunctivitis (ophthalmic)

CONTRAINDICATIONS:
Pregnancy **D** (3rd trimester), hypersensitivity, asthma, hepatic disease, peptic ulcer disease, CV bleeding

> **BLACK BOX WARNING:** Breastfeeding, severe renal disease, labor and delivery, perioperative pain in CABG, prior to major surgery, epidural/intrathecal administration, GI bleeding, hypovolemia

Precautions: Pregnancy **C**, GI/cardiac disorders, hypersensitivity to other antiinflammatory agents, CCr <25 ml/min

> **BLACK BOX WARNING:** Children, geriatric, bleeding, MI, stroke

DOSAGE AND ROUTES
Adult/adolescent >17 yr and ≥50 kg: PO continuation from **IM/IV** only 20 mg, then 10 mg q4-6hr prn, max 40 mg/day; nasal 1 spray (15.75 mg/spray) in each nostril (31.5 mg/spray) q6-8hr, max 4 doses/day × 5 days
Adult/adolescent >17 yr and <50 kg: IM (single dose) 30-60 mg, **IV** 15-30 mg; **IM/IV** (multiple dosing) 15-30 mg q6hr, max 60 mg/day × 5 day combined either **PO/IM/IV**; nasal 1 spray (15.75 mg/spray) in one nostril q6-8hr, max 4 doses/day × 5 days

Renal dose
Do not use in advanced renal disease

Ophthalmic route
Adult: 1 gtt (0.25 mg) qid × 7 days
Child: IV 1 mg/kg, then 0.5 mg/kg q6hr

Available forms: Inj 15, 30 mg/ml
(prefilled syringes); ophth 0.5% sol; tabs 10 mg;
nasal spray 15.75 mg/spray

Implementation
PO route
- Administer to patient crushed or whole
- **Max 5 days**
- Give with full glass of water; give with food or
milk to decrease gastric symptoms; give 30 min
before or 2 hr after meals; absorption may be
slowed

Nasal route
- Prime pump before using for the first time,
point away from person/pets, pump activator 5
times, no need to re-prime
- For single use only, discard 24 hr after open-
ing if not used
- Do not share with others
- Have patient blow nose, sit upright to spray

IM/IV route
- **IV** give undiluted ≥15 sec
- Give IM inj deeply into large muscle mass
- Store at room temperature, protect from light

Y-site compatibilities: Cisatracurium,
remifentanil, SUFentanil

Syringe incompatibilities: Morphine,
meperidine, promethazine, hydrOXYzine

Solution compatibilities: D$_5$W, 0.9%
NaCl, LR, D$_5$, plasmalate

ADVERSE EFFECTS
CNS: Dizziness, *drowsiness,* tremors,
seizures
CV: Hypertension, flushing, syncope, pallor,
edema, vasodilatation, **CV thrombotic events,
MI, stroke**
EENT: Tinnitus, hearing loss, blurred vision,
transient burning/stinging
GI: Nausea, anorexia, vomiting, diarrhea, constipation, flatulence, cramps, dry mouth, peptic
ulcer, **GI bleeding, perforation**, taste change,
hepatitis, hepatic failure
**GU: Nephrotoxicity: dysuria, hematuria,
oliguria, azotemia**
HEMA: Blood dyscrasias, prolonged
bleeding
INTEG: Purpura, rash, pruritus, sweating,
**angioedema, Stevens-Johnson syndrome,
toxic epidermal necrolysis**

Pharmacokinetics
Absorption	Rapidly, completely absorbed
Distribution	Bound to plasma proteins (99%)
Metabolism	Liver (<50%)
Excretion	Kidney, metabolites (92%); breast milk (6%); feces
Half-life	6 hr (IM); increased in renal disease

Pharmacodynamics
	IM	Ophth/PO
Onset	Up to 10 min	Unknown
Peak	50 min IM; 2-3 hr PO; 0.5-2 hr nasal	Unknown; 6-8 hr nasal
Duration	4-6 hr PO	Unknown

INTERACTIONS
Individual drugs
Alcohol, aspirin: increased GI effects
Aspirin: increased ketorolac levels, contraindicated
Cefamandole, cefoperazone, cefoTEtan, clopidogrel, eptifibatide, plicamycin, ticlopidine,
tirofiban, valproic acid: increased risk of
bleeding
CycloSPORINE, lithium, methotrexate, pentoxify-
line, probenecid: increased toxicity

Drug classifications
ACE inhibitors: increased renal impairment
Anticoagulants: increased effects
Antihypertensives: decreased antihypertensive
effect
Salicylates, SNRIs, SSRIs, thrombolytics:
increased risk of bleeding
Corticosteroids, NSAIDs, potassium products,
steroids: increased GI effects
Diuretics: decreased diuretic effect
NSAIDs (other): increased ketorolac levels;
contraindicated

Drug/lab test
Increased: AST, ALT, LDH, bleeding time

NURSING CONSIDERATIONS
Assessment

BLACK BOX WARNING: Monitor renal, hepatic, blood studies: BUN, creatinine, AST, ALT,
Hgb before treatment, periodically thereafter,
check for dehydration

• **Monitor for aspirin sensitivity,** asthma; these patients may be more likely to develop hypersensitivity to NSAIDs

• Assess patient's eyes: redness, swelling, tearing, itching

• **Monitor for pain:** type, location, intensity, ROM before and 1 hr after treatment

> **BLACK BOX WARNING:** Assess for GI bleeding: blood in sputum, emesis, stools

> **BLACK BOX WARNING:** Do not use epidurally, intrathecally; alcohol is present in the solution

> **BLACK BOX WARNING:** Assess for CV thrombotic events: MI, stroke; do not use for perioperative pain in CABG

Patient/family education

• Teach patient that product must be continued for prescribed time to be effective; to avoid aspirin, alcoholic beverages, other NSAIDs, acetaminophen

• Caution patient to report bleeding, bruising, fatigue, malaise, since blood dyscrasias do occur

• Instruct patient to use caution when driving; drowsiness, dizziness may occur

• Instruct patient to take with a full glass of water to enhance absorption

• Caution patient that this product may cause eye redness, burning if soft contact lenses are worn

• Advise to report use to all health care providers, not to use with other products unless approved by prescriber; use for ≤5 days

• Instruct patient to report change in urine pattern, weight increase, edema; pain in joints, fever, blood in urine (indicates nephrotoxicity); bruising, black tarry stools (indicates bleeding)

• Caution patient not to breastfeed

• Instruct patient to report if pregnancy is planned or suspected, pregnancy (C) systemic

• **Nasal:** Instruct patient to discard within 24 hr of opening; may cause irritation; may drink water after dose

> **BLACK BOX WARNING:** Instruct patient to report change in urine pattern, weight increase, edema, increased joint pain, fever, blood in urine (indicates nephrotoxicity); bruising, black tarry stools (indicates bleeding); pruritus, jaundice, nausea, right upper quadrant pain, abdominal pain (hepatotoxicity); to notify prescriber immediately

Evaluation

Positive therapeutic outcome

• Decreased pain

• Decreased inflammatory response

• Increased mobility

• Decreased ocular itching

ketorolac ophthalmic

See Appendix B

ketotifen ophthalmic

See Appendix B

labetalol (Rx)

(la-bet'a-lole)
Trandate
Func. class.: Antihypertensive, antianginal
Chem. class.: α- and β-blocker
Pregnancy category C

Do not confuse:
Trandate/Tridate

ACTION: Produces decreases in B/P without reflex tachycardia or significant reduction in heart rate through mixture of α-blocking, β-blocking effects; elevated plasma resins are reduced

Therapeutic outcome: Decreased B/P

USES: Mild to moderate hypertension; treatment of severe hypertension (**IV**)

Unlabeled uses: Hypertension in patients with pheochromocytoma, hypertension in clonidine withdrawal

CONTRAINDICATIONS:

Hypersensitivity to β-blockers, cardiogenic shock, heart block (2nd or 3rd degree), sinus bradycardia, CHF, bronchial asthma

Precautions: Pregnancy **C**, breastfeeding, geriatric, major surgery, diabetes mellitus, thyroid/renal/hepatic disease, COPD, well-compensated heart failure, CAD, nonallergic bronchospasm, peripheral vascular disease

> **BLACK BOX WARNING:** Abrupt discontinuation

DOSAGE AND ROUTES

Hypertension

Adult: PO 100 mg bid; may be given with a diuretic; may increase to 200 mg bid after 2 days; may continue to increase q1-3days; max 2400 mg/day in divided doses

Hypertensive crisis

Adult: **IV** intermittent 20 mg over 2 min, may repeat 20-80 mg over 2 min q10min, 200 mg

Available forms: Tabs 100, 200, 300 mg; inj 5 mg/ml in 20-ml ampules

Implementation

• Store in dry area at room temp; do not freeze
PO route
• Give before meals, at bedtime; tab may be crushed or swallowed whole; give with food to prevent GI upset, increase absorption

• Do not discontinue prior to surgery
• Store protected from light, moisture; place in cool environment

Direct IV route
• Give undiluted (5 mg/ml) over 2 min
Continuous IV infusion route
• Give after diluting in LR, D_5W, D_5 in 0.2%, 0.9%, 0.33% NaCl or Ringer's; infusion is titrated to patient's response; 200 mg of product/160 ml sol (1 mg/ml); 300 mg of product/240 ml sol (1 mg/ml); 200 mg of product/250 ml sol (2 mg/3 ml); use inf pump
• Keep patient recumbent during and for 3 hr after inf, monitor VS q5-15min

Y-site compatibilities: Amikacin, aminophylline, amiodarone, ampicillin, butorphanol, calcium gluconate, cefTAZidime, ceftizoxime, cimetidine, diltiazem, DOBUTamine, DOPamine, enalaprilat, EPINEPHrine, erythromycin, esmolol, famotidine, fentaNYL, gentamicin, HYDROmorphone, lidocaine, LORazepam, magnesium sulfate, meperidine, metroNIDAZOLE, midazolam, milrinone, morphine, niCARdipine, nitroglycerin, nitroprusside, norepinephrine, oxacillin, potassium chloride, potassium phosphate, propofol, ranitidine, sodium acetate, tobramycin, vancomycin, vecuronium

Y-site incompatibilities: Cefoperazone, nafcillin

ADVERSE EFFECTS

CNS: *Dizziness,* mental changes, drowsiness, *fatigue,* headache, catatonia, depression, anxiety, nightmares, paresthesias, lethargy
CV: *Orthostatic hypotension,* **bradycardia, CHF,** chest pain, **ventricular dysrhythmias,** AV block, scalp tingling
EENT: *Tinnitus,* vision changes, sore throat, double vision, dry burning eyes, floppy iris syndrome, nasal congestion
ENDO: Hyperkalemia
GI: *Nausea, vomiting, diarrhea,* dyspepsia, taste distortion, **hepatotoxicity**
GU: Impotence, dysuria, ejaculatory failure
HEMA: Agranulocytosis, thrombocytopenia, purpura (rare)
INTEG: Rash, alopecia, urticaria, pruritus, fever, **exfoliative dermatitis**
RESP: Bronchospasm, dyspnea, wheezing

Absorption	Bioavailability 25% (PO); complete (**IV**)
Distribution	Crosses placenta, CNS
Metabolism	Liver, extensively
Excretion	Breast milk, kidneys, bile
Half-life	6-8 hr

Pharmacodynamics

	PO	IV
Onset	30 min	2-5 min
Peak	1 hr	5-15 min
Duration	24 hr	2-4 hr

INTERACTIONS
Individual drugs
Alcohol (large amounts), cimetidine, nitroglycerin: increased hypotension
Lidocaine: decreased effect
Verapamil: increased myocardial depression

Drug classifications
Antidepressants, tricyclics: increased tremor
Antidiabetics: increased or decreased effect
Antihypertensives: increased hypotension
β-Blockers, bronchodilators, sympathomimetics, xanthines: decreased effects
Diuretics: increased hypotension
General anesthetics, hydantoins, class IC antidysrhythmics: increased myocardial depression
MAOIs: do not use within 2 wk
NSAIDs, salicylates: decreased antihypertensive effect
Theophyllines: decreased bronchodilatation

Drug/herb
Hawthorn: increased antihypertensive effect
Ephedra: decreased antihypertensive effect

Drug/lab test
Increased: ANA titer, blood glucose, alkaline phosphatase, LDH, AST, ALT, BUN, potassium, triglycerides, uric acid, serum lipoprotein
False increase: urinary catecholamines

NURSING CONSIDERATIONS
Assessment
• **Hypertension:** monitor B/P at beginning of treatment, periodically thereafter; pulse q4hr; note rate, rhythm, quality: apical/radial pulse before administration; notify prescriber of any significant changes (pulse <50 bpm)
• Check for baselines in renal, liver function tests before therapy begins

• **CHF:** assess for edema in feet, legs daily, monitor I&O, daily weight; check for jugular vein distention, crackles bilaterally, dyspnea

> **BLACK BOX WARNING:** Abrupt discontinuation: Product should be tapered to prevent adverse reactions

Patient/family education

> **BLACK BOX WARNING:** Teach patient not to discontinue product abruptly, precipitate angina might occur; taper over 2 wk

• Teach patient not to use OTC products containing α-adrenergic stimulants (such as nasal decongestants, cold preparations); to avoid alcohol, smoking; to limit sodium intake as prescribed
• Teach patient that product may mask symptoms of hypoglycemia; monitor blood glucose closely
• Teach patient how to take pulse and B/P at home; advise when to notify prescriber
• Instruct patient to comply with weight control, dietary adjustments, modified exercise program
• Advise patient to carry/wear emergency ID to identify products being taken, allergies; that product controls symptoms but does not cure the condition
• **Teach patient to report symptoms of CHF:** difficulty breathing, especially on exertion or when lying down, night cough, swelling of extremities, bradycardia, dizziness, confusion, depression, fever
• Teach patient to take product as prescribed, not to double or skip doses; take any missed doses as soon as remembered if at least 4 hr until next dose
• Advise patient to avoid driving or other hazardous activities until response is known; dizziness, drowsiness occurs
• Teach patient to take product at bedtime to prevent orthostatic hypotension, to rise slowly

Evaluation
Positive therapeutic outcome
• Decreased B/P in hypertension (after 1-2 wk)
• Absence of dysrhythmias

TREATMENT OF OVERDOSE:
Lavage, **IV** glucagon or atropine for bradycardia, **IV** theophylline for bronchospasm, digoxin, O_2, diuretic for cardiac failure, hemodialysis, **IV** glucose for hyperglycemia, **IV** diazepam (or phenytoin) for seizures

Adverse effects: *italics* = common; **bold** = life-threatening

lacosamide (Rx)

(la-koe′sa-mide)

Vimpat

Func. class.: Anticonvulsant

Chem. class.: Functionalized amino acid

Pregnancy category C

ACTION: May act through action at sodium channels; exact action is unknown

Therapeutic outcome: Decrease in severity of seizures

USES: Adjunctive therapy of partial seizures

CONTRAINDICATIONS:

Hypersensitivity

Precautions: Pregnancy **C,** breastfeeding, allergies, renal/hepatic disease, geriatric patients, child <17 yr, acute MI, atrial fibrillation/flutter, AV block, bradycardia, cardiac disease, congenital heart disease, dehydration, depression, dialysis, hazardous activity, electrolyte imbalance, heart failure, labor, PR prolongation, sick sinus syndrome, substance abuse, suicidal ideation, syncope, torsades de pointes

DOSAGE AND ROUTES

Adult and child ≥17 yr: PO 50 mg bid, may increase qwk by 100 mg bid to 200-400 mg/day; **IV** 50 mg 2 ×/day, infuse over 30-60 min, may be increased 100 mg/day weekly, up to 200-400 mg/day maintenance

Renal/hepatic dose

Adult: PO/**IV** max 300 mg/day in mild to moderate hepatic disease or CCr ≤30 ml/min

Available forms: Film-coated tabs 50, 100, 150, 200 mg; **IV** 20 ml single use vials (200 mg/20 ml), oral sol 10 mg/ml

Implementation

• Store PO products/IV vials at room temp; sol is stable for 24 hr when mixed with compatible diluents in glass or PVC bags at room temp

PO route

• **Tablet:** give without regard to meals

• **Oral sol:** measure with calibrated measuring device

IV route

• May give undiluted or mixed in 0.9% NaCl, D_5W, or LR

• Infuse over 30-60 min

• Do not use if discolored or particulates are present; discard unused portions

ADVERSE EFFECTS

CNS: Dizziness, syncope, tremor, vertigo, ataxia, drowsiness, fever, hypoesthesia, paresthesias, depression, fatigue, headache, confusion, irritability, psychological dependence, **suicidal ideation,** euphoria

CV: Atrial fibrillation/flutter, AV block, bradycardia, myocarditis, orthostatic hypotension, palpitations, **PR prolongation**

EENT: Diplopia, blurred vision, nystagmus, tinnitus

GI: Nausea, constipation, vomiting, **hepatitis,** diarrhea, dyspepsia

HEMA: Anemia, neutropenia, agranulocytosis

INTEG: Rash, erythema, inj site reaction, pruritus, xerostomia

MS: Asthenia, dysarthria, muscle cramps

SYST: Drug reaction with eosinophilia and systemic symptoms (DRESS)

Pharmacokinetics

Absorption	Unknown
Distribution	Protein binding <15%
Metabolism	Liver
Excretion	Kidneys (95%)
Half-life	13 hr (PO), elimination half-life 15-23 hr

Pharmacodynamics

	PO	IV
Onset	Unknown	Unknown
Peak	1-4 hr (PO)	30-60 min
Duration	Unknown	Unknown

INTERACTIONS

Individual drugs

Atazanavir, dronedarone, digoxin, lopinavir, ritonavir: increase PR prolongation

Drug classifications

β-blockers, calcium-channel blockers: increase PR prolongation

CYP2C19 inhibitors (fluconazole, isoniazid, miconazole): increase lacosamide effect

Drug/lab test

Increased: LFTs

NURSING CONSIDERATIONS

Assessment

⚠ **Assess for seizures: duration, type, intensity, precipitating factors**

• Monitor for renal function: albumin concentration

- Assess CV status: orthostatic hypotension, PR prolongation; monitor cardiac status throughout treatment
⚠ **Assess mental status: mood, sensorium, affect, memory (long, short), depression, suicidal ideation, psychological dependence**
- Assess for rash, hypersensitivity reactions
⚠ **Pregnancy: Enroll in UCB Antiepileptic Drugs Registry 1-888-537-7734**

Patient/family education
⚠ **Caution patient not to discontinue product abruptly, taper over 1 wk; seizures may occur**
- Advise patient to avoid hazardous activities until stabilized on product
- Instruct patient to carry emergency ID stating product use
⚠ **Advise patient to notify prescriber of suicidal thoughts or actions, syncope, cardiac changes**
- Instruct patient to notify prescriber if pregnancy is planned or suspected
- Teach patient that interactions with other medications may occur
- Give patient MediGuide for proper use and risks

Evaluation
Positive therapeutic outcome
- Decrease in severity of seizures

---

lactulose (Rx)
(lak'tyoo-lose)
Constulose, Enulose, Generlac, Kristalose
Func. class.: Laxative (hyperosmotic/ammonia detoxicant)
Chem. class.: Lactose synthetic derivative
Pregnancy category B

ACTION: Prevents absorption of ammonia in colon by acidifying stool; increases water, softens stool

Therapeutic outcome: Decreased constipation, decreased blood ammonia level

USES: Chronic constipation, portal-systemic encephalopathy in patients with hepatic disease

CONTRAINDICATIONS:
Hypersensitivity, low-galactose diet

Precautions: Pregnancy **B**, breastfeeding, geriatric and debilitated patient, diabetes mellitus

DOSAGE AND ROUTES
Constipation
Adult: PO 15-30 ml/day (10-20 g), may increase to 60 ml/day prn
Child (unlabeled): PO 7.5 ml/day

Hepatic encephalopathy
Adult: PO 30-45 ml (20-30 g) tid or qid until stools are soft; retention enema 300 ml diluted
Infant: PO 2.5-10 ml/day in divided doses
Child: PO 40-90 ml/day in divided doses given 3-4 ×/day

Available forms: Oral sol (encephalopathy) 10 g/15 ml; oral sol (constipation) 10 g/15 ml

Implementation
PO route
- Give with full glass of fruit juice, water, milk to increase palatability of oral form; for rapid effect, give on empty stomach; increase fluids by 2 L/day; do not give with other laxatives; if diarrhea occurs, reduce dosage
- Kristalose: dissolve contents of packet in 4 oz of water
Rectal route
- **Administer retention enema** by diluting 300 ml of lactulose/700 ml of water or of 0.9% NaCl; administer by rect balloon catheter; retain for 30-60 min; repeat if evacuated too quickly

ADVERSE EFFECTS
GI: *Nausea, vomiting, anorexia, abdominal cramps, diarrhea,* flatulence, *distention, belching*
META: Hypernatremia

Pharmacokinetics
Absorption	Poorly absorbed
Distribution	Not known
Metabolism	Colonic bacteria to acids
Excretion	Kidneys, unchanged
Half-life	Unknown

Pharmacodynamics
Unknown

INTERACTIONS
Individual drugs
Neomycin: decreased lactulose effect
NIFEdipine extended release tab: increased GI obstruction

Drug classifications
Antiinfectives (oral), antacids: decreased lactulose effect

Laxatives: do not use together (hepatic encephalopathy)

Drug/herb
Flax, senna: increased laxative effect

Drug/lab test
Blood glucose (diabetic patients): increase
Blood ammonia: decrease

NURSING CONSIDERATIONS
Assessment
• **Stool:** Assess for amount, color, consistency
• Monitor glucose levels in diabetic patients (increases)
• **Cause of constipation:** Determine whether fluids, bulk, or exercise is missing from lifestyle
• Monitor blood, urine, electrolytes if used often by patient; may cause diarrhea, hypokalemia, hypernatremia; check I&O ratio to identify fluid loss
• Assess cramping, rectal bleeding, nausea, vomiting; if these symptoms occur, product should be discontinued; identify cause of constipation: identify whether fluids, bulk, or exercise is missing from lifestyle
• **Hepatic encephalopathy:** Monitor blood ammonia level (30-70 mg/100 ml); monitor for clearing of confusion, lethargy, restlessness, irritability (hepatic encephalopathy); may decrease ammonia level by 50%

Patient/family education
• Discuss with patient that adequate fluid consumption is necessary
• Teach patient that normal bowel movements do not always occur daily
• Teach patient not to use in presence of abdominal pain, nausea, vomiting; tell patient to notify prescriber of unrelieved constipation or if symptoms of electrolyte imbalance occur: muscle cramps, pain, weakness, dizziness, excessive thirst
• Teach patient not to use laxatives for long-term therapy; bowel tone will be lost
• Do not give at bedtime as a laxative; may interfere with sleep
• Notify prescriber if diarrhea occurs; may indicate overdosage

Evaluation
Positive therapeutic outcome
• Decreased constipation
• Decreased blood ammonia level
• Clearing of mental state

lamiVUDine (3TC) (Rx)
(lam-i'vue-dine)
Epivir, Epivir-HBV, Heptovir ✿
Func. class.: Antiretroviral
Chem. class.: Nucleoside reverse transcriptase inhibitor (NRTI)
Pregnancy category C

Do not confuse:
lamiVUDine/LamoTRIgine

ACTION: Inhibits replication of HIV virus by incorporating into cellular DNA by viral reverse transcriptase, thereby terminating the cellular DNA chain

Therapeutic outcome: Improved symptoms of HIV infection

USES: HIV infection in combination with at least 2 other antiretrovirals; chronic hepatitis B (Epivir-HBV)

Unlabeled uses: Prophylaxis of HIV postexposure with indinavir and zidovudine

CONTRAINDICATIONS:
Hypersensitivity

> **BLACK BOX WARNING:** Lactic acidosis

Precautions: Pregnancy **C**, breastfeeding, children, geriatric, granulocyte count <1000/mm^3 or Hgb <9.5 g/dl, renal disease, pancreatitis, peripheral neuropathy

> **BLACK BOX WARNING:** Severe hepatic dysfunction

DOSAGE AND ROUTES
HIV infection
Adult and adolescent >16 yr: PO 150 mg bid or 300 mg/day
Child 3 mo-16 yr: PO 4 mg/kg bid; max 150 mg bid

Renal dose
Adult: PO CCr 30-49 ml/min: Epivir 150 mg/day; Epivir HBV 100 mg 1st dose, then 50 mg/day; CCr 15-29 ml/min: Epivir 150 mg 1st dose, then 100 mg/day; Epivir HBV 100 mg 1st dose, then 25 mg/day; CCr 5-14 ml/min: Epivir 150 mg 1st dose, then 50 mg/day; Epivir HBV 35 mg 1st dose, then 15 mg/day; CCr <5 ml/min: Epivir 50 mg 1st dose, then 25 mg/day; Epivir HBV 35 mg 1st dose, then 10 mg/day

Chronic hepatitis B
Adult: PO 100 mg/day
Child/adolescent 2-17 yr: PO 3 mg/kg/day, max 100 mg

Available forms: Oral sol **(Epivir)** 10 mg/ml, tabs 150, 300/mg; oral sol **(Epivir-HBV)** 5 mg/ml, tabs 100 mg

Implementation
• Epivir and Epivir-HBV are not interchangeable
• Administer PO daily, bid without regard to meals
• Give with other antiretrovirals only
• Store in cool environment; protect from light

ADVERSE EFFECTS
CNS: *Fever, headache, malaise, dizziness, insomnia, depression, fatigue, chills,* **seizures,** peripheral neuropathy, paresthesia
EENT: Taste change, hearing loss, photophobia
GI: *Nausea, vomiting, diarrhea,* anorexia, cramps, dyspepsia, **hepatomegaly with steatosis, pancreatitis**
HEMA: Neutropenia, anemia, **thrombocytopenia**
INTEG: *Rash*
MS: *Myalgia, arthralgia, pain*
RESP: *Cough*
SYST: Lactic acidosis, anaphylaxis, Stevens-Johnson syndrome

Pharmacokinetics
Absorption	Rapidly absorbed
Distribution	Extravascular space
Metabolism	Protein binding $<36\%$
Excretion	Unchanged in urine
Half-life	Terminal half-life 5-7 hr

Pharmacodynamics
Unknown

INTERACTIONS
Individual drugs
AMILoride, dofetilide, entecavir, metformin, memantine, procainamide, trospium, trimethoprim/sulfamethoxazole: increased level of lamiVUDine
Emtricitabine: do not combine, duplication
Zalcitabine: decreased both products, avoid concurrent use

Drug classifications
Interferons: decrease lamiVUDine

Drug/lab test
Increased: ALT, bilirubin
Decreased: Hgb, neutrophil, platelet count

NURSING CONSIDERATIONS
Assessment
• **HIV:** Test for HIV before starting treatment; monitor blood counts q2wk; watch for neutropenia, thrombocytopenia, Hgb, CD4, viral load, lipase, triglycerides periodically during treatment; if low, therapy may have to be discontinued and restarted after hematologic recovery; blood transfusions may be required; assess for lessening of symptoms; if HBV is present, a higher dose of Epivir-HBV is needed
• **Hepatitis B:** Assess for fatigue, anorexia, pruritus, jaundice during and for several months after discontinuation; monitor liver function tests: AST, ALT, bilirubin; amylase; bilirubin, triglycerides, lipase
• **Monitor children for pancreatitis:** abdominal pain, nausea, vomiting, neuropathy

> **BLACK BOX WARNING: Assess for lactic acidosis, severe hepatomegaly with steatosis:** obtain baseline liver function tests; if elevated, discontinue treatment; discontinue even if liver function tests are normal and symptoms of lactic acidosis, severe hepatomegaly develops; may be fatal

Patient/family education
• Teach patient that GI complaints and insomnia resolve after 3-4 wk of treatment
• Tell patient that product is not a cure for AIDS but will control symptoms; compliance is needed, take as directed, to complete full course of treatment even if feeling better
• Teach patient to notify prescriber of sore throat, swollen lymph nodes, malaise, fever, peripheral neuropathy; other infections may occur
• Teach patient that virus is still infective, may pass AIDS virus to others
• Encourage patient to continue follow-up visits since serious toxicity may occur; blood counts must be done q2wk
• Tell patient that other products may be necessary to prevent other infections
• Teach patient that product may cause fainting or dizziness
• Teach patient not to breastfeed; lamiVUDine is excreted in breast milk

Evaluation
Positive therapeutic outcome
• Absence of infection, symptoms of HIV infection

lamoTRIgine (Rx)

(lam-o-trye′geen)
Lamictal, Lamictal CD, Lamictal ODT, Lamictal XR
Func. class.: Anticonvulsant—miscellaneous
Chem. class.: Phenyltriazine
Pregnancy category C

Do not confuse:
lamoTRIgine/lamiVUDine,
LaMICtal/LamISIL/Lomotil

ACTION: May inhibit voltage-sensitive sodium channels, decreasing seizures

Therapeutic outcome: Decrease in intensity and number of seizures

USES: Adjunct in the treatment of partial, tonic-clonic seizures, children with Lennox-Gastaut syndrome, bipolar disorder

Unlabeled uses: Absence seizures

CONTRAINDICATIONS:
Hypersensitivity

Precautions: Pregnancy **C** (cleft lip/palate in 1st trimester), breastfeeding, geriatric, renal/hepatic/cardiac disease, severe depression, suicidal ideation, blood dyscrasias, children <16 yr, serious rash

DOSAGE AND ROUTES
Seizures: monotherapy
Adult and adolescent ≥16 yr: PO 50 mg/day for wk 1 and 2, then increase to 100 mg divided bid for wk 3 and 4; maintenance 300-500 mg/day; receiving enzyme inducing AEDs (carBAMazepine, PHENobarbital, phenytoin, primidone but not valproic acid); ext rel 50 mg/day × 1-2 wks, then 100 mg/day during wk 3-4, then 200 mg/day during wk 5, then 300 mg/day during wk 6, then 400 mg/day during wk 7; after wk 7 range is 400-600 mg/day
Adolescent <16 yr and child: PO 0.3 mg/kg/day wk 1 and 2, then 0.6 mg/kg/day wk 3 and 4; depends on use of AED; usual dosage 4.5-7.5 mg/kg/day, max 300 mg/day

Monotherapy for patients taking valproate
Adult/adolescent ≥16 yr: receiving lamoTRIgine and valproate, without enzyme-inducing drug PO (immediate-release) stabilize on valproate and target dose of 200 mg/day la-moTRIgine; if patient is not taking lamoTRIgine 200 mg/day, increase dose by 25-50 mg/day q1-2wk to reach 200 mg/day; while maintaining lamoTRIgine 200 mg/day, decrease valproate to 500 mg/day by ≤500 mg/day/wk, maintain valproate at 500 mg/day × 1 wk, then increase lamoTRIgine to 300 mg/day, while decreasing valproate 250 mg/day × 1 wk, then discontinue valproate and increase lamoTRIgine by 100 mg/day qwk to maintenance dosage of 500 mg/day

Seizures: multiple therapy with valproate
Adult and adolescent ≥16 yr: PO 25 mg every other day, then 25 mg/day wk 3-4, increase by 25-50 mg q1-2wk; maintenance 100-400 mg/day
Adolescent <16 yr and child: PO 0.1-0.2 mg/kg/day initially, then increase q2wk as needed to 1.5 mg/kg/day or 200 mg/day

Bipolar disorder (Escalation regimen in those not taking carBAMazepine, or other enzyme-inducing drugs or valproate)
Adult and adolescent ≥16 yr: PO wk 1-2 25 mg/day; wk 3-4 50 mg/day; wk 5 100 mg/day; wk 6-7 200 mg/day; for patients taking valproic acid: wk 1-2 25 mg every other day; wk 3-4 25 mg/day; wk 5 50 mg/day; wk 6 100 mg/day; wk 7 100 mg/day

Hepatic dose
Adult (moderate hepatic impairment or severe without ascites): PO reduce by 25%
Adult (severe hepatic impairment with ascites): PO reduce by 50%

Available forms: Tabs 25, 100, 150, 200 mg; chew tabs 5, 25 mg; oral disintegrating tab 25, 50, 100, 200 mg; oral disintegrating 25-50, 50-100, 25-50-100 mg titration kit; PO ext rel 25-50-100, 50-100-200 mg titration kit; PO 25-100 mg starter kit, ext rel 25, 50, 100, 250 mg

Implementation
PO route
• **Orange Starter Kit:** for those **NOT** taking carBAMazepine, phenytoin, PHENobarbital, primidone, rifampin, or valproate
• **Green Starter Kit:** for those taking carBAMazepine, phenytoin, PHENobarbital, primidone, rifampin but **NOT** valproate
• **Blue Starter Kit:** for those taking valproate
• Discontinue all products gradually ≥2 wk, abrupt discontinuation can increase seizures
• All forms may be given without regard to meals

• **Chewable dispersible tab:** may be swallowed whole, chewed, mixed in water or fruit juice; to mix add to small amount of liquid in a glass or spoon, tabs will dissolve in 1 min, then mix in more liquid and swirl and swallow immediately

• **Orally disintegrating tabs:** place on tongue, move around in mouth, when disintegrated, swallow; examine blister pack before use, do not use if blisters are torn or missing; do not cut tabs in half

• **Extended-release tabs:** swallow whole, do not cut, break

• Give correct starter kit: **severe side effects have occurred from incorrect starter kit**

• Give in divided doses with or after meals to decrease adverse effects

ADVERSE EFFECTS

CNS: Fever, insomnia, tremor, depression, anxiety, *dizziness,* ataxia, *headache,* **suicidal ideation**

EENT: Nystagmus, *diplopia, blurred vision*

GI: *Nausea, vomiting, anorexia,* abdominal pain, **hepatotoxicity**

GU: *Dysmenorrhea*

HEMA: Anemia, **DIC, leukopenia, thrombocytopenia**

INTEG: **Rash (potentially life-threatening),** alopecia

SYST: **Stevens-Johnson syndrome, angioedema, toxic epidermal necrolysis, DRESS**

Pharmacokinetics

Absorption	Well absorbed, rapid
Distribution	Protein binding 55%, crosses placenta
Metabolism	Glucuronic acid conjunction
Excretion	Excreted in breast milk
Half-life	Terminal 24 hr; 15 hr with enzyme inducers

Pharmacodynamics

Onset	Unknown
Peak	1.4-2.3 hr
Duration	Unknown

INTERACTIONS

Individual drugs

Acetaminophen, carBAMazepine, OXcarbazepine, PHENobarbital, phenytoin, primidone: decreased lamoTRIgine serum concentration

Valproic acid: decreased metabolic clearance of lamoTRIgine

Drug classifications

CYP3A4 inhibitors: decreased metabolic clearance of lamoTRIgine

Contraceptives (oral), estrogens, succinimides, rifamycins: decreased lamoTRIgine serum concentration

Drug/herb

Ginkgo: increased anticonvulsant effect

Ginseng, santonica: decreased anticonvulsant effect

NURSING CONSIDERATIONS

Assessment

⚠ Assess for rash (Stevens-Johnson syndrome or toxic epidermal necrolysis) in pediatric patients; product should be discontinued at first sign of rash

• **Assess for seizure activity:** duration, type, intensity, halo before seizure

• Assess for hypersensitive reactions

⚠ **Bipolar disorder: suicidal thoughts/ behaviors**

Patient/family education

• Caution patient not to discontinue product abruptly; seizures may occur

• Caution patient to avoid hazardous activities until stabilized on product

• Advise patient to notify prescriber of skin rash or increased seizure activity

• Instruct patient to report to prescriber if pregnancy is suspected or planned

• Teach patient to use sunscreen and protective clothing; photosensitivity occurs

• Advise patient to carry/wear emergency ID stating product use

⚠ **Advise patient to notify prescriber immediately of suicidal thoughts, behaviors**

⚠ **Teach patient to notify prescriber if pregnancy is planned or suspected, pregnancy (C), product decreases folate; avoid breastfeeding**

Evaluation

Positive therapeutic outcome

• Decrease in severity of seizures or severity of bipolar symptoms

lansoprazole (Rx, OTC)

(lan-soe'prah-zole)
Prevacid, Prevacid SoluTab
Func. class.: Anti-ulcer proton-pump inhibitor
Chem. class.: Benzimidazole
Pregnancy category B

Do not confuse:
Prevacid/Pravachol/Prinivil

ACTION: Suppresses gastric secretion by inhibiting hydrogen/potassium ATPase enzyme system in gastric parietal cell; characterized as gastric acid pump inhibitor since it blocks final step of acid production

Therapeutic outcome: Reduction in gastric pain, swelling, fullness

USES: Gastroesophageal reflux disease (GERD), severe erosive esophagitis, poorly responsive systemic GERD, pathologic hypersecretory conditions (Zollinger-Ellison syndrome, systemic mastocytosis, multiple endocrine adenomas); possibly effective for treatment of duodenal, gastric ulcers, maintenance of healed duodenal ulcers

CONTRAINDICATIONS:
Hypersensitivity

Precautions: Pregnancy **B**, breastfeeding, children

DOSAGE AND ROUTES
Frequent heartburn
Adult: PO 15 mg qd up to 14 days

Duodenal ulcer
Adult: PO 15 mg/day before meals for 4 wk, then 15 mg/day to maintain healing of ulcers; ulcers associated with *Helicobacter pylori:* 30 mg lansoprazole, 500 mg clarithromycin, 1 g amoxicillin bid × 14 days or 30 mg lansoprazole, 1 g amoxicillin tid × 14 days

Pathologic hypersecretory conditions
Adult: PO 60 mg/day, may give up to 90 mg bid, administer >120 mg/day in divided doses

GERD/esophagitis
Adult/adolescent: PO 15-30 mg/day × 8 wk
Child 1-11 yr (>30 kg): PO 30 mg/day ≤12 wk
Child 1-11 yr (≤30 kg): 15 mg/day ≤12 wk

Stress gastric prophylaxis
Adult: NG use 30 mg oral cap or 300 mg disintegrating tab

Available forms: del rel caps 15, 30 mg; orally disintegrating tabs 15, 30 mg

Implementation
PO route
• Swallow del rel cap whole; do not break, crush, chew, or open
• Administer before eating
• **Oral cap:** Open cap and pour ¼ of granules into NG feeding syringe with plunger removed, slowly add water and depress plunger, repeat until all granules are used, flush tube with 15 ml water
• Place on tongue, allow to dissolve, use without regard to water
• **Oral syringe:** Dissolve 15 mg/4 ml or 30 mg/10 ml water; use extra water in syringe to remove all of the product

NG tube
• **Oral disintegrating tab:** Mix 30 mg tab in 10 ml water, give via NG tube, flush tube with 10 ml sterile water, clamp for 60 min

ADVERSE EFFECTS
CNS: *Headache*
GI: Diarrhea, abdominal pain, vomiting, nausea, *constipation,* flatulence, acid regurgitation, anorexia, irritable colon, microscopic colitis
GU: **Hematuria,** glycosuria, impotence, kidney calculus, breast enlargement

Pharmacokinetics

Absorption	Rapid after granules leave stomach
Distribution	Protein binding 97%
Metabolism	Liver extensively
Excretion	Urine, feces; clearance decreased in geriatric, renal/hepatic disease
Half-life	Plasma 1.5 hr

Pharmacodynamics
Unknown

INTERACTIONS
Individual products
Octreotide, misoprostol: decreased lansoprazole effect
Extended release amphetamine/dextroamphetamine: decreased release of extended-release product

---

Calcium carbonate, iron salts, itraconazole, ketoconazole, atazanavir, ampicillin: decreased absorption of each specific product

FluvoxaMINE, voriconazole: increased lansoprazole toxicity

Sucralfate: delayed absorption of lansoprazole

Clopidogrel: decreased antiplatelet effect

Drug/herb
• Avoid use with red yeast rice, St. John's wort

Drug classifications
Loop/thiazide diuretics: increased hypomagnesemia

Antimuscarinics, H_2 blockers: decreased lansoprazole effect

NURSING CONSIDERATIONS
Assessment
• Assess GI system; bowel sounds q8hr, abdomen for pain, swelling, anorexia, blood in stool, emesis
• Monitor liver enzymes (AST, ALT, alkaline phosphatase) during treatment
• Monitor INR and pro-time when taking warfarin
• Low magnesium may occur

Patient/family education
• Instruct patient to report severe diarrhea; product may have to be discontinued
• Inform diabetic patient that hypoglycemia may occur
• Encourage patient to avoid hazardous activities; dizziness may occur
• Tell patient to avoid alcohol, salicylates, ibuprofen; may cause GI irritation

Evaluation
Positive therapeutic outcome
• Absence of gastric pain, swelling, fullness

⚠ HIGH ALERT

lapatinib (Rx)
(la-pa′tin-ib)
Tykerb
Func. class.: Antineoplastic—miscellaneous
Chem. class.: Biologic response modifier, signal transduction inhibitor (STIs)
Pregnancy category D

ACTION: Reversibly binds tyrosine kinase of both the epidermal growth factor receptor (ERbB1) and human epidermal receptor type 2 (HER2) (ERbB2), blocking downstream signaling for cell proliferation

Therapeutic outcome: Decrease in breast cancer progression

USES: Advanced/metastatic breast cancer patients with tumor that overexpresses HER2 protein and who have received previous chemotherapy

CONTRAINDICATIONS:
Pregnancy **D**, hypersensitivity, breastfeeding

Precautions: Geriatric, cardiac disease, bradycardia, hypertension, hypokalemia, hypomagnesemia, QT prolongation, pneumonitis, interstitial lung disease

> **BLACK BOX WARNING:** Hepatic disease

DOSAGE AND ROUTES
Advanced/metastatic breast cancer with HER2 overexpression who have received previous therapy
Adult: PO 1250 mg (5 tabs)/day 1 hr before or after food on days 1-21 plus capecitabine 2000 mg/m^2/day in 2 divided doses on days 1-14 in a repeating 21-day cycle; continue until therapeutic response or toxicity occurs

Metastatic breast cancer with HER2 overexpression for whom hormonal therapy is indicated
Adult: PO 1500 mg (6 tabs) 1 hr before food with letrozole 2.5/day

Hepatic dose
Adult (Child-Pugh C): PO 750 mg/day (with capecitabine); 1000 mg/day (with letrozole)

Available forms: Tabs 250 mg

Implementation
• Give once a day with water on an empty stomach, 1 hr before or after food
• Do not use with grapefruit products
• Store at room temperature away from heat

ADVERSE EFFECTS
CNS: Fatigue, insomnia, palmar-plantar erythrodysesthesia (hand/foot syndrome)
CV: **Heart failure,** palpitations, **QT prolongation**
GI: Anorexia, diarrhea, dyspepsia, mouth ulcerations, nausea, vomiting, xerosis
HEMA: **Anemia, neutropenia, thrombocytopenia**
INTEG: Rash
RESP: Dyspnea, pneumonitis

Pharmacokinetics

Absorption	Incomplete
Distribution	Steady state 6-7 days
Metabolism	Liver, extensively, by CYP3A4, CYP3A5; >99% protein bound
Excretion	Unknown
Half-life	Elimination 24 hr; increased in hepatic disease

Pharmacodynamics

Onset	Unknown
Peak	4 hr
Duration	Unknown

INTERACTIONS

Individual drugs
Arsenic trioxide, bepridil, chlorproMAZINE, chloroquine, grepafloxacin, halofantrine, haloperidol, levomethadyl, mesoridazine, pentamine, probucol, sparfloxacin, thioridazine: increased QT prolongation

Drug classifications
CYP3A4 inhibitors (amiodarone, amprenavir, aprepitant, atazanavir, chloramphenicol, clarithromycin, conivaptan, dalfopristin, danazol, darunavir, delavirdine, diltiazem, efavirenz, erythromycin, estradiol, fluconazole, fluvoxaMINE, imatinib, indinavir, isoniazid, itraconazole, ketoconazole, miconazole, mifepristone, nefazodone, nelfinavir, propoxyphene, quinupristin, ritonavir, RU-486, saquinavir, telithromycin, troleandomycin, verapamil, voriconazole, zafirlukast): increased effect of lapatinib; avoid concurrent use

CYP3A4 inhibitors (amiodarone, clarithromycin, erythromycin, telithromycin, troleandomycin), class IA, III antidysrhythmics: increased QT prolongation

CYP3A4 substrates (methadone, pimozide, QUEtiapine, quiNIDine, risperidone, terfenadine, ziprasidone): increased effect of these products, QT prolongation

NURSING CONSIDERATIONS

Assessment
• Assess cardiac status: EEG for QT prolongation, ejection fraction; chest pain, palpitations, dyspnea
• Assess hepatic status: liver function tests; jaundice of sclera, skin; dose should be reduced in hepatic disease
• Assess for skin toxicities NCI CTC grade 2 or greater; discontinue use in those with decreased left ventricular ejection fraction (LVEF) or for LVEF that drops below the institution's lower limit of normal; the product may be restarted after 2 wk if the LVEF recovers to normal at 1000 mg/day; restart at 1250 mg/day when toxicity improves to grade 1 or better

Patient/family education
• Instruct patient to take with a full glass of water, once a day, 1 hr before or after food; do not take with food or grapefruit products
• Advise patient to take as directed only; if a dose is missed, take as soon as remembered; if it is close to the next dose, take only that dose; do not double
• Teach patient to report to prescriber: chest pain, difficulty breathing, fever, chills, sore throat, bleeding, bruising, yellow skin or eyes, severe fatigue, dizziness, palpitations
• Advise patient of other side effects that can occur but do not need to be reported: nausea, diarrhea, heartburn, mouth sores, rash, numbness/pain in hands/feet
• Advise patient to use adequate contraception because this drug is teratogenic, pregnancy **D**

Evaluation
Positive therapeutic outcome
• Decrease in breast cancer progression

latanoprost ophthalmic
See Appendix B

leflunomide (Rx)
(leh-floo'noh-mide)
Arava
Func. class.: Antirheumatic (DMARDs)
Chem. class.: Immune modulator, pyrimidine synthesis inhibitor
Pregnancy category X

ACTION: Inhibits an enzyme involved in pyrimidine synthesis and has antiproliferative, antiinflammatory effect

Therapeutic outcome: Decreased pain, joint swelling, increased mobility

USES: Rheumatoid arthritis, to reduce disease process as well as symptoms

Unlabeled uses: Juvenile rheumatoid arthritis

CONTRAINDICATIONS:
Breastfeeding, hypersensitivity, jaundice, lactase deficiency, hepatic disease

Precautions: Children, renal disorders, vaccinations, infection, alcoholism, immunosuppression

DOSAGE AND ROUTES
Adult: PO loading dose 100 mg/day × 3 days, maintenance 20 mg/day; may be decreased to 10 mg/day if not well tolerated

Juvenile rheumatoid arthritis (unlabeled)
Adolescent and child >40 kg: PO 20 mg
Adolescent and child 20-40 kg: PO 15 mg
Adolescent and child 10-19.9 kg: PO 10 mg

Available forms: Tabs 10, 20, 100 mg

Implementation
• Give a loading dose of 100 mg/day × 3 days, then 200 mg/day, decrease to 100 mg/day if poorly tolerated
• Give with full glass of water to enhance absorption
• Give PO with food, milk, or antacids for GI upset
• **Drug elimination:** to eliminate product give cholestyramine 8 g tid × 11 days, check levels

ADVERSE EFFECTS
CNS: Dizziness, insomnia, depression, paresthesia, anxiety, migraine, neuralgia, headache
CV: Palpitations, hypertension, chest pain, angina pectoris, peripheral edema
EENT: Pharyngitis, oral candidiasis, stomatitis, dry mouth, blurred vision
GI: *Nausea, anorexia, vomiting, constipation, flatulence, diarrhea, increased liver function tests,* **hepatotoxicity**
HEMA: Anemia, ecchymosis, hyperlipidemia
INTEG: Rash, pruritus, alopecia, acne, hematoma, herpes infections
RESP: Pharyngitis, rhinitis, bronchitis, cough, respiratory infection, pneumonia, sinusitis, **interstitial lung disease**
SYST: Opportunistic/fatal infections, Stevens-Johnson syndrome

Pharmacokinetics
Absorption	Unknown
Distribution	Unknown
Metabolism	Liver
Excretion	Kidneys
Half-life	Unknown

Pharmacodynamics
Unknown

INTERACTIONS
Individual drugs
Activated charcoal, cholestyramine: decreased effect of leflunomide, use for overdose
Methotrexate: increased hepatotoxicity
Rifampin: increased leflunomide levels

Drug classifications
Hepatotoxic agents: increased side effects of leflunomide
Live virus vaccines: decreased antibody reaction
NSAIDs: increased NSAID effect

NURSING CONSIDERATIONS
Assessment

• Screen for latent TB before starting treatment; if TB is present, treat before using this product
• **Interstitial lung disease:** assess for worsening cough, dyspnea, fever; may need to be discontinued
• Monitor liver function tests: if ALT elevations are >2 times baseline, reduce dosage to 10 mg/day
• Obtain CBC with differential qmo × 6 mo, then q6-8wk thereafter, pregnancy test, electrolytes
• **Assess arthritic symptoms:** ROM, mobility, swelling of joints, baseline, during treatment
• **Assess for infection:** fatal opportunistic infections can occur

Patient/family education
• Teach patient that product must be continued for prescribed time to be effective, that up to a month may be required for improvement
• Instruct patient to take with food, milk, or antacids to avoid GI upset, take at same time of day
• Advise patient to use caution when driving; drowsiness, dizziness may occur
• Advise patient to take with a full glass of water to enhance absorption, may continue with correct prescribed treatment with other antiinflammatories
• Advise patient not to become pregnant (**X**) while taking this product

---

Adverse effects: *italics* = common; **bold** = life-threatening

- Inform patient that hair may be lost, review alternatives
- Advise patient to avoid live virus vaccinations during treatment

Evaluation
Positive therapeutic outcome
- Increased joint mobility without pain
- Decreased joint swelling

TREATMENT OF OVERDOSE:
Give cholestyramine 8 g tid × 11 days

---

letrozole (Rx)
(let'tro-zohl)
Femara
Func. class.: Antineoplastic, nonsteroidal aromatase inhibitor
Pregnancy category D

ACTION: Binds to the heme group of aromatase; inhibits conversion of androgens to estrogens to reduce plasma estrogen levels

Therapeutic outcome: Decreased spread of malignancy

USES: Early, advanced, or metastatic breast cancer in postmenopausal women who are hormone receptor positive

CONTRAINDICATIONS:
Pregnancy **D**, hypersensitivity, premenopausal females

Precautions: Hepatic disease, respiratory disease, osteoporosis

DOSAGE AND ROUTES
Adult: PO 2.5 mg/day

Available forms: Tabs 2.5 mg

Implementation
- May administer bisphosphates to increase bone density
- Give with food or fluids for GI upset
- Give in equal intervals q6hr

ADVERSE EFFECTS
CNS: Somnolence, dizziness, depression, anxiety, *headache, lethargy*
CV: Angina, **MI, CVA, thromboembolic events,** peripheral edema, hypertension
GI: *Nausea, vomiting, anorexia,* constipation, heartburn, diarrhea
GU: Endometrial cancer, vaginal bleeding, endometrial proliferation disorder

INTEG: *Rash, pruritus,* alopecia, sweating
MISC: Hot flashes, night sweats, **second malignancies, anaphylaxis, angioedema**
MS: Arthralgia, arthritis, bone fracture, myalgia, osteoporosis
RESP: Dyspnea, cough

Pharmacokinetics
Absorption	Well absorbed
Distribution	Widely distributed, steady state 2-6 wk
Metabolism	Liver
Excretion	Kidneys
Half-life	Terminal 48 hr

Pharmacodynamics
Onset	Unknown
Peak	2 days
Duration	Unknown

INTERACTIONS
Drug classifications
Estrogens, oral contraceptives: decreased letrozole effect

NURSING CONSIDERATIONS
Assessment
- Monitor temperature q4hr; may indicate beginning of infection
- Monitor LFTs before, during therapy (bilirubin, AST, ALT, LDH) as needed or monthly

Patient/family education
- Advise patient to avoid use of alcohol, which potentiates this product
- Tell patient that product may be taken without regard to meals
- Teach patient to report vaginal bleeding, diarrhea, chest/bone pain
- Advise patient to use adequate contraception in perimenopausal, recently menopausal women, pregnancy **D**

Evaluation
Positive therapeutic outcome
- Prevention of rapid division of malignant cells, postmenopausal cancer, prostate cancer

TREATMENT OF OVERDOSE:
Induce vomiting, provide supportive care

---

leucovorin (Rx)

(loo-koe-vor'in)

Func. class.: Vitamin/folic acid antagonist antidote

Chem. class.: Tetrahydrofolic acid derivative

Pregnancy category C

Do not confuse:

leucovorin/Leukeran/Leukine

ACTION: Needed for normal growth patterns; prevents toxicity during antineoplastic therapy by protecting normal cells

Therapeutic outcome: Reversal of severe toxic effects of folic acid antagonists

USES: Megaloblastic or macrocytic anemia caused by folic acid deficiency, overdose of folic acid antagonist, methotrexate toxicity, toxicity caused by pyrimethamine/trimethoprim/trimetrexate, pneumocystosis, toxoplasmosis

CONTRAINDICATIONS:

Hypersensitivity to this product or folic acid, benzyl alcohol, anemias other than megaloblastic not associated with vit B_{12} deficiency

Precautions: Pregnancy **C**, seizures, geriatric, neonates, stomatitis, vomiting, breastfeeding

DOSAGE AND ROUTES

Megaloblastic anemia caused by enzyme deficiency

Adult and child: PO/IM/**IV** up to 6 mg/day

Megaloblastic anemia caused by deficiency of folate

Adult and child: IM 1 mg or less/day until adequate response

Advanced colorectal cancer

Adult: **IV** 200 mg/m², then 5-fluorouracil 370 mg/m²; or leucovorin 20 mg/m², then 5-fluorouracil 425 mg/m²; give daily × 5 days q4-5wk

Methotrexate toxicity—leucovorin rescue

Adult and child: PO/IM/**IV (normal elimination)** given 6 hr after dose of methotrexate 10 mg/m² until methotrexate is $<5 \times 10^{-8}$ m, CCr has increased 50% above prior level, or methotrexate level is 5×10^{-8} m at 24 hr or at 48 hr level is $>9 \times 10^{-8}$ m; give leucovorin 100 mg/m² q3hr until level drops to $<10^{-8}$ m

Pyrimethamine/trimethoprim toxicity

Adult and child: PO/IM 5-15 mg/day

Available forms: Tabs 5, 10, 15, 25 mg; inj 3, 5 mg/ml; powder for inj 10 mg/ml

Implementation

• Instruct patient about leucovorin rescue; have patient drink 3 L of fluid each day of rescue

• Do not give concurrently with systemic methotrexate

PO route

• Use PO route only if patient is not vomiting

• Within 1 hr of folic acid antagonist, do not give concurrently with systemic methotrexate

• Increase fluid intake if used to treat folic acid inhibitor overdose

• Protect from light and heat

IM route

• Treatment of megaloblastic anemia uses IM dosing

• Give within 1 hr of folic acid antagonist, no reconstitution needed

• Give increased fluid intake if used to treat folic acid inhibitor overdose

• Provide protection from light and heat when storing ampules

IV route

• Reconstitute 50 mg/5 ml of bacteriostatic water or sterile water for inj (10 mg/ml) or 100 mg/10 ml; use immediately if sterile water for inj is used to reconstitute

Direct IV route

• Give over 160 mg/min or less (16 ml of 10 mg/ml sol/min)

Intermittent IV infusion route

• Give after diluting in 100-500 ml of 0.9% NaCl, D_5W, $D_{10}W$, LR, Ringer's

Syringe compatibilities: Bleomycin, CISplatin, cyclophosphamide, DOXOrubicin, fluorouracil, furosemide, heparin, methotrexate, metoclopramide, mitoMYcin, vinBLAStine, vinCRIStine

Y-site compatibilities: Acyclovir, alemtuzumab, alfentanil, allopurinol, amifostine, amikacin, aminocaproic acid, aminophylline, ampicillin, ampicillin-sulbactam, anidulafungin, argatroban, atenolol, atracurium, azithromycin, aztreonam, bivalirudin, bleomycin, bumetanide, buprenorphine, busulfan, butorphanol, calcium acetate/chloride/gluconate, carmustine, caspofungin, ceFAZolin, cefepime, cefotaxime, cefoTEtan, cefOXitin, cefTAZidime, ceftizoxime, cefuroxime, chloramphenicol, cimetidine, ciprofloxacin, cisatracurium, CISplatin, cladribine, clindamycin, codeine, cyclophosphamide, cycloSPORINE, cytarabine, DACTINomycin, DAPTOmycin, DAUNOrubicin liposome, dexamethasone, dexmedetomidine, dexrazoxane, digoxin, diltiazem, diphenhydrAMINE, DOBUTamine, DOCEtaxel, dolasetron, DOPamine, doxacurium, DOXOrubicin, DOXOrubicin liposomal, doxycycline, enalaprilat, ePHEDrine, EPINEPHrine, eptifibatide, ertapenem, erythromycin, esmolol, etoposide, etoposide phosphate, famotidine, fenoldopam, fentaNYL, filgrastim, fluconazole, fludarabine, fluorouracil, fosphenytoin, furosemide, gallium nitrate, ganciclovir, gatifloxacin, gemcitabine gentamicin, glycopyrrolate, granisetron, haloperidol, heparin, hydrALAZINE, hydrocortisone, HYDROmorphone, hydrOXYzine, IDArubicin, ifosfamide, imipenem-cilastatin, inamrinone, insulin (regular), irinotecan, isoproterenol, ketorolac, labetalol, lactated Ringer's injection, lepirudin, levofloxacin, lidocaine, linezolid injection, LORazepam, magnesium sulfate, mannitol, mechlorethamine, melphalan, meperidine, meropenem, mesna, metaraminol, methotrexate, methyldopate, metoclopramide, metoprolol, metroNIDAZOLE, midazolam, milrinone, minocycline, mitoMYcin, mitoXANtrone, mivacurium, morphine, mycophenolate mofetil, nafcillin, nalbuphine, nesiritide, niCARdipine, nitroglycerin, nitroprusside, norepinephrine, octreotide, ondansetron, oxaliplatin, oxytocin, PACLitaxel (solvent/surfactant), palonosetron, pancuronium, PEMEtrexed, pentazocine, PENTobarbital, PHENobarbital, phentolamine, phenylephrine piperacillin-tazobactam, polymyxin B, potassium acetate/chloride, procainamide, prochlorperazine, promethazine, propranolol, quiNIDine gluconate, ranitidine, remifentanil, riTUXimab, rocuronium, sodium acetate, sodium phosphates, streptozocin, succinylcholine, SUFentanil, sulfamethoxazole-trimethoprim, tacrolimus, teniposide, theophylline, thiotepa, ticarcillin, ticarcillin-clavulanate, tigecycline, tirofiban, TNA (3-in-1) Total Nutrient Admixture, tobramycin, TPN (2-in-1) Total Parenteral Nutrition Admixture, trastuzumab, trimethobenzamide, vasopressin, vecuronium, verapamil, vinBLAStine, vinCRIStine, vinorelbine, voriconazole, zidovudine

Additive compatibilities: CISplatin, CISplatin/floxuridine, floxuridine

ADVERSE EFFECTS

HEMA: Thrombocytosis (intraarterial)
INTEG: Rash, pruritus, erythema, urticaria
RESP: Wheezing

Pharmacokinetics

Absorption	Rapidly absorbed (PO); completely absorbed (**IV**)
Distribution	Widely distributed
Metabolism	Liver
Excretion	Kidney
Half-life	3½ hr

Pharmacodynamics

	PO/IM/IV
Onset	Up to 5 min
Peak	Unknown
Duration	4-6 hr

INTERACTIONS

Individual drugs

Sulfamethoxazole-trimethoprim: decreased effect
Capecitabine, floxuridine, fluorouracil: increased toxicity

Drug classifications

Barbiturates: increased metabolism of barbiturates
Hydantoins: increased metabolism of hydantoins

NURSING CONSIDERATIONS

Assessment

• Obtain CCr before leucovorin rescue and daily to detect nephrotoxicity, methotrexate level
• Monitor I&O, urine pH q6hr; maintain at >7 to prevent neurotoxicity; watch for nausea and vomiting; if vomiting occurs IM or **IV** route may be necessary
• Assess products currently taken: alcohol, hydantoins, trimethoprim may cause increased folic acid use by body
• Assess for allergic reactions: rash, dyspnea, wheezing
• Assess neurologic status (rescue), weakness, fatigue
• Monitor calcium levels
• Assess for megaloblastic anemia, plasma lactic acid, reticulocyte count, Hct, Hgb

Patient/family education

• **For leucovorin rescue:** Drink 3 L fluid day of rescue
• Advise patient to take product exactly as prescribed; to notify prescriber of side effects immediately
• Advise patient to report signs of hypersensitivity reaction immediately
• **Advise patient with folic acid deficiency** to eat folic acid–rich foods: bran, yeast, dried

beans, nuts, fruits, fresh green leafy vegetables, asparagus
• Advise patient to avoid breastfeeding

Evaluation
Positive therapeutic outcome
• Increased weight
• Improved orientation, well-being
• Absence of fatigue
• Reversal of toxicity: methotrexate, folic acid antagonist overdose

---

⚠ HIGH ALERT

leuprolide (Rx)
(loo-proe'lide)
Eligard, Lupron Depo, Lupron Depot-Ped, Viadur
Func. class.: Antineoplastic hormone
Chem. class.: Gonadotropin-releasing hormone
Pregnancy category X

Do not confuse:
Lupron/Lopurin/Nuprin

ACTION: Causes initial increase in circulating levels of LH, FSH; continuous administration results in decreased LH, FSH; in men testosterone is reduced to castration levels; in premenopausal women estrogen is reduced to menopausal levels

Therapeutic outcome: Prevention of rapidly growing malignant cells in prostate cancer, decreased pain in endometriosis, resolution of central precocious puberty (CPP)

USES: Metastatic prostate cancer (inj implant), management of endometriosis (depot), CPP, uterine leiomyomata (fibroids)

CONTRAINDICATIONS:
Pregnancy **X**, breastfeeding, hypersensitivity to GnRH or analogs, thromboembolic disorders, undiagnosed vaginal bleeding; Viadur implant or Eligard should not be used in women or children

Precautions: Edema, hepatic disease, CVA, MI, seizures, hypertension, diabetes mellitus, CHF, depression, osteoporosis, spinal cord compression, urinary tract obstruction

DOSAGE AND ROUTES
Prostate cancer
Adult: SUBCUT 1 mg/day; IM 7.5 mg/dose qmo; Viadur implant (72 mg) qyr; or IM 22.5 mg q3mo; or IM 30 mg q4mo; or IM 45 mg q6mo

Endometriosis/fibroids
Adult: IM 3.75 mg qmo for 6 mo, 11.25 mg q3mo for 6 mo, or IM 30 mg q4mo

Central precocious puberty
Child: SUBCUT 50 mcg/kg/day; increase as needed by 10 mcg/kg/day
Child >37.5 kg: IM 15 mg q4wk
Child 25-37.5 kg: IM 11.25 mg q4wk
Child ≤25 kg: 7.5 mg q4wk

Available forms: Powder for inj depot 1 mo 3.75 mg, depot 3 mo/1.25 mg, 22.5 mg; depot 4 mo 30 mg; depot-ped 7.5, 11.25, 15 mg; sol for inj 1 mg/0.2 ml; susp for inj 7.5, 22.5, 30, 45 mg; implant (Viadur) 65 mg

Implementation
• Store in tight container at room temp
• Use depot only IM; never give SUBCUT
• Unused vials may be stored at room temperature
Subcut route
• No dilution needed; if patient is self-administering make sure patient uses syringes provided by manufacturer
• **Viadur Duros implant:** Insert in inner aspect of arm, remove after 12 mo
• **Eligard subcut:** Bring to room temp, once mixed give within 30 min; prepare the 2 syringes for mixing, join the 2 syringes by pushing in and twisting until secure; mix the product by pushing the contents of both syringes back and forth between syringes until uniform, should be light tan to tan; hold syringes vertically with syringe B on the bottom, draw entire mixed product into syringe B (short, wide syringe) by depressing the syringe A plunger and slightly withdrawing syringe B plunger, uncouple syringe A while pushing down on syringe A plunger, small air bubbles will remain; hold syringe B upright, remove pink cap, attach needle cartridge to the end of syringe B, remove needle cover, give by subcut route
IM route
• **Give monthly:** reconstitute single-use vial with 1 ml of diluent; if multiple vials are used, withdraw 0.5 ml and inject into each vial (1 ml), withdraw all and inject at 90-degree angle (3.75 mg)
• **Give 3 month:** reconstitute microspheres using 1.5 ml of diluent and inject in vial, shake, withdraw and inject

Adverse effects: *italics* = common; **bold** = life-threatening

- **12-month:** inserted into upper arm; at the end of 12 months, implant must be removed
- Use syringe and product packaged together; give deep in large muscle mass; rotate sites

ADVERSE EFFECTS

CNS: Memory impairment, depression, **seizures**

CV: MI, pulmonary emboli, dysrhythmias, peripheral edema

GI: Anorexia, diarrhea, **GI bleeding,** nausea, vomiting

GU: Edema, hot flashes, impotence, decreased libido, amenorrhea, vaginal dryness, gynecomastia, **profuse vaginal bleeding**

INTEG: Alopecia

MS: Bone pain

Prostate cancer: Increased bone pain for the first 4 wk of treatment, those with metastases in spinal column might have severe back pain

RESP: Dyspnea, pulmonary fibrosis, interstitial lung disease

Pharmacokinetics

Absorption	Rapidly absorbed (SUBCUT); slowly absorbed (IM depot)
Distribution	Unknown
Metabolism	Unknown
Excretion	Unknown
Half-life	3-4 hr

Pharmacodynamics

Unknown

INTERACTIONS

Individual drugs

Flutamide, megestrol: increased antineoplastic action

Drug/herb

Do not confuse with black cohosh or chaste tree fruit, may interfere with treatment

NURSING CONSIDERATIONS

Assessment

- **Assess for symptoms of endometriosis/ fibroids** including lower abdominal pain, excessive vaginal bleeding, bloating if product is given for the diagnosis of endometriosis
- **For central precocious puberty (CPP):** the diagnosis should have been confirmed by development of secondary sex characteristics in children <9 yr; also included to confirm the diagnosis of CPP is estradiol/testosterone, GnRH test, tomography of head, adrenal steroid, cho-

rionic gonadotropin, wrist x-ray, height, weight; patients with CPP display the signs of testicular growth, facial, body hair (boys), breast development, menses (girls)
- Monitor liver function tests before, during therapy (bilirubin, AST, ALT, LDH) as needed or monthly; prostate-specific antigen in prostate cancer; calcium, testosterone, bone mineral density, blood glucose, HbA1c
- Monitor pituitary gonadotropic and gonadal function during therapy and 4-8 wk after therapy is decreased; check LH, FSH, acid phosphate at beginning of treatment
- **Tumor flare:** monitor worsening of signs and symptoms (normal during beginning therapy): fatigue, increased pulse, pallor, lethargy, edema in feet, joints, stomach pain, shaking
- Monitor renal status: I&O ratio, check for bladder distention daily during beginning therapy (renal obstruction)
- **Severe allergic reaction:** rash, pruritus, urticaria, purpuric skin lesions, itching, flushing

Patient/family education

- Advise patient to notify prescriber if menstruation continues (menstruation should stop); to use a nonhormonal method of contraception during therapy
- ⚠ **Teach patient to notify prescriber if pregnancy is planned or suspected (X), avoid breastfeeding**
- Instruct patient to report any complaints, side effects to nurse or prescriber; hot flashes may occur; record weight, report gain of 2 lb/day
- Teach patient how to prepare, administer; to rotate sites for SUBCUT inj; to keep accurate records of dosing (prostate cancer)
- Instruct patient that tumor flare may occur: increase in size of tumor, increased bone pain; tell patient that bone pain disappears after 1 wk; may take analgesics for pain
- Advise the patient not to breastfeed while taking this product
- Inform patient that voiding problems may increase in beginning of therapy, but will decrease in several weeks

Evaluation

Positive therapeutic outcome
- Decreased size, spread of malignancy
- Decreased pain in endometriosis, fibroids
- Decreased signs of CPP
- Increased follicle maturation

levalbuterol (Rx)
(lev-al-bute′er-ole)
Xopenex, Xopenex HFA
Func. class.: Bronchodilator
Chem. class.: Adrenergic β₂-agonist
Pregnancy category C

ACTION: Causes bronchodilatation by action on β₂ (pulmonary) receptors by increasing levels of cyclic adenosine monophosphate (AMP), which relaxes smooth muscle; produces bronchodilatation; CNS, cardiac stimulation, increased diuresis, and increased gastric acid secretion

Therapeutic outcome: Increased ability to breathe because of bronchodilatation

USES: Treatment or prevention of bronchospasm (reversible obstructive airway disease)

CONTRAINDICATIONS:
Hypersensitivity to sympathomimetics, this product, or albuterol

Precautions: Pregnancy **C,** breastfeeding, hyperthyroidism, diabetes mellitus, hypertension, prostatic hypertrophy, closed-angle glaucoma, seizures, renal disease, QT prolongation, tachydysrhythmias, severe cardiac disease, hypokalemia

DOSAGE AND ROUTES
Adult and child ≥12 yr: INH 0.63 mg tid, q6-8hr by nebulization; may increase to 1.25 mg q8hr
Adult/adolescent/child >4 yr: (HFA, metered dose) 90 mcg (2 INH) q4-6hr
Child 6-11 yr: INH 0.31 mg tid via nebulization, max 0.63 mg tid

Available forms: Inh pediatric 0.31 mg/3 ml; sol 0.63, 1.25 mg/3 ml; 45 mcg per actuation (HFA)

Implementation
• Give by nebulization q6-8hr; wait at least 1 min between inhalation of aerosols
• Use this medication before other medications and allow 5 min between each to prevent overstimulation
Inhalation route
• Shake well before use, use a spacer device, prime with 4 test sprays in new canister or when not used for >3 days

ADVERSE EFFECTS
CNS: *Tremors, anxiety,* insomnia, headache, dizziness, stimulation, *restlessness,* weakness, irritability
CV: Palpitations, tachycardia, hypertension, angina, hypotension, dysrhythmias, **QT prolongation**
EENT: Dry nose, irritation of nose and throat
GI: Heartburn, nausea, vomiting, diarrhea, rhinitis
INTEG: Rash
META: Hypokalemia, hyperglycemia
MS: Muscle cramps
RESP: Cough
SYST: Anaphylaxis, angioedema

Pharmacokinetics
Absorption	Unknown
Distribution	Unknown
Metabolism	Liver extensively, tissues
Excretion	Unknown, breast milk
Half-life	Unknown

Pharmacodynamics
	INH SOL	INH AEROSOL
Onset	5-15 min	4.5-10.2 min
Peak	1½ hr	76-78 min
Duration	5-6 hr	6 hr

INTERACTIONS
Individual drugs
Haloperidol, chloroquine, droperidol, pentamidine, arsenic trioxide, levomethadyl: increased QT prolongation

Drug classifications
Adrenergics: increased levalbuterol action
β-Adrenergic blockers: decreased levabuterol action, severe bronchospasm may occur
Bronchodilators (aerosol): increased action of bronchodilator
Class IA/III antidysrhythmics, some phenothiazines, beta agonists, local anesthetics, tricyclics, CYP3A4 inhibitors (amiodarone, clarithromycin, erythromycin, telithromycin, troleandomycin), CYP3A4 substrates (methadone, pimozide, QUEtiapine, quiNIDine, risperidone, ziprasidone): increased QT prolongation
MAOIs: increased levalbuterol action

Drug/herb
Cola nut, guarana, tea (black/green), coffee, yerba maté: increased stimulation

NURSING CONSIDERATIONS
Assessment
• Assess cardiac status: palpitations, increased or decreased B/P, dysrhythmias
• **QT prolongation:** Monitor ECG for QT prolongation, ejection fraction; assess for chest pain, palpitations, dyspnea
• **Assess respiratory function:** vital capacity, forced expiratory volume, ABGs, lung sounds, heart rate, rhythm (baseline, during therapy); character of sputum: color, consistency, amount
• Determine that patient has not received theophylline therapy before giving dose, to prevent additive effect; client's ability to self-medicate
• **Monitor for evidence of allergic reactions;** paradoxic bronchospasm, anaphylaxis, angioedema; withhold dose; notify prescriber

Patient/family education
• Tell patient not to use OTC medications before consulting prescriber; extra stimulation may occur; instruct patient to use this medication before other medications and allow at least 5 min between each to prevent overstimulation; to limit caffeine products such as chocolate, coffee, tea, and cola or herbs such as cola nut, guarana, yerba maté
⚠ **Teach patient that if paradoxical bronchospasm occurs to stop product immediately and notify prescriber**
• Teach patient to use this product first, if using other inhalers, wait 5 min or more between products; rinse mouth with water after each dose to prevent dry mouth

Evaluation
Positive therapeutic outcome
• Absence of dyspnea and wheezing after 1 hr
• Improved airway exchange
• Improved ABGs

TREATMENT OF OVERDOSE:
Administer a β_1-adrenergic blocker

---

levetiracetam (Rx)
(lev-ee-tye′ra-see-tam)
Keppra, Keppra XR
Func. class.: Anticonvulsant
Pregnancy category C

ACTION: Unknown; may inhibit nerve impulses by limiting influx of sodium ions across cell membrane in motor cortex

Therapeutic outcome: Absence of seizures

USES: Adjunctive therapy in partial-onset seizures, primary generalized tonic-clonic seizures, myoclonic seizures in juvenile patients

CONTRAINDICATIONS:
Hypersensitivity, breastfeeding

Precautions: Pregnancy **C**, children, geriatric, cardiac/renal disease, psychosis

DOSAGE AND ROUTES
Adjunctive treatment of partial seizures
Adult and adolescent ≥16 yr: IV 500 mg bid, may titrate by 1000 mg/day q2wk; max 3000 mg/day in divided doses; ext rel 1000 mg/day, may increase q2wk, max 3000 mg/day
Adolescent <16 yr/child/infant: PO 10 mg/kg bid, increase the daily dose q2wk, by 20 mg/kg to 30 mg/kg bid; if unable to tolerate, may reduce dose

Myoclonic seizures/tonic-clonic seizures/partial seizures
Adult and adolescent >16 yr: PO/IV 500 mg bid, may increase by 1000 mg/day q2wk; max 3000 mg/day

Renal dose
Adult: PO CCr 50-80 ml/min, 500-1000 mg q12hr, ext rel 1000-2000 q24hr, max 2000 mg/day; CCr 30-49 ml/min, 250-750 mg q12hr, ext rel 500-1500 mg q24hr, max 1500 mg/day; CCr <30 ml/min 250-500 mg q12hr, ext rel 500-1000 mg q24hr, max 1000 mg/day

Available forms: Tabs 250, 500, 750, 1000; oral sol 100 mg/ml; SOL for inj 100 mg/ml, ext rel tab 500, 750 mg; 1000 mg/100 ml 0.75% NaCl, 1500 mg/100 ml 0.54% NaCl, 500 mg/100 ml 0.82% NaCl

Implementation
PO route
• **Ext rel product should not be used in dialysis patients**
• Give with food, milk to decrease GI symptoms (rare)
• **Child <20 kg:** give oral sol, use calibrated device
• Store at room temperature (PO); diluted preparation stable for 24 hr at room temperature in polyvinyl bags

Intermittent IV route
• Single-use vials: dilute in 100 mg of 0.9% NaCl, D_5, LR; give over 15 min, discard unused vial contents, do not use product with particulates or discoloration

---

Additive compatibilities: Diazepam, LORazepam, valproate

ADVERSE EFFECTS

CNS: Dizziness, somnolence, asthenia, psychosis, **suicidal ideation,** non-psychotic behavioral symptoms, headache, ataxia
EENT: Diplopia, conjunctivitis
GI: Nausea, vomiting, anorexia, diarrhea, constipation, **hepatitis**
HEMA: Decreased Hct, Hgb, RBC, infection, leukopenia
INTEG: Pruritus, rash
MISC: Abdominal pain, pharyngitis, infection
SYST: **Stevens-Johnson syndrome, toxic epidermal necrolysis,** dehydration (child <4 yr)

Pharmacokinetics

Absorption	Rapidly absorbed
Distribution	Widely distributed, not protein bound
Metabolism	Liver, small amount
Excretion	Kidneys, 66% unchanged
Half-life	6-8 hr, longer in renal disease/geriatric

Pharmacodynamics

Unknown

INTERACTIONS

Individual drugs
Alcohol: avoid using
CarBAMazepine: increased carBAMazepine toxicity
Sevelamer: decreased levetiracetam absorption; separate by 1 hr before, 3 hr after sevelamer

Drug/lab test
Increased: eosinophils

NURSING CONSIDERATIONS

Assessment
• Monitor urine function tests (BUN, urine protein) periodically during treatments
⚠ **Assess seizure activity including type, location, duration, and character; provide seizure precautions**
• Assess blood studies: CBC, LFTs
⚠ **Assess mental status: mood, sensorium, affect, behavioral changes, suicidal thoughts/behaviors**

Patient/family education
• Teach patient to carry/wear emergency ID stating patient's name, products taken, condition, prescriber's name, phone number

• Caution patient to avoid driving, other activities that require alertness until stabilized on medication
• Teach patient not to discontinue medication quickly after long-term use
⚠ **Instruct patient to report suicidal thoughts**
• Teach patient to use a nonhormonal type of contraception to prevent harm to the fetus
• Teach patient to take exactly as prescribed, do not double or omit doses
• Advise not to breastfeed, excreted in breast milk

Evaluation
Positive therapeutic outcome
• Decreased seizure activity

levobetaxolol ophthalmic
See Appendix B

levobunolol ophthalmic
See Appendix B

levocabastine ophthalmic
See Appendix B

levocetirizine (Rx)
(lee-voh-she-teer'ah-zeen)
Xyzal
Func. class.: Antihistamine, low sedating
Chem. class.: H₁-histamine blocker
Pregnancy category B

ACTION: Acts on blood vessels, GI, respiratory system by competing with histamine for H₁-receptor site; decreases allergic response by blocking pharmacologic effects of histamine; minimal anticholinergic action

Therapeutic outcome: Absence of running or congested nose or rashes

USES: Perennial or seasonal rhinitis, allergy symptoms, chronic idiopathic urticaria

CONTRAINDICATIONS:
Breastfeeding; end-stage renal disease; dialysis; child 6-11 yr with renal disease; hypersensitivity to this product, cetirizine, hydroxyzine

Precautions: Pregnancy **B,** driving, renal disease

DOSAGE AND ROUTES
Adult and child ≥12 yr: PO 2.5-5 mg/day in the evening

Adverse effects: *italics* = common; **bold** = life-threatening

Child 6-11 yr: PO (oral SOL) 2.5 mg/day in the evening
Child 2-5 yr: PO (oral SOL) 1.25 mg/day in the evening
Geriatric: PO 2.5-5 mg/day in the evening

Renal dose
Adult: PO CCr 50-80 ml/min 2.5 mg/day; CCr 30-50 ml/min 2.5 mg every other day; CCr 10-30 ml/min 2.5 mg 2 ×/wk; CCr <10 ml/min, do not use

Available forms: Tabs 5 mg; oral sol 2.5 mg/5 ml

Implementation
• Give without regard to meals in the evening; tabs are scored and may be broken in half
• Store in tight, light-resistant container

ADVERSE EFFECTS
CNS: *Drowsiness, fatigue,* asthenia, dizziness
RESP: Pneumonia, cough

Pharmacokinetics

Absorption	Rapid
Distribution	Unknown
Metabolism	Protein binding 91%-92%
Excretion	Urine 85.4%, feces 12.9%
Half-life	8 hr

Pharmacodynamics

Onset	Unknown
Peak	0.9 hr
Duration	Unknown

INTERACTIONS
Individual drugs
Alcohol: increased CNS depression
Ritonavir: increased half-life; decreased clearance of levocetirizine

Drug classifications
MAOIs, phenothiazines, tricyclics: increased anticholinergic/sedative effect
Other CNS depressants: increased CNS depression

Drug/lab test
False negative: skin allergy tests

NURSING CONSIDERATIONS
Assessment
• Allergy symptoms: pruritus, urticaria, watering eyes, baseline, during treatment
• Respiratory status: rate, rhythm, increase in bronchial secretions, wheezing, chest tightness
• Liver function tests, serum creatinine, BUN

Patient/family education
• Teach patient all aspects of product use; to notify prescriber if confusion, sedation, hypotension occur, not to exceed recommended dose
• Advise patient to avoid driving, other hazardous activities if drowsiness occurs
• Advise patient to avoid alcohol, other CNS depressants
• Inform patient that product is not recommended during breastfeeding

Evaluation
Positive therapeutic outcome
• Absence of running or congested nose or rashes

TREATMENT OF OVERDOSE:
Administer diazepam, vasopressors, IV phenytoin

levodopa-carbidopa (Rx)
(lee-voe-doe′pa kar-bi-doe′pa)
Apo-Levocarb ✦, Atamet, Parcopa, Sinemet, Sinemet CR
Func. class.: Antiparkinsonism agent
Chem. class.: Catecholamine
Pregnancy category C ✷

ACTION: Decarboxylation of levodopa in periphery is inhibited by carbidopa; more levodopa is made available for transport to brain and conversion to dopamine in the brain

Therapeutic outcome: Absence of involuntary movements

USES: Parkinson's disease, parkinsonism resulting from carbon monoxide, chronic manganese intoxication, cerebral arteriosclerosis

Unlabeled uses: Restless legs syndrome

CONTRAINDICATIONS:
Hypersensitivity, malignant melanoma, history of malignant melanoma, or undiagnosed skin lesions resembling melanoma

Precautions: Pregnancy **C,** breastfeeding, diabetes, renal/cardiac/hepatic/respiratory disease, MI with dysrhythmias, open-angle glaucoma, seizures, peptic ulcer, depression

DOSAGE AND ROUTES
Beginning therapy for those not taking levodopa
Adult: PO 25 mg carbidopa/100 mg levodopa tid, may increase daily or every other day by 1

---

tab to desired response (8 tabs/day); ext rel tabs carbidopa 50 mg/levodopa 200 mg bid

For those not taking levodopa ER
Adult: PO 50 mg carbidopa/200 mg levodopa bid

For those taking levodopa ER
Adult: Begin treatment with 10% more levodopa/day given PO q4-8hr, may increase or decrease dose q3days

For those taking levodopa <1.5 g/day
Adult: PO 25 mg carbidopa/100 mg levodopa tid-qid, may increase daily to desired response

For those taking levodopa >1.5 g/day
Adult: PO 25 mg carbidopa/250 mg levodopa tid-qid, may increase daily to desired response

Restless legs syndrome (RLS) (unlabeled)
Adult: PO carbidopa 25 mg/levodopa 100 mg, 1 tab at bedtime, may repeat if awakening within 2 hr or 50 mg carbidopa/200 mg levodopa SUS REL tab 1-2 tabs 1 hr before bedtime

Available forms: Tabs 10 mg carbidopa/100 mg levodopa, 25 mg carbidopa/100 mg levodopa, 25 mg carbidopa/250 mg levodopa; ext rel tab 25 mg/100 mg, 50 mg/200 mg carbidopa/levodopa (Sinemet CR); oral disintegrating tab (Parcopa) 10 mg carbidopa/100 mg levodopa, 25 mg carbidopa/100 mg levodopa, 25 mg carbidopa/250 mg levodopa

Implementation
PO route
• Swallow **ext rel tabs** whole; do not break, crush, or chew
• **Oral disintegrating tab:** gently remove from bottle, place on tongue, swallow with saliva; after it dissolves, liquid is not necessary
• Give product until NPO before surgery; check with prescriber for continuing product
• Adjust dosage depending on patient response
• Give with meals or after meals to prevent GI symptoms; limit protein taken with product
• Give only after MAOIs have been discontinued for 2 wk; if previously on levodopa, discontinue for at least 8 hr before change to levodopa-carbidopa

ADVERSE EFFECTS
CNS: *Involuntary choreiform movements, hand tremors, fatigue, headache, anxiety, twitching, numbness, weakness, confusion, agitation, insomnia, nightmares,* psychosis, hallucination, hypomania, severe depression, dizziness, impulsive behaviors, **neuroleptic malignant syndrome**
CV: *Orthostatic hypotension,* tachycardia, hypertension, palpitation
EENT: Blurred vision, diplopia, dilated pupils
GI: *Nausea, vomiting, anorexia, abdominal distress, dry mouth, flatulence, dysphagia, bitter taste, diarrhea, constipation*
HEMA: Hemolytic anemia, leukopenia, agranulocytosis
INTEG: Rash, sweating, alopecia
MISC: Urinary retention, incontinence, weight change, dark urine

Pharmacokinetics

Absorption	Well absorbed (PO); ER dose slowly absorbed
Distribution	Widely distributed
Metabolism	Liver, extensively
Excretion	Kidneys, metabolites
Half-life	Levodopa (1 hr); carbidopa (1-2 hr)

Pharmacodynamics

	PO	PO-ER
Onset	Unknown	Unknown
Peak	1 hr	2½ hr
Duration	6-24 hr	Unknown

INTERACTIONS
Individual drugs
Metoclopramide: increased effects of levodopa
Papaverine, pyridoxine: decreased effects of levodopa

Drug classifications
Antacids: increased effects of levodopa
Anticholinergics, antipsychotics, benzodiazepines, hydantoins: decreased effects of levodopa
MAOIs: hypertensive crisis

Drug/food
Protein: decreased absorption of levodopa

Drug/lab test
Increased: AST, ALT, bilirubin, LDH, alkaline phosphatase, BUN, serum glucose
Decreased: BUN, creatinine, uric acid
False increase: urine protein
False positive: urine ketones (dipstick), Coombs' test
False negative: urine glucose

Adverse effects: *italics* = common; **bold** = life-threatening

NURSING CONSIDERATIONS
Assessment
- Assess for **parkinsonism:** shuffling gait, muscle rigidity, involuntary movements, pill rolling, muscle spasms, drooling before and during treatment
- Assess B/P, respiration, orthostatic B/P
- Monitor I&O ratio; retention commonly causes decreased urinary output, distention, frequency, incontinence; palpate bladder if retention occurs
- Assess for muscle twitching, blepharospasm that may indicate **toxicity**
- Monitor renal, liver, hematopoietic studies; also for diabetes, acromegaly during long-term therapy
- Monitor for constipation, cramping, pain in abdomen, abdominal distention; increase fluids, bulk, exercise if this occurs
- Assess for tolerance over long-term therapy; dose may have to be increased or changed
- Assess for mental status: affect, mood, CNS depression, worsening of mental symptoms during early therapy

Patient/family education
- Teach patient to change positions slowly to prevent orthostatic hypotension
- Teach patient to report side effects: twitching, eye spasms, grimacing, protrusion of tongue, personality changes that indicate overdose
- Instruct patient to use product exactly as prescribed; if product is discontinued abruptly, parkinsonian crisis may occur; do not double doses; take missed dose as soon as remembered up to 2 hr before next dose
- Teach patient that urine, sweat may darken and is harmless
- Advise patient to use physical activities to maintain mobility and lessen spasms
- Instruct patient that OTC medications should not be used unless approved by prescriber
- Advise patient that drowsiness, dizziness are common; to avoid hazardous activities until response is known
- Explain that sips of water, hard candy, or gum may lessen dry mouth
- Teach patient to take with meals to prevent GI symptoms; to limit protein intake, which impairs product's absorption

Evaluation
Positive therapeutic outcome
- Decrease in akathisia
- Improved mood
- Decreased involuntary movements

levofloxacin (Rx)
(lev-o-floks′a-sin)
Levaquin
Func. class.: Antiinfective
Chem. class.: Fluoroquinolone antibacterial
Pregnancy category C

ACTION: Interferes with conversion of intermediate DNA fragments into high molecular weight DNA in bacteria; DNA gyrase inhibitor; inhibits topoisomerase IV

Therapeutic outcome: Bacteriocidal action against the following: *Streptococcus pneumoniae, Haemophilus influenzae, Haemophilus parainfluenzae, Moraxella catarrhalis, Klebsiella pneumoniae, Mycoplasma pneumoniae, Escherichia coli, Serratia marcescens, Chlamydia pneumoniae, Legionella pneumophilia, Enterococcus faecalis, Staphylococcus epidermidis, Staphylococcus pyogenes*

USES: Acute sinusitis, acute chronic bronchitis, community-acquired pneumonia, uncomplicated skin infections, UTI, cellulitis, prostatitis, inhalational anthrax (postexposure), acute pyelonephritis, inhalation anthrax in children

CONTRAINDICATIONS:
Hypersensitivity to quinolones

Precautions: Pregnancy **C,** breastfeeding, children; photosensitivity, acute MI, atrial fibrillation, colitis, dehydration, diabetes, QT prolongation, myasthenia gravis, renal disease, seizure disorder, syphilis

> **BLACK BOX WARNING:** Tendon pain/rupture, tendinitis

DOSAGE AND ROUTES
Acute bacterial exacerbation of chronic bronchitis
Adult: PO/**IV** 500 mg q24hr × 7 days

Acute bacterial sinusitis
Adult: PO 500 mg q24hr × 10-14 days or 750 mg q24hr × 5 days

Mild-moderate UTI/acute pyelonephritis
Adult: PO/**IV** 750 mg q24hr × 5 days or 250 mg q24hr × 10 days

Chronic bacterial prostatitis
Adult: PO 500 mg q24hr × 28 days

Postexposure inhalational anthrax
Adult/adolescent/child >50 kg: PO/IV 500 mg q24hr × 60 days
Infant >6 mo and child <50 kg: IV 8 mg/kg q12hr × 60 days, max 250 mg/dose

Pneumonia, community acquired
Adult: PO/IV 500 mg q24hr × 7-14 days or 750 mg q24hr × 5 days

Pneumonia, nosocomial
Adult: PO/IV 750 mg q24hr × 7-14 days

SSSI, complicated
Adult: PO/IV 750 mg q24hr × 7-14 days

SSSI, uncomplicated
Adult: PO 500 mg q24hr × 7-10 days

UTI, complicated
Adult: PO/IV 750 mg q24hr × 5 days or 250 mg q24hr × 10 days

UTI, uncomplicated
Adult: PO 250 mg q24hr × 3 days

Plague *(Yersinia pestis)*
Adult: PO/IV 500 mg q24hr × 10-14 days (with pneumonia, 750 mg q24hr)
Adolescent/child <50 kg: PO/IV 8 mg/kg (max 250 mg/dose) q12hr × 10-14 days

Renal disease
Adult: PO/IV CCr 20-49 ml/min: for 750-mg dose, give 750 mg q48hr; for 500-mg dose, give 500 mg once, then 250 mg q24hr; for 250-mg dose, no adjustment; CCr 10-19 ml/min: for 750-mg dose, give 750 mg once, then 500 mg q48hr; for 500-mg dose, give 500 mg once, then 250 mg q48hr; for 250-mg dose, give 250 mg q48hr, except when treating complicated UTI, then no dose adjustment

Available forms: Single-use vials (500, 750 mg), premixed flexible container; 250 mg/50 ml D$_5$W, 500 mg/100 ml D$_5$W, 750 mg/150 ml D$_5$W; tabs 250, 500, 750 mg; oral sol 25 mg/ml

Implementation
• Obtain C&S before treatment and periodically
• Give PO 2 hr before or 2 hr after antacids, iron, calcium, zinc; give fluids
• Check for irritation, extravasation, phlebitis daily

Oral solution
• Give 1 hr prior to or 2 hr after food

Intermittent IV infusion route
• Discard any unused sol in the single-dose vial
• Visually inspect for particulate matter/discoloration prior to use

IV (single use vial)
• **500 mg/20 ml vials:** To prepare a dose of 500 mg, withdraw 10 ml from a 20-ml vial and dilute with a compatible IV solution (D$_5$W, NS) to a total volume of 50 ml. To prepare a 500-mg dosage, withdraw all 20 ml from the vial and dilute with a compatible IV solution to a total volume of 100 ml
• **750 mg/30 ml vials:** To prepare a dose of 750 mg, withdraw 30 ml from a 30-ml vial and dilute with a compatible intravenous solution (D$_5$W, NS) to a total volume of 150 ml
• The concentration of the diluted solution should be 5 mg/ml prior to administration. Solutions contain no preservatives; any unused portions must be discarded
• **Storage:** The diluted solution may be stored for up to 72 hours when stored at or below 25° C (77° F) or for 14 days when stored under refrigeration at 5° C (41° F) in plastic containers. Solutions may be frozen for up to 6 months (−20° C or −4° F) in glass bottles or plastic containers. Thaw frozen solutions at room temperature (25° C or 77° F) or in a refrigerator (8° C or 46° F). Do not force thaw by microwave or water bath immersion. Do not refreeze after initial thawing

Premixed IV solution
• No dilution is necessary

Intermittent IV injection
• Infuse doses of ≤500 mg IV over 60 minutes and doses of 750 mg IV over 90 minutes. Shorter infusions or bolus injections should be avoided because of the risk of hypotension

Y-site compatibilities: Alemtuzumab, alfentanil, amifostine, amikacin, aminocaproic acid, aminophylline, ampicillin, ampicillin-sulbactam, anidulafungin, argatroban, atenolol, atracurium, aztreonam, bivalirudin, bleomycin, bumetanide, buprenorphine, busulfan, butorphanol, caffeine citrate, calcium gluconate, CARBOplatin, carmustine, caspofungin, cefepime, cefoTEtan, ceftaroline, cefTAZidime, ceftizoxime, cefTRIAXone, cefuroxime, chlorproMAZINE, cimetidine, cisatracurium, CISplatin, clindamycin, codeine, cyclophosphamide, cycloSPORINE, cytarabine, dacarbazine, DACTINomycin, DAPTOmycin, DAUNOrubicin liposomal, dexamethasone, dexrazoxane, digoxin, diltiazem, diphenhydrAMINE, DOBUTamine, DOCEtaxel, dolasetron, DOPamine, doripenem, doxacurium, doxycycline, droperidol, enalaprilat, ePHEDrine, EPINEPHrine, epirubicin, ertapenem, erythromycin, esmolol, etoposide, etoposide phosphate, famotidine, fenoldopam, fentaNYL, filgrastim, floxuridine, fluconazole, fludarabine, foscarnet, fosphenytoin, gallium, gemcitabine, gemtuzumab, gentamicin, granisetron, haloperidol, hydrocortisone, HYDROmorphone, IDArubicin, ifosfamide, imipenem-cilastatin, irinotecan, isoproterenol, labetalol, lepirudin, leucovorin, levorphanol, lidocaine, linezolid, mannitol, mechlorethamine, meperidine, mesna, methylPREDNISolone, metoclopramide, metroNIDAZOLE, midazolam, milrinone, minocycline, mitoMYcin, mitoXANtrone, mivacurium, morphine, mycophenolate mofetil, nalbuphine, naloxone, nesiritide, netilmicin, niCARdipine, octreotide, ondansetron, oxacillin, oxaliplatin, oxytocin, PACLitaxel, palonosetron, pamidronate, pancuronium, PEMEtrexed, penicillin G sodium, pentamidine, phenylephrine, plicamycin, potassium acetate/chloride, promethazine, propranolol, quinupristin-dalfopristin, ranitidine, remifentanil, rocuronium, sargramostim, sodium bicarbonate, succinylcholine, SUFentanil, sulfamethoxazole-trimethoprim, tacrolimus, teniposide, theophylline, thiotepa, ticarcillin, ticarcillin-clavulanate, tigecycline, tirofiban, tobramycin, topotecan, trimethobenzamide, vancomycin, vasopressin, vecuronium, verapamil, vinBLAStine, vinCRIStine, vinorelbine, voriconazole, zidovudine, zoledronic acid

Solution compatibilities: 0.9% NaCl, D_5W, D_5/0.9% NaCl, D_5LR, D_5/0.45% NaCl, sodium lactate, plasma-lyte 56/D_5W

ADVERSE EFFECTS:

CNS: *Headache,* dizziness, *insomnia,* anxiety, **seizures,** *encephalopathy,* paresthesia, **pseudotumor cerebri**
CV: Chest pain, palpitations, vasodilatation, QT prolongation, hypotension (rapid infusion)
EENT: Dry mouth, visual impairment, tinnitus
GI: *Nausea,* flatulence, *vomiting,* diarrhea, abdominal pain, **pseudomembranous colitis, hepatotoxicity, esophagitis, pancreatitis**
GU: Vaginitis, crystalluria
HEMA: Eosinophilia, **hemolytic anemia,** lymphophemia
INTEG: Rash, pruritus, photosensitivity, **epidermal necrosis,** injection site reaction, edema
MISC: Hypoglycemia, hypersensitivity, tendon rupture, **rhabdomyolysis**
RESP: Pneumonitis

SYST: Anaphylaxis, multisystem organ failure, Stevens-Johnson syndrome, angioedema, toxic epidermal necrolysis

Pharmacokinetics

Absorption	Unknown
Distribution	Unknown
Excretion	Kidneys unchanged
Half-life	6-8 hr

Pharmacodynamics

Onset	Immediate
Peak	Infusion's end
Duration	Unknown

INTERACTIONS
Individual drugs
Calcium, iron, sucralfate, zinc: decreased absorption of levofloxacin
Foscarnet: increased CNS stimulation, seizures
Haloperidol, chloroquine, droperidol, pentamidine, arsenic trioxide, levomethadyl: increased QT prolongation
Magnesium: decreased levofloxacin absorption; do not use in same **IV** line
Probenecid: increased levofloxacin levels
Theophylline: decreased theophylline clearance; toxicity may result
Warfarin: increased bleeding

Drug classifications
Antacids (magnesium, aluminum): decreased absorption of levofloxacin

> **BLACK BOX WARNING:** Corticosteroids: increased tendon rupture

Class IA/III antidysrhythmics, some phenothiazines, beta agonists, local anesthetics, tricyclics, CYP3A4 inhibitors (amiodarone, clarithromycin, erythromycin, telithromycin, troleandomycin), CYP3A4 substrates (methadone, pimozide, QUETiapine, quiNIDine, risperidone, ziprasidone): increased QT prolongation
NSAIDs, cycloSPORINE: increased CNS stimulation, seizures

Drug/lab test
Increased: PT, INR
Decreased: glucose, lymphocytes

NURSING CONSIDERATIONS
Assessment
• Assess patient for previous sensitivity reaction to quinolones

---

- **Assess patient for signs and symptoms of infection,** including characteristics of wounds, sputum, urine, stool, WBC >10,000/mm^3, fever; baseline, during treatment
- Obtain C&S before beginning product therapy to identify if correct treatment has been initiated
- **QT prolongation:** Monitor for QT prolongation, ejection fraction; assess for chest pain, palpitations, dyspnea
- **Pseudomembranous colitis:** Assess for diarrhea, abdominal pain, fever, fatigue, anorexia; possible anemia, elevated WBC and low serum albumin; stop product and give usually either vancomycin or IV metroNIDAZOLE
- **Assess for allergic reactions and anaphylaxis:** rash, urticaria, pruritus, chills, fever, joint pain; may occur a few days after therapy begins; epinephrine and resuscitation equipment should be available for anaphylactic reaction
- Determine urine output; if decreasing, notify prescriber (may indicate nephrotoxicity); also check for increased BUN, creatinine
- Monitor blood tests: AST, ALT, CBC, Hct, bilirubin, LDH, alkaline phosphatase, Coombs' test monthly if patient is on long-term therapy
- Monitor electrolytes: potassium, sodium, chloride monthly if patient is on long-term therapy
- Monitor for bleeding: ecchymosis, bleeding gums, hematuria, stool guaiac daily if on long-term therapy
- **Assess for overgrowth of infection:** perineal itching, fever, malaise, redness, pain, swelling, drainage, rash, diarrhea, change in cough, sputum

> **BLACK BOX WARNING: Tendon rupture:** Discontinue product at first sign of tendon pain or inflammation; usually the Achilles tendon is affected, can occur up to a few months after treatment and may require surgical repair; steroids may increase risk

Patient/family education
- Teach patient to report sore throat, bruising, bleeding, joint pain; may indicate **blood dyscrasias (rare)**
- Advise patient to contact prescriber if vaginal itching, loose foul-smelling stools, furry tongue occur, may indicate superinfection; report itching, rash, pruritus, urticaria
- Instruct patient to take all medication prescribed for the length of time ordered; product must be taken around the clock to maintain blood levels; do not give medication to others

- Advise patient to notify prescriber of diarrhea with blood or pus
- Instruct patient to take 2 hr before antacids, iron, calcium, zinc products
- Tell patient to complete full course of therapy; to increase fluid intake to 2 L/day to prevent crystalluria
- Advise patient to avoid hazardous activities until response to product is known
- Instruct patient to rinse mouth frequently and use sugarless candy or gum for dry mouth
- Instruct patient to avoid taking other medications unless approved by prescriber
- Teach patient to monitor glucose (diabetes)
- Advise patient to avoid sun exposure or use sunscreen to prevent phototoxicity

> **BLACK BOX WARNING:** Teach patient to notify prescriber of tendon pain, inflammation, avoid corticosteroids with this product

Evaluation
Positive therapeutic outcome
- Absence of signs/symptoms of infection (WBC <10,000/mm^3, temp WNL)
- Reported improvement in symptoms of infection

levofloxacin ophthalmic
See Appendix B

levothyroxine (Rx)
(lee-voe-thye-rox′een)
Eltroxin ✦, Levothroid, Levoxyl, Synthroid, Tirosint, Unithroid
Func. class.: Thyroid hormone
Chem. class.: Levoisomer of thyroxine
Pregnancy category A

Do not confuse:
Synthroid/Symmetrel

ACTION: Controls protein synthesis; increases metabolic rate, cardiac output, renal blood flow, O$_2$ consumption, body temp, blood volume, growth, development at cellular level via action on thyroid hormone receptors

Therapeutic outcome: Correction of lack of thyroid hormone

USES: Hypothyroidism, myxedema coma, thyroid hormone replacement, thyrotoxicosis, congenital hypothyroidism, some types of thyroid cancer, pituitary TSH suppression

Adverse effects: *italics* = common; **bold** = life-threatening

CONTRAINDICATIONS:
Adrenal insufficiency, recent MI, thyrotoxicosis, hypersensitivity to beef, alcohol intolerance (inj only)

> **BLACK BOX WARNING:** Obesity treatment

Precautions: Pregnancy **A**, breastfeeding, geriatric, angina pectoris, hypertension, ischemia, cardiac disease, diabetes

DOSAGE AND ROUTES
Severe hypothyroidism
Adult ≤50 yr: PO 1.7 mcg/kg/day, 6-8 wk, average dose 100-200 mcg/day, max 200 mcg/day; IM/IV 50-100 mcg/day as a single dose or 50% of usual oral dosage

Adult >50 yr without heart disease or <50 yr with heart disease: PO 25-50 mcg/day, titrate q6-8wk

Adult >50 yr with heart disease: PO 12.5-25 mcg/day, titrate by 12.5-25 mcg q6-8wk

Child >12 yr: PO 2-3 mcg/kg/day given as a single dose AM

Child 6-12 yr: PO 4-5 mcg/kg/day given as a single dose AM

Child 1-5 yr: PO 5-6 mcg/kg/day given as a single dose AM

Child 6-12 mo: PO 6-8 mcg/kg/day given as a single dose AM

Child <6 mo: PO 8-10 mcg/kg/day given as a single dose AM

Myxedema coma
Adult: IV 200-500 mcg; may increase by 100-300 mcg after 24 hr; give oral medication as soon as possible

Subclinical hypothyroidism
Adult: PO 1 mcg/kg/day may be sufficient

Available forms: Powder for inj 200, 500 mcg/vial; tabs 25, 50, 88, 100, 112, 125, 137, 150, 175, 200, 300; cap (liquid filled) 13, 25, 50, 75, 88, 100, 112, 125, 137, 150 mcg

Implementation
• Store in tight, light-resistant container; sol should be discarded if not used immediately
• Withdraw medication 4 wk before RAIU test

PO route
• Give in AM if possible as a single dose to decrease sleeplessness; give at same time each day to maintain product level
• Give crushed and mixed with water, nonsoy formula, or breast milk for infants/children
• Give only for hormone imbalances; not to be used for obesity, male infertility, menstrual conditions, lethargy; give lowest dosage that relieves symptoms; lower dosage for geriatric and in cardiac disease
• Separate antacids, iron, calcium products by 4 hr

Direct IV route
• Give **IV** after diluting with provided diluent (0.9% NaCl), 500 mcg/5 ml, 200 mcg/2 ml; shake well; give through Y-tube or 3-way stopcock; give 100 mcg or less over 1 min; do not add to **IV** infusion; considered incompatible in syringe with all other products

ADVERSE EFFECTS
CNS: *Anxiety, insomnia, tremors,* headache, **thyroid storm,** excitability
CV: *Tachycardia, palpitations, angina, dysrhythmias,* hypertension, **cardiac arrest**
GI: Nausea, diarrhea, increased or decreased appetite, cramps
MISC: Menstrual irregularities, weight loss, sweating, heat intolerance, fever, alopecia, decreased bone mineral density

Pharmacokinetics
Absorption	Erratic (PO); complete (**IV**)
Distribution	Widely distributed
Metabolism	Liver; enterohepatic recirculation
Excretion	Feces via bile; breast milk (small amounts)
Half-life	6-7 days

Pharmacodynamics
	PO	IV
Onset	3-5 days	6-8 hr
Peak	12-48 hr	12-48 hr
Duration	Unknown	Unknown

INTERACTIONS
Individual drugs
Aluminum, calcium, iron, magnesium, sucralfate, rifampin, rifabutin: decreased levothyroxine effects
Orlistat, ferrous sulfate: decreased absorption of levothyroxine

Drug classifications
Antacids: decreased levothyroxine effects
Anticoagulants (oral): increased anticoagulant effect
Antidepressants (tricyclics): increased tricyclic effect
Bile acid sequestrants: decreased levothyroxine absorption

EPINEPHrine products: increased cardiac insufficiency risk

Estrogens: decreased thyroid hormone effects

Selective serotonin reuptake inhibitors: decreased levothyroxine effects

Sympathomimetics: increased sympathomimetic effect

Drug/herb
Soy: decreased thyroid hormone effect

Drug/lab test
Increased: CPK, LDH, AST, blood glucose
Decreased: thyroid function tests

NURSING CONSIDERATIONS
Assessment
• Determine if the patient is taking anticoagulants, antidiabetic agents; document on chart
• Take B/P, pulse before each dose; monitor I&O ratio and weight every day in same clothing, using same scale, at same time of day
• Monitor height, weight, psychomotor development, and growth rate if given to a child
• Monitor T_3, T_4, which are decreased; radioimmunoassay of TSH, which is increased; radioactive iodine uptake (RAIU), which is increased if patient's dosage of medication is too low
• Monitor pro-time (may require decreased anticoagulant); check for bleeding, bruising
• Assess for increased nervousness, excitability, irritability, which may indicate a too-high dosage of medication, usually after 1-3 wk of treatment
• Assess cardiac status: angina, palpitations, chest pain, change in VS; the geriatric patient may have undetected cardiac problems and baseline ECG should be completed before treatment

Patient/family education
• Teach patient that product is not a cure but controls symptoms and that treatment is long term
• Instruct patient to report excitability, irritability, anxiety, sweating, heat intolerance, chest pain, palpitations, which indicate overdose
• Advise patient not to switch brands unless approved by prescriber; bioavailability may differ; do not take with food; absorption will be decreased
• Teach patient that product may be discontinued after giving birth; thyroid panel will be evaluated after 1-2 mo
• Teach patient or parent that hyperthyroid child will show almost immediate behavior/personality change; that hair loss will occur in child but is temporary

• Caution patient that product is not to be taken to reduce weight
• Caution patient to avoid OTC preparations with iodine; read labels; other medications should not be used unless approved by prescriber
• Teach patient to avoid iodine-rich food: iodized salt, soybeans, tofu, turnips, high-iodine seafood, some bread

Evaluation
Positive therapeutic outcome
• Absence of depression
• Weight loss, increased diuresis, pulse, appetite
• Absence of constipation, peripheral edema, cold intolerance, pale, cool dry skin, brittle nails, alopecia, coarse hair, menorrhagia, night blindness, paresthesias, syncope, stupor, coma, rosy cheeks
• Improved levels of T_3, T_4 by laboratory tests
• Child: age-appropriate weight, height, and psychomotor development

TREATMENT OF OVERDOSE:
Withhold dose for up to 1 wk; acute overdose: gastric lavage or induced emesis, activated charcoal; provide supportive treatment to control symptoms

---

⚠ HIGH ALERT

lidocaine, parenteral (Rx)
(lye′doe-kane)
LidoPen Auto-Injector, Xylocaine, Xylocard ✚
Func. class.: Antidysrhythmic (class IB)
Chem. class.: Aminoacyl amide
Pregnancy category B

ACTION: Increases electrical stimulation threshold of ventricle and His-Purkinje system, which stabilizes cardiac membrane and decreases automaticity

Therapeutic outcome: Decreased ventricular dysrhythmia

USES: Ventricular tachycardia, ventricular dysrhythmias during cardiac surgery, MI, digoxin toxicity, cardiac catheterization

CONTRAINDICATIONS:
Hypersensitivity to amides, severe heart block, supraventricular dysrhythmias, Adams-Stokes syndrome, Wolff-Parkinson-White syndrome

---

Adverse effects: *italics* = common; **bold** = life-threatening

Precautions: Pregnancy **B**, breastfeeding, children, geriatric, renal/hepatic disease, CHF, respiratory depression, malignant hyperthermia, myasthenia gravis, weight <50 kg

DOSAGE AND ROUTES
Adult: **IV** BOL 50-100 mg (1-1.5 mg/kg) 25-50 mg/min, repeat q3-5min, max 300 mg in 1 hr; begin **IV** INF 1-4 mg/min (20-50 mcg/kg/min); IM 200-300 mg (4.3 mg/kg) in deltoid muscle, may repeat in 1-1½ hr if needed

Available forms: IV inf 0.2% (2 mg/ml), 0.4% (4 mg/ml), 0.8% (8 mg/ml); **IV** admixture 4% (40 mg/ml), 10% (100 mg/ml), 20% (200 mg/ml); **IV direct** 1% (10 mg/ml), 2% (20 mg/ml); **IM** 10% (300 mg/3 ml)

Implementation
IM route
• Administer in deltoid, aspirate to prevent **IV** administration
• Check site daily for extravasation

Direct IV route
• Give undiluted (1%, 2% only); give 6 mg or less over 1 min; if using an **IV** line, use port near insertion site, flush with 0.9% NaCl (50 ml)
• Store at room temperature; sol should be clear

Continuous IV infusion route
• Give after adding 1 g/250-1000 ml of D₅W; give 1-4 mg/min; use infusion pump for correct dosage; pediatric inf is 120 mg of lidocaine/100 ml of D₅W; 1-2.5 ml/kg/hr = 20-50 mcg/kg/min; use only 1%, 2% sol

Solution compatibilities: D₅W, D₅/0.9% NaCl, D₅/0.45% NaCl, D₅/LR, LR, 0.9% NaCl, 0.45% NaCl

Y-site compatibilities: Acetaminophen, alemtuzumab, alfentanil, alteplase, amikacin, aminocaproic acid, aminophylline, amiodarone, amphotericin B lipid/liposome, anidulafungin, argatroban, ascorbic acid injection, atenolol, atracurium, atropine, azithromycin, aztreonam, benztropine, bivalirudin, bleomycin, bumetanide, buprenorphine, butorphanol, calcium chloride/gluconate, CARBOplatin, carmustine, cefamandole, ceFAZolin, cefoperazone, cefotaxime, cefoTEtan, cefOXitin, ceftaroline, cefTAZidime, ceftizoxime, cefTRIAXone, cefuroxime, chloramphenicol, chlorproMAZINE, cimetidine, ciprofloxacin, cisatracurium, CISplatin, clarithromycin, clindamycin, cyanocobalamin, cyclophosphamide, cycloSPORINE, cytarabine, DACTINomycin, DAPTOmycin, DAUNOrubicin, dexamethasone, dexmedetomidine, dexrazoxane, digoxin, diltiazem, diphenhydrAMINE, DOBUTamine, DOCEtaxel, dolasetron, DOPamine, doxacurium, DOXOrubicin, DOXOrubicin liposomal, doxycycline, enalaprilat, EPINEPHrine, epirubicin, epoetin alfa, eptifibatide, ertapenem, erythromycin, esmolol, etomidate, etoposide, etoposide phosphate, famotidine, fenoldopam, fentaNYL, fluconazole, fludarabine, fluorouracil, folic acid, furosemide, gentamicin, granisetron, haloperidol, heparin, hydrocortisone, imipenem/cilastatin, inamrinone, insulin, isoproterenol, ketorolac, labetalol, levofloxacin, linezolid, LORazepam, magnesium sulfate, meperidine, methylPREDNISolone, metoclopramide, metoprolol, metroNIDAZOLE, micafungin, midazolam, morphine, nafcillin, niCARdipine, nitroglycerin, nitroprusside, norepinephrine, ondansetron, palonosetron, penicillin G potassium, phenylephrine, phytonadione, piperacillin/tazobactam, potassium chloride, procainamide, prochlorperazine, promethazine, propofol, propranolol, protamine, quinupristin/dalfopristin, ranitidine, remifentanil, sodium bicarbonate, tacrolimus, theophylline, ticarcillin/clavulanate, tigecycline, tirofiban, tobramycin, vancomycin, vasopressin, verapamil, vitamin B complex with C, voriconazole, warfarin

Y-site incompatibilities: Acyclovir, amphotericin B cholesteryl sulfate complex/colloidal, azaTHIOprine, caspofungin, diazepam, ganciclovir, lansoprazole, pantoprazole, phenytoin, thiopental, trimethoprim/sulfamethoxazole

ADVERSE EFFECTS
CNS: *Headache, dizziness,* involuntary movement, confusion, tremor, *drowsiness,* euphoria, **seizures,** shivering
CV: *Hypotension, bradycardia,* **heart block, cardiovascular collapse, arrest**
EENT: Tinnitus, blurred vision
GI: Nausea, vomiting, anorexia
HEMA: Methemoglobinemia
INTEG: Rash, urticaria, edema, swelling, petechiae, pruritus
MISC: Febrile response, phlebitis at inj site
RESP: Dyspnea, **respiratory depression**

Pharmacokinetics
Absorption	Complete bioavailability (**IV**)
Distribution	Erythrocytes, cardiovascular endothelium
Metabolism	Liver
Excretion	Kidneys
Half-life	Biphasic 8 min, 1-2 hr

Pharmacodynamics

	IV	IM
Onset	2 min	5-15 min
Peak	Unknown	½ hr
Duration	20 min	1½ hr

INTERACTIONS

Individual drugs

Amiodarone, phenytoin, procainamide, propranolol: increase cardiac depression, toxicity

Cimetidine, metoprolol, phenytoin: increased lidocaine effects

CycloSPORINE: decreased effect of cycloSPORINE

Tubocurarine: increased neuromuscular blockade

Drug classifications

Antihypertensives, MAOIs: increased hypotensive effects

β-blockers, protease inhibitors: increased lidocaine effects

Barbiturates: decreased lidocaine effects

Neuromuscular blockers: increased neuromuscular blockade

Drug/lab test

Increased: CPK

NURSING CONSIDERATIONS

Assessment

• Assess for oxygenation or perfusion deficit: decreased B/P, chest pain, dizziness, loss of consciousness

• Assess respiratory status: auscultate lung fields for bibasilar crackles in patients with advanced CHF

• Assess for urinary retention: check for pain, abdominal absorption, palpate bladder; check males with benign prostatic hypertrophy; anticholinergic reaction may cause retention

• Monitor I&O ratio, electrolytes (potassium, sodium, chloride); watch for decreasing urinary output, possible retention

• Monitor liver function tests: AST, ALT, bilirubin, alk phos

• Monitor ECG continuously to determine product effectiveness, measure PR, QRS, QT intervals, check for PVCs, other dysrhythmias; monitor B/P continuously for hypo/hypertension; check for rebound hypertension after 1-2 hr, prolonged PR/QT intervals, QRS complex; if QT or QRS increases by 50% or more, withhold next dose, notify prescriber

• Monitor for CNS symptoms: confusion, numbness, depression, involuntary movements; if these occur, product should be discontinued

• Monitor blood levels (therapeutic level 1.5-5 mcg/ml), notify prescriber of abnormal results

Patient/family education

• Teach patient or family reason for use of medication and expected results

⚠ Instruct patient in at-home use of Lidopen Auto-Injector; patient should call prescriber before use if heart attack is imminent

Evaluation

Positive therapeutic outcome

• Decreased B/P, dysrhythmias

• Decreased heart rate

• Normal sinus rhythm

TREATMENT OF OVERDOSE:

Oxygen, artificial ventilation, ECG, administer DOPamine for circulatory depression, diazepam or thiopental for seizures; decreased product or discontinuation may be required

lidocaine topical
See Appendix B

linaclotide
(lin'a-kloe'tide)
Linzess
Func. class.: Functional GI disorder agent
Chem. class.: Selective guanylate cyclase C agonist
Pregnancy category C

ACTION: Acts locally on the luminal surface of the intestinal epithelium; stimulates secretion of chloride and bicarbonate into the intestinal lumen; this action results in increased intestinal fluid and accelerated GI transit

Therapeutic outcome: Decreased constipation in IBS

USES: Irritable bowel syndrome (IBS) with constipation, chronic constipation not associated with IBS

CONTRAINDICATIONS:

Hypersensitivity, urticaria, infection, sinusitis, GI obstruction

> **BLACK BOX WARNING** Children <6 yr, infants, neonates

Precautions: Pregnancy (C), breastfeeding, diarrhea, abdominal pain, cholelithiasis, Crohn's

---

Adverse effects: *italics* = common; **bold** = life-threatening

disease, diverticulitis, fecal impaction, gastric cancer, GI disease, IBS

DOSAGE AND ROUTES
Constipation
Adult: PO 145 mcg/day on empty stomach, AM

Irritable bowel syndrome
Adult: PO 290 mcg/day on empty stomach, AM

Available forms: Caps 145, 290 mcg

Implementation
• Give on empty stomach, ≥30 min before first meal of day, swallow whole
• Store at room temperature

ADVERSE EFFECTS
CNS: Headache, fatigue
GI: Nausea, abdominal pain, diarrhea, flatulence, fecal incontinence, vomiting, GERD, GI bleeding

Pharmacokinetics

Absorption	Minimally absorbed, metabolized within the GI tract

INTERACTIONS
Drug classifications
Antidiarrheals: do not use with this agent
Antimuscarinics: decreased linaclotide effect

NURSING CONSIDERATIONS
Assessment

> **BLACK BOX WARNING** Neonates/infants/children <6 yr: Monitor carefully, product can cause serious effects, including death

• GI symptoms: Assess for nausea, abdominal pain, evidence of mechanical GI obstruction; check for other sources of constipation, determine stool quality and frequency

Patient/family education
• Teach patient to notify prescriber of GI symptoms, avoid antidiarrheals, if severe diarrhea occurs, stop product
• Advise patient not to crush, break, chew
• Pregnancy C: Teach patient to avoid use in pregnancy, breastfeeding

Evaluation
Positive therapeutic outcome
• Decreased constipation in IBS

---

linagliptin
(lin-a-glip′tin)
Tradjenta
Func. class.: Antidiabetic
Chem. class.: Dipeptidyl peptidase-4 inhibitor
Pregnancy category B

ACTION: Slows the inactivation of incretin hormones. Concentrations of the active, intact hormones are increased by linagliptin, thereby increasing and prolonging the action of these hormones. Incretin hormones are released by the intestine throughout the day, and levels are increased in response to a meal.

Therapeutic outcome: Decreasing blood glucose level, A1c; decreasing polydipsia, polyphagia

USES: Type 2 diabetes mellitus

CONTRAINDICATIONS:
Hypersensitivity to linagliptin, type 1 diabetes mellitus, diabetic ketoacidosis (DKA)

Precautions: Pregnancy category B, breastfeeding, adolescents or children <18 years old, debilitated physical condition, malnutrition, uncontrolled adrenal insufficiency, pituitary insufficiency, hypothyroidism, diarrhea, gastroparesis, GI obstruction, ileus, female hormonal changes, high fever, severe psychological stress, uncontrolled hypercortisolism, hyperthyroidism

DOSAGE AND ROUTES
Adult: PO 5 mg/day; when used with a sulfonylurea, a lower dose of the sulfonylurea or insulin may be necessary to minimize the risk of hypoglycemia

Available forms: Tab 5 mg

Implementation
• Given once daily; may give without regard to food
• Store at room temperature

ADVERSE EFFECTS
CNS: Headache
EENT: Nasopharyngitis
ENDO: Hyperuricemia, hypoglycemia
GI: Body weight loss, **pancreatitis**
INTEG: **Angioedema, exfoliative dermatitis,** hypersensitivity reactions, urticaria
MISC: Arthralgia, back pain
RESP: Bronchial hyperreactivity (with **bronchospasm**), cough, nasopharyngitis

---

Pharmacokinetics

Absorption	Rapidly, bioavailability 30%
Distribution	Extensive, tissues; protein binding concentration dependent
Metabolism	Weak CYP3A4 inhibitor
Excretion	90% unchanged, 80% enterohepatic, urine 5%
Half-life	Terminal >100 hr, effective 12 hr

Pharmacodynamics

Onset	Unknown
Peak	Unknown
Duration	Unknown

INTERACTIONS

Individual drugs
Alcohol, cisapride, lithium, metoclopramide, tegaserod: increased need for dosing change

Bumetanide, dextrothyroxine, ethacrynic acid, ethotoin, fosphenytoin, furosemide, glucagon, niacin (nicotinic acid), phenothiazine, phenytoin, torsemide, triamterene: decreased hypoglycemic effect

CloNIDine, dexfenfluramine, disopyramide, fenfluramine, fluoxetine, guanethidine, octreotide: increased hypoglycemia

Reserpine, β-blockers: increased masking the signs and symptoms of hypoglycemia

Drug classifications
Beta blockers, ACE inhibitors, angiotensin II receptor antagonists, fibric acid derivatives, monoamine oxidase inhibitors (MAOIs), salicylates, sulfonylureas: increased or prolonged hypoglycemia

Atypical antipsychotics (ARIPiprazole, cloZAPine, OLANZapine, QUEtiapine, risperidone, and ziprasidone), carbonic anhydrase inhibitors, estrogens, glucocorticoids, oral contraceptives, progestins, thiazide diuretics, thyroid hormones: decreased hypoglycemic effect

Androgens, quinolones: increased need for dosing change

CYP3A4 inducers (topiramate, rifabutin, pioglitazone, OXcarbazepine, carBAMazepine, nevirapine, modafinil, metyrapone, etravirine, efavirenz, bosentan, barbiturates, aprepitant, fosaprepitant): decreased effect of linagliptin

Drug/lab test
Increased: uric acid

NURSING CONSIDERATIONS

Assessment
• Monitor blood glucose, A1c, during treatment to determine diabetes control
• Monitor CBC baseline and periodically during treatment, report decreased blood counts

Patient/family education
• Teach patient the symptoms of hypo/hyperglycemia and what to do about each; to have glucagon emergency kit available, carry sugar packets
• Advise patient that product must be continued on a daily basis, explain consequences of discontinuing product abruptly; to take only as directed
• Direct patient to avoid OTC products unless approved by prescriber
• Teach patient that diabetes is a life-long illness, product will not cure diabetes
• Advise patient to carry emergency ID with prescriber, condition and medications taken
⚠ **Report immediately, skin disorders, swelling, difficulty breathing, or severe abdominal pain**

Evaluation
Positive therapeutic outcome
• Improving blood glucose level, A1c; decreasing polydipsia, polyphagia, polyuria, clear sensorium, absence of dizziness

---

lindane (OTC)
(lin-dane)
Hexit ♣
Func. class.: Scabicide/pediculicide
Chem. class.: Chlorinated hydrocarbon (synthetic)
Pregnancy category C

ACTION: Stimulates nervous system of arthropods, resulting in seizures, death of organism

Therapeutic outcome: Resolution of infestation

USES: Scabies, lice (head/pubic/body), nits in those intolerant to or who do not respond to other agents

CONTRAINDICATIONS:
Hypersensitivity; patients with known seizure disorders; Norwegian (crusted) scabies

---

BLACK BOX WARNING: Premature neonate; inflammation of skin, abrasions, or breaks in skin; seizure disorder

Precautions: Pregnancy **C,** breastfeeding, infants, children <10 yr; avoid contact with eyes

DOSAGE AND ROUTES
Lice
Adult and child: Shampoo using 30 ml, work into lather, rub for 5 min, rinse, dry with towel; use fine-toothed comb to remove nits; most require 1 oz, max 2 oz

Scabies
Adult and child: TOP cream/lotion wash area with soap and water, remove visible crusts; apply to skin surfaces; remove with soap, water 8-12 hr after application; may reapply in 1 wk if needed; TOP apply 1% cream/lotion to skin from neck to bottom of feet, toes; repeat in 1 wk if necessary; most require 1 oz, max 2 oz

Available forms: Lotion, shampoo, cream (1%)

Implementation
• Apply to body areas, scalp only; do not apply to face, lips, mouth, eyes, any mucous membrane, anus, or meatus
• Give topical corticosteroids as ordered to decrease contact dermatitis; provide antihistamines
• Apply menthol or phenol lotions to control itching
• Give topical antibiotics for infection
• Provide isolation until areas on skin, scalp have cleared and treatment is completed
• Remove nits by using a fine-toothed comb rinsed in vinegar after treatment; use gloves
• Caregivers applying these products to another person should wear gloves less permeable to lindane, thoroughly clean hands after application, avoid natural latex gloves
Cream/ointment/lotion
• Use for scabies only; skin should be clean without other products on it, wait 1 hr after bathing or showering before application, shake well, apply under fingernails after trimming, a toothbrush can be used to apply; after application wrap toothbrush in paper and discard, use only a single application, apply as a thin layer over all skin from neck down, close bottle with leftover and discard
• Do not cover, wash off after 8-12 hr using warm (not hot) water, do not leave on >12 hr

Shampoo
• For lice only, do not use other hair products before use, shake well, hair should be completely dry, use only enough shampoo to lightly wet the hair and scalp, work into hair, do not use water, allow to remain only 4 min, rinse and lather away, towel briskly

ADVERSE EFFECTS
CNS: Seizures, stimulation, dizziness
INTEG: *Pruritus, rash, irritation, contact dermatitis*

Pharmacokinetics
Absorption	20%
Distribution	Fat
Metabolism	Liver
Excretion	Kidneys
Half-life	18 hr

Pharmacodynamics
Onset	Rapid
Peak	Rapid
Duration	3 hr

INTERACTIONS
Oil-based hair dressing: increased absorption; wash, rinse, and dry hair before using lindane

NURSING CONSIDERATIONS
Assessment

BLACK BOX WARNING: Skin with abrasions, breaks, inflammation; do not use on these areas

• **Infestation:** Assess head, hair for lice and nits before, after treatment; if scabies are present, check all skin surfaces
• Identify source of infection: school, family members, sexual contacts

Patient/family education
• Advise patient to wash all inhabitants' clothing, using insecticide; preventive treatment may be required for all persons living in same house, using lotion or shampoo to decrease spread of infection; use rubber gloves when applying product
• Instruct patient that itching may continue for 4-6 wk; that product must be reapplied if accidently washed off, or treatment will be ineffective; remove after specified time to prevent toxicity
• Advise patient not to apply to face; if contact with eyes occurs, flush with water

- Advise patient that sexual contacts should be treated simultaneously

⚠ Inform the patient of CNS toxicity: dizziness, cramps, anxiety, nausea, vomiting, seizures

Evaluation
Positive therapeutic outcome
- Decreased crusts, nits, brownish trails on skin, itching papules in skinfolds
- Decreased itching after several wk

TREATMENT OF INGESTION:
Gastric lavage, saline laxatives, **IV** diazepam (Valium) for seizures (if taken orally)

---

linezolid (Rx)
(lih-nee′zoh-lid)
Zyvox
Func. class.: Broad-spectrum antiinfective
Chem. class.: Oxazolidinone
Pregnancy category C

Do not confuse:
Zyvox/Ziox/Zosyn

ACTION: Inhibits protein synthesis by interfering with translation; binds to bacterial 23S ribosomal RNA of the 50S subunit, preventing formation of the bacterial translation process in primarily gram-positive organisms

Therapeutic outcome: Negative blood cultures, absence of signs/symptoms of infection

USES: Vancomycin-resistant *Enterococcus faecium* infections, nosocomial pneumonia caused by *Staphylococcus aureus* or *Streptococcus pneumoniae,* uncomplicated or complicated skin and skin structure infections, community-acquired pneumonia, *Pasteurella multocida,* viridans Streptococcus

CONTRAINDICATIONS:
Hypersensitivity

Precautions: Pregnancy **C**, breastfeeding, children, thrombocytopenia, bone marrow suppression, hypertension, hyperthyroidism, pheochromocytoma, seizure disorder, ulcerative colitis, MI, PKU, renal/GI disease

DOSAGE AND ROUTES
Vancomycin-resistant *E. faecium* infections
Adult/adolescent/child ≥12 yr: **IV**/PO 600 mg q12hr × 14-28 days; max 1200 mg/day

Child <12 yr/infant/term neonate: **IV**/PO 10 mg/kg q8hr × 14-28 days

Nosocomial pneumonia/complicated skin infections/community-acquired pneumonia/concurrent bacterial infection
Adult: **IV**/PO 600 mg q12hr × 10-14 days; max 1200 mg/day
Child birth-11 yr: PO 10 mg/kg q8hr × 10-14 days

Uncomplicated skin infections
Adult: **IV**/PO 400 mg q12hr × 10-14 days; max 1200 mg/day
Adolescent: PO 600 mg q12hr × 10-14 days, max 1200 mg/day
Infant, preterm <7 days old: PO 10 mg/kg q12hr × 10-14 days

Available forms: Tabs 600 mg; oral susp 100 mg/5 ml; inj 2 mg/ml

Implementation
PO route
- Store reconstituted oral susp at room temperature, use within 3 wk
- Give over 30-120 min; do not use **IV** inf bag in series connections; do not use with additives in sol, do not use with another product, administer separately, flush line before and after use

Intermittent IV infusion route
- Do not use if particulate is present; yellow color is normal
- Premixed solutions are ready to use (2 mg/ml)

Y-site compatibilities: Acyclovir, alfentanil, amikacin, aminophylline, ampicillin, aztreonam, bretylium, buprenorphine, butorphanol, calcium gluconate, CARBOplatin, ceFAZolin, cefoperazone, cefoTEtan, cefOXitin, cefTAZidime, ceftizoxime, cefTRIAXone, cefuroxime, cimetidine, ciprofloxacin, cisatracurium, CISplatin, clindamycin, cyclophosphamide, cycloSPORINE, cytarabine, HYDROmorphone, ifosfamide, labetalol, leucovorin, levofloxacin, lidocaine, LORazepam, magnesium sulfate, mannitol, meperidine, meropenem, mesna, methotrexate, methylPREDNISolone, metoclopramide, metroNIDAZOLE, midazolam, minocycline, mitoXANtrone, morphine, nalbuphine, naloxone, nitroglycerin, ofloxacin, ondansetron, PACLitaxel, PENTobarbital, piperacillin, potassium chloride, prochlorperazine, promethazine, propranolol, ranitidine, remifentanil, theophylline, ticarcillin, tobramycin, vancomycin, vecuronium, verapamil, vinCRIStine, zidovudine

Solution compatibilities: D₅, 0.9% NaCl, LR

ADVERSE EFFECTS

CNS: *Headache*, dizziness, insomnia
GI: *Nausea, diarrhea*, increased ALT, AST, *vomiting*, taste change, tongue color change, **pseudomembranous colitis**
HEMA: Myelosuppression
MISC: Vaginal moniliasis, fungal infection, oral moniliasis, **lactic acidosis,** anaphylaxis, angioedema, **Stevens-Johnson syndrome**

Pharmacokinetics

Absorption	Rapid, excessive
Distribution	Protein binding 31%
Metabolism	Oxidation of the morpholine ring
Excretion	Unknown
Half-life	Unknown

Pharmacodynamics

Unknown

INTERACTIONS

Individual drugs

Amoxapine, cyclobenzaprine, maprotiline, methyldopa, mirtazapine, traZODone: increased hypertensive crisis, seizures, coma

Drug classifications

Adrenergic blockers: increased effects of adrenergics

Antidepressants (tricyclics): increased hypertensive crisis, seizures, coma

MAOIs or those that possess MAOI-like action (flurazolidone, isoniazid, procarbazine): do not use together; hypertensive crisis may occur

SSRIs, SNRIs: increased serotonin syndrome
Serotoninergic agents: increased effect

Drug/herb

Green tea, valerian, ginseng, yohimbe, kava: avoid use

Drug/food

Tyramine foods: avoid; increased pressor response

NURSING CONSIDERATIONS

Assessment

• Assess CNS symptoms: headache, dizziness
• Monitor liver function tests: AST, ALT
• Monitor CBC weekly, assess for myelosuppression (anemia, leukopenia, pancytopenia, thrombocytopenia)
⚠ **Pseudomembranous colitis:** Assess for **diarrhea, abdominal pain, fever, fatigue, anorexia; possible anemia, elevated WBC,** and low serum albumin; stop product and usually give either vancomycin or IV metroNIDAZOLE
⚠ **Serotonin syndrome:** at least 2 wk should elapse between continuing linezolid and start of serotonergic agents; assess for increased heart rate, shivering, sweating, dilated pupils, tremor, high B/P, hyperthermia, headache, confusion; if these occur stop linezolid; administer a serotonin antagonist if needed
⚠ **Lactic acidosis:** repeated nausea/vomiting, unexplained acidosis, low bicarbonate level: notify prescriber immediately
⚠ **Anaphylaxis/angioedema/Stevens-Johnson syndrome:** rash, pruritus, difficulty breathing, fever: have emergency equipment nearby
• **Diabetes mellitus:** Monitor those receiving insulin or oral antidiabetics for increased hypoglycemia

Patient/family education

• Advise patient if dizziness occurs, to ambulate and perform activities with assistance
• Advise patient to complete full course of product therapy
• Advise patient to contact prescriber if adverse reaction occurs
• Advise patient to avoid large amounts of tyramine-containing foods (give list)

Evaluation

Positive therapeutic outcome

• Decreased symptoms of infection, blood cultures negative

---

liothyronine (T$_3$) (Rx)

(lye-oh-thye′roe-neen)
Cytomel, Triostat
Func. class.: Thyroid hormone
Chem. class.: Synthetic T$_3$
Pregnancy category A

ACTION: Increases metabolic rates, cardiac output, O$_2$ consumption, body temp, blood volume, growth, development at cellular level; exact mechanism unknown

Therapeutic outcome: Correction of lack of thyroid hormone

USES: Hypothyroidism, myxedema coma, thyroid hormone replacement, nontoxic goiter, T$_3$ suppression test, congenital hypothyroidism

---

CONTRAINDICATIONS:
Adrenal insufficiency, MI, thyrotoxicosis, untreated hypertension

BLACK BOX WARNING: Obesity treatment

Precautions: Pregnancy **A,** breastfeeding, geriatric, angina pectoris, hypertension, ischemia, cardiac disease, diabetes

DOSAGE AND ROUTES
Adult: PO 25 mcg/day, increase by 12.5-25 mcg q1-2wk until desired response; maintenance dose 25-75 mcg/day; max 100 mcg/day
Geriatric: PO 5 mcg/day, increase by 5 mcg/day q1-2wk, maintenance 25-75 mcg/day

Congenital hypothyroidism
Child >3 yr: PO 50-100 mcg/day
Child <3 yr: PO 5 mcg/day, increase by 5 mcg q3-4day titrated to response; infant maintenance 20 mcg/day; 1-3 yr 50 mcg/day

Myxedema, severe hypothyroidism
Adult: PO 25-50 mcg, then may increase by 5-10 mcg q1-2wk; maintenance dose 50-100 mcg/day

Myxedema coma/precoma
Adult: IV 25-50 mcg initially; 5 mcg in geriatric; 10-20 mcg in cardiac disease; give doses q4-12hr

Nontoxic goiter
Adult: PO 5 mcg/day, increase by 12.5-25 mcg q1-2wk; maintenance dose 75 mcg/day

Suppression test (T₃)
Adult: PO 75-100 mcg daily × 1 wk; ¹³¹I is given before and after 1st wk dose

Available forms: Tabs 5, 25, 50 mcg; inj 10 mcg/ml

Implementation
PO route
• Give in AM if possible as a single dose to decrease sleeplessness; give at same time each day to maintain product level
• Do not take with food or absorption will be decreased
• Give only for hormone imbalances; not to be used for obesity, male infertility, menstrual conditions, lethargy; give lowest dose that relieves symptoms; give lower dose to geriatric and those with cardiac disease
• Store in airtight, light-resistant container

IV route
• Administer **IV** for myxedema coma and precoma; do not give IM or SUBCUT; give q4-12hr; use PO dose as soon as feasible

ADVERSE EFFECTS
CNS: *Insomnia, tremors,* headache, **thyroid storm**
CV: *Tachycardia, palpitations, angina, dysrhythmias,* hypertension, **cardiac arrest**
GI: Nausea, diarrhea, increased or decreased appetite, cramps
MISC: Menstrual irregularities, weight loss, sweating, heat intolerance, fever, alopecia

Pharmacokinetics
Absorption	Well (PO); complete (**IV**)
Distribution	Widely distributed; does not cross placenta
Metabolism	Liver
Excretion	Feces via bile, breast milk
Half-life	1-2 days

Pharmacodynamics
	PO/IV
Onset	Unknown
Peak	12-24 hr
Duration	72 hr

INTERACTIONS
Individual drugs
Cholestyramine, colestipol: decreased absorption of thyroid hormone

Drug classifications
Amphetamines, anticoagulants (oral), antidepressants (tricyclics), decongestants, sympathomimetics, vasopressors: increased effect of each specific product
Calcium, iron, aluminum, magnesium products: decreased absorption of liothyronine
Estrogens: decreased effects of liothyronine

Drug/herb
Soy: decreased thyroid hormone effect

Drug/lab test
Increased: CPK, LDH, AST, PBI, blood glucose
Decreased: thyroid function tests

NURSING CONSIDERATIONS
Assessment
• Determine if the patient is taking anticoagulants, antidiabetic agents; document on patient record

• Take B/P, pulse before each dose; monitor I&O ratio and weight every day in same clothing, using same scale, at same time of day
• Monitor height, weight, psychomotor development, and growth rate of child
• Monitor T_3, T_4, FTIs, which are decreased; radioimmunoassay of TSH, which is increased; radioactive iodine uptake, which is increased if medication dose is too low
• Monitor pro-time; may require decreased anticoagulant; check for bleeding, bruising
• Assess for increased nervousness, excitability, irritability, which may indicate a too-high dose, usually after 1-3 wk of treatment
• Assess cardiac status: angina, palpitations, chest pain, change in VS; geriatric may have undetected cardiac problems, and baseline ECG should be completed before treatment

Patient/family education
• Teach patient that product is not a cure but controls symptoms, treatment is long term
• Instruct patient to report excitability, irritability, anxiety, sweating, heat intolerance, chest pain, palpitations, which indicate overdose
• Advise patient not to switch brands unless approved by prescriber; bioavailability may differ
• Teach patient that product might be discontinued after giving birth; thyroid panel will be evaluated after 1-2 mo
• Teach patient that hyperthyroid child will show almost immediate behavior/personality change; that hair loss will occur in child but is temporary
• Caution patient that product is not to be taken to reduce weight
• Caution patient to avoid OTC preparations with iodine; read labels; other medications should not be used unless approved by prescriber
• Teach patient to avoid iodine-rich food: iodized salt, soybeans, tofu, turnips, high-iodine seafood, some bread

Evaluation
Positive therapeutic outcome
• Absence of depression
• Weight loss
• Increased diuresis, pulse, appetite
• Absence of constipation, peripheral edema, cold intolerance, pale cool dry skin, brittle nails, alopecia, coarse hair, menorrhagia, night blindness, paresthesias, syncope, stupor, coma, rosy cheeks
• Improved levels of T_3, T_4 by laboratory tests
• Child: age-appropriate weight, height, and psychomotor development

TREATMENT OF OVERDOSE:
Withhold dose for up to 1 wk; for acute overdose: gastric lavage or induce emesis, then activated charcoal; provide supportive treatment to control symptoms

---

liotrix (Rx)
(lye'oh-trix)
T₃/T₄, Thyrolar
Func. class.: Thyroid hormone
Chem. class.: Levothyroxine/liothyronine (synthetic T_4, T_3)
Pregnancy category A

Do not confuse:
Thyrolar/Thyrar

ACTION: Increases metabolic rates, cardiac output, O_2 consumption, body temp, blood volume, growth, development at cellular level; exact mechanism unknown

Therapeutic outcome: Correction of lack of thyroid hormone

USES: Hypothyroidism, thyroid hormone replacement

CONTRAINDICATIONS:
Adrenal insufficiency, MI, thyrotoxicosis

> **BLACK BOX WARNING:** Obesity treatment

Precautions: Pregnancy **A**, breastfeeding, geriatric, angina pectoris, hypertension, ischemia, cardiac disease, diabetes mellitus

DOSAGE AND ROUTES
Adult: PO a single dose of Thyrolar ¼ or ½ adult dose, adjust as needed at 2-wk intervals
Geriatric: PO ¼ tab initially, adjust q6-8wk

Available forms: Tabs levothyroxine 12.5 mcg/liothyronine 3.1 mcg; levothyroxine 25 mcg/liothyronine 6.25 mcg (Thyrolar-½); levothyroxine 50 mcg/liothyronine 12.5 mcg (Thyrolar-1); levothyroxine 100 mcg/liothyronine 25 mcg (Thyrolar-2); levothyroxine 150 mcg/liothyronine 37.5 mcg (Thyrolar-3)

Implementation
• Give in AM if possible as a single dose to decrease sleeplessness; give at same time each day to maintain product level
• Do not give with food or absorption will be decreased
• Give only for hormone imbalances; not to be used for obesity, male infertility, menstrual con-

---

ditions, lethargy; give lowest dose that relieves symptoms; give lower dose to the geriatric and those with cardiac disease
- Store in airtight, light-resistant container
- Remove medication 4 wk before RAIU test

ADVERSE EFFECTS

CNS: *Insomnia, tremors,* headache, **thyroid storm,** nervousness
CV: *Tachycardia, palpitations, angina, dysrhythmias,* hypertension, **cardiac arrest**
GI: Nausea, diarrhea, increased or decreased appetite, cramps, vomiting
MISC: Menstrual irregularities, weight loss, sweating, heat intolerance, fever

Pharmacokinetics

Absorption	50%-80% (T_4); 95% (T_3)
Distribution	Widely distributed; does not cross placenta
Metabolism	Liver, tissues
Excretion	Feces via bile; breast milk
Half-life	6-7 days (T_4); 2 days (T_3)

Pharmacodynamics

	PO (T_4)	PO (T_3)
Onset	Unknown	Unknown
Peak	Unknown	24-72 hr
Duration	Unknown	72 hr

INTERACTIONS

Individual drugs
CarBAMazepine, phenytoin, rifampin: decreased effects of liotrix
Cholestyramine: decreased absorption of thyroid hormone
Colestipol: decreased absorption of liotrix

Drug classifications
Amphetamines, decongestants, vasopressors: increased effect of each specific product
Anticoagulants (oral): increased effect of anticoagulants
Antidepressants (tricyclics): increased tricyclic effect
Catecholamines: increased catecholamine effect
Estrogens: decreased liotrix effect
Sympathomimetics: increased sympathomimetic effect

Drug/herb
Soy: decreased thyroid hormone effect

Drug/lab test
Increased: CPK, LDH, AST, PBI, blood glucose
Decreased: thyroid function tests

NURSING CONSIDERATIONS
Assessment
- Determine if the patient is taking anticoagulants, antidiabetic agents; document on chart
- Take B/P, pulse before each dose; monitor I&O ratio and weight every day in same clothing, using same scale, at same time of day
- Monitor height, weight, psychomotor development, and growth rate if given to a child
- Monitor T_3, T_4, FTIs, which are decreased; radioimmunoassay of TSH, which is increased; radioactive iodine uptake (RA international units), which is increased if medication dose is too low
- Monitor pro-time; may require decreased anticoagulant; check for bleeding, bruising
- Assess for increased nervousness, excitability, irritability, which may indicate a too-high dose of medication, usually after 1-3 wk of treatment
- Assess cardiac status: angina, palpitations, chest pain, change in VS; the geriatric patient may have undetected cardiac problems, and baseline ECG should be completed before treatment

Patient/family education
- Teach patient that product is not a cure but controls symptoms; treatment is long term
- Instruct patient to report excitability, irritability, anxiety, sweating, heat intolerance, chest pain, palpitations, which indicate overdose
- Advise patient not to switch brands unless approved by prescriber; bioavailability may differ
- Teach patient that product might be discontinued after giving birth; thyroid panel will be evaluated after 1-2 mo
- Teach patient that hyperthyroid child will show almost immediate behavior/personality change; that hair loss will occur in child but is temporary
- Caution patient that product is not to be taken to reduce weight
- Caution patient to avoid OTC preparations with iodine; read labels; other medications should not be used unless approved by prescriber
- Teach patient to avoid iodine-rich food: iodized salt, soybeans, tofu, turnips, high iodine seafood, some bread

Evaluation
Positive therapeutic outcome
- Absence of depression
- Weight loss
- Increased diuresis, pulse, appetite
- Absence of constipation, peripheral edema, cold intolerance, pale cool dry skin, brittle nails,

alopecia, coarse hair, menorrhagia, night blindness, paresthesias, syncope, stupor, coma, rosy cheeks
• Improved levels of T_3, T_4 by laboratory tests
• Child: age-appropriate weight, height, and psychomotor development

TREATMENT OF OVERDOSE:
Withhold dose for up to 1 wk; acute overdose: gastric lavage or induce emesis, then activated charcoal; provide supportive treatment to control symptoms

---

liraglutide (Rx)
(lir'a-gloo'tide)
Victoza
Func. class.: Antidiabetic agent
Chem. class.: Incretin mimetics
Pregnancy category C

ACTION: Improved glycemic control and potential weight loss via activation of the glucagon-like peptide-1 (GLP-1) receptor

Therapeutic outcome: Stable and improved serum glucose, HbA1C, weight loss

USES: Type 2 diabetes mellitus in combination with diet and exercise

CONTRAINDICATIONS:
Hypersensitivity, pancreatitis

Precautions: Alcoholism, breastfeeding, children, cholelithiasis, ketoacidosis, diarrhea, elderly, fever, gastroparesis, hepatic disease, hypoglycemia, infection, renal disease, surgery, thyroid disease, trauma, vomiting, pregnancy **C**

BLACK BOX WARNING: Medullary thyroid carcinoma (MTC), multiple endocrine neoplasia syndrome type 2 (MEN 2), thyroid cancer

---

DOSAGE AND ROUTES
Adult: Subcut 0.6 mg/day × 1 wk, then increase to 1.2 mg/day, max 1.8 mg/day

Available forms: Solution for injection 18mg/3 ml prefilled pen

Implementation
SUBCUT route
• Give by subcut only, inspect for particulate matter or discoloration, do not use if unusually viscous, cloudy, discolored, or if particles are present; give daily at any time without regard to meals; pen needles must be purchased separately, use Novo Nordisk needles, prime

before first use, see manual for directions; give in thigh, abdomen, or upper arm; lightly pinch fold of skin, insert needle at 90-degree angle or 45-degree angle if thin, release skin, aspiration is not needed, give over 6 seconds, rotate injection sites
• Storage: do not store pen with needle attached; avoid direct heat and sunlight, discard 30 days after first use, after first use may be stored at room temperature or refrigerated, do not freeze; if >3 days have elapsed since last dose, reinitiate at 0.6 mg, titrate
• If dose is missed, resume once daily dosing at next scheduled dose

ADVERSE EFFECTS
CNS: Dizziness, headache
CV: Hypertension
ENDO: Hypoglycemia
EENT: Sinusitis
GI: Abdominal pain, anorexia, constipation, diarrhea, dyspepsia, nausea, vomiting, **pancreatitis**
INTEG: **Angioedema**, erythema, injection site reaction, urticaria
MS: Back pain
SYST: Antibody formation, infection, influenza, **secondary thyroid malignancy, anaphylaxis, angioedema**

Pharmacokinetics

Absorption	Protein binding (98%)
Distribution	Binds to albumin, then released into circulation
Metabolism	Unknown
Excretion	Unknown
Half-life	12-13 hr

Pharmacodynamics

Onset	Unknown
Peak	Peak 8-12 hr
Duration	Unknown

INTERACTIONS
Individual drugs
Atorvastatin, acetaminophen, griseofulvin: increased or decreased effects of each specific drug
Baclofen, cycloSPORINE, tacrolimus, dextrothyroxine, diazoxide, phenytoin, fosphenytoin, ethotoin, isoniazid, niacin, nicotine: increased hyperglycemic reactions
Bortezomib, cloNIDine, alcohol, lithium, pentamidine: increased or decreased hypoglycemic reactions

---

Dexfenfluramine, fenfluramine, disopyramide, FLUoxetine, mecasermin, octreotide, pegvisomant, salicylates: increased hypoglycemic reactions
Digoxin: decreased digoxin levels

Drug classifications
Angiotensin II receptor antagonists, ACE inhibitors, other antidiabetics, β-blockers, fibric acid derivatives, MAOIs, salicylates: increased hypoglycemic reactions
Protease inhibitors, phenothiazines, atypical antipsychotics, corticosteroids, carbonic anhydrase inhibitors, estrogens, progestins, oral contraceptives, growth hormones, sympathomimetics: increased hyperglycemic reactions
Androgens, quinolones: decreased liraglutide effect

NURSING CONSIDERATIONS

> **BLACK BOX WARNING:** Thyroid C-cell tumors: monitor during treatment

Assessment
• Watch for hypoglycemic reactions that can occur soon after meals: hunger, sweating, weakness, dizziness, tremors, restlessness, tachycardia
• Assess for hypersensitivity to this product
• Monitor serum glucose, A1c, CBC during treatment
• **Assess for stress:** diabetic patients exposed to stress, surgery, fever, infections may require insulin administration temporarily
• **Assess for serious skin reactions:** angioedema; also pancreatitis, secondary thyroid malignancy

Patient/family education
• Teach patient the symptoms of hypo/hyperglycemia and what to do about each, to have glucagon emergency kit available, carry a carbohydrate source at all times
• Teach patient about side effects associated with therapy such as nausea and vomiting; upward dose titration can be delayed or ignored depending on tolerance
• Teach patient that diabetes is a life-long illness, product does not cure disease and must be continued on a daily basis
• Instruct patient to carry emergency ID with prescriber's phone number and medications taken
• Advise patient to continue with other recommendations: diet, exercise, hygiene

• Teach patient to test blood glucose using a blood glucose meter
• Advise patient to avoid other medications, herbs, supplements unless approved by prescriber
• Advise patient to report serious skin effects, abdominal pain with nausea/vomiting
• Provide patient with written instructions if self-administration is ordered

Evaluation
Positive therapeutic outcome
• Stable and improved serum glucose, A1C, weight loss

lisdexamfetamine (Rx)
(lis-dex'am-fet'a-meen)
Vyvanse
Func. class.: CNS stimulant
Chem. class.: Amphetamine
Pregnancy category C
Controlled substance schedule II

ACTION: Increases release of norepinephrine, DOPamine in cerebral cortex to reticular activating system

Therapeutic outcome: Ability to focus, decreased hyperactivity

USES: Attention-deficit disorder with hyperactivity (ADHD)

CONTRAINDICATIONS: Hyperthyroidism, hypertension, glaucoma, severe arteriosclerosis, CV disease, anxiety, breastfeeding, hypersensitivity to sympathomimetic amines

> **BLACK BOX WARNING:** Substance abuse

Precautions: Pregnancy **C**, children <6 yr, Tourette's syndrome, depression, anorexia nervosa, psychosis, seizure disorder, suicidal ideation, MI, heart failure, alcoholism, aortic stenosis, bipolar disorder

DOSAGE AND ROUTES
Child 6-12 yr: PO 30 mg/day in the AM, may increase by 20 mg/day at weekly intervals; max 70 mg/day

Available forms: Caps 30, 50, 70 mg

Implementation
• Provide gum, hard candy, frequent sips of water for dry mouth

> **BLACK BOX WARNING:** Before giving this product, identify substance abuse; there is a high potential for abuse

ADVERSE EFFECTS

CNS: *Hyperactivity, insomnia, restlessness, talkativeness,* dizziness, headache, dysphoria, irritability, aggressiveness, CNS tumor, dependence, addiction, mild euphoria, somnolence, lability, psychosis, mania, hallucinations, aggression
CV: *Palpitations, tachycardia,* hypertension, decrease in heart rate, **dysrhythmias,** MI, **cardiomyopathy**
EENT: Blurred vision, mydriasis, diplopia
ENDO: Growth inhibition
GI: *Anorexia,* dry mouth, diarrhea, weight loss
GU: Impotence, change in libido
INTEG: Urticaria, **angioedema, Stevens-Johnson syndrome, toxic epidermal necrolysis**

Pharmacokinetics

Absorption	Unknown
Distribution	Crosses placenta, breast milk
Metabolism	Liver
Excretion	Urine pH dependent
Half-life	<1 hr

Pharmacodynamics

Unknown

INTERACTIONS

Individual drugs

AcetaZOLAMIDE, sodium bicarbonate: increased lisdexamfetamine effect
Ascorbic acid, ammonium chloride: decreased lisdexamfetamine effect
Haloperidol, meperidine, modafinil, PHENobarbital, phenytoin: increased CNS effect
Melatonin: increased CNS stimulation
Phenytoin: decreased absorption

Drug classifications

Adrenergic blockers, antidiabetics: decreased effect
Antacids: increased lisdexamfetamine effect
⚠ **MAOIs or within 14 days of MAOIs: hypertensive crisis**
Phenothiazines, tricyclics: increased CNS effect
Urinary acidifiers: decreased lisdexamfetamine effect
Urinary alkalinizers: increased lisdexamfetamine effect

Drug/herb

Eucalyptus: decreased stimulant effect
Green tea, guarana, khat, melatonin: increased stimulant effect
St. John's wort: serotonin syndrome

Drug/food

Caffeine: increased amine effect

NURSING CONSIDERATIONS

Assessment

• Monitor VS, B/P; this product may reverse antihypertensives; check patients with cardiac disease often
• Monitor CBC, urinalysis; in diabetes: blood glucose; insulin changes may be required, since eating may decrease
• **Serotonin syndrome, neuroleptic malignant syndrome:** Assess for increased heart rate, shivering, sweating, dilated pupils, tremors, high B/P, hyperthermia, headache, confusion; if these occur, stop product, administer a serotonin antagonist if needed; at lease 2 wk should elapse between discontinuation of serotonergic agents and start of this product
• Monitor height, growth rate in children; growth rate may be decreased
• Assess mental status: mood, sensorium, affect, stimulation, insomnia, irritability
• Assess for tolerance or dependency: an increased amount may be used to get same effect; will develop after long-term use
• Assess for overdose: pain, fever, dehydration, insomnia, hyperactivity

Patient/family education

• Advise patient to decrease caffeine consumption (coffee, tea, cola, chocolate); may increase irritability, stimulation
• Advise patient to avoid OTC preparations unless approved by prescriber
• Teach patient to taper product over several weeks; depression, increased sleeping, lethargy
• Advise to take every day in AM
• Give without regard to meals
• Caps: may take whole or opened with contents dissolved in water and taken
• Avoid breastfeeding
• Advise to use as part of a comprehensive treatment program
• Caution patient to avoid alcohol ingestion
• Advise patient to avoid hazardous activities until stabilized on medication
• Instruct patient to get needed rest; patient will feel more tired at end of day
⚠ **Seizures: Product may decrease seizure threshold; those with a seizure disorder should notify prescriber if seizure occurs**

BLACK BOX WARNING: Serious CV effects may occur from increasing dose

Evaluation
Positive therapeutic outcome
• Ability to stay on task, decreased hyperactivity

TREATMENT OF OVERDOSE:
Administer fluids, antihypertensive for increased B/P, ammonium chloride for increased excretion, chlorproMAZINE to antagonize CNS effect

lisinopril (Rx)
(lyse-in′oh-pril)
Zestril
Func. class.: Antihypertensive, angiotensin converting enzyme (ACE) I inhibitor
Chem. class.: Enalaprilat lysine analog
Pregnancy category D

Do not confuse:
lisinopril/Risperdal/Lipitor,
Zestril/Zetia/Zipexa

ACTION: Selectively suppresses renin-angiotensin-aldosterone system; inhibits ACE; prevents conversion of angiotensin I to angiotensin II

Therapeutic outcome: Decreased B/P in hypertension, decreased preload, afterload in CHF

USES: Mild to moderate hypertension, adjunctive therapy of systolic CHF, acute MI

Unlabeled uses: Diabetic nephropathy/retinopathy, proteinuria, post MI

CONTRAINDICATIONS:
Hypersensitivity, angioedema

BLACK BOX WARNING: Pregnancy D (2nd/3rd trimesters)

Precautions: Pregnancy C (1st trimester), breastfeeding, renal disease, hyperkalemia, renal artery stenosis, CHF, aortic stenosis

DOSAGE AND ROUTES
Hypertension
Adult: PO 10-40 mg/day; may increase to 80 mg/day if required

Child ≥6 yr: PO 0.7 mg/kg/day, up to 5 mg/day; titrate q1-2wk up to 0.6 mg/kg/day or 40 mg/day
Geriatric: PO 2.5-5 mg/day, increase q7day

CHF
Adult: PO 5 mg initially with diuretics/digoxin, range 5-40 mg

Acute myocardial infarction
Adults who are hemodynamically stable: PO give 5 mg within 24 hr of onset of symptoms, then 5 mg after 24 hr, 10 mg after 48 hr, then 10 mg/day

Renal dose
Adult: PO CCr <30 ml/min reduce dose by 50%, initially 5 mg/day, max 40 mg/day; CCr <10 ml/min 2.5 mg/day, max 40 mg/day

Available forms: Tabs 2.5, 5, 10, 20, 30 40 mg

Implementation
• Store in airtight container at 86° F (30° C) or less
• Severe hypotension may occur after 1st dose of this medication; may be prevented by reducing or discontinuing diuretic therapy 3 days before beginning lisinopril therapy

ADVERSE EFFECTS
CNS: *Vertigo,* depression, **stroke,** insomnia, paresthesias, *headache,* fatigue, asthenia, *dizziness*
CV: Chest pain, *hypotension,* sinus tachycardia
EENT: Blurred vision, nasal congestion
GI: Nausea, vomiting, anorexia, constipation, flatulence, GI irritation, diarrhea, **hepatic failure, hepatic necrosis**
GU: **Proteinuria, renal insufficiency,** sexual dysfunction, impotence
HEMA: **Neutropenia, agranulocytosis**
INTEG: Rash, pruritus
MISC: Muscle cramps, *hyperkalemia*
RESP: Dry cough, dyspnea
SYST: **Angioedema, anaphylaxis, toxic epidermal necrolysis**

Pharmacokinetics

Absorption	Variable
Distribution	Unknown
Metabolism	Not metabolized
Excretion	Kidneys, unchanged
Half-life	12 hr

Adverse effects: *italics* = common; **bold** = life-threatening

Pharmacodynamics

Pharmacodynamics	
Onset	1 hr
Peak	6-8 hr
Duration	24 hr

INTERACTIONS

Individual drugs

Alcohol (large amounts), probenecid: increased hypotension

Allopurinol: increased hypersensitivity

Aspirin: decreased lisinopril effect

CycloSPORINE: increased hyperkalemia

Indomethacin: decreased antihypertensive effect

Lithium: increased levels of lithium, toxicity

Drug classifications

Antihypertensives, diuretics, nitrates, phenothiazines: increased hypotension

Diuretics, potassium-sparing, potassium salt substitutes, potassium supplements: increased hyperkalemia

NSAIDs: decreased lisinopril effect

Drug/food

High-potassium diet (bananas, orange juice, avocados, broccoli, nuts, spinach) should be avoided; hyperkalemia may occur

Drug/lab test

Interference: glucose/insulin tolerance tests, ANA titer

NURSING CONSIDERATIONS

Assessment

• Assess blood studies: platelets, WBC with differential: baseline, q3mo; if neutrophils are <1000/mm^3, discontinue treatment

• **Hypertension:** monitor B/P, check for orthostatic hypotension, syncope; if changes occur, dosage change may be required

• Establish baselines in renal/liver function tests before therapy begins

• Monitor renal/liver function tests: protein, BUN, creatinine; watch for increased levels that may indicate nephrotic syndrome and renal failure; monitor renal symptoms: polyuria, oliguria, frequency, dysuria

• Check potassium levels throughout treatment, although hyperkalemia rarely occurs

• **CHF:** check for edema in feet, legs daily, weight daily, dyspnea, wet crackles

• Assess for anaphylaxis, toxic epidermal necrolysis, angioedema, allergic reactions: rash, fever, pruritus, urticaria; facial swelling, dyspnea, tongue swelling (rare); product should be discontinued if antihistamines fail to help

Patient/family education

• Caution patient not to discontinue product abruptly; advise patient to inform all health care providers about taking this product

• Teach patient not to use OTC products (cough, cold, allergy) unless directed by prescriber; serious side effects can occur

• Teach patient the importance of complying with dosage schedule, even if feeling better; to continue with medical regimen to decrease B/P: exercise, cessation of smoking, decreasing stress, diet modifications

• Teach patient to notify prescriber of mouth sores, sore throat, fever, swelling of hands or feet, irregular heartbeat, chest pain, coughing, shortness of breath

• Caution patient to report excessive perspiration, dehydration, vomiting, diarrhea; may lead to fall in B/P

• Emphasize the need to rise slowly to sitting or standing position to minimize orthostatic hypotension; not to exercise in hot weather or increased hypotension can occur

• Caution patient that product may cause dizziness, fainting, light-headedness; may occur during 1st few days of therapy; to avoid activities that may be hazardous

• Teach patient how to take B/P, and normal readings for age-group; advise patient to take B/P regularly

• Instruct patient to avoid increasing potassium in the diet

> ⚠️ **BLACK BOX WARNING:** Advise patient to report if pregnancy is planned or suspected (pregnancy **D**), 2nd/3rd trimesters

Evaluation

Positive therapeutic outcome

• Decreased B/P in hypertension

• Decreased CHF symptoms

TREATMENT OF OVERDOSE:
0.9% NaCl **IV** inf, hemodialysis

lithium (Rx)
(li'thee-um)

Carbolith ✦, Duralith ✦, Lithobid

Func. class.: Antimanic, antipsychotic

Chem. class.: Alkali metal ion salt

Pregnancy category D

ACTION: May alter sodium, potassium ion transport across cell membrane in nerve, muscle cells; may balance biogenic amines of norepinephrine, serotonin in CNS areas involved in emotional responses

Therapeutic outcome: Stable mood

USES: Bipolar disorder (manic phase), prevention of bipolar manic-depressive psychosis

CONTRAINDICATIONS:
Pregnancy **D**, breastfeeding, children <12 yr, hepatic disease, brain trauma, organic brain syndrome, schizophrenia, severe cardiac/renal disease, severe dehydration

Precautions: Geriatric, thyroid disease, seizure disorders, diabetes mellitus, systemic infection, urinary retention

> **BLACK BOX WARNING:** Lithium level >1.5 mmol/L

DOSAGE AND ROUTES
Adult: PO 300-600 mg tid; maintenance 300 mg tid or qid; SLOW REL Tab 300 mg bid; dosage should be individualized to maintain blood levels at 0.5-1.5 mEq/L
Geriatric: PO 300 mg bid, increase q7day by 300 mg to desired dose
Child: PO 15-20 mg/kg/day in 3-4 divided doses; increase as needed; do not exceed adult doses; maintain blood levels at 0.4-0.5 mEq/L

Renal dose
Adult: PO CCr 10-50 ml/min 50%-75% of dose; CCr <10 ml/min 25%-50% of dose

Available forms: Caps 150, 300, 600 mg; tabs 300 mg; ext rel tabs 300, 450 mg; syr 300 mg/5 ml (8 mEq/5 ml); slow rel caps 150, 300 mg ✤

Implementation
• Do not break, crush, or chew caps and slow rel caps
• Administer reduced dosage to geriatric; give with meals to avoid GI upset
• Provide adequate fluids (2-3 L/day) to prevent dehydration during initial treatment, 1-2 L/day during maintenance
• Give list of products that interact with lithium

ADVERSE EFFECTS
CNS: *Headache, drowsiness, dizziness, tremors,* twitching, ataxia, **seizures,** slurred speech, restlessness, *confusion,* stupor, memory loss, clonic movements, *fatigue*
CV: *Hypotension,* ECG changes, **dysrhythmias, circulatory collapse, edema,** Brugada syndrome

EENT: Tinnitus, blurred vision
ENDO: Hypothyroidism, goiter, hyperglycemia, hyperthyroidism, hyponatremia
GI: *Dry mouth, anorexia, nausea, vomiting, diarrhea,* incontinence, abdominal pain, metallic taste
GU: **Polyuria, glycosuria, proteinuria, albuminuria,** urinary incontinence, polydipsia
HEMA: Leukocytosis
INTEG: Drying of hair, alopecia, rash, pruritus, hyperkeratosis, *acneiform rash, folliculitis*
MS: *Muscle weakness*

Pharmacokinetics
Absorption	Completely absorbed
Distribution	Reabsorbed by renal tubules (80%); crosses blood-brain barrier; crosses placenta
Metabolism	Unknown
Excretion	Urine, unchanged
Half-life	18-36 hr depending on age

Pharmacodynamics
Onset	Rapid
Peak	½-12 hr
Duration	Unknown

INTERACTIONS
Individual drugs
AcetaZOLAMIDE, aminophylline, mannitol, sodium bicarbonate: increased renal clearance
Calcium iodide, iodinated glycerol, potassium iodide: increased hypothyroid effect
CarBAMazepine, FLUoxetine, methyldopa, probenecid: increased lithium effect/toxicity
Haloperidol: increased neurotoxicity
Indomethacin, losartan: increased toxicity
Thioridazine: brain damage
Urea: decreased lithium effect

Drug classifications
Antithyroid agents: increased hypothyroid effects
β-Blockers used for lithium tremor: increase masking of lithium toxicity
Neuromuscular blocking agents: increased effect of neuromuscular blocking effects
NSAIDs, thiazides: increased lithium toxicity
Phenothiazines: increased effect of phenothiazines
Theophyllines, urinary alkalinizers: decreased effect of lithium

Drug/herb
Guarana, tea (black/green): decreased lithium effect
• Avoid use with kava, St. John's wort, valerian

Adverse effects: *italics* = common; **bold** = life-threatening

Drug/food
Significant changes in sodium intake will alter lithium excretion

Drug/lab test
Increased: potassium excretion, urine glucose, blood glucose, protein, BUN
Decreased: VMA, T_3, T_4, PBI, ^{131}I

NURSING CONSIDERATIONS
Assessment
• **Bipolar disorder:** manic symptoms, mood, behavior before and during treatment
• **Assess for lithium toxicity:** Vomiting, diarrhea, poor coordination, fine motor tremors, weakness, lassitude; major toxicity: coarse tremors, severe thirst, tinnitus, dilute urine

> **BLACK BOX WARNING:** Monitor serum lithium levels weekly initially, then q2mo (therapeutic level: 0.5-1.5 mEq/L; toxic level >1.5 mcg/L; twitching; toxicity and therapeutic levels are very close; toxicity may occur rapidly; blood levels are measured before the AM dose

• Assess weight daily; check for edema in legs, ankles, wrists; report if present; check skin turgor at least daily
• Monitor sodium intake; decreased sodium intake with decreased fluid intake may lead to lithium retention; increased sodium and fluids may decrease lithium retention
• Monitor urine for albuminuria, glycosuria, uric acid during beginning treatment, q2mo thereafter
• Assess neurologic status: LOC, gait, motor reflexes, hand tremors
• ECG in those >50 yr with CV disease; cardiology consult is recommended in those with risk factors

Patient/family education
• Provide patient with written information on symptoms of **minor toxicity:** vomiting, diarrhea, poor coordination, fine motor tremors, weakness, lassitude; **major toxicity:** coarse tremors, severe thirst, tinnitus, dilute urine
• Advise patient to monitor urine specific gravity; emphasize need for follow-up care to determine lithium effects
⚠ **Advise patient that contraception is necessary, since lithium may harm fetus, pregnancy D**
• Caution patient not to operate machinery until lithium levels are stable and response determined; that beneficial effects may take 1-3 wk

• Provide to the patient a list of products that interact with lithium and discuss need for adequate, stable intake of salt and fluid
• Advise patient to have lithium levels monitored to ensure effectiveness

Evaluation
Positive therapeutic outcome
• Decrease in excitement, poor judgment, insomnia (manic phase)
• Decreased mood swings and lability

TREATMENT OF OVERDOSE:
Induce emesis or lavage, maintain airway, respiratory function; dialysis for severe intoxication

Iodoxamide ophthalmic
See Appendix B

loperamide (OTC, Rx)
(loe-per'a-mide)
Anti-Diarrheal, Equaline Anti-Diarrheal ❖, Good Sense Anti-Diarrheal, Imodium, Imodium A-D, Rx Choice Loperamide, Select Brand Anti-Diarrheal, Top Care Anti-Diarrheal, Walgreens Anti-Diarrheal
Func. class.: Antidiarrheal
Chem. class.: Piperidine derivative
Pregnancy category C

Do not confuse:
Imodium/Indocin, **Loperimide**/furosemide

ACTION: Direct action on intestinal muscles to decrease GI peristalsis; reduces volume, increases bulk; electrolytes are not lost

Therapeutic outcome: Absence of diarrhea

USES: Diarrhea (cause undetermined), chronic diarrhea, to decrease amount of ileostomy discharge, traveler's diarrhea

CONTRAINDICATIONS:
Hypersensitivity, pseudomembranous colitis, constipation, dysentery, GI bleeding/obstruction/perforation, ileus, vomiting

Precautions: Pregnancy **C**, breastfeeding, children <2 yr, hepatic disease, gastroenteritis, toxic megacolon, geriatric patients, dehydration, bacterial disease, AIDS, severe ulcerative colitis

DOSAGE AND ROUTES

Adult: PO 4 mg, then 2 mg after each loose stool, max 16 mg/24 hr
Child 9-11 yr: PO 2 mg, then 1 mg after each loose stool, max 6 mg/24 hr
Child 6-8 yr: PO 2 mg, then 0.1 mg/kg after each loose stool, max 4 mg/day
Child 2-5 yr: PO 1 mg, then 0.1 mg/kg after each loose stool, max 4 mg/24 hr

Available forms: Caps 2 mg; liquid 1 mg/5 ml; tabs 2 mg; chew tabs 2 mg

Implementation

• Do not break, crush, or chew caps
• Store in airtight containers
• Do not mix oral sol with other sol

ADVERSE EFFECTS

CNS: Dizziness, drowsiness, fatigue
GI: *Nausea, dry mouth, vomiting, constipation,* abdominal pain, anorexia, **toxic megacolon,** bacterial enterocolitis, flatulence
INTEG: Rash
MISC: Hyperglycemia
SYST: Anaphylaxis, angioedema, toxic epidermal necrolysis

Pharmacokinetics

Absorption	Poor
Distribution	Unknown
Metabolism	Liver
Excretion	Feces, unchanged; small amount in urine
Half-life	9-14 hr

Pharmacodynamics

Onset	½-1 hr
Peak	Unknown
Duration	4-5 hr

INTERACTIONS

Individual drugs
Alcohol: increased CNS depression

Drug classifications
Antihistamines, analgesics (opioids), sedative/hypnotics: increased CNS depression

Drug/herb
Chamomile, hops, kava, skullcap, valerian: increased CNS depression
Nutmeg: increased antidiarrheal effect

NURSING CONSIDERATIONS

Assessment
• Monitor electrolytes (potassium, sodium, chloride) if patient is on long-term therapy; check fluid status, skin turgor
• **Stools:** Assess bowel pattern before, during treatment; check for rebound constipation after termination of medication; check bowel sounds
• Check response after 48 hr; if no response, product should be discontinued and other treatment initiated
• Assess for abdominal distention, toxic megacolon, which may occur in ulcerative colitis
• Assess for dehydration, CNS symptoms in children or those with hepatic disease

Patient/family education
• Caution patient to avoid alcohol and OTC products unless directed by prescriber; may cause increased CNS depression
• Advise patient not to exceed recommended dosage; product may be habit forming; ileostomy patient may take this product for extended time
• Advise patient that product may cause drowsiness and to avoid hazardous activities until response to product is determined
• Teach patient that dry mouth can be decreased by frequent sips of water, hard candy, sugarless gum

Evaluation
Positive therapeutic outcome
• Decreased diarrhea

---

loratadine (Rx, OTC)

(lor-a′ti-deen)
Alavert, Claritin, Children's Claritin RediTabs, Dimetapp, Equaline Non-Drowsy, Equate Allergy Relief, Good Sense Non-Drowsy, Leader Allergy Relief, Tavist ND, Wal-itin Aller-Melts, Wal-vert
Func. class.: Antihistamine (2nd generation)
Chem. class.: Selective histamine (H$_1$) receptor antagonist
Pregnancy category B

Do not confuse:
loratadine/lovastatin/LORazepam/losartan

ACTION: Binds to peripheral histamine receptors, which provides antihistamine action without sedation

Therapeutic outcome: Decreased nasal stuffiness, itching, swollen eyes

USES: Seasonal rhinitis, chronic idiopathic urticaria for those ≥2 yr

CONTRAINDICATIONS:
Hypersensitivity, acute asthma attacks, lower respiratory tract disease

Precautions: Pregnancy **B,** increased intra-ocular pressure, bronchial asthma, breastfeeding, hepatic/renal disease

DOSAGE AND ROUTES
Adult and child ≥6 yr: PO 10 mg/day
Child 2-5 yr: PO 5 mg/day

Renal dose
Adult: PO CCr <30 ml/min 10 mg every other day

Hepatic dose
Adult: PO 10 mg every other day

Available forms: Tabs 10 mg; rapid-disintegrating tabs 10 mg; orally disintegrating tabs 10 mg; syr 1 mg/ml; susp 5 mg/ml; ext rel tabs 10 mg

Implementation
• Give on an empty stomach, 1 hr before or 2 hr after meals to facilitate absorption
• **Rapid-disintegrating tabs:** Place rapidly disintegrating tabs on tongue, then swallow after disintegrated with or without water
• Use within 6 mo of opening pouch; immediately after opening blister pack
• Store in airtight, light-resistant container
• **Ext rel tab:** Do not break, crush, or chew

ADVERSE EFFECTS
CNS: Sedation (more common with increased dosages), headache, fatigue, restlessness
EENT: Dry mouth

Pharmacokinetics

Absorption	Well absorbed
Distribution	Unknown
Metabolism	Liver, extensively, to active metabolite desloratadine
Excretion	Kidneys
Half-life	17-28 hr

Pharmacodynamics

Onset	1-3 hr
Peak	8-12 hr
Duration	>24 hr

INTERACTIONS
Individual drugs
Alcohol: increased CNS depression
Cimetidine, ketoconazole: increased loratadine level

Drug classifications
Antidepressants, antihistamines (other), sedative-hypnotics: increased CNS depression
Macrolides (clarithromycin, erythromycin): increased loratadine level
MAOIs: increased antihistamine effects

Drug/lab test
False negative: skin allergy tests (discontinue antihistamine 3 days before testing)

NURSING CONSIDERATIONS
Assessment
• **Assess allergy:** hives, rash, rhinitis
• Assess respiratory status: rate, rhythm, increase in bronchial secretions, wheezing, chest tightness

Patient/family education
• Teach all aspects of product uses; to notify prescriber if confusion, sedation, hypotension occur; to avoid driving and other hazardous activity if drowsiness occurs; to avoid alcohol and other CNS depressants that may potentiate effect
• Teach patient to take 1 hr before or 2 hr after meals to facilitate absorption
• Advise patient to use sunscreen or stay out of the sun to prevent burns
• Caution patient not to exceed recommended dosage; dysrhythmias may occur
• Teach patient that hard candy, gum, frequent rinsing of mouth may be used for dryness

Evaluation
Positive therapeutic outcome
• Absence of runny or congested nose, other allergy symptoms

LORazepam (Rx)
(lor-az′e-pam)
Ativan
Func. class.: Sedative-hypnotic, antianxiety agent
Chem. class.: Benzodiazepine, short acting
Pregnancy category D
Controlled substance schedule IV

Do not confuse:
LORazepam/ALPRAZolam/clonazePAM

ACTION: Potentiates the actions of GABA, an inhibitory neurotransmitter, especially in the limbic system and reticular formation, which depresses the CNS

Therapeutic outcome: Decreased anxiety, relaxation

USES: Anxiety, irritability in psychiatric or organic disorders, preoperatively; adjunct in endoscopic procedures, status epilepticus

Unlabeled uses: Antiemetic before chemotherapy, rectal use, insomnia

CONTRAINDICATIONS:
Pregnancy **D**, breastfeeding, hypersensitivity to benzodiazepines/benzyl alcohol, closed-angle glaucoma, psychosis, history of drug abuse, COPD, sleep apnea

Precautions: Geriatric, debilitated patients, children <12 yr, renal/hepatic disease, addiction, suicidal ideation, abrupt discontinuation

DOSAGE AND ROUTES
Anxiety
Adult/adolescent: PO 2-3 mg/day in divided doses, max 10 mg/day
Geriatric: PO 1-2 mg/day in divided doses, or 0.5-1 mg at bedtime

Insomnia (unlabeled)
Adult: PO 2-4 mg at bedtime; only minimally effective after 2 wk continuous therapy
Geriatric: PO 0.5-1 mg initially

Preoperatively
Adult: IM 50 mcg/kg 2 hr before surgery; **IV** 44 mcg/kg 15-20 min before surgery, max 2 mg 15-20 min before surgery
Child ≥12 yr: IV 0.05 mg/kg

Status epilepticus
Neonate: IV 0.05 mg/kg
Child: IV 0.1 mg/kg up to 4 mg/dose; RECT (unlabeled) 0.05-0.1 mg × 2; wait 7 min before giving 2nd dose

Available forms: Tabs 0.5, 1, 2 mg; inj 2, 4 mg/ml; conc sol 2 mg/ml

Implementation
PO route
• Give largest dose before bedtime if giving in divided dose
• **Concentrate:** use calibrated dropper; add to food/drink, consume immediately
• Give with food or milk for GI symptoms; crush tab if patient is unable to swallow medication

whole; provide sugarless gum, hard candy, frequent sips of water for dry mouth
SUBCUT route
• Use by SUBCUT route for rapid response (investigational use)
IM route
• Give deep in muscle mass; if using for preoperative sedation, give 2 hr or more before surgical procedure
• Use this route when IV route is not feasible

Direct IV route
• Prepare immediately before use; short stability time
• Dilute with sterile water for inj, 0.9% NaCl, or D_5W just before using; give by Y-site or 3-way stopcock at 2 mg/min
• Do not use sol that is discolored or contains a precipitate
• **Do not use in neonates (benzyl alcohol)**

Y-site compatibilities: Acyclovir, albumin, allopurinol, amifostine, amikacin, amoxicillin, amoxicillin/clavulanate, amphotericin B cholesteryl, amsacrine, atenolol, atracurium, bivalirudin, bleomycin, bumetanide, butorphanol, calcium chloride/gluconate, CARBOplatin, ceFAZolin, cefepime, cefotaxime, cefoTEtan, cefOXitin, cefTAZidime, ceftizoxime, ceftobiprole, cefTRIAXone, cefuroxime, chloramphenicol, chlorproMAZINE, cimetidine, ciprofloxacin, cisatracurium, CISplatin, cladribine, clindamycin, cloNIDine, cyclophosphamide, cycloSPORINE, cytarabine, DACTINomycin, DAPTOmycin, dexamethasone, dexmedetomidine, diltiazem, DOBUTamine, DOCEtaxel, DOPamine, doripenem, DOXOrubicin, DOXOrubicin liposomal, droperidol, enalaprilat, ePHEDrine, EPINEPHrine, epirubicin, eptifibatide, erythromycin, esmolol, etomidate, famotidine, fenoldopam, fentaNYL, filgrastim, fluconazole, fludarabine, fosphenytoin, furosemide, ganciclovir, gatifloxacin, gemcitabine, gentamicin, glycopyrrolate, granisetron, haloperidol, heparin, hydrocortisone, HYDROmorphone, hydrOXYzine, ifosfamide, inamrinone, insulin (regular), irinotecan, isoproterenol, ketorolac, labetalol, lidocaine, linezolid, magnesium sulfate, mannitol, mechlorethamine, melphalan, meropenem, metaraminol, methadone, methotrexate, methyldopate, methylPREDNISolone, metoclopramide, metoprolol, metroNIDAZOLE, micafungin, midazolam, milrinone, minocycline, mitoXANtrone, morphine, mycophenolate, nafcillin, nalbuphine, naloxone, nesiritide, niCARdipine, nitroglycerin, nitroprusside, norepinephrine, octreotide, oxaliplatin, oxytocin, PACLitaxel, palonosetron, pamidronate, pancuronium,

PEMEtrexed, pentamidine, PENTobarbital, PHE-Nobarbital, piperacillin, piperacillin-tazobactam, polymyxin B, potassium chloride, propofol, ranitidine, remifentanil, tacrolimus, teniposide, theophylline, thiotepa, ticarcillin, ticarcillin-clavulanate, tigecycline, tirofiban, tobramycin, TPN, trastuzumab, trimethobenzamide, trimethoprim-sulfamethoxazole, vancomycin, vasopressin, vecuronium, verapamil, vinCRIStine, vinorelbine, voriconazole, zidovudine

Y-site incompatibilities: IDArubicin, ondansetron, sargramostim

ADVERSE EFFECTS

CNS: *Dizziness, drowsiness,* confusion, headache, anxiety, tremors, stimulation, fatigue, depression, insomnia, hallucinations, weakness, unsteadiness

CV: *Orthostatic hypotension,* **ECG changes, tachycardia,** hypotension, **apnea, cardiac arrest (IV, rapid)**

EENT: *Blurred vision,* tinnitus, mydriasis

GI: Constipation, dry mouth, nausea, vomiting, anorexia, diarrhea

INTEG: Rash, dermatitis, itching

MISC: Acidosis

Pharmacokinetics

Absorption	Well absorbed (PO); completely absorbed (IM)
Distribution	Widely distributed; crosses placenta, blood-brain barrier
Metabolism	Liver, extensively
Excretion	Kidneys, breast milk
Half-life	42 hr (neonates), 10.5 hr (older child), 12 hr (adult), 91% protein bound

Pharmacodynamics

	PO	IM	IV
Onset	½ hr	15-30 min	5-15 min
Peak	1-3 hr	1-1½ hr	Unknown
Duration	12-24 hr	6-8 hr	6-8 hr

INTERACTIONS

Individual drugs

Alcohol: increased CNS depression

Disulfiram: increased LORazepam effects

Oral contraceptives, valproic acid: decreased LORazepam effects

Drug classifications

CNS depressants: increased LORazepam effects

Drug/herb

Chamomile, hops, kava, lavender, valerian: increased CNS depression

Drug/lab test

Increased: AST, ALT

NURSING CONSIDERATIONS

Assessment

• **Assess degree of anxiety;** what precipitates anxiety and whether product controls symptoms; other signs of anxiety: dilated pupils, inability to sleep, restlessness, inability to focus

• **Assess for alcohol withdrawal symptoms,** including hallucinations (visual, auditory), delirium, irritability, agitation, fine to coarse tremors

• Monitor B/P (with patient lying/standing), pulse; check respiratory rate; if systolic B/P drops 20 mm Hg, hold product, notify prescriber; respirations q5-15min if given **IV**

• Monitor CBC during long-term therapy; blood dyscrasias have occurred (rare)

• Monitor for seizure control; type, duration, and intensity of seizures; what precipitates seizures

• Monitor hepatic studies: AST, ALT, bilirubin, creatinine, LDH, alkaline phosphatase

• Assess mental status: mood, sensorium, affect, sleeping pattern, drowsiness, dizziness, suicidal tendencies, and ability of product to control these symptoms; check for tolerance, withdrawal symptoms: headache, nausea, vomiting, muscle pain, weakness after long-term use

Patient/family education

A Teach patient to notify prescriber if pregnancy is planned or suspected; pregnancy (D), do not breastfeed

• Advise patient that product may be taken with food; that product is not to be used for everyday stress or used longer than 4 mo unless directed by a prescriber; to take no more than prescribed amount; may be habit forming

• Caution patient to avoid OTC preparations unless approved by prescriber; to avoid alcohol, other psychotropic medications unless prescribed by physician; not to discontinue medication abruptly after long-term use

• Inform patient to avoid driving and activities that require alertness; drowsiness may occur; to rise slowly or fainting may occur, especially in geriatric

• Inform patient that drowsiness may worsen at beginning of treatment

Evaluation
Positive therapeutic outcome
• Decreased anxiety, restlessness, insomnia

TREATMENT OF OVERDOSE:
Lavage, VS, supportive care

lorcaserin
(lor-ca-ser'in)
Belviq
Func. class.: Weight-control agent (anorexiant)
Chem. class.: Serotonin 2C (5-HT$_{2C}$) receptor agonist
Pregnancy category X

ACTION: Decreases food consumption and decreases hunger by selectively activating 5-HT$_{2C}$ receptors

Therapeutic outcome: Decrease in weight

USES: Obesity management

CONTRAINDICATIONS:
Pregnancy (X), breastfeeding, hypersensitivity, severe renal impairment

Precautions: Children, other organic causes of obesity, anemia, AV block, bradycardia, bundle branch block, depression, dialysis, liver/kidney disease, multiple myeloma, neutropenia, suicidal ideation, Peyronie's disease, pulmonary hypertension, sick sinus syndrome

DOSAGE AND ROUTES
Renal dose
Adult: PO 10 mg bid; do not exceed recommended dosage

Available forms: Tabs, film-coated 10 mg

Implementation
• Identify obesity if patient is on weight reduction program that includes dietary changes, exercise
• May give without regard to food

ADVERSE EFFECTS
CNS: Insomnia, depression, serotonin syndrome, anxiety, **suicidal ideation,** dizziness, headache, fatigue
CV: Bradycardia, hypertension
GI: Diarrhea, constipation, nausea
HEMA: Neutropenia, leukopenia, lymphopenia

INTEG: Rash
MS: Back pain

Pharmacokinetics
Absorption	Unknown
Distribution	70% protein binding
Metabolism	Unknown
Excretion	Unknown
Half-life	11 hr

Pharmacodynamics
Onset	Unknown
Peak	Unknown
Duration	Unknown

INTERACTIONS
Individual drugs
Linezolid, buPROPion, lithium, sibutramine, traMADol: increased life-threatening serotonin syndrome
Insulin: increased risk of hypoglycemia with this product

Drug classifications
SSRIs, SNRIs, serotonin receptor agonists, MAOIs, tricyclic antidepressants: increased life-threatening serotonin syndrome
Sulfonylureas: increased risk of hypoglycemia with this product

Drug/herb
St. John's wort: increased serotonin syndrome

NURSING CONSIDERATIONS
Assessment
• Monitor weight weekly; oral hypoglycemic dosage might need to be reduced in diabetic patients
• Monitor blood glucose, CBC with differential, Hct/Hgb, serum prolactin
• Pregnancy (X): do not use in pregnancy
• Suicidal ideation: use caution in psychiatric disorders with emotional lability; assess for depression, suicidal thoughts/behaviors

Patient/family education
• Advise patient to avoid hazardous activities until stabilized on medication
• Inform patient to discuss unpleasant side effects
• Teach patient to notify prescriber if pregnancy is planned or suspected, pregnancy X

Evaluation
Positive therapeutic outcome
• Decrease in weight

Adverse effects: *italics* = common; **bold** = life-threatening

losartan (Rx)

(low-sar'tan)

Cozaar

Func. class.: Antihypertensive

Chem. class.: Angiotensin II receptor (type AT₁)

Pregnancy category C (1st trimester), D (2nd/3rd trimesters)

Do not confuse:

losartan/valsartan, **Cozaar**/Zocor

ACTION: Blocks the vasoconstrictor and aldosterone-secreting effects of angiotensin II; selectively blocks the binding of angiotensin II to the AT_1 receptor found in tissues

Therapeutic outcome: Decreased B/P

USES: Hypertension, alone or in combination; nephropathy in type 2 diabetes, proteinuria, stroke prophylaxis in hypertensive patients with left ventricular hypertrophy

CONTRAINDICATIONS:

Hypersensitivity

> **BLACK BOX WARNING:** Pregnancy **D** (2nd/3rd trimesters)

Precautions: Pregnancy **C** (1st trimester), breastfeeding, children, geriatric, hypersensitivity to ACE inhibitors, hepatic disease, angioedema, renal artery stenosis, African descent, hyperkalemia, hypotension

DOSAGE AND ROUTES

Hypertension

Adult: PO 50 mg/day alone or 25 mg/day when used in combination with diuretic; maintenance 25-100 mg/day

Child ≥6 yr: PO 0.7 mg/kg/day, max 50 mg/day

Hepatic dose

Adult: PO 25 mg/day as starting dose/**volume depletion**

Hypertension with left ventricular hypertrophy (benefit does not apply to those of African descent)

Adult: PO 50 mg/day, add hydrochlorothiazide 12.5 mg/day and/or increase losartan to 100 mg/day, then increase hydrochlorothiazide to 25 mg/day

Nephropathy in type 2 diabetes patients

Adult: PO 50 mg/day, may increase to 100 mg/day

Available forms: Tabs 25, 50, 100 mg

Implementation

• Administer without regard to meals

ADVERSE EFFECTS

CNS: *Dizziness, insomnia,* anxiety, confusion, abnormal dreams, migraine, tremor, vertigo, headache, malaise, depression, fatigue

CV: Angina pectoris, 2nd-degree AV block, **CVA,** *hypotension,* **MI, dysrhythmias**

EENT: Blurred vision, burning eyes, conjunctivitis

GI: *Diarrhea, dyspepsia,* anorexia, constipation, dry mouth, flatulence, gastritis, vomiting

GU: Impotence, nocturia, urinary frequency, urinary tract infection, **renal failure**

HEMA: Anemia, **thrombocytopenia**

INTEG: Alopecia, dermatitis, dry skin, flushing, photosensitivity, rash, pruritus, sweating **angioedema**

META: Gout, hyperkalemia, hypoglycemia

MS: Cramps, myalgia, pain, stiffness

RESP: *Cough, upper respiratory infection,* congestion, dyspnea, bronchitis

Pharmacokinetics

Absorption	Well absorbed
Distribution	Bound to plasma proteins
Metabolism	Extensive
Excretion	Feces, urine
Half-life	Biphasic, 2 hr, 6-9 hr

Pharmacodynamics

Unknown

INTERACTIONS

Individual drugs

Fluconazole: increased antihypertensive effect

Lithium: increased toxicity

PHENobarbital, rifamycin: decreased antihypertensive effect

Drug classifications

ACE inhibitors, diuretics (potassium-sparing), potassium supplements: increased hyperkalemia

NSAIDs, salicylates: decreased antihypertensive effect

NURSING CONSIDERATIONS
Assessment
- Assess B/P with position changes, pulse q4hr; note rate, rhythm, quality
- Monitor electrolytes: potassium, sodium, chloride
- Obtain baselines for renal, electrolyte, liver function tests before therapy begins
- **CHF:** assess for jugular vein distention, weight daily, edema in feet, legs daily
- **Angioedema:** facial swelling, dyspnea, wheezing, may occur rapidly, tongue swelling (rare)
- **Blood dyscrasias:** thrombocytopenia, anemia (rare)

Patient/family education
- Teach patient to avoid sunlight or wear sunscreen if in sunlight; photosensitivity may occur
- Advise patient to comply with dosage schedule, even if feeling better
- Teach patient to notify prescriber of mouth sores, fever, swelling of hands or feet, irregular heartbeat, chest pain
- Advise patient that excessive perspiration, dehydration, vomiting, diarrhea may lead to fall in blood pressure, consult prescriber if these occur
- Inform patient that product may cause dizziness, fainting; light-headedness may occur, to avoid hazardous activities until reaction is known
- Caution patient to rise slowly to sitting or standing position to minimize orthostatic hypotension

> **BLACK BOX WARNING:** Advise patient to use contraception while taking this product, pregnancy **D** 2nd/3rd trimesters

Evaluation
Positive therapeutic outcome
- Decreased B/P

loteprednol ophthalmic
See Appendix B

lovastatin (Rx)
(loe'va-sta-tin)
Altoprev, Mevacor
Func. class.: Antilipemic
Chem. class.: HMG-CoA reductase inhibitor
Pregnancy category X

Do not confuse:
lovastatin/Lotensin/Leustatin,
Mevacor/mivacron

ACTION: By inhibiting HMG-CoA reductase, which reduces cholesterol synthesis

Therapeutic outcome: Decreased cholesterol levels and LDL, increased HDL

USES: As an adjunct in primary hypercholesterolemia (types IIa, IIb), atherosclerosis, heterozygous familial hypercholesterolemia (adolescents)

CONTRAINDICATIONS:
Pregnancy **X**, breastfeeding, hypersensitivity, active liver disease

Precautions: Past liver disease, alcoholism, severe acute infections, trauma, hypotension, uncontrolled seizure disorders, severe metabolic disorders, electrolyte imbalances, visual condition, children

DOSAGE AND ROUTES
Adult: PO 20 mg/day with evening meal; may increase to 20-40 mg/day in single or divided doses; max 40 mg/day; ext rel 20-60 mg/day at bedtime; max 40 mg/day

Heterozygous familial hypercholesterolemia
Adolescent 10-17 yr: PO 10-40 mg with evening meal

Renal dose
Adult: PO CCr <30 mg/min max 20 mg/day unless titrated

Available forms: Tabs 10, 20, 40 mg; ext rel tab (Altocor) 10, 20, 40, 60 mg

Implementation
- Give with evening meal; if dosage is increased, take with breakfast and evening meal
- Altroprev is not equivalent to Mevacor
- Store in cool environment in airtight, light-resistant container
- Do not crush or chew ext rel tab

ADVERSE EFFECTS

CNS: Dizziness, headache, tremor, insomnia, paresthesia
EENT: Blurred vision, lens opacities
GI: Nausea, constipation, diarrhea, dyspepsia, *flatus,* abdominal pain, heartburn, **liver dysfunction,** vomiting, acid regurgitation, dry mouth, dysgeusia
HEMA: Thrombocytopenia, hemolytic anemia, leukopenia
INTEG: Rash, pruritus, photosensitivity
MS: Muscle cramps, myalgia, **myositis, rhabdomyolysis;** leg, shoulder, or localized pain

Pharmacokinetics

Absorption	Poorly absorbed, erratic
Distribution	Crosses placenta, blood-brain barrier
Metabolism	Liver, extensively
Excretion	Feces (83%); kidneys, urine (10%)
Half-life	3-4 hr

Pharmacodynamics

Onset	Unknown
Peak	2-4 hr
Duration	Unknown

INTERACTIONS

Individual drugs

Bosentan, exonatide: decreased action of lovastatin
Clarithromycin, clofibrate, cycloSPORINE, dalfopristin, danazol, diltiazem, erythromycin, gemfibrozil, niacin, quinupristin, telithromycin, verapamil: increased myalgia, myositis, rhabdomyolysis; avoid concurrent use
Diltiazem: increased lovastatin effects
Warfarin: increased bleeding

Drug classifications

Azole antifungals, protease inhibitors: increased myositis, myalgia, rhabdomyolysis
Bile acid sequestrants: decreased lovastatin effects

Drug/herb

Pectin, St. John's wort: decreased effect
Red yeast rice: increased adverse reactions

Drug/food

Increased levels of lovastatin with food, must be taken with food
Grapefruit juice: increased toxicity
Oat bran: decreased absorption

Drug/lab test

Increased: CPK, liver function tests

NURSING CONSIDERATIONS

Assessment

• Assess nutrition: fat, protein, carbohydrates; nutritional analysis should be completed by dietitian before treatment
• Monitor bowel pattern daily; diarrhea may be a problem
• Monitor triglycerides, fasting cholesterol LDL, HDL at baseline, throughout treatment; watch LDL and VLDL closely; if increased, product should be discontinued
• Assess for muscle pain, tenderness, obtain CPK; if these occur, product may need to be discontinued
• **Rhabdomyolysis:** muscle pain, increased CPK, weakness, swelling of affected muscles; if these occur and if confirmed by CPK, product should be discontinued

Patient/family education

• Inform patient that compliance is needed for positive results to occur; not to double doses
• Inform patient that blood work and ophthalmic exam will be necessary during treatment
• Teach patient that risk factors should be decreased: high-fat diet, smoking, alcohol consumption, absence of exercise
⚠ **Advise patient to report if pregnancy is suspected, pregnancy X, do not breastfeed**
• Advise patient to notify prescriber if the GI symptoms of diarrhea, abdominal or epigastric pain, nausea, vomiting occur; or if chills, fever, sore throat, blurred vision, dizziness, headache, muscle pain, weakness occur
• Advise patient to stay out of the sun or use sunscreen to prevent burns
• Instruct patient that product should be taken with food, not to crush, chew ext rel product

Evaluation

Positive therapeutic outcome
• Decreased cholesterol, serum triglyceride levels
• Improved level of HDL

---

loxapine (Rx)

(lox'a-peen)
Adasuve, Loxapac ✹, Loxitane
Func. class.: Antipsychotic/neuroleptic
Chem. class.: Dibenzoxazepine
Pregnancy category C

Do not confuse:
Loxitane/Soriatane

ACTION: Depresses cerebral cortex, hypothalamus, limbic system, which control activity and aggression; blocks neurotransmission produced by DOPamine at synapse; exhibits strong α-adrenergic, anticholinergic blocking action; mechanism for antipsychotic effects is unclear

Therapeutic outcome: Decreased psychotic behavior

USES: Schizophrenia, bipolar disorder

Unlabeled uses: Depression, anxiety

CONTRAINDICATIONS:
Hypersensitivity, coma

> **BLACK BOX WARNING:** Acute bronchospasm, asthma, COPD, emphysema

Precautions: Pregnancy **C**, breastfeeding, children <16 yr, geriatric, seizure disorders, cardiac/renal/hepatic disease, prostatic hypertrophy, cardiac conditions

> **BLACK BOX WARNING: Dementia:** increased mortality in elderly patients with dementia-related psychosis

DOSAGE AND ROUTES
Adult: PO 10 mg bid-qid initially; may be rapidly increased depending on severity of condition; maintenance 60-100 mg/day; inhalation powder 10 mg as a single dose in 24 hr
Geriatric: PO 5-10 mg/day bid, increase q4-7day by 5-10 mg, max 250 mg/day

Available forms: Caps 5, 10, 25, 50 mg; tabs 5, 10, 25, 50 mg; inhalation powder

Implementation
• Give with food
PO route
• Administer product in liquid form mixed in glass of juice or soft drink if hoarding is suspected; do not mix in caffeine drinks, tannics, pectins
• Administer lowered dose in geriatric, since metabolism is slowed
• Administer with full glass of water or milk; or give with food to decrease GI upset
• Give antacids 2 hr before or after taking this product
• Store in airtight, light-resistant container, oral sol in amber bottle
Inhalation route
• Due to the risk of bronchospasm, loxapine for oral inhalation (Adasuve) is available only

through the Adasuve Risk Evaluation and Mitigation Strategy (ADASUVE REMS) program
• Only for use by a healthcare professional in a healthcare facility enrolled in the ADASUVE REMS program and with immediate on-site access to equipment and personnel trained to manage acute bronchospasm, including advanced airway management (intubation and mechanical ventilation)
• Prior to administration, all patients must be screened for history of asthma, COPD, or other pulmonary disease, and also for use of medications to treat airway disease; patients also must be examined (including chest auscultation) for respiratory abnormalities such as wheezing
• Each inhaler is for single use only; use only once in a 24-hr period
• *Step 1:* When ready to use, tear open pouch and remove inhaler; the indicator light on the inhaler should be off
• *Step 2:* Firmly pull the plastic tab from rear of inhaler and ensure that the green light turns on, which indicates that the inhaler is ready to use
• *Step 3:* Inform the patient that the inhaler may produce a flash of light and clicking sound and may become warm during use
• *Step 4:* Instruct the patient to hold the inhaler away from the mouth and exhale fully to empty the lungs
• *Step 5:* Instruct the patient to place the mouthpiece of the inhaler between the lips, close the lips, and inhale through the mouthpiece with a steady, deep breath
• *Step 6:* Instruct the patient to remove the inhaler from the mouth and hold his or her breath for as long as possible, up to 10 sec
• *Step 7:* Check that green light turns off, indicating that the dose was delivered; if the light remains on, then steps 4-6 should be repeated up to 2 additional times; if the green light does not turn off, discard the inhaler and use a new one
• Use inhaler within 15 min after removing the tab to prevent automatic deactivation
• The green light will turn off after use, at which time the inhaler is no longer usable
• After use, the patient must be monitored for signs and symptoms of bronchospasm or other respiratory distress, including a physical examination with chest auscultation, at least every 15 minutes for a minimum of 1 hr
• Refer to the Important Administration Instructions section

ADVERSE EFFECTS
CNS: *EPS: pseudoparkinsonism, akathisia, dystonia, tardive dyskinesia, drowsiness,*

headache, **seizures,** confusion, **neuroleptic malignant syndrome**
CV: *Orthostatic hypotension,* **cardiac arrest,** ECG changes, tachycardia
EENT: Blurred vision, glaucoma
ENDO: Hyperprolactinemia, galactorrhea, gynecomastia, menstrual irregularities
GI: *Dry mouth, nausea, vomiting, anorexia, constipation,* diarrhea, jaundice, weight gain
GU: Urinary retention, urinary frequency, enuresis, impotence, amenorrhea, gynecomastia
HEMA: **Anemia, leukopenia, leukocytosis, agranulocytosis**
INTEG: *Rash,* photosensitivity, dermatitis
RESP: Laryngospasm, dyspnea, **respiratory depression**

Pharmacokinetics

Absorption	Well absorbed (PO)
Distribution	Unknown
Metabolism	Liver, extensively; 96.6% protein binding
Excretion	Kidneys
Half-life	Biphasic 5 hr, 19 hr

Pharmacodynamics

	PO
Onset	½ hr
Peak	2-4 hr
Duration	12 hr

INTERACTIONS
Individual drugs
Alcohol: increased CNS depression
CarBAMazepine, guanadrel, guanethidine, levodopa: decreased effects
EPINEPHrine, lithium: increased toxicity
Metoclopramide: increased EPS

Drug classifications
Anticholinergics: increased anticholinergic effects
Antidepressants, MAOIs: increased CNS depression
Antipsychotics: increased EPS

NURSING CONSIDERATIONS
Assessment
• Assess mental status: orientation, mood, behavior, presence and type of hallucinations before initial administration, monthly; this product should significantly reduce psychotic behavior
• Check for swallowing of PO medication; check for hoarding or giving medication to other patients

• Monitor I&O ratio; palpate bladder if low urinary output occurs, especially in geriatric; urinalysis recommended before, during prolonged therapy, urinary retention may be cause
• Monitor bilirubin, CBC, LFTs monthly
• Assess affect, orientation, LOC, reflexes, gait, coordination, sleep pattern disturbances
• Monitor B/P with patient sitting, standing, and lying; take pulse and respirations q4hr during initial treatment; establish baseline before starting treatment; report drops of 30 mm Hg
• Check for dizziness, faintness, palpitations, tachycardia on rising; severe orthostatic hypotension is common
⚠ Identify neuroleptic malignant syndrome: hyperpyrexia, muscle rigidity, increased CPK, altered mental status; product should be discontinued
⚠ Bronchospasm: Monitor closely after use of inhalation powder
• **Assess for EPS,** including akathisia (inability to sit still, no pattern to movements), tardive dyskinesia (bizarre movements of the jaw, mouth, tongue, extremities), pseudoparkinsonism (ragged tremors, pill rolling, shuffling gait); an antiparkinsonian product should be prescribed
• Assess for constipation, urinary retention daily; if these occur, increase bulk, water in diet

Patient/family education
• Teach patient to use good oral hygiene; suggest frequent rinsing of mouth, sugarless gum for dry mouth; oral candidiasis can occur
• Caution patient to avoid hazardous activities until product response is determined; dizziness, blurred vision may occur
• Inform patient that orthostatic hypotension occurs often and to rise from sitting or lying position gradually; caution patient to avoid hot tubs, hot showers, tub baths, since hypotension may occur; tell patient that in hot weather heat stroke may occur; take extra precautions to stay cool
• Advise patient to avoid abrupt withdrawal of this product, or EPS may result; product should be withdrawn slowly
• Advise patient to avoid use with alcohol, CNS depressants; increased drowsiness may occur
• Advise patient to use a sunscreen and sunglasses to prevent burns
• Teach patient to take antacids 2 hr before or after taking this product
• Instruct patient to report sore throat, malaise, fever, bleeding, mouth sores; if these occur, CBC should be performed and product discontinued

---

⚠ Nurse Alert   ⭐ Key NCLEX® Drug

Evaluation
Positive therapeutic outcome
- Decrease in emotional excitement, hallucinations, delusions, paranoia
- Reorganization of patterns of thought, speech

TREATMENT OF OVERDOSE:
Lavage; barbiturates; provide airway, **IV** fluids; do not use EPINEPHrine, which may increase hypotension

lubiprostone (Rx)
(loo-bee-pros′tone)
Amitiza
Func. class.: Miscellaneous gastrointestinal agent
Pregnancy category C

ACTION: Locally acting chloride channel activator, enhances a chloride-rich intestinal fluid secretion without altering other electrolytes; increases motility in the intestine, increasing softening and passage of stool

Therapeutic outcome: Decreased constipation

USES: Chronic idiopathic constipation, constipation-predominant irritable bowel syndrome in women >18 yr, opiate agonist–induced constipation with chronic noncancer pain

CONTRAINDICATIONS:
Hypersensitivity, GI obstruction

Precautions: Pregnancy **C,** breastfeeding, children, diarrhea, IBD, abdominal pain, cholelithiasis, fecal inpaction, GI/hepatic disease

DOSAGE AND ROUTES
Chronic idiopathic constipation/ opiate agonist–induced constipation
Adult: PO 24 mcg bid with food/water

IBS with constipation (women)
Adult and adolescent ≥18 yr: PO 8 mcg bid with food and water

Hepatic dosage
Adult: For chronic constipation 16 mcg bid (Child-Pugh B); 8 mcg bid (Child-Pugh C); for irritable bowel: 8 mcg daily (Child-Pugh C), may be increased if tolerated

Available forms: Caps 8, 24 mcg

Implementation
- Give with food bid
- Store at room temperature

ADVERSE EFFECTS
CNS: *Headache,* dizziness, depression, fatigue, insomnia
CV: Hypertension, chest pain
GI: *Nausea, abdominal pain, eructation,* abdominal distention, constipation, diarrhea, dry mouth, dyspepsia, flatulence, viral gastroenteritis, gastroesophageal reflux disease, vomiting, fecal incontinence, fecal urgency
GU: UTI
MISC: Chest pain, peripheral edema, influenza, pyrexia, viral infection
MS: Back pain, arthralgia, muscle cramps, pain in extremities
RESP: Bronchitis; cough, dyspnea, nasopharyngitis, sinusitis, URI

Pharmacokinetics

Absorption	Unknown
Distribution	Protein binding 94%
Metabolism	Rapid in stomach, jejunum
Excretion	Unknown
Half-life	0.9-1.4 hr

Pharmacodynamics

Onset	Unknown
Peak	1.14 hr
Duration	Unknown

INTERACTIONS
Individual drugs
- Anticholinergics, antidiarrheals: decreased effects of lubiprostone
- Do not use with sodium phosphate monobasic monohydra, sodium phosphate dibasic anhydrous, with other laxative, purgatives, when evacuating the bowel before radiologic exam or surgery
- Possible GI obstruction with NIFEdipine extended rel tab

NURSING CONSIDERATIONS
Assessment
- Assess GI symptoms: nausea, abdominal pain
- Assess periodically for need for continued treatment

Patient/family education
- Teach patient to notify prescriber of GI symptoms, diarrhea, hypersensitivity reactions

---

Evaluation
Positive therapeutic outcome
• Decreased constipation

RARELY USED
lucinactant
(loo'sin-ak'tant)
Surfaxin
Func. class.: Synthetic lung surfactant

USES: Prevention of respiratory distress syndrome (RDS) in premature neonates

DOSAGE AND ROUTES
Premature neonate
Intratracheal 5.8 ml/kg birth weight divided in 4 doses; give each dose with neonate in a different position; provide positive pressure ventilation when stable; dosage may be repeated 4 times in first 48 hr

---

lurasidone (Rx)
(loo-ras'i-done)
Latuda
Func. class.: Atypical antipsychotic
Chem. class.: Benzoisothiazol derivative
Pregnancy category B

ACTION: May modulate central dopaminergic and serotoninergic activity, high affinity for dopamine-D_2 receptors, serotonin 5-HT_{2A} receptors, and partial agonist at serotonin 5-HT_{1A} receptor

Therapeutic outcome: Decreasing hallucinations, delusions, agitation, social withdrawal

USES: Schizophrenia

CONTRAINDICATIONS:
Hypersensitivity

Precautions: Abrupt discontinuation, ambient temperature increase, breast cancer, breastfeeding, cardiac disease, children, dehydration, diabetes, ketoacidosis, driving/operating machinery, dysphagia, geriatrics, heart failure, hematological/hepatic/renal disease, hypotension, hypovolemia, MI, infertility, obesity, Parkinson's disease, pregnancy **B**, seizures, strenuous exercise, stroke, substance abuse, suicidal ideation, syncope, tardive dyskinesia

---

BLACK BOX WARNING: Dementia: antipsychotics, such as lurasidone, are not approved for the treatment of dementia-related psychosis in geriatric patients and may increase the risk of death in this population

---

DOSAGE AND ROUTES
Adult: PO 40 mg/day, range 40-160 mg/day, those receiving CYP3A4 inhibitors (max 80 mg/day), do not use with strong CYP3A4 inducers/inhibitors

Hepatic/renal dose
Adult: PO Child-Pugh class B/C, CCr ≥10 ml/min-<50 ml/min max 40 mg/day

Available forms: 20, 40, 80, 120 mg tabs

Implementation
• Give with a meal of at least 350 calories
• Store at room temperature, protect from moisture

ADVERSE EFFECTS
CNS: Agitation, akathisia, anxiety, dizziness, drowsiness, fatigue, hyperthermia, insomnia, dystonic reactions; **neuroleptic malignant syndrome (rare)**, pseudoparkinsonism, restlessness, **seizures, suicidal ideation**, syncope, tardive dyskinesia, vertigo
CV: Angina, **AV block, bradycardia,** hypertension, orthostatic hypotension, **sinus tachycardia, stroke**
EENT: Blurred vision
ENDO: Diabetes mellitus, ketoacidosis, hyperglycemia, hyperprolactimemia
GI: Abdominal pain, diarrhea, dyspepsia, nausea, vomiting, gastritis, weight gain/loss
GU: Amenorrhea, breast enlargement, dysmenorrhea, impotence, dysuria, renal failure
HEMA: Agranulocytosis, anemia, leucopenia, neutropenia
INTEG: Pruritus, rash
MS: Back pain, dysarthria; **rhabdomyolysis (rare)**
SYST: Angioedema

Pharmacokinetics

Absorption	9%-19%
Distribution	99% protein binding
Metabolism	Unknown
Excretion	80% feces, 9% urine
Half-life	18 hr

Pharmacodynamics

Onset	Unknown
Peak	1-3 hr
Duration	Steady state 7 days

INTERACTIONS
Individual drugs
Metoclopramide: do not use concurrently

Drug classifications
Other CNS depressants, alcohol: increased sedation

Strong CYP3A4 inhibitors: increased lurasidone effect, do not use concurrently

SSRIs, SNRIs: increased serotonin syndrome, neuroleptic malignant syndrome

NURSING CONSIDERATIONS
Assessment
• **Assess for schizophrenia:** hallucinations, delusions, agitation, social withdrawal; monitor orientation, behavior, mood prior to and periodically during therapy
• **Assess for neuroleptic malignant syndrome (rare):** fever, dyspnea, tachycardia, seizures, sweating, hypertension, hypotension, muscle stiffness, pallor, report immediately
• **Monitor for blood dyscrasias:** CBC periodically, blood dyscrasias may occur
• **Monitor for serious cardiac symptoms:** AV block, stroke, bradycardia may occur
• **Assess for EPS:** restlessness, difficulty speaking, loss of balance, pill rolling, mask-like face, shuffling gait, rigidity, tremors, muscle spasms; monitor prior to and periodically during therapy; report tardive dyskinesia immediately

BLACK BOX WARNING: **Dementia:** This product is not approved for the elderly with dementia-related psychosis

• Monitor for weight gain, hyperglycemia, metabolic changes in diabetes

Patient/family education
• Explain reason for treatment and expected results
• Teach patient to report EPS, blood dyscrasias: sore throat, fever, unusual bleeding/bruising
• Teach patient that lab work will be needed regularly
• Advise patient to avoid hazardous activities until response is known
• Teach patient to avoid OTC products unless approved by prescriber
• Teach patient to report fast heart beat, extra beats

Evaluation
Positive therapeutic outcome
• Decreasing hallucinations, delusions, agitation, social withdrawal

lymphocyte immune globulin (antithymocyte) (Rx)
Atgam
Func. class.: Immune globulin immunosuppressant
Pregnancy category C

ACTION: Produces immunosuppression by inhibiting the function of T-lymphocytes

Therapeutic outcome: Absence of transplant rejection; hematologic remission (aplastic anemia)

USES: Renal organ transplants to prevent rejection, aplastic anemia

Unlabeled uses: Immunosuppressant in liver, bone marrow, heart and other organ transplants, stem cell transplant preparations

CONTRAINDICATIONS:
Hypersensitivity to this product or equine/porcine protein, acute viral illness

Precautions: Pregnancy C, breastfeeding, children, severe renal/hepatic disease, leukopenia, thrombocytopenia

BLACK BOX WARNING: Infection, neoplastic disease

DOSAGE AND ROUTES
Renal allograft
Adult/child: IV 10-15 mg/kg/day × 14 days, then every other day for 14 more days if needed up to 21 days total

Delay of renal allograft rejection
Adult: IV 15 mg/kg/day × 7-14 days, then every other day × 14 days for a total of 21 doses in 28 days

Aplastic anemia
Adult: IV 10-20 mg/kg/day × 8-14 days, then every other day for up to 21 total doses

Available forms: Inj 50 mg horse gamma globulin/ml

Implementation

IV route
- Use 0.2-1 micron in-line filter
- Do not infuse <4 hr
- Keep emergency equipment nearby for severe allergic reactions
- **Aplastic anemia:** Skin testing must be completed before treatment; use intradermal inj of 0.1 ml of a 1:1000 dilution (5 mcg of horse IgG) in 0.9% NaCl; if a wheal or rash or both >10 mm, use caution during inf
- Dilute in saline sol before inf; invert **IV** bag, so undiluted product does not contact the air inside; concentration should not be >1 mg/ml

ADVERSE EFFECTS

Renal transplant
CNS: Fever, chills, headache, dizziness, weakness, faintness, **seizures**
CV: Chest pain, hypo/hypertension, tachycardia
GI: Diarrhea, nausea, vomiting, epigastric pain, **GI bleeding**
INTEG: Rash, pruritus, urticaria, wheal
SYST: **Anaphylaxis**

Aplastic anemia
CNS: Fever, chills, headache, **seizures**, lightheadedness, encephalitis, postviral encephalopathy
CV: Bradycardia, myocarditis, irregularity
GI: Nausea, liver function test abnormality
HEMA: **Thrombocytopenia**

Pharmacokinetics

Absorption	Unknown
Distribution	Unknown
Metabolism	Unknown
Excretion	Unknown
Half-life	5.7 days

Pharmacodynamics

Onset	Rapid
Peak	Unknown
Duration	Unknown

NURSING CONSIDERATIONS

Assessment
- Assess for infection; if infection occurs, evaluation will be needed to continue treatment
- Monitor renal function tests: BUN, creatinine at least monthly during treatment, 3 mo after treatment
- Monitor liver function tests: alkaline phosphatase, AST, ALT, bilirubin

Patient/family education
- Advise patient to report fever, rash, chills, sore throat, fatigue, since serious infections may occur
- Caution patient to use contraceptive measures during treatment and for 12 wk after ending therapy; product is teratogenic
- Caution patient to avoid crowds and persons with known infections to reduce risk of infection

Evaluation
Positive therapeutic outcome
- Absence of graft rejection
- Hematologic recovery (aplastic anemia)

mafenide topical
See Appendix B

magaldrate (OTC)
(mag'al-drate)
Isopan, Losapan ✦, Riopan, Riopan Extra Strength ✦
Func. class.: Antacid
Chem. class.: Aluminum/magnesium hydroxide
Pregnancy category C

ACTION: Neutralizes gastric acidity; product is dissolved in gastric contents; this product is a combination of aluminum and magnesium

Therapeutic outcome: Decreased pain of ulcers

USES: Antacid, hiatal hernia, indigestion/heartburn, hyperacidity

Unlabeled uses: Duodenal and gastric ulcers, peptic ulcer disease (adjunct), reflex esophagitis

CONTRAINDICATIONS:
Hypersensitivity to this product or benzyl alcohol

Precautions: Pregnancy **C**, geriatric, fluid restriction, decreased GI motility, GI obstruction, dehydration, renal disease, sodium-restricted diets, bone disease, hypertension, appendicitis, diverticulitis, ulcerative colitis, neonates/infants, hypermagnesemia, hypophosphatemia

DOSAGE AND ROUTES
Adult/child/geriatric: SUSP 5-10 ml (480-1080 mg) with water between meals, at bedtime

Available forms: Susp 540 mg/5 ml

Implementation
• Take antacids 2 hr before or 2 hr after taking enteric-coated products
• Give laxatives or stool softeners if constipation occurs
• Give susp after shaking; give between meals and at bedtime
• Give when stomach is empty after meals and at bedtime

ADVERSE EFFECTS
GI: Constipation, diarrhea, anorexia
META: Hypermagnesemia, hypophosphatemia

Pharmacokinetics
Absorption	Not absorbed
Distribution	Not distributed
Metabolism	Not metabolized
Excretion	Kidneys
Half-life	Unknown

Pharmacodynamics
Onset	Unknown
Peak	½ hr
Duration	1 hr

INTERACTIONS
Individual drugs
ChlordiazePOXIDE, cimetidine, isoniazid, ketoconazole, phenytoin, tetracycline: decreased absorption of each specific product
Flecainide, quiNIDine: increased action when taken in large amounts

Drug classifications
Amphetamines: increased action when taken in large amounts
Anticholinergics, corticosteroids, fluoroquinolones, iron salts, phenothiazines, salicylates: decreased absorption of each specific product
Salicylates: decreased action when taken in large amounts

NURSING CONSIDERATIONS
Assessment
• **Antacid:** location of pain, intensity, characteristics, what aggravates, ameliorates pain; heartburn/indigestion; hematemesis
• Monitor serum magnesium, calcium, phosphate, potassium if using long term or with impaired renal function
• Assess for constipation: increase bulk in diet if needed or obtain order for stool softener

Patient/family education
• Advise patient to separate ingestion of enteric-coated products and antacid by 2 hr
• Advise patient to use product 2 wk or less; product should not be used for long periods
• Teach patient to notify prescriber immediately if coffee-ground emesis, emesis with frank blood, or black tarry stools occur

Evaluation
Positive therapeutic outcome
• Absence of abdominal pain
• Decreased acidity

M

magnesium salts
(mag-neez'ee-um)
magnesium chloride (Rx)
Mag-64
magnesium citrate (OTC)
magnesium gluconate (OTC)
Mag-G, Magtrate
magnesium hydroxide (OTC)
Freelax, Phillips Milk of Magnesia, MOM
magnesium oxide (OTC)
Mag-Ox 400, Uro-Mag
magnesium sulfate (OTC, Rx)
epsom salt, magnesium sulfate (IV)—HIGH ALERT

Func. class.: Electrolyte; anticonvulsant, laxative, saline; antacid

Pregnancy category A, B

ACTION: Increases osmotic pressure, draws fluid into colon, neutralizes HCl

Therapeutic outcome: Magnesium levels WNL, absence of constipation

USES: Constipation, bowel preparation before surgery or exam, electrolyte, anticonvulsant, in preeclampsia, eclampsia (magnesium sulfate)

CONTRAINDICATIONS:
Hypersensitivity, abdominal pain, nausea/vomiting, obstruction, acute surgical abdomen, rectal bleeding, heart block, myocardial damage

Precautions: Pregnancy **A, B** (magnesium sulfate), renal disease/cardiac disease

DOSAGE AND ROUTES
Laxative
Adult: PO 15-60 ml at bedtime (Milk of Magnesia)
Adult and child >12 yr: PO 15 g in 8 oz of H_2O (magnesium sulfate); PO 5-30 ml (Concentrated Milk of Magnesia); PO 5-10 oz at bedtime (magnesium citrate)
Child 2-6 yr: 5-15 ml/day (Milk of Magnesia)

Prevention of magnesium deficiency
Adult and child ≥10 yr: PO (male): 350-400 mg/day; (female): 280-300 mg/day; (breast-feeding): 335-350 mg/day; (pregnancy): 320 mg/day
Child 8-10 yr: PO 170 mg/day
Child 4-7 yr: PO 120 mg/day

Magnesium sulfate deficiency
Adult: PO 200-400 mg in divided doses tid-qid; IM 1 g q6hr × 4 doses; **IV** 5 g (severe)
Child 6-12 yr: 3-6 mg/kg/day in divided doses tid-qid

Preeclampsia/eclampsia magnesium sulfate
Adult: IM/**IV** INF 4-5 g; with 5 g IM in each gluteus, then 5 g q4hr or 4 g **IV** INF, then 1-2 g/hr cont INF, max 40 g/day or 20 g/48 hr in severe renal disease

Available forms: Chloride: sus rel tabs 535 mg (64 mg Mg); enteric tabs 833 mg (100 mg Mg); **hydroxide:** liquid 400 mg/5 ml (164 mg Mg/5 ml); conc liquid 800 mg/5 ml (328 mg Mg/5 ml); chew tabs 300, 600 mg; **oxide:** tabs 400 mg (241.3 mg Mg); caps 140 mg (84.5 mg Mg); **sulfate:** powder for oral; bulk packages; (epsom salts) bulk packages; inj 10, 12.5, 25, 50%; **citrate:** oral sol 240, 296, 300 ml bottles (77 mEq/100 ml)

Implementation
PO route
- Administer with 8 oz of water
- Refrigerate magnesium citrate before administration
- Shake susp before using
- Administer to patient crushed or whole; chewable tablets may be chewed
- Administer with food or milk to decrease gastric symptoms; give 30 min before or 2 hr after antacids
- Tablets should be chewed thoroughly before swallowing, give 4 oz of water afterward
- **Laxative:** give on empty stomach
IM route (magnesium sulfate)
- Give deeply in gluteal site
IV route (magnesium sulfate)
- Only when calcium gluconate available for magnesium toxicity
Direct IV route
- Dilute 50% solution to 20% or less give at ≤150 mg/min
Continuous IV INF route
- May dilute to 20% sol, infuse over 3 hr
- IV at less than 125 mg/kg/hr; circulatory collapse may occur; use inf pump

Y-site compatibilities: Acyclovir, aldesleukin, amifostine, amikacin, ampicillin, aztreonam, cefamandole, ceFAZolin, cefmetazole, cefoperazone, cefotaxime, cefOXitin, cephalothin, cephapirin, chloramphenicol, cisatracurium, DOBUTamine, doxycycline, DOXOrubicin liposome, enalaprilat, erythromycin, esmolol, famotidine, fludarabine, gallium, gentamicin, granisetron, heparin, HYDROmorphone, IDArubicin, insulin, kanamycin, labetalol, meperidine, metroNIDAZOLE, minocycline, morphine, moxalactam, nafcillin, ondansetron, oxacillin, PACLitaxel, penicillin G potassium, piperacillin, piperacillin/tazobactam, potassium chloride, propofol, remifentanil, sargramostim, thiotepa, ticarcillin, tobramycin, trimethoprim/sulfamethoxazole, vancomycin, vit B complex/C

ADVERSE EFFECTS

CNS: Muscle weakness, flushing, sweating, confusion, sedation, depressed reflexes, **flaccid paralysis, hypothermia**
CV: Hypotension, heart block, **circulatory collapse,** vasodilatation
GI: *Nausea, vomiting, anorexia, cramps,* diarrhea
HEMA: Prolonged bleeding time
META: Electrolyte, fluid imbalances
RESP: Respiratory depression/paralysis

Pharmacokinetics

Absorption	Unknown
Distribution	Unknown
Metabolism	Unknown
Excretion	Kidneys
Half-life	Unknown effective anticonvulsant levels 2.5-7.5 mEq/L

Pharmacodynamics

	PO	IM	IV
Onset	3-6 hr	1 hr	Unknown
Peak	Unknown	Unknown	Unknown
Duration	Unknown	4 hr	½ hr

INTERACTIONS
Individual products
Digoxin: decreased effect of digoxin
Nitrofurantoin: decreased absorption

Drug classifications
Antihypertensives: increased hypotension
Antiinfectives (fluoroquinolones), tetracyclines: decreased absorption
Neuromuscular blockers: increased effect

NURSING CONSIDERATIONS
Assessment
• Assess I&O ratio; check for decrease in urinary output
• **Laxative:** assess cause of constipation; lack of fluids, bulk, exercise
• Assess cramping, rectal bleeding, nausea, vomiting; product should be discontinued
⚠ **Assess magnesium toxicity: thirst, confusion, decrease in reflexes**
• Assess visual changes: blurring, halos, corneal and retinal damage
• Assess edema in feet, ankles, legs
• Assess prior product history; there are many product interactions
• Eclampsia: seizure precautions, BP, ECG (magnesium sulfate)

Patient/family education
• Teach not to use laxatives for long-term therapy; bowel tone will be lost
• Teach that chilling helps the taste of magnesium citrate
• Teach to shake suspension well
• Teach to not use at bedtime as a laxative; may interfere with sleep; MOM is usually given at bedtime
• Teach to give citrus fruit after administering to counteract unpleasant taste
• Teach reason for product, expected result

Evaluation
Positive therapeutic outcome
• Decreased constipation; absence of seizures (eclampsia), normal serum calcium levels

mannitol (Rx)
(man'i-tole)
Osmitrol, Resectisol
Func. class.: Diuretic-osmotic
Chem. class.: Hexahydric alcohol
Pregnancy category C

ACTION: Increases osmolarity of glomerular filtrate, which raises osmotic pressure of fluid in renal tubules; there is a decrease in reabsorption of water, electrolytes; increases in urinary output, sodium, chloride, potassium, calcium, phosphorus, uric acid, urea, magnesium

USES: Edema; promote systemic diuresis in cerebral edema, decrease intraocular pressure, improve renal function in acute renal failure, chemical poisoning, urinary bladder irrigation

M

CONTRAINDICATIONS:

Active intracranial bleeding, hypersensitivity, anuria, severe pulmonary congestion, edema, severe dehydration, progressive heart disease, renal failure, acute MI, aneurysm, stroke

Precautions: Pregnancy **C,** breastfeeding, geriatric, dehydration, severe renal disease, CHF, electrolyte imbalances

DOSAGE AND ROUTES

Oliguria, prevention

Adult: IV after initial test dose and if urine output is 30-50 mg/hr × 2 hr, give 20-100 g of a 15% or 20% SOL in a 24-hr period

Oliguria, treatment

Adult: IV after initial test dose, give balance of 50 g of a 20% SOL over 1 hr, then 5% via CONT IV INF to maintain output at 50 ml/hr
Child (unlabeled): IV 0.5-2 g/kg as a 15%-20% SOL, run over 30-60 min; maintenance 0.25-0.5 g/kg q4-6hr

Edema

Adult: IV after dose, use product 10%-20% at a rate of 25-75 ml/hr, give loop diuretics prior to mannitol
Child: IV (unlabeled) 0.5-2 g/kg of 15%-20% mannitol over 2-6 hr

Intraocular pressure

Adult: IV 1.5-2 g/kg of a 15%-25% SOL over 30-60 min

ICP

Adult: IV 1-2 g/kg, then 0.25-1 g/kg q4hr

Diuresis in product intoxication

Adult and child >12 yr: 5%-10% SOL continuously up to 200 g **IV,** while maintaining 100-500 ml urine output/hr

Available forms: Inj 5%, 10%, 15%, 20%, 25%; GU irrigation 5%

Implementation
Irrigation

• Use 100 ml of 25%/900 ml of sterile water for inj (2.5% sol)
• Administer potassium replacement if potassium level is <3 mg/ml

Intermittent/continuous IV route

• Change IV q24hr
• Precipitate may occur with PVC
• Use an in-line filter for 15%, 20%, 25%; give with inf pump; check **IV** patency at inf site before, during administration; do not use sol that is yellow or has a precipitate or crystals, use in-line filter, do not give as direct injection; to redissolve, run bottle under hot water and shake vigorously; cool to body temp before giving
• Run at 30-50 ml/hr in oliguria; run over 30-60 min in increased ICP; run over 30 min for intraocular pressure; 60-90 min after surgery
• **Test dose** with severe oliguria, 0.2 g/kg over 3-5 mins; if continued oliguria give 2nd test dose; if no response, reassess patient

Y-site compatibilities: Acyclovir, alemtuzumab, amifostine, amikacin, ampicillin, atropine, aztreonam, bivalirudin, bumetanide, calcium gluconate, caspofungin, ceFAZolin, cefotaxime, cefOXitin, cefTAZidime, ceftizoxime, chloramphenicol, cimetidine, cisatracurium, clindamycin, DAPTOmycin, dexmedetomidine, digoxin, diltiazem, diphenhydrAMINE, DOBUTamine, DOPamine, DOXOrubicin liposome, doxycycline, enalaprilat, EPINEPHrine, ertapenem, esmolol, famotidine, fenoldopam, fentaNYL, fluconazole, fludarabine, gentamicin, granisetron, heparin, HYDROmorphone, hydrOXYzine, IDArubicin, imipenem/cilastatin, insulin, isoproterenol, ketorolac, labetalol, levofloxacin, lidocaine, linezolid, LORazepam, meperidine, metoclopramide, metoprolol, metroNIDAZOLE, micafungin, midazolam, milrinone, morphine, nafcillin, niCARdipine, nitroglycerin, nitroprusside, norepinephrine, ondansetron, oxaliplatin, PACLitaxel, palonosetron, pantoprazole, penicillin G potassium, phenylephrine, piperacillin/tazobactam, potassium chloride, procainamide, prochlorperazine, promethazine, propofol, propranolol, protamine, quinupristin/dalfopristin, ranitidine, remifentanil, sargramostim, sodium bicarbonate, tacrolimus, thiotepa, ticarcillin/clavulanate, tirofiban, tobramycin, trimethoprim/sulfamethoxazole, vancomycin, vasopressin, verapamil, vitamin B complex with C, voriconazole

Y-site incompatibilities: Aminophylline, amphotericin B cholesteryl sulfate complex, calcium chloride, cefepime, cefTRIAXone, cefuroxime, ciprofloxacin, dexamethasone sodium phosphate, diazepam, drotrecogin, haloperidol, lansoprazole, methylPREDNISolone sodium succinate, phenytoin, phytonadione

ADVERSE EFFECTS

CNS: *Dizziness, headache,* **seizures, rebound increased ICP,** confusion
CV: Edema, hypotension, hypertension, **tachycardia, CHF,** thrombophlebitis, angina-like chest pains, fever, chills, **circulatory overload,** PVCs
EENT: Loss of hearing, blurred vision, nasal congestion, decreased intraocular pressure

---

⚠ Nurse Alert ✴ Key NCLEX® Drug

ELECT: Fluid, electrolyte imbalances, *acidosis,* electrolyte loss, dehydration, hyper/ hypokalemia
GI: *Nausea, vomiting,* dry mouth, diarrhea
GU: Marked diuresis, urinary retention, thirst
RESP: Pulmonary congestion, *cough,* dyspnea

Absorption	Complete
Distribution	Extracellular spaces
Metabolism	Minimal
Excretion	Renal
Half-life	100 min

Onset	½-1 hr
Peak	1 hr
Duration	6-8 hr

INTERACTIONS
Individual drugs
Lithium: increased elimination of mannitol
Imipramine: increased excretion of imipramine
Arsenic trioxide, levomethadyl: increased hypokalemia

Drug classifications
Salicylates, barbiturates, bromides: increased excretion of each specific product

Drug/food
Potassium foods: increased hyperkalemia

Drug/lab test
Interference: inorganic phosphorus, ethylene glycol

NURSING CONSIDERATIONS
Assessment
• Assess neurologic status: LOC, ICP reading, pupil size and reaction when product is given for increased ICP
• Assess for vision changes or eye discomfort or pain before, during treatment (increases intraocular pressure); neurologic checks, ICP during treatment (increased ICP)
• Assess patient for tinnitus, hearing loss, ear pain; periodic testing of hearing is needed when high doses of this product are given by **IV** route
• Assess fluid volume status: check I&O ratios and record hourly urine values, CVP, breath sounds, weight, distended red veins, crackles in lungs, color, quality, and specific gravity of urine, skin turgor, adequacy of pulses, moist mucous membranes (provide adequate fluids), bilateral lung sounds, peripheral pitting edema

• Assess for dehydration; symptoms of decreasing output, thirst, hypotension, dry mouth and mucous membranes should be reported
• Monitor electrolytes: potassium, sodium, calcium, magnesium; also include BUN, ABGs, CVP, PAP, CBC; regularly monitor serum and urine levels of sodium and potassium
• Assess B/P before, during therapy with patient lying, standing, and sitting as appropriate; orthostatic hypotension can occur rapidly
• Monitor for rebound ICP: headache, confusion

Patient/family education
• Teach patient reason for and method of treatment

Evaluation
Positive therapeutic outcome
• Decreased intraocular pressure
• Prevention of hypokalemia (diuretic use)
• Decreased edema
• Decreased ICP
• Increased diuresis of >30 ml/hr
• Increased excretion of toxic substances

TREATMENT OF OVERDOSE:
Discontinue infusion; correct fluid, electrolyte imbalances; hemodialysis; monitor hydration, CV, renal function

maraviroc (Rx)
(mah-rav′er-rock)
Selzentry
Func. class.: Antiretroviral
Chem. class.: Fusion inhibitor, CCR5-receptor antagonist
Pregnancy category B

ACTION: Interferes with entry into HIV-1 by inhibiting the fusion of the virus and cell membrane

Therapeutic outcome: Improvement in CD4, viral load, T-cell count

USES: CCR5-tropic HIV in combination with other antiretroviral agents in treating experienced patients

CONTRAINDICATIONS:
Hypersensitivity, dialysis, renal impairment

Precautions: Pregnancy **B**, breastfeeding, Asian patients, renal/hepatic/cardiac disease, electrolyte imbalance, dehydration, immune reconstitution syndrome, infection, MI, orthostatic hypotension, children, geriatric

> **BLACK BOX WARNING:** Hepatitis/hepato-
> toxicity, fever, serious rash; eosinophilia, or
> elevated IgE prior to hepatotoxicity may occur

DOSAGE AND ROUTES
Those not taking CYP3A inducers/inhibitors
Adult/adolescent ≥16 yr: PO 300 mg bid

Those taking CYP3A4 inhibitors with/without a CYP3A inducer
Adult/adolescent ≥16 yr: PO 150 mg bid

Those taking CYP3A4 inducers without a strong CYP3A inhibitor
Adult/adolescent ≥16 yr: PO 600 mg bid

Renal dose
Adult: PO ≤30 ml/min, reduce dose to 150 mg bid

Available forms: Tabs 150, 300 mg

Implementation
• May give without regard to meals, with 8 oz of water
• Store at room temperature

ADVERSE EFFECTS
CNS: Dizziness, depression, **viral meningitis**, disturbances in consciousness, peripheral neuropathy, paresthesia, dysesthesia, fever
CV: **MI, cardiac ischemia, orthostatic hypotension**
EENT: Gingival hyperplasia
GI: Diarrhea, constipation, dyspepsia, **pseudomembranous colitis, hepatotoxicity**
INTEG: Rash, urticaria, pruritus, folliculitis
MS: Joint pain, leg pain, muscle cramps
RESP: Cough, URI, sinusitis, bronchitis, pneumonia, **bronchospasm, obstruction**
SYST: Herpes virus

Pharmacokinetics
Absorption	Unknown
Distribution	Unknown
Metabolism	By P450 system, CYP3A metabolism
Excretion	Urine 20%, feces 76%
Half-life	Unknown

Pharmacodynamics
Unknown

INTERACTIONS
Drug classifications
CYP3A inhibitors (amiodarone, aprepitant, chloramphenicol, clarithromycin, conivaptan, cycloSPORINE, dalfopristin, danazol, diltiazem, erythromycin, estradiol, fluconazole, fluvoxaMINE, imatinib, isoniazid, itraconazole, ketoconazole, miconazole, nefazodone, niCARdipine, propoxyphene, RU-486, tamoxifen, telithromycin, troleandomycin, verapamil, voriconazole, zafirlukast); reduce dose: increased maraviroc levels
CYP3A4 inducers (aminoglutethimide, barbiturates, bexaroten, bosentan, carBAMazepine, dexamethasone, efavirenz, fosphenytoin, griseofulvin, modafinil, nafcillin, OXcarbazepine, phenytoin, rifabutin, rifamipin, rifapentine, topiramate, tipranavir): increase dose; decreased maraviroc effect

Drug/food
High-fat meal: decreased absorption 33%

Drug/herb
St. John's wort: decreased maraviroc effect

NURSING CONSIDERATIONS
Assessment
• **HIV:** CD_4, T-cell count, plasma HIV RNA, CCR5-tropic HIV-1; assess for change in symptoms, other infections during treatment
• Monitor renal tests: serum creatinine
• Assess bowel pattern before, during treatment
• **Allergies:** skin eruptions: rash, urticaria, itching; assess allergies before treatment and before each dose

> **BLACK BOX WARNING: Hepatitis:** assess
> for dark urine, abdominal pain, vomiting, yellowing of skin/eyes, hepatomegaly: if present, discontinue product; monitor LFTs

Patient/family education
• Advise patient to take as prescribed; if dose is missed, take as soon as remembered up to 1 hr before next dose; do not double dose
• Teach patient that product does not cure infection, just controls symptoms, and does not prevent infecting others
⚠ Teach patient to report sore throat, fever, fatigue; may indicate superinfection; yellow skin/eyes, abdominal pain, vomiting (hepatitis); itching, dyspnea (allergic reaction)
• Advise patient that product must be taken in equal intervals around the clock to maintain blood levels for duration of therapy

---

⚠ Nurse Alert ⭐ Key NCLEX® Drug

- Instruct patient to notify prescriber of side effects
- Advise patient to avoid driving or other hazardous activities until reaction is known; dizziness may occur
- Teach patient to make position changes slowly to prevent postural hypotension

⚠ **Inform patient to notify prescriber if pregnancy is planned or suspected, not to breastfeed**

Evaluation
Positive therapeutic outcome
- Improvement in CD4, viral load, T-cell count

mecasermin (Rx)
(mec-a′sir-men)
Increlex
Func. class.: Biologic response modifier; insulin-like growth factor
Pregnancy category C

ACTION: Stimulates growth; IGF-1 is the principal hormonal mediator of statural growth; GH binds to its receptor in the liver and other tissues

Therapeutic outcome: Increased height

USES: Growth failure in children with severe primary insulin-like growth factor-1 (IGF-1) deficiency (primary IGFD) or with growth hormone (GH) gene deletion who have developed neutralizing antibodies to GH

Unlabeled uses: ALS

CONTRAINDICATIONS:
Hypersensitivity, benzyl alcohol, closed epiphyses, active/suspected neoplasia, **IV** use

Precautions: Pregnancy **C,** breastfeeding, children <2 yr, diabetes mellitus, hypothyroidism, lymphoid tissue hypertrophy, increased ICP, malnutrition, scoliosis, sleep apnea

DOSAGE AND ROUTES
Child ≥2 yr: SUBCUT 0.04-0.08 mg/kg (40-80 mcg/kg) bid; if well tolerated for 1 wk, may increase by 0.04 mg/kg/dose, max 0.12 mg/kg bid

Available forms: Inj 10 mg/ml

Implementation
SUBCUT route
- Give within 20 min of a meal or snack; do not give if unable to eat or if vomiting

- Rotate inj site; use sterile, disposable syringe/needles; use small-volume syringe for accurate measurement
- Store in refrigerator before opening, avoid freezing; after opening, stable for 30 days after initial vial entry, store in refrigerator, do not use if particulate matter is present, avoid direct light, do not use after expiration date
- Do not double dose if a dose is missed

ADVERSE EFFECTS
CNS: Headache, *seizures,* dizziness, cardiac valvulopathy, **increased intracranial pressure**
CV: Cardiac murmur
EENT: Ear pain, otitis media, abnormal tympanometry, papilledema, visual impairment, tonsillar hypertrophy
ENDO: Hypoglycemia, ketosis, hypothyroidism, hypercholesterolemia, hypertriglyceridemia
GI: Vomiting, nausea
HEMA: Thymus hypertrophy
INTEG: Pruritus, urticaria, anaphylaxis, angioedema
MISC: Bruising, lipohypertrophy, hypersensitivity reactions, inj site reaction
MS: Arthralgia, joint pain, slipped upper femoral epiphysis
RESP: Snoring, apnea
SYST: Antibodies to growth hormone, secondary malignancy

Pharmacokinetics

Absorption	Near 100%
Distribution	Unknown
Metabolism	Liver/kidneys
Excretion	Unknown
Half-life	5.8 hr

Pharmacodynamics
Unknown

INTERACTIONS
Drug classifications
Antidiabetics, corticosteroids: increased hypoglycemia
Psychostimulants: decrease in growth suppression possible

NURSING CONSIDERATIONS
Assessment
- Monitor preprandial glucose at beginning of treatment and until well tolerated
- Monitor by funduscopic exam at beginning, periodically during treatment

- Assess for **allergic reactions;** if present, interrupt treatment and notify prescriber
- Assess growth rate of child at intervals during treatment

⚠ **Serious skin disorders: angioedema; anaphylaxis**

Patient/family education

- Teach patient that treatment may continue for years; regular assessments are required
- Advise patient to avoid hazardous activities, driving within 2-3 hr of dosing
- Teach patient correct administration and needle disposal

Evaluation

Positive therapeutic outcome
- Growth in children

---

meclizine (OTC, Rx)

(mek'li-zeen)
Antivert, Bonamine ✦, Bonine, Dramamine Less Drowsy Formula, Medivert, Travel Sickness, Wal-Dram II
Func. class.: Antiemetic, antihistamine, anticholinergic
Chem. class.: H_1-receptor antagonist, piperazine derivative
Pregnancy category B

ACTION: Acts centrally by blocking chemoreceptor trigger zone, which in turn acts on vomiting center

Therapeutic outcome: Decreased nausea in motion sickness; decreased vertigo

USES: Vertigo, motion sickness

CONTRAINDICATIONS:
Hypersensitivity to cyclizines, shock

Precautions: Pregnancy **B**, breastfeeding, children, geriatric, closed-angle glaucoma, glaucoma, prostatic hypertrophy, hypertension

DOSAGE AND ROUTES

Vertigo
Adult/adolescent: PO 25-100 mg/day in divided doses

Motion sickness
Adult/adolescent: PO 25-50 mg 1 hr before traveling; repeat dose q24hr prn

Available forms: Tabs 12.5, 25, 50 mg; chew tabs 25 mg; caps 25, 30 mg

Implementation

- May give without regard to food
- **Chew tab:** Give without regard to water or may be swallowed whole with water
- Give lowest possible dose in geriatric, anticholinergic effects

ADVERSE EFFECTS

CNS: *Drowsiness,* fatigue, restlessness, headache, insomnia
CV: Hypotension
EENT: Dry mouth, blurred vision
GI: Nausea, anorexia, constipation, increased appetite
GU: Urinary retention

Pharmacokinetics

Absorption	Well absorbed
Distribution	Unknown
Metabolism	Unknown
Excretion	Unknown
Half-life	6 hr

Pharmacodynamics

Onset	1 hr
Peak	Unknown
Duration	8-24 hr

INTERACTIONS

Individual drugs
Alcohol: increased effects
Atropine: increased anticholinergic effects

Drug classifications
Antihistamines, antidepressants, phenothiazines: increased anticholinergic effect
CNS depressants, opioids: increased CNS depression

Drug/herb
Hops, valerian, kava: increased sedative effect

Drug/lab test
False negative: allergy skin testing (allergen extracts)

NURSING CONSIDERATIONS

Assessment
- **Vertigo/motion sickness:** nausea, vomiting after 1 hr, assess vertigo periodically
- Monitor VS, B/P

⚠ **Assess for signs of toxicity of other products or masking of symptoms of disease: brain tumor, intestinal obstruction**
- Observe for drowsiness, dizziness, LOC

Patient/family education

• Teach patient that a false-negative result may occur with skin testing for allergies; these procedures should not be scheduled for 4 days after discontinuing use

• Teach patient to avoid hazardous activities, activities requiring alertness; dizziness may occur; instruct patient to request assistance with ambulation

• Teach patient to avoid alcohol, other depressants, breastfeeding

Evaluation

Positive therapeutic outcome

• Absence of dizziness, vomiting

---

medroxyPROGESTERone (Rx)

(me-drox-ee-proe-jess'te-rone)
Depo-Provera, Depo-subQ Provera, Gen-Medroxy ✿, Provera
Func. class.: Hormone: progestogen, contraceptive, antineoplastic
Chem. class.: Progesterone derivative
Pregnancy category X

Do not confuse:

medroxyPROGESTERone/methylPREDNISolone, **Provera**/Premarin/Covera

ACTION: Inhibits secretion of pituitary gonadotropins, which prevents follicular maturation and ovulation; antineoplastic action against endometrial cancer

Therapeutic outcome: Decreased abnormal uterine bleeding, absence of amenorrhea

USES: Uterine bleeding (abnormal), secondary amenorrhea, contraceptive, prevention of endometrial changes associated with estrogen replacement therapy (ERT), inoperable, recurrent, metastatic endometrial/renal cancer

CONTRAINDICATIONS:

Pregnancy **X,** hypersensitivity, reproductive cancer, genital bleeding (abnormal, undiagnosed), missed abortion, stroke, cerebrovascular disease, cervical cancer, hepatic disease, uterine/vaginal cancer

BLACK BOX WARNING: Breast cancer, MI, stroke, thromboembolic disease, thrombophlebitis

Precautions: Breastfeeding, hypertension, asthma, blood dyscrasias, gallbladder disease, CHF, diabetes mellitus, bone disease, depression, migraine headache, seizure disorders, renal/hepatic disease, family history of cancer of breast or reproductive tract, bone mineral density loss, ocular disorders, AIDS/HIV, alcoholism, children, hyperlipidemia

BLACK BOX WARNING: Use of this product has been shown to increase dementia in women ≥65 yr old; use may increase osteoporosis in long-term treatment, those at greater risk also smoke, adequate calcium and vitamin D should be taken

DOSAGE AND ROUTES

Secondary amenorrhea
Adult: PO 5-10 mg/day × 5-10 days

Uterine bleeding
Adult: PO 5-10 mg/day × 5-10 days starting on 16th or 21st day of menstrual cycle

With ERT
Adult: PO 5-10 mg qd × 10-14 or more days/mo (sequential estrogen); 2.5-5 mg qd (continuous estrogen)

Contraceptive
Adult: IM 150 mg q12wk; SUBCUT (depot SUBCUT Provera 104 inj) 104 mg q3mo

Endometrial/renal cancer
Adult: IM 400 mg-1 g (using 400 mg/ml depot inj susp) qwk

Available forms: Tabs 2.5, 5, 10 mg; inj susp 50, 150, 400 mg/ml; depot SUBCUT inj: 104 mg/0.65 ml

Implementation
PO route
• Give without regard to food
IM route
• Visually inspect particulate matter and discoloration prior to use
• Give titrated dose; use lowest effective dose; give oil sol deep in large muscle mass (IM); rotate sites; use after warming to dissolve crystals
Depo-Provera Contraceptive injection suspension:
• IM only, NEVER IV
• Instruct patient on risks and warnings associated with hormonal contraceptives (see Patient Information)
• The possibility of pregnancy should be excluded prior to giving the first dose of me-

M

droxyprogesterone or whenever more than 14 weeks have passed since the last dose
• Do not dilute
• Shake vigorously immediately before administration
• Inject deeply into the gluteal or deltoid muscle. Aspirate prior to injection to avoid injection into a blood vessel

Depo-Provera Sterile Aqueous Suspension, preserved:
• IM only, NEVER IV
• Instruct patient on risks and warnings associated with progestin use (see Patient Information)
• Shake vigorously immediately before use
• When multi-dose vials are used, take special care to prevent contamination
• Inject deeply into the gluteal or deltoid muscle. Aspirate prior to injection

Subcut route
Depo-subQ Provera 104 Contraceptive Injection Suspension ONLY:
• For subcut use only; NEVER give IM or IV
• Instruct patient on risks and warnings associated with hormonal contraceptives (see Patient Information)
• Shake vigorously for at least 1 min before use
• Inject the entire contents of the prefilled syringe subcut into the anterior thigh or abdomen, avoiding boney areas and the umbilicus. Gently grasp and squeeze a large area of skin in the chosen injection area, ensuring that the skin is pulled away from the body. Insert the needle at a 45-degree angle. Inject until the syringe is empty; this usually requires 5-7 seconds. Following use, press lightly on the injection site with a clean cotton pad for a few seconds; do not rub the area

ADVERSE EFFECTS

CNS: Dizziness, headache, migraine, depression, fatigue, nervousness
CV: Hypotension, thrombophlebitis, edema, **thromboembolism, stroke, pulmonary embolism, MI**
EENT: Diplopia
GI: *Nausea,* vomiting, anorexia, cramps, increased weight, **cholestatic jaundice,** abdominal pain
GU: Amenorrhea, cervical erosion, breakthrough bleeding, dysmenorrhea, vaginal candidiasis, breast changes, *gynecomastia, testicular atrophy, impotence,* endometriosis, **spontaneous abortion,** vaginitis, increased/decreased libido

INTEG: Rash, urticaria, acne, hirsutism, alopecia, oily skin, seborrhea, purpura, melasma, photosensitivity, injection site reaction
META: Hyperglycemia
MS: Decreased bone density
SYST: Angioedema, anaphylaxis

Pharmacokinetics
Unknown

Pharmacodynamics

	PO	IM
Onset	Unknown	Unknown
Peak	Unknown	Unknown
Duration	2-4 hr	Unknown

INTERACTIONS

Individual drugs
Aminoglutethimide, carBAMazepine, phenytoin, PHENobarbital, rifampin: decreased contraceptive effect

Drug categories
Anticoagulants, corticosteroids: decreased bone mineral density

Drug/lab test
Increased: LFTs, HDL, triglycerides
Decreased: GTT, HDL

NURSING CONSIDERATIONS

Assessment
• **Assess for symptoms indicating severe allergic reaction, angioedema;** have EPINEPHrine and resuscitative equipment available
• Monitor B/P at beginning of treatment and periodically; check weight daily; notify prescriber of weekly weight gain >5 lb; bone mineral density
• Monitor I&O ratio: be alert for decreasing urinary output, increasing edema, hypertension
• Assess liver function tests: ALT, AST, bilirubin, periodically during long-term therapy
• **Bone mineral density loss:** in those taking anticoagulants, corticosteroids with Depo-Provera or Depo-subQ Provera
• Assess for edema, hypertension, cardiac symptoms, jaundice
• Assess mental status: affect, mood, behavioral changes, depression

Patient/family education
• Advise patients to avoid sunlight or use sunscreen; photosensitivity and melasma (brown patches on the face) can occur
• Teach patient about cushingoid symptoms: weight gain, moon face, buffalo hump, acne

• Teach women patients to report breast lumps, vaginal bleeding, edema, jaundice, dark urine, clay-colored stools, dyspnea, headache, blurred vision, abdominal pain, sudden changes in speech/coordination, numbness or stiffness in legs, chest pain; teach men to report impotence or gynecomastia

⚠ Teach patient to report suspected pregnancy (X) immediately; fertility returns in 6-12 mo after discontinuing

> **BLACK BOX WARNING:** Long-term use decreases bone density; exercise, calcium supplements can help lessen osteoporosis

Evaluation
Positive therapeutic outcome
• Decreased abnormal uterine bleeding
• Absence of amenorrhea
• Prevention of pregnancy
• Arrested spread of malignant cells

medrysone ophthalmic
See Appendix B

megestrol (Rx)
(me-jess'trole)
Megace, Megace ES
Func. class.: Antineoplastic hormone
Chem. class.: Progestin
Pregnancy category D (tabs), X (susp)

Do not confuse:
Megace/Reglan

ACTION: Affects endometrium by antiluteinizing effect; this is thought to bring about cell death

Therapeutic outcome: Prevention of rapidly growing malignant cells; weight gain, increased appetite in AIDS

USES: Breast, endometrial cancer; increased weight, decreased cachexia and anorexia associated with AIDS

Unlabeled uses: Hot flashes, prostate cancer

CONTRAINDICATIONS:
Pregnancy **X** (susp), **D** (tabs), hypersensitivity

Precautions: Diabetes, thrombosis, adrenal insufficiency

DOSAGE AND ROUTES
Endometrial/ovarian carcinoma
Adult: PO 40-320 mg/day in divided doses

Breast carcinoma
Adult: PO 40 mg qid or 160 mg/day

AIDS
Adult: PO 800 mg/day (oral SUSP) or 625 mg/day (ES)

Hot flashes (unlabeled)
Adult: PO 20 mg bid

Available forms: Tabs 20, 40 mg; oral susp 40, 125 mg/ml

Implementation
• Administer with meals for GI symptoms
• Oral susp is usually used for AIDS patients; shake well
• Give tablets for carcinoma
• Give without regard to food

ADVERSE EFFECTS
CNS: Mood swings, insomnia, fever, lethargy, depression
CV: Thrombophlebitis, thromboembolism, hypertension
ENDO: Adrenal insufficiency
GI: Nausea, vomiting, diarrhea, abdominal cramps, weight gain, flatus, indigestion
GU: Gynecomastia, fluid retention, hypercalcemia, vaginal bleeding, discharge, impotence, decreased libido, menstruation disorders
INTEG: Alopecia, rash, pruritus, purpura, itching, sweating
META: Hyperglycemia
MISC: Tumor flare
RESP: Dyspnea

Pharmacokinetics

Absorption	Well absorbed; food increases oral sol
Distribution	Unknown
Metabolism	Liver, completely
Excretion	Feces, urine
Half-life	13-105 hr

Pharmacodynamics

Onset	Several wk to mo
Peak	Unknown

INTERACTIONS
Individual drugs
Dofetilide: do not use with megestrol

Drug/lab test
Increased: glucose

M

NURSING CONSIDERATIONS
Assessment
• PSA levels in men (prostate cancer); blood glucose, liver function studies, serum calcium, weight
• Monitor effects of alopecia on body image; discuss feelings about body changes
• In AIDS patients monitor calorie counts, weight, appetite
• **Assess for thrombophlebitis:** Homan's sign, pain, redness, swelling in calf, thigh; notify prescriber immediately if these occur

Patient/family education
• Teach patient to report any complaints or side effects to prescriber
• Advise patient that contraceptive measures must be used during and 4 mo after treatment; product is teratogenic: pregnancy **D** tabs, pregnancy **X** susp
• Explore with patient the need for wig or a hairpiece for hair loss
• Caution patient to report vaginal bleeding to prescriber
• Review with patient the need to comply with dosage schedule, not to miss or double doses; missed doses may be taken up to 1 hr before next dose
• Teach patient how to recognize signs of fluid retention, thromboembolism and report immediately
• Teach that gynecomastia and alopecia can occur; reversible after discontinuing treatment
• Advise to monitor blood glucose if diabetic

Evaluation
Positive therapeutic outcome
• Decreased spread of malignant cells
• Weight gain, increased appetite in AIDS patients
• Resolved dysfunctional uterine bleeding

⚠ HIGH ALERT

melphalan (Rx)
(mel′fa-lan)
Alkeran
Func. class.: Antineoplastic, alkylating agent
Chem. class.: Nitrogen mustard
Pregnancy category D

Do not confuse:
melphalan/myleran, **Alkeran**/Alferon

ACTION: Responsible for cross-linking DNA strands leading to cell death; activity is not cell cycle phase specific

Therapeutic outcome: Prevention of rapidly growing malignant cells

USES: Multiple myeloma, malignant melanoma, advanced ovarian cancer

Unlabeled uses: Breast, testicular, prostate carcinoma; osteogenic sarcoma, amyloidosis, chronic myelogenous leukemia, non-Hodgkin's lymphoma

CONTRAINDICATIONS:
Pregnancy **D,** breastfeeding, or other nitrogen mustards

> **BLACK BOX WARNING:** Hypersensitivity to this product

Precautions: Children, radiation therapy, infection, renal disease

> **BLACK BOX WARNING:** Bone marrow depression, secondary malignancy, radiation therapy: requires an experienced clinician

DOSAGE AND ROUTES
Multiple myeloma
Adult: PO 6 mg qd × 2-3 wk, adjust dose based on blood counts or, 10 mg qd × 7-10 days
Adult: IV INF 16 mg/m²; reduce in renal insufficiency; give over 15-20 min; give at 2-wk intervals × 4 doses, then at 4-wk intervals

Ovarian carcinoma
Adult: PO 200 mcg/kg/day × 5 days q4-5wk

Available forms: Tabs 2 mg; powder for inj 50 mg

Implementation
• Give fluids **IV** or PO before chemotherapy to hydrate patient
• Give antacid before oral agent; give product after evening meal, before bedtime; provide antiemetic 30-60 min before giving product and prn to prevent vomiting; give antibiotics for prophylaxis of infection
• Give in AM so product can be eliminated before bedtime
• Use a liquid diet: carbonated beverages; gelatin may be added if patient is not nauseated or vomiting

---

PO route
- Give 1 hr before or 2 hr after meals to prevent nausea/vomiting
- Protect from light, store refrigerated

Intermittent IV INF route
- Use gloves during administration; if skin exposure occurs, wash immediately with soap and water, use cytotoxic handling procedures
- Reconstitute with provided diluent (10 ml) to 5 mg/ml; shake until clear; further dilute with 0.9% NaCl to <0.45 mg/ml; give over ≥15 min, give within 1 hr, degrading of product occurs rapidly; make sure infusion is completed in time specified

Y-site compatibilities: Acyclovir, amikacin, aminophylline, ampicillin, aztreonam, bleomycin, bumetanide, buprenorphine, butorphanol, calcium gluconate, CARBOplatin, carmustine, ceFAZolin, cefepime, cefoperazone, cefotaxime, cefOTEtan, cefTAZidime, ceftizoxime, cefTRIAXone, cefuroxime, cimetidine, CISplatin, clindamycin, cyclophosphamide, cytarabine, dacarbazine, DACTINomycin, DAUNOrubicin, dexamethasone, diphenhydrAMINE, DOXO-rubicin, doxycycline, droperidol, enalaprilat, etoposide, famotidine, floxuridine, fluconazole, fludarabine, fluorouracil, furosemide, gallium, ganciclovir, gentamicin, granisetron, haloperidol, heparin, hydrocortisone sodium phosphate, hydromorphone, hydrOXYzine, IDArubicin, ifosfamide, imipenem-cilastatin, LORazepam, mannitol, mechlorethamine, meperidine, mesna, methylPREDNISolone, metoclopramide, methotrexate, metroNIDAZOLE, miconazole, minocycline, mitoMYcin, mitoXANtrone, morphine, nalbuphine, netilmicin, ondansetron, pentostatin, piperacillin, plicamycin, potassium chloride, prochlorperazine, promethazine, ranitidine, sodium bicarbonate, streptozocin, teniposide, thiotepa, ticarcillin, ticarcillin/clavulanate, tobramycin, trimethoprim/sulfamethoxazole, vancomycin, vinBLAStine, vinCRIStine, vinorelbine, zidovudine

ADVERSE EFFECTS
GI: *Nausea, vomiting,* stomatitis, diarrhea, **hepatitis**
GU: Amenorrhea, hyperuricemia, gonadal suppression
HEMA: Thrombocytopenia, neutropenia, leukopenia, anemia
INTEG: Rash, urticaria, alopecia, pruritus
RESP: Fibrosis, dysplasia, dyspnea, pneumonitis
SYST: Anaphylaxis, allergic reaction, **secondary malignancies,** edema

Absorption	Variable; incompletely absorbed
Distribution	Rapidly distributed, protein binding 80%-90%
Metabolism	Bloodstream
Excretion	Kidneys, unchanged (10%)
Half-life	1½ hr

Pharmacodynamics
Unknown

INTERACTIONS
Individual drugs
Sargramostim, GM-CSF, filgrastim, G-CSF: avoid administration 14 hr before or 24 hr after this product
Carmustine: increased pulmonary toxicity
CycloSPORINE: increased renal failure risk
Nalidixic acid: increased enterocolitis risk
Radiation: increased toxicity

Drug classifications
Anticoagulants, NSAIDs, salicylates, thrombolytics, platelet inhibitors: increased bleeding risk
Antineoplastics: increased toxicity
Live virus vaccines: increased adverse reactions; decreased antibody reaction

NURSING CONSIDERATIONS
Assessment

> **BLACK BOX WARNING:** Monitor CBC, differential, platelet count weekly; withhold product if WBC is <3000/mm³ or platelet count is <100,000/mm³; notify prescriber; recovery usually occurs in 6 wk

- **Hyperuricemia:** assess for increased uric acid levels, swelling, joint pain primarily in extremities; patient should be well hydrated to prevent urate deposits
- **Infection:** monitor for cold, fever, chills, sore throat
- **Assess for bleeding:** hematuria, guaiac, bruising or petechiae, from mucosa or orifices q8hr; no rectal temp
- **Assess for symptoms indicating severe allergic reaction:** rash, pruritus, urticaria, purpuric skin lesions, itching, flushing; assess allergy to chlorambucil; cross-sensitivity may occur

Patient/family education
- Teach patient to avoid use of products containing aspirin or ibuprofen, razors, commercial

mouthwash, since bleeding may occur; to report symptoms of bleeding (hematuria, tarry stools)
• Instruct patient to report signs of anemia (fatigue, headache, irritability, faintness, shortness of breath)
• Instruct patient to report any changes in breathing or coughing even several mo after treatment; to avoid crowds and persons with respiratory tract or other infections
• Tell patient hair loss is common; discuss the use of wigs or hairpieces
• Caution patient not to have any vaccinations without the advice of the prescriber, serious reactions can occur
⚠ **Advise patient to report suspected pregnancy, that contraception is needed during treatment and for several mo after the completion of therapy, pregnancy D**
• Teach patient to rinse mouth tid-qid with water, club soda; brush teeth bid-qid with soft brush or cotton-tipped applicators for stomatitis; use unwaxed dental floss

Evaluation
Positive therapeutic outcome
• Decreased size of tumor
• Decreased spread of malignancy

memantine (Rx)
(me-man'teen)
Ebixa ✦, Namenda, Namenda XR
Func. class.: Anti–Alzheimer's disease agent
Chem. class.: NMDA receptor antagonist
Pregnancy category B

ACTION: Antagonist action of CNS NMDA receptors that may contribute to the symptoms of Alzheimer's disease

Therapeutic outcome: Improved mood, orientation, decreasing confusion

USES: Moderate to severe dementia in Alzheimer's disease

Unlabeled uses: Vascular dementia

CONTRAINDICATIONS:
Hypersensitivity, children

Precautions: Pregnancy **B**, breastfeeding, renal disease, seizures, severe hepatic disease, GU conditions that raise urine pH, renal failure

DOSAGE AND ROUTES
Adult: PO 5 mg/day, may increase dose in 5-mg increments ≥1-wk intervals over a 3-wk period;

recommended target dose as 10 mg bid at week 4; ext rel 7 mg/day, increased by 7 mg ≤1 wk up to target dose of 28 mg/day

Available forms: Tabs 5, 10 mg; tab titration pak 5, 10 mg; oral sol 2 mg/ml, 10 mg/5 ml; cap ext rel 7, 14, 21, 28 mg

Implementation
• Can be taken without regard to meals
• Give twice a day if dose >5 mg
• Dosage is adjusted to response no more than q1wk
• Provide assistance with ambulation during beginning therapy; dizziness may occur
• **Extended Release Caps:** Do not crush, chew, divide; swallow whole or open and sprinkle on applesauce

ADVERSE EFFECTS
CNS: *Dizziness, confusion,* somnolence, headache, hallucinations, **stroke,** insomnia, depression, anxiety
CV: Hypertension, **heart failure, CHF**
GI: Vomiting, constipation
INTEG: Rash
MISC: Back pain, fatigue, pain, influenza-like symptoms
RESP: Coughing, dyspnea

Pharmacokinetics
Absorption	Rapidly absorbed PO
Distribution	44% protein binding
Metabolism	Very little
Excretion	57%-82% excreted unchanged in urine
Half-life	Terminal elimination half-life 60-80 hr

Pharmacodynamics
Unknown

INTERACTIONS
Individual drugs
Cimetidine, hydrochlorothiazide, nicotine, quiNIDine, ranitidine, triamterene: increased/decreased levels of both products
Ergot, levodopa: increased effect of each

Drug classifications
Drugs that make the urine alkaline (sodium bicarbonate, carbonic anhydrase inhibitors): decreased clearance
Use cautiously with amantadine, dextromethorphan, ketamine: reaction unknown

NURSING CONSIDERATIONS
Assessment
• Alzheimer's dementia: affect, mood, behavioral changes; hallucinations, confusion, attention, orientation, memory; monitor serum creatinine

Patient/family education
• Advise to report side effects: restlessness, psychosis, visual hallucinations, stupor, loss of consciousness; indicate overdose
• Advise patient to avoid alcohol, nicotine
• Advise to use product exactly as prescribed; product is not a cure
• Teach patient to avoid OTC, herbal products unless approved by prescriber

Evaluation
Positive therapeutic outcome
• Decrease in confusion, improved mood or ability to maintain function, even with no improvement in symptoms

---

⚠ HIGH ALERT

meperidine (Rx)
(me-per'i-deen)
Demerol, Meperitab
Func. class.: Opioid analgesic
Chem. class.: Phenylpiperidine derivative
Pregnancy category C
Controlled substance schedule II

Do not confuse:
meperidine/HYDROmorphone/meprobamate/morphine,
Demerol/Dilaudid/Desyrel/Demulen

ACTION: Depresses pain impulse transmission at the spinal cord level by interacting with opioid receptors

Therapeutic outcome: Relief of pain

USES: Moderate to severe pain, preoperatively, postoperatively

CONTRAINDICATIONS:
Hypersensitivity, severe respiratory insufficiency

Precautions: Pregnancy C, breastfeeding, children, geriatric, addictive personality, increased ICP, respiratory depression, renal/hepatic disease, seizure disorder, abrupt discontinuation, chronic pain, cardiac disease, adrenal insufficiency, alcoholism, angina, anticoagulant therapy, asthma, atrial flutter, biliary tract disease, bladder obstruction, cardiac dysrhythmias, COPD, CNS depression, coagulopathy, constipation, cor pulmonale, dehydration, diarrhea, driving epidural use, geriatrics, GI obstruction, head trauma, heart failure, hypotension, hypothyroidism, ileus, IBS, IM/intrathecal/IV use, labor, myxedema/thrombocytopenia, MAOI therapy

DOSAGE AND ROUTES
Moderate to severe pain
Adult: PO/SUBCUT/IM 50-150 mg q3-4hr prn
Child: PO/SUBCUT/IM 1-1.8 mg/kg q3-4hr prn, max single dose 150 mg

Preoperatively
Adult: IM/SUBCUT 50-100 mg 30-90 min before surgery
Child: IM/SUBCUT 1-2 mg/kg 30-90 min before surgery, max 100 mg

Renal dose
Adult: PO/SUBCUT/IM/IV, CCr 10-50 ml/min give 75% of dose; CCr <10 ml/min give 25%-50% of dose

Labor analgesia
Adult: SUBCUT/IM 50-100 mg given when contractions are regularly spaced, repeat q1-3hr prn

Available forms: Inj 10, 25, 50, 75, 100 mg/ml; tabs 50, 100 mg; syr 50 mg/5 ml

Implementation
• Give with antiemetic if nausea, vomiting occur
• Administer when pain is beginning to return; determine dosage interval by patient response; continuous dosing of medication is more effective given prn
• Medication should be slowly withdrawn after long-term use to prevent withdrawal symptoms
• Store in light-resistant container at room temperature
PO route
• May be given with food or milk to lessen GI upset
• Syr should be mixed with 4 oz of water
• **Oral liquid:** dilute in 4 oz water
IM/SUBCUT route
• Do not give if cloudy or a precipitate has formed
• Patient should remain recumbent for 1 hr after administration
• Inject IM into a large muscle mass; IM is preferred route for multiple injections
Direct IV route
• Give after diluting to 10 mg/ml with sterile water, 0.9% NaCl for inj; give slowly at ≤25 mg/

M

min; rapid administration may cause respiratory depression, hypotension, circulatory collapse
• Have emergency equipment and opiate antagonist on hand

Continuous IV infusion route
• Give after diluting to 1 mg/ml with D$_5$W, D$_{10}$W, dextrose/saline combinations, dextrose/Ringer's, inj combinations, 0.45% NaCl, 0.9% NaCl, Ringer's, LR; give by inf pump; titrate according to response

Syringe compatibilities: Butorphanol, chlorproMAZINE, cimetidine, dimenhyDRINATE, diphenhydrAMINE, droperidol, fentaNYL, glycopyrrolate, hydrOXYzine, ketamine, metoclopramide, midazolam, pentazocine, perphenazine, prochlorperazine, promazine, ranitidine, scopolamine

Syringe incompatibilities: Heparin, morphine, PENTobarbital

Y-site compatibilities: Amifostine, amikacin, atenolol, aztreonam, bumetanide, cefamandole, ceFAZolin, cefmetazole, cefotaxime, cefOXitin, cefTAZidime, ceftizoxime, cefTRIAXone, cefuroxime, cladribine, clindamycin, diltiazem, diphenhydrAMINE, DOBUTamine, DOPamine, doxycycline, droperidol, erythromycin lactobionate, famotidine, filgrastim, fluconazole, fludarabine, gallium, gentamicin, granisetron, hydrocortisone, regular insulin, kanamycin, labetalol, lidocaine, melphalan, methyldopate, metoclopramide, metoprolol, metroNIDAZOLE, ondansetron, oxytocin, PACLitaxel, penicillin G potassium, piperacillin, potassium chloride, propofol, propranolol, ranitidine, sargramostim, teniposide, thiotepa, ticarcillin, ticarcillin/clavulanate, tobramycin, vancomycin, verapamil, vinorelbine

Y-site incompatibilities: Cefoperazone, IDArubicin, imipenem/cilastatin, mezlocillin, minocycline

Continuous intrathecal infusion route
• Use controlled-infusion device, an implantable controlled-microinfusion device is used for highly concentrated infusion, monitor for several days after implantation
• Infusion reservoir should only be filled by those fully qualified
• To prevent pain, depletion of reservoir should be avoided

ADVERSE EFFECTS
CNS: Drowsiness, dizziness, confusion, headache, sedation, euphoria, **increased ICP, seizures,** serotonin syndrome

CV: Palpitations, bradycardia, hypotension, change in B/P, tachycardia (**IV**)
EENT: Tinnitus, blurred vision, miosis, diplopia, depressed corneal reflex
GI: Nausea, vomiting, anorexia, constipation, cramps, biliary spasm, paralytic ileus
GU: Urinary retention, dysuria
INTEG: Rash, urticaria, bruising, flushing, diaphoresis, pruritus
RESP: Respiratory depression
SYST: Anaphylaxis

Pharmacokinetics

Absorption	Well absorbed (IM, SUBCUT); 50% (PO)
Distribution	Widely distributed; crosses placenta; protein binding 65%-75%; toxic by-product accumulation can result from regular use or in renal disease
Metabolism	Liver, extensively to active/inactive metabolites
Excretion	Kidneys; breast milk
Half-life	3-4 hr

Pharmacodynamics

	PO	IM/SUBCUT	IV
Onset	15 min	10 min	5 min
Peak	1-1½ hr	½-1 hr	5-7 min
Duration	2-4 hr	2-4 hr	2 hr

INTERACTIONS
Individual drugs
Alcohol: increased respiratory depression, hypotension, sedation
Phenytoin: decreased meperidine effect
Procarbazine: fatal reaction, do not use together

Drug classifications
CNS depressants, opioids, sedative/hypnotics, antipsychotics, skeletal muscle relaxants: increased effects
SSRIs, SNRIs, serotonin-receptor agonists: increased serotonin syndrome, increased neuroleptic malignant syndrome
MAOIs: do not use for 2 wk before taking meperidine; may cause fatal reaction
Protease inhibitor antiretrovirals: increased adverse reactions

Drug/herb
St. John's wort: increased CNS depression

Drug/lab test
Increased: amylase, lipase

NURSING CONSIDERATIONS
Assessment
• **Assess pain:** location, duration, intensity before and 1 hr (IM, SUBCUT, PO), 5-10 min (**IV**) after administration
• Assess renal function before initiating therapy; poor renal function can lead to accumulation of toxic metabolite and seizures
• Monitor VS after parenteral route; note muscle rigidity, product history, liver, kidney function tests, respiratory dysfunction: respiratory depression, character, rate, rhythm; notify prescriber if respirations are <10/min
• Monitor CNS changes: dizziness, drowsiness, hallucinations, euphoria, LOC, pupil reaction; these are due to metabolite produced; CNS stimulation occurs with chronic or high doses
• Monitor allergic reactions: rash, urticaria
• Assess for constipation; increase fluids, bulk in diet; give stimulant laxatives if needed

Patient/family education
• Advise patients to avoid CNS depressants (alcohol, sedative/hypnotics) for at least 24 hr after taking this product
• Discuss with patient that dizziness, drowsiness, and confusion are common; to avoid getting up without assistance
• Discuss in detail with patient all aspects of the product, including its purpose and what to expect
• Caution patient to make position changes carefully to lessen orthostatic hypotension

Evaluation
Positive therapeutic outcome
• Decreased pain

TREATMENT OF OVERDOSE:
Naloxone 0.2-0.8 mg IV (caution in physically dependent patients), O_2, IV fluids, vasopressors

mercaptopurine (6-MP) (Rx)
(mer-kap-toe-pyoor′een)
Purinethol
Func. class.: Antineoplastic, antimetabolite
Chem. class.: Purine analog
Pregnancy category D

ACTION: Inhibits purine metabolism at multiple sites, which inhibits DNA and RNA synthesis S phase of cell cycle

Therapeutic outcome: Prevention of rapidly growing malignant cells

USES: Acute lymphocytic leukemia

Unlabeled uses: Ulcerative colitis; Crohn's disease

CONTRAINDICATIONS:
Pregnancy **D**, hypersensitivity, breastfeeding, patients with prior product resistance

Precautions: Renal/hepatic disease, tumor lysis syndrome, dental disease, herpes, radiation therapy, leukopenia, thrombocytopenia, anemia, requires an experienced clinician, secondary malignancy, infection, hypocalcemia, hyperuricemia, hyperphosphatemia, hyperkalemia

DOSAGE AND ROUTES
Acute lymphocytic leukemia
Adult: PO 2.5-5 mg/kg/day or 80-100 mg/m²/day, maintenance 1.5-2.5 mg/kg/day
Child: PO 2.5-5 mg/kg/day, maintenance 1.5-2.5 mg/kg/day or 70-100 mg/m²/day

Available forms: Tabs 50 mg

Implementation
• Give fluids IV or PO before chemotherapy to hydrate patient
• Give antiemetic 30-60 min before giving product and prn to prevent vomiting
• Give in PM on empty stomach
• Give entire dose at one time
• Provide liquid diet: carbonated beverages; gelatin may be added if patient is not nauseated or vomiting
• Tab may be crushed and added to fluids or food to facilitate swallowing

ADVERSE EFFECTS
CNS: Weakness
GI: *Nausea, vomiting, anorexia, diarrhea, stomatitis,* **hepatotoxicity** (with high doses), jaundice, gastritis, **pancreatitis**
GU: Renal failure, hyperuricemia, oliguria, crystalluria, **hematuria**
HEMA: Thrombocytopenia, leukopenia, myelosuppression, anemia
INTEG: *Rash,* dry skin, urticaria, alopecia

Pharmacokinetics

Absorption	Variable
Distribution	Widely, body water
Metabolism	Liver, extensively
Excretion	Kidneys unchanged (small amounts)
Half-life	Terminal 1-1.5 hr

M

Pharmacodynamics

Onset	Unknown
Peak	1-2 hr
Duration	Unknown

INTERACTIONS
Individual products

Allopurinol: increased effects of this agent; avoid use or decrease dose

Azathioprine, sulfamethoxazole-trimethoprim: avoid concurrent use—increased bone marrow depression

Balsalazide, mesalamine, olsalazine, sulfaSALAzine: decreased TPMT, rapid bone marrow suppression; use cautiously

Radiation: increased effects

Warfarin: increased effect of warfarin

Drug classifications

Anticoagulants, NSAIDs, platelet inhibitors, salicylates, thrombolytics: increased bleeding risk

Antineoplastics, immunosuppressants: increased effects

Live virus vaccines: decreased antibodies

NURSING CONSIDERATIONS
Assessment

• Assess buccal cavity for dryness, sores or ulceration, white patches, oral pain, bleeding, dysphagia; obtain prescription for viscous lidocaine (Xylocaine)

⚠ **Assess symptoms indicating severe allergic reaction: rash, pruritus, urticaria, purpuric skin lesions, itching, flushing, laryngeal edema**

• **Bone marrow suppression:** monitor CBC, differential, platelet count weekly; withhold product if WBC is <4000/mm³ or platelet count is <100,000/mm³; notify prescriber of results if WBC <20,000/mm³, platelets <150,000/mm³ or at first sign of abnormally large decrease in blood counts, unless bone marrow aplasia is the goal

⚠ **Thiopurine methyltransferase (TPMT) deficiency: individuals are prone to rapid bone marrow suppression; dosage reduction may be required in homozygous TPMT-deficient persons**

• Assess for increased uric acid levels, swelling, joint pain primarily in extremities; patient should be well hydrated to prevent urate deposits

• Monitor renal function tests: BUN, creatinine, serum uric acid, urine CCr before, during

therapy; check I&O ratio; report fall in urine output to <30 ml/hr

⚠ **Tumor lysis syndrome: monitor for increased potassium, uric acid, phosphate, decreased urine output, calcium**

• Monitor temp q4hr (may indicate beginning of infection)

⚠ **Monitor liver function tests before, during therapy (bilirubin, AST, ALT, LDH) as needed or monthly; check for yellowing of skin or sclera, dark urine, clay-colored stools, itchy skin, abdominal pain, fever, diarrhea; hepatic encephalopathy, toxic hepatitis, ascites: can be fatal**

• **Assess for bleeding:** hematuria, stool guaiac, bruising or petechiae, mucosa or orifices q8hr; check for inflammation of mucosa, breaks in skin, avoid IM injections if platelets are low; blood transfusions may be needed

Patient/family education

• Encourage patient to rinse mouth tid-qid with water, club soda; brush teeth bid-qid with soft brush or cotton-tipped applicators for stomatitis; use unwaxed dental floss

⚠ **Pregnancy: advise patient that contraceptive measures are recommended during therapy (D); serious teratogenic effects may occur, to avoid breast-feeding**

• Teach patient to avoid use of products containing aspirin or NSAIDs, razors, commercial mouthwash, since bleeding may occur; to report symptoms of bleeding (hematuria, tarry stools)

• Instruct patient to report signs of anemia (fatigue, headache, irritability, faintness, shortness of breath)

• Instruct patient to report any changes in breathing or coughing even several mo after treatment; to avoid crowds and persons with respiratory tract or other infections

• Caution patient not to have any vaccinations without the advice of the prescriber; serious reactions can occur

• Advise patient to take entire dose at one time

⚠ **Teach patient to notify prescriber of fever, chills, sore throat, nausea, vomiting, anorexia, diarrhea, bleeding, or bruising, which may indicate blood dyscrasias/ infection**

Evaluation
Positive therapeutic outcome

• Prevention of rapid division of malignant cells

---

meropenem (Rx)

(mer-oh-pen′em)
Merrem IV
Func. class.: Antiinfective—miscellaneous
Pregnancy category B

ACTION: Interferes with cell wall replication of susceptible organisms

Therapeutic outcome: Bactericidal action against the following: *Streptococcus pneumoniae,* group A β-hemolytic streptococci, *viridans* group streptococci, enterococcus; gram-negative organisms *Klebsiella, Proteus, Escherichia coli, Pseudomonas aeruginosa, Bacteroides fragilis, Bacteroides thetaiotamicron,* bacterial meningitis (>3 mo old)

USES: *Acinetobacter, Aeromonas hydrophila, Bacteroides distasonis, Bacteroides fragilis, Bacteroides ovatus, Bacteroides thetaiotaomicron, Bacteroides uniformis, Bacteroides ureolyticus, Bacteroides vulgatus, Campylobacter jejuni, Citrobacter diversus, Citrobacter freundii, Clostridium difficile, Clostridium perfringens, Enterobacter cloacae, Enterococcus faecalis, Escherichia coli, Eubacterium lentum, Fusobacterium, Haemophilus influenzae* (beta-lactamase negative), *Haemophilus influenzae* (beta-lactamase positive), *Hafnia alvei, Klebsiella oxytoca, Klebsiella pneumoniae, Moraxella catarrhalis, Morganella morganii, Neisseria meningitidis, Pasteurella multocida, Peptostreptococcus, Porphyromonas asaccharolytica, Prevotella bivia, Prevotella intermedia, Prevotella melaninogenica, Propionibacterium acnes, Proteus mirabilis, Proteus vulgaris, Pseudomonas aeruginosa, Salmonella, Serratia marcescens, Shigella, Staphylococcus aureus* (MSSA), *Staphylococcus epidermidis, Streptococcus agalactiae* (group B streptococci), *Streptococcus pneumoniae, Streptococcus pyogenes* (group A beta-hemolytic streptococci), *Viridans streptococci, Yersinia enterocolitica;* appendicitis, bacteremia, intraabdominal infections, meningitis, peritonitis, skin/skin structure infections, pseudomembranous colitis

Unlabeled uses: Febrile neutropenic, community-acquired pneumonia

CONTRAINDICATIONS:

Hypersensitivity to meropenem, carbapenems, cephalosporins, penicillins

Precautions: Pregnancy **B,** breastfeeding, geriatric, renal disease, seizure disorder, gram-negative infection, nosocomial pneumonia, pneumonia

DOSAGE AND ROUTES

Intraabdominal infections (complicated appendicitis, peritonitis)
Adult/adolescent/child >50 kg: IV 1 g q8hr or 500 mg q6hr
Adolescent/child ≤50 kg/infant ≥3 mo: IV 20 mg/kg q8hr

Complicated skin and skin structure infections
Adult/adolescent/child >50 kg: IV 500 mg q8hr
Adolescent/child ≤50 kg/infant ≥3 mo: IV 10 mg/kg q8hr

Bacterial meningitis
Adult: IV 2 g q8hr
Adolescent/child ≤50 kg/infant: IV 40 mg/kg q8hr

Renal dose
Adult: IV CCr 26-50 ml/min give dose q12hr; CCr 10-25 ml/min give ½ dose q12hr; CCr <10 ml/min give ½ dose q24hr

Available forms: Powder for inj 500 mg, 1 g

Implementation
Direct IV route
• Reconstitute 500 mg or 1 g vials with 10, 20 ml of sterile water for inj respectively, shake to dissolve and let stand until clear (average conc 50 mg/ml) reconstituted sol may be stored for 2 hr at room temperature or 12 hr refrigerated, inject up to 1 g in 5-20 ml over 3-5 min
Intermittent IV infusion route
• Vials may be directly constituted with compatible inf fluid (NS, D₅W) to 2.5-50 mg/ml vials; vials with 0.9% NaCl can be stored up to 2 hr at room temperature, or 18 hr refrigerated, D₅W may be stored up to 1 hr at room temperature or up to 8 hr refrigerated, infuse over 15-30 min
Continuous IV infusion route (unlabeled)
• **3 g/day continuous IV infusion:** Constitute a 1 g vial according to manufacturer's recommendations; further dilute in 50 ml or 250 ml of NS and run over 8 hr for cont inf, administer a new infusion bag q8hr
• **4 g/day continuous IV infusion:** Constitute a 1 g vial according to manufacturer recommendations. Further dilute in 100 ml of NS and administer over 6 hr. For cont inf, administer a new infusion bag q6hr
• **3 g/day IV continuous infusion in ambulatory infusion pump with freezer**

packs: Reconstitute 1 g vial according to manufacturer recommendations by adding 20 ml of NS into each vial. Add 3 g (60 ml) to a 100-ml medication cassette reservoir and bring the final volume to 100 ml (final concentration, 30 mg/ml) run over 24 hr

Y-site compatibilities: Alemtuzumab, aminocaproic acid, aminophylline, anidulafungin, argatroban, atenolol, atropine, azithromycin, bivalirudin, bleomycin, CARBOplatin, carmustine, caspofungin, cimetidine, CISplatin, cyclophosphamide, cycloSPORINE, cytarabine, DACTINomycin, DAPTOmycin, dexamethasone, dexmedetomidine, dexrazoxane, digoxin, diltiazem, diphenhydrAMINE, DOCEtaxel, doxacurium, DOXOrubicin liposomal, enalaprilat, eptifibatide, etoposide, etoposide phosphate, fluconazole, fludarabine, fluorouracil, foscarnet, furosemide, gallium, gatifloxacin, gemcitabine, gemtuzumab, gentamicin, granisetron, heparin sodium, HYDROmorphone, ifosfamide, insulin (regular), irinotecan, lepirudin, leucovorin, linezolid injection, LORazepam, mechlorethamine, methotrexate, metoclopramide, metroNIDAZOLE, milrinone, mitoXANtrone, morphine, nesiritide, norepinephrine, octreotide, oxaliplatin, oxytocin, PACLitaxel, palonosetron, pamidronate, pancuronium, PEMEtrexed, PHENobarbital, potassium acetate/chloride, rocuronium, teniposide, thiotepa, tigecycline, tirofiban, TNA (3-in-1) Total Nutrient Admixture, vancomycin, vasopressin, vecuronium, vinBLAStine, vinCRIStine, vinorelbine, voriconazole, zoledronic acid

Additive compatibilities: Aminophylline, atropine, cimetidine, dexamethasone, DOBUTamine, DOPamine, enalaprilat, fluconazole, furosemide, gentamicin, heparin, insulin (regular), magnesium sulfate, metoclopramide, morphine, norepinephrine, PHENobarbital, ranitidine, vancomycin

ADVERSE EFFECTS

CNS: Fever, somnolence, *seizures,* dizziness, weakness, *headache,* myoclonia, confusion, insomnia, agitation, confusion, drowsiness
CV: Hypotension, tachycardia
ENDO: Hypoglycemia
GI: Diarrhea, nausea, vomiting, **pseudomembranous colitis, hepatitis,** glossitis, jaundice
HEMA: Eosinophilia, neutropenia, decreased Hgb, Hct, **agranulocytosis**
INTEG: *Rash,* urticaria, *pruritus,* pain at inj site, phlebitis, erythema at inj site
RESP: Chest discomfort, dyspnea, hyperventilation, **pulmonary embolism**

SYST: Anaphylaxis, Stevens-Johnson syndrome, angioedema

Pharmacokinetics

Absorption	Complete bioavailability
Distribution	Widely distributed
Metabolism	Liver
Excretion	Kidneys
Half-life	1 hr; increased in renal disease

Pharmacodynamics

Onset	Rapid
Peak	Dose dependent
Duration	Unknown

INTERACTIONS

Individual drugs
Probenecid: increased meropenem levels
Valproic acid: decreased effect of valproic acid

Drug/herb
Do not use acidophilus with antiinfectives; separate by several hours

Drug/lab test
Increased: AST, ALT, LDH, BUN, alkaline phosphatase, bilirubin, creatinine
Decreased: prothrombin time
False positive: direct Coombs' test

NURSING CONSIDERATIONS

Assessment
• Assess patient for previous sensitivity reaction to carbapenem antiinfectives, penicillins, cephalosporins
• **Assess patient for signs and symptoms of infection,** including characteristics of wounds, sputum, urine, stool, WBC >10,000/100 mm^3, fever; obtain baseline information before, during treatment
• Complete C&S tests before beginning product therapy to identify if correct treatment has been initiated
A Seizures: may occur in those with brain lesions, seizure disorder, bacterial meningitis, or renal disease; stop product, notify prescriber if seizures occur
• Assess for allergic reactions, anaphylaxis: rash, urticaria, pruritus, chills, fever, joint pain; angioedema may occur a few days after therapy begins; epinephrine and resuscitation equipment should be available for anaphylactic reaction; **identify if there has been hypersensitivity to penicillins, cephalosporins, beta-lactams: cross-sensitivity may occur**

A Nurse Alert   ✳ Key NCLEX® Drug

- Identify urine output; if decreasing, notify prescriber (may indicate nephrotoxicity); also check for increased BUN, creatinine
- Monitor blood studies: AST, ALT, CBC, Hct, bilirubin, LDH, alkaline phosphatase, Coombs' test monthly if patient is on long-term therapy
- Monitor electrolytes: potassium, sodium, chloride monthly if patient is on long-term therapy
⚠ Assess bowel pattern daily; if severe diarrhea occurs, product should be discontinued; may indicate pseudomembranous colitis
- Monitor for bleeding: ecchymosis, bleeding gums, hematuria, stool guaiac daily if on long-term therapy
⚠ Assess for overgrowth of infection: perineal itching, fever, malaise, redness, pain, swelling, drainage, rash, diarrhea, change in cough, sputum

Patient/family education
- Teach patient to report sore throat, bruising, bleeding, joint pain; may indicate blood dyscrasias (rare)
- Advise patient to contact prescriber if vaginal itching, loose foul-smelling stools, furry tongue occur; may indicate superinfection; **seizures**
- Advise patient to avoid breastfeeding; product is excreted in breast milk
⚠ Advise patient to notify prescriber of diarrhea with blood or pus; may indicate pseudomembranous colitis

Evaluation
Positive therapeutic outcome
- Absence of signs/symptoms of infection (WBC <10,000/mm³, temp WNL, absence of red draining wounds)
- Reported improvement in symptoms of infection

TREATMENT OF ANAPHYLAXIS: EPINEPHrine, antihistamines, resuscitate if needed

mesalamine, 5-ASA (Rx)
(mez-al'a-meen)
Apriso, Asacol, Asacol HD, Canasa, Delzicol, Lialda, Pentasa, Rowasa, sf Rowasa, Salofalk ♥
Func class.: GI antiinflammatory
Chem. class.: 5-Aminosalicylic acid
Pregnancy category B

Do not confuse:
Asacol/Ansaid/Os-Cal

ACTION: May diminish inflammation by blocking cyclooxygenase, inhibiting prostaglandin production in colon, local action only

Therapeutic outcome: Decreased cramping, pain in GI conditions

USES: Mild to moderate active distal ulcerative colitis, proctosigmoiditis, proctitis

Unlabeled uses: Crohn's disease

CONTRAINDICATIONS:
Hypersensitivity to this product or salicylates, 5-aminosalicylates

Precautions: Pregnancy **B**, breastfeeding, children, geriatric, renal disease, sulfite sensitivity, pyloric stenosis

DOSAGE AND ROUTES
Treatment of ulcerative colitis
Adult: RECT 60 ml (4 g) at bedtime, retained for 8 hr × 3-6 wk; del rel tab (Lialda) 2.4-4.8 g/day × 8 wk; del rel tab (Asacol) 800 mg tid × 6 wk; cont rel cap (Pentasa) 1 g qid up to 8 wk, ext rel cap (Apriso) 1500 mg (4 caps) qd AM up to 6 mo; RECT SUPP 500 mg bid retained for 1-3 hr × 3-6 wk until remission, may increase to tid if needed; del rel cap (Delzicol) 800 mg tid ×6 wk

Maintenance of remission
Adult: PO (delayed release tabs: Asacol) 800 mg bid or 400 mg qid; (delayed release caps: Apriso) 1500 mg (4 caps) each AM; (delayed release tabs: Lialda) 2.4 g (2 tab)/day with a meal; del rel cap (Delzicol) 800 mg bid

Available forms: Enema 4 g/60 ml (Rowasa, ss Rowasa); del rel tabs 400 mg (Asacol); 800 mg (Asacol HD); ext rel tab 500 mg; ext rel cap 250 mg, 500 mg (Pentasa); del rel tab (Lialda) 1.2 g; 0.375 g (Apriso); rect supp 1000 mg; del rel cap (Delzicol) 400 mg

Implementation
PO route
- Do not break, crush, or chew del rel tabs
- **Lialda:** take with a meal
- **Apriso caps:** without regard to meals in AM
- **Delzicol caps:** give ≥1 hr before a meal or 2 hr after a meal
Rectal route (susp)
- Give at bedtime, retained until AM; empty bowel before insertion
- Store at room temperature
- Usual course of therapy is 3-6 wk
- Give after shaking bottle well

ADVERSE EFFECTS

CNS: *Headache, fever, dizziness,* insomnia, asthenia, weakness, fatigue
CV: Pericarditis, myocarditis, chest pain, palpitations
EENT: Sore throat, cough, pharyngitis, rhinitis
GI: *Cramps, gas, nausea, diarrhea,* rectal pain, constipation
GU: Nephrotoxicity, interstitial nephritis
INTEG: *Rash, itching,* acne
SYST: *Flulike symptoms, malaise,* back pain, peripheral edema, leg and joint pain, arthralgia, dysmenorrhea, **anaphylaxis,** acute intolerance syndrome

Pharmacokinetics

Absorption	20%-30% (PO), 10%-25% (RECT)
Distribution	Unknown
Metabolism	Unknown
Excretion	Feces
Half-life	1 hr; metabolite 5-10 hr

Pharmacodynamics

Unknown

INTERACTIONS

Individual drugs

Azathioprine, mercaptopurine: increased action of each product
Lactulose: decreased mesalamine absorption
Omeprazole: increased mesalamine absorption
Warfarin: decreased effect of warfarin

Drug classifications

H₂ blockers: do not give with Apriso
NSAIDs: increased nephrotoxicity
Antacids: decreased mesalamine absorption

Drug/lab test

Increased: AST, ALT, alkaline phosphatase, LDH, GGTP, amylase, lipase

NURSING CONSIDERATIONS

Assessment

• Assess for GI symptoms: cramping, gas, nausea, diarrhea, rectal pain, abdominal pain; if severe, the product should be discontinued
• Assess for allergy to salicylates, sulfonamides; if allergic reactions occur, discontinue product
• Assess renal function before, during treatment: BUN, creatinine periodically

Patient/family education

• Advise patient to notify prescriber if abdominal pain, cramping, diarrhea with blood, headache, fever, rash, chest pain occur; product should be discontinued
• Teach correct administration for PO or enema

Evaluation

Positive therapeutic outcome
• Absence of pain, bleeding from GI tract

---

metformin (Rx)
(met-for′min)
Fortamet, Glucophage, Glucophage XR, Glumetza, Riomet
Func. class.: Antidiabetic, oral
Chem. class.: Biguanide
Pregnancy category B

ACTION: Inhibits hepatic glucose production and increases sensitivity of peripheral tissue to insulin

Therapeutic outcome: Blood glucose at normal levels

USES: Type 2 diabetes mellitus

CONTRAINDICATIONS:

Creatinine ≥1.5 mg/ml (males); diabetic ketoacidosis

> **BLACK BOX WARNING:** History of lactic acidosis

Precautions: Pregnancy **B,** breastfeeding, geriatric, thyroid disease, previous hypersensitivity, CHF, hypersensitivity; hepatic disease; creatinine ≥1.4 (females); alcoholism; cardiopulmonary disease; acidemia; acute MI; cardiogenic shock; metabolic acidosis, renal disease

DOSAGE AND ROUTES

Type 2 diabetes mellitus

Adult: PO 500 mg bid or 850 mg/day initially, then 500 mg weekly or 850 mg q2wk up to 2000 mg/day in divided doses; dosage adjustment q2-3wk or 850 mg/day with morning meal with dosage increased every other week, max 2550 mg/day; ext rel (Glucophage XR) 500 mg qd with evening meal; may increase by 500 mg qwk, max 2000 mg/day; (Glumetza) 1000 mg qd with food, preferably with the PM meal, may increase by 500 mg qwk, max 2000 mg/day; (Fortamet) 500-1000 mg qd with PM meal, may increase by 500 mg qwk, max 2550 mg/day
Geriatric: PO use lowest effective dose

Available forms: Tabs 500, 850, 1000 mg; ext rel tabs 500, 750, 850, 1000 mg; oral sol (Riomet) 500 mg/5 ml

Implementation

• Conversion from other oral hypoglycemic agents; change may be made without gradual dosage change; monitor serum or urine glucose and ketones tid during conversion

• **Immediate rel:** give twice a day with meals to decrease GI upset and provide best absorption

• Give immediate rel tabs crushed and mixed with meal or fluids for patients with difficulty swallowing

• **Extended release product:** may also be taken as a single dose; titrate slowly to therapeutic response, side-effect tolerance

• Do not break, crush, or chew ext rel tabs

• Give in AM to prevent hypoglycemic reactions in PM

• Store in tight container in cool environment

ADVERSE EFFECTS:

CNS: *Headache, weakness, dizziness, drowsiness,* tinnitus, fatigue, vertigo, *agitation*
CV: **Heart failure**
ENDO: **Lactic acidosis,** hypoglycemia
GI: Nausea, vomiting, diarrhea, heartburn, anorexia, metallic taste
HEMA: **Thrombocytopenia,** decreased vit B_{12} levels
INTEG: Rash

Pharmacokinetics

Absorption	Unknown
Distribution	Unknown
Metabolism	Unknown
Excretion	Kidneys, unchanged (35%-50%)
Half-life	1½-6 hr

Pharmacodynamics

Onset	Unknown
Peak	1-2 hr (immediate rel); 7 hr (ext rel); 2.5 hr (sol)
Duration	Unknown

INTERACTIONS

Individual drugs

Cimetidine, digoxin, morphine, procainamide, quiNIDine, ranitidine, triamterone, vancomycin: increased metformin level
β-blockers, phenytoin: increased hyperglycemia
Digoxin: increased digoxin levels

Dofetilide: increased lactic acidosis, do not use together
Radiologic contrast media: do not give together; may cause renal failure

Drug classifications

Calcium channel blockers, contraceptives (oral), corticosteroids, diuretics, estrogens, phenothiazines, sympathomimetics: increased hypoglycemia

Drug/herb

Garlic, green tea: increased hypoglycemia
Glucosamine: increased hyperglycemia

Drug/lab test

Decreased: vitamin B_{12}

NURSING CONSIDERATIONS

Assessment

• Assess for hypoglycemic reactions (sweating, weakness, dizziness, anxiety, tremors, hunger), hyperglycemic reactions soon after meals; these occur rarely with this product

• Monitor CBC (baseline, q3mo) during treatment; check liver function tests (AST, LDH) and renal tests (BUN, creatinine) periodically during treatment; glucose, A1c; folic acid, vitamin B_{12} q1-2yr

• **Surgery:** product should be discontinued temporarily for surgical procedures when patient is NPO, or if contrast media is used; resume when patient is eating

> **BLACK BOX WARNING:** Monitor for lactic acidosis: malaise, myalgia, abdominal distress; risk increases with age, poor renal function; monitor electrolytes, lactate, pyruvate, blood pH, ketones, glucose; suspect in any diabetic patient with metabolic acidosis, with ketoacidosis; immediately stop product if hypoxemia, or significant renal dysfunction occurs

Patient/family education

• Teach patient to regularly self-monitor blood glucose using blood glucose meter

• Teach patient symptoms of hypo/hyperglycemia, what to do about each (rare)

• Advise patient that product must be continued on daily basis; explain consequence of discontinuing product abruptly

• Advise patient to take product in morning to prevent hypoglycemic reactions at night

• Advise patient to avoid OTC medications, alcohol unless approved by the prescriber

• Teach patient that diabetes is a lifelong illness; that this product controls symptoms, but does not cure the condition

BLACK BOX WARNING: Teach patient symptoms of lactic acidosis—hyperventilation, fatigue, malaise, myalgia, chills, somnolence—and to stop product/notify prescriber immediately

- Teach patient to carry/wear emergency ID and glucagon emergency kit for emergencies
- Advise patient that glucophage XR tab may appear in stool
- Advise patient to take with meals, not to break, crush, chew ext rel product

Evaluation
Positive therapeutic outcome
- Decrease in polyuria, polydipsia, polyphagia; clear sensorium; absence of dizziness; stable gait; blood glucose, A1c at normal level

⚠ HIGH ALERT

methadone (Rx)
(meth'a-done)
Dolophine, Metadol ✤, Methadose
Func. class.: Opioid analgesic
Chem. class.: Synthetic diphenylheptane derivative
Pregnancy category C
Controlled substance schedule II

Do not confuse:
methadone/methylphenidate

ACTION: Depresses pain impulse transmission at the spinal cord level by interacting with opioid receptors; produces CNS depression

Therapeutic outcome: Relief of pain; successful opioid withdrawal

USES: Severe pain, opiate withdrawal

Unlabeled uses: Bone pain

CONTRAINDICATIONS:
Hypersensitivity to this product, or hypersensitivity to chlorobutanol (inj route), asthma, ileus

BLACK BOX WARNING: Respiratory depression

Precautions: Pregnancy **C**, breastfeeding, children <18 yr, geriatric, addictive personality, increased ICP, MI (acute), severe heart disease, respiratory depression, renal/hepatic disease, respiratory insufficiency, torsades de pointes, pulmonary disease, COPD, seizures

BLACK BOX WARNING: QT prolongation, pain

DOSAGE AND ROUTES
Severe pain
Adult: PO/SUBCUT/IM 2.5-10 mg q8-12hr prn; IV dose approximately ½ PO dose

Opiate withdrawal
Adult including pregnant women: PO 20-30 mg initially, unless low opioid tolerance is expected, additional 5-10 mg q2-4hr as needed after initial dose, if symptoms continue may give for up to 5 days

Renal/hepatic dose
Adult: PO may need to be modified

Available forms: Inj 10 mg/ml; tabs 5, 10 mg; oral sol 5, 10 mg/5 ml, 10 mg/ml

Implementation
- Medication should be slowly withdrawn after long-term use to prevent withdrawal symptoms
PO route
- When using during a methadone maintenance program, use only PO according to NATA guidelines
- May be given with food or milk to lessen GI upset
- Store in light-resistant container at room temperature
IM/SUBCUT route
- Do not give if cloudy or a precipitate has formed
- Give deeply in large muscle mass (IM); rotate inj sites
- Pain and induration may occur at site

ADVERSE EFFECTS
CNS: *Drowsiness, dizziness, confusion, headache, sedation,* euphoria, **seizures**
CV: Palpitations, bradycardia, change in B/P, **cardiac arrest, shock,** hypotension, **torsades de pointes, QT prolongation**
EENT: Tinnitus, blurred vision, miosis, diplopia
GI: *Nausea, vomiting, anorexia, constipation, cramps,* biliary tract spasm
GU: Increased urinary output, dysuria, urinary retention, impotence
INTEG: *Rash,* urticaria, bruising, flushing, diaphoresis, pruritus
RESP: **Respiratory depression, respiratory arrest**

Pharmacokinetics

Absorption	Well absorbed (PO, SUBCUT, IM)
Distribution	Widely distributed; crosses placenta, half as active PO, as inj
Metabolism	Liver, extensively
Excretion	Kidneys, breast milk
Half-life	8-59 hr; extended interval with continued dosing

Pharmacodynamics

	PO	IM/SUBCUT
Onset	½-1 hr	20 min
Peak	1-1.5 hr	1½-2 hr
Duration	4-12 hr	4-6 hr

INTERACTIONS

Individual drugs

Alcohol: increased respiratory depression, hypotension, sedation

Nalbuphine, pentazine, phenytoin, rifampin: decreased analgesia

Selegiline: do not use within 2 wk of methadone

Drug classifications

Antipsychotics, opiates, sedative/hypnotics, skeletal muscle relaxants: increased respiratory depression, hypotension

Class IA antiarrhythmics (disopyramide, procainamide, quiNIDine), class III antiarrhythmics (amiodarone, bretylium, dofetilide, ibutilide, sotalol), astemizole, arsenic trioxide, bepridil, cisapride, chloroquine, clarithromycin, levomethadyl, pentamidine, some phenothiazines, pimozide, probucol, sparfloxacin, terfenadine: increased QT prolongation

CYP3A4 inducers (barbiturates, bosentan, carBAMazepine, efavirenz, phenytoins, nevirapine, rifabutin, rifampin): decreased methadone effect, withdrawal symptoms may occur

CYP3A4 inhibitors (aprepitant, antiretroviral protease inhibitors, clarithromycin, danazol, delavirdine, diltiazem, erythromycin, fluconazole, FLUoxetine, fluvoxaMINE, imatinib, ketoconazole, mibefradil, nefazodone, telithromycin, voriconazole): increased toxicity

MAOIs: do not use for 2 wk before taking methadone: unpredictable reactions

Drug/food

Avoid use with grapefruit juice

Drug/herb

Chamomile, hops, kava, valerian: increased CNS depression

St. John's wort: avoid use, withdrawal may result

Drug/lab test

Increased: amylase, lipase

NURSING CONSIDERATIONS

Assessment

• **Assess for pain:** type, location, intensity, grimacing before and 1½-2 hr after administration; use pain scoring

• Monitor VS after parenteral route; note muscle rigidity, product history, liver, kidney function tests

• Monitor CNS changes: dizziness, drowsiness, hallucinations, euphoria, LOC, pupil reaction

• Monitor allergic reactions: rash, urticaria

• Monitor opioid detoxification: no analgesia occurs, only prevention of withdrawal symptoms

> **BLACK BOX WARNING:** Monitor B/P, pulse, ECG: hypotension, palpitations may occur

• Monitor bowel changes; bulk, fluids, laxatives should be used for constipation

> **BLACK BOX WARNING:** Respiratory dysfunction: respiratory depression, character, rate, rhythm; notify prescriber if respirations <10/min

> **BLACK BOX WARNING: QT prolongation:** may be dose related or use with other products that increase QT

> **BLACK BOX WARNING: Accidental exposure:** make sure product is not accessible to children, pets

> **BLACK BOX WARNING: Overdose, poisoning:** advise persons involved in correct use

> **BLACK BOX WARNING: Substance abuse:** may occur but has less psychological dependence than other opiate agonists

Patient/family education

• Instruct patient to report any symptoms of CNS changes, allergic reactions; to avoid CNS depressants (alcohol, sedative-hypnotics) for at least 24 hr after taking this product

• Discuss with patient that dizziness, drowsiness, and confusion are common; to avoid getting up without assistance

M

- Discuss in detail with patient all aspects of the product
- Caution patient to make position changes slowly to prevent orthostatic hypotension
- Teach patient withdrawal symptoms may occur: nausea, vomiting, cramps, fever, faintness, anorexia
- Advise patient to maintain proper hydration, avoid alcohol use
- Teach patient to avoid use with other products without approval of prescriber; many drug interactions

Evaluation
Positive therapeutic outcome
- Decreased pain
- Successful opioid withdrawal

TREATMENT OF OVERDOSE:
Naloxone (Narcan) 0.2-0.8 mg **IV**, O$_2$, **IV** fluids, vasopressors

methimazole (Rx)
(meth-im′a-zole)
Tapazole
Func. class.: Thyroid hormone antagonist (antithyroid)
Chem. class.: Thioamide
Pregnancy category D

Do not confuse:
methimazole/metoprolol/minoxidil

ACTION: Inhibits synthesis of thyroid hormones by decreasing iodine use in the manufacture of thyroglobin and iodothyronine; does not affect already formed hormones, does not affect circulatory T$_4$, T$_3$

Therapeutic outcome: Decreased T$_4$ levels, hyperthyroid symptoms

USES: Hyperthyroidism, preparation for thyroidectomy, thyrotoxic crisis, thyroid storm when PTU is contraindicated

CONTRAINDICATIONS:
Pregnancy **D**, breastfeeding, hypersensitivity

Precautions: Infection, bone marrow depression, hepatic disease, bleeding disorders

DOSAGE AND ROUTES
Hyperthyroidism
Adult: PO 15 mg/day (mild hyperthyroidism); 30-40 mg/day (moderate-severe); 60 mg/day

(severe); maintenance dosage 5-15 mg/day, may be divided
Child: PO 0.4 mg/kg/day in divided doses q8hr; continue until euthyroid; maintenance dosage 0.2 mg/kg/day in divided doses q8hr, max 30 mg/24 hr, may be divided

Preparation for thyroidectomy
Adult and child: PO same as above; iodine may be added for 10 days before surgery

Thyrotoxic crisis
Adult and child: PO same as hyperthyroidism with iodine and propranolol

Available forms: Tabs 5, 10, 15, 20 mg

Implementation
- Give with meals to decrease GI upset; give at same time each day to maintain product level
- Give lowest dosage that relieves symptoms
- Store in light-resistant container
- Increase fluids to 3-4 L/day, unless contraindicated

ADVERSE EFFECTS
CNS: *Drowsiness, headache, vertigo, fever,* paresthesias, neuritis
ENDO: *Enlarged thyroid*
GI: *Nausea, diarrhea, vomiting, jaundice,* **hepatitis,** loss of taste
GU: **Nephritis**
HEMA: **Agranulocytosis, leukopenia, thrombocytopenia, hypothrombinemia, lymphadenopathy,** bleeding, vasculitis
INTEG: *Rash, urticaria, pruritus, alopecia, hyperpigmentation,* lupuslike syndrome
MS: Myalgia, arthralgia, nocturnal muscle cramps

Pharmacokinetics
Absorption	Rapidly absorbed
Distribution	Crosses placenta
Metabolism	Liver, extensively
Excretion	Kidneys, unchanged; breast milk
Half-life	5-13 hr

Pharmacodynamics
Onset	½ hr
Peak	Unknown
Duration	2-4 hr

INTERACTIONS
Individual drugs
Amiodarone, potassium iodide: decreased effectiveness
Digoxin: increased response

Radiation: increased bone marrow depression
Warfarin: decreased anticoagulant effect

Drug classifications

Antineoplastics: increased bone marrow depression

Drug/lab test

Increased: pro-time, AST, ALT, alkaline phosphatase

NURSING CONSIDERATIONS
Assessment

• **Hyperthyroidism:** palpitations, nervousness/loss of hair, insomnia, heat intolerance, weight loss, diarrhea

• **Hypothyroidism:** constipation, dry skin, weakness, fatigue, headache, intolerance to cold, weight gain; adjustment may be needed

• Monitor pulse, B/P, temp; check I&O ratio; check for edema (puffy hands, feet, periorbititis); indicates hypothyroidism

• Check weight daily; same clothing, scale, time of day

• Monitor T_3, T_4, which are increased; serum TSH, which is decreased; free thyroxine index, which is increased if dosage is too low; discontinue product 3-4 wk before radioactive iodine uptake

⚠ Monitor blood studies: CBC for blood dyscrasias (leukopenia, thrombocytopenia, agranulocytosis); if these occur, product should be discontinued and other treatment initiated; LFTs, may occur at higher doses

• **Assess for hypersensitivity** (rash, enlarged cervical lymph nodes); product may have to be discontinued

• **Assess for hypoprothrombinemia** (bleeding, petechiae, ecchymosis)

• Monitor clinical response: after 3 wk should include increased weight, pulse, decreased T_4

⚠ Assess for bone marrow depression: sore throat, fever, fatigue

Patient/family education

• Advise patient to abstain from breastfeeding after delivery; product appears in breast milk

• Instruct patient to take pulse daily; to keep graph of weight, pulse, mood

• Advise patient to report redness, swelling, sore throat, mouth lesions, which indicate blood dyscrasias

• Caution patient to avoid OTC products that contain iodine; that seafood and other iodine-containing products may be restricted by prescriber

• Caution patient not to discontinue this medication abruptly; thyroid crisis may occur; stress patient compliance

• Advise patient that response may take several mo if thyroid is large

• **Teach patient symptoms/signs of overdose:** periorbital edema, cold intolerance, mental depression; notify prescriber at once

• **Teach patient symptoms of inadequate dosage:** tachycardia, diarrhea, fever, irritability; prescriber should be notified to adjust

• Teach patient to take medication exactly as prescribed, not to skip or double doses; missed doses should be taken when remembered up to 1 hr before next dose

• Instruct patient to carry ID describing medication taken and condition being treated

Evaluation
Positive therapeutic outcome

• Decreased weight gain
• Decreased pulse
• Decreased T_4
• Decreased B/P

⚠ HIGH ALERT

methotrexate (Rx)
(meth-oh-trex′ate)
Rheumatrex, Trexall
Func. class.: Antineoplastic, antimetabolite
Chem. class.: Folic acid antagonist
Pregnancy category X

Do not confuse:
methotrexate/metolazone/mitoxantene

ACTION: Inhibits an enzyme that reduces folic acid, which is needed for nucleic acid synthesis in all cells; cell cycle specific (S phase); immunosuppressive

Therapeutic outcome: Prevention of rapidly growing malignant cells; immunosuppression

USES: Acute lymphocytic leukemia, in combination for breast, lung, head, neck carcinoma, lymphosarcoma, gestational choriocarcinoma, hydatidiform mole, psoriasis, rheumatoid arthritis, mycosis fungoides, osteosarcoma

CONTRAINDICATIONS:
Hypersensitivity, leukopenia ($<3500/mm^3$), thrombocytopenia ($<100,000/mm^3$), anemia,

---

psoriatic patients with severe renal disease, alcoholism, HIV infection

> **BLACK BOX WARNING:** Pregnancy **X**, hepatic disease

Precautions: Breastfeeding, children

> **BLACK BOX WARNING:** Renal disease, ascites, diarrhea, exfoliative dermatitis, infection, intrathecal administration, lymphoma, pleural effusion, pulmonary disease, radiation therapy, stomatitis, tumor lysis syndrome, ascites, renal impairment, stomatitis

DOSAGE AND ROUTES

Acute lymphocytic leukemia
Adult and child: PO/IM/IV 3.3 mg/m^2/day $\times$ 4-6 wk until remission, then 20-30 mg/m^2 PO/IM qwk in 2 divided doses or 2.5 mg/kg IV $\times$ 2 wk

Burkitt's lymphoma (stages I, II, III) (unlabeled)
Adult: PO 10-25 mg/day $\times$ 4-8 days with 7-day rest period

Lymphosarcoma (stage III)
Adult: PO/IM/IV 0.625-2.5 mg/kg/day

Meningeal leukemia
Adult and child: 12 mg/m^2 IT q2-5days until CSF is normal, then one additional dose, max 15 mg

Choriocarcinoma
Adult and child: PO/IM 15-30 mg/kg/day $\times$ 5 days, then off 1 wk; may repeat

Breast cancer
Adult: IV 40-60 mg/m^2 on day 1 of every 21-28 days with other antineoplastics

Epidermal head/neck cancer
Adult/child: IV 40 mg/m^2 on days 1 and 15, q21 days alone or in combination with bleomycin, CISplatin
Adult: PO 25-50 mg/m^2 q7 days
Child: PO 7.5-30 mg/m^2 q7-14 days

Rheumatoid arthritis
Adult: PO 7.5 mg/wk or divided doses of 2.5 mg q12hr $\times$ 3 given qwk, max 20 mg/wk

Polyarticular-course juvenile RA
Child: PO/IM 10 mg/m^2 qwk

Osteosarcoma
Adult and child: IV 12 g/m^2 given over 4 hr, then leucovorin rescue is given

Mycosis fungoides
Adult: PO 2.5-10 mg/day until cleared (may be many mo); IM 50 mg qwk or 15-37.5 mg 2 $\times$/wk

Psoriasis
Adult: PO/IM/IV 10-25 mg qwk or 2.5 mg PO q12hr $\times$ 3 doses qwk; may increase to 25 mg qwk

Available forms: Tabs 2.5, 5, 7.5, 10, 15 mg; inj 25 mg/ml; powder for inj 1 g

Implementation
• Avoid contact with skin, since product is very irritating; wash completely to remove
⚠ Leucovorin rescue: Administer leucovorin calcium within 24 hr of giving this product to prevent tissue damage; check agency policy; continue until methotrexate level <10^{-8} m
• Give antiemetic 30-60 min before giving product and prn to prevent vomiting; administer antibiotics for infection prophylaxis
• Give in AM so product can be eliminated before bedtime
• Provide liquid diet: carbonated beverages; gelatin may be added if patient is not nauseated or vomiting

PO route
• Give 1 hr before or 2 hr after meals to prevent vomiting
• Make sure product is taken weekly in RA, JRA

IM route
• Give deeply in large muscle mass
• Store in tightly closed container in cool environment; store inj, powder for inj in dark, dry area

Direct IV route
• Give **IV** after diluting 5 mg/2 ml of sterile water for inj; give through Y-tube or 3-way stopcock

Intermittent/continuous IV route
• Further dilute in D$_5$W, D$_5$/0.9% NaCl, 0.9% NaCl; prior to infusion check patency of vein, flush with 5-10 ml of D$_5$W, 0.9% NaCl, infuse at 4-20 mg/hr or prescribed rate

IV infusion
• Intermediate or high dose: 500 mg/m^2 over <4 hr or >1 g/m^2 over >4 hr; confirm WBC >15 mm^3, neutrophils >200 mm^3, platelets >75,000/mm^3, serum bilirubin <1.2 mg/dl, serum creatinine WNL, SGPT <450 U, creatinine clearance >60 ml/min
⚠ Give sodium bicarbonate tabs or IV fluids to prevent precipitation of product at high doses; urine pH should be >7; may need to reduce dose if BUN is 20-30 mg/dl or creati-

nine is 1.2-2 mg/dl; stop product if BUN >30 mg/dl or creatitine is >2 mg/dl

Syringe compatibilities: Bleomycin, CISplatin, cyclophosphamide, doxapram, DOXOrubicin, fluorouracil, furosemide, heparin, leucovorin, mitomycin, vinBLAStine, vinCRIStine

Syringe incompatibilities: Droperidol, ranitidine

Y-site compatibilities: Allopurinol, amifostine, asparaginase, aztreonam, bleomycin, cefepime, cefTRIAXone, cimetidine, CISplatin, cyclophosphamide, cytarabine, DAUNOrubicin, dexchlorpheniramine, diphenhydrAMINE, DOXOrubicin, etoposide, famotidine, filgrastim, fludarabine, fluorouracil, furosemide, gallium, ganciclovir, granisetron, heparin, HYDROmorphone, imipenem-cilastatin, leucovorin, LORazepam, melphalan, mesna, methylPREDNISolone, metoclopramide, mitoMYcin, morphine, ondansetron, oxacillin, PACLitaxel, piperacillin/tazobactam, prochlorperazine, ranitidine, sargramostim, teniposide, thiotepa, vinBLAStine, vinCRIStine, vinorelbine

Y-site incompatibilities: Droperidol, IDArubicin

Additive compatibilities: Cephalothin, cyclophosphamide, cytarabine, fluorouracil, hydrOXYzine, mercaptopurine, ondansetron, sodium bicarbonate, vinCRIStine

Additive incompatibilities: Bleomycin, prednisoLONE

Solution compatibilities: Amino acids, 4.25%/D_{25}, D_5W, sodium bicarbonate 0.05 mol/L, 0.9% NaCl

BLACK BOX WARNING: Intrathecal route: use preservative-free solutions, reconstitute with normal saline, the dose should be drawn into a 5-10 ml syringe after lumbar puncture, the volume of CSF should be withdrawn equal to volume of methotrexate, allow CSF to flow into syringe and mix, inject over 15-30 sec with bevel of needle upward

ADVERSE EFFECTS

CNS: Dizziness, **seizures,** headache, confusion, **encephalopathy,** hemiparesis, malaise, fatigue, chills, fever, **leukoencephalopathy; arachnoiditis** (intrathecal)
EENT: Blurred vision, optic neuropathy
GI: *Nausea, vomiting, anorexia, diarrhea, ulcerative stomatitis,* **hepatotoxicity,** cramps, ulcer, gastritis, **GI hemorrhage,** abdominal

pain, hematemesis, **hepatic fibrosis, acute toxicity**
GU: Urinary retention, **renal failure,** menstrual irregularities, defective spermatogenesis, **hematuria, azotemia, uric acid nephropathy**
HEMA: Leukopenia, thrombocytopenia, **myelosuppression, anemia**
INTEG: *Rash, alopecia,* dry skin, urticaria, photosensitivity, folliculitis, vasculitis, petechiae, ecchymosis, acne, alopecia, **severe fatal skin reactions**
RESP: Methotrexate-induced lung disease
SYST: **Sudden death,** *Pneumocystis jiroveci* pneumonia, **tumor lysis syndrome**

Pharmacokinetics

Absorption	Well absorbed (GI)
Distribution	Widely distributed; crosses placenta
Metabolism	Not metabolized
Excretion	Kidneys, unchanged; breast milk (minimal)
Half-life	Terminal 10-12 hr; increased in renal disease

Pharmacodynamics

	PO	IM/IV	IT
Onset	Unknown	Unknown	Unknown
Peak	1-4 hr	½-2 hr	Unknown
Duration	Unknown	Unknown	Unknown

INTERACTIONS
Individual drugs
Acitretin: increased hepatitis; avoid concurrent use
Alcohol, phenylbutazone, probenecid, radiation, theophylline: increased toxicity
Digoxin (PO), fosphenytoin, phenytoin: decreased effect of each specific product
Folic acid: decreased effect of methotrexate
Radiation: increased bone marrow suppression

Drug classifications
Anticoagulants (oral): increased hypoprothrombinemia
Antineoplastics, NSAIDs, penicillins, salicylates, sulfa products: increased toxicity
Live virus vaccines: decreased antibodies
Proton pump inhibitors: do not use concurrently

NURSING CONSIDERATIONS
Assessment
• Assess buccal cavity q8hr for dryness, sores or ulceration, white patches, oral pain, bleed-

ing, dysphagia; obtain prescription for viscous lidocaine (Xylocaine)

- **Assess symptoms indicating severe allergic reaction:** rash, pruritus, urticaria, purpuric skin lesions, itching, flushing
- Assess tachypnea, ECG changes, dyspnea, edema, fatigue; identify dyspnea, crackles, unproductive cough, chest pain, tachypnea

> **BLACK BOX WARNING: Infection:** those with active infections should be treated for infection prior to product use; monitor temperature, fever may indicate beginning of infection

- Monitor CBC, differential, platelet count weekly; avoid use until WBC is $>1500/mm^3$ or platelet count is $>75,000/mm^3$, neutrophils $>200/mm^3$, notify prescriber of results if WBC $<20,000/mm^3$, platelets $<150,000/mm^3$; WBC, platelet nadirs occur on day 7; monitor
- Assess for increased uric acid levels, swelling, joint pain primarily in extremities; patient should be well hydrated to prevent urate deposits
- Make sure drug-drug interacting products are discontinued prior to therapy, and do not resume until methotrexate level is safe

> **BLACK BOX WARNING: Renal disease:** avoid use in renal failure; monitor renal function studies: BUN, creatinine, serum uric acid, urine CCr before, during therapy; check I&O ratio; report fall in urine output to <30 ml/hr

> **BLACK BOX WARNING: Hepatotoxicity:** monitor liver function tests before, during therapy (bilirubin, AST, ALT, LDH) as needed or monthly; check for jaundice of skin and sclera, dark urine, clay-colored stools, itchy skin, abdominal pain, fever, diarrhea (hepatotoxicity)

- Assess for bleeding: hematuria, stool guaiac, bruising or petechiae, mucosa or orifices; check for inflammation of mucosa, breaks in skin
- Identify effects of alopecia on body image; discuss feelings about body changes
- Identify edema in feet, joint and stomach pain, shaking; prescriber should be notified
- Monitor methotrexate levels, adjust leucovorin dose based on the level

> **BLACK BOX WARNING: Pulmonary toxicity:** those with ascites or pleural effusions are at greater risk for toxicity, fluid should be removed before treatment, monitor plasma methotrexate level

> **BLACK BOX WARNING: Tumor lysis syndrome:** hyperkalemia, hyperphosphatemia, hyperuricemia, hypocalcemia, decreased urine output; use aggressive hydration and allopurinol to correct severe electrolyte imbalances, renal toxicity

> **BLACK BOX WARNING: Serious skin reaction:** Stevens-Johnson syndrome, exfoliative dermatitis, skin necrosis, erythema multiforme may occur within days of receiving product by any route; product should be discontinued

- ⚠ **Stroke-like encephalopathy: common in high-dose therapy; assess for confusion, hemiparesis, seizures, coma; usually transient**
- **Rheumatoid arthritis:** ROM, pain, joint swelling, prior to and during treatment
- **Psoriasis:** assess skin lesions prior to and during treatment

Patient/family education

- Encourage patient to rinse mouth tid-qid with water, club soda; brush teeth bid-qid with soft brush or cotton-tipped applicators for stomatitis; use unwaxed dental floss

> **BLACK BOX WARNING:** Advise patient that contraceptive measures for women and men are recommended during therapy; product is teratogenic; contraception should be used for 3 mo (male) and 4-6 wk (female); to discontinue breastfeeding; toxicity to infant may occur (X)

> **BLACK BOX WARNING:** Teach patient to avoid use of products containing aspirin or NSAIDs, razors, commercial mouthwash, since bleeding may occur; to report symptoms of bleeding (hematuria, tarry stools)

- Caution patient to report signs of anemia (fatigue, headache, irritability, faintness, shortness of breath); seizures
- Advise patient to report any changes in breathing or coughing even several mo after treatment; to avoid crowds and persons with respiratory tract or other infections
- Advise patient to report stomatitis: any bleeding, white spots, ulcerations in mouth to prescriber; tell patient to examine mouth daily, report symptoms, use good oral hygiene
- Teach patient that hair may be lost during treatment; a wig or hairpiece may make patient feel better; new hair may be different in color, texture

---

- Caution patient not to have any vaccinations without the advice of the prescriber; serious reactions can occur
- Advise patient to use sunblock or protective clothing to prevent burns
- Teach patient to use good dental care, to prevent overgrowth of infection in the mouth
- Teach patient how to use this product with leucovorin rescue
- Teach patient to continue leucovorin until told it is safe to stop
- Teach patient to report CNS symptoms, vision changes
- Teach patient to report fever, other symptoms of infection
- Teach patient to report decreased urine output

Evaluation

Positive therapeutic outcome
- Prevention of rapid division of malignant cells
- Decreased joint inflammation in RA

methyldopa/methyldopate (Rx)

(meth-ill-doe'pa)
Func. class.: Antihypertensive
Chem. class.: Centrally acting
α-adrenergic inhibitor
Pregnancy category B (PO) C (IV)

Do not confuse:
methyldopa/ʟ-dopa (levodopa)

ACTION: Stimulates central inhibitory α_2-adrenergic receptors or acts as false transmitter, resulting in reduction of arterial pressure

Therapeutic outcome: Decreased B/P in hypertension

USES: Hypertension, hypertensive crisis

CONTRAINDICATIONS:
Active hepatic disease, hypersensitivity, MAOI therapy

Precautions: Pregnancy **B**, geriatric patients, cardiac disease, autoimmune disease, depression, dialysis, hemolytic anemia, Parkinson's disease, pheochromocytoma, sulfite hypersensitivity

DOSAGE AND ROUTES
Adult: PO 250-500 mg bid or tid, then adjusted q2day prn, 0.5-2 g/day in 2-4 divided doses (maintenance), max 3 g/day; **IV** 250-500 mg in 100 ml D_5W q6hr, run over 30-60 min, max 1 g q6hr, switch to PO as soon as possible
Geriatric: PO 125 mg bid/tid, increase q2day as needed, max 3 g/day
Child: PO 10 mg/kg/day in 2-4 divided doses, max 65 mg/kg or 3 g/day, whichever is less; **IV** 20-40 mg/kg/day in 4 divided doses, max 65 mg/kg or 3 g, whichever is less

Renal dose
Adult: PO CCr 10-50 ml/min dose q8-12hr; CCr <10 ml/min dose q12-24hr

Available forms: Methyldopa: tabs 250, 500 mg; methyldopate: inj 50 mg/ml (250 mg/5 ml)

Implementation
PO route
- Give before meals
- Shake susp before using
- Store in airtight container at room temperature
- Increase in dose should be done in the evening to minimize drowsiness

Intermittent IV infusion route
- Give after diluting in 100 ml of 0.9% NaCl, D_5W, D_5/0.9% NaCl, 5% sodium bicarbonate, Ringer's; administer over 30-60 min

Y-site compatibilities: Alfentanil, amikacin, aminophylline, anidulafungin, ascorbic acid, atenolol, atracurium, atropine, aztreonam, benztropine, bivalirudin, bleomycin, bumetanide, buprenorphine, butorphanol, calcium chloride/gluconate, caspofungin, cefamandole, ceFAZolin, cefmetazole, cefonicid, cefotaxime, cefoTEtan, cefOXitin, cefTAZidime, ceftizoxime, cefTRIAXone, cefuroxime, cephalothin, chlorproMAZINE, cimetidine, clindamycin, cyanocobalamin, cycloSPORINE, DACTINomycin, DAPTOmycin, dexamethasone, digoxin, diltiazem, diphenhydrAMINE, DOCEtaxel, DOPamine, doxycycline, enalaprilat, ePHEDrine, EPINEPHrine, epoetin alfa, ertapenem, erythromycin, esmolol, etoposide, etoposide phosphate, famotidine, fenoldopam, fentaNYL, fluconazole, fludarabine, gatifloxacin, gemcitabine, gentamicin, glycopyrrolate, granisetron, heparin, hydrocortisone, HYDROmorphone, hydrOXYzine, IDArubicin, insulin (regular), irinotecan, isoproterenol, labetalol, lidocaine, linezolid, LORazepam, magnesium sulfate, mannitol, mechlorethamine, meperidine, metaraminol, methicillin, methoxamine, methylPREDNISolone, metoclopramide, metoprolol, metroNIDAZOLE, mezlocillin, miconazole, midazolam, milrinone, minocycline, mitoXANtrone, morphine, moxalactam, multiple vitamins, mycophenolate mofetil, nafcillin, nalbuphine, naloxone, netilmicin, nitroglycerin, nitroprusside, norepinephrine, octreotide, ondansetron, oxacillin, oxaliplatin, oxytocin, PACLitaxel, palonosetron, pamidronate, pancuronium, pantoprazole, papaverine, PEMEtrexed, penicillin G potassium/sodium, pentazocine, phentolamine, phenylephrine, phytonadione, piperacillin, polymyxin B, potassium chloride, procainamide, prochlorperazine, promethazine, propranolol, protamine, pyridoxine, quiNIDine, ranitidine, ritodrine, sodium bicarbonate, succinylcholine, SUFentanil, tacrolimus, teniposide, theophylline, thiamine, thiotepa, ticarcillin, ticarcillin-clavulanate, tigecycline, tirofiban, tobramycin, tolazoline, trimetaphan, urokinase, vancomycin, vasopressin, vecuronium, verapamil, vinorelbine, voriconazole, zoledronic acid

Additive compatibilities: Aminophylline, ascorbic acid, chloramphenicol, diphenhydrAMINE, heparin, magnesium sulfate, multivitamins, netilmicin, potassium chloride, promazine, sodium bicarbonate, succinylcholine, verapamil, vit B/C

Additive incompatibilities: Amphotericin B, barbiturates, methohexital, sulfonamides

Solution compatibilities: D_5W, $D_5/0.9\%$ NaCl, Ringer's, sodium bicarbonate 5%, 0.9% NaCl, amino acids 4.25%/D_{25}, Dextran$_6$/0.9% NaCl, Normosol R, Normosol M/D_5W

ADVERSE EFFECTS

CNS: *Drowsiness, weakness, dizziness, sedation, headache,* depression, psychosis, paresthesias, parkinsonism, Bell's palsy, nightmares
CV: Bradycardia, **myocarditis,** orthostatic hypotension, angina, edema, weight gain, **CHF,** paradoxical pressor response (**IV** use)
EENT: Nasal congestion
ENDO: Breast enlargement, gynecomastia, amenorrhea
GI: Nausea, vomiting, diarrhea, constipation, **hepatic dysfunction,** sore or "black" tongue, **pancreatitis,** colitis, flatulence
GU: Impotence, failure to ejaculate
HEMA: Leukopenia, **thrombocytopenia, hemolytic anemia, granulocytopenia,** positive Coombs' test
INTEG: Lupus-like syndrome, rash, **toxic epidural necrolysis**

Pharmacokinetics

Absorption	50% (PO)
Distribution	Crosses placenta, blood-brain barrier
Metabolism	Liver, moderately
Excretion	Kidneys, unchanged (partially)
Half-life	1½ hr

Pharmacodynamics

	PO	IV
Onset	Unknown	Unknown
Peak	4-6 hr	2 hr
Duration	12-24 hr	10-16 hr

INTERACTIONS

Individual drugs
Alcohol: CNS depression
Haloperidol: increased psychosis
Iron: decreased methyldopa absorption
Levodopa: increased CNS toxicity, hypotension
Lithium: increased lithium toxicity
TOLBUTamide: increased hypoglycemia

Drug classifications
Amphetamines, antidepressants (tricyclics), barbiturates, NSAIDs, phenothiazines: decreased antihypertensive effect
Analgesics, antidepressants, antihistamines, sedative/hypnotics: increased CNS depression
Antihypertensives, diuretics: increased hypotension
β-Adrenergic blockers: increased B/P
MAOIs: increased pressor effect, do not use concurrently
Sympathomimetic amines: increased pressor effect

Drug/lab test
Increased: creatinine, LFTs
Decreased: platelets, WBC, Hgb/Hct
Interference: urinary uric acid, serum creatinine, AST
False increase: urinary catecholamines

NURSING CONSIDERATIONS

Assessment
• **Hemolytic anemia:** monitor blood tests: CBC, neutrophils, decreased platelets; direct Coombs' test before, after 6, 12 mo of therapy; a positive test may indicate hemolytic anemia; usually reverses within weeks to months after discontinuing treatment, monitor Hgb/Hct and RBC, do not start therapy in those with hemolytic anemia

---

- Monitor renal studies: protein, BUN, creatinine; watch for increased levels that may indicate nephrotic syndrome: polyuria, oliguria, frequency; report weight gain >5 lb
- **Product tolerance:** may occur within 3 mo of starting treatment; dosage change and other products may be needed
- Obtain baselines in renal, liver function tests before therapy begins; check potassium levels, although hyperkalemia rarely occurs
- Monitor B/P, pulse if the product is being used for hypertension; notify prescriber of changes
- Monitor edema in feet, legs daily; monitor I&O; check weight for decreasing output
- Assess for allergic reaction: rash, fever, pruritus, urticaria; product should be discontinued if antihistamines fail to help
- Monitor CNS symptoms, especially in the geriatric; depression; change in mental status

Patient/family education
- Instruct patient not to discontinue product abruptly, or withdrawal symptoms may occur: anxiety, increased B/P, headache, insomnia, increased pulse, tremors, nausea, sweating
- Caution patient not to use OTC (cough, cold, or allergy) products unless directed by prescriber
- Teach patient about excessive perspiration, dehydration, vomiting, diarrhea; may lead to fall in B/P; consult prescriber if these occur
- Advise patient that product may cause dizziness, fainting; light-headedness may occur during 1st few days of therapy; that product may cause dry mouth, use hard candy, saliva product, or frequent rinsing of mouth; caution patient to change position slowly, to rise slowly to sitting or standing position to minimize orthostatic hypotension, especially geriatric
- Caution patient that compliance is necessary; not to skip or stop product unless directed by prescriber
- Teach patient that product may cause skin rash
- Teach patient to avoid hazardous activities, since product may cause drowsiness, dizziness

Evaluation
Positive therapeutic outcome
- Decreased B/P

TREATMENT OF OVERDOSE:
Gastric evacuation, sympathomimetics may be indicated if severe; hemodialysis

---

methylergonovine (Rx)
(meth-ill-er-goe-noe′veen)
Methergine
Func. class.: Oxytocic
Chem. class.: Ergot alkaloid
Pregnancy category C

ACTION: Stimulates uterine and vascular smooth muscle, causing contractions, decreased bleeding, arterial vasoconstriction

Therapeutic outcome: Absence of hemorrhage

USES: Treatment of hemorrhage postpartum or after abortion, uterine contractions

CONTRAINDICATIONS:
Pregnancy (4th stage of labor [other than obstetric delivery/abortion]), hypersensitivity to ergot preparations, preeclampsia, eclampsia, elective induction of labor

Precautions: Severe renal/hepatic disease, jaundice, diabetes mellitus, seizure disorders, sepsis, CAD, last stage of labor

DOSAGE AND ROUTES
Adult: PO 200 mcg tid-qid up to 7 days; IM/IV 200 mcg q2-4hr for 1-5 doses

Available forms: Inj 200 mcg/ml; tabs 200 mcg

Implementation
PO route
- PO is the preferred route
- Do not exceed dosage limits
- Store tabs at room temperature
- Give with water

IM route
- Give inj deeply in large muscle mass, aspirate
- Protect from light

Direct IV route
- Give by this route for severe, life-threatening hemorrhage
- Give directly undiluted or diluted with 5 ml of 0.9% NaCl given through Y-site or 3-way stopcock; give 0.2 mg/min; use clear, colorless sol
- Store up to 2 mo if unused

Y-site compatibilities: Heparin, hydrocortisone sodium succinate, potassium chloride, vit B/C

M

Adverse effects: *italics* = common; **bold** = life-threatening

ADVERSE EFFECTS
CNS: *Headache, dizziness,* **seizures,** hallucinations, **stroke (IV)**
CV: **Hypotension,** chest pain, palpitations, *hypertension,* dysrhythmias; **CVA (IV)**
EENT: Tinnitus
GI: *Nausea, vomiting*
GU: Cramping
INTEG: Sweating, rash, allergic reactions
MS: Leg cramps
RESP: *Dyspnea*

Pharmacokinetics

Absorption	Well absorbed (PO, IM)
Distribution	Unknown
Metabolism	Liver, possibly
Excretion	Unknown
Half-life	½-2 hr

Pharmacodynamics

	PO	IM	IV
Onset	5-15 min	5 min	Immediate
Peak	Unknown	Unknown	Unknown
Duration	3 hr	3 hr	Unknown

INTERACTIONS
Individual drugs
Smoking: increased vasoconstriction

Drug classifications
CYP3A4 inhibitors: increased ergot toxicity, do not use together
Vasopressors, ergots, anesthetics (regional): increased vasoconstriction

NURSING CONSIDERATIONS
Assessment
• Monitor B/P, pulse; watch for change that may indicate hemorrhage
• Assess fundal tone, nonphasic contractions; check for relaxation or severe cramping
• **Assess for ergotism or overdose:** nausea, vomiting, weakness, muscular pain, insensitivity to cold, paresthesia of extremities; product should be decreased or infusion discontinued
• Before administering ergonovine, check calcium levels; if hypocalcemia is present, correction should be made to increase effectiveness of this product
• Monitor prolactin levels and for decreased breast milk production

Patient/family education
• Inform patient that abdominal cramps are a side effect of this medication

• Instruct patient to notify prescriber if chest pain, nausea, vomiting, headache, muscle pain, weakness, or cold, numb extremities occur

Evaluation
Positive therapeutic outcome
• Prevention of hemorrhage

methylnaltrexone (Rx)
(meth-il-nal-trex′one)
Relistor
Func. class.: Opioid antagonist
Pregnancy category B

ACTION: Peripheral mu-opioid receptor antagonist that reduces constipation associated with opiate agonists

Therapeutic outcome: Decreased constipation

USES: Treatment of opioid-induced constipation in patients with advanced illness who are receiving palliative care when response to laxative therapy has been insufficient

CONTRAINDICATIONS:
Hypersensitivity, GI obstruction, **IV** route

Precautions: Pregnancy **B**, breastfeeding, renal disease, children, diarrhea, driving, operating machinery, geriatric patients, neoplastic disease, Crohn's disease, peptic ulcer, ulcerative colitis

DOSAGE AND ROUTES
Opiate-agonist induced constipation
Adult >114 kg: SUBCUT 0.15 mg/kg every other day prn
Adult 62-114 kg: SUBCUT 12 mg every other day prn, max 12 mg/24 hr
Adult 38-62 kg: SUBCUT 8 mg every other day prn, max 8 mg/24 hr
Adult <38 kg: SUBCUT 0.15 mg/kg every other day prn, max 0.15 mg/kg/24 hr

Renal dose
Adult: SUBCUT CCr <30 ml/min, reduce normal adult dose by 50%

Available forms: Solution for inj 12 mg/0.6 ml, 8 mg/0.4 ml

Implementation
• Give SUBCUT only; oral dose is investigational and not currently available
• Do not give IV; IV dosing for urinary retention is investigational

- Store at 15°-30° C (59°-86° F); do not freeze
- Store away from light

SUBCUT route

- Inspect the solution before use; it should be a clear, colorless to pale yellow aqueous solution; do not use if particulate matter or discoloration are present
- Withdraw the needed amount of solution into a sterile syringe; if immediate administration is impossible, the syringe may be kept at room temperature for up to 24 hr; the syringe does not need to be kept away from light during the 24-hr period; immediately discard any unused portion in the vial; no preservatives are present
- Administer into the upper arm, abdomen, or thigh no more than 1 ×/24 hr; rotate inj sites; do not inject the same spot each time; do not inject into areas where skin is tender, bruised, red, or hard; avoid areas with scars or stretch marks
- If using with retractable needle, slowly push down on the plunger past the resistance point until the syringe is empty and a click is heard

ADVERSE EFFECTS

CNS: Dizziness
GI: Nausea, vomiting, diarrhea, flatulence, abdominal pain, **GI perforation**
INTEG: Hyperhidrosis

Pharmacokinetics

Absorption	Unknown
Distribution	Protein binding 11%-15.3%
Metabolism	Unknown
Excretion	Unknown
Half-life	Terminal 8 hr

Pharmacodynamics

Onset	Unknown
Peak	30 min (SUBCUT)
Duration	Unknown

NURSING CONSIDERATIONS

Assessment

- Monitor serum creatinine
- **Opioid-induced constipation:** assess for stool characteristics: amount, consistency; bowel sounds during treatment

Patient/family education

- Teach patient that after 30 min, toilet facilities should be nearby, bowel relaxation occurs, not to use more than one dose in 24 hr
- Advise patient to notify prescriber of abdominal pain, continuous or severe diarrhea, nausea or vomiting

- Teach patient to avoid use in pregnancy unless absolutely necessary; avoid in breastfeeding

Evaluation

Positive therapeutic outcome
- Decreased constipation

---

methylphenidate (Rx)

(meth-ill-fen′i-date)
Biphentin ✦, Concerta, Daytrana, Metadate CD, Methidate, Methylin, Ritalin, Ritalin LA, Ritalin SR
Func. class.: Cerebral stimulant
Chem. class.: Piperidine derivative
Pregnancy category C
Controlled substance schedule II

Do not confuse:
methylphenidate/methadone

ACTION: Increases release of norepinephrine and dopamine in cerebral cortex to reticular activating system; exact action not known

Therapeutic outcome: Increased alertness, decreased fatigue, ability to stay awake (narcolepsy), increased attention span, decreased hyperactivity (ADHD)

USES: Attention deficit disorder with hyperactivity (ADHD), narcolepsy (except Concerta, Metadate CD, Ritalin LA), attention deficit disorder (ADD)

CONTRAINDICATIONS:
Hypersensitivity, anxiety, history of Tourette's syndrome, children <6 yr, glaucoma, anorexia nervosa, tartrazine dye hypersensitivity, glaucoma

Precautions: Pregnancy **C**, breastfeeding, hypertension, depression, seizures

BLACK BOX WARNING: Substance abuse

DOSAGE AND ROUTES

Attention-deficit/hyperactivity disorder (ADHD) initial treatment (not currently on methylphenidate)
Regular release: Ritalin, Methylin, Methylin oral sol, Methylin chew tabs
Adult: PO 20-30 mg/day, range 10-60 mg/day in 2-3 divided doses, 30-45 min before meals
Child ≥6 yr: PO 5 mg bid initially, increase 5-10 mg/day qwk, usual dose 0.3-2 mg/kg/day, max 60 mg/day

Extended release: Ritalin SR, Metadate ER, Methylin ER

Adult/adolescent/child ≥6 yr: **PO** max 20-30 mg tid

Extended-release once-daily tabs: Concerta

Adult: **PO** 18-36 mg/day initially, then adjust by 18 mg q wk, max 72 mg/day

Adolescent: **PO** 18 mg/day initially, then adjust by 18 mg q wk, max 72 mg/day

Child ≥6 yr: **PO** 18 mg/day initially, then adjust by 18 mg q wk, max 54 mg/day

Extended-release once-daily capsules: Ritalin LA

Adult/adolescent/child ≥6 yr: **PO** 20 mg/day in AM initially, adjust by 10 mg qwk, max 60 mg/day

Extended-release once-daily capsules: Metadate CD

Adult/adolescent/child ≥6 yr: **PO** 20 mg/day in AM, adjust by 20 mg qwk, max 60 mg/day

Transdermal: Daytrana

Adolescent/child ≥6 yr: **TD** wk 1: 10 mg/day (9-mg patch); wk 2: 15 mg/day (9-mg patch); wk 3: 20 mg/day (9-mg patch); wk 4: 30 mg/day (9-mg patch)

Conversion to once-daily from other forms for ADHD

Extended-release once-daily capsules: Metadate CD

Adult/adolescent/child ≥6 yr: **PO** give no more than total daily dose of other forms, may adjust by 20 mg qwk, max 60 mg/day

Extended-release once-daily capsules: Ritalin LA

Adult/adolescent/child ≥6 yr: **PO** give no more than total daily dose of other forms, may adjust by 10 mg qwk, max 60 mg/day

Extended-release once-daily tablets: Concerta

Adult/adolescent/child ≥6 yr (currently receiving 10-15 mg/day): **PO** 18 mg q AM initially, adjust by 18 mg qwk, max 72 mg/day (adult); max 72 mg/day, 2 mg/kg/day (adolescent); 54 mg/day (child)

Adult/adolescent/child ≥6 yr (currently receiving 20-30 mg/day): **PO** 36 mg q AM, adjust by 18 mg qwk, max 72 mg/day (adult); 72 mg/day, 2 mg/kg/day (adolescent); 54 mg/day (child)

Adult/adolescent/child ≥6 yr (currently receiving 30-45 mg/day): **PO** 54 mg q AM, adjust by 18 mg qwk, max 72 mg/day (adult); 72 mg/day, 2 mg/kg/day (adolescent); 54 mg/day (child)

Adult/adolescent/child ≥6 yr (currently receiving 40-60 mg/day): **PO** 72 mg q AM, 72 mg/day

Transdermal: Daytrana

Adolescent and child ≥6 yr: **TD** wk 1: 10 mg/day (9-mg patch); wk 2: 15 mg/day (9-mg patch); wk 3: 20 mg/day (9-mg patch); wk 4: 30 mg/day (9-mg patch)

Narcolepsy

Immediate release: Ritalin, Methylin oral sol, Methylin chew tabs

Adult: **PO** 20-30 mg/day, range 10-60 mg/day in 2-3 divided doses

Child ≥6 yr: **PO** 5 mg bid, may increase by 5-10 mg qwk, max 60 mg/day

Extended-release tabs: Ritalin SR, Metadate ER

Adult/adolescent/child ≥6 yr: **PO** max 20 mg tid

Poststroke depression; major depression (unlabeled)

Adult and geriatric: **PO** (immediate rel tabs) 2.5 mg bid, may increase by 2.5-5 mg q2-3days

Available forms: Tabs 5, 10, 20 mg; ext rel tabs 10, 20, mg; ext rel tabs (Concerta) 18, 27, 36, 54 mg; ext rel caps 10, 20, 30, 40 mg; oral sol 5 mg, 10 mg/ml; chew tabs (Methylin) 2.5, 5, 10 mg; transdermal patch 12.5 cm^2 (10 mg), 18.75 cm^2 (15 mg), 25 cm^2 (20 mg), 37.5 cm^2 (30 mg)

Implementation
PO route

• Do not chew, crush time rel tabs; caps may be opened and beads sprinkled over spoonful of applesauce

• Give at least 6 hr before bedtime (regular release); at least 10 hr (ext rel) to avoid sleeplessness; titrate to patient's response; lowest dosage should be used to control symptoms

• Give gum, hard candy, frequent sips of water for dry mouth at beginning of treatment; these symptoms tend to lessen with time

• Avoid Metadate CD on day of surgery

Transdermal route

• Place on clean, dry area of the hip; avoid waist; removal is 9 hr after application; fold after removal and flush down toilet

• If patch falls off, apply a new patch to a different site; total wear time should be 9 hr

ADVERSE EFFECTS

CNS: *Hyperactivity, insomnia, restlessness, talkativeness,* dizziness, headache, akathisia, dyskinesia, masking or worsening of Tourette's

---

⚠ Nurse Alert   ⭐ Key NCLEX® Drug

syndrome, **seizures,** drowsiness, toxic psycho-sis, hallucinations, **neuroleptic malignant syndrome, aggression, cerebral vasculitis, hemorrhage, stroke (rare)**
CV: *Palpitations, tachycardia,* B/P changes, angina, **dysrhythmias**
ENDO: Growth retardation
GI: Nausea, anorexia, dry mouth, weight loss, abdominal pain
HEMA: Leukopenia, anemia, thrombocytopenic purpura
INTEG: Exfoliative dermatitis, urticaria, rash, erythema multiforme, **hypersensitivity reactions**
MISC: Fever, arthralgia, scalp hair loss

Pharmacokinetics

Absorption	Well absorbed (PO); delayed (ext rel)
Distribution	Widely distributed; crosses placenta
Metabolism	Liver
Excretion	Kidneys
Half-life	1-3 hr

Pharmacodynamics

	PO	PO–ext rel
Onset	½-1 hr	2 hr
Peak	1-3 hr	4 hr
Duration	4-6 hr	6-8 hr

INTERACTIONS
Individual drugs
Guanethidine: decreased effect of guanethidine

Drug classifications
Anticonvulsants, antidepressants (tricyclics), SNRIs, CNS stimulants, selective serotonin reuptake inhibitors (SSRIs): increased effects
MAOIs (or within 14 days of MAOIs), vasopressors: hypertensive crisis
Antihypertensives: decreased effects of antihypertensives

Drug/herb
Cola nut, guarana, horsetail, yerba maté, yohimbe: increased CNS stimulation
Melatonin: synergistic effect

Drug/food
Caffeine: increased stimulation

NURSING CONSIDERATIONS
Assessment
• **ADHD:** In children or adults with ADHD, monitor for improved organizational skills, attention span, attending to tasks, impulse control,

socialization, and ability to get along better with others

> **BLACK BOX WARNING: Substance abuse:** there is a high potential for abuse, use caution in those with history of substance abuse

• Monitor VS, B/P, since this product may reverse antihypertensives; check patients with cardiac disease more often for increased B/P
• Perform CBC, urinalysis; for diabetic patients monitor blood glucose, urine glucose; insulin changes may be required, since eating will decrease, but decreased growth will resume when product is discontinued
• Monitor height and weight q3mo since growth rate in children may be decreased; appetite is suppressed, weight loss is common during the first few mo of treatment
• Monitor mental status: mood, sensorium, affect, stimulation, insomnia; aggressiveness may occur; depression with crying spells may occur after product has worn off
• Assess for tolerance; should not be used for extended time except in ADHD; dosage should be discontinued gradually to prevent withdrawal symptoms
• **Assess for narcoleptic symptoms** before medication and after; ability to stay awake should increase significantly
⚠ **Assess for withdrawal symptoms: headache, nausea, vomiting, muscle pain, weakness; product tolerance will develop after long-term use; dosage should not be increased if tolerance develops, usually not associated with drug holidays**
• Assess appetite, sleep, speech patterns

Patient/family education
• Teach patient to decrease caffeine consumption (coffee, tea, cola, chocolate); not to use guarana, cola nut, yerba maté, which may increase irritability and stimulation; to avoid OTC preparations unless approved by prescriber; to avoid alcohol ingestion; these may cause serious product interactions
• Advise patient to taper off product over several wk, or depression, increased sleeping, lethargy may occur
• Notify prescriber if skin irritation or rash occurs
• Caution patient to avoid hazardous activities until stabilized on medication
• Instruct patient not to double doses if medication is missed; prescriber may suggest product holidays (ADHD) during the school year to assess progress and determine continued product necessity

M

• Instruct patient/family to notify presciber if significant side effects occur: tremors, insomnia, palpitations, restlessness; product changes may be needed
• Inform patient that if dry mouth occurs to use frequent sips of water, sugarless gum, hard candy during beginning therapy; dry mouth lessens with continued treatment
• Encourage patient to get needed rest; patient will feel more tired at end of day; to take last dose at least 6 hr before bedtime to avoid insomnia
• Advise patient that shell of Concerta tab may appear in stools

Evaluation
Positive therapeutic outcome
• Decreased hyperactivity in ADHD
• Improved attention span in ADHD
• Absence of sleeping during day in narcolepsy

TREATMENT OF OVERDOSE:
Administer fluids, hemodialysis, peritoneal dialysis, antihypertensives for increased B/P; administer short-acting barbiturate before lavage

---

methylPREDNISolone (Rx)
(meth-ill-pred-niss'oh-lone)
A-Methapred, Depo-Medrol, Medrol, Solu-Medrol
Func. class.: Corticosteroid, synthetic
Chem. class.: Glucocorticoid, immediate acting
Pregnancy category C

Do not confuse:
methylPREDNISolone/medroxyPROGESTERone/predniSONE/methylTESTOSTERone

ACTION: Decreases inflammation by suppression of migration of polymorphonuclear leukocytes, fibroblasts; reverses increased capillary permeability and lysosomal stabilization

Therapeutic outcome: Decreased inflammation

USES: Severe inflammation, shock, adrenal insufficiency, collagen disorders, management of acute spinal cord injury, multiple sclerosis

CONTRAINDICATIONS:
Hypersensitivity, intrathecal use, neonates

Precautions: Pregnancy **C,** breastfeeding, diabetes mellitus, glaucoma, osteoporosis, seizure disorders, ulcerative colitis, CHF, myasthenia gravis, renal disease, esophagitis, peptic ulcer, tartrazine, benzyl alcohol, corticosteroid hypersensitivity, viral infection, TB, traumatic brain injury, Cushing's syndrome, measles, varicella, fungal infections

DOSAGE AND ROUTES
Adrenal insufficiency/inflammation
Adult: PO 4-48 mg in 4 divided doses; IM 10-80 mg (acetate); IM/IV 10-250 mg (succinate); intraarticular 4-80 mg (acetate)
Child: IV 0.5-1.7 mg/kg in 3-4 divided doses (succinate)

Multiple sclerosis
Adult: PO 160 mg/day × 1 wk, then 64 mg every other day × 30 days

Available forms: Tabs 2, 4, 6, 8, 16, 24, 32 mg; inj 20, 40, 80 mg/ml acetate; inj 40, 125, 500, 1000, 2000 mg/vial succinate

Implementation
PO route
• Give with food or milk to decrease GI symptoms
• Single daily dose should be given in AM to coincide with body's normal cortisol secretion
IM route
• Give IM inj deep in large muscle mass; rotate sites; avoid deltoid; use 21-G needle; injection site reaction may occur (induration, pain at site, atrophy)
• Give in one dose in AM to prevent adrenal suppression; avoid SUBCUT administration; may damage tissue

IV route
• Use only methylPREDNISolone sodium succinate (Solu-Medrol) IV, never use methylPREDNISolone acetate suspension IV
• Give after diluting with provided diluent, agitate slowly; give directly over 3-15 min; doses ≥2 mg/kg or 250 mg should be given by intermittent IV infusion unless potential benefits outweigh potential risks
Intermittent/continuous IV infusion route
• Dilute further in D_5W, 0.9% NaCl, D_5NS, haze may form, give over 15-60 min, large doses (≥500 mg) give over 30-60 min
• Give after shaking susp (parenteral)
• Give titrated dosage; use lowest effective dosage

Syringe compatibilities: Granisetron, metoclopramide

Y-site compatibilities: Acyclovir, amifostine, aztreonam, cefepime, CISplatin, cladribine, cyclophosphamide, cytarabine, DOPamine, DOXOrubicin, enalaprilat, famotidine, fludarabine, granisetron, heparin, inamrinone, melphalan, meperidine, methotrexate, metroNIDAZOLE, midazolam, morphine, piperacillin/tazobactam, sodium bicarbonate, tacrolimus, teniposide, theophylline, thiotepa, vit B with C

Y-site incompatibilities: Ondansetron, PACLitaxel, sargramostim, vinorelbine

Inhalation route
• Give inh with water to decrease possibility of fungal infections
• Give titrated dosage; use lowest effective dosage
• Clean aerosol topically daily with warm water; dry thoroughly
• Store in cool environment; do not puncture or incinerate container

Topical route
• Cleanse area before applying product
• Apply only to affected areas; do not get in eyes
• Apply medication, then cover with occlusive dressing (only if prescribed); seal to normal skin; change q12hr; systemic absorption may occur
• Apply only to dermatoses; do not use on weeping, denuded, or infected area
• Apply treatment for a few days after area has cleared
• Store at room temperature

ADVERSE EFFECTS

CNS: Depression, flushing, sweating, headache, mood changes
CV: Hypertension, **circulatory collapse, thrombophlebitis, embolism,** tachycardia
EENT: Fungal infections, increased intraocular pressure, blurred vision, cataracts
GI: Diarrhea, nausea, abdominal distention, **GI hemorrhage,** increased appetite, **pancreatitis**
HEMA: Thrombocytopenia
INTEG: Acne, poor wound healing, ecchymosis, petechiae
MS: Fractures, osteoporosis, weakness

Pharmacokinetics

Absorption	Well absorbed (PO); systemic (topical)
Distribution	Crosses placenta
Metabolism	Liver, extensively
Excretion	Kidney
Half-life	3-5 hr (plasma) 18-36 hr (tissue); adrenal suppression 3-4 days

Pharmacodynamics

	PO	IM	IV	Topical
Onset	Unknown	Unknown	Rapid	Min to hr
Peak	2 hr	4-8 days	Unknown	Hr to days
Duration	1½ days	1-4 wk	Unknown	Hr to days

INTERACTIONS

Individual drugs
Amphotericin B: increased side effects
Insulin: increased need for insulin
Phenytoin, rifampin: decreased action; increased metabolism
Somatrem: decreased effect

Drug classifications
Contraceptives, oral: increased methylPREDNISolone action
CYP3A4 inducers (barbiturates, bosentan, carBAMazepine, efavirenz, phenytoins, nevirapine, rifabutin, rifampin): decreased methylPREDNISolone effect
CYP3A4 inhibitors (aprepitant, antiretroviral protease inhibitors, clarithromycin, danazol, delavirdine, diltiazem, erythromycin, fluconazole, FLUoxetine, fluvoxaMINE, imatinib, ketoconazole, mibefradil, nefazodone, telithromycin, voriconazole): increased adrenal suppression
Diuretics: increased side effects
Hypoglycemic agents: increased need for hypoglycemic agents
Vaccines: decreased effects of vaccines

Drug/herb
St. John's wort: avoid use

Drug/food
Grapefruit juice: increased methylPREDNISolone level; do not use concurrently

Drug/lab test
Increased: cholesterol, blood glucose
Decreased: calcium, potassium, T_4, T_3, thyroid radioactive iodine uptake test, urine 17-OHCS, 17-KS
False negative: skin allergy tests

NURSING CONSIDERATIONS

Assessment
• **Adrenal insufficiency:** assess for weight loss, nausea, vomiting, confusion, anxiety, hypotension, weakness
• Monitor plasma cortisol levels during long-term therapy (normal level 138-635 nmol/L when drawn at 8 AM)

Adverse effects: *italics* = common; **bold** = life-threatening

- Monitor potassium, blood glucose, urine glucose while patient is on long-term therapy; hypokalemia and hyperglycemia
- Monitor weight daily; notify prescriber of weekly gain >5 lb
- Monitor B/P q4hr, pulse; notify prescriber if chest pain occurs
- Monitor I&O ratio; be alert for decreasing urinary output and increasing edema
- Monitor adrenal function periodically for hypothalamic-pituitary-adrenal axis suppression
- **Assess for infection:** increased temp, WBC even after withdrawal of medication; product masks infection symptoms
- Assess for potassium depletion: paresthesias, fatigue, nausea, vomiting, depression, polyuria, dysrhythmias, weakness
- Assess for edema, hypertension, cardiac symptoms
- Assess mental status: affect, mood, behavioral changes, aggression
- Check temp; if fever develops, product should be discontinued
- Assess for systemic absorption: increased temp, inflammation, irritation (topical)

Patient/family education
- Teach patient that emergency ID as corticosteroid user should be carried/worn
- Advise patient to notify prescriber if therapeutic response decreases; dosage adjustment may be needed
- ⚠ **Caution patient not to discontinue abruptly; adrenal crisis can result**
- Teach patient to take PO with food, milk, to decrease GI symptoms
- Caution patient to avoid OTC products: salicylates, alcohol in cough products, cold preparations unless directed by prescriber
- Teach patient all aspects of product use including cushingoid symptoms
- Teach patient symptoms of **adrenal insufficiency:** nausea, anorexia, fatigue, dizziness, dyspnea, weakness, joint pain
- Inform patient that long-term therapy may be needed to clear infection (1-2 mo depending on type of infection)

Nasal route
- Advise patient to clear nasal passages if sneezing attack occurs; repeat dose
- Advise patient to continue using product even if mild nasal bleeding occurs; is usually transient
- Teach patient method of instillation after providing written instructions from manufacturer
- Teach patient to recognize **Cushingoid symptoms:** buffalo hump, moon face, rapid weight gain, excess sweating

- **Infection:** Teach patient to avoid persons with known infections; corticosteroids can mask symptoms of infection

Topical route
- Advise patient to avoid sunlight on affected area; burns may occur

Evaluation

Positive therapeutic outcome
- Ease of respirations, decreased inflammation
- Absence of severe itching, patches on skin, flaking (top)

metipranolol ophthalmic
See Appendix B

metoclopramide (Rx)
(met-oh-kloe-pra'mide)
Apo-Metoclop ✦, Metozolv ODT, Reglan
Func. class.: Cholinergic, antiemetic
Chem. class.: Central dopamine receptor antagonist
Pregnancy category B

Do not confuse:
metoclopramide/metolazone,
Reglan/Megace/Renagel

ACTION: Enhances response to acetylcholine of tissue in upper GI tract, which causes contraction of gastric muscle, relaxes pyloric, duodenal segments, increases peristalsis without stimulating secretions, blocks dopamine in chemoreceptor trigger zone of CNS

Therapeutic outcome: Decreased symptoms of delayed gastric emptying, decreased nausea, vomiting

USES: Prevention of nausea, vomiting induced by chemotherapy, radiation; delayed gastric emptying, gastroesophageal reflux

CONTRAINDICATIONS: Hypersensitivity to this product or procaine or procainamide, seizure disorder, pheochromocytoma, breast cancer (prolactin dependent), GI obstruction

Precautions: Pregnancy **B**, breastfeeding, GI hemorrhage, CHF, Parkinson's disease

BLACK BOX WARNING: Tardive dyskinesia

DOSAGE AND ROUTES

Nausea/vomiting (chemotherapy)
Adult: IV 1-2 mg/kg 30 min before administration of chemotherapy, then q2hr × 2 doses, then q3hr × 3 doses
Child (unlabeled): IV 1-2 mg/kg/dose

Facilitation of small bowel intubation in radiologic exams
Adult and child >14 yr: IV 10 mg over 1-2 min
Child 6-14 yr: IV 2.5-5 mg
Child <6 yr: IV 0.1 mg/kg

Diabetic gastroparesis
Adult: PO 10 mg 30 min before meals, at bedtime × 2-8 wk
Geriatric: PO 5 mg ½ hr before meals, at bedtime, increase to 10 mg if needed

Gastroesophageal reflux
Adult: PO 10-15 mg qid 30 min before meals and at bedtime
Child: PO 0.4-0.8 mg/kg/day divided in 4 doses

Renal dose
Adult: IV CCr <40 ml/min 50% of dose

Available forms: Tabs 5, 10 mg; syr 5 mg/5 ml; inj 5 mg/ml, conc sol 10 mg/ml, orally disintegrating tab 5, 10 mg

Implementation
PO route
• Use gum, hard candy, frequent rinsing of mouth for dryness of oral cavity
• Give ½-1 hr before meals for better absorption
• **Oral disintegrating:** place on tongue, allow to dissolve, swallow, remove from bottle immediately before use
IM route
• Give for postop nausea and vomiting before end of surgery
Direct IV route
• Give **IV** undiluted if dose is ≤10 mg; give over 2 min
• Give diphenhydrAMINE **IV** or benztropine IM for EPS
• Discard open ampules
Intermittent IV infusion route
• Dilute more than 10 mg in 50 ml or more D₅W, NaCl, Ringer's, LR and give over 15 min or more

Y-site compatibilities: Acyclovir, aldesleukin, alfentanil, amifostine, amikacin, aminophylline, ascorbic acid, atracurium, atropine, azaTHIOprine, aztreonam, bivalirudin, bleomycin, bumetanide, buprenorphine, butorphanol, calcium chloride/gluconate, CARBOplatin, caspofungin, ceFAZolin, cefonicid, cefoperazone, cefotaxime, cefoTEtan, cefOXitin, cefTAZidime, ceftizoxime, cefTRIAXone, cefuroxime, chloramphenicol, chlorproMAZINE, cimetidine, ciprofloxacin, cisatracurium, CISplatin, cladribine, clindamycin, cyanocobalamin, cyclophosphamide, cycloSPORINE, cytarabine, DACTINomycin, DAPTOmycin, dexamethasone, dexmedetomidine, digoxin, diltiazem, diphenhydrAMINE, DOBUTamine, DOCEtaxel, DOPamine, doripenem, doxapram, DOXOrubicin hydrochloride, doxycycline, droperidol, enalaprilat, ePHEDrine, EPINEPHrine, epirubicin, epoetin alfa, ertapenem, erythromycin, esmolol, etoposide, etoposide phosphate, famotidine, fenoldopam, fentaNYL, filgrastim, fluconazole, fludarabine, folic acid, foscarnet, gallium nitrate, gemcitabine, gentamicin, glycopyrrolate, granisetron, heparin, hydrocortisone, HYDROmorphone, IDArubicin, ifosfamide, imipenem/cilastatin, indomethacin, insulin, isoproterenol, ketorolac, labetalol, leucovorin, levofloxacin, lidocaine, linezolid, LORazepam, magnesium sulfate, mannitol, mechlorethamine, melphalan, meperidine, meropenem, metaraminol, methadone, methotrexate, methoxamine, methyldopate, methylPREDNISolone, metoprolol, metroNIDAZOLE, miconazole, midazolam, milrinone, minocycline, mitoMYcin, morphine, moxalactam, multiple vitamins, nafcillin, nalbuphine, naloxone, nesiritide, nitroglycerin, nitroprusside, norepinephrine, octreotide, ondansetron, oxaliplatin, oxytocin, PACLitaxel, palonosetron, pantoprazole, papaverine, PEMEtrexed, penicillin G, pentamidine, pentazocine, PENTobarbital, PHENobarbital, phentolamine, phenylephrine, phytonadione, piperacillin/tazobactam, potassium chloride, procainamide, prochlorperazine, promethazine, propranolol, protamine, pyridoxine, quinupristin/dalfopristin, ranitidine, remifentanil, riTUXimab, rocuronium, sargramostim, sodium acetate/bicarbonate, succinylcholine, SUFentanil, tacrolimus, teniposide, theophylline, thiamine, thiotepa, ticarcillin/clavulanate, tigecycline, tirofiban, tobramycin, tolazoline, topotecan, trastuzumab, trimethaphan, urokinase, vancomycin, vasopressin, vecuronium, verapamil, vinBLAStine, vinCRIStine, vinorelbine, voriconazole, zidovudine

Y-site incompatibilities: Amphotericin B cholesteryl/colloidal, amphotericin B liposome, amsacrine, cefepime, dantrolene, diazepam, diazoxide, DOXOrubicin liposome, ganciclovir, inamrinone, phenytoin, propofol, trimethoprim/sulfamethoxazole

ADVERSE EFFECTS

CNS: *Sedation, fatigue, restlessness, headache, sleeplessness, dystonia,* dizziness, drowsiness, **suicidal ideation, seizures,** EPS, **neuroleptic malignant syndrome; tardive dyskinesia** ($>$3 mo, high doses)

CV: Hypotension, **supraventricular tachycardia**

GI: Dry mouth, constipation, nausea, anorexia, vomiting, diarrhea

GU: Decreased libido, prolactin secretion, amenorrhea, galactorrhea

HEMA: Neutropenia, leukopenia, agranulocytosis

INTEG: Urticaria, rash

Pharmacokinetics

Absorption	Well absorbed (PO)
Distribution	Widely distributed; crosses blood-brain barrier, placenta
Metabolism	Liver, minimally
Excretion	Kidneys, breast milk
Half-life	4 hr

Pharmacodynamics

	PO	IM	IV
Onset	½-1 hr	10-15 min	1-3 min
Peak	Unknown	Unknown	Unknown
Duration	1-2 hr	1-2 hr	1-2 hr

INTERACTIONS

Individual drugs

Alcohol: increased sedation
Haloperidol: increased extrapyramidal reaction

Drug classifications

Anticholinergics, opiates: decreased action of metoclopramide
CNS depressants: increased sedation
MAOIs: avoid use
Phenothiazines: increased extrapyramidal reaction

Drug/lab test

Increased: prolactin, aldosterone, thyrotropin

NURSING CONSIDERATIONS

Assessment

• Assess GI complaints: nausea, vomiting, anorexia, constipation, abdominal distention before, after administration

BLACK BOX WARNING: Assess for EPS and tardive dyskinesia (more likely to occur in treatment >3 mo, geriatric): rigidity, grimacing, shuffling gait, tremors, rhythmic involuntary movements of tongue, mouth, jaw, feet, hands; these side effects should be reported to prescriber immediately; some effects may be irreversible; assess for involuntary movements frequently

• Assess mental status: depression, anxiety, irritability during treatment

⚠ Neuroleptic malignant syndrome: assess for hyperthermia, change in B/P, pulse, tachycardia, sweating, rigidity, altered consciousness

Patient/family education

• Instruct patient to avoid driving, other hazardous activities until stabilized on this medication
• Advise patient to avoid alcohol and other CNS depressants that enhance sedating properties of this product
• Advise patient to notify prescriber if involuntary movements occur

Evaluation

Positive therapeutic outcome
• Absence of nausea, vomiting, anorexia, fullness

---

metolazone (Rx)

(me-tole′a-zone)
Zaroxolyn
Func. class.: Diuretic, antihypertensive
Chem. class.: Thiazide-like quinazoline derivative
Pregnancy category B

Do not confuse:

metolazone/methotrexate/metoclopramide

ACTION: Acts on the distal tubule and cortical thick ascending limb of the loop of Henle in the kidney, increasing excretion of sodium, water, chloride, magnesium, potassium, and bicarbonate, decreases GFR

Therapeutic outcome: Decreased B/P, decreased edema in lung tissue and peripherally

USES: Edema, hypertension

CONTRAINDICATIONS:

Pregnancy (D) (preeclampsia, intrauterine growth retardation), hypersensitivity to thia-

---

zides or sulfonamides, anuria, coma, hepatic encephalopathy

Precautions: Pregnancy **B**, breastfeeding, geriatric, hypokalemia, renal/hepatic disease, gout, COPD, lupus erythematosus, diabetes mellitus, hypotension, history of pancreatitis, hypersensitivity to sulfonamides, thiazides, electrolyte imbalance

DOSAGE AND ROUTES
Edema
Adult: PO 5-10 mg/day; max 20 mg/day

Hypertension
Adult: PO 2.5-5 mg/day
Child: PO 0.2-0.4 mg/kg/day in divided doses q12-24hr

Available forms: Tabs 2.5, 5, 10 mg

Implementation
• Give in AM to avoid interference with sleep
• Provide potassium replacement if potassium level is 3.0; product may be crushed if patient is unable to swallow
• Give with food; if nausea occurs, absorption may be increased

ADVERSE EFFECTS
CNS: Anxiety, depression, headache, *dizziness, fatigue, weakness*
CV: *Orthostatic hypotension,* palpitations, volume depletion, chest pain, hypotension
EENT: Blurred vision
ELECT: *Hypokalemia,* hypercalcemia, hyponatremia
GI: *Nausea, vomiting, anorexia,* constipation, diarrhea, cramps, **pancreatitis,** GI irritation, dry mouth, jaundice, **hepatitis**
GU: *Frequency,* polyuria, **uremia,** glucosuria, nocturia, impotence
HEMA: Aplastic anemia, **hemolytic anemia, leukopenia, agranulocytosis, neutropenia**
INTEG: *Rash,* urticaria, purpura, photosensitivity, fever, dry skin, **toxic epidermal necrolysis, Stevens-Johnson syndrome**
META: *Hyperglycemia,* increased creatinine, BUN
MS: Muscle cramps, joint pain, swelling

Pharmacokinetics
Absorption	GI tract (10%-20%)
Distribution	Crosses placenta; protein binding 33%
Metabolism	Urine, unchanged
Excretion	Breast milk
Half-life	8 hr (extended); 14 hr (prompt)

Pharmacodynamics
Onset	Unknown
Peak	8 hr
Duration	12-24 hr

INTERACTIONS
Individual drugs
Alcohol: increased hypotension (large amounts)
Amphotericin B, digoxin, mezlocillin, piperacillin: increased hypokalemia
Lithium: increased toxicity

Drug classifications
Antidiabetics: increased hyperglycemia
Antihypertensives: increased antihypertensive effect
Barbiturates, nitrates, opioids: increased hypotension
Diuretics (loop): increased metolazone effect
Glucocorticoids, laxatives (stimulant): increased hypokalemia
NSAIDs, salicylates: decreased action of metolazone

Drug/food
Licorice: increased severe hypokalemia

Drug/herb
Ephedra (ma huang): decreased antihypertensive effect
Hawthorn: increased antihypertensive effect

NURSING CONSIDERATIONS
Assessment
• **Hypertension:** assess B/P before, during therapy with patient lying, standing, and sitting as appropriate; orthostatic hypotension can occur rapidly
• Monitor blood glucose if patient is diabetic
• **CHF:** assess for improvement in feet, legs, sacral area daily if medication is being used
• Check for rashes, temp elevation daily
• Monitor patients receiving cardiac glycosides for increased hypokalemia
• **Hypokalemia:** assess for postural hypotension, malaise, fatigue, tachycardia, leg cramps, weakness

BLACK BOX WARNING: Hepatic encephalopathy: do not use in hepatic coma or precoma, fluctuations in electrolytes can occur rapidly and precipitate hepatic coma, use caution in those with impaired hepatic function

- Assess and record fluid volume status: I&O ratios; monitor weight, distended red veins, crackles in lung, color, quality, and specific gravity of urine; skin turgor, adequacy of pulses, moist mucous membranes, bilateral lung sounds, peripheral pitting edema; dehydration symptoms of decreasing output, thirst, hypotension, dry mouth and mucous membranes should be reported
- Monitor electrolytes: potassium, sodium, calcium, magnesium; also include BUN, blood pH, ABGs, uric acid, CBC, blood glucose

Patient/family education
- Teach patient to take the medication early in the day to prevent nocturia
- Instruct patient to take with food or milk if GI symptoms of nausea and anorexia occur
- Teach patient to maintain a weekly record of weight and notify prescriber of weight loss >5 lb
- Caution patient that this product causes a loss of potassium, so foods rich in potassium should be added to the diet; refer to a dietitian for assistance in planning
- Caution the patient to rise slowly from sitting or reclining positions, not to exercise in hot weather or stand for prolonged periods, since orthostatic hypotension will be enhanced; lie down if dizziness occurs
- Teach patient not to use alcohol or any OTC medications without prescriber's approval; serious product reactions may occur
- Emphasize the need to contact prescriber immediately if muscle cramps, weakness, nausea, dizziness, or numbness occur
- Teach patient to take own B/P and pulse and record
- Advise patient to use sunscreen to prevent burns
- Teach patient to continue taking medication even if feeling better; this product controls symptoms but does not cure the condition
- Advise patient with hypertension to continue other medical regimen (exercise, weight loss, relaxation techniques, smoking cessation)
- Do not stop product abruptly

Evaluation
Positive therapeutic outcome
- Decreased edema
- Decreased B/P

TREATMENT OF OVERDOSE:
Lavage if taken orally, monitor electrolytes; administer dextrose in saline; monitor hydration, CV, renal status

metoprolol (Rx)
(met-oh-proe'lole)
Lopressor, Nu-Metop ✦, Toprol-XL
Func. class.: Antihypertensive, antianginal
Chem. class.: β_1-Adrenergic blocker
Pregnancy category C

Do not confuse:
metoprolol/misoprostol

ACTION: Lowers B/P by β-blocking effects; reduces elevated renin plasma levels; blocks β_2-adrenergic receptors in bronchial, vascular smooth muscle only at high doses, negative chronotropic effect

Therapeutic outcome: Decreased B/P, heart rate, AV conduction

USES: Mild to moderate hypertension, acute MI to reduce cardiovascular mortality, angina pectoris, New York Heart Association class II, III heart failure, cardiomyopathy

CONTRAINDICATIONS:
Hypersensitivity to β-blockers, cardiogenic shock, heart block (2nd and 3rd degree), sinus bradycardia, pheochromocytoma, sick sinus syndrome

Precautions: Pregnancy **C,** breastfeeding, geriatric, major surgery, diabetes mellitus, thyroid/renal/hepatic disease, COPD, CAD, nonallergic bronchospasm, CHF, bronchial asthma, CVA, children, depression, vasospastic angina

BLACK BOX WARNING: Abrupt discontinuation

DOSAGE AND ROUTES
Hypertension
Adult: PO 50 mg bid, or 100 mg/day; may give 200-450 mg in divided doses; ext rel 25-100 mg qd, titrate at weekly intervals, max 400 mg/day
Child/adolescent 6-16 yr: PO ext rel 1 mg/kg up to 50 mg qd
Geriatric: PO 25 mg/day initially, increase weekly as needed

⚠ Nurse Alert　　　✳ Key NCLEX® Drug

Myocardial infarction
Adult: IV BOL (early treatment) 5 mg q2min × 3 doses, then 50 mg PO 15 min after last dose and q6hr × 48 hr (late treatment); PO maintenance 50-100 mg bid for 1-3 yr

Heart failure (NYHA class II/III)
Adult: PO ext rel 25 mg qd × 2 wk (class II); 12.5 mg qd (class III)

Angina
Adult: PO 100 mg/day as a single dose or in 2 divided doses, increase qwk as needed, or 100 mg ext rel tab daily, max 400 mg/day ext rel

Migraine prevention (unlabeled)
Adult: PO 25-100 mg bid-qid; 50-200 mg daily (XL)

Available forms: Tabs 25, 50, 100 mg; inj 1 mg/ml; ext rel tabs (tartrate) 100 mg; ext rel tabs (succinate) (XL) 25, 50, 100, 200 mg

Implementation
PO route
• Do not break, crush, or chew ext rel tabs
• Give regular release tab before meals, at bedtime; tab may be crushed or swallowed whole; give with food to prevent GI upset; reduced dosage in renal dysfunction; give at same time each day
• Store in dry area at room temp; do not freeze

Direct IV route
• Give 5 mg/2 min or more × 3 doses at 2 min intervals, start PO 15 min after last **IV** dose

Y-site compatibilities: Abciximab, acyclovir, alemtuzumab, alfentanil, alteplase, amikacin, aminophylline, amiodarone, amphotericin B liposome, anidulafungin, argatroban, ascorbic acid, atracurium, atropine, azaTHIOprine, aztreonam, benztropine, bivalirudin, bleomycin, bumetanide, buprenorphine, butorphanol, calcium chloride/gluconate, CARBOplatin, caspofungin, ceFAZolin, cefonicid, cefoperazone, cefotaxime, cefoTEtan, cefOXitin, cefTAZidime, ceftizoxime, cefTRIAXone, cefuroxime, chloramphenicol, chlorproMAZINE, cimetidine, CISplatin, clindamycin, cyanocobalamin, cyclophosphamide, cycloSPORINE, cytarabine, DACTINomycin, DAPTOmycin, dexamethasone, dexmedetomidine, digoxin, diltiazem, diphenhydrAMINE, DOBUTamine, DOCEtaxel, DOPamine, doxacurium, DOXOrubicin, doxycycline, enalaprilat, ePHEDrine, EPINEPHrine, epirubicin, epoetin alfa, eptifibatide, esmolol, etoposide, etoposide phosphate, famotidine, fenoldopam, fentaNYL, fluconazole, fludarabine, fluorouracil, folic acid, furosemide, ganciclo-

vir, gemcitabine, gentamicin, glycopyrrolate, granisetron, heparin, hydrocortisone, HYDROmorphone, IDArubicin, ifosfamide, imipenem/cilastatin, indomethacin, insulin, isoproterenol, ketorolac, labetalol, linezolid, LORazepam, magnesium sulfate, mannitol, mechlorethamine, meperidine, metaraminol, methotrexate, methoxamine, methyldopate, methylPREDNISolone, metoclopramide, metroNIDAZOLE, midazolam, milrinone, mitoXANtrone, morphine, multivitamins, nafcillin, nalbuphine, naloxone, nitroprusside, norepinephrine, octreotide, ondansetron, oxacillin, oxaliplatin, oxytocin, PACLitaxel, palonosetron, pancuronium, papaverine, PEMEtrexed, penicillin G, pentamidine, pentazocine, PENTobarbital, PHENobarbital, phentolamine, phenylephrine, phytonadione, piperacillin/tazobactam, potassium chloride, procainamide, prochlorperazine, promethazine, propranolol, protamine, pyridoxime, quinupristin/dalfopristin, ranitidine, rocuronium, sodium bicarbonate, succinylcholine, SUFentanil, tacrolimus, teniposide, theophylline, thiamine, thiotepa, ticarcillin/clavulanate, tigecycline, tirofiban, tobramycin, tolazoline, trimetaphan, urokinase, vancomycin, vasopressin, vecuronium, verapamil, vinCRIStine, vinorelbine, voriconazole

Y-site incompatibilities: Allopurinol, amphotericin B cholesteryl/colloidal/lipid complex, dantrolene, diazepam, diazoxide, lepirudin, pantoprazole, phenytoin, trimethoprim/sulfamethoxazole

ADVERSE EFFECTS
CNS: *Insomnia, dizziness,* mental changes, hallucinations, depression, anxiety, headaches, nightmares, confusion, fatigue
CV: CHF, *palpitations,* dysrhythmias, **cardiac arrest, AV block,** *hypotension,* **bradycardia, pulmonary/peripheral edema, chest pain**
EENT: Sore throat, dry burning eyes
GI: *Nausea, vomiting,* colitis, cramps, *diarrhea,* constipation, flatulence, dry mouth, *hiccups*
GU: Impotence
HEMA: Agranulocytosis, eosinophilia, thrombocytopenic purpura
INTEG: Rash, purpura, alopecia, dry skin, urticaria, pruritus
RESP: Bronchospasm, dyspnea, wheezing

M

Pharmacokinetics

Absorption	Well absorbed (PO); completely absorbed (**IV**)
Distribution	Crosses blood-brain barrier, placenta
Metabolism	Liver, extensively
Excretion	Kidneys, breast milk
Half-life	3-4 hr

Pharmacodynamics

	PO	IV
Onset	15 min	Immediate
Peak	2-4 hr	20 min
Duration	6-19 hr	5-8 hr

INTERACTIONS

Individual drugs
Cimetidine: increased metoprolol level
EPINEPHrine, hydrALAZINE, methyldopa prazosin, reserpine: increased hypotension, bradycardia
Insulin: increased hypoglycemia

Drug classifications
Antidiabetics (oral): increased hypoglycemia
Amphetamines, calcium channel blockers, histamine H$_2$ antagonists: increased hypotension, bradycardia
Barbiturates: decreased metoprolol level
MAOIs: do not use together
NSAIDs, salicylates: decreased antihypertensive effect
Xanthines: decreased effects of xanthines

Drug/food
Increased: absorption with food

Drug/lab test
Increased: BUN, potassium, ANA titer, serum lipoprotein, triglycerides, uric acid, alkaline phosphatase, LDH, AST, ALT

NURSING CONSIDERATIONS
Assessment

> **BLACK BOX WARNING:** Abrupt withdrawal: may cause MI, ventricular dysrhythmias, myocardial ischemia; taper dose over 7-14 days

• **Hypertension/angina:** monitor ECG directly when giving IV during initial treatment
• Monitor B/P during beginning treatment, periodically thereafter; pulse q4hr; note rate, rhythm, quality; check apical/radial pulse before administration; notify prescriber of any significant changes (pulse <60 bpm)

• Check for baselines in renal, liver function tests before therapy begins and periodically thereafter
• Assess for edema in feet, legs daily; monitor I&O, daily weight; check for jugular vein distention, crackles bilaterally, dyspnea (CHF)

Patient/family education

> **BLACK BOX WARNING:** Teach patient not to discontinue product abruptly; taper over 2 wk; may cause precipitate angina if stopped abruptly

• Teach patient not to use OTC products containing α-adrenergic stimulants (such as nasal decongestants, cold preparations); to avoid alcohol, smoking and to limit sodium intake as prescribed
• Teach patient how to take pulse and B/P at home; advise when to notify prescriber
• Instruct patient to comply with weight control, dietary adjustments, modified exercise program
• Tell patient to carry/wear emergency ID to identify product being taken, allergies; tell patient product controls symptoms but does not cure
• Caution patient to avoid hazardous activities if dizziness, drowsiness is present, to avoid driving until product response is known
• Teach patient to report symptoms of CHF; difficult breathing, especially with exertion or when lying down, night cough, swelling of extremities or bradycardia, dizziness, confusion, depression, fever, decreased vision
• Teach patient to take product as prescribed, not to double doses or skip doses; take any missed doses as soon as remembered if at least 4 hr until next dose
• Advise to monitor blood glucose closely if diabetic
• Advise to report Raynaud's symptoms

Evaluation
Positive therapeutic outcome
• Decreased B/P in hypertension (after 1-2 wk)
• Absence of dysrhythmias
• Decreased anginal pain

TREATMENT OF OVERDOSE:
Lavage, **IV** atropine for bradycardia, **IV** theophylline for bronchospasm, digoxin, O$_2$, diuretic for cardiac failure, hemodialysis, **IV** glucose for hyperglycemia, **IV** diazepam (or phenytoin) for seizures

---

metroNIDAZOLE (Rx)

(me-troe-ni′da-zole)
**Flagyl, Flagyl ER, Flagyl IV,
Flagyl IV RTU, Florazone ER ✦,
Novonidazole ✦**
Func. class.: Antiinfective, miscellaneous
Chem. class.: Nitroimidazole derivative
Pregnancy category B (2nd, 3rd trimesters)

ACTION: Direct-acting amebicide/trichomonacide; binds, degrades DNA structure, inhibiting bacterial nucleic acid synthesis

Therapeutic outcome: Trichomonacidal, amebicidal, bactericidal for the following susceptible organisms: *Bacteroides, Clostridium, Trichomonas vaginalis, Giardia lamblia, Entamoeba histolytica*

USES: Intestinal amebiasis, amebic abscess, trichomoniasis, refractory trichomoniasis, bacterial anaerobic infections, giardiasis; septicemia, endocarditis, bone, joint, and lower respiratory tract infections, rosacea

Unlabeled uses: Crohn's disease

CONTRAINDICATIONS:

Pregnancy (1st trimester), breastfeeding, hypersensitivity to this product

Precautions: Pregnancy **B** (2nd/3rd trimesters), candidal infections, heart failure, fungal infection, geriatric, dental disease, bone marrow suppression, hematologic disease, renal/hepatic/GI disease, contracted visual or color fields, blood dyscrasias, CNS disorders

> **BLACK BOX WARNING:** Secondary malignancy

DOSAGE AND ROUTES
Trichomoniasis
Adult: PO 500 mg bid × 7 days or 2 g in single dose; do not repeat treatment for 4-6 wk
Child ≥45 kg (unlabeled): PO 2 g once
Child <45 kg (unlabeled): PO 15 mg/kg/day divided in 3 doses × 7-10 days

Amebic hepatic abscess
Adult: PO 750 mg tid × 7-10 days
Child: PO 35-50 mg/kg/day in 3 divided doses × 7-10 days

Intestinal amebiasis
Adult: PO 750 mg tid × 7-10 days
Child: PO 35-50 mg/kg/day in 3 divided doses × 7-10 days; then oral iodoquinol

Anaerobic bacterial infections
Adult: IV INF 15 mg/kg/over 1 hr, then 7.5 mg/kg IV or PO q6hr, max 4 g/day; first maintenance dose should be administered 6 hr after loading dose

Bacterial vaginosis
Adult: PO reg rel 500 mg bid or 250 mg tid × 7 days; ext rel 750 mg/day × 7 days

Giardiasis (unlabeled)
Adult: PO 250 mg tid × 5-7 days
Child: PO 5 mg/kg divided tid × 5 days

Antibiotic-associated pseudomembranous colitis
Adult (unlabeled): PO 250-500 mg 3-4 ×/day × 7-14 days
Child: PO 20 mg/kg/day (max 2 g) divided q6hr

Available forms: Tabs 250, 500 mg; ext rel tabs 750 mg; caps 375 mg; inj 500 mg/100 ml; inj sol 5 mg/ml

Implementation
• Store in light-resistant container; do not refrigerate
PO route
• Give with or after a meal to avoid GI symptoms, metallic taste; crush tab if needed, give on empty stomach
Topical route
• A thin coating should be applied to affected area after cleaning with soap and water and patting dry

IV route
• Give intermittent **IV** prediluted; for Flagyl **IV** dilute with 4.4 ml of sterile water or 0.9% NaCl; must be diluted further with ≤8 mg/ml 0.9% NaCl, D₅W, or LR; must neutralize with 5 mEq of $NaCO_3$/500 mg; CO_2 gas will be generated and may require venting; run over 1 hr or more; primary **IV** must be discontinued; may be given as cont inf; do not use aluminum products; **IV** may require venting

Y-site compatibilities: Acyclovir, alemtuzumab, alfentanil, allopurinol, amifostene, amikacin, aminophylline, amiodarone, ampicillin, ampicillin/sulbactam, anidulafungin, atracurium, bivalirudin, bumetanide, buprenor-

M

phine, busulfan, butorphanol, calcium acetate/ chloride/gluconate, CARBOplatin, ceFAZolin, cefepime, cefoperazone, cefoTEtan, cefotaxime, cefTRIAXone, cefuroxime, chloramphenicol, chlorproMAZINE, cimetidine, ciprofloxacin, cisatracurium, CISplatin, clindamycin, codeine, cyclophosphamide, cycloSPORINE, cytarabine, DACTINomycin, dexamethasone, dexmedetomidine, dexrazoxane, digoxin, diltiazem, dimenhyDRINATE, diphenhydrAMINE, DOBUTamine, DOCEtaxel, DOPamine, doripenem, doxacurium, doxapram, DOXOrubicin, DOXOrubicin liposome, doxycycline, droperidol, enalaprilat, ePHEDrine, EPINEPHrine, epirubicin, eptifibatide, ertapenem, erythromycin, esmolol, etoposide, etoposide phosphate, famotidine, fenoldopam, fentaNYL, fluconazole, fludarabine, fluorouracil, foscarnet, fosphenytoin, furosemide, gemcitabine, gentamicin, glycopyrrolate, granisetron, haloperidol, heparin, hydrALAZINE, hydrocortisone, HYDROmorphone, IDArubicin, ifosfamide, imipenem/cilastatin, inamrinone, insulin, isoproterenol, ketorolac, labetalol, leucovorin, levofloxacin, lidocaine, linezolid, LORazepam, magnesium sulfate, mannitol, mechlorethamine, melphalan, meperidine, meropenem, mesna, metaraminol, methotrexate, methyldopate, methylPREDNISolone, metoclopramide, metoprolol, midazolam, milrinone, mitoXANtrone, morphine, nafcillin, nalbuphine, naloxone, nesiritide, niCARdipine, nitroglycerin, nitroprusside, norepinephrine, octreotide, ondansetron, oxaliplatin, oxytocin, PACLitaxel, palonosetron, pancuronium, pentamidine, pentazocine, PENTobarbital, perphenazine, PHENobarbital, phentolamine, phenylephrine, piperacillin/tazobactam, potassium chloride/ phosphates, prochlorperazine, promethazine, propranolol, ranitidine, remifentanil, riTUXimab, rocuronium, sargramostim, sodium acetate/bicarbonate/phosphates, streptozocin, succinylcholine, SUFentanil, tacrolimus, teniposide, theophylline, thiopental, thiotepa, ticarcillin/ clavulanate, tigecycline, tirofiban, tobramycin, trastuzumab, trimethobenzamide, trimethoprim/ sulfamethoxazole, vancomycin, vasopressin, vecuronium, verapamil, vinCRIStine, vinorelbine, voriconazole, zidovudine, zoledronic acid

Y-site incompatibilities: Amphotericin B cholesteryl/colloidal/liposome, aztreonam, dantrolene, DAPTOmycin, diazepam, drotrecogin, filgrastim, ganciclovir, pantoprazole, PEMEtrexed, phenytoin, procainamide, quinupristin/ dalfopristin

ADVERSE EFFECTS
CNS: *Headache, dizziness,* confusion, irritability, restlessness, ataxia, depression, fatigue, drowsiness, insomnia, paresthesia, peripheral neuropathy, **seizures,** incoordination, depression, encephalopathy, **aseptic meningitis**
CV: Flat $\top$-waves
EENT: Blurred vision, sore throat, retinal edema, dry mouth, metallic taste, furry tongue, glossitis, stomatitis, photophobia, optic neuritis
GI: *Nausea, vomiting, diarrhea,* epigastric distress, *anorexia,* constipation, *abdominal cramps,* **pseudomembranous colitis,** xerostomia, metallic taste, abdominal pain, **pancreatitis**
GU: Darkened urine, vaginal dryness, polyuria, **albuminuria,** dysuria, cystitis, decreased libido, **nephrotoxicity,** incontinence, dyspareunia, candidiasis, increased urinary frequency
HEMA: Leukopenia, bone marrow depression, aplasia, thrombocytopenia
INTEG: Rash, pruritus, urticaria, flushing, phlebitis at injection site, **toxic epidermal necrolysis**

Pharmacokinetics

Absorption	80% (PO)
Distribution	Widely distributed, crosses placenta
Metabolism	Liver
Excretion	Urine, unchanged; feces
Half-life	6-11 hr

Pharmacodynamics

	PO	IV
Onset	Rapid	Immediate
Peak	1-2 hr	Infusion's end
Duration	Unknown	Unknown

INTERACTIONS
Individual drugs
Alcohol, oral ritonavir, any product with alcohol: increased disulfiram-like reaction
AzaTHIOprine, fluorouracil: increased leukopenia
Amprenavir, disulfiram: do not use bortezomib; norfloxacin, zalcitabine: avoid use
Busulfan: increased busulfan toxicity, avoid concurrent use
Cholestyramine: decreased metroNIDAZOLE, toxicity
Fosphenytoin, lithium, phenytoin, warfarin: increased action of these drugs

---

Drug classifications
Barbiturates: decreased metroNIDAZOLE
half-life
CYP3A4 substrates: increased levels

Drug/lab test
Altered: AST, ALT, LDH
Decrease: WBC, neutrophils
False decrease: triglycerides

NURSING CONSIDERATIONS
Assessment
• **Assess patient for signs and symptoms of infection** including characteristics of wounds, WBC >10,000/mm^3, vaginal secretions, fever; obtain baseline information and during treatment
• Obtain C&S before beginning product therapy to identify if correct treatment has been initiated
• **Assess for allergic reactions:** rash, urticaria, pruritus
• Identify urine output; if decreasing, notify prescriber **(may indicate nephrotoxicity)**; also check for increased BUN, creatinine
• Assess bowel pattern daily; if severe diarrhea occurs, product should be discontinued
• Assess for overgrowth of infection: perineal itching, fever, malaise, redness, pain, swelling, drainage, rash, diarrhea, change in cough, sputum
• Teach patient to notify prescriber if pregnancy is planned or suspected, pregnancy (B) 2nd/3rd trimester in trichomoniasis

> **BLACK BOX WARNING: Secondary malignancy:** use only when indicated, avoid unnecessary use

Patient/family education
• Teach patient to report sore throat, bruising, bleeding, joint pain; may indicate blood dyscrasias (rare)
• Advise patient to contact prescriber if vaginal itching, loose foul-smelling stools, furry tongue occur; may indicate superinfection
• Advise patient to notify physician of numbness or tingling of extremities
• Teach trichomoniasis patient that both partners need to be treated; condoms should be used during intercourse to prevent reinfection
• Advise patient of disulfiram-like reaction to alcohol ingestion; alcohol should not be used within 48 hr of this product
• Inform patient product has a metallic taste and urine may turn dark
• Advise patient to contact prescriber if pregnancy is suspected

• Advise patient to use sips of water, sugarless gum, candy for dry mouth

Evaluation
Positive therapeutic outcome
• Decreased symptoms of infection

metroNIDAZOLE topical
See Appendix B

micafungin (Rx)
(my-ca-fun′gin)
Mycamine
Func. class.: Antifungal, systemic
Chem. class.: Echinocandin
Pregnancy category C

ACTION: Inhibits an essential component in fungal cell walls; causes direct damage to fungal cell wall

Therapeutic outcome: Prevention of *Candida* infection in hematopoietic stem cell transplantation (HSCT); or decreased symptoms of *Candida* infection, negative culture

USES: Treatment of esophageal candidiasis; prophylaxis of *Candida* infections in patients undergoing HSCT; susceptible *Candida* species: *C. albicans, C. glabrata, C. krusei, C. parapsilosis, C. tropicalis,* prophylaxis of HIV-related esophageal candidiasis

CONTRAINDICATIONS:
Hypersensitivity to this product or other echinocandins

Precautions: Pregnancy **C**, breastfeeding, children, geriatric, severe hepatic disease, renal impairment, hemolytic anemia

DOSAGE AND ROUTES
Candidemia/acute disseminated candidiasis, abscess, peritonitis
Adult: IV 100 mg/day over 1 hr

Esophageal candidiasis
Adult: IV 150 mg/day, given over 1 hr

Prophylaxis of *Candida* infections
Adult: IV 50 mg/day, given over 1 hr

Available forms: Powder for injection 50 mg, in single-dose vials; 50, 100 mg vial

Implementation
• Protect diluted sol from light
• Do not use if cloudy or precipitated; do not admix product

M

- Flush line before, after administration with 0.9% NaCl

IV route
- For *Candida* **prevention:** reconstitute with provided diluent 0.9% NaCl without bacteriostatic product; 50 mg vial/5 ml (10 mg/ml), swirl to dissolve, do not shake; further dilute with 100 ml 0.9% NaCl, only; run over 1 hr
- For *Candida* **infection:** reconstitute with provided diluent 50 mg/5 ml (10 mg/ml); further dilute 3 reconstituted vials in 100 ml of 0.9% NaCl, run over 1 hr
- Store at room temperature, away from light; do not freeze; discard unused solution

Y-site compatibilities: Aminophylline, bumetanide, calcium chloride/gluconate, cycloSPORINE, DOPamine, eptifibatide, esmolol, fenoldopam, furosemide, heparin, HYDROmorphone, lidocaine, LORazepam, magnesium sulfate, milrinone, nitroglycerin, nitroprusside, norepinephrine, phenylephrine, potassium chloride, potassium phosphate, tacrolimus, vasopressin

Y-site incompatibilities: Albumin, amiodarone, cisatracurium, diltiazem, DOBUTamine, EPINEPHrine, insulin, labetalol, meperidine, midazolam, morphine, mycophenolate mofetil, nesiritide, niCARdipine, octreotide, ondansetron, phenytoin, telavancin, vecuronium

ADVERSE EFFECTS
CNS: Convulsions, dizziness, *headache, somnolence,* fever, anxiety
CV: Flushing, hypertension, phlebitis, tachycardia, **atrial fibrillation**
GI: Abdominal pain, *nausea, anorexia, vomiting, diarrhea,* **hepatitis**
GU: Renal failure
HEMA: Neutropenia, thrombocytopenia, leukopenia, coagulopathy, anemia, hemolytic anemia
INTEG: *Rash, pruritus, inj site pain*
META: Hypokalemia, hypocalcemia, hypomagnesemia
MS: *Rigors*

Pharmacokinetics	
Absorption	Unknown
Distribution	Protein binding 99%
Metabolism	Liver
Excretion	Feces, urine
Half-life	Terminal 14-17.2 hr

Pharmacodynamics
Unknown

INTERACTIONS
Individual drugs
Itraconazole, sirolimus, NIFEdipine: increased plasma concentrations; may need dosage reduction

Drug/lab test
Increased: ALT/AST, alk phos, bilirubin
Decreased: blood glucose, potassium sodium

NURSING CONSIDERATIONS
Assessment
- Assess for signs and symptoms of infection, clearing of cultures during treatment; obtain culture baseline, throughout; product may be started as soon as culture is taken (esophageal candidiasis); monitor cultures during HSCT, for prevention of *Candida* infections
- Monitor CBC (RBC, Hct, Hgb), differential, platelet count periodically; notify prescriber of results
- Monitor renal studies: BUN, urine CCr, electrolytes before, during therapy
- Monitor hepatic studies before, during treatment: bilirubin, AST, ALT, alkaline phosphatase, as needed
- Assess for bleeding: hematuria, heme-positive stools, bruising or petechiae of mucosa or orifices; blood dyscrasias can occur
- Assess for hypersensitivity: rash, pruritus, facial swelling; also for phlebitis
- Assess for hemolytic anemia
- Assess **GI symptoms:** frequency of stools, cramping; if severe diarrhea occurs, electrolytes may need to be given

Patient/family education
- Advise patient to notify prescriber if pregnancy is suspected or planned
- Teach patient to avoid breastfeeding while taking this product
- Teach patient to inform prescriber of renal or hepatic disease
- Teach patient to report bleeding, facial swelling, wheezing, difficulty breathing, itching, rash, hives, increasing warmth, flushing
- Instruct patient to report signs of infection: increased temp, sore throat, flulike symptoms
- Advise patient to notify prescriber of nausea, vomiting, diarrhea, jaundice, anorexia, clay-colored stools, dark urine; hepatotoxicity may occur

Evaluation
Positive therapeutic outcome
- Prevention of *Candida* infection in HSCT; decreased symptoms of *Candida* infection, negative culture

miconazole (Rx, OTC)
(mi-kon′a-zole)
Oravig
miconazole nitrate
Femizole-M, Monistat, Monistat 3, Monistat 7, Monistat-Derm, Monistat Dual-Pak, M-Zole 7 Dual Pack, topical: Micatin, Micatin Liquid, miconazole nitrate
Func. class.: Antifungal
Chem. class.: Imidazole
Pregnancy category C

ACTION: Alters cell membranes, inhibits fungal enzymes, inhibits sterols so intracellular contents are lost, prevents biosynthesis of phospholipids/triglycerides

Therapeutic outcome: Fungistatic/fungicidal against *Aspergillus, Coccidioides, Cryptococcus, Candida, Dermatophytes, Histoplasma*

USES: Coccidioidomycosis, candidiasis, cryptococcosis, paracoccidioidomycosis, chronic mucocutaneous candidiasis, fungal meningitis; **IV** used for severe infections only; topical for tinea pedis, tinea cruris, tinea corporis, tinea versicolor, vaginal or vulva candidal infections

CONTRAINDICATIONS:
Hypersensitivity

Precautions: Pregnancy **C**, renal/hepatic disease

DOSAGE AND ROUTES
Oropharyngeal candidiasis (thrush)
Adult/adolescent ≥16 yr: Buccal apply 1 tab (50 mg) to upper gum region just above incisor tooth q day × 14 days
Adult: **IV** INF 200-3600 mg/day; may be divided in 3 INF at 200-1200 mg/INF; may have to repeat course; IT 20 mg given simultaneously with **IV** for fungal meningitis q1-2day
Child: **IV** 20-40 mg/kg/day, max 15 mg/kg/day
Adult and child: TOP apply to affected area bid × 2-4 wk
Adult: Intravaginal 200 mg SUPP at bedtime × 3 days or 100 mg SUPP × 1 wk

Available forms: Inj 10 mg/ml; aerosol 2%; cream 2%; lotion 2%; powder 2%; spray 2%; vag cream 2%; vag supp 100, 200 mg; buccal tab 50 mg

Implementation
• Have adrenalin, suction, tracheostomy set, endotracheal intubation equipment available
Transmucosal use (adhesive buccal tablet)
• Apply tab in the morning after brushing the teeth; use dry hands
• Place the rounded surface of the tab against the upper gum just above the incisor tooth; hold in place with a slight pressure over the upper lip for 30 seconds to ensure adhesion
• Although the tab is rounded on one side for comfort, the flat side may also be applied to the gum
• The tab will gradually dissolve
• Administration of subsequent tabs should be made to alternating sides of the mouth
• Before applying the next tab, clear away any remaining tab material
• Do not crush, chew or swallow; food and drink can be taken normally; avoid chewing gum
• If tab does not adhere or falls off within the first 6 hr, the same tab should be repositioned immediately. If the tab still does not adhere, a new tab should be used
• If the tab falls off or is swallowed after it was in place for 6 hr or more, a new tab should not be applied until the next regularly scheduled dose
Topical route
• Apply after cleansing area with soap and water before each application; use enough medication to cover lesions completely; dry well
• Store at room temperature in dry place
Vaginal route
• Administer 1 applicator full every night high into the vagina
• Store at room temperature in dry place
IV route
• Give 200 mg initially to prevent severe hypersensitive reaction
• Give **IV** after diluting in ≤1 g/10 ml of sterile water, D$_5$W, or 0.45% NaCl for 3-5 min
• Give by intermittent **IV** after diluting in 200 ml or more D$_5$W or 0.9% NaCl; give over 30-60 min
• Store at room temperature; reconstituted sol is stable for 24 hr refrigerated

Y-site compatibilities: Allopurinol, filgrastim, foscarnet, granisetron, melphalan, ondansetron, propofol, sargramostim, teniposide, thiotepa, vinorelbine

Y-site incompatibilities: Fludarabine

M

ADVERSE EFFECTS

CNS: Drowsiness, headache, lethargy
CV: Tachycardia, **dysrhythmias** (rapid **IV**)
GI: Nausea, vomiting, anorexia, diarrhea, cramps
GU: Vulvovaginal burning, itching, hyponatremia, pelvic cramps (topical forms)
HEMA: Decreased Hct, thrombocytopenia, hyperlipidemia
INTEG: Pruritus, rash, fever, flushing, hives
SYST: Anaphylaxis

Pharmacokinetics

Absorption	Poorly absorbed (PO)
Distribution	Widely distributed (**IV**); bound to serum proteins (90%)
Metabolism	Liver, extensively
Excretion	Unknown
Half-life	Triphasic: 0.4, 2.1, 24 hr

Pharmacodynamics

	IV	Topical	Vag
Onset	Rapid	Unknown	Unknown
Peak	Infusion's end	Unknown	Unknown
Duration	Unknown	Unknown	Unknown

INTERACTIONS

Individual drugs

Amphotericin B: decreased effect of amphotericin B
Amphotericin B, isoniazid, rifampin: decreased effect of miconazole
Phenytoin: increased effect
Warfarin: increased anticoagulant effect

Drug classifications

Sulfonylureas: increased effect

Drug/lab test

False positive: urine glucose, urine protein

NURSING CONSIDERATIONS

Assessment

• Assess for signs and symptoms of infection: drainage, sore throat, urinary pain, hematuria, fever
• Obtain C&S before beginning treatment; therapy may be started after culture is taken; monitor signs of infection before, throughout treatment
• Monitor bowel pattern before, during treatment; diarrhea may occur
• Monitor cardiac system: B/P, pulse; watch for increasing pulse, cardiac dysrhythmias; product should be discontinued
• Monitor blood studies: WBC, RBC, Hgb, Hct, bleeding time; patients taking anticoagulants may need a decreased dosage; monitor liver and renal studies periodically for patients on long-term therapy
• Monitor I&O ratio; watch for decreasing urinary output, change in specific gravity; discontinue product to prevent renal damage; patients with renal disease may require lowered dose
• Monitor **IV** site for thrombophlebitis; site should be changed q48-72hr
• Monitor for allergies before initiation of treatment and reaction to each medication; highlight allergies on chart; check for allergic reaction: burning, stinging, swelling, redness (topical); observe for skin eruptions after administration of product to 1 wk after discontinuing product

Patient/family education

• Inform patient that culture may be performed after completed course of medication
• Advise patient to notify nurse of diarrhea, symptoms of candidal vaginitis

Topical route

• Teach patient to use medical asepsis (hand washing) before, after each application; to apply with glove to prevent further infection; to avoid contact with eyes; not to use occlusive dressings
• Caution patient to avoid use of OTC creams, ointments, lotions unless directed by prescriber
• Instruct patient to notify prescriber if condition does not improve in 4 wk or if symptoms return in 2 mo; pregnancy or a serious medical condition may be the cause
• Teach patient to use for full prescribed treatment time, or reinfection may occur

Vaginal route

• Instruct patient in asepsis (hand washing) before, after each application
• Teach patient to apply with applicator only; to avoid use of any other vaginal product unless directed by prescriber; sanitary napkin may prevent soiling of undergarments; to abstain from sexual intercourse until treatment is completed or reinfection and irritation may occur; not to use tampons, douches, spermicides; not to engage in sexual activity; product may damage condoms, diaphragms, cervical caps
• Instruct patient to notify prescriber if symptoms persist

⚠ Nurse Alert   ✷ Key NCLEX® Drug

Evaluation
Positive therapeutic outcome
• Decreasing oral candidiasis, fever, malaise, rash
• Negative C&S for infectious organism
• Decrease in size, number of lesions
• Decrease in itching or white discharge (vaginal)

TREATMENT OF OVERDOSE:
Withdraw product; maintain airway; administer EPINEPHrine, aminophylline, O₂, **IV** corticosteroids for anaphylaxis

miconazole topical
See Appendix B

miconazole vaginal antifungal
See Appendix B

midazolam (Rx)
(mid′ay-zoe-lam)
Func. class.: Sedative/hypnotic, antianxiety
Chem. class.: Benzodiazepine, short-acting
Pregnancy category D
Controlled substance schedule IV

ACTION: Depresses subcortical levels in CNS; may act on limbic system, reticular formation; may potentiate GABA by binding to specific benzodiazepine receptors

Therapeutic outcome: Sedation for anesthesia induction and procedures

USES: Preoperative sedation, general anesthesia induction, sedation for diagnostic endoscopic procedures, intubation, anxiety

Unlabeled uses: Refractory status epilepticus, alcohol withdrawal, agitation

CONTRAINDICATIONS:
Pregnancy **D**, hypersensitivity to benzodiazepines, acute closed-angle glaucoma, epidural/intrathecal use

Precautions: Breastfeeding, children, geriatric, COPD, CHF, chronic renal failure, chills, debilitated, hepatic disease, shock, coma, alcohol intoxication, status asthmaticus

BLACK BOX WARNING: Neonates (contains benzyl alcohol), **IV** administration, respiratory depression/insufficiency

DOSAGE AND ROUTES
Preoperative sedation/amnesia induction
Adult and child ≥12 yr: IM 0.07-0.08 mg/kg 30-60 min before general anesthesia
Child 6 mo-5 yr: IV 0.05-0.1 mg/kg, a total dose of 0.6 mg/kg may be needed
Child 6-12 yr: IV 0.025-0.05 mg/kg, a total dose of 0.4 mg/kg may be needed

Induction of general anesthesia
Adult >55 yr: (ASA I/II) **IV** 150-300 mcg/kg over 30 sec; (ASA III/IV) limit dose to 250 mcg/kg (nonpremedicated) or 150 mcg/kg (premedicated)
Adult <55 yr: IV 200-350 mcg/kg over 20-30 sec; if patient has not received premedication, may repeat by giving 20% of original dose; if patient has received premedication reduce dosage by 50 mcg/kg
Child: No safe and effective dosage is established; however, doses of 50-200 mcg/kg **IV** have been used

Continuous infusion for mechanical ventilation (critical care)
Adult: IV 0.01-0.05 mg/kg over several min; repeat at 10-15 min intervals until adequate sedation, then 0.02-0.10 mg/kg/hr maintenance; adjust as needed
Child: IV 0.05-0.2 mg/kg over 2-3 min, then 0.06-0.12 mg/kg/hr by CONT INF; adjust as needed
Neonate: IV 0.03-0.06 mg/kg/hr titrate using lowest dose

Alcohol withdrawal (unlabeled)
Adult: IV 1-5 mg q1-2hr (mild-moderate symptoms); cont IV inf 1-20 mg q1-2hr (delirium tremens)

Available forms: Inj 1, 5 mg/ml, 25 mg/5 ml, 50 mg/10 ml; syr 2 mg/ml

Implementation
• Store at room temperature; protect from light
PO route
• Remove cap of press-in bottle adaptor and push adaptor into neck of bottle; close with cap, remove cap, and insert tip of dispenser and insert into adaptor; turn upside-down and withdraw correct dose; place in mouth
IM route
• Give inj deep into large muscle mass

M

Adverse effects: *italics* = common; **bold** = life-threatening

IV route
• Give **IV** undiluted or after diluting with D₅W or 0.9% NaCl to a conc of 0.25 mg/ml; give over 2 min (conscious sedation) or over 30 sec (anesthesia induction)
• Ensure immediate availability of resuscitation equipment, O₂ to support airway; do not give by rapid bol

Syringe compatibilities: Alfentanil, atracurium, atropine, benzquinamide, buprenorphine, butorphanol, chlorproMAZINE, cimetadine, cisatracurium, diphenhyDRAMINE, droperidol, fentaNYL, glycopyrrolate, hydromorphine, hydrOXYzine, ketamine, meperidine, metoclopramide, morphine, nalbuphine, promazine, promethazine, remifentanil, scopolamine, SUFentanil, thiethylperazine, trimethobenzamide

Syringe incompatibilities: DimenhyDRINATE, PENTobarbital, perphenazine, prochlorperazine, ranitidine

Y-site compatibilities: Abcixmab, alfentamil, amikacin, amiodarone, argatroban, atracurium, atropine, aztreonam, benzotropine, calcium gluconate, ceFAZolin, cefotaxime, cefOXitine, cefTRIAXone, cimetidine, ciprofloxacin, CISplatin, clindamycin, cloNIDine, cyanocobalamin, cycloSPORINE, DACTINomycin, digoxin, diltiazem, diphenhydrAMINE, DOCEtaxal, DOPamine, doxycycline, enalaprilat, EPINEPHrine, erythromycin, esmolol, etomidate, etoposide, famotidine, fentaNYL, fluconazole, folic acid, gatifloxacin, gemcitabine, gentamicin, glycopyrrolate, granisetron, heparin, hetastarch, HYDROmorphone, hydrOXYzine, inamrinone, isoproterenol, labetalol, lactated Ringer's, levofloxacin, lidocaine, linezolid, LORazepam, magnesium, mannitol, meperidine, methadone, methyldopa, methylPREDNISolone, metoclopramide, metomolol, metroNIDAZOLE, milrinone, morphine, nalbuphine, naloxone, niCARdipine, nitroglycerin, nitroprusside, norepinephrine, ondansetron, oxacillin, oxytocin, PACLitaxel, palonosetron, pancuronium, papaverin, phentolamine, phytonadione, piperacillin, potassium chloride, propanolol, protamine, pyridoxine, ranitidine, remifentanil, sodium nitroprusside, streptokinase, succinylcholine, SUFentanil, teniposide, theophylline, thiotepa, ticarcillin, tobramycin, vancomycin, vasopressin, vecuronium, verapamil, voriconazole

Y-site incompatibilities: Foscarnet

ADVERSE EFFECTS
CNS: Retrograde amnesia, euphoria, confusion, headache, anxiety, insomnia, slurred speech, paresthesia, tremors, weakness, chills, agitation, paradoxical reactions
CV: Hypotension, PVCs, tachycardia, bigeminy, nodal rhythm, **cardiac arrest**
EENT: Blurred vision, nystagmus, diplopia, loss of balance
GI: *Nausea, vomiting,* increased salivation, hiccups
INTEG: Urticaria, pain at injection site, swelling at inj site, rash, pruritus at injection site
RESP: Coughing, **apnea, bronchospasm, laryngospasm,** dyspnea, **respiratory depression**

Pharmacokinetics
Absorption	Well absorbed
Distribution	Crosses placenta, blood-brain barrier; protein binding 97%
Metabolism	Liver; by CYP3A4 to metabolites excreted in urine
Excretion	Kidneys, breast milk
Half-life	1-5 hr

Pharmacodynamics
	PO	IM	IV
Onset	10-30 min	15 min	1.5-5 min
Peak	Unknown	½-1 hr	Unknown
Duration	Unknown	2-3 hr	<2 hr

INTERACTIONS
Individual drugs
Alcohol: increased respiratory depression
Cimetidine, erythromycin, ranitidine, theophylline: decreased midazolam metabolism
FluvoxaMINE, indinavir, ritonavir, verapamil, protease inhibitors: increased respiratory depression

Drug classifications
Antihypertensives, nitrates, opiates: increase in hypotension
Barbiturates, opiate analgesics, other CNS depressants: increased respiratory depression
CYP3A4 inducers (azole antifungals, theophylline): increased half-life of midazolam
CYP3A4 inhibitors: increased levels of midazolam

Drug/herb
Kava, valerian: increased sedation
St. John's wort: decreased midazolam

⚠ Nurse Alert   ✷ Key NCLEX® Drug

Drug/food
Grapefruit juice: increased midazolam effect
(PO)

NURSING CONSIDERATIONS
Assessment
• Monitor B/P, pulse, respiration during **IV**; O_2 and emergency equipment should be nearby
• Monitor inj site for redness, pain, swelling
• Assess degree of amnesia in geriatric; may be increased
• Assess anterograde amnesia
• Assess vital signs for recovery period in obese patient, since half-life may be extended
• **Respiratory depression/insufficiency:** assess for apnea, respiratory depression, which may be increased in the geriatric

Patient/family education
• Inform patient that amnesia occurs; events might not be remembered
• Caution patient to avoid CNS depressants including alcohol for 24 hr after taking this product

Evaluation
Positive therapeutic outcome
• Induction of sedation, amnesia

TREATMENT OF OVERDOSE:
O_2, flumazenil

miglitol (Rx)
(mig′le-tol)
Glyset
Func. class.: Oral hypoglycemic
Chem. class.: α-Glucosidase inhibitor
Pregnancy category B

ACTION: Delays the digestion/absorption of ingested carbohydrates, results in a smaller rise in blood glucose after meals; does not increase insulin production

Therapeutic outcome: Decreased blood glucose levels in diabetes mellitus

USES: Type 2 diabetes mellitus

Unlabeled uses: Type 1 diabetes mellitus

CONTRAINDICATIONS:
Hypersensitivity, diabetic ketoacidosis, cirrhosis, IBD, colonic ulceration, partial intestinal obstruction, chronic intestinal disease, ileus

Precautions: Pregnancy **B,** breastfeeding, children, diarrhea, hiatal hernia, hypoglycemia, renal disease, Type 1 diabetes, vomiting

DOSAGE AND ROUTES
Initial dose
Adult: PO 25 mg tid initially, with first bite of meal

Maintenance dose
Adult: PO may be increased to 50 mg tid; may increase to 100 mg tid if needed with dosage adjustment at 4-8 wk intervals

Available forms: Tabs 25, 50, 100 mg

Implementation
• Give tid with first bite of each meal
• Provide storage in airtight container at room temperature

ADVERSE EFFECTS
GI: *Abdominal pain, diarrhea, flatulence,* **hepatotoxicity**
HEMA: Low iron
INTEG: Rash

Pharmacokinetics
Absorption	Unknown
Distribution	Unknown
Metabolism	Not metabolized
Excretion	Kidneys, unchanged product
Half-life	2 hr

Pharmacodynamics
Onset	Unknown
Peak	2-3 hr
Duration	Unknown

INTERACTIONS
Individual drugs
Digoxin: decreased levels of digoxin
Propranolol: decreased levels of propranolol
Ranitidine: decreased levels of ranitidine

Drug classifications
Adsorbents (intestinal), enzymes (digestive): decreased miglitol levels; do not use together

Drug/food
Carbohydrates: increased diarrhea

NURSING CONSIDERATIONS
Assessment
• Assess for hypo/hyperglycemia; even though this product does not cause hypoglycemia, if taking a sulfonylurea or insulin, hypoglycemia may be additive (rare)

M

• Monitor blood glucose levels, A1c, liver function tests; if hypoglycemia occurs with monotherapy, treat with glucose

Patient/family education
• Teach patient the symptoms of hypo/hyperglycemia and what to do about each
• Instruct that medication must be taken as prescribed; explain consequences of discontinuing the medication abruptly; that during periods of stress, infection, surgery, insulin may be required
• Tell patient to avoid OTC medications unless approved by prescriber
• Teach patient that diabetes is a lifelong illness; product will not cure condition
• Instruct patient to carry/wear emergency ID as diabetic
• Teach patient that diet and exercise regimen must be followed
• Teach patient GI side effects and what to do about them

Evaluation
Positive therapeutic outcome
• Decreased signs, symptoms of diabetes mellitus (polyuria, polydipsia, polyphagia, clear sensorium, absence of dizziness, stable gait)
• Improved blood glucose, A1c

⚠ HIGH ALERT

milrinone (Rx)
(mill-re′none)
Func. class.: Inotropic/vasodilator agent with phosphodiesterase activity
Chem. class.: Bipyridine derivative
Pregnancy category C

ACTION: Positive inotropic agent with vasodilator properties; increases contractility of cardiac muscle; reduces preload and afterload by direct relaxation of vascular smooth muscle; increases myocardial contractility

Therapeutic outcome: Increased inotropic effect resulting in increased cardiac output

USES: Short-term management of advanced CHF that has not responded to other medication

CONTRAINDICATIONS:
Hypersensitivity to this product, severe aortic disease, severe pulmonic valvular disease, acute MI

Precautions: Pregnancy **C,** breastfeeding, children, geriatric, renal/hepatic disease, atrial flutter/fibrillation

DOSAGE AND ROUTES
Adult: **IV** BOL 50 mcg/kg given over 10 min; start INF of 0.375-0.75 mcg/kg/min; reduce dosage in renal impairment

Renal dose
Adult: IV CCr 41-50 ml/min 0.43 mcg/kg/min, titrate up; CCr 31-40 ml/min 0.38 mcg/kg/min, titrate up; CCr 21-30 ml/min 0.33 mcg/kg/min, titrate up; CCr 11-20 ml/min 0.08 mcg/kg/min; CCr 6-10 ml/min 0.23 mcg/kg/min; CCr <6 ml/min 0.20 mcg/kg/min; max all dosages 0.75 mcg/kg/min

Available forms: Inj 1 mg/ml; premixed inj 200 mcg/ml in D₅W

Implementation
Direct IV route
• Give **IV** loading dose undiluted over 10 min; use controlled-rate device
• Administer by direct **IV** into inf through Y-connector or directly into tubing
Continuous IV infusion route
• Dilute 20 mg vial with 80, 112, 180 ml of 0.45% NaCl, 0.9% NaCl, or D₅W to a concentration of 200, 150, 100 mcg/ml respectively
• Do not mix directly with glucose sol (chemical reaction occurs over 24 hr) precipitate forms if milrinone and furosemide come into contact
• Titrate rate based on hemodynamic and clinical response, use controlled device
• Administer potassium supplements if ordered for potassium levels <3.0 mg/dl

Y-site compatibilities: Acyclovir, alfentanil, allopurinol, amifostine, amikacin, aminocaproic acid, aminophylline, amiodarone, amphotericin B liposome, ampicillin, ampicillin-sulbactam, anidulafungin, argatroban, atenolol, atracurium, aztreonam, bivalirudin, bleomycin, bumetanide, buprenorphine, busulfan, butorphanol, calcium chloride/gluconate, CARBOplatin, caspofungin, ceFAZolin, cefepime, cefotaxime, cefoTEtan, cefOXitin, cefTAZidime, ceftizoxime, cefTRIAXone, cefuroxime, chloramphenicol, chlorproMAZINE, cimetidine, ciprofloxacin, cisatracurium, CISplatin, clindamycin, cyclophosphamide, cycloSPORINE, cytarabine, DACTINomycin, DAPTOmycin, dexamethasone, digoxin, diltiazem, DOBUTamine, DOCEtaxel, DOPamine, doripenem, doxacurium, DOXOrubicin, doxycycline, droperidol, enalaprilat, ePHEDrine, EPINEPHrine, epirubicin, eptifibatide, ertapenem, erythromycin, etoposide, famotidine, fenoldopam, fentaNYL, fluconazole, fludarabine, fluorouracil, gallium, ganciclovir, gatifloxacin, gemcitabine, gentamicin, glycopyrrolate, granisetron, haloperidol, heparin, hydrALAZINE, hydrocortisone, HYDROmorphone, IDArubicin, ifosfamide, insulin (regular), irinotecan, isoproterenol, ketorolac, labetalol, levofloxacin, linezolid, LORazepam, magnesium sulfate, mannitol, mechlorethamine, melphalan, meperidine, meropenem, methohexital, methotrexate, methyldopate, methylPREDNISolone, metoclopramide, metoprolol, metroNIDAZOLE, micafungin, midazolam, mitoXANtrone, morphine, mycophenolate, nafcillin, nalbuphine, naloxone, nesiritide, norepinephrine, octreotide, oxacillin, oxaliplatin, oxytocin, PACLitaxel, palonosetron, pamidronate, pancuronium, PEMEtrexed, pentamidine, pentazocine, PENTobarbital, PHENobarbital, phenylephrine, piperacillin, piperacillin-tazobactam, polymyxin B, potassium chloride/phosphates, prochlorperazine, promethazine, propofol, propranolol, quiNIDine, quinupristin-dalfopristin, ranitidine, remifentanil, rocuronium, sodium acetate/bicarbonate/phosphates, streptozocin, succinylcholine, SUFentanil, sulfamethoxazole-trimethoprim, tacrolimus, teniposide, theophylline, thiopental, thiotepa, ticarcillin, ticarcillin-clavulanate, tigecycline, tirofiban, tobramycin, torsemide, vancomycin, vasopressin, vecuronium, verapamil, vinCRIStine, vinorelbine, voriconazole, zidovudine, zoledronic acid

ADVERSE EFFECTS

CV: Dysrhythmias, hypotension, chest pain, PVCs
GI: Nausea, vomiting, anorexia, abdominal pain, **hepatotoxicity,** jaundice
HEMA: Thrombocytopenia
MISC: Headache, hypokalemia, tremor, injection site reactions

Pharmacokinetics

Absorption	Completely absorbed
Distribution	Unknown
Metabolism	Liver (50%)
Excretion	Kidney, unchanged (83%), metabolites (12%)
Half-life	2.4 hr; increased in CHF

Pharmacodynamics

Onset	2-5 min
Peak	10 min
Duration	Variable

INTERACTIONS
Drug classifications
Antihypertensives, diuretics: increased effects

NURSING CONSIDERATIONS
Assessment
• Monitor for hypokalemia: acidic urine, reduced urine, osmolality, nocturia; hypotension, broad T-wave, U-wave, ectopy, tachycardia, weak pulse; muscle weakness, altered LOC, drowsiness, apathy, lethargy, confusion, depression; anorexia, nausea, cramps, constipation, distention, paralytic ileus; hypoventilation, respiratory muscle weakness
• Assess fluid volume status: complete I&O ratio and record; note weight, distended red veins, crackles in lung; color, quality, and specific gravity of urine; skin turgor, adequacy of pulses, moist mucous membranes, bilateral lung sounds, peripheral pitting edema; dehydration symptoms of decreasing output, thirst, hypotension, dry mouth and mucous membranes should be reported
• Monitor electrolytes: potassium, sodium, calcium, magnesium; also include BUN, blood pH, ABGs
⚠ Monitor B/P and pulse, ECG continuously during IV; ventricular dysrhythmia can occur; PCWP, CVP, index often during inf; if B/P drops 30 mm Hg, stop inf and call prescriber
• Monitor ALT, AST, bilirubin daily; if these are elevated, hepatotoxicity is suspected
• Monitor platelets; if <150,000/mm³, product is usually discontinued and another product started
• Assess for extravasation: change site q48hr

Patient/family education
• Teach patient reason for medication and expected results
• Instruct patient to make position changes slowly; orthostatic hypotension may occur
• Teach patient signs and symptoms of hypersensitivity reactions and hypokalemia

Evaluation
Positive therapeutic outcome
• Increased cardiac output
• Decreased PCWP, adequate CVP
• Decreased dyspnea, fatigue, edema, ECG

TREATMENT OF OVERDOSE:
Discontinue product, support circulation

M

minocycline (Rx)
(min-oh-sye′kleen)
Arestin, Dynacin, Minocin, Solodyn
Func. class.: Broad-spectrum antiinfective
Chem. class.: Tetracycline
Pregnancy category D

ACTION: Inhibits protein synthesis and phosphorylation in microorganisms by binding to 30S ribosomal subunits and reversibly binding to 50S ribosomal subunits; bacteriostatic

Therapeutic outcome: Bactericidal action against susceptible organisms, including *Neisseria meningitidis, Neisseria gonorrhoeae, Treponema pallidum, Chlamydia trachomatis, Ureaplasma urealyticum, Mycoplasma pneumoniae, Nocardia, Rickettsia*

USES: Syphilis, chlamydial infection, gonorrhea, lymphogranuloma venereum, rickettsial infections, inflammatory acne, meningitis carriers, periodontitis, methicillin-resistant *Staphylococcus aureus* (MRSA) infections, nonnodular moderate to severe acne vulgaris, *Rickettsia* sp.

Unlabeled uses: Rheumatoid arthritis

CONTRAINDICATIONS:
Pregnancy **D**, hypersensitivity to tetracyclines, children <8 yr

Precautions: Breastfeeding, hepatic disease

DOSAGE AND ROUTES
Adult: PO/IV 200 mg, then 100 mg q12hr, max 400 mg/24 hr **IV;** subgingival insert into periodontal pocket
Child >8 yr: PO/IV 4 mg/kg then 4 mg/kg/day PO in divided doses q12hr

Rickettsial infections
Adult: PO/IV 200 mg, then 100 mg q12hr
Adolescent/child ≥8 yr: PO/IV 4 mg/kg, then 2 mg kg q12hr, max adult dose

Gonorrhea
Adult: PO 200 mg, then 100 mg q12hr × 4 days or more

C. trachomatis infection
Adult: PO 100 mg bid × 7 days

Syphilis
Adult: PO 200 mg, then 100 mg q12hr × 10-15 days

Uncomplicated gonococcal urethritis in men
Adult: PO 100 mg q12hr × 5 days

Rheumatoid arthritis (unlabeled)
Adult: PO 100 mg bid for ≤48 wk

Acne vulgaris (solodyn only)
Adult/adolescent/child ≥12 yr: ext rel 1 mg/kg/day × 12 wk or those weighing 126-136 kg: 135 mg/day; 111-125 kg: 115 mg/day; 97-110 kg: 105 mg/day; 85-96 kg: 90 mg/day; 72-84 kg: 80 mg/day; 60-71 kg: 65 mg/day; 50-59 kg: 55 mg/day; 45-49 kg: 45 mg/day

Acne vulgaris (all except solodyn)
Adult/adolescent/child ≥12 yr: ext rel 1 mg/kg × 12 wk or 91-136 kg/135 mg/day; 60-90 kg 90 mg/day; 45-59 kg 45 mg/day

Available forms: Caps 50, 75, 100 mg; powder for inj 100 mg; pellet-filled caps 50, 100 mg; tabs 50, 75, 100 mg; ext rel tabs 45, 55, 65, 80, 90, 105, 115, 135 mg

Implementation
• Store in airtight, light-resistant container at room temp
PO route
• Give around the clock to maintain proper blood levels; give with food to increase absorption of product; do not give within 3 hr of other agents; product interactions may occur
• Give with 8 oz of water 1 hr before bedtime to prevent ulceration
• Shake liquid preparation well before giving; use calibrated device for proper dosing
• Do not give with iron, calcium, magnesium products, or antacids, which decrease absorption and form insoluble chelate

IV route
• Check for irritation, extravasation, phlebitis daily; change site q72hr
• For intermittent inf, dilute each 100 mg/10 ml of 0.9% NaCl, sterile water for inj; further dilute in 500-1000 ml of 0.9% NaCl, D₅W, Ringer's, LR, D₅/LR; give over 6 hr

Y-site compatibilities: Alfentanil, amikacin, atracurium, benztropine, bretylium, buprenorphine, butorphanol, calcium chloride, CARBOplatin, caspofungin, cefonicid, chlorproMAZINE, cimetidine, codeine, cyclophosphamide, cycloSPORINE, cytarabine, DACTINomycin, dexmedetomidine, diltiazem, diphenhydrAMINE, DOBUTamine, DOCEtaxel, doxacurium, doxycycline, enalaprilat, ePHEDrine, EPINEPHrine, eptifibatide, etoposide, fenoldopam, fentaNYL, fludarabine, gatifloxacin, gemcitabine, gentamicin, glycopyrrolate, granisetron, heparin, hetastarch, IDArubicin, ifosfamide, inamrinone, isoproterenol, labetalol, levofloxacin, lidocaine, linezolid, LORazepam, magnesium sulfate, mannitol, melphalan, metaraminol, methotrexate, methyldopa, metoclopramide, metoprolol, midazolam, mito-XANtrone, nalbuphine, naloxone, perphenazine, potassium chloride, sargramostim, sodium succinate, vinorelbine, vit B/C

Y-site incompatibilities: Aztreonam, filgrastim, HYDROmorphone, meperidine, morphine, teniposide

ADVERSE EFFECTS
CNS: *Dizziness,* fever, light-headedness, vertigo, seizures, **increased intracranial pressure**
CV: Pericarditis
EENT: Dysphagia, glossitis, decreased calcification, permanent discoloration of teeth, oral candidiasis
GI: *Nausea,* abdominal pain, *vomiting, diarrhea,* anorexia, enterocolitis, **hepatotoxicity,** flatulence, abdominal cramps, epigastric burning, stomatitis, **pseudomembranous colitis**
GU: Increased BUN, polyuria, polydipsia, **renal failure, nephrotoxicity**
HEMA: **Eosinophilia, neutropenia, thrombocytopenia, hemolytic anemia,** pancytopenia
INTEG: *Rash, urticaria, photosensitivity, increased pigmentation,* **exfoliative dermatitis,** pruritus, blue-gray color of skin and mucous membranes
MS: Myalgia, arthritis, bone discoloration, joint stiffness
SYST: **Angioedema, Stevens-Johnson syndrome**

Pharmacokinetics
Absorption	Well absorbed (PO)
Distribution	Widely distributed (70%-75% protein bound); some distribution in CSF, crosses placenta
Metabolism	Liver, some
Excretion	Kidneys, unchanged (20%), bile, feces
Half-life	11-17 hr

Pharmacodynamics
	PO	IV
Onset	Rapid	Rapid
Peak	2-3 hr	Infusion's end
Duration	Unknown	Unknown

INTERACTIONS
Individual drugs
Calcium: forms chelates, decreased absorption
CarBAMazepine, phenytoin: decreased effect
Digoxin: increased effect
Insulin: increased effect
Kaolin/pectin, sodium bicarbonate, cimetidine, quinapril, sucralfate, iron: decreased minocycline effect
Theophylline: increased effect
Warfarin: increased effect

Drug classifications
Alkali products, antacids: decreased minocycline effect
Anticoagulants (oral neuromuscular blockers): increased effect
Barbiturates, penicillins: decreased effect
Oral contraceptives: decreased effect of oral contraception
Retinoids: increased chance of pseudomotor cerebri, do not use concurrently

Drug/lab test
False negative: urine glucose with Clinistix, Tes-Tape

NURSING CONSIDERATIONS
Assessment
• Assess patient for previous sensitivity reaction
• **Assess patient for signs and symptoms of infection** including characteristics of wounds, sputum, urine, stool, WBC >10,000/mm³, fever; obtain baseline information before, during treatment
• Obtain C&S before beginning product therapy to identify if correct treatment has been initiated
• **Assess for allergic reactions:** rash, urticaria, pruritus, angioedema
• Monitor blood studies: AST, ALT, CBC, Hct, bilirubin, alkaline phosphatase, amylase monthly if patient is on long-term therapy
• **Pseudomembranous colitis:** assess bowel pattern daily; if severe diarrhea occurs, product should be discontinued
• Monitor for bleeding: ecchymosis, bleeding gums, hematuria, stool guaiac daily if on long-term therapy; blood dyscrasias may occur
• **Assess for overgrowth of infection:** perineal itching, fever, malaise, redness, pain, swelling, drainage, rash, diarrhea, change in cough, sputum; black, furry tongue

Patient/family education
• Teach patient to use sunscreen when outdoors to decrease photosensitivity reaction

M

- Teach patient to report sore throat, bruising, bleeding, joint pain; may indicate blood dyscrasias (rare)
- Advise patient to contact prescriber if vaginal itching, loose foul-smelling stools, furry tongue occur; may indicate superinfection; report itching, rash, pruritus, urticaria
- Instruct patient to take all medication prescribed for the length of time ordered; product must be taken around the clock to maintain blood levels; do not give medication to others; take with a full glass of water; may take with food; not to use outdated product, Fanconi's syndrome may occur
- Advise patient to use a form of contraception other than hormonal

Evaluation
Positive therapeutic outcome
- Absence of signs/symptoms of infection (WBC <10,000/mm^3, temp WNL, absence of red, draining wounds)
- Reported improvement in symptoms of infection

minoxidil (Rx, OTC)
(mi-nox′i-dill)
Rogaine (TOP)
Func. class.: Antihypertensive, hair growth stimulant
Chem. class.: Vasodilator, peripheral
Pregnancy category C

Do not confuse:
minoxidil/Monopril

ACTION: Directly relaxes arteriolar smooth muscle, causing vasodilatation; reduces peripheral vascular resistance, decreases B/P; increased cutaneous blood flow; stimulation of hair follicles

Therapeutic outcome: Decreased B/P in hypertension; hair growth

USES: Severe hypertension unresponsive to other therapy (use with diuretic and β-blocker); topically to treat alopecia, anal fissures

CONTRAINDICATIONS:
Dissecting aortic aneurysm, hypersensitivity, pheochromocytoma

> **BLACK BOX WARNING:** Acute MI

Precautions: Pregnancy C, breastfeeding, children, geriatric, renal disease, CVD

> **BLACK BOX WARNING:** CAD, CHF, cardiac disease, cardiac tamponade, edema, hypotension, orthostatic hypotension, pericardial effusion

DOSAGE AND ROUTES
Severe hypertension
Adult: PO 2.5-5 mg/day in 1-2 divided doses, max 100 mg/day; usual range 10-40 mg/day in single doses
Geriatric: PO 2.5 mg/day, may be increased gradually
Child <12 yr: PO initial 0.1-0.2 mg/kg/day; effective range, 0.25-1 mg/kg/day; max, 50 mg/day

Alopecia
Adult: TOP 1 ml bid, rub into scalp daily, max 2 ml/day

Renal dose
Adult: PO CCr 10-15 ml/min extend interval to q24hr; CCr <10 ml/min not recommended

Anal fissures (unlabeled)
Adult/adolescent: TOP (0.5% minoxidil in white paraffin base) 0.5 g each compounded minoxidil and lignocaine ointment q8hr

Available forms: Tabs 2.5, 10 mg; topical 2%, 5% sol, topical foam 5%

Implementation
PO route
- Administer without regard to meals
- Give with β-blockers and/or diuretic for hypertension
- Store protected from light and heat
Topical route
- Administer 1 ml dose no matter how much balding has occurred; increasing dose does not speed hair growth
- Treatment must continue long term or new hair will be lost again

ADVERSE EFFECTS
Systemic
CNS: Headache, fatigue
CV: *Severe rebound hypertension (on withdrawal in children)*, tachycardia, angina, increased T-wave, **CHF, pulmonary edema, pericardial effusion**, edema, sodium retention, water retention, *hypotension*
GI: Nausea, vomiting
GU: Breast tenderness

HEMA: Hct, Hgb, erythrocyte count may decrease initially, leukopenia
INTEG: Pruritus, **Stevens-Johnson syndrome,** rash, hirsutism, contact dermatitis

Pharmacokinetics

Absorption	Well absorbed (PO); minimally absorbed (topical)
Distribution	Widely distributed, protein binding minimal
Metabolism	Liver
Excretion	Kidneys, breast milk
Half-life	4.2 hr

Pharmacodynamics

	PO	Topical
Onset	½ hr	4 mo
Peak	2-3 hr	Unknown
Duration	75 hr	4 mo

INTERACTIONS

Individual
Guanethidine, nitroprusside: increased hypotension

Drug classifications
Antihypertensives, MAOIs, nitrates: increased hypotension
Estrogens, NSAIDs, salicylates: decreased antihypertensive effect

Drug/herb
Hawthorn: increased antihypertensive effect

Drug/lab test
Increased: renal function tests
Decreased: Hgb, Hct, RBC

NURSING CONSIDERATIONS

Assessment
⚠ **Monitor closely; usually given with β-blocker to prevent tachycardia and increased myocardial workload; usually given with diuretic to prevent serious fluid accumulation; patient should be hospitalized during beginning treatment**
• Monitor B/P, pulse, jugular venous distention periodically throughout treatment
• Monitor electrolytes, blood studies: potassium, sodium, chloride, CBC, serum glucose
⚠ **Monitor weight daily, I&O; assess edema in feet, legs daily; check skin turgor, dryness of mucous membranes for hydration status**
• Assess for crackles, dyspnea, orthopnea, peripheral edema, fatigue, weight gain, jugular vein distention (CHF)

• Assess for signs of hyperglycemia: acetone breath, increased urinary output, severe thirst, lethargy, dizziness

Patient/family education
Topical route
• Teach patient that new hair will be soft and hardly visible, use on clean, dry scalp before styling aids, wash hands after each use
• Caution patient not to use on other parts of the body; product is to be used on the scalp only
• Instruct patient that hair should be clean before applying medication; do not get on clothing
• Caution patient not to get medication near mucous membranes (mouth, nose, eyes) and to contact prescriber if burning, stinging, or rash occurs

Evaluation
Positive therapeutic outcome
• Decreased B/P in hypertension
• Hair growth (TOP)

---

mirabegron
(mir'a-beg'ron)
Myrbetriq
Func. class.: Bladder antispasmodic
Chem. class.: β_2-Adrenergic receptor agonist
Pregnancy category C

ACTION: Relaxes smooth muscles in urinary tract

Therapeutic outcome: Decreasing dysuria, frequency, nocturia, incontinence

USES: Overactive bladder (urinary frequency, urgency), urinary incontinence

CONTRAINDICATIONS:
Hypersensitivity

Precautions: Pregnancy (C), breastfeeding, children, kidney/liver disease, bladder obstruction, dialysis, hypertension

DOSAGE AND ROUTES
Adult: PO 25 mg/day, may increase to 50 mg/day if needed

Hepatic/renal dose
Adult: PO Child–Pugh B or (CCr 15-29 ml/min, max 25 mg/day; Child–Pugh C or CCr 15 ml/min, not recommended

Available forms: Tabs ext rel 25, 50 mg

Adverse effects: *italics* = common; **bold** = life-threatening

Implementation
• Give whole; take with liquids; do not crush, chew, or break ext rel product; use without regard to meals

ADVERSE EFFECTS
CNS: Fatigue, dizziness, headache
CV: Hypertension
EENT: Xerophthalmia, blurred vision
GI: Nausea, vomiting, anorexia, abdominal pain, constipation, diarrhea, dyspepsia
GU: Dysuria, urinary retention, frequency, UTI, bladder discomfort
INTEG: Rash, pruritus
MISC: Arthralgia, back pain
RESP: Pharyngitis
SYST: Stevens–Johnson syndrome

Pharmacokinetics

Absorption	Unknown
Distribution	71% protein binding
Metabolism	Unknown
Excretion	25% unchanged in urine
Half-life	Terminal 50 hr

Pharmacodynamics

Onset	Unknown
Peak	3.5 hr
Duration	Unknown

INTERACTIONS
Individual drugs
Digoxin, warfarin, desipramine, thioridazine, flecainide, propafenone: increased effect of these agents

Drug classifications
Antimuscarinic agents (e.g., atropine, scopolamine): increased risk of urinary retention

NURSING CONSIDERATIONS
Assessment
• Urinary patterns: Assess for distention, nocturia, frequency, urgency, incontinence
• Monitor LFTs at baseline, periodically
• Monitor B/P

Patient/family education
• Teach patient to avoid hazardous activities; dizziness can occur
• Advise patient not to drink liquids before bedtime
• Inform patient about the importance of bladder maintenance

Evaluation
Positive therapeutic outcome
• Decreasing dysuria, frequency, nocturia, incontinence

---

mirtazapine (Rx)
(mer-ta′za-peen)
Remeron, Remeron Soltab
Func. class.: Antidepressant
Chem. class.: Tetracyclic
Pregnancy category C

ACTION: Blocks reuptake of norepinephrine, serotonin into nerve endings, increasing action of norepinephrine, serotonin in nerve cells; antagonist of central α_2-receptors, blocks histamine receptors; has anticholinergic action

Therapeutic outcome: Decreased symptoms of depression after 2-3 wk

USES: Depression, dysthymic disorder, bipolar disorder: depression, agitated depression

CONTRAINDICATIONS:
Hypersensitivity to tricyclics, recovery phase of MI, agranulocytosis, jaundice

Precautions: Pregnancy C, geriatric, suicidal patients, severe depression, increased intraocular pressure, closed-angle glaucoma, urinary retention, cardiac/renal/hepatic disease, hypo/hyperthyroidism, electroshock therapy, elective surgery, seizure disorder, bone marrow suppression, thrombocytopenia

> **BLACK BOX WARNING:** Suicidal ideation, children

DOSAGE AND ROUTES
Adult: PO 15 mg/day at bedtime, maintenance to continue for 6 mo, titrate up to 45 mg/day; orally disintegrating tabs open blister pack, place tab on tongue, allow to disintegrate, swallow
Geriatric: PO 7.5 mg nightly, increase by 7.5 mg q1-2wk to desired dose, max 45 mg/day

Available forms: Tabs 15, 30, 45 mg; orally disintegrating tabs (Soltab) 15, 30, 45 mg

Implementation
• Administer without regard to meals; crush if patient is unable to swallow medication whole
• Give dose at bedtime if oversedation occurs during day; may take entire dose at bedtime; geriatric may not tolerate once/day dosing

---

🛆 Nurse Alert   ✳ Key NCLEX® Drug

- Store in tight container at room temperature; do not freeze
- Allow **orally disintegrating tablets** to dissolve on tongue; no water needed; do not split; contain phenylalanine
- **Serotonin syndrome, neuroleptic malignant syndrome:** assess for increased heart rate, shivering, sweating, dilated pupils, tremors, high B/P, hyperthermia, headache, confusion; if these occur, stop product, administer a serotonin antagonist if needed; at least 2 wk should elapse between discontinuation of serotoninergic agents and start of this product

ADVERSE EFFECTS

CNS: *Dizziness, drowsiness,* confusion, headache, anxiety, tremors, stimulation, weakness, nightmares, EPS (geriatric), increased psychiatric symptoms, **seizures**
CV: *Orthostatic hypotension, ECG changes, tachycardia, hypertension,* palpitations
EENT: *Blurred vision,* tinnitus, mydriasis
GI: *Diarrhea, dry mouth,* nausea, vomiting, **paralytic ileus,** increased appetite, cramps, epigastric distress, **jaundice, hepatitis,** stomatitis, constipation, weight gain
GU: *Retention,* **acute renal failure,** urinary frequency
HEMA: Agranulocytosis, thrombocytopenia, eosinophilia, leukopenia
INTEG: Rash, urticaria, sweating, pruritus, photosensitivity
MS: Back pain, myalgia
RESP: Cough
SYST: Flulike symptoms, increased lipid levels

Pharmacokinetics

Absorption	Slow, complete
Distribution	Widely distributed; crosses placenta
Metabolism	Liver, extensively
Excretion	Feces; breast milk
Half-life	20-40 hr

Pharmacodynamics

Onset	Unknown
Peak	2 hr
Duration	Unknown

INTERACTIONS

Individual drugs
Alcohol: increased CNS depression
CloNIDine: decreased effects
Fenfluramine, dexfenfluramine, sibutramine, nefazodone: increased serotonin syndrome

Drug classifications
Barbiturates, benzodiazepines, CNS depressants (other): increased effects
MAOIs: hypertensive episode, seizures, hyperpyretic crisis
Sympathomimetics, indirect acting (ePHEDrine): decreased effects
SSRIs, SNRIs, serotonin-receptor agonists: increased serotonin syndrome

Drug/herb
Kava: increased CNS depression
St. John's wort, SAM-e: serotonin syndrome

Drug/lab test
Increased: serum bilirubin, blood glucose, alkaline phosphatase
Decreased: VMA, 5-HIAA
False increase: urinary catecholamines

NURSING CONSIDERATIONS

Assessment
- Monitor B/P (with patient lying, standing), pulse q4hr during beginning treatment; if systolic B/P drops 20 mm Hg, hold product, notify prescriber; take VS q4hr in patients with CV disease
- Monitor blood studies: CBC, leukocytes, differential, cardiac enzymes if patient is receiving long-term therapy, LFTs, serum creatinine/BUN
- Monitor liver function tests: AST, ALT, bilirubin
- Check weight weekly; product may increase appetite
- ⚠ Assess ECG for flattening of T-wave, bundle branch block, AV block, dysrhythmias in cardiac patients
- Assess for EPS primarily in geriatric: rigidity, dystonia, akathisia
- Assess mental status: mood, sensorium, affect, suicidal tendencies; assess increase in psychiatric symptoms: depression, panic
- Identify alcohol consumption; if alcohol is consumed, hold dose until AM

Patient/family education
- Inform patient that therapeutic effects may take 2-3 wk; take at bedtime, do not discontinue abruptly
- Advise patient to use caution in driving and other activities requiring alertness because of drowsiness, dizziness, blurred vision; to avoid rising quickly from sitting to standing, especially geriatric
- Caution patient to avoid alcohol ingestion, other CNS depressants
- Teach patient to increase fluids, bulk in diet if constipation, urinary retention occur, especially geriatric

• Teach patient to use gum, hard sugarless candy, or frequent sips of water for dry mouth
• Advise not to use within 14 days of MAOIs

> **BLACK BOX WARNING:** Notify prescriber of suicidal thoughts, behavior

Evaluation
Positive therapeutic outcome
• Decrease in depression
• Absence of suicidal thoughts

TREATMENT OF OVERDOSE:
ECG monitoring, lavage, activated charcoal, administer anticonvulsant

---

misoprostol (Rx)
(mye-soe-prost'ole)
Cytotec
Func. class.: Gastric mucosa protectant; antiulcer
Chem. class.: Prostaglandin E₁ analog
Pregnancy category X

Do not confuse:
misoprostol/metoprolol, **Cytotec**/Cytoxan

ACTION: Inhibits gastric acid secretion; may protect gastric mucosa; can increase bicarbonate, mucus production

Therapeutic outcome: Prevention of gastric ulcers

USES: Prevention of NSAID-induced gastric ulcers

CONTRAINDICATIONS:
Hypersensitivity to this product or prostaglandins

> **BLACK BOX WARNING:** Pregnancy **X**, females

Precautions: Breastfeeding, children, geriatric, renal disease, CV disease, abnormal fetal position, cardiac/renal/inflammatory bowel disease, C-section, dehydration, diarrhea, fever, ectopic pregnancy, fetal distress, sepsis, vaginal bleeding

DOSAGE AND ROUTES
Adult: PO 200 mcg qid with food for duration of NSAID therapy with last dose at bedtime; if 200 mcg is not tolerated, 100 mcg may be given

Available forms: Tabs 100, 200 mcg

Implementation
• Give with meals for prolonged product effect; avoid use of magnesium antacids
• Store at room temp

ADVERSE EFFECTS
GI: *Diarrhea*, nausea, vomiting, flatulence, constipation, dyspepsia, abdominal pain
GU: Spotting, cramps, hypermenorrhea, menstrual disorders

Pharmacokinetics
Absorption	Well absorbed
Distribution	Unknown
Metabolism	Liver
Excretion	Kidneys
Half-life	½-1 hr

Pharmacodynamics
Onset	½ hr
Peak	Unknown
Duration	3 hr

INTERACTIONS
Drug/food
Maximum concentrations when taken with food

NURSING CONSIDERATIONS
Assessment
• **NSAID-induced ulcer prophylaxis:** monitor patient for GI symptoms: hematemesis, occult or frank blood in stools, also severe abdominal pain, cramping, severe diarrhea

> **BLACK BOX WARNING:** Pregnancy **X**: obtain a negative pregnancy test in women of childbearing age before starting medication; miscarriages are common

Patient/family education
• Advise patient to avoid black pepper, caffeine, alcohol, harsh spices, extremes in temperature of food, which may aggravate condition
• Caution patient to avoid OTC preparations: aspirin, cough, cold preparations; condition may worsen
• Teach patient that product must be continued for prescribed time to be effective and taken exactly as prescribed; doses are not to be doubled
• Instruct patient to report to prescriber diarrhea, black tarry stools, abdominal pain, cramping, menstrual disorders

> **BLACK BOX WARNING:** Caution patient to prevent pregnancy while taking this product; spontaneous abortion may occur, pregnancy **X**

⚠ Nurse Alert   ✴ Key NCLEX® Drug

Evaluation

Positive therapeutic outcome
• Prevention of ulcers

⚠ HIGH ALERT

mitoMYcin (Rx)
(mye-toe-mye′sin)
Mitosyl
Func. class.: Antineoplastic, antibiotic
Pregnancy category D

Do not confuse:
mitoMYcin/mithramycin/mitotane/mitoXANtrone

ACTION: Inhibits DNA synthesis, primarily; derived from *Streptomyces caespitosus;* appears to cause cross-linking of DNA; a vesicant

Therapeutic outcome: Prevention of rapidly growing malignant cells

USES: Pancreas, stomach, colorectal, bladder cancer

CONTRAINDICATIONS:
Pregnancy **D** (1st trimester), breastfeeding, hypersensitivity, as a single agent, coagulation disorders

BLACK BOX WARNING: Thrombocytopenia

Precautions: Accidental exposure, acute bronchospasm, anemia, children, dental disease/work, extravasation, females, hemolytic-uremic syndrome, infection, radiation therapy, surgery, vaccines, renal/respiratory disease

BLACK BOX WARNING: Bone marrow suppression, hemolytic uremic syndrome

DOSAGE AND ROUTES
Adult: **IV** 10-20 mg/m^2 q6-8wk

Available forms: Inj 5, 20, 40 mg/vial

Implementation

Direct IV route
• Use cytotoxic handling procedures
• Give antiemetic 30-60 min before product to prevent vomiting
• Use port or central line if possible, product is very irritating to tissues
• Reconstitute 5 mg/10 ml; 20 mg/40 ml; 40 mg/80 ml of sterile water for injection (0.5 mg/ml); shake to dissolve, let stand until completely dissolved; stable for 1 wk at room temperature,

2 wk refrigerated, can be further diluted to 20-40 mcg/ml
• Inject reconstituted injection slowly over 5-10 min **IV** push into free-flowing **IV** infusion of 0.9% NaCl or D$_5$W
• Avoid excessive heat, store reconstituted product in refrigerator, discard after 2 wk, store unreconstituted product at room temp

Syringe compatibilities: Bleomycin, CISplatin, cyclophosphamide, DOXOrubicin, droperidol, fluorouracil, furosemide, heparin, leucovorin, methotrexate, metoclopramide, vinBLAStine, vinCRIStine

Y-site compatibilities: Allopurinol, amifostine, amphotericin B lipid complex, amphotericin B liposome, anidulafungin, argatroban, atenolol, bivalirudin, bleomycin, caspofungin, CISplatin, cyclophosphamide, DACTINomycin, dolasetron, DOXOrubicin, droperidol, epirubicin, ertapenem, fluorouracil, furosemide, granisetron, heparin, leucovorin, melphalan, methotrexate, metoclopramide, nesiritide, octreotide, ondansetron, oxaliplatin, PACLitaxel, palonosetron, PEMEtrexed, riTUXimab, teniposide, thiotepa, tigecycline, tirofiban, trastuzumab, vinBLAStine, vinCRIStine, voriconazole, zoledronic acid

Y-site incompatibilities: Sargramostim, vinorelbine

ADVERSE EFFECTS
CNS: Fever, headache, confusion, drowsiness, syncope, fatigue
EENT: Blurred vision
GI: *Nausea, vomiting, anorexia, stomatitis,* **hepatotoxicity,** diarrhea
GU: Urinary retention, **renal failure,** edema
HEMA: **Thrombocytopenia, leukopenia, anemia**
INTEG: *Rash,* alopecia, **extravasation,** nail discoloration
MISC: **Hemolytic uremic syndrome, CHF**
RESP: **Fibrosis, pulmonary infiltrate,** dyspnea

Pharmacokinetics

Absorption	Complete bioavailability
Distribution	Widely distributed; concentrates in tumor
Metabolism	Liver, extensively
Excretion	Kidneys, unchanged
Half-life	1 hr

Pharmacodynamics

Unknown

Adverse effects: *italics* = common; **bold** = life-threatening

INTERACTIONS
Individual drugs
Radiation: increased toxicity

Drug classifications
Anticoagulants, NSAIDs: increased bleeding risk
Antineoplastics: increased toxicity
Vaccines: avoid concurrent use

Drug/herb
Black cohosh: avoid use

NURSING CONSIDERATIONS
Assessment

> **BLACK BOX WARNING:** Assess for fatal hemolytic uremic syndrome: hypertension, thrombocytopenia, microangiopathic hemolytic anemia; occurs during long-term therapy

• Assess buccal cavity q8hr for dryness, sores or ulceration, white patches, oral pain, bleeding, dysphagia; obtain prescription for viscous lidocaine (Xylocaine)
• Assess symptoms indicating severe allergic reaction: rash, pruritus, urticaria, purpuric skin lesions, itching, flushing

> **BLACK BOX WARNING:** Bone marrow suppression: Monitor CBC, differential, platelet count weekly; withhold product if WBC is <4000/mm³ or platelet count is <100,000/mm³ or serum creatinine >1.7 mg/dl; notify prescriber; bleeding: hematuria, guaiac, bruising, petechiae, mucosa, or orifices

• Monitor renal function tests: BUN, creatinine, serum uric acid, urine CCr before, during therapy; check I&O ratio; report fall in urine output to <30 ml/hr; adjust dose based on renal function
⚠ Assess for pulmonary fibrosis, bronchospasm, dyspnea, crackles, unproductive cough, chest pain, tachypnea, fatigue, increased pulse, pallor, lethargy
• Monitor temp q4hr (may indicate beginning of infection)
• Monitor liver function tests before, during therapy (bilirubin, AST, ALT, LDH) as needed or monthly; check for jaundiced skin and sclera, dark urine, clay-colored stools, itchy skin, abdominal pain, fever, diarrhea
• Assess for bleeding: hematuria, stool guaiac, bruising or petechiae, mucosa or orifices q8hr
• Identify effects of alopecia on body image; discuss feelings about body changes
• Identify edema in feet, joint pain, stomach pain, shaking; check for inflammation of mucosa, breaks in skin

Patient/family education
• Advise patient to get adequate fluids 2-3 L/day unless contraindicated
• Encourage patient to rinse mouth tid-qid with water, club soda, brush teeth bid-qid with soft brush or cotton-tipped applicators for stomatitis, use unwaxed dental floss
• Teach patient to avoid use of products containing aspirin or ibuprofen, razors, commercial mouthwash, since bleeding may occur; to report symptoms of bleeding (hematuria, tarry stools)
• Caution patient to report signs of anemia (fatigue, headache, irritability, faintness, shortness of breath)
• Advise patient to report any changes in breathing or coughing even several mo after treatment; to avoid crowds and persons with respiratory tract or other infections
⚠ Teach patient to report signs of IV site reaction, redness, inflammation, burning, pain
• Inform patient that hair may be lost during treatment; a wig or hairpiece may make patient feel better; new hair may be different in color, texture
⚠ Infection: teach patient to report fever, flulike symptoms, sore throat
• Advise patient not to have any vaccinations without the advice of the prescriber; serious reactions can occur
• Teach patient that contraception is needed during treatment and for several mo after completion of therapy
• Teach patient to report immediately urine retention, absence of urine, dyspnea, bleeding, jaundice, **signs of pulmonary toxicity**

Evaluation
Positive therapeutic outcome
• Prevention of rapid division of malignant cells

> **⚠ HIGH ALERT**
>
> ## mitoXANtrone (Rx)
> (mye-toe-zan′trone)
> **Novantrone**
> *Func. class.:* Antineoplastic-antibiotic, immunomodulator
> *Chem. class.:* Synthetic anthraquinone
> **Pregnancy category D**

Do not confuse:
mitoXANtrone/mitoMYcin/mithramycin/mitotane

ACTION: DNA reactive agent; cytocidal effect on both proliferating and nonproliferating cells; topoisomerase II inhibitor; a vesicant

Therapeutic outcome: Prevention of rapidly growing malignant cells

USES: Acute myelogenous leukemia (adult), relapsed leukemia, breast cancer, multiple sclerosis; used with steroids to treat bone pain (advanced prostate cancer); multiple sclerosis

Unlabeled uses: Liver malignancies, non-Hodgkin's lymphoma, breast cancer, ALL, bone marrow ablation, CLL, hepatocellular cancer, ovarian cancer, pleural effusion, stem cell transplant preparation

CONTRAINDICATIONS:
Pregnancy **D**, hypersensitivity

Precautions: Breastfeeding, children, myelosuppression, cardiac/renal/hepatic disease, gout

> **BLACK BOX WARNING:** Secondary malignancy, neutropenia, intrathecal administration, extravasation, heart failure

DOSAGE AND ROUTES
Acute nonlymphatic leukemia/induction
Adult: IV INF 12 mg/m^2/day on days 1-3, and 100 mg/m^2 cytosine arabinoside × 7 days as a CONT 24-hr INF

Consolidation
Adult: IV INF 12 mg/m^2 given as a short 5-15 min INF for 2 days with cytarabine × 5 days

Advanced prostate cancer
Adult: IV 12-14 mg/m^2 as a single dose or short INF q21day

Multiple sclerosis, relapsing
Adult: IV INF 12 mg/m^2 as a 5-15 min INF q3mo, cumulative lifetime dose 140 mg/m^2

Available forms: Inj 2, 10, 12.5, 15 mg/ml

Implementation
⚠ Do not mix with any other product
• Avoid contact with skin, since medication is very irritating; wash completely to remove
• Give fluids IV or PO before chemotherapy to hydrate patient
• Give antacid before oral agent; give product after evening meal, before bedtime; provide antiemetic 30-60 min before giving product and prn to prevent vomiting; administer antibiotics for prophylaxis of infection
• Give topical or systemic analgesics for pain
• Liquid diet: carbonated beverages; gelatin may be added if patient is not nauseated or vomiting
• Sol should be prepared by qualified personnel only under controlled conditions in a biological cabinet using mask, gloves, gown
• Use Luer-Lok tubing to prevent leakage; do not let sol come in contact with skin; if contact occurs, wash well with soap and water

Direct IV route
• Give after diluting with 50 ml or more of 0.9% NaCl or D$_5$W; give over 3-5 min into running IV of D$_5$W or 0.9% NaCl
Intermittent IV infusion route
• May be diluted further in D$_5$W, 0.9% NaCl and run over 15-30 min; check for extravasation
Continuous IV infusion route
• Give over 24 hr

Y-site compatibilities: Acyclovir, alemtuzumab, alfentanil, allopurinol, amikacin, aminocaproic acid, aminophylline, amiodarone, anidulafungin, argatroban, atracurium, bivalirudin, bleomycin, bretylium, bumetanide, buprenorphine, butorphanol, calcium chloride, calcium gluconate, CARBOplatin, carmustine, caspofungin, cefoTEtan, ceftizoxime, chloramphenicol, chlorproMAZINE, cimetidine, ciprofloxacin, cisatracurium, CISplatin, cladribine, codeine, cyclophosphamide, cycloSPORINE, cytarabine, DACTINomycin, DAPTOmycin, DAUNOrubicin citrate liposome, dexmedetomidine, dexrazoxane, diltiazem, diphenhydrAMINE, DOBUTamine, DOCEtaxel, dolasetron, DOPamine, doxacurium, doxycycline, droperidol, enalaprilat, ePHEDrine, EPINEPHrine, erythromycin l, esmolol, etoposide, etoposide phosphate, famotidine, fenoldopam, fentaNYL, filgrastim, fluconazole, fludarabine, fluorouracil, ganciclovir, gatifloxacin, gemcitabine, gentamicin, glycopyrrolate, granisetron, haloperidol, hydrALAZINE, hydrocortisone sodium succinate, HYDROmorphone, hydrOXYzine, ifosfamide, imipenem-cilastatin, inamrinone, insulin, regular, irinotecan, isoproterenol, ketorolac, labetalol, leucovorin, levofloxacin, levorphanol, lidocaine, linezolid, LORazepam, magnesium sulfate, mannitol, melphalan, meperidine, meropenem, mesna, metaraminol, methohexital, methotrexate, methyldopate, metoclopramide, metoprolol, metroNIDAZOLE, midazolam, milrinone, minocycline, mivacurium, morphine sulfate, nalbuphine, naloxone, nesiritide, niCARdipine, nitroglycerin, norepinephrine, octreotide, ondansetron, oxaliplatin, palonosetron, pamidronate, pancuronium, pentamidine, pentazocine, PENTobarbital, PHENobarbital, phentolamine, phenylephrine, polymyxin B, potassium acetate, potassium chloride, procainamide, prochlorperazine, promethazine hydrochloride, propranolol, quiNIDine gluconate, quinupristin-dalfopristin, ranitidine, remifentanil, riTUXimab, rocuronium, sargramostim, sodium acetate, sodium bicarbonate, succinylcholine, SUFentanil, sulfamethoxazole-trimethoprim, tacrolimus, teniposide, theophylline, thiopental, thiotepa, tigecycline, tirofiban, tobramycin, tolazoline, trastuzumab, trimethobenzamide, vancomycin, vasopressin, vecuronium, verapamil, vinCRIStine, vinorelbine, zidovudine, zoledronic acid

Y-site incompatibilities: PACLitaxel

Additive compatibilities: Cyclophosphamide, cytarabine, fluorouracil, hydrocortisone, potassium chloride

Additive incompatibilities: Heparin

Solution compatibilities: D_5/0.9 NaCl, D_5W, 0.9% NaCl

ADVERSE EFFECTS

CNS: Headache, **seizures**, fatigue
CV: CHF, cardiomyopathy, dysrhythmias
EENT: Conjunctivitis, blue-green sclera, blurred vision
GI: *Nausea, vomiting, diarrhea, anorexia, mucositis, hepatotoxicity*, abdominal pain, constipation, jaundice
GU: Amenorrhea, menstrual disorders
HEMA: Thrombocytopenia, leukopenia, myelosuppression, anemia, secondary leukemia
INTEG: *Rash, necrosis at inj site*, alopecia, dermatitis, thrombophlebitis at inj site
MISC: Fever, hyperuricemia, infections
RESP: Cough, dyspnea
SYST: Tumor lysis syndrome, sepsis

Pharmacokinetics

Absorption	Completely absorbed
Distribution	Widely distributed, protein binding 78%
Metabolism	Liver
Excretion	Bile; kidneys, unchanged ($<10\%$)
Half-life	23-215 hr

Pharmacodynamics

Unknown

INTERACTIONS
Individual drugs
Digoxin, phenytoin: increased mitoXANtrone effects
Radiation: increased toxicity, bone marrow suppression
Trastuzumab: increased adverse reactions

Drug classifications
Anticoagulants, NSAIDs: increased bleeding risk
Antineoplastics: increased toxicity, bone marrow suppression
Live virus vaccines: increased adverse reactions

Drug/herb
Black cohosh, dong quai: avoid use

Drug/lab test
Increased: LFTs, uric acid
Decreased: Hct/Hgb, platelets, WBC

NURSING CONSIDERATIONS
Assessment
• **Multiple sclerosis:** obtain baseline multigated angiogram, left ventricular ejection fraction (LVEF) if symptoms of CHF occur, repeat LVEF or if cumulative dose is >100 mg/m²; do not administer to patients who have received a lifetime dose of ≥140 mg/m² or if LVEF is $<50\%$ or significant decrease in LVEF
• Do not administer in multiple sclerosis if neutrophils <1500/mm³
• Obtain pregnancy test in all women of childbearing age

> **BLACK BOX WARNING:** Monitor ECG; watch for ST-T wave changes, low QRS and T, possible dysrhythmias (sinus tachycardia, heart block, PVCs); also monitor ECHO, MUGA, chest x-ray, RAI angiography to assess ejection fraction before, during treatment; product is cardiotoxic: may develop during treatment or months to years after treatment

• Assess buccal cavity q8hr for dryness, sores or ulceration, white patches, oral pain, bleeding, dysphagia; obtain prescription for viscous lidocaine (Xylocaine)
• **Assess symptoms indicating severe allergic reaction:** rash, pruritus, urticaria, purpuric skin lesions, itching, flushing
• Assess tachypnea, ECG changes, dyspnea, edema, fatigue
• Monitor CBC, differential, platelet count weekly; withhold product if WBC is <1500/mm³; leukopenia, neutropenia, thrombocytopenia are expected—leukocyte nadir 10-14 days, recovery in 2-3 wk

---

• Assess for increased uric acid levels, swelling, joint pain primarily in extremities; patient should be well hydrated to prevent urate deposits

• Monitor renal function tests: BUN, creatinine, urine CCr before, during therapy; determine I&O ratio

• Monitor temp q4hr: may indicate beginning of infection

• **Hepatotoxicity:** monitor liver function tests before, during therapy (bilirubin, AST, ALT, LDH) as needed or monthly; dose reduction needed in hepatic disease; check for jaundiced skin and sclera, dark urine, clay-colored stools, itchy skin, abdominal pain, fever, diarrhea

• **Assess for bleeding:** hematuria, stool guaiac, bruising or petechiae, mucosa or orifices q8hr; check for inflammation of mucosa, breaks in skin

• Identify effects of alopecia on body image; discuss feelings about body changes

⚠ Assess for multiple sclerosis: obtain MUGA, LVEF baselines; repeat LVEF if symptoms of CHF occur or if cumulative dose is >100 mg/m²; do not give to patients who have received a lifetime dose of ≥140 mg/m² or if LVEF is <50% or significant LVEF

> **BLACK BOX WARNING:** Assess for secondary acute myelogenous leukemia (AML), which can develop after taking this product

Patient/family education
• Encourage patient to rinse mouth tid-qid with water, club soda; brush teeth bid-qid with soft brush or cotton-tipped applicators for stomatitis; use unwaxed dental floss

• Teach patient to avoid use of products containing aspirin or NSAIDs, razors, commercial mouthwash, since bleeding may occur; to report symptoms of bleeding (hematuria, tarry stools)

• Caution patient to report signs of anemia (fatigue, headache, irritability, faintness, shortness of breath)

• Inform patient that hair may be lost during treatment; a wig or hairpiece may make patient feel better; new hair may be different in color, texture

• Caution patient not to have any vaccinations without the advice of the prescriber; serious reactions can occur

• Advise patient that contraception is needed during treatment and for several mo after completion of therapy

> **BLACK BOX WARNING:** Teach patient to notify prescriber if pregnancy is planned or suspected

• Advise patient that sclera, urine may turn blue or green

• Advise patient to increase fluids to 2-3 L/day unless contraindicated

• Teach patient to avoid crowds, persons with infections

• Teach patient to report immediately bleeding, dyspnea, possible infections, seizure, jaundice, fever, cough or dyspnea

Evaluation
Positive therapeutic outcome
• Prevention of rapid division of malignant cells

modafinil (Rx)
(mo-daf′i-nil)
Alertec ✦, Provigil
Func. class.: CNS stimulant
Chem. class.: Racemic compound
Pregnancy category C
Controlled substance IV

M

ACTION: Similar action as sympathomimetics; does not alter release of dopamine, norepinephrine

Therapeutic outcome: Ability to stay awake

USES: Narcolepsy, shift work sleep disturbance, obstructive sleep apnea

Unlabeled uses: Fatigue in MS, ADHD

CONTRAINDICATIONS:
Hypersensitivity, ischemic heart disease, left ventricular hypertrophy, chest pain, dysrhythmias

Precautions: Pregnancy **C**, breastfeeding, child <16 yr, geriatric, unstable angina, history of MI, severe hepatic disease

DOSAGE AND ROUTES
To improve wakefulness with day-time sleepiness
Adult/adolescent ≥16 yr: PO 200 mg qd

Hepatic dose (severe hepatic disease)
Adult: PO 100 mg qd

Multiple sclerosis (unlabeled)
Adult/elderly/child ≥6 yr: PO 200-400 mg/day in the AM

Available forms: Tabs 100, 200 mg

Implementation

- Give 1 hr before start of shift work, or in the AM for those with narcolepsy or sleep apnea
- Store at room temperature

ADVERSE EFFECTS

CNS: *Headache,* anxiety, cataplexy, depression, dizziness, insomnia, amnesia, confusion, ataxia, tremors, paresthesia, dyskinesia, **suicidal ideation**
CV: Dysrhythmias, hyper/hypotension, chest pain, vasodilation
EENT: Change in vision, *rhinitis,* pharyngitis, epistaxis
GI: Nausea, vomiting, changes in LFTs, anorexia, diarrhea, thirst, mouth ulcers
GU: Ejaculation disorder, urinary retention, albuminuria
HEMA: Eosinophilia
INTEG: Rash, dry skin, herpes simplex, **Stevens-Johnson syndrome**
MISC: Infection, hyperglycemia, neck pain
RESP: *Dyspnea,* lung changes

Pharmacokinetics

Absorption	Rapid
Distribution	60% protein binding
Metabolism	Liver (90%)
Excretion	Unknown
Half-life	15 hr

Pharmacodynamics

Onset	Unknown
Peak	2-4 hr
Duration	Unknown

INTERACTIONS

Individual drugs

CycloSPORINE, theophylline: decreased effects of these drugs
Methylphenidate: delayed effect of modafinil by 1 hr

Drug classifications

Antidepressants (tricyclics): increased effects
CYP3A4 inhibitors (azole antibiotics, some SSRIs): altered levels of these agents, reaction difficult to predict
CYP2C19 substrates (diazepam, phenytoin, some tricyclics): increased levels of these agents
CYP3A4 inducers (carBAMazepine, phenytoin, rifampin; cycloSPORINE, theophylline): altered levels of these agents
Hormonal contraceptives: decreased effects

Drug/herb

Coffee, cola nut, guarana, mate, tea: increased stimulation

Drug/lab test

Increased: eosinophils, glucose, LFTs

NURSING CONSIDERATIONS

Assessment

- For narcolepsy, shift work, history of sleep apnea
- For depression, suicidal ideation
- Monitor B/P in those with hypertension

Patient/family education

- Advise patient to take only as directed; may be taken with or without food
- **⚠ Advise patient to use other form of contraception during and at least 30 days after discontinuing medication, if using hormonal birth control; advise patient to notify prescriber if pregnancy is planned or suspected or if breastfeeding**
- Advise patient to notify prescriber of allergic reaction, tremors, confusion
- Teach patient to avoid all OTC medications unless approved by prescriber
- Teach patient to avoid hazardous activities until drug effect is known

Evaluation

Positive therapeutic outcome
- Ability to stay awake

---

montelukast (Rx)

(mon-teh-loo′kast)
Singulair
Func. class.: Bronchodilator
Chem. class.: Leukotriene antagonist, cysteinyl
Pregnancy category B

ACTION: Inhibits leukotriene (LTD_4) formation; leukotrienes exert their effects by increasing neutrophil, eosinophil migration; aggregation of neutrophils, monocytes; smooth muscle contraction, capillary permeability; these actions further lead to bronchoconstriction, inflammation, edema

Therapeutic outcome: Ability to breathe with ease

USES: Chronic asthma in adults and children, seasonal allergic rhinitis, bronchospasm prophylaxis

Unlabeled uses: Chronic urticaria

CONTRAINDICATIONS:
Hypersensitivity

Precautions: Pregnancy **B,** breastfeeding, children <6 yr, acute attacks of asthma, alcohol consumption, severe hepatic disease, corticosteroid withdrawal, phenylketonuria, suicidal ideation, depression

DOSAGE AND ROUTES
Asthma
Adult and child ≥15 yr: PO 10 mg/day PM
Child 6-14 yr: PO 5 mg chew tabs/day PM
Child 2-5 yr: PO (chew tabs, granules) 4 mg/day
Child 12-23 mo: PO 1 packet of granules taken PM

Exercise-induced bronchoconstriction
Adult/child ≥6 yr: PO 10 mg 2 hr prior to exercise; do not take another dose within 24 hr

Available forms: Tabs 10 mg; chewable tabs 4, 5 mg; oral granules 4 mg/packet

Implementation
PO route
• Give PO in PM daily for all uses except exercise-induced bronchoconstriction; then take 2 hr prior to exercise
• Do not open packet until ready to use; mix whole dose, give within 15 min
• Granules may be given directly in mouth or mixed with a spoonful of soft food (carrots, applesauce, ice cream, rice)

ADVERSE EFFECTS
CNS: Dizziness, fatigue, headache, behavior changes, **seizures,** agitation, anxiety, depression, fever, hallucinations, drowsiness, **suicidal ideation,** memory impairment, hostility, somnambulism
GI: Abdominal pain, dyspepsia, nausea, vomiting, diarrhea, **pancreatitis**
HEMA: Thrombocytopenia
INTEG: Rash, pruritus, erythema
MS: Asthenia, myalgia, muscle cramps
RESP: Influenza, cough, nasal congestion
SYST: Anaphylaxis, angioedema, Churg-Strauss syndrome, Stevens-Johnson syndrome, toxic epidermal necrolysis

Absorption	Rapidly absorbed
Distribution	Protein binding 99%
Metabolism	Liver
Excretion	Bile
Half-life	2.7-5.5 hr

Onset	Unknown
Peak	3-4 hr
Duration	Unknown

INTERACTIONS
Individual drugs
Rifabutin, rifapentine, carBAMazepine, fosphenytoin, phenytoin, rifampin: decreased montelukast levels

Drug classifications
Barbiturates: decreased montelukast levels

Drug/herb
Tea (green, black), guarana: increased stimulation

Drug/lab test
Increased: ALT, AST

NURSING CONSIDERATIONS
Assessment
⚠ Assess adult patients carefully for symptoms of Churg-Strauss syndrome (rare), including eosinophilia, vasculitic rash, worsening pulmonary symptoms, cardiac complications and/or neuropathy
• Monitor CBC, blood chemistry during treatment
• Assess allergic reactions: rash, urticaria; product should be discontinued
• Assess for behavior changes and suicidal ideation, other neuropsychiatric reactions
• **Severe hepatic disease:** use cautiously

Patient/family education
• Advise patient to avoid hazardous activities; dizziness may occur
• Teach patient that product is not to be used for acute asthma attacks
• Advise patient to avoid NSAIDs if sensitive to aspirin
• Advise patient to continue to use inhaled β-agonists if exercise-induced asthma occurs
• **Granules:** instruct patient to take directly by mouth or mixed in a spoonful of room temperature soft food (use only applesauce, carrots, rice, or ice cream); use within 15 min of opening packet, discard used portions

Evaluation
Positive therapeutic outcome
• Increased ease of breathing
• Decreased bronchospasm

M

⚠ HIGH ALERT

morphine (Rx)

(mor'feen)

Astramorph PF, AVINza, Depo Dur, Infumorph PF, Kadian, M.O.S. ✦, MS Contin, MSIR ✦, Oramorph SR

Func. class.: Opioid analgesic
Chem. class.: Alkaloid
Pregnancy category C
Controlled substance schedule II 🌟

Do not confuse:
morphine/HYDROmorphone,
MS Contin/oxyCONTIN

ACTION: Depresses pain impulse transmission at the spinal cord level by interacting with opioid receptors

Therapeutic outcome: Decreased pain

USES: Moderate to severe pain

Unlabeled uses: Agitation, bone/dental pain, dyspnea in end-stage cancer or pulmonary disease, sedation induction, rapid-sequence intubation

CONTRAINDICATIONS:
Hypersensitivity, addiction (opioid/alcohol), hemorrhage, bronchial asthma, increased ICP, paralytic ileus, hypovolemic shock, MAOI therapy

BLACK BOX WARNING: Respiratory depression

Precautions: Pregnancy **C**, breastfeeding, children <18 yr, geriatric, addictive personality, acute MI, severe heart disease, renal/hepatic disease, bowel impaction, abrupt discontinuation, seizures

BLACK BOX WARNING: Accidental exposure, epidural/intrathecal/IM/subcut administration, opioid-naive patients, substance abuse

DOSAGE AND ROUTES
Acute moderate to severe pain
PO regular-release
Adult ≥50 kg: Initially, 10-30 mg q3-4hr as needed
Adult <50 kg/geriatric patient: May require lower doses and/or extended dosing intervals; doses should be titrated carefully

Child/infant ≥6 mo: 0.2-0.5 mg/kg q4-6hr as needed
Infant <6 mo/neonate: 0.1 mg/kg PO q3-4hr

IV/IM/subcut
Adult ≥50 kg: 2.5-15 mg q2-6hr as needed, titrate or a loading dose of 0.05-0.1 mg/kg **IV**, followed by 0.8-10 mg/hr **IV**, titrate
Adult <50 kg/geriatric patient: May require lower doses and/or extended dosing intervals 0.1 mg/kg q3-4hr, titrate
Child/infant ≥6 mo: 0.05-0.2 mg/kg q2-4hr, titrate to relief max initial doses 15 mg/dose
Neonate/infant <6 mo: 0.03-0.05 mg/kg q3-8hr, titrate to relief

Epidural (morphine sulfate injection, but NOT DepoDur)
Adult: Initially, 5 mg in the lumbar region; if pain relief does not occur in 1 hr, give 1-2 mg epidurally; max 10 mg/24 hr; **continuous epidural infusion,** 2-4 mg/24 hr; may give another 1-2 mg

Intrathecal dosage (morphine sulfate injection, but NOT DepoDur)
Do not inject >2 ml of the 0.5 mg/ml or 1 ml of the 1 mg/ml ampule
Adult: 0.2-1 mg in the lumbar area as a single dose or to establish dosage for continuous intrathecal infusion; repeated injections are not recommended

Rectal dosage
Adult: 10-20 mg PR q4hr, as needed
Child: Individualize

Chronic moderate and severe pain
⚠ Do not use extended-release cap or tab as prn analgesics, for acute pain, or if the pain is mild or not expected to persist for an extended period of time. Use for postoperative pain only if the patient is receiving chronic opioid therapy prior to surgery or if the postoperative pain is expected to be moderate to severe and persist for an extended period of time. Do not use controlled-release tablets (MS Contin) immediately after surgery (for the first 24 hr) in patients not previously taking the drug
⚠ Do not use in opioid-naive patients: 90 mg, 120 mg morphine biphasic-release capsules (AVINza); 100 mg, 130 mg, 150 mg, 200 mg morphine extended-release capsules (Kadian), 100 mg, 200 mg morphine control-release tablets (MS Contin); patients considered opioid tolerant are those who are taking at least 60 mg/day oral morphine, 30 mg/day of oral oxyCODONE, 8 mg/day

oral HYDROmorphone, or an equal dose of another opioid, for a wk or longer

PO [extended-release tab (MS Contin, Oramorph SR) or caps (Kadian, AVINza)] (opiate naïve)

Adult: 15-30 mg q12hr (tabls); 10 mg bid or 20 mg/day (Kadian); or 30 mg/day (AVINza), titrate; AVINza should be adjusted in increments ≤30 mg q4 days; Kadian should be increased ≤20 mg q1-2 days, taper gradually; to discontinue, gradually decrease AVINza and Kadian over 2-4 days

Child (unlabeled): 0.3-0.6 mg/kg q12hr (tablets)

IV/subcut route (opiate naïve)

Adult: IV 2-10 mg loading dose, then 0.8-10 mg/hour **IV**, titrate; maintenance 0.8-80 mg/ hour **IV**

Child/infant ≥6 mo: IV Initially, 0.04-0.07 mg/kg/hr (range: 0.025-2.6 mg/kg/hr), **Subcut inf** 0.025-1.79 mg/kg/hr

Infant <6 mo/neonate: IV 0.01 mg/kg/hour **IV**, initially, infusion rates max 0.015-0.02 mg/ kg/hour **IV**

Breakthrough pain in patients receiving long-acting or continuous infusion morphine

PO (regular-release)

Adult/child: The dose is usually one-fourth to one-third the 8- to 12-hour extended-release dose q4-6hr as needed

Adult/child: For PCA, intermittent dose is usually 25%-30% of the hourly rate IV/SC q6-15min as needed; intermittent IV injection dosage is 25%-30% of the hourly rate given IV/SC q1-2hr as needed

Available forms: Inj 0.5, 1, 2, 3, 4, 5, 8, 10, 15, 25, 50 mg/ml; oral sol 10, 20 mg/5 ml, 10 mg/0.5 ml; oral tabs 15, 30 mg; rect supp 5, 10, 20, 30 mg; ext rel tabs 15, 30, 60, 100, 200 mg; caps 15, 30 mg; syr 1, 5 mg/ml; cont rel cap pellets (Kadian) 10, 20, 30, 50, 60, 100, 200 mg; ext rel caps (Avinza) 30, 60, 90, 120 mg

Implementation

PO route

• Give with food or milk to minimize GI effects
Immediate-release cap
• May swallow whole, or opened and contents sprinkled on cool food (pudding or apple-sauce), or added to juice (given immediately) or delivered via gastric or NG tube by either adding to or following with liquid

Extended-release and controlled-release tabs
• Swallow whole; do not crush, break, dissolve, or chew.
• The use of MS Contin 100 mg or 200 mg tabs should be limited to opioid-tolerant patients requiring oral doses equivalent to ≥200 mg/ day. Use of the 100 mg or 200 mg tablet is only recommended for patients who have already been titrated to a stable analgesic regimen using lower strengths of MS Contin or other opioids
Sustained-release caps
• Swallow; do not chew, crush, or dissolve
• Caps may be opened and contents sprinkled on applesauce (at room temperature or cooler) immediately prior to ingestion. Do not chew, crush, or dissolve the pellets/beads inside the cap. The applesauce should be swallowed without chewing. If the pellets/beads are chewed, an immediate release of a potentially fatal morphine dose may be delivered. Rinse mouth to ensure all the pellets/beads have been swallowed. Do not separate applesauce into separate doses; the entire portion should be taken. Discard unused portion
• Kadian caps may be given through a 16 French gastrostomy tube; flush with water, and sprinkle the cap contents into 10 ml of water. Using a funnel and a swirling motion, pour the pellets and water into the tube. Rinse the beaker with 10 ml of water, and pour the water into the funnel. Repeat until no pellets remain in the beaker
⚠ Do NOT administer AVINza tabs through a gastrostomy tube. Do NOT administer Kadian or AVINza through a nasogastric tube
⚠ Avoid concurrent administration of AVINza with prescription or nonprescription medications that contain alcohol. Consumption of alcohol while taking the ext rel capsules may result in the rapid release and absorption of a potentially fatal dose of morphine
⚠ AVINza ≥90 mg or Kadian 100 mg, 130 mg, 150 mg or 200 mg caps should be given only to opioid tolerant patients
• Begin with immediate release products and titrate to correct dose and convert to a sustained release product
Oral liquid
• Check dose prior to use; many concentrations of oral sol are available; may be diluted in fruit juice; protect from light

• Visually inspect for particulate matter and discoloration before use; do not use if a precipitate is present after shaking; do not use the Duramorph solution if a precipitate is present or if the color is darker than pale yellow

IV route
• Prior or to use, an opiate antagonist and emergency facilities should be available
⚠️ **Do not use the highly concentrated morphine injections (i.e., 10-25 mg/ml) for IV, IM, or SC administration of single doses. These injection solutions are intended for use via continuous, controlled-microinfusion devices**

Direct IV route
• Dilute dose with ≥5 ml of sterile water for injection or NS injection
• Inject 2.5-15 mg directly into a vein or into the tubing of a freely flowing IV solution over 4-5 min; do not give rapidly

Continuous IV infusion
• Dilute in 5% dextrose; use a controlled-infusion device
• Adjust dose and rate based on patient response

Patient-controlled analgesia (PCA)
• A compatible patient-controlled infusion device must be used
• Dilute solutions to obtain a concentration of 1 or 10 mg/ml for ease in calculations and programming of PCA pumps
• Adjust dose and rate based on patient response. Consult the patient-controlled infusion device manual for directions on rate of infusion

Subcut route
• Inject taking care not to inject intradermally

Continuous SC infusion
• Morphine is not approved by the FDA for subcut use
• Dilute to an appropriate concentration in D_5W; administer using a portable, controlled, subcut device; adjust rate based on patient response and tolerance
• Max subcut rate 2 ml/hr/site

Intrathecal/epidural route
⚠️ **Morphine sulfate injection is not interchangeable with morphine sulfate extended-release liposome injection (DepoDur), DepoDur is only for epidural administration**
⚠️ **Do not use Infumorph (10 mg/ml or 25 mg/ml) for single-dose neuraxial injection because lower doses can be more reliably administered with Duramorph (0.5 mg/ml or 1 mg/ml)**

• Moisten the suppository with water prior to insertion. If suppository is too soft, chill in the refrigerator for 30 min or run cold water over it before removing the wrapper

Immediate-release capsules administration
• May be swallowed whole or opened and the contents sprinkled on cool food such as pudding or applesauce
• Capsule contents may be added to juice and administered immediately or delivered via gastric or NG tube by either adding to or following with liquid

• Swallow whole; do not crush, break, dissolve, or chew
• The use of MS Contin 100 mg or 200 mg tablets should be limited to opioid-tolerant patients requiring oral doses equivalent to ≥200 mg/day. Use of the 100 mg or 200 mg tablet is only recommended for patients who have already been titrated to a stable analgesic regimen using lower strengths of MS Contin or other opioids

Sustained-release capsule administration
• Capsules should be swallowed; do not chew, crush, or dissolve
• Capsules may be opened and the contents sprinkled on applesauce (at room temperature or cooler) immediately prior to ingestion; no other food has been tested. Do not chew, crush, or dissolve the pellets/beads inside the capsule. The applesauce needs to be swallowed without chewing. If the pellets/beads are chewed, an immediate release of a potentially fatal morphine dose may be delivered. Rinse mouth to ensure all the pellets/beads have been swallowed. Do not separate applesauce into separate doses; the entire portion should be taken. Discard any unused portion of the capsules after the contents have been sprinkled on the applesauce
• Kadian capsules may be administered through a 16 French gastrostomy tube. Flush the tube with water, and sprinkle the capsule contents into 10 ml of water. Using a funnel and a swirling motion, pour the pellets and water into the tube. Rinse the beaker with 10 ml of water, and pour the water into the funnel. Repeat until no pellets remain in the beaker
⚠️ **Do NOT administer AVINza tablets through a gastrostomy tube. Do NOT administer Kadian or AVINza through a nasogastric tube**

⚠️ Nurse Alert ⭐ Key NCLEX® Drug

⚠ Avoid concurrent administration of AVINza with prescription or non-prescription medications that contain alcohol. Consumption of alcohol while taking the extended-release capsules may result in the rapid release and absorption of a potentially fatal dose of morphine

⚠ The use of AVINza ≥90 mg or Kadian 100 mg, 130 mg, 150 mg or 200 mg capsules should be limited to opioid tolerant patients

Oral liquid formulations

Oral solution administration
• Carefully check dose prior to dispensing medication as many concentrations of morphine oral solution are available
• May be diluted in fruit juice prior to administration
• Protect from light

Injectable administration
• Visually inspect parenteral products for particulate matter and discoloration prior to administration whenever solution and container permit. Unopened solutions should be discarded if a precipitate is present that does not disappear with shaking. Do not use the Duramorph solution if a precipitate is present or if the color is darker than pale yellow

Intravenous administration
• Prior to administration, an opiate antagonist and facilities for administration of oxygen and control of respiration should be available

⚠ Do not use the highly concentrated morphine injections (i.e., 10-25 mg/ml) for IV, IM, or SC administration of single doses. These injection solutions are intended for use via continuous, controlled-microinfusion devices

Direct IV injection
• Dilute appropriate dose with at least 5 ml of sterile water for injection or NS injection
• Inject 2.5-15 mg directly into a vein or into the tubing of a freely flowing IV solution over 4-5 minutes. Rapid IV injection of morphine may result in an increased frequency of adverse effects. For example, the maximum CNS effects occur 30 minutes after administration. Rapid intravenous administration could result in an overdose

Continuous IV infusion
• Dilute in 5% dextrose
• Administer using a controlled-infusion device
• Adjust dose and rate based on patient response

Patient-controlled analgesia (PCA)
• A compatible patient-controlled infusion device must be used
• Dilute solutions to obtain morphine concentration of 1 or 10 mg/ml for ease in calculations and programming of PCA pumps
• Adjust dose and rate based on patient response. Consult the patient-controlled infusion device operator's manual for directions on administering the drug at the desired rate of infusion

Subcutaneous administration
• Inject subcutaneously taking care not to inject intradermally

Continuous SC infusion
• Morphine is not approved by the FDA for subcutaneous administration
• Dilute to an appropriate concentration in D_5W and administer using a portable, controlled, subcutaneous infusion device. Adjust rate based on patient response and tolerance
• Maximum SC rate of infusion is 2 ml/hour/site

Intrathecal administration

⚠ Intrathecal dose is approximately one-tenth (1/10) the epidural dose

⚠ Morphine sulfate injection is not interchangeable with morphine sulfate extended-release liposome injection (DepoDur). DepoDur is only for epidural administration (see below)

⚠ Do not use Infumorph (10 mg/ml or 25 mg/ml) for single-dose neuraxial injection because lower doses can be more reliably administered with Duramorph (0.5 mg/ml or 1 mg/ml)

• Epidural or intrathecal administration should only be used by specially trained healthcare professionals
• May be given as intermittent bolus, continuous infusion, or as patient-controlled epidural analgesia. Infumorph is only indicated for intrathecal or epidural infusion; Infumorph is not recommended for single-dose intravenous, intramuscular, or subcutaneous administration because of the very large amount of morphine in the ampul and the associated overdosage risk
• Prior to administration, an opiate antagonist and facilities for administration of oxygen and control of respiration should be available. The patient should be in a setting where adequate monitoring is possible. Immediate availability of naloxone injection and resuscitative equipment is also needed during Infumorph reservoir refilling or reservoir manipulation

M

• Placement of epidural catheter and administration should be at a site near the dermatomes covering the field of pain to decrease dose requirements and increase specificity. For example, for thoracic surgery placement at T2-T8, upper abdominal surgery, T4-L1, lower abdominal surgery, T10-L3, upper extremity surgery, C2-C8 and lower extremity surgery, T12-L3

• Visually inspect parenteral products for particulate matter and discoloration prior to administration whenever solution and container permit. Unopened Infumorph solution should be discarded if a precipitate is present that does not disappear with shaking or if it is not colorless or pale yellow. Do not use the Duramorph solution if a precipitate is present or if the color is darker than pale yellow

Intrathecal injection (morphine sulfate injection)

• No more than 2 or 1 ml of the injection containing 0.5 or 1 mg/ml, respectively, should be injected intrathecally

• After ensuring proper placement of the needle or catheter, inject appropriate dose intrathecally. Monitor patient in a fully equipped and staffed environment for at least 24 hr after each dose, as severe respiratory depression may occur up to 24 hr after drug administration. Repeated intrathecal injections are not recommended other than for establishing initial intrathecal dosage for continuous intrathecal infusion

Continuous intrathecal infusion (morphine sulfate injection)

⚠ Intrathecal dose is approximately one-tenth (1/10) the epidural dose. Epidural dose is usually considered to be one-tenth (1/10) the IV dose

• A controlled-infusion device must be used. For highly concentrated injections, an implantable controlled-microinfusion device is used. Patients should be monitored in a fully equipped and staffed environment for several days following implantation of the device

• If dilution of the injection is necessary, NS injection is recommended

• The infusion device reservoir should only be filled by fully trained and qualified healthcare professionals. Strict aseptic technique must be used. Withdraw dose from the ampul through a 5-µm (or smaller pore diameter) microfilter to avoid contamination with glass or other particles. Ensure proper placement of the needle when filling the reservoir to avoid accidental overdosage

• To avoid exacerbation of severe pain and/or reflux of CSF into the reservoir, depletion of the reservoir should be avoided

Other injectable administration

Epidural administration

⚠ Intrathecal dose is approximately one-tenth (1/10) the epidural dose. Epidural dose is usually considered to be one-tenth (1/10) the IV dose

⚠ Morphine sulfate injection is not interchangeable with morphine sulfate extended-release liposome injection (DepoDur). DepoDur is only for epidural administration (see below)

⚠ Do not use Infumorph (10 mg/ml or 25 mg/ml) for single-dose neuraxial injection because lower doses can be more reliably administered with Duramorph (0.5 mg/ml or 1 mg/ml)

• Epidural administration should only be used by specially trained healthcare professionals

• May be given as intermittent bolus, cont inf, or as patient-controlled epidural analgesia. Infumorph is only indicated for intrathecal or epidural infusion; Infumorph is not recommended for single-dose intravenous, intramuscular, or subcutaneous administration because of the very large amount of morphine in the ampul and the associated overdosage risk

• Prior to administration, an opiate antagonist and facilities for administration of oxygen and control of respiration should be available. The patient should be in a setting where adequate monitoring is possible. Immediate availability of naloxone injection and resuscitative equipment is also needed during Infumorph reservoir refilling or reservoir manipulation

• Placement of epidural catheter and administration should be at a site near the dermatomes covering the field of pain to decrease dose requirements and increase specificity. For example, for thoracic surgery placement at T2-T8, upper abdominal surgery, T4-L1, lower abdominal surgery, T10-L3, upper extremity surgery, C2-C8 and lower extremity surgery, T12-L3

Epidural injection (morphine sulfate injection)

• After ensuring proper placement of the needle or catheter, inject appropriate dose into the epidural space. Monitor patient in a fully equipped and staffed environment for at least 24 hr after each dose, as severe respiratory depression may occur up to 24 hr after drug administration

Continuous epidural infusion (morphine sulfate injection)

⚠️ **Intrathecal dose is approximately one-tenth (1/10) the epidural dose. Epidural dose is usually considered to be one-tenth (1/10) the IV dose**

• A controlled-infusion device must be used. For highly concentrated injections, an implantable controlled-microinfusion device is used. Patients should be monitored in a fully equipped and staffed environment for several days following implantation of the device
• If dilution of the injection is necessary, NS injection is recommended
• The infusion device reservoir should only be filled by fully trained and qualified healthcare professionals. Strict aseptic technique must be used. Withdraw dose from the ampul through a 5-μm (or smaller pore diameter) microfilter to avoid contamination with glass or other particles. Ensure proper placement of the needle when filling the reservoir to avoid accidental overdosage
• To avoid exacerbation of severe pain and/or reflux of CSF into the reservoir, depletion of the reservoir should be avoided

Epidural administration (morphine sulfate extended-release liposome injection [DepoDur] ONLY)

⚠️ **Morphine sulfate ext rel liposome injection (DepoDur) is not interchangeable with other morphine sulfate injections**

• DepoDur is only for epidural administration. Do not administer by any other parenteral route
• Epidural administration should only be used by specially trained healthcare professionals
• Prior to administration, an opiate antagonist and facilities for administration of oxygen and control of respiration should be available. The patient should be in a setting where adequate monitoring is possible. Monitor patient in a fully equipped and staffed environment for at least 48 hr after each dose, as severe respiratory depression may occur
• Invert the vial to resuspend particles immediately before withdrawal. Administer DepoDur within 4 hr after withdrawal from the vial when kept at controlled room temperature 59-86° F (15-30° C). The product does not contain any bacteriostatic agents or preservatives. Do not heat- or gas-sterilize

Epidural injection [morphine sulfate extended-release liposome injection (DepoDur)]

• Placement of epidural needle or catheter and administration should be at the lumbar level.

Due to lack of study data, administration of DepoDur at the thoracic level or higher is not recommended
• Determine proper needle or catheter placement by aspiration to check for blood or cerebrospinal fluid and/or by administration of a test dose of 3 ml of 1.5% preservative-free lidocaine and EPINEPHrine (1:200,000). If tachycardia or sudden onset of segmental anesthesia occurs, the needle or catheter is in the intrathecal space and thus, needs to be repositioned. If a test dose is given, flush the catheter with 1 ml of preservative-free normal saline injection and wait at least 15 minutes after test dose administration before administration of DepoDur
• Inject DepoDur at the lumbar level undiluted or diluted up to 5 ml total volume with preservative-free normal saline. During administration, do not use an inline filter or mix DepoDur with any medication. Additionally, do not administer any medication into the epidural space within 48 hr of DepoDur receipt

Rectal administration

• Instruct patient on proper use of suppository (see Patient Information)
• Moisten the suppository with water prior to insertion. If suppository is too soft because of storage in a warm place, chill in the refrigerator for 30 minutes or run cold water over it before removing the wrapper

Syringe compatibilities: Atropine, bupivacaine, butorphanol, cimetidine, dimenhyDRINATE, diphenhydrAMINE, droperidol, fentaNYL, glycopyrrolate, hydrOXYzine, ketamine, metoclopramide, milrinone, pentazocine, perphenazine, promazine, ranitidine, scopolamine

Syringe incompatibilities: Meperidine, thiopental

Y-site compatibilities: Allopurinol, amifostine, amikacin, aminophylline, amiodarone, atenolol, atracurium, aztreonam, bumetanide, calcium chloride, cefamandole, ceFAZolin, cefotaxime, cefoTEtan, cefOXitin, cefTAZidime, ceftizoxime, cefTRIAXone, cefuroxime, cephalothin, chloramphenicol, cladribine, clindamycin, cyclophosphamide, cytarabine, dexamethasone, digoxin, diltiazem, DOBUTamine, DOPamine, doxycycline, enalaprilat, EPINEPHrine, erythromycin, esmolol, etomidate, famotidine, fentaNYL, filgrastim, fluconazole, fludarabine, foscarnet, gentamicin, granisetron, heparin, hydrocortisone, HYDROmorphone, kanamycin, labetalol, lidocaine, LORazepam, magnesium sulfate, melphalan, meropenem, methotrexate, methyldopa, methylPREDNISolone,

M

metoclopramide, metoprolol, metroNIDAZOLE, midazolam, milrinone, nafcillin, niCARdipine, nitroglycerin, norepinephrine, ondansetron, oxacillin, oxytocin, PACLitaxel, pancuronium, penicillin G potassium, piperacillin, piperacillin/tazobactam, potassium chloride, propranolol, ranitidine, sodium bicarbonate, teniposide, thiotepa, ticarcillin, ticarcillin/clavulanate, tobramycin, vancomycin, vecuronium, vinorelbine, vit B/C, warfarin, zidovudine

Y-site incompatibilities: Furosemide, minocycline, tetracycline

ADVERSE EFFECTS

CNS: Drowsiness, dizziness, *confusion,* headache, *sedation,* euphoria, insomnia, **seizures**
CV: Palpitations, **bradycardia**, change in B/P, **shock, cardiac arrest,** chest pain, hyper/hypotension, edema, **tachycardia**
EENT: Blurred vision, miosis, diplopia
ENDO: Gynecomastia
GI: Nausea, vomiting, anorexia, *constipation,* cramps, biliary tract pressure
GU: Urinary retention, impotence, gonadal suppression
HEMA: Thrombocytopenia
INTEG: Rash, urticaria, bruising, flushing, diaphoresis, pruritus
RESP: Respiratory depression, respiratory arrest, apnea

Pharmacokinetics

Absorption	Variably absorbed (PO); well absorbed (IM, SUBCUT, RECT); completely absorbed (**IV**)
Distribution	Widely distributed; crosses placenta
Metabolism	Liver, extensively
Excretion	Kidneys
Half-life	1½-2 hr; IM 3-4 hr; AVINza 24 hr; Kadian 11-13 hr

INTERACTIONS

Individual drugs
Alcohol: increased effects with other CNS depressants
Rifampin: decreased analgesic action

Drug classifications
Antipsychotics, opiates, sedative-hypnotics, skeletal muscle relaxants: increased effects with other CNS depressants
MAOIs: unpredictable reaction may occur; avoid use

Drug/herb
Chamomile, hops, kava, St. John's wort, valerian: increased CNS depression

Drug/lab test
Increased: amylase

NURSING CONSIDERATIONS

Assessment
• Assess pain: location, type, character, intensity; give dose before pain becomes extreme
• Monitor I&O ratio; check for decreasing output; may indicate urinary retention; check for constipation; increase fluids, bulk in diet if needed, or stimulant laxatives may be prescribed; monitor serum sodium

> **BLACK BOX WARNING:** Abrupt discontinuation: gradually taper to prevent withdrawal symptoms; decrease by 50% q1-2 days, avoid use of narcotic antagonist

• Monitor CNS changes: dizziness, drowsiness, hallucinations, euphoria, LOC, pupil reactions
• Monitor allergic reactions: rash, urticaria

> **BLACK BOX WARNING:** Accidental exposure: if Duramorph or Infamorph gets on skin, remove contaminated clothing and rinse affected area with water

Pharmacodynamics

	PO	PO EXT REL	IM	SUBCUT	RECT	IV	IT
Onset	Variable	Unknown	10-30 min	20 min	Unknown	Rapid	Rapid
Peak	1 hr	Unknown	50-90 min	1-1½ hr	½-1 hr	20 min	Unknown
Duration	4-5 hr	8-12 hr	3-7 hr	4-5 hr	4-5 hr	4-5 hr	Ext

Patient/family education
• Advise patient to report any symptoms of CNS changes, allergic reactions
• Caution patients to avoid CNS depressants (alcohol, sedative/hypnotics) for at least 24 hr after taking this product
• Discuss with patient that dizziness, drowsiness, and confusion are common; to avoid getting up without assistance
• Discuss in detail all aspects of the product and expected response

Evaluation
Positive therapeutic outcome
• Decreased pain

TREATMENT OF OVERDOSE:
Naloxone (Narcan) 0.2-0.8 **IV** (caution with opioid-tolerant individuals), O₂, **IV** fluids, vasopressors

moxifloxacin (Rx)
(mox-i-floks′a-sin)
Avelox, Avelox IV
Func. class.: Antiinfective
Chem. class.: Fluoroquinolone
Pregnancy category C

ACTION: Interferes with conversion of intermediate DNA fragments into high molecular weight DNA in bacteria; DNA gyrase inhibitor

Therapeutic outcome: Bactericidal action against the following: *Staphylococcus aureus, Streptococcus pneumoniae, Haemophilus influenzae, Haemophilus parainfluenzae, Moraxella catarrhalis, Klebsiella pneumoniae, Mycoplasma pneumoniae, Chlamydia pneumoniae; Streptococcus pyogenes, Escherichia coli, Bacteroides fragilis, Streptococcus arginosus, Streptococcus constellatus, Enterococcus faecalis, Proteus mirabilis, Clostridium perfringens, Bacteroides thetalomicron, Peptostreptococcus, Enterobacter cloacae*

USES: Acute bacterial sinusitis, acute bacterial exacerbation of chronic bronchitis, community-acquired pneumonia (mild to moderate), uncomplicated skin/skin structure infections, complicated intraabdominal infections including polymicrobial infections, complicated skin/skin structure infections

Unlabeled uses: Anthrax treatment/prophylaxis, gastroenteritis, MAC, nongonococcal urethritis, shigellosis, surgical infection prophylaxis, TB

CONTRAINDICATIONS:
Hypersensitivity to quinolones

Precautions: Pregnancy **C**, breastfeeding, children, renal/hepatic/cardiac disease, epilepsy, uncorrected hypokalemia, prolonged QT interval, patients receiving class IA, III antidysrhythmics, GI disease, seizure disorder, pseudomembranous colitis, diabetes mellitus

DOSAGE AND ROUTES
Acute bacterial sinusitis
Adult: PO/**IV** 400 mg q24hr × 10 days

Acute bacterial exacerbation of chronic bronchitis
Adult: PO/**IV** 400 mg q24hr × 5 days

Community-acquired pneumonia
Adult: PO/**IV** 400 mg q24hr × 7-14 days

Uncomplicated skin/skin structure infections
Adult: PO/**IV** 400 mg q24hr × 7 days

Complicated intraabdominal infections
Adult: **IV** 400 mg/day × 5-14 days

Complicated skin/skin structure infections
Adult: PO/**IV** 400 mg/day × 7-21 days

Available forms: Tabs 400 mg; inj premix 400 mg/250 ml

Implementation
• Do not use theophylline with this product; may cause toxicity
PO route
• Give once a day for 5-10 days depending on condition
• Give without regard to food
• Store at room temperature

IV route
• Discontinue primary **IV** while administering moxifloxacin, give over 60 min
• Do not give SUBCUT, IM
• Available as premixed sol, may be diluted at ratios from 1:10 to 10:1, do not refrigerate, give

by direct infusion or through Y-type infusion set, do not add other medications to sol or infuse through same IV line at same time

• Do not refrigerate
• Flush line with compatible sol before and after use
• Do not admix

Solution compatibilities: 0.9% NaCl, D$_5$, D$_{10}$, LR, sterile water for inj

ADVERSE EFFECTS

CNS: Headache, dizziness, fatigue, insomnia, depression, restlessness, **seizures**, confusion, **increased intracranial pressure,** peripheral neuropathy, **pseudotumor cerebri,** fever
CV: Prolonged QT interval, dysrhythmias, torsades de pointes, tachycardia
EENT: Blurred vision, tinnitus, taste changes
GI: Nausea, increased ALT, AST, flatulence, heartburn, vomiting, diarrhea, oral candidiasis, dysphagia, **pseudomembranous colitis,** abdominal pain, dyspepsia, constipation, gastroenteritis, xerostomia
GU: Renal failure
INTEG: Rash, pruritus, urticaria, photosensitivity, flushing, fever, chills, injection site reactions
MISC: Candidiasis vaginitis
MS: Tremor, arthralgia, **tendon rupture,** myalgia
SYST: Anaphylaxis, Stevens-Johnson syndrome, angioedema, toxic epidermal necrolysis

Pharmacokinetics

Absorption	Well absorbed (75%) (PO)
Distribution	Widely distributed
Metabolism	Liver
Excretion	Kidneys
Half-life	Increased in renal disease

Pharmacodynamics

	PO
Onset	Rapid
Peak	1 hr
Duration	Unknown

INTERACTIONS

Individual drugs

Aluminum hydroxide, calcium, didanosine, iron, sucralfate, zinc sulfate: decreased absorption of moxifloxacin
CycloSPORINE: increased cycloSPORINE effect

Haloperidol, chloroquine, droperidol, pentamidine; arsenic trioxide, levomethadyl: increased QT prolongation
Probenecid: increased blood levels
Warfarin: increased warfarin effect

Drug classifications

Antacids (magnesium), iron salts: decreased absorption of moxifloxacin
Class IA/III antidysrhythmics, some phenothiazines, β-agonists, local anesthetics, tricyclics, CYP3A4 inhibitors (amiodarone, clarithromycin, erythromycin, telithromycin, troleandomycin), CYP3A4 substrates (methadone, pimozide, QUEtiapine, quiNIDine, risperidone, ziprasidone): increased QT prolongation
NSAIDs: increased seizure risk

> **BLACK BOX WARNING:** Corticosteroids: increased tendon rupture

Drug/food

Enteral feeding: decreased absorption of moxifloxacin
Increased: QT prolongation in drugs that interval QT

Drug/lab test

Increased: glucose, amylase, lipids, triglycerides, uric acid, LDH
Decreased: potassium

NURSING CONSIDERATIONS

Assessment

• Assess patient for previous sensitivity reaction
• Assess patient for signs and symptoms of infection including characteristics of wounds, sputum, urine, stool, WBC >10,000/mm^3, fever baseline, during treatment
• Obtain C&S before beginning product therapy to identify if correct treatment has been initiated
• **Assess for allergic reactions, Stevens-Johnson syndrome, toxic epidermal necrolysis, and anaphylaxis:** rash, urticaria, pruritus, chills, fever, joint pain; may occur a few days after therapy begins; epinephrine and resuscitation equipment should be available for anaphylactic reaction
• Assess for CNS symptoms: headache, dizziness, fatigue, insomnia, depression, **seizures**
• Identify urine output; if decreasing, notify prescriber (may indicate nephrotoxicity); also check for increased BUN, creatinine, electrolytes
• Monitor blood tests: AST, ALT, CBC, Hct, bilirubin, LDH, alkaline phosphatase, Coombs' test monthly if patient is on long-term therapy

- Monitor electrolytes: potassium, sodium chloride monthly if patient is on long-term therapy
- **Pseudomembranous colitis:** assess for diarrhea, abdominal pain, fever, fatigue, anorexia; possible anemia, elevated WBC and low serum albumin; stop product and usually give either vancomycin or IV metroNIDAZOLE
- Monitor for bleeding: ecchymosis, bleeding gums, hematuria, stool guaiac daily if on long-term therapy
- Assess for overgrowth of infection: perineal itching, fever, malaise, redness, pain, swelling, drainage, rash, diarrhea, change in cough, sputum

> **BLACK BOX WARNING:** Assess for tendon pain, rupture, tendinitis; if tendon becomes inflamed, drug should be discontinued, more common in achilles tendon

⚠ **QT prolongation: Monitor ECG for QT prolongation, ejection fraction; assess for chest pain, palpitations, dyspnea**

Patient/family education

> **BLACK BOX WARNING:** Notify prescriber of tendon pain, inflammation, stop drug

- Teach patient to report sore throat, bruising, bleeding, joint pain; may indicate blood dyscrasias (rare)
- Advise patient to contact prescriber if vaginal itching, loose foul-smelling stools, furry tongue occur; may indicate superinfection; report itching, rash, pruritus, urticaria
- Instruct patient to take all medication prescribed for the length of time ordered; not to give medication to others
- Advise patient to notify prescriber of diarrhea with blood or pus
- Advise patient to rinse mouth frequently, use sugarless candy or gum for dry mouth
- Advise patient to take as prescribed, not to double or miss doses

Evaluation

Positive therapeutic outcome
- Absence of signs/symptoms of infection (WBC <10,000/mm^3, temp WNL)
- Reported improvement in symptoms of infection

moxifloxacin ophthalmic
See Appendix B

mupirocin topical
See Appendix B

mycophenolate (Rx)
(mie-koe-feen'oh-late)
Mycophenolate Mofetil CellCept, Myfortic (Rx)
Func. class.: Immunosuppressant
Pregnancy category C

ACTION: Inhibits inflammatory responses that are mediated by the immune system; prolongs survival of allogenic transplants

Therapeutic outcome: Absence of graft rejection

USES: Organ transplants to prevent rejection (renal); prophylaxis of rejection in allogenic cardiac, hepatic, renal transplants

Unlabeled uses: Refractory uveitis, 2nd-line therapy for Churg-Strauss syndrome, diffuse proliferative lupus nephritis (in combination), rheumatoid arthritis, psoriasis

CONTRAINDICATIONS:
Hypersensitivity to this product or mycophenolic acid

> **BLACK BOX WARNING:** Pregnancy **D**

Precautions: Breastfeeding, lymphomas, neutropenia, renal disease, accidental exposure, anemia

> **BLACK BOX WARNING:** Infection, neoplastic disease

DOSAGE AND ROUTES
Renal transplant (to prevent organ rejection)
Adult: PO 1 g or 720 mg bid given to renal transplant patients in combination with corticosteroids and cycloSPORINE; mycophenolate mofetil 1 g or 720 mg mycophenolate sodium
Child: PO-ER 400 mg/m^2 bid, max 720 mg bid

Renal dose
Adult: PO/IV GFR <25 ml/min, max 2 g/day

Cardiac transplant (to prevent organ rejection)
Adult: PO/IV 1.5 g bid, **IV** can be started ≤24 hr after transplant, switch to PO when able

Hepatic transplant (to prevent organ rejection)
Adult: PO 1.5 g bid, **IV** 1 g over ≥2 hr

Available forms: Caps 250 mg; tabs 500 mg; inj (powder) 500 mg/20 ml vial; powder for oral susp 200 mg/ml; ext rel tab (Myfortic) 180, 360 mg

Implementation
• May be given in combination with corticosteroids and cycloSPORINE

PO route
• Do not crush, chew tabs; do not open caps; avoid inhalation or direct contact with skin, mucous membranes; tetratogenic in animals
• Give alone for better absorption
• Delayed rel tabs and caps; oral **susp** and tab are not interchangeable

Intermittent IV infusion route
• Reconstitute each vial with 14 ml D_5W, shake gently, further dilute to 6 mg/ml, dilute 1-g doses in 140 ml D_5W, and 1.5-g doses in 210 ml D_5W, give by slow **IV** infusion ≥2 hr, never give by bolus or rapid **IV** injection
• Do not give with other medications or solutions

Y-site compatibilities: Alemtuzumab, alfentanil, amikacin, anidulafungin, argatroban, bivalirudin, caspofungin, cefepime, DAPTOmycin, DOPamine, norepinephrine, octreotide, oxytocin, tacrolimus, tigecycline, tirofiban, vancomycin

Y-site incompatibilities: Acyclovir, allopurinol, amifostine, aminocaproic acid, aminophylline, amphotericin B, colloidal/lipid complex/liposome, ampicillin, atenolol, azithromycin, aztreonam

ADVERSE EFFECTS
CNS: *Tremor, dizziness, insomnia, headache, fever,* **progressive multifocal leukoencephalopathy,** asthenia, paresthesia, anxiety, pain
CV: *Hypertension, chest pain,* hypotension, edema
GI: *Nausea, vomiting,* stomatitis, *diarrhea, constipation,* **GI bleeding,** abdominal pain, anorexia, dyspepsia
GU: *UTI, hematuria,* **renal tubular necrosis, polyomavirus-associated nephropathy**
HEMA: **Leukopenia, thrombocytopenia, anemia, pancytopenia,** pure red cell aplasia, neutropenia
INTEG: *Rash*
META: *Peripheral edema, hypercholesterolemia, hypophosphatemia, edema, hypo/hyperkalemia, hyperglycemia,* hypocalcemia, hypomagnesemia
MS: Arthralgia, muscle wasting, back pain, weakness

RESP: *Dyspnea, respiratory infection, increased cough, pharyngitis, bronchitis, pneumonia,* **pleural effusion, pulmonary fibrosis**
SYST: **Lymphoma, nonmelanoma skin carcinoma, sepsis**

Pharmacokinetics

Absorption	Rapid and complete
Distribution	Unknown
Metabolism	To active metabolite (MPA)
Excretion	Urine, feces
Half-life	Unknown

Pharmacodynamics
Unknown

INTERACTIONS
Individual drugs
Acyclovir, ganciclovir, valcyclovir: increased toxicity
AzaTHIOprine: increased bone marrow suppression
Cholestyramine, cycloSPORINE, rifamycin: decreased levels of mycophenolate
Phenytoin: increased effects; decreased protein binding of phenytoin
Probenecid: increased levels of mycophenolate
Theophylline: increased effects; decreased protein binding of theophylline

Drug classifications
Antacids (magnesium, aluminum): decreased levels of mycophenolate
Anticoagulants, NSAIDs, thrombolytics, salicylates: increased risk of bleeding
Contraceptives (oral), live attenuated vaccines: decreased effects
Immunosuppressives, salicylates: increased levels of mycophenolate

Drug/herb
Astragalus, echinacea, melatonin: interferes with immunosuppression

Drug/food
Decreased absorption if taken with food

Drug/lab test
Increased: serum creatinine, BUN, potassium, cholesterol, glucose, abnormal LFTs
Decreased: WBC, platelets, neutrophils

NURSING CONSIDERATIONS
Assessment
• **Progressive multifocal leukoencephalopathy; may be fatal:** ataxia, confusion,

---

apathy, hemiparesis, visual problems, weakness; side effects should be reported to the FDA

> **BLACK BOX WARNING: Infection/lymphoma:** may occur from immunosuppressives, increased infections including BK virus, and may cause kidney graft loss

- Monitor blood tests: CBC monthly during treatment
- Monitor liver function tests: alkaline phosphatase, AST, ALT, bilirubin
- Monitor renal studies: BUN, CCr, electrolytes
⚠ **Obtain pregnancy test within 1 wk prior to initiation of treatment; confirm negative pregnancy test**

Patient/family education
⚠ **Teach patient to report fever, rash, severe diarrhea, chills, sore throat, fatigue, since serious infections may occur**

- Instruct patient to avoid crowds to reduce risk of infection
- Advise patient that repeated lab tests are necessary
⚠ **Instruct patient to notify prescriber if pregnancy is planned or suspected (D), to use two forms of contraception before, during, and 6 wk after therapy**

> **BLACK BOX WARNING:** Advise patient that infection and lymphomas may occur

- Teach patient to take on empty stomach, not to crush, chew, break ext rel caps

Evaluation
Positive therapeutic outcome
- Absence of graft rejection

M

nabumetone (Rx)

(na-byoo'me-tone)
Apo-Nabumetone ✦,
Gen-Nabumetone ✦, Relafen ✦
Func. class.: Nonsteroidal antiinflammatory
Chem. class.: Acetic acid derivative
Pregnancy category C

ACTION: Metabolite inhibits COX-1, COX-2 by blocking arachidonate; analgesic, antiinflammatory, antipyretic

Therapeutic outcome: Decreased pain, swelling of joints

USES: Osteoarthritis, rheumatoid arthritis, acute or chronic treatment

CONTRAINDICATIONS:

Hypersensitivity to this product or aspirin, NSAIDs

> **BLACK BOX WARNING:** Perioperative pain in CABG surgery

Precautions: Pregnancy **C**, breastfeeding, children, geriatric, bleeding disorders, GI/cardiac/renal disorders, hepatic dysfunction, asthma, bone marrow suppression, lupus (SLE), ulcerative colitis, blood dyscrasias

> **BLACK BOX WARNING:** MI, stroke, GI bleeding

DOSAGE AND ROUTES

Adult: PO 1 g as a single dose or divided bid; may increase to 2 g/day if needed; max 2 g/day if needed (as a divided dose)

Renal dose

Adult: PO CCr 31-49 ml/min, 750 mg daily, max 1500 mg/day; CCr <30 ml/min, 500 mg daily, max 1000 mg/day

Available forms: Tabs 500, 750 mg

Implementation

• Administer tab to patient crushed or whole
• Give with food or milk to decrease gastric symptoms
• Patient should take with a full glass of water and sit upright
• Store at room temp

ADVERSE EFFECTS

CNS: Dizziness, headache, drowsiness, fatigue, tremors, confusion, insomnia, anxiety, depression, nervousness
CV: Tachycardia, peripheral edema, palpitations, **dysrhythmias, CHF, MI, stroke**
EENT: Tinnitus
GI: Nausea, anorexia, vomiting, diarrhea, jaundice, cholestatic hepatitis, constipation, flatulence, cramps, dry mouth, peptic ulcer, gastritis, **ulceration, perforation,** bleeding
GU: **Nephrotoxicity, dysuria, hematuria, azotemia,** cystitis
HEMA: Thrombocytopenia
INTEG: Purpura, rash, pruritus, sweating, photosensitivity
RESP: Dyspnea, pharyngitis, **bronchospasm**
SYST: **Anaphylaxis, angioedema, Stevens-Johnson syndrome**

Pharmacokinetics

Absorption	Well absorbed
Distribution	Protein binding >99%
Metabolism	Liver, extensively, to inactive metabolite
Excretion	Unknown
Half-life	24 hr

Pharmacodynamics

Onset	Unknown
Peak	2½-4 hr
Duration	Unknown

INTERACTIONS

Individual drugs

Alcohol, potassium: increased GI reactions
Cidofovir, lithium, methotrexate: increased effect of each
Clopidogrel, eptifibatide, ticlopidine: increased risk of bleeding
Radiation: increased risk of hematologic reactions

Drug classifications

Anticoagulants, thrombolytics, SSRIs, SNRIs: increased risk of bleeding
Antihypertensives: decreased effect of antihypertensives
Antineoplastics: increased risk of hematologic reactions
Corticosteroids, NSAIDs, potassium supplements, salicylates: increased GI reactions
Diuretics: decreased effectiveness of diuretics

Drug/herb
Arginine, gossypol: increased gastric irritation
Bearberry, bilberry: increased NSAID effect
Garlic, ginger, ginkgo: increased bleeding risk

Drug/lab test
Increased: bleeding time, K, BUN, AST, ALT, LDH, alkaline phosphatase, creatinine
Decreased: CCr, blood glucose, Hct, Hgb

NURSING CONSIDERATIONS
Assessment

> **BLACK BOX WARNING: Cardiac status:** CV thrombic events, MI, stroke; may be fatal, not to be used in perioperative pain after CABG

> **BLACK BOX WARNING: GI status:** ulceration, bleeding, perforation; may be fatal

• **Assess for pain:** frequency, characteristics, location, duration, intensity, relief of pain after medication; and for inflammation of joints, ROM
• Monitor blood counts during therapy; watch for decreasing platelets; if low, therapy may need to be discontinued, restarted after hematologic recovery; check for blood dyscrasias (thrombocytopenia): bruising, fatigue, bleeding, poor healing; monitor liver function tests: AST, ALT, alkaline phosphatase; LDH, blood glucose, WBC, CCr
• Assess for asthma, aspirin sensitivity, nasal polyps; increased hypersensitivity reactions

Patient/family education
• Tell patient that product must be continued for prescribed time to be effective; to avoid aspirin, alcoholic beverages, NSAIDs, and OTC medications unless approved by prescriber
• Caution patient to report bleeding, bruising, fatigue, malaise, since blood dyscrasias do occur
• Instruct patient to use caution when driving; drowsiness, dizziness may occur
• Advise patient to use sunscreen, hat, and other protective clothing to prevent burns
• Advise patient to report dark stools, a change in urine pattern, increased weight, edema, increased pain in joints, fever, blood in urine, blurred vision, ringing or roaring in ears
• Advise to report use to all health care providers

Evaluation
Positive therapeutic outcome
• Decreased pain
• Decreased inflammation
• Increased mobility

---

nadolol (Rx)
(nay-doe'lole)
Corgard
Func. class.: Antihypertensive, antianginal
Chem. class.: β-Adrenergic receptor blocker
Pregnancy category C

Do not confuse:
Corgard/Cognex/Coreg

ACTION: Long-acting, nonselective β-adrenergic receptor blocking agent, blocks β_1 in the heart and β_2 in the lungs, uterus, and circulatory system; mechanism is similar to that of propranolol

Therapeutic outcome: Decreased B/P, heart rate

USES: Chronic stable angina pectoris, mild to moderate hypertension, atrial fibrillation

Unlabeled uses: Tachydysrhythmias, anxiety, tremors, esophageal varices (rebleeding only), prophylaxis of migraine headaches

CONTRAINDICATIONS:
Hypersensitivity to this product, cardiac failure, cardiogenic shock, 2nd- or 3rd-degree heart block, bronchospastic disease, sinus bradycardia, CHF, COPD

Precautions: Pregnancy C, breastfeeding, diabetes mellitus, renal disease, hyperthyroidism, peripheral vascular disease, myasthenia gravis, major surgery, nonallergic bronchospasm

> **BLACK BOX WARNING:** Abrupt discontinuation

DOSAGE AND ROUTES
Adult: PO 40 mg/day; increase by 40-80 mg q2-14 days; maintenance 40-240 mg/day for angina, 40-320 mg/day for hypertension
Geriatric: PO 20 mg/day, may increase by 20 mg until desired dose

Renal dose
Adult: PO CCr 31-50 ml/min give q24-36hr; CCr 10-30 ml/min give q24-48hr; CCr <10 ml/min give q40-60hr

Migraine prevention (unlabeled)
Adult: PO 40-240 mg/day × 2-18 mo

Available forms: Tabs 20, 40, 80 mg

Adverse effects: *italics* = common; **bold** = life-threatening

Implementation
• Give at bedtime; tab may be crushed or swallowed whole; give with food to prevent GI upset; give reduced dosage in renal dysfunction; check apical pulse prior to use, if <60 bpm, withhold dose and contact prescriber
• Store protected from light, moisture; place in cool environment
• Give without regard to food

ADVERSE EFFECTS
CNS: Depression, *dizziness,* fatigue, lethargy, paresthesia, headache, *weakness,* insomnia, memory loss, nightmares
CV: *Bradycardia, hypotension,* **CHF,** palpitations, AV block, chest pain, peripheral ischemia, flushing, edema, vasodilatation, conduction disturbances
EENT: Blurred vision, dry eyes, nasal congestion
ENDO: Hyperglycemia, hypoglycemia
GI: Nausea, vomiting, diarrhea, colitis, constipation, cramps, dry mouth, flatulence, hepatomegaly, **pancreatitis,** taste distortion
GU: *Impotence,* decreased libido
HEMA: **Agranulocytosis, thrombocytopenia**
INTEG: Rash, pruritus, fever, alopecia
RESP: Dyspnea, respiratory dysfunction, **bronchospasm,** cough, wheezing, pharyngitis, **laryngospasm, pulmonary edema**

Pharmacokinetics
Absorption	Variably absorbed
Distribution	Crosses placenta; minimal concentration in CNS, protein binding 30%
Metabolism	Unknown
Excretion	Kidneys, unchanged
Half-life	10-24 hr; increased in renal disease

Pharmacodynamics
Onset	Variable
Peak	3-4 hr
Duration	10-24 hr

INTERACTIONS
Individual drugs
CloNIDine, EPINEPHrine: increased hypotension, bradycardia
Digoxin: increased bradycardia
Thyroid: decreased β-blocking effect

Drug classifications
Antihypertensives: increased hypotension
Ergots: peripheral ischemia
MAOIs: increased bradycardia; do not use together
NSAIDs: decreased antihypertensive effect
Phenothiazines: increased hypotensive effects

Drug/lab test
Increased: serum potassium, serum uric acid, ALT, AST, alkaline phosphatase, LDH, blood glucose, cholesterol, ANA, triglycerides

NURSING CONSIDERATIONS
Assessment
• **Pain:** assess for duration, time started, activity being performed, location, character
• Monitor B/P at beginning of treatment, periodically thereafter; note rate, rhythm, quality of apical/radial pulse before administration; notify prescriber of any significant changes (pulse <60 bpm), orthostatic hypotension
• Check for baselines in renal, liver function tests before therapy begins
• Assess for edema in feet, legs daily; monitor I&O, daily weight; check for jugular vein distention and crackles bilaterally, dyspnea **(CHF)**
• Headache, light-headedness, decreased B/P; may indicate a need for decreased dosage

> **BLACK BOX WARNING:** Abrupt discontinuation: can result in MI, myocardial ischemia, ventricular dysrhythmias, severe hypertension, withdraw slowly by tapering over 2 wk

Patient/family education
• Teach patient not to discontinue product abruptly; taper over 2 wk; may cause precipitate angina, serious dysrhythmias if stopped abruptly
• Teach patient not to use OTC products containing α-adrenergic stimulants (such as nasal decongestants, cold preparations); to avoid alcohol and smoking and to limit sodium intake as prescribed
• Teach patient how to take pulse and B/P at home; to hold dose if pulse is ≤50 bpm, systolic B/P <90 mm Hg; advise when to notify prescriber; to take missed dose as soon as possible if less than 8 hr
• **Hypertension:** instruct patient to comply with weight control, dietary adjustments, modified exercise program; to report weight gain >5 lb, swelling, unusual bruising, bleeding
• Advise patient to carry/wear emergency ID to identify product being taken, allergies; teach patient product controls symptoms but does not cure condition

---

⚠ Nurse Alert   ✷ Key NCLEX® Drug

- Caution patient to avoid hazardous activities if dizziness, drowsiness are present; to rise slowly to prevent orthostatic hypotension
- **Teach patient to report symptoms of CHF:** difficult breathing, especially on exertion or when lying down, night cough, swelling of extremities or bradycardia, dizziness, confusion, depression, fever
- Teach patient to take product as prescribed, not to double doses, skip doses; take any missed doses as soon as remembered if at least 4 hr until next dose

Evaluation
Positive therapeutic outcome
- Decreased B/P in hypertension

---

nafcillin (Rx)

(naf-sill'in)
Func. class.: Antiinfective, broad-spectrum
Chem. class.: Penicillinase-resistant penicillin

Pregnancy category B

ACTION: Interferes with cell wall replication of susceptible organisms; osmotically unstable cell wall swells, bursts from osmotic pressure

Therapeutic outcome: Bactericidal effects for gram-positive cocci *Staphylococcus aureus, Streptococcus viridans, Streptococcus pneumoniae* and infections caused by penicillinase-producing *Staphylococcus*

USES: Infections caused by penicillinase-producing staphylococci, streptococci; respiratory tract, skin, skin structure, urinary tract, bone, joint infections; sinusitis; endocarditis; septicemia; meningitis

CONTRAINDICATIONS:
Hypersensitivity to penicillins or corn

Precautions: Pregnancy **B**, breastfeeding, neonates, GI disease, asthma, hypersensitivity to cephalosporins or carbapenems, electrolyte imbalances, hepatic/renal disease, pseudomembranous colitis

DOSAGE AND ROUTES
Adult: IV 500-2000 mg q4hr; IM 500 mg q6-8hr, max 12 g/day
Infant and child >1 mo: IV 150-200 mg/kg/day in divided doses q4-6hr
Neonate >7 days (weight >2 kg): IV 25 mg/kg q6hr

Neonate ≤7 days (weight ≤2 kg): IV 25 mg/kg q8hr

Available forms: Powder for inj 1, 2, 10 premixed or Add-Vantage vials (1-2 g)

Implementation
IM route
- Give deep in large muscle mass

IV route
- Reconstitute vials: add 1.7 (1.8 nafcil), 3, 4, or 6.4 ml (6.6 ml NaCl) sterile water for inj, 0.9% NaCl, bacteriostatic water for inj with benzyl alcohol or parabens to vials with 500 mg, 1 g, 2 g of nafcillin, respectively (250 mg/ml); pharmacy bulk pack reconstitute 10 g/93 ml sterile water inj or 0.9% NaCl (100 mg/ml)
- **Nallpen piggyback units:** reconstitute 1 or 2 g with 50-100 ml or 99 ml, respectively, of sterile water for inj, 0.45% NaCl, 0.9% NaCl
- **Unipen piggyback units:** reconstitute according to manufacturer

Direct intermittent IV INJ route
- Further dilute the reconstituted sol in 15-30 ml of sterile water for inj, 0.45% NaCl, 0.9% NaCl; inj slowly over 5-10 min into the tubing of a free-flowing compatible IV solution

Intermittent IV infusion route
- Vials, further dilute reconstituted solution to 2-40 mg/ml, for peripheral vein inf ≤20 mg/ml (preferred); piggyback unit no further dilution needed; infuse ≥30-60 min, make sure entire dose is given before 10% or more of solution is inactivated
- Extravasation management with cold packs, hyaluronidase

Y-site compatibilities: Acyclovir, alfentanil, amikacin, aminophylline, amphotericin B lipid complex (Abelcet), anidulafungin, argatroban, ascorbic acid injection, atenolol, atracurium, atropine, aztreonam, benztropine, bivalirudin, bleomycin, bretylium, bumetanide, buprenorphine, butorphanol, calcium chloride/gluconate, CARBOplatin, carmustine, cefamandole, ceFAZolin, cefoperazone, cefotaxime, cefoTEtan, cefOXitin, cefTAZidime, ceftizoxime, cefTRIAXone, cefuroxime, chlorproMAZINE, cimetidine, CISplatin, clindamycin, cyanocobalamin, cyclophosphamide, cycloSPORINE, DACTINomycin, DAPTOmycin, DAUNOrubicin liposome, dexamethasone, digoxin, DOBUTamine, DOCEtaxel, DOPamine, DOXOrubicin liposomal, enalaprilat, ePHEDrine, EPINEPHrine, epoetin alfa, erythromycin, etoposide, etoposide phosphate, famotidine, fenoldopam, fentaNYL, fluconazole, fludarabine, foscarnet, furosemide, gallium, ganciclovir, gatifloxacin, gemtu-

N

Adverse effects: *italics* = common; **bold** = life-threatening

zumab, gentamicin, glycopyrrolate, granisetron, heparin, hydrocortisone, HYDROmorphone, imipenem-cilastatin, indomethacin, isoproterenol, ketorolac, lactated Ringer's, lepirudin, leucovorin, lidocaine, linezolid injection, LORazepam, magnesium sulfate, mannitol, methyldopate, methylPREDNISolone, metoclopramide, metoprolol, metroNIDAZOLE, milrinone, morphine, multiple vitamins injection, naloxone, niCARdipine, nitroglycerin, nitroprusside, norepinephrine, octreotide, ondansetron, oxacillin, oxaliplatin, oxytocin, PACLitaxel (solvent/surfactant), pamidronate, pancuronium, pantoprazole, PEMEtrexed, penicillin G potassium/sodium, PENTobarbital, perphenazine, PHENobarbital, phentolamine, phenylephrine, phytonadione, piperacillin, polymyxin B, potassium acetate/chloride, procainamide, prochlorperazine, propofol, propranolol, ranitidine, ringer's injection, sodium bicarbonate, SUFentanil, tacrolimus, teniposide, theophylline, thiamine, thiotepa, ticarcillin, ticarcillin clavulanate, tigecycline, tirofiban, TNA (3-in-1), tobramycin, tolazoline, TPN (2-in-1), urokinase, vasopressin, vinBLAStine, voriconazole, zidovudine, zoledronic acid

Y-site incompatibilities: Droperidol, fentaNYL/droperidol, labetalol, nalbuphine, pentazocine, regular insulin, verapamil

ADVERSE EFFECTS

CNS: Lethargy, hallucinations, anxiety, depression, muscle twitching, **coma, seizures**
GI: *Nausea, vomiting, diarrhea,* increased AST, ALT, abdominal pain, glossitis, **pseudomembranous colitis**
GU: Oliguria, **proteinuria, hematuria,** vaginitis, moniliasis, **glomerulonephritis, interstitial nephritis**
HEMA: Anemia, increased bleeding time, **bone marrow depression, neutropenia, agranulocytosis**
INTEG: Tissue necrosis, extravasation injury at injection site
SYST: Anaphylaxis, serum sickness, Stevens-Johnson syndrome

Pharmacokinetics

Absorption	Well absorbed (IM); erratic (PO)
Distribution	Widely distributed; crosses placenta, 90% protein bound
Metabolism	Liver; 70%
Excretion	Kidneys, unchanged; breast milk
Half-life	30-90 min; increased in renal disease

Pharmacodynamics

	PO	IM	IV
Onset	½ hr	½ hr	Immediate
Peak	1-2 hr	1-2 hr	Infusion end
Duration	Unknown	Unknown	Unknown

INTERACTIONS
Individual drugs
CycloSPORINE: decreased effect of cycloSPORINE
NDR: decrease: effect of cycloSPORINE: warfarin
Probenecid: increased nafcillin levels

Drug classifications
Tetracyclines, aminoglycosides: avoid use

Drug/food
Food, carbonated drinks, citrus fruit juices: decreased absorption

Drug/lab test
False positive: urine glucose, urine protein
Decreased: potassium, Hgb/Hct, neutrophils

NURSING CONSIDERATIONS
Assessment
• Assess patient for previous sensitivity reaction to penicillins or other cephalosporins; cross-sensitivity between penicillins and cephalosporins is common
• Assess patient for signs and symptoms of infection including characteristics of wounds, sputum, urine, stool, WBC $>10,000/mm^3$, earache, fever; obtain information baseline, during treatment
• Obtain C&S before beginning product therapy to identify if correct treatment has been initiated
• **Assess for allergic reactions, anaphylaxis:** rash, urticaria, pruritus, chills, fever, dyspnea, laryngeal edema, joint pain; angioedema may occur a few days after therapy begins; cross-sensitivity with cephalosporins may occur; EPINEPHrine, resuscitation equipment should be available for anaphylactic reaction
• Assess renal function tests: urinalysis, protein, blood, BUN, creatinine; abnormal urinalysis may indicate nephrotoxicity
⚠ **Identify urine output; if decreasing, notify prescriber (may indicate nephrotoxicity)**
• Monitor blood studies: AST, ALT, CBC, Hct, bilirubin, LDH, alkaline phosphatase, Coombs'

test monthly if patient is on long-term therapy, electrolytes
• Monitor electrolytes: potassium, sodium, chloride monthly if patient is on long-term therapy
• **Pseudomembranous colitis:** assess for diarrhea, abdominal pain, fever, fatigue, anorexia; possible anemia, elevated WBC and low serum albumin; stop product and usually give either vancomycin or IV metroNIDAZOLE
• Monitor for bleeding: ecchymosis, bleeding gums, hematuria, stool guaiac daily if on long-term therapy
• Assess for overgrowth of infection: perineal itching, fever, malaise, redness, pain, swelling, drainage, rash, diarrhea, change in cough, sputum
• **IV site:** assess for redness, swelling, pain at site

Patient/family education
• Teach patient to report sore throat, bruising, bleeding, joint pain; may indicate blood dyscrasias (rare)
• Advise patient to contact prescriber if vaginal itching, loose foul-smelling stools, furry tongue occur; may indicate superinfection
• Instruct patient to take all medication prescribed for the length of time ordered
• Advise patient to notify prescriber of diarrhea with blood or pus, which may indicate pseudomembranous colitis
• Advise patient to carry/wear emergency ID if allergic to penicillins
• Teach patient to avoid use with other products unless approved by prescriber

Evaluation
Positive therapeutic outcome
• Absence of signs/symptoms of infection (WBC <10,000/mm^3, temp WNL, absence of red, draining wounds, earache)
• Reported improvement in symptoms of infection

TREATMENT OF ANAPHYLAXIS:
Withdraw product, maintain airway, administer EPINEPHrine, aminophylline, O$_2$, **IV** corticosteroids

---

⚠ HIGH ALERT
nalbuphine (Rx)
(nal'byoo-feen)
Func. class.: Opioid analgesic
Chem. class.: Synthetic opioid agonist/antagonist
Pregnancy category C

ACTION: Depresses pain impulse transmission at the spinal cord level by interacting with opioid receptors

Therapeutic outcome: Relief of pain

USES: Moderate to severe pain, supplement to anesthesia

CONTRAINDICATIONS:
Hypersensitivity to this product or parabens, addiction (opioid)

Precautions: Pregnancy **B**, breastfeeding, addictive personality, increased ICP, MI (acute), severe heart disease, respiratory depression, renal/hepatic disease, bowel impaction, abrupt discontinuation

DOSAGE AND ROUTES
Analgesic
Adult: SUBCUT/IM/**IV** max 10 mg q3-6hr prn, max 160 mg/day

Balanced anesthesia adjunct
Adult: **IV** 0.3-3 mg/kg given over 10-15 min; may give 0.25-0.5 mg/kg as needed (maintenance)

Available forms: Inj 10, 20 mg/ml

Implementation
• Give by inj (IM, **IV**), only with resuscitative equipment available; give slowly to prevent rigidity
• Store in light-resistant area at room temperature

IM route
• Give inj deeply in large muscle mass; rotate inj sites; protect vial from light

Direct IV route
• Give direct **IV** undiluted 10 mg or less over 3-5 min or more into free-flowing IV line of D$_5$W, NS, LR

Syringe compatibilities: Atropine, cimetidine, diphenhydrAMINE, droperidol, glycopyrrolate, hydrOXYzine, lidocaine, midazolam, prochlorperazine, promethazine, ranitidine, scopolamine, trimethobenzamide

---

Syringe incompatibilities: Diazepam, PENTobarbital

Y-site compatibilities: Amifostine, aztreonam, cladribine, filgrastim, fludarabine, granisetron, melphalan, PACLitaxel, propofol, teniposide, thiotepa, vinorelbine

Y-site incompatibilities: Nafcillin, sargramostim

ADVERSE EFFECTS

CNS: *Drowsiness, dizziness, confusion, headache, sedation, euphoria,* dysphoria (high doses), hallucinations, increased dreaming, tolerance, physical and psychological dependency
CV: Bradycardia, change in B/P, **cardiac arrest**
EENT: Blurred vision, miosis, diplopia
GI: *Nausea, vomiting, anorexia, constipation, cramps,* abdominal pain, dyspepsia, xerostomia, bitter taste
GU: Urinary urgency
INTEG: *Rash,* urticaria, flushing, *diaphoresis,* pruritus
RESP: **Respiratory depression/arrest,** pulmonary edema

Pharmacokinetics	
Absorption	Well absorbed (SUBCUT, IM); completely absorbed (**IV**)
Distribution	Crosses placenta
Metabolism	Liver, extensively
Excretion	Feces, kidneys, unchanged (small amounts); breast milk
Half-life	3-6 hr

Pharmacodynamics			
	IM	SUBCUT	IV
Onset	Up to 15 min	Up to 15 min	2-3 min
Peak	1 hr	Unknown	½ hr
Duration	3-6 hr	3-6 hr	3-6 hr

INTERACTIONS
Individual drugs
Alcohol: increased respiratory depression, hypotension, sedation

Drug classifications
Antipsychotics, CNS depressants, sedative/hypnotics, skeletal muscle relaxants: increased respiratory depression, hypotension
Opiates: increased effects with other CNS depressants

NURSING CONSIDERATIONS
Assessment
• **Assess pain characteristics** (location, intensity, type) before medication administration, 30-60 min after treatment, titrate upward by 25%-50% until pain is reduced by 50%
• Assess bowel status; constipation is common, may need laxative or stool softener
• Monitor VS after parenteral route; note muscle rigidity, product history, liver, kidney function tests; **respiratory dysfunction: respiratory depression, character, rate, rhythm; notify prescriber if respirations are <10/min**
• **Monitor CNS changes:** dizziness, drowsiness, hallucinations, euphoria, LOC, pupil reaction
• Monitor allergic reactions: rash, urticaria

Patient/family education
• Instruct patient to report any symptoms of CNS changes, allergic reactions
• Teach patient that physical dependency can result from long-term use, although there is a low potential for dependency, profuse sweating, twitching; without treatment, symptoms resolve in 5-14 days; chronic abstinence syndrome may last 2-6 mo
• Caution patients to avoid CNS depressants: alcohol, sedative/hypnotics for at least 24 hr after taking this product
• Discuss with patient that dizziness, drowsiness, confusion are common; to avoid getting up without assistance
• Discuss in detail all aspects of the product: reason for taking product and expected results
• Instruct patient to change position slowly to prevent orthostatic hypotension

Evaluation
Positive therapeutic outcome
• Relief of pain without respiratory depression

TREATMENT OF OVERDOSE:
Naloxone (Narcan) 0.2-0.8 **IV**, O_2, **IV** fluids, vasopressors

---

naloxone (Rx)
(nal-oks′one)
naloxone HCl
Func. class.: Opioid antagonist, antidote
Chem. class.: Thebaine derivative
Pregnancy category C

Do not confuse:
naloxone/naltrexone

ACTION: Competes with opioids at opioid-receptor sites

Therapeutic outcome: Absence of opioid overdose

USES: Respiratory depression induced by opioids; refractory circulatory shock, asphyxia neonatorum, coma, hypotension, opiate agonist overdose

Unlabeled uses: IBS, opiate agonist dependence, opiate agonist-induced constipation, pruritus

CONTRAINDICATIONS:
Hypersensitivity

Precautions: Pregnancy **B**, breastfeeding, neonates, children, CV disease, opioid dependency, seizure disorder, drug dependency, hepatic disease

DOSAGE AND ROUTES
Opioid-induced respiratory depression (known or suspected opiate agonist overdose)
Adult: IV/SUBCUT/IM 0.4-2 mg; repeat q2-3min if needed, max 10 mg; IV infusion loading dose 0.005 mg/kg, then 0.0025 mg/kg/hr
Child <5 yr or ≤20 kg: IV/intraosseous 0.01 mg/kg slowly followed by 0.1 mg/kg if needed; IV infusion (PALS) 0.04-0.16 mg/kg/hr, titrate

Postoperative opioid-induced respiratory depression
Adult: IV 0.1-0.2 mg q2-3min prn
Child: IV 0.005-0.01 mg/kg q2-3min prn

Nausea/vomiting from continuous morphine infusion/urinary retention (unlabeled)
Adult: IV 0.2 mg

Available forms: Inj 0.02, 0.4, 1 mg/ml

Implementation
• Store at room temperature and protect from light

Direct IV route
• Give undiluted; give 0.4 mg or less over 15 sec or titrate inf to response
Continuous IV infusion route
• Dilute 2 mg/500 ml 0.9% NaCl or D₅W (4 mcg/ml), titrate to response
• Give only with resuscitative equipment, O₂ nearby
• Use only sol prepared within 24 hr

Y-site compatibilities: Acyclovir, alfentanil, amikacin, aminocaproic acid, aminophylline, anidulafungin, ascorbic acid, atenolol, atracurium, atropine, azaTHIOprine, aztreonam, benztropine, bivalirudin, bleomycin, bumetanide, buprenorphine, butorphanol, calcium chloride/gluconate, CARBOplatin, caspofungin, cefamandole, ceFAZolin, cefmetazole, cefonicid, cefoperazone, cefotaxime, cefoTEtan, cefOXitin, cefTAZidime, ceftizoxime, cefTRIAXone, cefuroxime, cephalothin, cephapirin, chloramphenicol, chlorproMAZINE, cimetidine, CISplatin, clindamycin, cyanocobalamin, cyclophosphamide, cycloSPORINE, cytarabine, DACTINomycin, DAPTOmycin, dexamethasone, digoxin, diltiazem, diphenhydrAMINE, DOBUTamine, DOCEtaxel, DOPamine, doxacurium, DOXOrubicin, doxycycline, enalaprilat, ePHEDrine, EPINEPHrine, epirubicin, epoetin alfa, eptifibatide, ertapenem, erythromycin, esmolol, etoposide, etoposide phosphate, famotidine, fenoldopam, fentaNYL, fluconazole, fludarabine, fluorouracil, folic acid, furosemide, ganciclovir, gatifloxacin, gemcitabine, gentamicin, glycopyrrolate, granisetron, heparin, hydrocortisone, hydrOXYzine, IDArubicin, ifosfamide, imipenem-cilastatin, inamrinone, indomethacin, insulin (regular), irinotecan, isoproterenol, ketorolac, labetalol, levofloxacin, lidocaine, linezolid, LORazepam, mannitol, mechlorethamine, meperidine, metaraminol, methicillin, methotrexate, methyldopate, methylPREDNISolone, metoclopramide, metoprolol, metroNIDAZOLE, mezlocillin, miconazole, midazolam, milrinone, minocycline, mitoXANtrone, morphine, multiple vitamins, mycophenolate, nafcillin, nalbuphine, nesiritide, netilmicin, nitroglycerin, nitroprusside, norepinephrine, octreotide, ondansetron, oxacillin, oxaliplatin, oxytocin, PACLitaxel, palonosetron, pamidronate, pancuronium, papaverine, PEMEtrexed, penicillin G potassium/sodium, pentamidine, pentazocine, PENTobarbital, PHENobarbital, phentolamine, phenylephrine, phytonadione, piperacillin, piperacillin-tazobactam, polymyxin B, potassium chloride, procainamide, prochlorperazine, promethazine, propofol, propranolol, protamine, pyridoxine, quiNIDine, quinupristin-dalfopristin, ranitidine, rocuronium, sodium acetate/bicarbonate, succinylcholine, SUFentanil, tacrolimus, teniposide, theophylline, thiamine, ticarcillin, ticarcillin-clavulanate, tigecycline, tirofiban, tobramycin, tolazoline, urokinase, vancomycin, vasopressin, vecuronium, verapamil, vinCRIStine, vinorelbine, voriconazole, zoledronic acid

N

ADVERSE EFFECTS

CNS: Nervousness, **seizures,** tremor, opioid withdrawal symptoms

CV: Rapid pulse, **ventricular tachycardia, fibrillation,** increased systolic B/P (high doses), hypo/hypertension, **cardiac arrest, sinus tachycardia**

GI: Nausea, vomiting

RESP: Pulmonary edema, dyspnea

Pharmacokinetics

Absorption	Well absorbed (SUBCUT, IM); completely absorbed (**IV**)
Distribution	Rapidly distributed; crosses placenta
Metabolism	Liver
Excretion	Kidneys
Half-life	1 hr; up to 3 hr (neonates)

Pharmacodynamics

	IV	IM/SUBCUT
Onset	1 min	2-5 min
Peak	Unknown	Unknown
Duration	45 min	30-81 min

INTERACTIONS

Individual drugs

TraMADol: increased seizures, overdose

Drug classifications

Analgesics (opioids): decreased effects of opioid analgesics

Drug/lab test

Interference: urine VMA, 5-HIAA, urine glucose

NURSING CONSIDERATIONS

Assessment

• **Assess for signs of opioid withdrawal** in drug-dependent individuals: cramping, hypertension, anxiety, vomiting; may occur up to 2 hr after administration

• Monitor VS q3-5min; ABGs including Po$_2$, Pco$_2$

• Assess cardiac status: tachycardia, hypertension; monitor ECG

• **Assess for pain:** duration, intensity, location before, after administration; may be used for respiratory depression

• **Assess for respiratory dysfunction:** respiratory depression, character, rate, rhythm; if respirations are <10/min, probably due to opioid overdose, administer naloxone; monitor LOC

Patient/family education

• Explain reason for and expected results of medication when patient is alert

Evaluation

Positive therapeutic outcome

• Reversal of respiratory depression

• LOC: alert

---

naphazoline nasal
See Appendix B

naphazoline ophthalmic
See Appendix B

naproxen
(na-prox′en)

Aleve, Anaprox, Anaprox DS, Apo-Napro-Na ✦, EC-Naprosyn, Equaline All Day Relief, Good Sense All Day Pain Relief, Midol Extended Relief, Nu-Naprox ✦, Top Care All Day Pain Relief, Wal-Proxen

Func. class.: Nonsteroidal antiinflammatory, nonopioid analgesic

Chem. class.: Propionic acid derivative

Pregnancy category B (1st trimester), D (2nd/3rd trimesters) ✳

Do not confuse:
Naprosyn/Natacyn/Naprelan

ACTION: Completely inhibits COX-1, COX-2 by blocking arachidonate; analgesic, antiinflammatory, antipyretic

Therapeutic outcome: Decreased pain, inflammation

USES: Mild to moderate pain, osteoarthritis, rheumatoid arthritis, gouty arthritis, primary dysmenorrhea, tendinitis, ankylosing spondylitis, bursitis, myalgia, dental pain, juvenile rheumatoid arthritis

CONTRAINDICATIONS:

Pregnancy **C** (2nd/3rd trimesters), hypersensitivity to NSAIDs, salicylates

BLACK BOX WARNING: Perioperative pain in CABG surgery

Precautions: Pregnancy **C** (1st trimester), breastfeeding, children <2 yr, geriatric, bleeding disorders, GI/cardiac disorders, hypersensi-

---

tivity to other antiinflammatory agents, CCr <30 ml/min, asthma, renal failure, hepatic disease

> **BLACK BOX WARNING:** MI, GI bleeding, stroke

DOSAGE AND ROUTES
200 mg base = 220 mg naproxen sodium

Antiinflammatory/analgesic/antidysmenorrheal
Adult: PO 250-500 mg bid, max 1250 mg/day; DEL REL TAB 375-500 mg bid
Child ≥2 yr: PO 7 mg/kg/12 hr

Antigout
Adult: PO 750 mg, then 250 mg q8hr

OTC use
Adult: PO 220 mg q8-12hr or 440 mg, then 220 mg q12hr, max 660 mg/24 hr, taken no longer than 10 days
Geriatric >65 yr: PO max 220 mg q12hr

Available forms: Naproxen: tabs: 250, 375, 500 mg; del rel tabs (EC-Naprosyn, Naprosyn-E) 250♣, 375, 500 mg; oral susp 125 mg/5 ml; ext rel tabs (CR) 375, 500, 750 mg♣; naproxen sodium; tabs 220, 275, 550 mg; ext rel tab 220 mg

Implementation
• Store at room temp
• Administer to patient crushed or whole (**regular release**); do not crush, break, or chew **extended rel tab**
• Give OTC for 10 days or less unless approved by prescriber
• Adequately hydrate those taking angiotensin receptor blockers/angiotensin-converting enzyme inhibitors
• Give with food or milk to decrease gastric symptoms; give ½ hr before or 2 hr after meals for better absorption
• Patient should take with 8 oz of water and sit upright for 30 min after dose to prevent ulceration

ADVERSE EFFECTS
CNS: Dizziness, drowsiness, fatigue, tremors, confusion, insomnia, anxiety, depression
CV: Tachycardia, peripheral edema, palpitations, **dysrhythmias, MI, stroke**
EENT: Tinnitus, hearing loss, blurred vision
GI: Nausea, anorexia, vomiting, diarrhea, jaundice, **hepatitis,** constipation, flatulence, cramps, peptic ulcer, **GI ulceration, bleeding, perforation**
GU: Nephrotoxicity: dysuria, hematuria, oliguria, azotemia
HEMA: Blood dyscrasias
INTEG: Purpura, rash, pruritus, sweating
SYST: Anaphylaxis, Stevens-Johnson syndrome

Pharmacokinetics
Absorption	Completely absorbed
Distribution	Crosses placenta, 99% protein binding
Metabolism	Liver, extensively
Excretion	Breast milk
Half-life	10-20 hr

Pharmacodynamics
Onset	1 hr
Peak	2-4 hr
Duration	<7 hr

INTERACTIONS
Individual drugs
Adefovir, cidofovir: increased nephrotoxicity, avoid concurrent use
Alcohol, aspirin: increased risk of GI side effects
Clopidogrel, eptifibatide, plicamycin, ticlopidine, tirofiban: increased bleeding risk
Lithium, methotrexate, probenecid, radiation: increased toxicity
Cholestyramine, sucralfate: decreased/delayed absorption of naproxen

Drug classifications
ACE inhibitors: possible renal impairment
Antacids: decreased/delayed absorption of naproxen
Anticoagulants, SSRIs, SNRIs, thrombolytics, tricyclics: increased risk of bleeding
Antihypertensives: decreased effect of antihypertensives
Antineoplastics: increased risk of hematologic toxicity
Corticosteroids, NSAIDs: increased risk of GI adverse reactions
Diuretics: decreased effectiveness of diuretics

Drug/herb
Fenugreek, feverfew, garlic, ginger, ginkgo, ginseng *(Panax)*, licorice: increased bleeding risk

Drug/lab test
Increased: BUN, alkaline phosphatase, LFTs, potassium, glucose, cholesterol
Decreased: potassium, sodium
False: increased 5-HIAA, 17KS

NURSING CONSIDERATIONS
Assessment

> **BLACK BOX WARNING: Cardiac status:** CV thrombotic events, MI, stroke; may be fatal; not to be used in CABG

> **BLACK BOX WARNING: GI status:** ulceration, bleeding, perforation; may be fatal

• Monitor liver function, renal function, other blood tests: AST, ALT, bilirubin, creatinine, BUN, CBC, Hct, Hgb, pro-time, LDH, blood glucose, WBC, platelets; if patient is on long-term therapy
• Check I&O ratio; decreasing output may indicate renal failure (long-term therapy)
• **Assess hepatotoxicity:** dark urine, clay-colored stools, yellowing of the skin and sclera, itching, abdominal pain, fever, diarrhea if patient is on long-term therapy
• Assess for allergic reactions: rash, urticaria; if these occur, product may have to be discontinued
• **Assess for ototoxicity:** tinnitus, ringing, roaring in ears; audiometric testing needed before, after long-term therapy
• Assess for vision changes: blurring, halos if taking long term; may indicate corneal, retinal damage
• Check for edema in feet, ankles, legs
• Identify prior product history; there are many product interactions
• **Monitor pain:** location, frequency, duration, characteristics, type, intensity before dose and 1 hour after
• **Arthritis:** Assess ROM, pain, swelling before and 1-2 hr after use
• **Fever:** Assess before use and 1 hr after use
• Assess for asthma, aspirin hypersensitivity, or nasal polyps, increased risk of hypersensitivity

Patient/family education
• Teach patient to report any symptoms of renal/hepatic toxicity, vision changes, ototoxicity, allergic reactions, bleeding (long-term therapy); to report use to all health care providers
• Caution patient not to exceed recommended dosage; acute poisoning may result; to take as prescribed, do not double dose
• Teach patient to read label on other OTC products; many contain other antiinflammatories; caution patient to avoid alcohol ingestion; GI bleeding may occur
• Inform patient that the therapeutic response takes 2 wk (arthritis)
• Teach patient to report tinnitus, confusion, diarrhea, sweating, hyperventilation, blurred vision, fever, joint aches, black stools, flulike symptoms
• Teach patient to notify prescriber if pregnancy is planned or suspected, pregnancy (**C**), avoid breastfeeding

Evaluation
Positive therapeutic outcome
• Decreased pain
• Decreased inflammation
• Increased mobility

---

naratriptan (Rx)
(nair′ah-trip-tan)
Amerge
Func. class.: Antimigraine agent
Chem. class.: 5-HT₁-like receptor agonist
Pregnancy category C

Do not confuse:
Amerge/Altace/Amaryl

ACTION: Binds selectively to the vascular 5-HT₁ receptor subtype, exerts antimigraine effect; causes vasoconstriction in cranial arteries

Therapeutic outcome: Decreased intensity and incidence of migraines

USES: Acute treatment of migraine with or without aura

CONTRAINDICATIONS:
Angina pectoris, history of MI, documented silent ischemia, ischemic heart disease, concurrent ergotamine-containing preparations, uncontrolled hypertension, hypersensitivity, severe renal disease (CCr <15 ml/min), severe hepatic disease (Child-Pugh grade C), CV syndromes, hemiplegic or basilar migraines

Precautions: Pregnancy **C**, breastfeeding, children, geriatric, postmenopausal women, men >40 yr, risk factors for CAD, hypercholesterolemia, obesity, diabetes, impaired renal/hepatic function, peripheral vascular disease

DOSAGE AND ROUTES
Adult: PO 1 or 2.5 mg with fluids; if headache returns, repeat once after 4 hr, max 5 mg/24 hr

Renal/hepatic dose
Adult: PO CCr 15-39 ml/min
Max 2.5 mg/24 hr

Available forms: Tabs 1, 2.5 mg

Implementation
- Do not use product if another 5-HT$_1$ agonist or an ergot preparation has been used in past 24 hr
- Give with fluids as soon as symptoms appear; may take another dose after 4 hr; max 5 mg in any 24-hr period
- Provide a quiet, calm environment with decreased stimulation, including noise, bright light, excessive talking

ADVERSE EFFECTS
CNS: Dizziness, sedation, fatigue
CV: Increased B/P, palpitations, **tachydys-rhythmias, PR and QT$_C$ prolongation, ST/T wave changes, PVCs, atrial flutter, fibrillation, coronary vasospasm**
EENT: EENT infections, photophobia
GI: *Nausea, vomiting*
MISC: Temp change sensations, tightness, pressure sensations
MS: *Weakness, neck stiffness,* myalgia

Pharmacokinetics
Absorption	Unknown
Distribution	28%-31% protein binding
Metabolism	Liver (metabolite)
Excretion	Urine/feces
Half-life	6 hr

Pharmacodynamics
Onset	Unknown
Peak	2-3 hr
Duration	Unknown

INTERACTIONS
Individual drugs
Sibutramine: increased serotonin syndrome risk

Drug classifications
5-HT$_1$ agonists, ergot derivatives: increased vasospastic effect
MAOIs: increased risk of adverse reactions, do not use together
SSRIs (FLUoxetine, fluvoxaMINE, PARoxetine, sertraline), SNRIs, serotonin receptor agonists, sibutramine: increased serotonin syndrome, neuroleptic malignant syndrome

Drug/herb
SAMe, St. John's wort: increased serotonin syndrome

NURSING CONSIDERATIONS
Assessment
- **Serotonin syndrome, neuroleptic malignant syndrome:** assess for increased heart rate, shivering, sweating, dilated pupils, tremors, high B/P, hyperthermia, headache, confusion; if these occur, stop product, administer a serotonin antagonist if needed; at least 2 wk should elapse between discontinuing serotoninergic agents and starting this product
- **Migraines:** assess for aura, duration, effect of lifestyle, aggravating/alleviating factors
- Cardiac status: ECG, increased B/P, dysrhythmias, monitor for PR, QT prolongation, ST-T wave changes, PVCs in those with cardiac disease
- Assess for stress level, activity, recreation, coping mechanisms
- Assess neurologic status: LOC, blurred vision, nausea, tics preceding headache

Patient/family education
- Teach patient to report pain, tightness in chest, neck, throat, or jaw; notify prescriber immediately if sudden, severe abdominal pain occurs
- Teach patient to use contraception while taking product, to notify prescriber if pregnancy is planned or suspected
- Teach patient not to use if another 5-HT$_1$ agonist or an ergot preparation has been used in the past 24 hr; avoid using >2 days/wk, rebound headache may occur

Evaluation
Positive therapeutic outcome
- Absence of migraine headaches

---

natalizumab (Rx)
(na-ta-liz'u-mab)
Tysabri
Func. class.: Biological response modifier, immunoglobulins, monoclonal antibody
Pregnancy category C

ACTION: Biological response modifying properties mediated through specific receptors on cells, may be secondary to blockade of the interaction by inflammatory cells on vascular endothelial cells

Therapeutic outcome: Decreased symptoms of multiple sclerosis

USES: Ambulatory patients with relapsing-remitting multiple sclerosis who have not responded to other treatment, moderate to severe Crohn's disease

CONTRAINDICATIONS:

Hypersensitivity, immunocompromised individuals (HIV, AIDS, leukemia, lymphoma, transplants), PML, murine (mouse) protein allergy

> **BLACK BOX WARNING:** Progressive multifocal leukoencephalopathy, incidence increases with number of doses, over 2 yr immunosuppressants and anti-JC virus antibody; consider testing for the anti-JC virus and periodically retest

Infection: report serious opportunistic infections to the manufacturer, those with Crohn's disease and chronic oral corticosteroids may be at greater risk of infection

Precautions: Pregnancy **C**, breastfeeding, geriatric, chronic progressive multiple sclerosis, depression, mental disorders, diabetes, TB, active infections, hepatotoxicity

DOSAGE AND ROUTES

Adult: **IV** INF 300 mg q4wk, give over 1 hr, observe during and for 1 hr after inf

Available forms: Single-use vial, 300 mg/100 ml 0.9% NaCl

Implementation

• Give acetaminophen for fever, headache
• Give only after being enrolled in the TOUCH Prescribing Program

Intermittent IV INF route
• Use only clear, colorless solution, without particulates
• Withdraw 15 ml from the vial using aseptic technique: inject conc into 100 ml 0.9% NaCl; do not use other diluents; mix completely; do not shake; infuse immediately or refrigerate for up to 8 hr; warm to room temperature before using; flush with 0.9% NaCl before, after inf; do not admix or use in same line with other agents
• Withhold product at first sign of PML
• Prescribers must be registered in the TOUCH prescribing program (1-800-456-2255)
• Store solution in refrigerator; do not freeze or shake; protect from light

ADVERSE EFFECTS

CNS: *Headache, fatigue,* rigors, syncope, tremors, *depression,* **PML (progressive multifocal leukoencephalopathy), suicidal ideation,** anxiety

CV: Chest discomfort, hyper/hypotension, tachycardia
GI: *Abdominal discomfort,* abnormal liver function tests, gastroenteritis, **severe hepatic injury**
GU: Amenorrhea, *UTI, irregular menses,* vaginitis, urinary frequency
INTEG: *Rash,* dermatitis, pruritus, **skin melanoma,** infusion-related reactions
MS: *Arthralgia,* myalgia
RESP: *Lower respiratory tract infection,* dyspnea
SYST: **Anaphylaxis, angioedema**

Pharmacokinetics

Absorption	Unknown
Distribution	Unknown
Metabolism	Unknown
Excretion	Unknown
Half-life	Approximately 11 days

Pharmacodynamics

Unknown

INTERACTIONS

Drug classifications
Do not use with vaccines
Immunosuppressants, antineoplastics, immunomodulators, tumor-necrosis factors: increased infection

NURSING CONSIDERATIONS

Assessment

> **BLACK BOX WARNING:** Assess for progressive multifocal leukoencephalopathy (weakness, paralysis, vision loss, impaired speech, cognitive deterioration), notify prescriber immediately

⚠ **Infection: report serious opportunistic infections to the manufacturer, those with Crohn's disease and taking chronic oral corticosteroids are at greater risk**
• Monitor blood, renal, hepatic tests: CBC, differential, platelet counts, BUN, creatinine, ALT, urinalysis, for hypersensitivity reactions
• Assess CNS symptoms: headache, fatigue, depression, rigors, tremors
• Assess GI status: abdominal discomfort
• Assess mental status: depression, depersonalization, suicidal thoughts, insomnia
• **Assess for multiple sclerosis symptoms;** this product should only be used in patients who have not responded to other treatments

---

⚠ Assess for anaphylaxis: shortness of breath, hives; swelling, tightness in throat, chest pain; usually within 2 hr of inf
• Monitor using gadolinium-enhanced MRI scan of the brain, possibly CSF for JC viral DNA

Patient/family education
• Provide patient or family member with written, detailed information about the product (med guide)
• Teach female patients they may experience irregular menses, amenorrhea
• Instruct patient to notify prescriber if pregnancy is suspected; if pregnant, call the Tysabri Pregnancy Exposure Registry (1-800-456-2255)
• Teach patient that continuing follow-up will be needed at 3, 6 mo after first dose, then every 6 mo
• Teach patient to inform all prescribers of product use
• Instruct patient to avoid breastfeeding while taking this product
• Instruct patient to notify prescriber of possible infection: sore throat, cough, increased temp, may worsen over several days

Evaluation
Positive therapeutic outcome
• Decreased symptoms of multiple sclerosis

natamycin ophthalmic
See Appendix B

nebivolol (Rx)
(ne-biv′oh-lol)
Bystolic
Func. class.: Antihypertensive
Chem. class.: β₁-Blocker
Pregnancy category C

ACTION: Competitively blocks stimulation of β-adrenergic receptors within vascular smooth muscle; decreases rate of SA node discharge, increases recovery time, slows conduction of AV node resulting in decreased heart rate (negative chronotropic effect), which decreases O₂ consumption in myocardium due to β₁-receptor antagonism; also decreases renin-aldosterone-angiotensin system at high doses, inhibits β₂-receptors in bronchial system (high doses)

Therapeutic outcome: Decreased B/P after 1-2 wk

USES: Hypertension alone or in combination

Unlabeled uses: Heart failure

CONTRAINDICATIONS:
Cardiogenic shock, acute sick sinus syndrome, AV heart block, hypersensitivity to this agent or β-blockers, heart failure, severe hepatic disease, severe bradycardia

Precautions: Pregnancy C, breastfeeding, children, major surgery, peripheral vascular disease, diabetes mellitus, thyrotoxicosis, COPD, asthma, well-compensated heart failure, renal/hepatic disease, abrupt discontinuation, acute bronchospasm

DOSAGE AND ROUTES
Hypertension
Adult: PO 5 mg/day, may be increased to desired response q2wk; max 40 mg/day
Geriatric: PO max 40 mg/day

Renal dose
Adult: PO CCr <30 ml/min, 2.5 mg/day; may increase cautiously

Hepatic dose
Adult: PO (Child-Pugh class B) 2.5 mg qd; use dose escalation cautiously

Heart failure (unlabeled)
Adult: PO 1.25 mg titrated to max 10 mg/day

Available forms: Tabs 2.5, 5, 10, 20 mg

Implementation
PO route
• Give without regard for meals; tab may be crushed or swallowed whole; give with food to prevent GI upset
• Store protected from light, moisture; place in cool environment

ADVERSE EFFECTS
CNS: *Insomnia, fatigue, dizziness, mental changes,* drowsiness, **headache**
CV: **Bradycardia, MI,** AV heart block, edema
GI: *Nausea, diarrhea,* vomiting, abdominal pain
GU: *Impotence*
HEMA: **Thrombocytopenia**
INTEG: Rash, pruritus, vasculitis, urticaria, psoriasis, **angioedema**
MISC: **Renal failure, pulmonary edema,** hyperuricemia, hypercholesterolemia, withdrawal symptoms
RESP: **Bronchospasm,** dyspnea

N

Adverse effects: *italics* = common; **bold** = life-threatening

Pharmacokinetics

Absorption	Unknown
Distribution	Unknown
Metabolism	In liver by CYP2D6
Excretion	38% excreted in urine, 44% in feces
Half-life	12 hr

Pharmacodynamics

Onset	Unknown
Peak	1.5-4 hr
Duration	Unknown

INTERACTIONS

Individual drugs
Cimetidine: increased nebivolol action
Mefloquine: do not give
Sildenafil: decreased nebivolol action

Drug classifications
β-blockers, others: do not use concurrently
Calcium channel blockers (nondihydro-pyridine), CYP2D6 inhibitors (amiodarone, buPROPion, chloroquine, chlorpheniramine, chlorproMAZINE, cinacalcet, diphenhydrAMINE, DULoxetine, FLUoxetine, haloperidol, imatinib, PARoxetine, promethazine, propoxyphene, quiNIDine, quiNINE, ritonavir, terbinafine, thioridazine): increased nebivolol action
CYP2D6 inducers (rifampin): decreased nebivolol action

Drug/herb
Hawthorn: may increase nebivolol effect
Ephedra: decreased nebivolol effect

Drug/lab test
Increased: serum lipoprotein levels, BUN, potassium, triglyceride, uric acid, LDH, AST, ALT, alkaline phosphatase
Decreased: platelets

NURSING CONSIDERATIONS

Assessment
• **Hypertension:** monitor B/P during beginning treatment, periodically thereafter; assess apical/radial pulse before administration; notify prescriber of any significant changes (pulse <50 bpm); **signs of CHF** (dyspnea, crackles, weight gain, jugular vein distention)
• Assess baselines in renal/hepatic studies before therapy begins and periodically, **do not use in Child-Pugh class >B**
• Monitor I&O, edema in feet, legs daily

• Monitor skin turgor, dryness of mucous membranes for hydration status, especially geriatric patients
• Assess blood glucose in diabetics

Patient/family education
⚠ Caution patient not to discontinue product abruptly; severe cardiac reactions may occur; taper over 2 wk; do not double dose; if a dose is missed, take as soon as remembered up to 4 hr before next dose
• Inform patient product may mask signs of hypoglycemia or alter blood glucose levels
• Advise patient not to use OTC products containing α-adrenergic stimulants (such as nasal decongestants, OTC cold preparations) unless directed by prescriber
• Instruct patient to report low pulse, dizziness, confusion, depression, fever
• Teach patient to take pulse, B/P at home; advise when to notify prescriber
• Advise patient to comply with weight control, dietary adjustments, modified exercise program
• Instruct patient to carry emergency ID to identify product, allergies
• Caution patient to avoid hazardous activities if dizziness, drowsiness are present
• **Instruct patient to report symptoms of CHF:** difficulty breathing, especially on exertion or when lying down, night cough, swelling of extremities
• Teach patient to continue with required lifestyle changes (exercise, diet, weight loss, stress reduction)

Evaluation
Positive therapeutic outcome
• Decreased B/P after 1-2 wk
• Decreased dysrhythmias

TREATMENT OF OVERDOSE:
Lavage, **IV** atropine for bradycardia, **IV** theophylline for bronchospasm, digoxin, O₂, diuretic for cardiac failure, **IV** glucose for hypoglycemia, **IV** diazepam (or phenytoin) for seizures, **IV** fluids, **IV** pressors

---

nelfinavir (Rx)
(nell-fin′a-veer)
Viracept
Func. class.: Antiretroviral
Chem. class.: Protease inhibitor
Pregnancy category B

ACTION: Inhibits HIV-1 protease, which prevents maturation of the infectious virus

---

USES: HIV-1 in combination with other antiretrovirals

CONTRAINDICATIONS:
Hypersensitivity to protease inhibitors

Precautions: Pregnancy **B**, breastfeeding, hemophilia, PKU, renal/hepatic disease, pancreatitis, diabetes, infection

DOSAGE AND ROUTES
HIV infection
Adult and child >13 yr: PO 750 mg tid or 1250 mg bid
Child 2-13 yr: PO 25-30 mg/kg tid, max 2500 mg/day

Prevention of HIV infection after exposure (unlabeled)
Adult: PO 1250 mg bid with two other antiretroviral agents × 4 wk

Available forms: Tabs 250, 625 mg; oral powder 50 mg/g/scoop

Implementation
• Administer with food
• Oral powder can be mixed with fluids; do not mix with juice or acidic fluids; stable mixed for 6 hr, may use in child unable to take tabs; do not mix with water in original bottle

ADVERSE EFFECTS
CNS: Headache, asthenia, poor concentration, **seizures, suicidal ideation**
CV: Bleeding
ENDO: Hyperglycemia, hyperlipidemia
GI: Diarrhea, nausea, anorexia, dyspepsia, *flatulence*, **hepatitis, pancreatitis**
HEMA: **Anemia, leukopenia, thrombocytopenia, Hgb abnormalities**
INTEG: Rash, dermatitis, **anaphylaxis**
MS: Pain, arthralgia, myalgia, myopathy
OTHER: **Hypoglycemia**, redistribution/accumulation of body fat, **immune reconstitution syndrome**

Pharmacokinetics

Absorption	Unknown
Distribution	98% protein binding
Metabolism	Liver (minimal)
Excretion	Feces/urine
Half-life	3½-5 hr

Pharmacodynamics

Onset	Unknown
Peak	2-4 hr
Duration	Unknown

INTERACTIONS
Individual drugs
Amiodarone, lovastatin, midazolam, pimozide, quiNIDine, salmeterol, simvastatin, triazolam: increased serious dysrhythmias

Alfentanil, alosetron, atorvastatin, azithromycin, bortezomib, buprenorphine, busPIRone, cilostazol, cycloSPORINE, disopyramide, DOCEtaxel, dofetilide, donepezil, ethosuximide, fentaNYL, galantamine, gefitinib, halofantrine, indinavir, levomethadyl, systemic lidocaine, PACLitaxel, rifabutin, saquinavir, sibutramine, sildenafil, sirolimus, SUFentanil, tacrolimus, traZODone, ziprasidone, zonisamide: increased effect of each product

CarBAMazepine, nevirapine, PHENobarbital, phenytoin, rifamycin: decreased nelfinavir levels

Delavirdine: increased protease inhibitor levels

Didanosine, methadone, phenytoin: decreased effect

Indinavir, ketoconazole, ritonavir: increased nelfinavir levels

Drug classifications
Calcium channel blockers, tricyclic antidepressants, vinca alkaloids: increased effects
Contraceptives (oral): decreased effect
Ergots: increased serious dysrhythmias
HIV protease inhibitors: increased protease inhibitor levels

Drug/herb
St. John's wort: decreased antiretroviral effect, do not use concurrently

Drug/food
Increased: absorption with food

Drug/lab test
Increased: AST, ALT, alkaline phosphatase, total bilirubin, CPK, LDH, lipids, uric acid
Decreased: WBC, platelets

NURSING CONSIDERATIONS
Assessment
• Assess resistance testing at initiation and failure of treatment
• Assess signs of infection, anemia
• Monitor liver function tests: ALT, AST
• Assess bowel pattern before, during treatment; if severe abdominal pain with bleeding occurs, product should be discontinued; monitor hydration
• **Anaphylaxis, hypersensitivity reaction:** assess for wheezing, flushing, swelling of lips, tongue, throat, skin eruptions, rash, urticaria, itching

N

Adverse effects: *italics* = common; **bold** = life-threatening

• **HIV:** Monitor blood studies: serum lipid profile, plasma HIV RNA, blood glucose, viral load, CD4 cell counts baseline, throughout treatment
• **Immune reconstitution syndrome:** occurs with combination therapy; includes MAC, CMV, PCP, TB that require treatment
• **Phenylketonuria:** powder contains phenylalanine

Patient/family education
• Advise patient to take with meal or snack; if dose is missed, take as soon as remembered up to 1 hr before next dose; do not double dose
• Advise patient to avoid taking with other medications, unless directed by prescriber
• Teach patient that diarrhea is the most common side effect; may use loperamide to control
• Teach patient that product does not cure, but manages symptoms; does not prevent transmission of HIV to others
• Teach patient to use nonhormonal form of contraception while taking this product if using contraceptives
• Teach to report symptoms of hyperglycemia

Evaluation
Positive therapeutic outcome
• Decreasing symptoms of HIV
• Improving viral load and CD4 cell counts

---

neomycin topical
See Appendix B

---

nepafenac ophthalmic
See Appendix B

⚠ HIGH ALERT

nesiritide (Rx)
(nes-eer′ih-tide)
Natrecor
Func. class.: Vasodilator
Chem. class.: Human B-type natriuretic peptide
Pregnancy category C

ACTION: Uses DNA technology; human B-type natriuretic peptide binds to the receptor in vascular smooth muscle and endothelial cells, leading to smooth muscle relaxation

Therapeutic outcome: Improvement in symptoms of CHF

USES: Acutely decompensated CHF

CONTRAINDICATIONS:
Hypersensitivity to this product or *E. coli* protein, cardiogenic shock or B/P <90 mm Hg as primary therapy

Precautions: Pregnancy C, breastfeeding, children, mitral stenosis; significant valvular stenosis, restriction, or obstructive cardiomyopathy, or any condition that depends on venous return; renal disease, constrictive pericarditis

DOSAGE AND ROUTES
Adult: BOL **IV** 2 mcg/kg, then CONT **IV** INF 0.01 mcg/kg/min

Available forms: Powder for inj, 1.5 mg single-use vial

Implementation
IV route
• Do not administer nesiritide through a central heparin-coated catheter; heparin should be administered through a separate catheter
• Reconstitute one 1.5 mg vial/5 ml of diluent from prefilled 250 ml plastic **IV** bag with diluent of choice (D_5, 0.9% NaCl, D_5/0.9% NaCl, D_5/0.2% NaCl); do not shake vial, roll gently; use only clear sol
• Withdraw all contents of reconstituted vial and add to the 250-ml plastic **IV** bag (6 mcg/ml); invert bag several times
• Use within 24 hr of reconstituting
Direct IV route
• Prime tubing with 5 ml of inf sol, calculate dose based on patients' weight, 0.33 × patient weight (kg) = bolus vol (ml) (6 mcg/ml), withdraw prescribed bolus dose (volume) from prepared inf bag; give over 1 min through IV port
Intermittent IV INF route
• After bolus dose, use inf, give at 0.1 ml/kg/hr (0.01 mcg/kg/min)

Y-site compatibilities: Acyclovir, alfentanil, allopurinol, amifostine, aminocaproic acid, aminophylline, amiodarone, amphotericin B colloidal, amphotericin B lipid complex, amphotericin B liposome, anidulafungin, argatroban, atenolol, atracurium, azithromycin, aztreonam, bivalirudin, bleomycin, buprenorphine, busulfan, butorphanol, calcium acetate/chloride/gluconate, CARBOplatin, carmustine, ceFAZolin, cefotaxime, cefoTEtan, cefOXitin, cefTAZidime, ceftizoxime, cefTRIAXone, cefuroxime, chloramphenicol, cimetidine, ciprofloxacin, cisatracurium, CISplatin, clindamycin, cyclophosphamide, cycloSPORINE, cytarabine,

---

dacarbazine, DACTINomycin, DAUNOrubicin, digoxin, diltiazem, diphenhydrAMINE, DOCEtaxel, dolasetron, doxacurium, DOXOrubicin, doxycycline, droperidol, ePHEDrine, epirubicin, ertapenem, erythromycin, esmolol, etoposide, etoposide phosphate, famotidine, fenoldopam, fentaNYL, filgrastim, fluconazole, fludarabine, fluorouracil, foscarnet, fosphenytoin, ganciclovir, gatifloxacin, gemcitabine, gemtuzumab, glycopyrrolate, granisetron, haloperidol, hydrocortisone, HYDROmorphone, hydrOXYzine, IDArubicin, ifosfamide, imipenem-cilastatin, irinotecan, ketorolac, leucovorin, levofloxacin, lidocaine, linezolid, LORazepam, magnesium sulfate, mannitol, mechlorethamine, melphalan, meropenem, mesna, metaraminol, methohexital, methotrexate, methylPREDNISolone, metoclopramide, metroNIDAZOLE, midazolam, milrinone, minocycline, mitoMYcin, mitoXANtrone, mivacurium, moxifloxacin, mycophenolate, nalbuphine, naloxone, niCARdipine, nitroglycerin, nitroprusside, octreotide, ondansetron, oxaliplatin, oxytocin, PACLitaxel, palonosetron, pamidronate, pancuronium, PEMEtrexed, pentamidine, PENTobarbital, PHENobarbital, phentolamine, phenylephrine, polymyxin B sulfate, potassium chloride/phosphates, prochlorperazine, propranolol, quiNIDine, quinupristin-dalfopristin, ranitidine, remifentanil, rocuronium, sodium acetate/bicarbonate/phosphates, streptozocin, succinylcholine, SUFentanil, tacrolimus, teniposide, theophylline, thiotepa, ticarcillin, tigecycline, tirofiban, tolazoline, topotecan, torsemide, trimethobenzamide, vancomycin, vasopressin, vecuronium, verapamil, vinBLAStine, vinCRIStine, vinorelbine, zidovudine, zoledronic acid

ADVERSE EFFECTS

CNS: Headache, insomnia, dizziness, anxiety, confusion, paresthesia, tremor
CV: *Hypotension,* **tachycardia,** dysrhythmias, bradycardia, ventricular tachycardia, ventricular extrasystoles, **atrial fibrillation**
GI: Vomiting, nausea
INTEG: Rash, sweating, pruritus, inj site reaction
MISC: Back pain, abdominal pain
RESP: Increased cough, hemoptysis, **apnea**

Pharmacokinetics

Absorption	Vascular smooth muscle and endothelial cells
Distribution	Unknown
Metabolism	Unknown
Excretion	Bound to cell surfaces, internalized, and proteolyzed; cleaved by endopeptidases on vascular lumenal surface; renal filtration
Half-life	18 min

Pharmacodynamics

Onset	15 min
Peak	1 hr
Duration	Unknown

INTERACTIONS

Drug classifications

ACE inhibitors, antihypertensives, inotropes, **IV** nitrates: increased symptomatic hypotension

NURSING CONSIDERATIONS

Assessment
• Assess PCWP, RAP, cardiac index, MPAP, B/P, pulse during treatment until stable
• Monitor I&O, daily weight, serum creatinine, BUN
• **Assess for CHF:** weight gain, dyspnea, crackles, I&O ratios, peripheral edema

Patient/family education
• Explain purpose of medication and expected results
• Instruct patient to report pain at IV site

Evaluation

Positive therapeutic outcome
• Improvement in CHF with improved PCWP, RAP, MPAP

nevirapine (Rx)
(ne-veer′a-peen)
Viramune, Viramune XR
Func. class.: Antiretroviral
Chem. class.: Non-nucleoside reverse transcriptase inhibitor (NNRTI)
Pregnancy category B

Do not confuse:
nevirapine/nelfinavir, **Viramune**/Viracept

ACTION: Binds directly to reverse transcriptase and blocks RNA, DNA, causing a disruption of the enzyme's site

Therapeutic outcome: Improvement of HIV-1 infection

USES: HIV-1 in combination with other highly active antiretroviral treatments (HAART)

CONTRAINDICATIONS:

> **BLACK BOX WARNING:** Hypersensitivity, hepatic disease

Precautions: Pregnancy **B**, breastfeeding, children, renal disease, Hispanic patients

> **BLACK BOX WARNING:** Females, hepatitis

DOSAGE AND ROUTES
Treatment of HIV infection in combination with other antiretrovirals
Adult and adolescent: PO 200 mg/day × 2 wk, then 200 mg bid in combination; ext rel tab (adults not currently taking immediate release nevirapine) 200 mg/day (immediate rel tab) × 14 days with other antiretrovirals; if rash develops during lead-in period and persists beyond 14 days, do not use ext rel tab; if no consistent rash is present then give 400 mg/day ext rel tab with other antiretrovirals; if interrupted > 7 days, restart 14-day lead-in dosing; adults switched from immediate-release tab, 400 mg/day ext rel tab
Neonate ≥15 days old/infant/child: PO 150 mg/m²/day × 14 days, then 150 mg/m² bid; max 400 mg/day

Perinatal transmission prophylaxis (unlabeled)
Females with no previous antiretroviral therapy: PO 200 mg as a single dose at onset of labor with zidovudine 2 mg/kg over 1 hr followed by zidovudine 1 mg/kg/hr until delivery
Neonate ≥34 wk gestation: PO nevirapine 2 mg/kg as a single dose at age 48-72 hr and PO zidovudine 2 mg/kg q6hr for 6 wk

Hepatic dose
Adult: PO do not use in Child-Pugh B or C

Available forms: Tabs 200 mg; oral susp 50 mg/5 ml; ext rel tabs: 400 mg

Implementation
• Do not initiate treatment in females when CD4 counts >250 cells/mm³, or in males when >400 cells/mm³ unless benefit outweighs risks
• Give without regard to meals
• Use in combination with at least 1 other antiretroviral

• Give at equal intervals around the clock to maintain blood levels

ADVERSE EFFECTS
CNS: *Paresthesia, headache, fever, peripheral neuropathy*
GI: *Diarrhea,* abdominal pain, *nausea, stomatitis,* **hepatotoxicity, hepatic failure**
HEMA: **Neutropenia, anemia, thrombocytopenia**
INTEG: *Rash,* **toxic epidermal necrolysis**
MISC: **Stevens-Johnson syndrome, anaphylaxis**
MS: Pain, myalgia, **rhabdomyolysis**

Pharmacokinetics

Absorption	Rapid
Distribution	Protein binding 60%
Metabolism	Liver, by P450 enzyme system
Excretion	91% urine
Half-life	25-30 hr 50% removed by peritoneal dialysis; slower clearance rate in Hispanics, African Americans

Pharmacodynamics

Onset	Unknown
Peak	4 hr
Duration	Unknown

INTERACTIONS
Individual drugs
Cimetidine: increased nevirapine levels
ClonazePAM, diazepam, warfarin: decreased nevirapine level
Itraconazole: decreased effect of itraconazole
Ketoconazole: decreased effect of ketoconazole
Methadone: decreased effect of methadone

Drug classifications
Anticonvulsants, rifamycins: decreased nevirapine levels
Antiinfectives, macrolides: increased nevirapine levels
Oral contraceptives, protease inhibitors: decreased action

Drug/herb
St. John's wort: decreased nevirapine levels, do not use together

Drug/lab test
Increased: ALT, AST, GGT, bilirubin, Hgb
Decreased: neutrophil count

NURSING CONSIDERATIONS
Assessment
• Use resistance testing before starting and when therapy fails
• **Assess signs of infection,** anemia, hepatotoxicity, immune reconstitution syndrome
• **HIV:** Assess liver, renal, blood tests: ALT, AST, viral load, CD4, plasma HIV RNA, glucose levels in diabetic patients; if liver function tests are elevated significantly, product should be withheld; if treatment is interrupted by >1 wk, restart at initial dose
• Assess bowel pattern before, during treatment; if severe abdominal pain with bleeding occurs, product should be discontinued; monitor hydration
⚠ **Assess skin eruptions; rash, urticaria, itching; if rash is severe or systemic symptoms occur, discontinue immediately**
• Assess allergies before treatment, reaction to each medication
• **Rhabdomyolysis:** assess for pain, tenderness, weakness, edema; product should be discontinued
⚠ **Stevens-Johnson syndrome, toxic epidermal necrolysis, assess for allergies before treatment, reaction to each medication; skin eruptions; rash, urticaria, itching; if rash is severe or systemic symptoms occur, discontinue immediately**

Patient/family education
• Instruct patient to report immediately any right quadrant pain, yellowing of eyes/skin, dark urine, nausea, anorexia, muscle pain/tenderness, rash
• Inform patient that product may be taken with food, antacids
• Advise patient to take as prescribed; if dose is missed, take as soon as remembered up to 1 hr before next dose; do not double dose
• Advise patient that product must be taken in equal intervals around the clock to maintain blood levels for duration of therapy
• Advise patient that product is not a cure, controls symptoms of HIV, does not prevent transmission
• Instruct patient to avoid OTC agents unless approved by prescriber
• Advise patients who are using contraceptives to use a nonhormonal form of contraception during treatment

Evaluation
Positive therapeutic outcome
• Improving viral load and CD4 cell counts
• Absence of AIDS-defining symptoms
• Improvement in quality of life

---

niacin (Rx, OTC)
(nye′a-sin)
Equaline Niacin, Niaspan, Ni-Odan ✦, Slo-Niacin
niacinamide (Rx, OTC)
(nye-a-sin′a-mide)
Func. class.: Vitamin B₃ lipid-lowering product
Chem. class.: Water-soluble vitamin
Pregnancy category C

ACTION: Needed for conversion of fats, protein, carbohydrates by oxidation-reduction; acts directly on vascular smooth muscle, causing vasodilatation; reduces LDL, VLDL, total cholesterol, triglycerides, increases HDL

Therapeutic outcome: Decreasing cholesterol and LDL levels, B₃ supplementation

USES: Pellagra, hyperlipidemias (types IV, V), peripheral vascular disease that presents a risk for pancreatitis

CONTRAINDICATIONS:
Breastfeeding, hypersensitivity, peptic ulcer, hepatic disease, hemorrhage, severe hypotension

Precautions: Pregnancy **C**, breastfeeding, glaucoma, CV disease, CAD, diabetes mellitus, gout, schizophrenia

DOSAGE AND ROUTES
Niacin deficiency
Adult: PO 100-500 mg/day in divided doses; IM/SUBCUT 5-100 mg 5 or more times a day; **IV** 25-100 mg bid or tid
Child: PO up to 300 mg/day in divided doses

Adjunct in hyperlipidemia
Adult: 250 mg after evening meal, may increase dosage at 1-4 wk intervals to 1-2 g tid, max 6 g/day; ext rel 500 mg at bedtime, ×4 wk, then 1000 mg at bedtime for wk 5-8, do not increase by more than 500 mg q4wk, max 2000 mg/day

Pellagra
Adult: PO 300-500 mg/day in divided doses, IM 50-100 mg 5 ×/day or IV 25-100 mg bid by slow IV INF
Child: PO 100-300 mg/day in divided doses; IV up to 300 mg/day by slow IV/INF

Peripheral vascular disease (unlabeled)
Adult: PO 250-800 mg/day in 3-5 divided doses

Adverse effects: *italics* = common; **bold** = life-threatening

Available forms: Niacin: tabs 50, 100, 250, 500 mg; ext rel caps 250, 500 mg; ext rel tabs 250, 500, 750, 1000 mg; niacinamide: tabs 100, 500 mg

Implementation
PO route
- Do not break, crush, or chew ext rel products
- Give with meals or milk for GI symptoms, with 81-325 mg of aspirin or NSAIDs ½ hr before dose to decrease flushing

ADVERSE EFFECTS
CNS: Paresthesias, headache, dizziness, anxiety
CV: Postural hypotension, vasovagal attacks, dysrhythmias, vasodilatation
EENT: Blurred vision, ptosis
GI: Nausea, vomiting, anorexia, *jaundice,* diarrhea, peptic ulcer, **hepatotoxicity,** dyspepsia, **hepatitis**
GU: Hyperuricemia, **glycosuria, hypoalbuminemia**
INTEG: Flushing, dry skin, rash, pruritus, itching, tingling

Pharmacokinetics

Absorption	Well absorbed (PO)
Distribution	Widely distributed
Metabolism	Converted to niacinamide
Excretion	Urine, unchanged (30%); breast milk
Half-life	45 min

Pharmacodynamics

	PO	IV
Onset	Unknown	Unknown
Peak	30-70 min	Unknown
Duration	Unknown	Unknown

INTERACTIONS
Individual drugs
Alcohol: increased flushing, pruritus, avoid use

Drug classifications
Ganglionic blockers: increased postural hypotension
HMG-CoA reductase inhibitors: increased myopathy, rhabdomyolysis

Drug/herb
Red yeast rice: increased myopathy, rhabdomyolysis

Drug/lab test
Increased: bilirubin, alkaline phosphatase, liver enzymes, LDH, uric acid, glucose

Decreased: cholesterol
False increase: urinary catecholamines
False positive: urine glucose

NURSING CONSIDERATIONS
Assessment
- **Assess for niacin deficiency (pellagra):** nausea, vomiting, stomatitis, confusion, hallucinations before, throughout treatment
- **Hyperlipidemia:** assess for lipid, triglyceride, cholesterol level, if using for hyperlipidemia
- Assess nutrition: fat, protein, carbohydrates, nutritional analysis should be completed by dietitian
- **Hepatotoxicity:** monitor liver function tests: AST, ALT, bilirubin, uric acid, alkaline phosphatase; blood glucose before, during treatment; liver dysfunction: clay-colored stools, itching, dark urine, jaundice
- Monitor niacin levels during administration of this product
- Monitor cardiac status: rate, rhythm, quality; postural hypotension, dysrhythmias
- Monitor nutritional status: liver, yeast, legumes, organ meat, lean poultry; high-level niacin products should be included in the diet
- Assess for CNS symptoms: headache, paresthesias, blurred vision

Patient/family education
- Advise patient that flushing and increase in feelings of warmth will occur several hr after taking product (PO); after 2 wk of therapy these side effects diminish
- Instruct patient to remain recumbent if postural hypotension occurs; to rise slowly from sitting or recumbency
- Caution patient to abstain from alcohol if product is prescribed for hyperlipidemia
- Caution patient to avoid sunlight if skin lesions are present
- **Hepatotoxicity:** Advise patient to report clay-colored stools, anorexia, yellow eyes/skin, dark urine

Evaluation
Positive therapeutic outcome
- Decreased lipid levels
- Warm extremities
- Absence of numbness in extremities

---

niCARdipine (Rx)

(nye-card'i-peen)

Cardene IV, Cardene SR

Func. class.: Calcium channel blocker, antianginal, antihypertensive

Chem. class.: Dihydropyridine

Pregnancy category C

Do not confuse:

niCARdipine/NIFEdipine, **Cardene**/Cardizem, **Cardene SR**/Cardizem SR

ACTION: Inhibits calcium ion influx across cell membrane during cardiac depolarization, produces relaxation of coronary vascular smooth muscle and peripheral vascular smooth muscle, dilates coronary arteries, increases myocardial oxygen delivery in patients with vasospastic angina

Therapeutic outcome: Decreased angina pectoris, decreased B/P in hypertension

USES: Chronic stable angina pectoris, hypertension

CONTRAINDICATIONS:

Sick sinus syndrome, 2nd- or 3rd-degree heart block, hypersensitivity to this product or dihydropyridine, advanced aortic stenosis

Precautions: Pregnancy **C**, breastfeeding, children, geriatric, CHF, hypotension, hepatic injury, renal disease

DOSAGE AND ROUTES

Hypertension

Adult: PO 20 mg tid initially; may increase after 3 days (range 20-40 mg tid) or SUS REL 30 mg bid; may increase to 60 mg bid **IV** 5 mg/hr; may increase by 2.5 mg/hr q15min; max 15 mg/hr

Angina

Adult: PO 20 mg tid, may be adjusted q3day, may use 20-40 mg tid

Renal dose

Adult: PO 20 mg tid or SUS REL 30 mg bid

Hepatic dose

Adult: PO 20 mg bid

Available forms: Caps 20, 30 mg; sus rel caps 30, 45, 60 mg; inj 2.5 mg/ml, premixed 20 mg/200 ml, 40 mg/200 ml

Implementation

PO route

• Do not break, crush, chew, or open sus rel caps

• Give without regard to meals

• Store in airtight container at room temperature

IV route

• Dilute each 25 mg/240 ml of compatible sol (0.1 mg/ml), give slowly, titrate to patient's response, stable for 24 hr at room temperature, change IV site q30min

Solution compatibilities: D₅W, D₅/0.45% NaCl, D₅/0.9% NaCl

Y-site compatibilities: Alemtuzumab, amikacin, aminophylline, aztreonam, bivalirudin, butorphanol, calcium gluconate, CARBOplatin, caspofungin, ceFAZolin, ceftizoxime, chloramphenicol, cimetidine, CISplatin, clindamycin, cytarabine, DAPTOmycin, dexmedetomidine, diltiazem, DOBUTamine, DOCEtaxel, DOPamine, DOXOrubicin hydrochloride, enalaprilat, EPINEPHrine, epirubicin, erythromycin, esmolol, famotidine, fenoldopam, fentaNYL, gentamicin, hydrocortisone, HYDROmorphone, labetalol, lidocaine, linezolid, LORazepam, magnesium sulfate, mechlorethamine, methylPREDNISolone, metroNIDAZOLE, midazolam, milrinone, morphine, nafcillin, nesiritide, nitroglycerin, nitroprusside, norepinephrine, octreotide, oxaliplatin, oxytocin, palonosetron, penicillin G potassium, potassium chloride/phosphate, quinupristin-dalfopristin, ranitidine, rocuronium, tacrolimus, tirofiban, tobramycin, trimethoprim/sulfamethoxazole, vancomycin, vasopressin, vecuronium, vinCRIStine, voriconazole, zoledronic acid

Y-site incompatibilities: Amphotericin B liposome/lipid complex, ampicillin, ampicillin/sulbactam, cefepime, cefoperazone, ertapenem, fluorouracil, furosemide, methotrexate, micafungin, pantoprazole, PEMEtrexed, thiopental, thiotepa, tigecycline

ADVERSE EFFECTS

CNS: *Headache, dizziness,* anxiety, depression, confusion, paresthesia, somnolence, *flushing*

CV: Edema, bradycardia, hypotension, palpitations, **pulmonary edema,** chest pain, tachycardia, increased angina, **arrhythmias, CHF**

GI: Nausea, vomiting, gastric upset, constipation, **hepatitis,** abdominal cramps, dry mouth, sore throat

N

Adverse effects: *italics* = common; **bold** = life-threatening

GU: Nocturia, polyuria
INTEG: Rash, infusion site discomfort, **Stevens-Johnson syndrome**
MISC: Blurred vision, flushing, sweating, SOB, impotence

Pharmacokinetics

Absorption	Well absorbed (PO); bioavailability poor
Distribution	Unknown
Metabolism	Liver, extensively
Excretion	Kidneys 60%, feces 35%
Half-life	2-5 hr

Pharmacodynamics

	PO	PO SUS REL
Onset	½ hr	Unknown
Peak	1-2 hr	2-6 hr
Duration	8 hr	10-12 hr

INTERACTIONS

Individual drugs

Alcohol: increased hypotension
CarBAMazepine, cycloSPORIINE, prazosin, propranolol, quiNIDine: increased risk of toxicity
Cimetidine: increased niCARdipine effects
Digoxin, quiNIDine, theophylline: increased effects
Rifampin: decreased antihypertensive effect

Drug classifications

Antihypertensives, neuromuscular blocking agents, nitrates: increased hypotension
NSAIDs: decreased antihypertensive effect

Drug/herb

Ginkgo, ginseng, hawthorn: increased effect
Ephedra, melatonin, St. John's wort, yohimbe: decreased effect

Drug/food

Grapefruit juice: increased hypotensive effect

Drug/lab test

Increased: LFTs
Decreased: potassium (IV), phosphate, platelets

NURSING CONSIDERATIONS

Assessment

• Assess fluid volume status (I&O ratio) and record weight, color, quality, and specific gravity of urine, skin turgor, adequacy of pulses, moist mucous membranes, bilateral lung sounds, peripheral pitting edema; dehydration symptoms of decreasing output, thirst, hypotension, dry mouth, and mucous membranes should be reported

• **Monitor for CHF:** weight gain, crackles, jugular venous distention, dyspnea

• **Hypertension:** assess for decreasing B/P; salt in diet, smoking, exercise, diet, weight, monitor B/P often

• **Assess anginal pain:** intensity, location, duration, alleviating factors

• Monitor potassium, renal/liver function tests, periodically

Patient/family education

• Advise patient to avoid hazardous activities until stabilized on product and dizziness is no longer a problem

• Instruct patient to limit caffeine consumption; to avoid alcohol and OTC products unless directed by a prescriber, to take without regard to food, avoid high-fat foods, to swallow sus rel product whole

A Hypertension: instruct patient to comply with all areas of medical regimen: diet, exercise, stress reduction, product therapy

• Instruct patient to notify prescriber of irregular heartbeat, shortness of breath, swelling of feet and hands, pronounced dizziness, constipation, nausea, hypotension, change in severity/pattern/incidence of angina

• Teach patient to use medication as directed even if feeling better; may be taken with other cardiovascular products (nitrates, β-blockers)

• Teach patient to take medication exactly as prescribed

• Advise patient to contact prescriber if anginal attacks continue or become worse

Evaluation

Positive therapeutic outcome

• Decreased angina attacks
• Decreased B/P

TREATMENT OF OVERDOSE:

Defibrillation, atropine for AV block, vasopressor for hypotension

nicotinamide
See niacin

nicotine
(nik′o-teen)

nicotine chewing gum
CVS Nicotine Polacrilex, Equate Nicotine, Good Sense Nicotine, Leader Nicotine Gum, GNP Nicotine, NICO-relief, Nicorette, Publix Stop Smoking Aid, TopCare Nicotine, Walgreens Nicotine

nicotine inhaler (OTC, Rx)
Nicotrol Inhaler

nicotine lozenge (OTC)
CVS Nicotine Polacrilex, GNP Nicotine Polacrilex, Good Sense Nicotine, Polacrilex, TopCare Nicotine Polacrilex Lozenge, Walgreens Nicotine Polacrilex Lozenge

nicotine nasal spray (Rx)
Nicotrol NS

nicotine transdermal (OTC, Rx)
CVS Nicotine Transdermal System, Equate Nicotine Transdermal System, Habitrol ♣, Leader Nicotine Transdermal Patch, Nicoderm CQ, Sunmark Nicotine Transdermal System, Walgreens Nicotine Transdermal Patch

Func. class.: Smoking deterrent
Chem. class.: Ganglionic cholinergic agonist
Pregnancy category D (transdermal), C (gum)

ACTION: Agonist at nicotinic receptors in the peripheral and central nervous systems; acts at sympathetic ganglia, on chemoreceptors of the aorta and carotid bodies; also affects adrenalin-releasing catecholamines

Therapeutic outcome: Decreased withdrawal effects when smoking cessation is attempted

USES: Deter cigarette smoking

Unlabeled uses: Tourette's syndrome

CONTRAINDICATIONS:
Pregnancy **D** (transdermal, inhaler), hypersensitivity, immediate post-MI recovery period, severe angina pectoris

Precautions: Pregnancy **C** (gum), breast-feeding, vasospastic disease, dysrhythmias, diabetes mellitus, hyperthyroidism, pheochromocytoma, coronary disease, esophagitis, peptic ulcer, renal/hepatic disease; MRI (patch)

DOSAGE AND ROUTES
Nicotine chewing gum
Adult: If patient smokes ≤25 cigarettes/day, start with 2 mg gum; if >25 cigarettes/day, start with 4 mg gum; then 1 piece of gum q1-2hr × 6 wk, then 1 piece of gum q2-4hr × 2 wk, then 1 piece of gum q4-8hr × 2 wk, then discontinue; max 24/day

Nicotine inhaler
Adult: Inhale 6 cartridges/day for first 3-6 wk, max 16/day × 12 wk

Nicotine lozenge
Adult: If cigarette is desired >30 min after awakening, start with 1-2–mg lozenge; if <30 min after awakening, start with 4-mg lozenge; then 1 q1-2hr, max 20 lozenges/day or 5 lozenges/6 hr × 6 wk, then 1 lozenge q2-4hr × 2 wk, then 1 lozenge q4-8hr × 2 wk, then discontinue

Nicotine nasal spray
Adult: 1 spray in each nostril 1-2 ×/hr, max 5 ×/hr or 40 ×/day, max 3 mo

Nicotine transdermal/inhaler system

Habitrol ♣, NicoDerm
Adult: 21 mg/day × 4-8 wk; 14 mg/day × 2-4 wk; 7 mg/day × 2-4 wk

Nicotrol
Adult: 15 mg/day × 12 wk; 10 mg/day × 2 wk; 5 mg/day × 2 wk

Nicotrol inhaler
Adult: Delivers 30% of what a smoker receives from an actual cigarette

Tourette's syndrome (unlabeled)
Adult and child: Chewing gum 2 mg chewed × ½ hr bid × 1-6 mo; transdermal 7 or 10 mg patch daily × 2 days

Available forms: Gum: 2, 4 mg/piece; nicotine transdermal system (Habitrol ♣, NicoDerm, Nicotine Transdermal System); 7, 14, 21 mg/day delivered; (NicoDerm) 5, 10, 15 mg/day; nicotine inhaler: 4 mg delivered; nasal spray: 0.5 mg of nicotine/actuation; lozenge: 2 mg, 4 mg

N

Adverse effects: *italics* = common; **bold** = life-threatening

Implementation
- Give only prescribed amount, or toxicity may occur
- **Gum:** chew gum slowly for 30 min to promote buccal absorption of the product; do not chew > 45 min
- Begin product withdrawal after 3 mo of use; do not exceed 6 mo
- **Transdermal patch:** apply once a day to a nonhairy, clean, dry area of skin on upper body or upper outer arm; rotate sites to prevent skin irritation
- **Inhaler:** puffing on mouthpiece delivers nicotine through the mouth

ADVERSE EFFECTS
CNS: Dizziness, vertigo, insomnia, headache, confusion, **seizures,** depression, euphoria, numbness, tinnitus, strange dreams
CV: Dysrhythmias, tachycardia, palpitations, edema, flushing, hypertension
EENT: Jaw ache, irritation in buccal cavity
GI: *Nausea, vomiting, anorexia, indigestion,* diarrhea, abdominal pain, constipation, eructation, irritation
RESP: Breathing difficulty, cough, hoarseness, sneezing, wheezing, bronchial spasm

Pharmacokinetics

Absorption	Slowly absorbed, buccal cavity
Distribution	Unknown
Metabolism	Liver; some by lungs, kidneys
Excretion	Kidneys, unchanged (20%); breast milk
Half-life	1-2 hr

Pharmacodynamics

Onset	Rapid
Peak	½ hr
Duration	Unknown

INTERACTIONS
Individual drugs
Bromocriptine, cabergoline: increased vasoconstriction
Adenosine: increased effects
BuPROPion: increased B/P
Insulin: decreased effect
Cimetidine: decreased nicotine clearance

Drug classifications
Ergots: increased vasoconstriction
α-Blockers: decreased effect

Drug/food
Acidic foods (colas, coffee): avoid use of gum with and for 15 min after

NURSING CONSIDERATIONS
Assessment
- **Assess for adverse reaction to gum:** irritation of buccal cavity, dislike of taste, jaw ache
- **Assess for withdrawal symptoms:** headache, fatigue, drowsiness, restlessness, irritability, severe cravings for nicotine products before, during, and after treatment
- **Smoking:** obtain a nicotine assessment: brand of cigarettes, chewing tobacco, cigars, number of each used per day; what increases need or activities performed when each is used
- Gum should not be used if temporomandibular condition exists
- **Assess for nicotine toxicity:** GI symptoms (nausea, vomiting, diarrhea), cardiopulmonary symptoms (decreased B/P, dyspnea, change in pulse), weakness, abdominal cramping, headache, blurred vision, tinnitus; product should be discontinued

Patient/family education
- Advise patient to begin product withdrawal after 3 mo use; max 6 mo
- Teach patient all aspects of product; give package insert to patient and explain; caution patient not to exceed prescribed dose
- Caution patient not to use during pregnancy; birth defects may occur
Gum
- Advise patient to chew gum slowly for 30 min to promote buccal absorption of the product; do not chew over 45 min
- Inform patient that gum will not stick to dentures, dental appliances
- Caution patient that gum is as toxic as cigarettes; it is to be used only to deter smoking
Transdermal patch
- Caution patient that patch is as toxic as cigarettes; to be used only to deter smoking
- Caution patient not to use during pregnancy; birth defects may occur
- Instruct patient to keep used and unused system out of reach of children and pets
- Instruct patient to apply once a day to a nonhairy, clean, dry area of skin on upper body or upper outer arm; to rotate sites to prevent skin irritation
- Instruct patient to stop smoking immediately when beginning patch treatment
- Teach patient to apply promptly after removing from protective pouch; system may lose strength

- **Nasal spray:** tilt head back, do not swallow or inhale during administration; after smoking is stopped, use spray up to 8 wk, then discontinue over 6 wk by tapering
- **Lozenges:** allow to dissolve, avoid swallowing
- **Inhalation:** use the inhaler for 20 min
- Advise patient that puffing on mouthpiece delivers nicotine through the mouth lining

Evaluation
Positive therapeutic outcome
- Decrease in urge to smoke
- Decreased need for gum after 3-6 mo

NIFEdipine (Rx)
(nye-fed′i-peen)
**Adalat CC, Afedtab CR,
Apo-Nifed ✦, Apo-Nifed PA ✦,
Nifediac CC, Nifedical XL, Procardia,
Procardia XL**
Func. class.: Calcium channel blocker, antianginal, antihypertensive
Chem. class.: Dihydropyridine
Pregnancy category C

Do not confuse:
NIFEdipine/niCARdipine/niMODipine

ACTION: Inhibits calcium ion influx across cell membrane during cardiac depolarization, produces relaxation of coronary vascular smooth muscle, dilates coronary vascular arteries, increases myocardial oxygen delivery in patients with vasospastic angina, dilates peripheral arteries

Therapeutic outcome: Decreased angina pectoris, decreased B/P in hypertension

USES: Chronic stable angina pectoris, variant angina, hypertension, migraine prophylaxis

CONTRAINDICATIONS:
Hypersensitivity to this product or dihydropyridine, cardiogenic shock

Precautions: Pregnancy C, breastfeeding, children, hypotension, sick sinus syndrome, 2nd- or 3rd-degree heart block, hypotension less than 90 mm Hg systolic, hepatic injury, renal disease, acute MI, aortic stenosis, GERD, heart failure

DOSAGE AND ROUTES
Adult: PO immediate release, 10 mg tid; increase in 10-mg increments q7-14day, max 180 mg/24 hr or single dose of 30 mg; sus rel 30-60 mg/day; may increase q7-14day; doses >120 mg not recommended

Hypertension
Adult: PO ext rel 30-60 mg qd, titrate upward as needed; max 90 mg/day (Adalat CC); 120 mg/day (Procardia XL)
Adolescent/child (unlabeled): PO ext rel 0.25-0.5 mg/kg/day, max 3 mg/kg/day

Hiccups (unlabeled)
Adult: PO 10-20 mg tid

Available forms: Caps 10, 20 mg; ext rel tabs (CC, XL) 30, 60, 90 mg

Implementation
PO route
- Do not use immediate release caps within 7 days of MI, coronary syndrome
- Give without regard to meals
- Store in airtight container at room temperature
- Protect caps from direct light, keep in dry area, do not freeze
Sublingual route
- Using a sterile needle, puncture the cap and squeeze medication in buccal/sublingual area (not an FDA-approved use)

ADVERSE EFFECTS
CNS: *Headache,* fatigue, drowsiness, *dizziness,* anxiety, depression, weakness, insomnia, *light-headedness,* paresthesia, tinnitus, blurred vision, nervousness, tremor, flushing
CV: **Dysrhythmias,** edema, hypotension, palpitations, tachycardia
GI: *Nausea,* vomiting, diarrhea, gastric upset, constipation, increased LFTs, dry mouth, flatulence, gingival hyperplasia
GU: Nocturia, polyuria
HEMA: Bruising, bleeding, petechiae
INTEG: Rash, pruritus, *flushing,* hair loss, **Stevens-Johnson syndrome, toxic epidermal necrolysis, exfoliative dermatitis**
MISC: Sexual difficulties, cough, fever, chills

Pharmacokinetics
Absorption	Well absorbed (PO)
Distribution	Protein binding 92%
Metabolism	Liver, extensively
Excretion	Unknown
Half-life	2-5 hr

Adverse effects: *italics* = common; **bold** = life-threatening

Pharmacodynamics

	PO	PO EXT REL
Onset	30 min-1 hr	Unknown
Peak	2 hr	Unknown
Duration	6-8 hr	24 hr

INTERACTIONS

Individual drugs
Cimetidine, ranitidine: increased risk of toxicity
CarBAMazepine, cycloSPORINE, phenytoin, prazosin, digoxin: increased levels of each product
QuiNIDine: decreased effects
Smoking: decreased NIFEdipine level

Drug classifications
Strong CYP3A4 inducers: use is contraindicated
Antihypertensives, β-adrenergic blockers: increased effects
NSAIDs: decreased antihypertensive effect

Drug/herb
Ginkgo biloba, ginseng, hawthorn: increased effect
Ephedra, melatonin, St. John's wort, yohimbe: decreased effect

Drug/food
Grapefruit juice: increased NIFEdipine level

Drug/lab test
Positive: ANA titer, direct Coombs' test
Increased: CPK, LDH, AST

NURSING CONSIDERATIONS

Assessment
• **Assess anginal pain:** location, intensity, duration, character, alleviating, aggravating factors
• Assess for bruising, petechiae, bleeding
• Monitor potassium, renal/liver function tests periodically during treatment; in those taking antihypertensives, beta blockers, monitor B/P often
• **Serious skin disorders:** rash starts suddenly, assess for fever, cutaneous lesions, may have pustules; discontinue product
• Assess fluid volume status (I&O ratio) and record weight, distended red veins, crackles in lung, color, quality, and specific gravity of urine, skin turgor, adequacy of pulses, moist mucous membranes, bilateral lung sounds, peripheral pitting edema; dehydration symptoms of decreasing output, thirst, hypotension, dry mouth, and mucous membranes should be reported
• Monitor cardiac status: B/P, pulse, respirations, ECG

⚠ GI obstruction: ext rel products have been associated with rare reports of obstruction in those with strictures, and no known GI disease

Patient/family education
• Advise patient to avoid hazardous activities until stabilized on product and dizziness is no longer a problem
• Instruct patient to limit caffeine consumption; to avoid alcohol and OTC products unless directed by prescriber
• Advise patient that empty tab shells may appear in stools and are not significant
• Give without regard to meals (exception: Adelat CC should be taken on empty stomach)
• **Hypertension:** instruct patient to comply in all areas of medical regimen: diet, exercise, stress reduction, product therapy
• Tell patient to notify prescriber of irregular heartbeat, SOB, swelling of feet and hands, pronounced dizziness, constipation, nausea, hypotension, severe rash, changes in pattern/frequency/severity of angina
• Teach patient to use as directed even if feeling better; may be taken with other cardiovascular products (nitrates, β-blockers)
• Advise patient to increase fluid intake to prevent constipation
• Teach patient to check for gingival hyperplasia and report promptly
• Teach patient not to discontinue abruptly; gradually taper

Evaluation

Positive therapeutic outcome
• Decreased angina attacks
• Decreased B/P

TREATMENT OF OVERDOSE:
Defibrillation, atropine for AV block, vasopressor for hypotension

nilotinib (Rx)
(nye-loe'ti-nib)
Tasigna
Func. class.: Antineoplastic—miscellaneous
Chem. class.: Protein-tyrosine kinase inhibitor
Pregnancy category D

ACTION: Inhibits BCR-ABL tyrosine kinase created in chronic myeloid leukemia (CML)

Therapeutic outcome: Decrease in progression of disease

USES: Chronic phase/accelerated phase Philadelphia chromosome–positive chronic myelogenous leukemia that is resistant/intolerant to imatinib

CONTRAINDICATIONS:
Pregnancy **D**, breastfeeding, hypersensitivity

> **BLACK BOX WARNING:** Hypokalemia, hypomagnesemia, QT prolongation

Precautions: Children, women, geriatric patients, active infections, anemia, cardiac disease, bone marrow suppression, cholestasis, diabetes, gelatin hypersensitivity, infertility, galactose-free diet, lactase deficiency, neutropenia, pancreatitis, thrombocytopenia

> **BLACK BOX WARNING:** Hepatic disease

DOSAGE AND ROUTES
Adult: PO 400 mg q12h; continue until disease progression or unacceptable toxicity

Escalation regimen for those taking a strong CYP3A4 inducer
Adult: PO increase dose as required

Adjustment following discontinuation of a strong CYP3A4 inducer
Adult: PO reduce to 400 mg/bid

For those taking a strong CYP3A4 inhibitor
Adult: PO reduce dose to 400 mg/day

QT prolongation
QTcF >480 msec: Withhold dose

Myelosuppression
ANC 1 × 10⁹/L or platelets <50 × 10⁹/L: Withhold dose

Hepatic Dose
Adult: PO (Child-Pugh classes A-C): newly diagnosed CML 200 mg bid, then escalation to 300 mg bid initially

Available forms: Caps 150, 200 mg

Implementation
• Do not break, crush, or chew caps; if a whole capsule cannot be swallowed, disperse capsule contents in 1 tsp of applesauce
• Give without regard to meals; separate doses by 12 hr; a make-up dose should not be taken if a dose is missed
• Store at 15°-30° C (59°-86° F)

ADVERSE EFFECTS
CNS: Headache, dizziness, fatigue, fever, flushing, paresthesia
CV: QT prolongation, palpitations, **torsades de pointes,** AV block
GI: *Nausea,* **hepatotoxicity, vomiting,** *dyspepsia, anorexia, abdominal pain,* constipation, **pancreatitis,** diarrhea, xerostomia
HEMA: Neutropenia, thrombocytopenia, anemia, pancytopenia
INTEG: *Rash,* alopecia, erythema
META: Hyperamylasemia, hyperbilirubinemia, hyperglycemia, hyperkalemia, hypocalcemia, hyponatremia, hypomagnesemia
MISC: Diaphoresis, anxiety
MS: Arthralgia, myalgia, back/bone pain, muscle cramps
RESP: Cough, dyspnea
SYST: Bleeding, tumor lysis syndrome

Pharmacokinetics

Absorption	Unknown
Distribution	Protein binding 98%, plasma levels 3 hr
Metabolism	By CYP3A4
Excretion	Unknown
Half-life	Elimination 17 hr

Pharmacodynamics
Unknown

INTERACTIONS
Individual drugs
• Product interactions are numerous
Acetaminophen: increased hepatotoxicity
CarBAMazepine, dexamethasone, PHENobarbital, phenytoin, rifampin: decreased concentrations
Clarithromycin, erythromycin, itraconazole, ketoconazole: increased concentrations
Haloperidol, chloroquine, droperidol, pentamidine, arsenic trioxide, levomethadyl: increased QT prolongation
Pimozide, ziprasidone: do not use concurrently
Simvastatin: increased plasma concentrations
Warfarin: increased plasma concentration; avoid use with warfarin, use low-molecular-weight anticoagulants instead

Drug classifications
Class IA/III antidysrhythmics, some phenothiazines, β-agonists, local anesthetics, tricyclics, CYP3A4 inhibitors (amiodarone, clarithromycin, erythromycin, telithromycin, troleandomycin), CYP3A4 substrates (methadone, pimozide, QUEtiapine, quiNIDine,

N

risperidone, ziprasidone): increased QT prolongation
Calcium channel blockers: increased plasma concentrations
Phenothiazines: do not use concurrently

Drug/herb
St. John's wort: decreased concentration

Drug/food
Grapefruit juice: increased plasma concentrations

NURSING CONSIDERATIONS
Assessment
• Assess ANC and platelets; if ANC $<1 \times 10^9$/L and/or platelets $<50 \times 10^9$/L, stop until ANC $>1.5 \times 10^9$/L and platelets $>75 \times 10^9$/L
• Monitor CV status: hypertension, QT prolongation can occur; monitor left ventricular ejection fraction (LVEF) baseline periodically
• Assess for renal toxicity: if bilirubin $>3 \times$ IULN, withhold until bilirubin levels return to $<1.5 \times$ IULN
• **Assess for hepatotoxicity:** monitor hepatic function tests, before treatment and qmo; if liver transaminases $>5 \times$ IULN, withhold until transaminase levels return to $<2.5 \times$ IULN
• **Myelosuppression:** Monitor CBC, differential, platelet count weekly; withhold product if WBC is <3500/mm^3 or platelet count $<100,000$/mm^3; notify prescriber of these results; product should be discontinued
• Monitor for bleeding: epistaxis, rectal, gingival, upper GI, genital, and wound bleeding; tumor-related hemorrhage may occur rapidly
⚠ Tumor lysis syndrome: maintain hydration, correct uric acid prior to use of this product
• **Monitor electrolytes:** calcium, potassium, magnesium, sodium; lipase, phosphate; hypokalemia, hypomagnesemia should be corrected prior to use
• **QT prolongation:** ECG for QT prolongation, ejection fraction; assess for chest pain, palpitations, dyspnea

Patient/family education
• Instruct patient to report adverse reactions immediately: SOB, bleeding
• Inform patient reason for treatment, expected result
• Advise patient that many adverse reactions may occur
• Teach patient to avoid persons with known upper respiratory infections; immunosuppression is common

• Instruct in signs/symptoms of low potassium or magnesium

Evaluation
Positive therapeutic outcome
• Decrease in progression of disease

---

niMODipine (Rx)
(ni-moe′dip-een)
Nimotop
Func. class.: Calcium channel blocker
Chem. class.: Dihydropyridine
Pregnancy category C

ACTION: Unknown, may have greater effect on cerebral arteries

Therapeutic outcome: Prevention of vascular spasm (subarachnoid hemorrhage)

USES: Prevention of cerebrovascular spasm in subarachnoid hemorrhage

CONTRAINDICATIONS:
Sick sinus syndrome, 2nd- or 3rd-degree heart block, hypotension less than 90 mm Hg systolic, hypersensitivity

Precautions: Pregnancy **C**, breastfeeding, children, geriatric, CHF, hypotension, hepatic injury, renal disease

DOSAGE AND ROUTES
Adult: PO begin therapy within 96 hr, 60 mg q4hr × 21 days

Available forms: Caps 30 mg

Implementation
• May puncture cap and dilute in water and give through nasogastric tube; flush tube with 0.9% NaCl
• Store in airtight container at room temperature

ADVERSE EFFECTS
CNS: Headache, fatigue, drowsiness, dizziness, anxiety, depression, weakness, insomnia, confusion, paresthesia, somnolence
CV: Dysrhythmia, edema, CHF, bradycardia, hypotension, palpitations, **MI, pulmonary edema**
GI: Nausea, vomiting, diarrhea, gastric upset, constipation, **hepatitis,** abdominal cramps
GU: Nocturia, polyuria, **acute renal failure**
INTEG: Rash, pruritus, urticaria, photosensitivity, hair loss
MISC: Blurred vision, flushing, nasal congestion, sweating, shortness of breath, gynecomastia, hyperglycemia, sexual difficulties

---

Pharmacokinetics

Absorption	Well absorbed, poor bioavailability
Distribution	Crosses blood-brain barrier
Metabolism	Liver, extensively
Excretion	Kidneys
Half-life	1-2 hr

Pharmacodynamics

Onset	Unknown
Peak	1 hr
Duration	Unknown

INTERACTIONS

Individual drugs
Alcohol: increased hypotension
Digoxin: increased digoxin levels, bradycardia
PHENobarbital, phenytoin: decreased effectiveness
Propranolol: increased toxicity

Drug classifications
Antihypertensives: increased hypotension
β-Adrenergic blockers: increased bradycardia
Nitrates: increased nitrates

Drug/herb
Barberry, betel palm, burdock, goldenseal, khat, khella, lily of the valley, plantain: increased effect
Yohimbe: decreased effect

NURSING CONSIDERATIONS

Assessment
• Assess fluid volume status (I&O ratio) and record weight; distended red veins; crackles in lung; color, quality, and specific gravity of urine; skin turgor; adequacy of pulses; moist mucous membranes; bilateral lung sounds; peripheral pitting edema; dehydration symptoms of decreasing output, thirst, hypotension, dry mouth and mucous membranes should be reported
• Monitor B/P and pulse; if B/P drops 30 mm Hg, call prescriber
• Monitor ALT, AST, bilirubin daily; if these are elevated, hepatotoxicity is suspected

Nursing diagnoses
• Injury, risk for (uses)
• Knowledge, deficient (teaching)

Evaluation
Positive therapeutic outcome
• Prevention of neurologic damage from subarachnoid hemorrhage

nisoldipine (Rx)

(nye′sol-dye-peen)
Sular
Func. class.: Antihypertensive, calcium channel blocker
Chem. class.: Dihydropyridine
Pregnancy category C

Do not confuse:
nisoldipine/NIFEdipine/niMODipine

ACTION: Inhibits calcium ion influx across cell membrane, resulting in dilatation of peripheral arteries

Therapeutic outcome: Decreased B/P in hypertension

USES: Essential hypertension, alone or with other antihypertensives

CONTRAINDICATIONS:
Hypersensitivity to this product or dihydropyridines, sick sinus syndrome, 2nd- or 3rd-degree heart block, aortic stenosis

Precautions: Pregnancy **C,** breastfeeding, children, geriatric, CHF, hypotension <90 mm Hg systolic, hepatic injury, renal disease, acute MI, unstable angina, CAD, cardiogenic shock

DOSAGE AND ROUTES
Adult: PO 17 mg/day initially, may increase by 8.5 mg/wk, usual dose 17-34 mg/day, max 34 mg/day
Geriatric dose: PO 8.5 mg/day, increase based on response

Hepatic dose
Adult: PO 8.5 mg/day

Available forms: Ext rel tabs 8.5, 17, 20, 25.5, 30, 34, 40 mg

Implementation
PO route
• Give once a day, with food to decrease GI symptoms; avoid high-fat foods, grapefruit

ADVERSE EFFECTS
CNS: Headache, fatigue, drowsiness, dizziness, anxiety, depression, nervousness, insomnia, light-headedness, paresthesia, tinnitus, psychosis, somnolence, ataxia, confusion, malaise, migraine, flushing
CV: Dysrhythmias, edema, **CHF,** hypotension, palpitations, **MI, pulmonary edema,** tachycardia, syncope, AV block, angina, chest pain, ECG abnormalities

GI: Nausea, vomiting, diarrhea, gastric upset, constipation, elevated liver function tests, dry mouth, dyspepsia, dysphagia, flatulence
GU: Nocturia, hematuria, dysuria
HEMA: Anemia, leukopenia, petechiae
INTEG: Rash, pruritus
MISC: Sexual difficulties, gingival hyperplasia, chills, fever, gout, sweating, cough, nasal congestion, shortness of breath, wheezing, epistaxis, dyspnea

Pharmacokinetics

Absorption	Well absorbed
Distribution	Highly protein bound
Metabolism	Liver
Excretion	Kidneys
Half-life	Unknown

Pharmacodynamics

Onset	Unknown
Peak	6-12 hr
Duration	Unknown

INTERACTIONS
Individual drugs
Cimetidine, ranitidine: increased nisoldipine level
Digoxin: increased effects

Drug classifications
Antifungals (azole), CYP3A4 inhibitors: increased nisoldipine level
Antihypertensives: increased hypotension
β-Adrenergic blockers: increased effects
Hydantoins, CYP3A4 inducers: decreased nisoldipine effect

Drug/herb
Ephedra, melatonin: increased B/P
Hawthorn: decreased B/P
St. John's wort, ginseng, ginkgo biloba: decreased effect

Drug/food
Grapefruit juice: increased hypotension
High-fat foods: increased nisoldipine level

NURSING CONSIDERATIONS
Assessment
• Assess fluid volume status: I&O ratio and record; weight; skin turgor; adequacy of pulses; moist mucous membranes; bilateral lung sounds; peripheral pitting edema; dehydration symptoms of decreasing output, thirst, hypotension, dry mouth and mucous membranes should be reported

• **Angina:** assess frequency, severity of attacks; if angina worsens, report immediately
• Monitor ALT, AST, bilirubin daily if these are elevated and hepatotoxicity is suspected
• Monitor cardiac status: B/P, pulse, respiration, ECG

Patient/family education
• Caution patient to avoid hazardous activities until stabilized on product and dizziness is no longer a problem
• Instruct patient to limit caffeine consumption; to avoid alcohol and OTC products unless directed by prescriber
• Urge patient to comply in all areas of medical regimen: diet, exercise, stress reduction, product therapy; to notify prescriber of irregular heartbeat, SOB, swelling of feet and hands, pronounced dizziness, constipation, nausea, hypotension
• Teach patient to use as directed even if feeling better; may be taken with other cardiovascular products (nitrates, β-blockers)
• Advise patient to rise slowly to prevent orthostatic hypotension
• Teach patient to report nausea, dizziness, edema, SOB, palpitations

Evaluation
Positive therapeutic outcome
• Decreased B/P

---

nitazoxanide (Rx)
(nye-taz-ox′a-nide)
Alinia
Func. class.: Antiprotozoal
Pregnancy category B

ACTION: Interferes with DNA/RNA synthesis in protozoa

Therapeutic outcome: C&S negative for organism

USES: Diarrhea caused by *Cryptosporidium parvum* or *Giardia lamblia*

CONTRAINDICATIONS:
Hypersensitivity

Precautions: Pregnancy **B,** breastfeeding, children <1 yr or >11 yr, renal/hepatic disease, diabetes mellitus (contains sucrose), HIV, immunocompromised patients

---

DOSAGE AND ROUTES
Adult: PO 500 mg q12hr × 3 days
Child 4-11 yr: **PO** 10 ml (200 mg) q12hr × 3 days
Child 12-47 mo: **PO** 5 ml (100 mg) q12hr × 3 days

Available forms: Powder for oral susp 100 mg/5 ml; tab 500 mg

Implementation
PO route
• Give with food
• Shake oral susp before giving, discard after 1 wk

ADVERSE EFFECTS
CNS: *Dizziness, fever, headache*
CV: Hypotension
GI: *Nausea,* anorexia, flatulence, increased appetite, enlarged salivary glands, abdominal pain, diarrhea, vomiting
HEMA: Anemia, **leukopenia,** neutropenia
INTEG: Pruritus, sweating
MISC: Increased creatinine, pale yellow eye discoloration, rhinitis, discolored urine, infection, malaise

Pharmacokinetics
Absorption	Unknown
Distribution	Metabolite protein binding >99%
Metabolism	Hydrolyzed to active metabolite, undergoes conjugation
Excretion	Urine, bile, feces
Half-life	Unknown

Pharmacodynamics
Unknown

INTERACTIONS
Drug classifications
Other highly protein-bound products (phenytoin, aspirin): competes for binding sites

Drug/lab test
Increase: creatinine, GPT

NURSING CONSIDERATIONS
Assessment
• Assess for signs of infection
• Assess bowel pattern before, during treatment

Patient/family education
• Advise to take with food; shake susp well before each dose

Evaluation
Positive therapeutic outcome
• C&S negative for organism
• Decreased diarrhea

---

nitrofurantoin (Rx)
(nye-troe-fyoor′an-toyn)
Furadantin, Macrobid, Macrodantin, Novo-Furantoin ✦
Func. class.: Urinary tract antiinfective
Chem. class.: Synthetic nitrofuran derivative
Pregnancy category B

ACTION: Inhibits bacterial acetyl-CoA from interfering with carbohydrate metabolism

Therapeutic outcome: Resolution of infection

USES: Urinary tract infections caused by *Escherichia coli, Klebsiella, Pseudomonas, Proteus vulgaris, Proteus morganii, Serratia, Citrobacter, Staphylococcus aureus, Staphylococcus epidermidis, Enterococcus, Salmonella, Shigella*

CONTRAINDICATIONS: Infants <1 mo, hypersensitivity, anuria, severe renal disease, CCr <60 ml/min, at term pregnancy (38-42 wk), labor, delivery, cholestatic jaundice due to nitrofurantoin therapy

Precautions: Pregnancy **B,** breastfeeding, geriatric, G6PD deficiency, GI disease, diabetes

DOSAGE AND ROUTES
Active infections
Adult: PO 50-100 mg qid after meals or 50-100 mg at bedtime for long-term treatment
Child: PO 5-7 mg/kg/day in 4 divided doses; 1-2 mg/kg/day for long-term treatment; max 7 mg/kg/day

Chronic suppression
Adult: PO 50-100 mg qPM
Child: PO 2 mg/kg/day qPM or 0.5-1 mg/kg q12hr if dose is not well tolerated

Available forms: Caps 25, 50, 100 mg; susp 25 mg/ml; macrocrystal caps (Macrodantin) 25, 50, 100 mg; cap (Macrobid) 100 mg (25 macrocrystals, 75 monohydrate)

Implementation
• Give with meals
• Do not break, crush, chew, or open tabs, caps; store in original container

- Give after clean-catch urine for C&S
- Give two daily doses if urine output is high or if patient has diabetes

ADVERSE EFFECTS

CNS: *Dizziness, headache,* drowsiness, peripheral neuropathy, chills, confusion, vertigo
CV: Bundle branch block, chest pain
GI: *Nausea, vomiting, abdominal pain, diarrhea,* **cholestatic jaundice,** loss of appetite, **pseudomembranous colitis, hepatitis,** pancreatitis
HEMA: Anemia, agranulocytosis, hemolytic anemia, leukopenia, thrombocytopenia
INTEG: Pruritus, rash, urticaria, **angioedema,** alopecia, tooth staining, **exfoliative dermatitis**
MS: Arthralgia, myalgia, numbness, peripheral neuropathy
RESP: Cough, dyspnea, pneumonitis, pulmonary fibrosis/infiltrate
SYST: Stevens-Johnson syndrome, superinfection, SLE-like syndrome

Pharmacokinetics

Absorption	Readily absorbed
Distribution	Crosses placenta, excreted in breast milk
Metabolism	Liver, partially
Excretion	Kidneys, 30%-50% unchanged
Half-life	20-60 min

Pharmacodynamics

Onset	Unknown
Peak	30 min
Duration	6-12 hr

INTERACTIONS

Individual products

Magnesium trisilicate: decreased absorption
Norfloxacin: antagonist effect
Probenecid: increased nitrofurantoin levels

Drug/lab test

Increased: BUN, alkaline phosphatase, bilirubin, creatinine, blood glucose

NURSING CONSIDERATIONS

Assessment

⚠ **Pseudomembranous colitis: assess for diarrhea with mucus, abdominal pain, fever, fatigue, anorexia; may be treated with vancomycin or metroNIDAZOLE**

- Monitor blood count during chronic therapy
- Assess CNS symptoms: insomnia, vertigo, headache, drowsiness, seizures
- Assess allergy: fever, flushing, rash, urticaria, pruritus
- **Urinary tract infection:** assess for burning, pain on urination, fever; cloudy, foul-smelling urine; I&O ratio; C&S before treatment, after completion; serum creatinine, BUN
- **Hepatotoxicity:** assess for yellowing of skin, eyes, dark urine, clay-colored stools; monitor AST, ALT
- **Pulmonary fibrosis, pneumonitis:** assess for dyspnea, tachypnea, persistent cough
- **Serious skin disorders:** assess for fever, flushing, rash, urticaria, pruritus
- **Peripheral neuropathy:** assess for paresthesias (more common in diabetes mellitus, electrolyte imbalances, vit B deficiency, debilitated patients)
- **Pseudomembranous colitis:** assess for diarrhea, abdominal pain, fever, fatigue, anorexia; possible anemia, elevated WBC and low serum albumin; stop product and usually give either vancomycin or IV metroNIDAZOLE

Patient/family education

- Teach patient to take with food or milk; avoid alcohol
- Teach patient to protect susp from freezing and shake well before taking
- Teach patient that product may cause drowsiness; instruct client to seek aid in walking and other activities; advise patient not to drive or operate machinery while on medication
- Teach patient that diabetics should monitor blood glucose level
- Teach patient that product may turn urine rust-yellow to brown
⚠ **Teach patient to notify prescriber of symptoms of pseudomembranous colitis: fever, diarrhea with mucous, pus, or blood; report immediately**

Evaluation

Positive therapeutic outcome

- Decreased dysuria, fever; negative C&S

nitrofurazone topical
See Appendix B

nitroglycerin (Rx)
(nye-troe-gli′ser-in)
extended release caps (Rx)
Nitro-Time
translingual spray (Rx)
Nitrolingual
sublingual (Rx)
Nitrostat
rectal ointment
Rectiv
topical ointment (Rx)
Nitro-Bid
transdermal (Rx)
Minitran, Nitro-Dur
Func. class.: Coronary vasodilator, antianginal
Chem. class.: Nitrate
Pregnancy category C

Do not confuse:
Nitro-Bid/Nicobid

ACTION: Decreases preload and afterload, which thus decreases left ventricular end-diastolic pressure and systemic vascular resistance; dilates coronary arteries and improves blood flow through coronary vasculature, dilates arterial, venous beds systemically

Therapeutic outcome: Prevention of anginal attack

USES: Chronic stable angina pectoris, prophylaxis of angina pain, CHF associated with acute MI, controlled hypotension in surgical procedures, anal fissures

CONTRAINDICATIONS:
Hypersensitivity to this product or nitrites, severe anemia, increased ICP, cerebral hemorrhage, closed-angle glaucoma, cardiac tamponade, cardiomyopathy, constrictive pericarditis

Precautions: Pregnancy **C**, breastfeeding, children, postural hypotension, severe renal/hepatic disease, acute MI, abrupt discontinuation, hyperthyroidism

DOSAGE AND ROUTES
Adult: SL dissolve tab under tongue when pain begins; may repeat q5min until relief occurs; take no more than 3 tab/15 min; use 1 tab prophylactically 5-10 min before activities; SUS REL cap q6-12hr on empty stomach; TOP 1-2 in q8hr; increase to 4 in q4hr as needed; **IV** 5 mcg/min, then increase by 5 mcg/min q3-5min; if no response after 20 mcg/min, increase by 10-20 mcg/min until desired response; transdermal apply a pad daily to a site free from hair; remove patch at bedtime to provide 10-12 hr nitrate-free interval to avoid tolerance
Child: **IV** initial 0.25-0.5 mcg/kg/min, titrate to patient response, usual dose 1-3 mcg/kg/min transmucosal

Anal fisures (Rectiv)
Adult: rectal apply 1 in of 0.4% ointment q12hr × 3 wk

Available forms: Translingual aerosol 0.4 mg/m spray; sus rel caps 2.5, 6.5, 9, 13 mg; sus rel tabs 2.6, 6.5, 9 mg; SL tabs 0.3, 0.4, 0.6 mg; topical joint 2%; trans syst 0.1, 0.2, 0.3, 0.4, 0.6, 0.8 mg/hr; inj 25 mg/250 ml, 50 mg/250 ml, 100 mg/250 ml, 50 mg/500 ml, 100 mg/500 ml, 200 mg/500 ml; rectal ointment 0.4% (Rectiv)

Implementation
PO route
• Swallow sus rel tabs whole; do not break, crush, or chew sus rel tabs
• Give 1 hr before or 2 hr after meals with 8 oz of water
SL route
• Should be dissolved under tongue, not swallowed
Aerosol route
• Sprayed under tongue (nitrolingual); not inhaled, prime before 1st-time use or if product has not been used in > 6 wk; press valve head with forefinger
Transmucosal route
• Tab should be placed between cheek and gum line
• Do not take anything PO when tab is in place
Topical ointment route
• Apply ointment using dose-measuring papers supplied; apply to an area without hair; ointment should cover 2-3–inch area; may apply an occlusive dressing as directed
Transdermal route
• Apply transdermal patches to area without hair; press hard to adhere; if patch becomes dislodged, apply a new one
SL route
• Keep tab in original container
• If 3 SL tab in 15 min do not relieve pain, consider diagnosis of MI
• SL tab should be held under tongue until dissolved (a few min); do not take anything by mouth when SL tab is in place

Rectal route
• Cover finger with plastic wrap, disposable glove or finger cot, lay finger alongside 1 inch dosing line on carton, squeeze tube until equal to 1 inch dosing line, insert covered finger no further than 1st finger joint gently into anal canal and on sides, wash hands thoroughly, if too painful, apply directly to outside of anus

Continuous IV infusion route
• Diluted in D_5, D_5W, 0.9% NaCl for inf to 200-400 mcg/ml depending on patient's fluid status, common dilution is 50 mg/250 ml, use controlled inf device; use glass inf bottles, non–polyvinyl chloride inf tubing; titrate to patient response; do not use filters

Y-site compatibilities: Acyclovir, alfentanil, amikacin, aminocaproic acid, aminophylline, amiodarone, amphotericin B lipid complex, amphotericin B liposome, anidulafungin, argatroban, ascorbic acid, atenolol, atracurium, atropine, azaTHIOprine, aztreonam, benztropine, bivalirudin, bleomycin, bumetanide, buprenorphine, butorphanol, calcium chloride/gluconate, CARBOplatin, caspofungin, cefamandole, ceFAZolin, cefmetazole, cefonicid, cefoperazone, cefotaxime, cefoTEtan, cefOXitin, cefTAZidime, ceftizoxime, cefTRIAXone, cefuroxime, cephalothin, cephapirin, chloramphenicol, chlorproMAZINE, cimetidine, cisatracurium, CISplatin, clindamycin, cloNIDine, cyanocobalamin, cyclophosphamide, cycloSPORINE, cytarabine, DACTINomycin, dexamethasone, digoxin, diltiazem, diphenhydrAMINE, DOBUTamine, DOCEtaxel, DOPamine, doxacurium, DOXOrubicin, doxycycline, drotrecogin alfa, enalaprilat, ePHEDrine, EPINEPHrine, epirubicin, epoetin alfa, eptifibatide, ertapenem, erythromycin, esmolol, etoposide, famotidine, fenoldopam, fentaNYL, fluconazole, fludarabine, fluorouracil, folic acid, ganciclovir, gatifloxacin, gemcitabine, gemtuzumab, gentamicin, glycopyrrolate, granisetron, heparin, hydrocortisone, HYDROmorphone, hydrOXYzine, IDArubicin, ifosfamide, imipenem-cilastatin, indomethacin, insulin (regular), irinotecan, isoproterenol, ketorolac, labetalol, lidocaine, linezolid, LORazepam, magnesium sulfate, mannitol, mechlorethamine, meperidine, metaraminol, methicillin, methotrexate, methoxamine, methyldopate, methylPREDNISolone, metoclopramide, metroNIDAZOLE, mezlocillin, micafungin, miconazole, midazolam, milrinone, minocycline, mitoXANtrone, morphine, moxalactam, mycophenolate, nafcillin, nalbuphine, naloxone, nesiritide, netilmicin, octreotide, ondansetron, oxacillin, oxaliplatin, oxytocin, PACLitaxel, palonosetron, pamidronate, pancuronium, pantoprazole, papaverine, PEMEtrexed, penicillin G potassium/sodium, pentamidine, pentazocine, PENTobarbital, PHENobarbital, phentolamine, phenylephrine, phytonadione, piperacillin, piperacillin-tazobactam, polymyxin B, potassium chloride, procainamide, prochlorperazine, promethazine, propofol, propranolol, protamine, pyridoxine, quiNIDine, quinupristin-dalfopristin, ranitidine, remifentanil, ritodrine, rocuronium, sodium bicarbonate, succinylcholine, SUFentanil, tacrolimus, teniposide, theophylline, thiamine, thiopental, thiotepa, ticarcillin, ticarcillin-clavulanate, tigecycline, tirofiban, tobramycin, tolazoline, trimetaphan, urokinase, vancomycin, vasopressin, vecuronium, verapamil, vinCRIStine, vinorelbine, voriconazole, warfarin, zoledronic acid

Y-site incompatibilities: Alteplase

ADVERSE EFFECTS
CNS: *Headache, flushing, dizziness*
CV: *Postural hypotension,* tachycardia, **collapse,** syncope, palpitations
GI: Nausea, vomiting
INTEG: Pallor, sweating, rash

Pharmacokinetics

Absorption	Well absorbed (PO, buccal, SL)
Distribution	Unknown
Metabolism	Liver, extensively
Excretion	Kidney
Half-life	1-4 min

Pharmacodynamics

	SUS REL	SL	TD	IV	TRANS-MUCOSAL	AEROSOL	TOPICAL OINT
Onset	20-45 min	1-3 min	½-1 hr	1-2 min	1-2 min	2 min	½-1 hr
Peak	Unknown	Unknown	Unknown	Unknown	Unknown	Unknown	Unknown
Duration	3-8 hr	½ hr	12-24 hr	3-5 min	3-5 hr	½-1 hr	2-12 hr

INTERACTIONS
Individual drugs
Alcohol: increased hypotension, CV collapse

Aspirin: increased nitrate level

Heparin: decreased effects (with IV nitroglycerin)

Sildenafil, tadalafil, vardenafil: increased fatal hypotension, do not use together

Drug classifications
Antihypertensives, β-adrenergic blockers, calcium channel blockers, diuretics: increased hypotension

Drug/lab test
Increased: urine catecholamine, urine VMA

False increase: cholesterol

NURSING CONSIDERATIONS
Assessment
- Monitor orthostatic B/P, pulse
- **Assess pain:** duration, time started, activity being performed, character; check for tolerance if taken over long period
- Monitor for headache, light-headedness, decreased B/P; may indicate a need for decreased dosage

Patient/family education
- Instruct patient to avoid alcohol
- Advise patient that product may cause headache; tolerance usually develops; use nonopioid analgesic
- Teach patient that product may be taken before stressful activity, exercise, sexual activity
- Inform patient that SL tab may sting when product comes in contact with mucous membranes
- Caution patient to avoid hazardous activities if dizziness occurs
- Instruct patient to comply with complete medical regimen
- Advise patient to make position changes slowly to prevent fainting
- ⚠ **Advise patient to never use erectile dysfunction products (sildenafil, tadalafil, vardenafil); may cause severe hypotension, death**

Evaluation
Positive therapeutic outcome
- Decreased, prevention of anginal pain

⚠ HIGH ALERT

nitroprusside (Rx)
(nye-troe-pruss′ide)
Nitropress
Func. class.: Antihypertensive, vasodilator
Pregnancy category C

ACTION: Directly relaxes arteriolar, venous smooth muscle, resulting in reduction in cardiac preload, afterload

Therapeutic outcome: Decreased B/P in hypertensive crisis, decreased preload, afterload

USES: Hypertensive crisis/urgency/induction, to decrease bleeding by creating hypotension during surgery, acute CHF

CONTRAINDICATIONS:
Hypersensitivity, hypertension (compensatory) due to aortic coarctation or AV shunting, acute CHF associated with reduced peripheral vascular resistance, AV shunt, Leber's disease, toxic amblyopia

BLACK BOX WARNING: Cyanide toxicity

Precautions: Pregnancy C, breastfeeding, children, geriatric, fluid, electrolyte imbalances, renal/hepatic disease, hypothyroidism, anemia, increased intracranial pressure, hypovolemia

BLACK BOX WARNING: Hypotension

DOSAGE AND ROUTES
Adult and child: **IV** INF 0.25-1.0 mcg/kg/min; max 10 mcg/kg/min

Renal dose
Adult: **IV INF** CCr <60 ml/min maintain doses <3 mcg/kg/min to reduce thiocyanate accumulation

Available forms: Inj 50 mg 12 ml

Implementation
Continuous IV infusion route
- Depending on B/P reading q15min
- Reconstitute 50 mg/2-3 ml of D₅W, further dilute in 250, 500, or 1000 ml of D₅W to 200, 100, 50 mcg/ml respectively; use an infusion pump only; wrap bottle with aluminum foil to protect from light; observe for color change in the inf; discard if highly discolored (blue, green, dark red); titrate to patient response, protect from light

---

Y-site compatibilities: Alfentanil, alprostadil, amikacin, aminocaproic acid, aminophylline, amphotericin B lipid complex, amphotericin B liposome, anidulafungin, argatroban, atenolol, atropine, aztreonam, benztropine, bivalirudin, bleomycin, bumetanide, buprenorphine, butorphanol, calcium chloride/gluconate, CARBOplatin, cefamandole, ceFAZolin, cefmetazole, cefonicid, cefoperazone, cefotaxime, cefoTEtan, cefOXitin, cefTAZidime, ceftizoxime, cefTRIAXone, cefuroxime, cephalothin, chloramphenicol, cimetidine, CISplatin, clindamycin, cyanocobalamin, cyclophosphamide, cycloSPORINE, cytarabine, DACTINomycin, DAPTOmycin, dexamethasone, digoxin, diltiazem, DOCEtaxel, DOPamine, doxacurium, DOXOrubicin, doxycycline, enalaprilat, ePHEDrine, EPINEPHrine, epirubicin, epoetin alfa, eptifibatide, ertapenem, esmolol, etoposide, famotidine, fenoldopam, fentaNYL, fluconazole, fludarabine, fluorouracil, folic acid, furosemide, ganciclovir, gatifloxacin, gemcitabine, gemtuzumab, gentamicin, glycopyrrolate, granisetron, heparin, hydrocortisone, HYDROmorphone, IDArubicin, ifosfamide, inamrinone, indomethacin, insulin (regular), isoproterenol, ketorolac, labetalol, lidocaine, linezolid, LORazepam, magnesium sulfate, mannitol, mechlorethamine, meperidine, metaraminol, methicillin, methoxamine, methyldopa, methylPREDNISolone, metoclopramide, metoprolol, metroNIDAZOLE, mezlocillin, micafungin, miconazole, midazolam, milrinone, minocycline, morphine, moxalactam, multiple vitamins injection, nafcillin, nalbuphine, naloxone, nesiritide, netilmicin, niCARdipine, nitroglycerin, norepinephrine, octreotide, ondansetron, oxacillin, oxaliplatin, oxytocin, PACLitaxel, palonosetron, pamidronate, pancuronium, pantoprazole, penicillin G potassium/sodium, pentamidine, PENTobarbital, PHENobarbital, phentolamine, phenylephrine, phytonadione, piperacillin, piperacillin-tazobactam, polymyxin B, potassium chloride/phosphates, procainamide, propofol, propranolol, protamine, pyridoxine, ranitidine, ritodrine, rocuronium, sodium acetate/bicarbonate, succinylcholine, SUFentanil, tacrolimus, teniposide, theophylline, thiamine, ticarcillin, ticarcillin-clavulanate, tigecycline, tirofiban, tobramycin, tolazoline, trimetaphan, urokinase, vancomycin, vasopressin, vecuronium, verapamil, vinCRIStine, zoledronic acid

ADVERSE EFFECTS
CNS: *Dizziness, headache,* agitation, twitching, decreased reflexes, *restlessness*

CV: *Bradycardia,* ECG changes, tachycardia, *hypotension*
GI: Nausea, vomiting, abdominal pain
INTEG: Pain, irritation at inj site, sweating
MISC: **Cyanide, thiocyanate toxicity,** flushing, hypothyroidism

Pharmacokinetics
Absorption	Complete bioavailability
Distribution	Not known
Metabolism	RBCs, tissues
Excretion	Kidneys
Half-life	2 min

Pharmacodynamics
Onset	1-2 min
Peak	Rapid
Duration	1-10 min

INTERACTIONS
Individual drugs
Enflurane, halothane; severe hypotension

Drug classifications
Circulatory depressants, ganglionic blockers, volatile liquid anesthetics: severe hypotension

Drug/herb
Hawthorn: increased antihypertensive effect

NURSING CONSIDERATIONS
Assessment

> **BLACK BOX WARNING: Hypotension:** monitor B/P q5min × 2 hr, then qhr × 2 hr; monitor pulse q4hr; monitor jugular venous distention q4hr; ECG should be monitored continuously; monitor PCWP; rebound hypertension may occur after nitroprusside is discontinued, give only with emergency equipment nearby, rapid decrease in B/P may occur

• Monitor electrolytes, blood studies: potassium, sodium, chloride, CO_2, CBC, serum glucose, serum methemoglobin if pulmonary oxygen levels are decreased, ABGs
• Check weight, I&O, edema in feet and legs daily; assess skin turgor, dryness of mucous membranes for hydration status
• Assess for signs of CHF: dyspnea, edema, wet crackles
⚠ Monitor for increased lactate, cyanide, thiocyanate levels if on long-term treatment; thiocyanate level should be ≤1 millimole/L

- Monitor for decrease in bicarbonate, P_{CO_2}, and blood pH; acidosis may occur with this product

Patient/family education
- Teach patient to report headache, dizziness, loss of hearing, blurred vision, dyspnea, faintness; may indicate adverse reactions, pain at IV site

Evaluation
Positive therapeutic outcome
- Decreased B/P in hypertension
- Absence of bleeding in surgery

TREATMENT OF OVERDOSE:
Administer amyl nitrate inh until 3% sodium nitrate sol can be prepared for **IV** administration, then inject sodium thiosulfate **IV**; correct drop in B/P with vasopressor

---

⚠ HIGH ALERT

norepinephrine
(nor-ep-i-nef′rin)
Levophed
Func. class.: Adrenergic
Chem. class.: Catecholamine
Pregnancy category C

Do not confuse:
norepinephrine/EPINEPHrine

ACTION: Causes increased contractility and heart rate by acting on β-receptors in heart; also acts on a-receptors, thereby causing vasoconstriction in blood vessels; B/P is elevated, coronary blood flow improves, and cardiac output increases

Therapeutic outcome: Increased B/P with stabilization; adequate tissue perfusion

USES: Acute hypotension, shock

CONTRAINDICATIONS:
Hypersensitivity to this product or cyclopropane/halothane anesthesia; ventricular fibrillation, tachydysrhythmias, pheochromocytoma, hypotension, hypovolemia

BLACK BOX WARNING: Extravasation

Precautions Pregnancy C, breastfeeding, geriatric patients, arterial embolism, peripheral vascular disease, hypertension, hyperthyroidism, cardiac disease

DOSAGE AND ROUTES
Adult: IV INF 0.5-1 mcg/min titrated to B/P; maintenance 2-4 mcg/min; max 30 mcg/min
Child: IV INF 0.1-0.2 mcg/kg/min titrated to B/P; max 2 mcg/kg/min

Available forms: Inj 1 mg/ml

Implementation
CONT IV INF route
- Dilute with 500-1000 ml D_5W or $D_5/0.9\%$ NaCl; average dilution 4 mg/1000 ml diluent (4 mcg base/ml); give as inf 2-3 ml/min; titrate to response
- Store reconstituted sol in refrigerator <24 hr, protect from light, store unopened product at room temp, do not use discolored sol

Y-site compatibilities: Alfentanil, amikacin, amiodarone, anidulafungin, argatroban, ascorbic acid, atenolol, atracurium, atropine, aztreonam, benztropine, bivalirudin, bleomycin, bumetanide, buprenorphine, butorphanol, calcium chloride/gluconate, CARBOplatin, caspofungin, cefamandole, ceFAZolin, cefmetazole, cefonicid, cefoperazone, cefotaxime, cefoTEtan, cefOXitin, cefTAZidime, ceftizoxime, ceftobiprole, cefTRIAXone, cefuroxime, cephalothin, chloramphenicol, chlorproMAZINE, cimetidine, cisatracurium, CISplatin, clindamycin, cloNIDine, cyanocobalamin, cyclophosphamide, cycloSPORINE, cytarabine, DAPTOmycin, dexamethasone, digoxin, diltiazem, diphenhydrAMINE, DOBUTamine, DOCEtaxel, DOPamine, doripenem, doxycycline, enalaprilat, ePHEDrine, EPINEPHrine, epirubicin, epoetin alfa, ertapenem, erythromycin, esmolol, etoposide, famotidine, fenoldopam, fentaNYL, fluconazole, fludarabine, gatifloxacin, gemcitabine, gentamicin, glycopyrrolate, granisetron, heparin, hydrocortisone, HYDROmorphone, hydrOXYzine, IDArubicin, ifosfamide, imipenemcilastatin, irinotecan, isoproterenol, ketorolac, labetalol, lidocaine, linezolid, LORazepam, magnesium sulfate, mannitol, mechlorethamine, meperidine, meropenem, metaraminol, methicillin, methotrexate, methoxamine, methyldopate, methylPREDNISolone, metoclopramide, metoprolol, metroNIDAZOLE, mezlocillin, micafungin, miconazole, midazolam, milrinone, minocycline, mitoXANtrone, morphine, moxalactam, multiple vitamins injection, mycophenolate, nafcillin, nalbuphine, naloxone, netilmicin, niCARDipine, nitroglycerin, nitroprusside, octreotide, ondansetron, oxacillin, oxaliplatin, oxytocin, PACLitaxel, palonosetron, pamidronate, pancuronium, papaverine, PEMEtrexed,

*Adverse effects: italics = common; **bold** = life-threatening*

penicillin G potassium/sodium, pentamidine, pentazocine, phenylephrine, phytonadione, piperacillin, piperacillin-tazobactam, polymyxin B, potassium chloride, procainamide, prochlorperazine, promethazine, propofol, propranolol, protamine, pyridoxine, quiNIDine, ranitidine, remifentanil, ritodrine, succinylcholine, SUFentanil, tacrolimus, teniposide, theophylline, thiamine, thiotepa, ticarcillin, ticarcillin-clavulanate, tigecycline, tirofiban, tobramycin, tolazoline, trimetaphan, urokinase, vancomycin, vasopressin, vecuronium, verapamil, vinCRIStine, vinorelbine, vitamin B complex with C, voriconazole, zoledronic acid

ADVERSE EFFECTS

CNS: *Headache,* anxiety, dizziness, insomnia, restlessness, tremor, **cerebral hemorrhage**
CV: *Palpitations, tachycardia, hypertension, ectopic beats, angina*
GI: *Nausea, vomiting*
GU: Decreased urine output
INTEG: Necrosis, tissue sloughing with extravasation, **gangrene**
RESP: Dyspnea
SYST: Anaphylaxis

Pharmacokinetics

Absorption	Complete
Distribution	Crosses placenta
Metabolism	Liver
Excretion	Urine

Pharmacodynamics

Onset	Immediate
Peak	Rapid
Duration	1 min

INTERACTIONS

Individual drugs
Bicarbonate, sodium: incompatible with alkaline solutions
⚠ Guanethidine, methyldopa: do not use norepinephrine within 2 wk of using these drugs because hypertensive crisis may result

Drug classifications
α-blockers: decreased norepinephrine action
⚠ Antihistamines, ergots, MAOIs, oxytocics, tricyclics: do not use norepinephrine within 2 wk of using these drugs because hypertensive crisis may result
Oxytocics: Increased B/P
MAOIs, tricyclics: increased pressor effect

NURSING CONSIDERATIONS

Assessment
• Assess I&O ratio; notify prescriber if output <30 ml/hr
• Assess B/P, pulse q2-3min after parenteral route, ECG during administration continuously; if B/P increases, product is decreased, CVP or PWP during inf if possible
• Assess paresthesias and coldness of extremities; peripheral blood flow may decrease

---

BLACK BOX WARNING: Extravasation: inj site: tissue sloughing

• Assess for sulfite sensitivity, which may be life-threatening

Patient/family education
• Teach patient about the reason for product administration
• Advise family to report dyspnea, dizziness, chest pain

Evaluation
Positive therapeutic outcome
• Increased B/P with stabilization
• Adequate tissue perfusion

TREATMENT OF OVERDOSE:
Administer fluids, electrolyte replacement

norfloxacin ophthalmic
See Appendix B

nortriptyline (Rx)
(nor-trip'ti-leen)
Arentyl ✦, Pamelor
Func. class.: Antidepressant, tricyclic
Chem. class.: Dibenzocycloheptene, secondary amine
Pregnancy category D

Do not confuse:
nortriptyline/amitriptyline

ACTION: Blocks reuptake of norepinephrine, serotonin into nerve endings, increasing action of norepinephrine, serotonin in nerve cells; has anticholinergic effects

Therapeutic outcome: Decreased symptoms of depression after 2-3 wk

USES: Major depression

Unlabeled uses: Chronic pain management

CONTRAINDICATIONS:

Hypersensitivity to tricyclics, recovery phase of MI, seizure disorders, prostatic hypertrophy

Precautions: Breastfeeding, suicidal ideation, severe depression, increased intraocular pressure, closed-angle glaucoma, urinary retention, cardiac/hepatic disease, hyperthyroidism, electroshock therapy, elective surgery, pregnancy (**C**), carBAMazepine hypersensitivity

> **BLACK BOX WARNING:** Children, suicidal ideation

DOSAGE AND ROUTES

Adult: PO 25 mg tid or qid; may increase to 150 mg/day; may give daily dose at bedtime
Adolescent: PO 1-3 mg/kg/day in 3-4 divided doses or qd at bedtime; max 150 mg/day
Geriatric: PO 10-25 mg nightly, increase by 10-25 mg at weekly intervals to desired dose; usual maintenance 75 mg/day, max 150 mg/day

Available forms: Caps 10, 25, 50, 75 mg; sol 10 mg/5 ml

Implementation

• Give with food or milk to decrease GI symptoms; mix conc with water, milk, fruit juice to disguise taste
• Give dose at bedtime if oversedation occurs during day; may take entire dose at bedtime; geriatric may not tolerate once/day dosing
• Store in tight, light-resistant container at room temp; do not freeze

ADVERSE EFFECTS

CNS: *Dizziness, drowsiness,* confusion, headache, anxiety, tremors, stimulation, weakness, insomnia, nightmares, EPS (geriatric), increased psychiatric symptoms, **seizures**
CV: *Orthostatic hypotension,* **ECG changes,** *tachycardia,* **hypertension,** palpitations, **dysrhythmias**
EENT: Blurred vision, tinnitus, mydriasis, dry eyes
ENDO: SIADH, hyponatremia, hypothyroidism
GI: *Constipation, dry mouth,* nausea, vomiting, **paralytic ileus,** increased appetite, cramps, epigastric distress, jaundice, **hepatitis,** stomatitis, weight gain
GU: *Retention,* **acute renal failure,** sexual dysfunction
HEMA: **Agranulocytosis, thrombocytopenia, eosinophilia, leukopenia**

INTEG: Rash, urticaria, sweating, pruritus, photosensitivity
SYST: Serotonin syndrome

Pharmacokinetics

Absorption	Well absorbed
Distribution	Widely distributed; crosses placenta
Metabolism	Liver, extensively
Excretion	Kidneys, breast milk
Half-life	18-28 hr; steady state 4-19 days

Pharmacodynamics

Unknown

INTERACTIONS

Individual drugs

Alcohol: increased CNS depression
CloNIDine, guanethidine: decreased effects
Smoking (heavy): decreased product effect
Haloperidol, chloroquine, droperidol, pentamidine, arsenic trioxide, levomethadyl: increased QT prolongation

Drug classifications

Barbiturates, benzodiazepines, CNS depressants: increased effects
MAOIs: hypertensive episode, hyperpyretic crisis, seizures
SSRIs, SNRIs, serotonin-receptor agonists: increased serotonin syndrome, neuroleptic malignant syndrome
Class IA/III antidysrhythmics, some phenothiazines, β-agonists, local anesthetics, tricyclics, CYP3A4 inhibitors (amiodarone, clarithromycin, erythromycin, telithromycin, troleandomycin), CYP3A4 substrates (methadone, pimozide, QUEtiapine, quiNIDine, risperidone, ziprasidone): increased QT prolongation
Sympathomimetics (direct-acting), products increasing QT interval: increased effects
Sympathomimetics (indirect-acting): decreased effects

Drug/herb

Kava, valerian: increased CNS effect
St. John's wort: decreased nortriptyline level

Drug/lab test

Increased: serum bilirubin, blood glucose, alkaline phosphatase
Decreased: VMA, 5-HIAA
False increase: urinary catecholamines

NURSING CONSIDERATIONS
Assessment

> **BLACK BOX WARNING: Suicidal thoughts/
> behaviors in children/young adults:** not
> approved for children; monitor for suicidal ide-
> ation in depression, adolescents, young adults

- Monitor B/P (with patient lying, standing),
pulse q4hr; if systolic B/P drops 20 mm Hg,
hold product, notify prescriber; take VS q4hr of
patients with CV disease
- Monitor blood studies: thyroid function tests,
LFTs, serum nortriptyline level/target 50-150 ng/
ml if patient is receiving long-term therapy
- Monitor liver function tests: AST, ALT, bilirubin
- Check weight weekly; appetite may increase
- **QT prolongation:** assess for chest pain,
palpitations, dyspnea
- Assess ECG for flattening of T-wave, bundle
branch block, AV block, dysrhythmias in cardiac
patients
- Assess for EPS primarily in geriatric: rigidity,
dystonia, akathisia
- Assess mental status: mood, sensorium, affect,
suicidal tendencies; increase in psychiatric
symptoms: depression, panic
- Monitor urinary retention, constipation;
constipation is more likely to occur in children
or geriatric
- ⚠ **Assess for withdrawal symptoms:
headache, nausea, vomiting, muscle pain,
weakness; do not usually occur unless
product was discontinued abruptly**
- Monitor for glaucoma exacerbation and
paralytic ileus
- Identify alcohol consumption; if alcohol is
consumed, hold dose until AM
- **Serotonin syndrome, neuroleptic malignant syndrome:** assess for increased heart
rate, shivering, sweating, dilated pupils, tremors,
high B/P, hyperthermia, headache, confusion;
if these occur, stop product, administer a serotonin antagonist if needed (rare)

Patient/family education
- Teach patient that therapeutic effects may take
2-3 wk
- Teach patient to use caution in driving and
other activities requiring alertness because of
drowsiness, dizziness, blurred vision; to avoid
rising quickly from sitting to standing, especially
geriatric
- Teach patient to avoid alcohol ingestion,
MAOIs within 14 days, other CNS depressants;
teach patient not to discontinue medication
quickly after long-term use; may cause nausea,
headache, malaise

- Teach patient to wear sunscreen or large hat
to avoid burns, because photosensitivity occurs
- Teach patient to increase fluids, bulk in diet
if constipation, urinary retention occur, especially geriatric, worsening depression, suicidal
thoughts/behavior
- Teach patient to take gum, hard sugarless
candy, or frequent sips of water for dry mouth

Evaluation
Positive therapeutic outcome
- Decrease in depression
- Absence of suicidal thoughts

TREATMENT OF OVERDOSE:
ECG monitoring, lavage, activated charcoal,
administer anticonvulsant

nystatin (Rx, OTC)
(nis'ta-tin)
**Bio-Statin, Nyamyc, Pediaderm AF,
Pedi-Dri**
Func. class.: Antifungal
Chem. class.: Amphoteric polyene
Pregnancy category C

ACTION: Interferes with fungal DNA replication; binds sterols in fungal cell membrane,
which increases permeability, resulting in leaking of cell nutrients

Therapeutic outcome: Fungistatic/fungi-
cidal against *Candida* organisms

USES: *Candida* species causing oral,
vaginal, intestinal infections

CONTRAINDICATIONS:
Hypersensitivity

Precautions: Pregnancy **C**

DOSAGE AND ROUTES
Oral infection
Adult/adolescent/child: Susp 400,000-
600,000 units qid, use ½ dose in each side of
mouth, swish and swallow, use for at least 48 hr
after symptoms are resolved
Infant: SUSP 200,000 units qid (100,000 units
in each side of mouth)

Newborn and premature infant:
SUSP 100,000 units qid
Adult and child: Troches 200,000-400,000
units qid × up to 2 wk

GI infection
Adult: PO 500,000-1,000,000 units tid

Cutaneous candidiasis
Adult/child:
Top cream/ointment
Apply to affected area bid
Powder
Apply to affected area bid-tid

Available forms: Tabs 500,000 units; oral caps 500,000, 1,000,000 units, bulk powder

Implementation
• Store oral susp at room temp; store tabs in tight, light-resistant containers at room temp
PO route
• Give oral susp dose by placing ½ in each cheek, swish for several min, then swallow; shake susp before use
• Store oral susp at room temp, tab in airtight, light-resistant containers at room temp
Topical route
• Administer by moistening lesions with a swab coated with cream or ointment; use enough medication to cover lesions completely; give after cleansing with soap, water before each application; dry well; very moist lesions are best treated with topical powder
Vaginal route
• Insert vag tab high into vagina with applicator provided; administer in gravid client 3-6 wk before term to decrease candidiasis in the newborn
• Store at room temperature in dry place; protect from light, air, heat

ADVERSE EFFECTS
GI: Nausea, vomiting, anorexia, diarrhea, cramps
INTEG: Rash, urticaria (rare)

Pharmacokinetics

Absorption	Poorly absorbed
Distribution	Unknown
Metabolism	Not metabolized
Excretion	Feces, unchanged
Half-life	Unknown

Pharmacodynamics

Onset	Rapid
Peak	Unknown
Duration	6-12 hr

NURSING CONSIDERATIONS
Assessment
• **Assess for allergic reaction:** rash, urticaria; product may have to be discontinued
• Assess for predisposing factors for candidal infection: antibiotic therapy, pregnancy, diabetes mellitus, sexual partner infection (vag infections), AIDS
• Obtain culture and histologic tests to confirm organism

Patient/family education
• Instruct patient that long-term therapy may be needed to clear infection; to complete entire course of medication
• Teach patient proper hygiene: use no commercial mouthwashes for mouth infection
• Advise patient to avoid getting preparation on hands
• Instruct patient to wear light-day pad for vag preparations to avoid soiling clothing; to avoid sexual contact during treatment to minimize reinfection
• Instruct patient to notify prescriber if irritation occurs; product may have to be discontinued
• Inform patient that relief from itching may occur after 24-72 hr
Topical route
• Advise patient to discontinue use and notify prescriber if irritation occurs
• Teach patient to apply with glove to prevent further infection; product may stain
• Caution patient not to use occlusive dressings; to avoid use of OTC creams, ointments, lotions unless directed by prescriber

Evaluation
Positive therapeutic outcome
• Culture negative for *Candida*
• Decrease in size, number of lesions
• Decreased itching, white patches on vulva (vaginal)

nystatin topical
See Appendix B

nystatin vaginal antifungal
See Appendix B

N

ocriplasmin
(ok-ri-plas′min)
Jetrea
Func. class.: Ophthalmic agent
Pregnancy category C

USES: Symptomatic vitreomacular adhesion

DOSAGE AND ROUTES
Adult: Intravitreal **INJ** 0.125 mg (0.1 ml of diluted solution) by intravitreal injection to the affected eye once as a single dose

octreotide (Rx)
(ok-tree′o-tide)
Sandostatin, Sandostatin LAR Depot
Func. class.: Growth hormone, antidiarrheal
Chem. class.: Synthetic octapeptide
Pregnancy category B

ACTION: A potent growth hormone similar to somatostatin

Therapeutic outcome: Decreased diarrhea; decreased symptoms of acromegaly, carcinoid tumors, vasoactive intestinal peptide tumors (VIPomas)

USES: Sandostatin: acromegaly, carcinoid tumors, VIPomas; **LAR Depot:** long-term maintenance of acromegaly, carcinoid tumors, VIPomas, short bowel syndrome, insulinoma, hepatorenal syndrome

Unlabeled uses: GI fistula, variceal bleeding, diarrheal conditions, pancreatic fistula, IBS, dumping syndrome

CONTRAINDICATIONS:
Hypersensitivity

Precautions: Pregnancy **B,** breastfeeding, children, geriatric, diabetes mellitus, hypothyroidism, renal disease

DOSAGE AND ROUTES
Acromegaly
Adult: SUBCUT/**IV** 50-100 mcg bid-tid, adjust q2wk based on growth hormone levels (Sandostatin) or IM 20 mg q4wk × 3 mo, adjust by growth hormone levels (Sandostatin LAR)

VIPomas
Adult: SUBCUT/**IV** 200-300 mcg/day in 2-4 doses for 2 wk, max 450 mcg/day; (Sandostatin) or IM 20 mg q2wk × 2 mo, adjust dose (Sandostatin LAR)

Flushing/diarrhea in carcinoid tumors
Adult: SUBCUT/**IV** 100-600 mcg/day in 2-4 doses for 2 wk, titrated to patient response (Sandostatin) or IM 20 mg q4wk × 2 mo, adjust dose (Sandostatin LAR)

GI fistula
Adult: SUBCUT 50-200 mcg q8hr

Antidiarrheal in AIDS patients (unlabeled)
Adult: SUBCUT 50 mcg q8h PRN, increase to 500 mcg q8h

Irritable bowel syndrome (unlabeled)
Adult: SUBCUT 100 mcg single dose to 125 mcg bid

Dumping syndrome (unlabeled)
Adult: SUBCUT 50-150 mcg/day

Variceal bleeding (unlabeled)
Adult: **IV** 25-50 mcg/hr CONT **IV** INF for 18 hr-5 days

Available forms: Sandostatin: inj 0.05, 0.1, 0.2, 0.5, 1 mg/ml; LAR Depot: inj powder for susp 10 mg, 20, 30 mg/5 ml

Implementation
• Store in refrigerator for unopened amps, vials, or at room temp for 2 wk; protect from light; do not use discolored or cloudy sol
IM route
• Reconstitute with diluent provided; give into gluteal
SUBCUT route
• Rotate inj sites; use hip, thigh, abdomen
• Avoid using medication that is cold; allow to reach room temperature; do not use LAR Depot

Direct IV route
• Give over 3 min; in an emergency carcinoid crisis, give rapid bolus
Intermittent IV INF route
• Dilute in 50-200 ml D_5W, 0.9% NaCl; give over 15-30 min

Y-site compatibilities: Acyclovir, alfentanil, allopurinol, amifostine, amikacin, aminocaproic acid, aminophylline, amiodarone, amphotericin B colloidal, amphotericin B lipid complex, amphotericin B liposome,

---

ampicillin, ampicillin-sulbactam, anidulafungin, argatroban, arsenic trioxide, atenolol, atracurium, azithromycin, aztreonam, bivalirudin, bleomycin, bumetanide, buprenorphine, busulfan, butorphanol, calcium chloride/gluconate, capreomycin, CARBOplatin, carmustine, caspofungin, ceFAZolin, cefepime, cefotaxime, cefoTEtan, cefOXitin, cefTAZidime, ceftizoxime, cefTRIAXone, cefuroxime, chloramphenicol, chlorproMAZINE, cimetidine, ciprofloxacin, cisatracurium, CISplatin, clindamycin, cyclophosphamide, cycloSPORINE, cytarabine, dacarbazine, DACTINomycin, DAPTOmycin, DAUNOrubicin, DAUNOrubicin liposome, dexamethasone, digoxin, diltiazem, diphenhydrAMINE, DOBUTamine, DOCEtaxel, dolasetron, DOPamine, DOXOrubicin, DOXOrubicin liposomal, doxycycline, droperidol, enalaprilat, ePHEDrine, EPINEPHrine, epirubicin, eptifibatide, ertapenem, erythromycin, esmolol, etoposide, famotidine, fenoldopam, fentaNYL, fluconazole, fludarabine, fluorouracil, foscarnet, fosphenytoin, furosemide, gallium nitrate, ganciclovir, gatifloxacin, gemcitabine, gentamicin, glycopyrrolate, granisetron, haloperidol, heparin, hydrALAZINE, hydrocortisone, HYDROmorphone, hydrOXYzine, IDArubicin, ifosfamide, imipenem-cilastatin, insulin (regular), irinotecan, isoproterenol, ketorolac, labetalol, lansoprazole, leucovorin, levofloxacin, lidocaine, linezolid, LORazepam, magnesium sulfate, mannitol, mechlorethamine, melphalan, meperidine, meropenem, mesna, methohexital, methotrexate, methyldopate, methylPREDNISolone, metoclopramide, metoprolol, metroNIDAZOLE, midazolam, milrinone, minocycline, mitoMYcin, mitoXANtrone, mivacurium, morphine, moxifloxacin, mycophenolate, nafcillin, nalbuphine, naloxone, nesiritide, niCARdipine, nitroglycerin, nitroprusside, norepinephrine, ondansetron, oxaliplatin, PACLitaxel, palonosetron, pamidronate, pancuronium, PEMEtrexed, pentamidine, pentazocine, PENTobarbital, PHENobarbital, phenylephrine, piperacillin, piperacillin-tazobactam, polymyxin B, potassium acetate/chloride/phosphates, procainamide, prochlorperazine, promethazine, propranolol, quiNIDine, quinupristin-dalfopristin, ranitidine, remifentanil, rocuronium, sodium acetate/bicarbonate/phosphates, streptozocin, succinylcholine, SUFentanil, sulfamethoxazole-trimethoprim, tacrolimus, teniposide, thiopental, thiotepa, ticarcillin, ticarcillin-clavulanate, tigecycline, tirofiban, tobramycin, topotecan, vancomycin, vasopressin, vecuronium, verapamil, vinBLAStine, vinCRIStine, vinorelbine, voriconazole, zidovudine, zoledronic acid

ADVERSE EFFECTS

CNS: *Headache, dizziness, fatigue, weakness,* depression, anxiety, tremors, **seizures,** paranoia

CV: *Sinus bradycardia, conduction abnormalities,* **dysrhythmias,** chest pain, shortness of breath, thrombophlebitis, ischemia, **CHF,** hypertension, palpitations, **QT prolongation, ST-T wave changes**

ENDO: *Hypo/hyperglycemia, ketosis, hypothyroidism,* galactorrhea, diabetes insipidus

GI: *Diarrhea, nausea, abdominal pain, vomiting, flatulence, distension, constipation,* **hepatitis,** elevated liver function tests, **GI bleeding, pancreatitis,** cholelithiasis, ileus

GU: UTI

HEMA: Hematoma of inj site, bruise

INTEG: Rash, urticaria, pain, inflammation at inj site

MS: Joint and muscle pain

Pharmacokinetics

Absorption	Rapidly, completely absorbed
Distribution	Unknown
Metabolism	Little
Excretion	Urine, unchanged
Half-life	1.7 hr

Pharmacodynamics

	Subcut/IV	IM
Onset	Unknown	Unknown
Peak	½ hr	2-4 wk
Duration	12 hr	Unknown

INTERACTIONS

Individual drugs

Other products that prolong QT: increased QT prolongation

CycloSPORINE: decreased effect of cycloSPORINE

Haloperidol, chloroquine, droperidol, pentamidine, arsenic trioxide, levomethadyl: increased QT prolongation

Drug classifications

Class IA/III antidysrhythmics, some phenothiazines, β-agonists, local anesthetics, tricyclics, CYP3A4 inhibitors (amiodarone, clarithromycin, erythromycin, telithromycin, troleandomycin), CYP3A4 substrates (methadone, pimozide, QUEtiapine, quiNIDine, risperiDONE, ziprasidone): increased QT prolongation

Drug/food
Decreased: absorption of dietary fat, vit B$_{12}$ levels

Drug/lab test
Increased: glucose
Decreased: T$_4$, thyroid function tests, Vit B$_{12}$, glucose

NURSING CONSIDERATIONS
Assessment
• Identify growth hormone antibodies, IGF-1, 1-4 hr intervals for 8-12 hr after dose in acromegaly; 5-HIAA; blood glucose, serotonin levels (carcinoid tumors), plasma substance P, plasma vasoactive intestinal peptide (VIP) (VIPomas)
• Monitor for fecal fat, serum carotene, somatomedin-C q14 days, glucose; plasma serotonin levels (carcinoid tumors); plasma vasoactive intestinal peptide levels (VIPoma); serum growth hormone, serum IGF-1 baseline and periodically, diabetes to monitor blood glucose
• Monitor thyroid function tests: T$_3$, T$_4$, T$_7$, TSH to identify hypothyroidism
• Assess for allergic reaction: rash, itching, fever, nausea, wheezing
• **Assess for cardiac status:** bradycardia, conduction abnormalities, dysrhythmias; monitor ECG for QT prolongation, low voltage, axis shifts, early repolarization, R/S transition, early wave progression
• **Allergic reaction:** assess for rash, itching, fever, nausea, wheezing
• Gallbladder disease, pancreatitis: monitor closely

Patient/family education
• Explain reason for medication and expected results
• Advise patient that routine follow-up is needed
• Instruct parents on procedure for medication preparation and inj use; request demonstration, return demonstration; provide written instructions
• Advise patient that dizziness, drowsiness, weakness may occur; to avoid hazardous activities if these occur; to report abdominal pain immediately
• Teach patient that pregnancy may occur in acromegaly since fertility may be restored
• Teach diabetic patients to monitor glucose regularly

Evaluation
Positive therapeutic outcome
• Decreased symptoms of acromegaly, carcinoid, VIPoma
• Decreased diarrhea in AIDS

---

ofloxacin (Rx)
(o-flox′a-sin)
Func. class.: Antiinfective
Chem. class.: Fluoroquinolone
Pregnancy category C

ACTION: Interferes with conversion of intermediate DNA fragments into high molecular weight DNA in bacteria, inhibits DNA gyrase

Therapeutic outcome: Bactericidal action against gram-positive pathogens *Staphylococcus epidermidis,* methicillin-resistant strains of *Staphylococcus aureus, Streptococcus pyogenes, Streptococcus pneumoniae;* gram-negative pathogens *Escherichia coli, Klebsiella* species, *Enterobacter, Salmonella, Shigella, Proteus vulgaris, Proteus rettgeri, Providencia stuartii, Morganella morganii, Pseudomonas aeruginosa, Serratia, Haemophilus* species, *Acinetobacter, Neisseria gonorrhoeae, Neisseria meningitidis, Yersinia, Vibrio, Brucella, Campylobacter,* and *Aeromonas* species; anaerobic pathogens *Bacteroides fragilis intermedius, Clostridium perfringens, Gardnerella vaginalis, Peptococcus niger, Peptostreptococcus* species; *Chlamydia pneumoniae, Chlamydia trachomatis, Legionella pneumoniae, Mycobacterium tuberculosis, Mycoplasma pneumoniae*

USES: Treatment of lower respiratory tract infections (pneumonia, bronchitis), genitourinary infections (prostatitis, UTIs), skin and skin structure infections, gonorrhea, otitis media, conjunctivitis (ophth)

CONTRAINDICATIONS:
Hypersensitivity to quinolones, QT prolongation, TB

Precautions: Pregnancy **C,** breastfeeding, children, geriatric, renal disease, seizure disorders, excessive sunlight, hypokalemia, colitis

> **BLACK BOX WARNING:** Tendon pain/rupture, tendinitis, myasthenia gravis

DOSAGE AND ROUTES
Lower respiratory tract infection/ skin and skin structure infections
Adult: PO 400 mg q12hr × 10 days

Prostatitis from *E. Coli*
Adult: PO 300 mg q12hr × 6 wk

Urinary tract infection
Adult: PO 200 mg q12hr × 10 days

Renal dose
Adult: PO CCr 20-50 ml/min give q24hr; CCr <20 ml/min give ½ of dose q24hr

Hepatic dose
Adult (Child-Pugh class C): PO max 400 mg/day

Available forms: Tabs 200, 300, 400 mg

Implementation
• Store at room temp, protect from light
PO route
• Give in equal intervals q12hr around the clock to maintain proper blood levels; do not give within 2 hr of other agents, since product interactions are possible: give with 8 oz of water
• Do not give with iron, aluminum, zinc products or antacids, which decrease absorption and form insoluble chelate

ADVERSE EFFECTS
CNS: Dizziness, headache, fatigue, somnolence, depression, insomnia, lethargy, malaise, **seizures**, vertigo
CV: QT prolongation, **dysrhythmias**, chest pain
EENT: Visual disturbances, pharyngitis
GI: Diarrhea, nausea, vomiting, anorexia, flatulence, heartburn, dry mouth, increased AST, ALT, abdominal pain, constipation, **pseudomembranous colitis**, abnormal taste, xerostomia
HEMA: Blood dyscrasias
INTEG: Rash, pruritus, photosensitivity
MS: Tendinitis, **tendon rupture, rhabdomyolysis**
SYST: Anaphylaxis, **Stevens-Johnson syndrome, toxic epidermal necrosis**

Pharmacokinetics
Absorption	Well absorbed (PO)
Distribution	Widely distributed
Metabolism	Unknown
Excretion	Kidneys, unchanged; breast milk
Half-life	5-9 hr; increased in renal disease

Pharmacodynamics
	PO	Ophth
Onset	Rapid	Unknown
Peak	1-2 hr	Unknown
Duration	Unknown	Unknown

INTERACTIONS
Individual drugs
Chloroquine, clarithromycin, droperidol, erythromycin, haloperidol, methadone, pentamidine: increased QT prolongation
Sevelamer: decreased ofloxacin effect
Sucralfate, zinc sulfate: decreased absorption of ofloxacin, separate by 2 hr
Theophylline: possible toxicity
Warfarin: increased anticoagulation

Drug classifications
Antacids with aluminum, iron salts, magnesium: decreased absorption of ofloxacin, separate by 2 hr
Antidiabetics: altered blood glucose levels
β-agonists, class IA/III antidysrhythmics, local anesthetics, some phenothiazines, tricyclics: increased QT prolongation

> **BLACK BOX WARNING: Corticosteroids:** Increased tendon rupture/tendinitis

NSAIDs: increased CNS stimulation, seizures

Drug/lab test
Increased: INR

NURSING CONSIDERATIONS
Assessment
• Assess patient for previous sensitivity reaction
• Assess patient for signs and symptoms of infection including characteristics of wounds, sputum, urine, stool, WBC >10,000/mm^3, fever; obtain baselines and monitor during treatment
• Obtain C&S before beginning product therapy to identify if correct treatment has been initiated
• **QT prolongation:** assess ECG for QT prolongation, ejection fraction; assess for chest pain, palpitations, dyspnea
• **Pseudomembranous colitis:** assess for diarrhea, abdominal pain, fever, fatigue, anorexia; possible anemia, elevated WBC and low serum albumin; stop product and usually give either vancomycin or IV metroNIDAZOLE
• **Rhabdomyolysis:** assess muscle pain, increased CPK, weakness, swelling of affected muscles; if these occur and if confirmed by CPK, product should be discontinued

> **BLACK BOX WARNING:** Assess for allergic reactions: rash, urticaria, pruritus; stop product if these occur

• Monitor blood studies: AST, ALT, CBC, serum glucose monthly if patient is on long-term therapy; INR (warfarin use)

• Assess for overgrowth of infection in long-term treatment: perineal itching, fever, malaise, redness, pain, swelling, drainage, rash, diarrhea, change in cough, sputum
• Assess for CNS symptoms: seizures, vertigo, drowsiness, agitation, confusion, tremors

> **BLACK BOX WARNING: Myasthenia gravis:** product may increase weakness; avoid use

Patient/family education
• Instruct patient to take all medication prescribed for the length of time ordered; product must be taken around the clock to maintain blood levels; do not give medication to others
• Teach patient to use sunscreen when outdoors to decrease phototoxicity
• Teach patient that allergic reactions usually occur after first dose, but may occur later; stop product if a reaction occurs
• Advise patient to increase fluids to 2 L/day to prevent crystalluria
• Caution patient to avoid driving and other hazardous activities until response is known; dizziness, confusion, drowsiness may occur
• Teach patient to take without regard to meals
• Teach patient to avoid use with other products unless approved by prescriber

Evaluation
Positive therapeutic outcome
• Absence of signs/symptoms of infection
• Reported improvement in symptoms of infection
• Absence of red or itching eyes (ophth)

ofloxacin ophthalmic
See Appendix B

OLANZapine (Rx)
(oh-lanz′a-peen)
Zyprexa, Zyprexa Intramuscular, Zyprexa Relprevv, Zyprexa Zydis
Func. class.: Antipsychotic/neuroleptic
Chem. class.: Thienobenzodiazepine
Pregnancy category C

Do not confuse:
OLANZapine/osalazine,
Zyprexa/Celexa/Zyrtec

ACTION: May mediate antipsychotic activity by both DOPamine and serotonin type 2 (5-HT$_2$) antagonism; also, may antagonize muscarinic, histaminic (H$_1$), and α-adrenergic receptors

Therapeutic outcome: Decreased psychotic symptoms

USES: Schizophrenia, acute manic episodes in bipolar disorder, acute agitation

Unlabeled uses: Dementia related to Alzheimer's disease, OCD, acute psychosis

CONTRAINDICATIONS:
Hypersensitivity

Precautions: Pregnancy C, breastfeeding, geriatric, hypertension, cardiac/renal/hepatic disease, diabetes, agranulocytosis, abrupt discontinuation, Asian patients, closed-angle glaucoma, coma, leukopenia, QT prolongation, tardive dyskinesia, torsades de pointes, suicidal ideation, stroke history, TIA

> **BLACK BOX WARNING:** Dementia, postinjection delirium/sedation syndrome

DOSAGE AND ROUTES
Schizophrenia
Adult: PO 5-10 mg/day initially, may increase dosage by 5 mg at ≥1 wk intervals; orally disintegrating tabs: open blister pack, place tab on tongue, let disintegrate, swallow; max 20 mg/day; ext rel inj (Zyprexa Relprevv) IM 150-300 mg q2wk or 405 mg q4wk
Geriatric: PO 5 mg, may increase cautiously at 1 wk intervals, max 20 mg/day
Adolescent: PO 2.5 mg or 5 mg/day, target 10 mg/day

Bipolar mania
Adult: PO 10-15 mg/day, may increase dose after 24 hr by 5 mg, max 20 mg/day
Adolescent: PO 2.5 or 5 mg/day, target 10 mg/day

Agitation associated with schizophrenia, bipolar I mania
Adult: IM (reg rel) 10 mg once
Geriatric: IM (reg rel) 2.5-5 mg once

Available forms: Tabs 2.5, 5, 7.5, 10, 15, 20 mg; **orally disintegrating tabs** 5, 10, 15, 20 mg (Zyprexa Zydis); **powder for injection** 10 mg

Implementation
• Give antiparkinsonian agent for EPS
• Give decreased dose in geriatric
PO route
• Give with full glass of water/milk or with food to decrease GI upset

---

• **Orally disintegrating tabs:** open blister pack; place tab on tongue until dissolved; swallow; no water needed, do not break, crush, chew

• Store in tight, light-resistant container

IM route (Zyprexa Intramuscular)

• Dissolve contents of vials with 2.1 ml sterile water for injection (5 mg/ml), use immediately

• Do not use IV or SUBCUT

• Inject slowly, deep into muscle mass

IM route (Zyprexa Relprevv)

> **BLACK BOX WARNING:** Available only through restricted distribution program due to postinjection delirium/sedation syndrome; give at a facility with emergency services

• Use deep IM gluteal inj only

• Use only diluent provided in kit; give q2-4wk using 19G 1.5-inch needle in kit, in obesity use 19G 2-inch or larger needle

• Provide supervised ambulation until stabilized on medication; do not involve in strenuous exercise program because fainting is possible; patients should not stand still for long periods

• Give increased fluids to prevent constipation

• Give sips of water, candy, gum for dry mouth

• Store in airtight, light-resistant container

• Give orally disintegrating tabs: open blister pack, place tab on tongue until dissolved, swallow; no water needed

ADVERSE EFFECTS

CNS: EPS (pseudoparkinsonism, akathisia, dystonia, tardive dyskinesia), **seizures,** headache, **neuroleptic malignant syndrome (rare),** agitation, nervousness, hostility, dizziness, hypertonia, tremor, euphoria, confusion, *drowsiness,* fatigue, *abnormal gait, insomnia, fever*

CV: Hypotension, tachycardia, chest pain, **heart failure, sudden death (geriatric, IM),** orthostatic hypotension, peripheral edema

ENDO: Increased prolactin levels, hyperglycemia, hypoglycemia

GI: Dry mouth, nausea, vomiting, anorexia, constipation, abdominal pain, weight gain, appetite, dyspepsia, jaundice, **hepatitis**

GU: Urinary retention, urinary frequency, enuresis, impotence, amenorrhea, gynecomastia, breast engorgement, premenstrual syndrome

HEMA: Neutropenia

INTEG: Rash

MISC: Peripheral edema, accidental injury, hypertonia, hyperlipidemia

MS: Joint pain, twitching

RESP: *Cough, pharyngitis,* **fatal pneumonia (geriatric, IM)**

Pharmacokinetics

Absorption	Well absorbed
Distribution	93% plasma protein binding
Metabolism	Liver
Excretion	Kidneys
Half-life	Unknown

Pharmacodynamics

Onset	Unknown
Peak	PO 6 hr, IM 15-45 min
Duration	Unknown

INTERACTIONS

Individual drugs

Alcohol: increased sedation, hypotension

Bromocriptine, levodopa: decreased antiparkinson activity

CarBAMazepine, omeprazole, rifampin: decreased levels of OLANZapine

Diazepam: increased hypotension

FluvoxaMINE: increased OLANZapine levels

Drug classifications

SSRIs, SNRIs: increased serotonin syndrome, increased neuroleptic malignant syndrome

Anesthetics (barbiturates), antidepressants, antihistamines, CNS depressants, sedative/hypnotics: increased sedation

Anticholinergics: increased anticholinergic effects

Antihypertensives: increased hypotension

DOPamine agonists: decreased antiparkinson activity

Drug/lab test

Increased: liver function tests, prolactin, CPK

NURSING CONSIDERATIONS

Assessment

> **BLACK BOX WARNING:** Postinjection delirium/sedation syndrome (Zyprexa Relprevv): monitor continuously for ≥3 hr after injection; this patient must be accompanied when leaving: sedation, coma, delirium, EPS, slurred speech, altered gait, aggression, dizziness, weakness, hypertension, seizures; before leaving, confirm the patient is alert, oriented, and free of any other symptoms

• Assess mental status, orientation, mood, behavior, presence of hallucinations and type before initial administration and monthly

Adverse effects: *italics* = common; **bold** = life-threatening

• Monitor I&O ratio; palpate bladder if low urinary output occurs, especially in geriatric
• Monitor bilirubin, CBC
• Monitor urinalysis; recommended before, during prolonged therapy
• Assess affect, orientation, LOC, reflexes, gait, coordination, sleep pattern disturbances
• Monitor B/P sitting, standing, lying; take pulse and respirations q4hr during initial treatment; establish baseline before starting treatment; report drops of 30 mm Hg; obtain baseline ECG
• **Serotonin syndrome:** assess for increased heart rate, shivering, sweating, dilated pupils, tremors, high B/P, hyperthermia, headache, confusion; if these occur, stop product, administer a serotonin antagonist if needed
• Assess dizziness, faintness, palpitations, tachycardia on rising
• **Assess for neuroleptic malignant syndrome:** hyperpyrexia, muscle rigidity, increased CPK, altered mental status, for acute dystonia (cheek chewing, swallowing, eyes, pill rolling)
• **EPS** including akathisia (inability to sit still, no pattern to movements), tardive dyskinesia (bizarre movements of the jaw, mouth, tongue, extremities), pseudoparkinsonism (rigidity, tremors, pill rolling, shuffling gait)
• Monitor constipation, urinary retention daily; increase bulk, water in diet

Patient/family education

BLACK BOX WARNING: Teach patient about postinjection delirium/sedation syndrome; teach about all symptoms

• Teach patient to use good oral hygiene; frequent rinsing of mouth, candy, ice chips, sugarless gum for dry mouth
• Advise patient to avoid hazardous activities until product response is determined
• Advise patient that orthostatic hypotension occurs often and to rise from sitting or lying position gradually
• Advise patient to avoid hot tubs, hot showers, tub baths, since hypotension may occur
• Advise patient to avoid abrupt withdrawal of this product, or EPS may result; product should be withdrawn slowly
• Advise patient to avoid OTC preparations (cough, hay fever, cold) unless approved by prescriber, since serious product interactions may occur; avoid use with alcohol, CNS depressants, increased drowsiness may occur
• Advise patient that in hot weather, heat stroke may occur; take extra precautions to stay cool

Evaluation
Positive therapeutic outcome
• Decrease in emotional excitement, hallucinations, delusions, paranoia, reorganization of patterns of thought, speech

TREATMENT OF OVERDOSE:
Lavage if orally ingested; provide airway; do not induce vomiting or use epinephrine

olmesartan (Rx)
(ol-meh-sar′tan)
Benicar
Func. class.: Antihypertensive
Chem. class.: Angiotensin II receptor (type AT$_1$) antagonist
Pregnancy category C (1st trimester), D (2nd/3rd trimesters)

Do not confuse:
Benicar/Mevacor

ACTION: Blocks the vasoconstrictor and aldosterone-secreting effects of angiotensin II; selectively blocks the binding of angiotensin II to the AT$_1$ receptor found in tissues

Therapeutic outcome: Decreased B/P

USES: Hypertension, alone or in combination with other antihypertensives

CONTRAINDICATIONS:
Hypersensitivity, pregnancy **D** (2nd/3rd trimesters)

Precautions: Breastfeeding, children, geriatric, hepatic disease, CHF, renal artery stenosis, African descent, hyperkalemia

DOSAGE AND ROUTES
Adult: PO single agent 20 mg/day initially in patients who are not volume depleted; may be increased to 40 mg/day if needed after 2 wk
Adolescent ≤16 yr/child ≥6 yr weighing ≥35 kg: PO 20 mg/day, may increase to max 40 mg/day after 2 wk
Adolescent ≤16 yr/child ≥6 yr weighing 20-<35 kg: PO 10 mg/day, may increase to max 20 mg/day after 2 wk

Available forms: Tabs 5, 20, 40 mg

Implementation
• Give without regard to meals

ADVERSE EFFECTS

CNS: *Dizziness,* fatigue, insomnia, syncope
CV: Chest pain, peripheral edema, tachycardia, *hypotension*
EENT: Sinusitis, rhinitis, pharyngitis
GI: *Diarrhea,* abdominal pain
META: Hyperkalemia
MS: Arthralgia, pain, rhabdomyolysis
RESP: *Upper respiratory infection,* bronchitis
SYST: Angioedema

Pharmacokinetics

Absorption	Unknown
Distribution	Unknown
Metabolism	Unknown
Excretion	Urine, feces
Half-life	Unknown

Pharmacodynamics

Onset	Unknown
Peak	1-2 hr
Duration	Unknown

INTERACTIONS

Individual drugs

Lithium, ACE inhibitors: increased effect

Drug classifications

Antihypertensives (other), diuretics: increased antihypertensive effects
NSAIDs: decreased antihypertensive effect
Antioxidants: increased effects
Potassium supplements, potassium-sparing diuretics: increased hyperkalemia

Drug/herb

Aconite: increased toxicity, death
Astragalus, cola tree: increased or decreased antihypertensive effect
Hawthorn: increased antihypertensive effect
Ephedra: decreased antihypertensive effect

NURSING CONSIDERATIONS

Assessment

> **BLACK BOX WARNING: Assess for pregnancy;** this product can cause fetal death when given in pregnancy, 2nd/3rd trimester

• Assess response and adverse reactions, especially in renal disease, monitor renal function
• Monitor B/P, pulse q4hr; note rate, rhythm, quality; electrolytes: sodium, potassium, chloride; baselines in renal, liver function tests before therapy begins

• Hypotension: place supine; may occur with hyponatremia or in those with volume depletion; more common in those also taking a diuretic

Patient/family education

• Advise to comply with dosage schedule, even if feeling better
• Advise patient to notify prescriber of mouth sores, fever, swelling of hands or feet, irregular heartbeat, chest pain
• Teach that excessive perspiration, dehydration, vomiting, diarrhea may lead to fall in B/P; to consult prescriber if these occur, maintain adequate hydration
• Teach that product may cause dizziness, fainting; light-headedness may occur, avoid hazardous activities
• Advise to rise slowly to sitting or standing position to minimize orthostatic hypotension

> **BLACK BOX WARNING:** Teach to notify prescriber immediately if pregnant; not to use during breastfeeding

• Advise to avoid all OTC medications, unless approved by prescriber
• Teach patient that blood glucose may increase and antidiabetic product may need dosage change
• Advise to inform all health care providers of medication use
• Advise to use proper technique for obtaining B/P and acceptable parameters

Evaluation

Positive therapeutic outcome
• Decreased B/P

---

olopatadine ophthalmic
See Appendix B

---

olsalazine (Rx)
(ohl-sal′ah-zeen)
Dipentum
Func. class.: Antiinflammatory
Chem. class.: Salicylate derivative
Pregnancy category C

Do not confuse:
olsalazine/OLANZapine

ACTION: Bioconverted to 5-aminosalicylic acid, which decreases inflammation

Therapeutic outcome: Lessening of loose diarrhea stools and cramping

USES: Maintenance of remission of ulcerative colitis in patients intolerant to sulfasalazine

CONTRAINDICATIONS:
Hypersensitivity to this product or salicylates

Precautions: Pregnancy **C**, breastfeeding, children <14 yr, impaired renal/hepatic function, severe allergy, bronchial asthma

DOSAGE AND ROUTES
Adult: PO 500 mg bid, max 3 g/day

Available forms: Caps 250 mg

Implementation
• Give total daily dose evenly spaced to minimize GI intolerance, give with food
• Store in tight, light-resistant container at room temperature

ADVERSE EFFECTS
CNS: Headache, hallucinations, depression, vertigo, fatigue, dizziness
GI: Nausea, vomiting, abdominal pain, **hepatitis**, diarrhea, bloating, **pancreatitis**
HEMA: Leukopenia, neutropenia, thrombocytopenia, agranulocytosis, anemia
INTEG: Rash, dermatitis, urticaria

Pharmacokinetics

Absorption	Colon 99% converted to mesalamine
Distribution	Colon
Metabolism	Liver
Excretion	Feces
Half-life	0.9 hr

Pharmacodynamics

Onset	Unknown
Peak	1 hr
Duration	12 hr

INTERACTIONS
Individual drugs
AzaTHIOprine: increased toxicity
Mercaptopurine, thioguanine: increased myelosuppression
Warfarin: increased pro-time, INR

Drug/lab test
Increased: AST, ALT

NURSING CONSIDERATIONS
Assessment
⚠ Assess for blood dyscrasias: skin rash, fever, sore throat, bruising, bleeding, fatigue, joint pain (rare)

• **Assess for allergic reaction:** rash, dermatitis, urticaria, pruritus, dyspnea, bronchospasm
• **Colitis:** assess bowel pattern, number of stools, consistency, frequency, pain, mucus before treatment and periodically

Patient/family education
• Advise patient to take as prescribed, take missed dose as soon as remembered
• Inform patient not to operate machinery or drive until effects are known, may cause dizziness
• Advise patient to notify prescriber if symptoms do not improve or if allergic reaction or sore throat occurs
• Teach patient to report diarrhea, rash, bleeding, bruising, fever, hallucinations

Evaluation
Positive therapeutic outcome
• Absence of fever, mucus in stools

omacetaxine
(oh′ma-set-ax′een)
Synribo
Func. class.: Antineoplastic miscellaneous
Chem. class.: Cephalotaxine ester (derived from the evergreen tree *Cephalotaxus harringtonia*)
Pregnancy category D

ACTION: Inhibits protein synthesis by binding to site of large ribosome subunit, it reduces Bcr-Abl and Mcl-1 independent of direct Bcr-Abl binding, inducing apoptosis

Therapeutic outcome: Decreased CML, positive hematologic response

USES: Chronic or accelerated phase chronic myelogenous leukemia (CML) with resistance or/and intolerance to 2 or more tyrosine kinase inhibitors

CONTRAINDICATIONS:
Pregnancy (D), breastfeeding, hypersensitivity

Precautions: Children, bleeding, diabetes mellitus, female patients, geriatric patients, hyperglycemia, hyperosmolar hyperglycemic state (HHS), infection, anemia, neutropenia, thrombocytopenia

DOSAGE AND ROUTES
Adult: SUBCUT 1.25 mg/m^2 bid × 14 days every 28 days
Grade 4 neutropenia (absolute neutrophil count [ANC] < 0.5 × 10^9/L) or grade 3 thrombo-

cytopenia (platelet count < 50 × 10⁹/L): Do not start the next cycle until the ANC is ≥1 × 10⁹/L and platelets are 50 × 10⁹/L; when therapy is resumed, reduce the number of dosing days by 2 days/cycle (initial cycles, from 14 to 12 days; maintenance cycles, from 7 to 5 days)

Available forms: Powder for injection 3.5 mg

Implementation
SUBCUT route
• Reconstitution: Add 1 ml of 0.9% saline for injection/vial to 3.5 mg/ml, gently swirl until the solution is clear and completely dissolved, visually inspect for particulate matter and discoloration before use, protect from light
• Administration: Calculate dose, withdraw into a syringe, and give as a SUBCUT injection; discard unused portion, use 12 hr at room temperature, 24 hr when refrigerated

ADVERSE EFFECTS
CNS: *Seizures,* weakness, agitation, anxiety, chills, fever, confusion, depression, dizziness, fatigue, headache, insomnia, lethargy, night sweats, tremor
CV: Hypotension, peripheral edema, sinus tachycardia
EENT: Blurred vision, change in taste (dysgeusia)
GI: Nausea, vomiting, diarrhea, abdominal pain, stomatitis
HEMA: **Neutropenia, leukopenia, thrombocytopenia, anemia, bleeding**
INTEG: Alopecia, rash, skin hyperpigmentation, stomatitis, skin ulcer, purpura, petechiae, pruritus
MISC: Fever
MS: Arthralgia, gout, myalgia, back pain
RESP: Dyspnea, cough, rales, sinus congestion
SYST: Infections

Pharmacokinetics
Absorption	Unknown
Distribution	Protein binding 50%
Metabolism	Unknown
Excretion	Unknown
Half-life	6 hr

Pharmacodynamics
Onset	Unknown
Peak	30 min
Duration	Unknown

INTERACTIONS
Drug classifications
Anticoagulants, salicylates, NSAIDs, avoid use when platelets are 50,000 cells/mL: Increased bleeding risk

NURSING CONSIDERATIONS
Assessment

> **BLACK BOX WARNING:** Monitor CBC, differential, platelet count before treatment and weekly, during induction/maintenance, then every 2 wk as needed

⚠ **Pregnancy D: assess for pregnancy before starting treatment**
• Infection: monitor temp every 4 hr; fever might indicate beginning of infection
• CV status: Monitor B/P, edema, flushing
• CNS changes: Monitor confusion, paresthesias, dysesthesia, pain, weakness
⚠ **Hypersensitive reactions, anaphylaxis: Assess for hypotension, dyspnea, angioedema, generalized urticaria; discontinue infusion immediately**
⚠ **Bone marrow depression/bleeding: Assess for hematuria, guaiac, bruising or petechiae, mucosa or orifices every 8 hr; obtain prescription for viscous lidocaine (Xylocaine); avoid invasive procedures**
• Assess for effects of alopecia on body image; discuss feelings about body changes
• **Diabetes mellitus:** avoid this product in poorly controlled disease, monitor blood glucose levels frequently

Patient/family education
• Teach patient to report signs of infection: fever, sore throat, flulike symptoms
• Teach patient to report signs of anemia: fatigue, headache, faintness, SOB, irritability
• Teach patient to report bleeding; to avoid use of razors, commercial mouthwash; to avoid use of aspirin, ibuprofen
• Advise patient that hair may be lost during treatment; that a wig or hairpiece might make patient feel better; that new hair may be different in color and texture
• Inform patient that pain in muscles and joints 2–5 days after infusion is common
⚠ **Advise patient to use barrier contraception during and for several mo after treatment, pregnancy D; to avoid breastfeeding**
• Teach patient to avoid receiving vaccinations while taking product

Evaluation
Positive therapeutic outcome
• Decreased CML, positive hematologic response

---

omalizumab (Rx)
(oh-mah-lye-zoo′mab)
Xolair
Func. class.: Antiasthmatic
Chem. class.: Monoclonal antibody
Pregnancy category B

ACTION: Recombinant DNA-derived humanized IgG murine monoclonal antibody that selectively binds to IgE to limit the release of mediators in the allergic response

Therapeutic outcome: Ability to breathe more easily

USES: Moderate to severe persistent asthma

Unlabeled uses: Seasonal allergic rhinitis, food allergy

CONTRAINDICATIONS:
Hypersensitivity to hamster protein

> **BLACK BOX WARNING:** Hypersensitivity to this product

Precautions: Pregnancy **B,** breastfeeding, children <12 yr, acute attacks of asthma, lymphoma, nephrotic disease, bronchospasm, neoplastic disease, status asthmaticus

DOSAGE AND ROUTES
Adult/adolescent/child ≥12 yr: SUBCUT 150-375 mg × 2-4 wk, divide inj into 2 sites, if dose is >150 mg; dose is adjusted based on IgE levels and significant changes in body weight

Available forms: Powder for inj, lyophilized 202.5 mg (150 mg/1.2 ml after reconstitution)

Implementation
SUBCUT route
• Reconstitute using 1.4 ml sterile water for inj (150 mg/1.2 ml or 125 mg/ml); gently swirl to dissolve; allow vial to stand and q5min gently swirl for 5-10 sec to dissolve, some vials take ≥20 min, do not use if contents do not dissolve within 40 min, should be clear or slightly opalescent; use large-bore needle to withdraw medication; replace needle with small-bore needle

• Given q2-4wk; product is viscous; if >150 mg is given, divide into two sites; the inj may take 5-10 sec to administer
• Do not give more than 150 mg/inj site

ADVERSE EFFECTS
CV: Heart failure, cardiomyopathy, hypotension
HEMA: Serious systemic eosinophilia
INTEG: Pruritus, dermatitis, inj site reactions, rash
MISC: Earache, dizziness, fatigue, pain, **malignancies,** viral infections, **anaphylaxis, thrombocytopenia,** headache
MS: Arthralgia, fracture, leg, arm pain
RESP: Sinusitis, upper respiratory tract infections, pharyngitis, pulmonary hypertension, **bronchospasm**

Pharmacokinetics
Absorption	Slow
Distribution	Unknown
Metabolism	Degradation by liver
Excretion	In bile
Half-life	26 days

Pharmacodynamics
Onset	Unknown
Peak	7-8 days
Duration	Unknown

INTERACTIONS
Drug classifications
Vaccines (live virus): use cautiously

Drug/lab test
Increased: IgE

NURSING CONSIDERATIONS
Assessment
• Monitor respiratory rate, rhythm, depth; auscultate lung fields bilaterally; notify prescriber of abnormalities; monitor pulmonary function tests; serum IgE

> **BLACK BOX WARNING: Assess for anaphylaxis, allergic reactions:** rash, urticaria, inability to breathe, edema of throat; observe for 2 hr, reaction can occur up to 24 hr; have emergency equipment available; product should be discontinued

Patient/family education
• Advise patient that improvement will not be immediate

- Teach patient not to stop taking or decrease current asthma medications unless instructed by prescriber

> **BLACK BOX WARNING:** Instruct patient to report signs of allergic reaction

Evaluation
Positive therapeutic outcome
- Ability to breathe more easily

---

omeprazole (Rx, OTC)
(oh-mep′ra-zole)
Good Sense Omeprazole, Losec ✖,
PriLOSEC, PriLOSEC OTC
Func. class.: Antiulcer, proton pump inhibitor
Chem. class.: Benzimidazole
Pregnancy category C

Do not confuse:
PriLOSEC/Prinivil/predniSONE/PROzac

ACTION: Suppresses gastric secretion by inhibiting hydrogen/potassium ATPase enzyme system in the gastric parietal cell; characterized as a gastric acid pump inhibitor, since it blocks the final step of acid production

Therapeutic outcome: Absence of duodenal ulcers; decreased gastroesophageal reflux

USES: Gastroesophageal reflux disease (GERD), severe erosive esophagitis, poorly responsive systemic GERD, pathologic hypersecretory conditions (Zollinger-Ellison syndrome, systemic mastocytosis, multiple endocrine adenomas); possibly effective for treatment of duodenal ulcers with or without antiinfectives for *Helicobacter pylori*

CONTRAINDICATIONS:
Hypersensitivity

Precautions: Pregnancy **C**, breastfeeding, children

DOSAGE AND ROUTES
Active duodenal ulcers
Adult: PO 20 mg/day × 4-8 wk; associated with *H. pylori* 40 mg qAM and clarithromycin 500 mg tid on days 1-14, then 20 mg/day days 15-28

Severe erosive esophagitis/poorly responsive GERD
Adult: PO (DEL REL cap/SUSP) 20 mg/day × 4-8 wk

Pathologic hypersecretory conditions
Adult: PO 60 mg/day; may increase to 120 mg tid; daily doses >80 mg should be divided

Gastric ulcer
Adult: PO 40 mg/day × 4-8 wk
Geriatric: PO max 20 mg/day

Heartburn (OTC)
Adult: PO 1 DEL REL tab (20 mg) daily before AM meal with glass of water

Available forms: Del rel caps 10, 20, 40 mg, del rel tabs (PriLOSEC OTC) 20 mg; granules for oral susp 2.5, 10 mg (del rel)

Implementation
- Swallow sus rel caps whole; do not break, crush, chew, or open
- Give before patient eats; may give with antacids

ADVERSE EFFECTS
CNS: *Headache, dizziness, asthenia*
CV: Chest pain, angina, tachycardia, bradycardia, palpitations, peripheral edema, **heart failure**
EENT: Tinnitus, taste perversion
GI: *Diarrhea, abdominal pain, vomiting, nausea, constipation, flatulence, acid regurgitation,* abdominal swelling, anorexia, irritable colon, esophageal candidiasis, dry mouth, **hepatic failure**
GU: UTI, frequency, increased creatinine, **proteinuria, hematuria,** testicular pain, glycosuria
HEMA: Pancytopenia, thrombocytopenia, neutropenia, leukocytosis, anemia
INTEG: Rash, dry skin, urticaria, pruritus, alopecia
META: Hypoglycemia, increased hepatic enzymes, weight gain, hypomagnesemia, hyponatremia, vit B_{12} deficiency
MISC: *Back pain,* fever, fatigue, malaise
RESP: *Upper respiratory tract infections, cough,* epistaxis, **pneumonia**
SYST: Angioedema, exfoliative dermatitis, Stevens-Johnson syndrome, toxic epidermal necrolysis

Pharmacokinetics

Absorption	Rapidly absorbed
Distribution	Protein binding (95%); gastric parietal cells
Metabolism	Liver, extensively; by CYP450 enzyme system
Excretion	Kidneys, feces
Half-life	½-1 hr; increased in the geriatric, hepatic disease

---

Pharmacodynamics

Onset	1 hr
Peak	½-3½ hr
Duration	3-4 days

INTERACTIONS

Individual drugs

Ampicillin: decreased effect of ampicillin

Calcium carbonate: decreased absorption of calcium carbonate

Cyanocobalamin: decreased absorption of cyanocobalamin

CycloSPORINE: increased cycloSPORINE levels

Diazepam: increased serum levels of diazepam

Digoxin: increased serum levels, delayed absorption of digoxin

Disulfiram: increased disulfiram levels

Flurazepam: increased flurazepam level

Gefitinib: decreased effect of gefitinib

Indinavir: decreased effect of indinavir

Iron salts: decreased absorption

Ketoconazole: decreased absorption of keto-conazole

Phenytoin: increased serum levels of phenytoin

Triazolam: increased triazolam level

Warfarin: increased bleeding tendencies

Drug classifications

Iron products: decreased absorption of iron

Drug/lab test

Increased: alkaline phosphatase, AST, ALT, bilirubin, gastrin

NURSING CONSIDERATIONS

Assessment

• **Electrolyte imbalances:** hyponatremia, hypomagnesemia in those using this product 3 mo-1 yr; if hypomagnesemia occurs, use of magnesium supplement may be sufficient; if severe, discontinue use

• **Serious skin reactions:** toxic epidermal necrolysis, **Stevens-Johnson syndrome,** angioedema, exfoliative dermatitis; assess for fever, sore throat, fatigue, thin ulcers, lesions in mouth, lips; discontinue product

• **Assess GI system:** bowel sounds q8hr, abdomen for pain and swelling, anorexia

• **Monitor hepatic enzymes:** AST, ALT, increased alkaline phosphatase during treatment; blood studies; CBC, differential during treatment, blood dyscrasias may occur; vitamin B_{12} in long-term treatment

• Teach patient to take as directed, even if feeling better; to take missed dose as soon as remembered; not to double; PriLOSEC OTC can take up to 4 days for full effect

Patient/family education

• Advise patient to report severe diarrhea; black, tarry stools; abdominal cramps/pain, continuing headache; product may have to be discontinued

• Caution patient to avoid driving and other hazardous activities until response to product is known

• Caution patient to avoid alcohol, salicylates, ibuprofen; may cause GI irritation

Evaluation

Positive therapeutic outcome

• Absence of epigastric pain, swelling, fullness

---

ondansetron (Rx)

(on-dan′sa-tron)

Zofran, Zofran ODT, Zuplenz

Func. class.: Antiemetic

Chem. class.: 5-HT receptor antagonist

Pregnancy category B

Do not confuse:
Zofran/Zantac

ACTION: Prevents nausea, vomiting by blocking serotonin (5-HT) peripherally, centrally, and in the small intestine

Therapeutic outcome: Control of nausea, vomiting

USES: Prevention of nausea, vomiting associated with cancer chemotherapy, radiotherapy, and prevention of postoperative nausea, vomiting

Unlabeled uses: Bulimia, pruritus (rectal use), alcoholism, hyperemesis gravidarum

CONTRAINDICATIONS: Hypersensitivity; phenylketonuric hypersensitivity (oral disintegrating tab), torsades de pointes

Precautions: Pregnancy **B**, breastfeeding, children, geriatric, granisetron hypersensitivity, QT prolongation, torsades de pointes

DOSAGE AND ROUTES

Prevention of nausea/vomiting (cancer chemotherapy)

Adult and child 4-18 yr: **IV** 0.15 mg/kg infused over 15 min, 30 min before start of cancer chemotherapy, max 16 mg/dose; 0.15 mg/kg is given 4 hr and 8 hr after first dose or 16 mg as a single dose; dilute in 50 ml of D_5 or 0.9% NaCl before giving; **RECT** (unlabeled) 16 mg daily 2

---

hr before chemotherapy; PO 8 mg ½ hr prior to chemotherapy, repeat 4, 8 hr after 1st dose
Child ≥4 yr: PO 4 mg ½ hr prior to chemotherapy

Prevention of nausea/vomiting (radiotherapy)
Adult: PO 8 mg tid, may repeat q8hr

Prevention of postoperative nausea/vomiting
Adult: IV/IM 4 mg undiluted over >30 sec prior to induction of anesthesia
Child 2-12 yr: IV 0.1 mg/kg (≤40 kg); 4 mg (≥40 kg), give ≥30 sec

Hepatic dose
Adult: PO/IM/IV max dose 8 mg daily

Hyperemesis gravidarum (unlabeled)
Adult: PO/IV 4-8 mg bid-tid

Pruritus (unlabeled)
Adult: PO 4 mg bid

Alcoholism (unlabeled)
Adult: PO 4 mcg/kg bid

Available forms: Inj 2 mg/ml, 32 mg/50 ml (premixed); tabs 4, 8 mg; oral sol 4 mg/5 ml; oral disintegrating tabs 4, 8 mg; oral dissolving film 4.8 mg

Implementation
PO route
• **Oral disintegrating tab:** do not push through foil; gently remove and immediately place on tongue to dissolve, swallow with saliva
• **Oral dissolving film:** fold pouch along dotted line to expose near notch; while folded, tear and remove film, place film on tongue until dissolved, swallow after dissolved; to reach desired dose, administer successive films, allowing each to dissolve before using another
• Check for discoloration or particulate; if particulate is present, shake to dissolve
IM route
• Visually inspect for particulate or discoloration
• May give 4 mg undiluted IM; inject deeply in large muscle mass, aspirate

Direct IV route
• Give **IV** after diluting a single dose in 50 ml of 0.9% NaCl or D₅W, 0.45% NaCl; give over 15 min
• Store at room temperature for 48 hr after dilution
• Do not use IV 32-mg dose in chemotherapy; nausea/vomiting due to QT prolongation, max 16 mg/dose (adult)

Y-site compatibilities: Aldesleukin, amifostine, amikacin, aztreonam, bleomycin, CARBOplatin, carmustine, ceFAZolin, ceforanide, cefotaxime, cefOXitin, cefTAZidime, ceftizoxime, cefuroxime, chlorproMAZINE, cimetidine, cisatracurium, CISplatin, cladribine, clindamycin, cyclophosphamide, cytarabine, dacarbazine, DACTINomycin, DAUNOrubicin, dexamethasone, diphenhydrAMINE, DOXOrubicin, DOXOrubicin liposome, doxycycline, droperidol, etoposide, famotidine, filgrastim, floxuridine, fluconazole, fludarabine, gentamicin, haloperidol, heparin, hydrocortisone, HYDROmorphone, hydrOXYzine, ifosfamide, imipenem/cilastatin, magnesium sulfate, mannitol, mechlorethamine, melphalan, meperidine, mesna, methotrexate, metoclopramide, miconazole, mitoMYcin, mitoXANtrone, morphine, PACLitaxel, pentostatin, potassium chloride, prochlorperazine, ranitidine, remifentanil, streptozocin, teniposide, thiotepa, ticarcillin, ticarcillin/clavulanate, vancomycin, vinBLAStine, vinCRIStine, vinorelbine, zidovudine

Y-site incompatibilities: Acyclovir, aminophylline, amphotericin B, ampicillin, ampicillin/sulbactam, cefoperazone, furosemide, ganciclovir, LORazepam, methylPREDNISolone, mezlocillin, piperacillin, sargramostim, sodium bicarbonate

ADVERSE EFFECTS
CNS: *Headache,* dizziness, drowsiness, fatigue, EPS
GI: *Diarrhea, constipation, abdominal pain,* dry mouth
MISC: Rash, **bronchospasm** (rare), *musculoskeletal pain, wound problems, shivering, fever, hypoxia, urinary retention*

Pharmacokinetics

Absorption	Completely absorbed (**IV**)
Distribution	Unknown
Metabolism	Liver, extensively
Excretion	Kidneys
Half-life	3.5-4.7 hr

Pharmacodynamics
Unknown

INTERACTIONS
Individual drugs
Apomorphine: increased unconsciousness, hypotension: do not use together
CarBAMazepine, phenytoin, rifampin: decreased ondansetron effect

---

Drug classifications
Increased QT prolongation with other products that prolong QT

Drug/lab test
Increased: LFTs

NURSING CONSIDERATIONS

Assessment
• Assess for absence of nausea, vomiting during chemotherapy
• Assess for hypersensitivity reaction: rash, bronchospasm
• **Assess for EPS** shuffling gait, tremors, grimacing, rigidity
• **QT prolongation:** monitor ECG in those with cardiac disease and those receiving other products that increase QT

Patient/family education
• Instruct patient to report diarrhea, constipation, rash, changes in respirations, or discomfort at insertion site
• Teach patient reason for medication and expected results

Evaluation
Positive therapeutic outcome
• Absence of nausea, vomiting during cancer chemotherapy

---

orlistat (Rx, OTC)
(or-li'stat)
Alli, Xenical
Chem. class.: Weight control agent, lipase inhibitor
Pregnancy category B

ACTION: Inhibits the absorption of dietary fat

Therapeutic outcome: Decrease in weight

USES: Obesity management

CONTRAINDICATIONS:
Hypersensitivity, chronic malabsorption syndrome, cholestasis, pregnancy (**X**)

Precautions: Children, hypothyroidism, other organic causes of obesity, anorexia nervosa, bulimia, nephrolithiasis, GI disease, diabetes, fat-soluble vitamin deficiency, breastfeeding

DOSAGE AND ROUTES
Adult: PO 60 mg (Alli)-120 mg (Xenical) tid with each main meal containing fat, max 360 mg/day

Available forms: Caps 60 mg (Alli), 120 mg (Xenical)

Implementation
• Patient should be on a diet with 30% of calories from fat; omit dose of orlistat if a meal contains no fat

ADVERSE EFFECTS
CNS: *Insomnia,* dizziness, headache, depression, anxiety, fatigue
GI: *Oily spotting, flatus with discharge, fecal urgency, fatty/oily stool, oily evacuation, fecal incontinence,* frequent defecation, nausea, vomiting, abdominal pain, infectious diarrhea, rectal pain, tooth disorder, hypovitaminosis, **hepatic failure, hepatitis, pancreatitis**
GU: UTI, vaginitis, menstrual irregularity
INTEG: Dry skin, rash
MS: Back pain, arthritis, myalgia, tendinitis
RESP: Influenza, upper, lower respiratory tract infection, EENT symptoms

Pharmacokinetics
Absorption	Minimal
Distribution	99% protein binding
Metabolism	Unknown
Excretion	Feces
Half-life	1-2 hr

Pharmacodynamics
Onset	Unknown
Peak	8 hr
Duration	Unknown

INTERACTIONS
Individual drugs
CycloSPORINE: decreased absorption
Pravastatin: increased lipid-lowering effect
Warfarin: increased effects of warfarin

Drug classifications
Fat-soluble vitamins: decreased absorption

NURSING CONSIDERATIONS
Assessment
• **Weight status:** before starting therapy, obtain testing to rule out physiologic reactions for weight; obtain thyroid testing, BMI, glucose
• Monitor weight weekly, diabetic patients may need reduction in oral hypoglycemics

---

• Assess for misuse in certain populations (anorexia nervosa, bulimia)
• **Hepatotoxicity/pancreatitis:** assess for liver injury: jaundice, weakness, abdominal pain (rare)

Patient/family education
• Advise patient that 60 mg cap can be obtained OTC; 60 mg tid is the highest OTC dose
• Warn patient that safety and effectiveness beyond 2 yr have not been determined
• Instruct patient to read patient's information sheet, discuss unpleasant GI side effects
• Advise patient to avoid hazardous activities until stabilized on medication
• Instruct patient to take a multivitamin containing fat-soluble vitamins, take 2 hr before or after orlistat; psyllium taken with each dose or at bedtime may decrease GI symptoms
• Instruct patient/family to notify prescriber if significant side effects occur
⚠ Advise prescriber if pregnancy is planned or suspected; pregnancy (X), if breastfeeding, take proper fat-soluble vitamins
• **Hepatotoxicity/pancreatitis:** advise patient to report yellowing skin/eyes, dark urine, weakness, abdominal pain

Evaluation
Positive therapeutic outcome
• Decreased weight

---

oseltamivir (Rx)
(oh-sell-tam'ih-ver)
Tamiflu
Func. class.: Antiviral
Chem. class.: Neuramidase inhibitor
Pregnancy category C

ACTION: Inhibits influenza virus neuraminidase with possible alteration of virus particle aggregation and release

Therapeutic outcome: Decreased symptoms of influenza type A

USES: Prevention/treatment of influenza type A or B

Unlabeled uses: Avian influenzae (H5N1), swine flu (H1N1), encephalitis

CONTRAINDICATIONS:
Hypersensitivity

Precautions: Pregnancy **C**, geriatric, renal/hepatic/pulmonary/cardiac disease, infants,

children, neonates, psychosis, viral infection, breastfeeding

DOSAGE AND ROUTES
Treatment
Adult and child >40 kg: PO 75 bid mg × 5 days, begin treatment within 2 days of onset of symptoms
Child 23-40 kg and ≥1 yr: PO 60 mg bid
Child 15-23 kg and ≥1 yr: PO 45 mg bid
Child ≤15 kg and ≥1 yr: PO 30 mg bid

Prevention
Adult and child ≥13 yr: PO 75 mg/day × ≥7 days; begin treatment within 2 days of contact, max use 6 wk

Renal dose
Adult: PO CCr 10-30 ml/min 75 mg/day × 5 days (treatment); 75 mg every other day or 30 mg/day (prophylaxis)

H1N1 influenzae A virus (unlabeled)
Adult/adolescent/child >40 kg: PO 75 mg bid × 5 days
Child/adolescent 24-40 kg: PO 60 mg bid × 5 days
Child >1 yr and 15-23 kg: PO 45 mg bid × 5 days
Child >1 yr and <15 kg: PO 30 mg bid × 5 days

Available forms: Caps 30, 45, 75 mg; powder for oral susp 6 mg/ml

Implementation
• Give within 2 days of symptoms of influenza; continue for 5 days
• Give at least 4 hr before bedtime to prevent insomnia
• 12 mg/ml concentration will be available for a limited time, new product is 6 mg/ml concentration, take care to give correct dose
• Give without regard to food, give with food for GI upset, take with full glass of water
• **Oral susp:** loosen powder from side of bottle 55 ml shake well (6 mg/ml); remove child-resistant cap and push bottle adapter into neck of bottle, close tightly with child-resistant cap to ensure sealing; use within 17 days of preparation when refrigerated or 10 days at room temperature, write expiration date on bottle, shake well before use, use oral syringe provided but only with markings for 30, 45, 60 mg, confirm dosing instructions are in same units as syringe provided
• Store in airtight, dry container

Adverse effects: *italics* = common; **bold** = life-threatening

ADVERSE EFFECTS

CNS: Headache, fatigue, insomnia, dizziness, delirium, **self-injury (children)**
ENDO: Hyperglycemia
GI: *Nausea, vomiting,* diarrhea, abdominal pain
INTEG: Toxic epidermal necrolysis, Stevens-Johnson syndrome, erythema multiforme
RESP: Cough

Pharmacokinetics

Absorption	Rapidly absorbed
Distribution	Protein binding 3%
Metabolism	Converted to oseltamivir carboxylate (active form)
Excretion	Eliminated by conversion, urine 99%
Half-life	1-3 hr (active form)

Pharmacodynamics

Unknown

INTERACTIONS

Avoid use with H1N1 virus vaccine, intranasal influenza vaccine

NURSING CONSIDERATIONS

Assessment

• **Influenza:** assess for symptoms of influenza A: increased temperature, malaise, aches and pains

Patient/family education

• Teach patient about aspects of product therapy
• Teach patient to avoid hazardous activities if dizziness occurs
• Advise patient to take as soon as symptoms appear, to take full course, even if feeling better
• Advise patient to take missed dose as soon as remembered if within 2 hr of next dose
• Teach patient to stop product immediately and report to prescriber skin rash, delirium, psychosis, hallucinations (child)
• Advise patient that product is not a substitute for a flu shot
• Inform patient to avoid other products without approval of prescriber

Evaluation

Positive therapeutic outcome

• Absence of fever, malaise, cough, dyspnea in influenza A

⚠ HIGH ALERT

oxaliplatin (Rx)

(ox-al-i′plat-in)
Eloxitin
Func. class.: Antineoplastic
Chem. class.: 3rd generation platinum analog
Pregnancy category D

ACTION: Forms cross links, inhibiting DNA replication and transcription, cell-cycle nonspecific

Therapeutic outcome: Decreased size of tumor, spread of malignancy

USES: Metastatic carcinoma of the colon or rectum in combination with 5-FU/leucovorin

Unlabeled uses: Relapsed or refractory non-Hodgkin's lymphoma, advanced ovarian cancer

CONTRAINDICATIONS:

Pregnancy **D**, breastfeeding, radiation therapy or chemotherapy within 1 mo, thrombocytopenia, smallpox vaccination

> **BLACK BOX WARNING:** Hypersensitivity to this product or other platinum products

Precautions: Children, geriatric, pneumococcus vaccination, renal disease

DOSAGE AND ROUTES

Colorectal cancer

Dosage protocols may vary
Adult: IV INF *Day 1:* oxaliplatin 85 mg/m^2 in 250-500 ml D$_5$W and leucovorin 200 mg/m^2 in D$_5$W, give both over 2 hr at the same time in separate bags using a Y-line, followed by 5-FU 400 mg/m^2 **IV** BOL over 2-4 min, then 5-FU 600 mg/m^2 **IV** INF in 500 ml D$_5$W as a 22-hr CONT INF; *Day 2:* leucovorin 200 mg/m^2 **IV** INF over 2 hr, then 5-FU 400 mg/m^2 **IV** BOL over 2-4 min, then 5-FU 600 mg/m^2 **IV** INF in 500 ml D$_5$W as a 22-hr CONT INF; repeat cycle q2wk

Renal dose

Adult: IV CCr <30 ml/min: reduce starting dose to 65 mg/m^2

Available forms: Powder for inj 50, 100 mg single-use vials (5 mg/ml); solution for inj 50 mg/10 ml, 100 mg/20 ml, 200 mg/40 ml

---

Implementation

Intermittent IV INF route

• Premedicate with antiemetics including 5-HT$_3$ blockers, with or without dexamethasone, prehydration is not needed

• Do not reconstitute or dilute with sodium chloride or any chloride-containing solutions, do not use aluminum equipment during any preparation or administration, will degrade platinum; do not refrigerate unopened powder or solution; do not freeze; protect from light

• Use cytotoxic handling procedures; prepare in biological cabinet using gown, gloves, mask; do not allow product to come in contact with skin; use soap and water if contact occurs

• EPINEPHrine, antihistamines, corticosteroids for hypersensitivity reaction

• **Lyophilized powder:** reconstitute vial 50 mg/10 ml, or 100 mg/20 ml sterile water for inj or D$_5$W, after reconstitution, solution may be stored for ≤24 hr in refrigerator, after dilution in 250-500 ml D$_5$W, may store ≤24 hr in refrigerator or 6 hr at room temp, infuse over 2 hr

• **Aqueous solution:** dilute in 250-500 ml of D$_5$W, after dilution may store ≤24 hr refrigerator, 6 hr at room temp, infuse over 2 hr

Y-site compatibilities: Alfentanil, amifostine, amikacin, aminocaproic acid, amiodarone, amphotericin B colloidal, amphotericin B lipid complex, amphotericin B liposome, ampicillin, ampicillin-sulbactam, anidulafungin, atenolol, atracurium, azithromycin, aztreonam, bivalirudin, bleomycin, bumetanide, buprenorphine, butorphanol, calcium chloride/gluconate, CARBOplatin, caspofungin, ceFAZolin, cefotaxime, cefoTEtan, cefOXitin, cefTAZidime, ceftizoxime, cefTRIAXone, cefuroxime, chloramphenicol, chlorproMAZINE, cimetidine, ciprofloxacin, cisatracurium, CISplatin, clindamycin, cyclophosphamide, cycloSPORINE, cytarabine, dacarbazine, DACTINomycin, DAPTOmycin, DAUNOrubicin, dexamethasone, digoxin, diltiazem, diphenhydrAMINE, DOBUTamine, DOCEtaxel, dolasetron, DOPamine, doxacurium, DOXOrubicin, doxycycline, droperidol, enalaprilat, ePHEDrine, EPINEPHrine, epirubicin, ertapenem, erythromycin, esmolol, etoposide, famotidine, fenoldopam, fentaNYL, fluconazole, fludarabine, foscarnet, fosphenytoin, furosemide, gatifloxacin, gemcitabine, gemtuzumab, gentamicin, glycopyrrolate, granisetron, haloperidol, heparin, hydrALAZINE, hydrocortisone, HYDROmorphone, hydrOXYzine, IDArubicin, ifosfamide, imipenem-cilastatin, inamrinone, insulin (regular), irinotecan, isoproterenol, ketorolac, labetalol, leucovorin, levofloxacin, levorphanol, lidocaine, linezolid, LORazepam, magnesium sulfate, mannitol, meperidine, meropenem, mesna, metaraminol, methyldopate, methylPREDNISolone, metoclopramide, metoprolol, metroNIDAZOLE, midazolam, milrinone, minocycline, mitoMYcin, mitoXANtrone, mivacurium, morphine, nafcillin, nalbuphine, naloxone, nesiritide, niCARdipine, nitroglycerin, nitroprusside, norepinephrine, octreotide, ondansetron, PACLitaxel, palonosetron, pancuronium, PEMEtrexed, pentamidine, pentazocine, phenylephrine, piperacillin, polymyxin B, potassium chloride/phosphates, procainamide, prochlorperazine, promethazine, propranolol, quiNIDine, quinupristin-dalfopristin, ranitidine, rocuronium, sodium acetate/phosphates, succinylcholine, SUFentanil, sulfamethoxazole-trimethoprim, tacrolimus, teniposide, theophylline, thiotepa, ticarcillin, ticarcillin-clavulanate, tigecycline, tirofiban, tobramycin, tolazoline, topotecan, trimethobenzamide, vancomycin, vasopressin, vecuronium, verapamil, vinBLAStine, vinCRIStine, vinorelbine, voriconazole, zidovudine, zoledronic acid

ADVERSE EFFECTS

CNS: Peripheral neuropathy, fatigue, headache, dizziness, insomnia
CV: Cardiac abnormalities, **thromboembolism**
EENT: *Decreased visual acuity, tinnitus, hearing loss*
GI: *Severe nausea, vomiting, diarrhea, weight loss,* stomatitis, anorexia, gastroesophageal reflux, constipation, dyspepsia, mucositis, flatulence
GU: Hematuria, dysuria, creatinine
HEMA: Thrombocytopenia, leukopenia, pancytopenia, neutropenia, anemia, hemolytic uremic syndrome
INTEG: *Alopecia,* rash, flushing, extravasation, redness, swelling, pain at inj site
META: Hypokalemia
RESP: Fibrosis, dyspnea, cough, rhinitis, URI, pharyngitis
SYST: Anaphylaxis, angioedema

Pharmacokinetics

Absorption	Unknown
Distribution	15% of platinum in systemic circulation; 85% is either in tissues or being eliminated in urine
Metabolism	Liver
Excretion	Urine
Half-life	40 days

Adverse effects: *italics* = common; **bold** = life-threatening

Pharmacodynamics
Unknown

INTERACTIONS
Individual drugs
Alcohol, aspirin: increased risk of bleeding
Radiation: increased myelosuppression

Drug classifications
Aminoglycosides, diuretics (loop): increased nephrotoxicity
Anticoagulants, NSAIDs, platelet inhibitors, thrombolytics, salicylates: increased risk of bleeding
Live virus vaccines: decreased antibody response
Myelosuppressives: increased myelosuppression
Tannins: increased oxaliplatin toxicity

Drug/lab test
Increased: ALT, AST, bilirubin, creatinine
Decreased: potassium, neutrophils, WBC, platelets

NURSING CONSIDERATIONS
Assessment
• **Bone marrow depression:** monitor CBC, differential, platelet count weekly; withhold product if WBC is <4000 or platelet count is <100,000; notify prescriber of results
• Monitor renal function tests: BUN, creatinine, serum uric acid, urine CCr before, electrolytes during therapy; dose should not be given if BUN >19 mg/dl; creatinine <1.5 mg/dl; I&O ratio; report fall in urine output of <30 ml/hr

> **BLACK BOX WARNING: Assess for anaphylaxis:** wheezing, tachycardia, facial swelling, fainting; discontinue product and report to prescriber; resuscitation equipment should be nearby

• Monitor temp (may indicate beginning infection)
• Monitor liver function tests before, during therapy (bilirubin, AST, ALT, LDH) as needed or monthly
• **Assess for bleeding:** hematuria, guaiac, bruising or petechiae, mucosa or orifices q8hr; obtain prescription for viscous lidocaine (Xylocaine)
• Assess effects of alopecia on body image; discuss feelings about body changes
• Assess for jaundice of skin, sclera; dark urine; clay-colored stools; itchy skin; abdominal pain; fever; diarrhea
• Assess for edema in feet, joint pain, stomach pain, shaking

• **Pulmonary fibrosis:** assess for cough, crackles, dyspnea, pulmonary infiltrate; discontinue immediately; may be fatal

Patient/family education
• **Advise patient to report signs of infection:** increased temp, sore throat, flulike symptoms
• **Advise patient to report signs of anemia:** fatigue, headache, faintness, shortness of breath, irritability
• **Advise patient to report bleeding;** avoid use of razors, commercial mouthwash
• Advise patient to avoid aspirin, ibuprofen, NSAIDs, alcohol; may cause GI bleeding
• Advise patient to report any changes in breathing, coughing
• Advise patient that hair may be lost during treatment; a wig or hairpiece may make patient feel better; new hair may be different in color, texture
• Advise patient to report numbness, tingling in face or extremities, poor hearing or joint pain, swelling
• Advise patient not to receive vaccines during treatment
• Advise patient to use contraception during treatment and 4 mo after; this product may cause infertility, pregnancy **D**
• Teach patient to avoid contact with cold (air, ice, liquid); causes acute dysesthesias

Evaluation
Positive therapeutic outcome
• Decreased tumor size, spread of malignancy

---

oxazepam (Rx)
(ox-az′e-pam)
Func. class.: Sedative-hypnotic; antianxiety
Chem. class.: Benzodiazepine, short-acting
Pregnancy category D
Controlled substance schedule IV

ACTION: Depresses subcortical levels of CNS, including limbic system, reticular formation; potentiates GABA

Therapeutic outcome: Decreased anxiety, successful alcohol withdrawal, relaxation

USES: Anxiety, alcohol withdrawal
Unlabeled uses: Insomnia

CONTRAINDICATIONS:

Pregnancy **D**, breastfeeding, children <6 yr, hypersensitivity to benzodiazepines, closed-angle glaucoma, psychosis

Precautions: Geriatric, debilitated, renal/hepatic disease, depression, suicidal ideation, dementia, sleep apnea, seizure disorder, respiratory depression

DOSAGE AND ROUTES
Anxiety
Adult: PO 15-30 mg tid-qid, max 120 mg/day
Geriatric: PO 10 mg daily bid-tid, max 60 mg/day

Alcohol withdrawal
Adult: PO 15-30 mg tid-qid

Available forms: Caps 10, 15, 30 mg

Implementation
• Give with food or milk for GI symptoms; tab may be crushed if patient is unable to swallow medication whole

ADVERSE EFFECTS

CNS: *Dizziness, drowsiness,* confusion, headache, anxiety, tremors, fatigue, depression, insomnia, hallucinations, paradoxical excitement, transient amnesia
CV: *Orthostatic hypotension,* **ECG changes, tachycardia,** hypotension
EENT: *Blurred vision,* tinnitus, mydriasis
GI: Nausea, vomiting, anorexia
HEMA: Leukopenia
INTEG: Rash, dermatitis, itching
SYST: Dependence

Pharmacokinetics

Absorption	Well absorbed
Distribution	Widely distributed; crosses placenta, blood-brain barrier
Metabolism	Liver
Excretion	Kidneys, breast milk
Half-life	5-15 hr

Pharmacodynamics

Onset	½-1½ hr
Peak	Unknown
Duration	6-12 hr

INTERACTIONS
Individual drugs
Alcohol: increased CNS depression
Disulfiram: increased oxazepam effects

Levodopa: decreased effects of levodopa
Phenytoin, theophylline, valproic acid: decreased oxazepam effects

Drug classifications
CNS depressants: increased oxazepam effects
Oral contraceptives: increased or decreased oxazepam effect

Drug/herb
Kava, melatonin, valerian: increased CNS depression

Drug/lab test
Increased: AST, ALT, serum bilirubin
Decreased: WBC

NURSING CONSIDERATIONS
Assessment
• Assess mental status: mood, sensorium, anxiety, affect, sleeping pattern, drowsiness, dizziness, **suicidal thoughts, behavior; physical dependency, withdrawal symptoms:** anxiety, panic attacks, agitation, seizures, headache, nausea, vomiting, muscle pain, weakness; suicidal thoughts, behavior; indications of increasing tolerance and abuse
• Monitor B/P with patient lying, standing; pulse; if systolic B/P drops 20 mm Hg, hold product, notify prescriber

Patient/family education
• Teach patient that product may be taken without regard to food or fluids; tab may be crushed or swallowed whole
• Caution patient not to use for everyday stress or longer than 4 mo unless directed by prescriber; not to take more than prescribed amount; not to double doses or skip doses
• Advise patient to avoid OTC preparations unless approved by prescriber; alcohol and CNS depressants will increase CNS depression
• Caution patient to avoid driving and activities that require alertness, since drowsiness may occur; to avoid alcohol and other psychotropic medications; to rise slowly or fainting may occur, especially geriatric; that drowsiness may worsen at beginning of treatment
• Caution patient not to discontinue medication abruptly after long-term use; withdrawal symptoms include vomiting, cramping, tremors, seizures
• Advise patient to use sugarless gum, hard candy, frequent sips of water for dry mouth
• Teach patient that drowsiness may worsen at beginning of treatment
⚠ Teach patient to notify prescriber if pregnancy is planned or suspected, pregnancy (D)

Adverse effects: *italics* = common; **bold** = life-threatening

Evaluation
Positive therapeutic outcome
• Decreased anxiety, restlessness, sleeplessness (short-term treatment only)

TREATMENT OF OVERDOSE:
Lavage, VS, supportive care

OXcarbazepine (Rx)
(ox′kar-baz′uh-peen)
Oxtellar XR, Trileptal
Func. class.: Anticonvulsant
Pregnancy category C

ACTION: May inhibit nerve impulses by limiting influx of sodium ions across cell membrane in motor cortex

Therapeutic outcome: Absence of seizures

USES: Partial seizures

Unlabeled uses: Trigeminal neuralgia, atypical panic disorder, bipolar disorder

CONTRAINDICATIONS:
Hypersensitivity

Precautions: Pregnancy **C**, breastfeeding, children <4 yr, hypersensitivity to carbamazepine, renal disease, fluid restriction, hyponatremia, abrupt discontinuation, suicidal ideation

DOSAGE AND ROUTES
Seizures adjunctive therapy
Adult: PO 300 mg bid, may be increased by 600 mg/day in divided doses bid at weekly intervals; maintenance 1200 mg/day; ext rel 600 mg/day × 1 wk, increase weekly in 600 mg/day increments to 1200-2400 mg/day
Child 4-16 yr: PO 8-10 mg/kg/day divided bid, dose is determined by weight, increase by 5 mg/kg/day q3 days, max doses are weight dependent

Conversion to monotherapy in partial seizures
Adult: PO 300 mg bid with reduction in other anticonvulsants, increase OXcarbazepine by 600 mg/day qwk over 2-4 wk; withdraw other anticonvulsants over 3-6 wk, max 2400 mg/day

Initiation of monotherapy in partial seizures
Adult: PO 300 mg bid, increase by 300 mg/day q3day to 1200 mg divided bid, max 2400 mg/day

Renal dose
Adult: PO CCr <30 ml/min 150 mg bid and increase slowly

Available forms: Film-coated tabs 150, 300, 600 mg; oral susp 300 mg/5 ml; ext rel tab 150, 300, 600 mg

Implementation
• Store product at room temperature
• Provide assistance with ambulation during early part of treatment; dizziness may occur
• Give product with food, milk to decrease GI symptoms
• **Oral susp:** shake well, use calibrated oral syringe provided, use or discard within 7 days of opening
• **Ext rel:** do not crush, break, or chew

ADVERSE EFFECTS
CNS: *Headache, dizziness, confusion, fatigue,* feeling abnormal, ataxia, abnormal gait, tremors, anxiety, agitation, **worsening of seizures, suicidal ideation/behavior**
CV: *Hypotension,* chest pain, edema, bradycardia, syncope
EENT: *Blurred vision, diplopia, nystagmus,* rhinitis, sinusitis
ENDO: Hypothyroidism, hot flashes
GI: *Nausea, constipation, diarrhea,* anorexia, vomiting, abdominal pain, gastritis
GU: Urinary frequency, hematuria, menses change
INTEG: Purpura, rash, acne
META: Hyponatremia
RESP: Flulike symptoms
SYST: Angioedema, anaphylaxis, Stevens-Johnson syndrome, toxic epidermal necrolysis, drug reaction with eosinophilia and systemic symptoms (DRESS)

Pharmacokinetics
Absorption	Unknown
Distribution	Unknown
Metabolism	Liver; 95% renal extraction
Excretion	Unknown
Half-life	Unknown

Pharmacodynamics
Onset	Unknown
Peak	4-6 hr
Duration	Unknown

INTERACTIONS
Individual products
Alcohol: increased CNS depression
CarBAMazepine: decreased carBAMazepine level, decreased OXcarbazepine levels
Felodipine: decreased effects of felodipine
Nisoldipine, ranolazine: do not use concurrently
PHENobarbital, valproic acid, verapamil: decreased OXcarbazepine level
Phenytoin: decreased OXcarbazepine level

Drug classifications
Contraceptives (oral): decreased oral contraceptive level
MAOIs: do not use concurrently

Drug/herb
Ginkgo: increased anticonvulsant effect
Ginseng, santonica: decreased anticonvulsant effect

Drug/lab test
Decreased: sodium

NURSING CONSIDERATIONS
Assessment
• **Assess seizure activity,** including frequency, duration, and aura; provide seizure precautions
• Assess mental status including mood, sensorium, affect, behavioral changes, suicidal thoughts, behavior; if mental status changes, notify prescriber; usually occurs within the first 3 mo of treatment, but may occur ≤1 yr; if this product is being used with other products that decrease sodium, monitor sodium levels
• Assess eye problems: ophthalmic examinations (slit lamp, funduscopy, tonometry) are needed before, during, after treatment
• Assess patient for hypersensitivity to carBAMazepine
• **Assess for serious skin reactions:** angioedema, anaphylaxis, Stevens-Johnson syndrome
• **Pregnancy:** lack of seizure control due to MHD, a metabolite of OXcarbazepine; monitor seizure control
• May monitor target serum level 12-30 mcg/ml to identify compliance/toxicity

Patient/family education
• Caution patient to avoid driving, other activities that require alertness
• Instruct patient to take twice a day at same intervals
• Advise patient not to discontinue medication quickly after long-term use, seizures may increase
• Instruct patient to avoid use of alcohol while taking this medication
• Instruct patient to use alternative contraception if using hormonal method, to report if pregnancy is planned or suspected, pregnancy (**C**)
⚠ **Teach patient to report skin rashes immediately; serious skin reactions can occur**
• Instruct patient to inform prescriber if allergic to carBAMazepine; multisystem hypersensitivity may occur, to report fever, other allergic symptoms
⚠ **Instruct patient to report suicidal thoughts/behavior immediately**

Evaluation
Positive therapeutic outcome
• Decreased seizure activity

TREATMENT OF OVERDOSE:
Activated charcoal, give 0.9% NaCl (hypotensive state), atropine (bradycardia); use benzodiazepines, barbiturates for seizures

oxybutynin (Rx, OTC)
(ox-i-byoo′ti-nin)
Ditropan, Ditropan XL, Gelnique, Oxytrol ✷, Oxytrol Transdermal, Uromax ✷
Func. class.: Anticholinergic
Chem. class.: Synthetic tertiary amine
Pregnancy category B

Do not confuse:
Ditropan/diazepam

ACTION: Relaxes smooth muscles in urinary tract by inhibiting acetylcholine at postganglionic sites

Therapeutic outcome: Decreased symptoms of urgency, nocturia, incontinence

USES: Antispasmodic for neurogenic bladder, overactive bladder in females (OTC)

CONTRAINDICATIONS:
Hypersensitivity, GI obstruction, urinary retention, glaucoma, severe colitis, myasthenia gravis, unstable CV, infants

Precautions: Pregnancy **B**, breastfeeding, children <12 yr, geriatric, suspected glaucoma, cardiac disease, dementia

Adverse effects: *italics* = common; **bold** = life-threatening

DOSAGE AND ROUTES

Adult: PO 5 mg bid-tid, max 5 mg qid; ext rel tabs 5-10 mg/day, may increase by 5 mg, max 30 mg/day; transdermal apply one patch to abdomen, hip, buttock 2 ×/wk (q3-4day); GEL apply contents of 1 packet to abdomen, upper arms, shoulders, thighs daily

Geriatric: PO 2.5-5 mg bid-tid, increase by 2.5 mg q several days

Child ≥6 yr: PO 5 mg bid, not to exceed 5 mg tid; ext rel 5 mg/day, max 20 mg/day

Child 1-5 yr: PO 0.2 mg/kg/dose 2-3 ×/day

Available forms: Syr 5 mg/5 ml; tabs 5 mg; ext rel tabs 5, 10, 15 mg; transdermal 3.9 mg/day; top gel 10% (Gelnique)

Implementation

PO route

- Do not break, crush, or chew ext rel tabs
- May be given with meals or fluids or on an empty stomach

Topical route

- Wash hands, apply to clean, dry, intact skin on abdomen, upper arms/shoulders, thighs, avoid navel, rotate sites
- Squeeze contents in palm of hand or directly on this site, rub gently
- Do not bathe, exercise, swim for 1 hr after application
- Allow to dry before putting on clothing
- Do not be near flame, fire, or smoke until gel has dried
- Delivers 100 mg

Transdermal route

- Apply to clean, dry, intact skin on the abdomen, hip, buttock, use firm pressure, not affected by showering/bathing; rotate sites
- Delivers 3.9 mg/day

ADVERSE EFFECTS

CNS: *Anxiety, restlessness, dizziness,* somnolence, insomnia, nervousness, **seizures,** headache, drowsiness, confusion

CV: *Palpitations, sinus tachycardia,* hypertension, peripheral edema, **QT prolongation**

EENT: Blurred vision, increased intraocular tension; dry mouth, throat, dry eyes

GI: *Nausea, vomiting, anorexia,* abdominal pain, constipation, *dyspepsia,* diarrhea, taste perversion, GERD

GU: Dysuria, impotence, retention, hesitancy

MISC: **Hyperthermia, anaphylaxis, angioedema**

Pharmacokinetics

Absorption	Rapidly absorbed
Distribution	Unknown
Metabolism	Liver
Excretion	Unknown
Half-life	Unknown

Pharmacodynamics

Onset	½-1 hr
Peak	3-4 hr
Duration	6-10 hr

INTERACTIONS

Individual drugs

Acetaminophen: decreased levels of acetaminophen

Amantadine: increased anticholinergic effects

Atenolol: increased levels of atenolol

Digoxin: increased levels of digoxin

Haloperidol, chloroquine, droperidol, pentamidine, arsenic trioxide, levomethadyl: increased QT prolongation

Levodopa: decreased levels of levodopa

Nitrofurantoin: increased levels of nitrofurantoin

Drug classifications

Antihistamines, other anticholinergics: increased anticholinergic effects

Benzodiazepines, sedatives, hypnotics, opioids: increased CNS depression

Class IA/III antidysrhythmics, some phenothiazines, β-agonists, local anesthetics, tricyclics, CYP3A4 inhibitors (amiodarone, clarithromycin, erythromycin, telithromycin, troleandomycin), CYP3A4 substrates (methadone, pimozide, QUEtiapine, quiNIDine, risperiDONE, ziprasidone): increased QT prolongation

NURSING CONSIDERATIONS

Assessment

- **Assess for allergic reactions:** rash, urticaria; if these occur, product should be discontinued
- **Assess urinary patterns:** distention, nocturia, frequency, urgency, incontinence; catheterization may be required to remove residual urine; urinary tract infections should be treated
- **QT prolongation:** assess ECG for QT prolongation, ejection fraction; assess for chest pain, palpitations, dyspnea

Patient/family education

- Advise patient to avoid hazardous activities until response to product is known; dizziness, blurred vision may occur

---

- Caution patient to avoid OTC medication with alcohol or other CNS depressants
- Teach patient to use frequent rinsing of mouth, sips of water for dry mouth
- Teach patient to stay cool; avoid hot weather, strenuous activity since overheating may occur; product decreases perspiration
- Advise patient to report CNS effects: confusion, anxiety, anticholinergic effect in the geriatric

Transdermal
- Instruct patient to change patch 2×/wk and not to use same site within 7 days
- Instruct patient to use container that is not accessible to pets/children and to dispose of container after use
- Instruct patient to open patch immediately before using
- Instruct patient to remove patch during MRI

Topical gel
- **Instruct patient to rotate sites**
- Instruct patient to apply to clean, dry skin on abdomen, upper arm/shoulders/thighs
- Teach patient that gel is flammable

Evaluation
Positive therapeutic outcome
- Absence of dysuria, frequency, nocturia, incontinence

> **⚠ HIGH ALERT**
>
> ## oxyCODONE (Rx)
> (ox-i-koe′done)
> **ETH-Oxydose, Oxecta, OxyCONTIN, OxyFast, Roxicodone, Supeudol ✦**
> ## oxyCODONE/acetaminophen (Rx)
> **Magnacet, Percocet, Primalev, Roxicet, Tylox, Xolox**
> ## oxyCODONE/aspirin (Rx)
> **Endodan ✦, Percodan**
> ## oxyCODONE/ibuprofen (Rx)
> *Func. class.:* Opiate analgesic
> *Chem. class.:* Semisynthetic derivative
> **Pregnancy category B**
> **Controlled substance schedule II**

Do not confuse:
oxyCODONE/HYDROcodone/OxyCONTIN, Percodan/Decadron, Roxicet/Roxanol, Roxicodone/Roxanol, Tylox/Trimox/Wymox/Xanax

ACTION: Inhibits ascending pain pathways in CNS, increases pain threshold, alters pain perception

Therapeutic outcome: Decreased pain

USES: Moderate to severe pain

Unlabeled uses: Postherpetic neuralgia (cont rel)

CONTRAINDICATIONS:
Hypersensitivity, addiction (opiate), asthma, ileus

> **BLACK BOX WARNING:** Respiratory depression

Precautions: Pregnancy **B**, breastfeeding, children <18 yr, addictive personality, increased ICP, MI (acute), severe heart disease, renal/hepatic disease, bowel impaction

> **BLACK BOX WARNING:** Opioid-naïve patients, substance abuse, accidental exposure, potential for overdose/poisoning, status asthmaticus

DOSAGE AND ROUTES
Adult: PO 10-30 mg q4hr (5-15 mg q4-6hr for opiate naive patients); **OxyFast CONC SOL is extremely concentrated, do not use interchangeably;** CONT REL 10 mg q12hr in opiate-naïve patients

Available forms: OxyCODONE: cont rel tabs (OxyCONTIN) 10, 15, 20, 30, 40, 80, 160 mg; immediate rel tabs 5, 7.5, 10, 15, 20, 30 mg; immediate rel caps 5 mg; oral sol 5 mg/5 ml, 20 mg/ml; oxyCODONE with acetaminophen: tabs 2.5 mg/300 mg, 2.5 mg/325 mg, 5 mg/300 mg, 5 mg/325 mg; 7.5 mg/325 mg, 7.5 mg/500 mg, 10 mg/325 mg, 10 mg/400 mg, 10 mg/650 mg; caps 5 mg/500 mg; oral sol 5 mg/325 mg/5 ml; oxyCODONE with aspirin: 4.88 mg/325 mg oxyCODONE with ibuprofen: 5 mg/400 mg

Implementation
- OxyCODONE should be titrated from the initial recommended dosage to the dose required to relieve pain
- There is no maximum dose of oxyCODONE; however, careful titration is required until tolerance develops to some of the side effects (drowsiness and respiratory depression)
- Store in light-resistant area at room temp

Immediate-release tablets
- May be administered with food or milk to minimize GI irritation

---

Adverse effects: *italics* = common; **bold** = life-threatening

• Oxecta brand tablets: Swallow whole; do not crush or dissolve. Due to the nature of this formulation do not pre-soak, lick, or otherwise wet tablet prior to dose administration. Administer 1 tablet at a time; allow patient to swallow each tablet separately with sufficient liquid to ensure prompt and complete transit through the esophagus. Do not use this brand for administration via nasogastric, gastric, or other feeding tubes as it may cause obstruction of feeding tubes

Controlled-release tablets (OxyCONTIN)

• Administer whole; do not crush, chew, or break in half. Taking chewed, broken, or crushed controlled-release tabs could lead to the rapid release and absorption of a potentially toxic dose of oxyCODONE

• OxyCONTIN brand tablets: Due to hydro-gelling nature of the 2010 reformulation, do not pre-soak, lick, or otherwise wet tab prior to dose administration. Administer 1 tab at a time; allow patient to swallow each tab separately with sufficient liquid to ensure prompt and complete transit through the esophagus

• OxyCODONE controlled-release (OxyCONTIN) 60 mg and 80 mg tablets are for use ONLY in opioid-tolerant patients

• May be administered with or without food

Oral concentrate solution route

• As OxyFast is a highly concentrated solution (20 mg oxyCODONE/ml), care should be taken in dispensing and administering this medication. For ease of administration, the solution may be added to 30 ml of a liquid or semisolid food. If the medication is placed in liquid or food, the patient needs to consume immediately; do not store diluted oxyCODONE for future use

PO route

• Do not break, crush, or chew cont rel tabs; give q12hr, no more frequently

• May be given with food or milk to lessen GI upset

• Use 80, 160 mg cont rel tabs (oxyCONTIN) only in opioid-tolerant patients

ADVERSE EFFECTS

CNS: *Drowsiness, dizziness, confusion, headache, sedation, euphoria,* fatigue, abnormal dreams, thoughts, hallucinations
CV: Palpitations, bradycardia, change in B/P
EENT: Tinnitus, blurred vision, miosis, diplopia
GI: *Nausea, vomiting, anorexia, constipation, cramps,* gastritis, dyspepsia, biliary spasms
GU: Increased urinary output, dysuria, urinary retention

INTEG: *Rash,* urticaria, bruising, flushing, diaphoresis, pruritus
RESP: Respiratory depression

Pharmacokinetics

Absorption	Well absorbed
Distribution	Widely distributed; crosses placenta, protein binding 45%
Metabolism	Liver, extensively
Excretion	Kidneys, breast milk
Half-life	3-5 hr

Pharmacodynamics

	PO	RECT
Onset	15-30 min	Unknown
Peak	½-1 hr	Unknown
Duration	Reg rel 2-6 hr, cont rel 12 hr	4-6 hr

INTERACTIONS
Individual drugs
Alcohol: increased respiratory depression, hypotension, sedation
Cimetidine: increased toxicity

Drug classifications
Antipsychotics, CNS depressants, opioids, sedative/hypnotics, skeletal muscle relaxants: increased respiratory depression, hypotension
CYP3A4 inhibitors: increased oxyCODONE level
MAOIs: increased toxicity

Drug/herb
St. John's wort, valerian: increased sedative effect

Drug/lab test
Increased: amylase, lipase

NURSING CONSIDERATIONS
Assessment
• **Pain:** assess intensity, location, type, characteristics; need for pain medication by pain/sedation scoring; physical dependence
• Monitor I&O ratio; check for decreasing output; may indicate urinary retention
• **CNS changes:** assess for dizziness, drowsiness, hallucinations, euphoria, LOC, pupil reaction
• **Allergic reactions:** assess for rash, urticaria

> **BLACK BOX WARNING: Respiratory dysfunction:** assess for respiratory depression, character, rate, rhythm; notify prescriber if respirations are <10/min; also B/P, pulse

• **Bowel status:** assess for constipation; stimulate laxative may be needed with fluids, fiber
• Monitor VS after parenteral route; note muscle rigidity, product history, renal, liver function tests, respiratory dysfunction: respiratory depression, character, rate, rhythm; notify prescriber if respirations are <10/min

BLACK BOX WARNING: **Substance abuse:** assess for substance abuse in patient/family/friends before prescribing; monitor for abuse

BLACK BOX WARNING: **Accidental exposure:** dispose of properly away from pets, children

Patient/family education
• Advise patients to avoid CNS depressants: alcohol, sedative/hypnotics
• Discuss with patient that dizziness, drowsiness, and confusion are common; to avoid getting up without assistance
• Discuss in detail all aspects of the product, including purpose and what to expect
• Advise patient to make position changes slowly to lessen orthostatic hypotension
• Advise patient to avoid CNS depressants, alcohol
• Advise patient to avoid operating machinery, driving if drowsiness occurs
• Teach patient that withdrawal symptoms may occur after long-term use: nausea, vomiting, cramps, fever, faintness, anorexia

Evaluation
Positive therapeutic outcome
• Decreased pain

TREATMENT OF OVERDOSE:
Naloxone 0.2-0.8 **IV**, O$_2$, **IV** fluids, vasopressors; caution with patients physically dependent on opioids

oxymetazoline nasal agent
See Appendix B

oxymetazoline ophthalmic
See Appendix B

⚠ **HIGH ALERT**

oxymorphone (Rx)
(ox-i-mor'fone)
Opana, Opana ER
Func. class.: Opiate analgesic
Chem. class.: Semisynthetic phenanthrene derivative
Pregnancy category B
Controlled substance schedule II

Do not confuse:
oxymorphone/oxyCODONE

ACTION: Depresses pain impulse transmission at the spinal cord level by interacting with opioid receptors, increases pain threshold, alters pain perception

Therapeutic outcome: Decreased pain

USES: Moderate to severe pain

CONTRAINDICATIONS:
Hypersensitivity, addiction (opioid), asthma, hepatic disease, ileus, intrathecal use, surgery

BLACK BOX WARNING: Respiratory depression

Precautions: Pregnancy **B** (short-term), breastfeeding, children <18 yr, addictive personality, increased ICP, MI (acute), severe heart disease, respiratory depression, renal/hepatic disease, bowel impaction

BLACK BOX WARNING: Alcoholism, opioid-naïve patients, substance abuse

DOSAGE AND ROUTES
Adult: IM/SUBCUT 1-1.5 mg q4-6hr prn; **IV** 0.5 mg q4-6hr prn; PO (immediate release only) 5-20 mg q4-6hr prn; PO-ER 5 mg q12hr in those requiring around the clock dosing

Labor analgesia
Adult: IM 0.5-1 mg

Available forms: Inj 1, 1.5 mg/ml; supp 5 mg; ER tab 5, 10, 20, 40 mg; ER tab, crush resistant 5, 10, 20, 30, 40 mg; tabs 5, 10 mg

Implementation
• Give 1 hr before or 2 hr after food (PO)
• Give with antiemetic if nausea, vomiting occur
• Do not break, crush, chew ER product
• Give when pain is beginning to return; determine dosage interval by patient response;

Adverse effects: *italics* = common; **bold** = life-threatening

continuous dosing of medication is more effective than when given prn
• Medication should be slowly withdrawn after long-term use to prevent withdrawal symptoms
• Store in light-resistant area at room temp

CONTROLLED REL
• **Opiate naive:** start with lowest dose, titrate upward in 5-10 mg q12hr q3-7days to therapeutic response
• When converting from immediate release to ext rel, give ½ daily dose of ER product q12hr

Direct IV route
• Give undiluted over 2-3 min

Syringe compatibilities: Glycopyrrolate, hydrOXYzine, ranitidine

ADVERSE EFFECTS

CNS: *Drowsiness, dizziness, confusion, headache, sedation, euphoria (geriatric),* **seizures,** hallucinations, **increased ICP**
CV: Palpitations, **bradycardia,** change in B/P, hypotension
EENT: Tinnitus, blurred vision, miosis, diplopia
GI: *Nausea, vomiting, anorexia, constipation, cramps*
GU: Dysuria, urinary retention
INTEG: *Rash,* urticaria, bruising, flushing, diaphoresis, pruritus
RESP: Respiratory depression

Pharmacokinetics

Absorption	Well absorbed (RECT, IM, SUBCUT); completely absorbed (**IV**)
Distribution	Widely distributed; crosses placenta
Metabolism	Liver, extensively
Excretion	Kidneys
Half-life	PO: 7-9 hr, ER: 9-11 hr

Pharmacodynamics

	IM/SUB-CUT	IV	RECT
Onset	15 min	10 min	30 min
Peak	1-1½ hr	15-30 min	Unknown
Duration	3-6 hr	3-4 hr	3-6 hr

INTERACTIONS

Individual drugs
Alcohol: increased respiratory depression, hypotension, sedation

Drug classifications
CNS depressants, opiates, antipsychotics, skeletal muscle relaxants, sedative/hypnotics: increased respiratory depression, hypotension
MAOIs: do not use 2 wk before oxymorphone; unpredictable effects

Drug/herb
Kava, St. John's wort, valerian: increased sedative effect

Drug/lab test
Increased: amylase

NURSING CONSIDERATIONS

Assessment
• **Pain:** assess location, intensity, type, other characteristics, before and 1 hr after (IM) IV 30 min; need for pain medication, physical dependence, give 25%-50% until there is pain reduction of 50% on pain rating scale, repeat dose may be given at time of peak, if previous dose does not control pain, and respiratory depression has not occurred; give short-acting opioids for breakthrough pain if on controlled rel product

BLACK BOX WARNING: Respiratory dysfunction: Assess for respiratory depression, character, rate, rhythm; notify prescriber if respirations are <10/min

BLACK BOX WARNING: Accidental exposure: Dispose of properly, away from children/pets

BLACK BOX WARNING: Overdose/poisoning: Avoid alcohol ingestion; do not crush, chew, snort, or inject tabs, high abuse potential

BLACK BOX WARNING: Opioid-naive patients: Ext rel tabs are not to be used immediately post-op (12-24 hr after surgery) in these patients

• **Assess bowel/bladder status:** constipation, may need stimulant laxative; I&O ratio for decreasing output, may indicate urinary retention
• Monitor VS after parenteral route; note muscle rigidity, product history, liver, kidney function tests
• Monitor CNS changes: dizziness, drowsiness, hallucinations, euphoria, LOC, pupil reaction
• Monitor allergic reactions: rash, urticaria

⚠ Nurse Alert   ✳ Key NCLEX® Drug

Patient/family education
- Advise patient not to use other CNS depressants: alcohol, sedative/hypnotics
- Discuss with patient that dizziness, drowsiness, and confusion are common; to avoid getting up without assistance
- Discuss in detail all aspects of the product, including purpose and what to expect
- Advise patient to make position changes slowly to lessen orthostatic hypotension
- Advise patient not to drive, operate machinery if drowsiness occurs

Evaluation
Positive therapeutic outcome
- Decreased pain

TREATMENT OF OVERDOSE:
Naloxone (Narcan) 0.2-0.8 mg **IV**, O$_2$, **IV** fluids, vasopressors (caution with patients physically dependent on opioids)

⚠ HIGH ALERT

oxytocin (Rx)
(ox-i-toe′sin)
Pitocin
Func. class.: Oxytocic hormone
Pregnancy category N/A

ACTION: Acts directly on myofibrils, producing uterine contraction; stimulates breast milk letdown, vasoactive antidiuretic effect

Therapeutic outcome: Stimulation of labor, control of bleeding; stimulation of milk letdown

USES: Stimulation, induction of labor; missed or incomplete abortion; postpartum bleeding

CONTRAINDICATIONS:
Hypersensitivity, serum toxemia, cephalopelvic disproportion, fetal distress, hypertonic uterus, prolapsed umbilical cord, active genital herpes

Precautions: Cervical/uterine surgery, uterine sepsis, primipara >35 yr, 1st/2nd stage of labor

BLACK BOX WARNING: Elective induction of labor

DOSAGE AND ROUTES
Labor induction
Adult: IV 1-2 milliunit/min, increase by 1-2 milliunit q15-60min until regular contractions occur, then decrease dosage

Postpartum hemorrhage
Adult: IV 10-40 units in 1000 ml nonhydrating diluent infused at 20-40 milliunit/min
Adult: IM 3-10 units after placenta delivery

Incomplete abortion
Adult: IV INF 10 units/500 ml D$_5$W or 0.9% NaCl run at 10-20 milliunit/min; max 30 units/12 hr

Fetal stress test
Adult: IV 0.5 milliunit/min; increase q20min until 3 contractions occur at 10 min

Available forms: Inj 10 units/ml

Implementation
IV route
- Use an inf pump; rotate sol for mixing; have magnesium sulfate available
Labor induction
- Give after diluting 10 units/1000 ml of 0.9% NS or D$_5$ NS run at 1-2 mU/min at 15-30 min intervals to begin normal labor; dilute 10-40 mU/min; titrate to control postpartum bleeding; dilute 10 units/500 ml sol; run 10 units-20 mU/ml; administer by only 1 route at a time; use inf pump; rotate inf to provide mixing; do not shake
Control of postpartum bleeding
- Dilute 10-40 units/1000 ml of sol; run at 10-20 mU/min; adjust rate as needed
- Have crash cart available on unit (magnesium sulfate at bedside)
Incomplete, inevitable, elective abortion
- Dilute 10 units/500 ml compatible IV solution

Y-site compatibilities: Heparin, hydrocortisone, insulin (regular), meperidine, morphine, potassium chloride, vit B/C, warfarin

ADVERSE EFFECTS
CNS: *Seizures, tetanic contractions*
CV: Hypo/hypertension, dysrhythmias, increased pulse, bradycardia, tachycardia, premature ventricular contractions
FETUS: Dysrhythmias, jaundice, hypoxia, **intracranial hemorrhage**
GI: Anorexia, nausea, vomiting, constipation
GU: **Abruptio placentae, decreased uterine blood flow**
HEMA: Increased hyperbilirubinemia
INTEG: Rash
RESP: *Asphyxia*
SYST: Water intoxication of mother

Adverse effects: *italics* = common; **bold** = life-threatening

Absorption	Well absorbed (nasal); completely absorbed (**IV**)
Distribution	Widely distributed (extra-cellular fluid)
Metabolism	Liver, rapidly
Excretion	Kidneys
Half-life	3-12 min

	Nasal	IV	IM
Onset	5 min	Rapid	3-7 min
Peak	Un-known	Un-known	Un-known
Duration	20 min	1 hr	1 hr

INTERACTIONS
Drug classifications
Vasopressors: increased hypertension

Drug/herb
Ephedra: hypertension

NURSING CONSIDERATIONS
Assessment
• Assess labor contractions: fetal heart tones, frequency, duration, intensity of contractions; if fetal heart tones increase or decrease significantly or if contractions are longer than 1 min, notify prescriber; turn patient on left side to increase oxygen to fetus

⚠ **Assess for water intoxication: confusion, anuria, drowsiness, headache; notify prescriber**

• Watch for fetal distress, acceleration, deceleration, fetal presentation, pelvic dimensions
• Monitor B/P, pulse, respiratory rate, rhythm, depth
• Monitor I&O ratio
• Provide an environment conducive to letdown reflex

Patient/family education
• Teach patient to report increased blood loss, abdominal cramps, increased temp or foul-smelling lochia
• Advise patient that contractions will be similar to menstrual cramps, gradually increasing in intensity

Evaluation
Positive therapeutic outcome
• Stimulation of milk letdown (nasal)
• Induction of labor
• Decreased postpartum bleeding

PACLitaxel (Rx)
(pa-kli-tax'el)
PACLitaxel protein-bound particles (Rx)
Abraxane
Func. class.: Antineoplastic—miscellaneous
Chem. class.: Taxane
Pregnancy category D

Do not confuse:
PACLitaxel/PARoxetine/Paxil

ACTION: Inhibits the reorganization of the microtubule network needed for interphase and mitotic cellular functions; also causes abnormal bundles of microtubules during cell cycle and multiple esters of microtubules during mitosis

Therapeutic outcome: Prevention of rapidly growing malignant cells

USES: Taxol: metastatic carcinoma of the ovary, breast carcinoma, AIDS-related Kaposi's sarcoma (second line), non–small cell lung cancer (first line), adjuvant treatment for node-positive breast cancer

Unlabeled uses: Advanced head, neck, small cell lung cancer; non-Hodgkin's lymphoma, adenocarcinoma of the upper GI tract, hormone-refractory prostate cancer

CONTRAINDICATIONS:
Pregnancy **D**, hypersensitivity to paclitaxel or other products with polyoxyethylated castor oil, albumin

> **BLACK BOX WARNING:** Neutropenia (neutrophils <1500/mm³)

Precautions: Breastfeeding, children, CV/hepatic disease, CNS disorder, renal disease, bone marrow suppression, dental disease/work, extravasation, females, geriatric patients, herpes, infection, infertility, jaundice, ocular exposure, radiation therapy, thrombocytopenia, vaccination

> **BLACK BOX WARNING:** Taxane hypersensitivity, requires a specialized care setting and an experienced clinician

DOSAGE AND ROUTES
PACLitaxel
Ovarian carcinoma
Adult: **IV** INF 135 mg/m² given over 24 hr q3wk, then CISplatin 75 mg/m² or 175 mg/m² over 3 hr q3wk or 175 mg/m² over 3 hr

Advanced ovarian carcinoma
Adult: **IV** INF 175 mg/m² with CISplatin 75 mg/m² over 3 hr q3wk

Breast carcinoma
Adult: **IV** INF 175 mg/m² over 3 hr q3wk × 4 courses

AIDS-related Kaposi's sarcoma
Adult: **IV** INF 135 mg/m² over 3 hr q3wk or 100 mg/m² over 3 hr q2wk

1st line non–small cell lung cancer
Adult: **IV** INF 135 mg/m²/24 hr with CISplatin 75 mg/m² × 3 wk

PACLitaxel protein-bound particles
Adult: **IV** 260 mg/m² q3wk

Hepatic dose
Adult, for 135 mg/m² 24 hr IV inf: AST/ALT 2-10 × ULN, total bilirubin ≤1.5 mg/dl: 100 mg/m²; AST/ALT <10 × ULN, total bilirubin 1.6-7.5 mg/dl: 50 mg/m²; AST/ALT ≥10 × ULN or total bilirubin >7.5 mg/dl: avoid use

Adult, for 175 mg/m² 3 hr IV inf: AST/ALT <10 × ULN, total bilirubin 1.26-2 × ULN: 135 mg/m²; AST/ALT <10 × ULN, total bilirubin 2.01-5 × ULN: 90 mg/m²; AST/ALT ≥10 × ULN or total bilirubin >5 × ULN: avoid use

Available forms: Inj 6 mg/ml, 30 mg/5-ml vial, 100 mg/16.7-ml vial, 150 mg/25-ml vial, 300 mg/50-ml vials; powder for inj, lyophilized 100 mg in single-use vials (Abraxane)

Implementation
• Monitor CBC, differential, platelet count weekly; withhold product if WBC is <1500/mm³ or platelet count is <100,000/mm³, notify prescriber of results
• If CISplatin is given, use after taxane

Continuous IV INF route
• After premedicating with dexamethasone 20 mg PO 12 hr and 6 hr before paclitaxel, diphenhydrAMINE 50 mg IV ½-1 hr before PACLitaxel and cimetidine 300 mg or ranitidine 50 mg IV ½-1 hr before PACLitaxel
• For extravasation if given by regular IV, not port

P

PACLitaxel

- After diluting in 0.9% NaCl, D_5, D_5 and 0.9% NaCl, D_5LR (0.3-1.2 mg/ml) chemo dispensing pin or similar devices with spikes should not be used in vials of Taxol, use in-line filter ≤0.22 micron, may be given as 3 hr or 24 hr inf
- Use only glass bottles, polypropylene, polyolefin bags and administration sets; do not use PVC inf bags or sets

Y-site compatibilities: Acyclovir, amikacin, aminophylline, ampicillin/sulbactam, bleomycin, butorphanol, calcium chloride, CARBOplatin, cefepime, cefoTEtan, cefTAZidime, cefTRIAXone, cimetidine, CISplatin, cladribine, cyclophosphamide, cytarabine, dacarbazine, dexamethasone, diphenhydrAMINE, DOXOrubicin, droperidol, etoposide, famotidine, floxuridine, fluconazole, fluorouracil, furosemide, ganciclovir, gentamicin, granisetron, haloperidol, heparin, hydrocortisone, HYDROmorphone, ifosfamide, LORazepam, magnesium sulfate, mannitol, meperidine, mesna, methotrexate, metoclopramide, morphine, nalbuphine, ondansetron, pentostatin, potassium chloride, prochlorperazine, propofol, ranitidine, sodium bicarbonate, thiotepa, vancomycin, vinBLAStine, vinCRIStine, zidovudine

Abraxane

Intermittent IV INF route
- Reconstitute vial by injecting 20 ml of 0.9% NaCl; slowly inject the 20 ml of 0.9% NaCl over at least 1 min to direct the sol flow on wall of vial; do not inject 0.9% NaCl directly onto lyophilized cake (foaming will occur); allow vial to sit for at least 5 min to ensure proper wetting of lyophilized cake; gently swirl or invert vial slowly for at least 2 min until completely dissolved
- Calculate dosing by dosing vol/ml = total dose (mg) ÷ 5 (mg/ml)

ADVERSE EFFECTS

CNS: Peripheral neuropathy
CV: *Bradycardia, hypotension, abnormal ECG,* supraventricular tachycardia (SVT)
GI: *Nausea, vomiting, diarrhea, mucositis; increased bilirubin, alkaline phosphatase, AST*
HEMA: **Neutropenia, leukopenia, thrombocytopenia, anemia,** bleeding, infections
INTEG: Alopecia, tissue necrosis, generalized urticaria, flushing
MS: *Arthralgia, myalgia*
RESP: **Pulmonary embolism,** dyspnea
SYST: *Hypersensitivity reactions,* **anaphylaxis, Stevens-Johnson syndrome, toxic epidermal necrolysis, angioedema**

Pharmacokinetics

Absorption	Completely absorbed
Distribution	89%-98% protein binding
Metabolism	Liver, extensively
Excretion	Unknown
Half-life	5-17 hr

Pharmacodynamics

Onset	Unknown
Peak	1-2 wk
Duration	3 wk

INTERACTIONS
Individual drugs
CycloSPORINE, dexamethasone, diazepam, etoposide, quiNIDine, teniposide, testosterone, verapamil, vinCRIStine: decreased metabolism of PACLitaxel
DOXOrubicin: increased levels of DOXOrubicin
Ketoconazole: increased toxicity, decreased metabolism; avoid concurrent use
Radiation: increased myelosuppression

Drug classifications
Anticoagulants, NSAIDs: increased bleeding risk
Antineoplastics: increased myelosuppression
CYP2C8, CYP2C9 inducers: decreased PACLitaxel level
Vaccines (live virus): decreased immune response

Drug/lab test
Increased: AST/ALT
Decreased: neutrophils, platelets, WBCs, Hgb

NURSING CONSIDERATIONS
Assessment
- Assess CNS changes: confusion, paresthesias, psychosis, tremors, seizures, neuropathies; product should be discontinued
- Check buccal cavity q8hr for dryness, sores or ulceration, white patches, oral pain, bleeding, dysphagia; obtain prescription for viscous lidocaine (Xylocaine) to use in mouth

> **BLACK BOX WARNING:** Requires a specialized care setting such as a hospital or facility capable of managing complications; should be used by a clinician experienced in cytotoxic agents

- **Cardiovascular status:** monitor ECG continuously in CV conditions; monitor for hypotension, sinus bradycardia/tachycardia
- **Peripheral neuropathy:** assess for paresthesias, numbness; during inf use ice packs on

extremities to lessen continued neuropathy; use ice on extremities when infusing
• **Arthralgia, myalgia:** may begin 2-3 days after infusion and continue for 4-5 days, may use analgesics
• **Nausea, vomiting:** premedicate with antiemetics, nausea and vomiting occur often
• Monitor renal function tests: BUN, creatinine, serum uric acid, urine CCr before, during therapy; check I&O ratio; report fall in urine output to <30 ml/hr
• Monitor temp q4hr (may indicate beginning of infection)
• Monitor liver function tests before, during therapy (bilirubin, AST, ALT, LDH) as needed or monthly; check for jaundice of skin and sclera, dark urine, clay-colored stools, itchy skin, abdominal pain, fever, diarrhea
• Assess for bleeding: hematuria, stool guaiac, bruising or petechiae, mucosa or orifices q8hr; check for inflammation of mucosa, breaks in skin
• Assess effects of alopecia on body image; discuss feelings about body changes
• VS during 1st hr of inf, check IV site for signs of infiltration
⚠ **Hypersensitive reactions, anaphylaxis, hypotension, dyspnea, angioedema, generalized urticaria; discontinue inf immediately; keep emergency equipment available, monitor continuously during first 30-60 min, then periodically**
• **Flush:** for mild to moderate flush, may continue diphenhydrAMINE for up to 48 hr
• Effects of alopecia on body image; discuss feelings about body changes

Patient/family education
⚠ **Teach patient to notify prescriber if pregnancy is planned or suspected (D), do not breastfeed**
• Teach patient to avoid use of products containing aspirin or ibuprofen, razors, commercial mouthwash, since bleeding may occur; to report symptoms of bleeding (hematuria, tarry stools)
• Instruct patient to report signs of anemia (fatigue, headache, irritability, faintness, shortness of breath) and CNS reactions (confusion, psychosis, nightmares, seizures, severe headaches)
• Teach patient to rinse mouth tid-qid with water, club soda; brush teeth bid-qid with soft brush or cotton-tipped applicators for stomatitis; use unwaxed dental floss
• Inform patient that hair may be lost during treatment; a wig or hairpiece may make patient feel better; new hair may be different in color, texture

• Inform patient that receiving vaccinations during therapy may cause serious reactions

Evaluation
Positive therapeutic outcome
• Prevention of rapid division of malignant cells

---

paliperidone (Rx)
(pal-ee-per′i-done)
Invega, Invega Sustenna
Func. class.: Antipsychotic
Chem. class.: Benzisoxazole derivative
Pregnancy category C

Do not confuse:
Invega/Iveegan, **paliperidone**/risperidone

ACTION: Mediated through both dopamine type 2 (D_2) and serotonin type 2 (5-HT$_2$) antagonism

Therapeutic outcome: Decrease in emotional excitement, hallucinations, delusions, paranoia; reorganization of patterns of thought, speech

USES: Schizophrenia, schizoaffective disorder

Unlabeled uses: Agitation

CONTRAINDICATIONS:
Breastfeeding, seizure disorders, AV block, geriatric, QT prolongation, torsades de pointes, hypersensitivity to this product or risperidone

Precautions: Pregnancy C, children, renal/hepatic disease, obesity, Parkinson's disease, suicidal ideation, diabetes mellitus, hematologic disease

BLACK BOX WARNING: Mortality-related psychosis in dementia

DOSAGE AND ROUTES
Adult: PO 6 mg/day; max 12 mg/day; IM 234 mg on day 1, then 156 mg 1 wk later; after 2nd dose, give 117 mg qmo, range 39-234 mg
Child/adolescent ≥12 yr and ≥51 kg: PO 3 mg/day, may increase if needed by 3 mg/day in intervals >5 days up to max 12 mg/day; <51 kg max 6 mg/day

Renal dose
Adult: PO CCr 50-79 ml/min, 3 mg/day, max 6 mg/day; ext rel/IM 156 mg on day 1, 117 mg 1 wk later, then 78 mg each mo CCr 10-49 ml/

min, 1.5 mg/day, max 3 mg/day; **IM not recommended**

Available forms: Ext rel tabs 1.5, 3, 6, 9 mg; ext rel susp for inj 39 mg/0.25 ml, 78 mg/0.5 ml, 117 mg/0.75 ml, 156 mg/1 ml, 234 mg/1.5 ml

Implementation
PO route
- Do not break, crush, or chew ext rel tabs, use plenty of water
- Give without regard for food
- Give a reduced dose to the geriatric patient
- Give antiparkinsonian agent on order from prescriber; to be used for EPS
- Avoid use with CNS depressants
- Supervise ambulation until patient is stabilized on medication; do not involve in strenuous exercise program, because fainting is possible; patient should not stand still for a long time
- Increase fluids to prevent constipation
- Decrease stimulus by dimming lights, avoiding loud noise
- Provide sips of water, candy, gum for dry mouth
- Store in airtight, light-resistant container

IM route
- Use for IM only, do not use IV or SUBCUT, injection kits contain a prefilled syringe and 2 safety needles, for single use only, shake for 10 secs
- **Deltoid injection:** ≥ 90 kg use 1.5 inch, 22 G needle; < 90 kg use 1 inch, 23 G needle, alternate injections between deltoid muscles
- **Gluteal injection:** use 1.5 inch, 22 G needle; while holding syringe upright, twist rubber tip clockwise to remove, peel safety needle pouch half way open, grasp needle sheath using plastic peel pouch, attach needle to luer connection in clockwise motion, pull needle sheath away using straight pull, bring syringe with attached needle upright to de-aerate, de-aerate, inject; after injection, use finger, thumb or flat surface to activate needle protection system, until click heard, use deltoid × 2 dosages

ADVERSE EFFECTS
CNS: *EPS, pseudoparkinsonism, akathisia, dystonia, tardive dyskinesia; drowsiness, insomnia, agitation, anxiety, headache,* **seizures, neuroleptic malignant syndrome,** dizziness

CV: Orthostatic hypotension, **tachycardia, heart failure, QT prolongation,** heart block, dysrhythmias

EENT: Blurred vision, cough
ENDO: Insulin increase, hyperinsulinemia, diabetes mellitus, weight gain, hyperglycemia, dyslipidemia
GI: *Nausea,* vomiting, *anorexia, constipation,* weight gain in adolescents, xerostomia
GU: Menstrual irregularities
HEMA: Agranulocytosis

Pharmacokinetics

Absorption	Unknown
Distribution	Unknown, protein binding >74%
Metabolism	Unknown
Excretion	80% urine, 11% feces
Half-life	Elimination 23 hr

Pharmacodynamics

Onset	Unknown
Peak	24 hr
Duration	Unknown

INTERACTIONS
Individual drugs
Abarelix, alfuzosin, amoxapine, apomorphine, chloroquine, dasatinib, dolasetron, droperidol, flecainide, pimozide: increased QT prolongation
Alcohol: increased sedation
Levodopa: decreased levodopa effect
Lithium: increased neurotoxicity
Paliperidone: decreased effect

Drug classifications
Azole antifungals; β-blockers; class IA, III antidysrhythmics; halogenated anesthetics; some antipsychotics; some phenothiazines; tricyclics (high doses): increased QT prolongation
SSRIs, SNRIs: increased serotonin syndrome, increased neuroleptic malignant syndrome
Other antipsychotics: increased EPS
Other CNS depressants, sedatives/hypnotics, opiates: increased sedation

Drug/herb
Betel palm, kava: increased EPS
Cola tree, hops, nettle, nutmeg: increased action
Kava: increased CNS depression

Drug/lab test
Increased: prolactin levels

NURSING CONSIDERATIONS
Assessment

> **BLACK BOX WARNING:** Assess mental status; mood, behavior, confusion, orientation, suicidal thoughts/behaviors; dementia especially in geriatric patients before initial administration

- **QT prolongation:** monitor ECG for QT prolongation, ejection fraction; assess for chest pain, palpitations, dyspnea
- Monitor for swallowing of PO medication; check for hoarding or giving of medication to other patients
- Monitor I&O ratio; palpate bladder if urinary output is low
- Assess affect, orientation, LOC, reflexes, gait, coordination, sleep pattern disturbances
- Monitor B/P standing and lying; also pulse, respirations; take these q4hr during initial treatment; establish baseline before starting treatment; report drops of 30 mm Hg; watch for ECG changes
- Assess for dizziness, faintness, palpitations, tachycardia on rising
- **Hyperprolactinemia:** assess for sexual dysfunction, decreased menstruation, breast pain
- **Assess for EPS,** including akathisia, tardive dyskinesia (bizarre movements of the jaw, mouth, tongue, extremities), pseudoparkinsonism (rigidity, tremors, pill rolling, shuffling gait)
- ⚠ **Assess for serious reactions in the geriatric patient**
- ⚠ **Serotonin syndrome, neuroleptic malignant syndrome: assess for increased heart rate, shivering, sweating, dilated pupils, tremors, high B/P, hyperthermia, headache, confusion; if these occur, stop product, administer a serotonin antagonist if needed**
- Assess skin turgor daily
- Assess for constipation, urinary retention daily; if these occur, increase bulk and water in diet; monitor for weight gain in adolescents

Patient/family education

- Advise patient that orthostatic hypotension may occur and to rise from sitting or lying position gradually
- Advise patient to avoid hot tubs, hot showers, tub baths; hypotension may occur
- Caution patient to avoid abrupt withdrawal of this product; EPS may result; product should be withdrawn slowly
- Teach patient to avoid OTC preparations (cough, hay fever, cold) unless approved by prescriber; serious product interactions may occur; avoid use of alcohol; increased drowsiness may occur
- Advise patient to avoid hazardous activities if drowsy or dizzy
- Teach patient compliance with product regimen; non-absorbable tab shell is expelled in stool
- Teach patient to report impaired vision, tremors, muscle twitching
- Caution patient that heat stroke may occur in hot weather; take extra precautions to stay cool
- Teach patient to use contraception, inform prescriber if pregnancy is planned or suspected

> **BLACK BOX WARNING:** Teach patient to notify prescriber of suicidal thoughts, behaviors, or other changes in behavior

Evaluation
Positive therapeutic outcome
- Decrease in emotional excitement, hallucinations, delusions, paranoia; reorganization of patterns of thought, speech

TREATMENT OF OVERDOSE:
Lavage if orally ingested; provide airway; *do not induce vomiting*

palonosetron (Rx)
(pa-lone-o'se-tron)
Aloxi
Func. class.: Antiemetic
Chem. class.: 5-HT₃ receptor antagonist
Pregnancy category B

ACTION: Prevents nausea, vomiting by blocking serotonin peripherally, centrally, and in the small intestine at the 5-HT₃ receptor

Therapeutic outcome: Decreased nausea, vomiting during chemotherapy

USES: Prevention of nausea, vomiting associated with cancer chemotherapy; postoperative nausea/vomiting

CONTRAINDICATIONS:
Hypersensitivity

Precautions: Pregnancy **B**, breastfeeding, children, geriatric, with hypokalemia, hypomagnesemia, patients taking diuretics

DOSAGE AND ROUTES
Adult: PO 0.5 mg as a single dose 1 hr prior to chemotherapy; **IV** 0.25 mg as a single dose over 30 sec, 30 min prior to chemotherapy, max 0.25 mg **IV** over q 7 days

Postoperative nausea/vomiting prophylaxis for up to 24 hr after surgery

Adult: IV 0.075 mg given over 10 sec immediately before induction

Available forms: Inj 0.25 mg/5 ml, caps 0.5 mg

Implementation

Direct IV route
• Do not mix with other products; flush **IV** line before, after administration
• Store at room temperature
• **Chemotherapy nausea/vomiting:** give as a single dose over 30 seconds
• **Postoperative nausea/vomiting:** give over 10 seconds immediately prior to anesthesia induction

Syringe compatibilities: Dexamethasone

Y-site compatibilities: Alemtuzumab, alfentanil, amikacin, aminocaproic acid, aminophylline, amiodarone, amphotericin B liposome, ampicillin, ampicillin/sulbactam, atracurium, atropine, azithromycin, aztreonam, bivalirudin, bleomycin, bumetanide, buprenorphine, busulfan, butorphanol, calcium acetate/chloride/gluconate, CARBOplatin, carmustine, caspofungin, ceFAZolin, cefepime, cefotaxime, cefoTEtan, cefOXitin, cefTAZidime, ceftizoxime, cefTRIAXone, cefuroxime, chloramphenicol, chlorproMAZINE, cimetidine, ciprofloxacin, cisatracurium, CISplatin, clindamycin, cyclophosphamide, cycloSPORINE, cytarabine, dacarbazine, DACTINomycin, dantrolene, DAPTOmycin, DAUNOrubicin, dexamethasone, dexmedetomidine, dexrazoxane, digoxin, diltiazem, diphenhydrAMINE, DOBUTamine, DOCEtaxel, DOPamine, doxacurium, DOXOrubicin hydrochloride, droperidol, enalaprilat, ePHEDrine, EPINEPHrine, epirubicin, eptifibatide, erythromycin, esmolol, etoposide, etoposide phosphate, famotidine, fenoldopam, fentaNYL, fluconazole, fludarabine, fluorouracil, foscarnet, fosphenytoin, furosemide, gemcitabine, gentamicin, glycopyrrolate, haloperidol, heparin, hydrALAZINE, hydrocortisone, HYDROmorphone, IDArubicin, ifosfamide, inamrinone, insulin, irinotecan, isoproterenol, ketorolac, labetalol, leucovorin, levofloxacin, lidocaine, linezolid, LORazepam, magnesium sulfate, mannitol, mechlorethamine, melphalan, meperidine, meropenem, mesna, metaraminol, methotrexate, methyldopate, metoclopramide, metoprolol, metroNIDAZOLE, midazolam, milrinone, mitoMYcin, mitoXANtrone, mivacurium, morphine, nalbuphine, naloxone, neostigmine, nesiritide, niCARdipine, nitroglycerin, nitroprusside, norepinephrine, octreotide, oxaliplatin, oxytocin, PACLitaxel, pamidronate, pancuronium, pentazocine, PHENobarbital, phentolamine, phenylephrine, piperacillin/tazobactam, potassium acetate/chloride/phosphates, procainamide, prochlorperazine, promethazine, propranolol, quinupristin/dalfopristin, ranitidine, remifentanil, rocuronium, sodium acetate/bicarbonate/phosphates, streptozocin, succinylcholine, SUFentanil, tacrolimus, teniposide, theophylline, thiotepa, ticarcillin/clavulanate, tigecycline, tirofiban, tobramycin, topotecan, trimethobenzamide, trimethoprim/sulfamethoxazole, vancomycin, vasopressin, vecuronium, verapamil, vinBLAStine, vinCRIStine, vinorelbine, zidovudine

Y-site incompatibilities: Acyclovir, allopurinol, amphotericin B colloidal, diazepam, doxycycline, ganciclovir, imipenem/cilastatin, methylPREDNISolone, minocycline, nafcillin, pantoprazole, pentamidine, PENTobarbital, phenytoin, thiopental

ADVERSE EFFECTS

CNS: *Headache, dizziness, drowsiness, fatigue, insomnia*

GI: *Diarrhea, constipation,* abdominal pain

MISC: Weakness, hyperkalemia, anxiety, rash, **bronchospasm** (rare), arthralgia, *fever, urinary retention*

Pharmacokinetics

Absorption	Unknown
Distribution	62% protein bound
Metabolism	Liver
Excretion	Unchanged product and metabolites excreted by kidney
Half-life	40 hr

Pharmacodynamics

Unknown

INTERACTIONS

Individual drugs

Chloroquine, clarithromycin, droperidol, erythromycin, grepafloxacin, halofantrine, haloperidol, levomethadyl, methadone, pentamidine: possible QT prolongation

Drug classifications

Class 1A antidysrhythmics (disopyramide, procainamide, quiNIDine), class III antidysrhythmics (amiodarone, dofetilide,

---

ibutilide), diuretics (except potassium sparing), some phenothiazines: possible QT prolongation

NURSING CONSIDERATIONS
Assessment
⚠ Monitor for absence of nausea, vomiting during chemotherapy
⚠ Assess hypersensitivity reaction: rash, bronchospasm
• Cardiac disease: check ECG before use
• Hyperkalemia: monitor potassium

Patient/family education
• Teach to report diarrhea, constipation, rash, or changes in respirations or discomfort at insertion site
• Advise patient to avoid alcohol, barbiturates
• Teach patient to use other antiemetics if nausea occurs

Evaluation
Positive therapeutic outcome
• Absence of nausea, vomiting during cancer chemotherapy

pamidronate (Rx)
(pam-i-drone'ate)
Aredia
Func. class.: Bone resorption inhibitor, electrolyte modifier
Chem. class.: Bisphosphonate
Pregnancy category D

Do not confuse:
Aredia/Adriamycin

ACTION: Inhibits bone resorption, apparently without inhibiting bone formation and mineralization; absorbs calcium phosphate crystals in bone and may directly block dissolution of hydroxyapatite crystals of bone

Therapeutic outcome: Serum calcium at normal level

USES: Moderate to severe Paget's disease, hypercalcemia, osteolytic bone metastases in breast cancer patients, multiple myeloma

Unlabeled uses: Postmenopausal osteoporosis, hyperparathyroidism

CONTRAINDICATIONS:
Pregnancy **D**, hypersensitivity to bisphosphonates

Precautions: Children, nursing mothers, renal dysfunction, poor dentition

DOSAGE AND ROUTES
Hypercalcemia of malignancy
Adult: IV INF 60-90 mg as a single dose in moderate hypercalcemia, 90 mg in severe hypercalcemia given over 2-24 hr; dose should be diluted in 1000 ml 0.45% NaCl, 0.9% NaCl, or D$_5$W; wait 7 days before 2nd course

Osteolytic lesions
Adult: IV 90 mg/500 ml of D$_5$W, 0.45% NaCl, or 0.9% NaCl given over 4 hr on a monthly basis (multiple myeloma) or over 2 hr q3-4wk (breast carcinoma)

Paget's disease
Adult: IV INF 30 mg/day given over 4 hr × 3 days

Available forms: Powder for inj 30, 90 mg/vial; inj 3, 6, 9 mg/ml

Implementation
IV route
• After reconstituting by adding 10 ml of sterile water for inj to each vial (30 mg/10 ml or 90 mg/10 ml depending on vial used); add to 1000 ml of sterile 0.45%, 0.9% NaCl, D$_5$W, run over 2-24 hr **(hypercalcemia)**; dilute reconstituted sol in 500 ml of 0.9% NaCl, 0.45% NaCl, or D$_5$W, give over 4 hr **(multiple myeloma, Paget's disease)**; dilute reconstituted sol in 250 ml of 0.9% NaCl, 0.45% NaCl or D$_5$W, give over 2 hr **(osteolytic bone metastases of breast cancer)**
• Store inf sol for up to 24 hr at room temperature
• Reconstituted sol with sterile water may be stored under refrigeration for up to 24 hr
• Do not mix with calcium-containing inf sol such as Ringer's sol

Y-site compatibilities: Acyclovir, alfentanil, allopurinol, amifostine, amikacin, aminocaproic acid, aminophylline, amphotericin B lipid complex, amphotericin B liposome, ampicillin, anidulafungin, atenolol, atracurium, azithromycin, aztreonam, bivalirudin, bleomycin, bumetanide, buprenorphine, butorphanol, CARBOplatin, carmustine, ceFAZolin, cefepime, cefoperazone, cefotaxime, cefoTEtan, cefOXitin, cefTAZidime, ceftizoxime, cefTRIAXone, cefuroxime, chloramphenicol, chlorproMAZINE, cimetidine, ciprofloxacin, cisatracurium, CISplatin, clindamycin, cyclophosphamide, cycloSPORINE, cytarabine, dacarbazine, DAPTOmycin, dexamethasone, dexmedetomidine, dexrazoxane, digoxin, diltiazem, diphenhy-drAMINE, DOBUTamine, DOCEtaxel, dolasetron, DOPamine, doxacurium, DOXOrubicin, doxycycline, droperidol, enalaprilat, ePHEDrine, EPINEPHrine, epirubicin, ertapenem, erythromycin, esmolol, etoposide, famotidine, fenoldopam, fentaNYL, fluconazole, fludarabine, fluorouracil, foscarnet, fosphenytoin, furosemide, gallium, ganciclovir, gatifloxacin, gemcitabine, gentamicin, glycopyrrolate, granisetron, haloperidol, heparin, hetastarch 6%, hydrALAZINE, hydrocortisone, HYDROmorphone, hydrOXYzine, ifosfamide, imipenem-cilastatin, inamrinone, insulin (regular), isoproterenol, ketorolac, labetalol, levofloxacin, levorphanol, lidocaine, linezolid, LORazepam, magnesium sulfate, mannitol, mechlorethamine, melphalan, meperidine, meropenem, mesna, metaraminol, methotrexate, methyldopate, methylPREDNISolone, metoclopramide, metoprolol, metroNIDAZOLE, midazolam, milrinone, minocycline, mitoXANtrone, mivacurium, morphine, mycophenolate, nafcillin, nalbuphine, naloxone, nesiritide, niCARdipine, nitroglycerin, nitroprusside, norepinephrine, octreotide, ondansetron, oxytocin, PACLitaxel, palonosetron, pancuronium, PEMEtrexed, pentamidine, pentazocine, PENTobarbital, PHENobarbital, phenylephrine, piperacillin, polymyxin B, potassium chloride/phosphates, procainamide, prochlorperazine, promethazine, propranolol, quiNIDine, quinupristin-dalfopristin, ranitidine, remifentanil, rocuronium, sodium acetate/bicarbonate/phosphates, succinylcholine, SUFentanil, sulfamethoxazole-trimethoprim, teniposide, theophylline, thiopental, thiotepa, ticarcillin, ticarcillin-clavulanate, tigecycline, tirofiban, tobramycin, tolazoline, topotecan, trimethobenzamide, vancomycin, vasopressin, vecuronium, verapamil, vinBLAstine, vinCRIStine, vinorelbine, voriconazole, zidovudine

ADVERSE EFFECTS

CNS: Fatigue, *fever*
CV: *Hypertension,* **atrial fibrillation**
EENT: Ocular pain, inflammation, vision impairment
GI: *Abdominal pain, anorexia, constipation, nausea, vomiting,* dyspepsia
GU: Renal failure
HEMA: **Thrombocytopenia, anemia, leukopenia**
INTEG: Redness, swelling, induration, pain on palpation at site of catheter insertion
META: Hypokalemia, hypomagnesemia, hypophosphatemia, hypocalcemia, hypothyroidism

MS: *Severe bone pain,* myalgia, **osteonecrosis of the jaw**
RESP: Coughing, dyspnea, URI
SYST: **Angioedema, anaphylaxis**

Pharmacokinetics

Absorption	Rapidly cleared from circulation
Distribution	Mainly to bones, primarily in areas of high bone turnover
Metabolism	Unknown
Excretion	Kidneys, unchanged (50%)
Half-life	Biphasic 27 hr; from bone to 300 days

Pharmacodynamics

Onset	1 day
Peak	1 wk
Duration	Unknown

INTERACTIONS

Individual drugs
Calcium, vitamin D: decreased pamidronate effect
CycloSPORINE, tacrolimus, vancomycin: increased nephrotoxicity
Entecavir: increased effect of entecavir

Drug classifications
Aminoglycosides, NSAIDs, radiopaque contrast agents: increased nephrotoxicity
Loop diuretics: increased hypokalemia

Drug/lab test
Increased: creatinine
Decreased: potassium, magnesium, phosphate, calcium, WBC, platelets

NURSING CONSIDERATIONS

Assessment
• **Dental health:** give antiinfectives for dental extractions
• Monitor WBCs, platelets, electrolytes, creatinine, BUN, Hgb/Hct prior to beginning treatment
• Temperature may be elevated during the first 3 days after a dose; risk of fever increases as dose increases
⚠ Renal disease: max 90 mg single dose, longer infusions >2 hr may increase risk for renal toxicity
• **Hypocalcemia:** assess for nausea, vomiting, constipation, thirst, dysrhythmias, hypocalcemia, paresthesia, twitching, laryngospasm,

Chvostek's, Trousseau's signs; **hypercalcemia:** thirst, nausea, vomiting, dysrhythmias
• **Dehydration/hypovolemia:** should be corrected during treatment of hypercalcemia, prior to therapy; maintain adequate urine output
• Assess for atrial fibrillation
• Assess fluid volume status: check I&O ratio and record, assess for distended red veins, crackles in lung, color, quality, and specific gravity of urine, skin turgor, adequacy of pulses, moist mucous membranes, bilateral lung sounds, peripheral pitting edema
• Monitor electrolytes: phosphorus, potassium, sodium, calcium, magnesium; also include BUN, creatinine, CBC, platelets, hemoglobin
• Assess B/P before, during therapy
• Assess for pain: in joints or on exertion, duration and characteristics; analgesics may be ordered
• Assess for phlebitis at **IV** site: swelling, redness, pain, warmth

Patient/family education
• Advise patient to report hypercalcemic relapse: nausea, vomiting, bone pain, thirst; unusual muscle twitching, muscle spasms, severe diarrhea, constipation, ocular symptoms
• Advise patient to continue with dietary recommendations, including calcium and vit D
• To obtain an analgesic from provider for bone pain
• Advise patient that small, frequent meals may help nausea/vomiting
⚠ Teach patient to notify prescriber if pregnancy (D) is planned or suspected

Evaluation
Positive therapeutic outcome
• Decreased calcium levels to normal

---

pancrelipase (Rx)
(pan-kre-li′pase)
Creon, DMH ✢, Pancrease ✢, Pancreaze, Pancrecarb MS, Ultrase MT, VioKase, Zenpep
Func. class.: Digestant
Chem. class.: Pancreatic enzyme (bovine/porcine)
Pregnancy category B

ACTION: Pancreatic enzyme needed for breakdown of substances released from the pancreas

Therapeutic outcome: Increases protein, fat, carbohydrate digestion

USES: Exocrine pancreatic secretion insufficiency, cystic fibrosis (digestive aid), steatorrhea, pancreatic enzyme deficiency

CONTRAINDICATIONS:
Allergy to pork

Precautions: Pregnancy **B**, ileus, pancreatitis, Crohn's disease, diabetes mellitus

DOSAGE AND ROUTES
Many products listed above are not interchangeable

Del rel caps—Creon caps, Zenpep caps, Pancreaze caps
Adult/adolescent/child ≥4 yr: PO 500 lipase units/kg/meal, titrate based on response, max 2500 lipase units/kg/meal
Child 1<4 yr: PO 1000 lipase units/kg/meal, titrate based on response, max 2500 lipase units/kg/meal

Available forms: Tabs (VioKase) 10, 204 units; cap, del rel 4, 8, 154 units (Pancrecarb MS), 12, 18, 20 units (Ultrase MT), Ultrase; cap 3000, 4200, 5000, 6000, 8000, 10,500, 12,000, 15,000, 16,000, 16,800, 24,000, 25,000 units

Implementation
• Give after antacid or cimetidine; decreased pH inactivates product
• Administer low-fat diet to decrease GI symptoms
• Provide adequate hydration
• Store in airtight container at room temperature
• Do not crush, chew del rel products, caps

ADVERSE EFFECTS
ENDO: Hyperglycemia, hypoglycemia
GI: Anorexia, nausea, vomiting, diarrhea, cramping, bloating
GU: Hyperuricuria, hyperuricemia

Pharmacokinetics
Unknown

Pharmacodynamics
Unknown

INTERACTIONS
Individual drugs
Acarbose, miglitol: decreased effects of each specific drug
Cimetidine, iron (oral): decreased absorption of pancrelipase

Drug classifications
Antacids: decreased absorption of pancrelipase

NURSING CONSIDERATIONS
Assessment
- Monitor I&O ratio; watch for increasing urinary output
- Monitor fecal fat, nitrogen, pro-time during treatment
- Monitor for polyuria, polydipsia, polyphagia (may indicate diabetes mellitus); monitor glucose level more frequently
- Assess for allergy to pork; patient may also be sensitive to this product
- Assess for appropriate weight, height, development; there may be a developmental lag
- Check stools for steatorrhea, which signifies undigested fat content

Patient/family education
- Teach patient to always take with food, not to crush, chew del rel product, caps
- Instruct patient to store at room temperature, away from moisture
- Teach patient to take tab with 8 oz or more water, not to let tab sit in mouth; have patient take tab sitting up only
- Advise patient to notify prescriber of allergic reactions, abdominal pain, cramping, or hematuria

Evaluation
Positive therapeutic outcome
- Absence of steatorrhea
- Improved digestion of carbohydrates, proteins, fat

⚠ HIGH ALERT
pancuronium (Rx)
(pan-cure-oh'nee-yum)
Func. class.: Neuromuscular blocker (nondepolarizing)
Chem. class.: Synthetic curariform
Pregnancy category C

ACTION: Inhibits transmission of nerve impulses by binding with cholinergic receptor sites, antagonizing action of acetylcholine

Therapeutic outcome: Paralysis of all skeletal muscles

USES: Facilitation of endotracheal intubation, skeletal muscle relaxation during mechanical ventilation, surgery, or general anesthesia

CONTRAINDICATIONS:
Hypersensitivity to bromide ion

Precautions: Pregnancy **C**, breastfeeding, children <2 yr, renal/hepatic/cardiac/neuromuscular disease, electrolyte imbalances, dehydration, previous anaphylactic reactions (other neuromuscular blockers)

> **BLACK BOX WARNING:** Respiratory insufficiency

DOSAGE AND ROUTES
Adult/child/infant >1 mo: IV 0.04-0.1 mg/kg initially or 0.05 mg/kg after initial dose of succinylcholine; maintenance 0.01 mg/kg 60-100 min after initial dose, then 0.01 mg/kg q25-60min as needed; in obese patients, use ideal body weight

Neonate <1 mo: IV test dose 0.02 mg/kg, then 0.03 mg/kg/dose initially, repeat 2 × as needed at 5-10 min intervals; maintenance 0.03-0.09 mg/kg/dose q30min-4hr as needed

Available forms: Inj 1, 2 mg/ml

Implementation
- Use peripheral nerve stimulator (anesthesiologist) to determine neuromuscular blockade; deep tendon reflexes should be monitored during extended periods

Direct IV route
- Give undiluted over 1-2 min (1 mg/ml [10 ml vial], 2 mg/ml [2, 5 ml vial])

Intermittent IV infusion route
- Add 100 mg of product to 250 ml D$_5$W, 0.9% NaCl, or LR (0.4 mg/ml)
- Store in light-resistant area
- Give anticholinesterase to reverse neuromuscular blockade

Y-site compatibilities: Aminophylline, ceFAZolin, cefuroxime, cimetidine, DOBUTamine, DOPamine, EPINEPHrine, esmolol, fentaNYL, fluconazole, gentamicin, heparin, hydrocortisone, isoproterenol, LORazepam, midazolam, morphine, nitroglycerin, nitroprusside, ranitidine, sulfamethoxazole/trimethoprim, vancomycin

Y-site incompatibilities: Diazepam

Additive compatibilities: Verapamil

Additive incompatibilities: Barbiturates

ADVERSE EFFECTS
CV: Bradycardia, tachycardia, increased, decreased B/P, ventricular extrasystoles, edema, hypotension

---

EENT: Increased secretions
INTEG: Rash, flushing, pruritus, urticaria, sweating, salivation
MS: Weakness to prolonged skeletal muscle relaxation
RESP: Prolonged apnea, bronchospasm, cyanosis, respiratory depression, dyspnea
SYST: Anaphylaxis

Pharmacokinetics

Absorption	Complete bioavailability
Distribution	Extracellular space; crosses placenta
Metabolism	Plasma
Excretion	Kidneys, unchanged
Half-life	2 hr

Pharmacodynamics

Onset	3-5 min, dose dependent
Peak	3-5 min
Duration	35-40 min

INTERACTIONS
Individual products
Clindamycin, enflurane, isoflurane, lincomycin, lithium, quiNIDine: increased neuromuscular blockade
Theophylline: dysrhythmias

Drug classifications
Aminoglycosides, anesthetics (local), analgesics (opioid), polymyxin antiinfectives, thiazides: increased neuromuscular blockade

Drug/lab test
Decreased: cholinesterase

NURSING CONSIDERATIONS
Assessment
• Monitor vital signs (B/P, pulse, respirations, airway) until fully recovered; note rate, depth, pattern of respirations, strength of hand grip; patient should be intubated before use
• Monitor for electrolyte imbalances (potassium, magnesium) before product is used; electrolyte imbalances may lead to increased action of this product
• **Monitor for recovery:** decreased paralysis of face, diaphragm, leg, arm, rest of body; residual weakness and respiratory problems may occur during recovery period
⚠ **Assess for hypersensitive reactions, anaphylaxis: rash, fever, respiratory distress, pruritus; product should be discontinued**

Patient/family education
• Provide reassurance if communication is difficult during recovery from neuromuscular blockade
• Provide explanation to patients regarding all procedures or treatments; patient will remain conscious if anesthesia is not given also

Evaluation
Positive therapeutic outcome
• Paralysis of jaw, eyelid, head, neck, rest of body as evaluated by peripheral nerve stimulator

TREATMENT OF OVERDOSE:
Neostigmine, atropine; monitor VS; may require mechanical ventilation

panitumumab (Rx)
(pan-i-tue′moo-mab)
Vectibix
Func. class.: Antineoplastic—miscellaneous
Chem. class.: Multikinase inhibitor, signal transduction inhibitor
Pregnancy category C

ACTION: Decreases growth and survival of cancer cells by competitive inhibition of EGF receptor

Therapeutic outcome: Decrease in colon carcinoma progression

USES: EGFR expressing metastatic colorectal cancer, not beneficial in *KRAS* mutations in codon 12 or 13

CONTRAINDICATIONS:
Hypersensitivity

Precautions: Pregnancy **C,** breastfeeding, children, hepatic disease, acute bronchospasm, diarrhea, hamster protein allergy, hypomagnesemia, hypotension, pulmonary fibrosis, sepsis, *KRAS* mutations, soft-tissue toxicities

> **BLACK BOX WARNING:** Exfoliative dermatitis, infusion-related reactions

DOSAGE AND ROUTES
Adult: IV INF 6 mg/kg over 60 min q2wk; doses > 1000 mg over 90 min

Available forms: Sol for inj 20 mg/ml (100 mg/5 ml, 400 mg/20 ml)

Implementation

Intermittent IV infusion route

- Give in hospital or clinic setting with full resuscitation equipment
- Give only as IV inf using controlled IV inf pump; do not give **IV** push or bolus; use low-protein binding 0.2 or 0.22 micron in-line filter; flush line with 0.9% NaCl before, after administration
- Give over 60 min through a peripheral line or in-dwelling catheter; inf doses of >1000 mg over 90 min
- Dilute in 100 ml of 0.9% NaCl; dilute doses >1000 mg in 150 ml of 0.9% NaCl; mix by inverting; max 10 mg/ml; use within 6 hr if stored at room temperature; can be stored between 2°-8° C for up to 24 hr
- Store unopened vials in refrigerator; do not shake; protect from direct sunlight; do not freeze

Dosage adjustment for infusion/dermatologic reaction

⚠ **Grade 1/2: reduce infusion by 50%; Grade 3/4: terminate, permanently discontinue depending on severity/resistance**

ADVERSE EFFECTS

CNS: Fatigue
CV: Peripheral edema
EENT: Ocular irritation, **ocular toxicity**
GI: *Nausea, diarrhea, vomiting,* anorexia, mouth ulceration, abdominal pain, constipation
HEMA: Thrombophlebitis
INTEG: *Rash,* pruritus, **exfoliative dermatitis,** skin fissure, **angioedema, severe/fatal infusion reactions**
META: Hypocalcemia, hypomagnesemia, antibody formation
RESP: **Bronchospasm, cough,** dyspnea, **hypoxia, pulmonary fibrosis/embolism,** pneumonitis, wheezing, interstitial lung disease

Pharmacokinetics

Absorption	38%-49%, high-fat meal decreases absorption
Distribution	Protein binding 99.5%
Metabolism	Liver, oxidative metabolism by CYP3A4, glucuronidation by UGT1A9, some Asian patients (15%-20%) are poor metabolizers
Excretion	Feces 77%
Half-life	Elimination 7.5 day

Pharmacodynamics

Onset	Unknown
Peak	3 hr
Duration	Unknown

INTERACTIONS

Drug classifications

Antineoplastics, other: do not use with other products

NURSING CONSIDERATIONS

Assessment

- **Pulmonary fibrosis:** assess for dyspnea, cough, wheezing, may need to discontinue

> **BLACK BOX WARNING: Serious skin disorders:** assess for fever, sore throat, fatigue, then lesions in mouth, lips; withhold product, notify prescriber

- Monitor serum electrolytes periodically (calcium, magnesium)
- Assess for signs of infection: increased temperature

> **BLACK BOX WARNING:** Assess for signs of infusion reactions: bronchospasm, fever, chills, hypotension; may require discontinuation; have emergency equipment available

- **Assess for signs of ocular toxicity:** ocular irritation, hyperemia

Patient/family education

⚠ **Instruct patient to report adverse reactions immediately: difficulty breathing, mouth sores, skin rash, ocular toxicity**
- Teach patient reason for treatment, expected results, adverse reactions
- Teach males/females to use contraception while taking this product and for 6 mo after treatment; do not breastfeed for at least 2 mo after treatment
- Advise to use sunscreen while taking, 2 mo after

Evaluation

Positive therapeutic outcome
- Decrease in colon carcinoma progression

pantoprazole (Rx)

(pan-toe-pray'zole)

Panto ✤, **Pantoloc** ✤, **Protonix, Protonix IV**

Func. class.: Proton pump inhibitor
Chem. class.: Benzimidazole
Pregnancy category C

ACTION: Suppresses gastric secretion by inhibiting hydrogen/potassium ATPase enzyme system in gastric parietal cell; characterized as gastric acid pump inhibitor, since it blocks final step of acid production

Therapeutic outcome: Absence of epigastric fullness, pain, swelling

USES: Gastroesophageal reflux disease (GERD), severe erosive esophagitis, maintenance, long-term pathological hypersecretory conditions including Zollinger-Ellison syndrome

CONTRAINDICATIONS: Hypersensitivity to this product or benzimidazole

Precautions: Pregnancy C, breastfeeding, children, proton pump hypersensitivity

DOSAGE AND ROUTES

GERD

Adult: PO 40 mg/day × 8 wk, may repeat course

Erosive esophagitis

Adult: **IV** 40 mg/day × 7-10 days; PO 40 mg/day × 8 wk; may repeat PO course

Pathologic hypersecretory conditions

Adult: PO 40 mg bid; **IV** 80 mg q12hr; max 240 mg/day

Available forms: Del rel tabs 20, 40 mg; powder for inj 40 mg/vial; del rel granules for susp 40 mg

Implementation

• Swallow del rel tabs whole; do not break, crush, or chew
• May take with or without food
• **Suspension:** give in apple juice 30 minutes before a meal or sprinkled on 1 tbsp of applesauce
• **NG tube:** empty contents of packet of granules into barrel of a 60-ml catheter tip syringe (plunger removed) connected to ≥16F NG tube; add 10 ml apple juice and tap or shake barrel of syringe to empty into the tube; add another 10 ml of apple juice; rinse with additional apple juice until syringe is clear

IV route

• Use of Protonix IV vials with spiked IV system adaptors is not recommended
• Visually inspect for particulate matter and discoloration prior to use
• Give as an IV infusion over 15 min either through a dedicated line or a Y-site; a 2-min slow injection regimen is also approved; do not give fast IV push
• When using a Y-site, immediately stop use if a precipitation or discoloration occurs

Reconstitution of vial:
• Use 40 mg vial/10 ml NS; do not freeze

2-minute slow intravenous (IV) infusion injection:
• Dilute one or two 40-mg vials with 10 ml NS per vial to 4 mg/ml, store up to 24 hr at room temperature prior to use; infuse slowly over at least 2 min; do not give with other IV fluids or medications; flush line with D_5W, NS, or LR before and after each dose

15-minute intravenous (IV) infusion:
• Dilute each 40 mg dose with 10 ml NS; the reconstituted vial should be further admixed with 100 ml (for one vial) or 80 ml (for 2 vials) of D_5W, NS, or LR (to 0.4 mg/ml or 0.8 mg/ml, respectively), store up to 6 hr at room temperature prior to further dilution; the admixed solution (0.4 mg/ml or 0.8 mg/ml) may be stored at room temperature and must be used within 24 hr from the time of initial reconstitution; infuse over 15 min at 7 ml/min; do not administer with other IV fluids or medications; flush the IV line with D_5W, NS, or LR before and after each dose

ADVERSE EFFECTS

CNS: *Headache,* insomnia, asthenia, fatigue, malaise, insomnia, somnolence
GI: *Diarrhea, abdominal pain,* flatulence, **pancreatitis,** weight changes
INTEG: *Rash*
META: Hyperglycemia, weight gain/loss, hyponatremia, hypomagnesemia
MS: Rhabdomyolysis, myalgia
RESP: Pneumonia
SYST: Stevens-Johnson syndrome, toxic epidermal necrolysis, anaphylaxis, angioedema

Pharmacokinetics

Absorption	Unknown
Distribution	Protein binding 97%
Metabolism	Unknown
Excretion	Urine-metabolites, feces, decreased rate in geriatric
Half-life	1½ hr

Pharmacodynamics

Onset	Unknown
Peak	2.4 hr
Duration	>24 hr

INTERACTIONS
Individual drugs
Calcium carbonate, sucralfate, vit B$_{12}$, ketoconazole, itraconazole, atazanair, ampicillin, iron salts: decreased absorption of these products

Clarithromycin, diazepam, flurazepam, phenytoin, triazolam: increased levels of pantoprazole

Clopidogrel: decreased clopidogrel effect

Warfarin: increased risk of bleeding

Drug/herb
St. John's wort: decreased effect of pantoprazole

NURSING CONSIDERATIONS
Assessment
• **Rhabdomyolysis:** muscle pain, increased CPK, weakness, swelling of affected muscles; if these occur and if confirmed by CPK, product should be discontinued

• Assess GI system: bowel sounds q8hr, abdomen for pain, swelling, anorexia

• Monitor hepatic enzymes: AST, ALT, alkaline phosphatase during treatment

• **Serious skin reactions:** assess for toxic epidermal necrolysis, **Stevens-Johnson syndrome,** exfoliative dermatitis; fever, sore throat, fatigue, thin ulcers, lesions in the mouth, lips

• **Electrolytic imbalances:** hyponatremia; hypomagnesemia in those using this product (3 mo-1 yr) if hypomagnesemia occurs, use of magnesium supplements may be sufficient; if severe, discontinuation of this product may be required

Patient/family education
• Advise patient to report severe diarrhea; product may have to be discontinued

• Advise patient with diabetes that hyperglycemia may occur

• Advise patient to avoid hazardous activities; dizziness may occur

• Advise patient to avoid alcohol, salicylates, ibuprofen; may cause GI irritation

Evaluation
Positive therapeutic outcome
• Absence of epigastric pain, swelling, fullness

PARoxetine (Rx)
(par-ox′ e-teen)
Paxil, Paxil CR, Pexeva, PMS
Func. class.: Antidepressant, selective serotonin reuptake inhibitor (SSRI)
Chem. class.: Phenylpiperidine derivative
Pregnancy category D

Do not confuse:
**PARoxetine/PACLitaxel,
Paxil/PACLitaxel/Taxol**

ACTION: Inhibits CNS neuron reuptake of serotonin but not of norepinephrine or DOPamine

Therapeutic outcome: Relief of depression

USES: Major depressive disorder, obsessive-compulsive disorder, panic disorder, generalized anxiety disorder, posttraumatic stress disorder, premenstrual disorders, social anxiety disorder

Unlabeled uses: Premature ejaculation

CONTRAINDICATIONS:
Pregnancy **D,** hypersensitivity, MAOI use, alcohol use

Precautions: Breastfeeding, geriatric, seizure history, patients with history of mania, renal/hepatic disease

> **BLACK BOX WARNING:** Children, suicidal ideation

DOSAGE AND ROUTES
Depression
Adult: PO 20 mg/day in AM; after 4 wk if no clinical improvement is noted, dosage may be increased by 10 mg/day weekly to desired response; max 50 mg/day; or CONT REL 25 mg/day, may increase by 12.5 mg/day weekly up to 62.5 mg/day

Geriatric: PO 10 mg/day, increase by 10 mg to desired dose, max 40 mg/day

Obsessive-compulsive disorder
Adult: PO 40 mg/day in AM; start with 20 mg/day, increase 10 mg/day increments, max 60 mg/day

Panic disorder
Adult: Start with 10 mg/day and increase in 10 mg/day increments to 40 mg/day, max 60 mg/day; or CONT REL 12.5 mg/day max 75 mg/day

Generalized anxiety disorder
Adult: PO 20 mg/day in AM, range 20-50 mg/day

Posttraumatic stress disorder
Adult: PO 20 mg/day, range 20-60 mg/day

Premenstrual disorders
Adult: CONT REL 12.5 mg/day in AM

Renal dose
Adult: PO CCr 30-60 ml/min lower doses may be needed, CCr <30 ml/min 10 mg/day in AM, may increase by 10 mg/day qwk, max 40 mg/day; or CONT REL 12.5 mg/day max 50 mg/day

Hepatic dose
Adult: PO 10 mg/day initially, max 40 mg regular release, CONT REL 12.5 mg/day initially, max 50 mg/day

Available forms: Tabs 10, 20, 30, 40 mg; oral susp 10 mg/5 ml; cont rel 12.5, 25, 37.5 mg

Implementation
• Give with food or milk for GI symptoms; store at room temperature; do not freeze
• Give crushed if patient is unable to swallow whole, regular release only
• Use gum, hard candy, frequent sips of water for dry mouth
• Avoid use with other CNS depressants
• **Oral susp:** shake, measure with oral syringe or calibrated measuring device
• **Cont rel tab:** do not cut, chew, crush; do not give concurrently with antacids

ADVERSE EFFECTS
CNS: *Headache, nervousness, insomnia, drowsiness, anxiety, tremor, dizziness, fatigue, sedation,* abnormal dreams, agitation, apathy, euphoria, hallucinations, delusions, psychosis, **seizures, malignant neuroleptic syndrome–like reactions,** restless legs syndrome
CV: Vasodilatation, postural hypotension, palpitations, bleeding
EENT: Visual changes
GI: *Nausea, diarrhea, constipation, dry mouth, anorexia,* dyspepsia, vomiting, taste changes, flatulence, decreased appetite, cramps
GU: Dysmenorrhea, decreased libido, urinary frequency, UTI, amenorrhea, cystitis, impotence, decreased sperm quality, decreased fertility, *abnormal ejaculation* (male)
INTEG: *Sweating,* rash
MS: Pain, arthritis, myalgia, myopathy, myasthenia

RESP: Infection, pharyngitis, nasal congestion, sinus headache, sinusitis, cough, dyspnea, yawning
SYST: Asthenia, fever, abrupt withdrawal syndrome

Pharmacokinetics
Absorption	Well absorbed
Distribution	Widely distributed; crosses blood-brain barrier, protein-binding 95%
Metabolism	Liver, mostly by CYP2D6 enzyme system
Excretion	Kidneys, unchanged (2%); breast milk
Half-life	21 hr (reg rel); 15-20 hr (cont rel)

Pharmacodynamics
Onset	Unknown
Peak	5.2 hr
Duration	Unknown

INTERACTIONS
Individual drugs
Methylphenidate, traMADol: increased serotonin syndrome
Cimetidine: increased PARoxetine levels
Digoxin: decreased effect of digoxin
L-tryptophan: increased agitation
PHENobarbital: decreased PARoxetine levels
Phenytoin: decreased effect of PARoxetine
⚠ **Pimozide: potentially fatal reactions**
Theophylline: increased theophylline levels
⚠ **Thioridazine: do not use with PARoxetine; hypertensive crisis, seizures, potentially fatal reactions can occur**
Warfarin: increased bleeding

Drug classifications
CYP2D6 inhibitors (aprepitant, delavirdine, imatinib, nefazodone): increased toxicity
Highly protein-bound products: increased side effects
⚠ **MAOIs: hypertensive crisis, seizures; do not use together; potentially fatal reactions can occur**
SSRIs, SNRIs, atypical antipsychotics, serotonin-receptor agonists, tricyclics, amphetamines: increased serotonin syndrome
NSAIDs, thrombolytics, salicylates, platelet inhibitors, anticoagulants: increased bleeding

Drug/herb
Ephedra: hypertensive crisis
Kava: avoid use

P

Adverse effects: *italics* = common; **bold** = life-threatening

St. John's wort: possible serotonin syndrome, avoid use

NURSING CONSIDERATIONS
Assessment

> **BLACK BOX WARNING: Depression/OCD/ anxiety/panic attacks:** assess mental status: mood, sensorium, affect, suicidal tendencies (especially in child/young adult), increase in psychiatric symptoms, increasing obsessive thoughts, compulsive behaviors, restrict amount available

• **Postural hypotension:** monitor B/P (lying/ standing), pulse q4hr; if systolic B/P drops 20 mm Hg, hold product, notify prescriber; take vital signs q4hr in patients with CV disease
• **Renal status:** monitor BUN, creatinine, urinary retention
• **Withdrawal symptoms:** assess for headache, nausea, vomiting, muscle pain, weakness; not usual unless product discontinued abruptly, taper over 1-2 wk
⚠ **Serotonin, neuroleptic malignant syndrome: assess for hallucinations, coma, headache, agitation, shivering/sweating, tachycardia, diarrhea, tremor, hypertension, hyperthermia, rigidity, delirium, coma, myoclonus, agitation, nausea, vomiting**
• Monitor blood studies: CBC, leukocytes, differential, cardiac enzymes if patient is receiving long-term therapy
• Monitor hepatic studies: AST, ALT, bilirubin
• Check weight weekly; appetite may increase with product
• Assess ECG for flattening of T-wave, bundle branch block, AV block, dysrhythmias in cardiac patients
• Assess for EPS primarily in geriatric: rigidity, dystonia, akathisia
• Monitor urinary retention, constipation; constipation is more likely to occur in children or geriatric
• Identify alcohol consumption; if alcohol is consumed, hold dose until AM

Patient/family education
• Advise patient that therapeutic effects may take 1-4 wk
• Teach patient to use caution in driving and other activities requiring alertness because of drowsiness, dizziness, blurred vision; to avoid rising quickly from sitting to standing, especially geriatric
• Caution patient to avoid alcohol ingestion, other CNS depressants, and OTC medication unless prescribed

• Caution patient not to discontinue medication quickly after long-term use; may cause nausea, anxiety, headache, malaise; do not double doses if one is missed
• Advise patient to use gum, hard sugarless candy, or frequent sips of water for dry mouth; if dry mouth continues an artificial saliva product may be used

> **BLACK BOX WARNING:** Advise patient that depression may worsen, suicidal thoughts/ behavior may occur (especially in child/young adult), to notify prescriber

• Advise patient to discuss sexual side effects: impotence, possible male infertility while taking this product

Evaluation
Positive therapeutic outcome
• Decrease in depression
• Absence of suicidal thoughts

TREATMENT OF OVERDOSE:
Activated charcoal, gastric lavage, maintain airway; for seizures give diazepam, symptomatic treatment

---

pazopanib
(paz-oh'pa-nib)
Votrient
Func. class.: Antineoplastic biologic response modifier/multikinase angiogenesis inhibitor
Chem. class.: Signal transduction inhibitor (STI)
Pregnancy category D

ACTION: Targets vascular endothelial growth factor receptors; a multikinase angiogenesis inhibitor

Therapeutic outcome: Decrease in size, spread of tumor

USES: Advanced renal cell carcinoma; soft-tissue sarcoma patients who have received prior chemotherapy

CONTRAINDICATIONS:
Pregnancy (D), hypothyroidism, QT prolongation, MI, wound dehiscence, hypertension

Precautions: Breastfeeding, children, cardiac/renal/hepatic/dental disease, GI bleeding

> **BLACK BOX WARNING:** Hepatic disease

DOSAGE AND ROUTES

Adult: **PO** 800 mg/day without food (1 hr before, 2 hr after a meal), may decrease to 400 mg/day if not tolerated (renal cell cancer); or adjust in 200-mg increments based on toxicity (soft-tissue sarcoma)

Available forms: Tabs 200 mg

Implementation
• Give on an empty stomach (1 hr before or 2 hr after a meal); separate doses by 24 hr
• Do not crush tablets, can lead to an increased rate of absorption, which can affect systemic exposure; only intact, whole tablets should be used
• If a dose is missed, it should not be taken if it is ≤12 hr until the next dose
• Store at 77°F (25°C)

ADVERSE EFFECTS

CNS: Intracranial bleeding, headache
CV: **Heart failure,** hypertension, **hypertensive crisis,** chest pain, **MI, QT prolongation, torsades de pointes**
GI: Nausea, **hepatotoxicity,** vomiting, dyspepsia, GI hemorrhage, anorexia, abdominal pain, **GI perforation, pancreatitis,** diarrhea
HEMA: **Neutropenia, thrombocytopenia, bleeding**
INTEG: Rash, alopecia
MISC: Fatigue, epistaxis, pyrexia, hot sweats, increased weight, flulike symptoms, hypothyroidism, **hand–foot syndrome**

Pharmacokinetics

Absorption	Unknown
Distribution	Protein binding 99%
Metabolism	Unknown
Excretion	Unknown
Half-life	Unknown

Pharmacodynamics

Onset	Unknown
Peak	Unknown
Duration	Unknown

INTERACTIONS

Individual drugs
Arsenic trioxide, levomethadyl, haloperidol, chloroquine, droperidol, pentamidine: increased QT prolongation, pazopanib concentrations
Simvastin: increased plasma concentrations of this agent

Warfarin: avoid use with warfarin; use low-molecular-weight anticoagulants instead; increased plasma concentration of warfarin

Drug classifications
Class IA/III antidysrhythmics, some phenothiazines, Beta-agonists, local anesthetics, tricyclics, CYP3A4 inhibitors (amiodarone, clarithromycin, erythromycin, telithromycin, ketoconazole, troleandomycin); CYP3A4 substrates (methadone, pimozide, QUEtiapine, quiNIDine, risperiDONE, ziprasidone): increased QT prolongation, increased pazopanib concentrations
Calcium-channel blockers, ergots: increased plasma concentrations of these agents
CYP3A4 inducers (dexamethasone, phenytoin, carBAMazepine, rifampin, PHENobarbital): decreased pazopanib concentrations

Drug/food
Grapefruit juice: avoid use; increased prazopanib effect

Drug/herb
St. John's wort: decreased pazopanib concentration

NURSING CONSIDERATIONS

Assessment

> **BLACK BOX WARNING:** Hepatic disease: fatal hepatotoxicity can occur; obtain LFTs baseline and at least every 2 wk × 2 mo, then monthly

> **BLACK BOX WARNING:** Fatal bleeding: from GI, respiratory, GU tracts, permanently discontinue in those with severe bleeding

⚠ **Palmar-plantar erythrodysesthesia (hand–foot syndrome): more common in those previously treated; assess for swelling, numbness, desquamation on palms and soles**
⚠ **GI perforation/fistula: discontinue if this occurs, assess for pain in epigastric area, dyspepsia, flatulence, fever, chills**
⚠ **Hypertension/hypertensive crisis: hypertension usually occurs in the first cycle; in those with preexisting hypertension, do not start treatment until B/P is controlled; monitor B/P every wk × 6 wk, then at start of each cycle or more often if needed, temporarily or permanently discontinue for severe uncontrolled hypertension**

Patient/family education
• Advise patient to report adverse reactions immediately: bleeding
• Teach patient about reason for treatment, expected results
• Inform patient that effect on male fertility is unknown

Evaluation
Positive therapeutic outcome
• Decrease in size, spread of tumor

pegaptanib (Rx)
(peg-ap′ta-nib)
Macugen
Func. class: Ophthalmic agent—miscellaneous
Pregnancy category B

ACTION: Binds to vascular endothelial growth factor (VEGF), thereby inhibiting angiogenesis

Therapeutic outcome: Stabilization of vision in macular degeneration

USES: Treatment of neovascular (wet) age-related macular degeneration; may be used alone or with photodynamic therapy (PDT)

CONTRAINDICATIONS:
Hypersensitivity, ocular or periocular infections

Precautions: Pregnancy **B**, inflammatory eye disease, ocular hypertension

DOSAGE AND ROUTES
Adult: Intravitreal inj 0.3 mg inj q6wk

Available forms: Inj 0.3 mg, single glass syringes

Implementation
• Administer anesthesia and a broad-spectrum antiinfective prior to injection
• The inj should be done under aseptic conditions
• Remove all air bubbles prior to use
• Store at 36°-46° F, do not freeze or shake vigorously

ADVERSE EFFECTS
EENT: *Anterior chamber inflammation, blurred vision, conjunctival hemorrhage, corneal edema, cataract, eye discharge, eye pain, increased intraocular pressure, punctate keratitis, reduced visual acuity, vitreous floaters, vitreous opacities, blepharitis, conjunctivitis, photophobia,* retinal detachment, iatrogenic traumatic cataract

Pharmacokinetics
Absorption	Unknown
Distribution	Unknown
Metabolism	Unknown
Excretion	Unknown
Half-life	87-100 hr in vitreous humor of the monkey

Pharmacodynamics
Onset	Unknown
Peak	Unknown
Duration	May remain fully active in the eye for 7-28 days

NURSING CONSIDERATIONS
Assessment
• Test visual acuity periodically
• Assess treated eye for increased intraocular pressure, infection, endophthalmitis
• Monitor perfusion of the optic nerve head immediately after injection, tonometry ½ hr after inj, biomicroscopy 2-7 days after inj

Patient/family education
• Instruct patient to report any inflammation, bleeding, eye discharge, opacities to prescriber
• Instruct patient to continue with follow-up care during treatment

Evaluation
Positive therapeutic outcome
• Macular degeneration stabilized

pegfilgrastim (Rx)
(peg-fill-grass′stim)
Neulasta
Func. class.: Hematopoietic agent
Pregnancy category C

ACTION: Stimulates proliferation and differentiation of neutrophils

Therapeutic outcome: Absence of infection

USES: To decrease infection in patients receiving antineoplastics that are myelosuppressive; to increase WBC in patients with product-induced neutropenia

CONTRAINDICATIONS:
Hypersensitivity to proteins of *E. coli,* filgrastim

Precautions: Pregnancy **C**, breastfeeding, child <45 kg, adolescents, myeloid malignancies, sickle cell disease, leukocytosis, splenic rupture, allergic-type reactions, ARDS, peripheral blood stem cell mobilization (PBSC)

DOSAGE AND ROUTES
Adult: SUBCUT 6 mg give once per chemotherapy cycle

Available forms: Sol for inj 10 mg/0.6 ml

Implementation
SUBCUT route
• Give using single-use vials; after dose is withdrawn, do not reenter vial
• Do not use 6-mg fixed dose in infants, children, or others <45 kg
• Inspect sol for discoloration, particulates; if present, do not use
• Do not administer in the period 14 days before and 24 hr after cytotoxic chemotherapy
• Store in refrigerator; do not freeze; may store at room temp up to 6 hr, avoid shaking, protect from light

ADVERSE EFFECTS
CNS: Fever, fatigue, headache, dizziness, insomnia, peripheral edema
GI: *Nausea*, vomiting, diarrhea, mucositis, anorexia, constipation, dyspepsia, abdominal pain, stomatitis, **splenic rupture**
HEMA: Leukocytosis, granulocytopenia, sickle cell crisis, hemoglobin S disease with crisis
INTEG: Alopecia
MISC: Chest pain, hyperuricemia, **anaphylaxis, flulike syndrome, angioedema, antibody formation**
MS: Skeletal pain
RESP: Respiratory distress syndrome

Pharmacokinetics

Absorption	Unknown
Distribution	Unknown
Metabolism	Unknown
Excretion	Unknown
Half-life	15-80 hr; 20-38 hr (child)

Pharmacodynamics
Unknown

INTERACTIONS
Individual drug
Lithium: increased release of neutrophils

Drug classifications
Cytotoxic chemotherapy agents: do not use this product concomitantly or 2 wk before or 24 hr after administration of cytotoxics

Drug/lab test
Increased: uric acid, LDH, alkaline phosphatase

NURSING CONSIDERATIONS
Assessment
• **Assess for allergic reactions, anaphylaxis:** rash, urticaria; discontinue this product, have emergency equipment nearby
• Monitor blood studies: CBC, platelet count before treatment and twice weekly; neutrophil counts may be increased for 2 days after therapy
• **ARDS:** assess for dyspnea, fever, tachypnea, occasional confusion; obtain ABGs, chest x-ray, product may need to be discontinued
• Monitor B/P, respirations, pulse before, during therapy
• **Assess for bone pain,** give mild analgesics

Patient/family education
• Teach the technique for self-administration: dose, side effects, disposal of containers and needles; provide instruction sheet

Evaluation
Positive therapeutic outcome
• Absence of infection

⚠ HIGH ALERT

PEMEtrexed (Rx)
(pem-ah-trex′ed)
Alimta
Func. class.: Antineoplastic-antimetabolite
Chem. class.: Folic acid antagonist
Pregnancy category D

ACTION: Inhibits multiple enzymes that reduce folic acid, which is needed for cell replication

Therapeutic outcome: Decreased spread of mesothelioma, decreased tumor size

USES: Malignant pleural mesothelioma in combination with CISplatin; non–small cell lung cancer as a single agent; non-squamous non–small cell lung cancer (first-line treatment)

CONTRAINDICATIONS:
Pregnancy **D**, hypersensitivity, ANC <1500 cells/mm^3, CCr <45 ml/min, thrombocytopenia (<100,000/mm^3), anemia

Adverse effects: *italics* = common; **bold** = life-threatening

Precautions: Breastfeeding, children, renal/hepatic disease

DOSAGE AND ROUTES
Adult: **IV** INF 500-600 mg/m² given over 10 min on day 1 of a 21-day cycle with CISplatin 75 mg/m² INF over 2 hr beginning ½ hr after end of PEMEtrexed INF

Renal dose
Adult: IV infusion CCr <45 ml/min, not recommended

Available forms: Inj, single-use vials, 100, 500 mg

Implementation
• Administer vit B_{12} and low-dose folic acid as a prophylactic measure to treat related hematologic, GI toxicity; at least 5 daily doses of folic acid must be taken in the 7 days preceding first dose
• Premedicate with a corticosteroid (dexamethasone) given PO bid the day before, day of, and day after administration of PEMEtrexed
• **Neurotoxicity:** assess for CTC grade 2: withhold until resolution to at least pretherapy value/condition, reduce CISplatin by 50%; CTC grade 3/4; immediately discontinue this product and CISplatin if given in combination
• **Mucositis:** assess for CTC 3-4; withhold until resolution to at least pretherapy value/condition, reduce dose by 50%, if grade 3-4 occurs after 2 dosage reductions, discontinue this product and CISplatin
• **Bleeding:** assess for bleeding time, coagulation time during treatment; bleeding; hematuria, guaiac, brusing or petechiae, mucosa or orifices q8hr
• Use a liquid diet: carbonated beverage, gelatin; dry toast, crackers may be added when patient is not nauseated or vomiting
• Assist patient with rinsing of mouth tid-qid with water, club soda; brushing of teeth bid-tid with soft brush or cotton-tipped applicators for stomatitis; use unwaxed dental floss

IV route
• Use cytotoxic handling procedures
• Reconstitute 500-mg vial/20 ml 0.9% NaCl inj (preservative free) = 25 mg/ml, swirl until dissolved, further dilute with 100 ml 0.9% NaCl inj (preservative free), give as IV inf over 10 min
• Use only 0.9% NaCl inj (preservative free) for reconstitution, dilution
• Store at 77° F, excursions permitted 59°-86°F, not light sensitive, discard unused portions

Dosage adjustments
Do not begin a new cycle unless neutrophils (ANC) ≥1500 cells/mm³, platelets ≥100,000 cells/mm³, CCr is ≥45 ml/min
• **Platelet nadir <50,000/mm³ regardless of the ANC:** If necessary, delay until platelet count recovery, reduce PEMEtrexed and CISplatin, by 50%; if grade 3/4 toxicity occurs after 2 reductions, discontinue both products
• **ANC nadir <500/mm³ when platelet nadir is ≥50,000/mm³:** If necessary, delay until ANC recovery, reduce PEMEtrexed and CISplatin, by 75%; if grade 3/4 toxicity occurs after 2 reductions, discontinue both products
• **CTC Grade 3/4 nonhematologic toxicity including diarrhea requiring hospitalization and excluding neurotoxicity, mucositis, and grade 3 transaminase elevations:** Withhold therapy until pre-therapy value or condition, reduce by 75% both products, if grade 3 or 4 toxicity occurs after 2 reductions, discontinue both products
• **CTC grade 3/4 mucositis:** Withhold therapy until pre-therapy condition, reduce 50% of PEMEtrexed, if grade 3 or 4 mucositis occurs after 2 dosage reductions, discontinue both products
• **CTC grade 2 neurotoxicity:** Withhold therapy until pre-therapy value or condition, reduce dose of CISplatin by 50%
• **CTC grade 3/4 neurotoxicity:** discontinue both products

Y-site compatibilities: Acyclovir sodium, alfentanil, allopurinol, amifostine, amikacin, aminocaproic acid, aminophylline, amiodarone, amphotericin B lipid complex, amphotericin B liposome, ampicillin, ampicillin-sulbactam, atenolol, atracurium, azithromycin, aztreonam, bivalirudin, bleomycin, bumetanide, buprenorphine, butorphanol, CARBOplatin, carmustine, ceftizoxime, cefTRIAXone, cefuroxime, cimetidine, cisatracurium, CISplatin, clindamycin, cyclophosphamide, cycloSPORINE, cytarabine, DACTINomycin, DAPTOmycin, dexamethasone, digoxin, diltiazem, diphenhydrAMINE, DOCEtaxel, dolasetron, DOPamine, doxacurium, enalaprilat, ePHEDrine, EPINEPHrine, eptifibatide, ertapenem, esmolol, etoposide, famotidine, fenoldopam, fentaNYL, fluconazole, fludarabine, fluorouracil, foscarnet, fosphenytoin, furosemide, ganciclovir, gatifloxacin, glycopyrrolate, granisetron, haloperidol, heparin, hydrocortisone, HYDROmorphone, hydrOXYzine, ifosfamide, imipenem-cilastatin, insulin (regular), isoproterenol, ketorolac, labetalol, leucovorin, levofloxacin, lidocaine, linezolid,

LORazepam, magnesium, mannitol, meperidine, meropenem, mesna, methyldopate, methyl-PREDNISolone, metoclopramide, metoprolol, midazolam, milrinone, mitoMYcin, mivacurium, morphine, moxifloxacin, nafcillin, naloxone, nesiritide, nitroglycerin, norepinephrine, octreotide, oxaliplatin, PACLitaxel, pamidronate, pancuronium, PENTobarbital, PHENobarbital, piperacillin-tazobactam, polymyxin B, potassium chloride/phosphates, procainamide, promethazine, propranolol, ranitidine, remifentanil, rocuronium, sodium acetate/bicarbonate/phosphates, succinylcholine, SUFentanil, sulfamethoxazole-trimethoprim, tacrolimus, theophylline, thiopental, thiotepa, ticarcillin, ticarcillin-clavulanate, tigecycline, tirofiban, trimethobenzamide, vancomycin, vecuronium, verapamil, vinBLAStine, vinCRIStine, vinorelbine, zidovudine, zoledronic acid

ADVERSE EFFECTS

CNS: *Fatigue, fever, mood alteration, neuropathy*
CV: Thrombosis/embolism, *chest pain,* arrhythmia exacerbation
GI: *Nausea, vomiting, anorexia, diarrhea, ulcerative stomatitis, constipation, dysphagia, dehydration*
GU: Renal failure, *creatinine elevation*
HEMA: Neutropenia, leukopenia, thrombocytopenia, myelosuppression, anemia
INTEG: *Rash, desquamation*
RESP: *Dyspnea*
SYST: Infection with/without neutropenia, radiation recall reaction

Pharmacokinetics

Absorption	Unknown
Distribution	81% protein binding
Metabolism	Not metabolized
Excretion	Excreted in urine (unchanged 70%-90%) Not known if it is excreted in breast milk
Half-life	3.5 hr

Pharmacodynamics

Unknown

INTERACTIONS

Drug classifications

Anticoagulants, NSAIDs, platelet inhibitors, salicylates, thrombolytics: increased bleeding risk
Nephrotoxic products (NSAIDs): decreased PEMEtrexed clearance

NURSING CONSIDERATIONS

Assessment

⚠ Bone marrow depression: monitor CBC, differential, platelet count; monitor for nadir and recovery; a new cycle should not begin if ANC < 1500 cells/mm³, platelets are < 100,000 cells/mm³, creatinine clearance < 45 ml/min
• Monitor renal tests: BUN, serum uric acid, urine CCr, electrolytes before, during therapy
• For previous radiation treatments; radiation recall reactions have occurred (erythema, exfoliative dermatitis, pain, burning)
• Monitor I&O ratio; report fall in urine output to <30 ml/hr
• Monitor temp q4hr; fever may indicate beginning infection; no rectal temps
• Assess bleeding time, coagulation time during treatment; bleeding: hematuria, guaiac, bruising or petechiae, mucosa or orifices q8hr
• Assess buccal cavity q8hr for dryness, sores, ulceration, white patches, oral pain, bleeding, dysphagia
⚠ Assess for symptoms indicating severe allergic reaction/toxic epidermal necrolysis: rash, urticaria, itching, flushing
• **Neurotoxicity:** CTC grade 2: withhold until resolution to at least pretherapy value/condition; reduce CISplatin by 50%; CTC grade 3-4; immediately discontinue product and CISplatin if given in combination
• **Mucositis:** CTC grade 3-4: withhold until resolution to at least pretherapy value/condition; reduce dose by 50%; if grade 3-4 occurs after 2 dosage reductions, discontinue product and CISplatin

Patient/family education

• Instruct patient to report any complaints, side effects to nurse or prescriber: black tarry stools, chills, fever, sore throat, bleeding, bruising, cough, shortness of breath, dark or bloody urine
• Instruct patient to avoid foods with citric acid, hot or rough texture if stomatitis is present
• Instruct patient to report stomatitis: any bleeding, white spots, ulcerations in mouth to prescriber; tell patient to examine mouth daily, report symptoms to nurse, use good oral hygiene
• Advise patient that contraceptive measures are recommended during therapy and for at least 8 wk following cessation of therapy, to discontinue breastfeeding; toxicity to infant may occur
• Advise patient to avoid alcohol, salicylates, live vaccines

- Advise patient to avoid use of razors, commercial mouthwash
- Teach to eat foods high in folic acid and take supplements as prescribed

Evaluation
Positive therapeutic outcome
- Decreased spread of malignancy

penciclovir topical
See Appendix B

PENICILLINS
penicillin G benzathine (Rx)
(pen-i-sill'in)
Bicillin L-A
penicillin G (Rx)
Pfizerpen
penicillin G procaine (Rx)
penicillin V (Rx)
Apo-Pen-VK ❖, Penicillin VK
Func. class.: Broad-spectrum antiinfective
Chem. class.: Natural penicillin
Pregnancy category B

ACTION: Interferes with cell wall replication of susceptible organisms; osmotically unstable cell wall swells and bursts from osmotic pressure, resulting in cell death

Therapeutic outcome: Bactericidal effects on the gram-positive cocci *Staphylococcus, Streptococcus pyogenes, Streptococcus viridans, Streptococcus faecalis, Streptococcus bovis, Streptococcus pneumoniae;* gram-negative cocci *Neisseria gonorrhoeae;* gram-positive bacilli *Actinomyces, Bacillus anthracis, Clostridium perfringens, Clostridium tetani, Corynebacterium diphtheriae, Listeria monocytogenes;* gram-negative bacilli *Escherichia coli, Proteus mirabilis, Salmonella, Shigella, Enterobacter, Streptobacillus moniliformis;* spirochete *Treponema pallidum*

USES: Respiratory tract infections, scarlet fever, erysipelas, otitis media, pneumonia, skin and soft tissue infections, gonorrhea

CONTRAINDICATIONS:
Hypersensitivity to penicillins, corn

Precautions: Pregnancy **B**, breastfeeding, hypersensitivity to cephalosporins/carbapenem/sulfite, severe renal disease, GI disease, asthma

DOSAGE AND ROUTES
Penicillin G benzathine
Early syphilis
Adult: IM 2.4 million units in single dose
Congenital syphilis
Child <2 yr: IM 50,000 units/kg in single dose, max 2.4 million units as a single inj
Prophylaxis of rheumatic fever, glomerulonephritis
Adult and child: IM 1.2 million units in single dose
Upper respiratory tract infections (group A streptococcal)
Adult: IM 1.2 million units in single dose
Child >27 kg: IM 900,000 units in single dose
Child <27 kg: IM 300,000-600,000 units in single dose

Available forms: Inj 300,000 units/ml; 600,000 units/ml

Penicillin G
Pneumococcal/streptococcal infections (serious)
Adult: IM/IV 5-24 million units in divided doses q4-6hr
Child <12 yr: IV 150,000-300,000 units/kg/day in 4-6 divided doses; max 24 million units/day
Renal dose
CCr <10 ml/min, give full loading dose, then ½ of loading dose q8-10hr

Available forms: Inj 1, 2, 3 million units/50 ml; powder for inj 1, 5, 20 million units/vial

Penicillin G procaine
Moderate to severe pneumococcal infections
Adult and child: IM 600,000-1.2 million units in 1 or 2 doses/day for 10 days to 2 wk
Newborn: Avoid use in newborns
Pneumococcal pneumonia
Adult and child >12 yr: IM 600,000-1.2 million units/day × 7-10 days

Available forms: Inj 600,000, 1,200,000 units/dose

Moderately severe group A streptococcal/staphylococcal pneumonia
Adult, adolescent, child ≥60 lb: IM 600,000-1 million units/day
Adolescent and child <60 lb: IM 300,000 units/day

🅰 Nurse Alert   🅺 Key NCLEX® Drug

Penicillin V

Pneumococcal/staphylococcal infections

Adult: PO 250-500 mg q6hr
Child <12 yr/adolescent/child >12 yr: PO 25-50 mg/kg/day in divided doses q6-8hr, max 3 g/day

Streptococcal infections

Adult/adolescent/child >12 yr: PO 125 mg q6-8hr × 10 days
Child <12 yr and >27 kg: PO 500 mg q8hr or 12hr × 10 days
Child <12 yr and ≤27 kg: PO 250 mg q8hr or q12hr or 40 mg/kg/day in 3 divided doses × 10 days

Prevention of recurrence of rheumatic fever/chorea

Adult: PO 125-250 mg bid continuously

Vincent's gingivitis/pharyngitis

Adult: PO 250 mg q6-8hr

Renal dose

CCr <50 ml/min dosage reduction indicated based on clinical response, degree of impairment

Available forms: Tabs 250, 500 mg; powder for oral sol 125, 250 mg/5 ml

Implementation

Penicillin G benzathine

IM route
• No dilution needed, shake well, give deeply IM in large muscle mass, avoid intravascular inj; aspirate; do not give **IV**

Penicillin G

• Penicillin G sodium or potassium can be given IM or IV, vials containing 10 or 20 million units are not for IM use

Intermittent IV infusion route
• Vials/bulk packages; dilute according to manufacturer's directions
• Frozen bags: thaw at room temp, do not force thaw, no reconstitution needed
• Final conc (100,000-500,000 units/ml, adults; 50,000 units/ml, neonate/infant)
• Total daily dose divided q4-6hr and given over 1-2 hr (adult), 15 min (infant/neonate)

Penicillin G potassium

Y-site compatibilities: Acyclovir, amiodarone, cyclophosphamide, diltiazem, enalaprilat, esmolol, fluconazole, foscarnet, heparin, HYDROmorphone, labetalol, magnesium sulfate, meperidine, morphine, perphenazine, potassium chloride, tacrolimus, theophylline, verapamil, vit B/C

Penicillin G procaine

• No dilution needed, give deep IM inj; avoid intravascular inj; aspirate; do not give IV
• Do not give **IV**
• Give deeply in large muscle mass
• Reconstitute with 0.9% NaCl, sterile water for inj, D_5W; refrigerate unused portion
• Shake medication before administering
• IM route may include procaine reactions: fear of death, depression, seizures, anxiety, confusion, hallucinations

Penicillin V

• Orally on empty stomach for best absorption
• Oral susp: tap bottle to loosen, add ½ total amount of water, shake, add remaining water, shake; final conc (125 or 250); store in refrigerator after reconstitution, discard after 14 days
• Give in even doses around the clock; if GI upset occurs, give with food; product must be given for 10-14 days to ensure organism death and prevent superinfection; store in tight container
• Shake susp; store in refrigerator for 2 wk or for 1 wk at room temperature

ADVERSE EFFECTS

CNS: Lethargy, hallucinations, anxiety, depression, twitching, **coma, seizures,** hyperreflexia
GI: *Nausea, vomiting, diarrhea,* increased AST, ALT, abdominal pain, glossitis, colitis, **pseudomembranous colitis**
GU: **Oliguria, proteinuria, hematuria,** *vaginitis, moniliasis,* **glomerulonephritis,** renal tubular damage
HEMA: Anemia, increased bleeding time, **bone marrow depression, granulocytopenia,** hemolytic anemia
META: Hyperkalemia, hypokalemia, alkalosis, hypernatremia
MISC: Local pain, tenderness and fever with IM inj, **anaphylaxis serum sickness, Stevens-Johnson syndrome**

Penicillin G benzathine

Pharmacokinetics

Absorption	Delayed; prolonged drug levels
Distribution	Widely distributed; crosses placenta
Metabolism	Liver, minimally
Excretion	Kidneys, unchanged; breast milk
Half-life	½-1 hr

Adverse effects: *italics* = common; **bold** = life-threatening

Pharmacodynamics

Onset	Slow
Peak	12-24 hr
Duration	1-4 wk

Pharmacokinetics

Absorption	Variably absorbed (PO); well absorbed (IM)
Distribution	Widely distributed; crosses placenta
Metabolism	Liver, minimally
Excretion	Kidneys, unchanged; breast milk
Half-life	½-1 hr

Pharmacodynamics

	PO	IM	IV
Onset	Rapid	Rapid	Rapid
Peak	1 hr	¼-½ hr	Immediate
Duration	Unknown	Unknown	Unknown

Pharmacokinetics

Absorption	Delayed; prolonged drug levels
Distribution	Widely distributed; crosses placenta
Metabolism	Liver, minimally
Excretion	Kidneys, unchanged; breast milk
Half-life	½-1 hr

Pharmacodynamics

Onset	Slow
Peak	1-4 hr
Duration	15 hr

Pharmacokinetics

Absorption	Widely absorbed
Distribution	Widely distributed; crosses placenta
Metabolism	Liver, minimally
Excretion	Kidneys, unchanged; breast milk
Half-life	½-1 hr

Pharmacodynamics

Onset	Rapid
Peak	½ hr
Duration	Unknown

INTERACTIONS
Individual drugs
Aspirin, probenecid: increased penicillin levels
Heparin: increased effect of heparin
Methotrexate: increased effect of methotrexate
Typhoid vaccine: decreased effect of toxoid vaccine

Drug classifications
Contraceptives (oral): decreased contraceptive effectiveness
Tetracyclines: decreased antimicrobial effectiveness of penicillin

Drug/lab test
False positive: urine glucose, urine protein

NURSING CONSIDERATIONS
Assessment
• Assess patient for previous sensitivity reaction to penicillins or cephalosporins; cross-sensitivity between penicillins and cephalosporins is common
• **Assess patient for signs and symptoms of infection** including characteristics of wounds, sputum, urine, stool, WBC >10,000/mm^3, earache, fever; obtain information baseline, during treatment
• Obtain C&S before beginning drug therapy to identify if correct treatment has been initiated
⚠ Assess for allergic reactions: rash, urticaria, pruritus, chills, fever, joint pain; angioedema may occur a few days after therapy begins; epinephrine, resuscitation equipment should be available for anaphylactic reaction
⚠ Pseudomembranous colitis: Assess for diarrhea, abdominal pain, fever, fatigue, anorexia; possible anemia, elevated WBC and low serum albumin; stop product and usually give either vancomycin or IV metroNIDAZOLE
⚠ Identify urine output; if decreasing, notify prescriber (may indicate nephrotoxicity); also check for increased BUN, creatinine
• Monitor blood studies: AST, ALT, CBC, Hct, bilirubin, LDH, alkaline phosphatase, Coombs' test monthly if patient is on long-term therapy
• Monitor electrolytes: potassium, sodium, chloride monthly if patient is on long-term therapy

• Assess bowel pattern daily; if severe diarrhea occurs, product should be discontinued; may indicate pseudomembranous colitis
• Monitor for bleeding: ecchymosis, bleeding gums, hematuria, stool guaiac daily if on long-term therapy
• **Assess for overgrowth of infection:** perineal itching, fever, malaise, redness, pain, swelling, drainage, rash, diarrhea, change in cough, sputum

Patient/family education
• Teach patient to report sore throat, bruising, bleeding, joint pain; may indicate **blood dyscrasias (rare)**
• Advise patient to contact prescriber if vaginal itching, loose foul-smelling stools, furry tongue occur; may indicate **superinfection**
• Instruct patient to take all medication prescribed for the length of time ordered
• Advise patient to notify prescriber of diarrhea with blood or pus, which may indicate **pseudomembranous colitis**

Evaluation
Positive therapeutic outcome
• Absence of signs/symptoms of infection (WBC <10,000/mm^3, temp WNL, absence of red, draining wounds, earache)
• Reported improvement in symptoms of infection

TREATMENT OF ANAPHYLAXIS:
Withdraw product, maintain airway, administer EPINEPHrine, aminophylline, O$_2$, **IV** corticosteroids

pentamidine (Rx)
(pen-tam′i-deen)
Nebupent, Pentam 300
Func. class.: Antiprotozoal
Chem. class.: Aromatic diamide derivative
Pregnancy category C

ACTION: Interferes with DNA/RNA synthesis in protozoa; has direct effect on islet cells in the pancreas

Therapeutic outcome: Protozoa death

USES: Treatment/prevention of *Pneumocystis jiroveci* infections

Unlabeled uses: Leishmaniasis, African trypanosomiasis

CONTRAINDICATIONS:
Hypersensitivity

Precautions: Pregnancy **C**, breastfeeding, children, blood dyscrasias, cardiac/renal/hepatic disease, diabetes mellitus, hypocalcemia, hyper/hypotension, anemia

DOSAGE AND ROUTES
Adult and child ≥4 mo: IV/IM 4 mg/kg/day × 2-3 wk; NEB 300 mg via specific nebulizer given q4wk for prevention

Available forms: Inj; aerosol 300 mg/vial; sol for aerosol 60 mg/vial ♣

Implementation
Inhalation route
• Through nebulizer, using Raspirgard II jet nebulizer; mix contents in 6 ml of sterile water; do not use low pressure (<20 psi); flow rate should be 5-7 L/min (40-50 psi) air or O$_2$ source over 30-45 min until chamber is empty
IM route
• 300 mg diluted in 3 ml sterile water; give deep IM by Z-track; painful by this route, rotate inj site

Intermittent IV infusion route
• 300 mg/3-5 ml of sterile water for inj, D$_5$W; withdraw dose and further dilute in 50-250 ml of D$_5$W; diluted sol is stable for 48 hr; discard unused sol; give over 1 hr or more

Y-site compatibilities: Alfentanil, atracurium, atropine, benztropine, buprenorphine, calcium gluconate, CARBOplatin, caspofungin, chlorpromazine, cimetidine, CISplatin, cyclophosphamide, cycloSPORINE, cytarabine, DACTINomycin, diltiazem, gatifloxacin, zidovudine

Y-site incompatibilities: Foscarnet, fluconazole

ADVERSE EFFECTS
CNS: Disorientation, hallucinations, dizziness, confusion, drowsiness
CV: Hypotension, ventricular tachycardia, **QT prolongation, dysrhythmias**
GI: *Nausea, vomiting, anorexia,* increased AST, ALT, **acute pancreatitis,** metallic taste
GU: Acute renal failure, increased serum creatinine, renal toxicity, decreased urination
HEMA: Anemia, **leukopenia, thrombocytopenia**
INTEG: Sterile abscess, pain at inj site, pruritus, urticaria, rash
META: Hyperkalemia, hypocalcemia, *hypoglycemia,* hypomagnesemia
MISC: Fatigue, fever, chills, night sweats, **anaphylaxis, Stevens-Johnson syndrome**

P

RESP: Cough, shortness of breath, **broncho-spasm** (with aerosol), sore throat

Pharmacokinetics

Absorption	Well absorbed (IM); minimally absorbed (INH); completely absorbed (**IV**)
Distribution	Widely distributed; does not appear in CSF
Metabolism	Not known
Excretion	Kidneys, unchanged (up to 30%)
Half-life	6½-9½ hr; increased in renal disease

Pharmacodynamics

	IM	IV	INH
Onset	Un-known	Un-known	Un-known
Peak	½-1 hr	Inf end	Un-known
Duration	Un-known	Un-known	Un-known

INTERACTIONS

Individual drugs

Amphotericin B, CISplatin, vancomycin: increased nephrotoxicity

⚠ Erythromycin IV: fatal dysrhythmias

Haloperidol, chloroquine, droperidol, pentamidine; arsenic trioxide, levomethadyl: increased QT prolongation

Radiation: bone marrow suppression

Drug classifications

Aminoglycosides NSAIDs: increased nephrotoxicity

Antineoplastics: increased bone marrow depression

Class IA/III antidysrhythmics, some phenothiazines, β-agonists, local anesthetics, tricyclics, CYP3A4 inhibitors (amiodarone, clarithromycin, erythromycin, telithromycin, troleandomycin), CYP3A4 substrates (methadone, pimozide, QUEtiapine, quiNIDine, risperidone, ziprasidone): increased QT prolongation

Drug/lab test

Decrease: WBC, platelets, Hbg, Hct
Increase: BUN, creatinine

NURSING CONSIDERATIONS

Assessment

⚠ Assess any patient with compromised renal system: product is excreted slowly

in poor renal system function; toxicity may occur rapidly

• **QT prolongation:** ECG for QT prolongation, ejection fraction; assess for chest pain, palpitations, dyspnea

• **Assess patient for infection,** including increased temp, thick sputum, WBC >10,000/mm^3; monitor these signs of infection throughout treatment; obtain C&S before beginning therapy; treatment may begin after culture is obtained

• Assess respiratory system including rate, rhythm, bilateral lung sounds, SOB, wheezing, dyspnea

• Monitor ECG for cardiac dysrhythmias; ECG and pulse should be checked frequently during treatment, since cardiotoxicity can occur

• Assess for hypoglycemia including nausea, tremors, anxiety, chills, diaphoresis, headache, hunger, cold, pale skin; this side effect can last for several mo after treatment is completed

• Monitor for hyperglycemia including flushed, dry skin, acetone breath, thirst, anorexia, drowsiness, polyuria; this side effect can last for several mo after treatment is completed

• Monitor renal function tests including BUN, urinalysis, creatinine; obtain at baseline and frequently during treatment; nephrotoxicity may occur; check I&O, report hematuria, oliguria

• Monitor blood studies including blood glucose, CBC, platelets; blood glucose fluctuations are common; anemia, leukopenia, thrombocytopenia can occur

• Monitor liver function studies including AST, ALT, alkaline phosphatase, bilirubin before beginning treatment and every 3 days during therapy

• Monitor calcium and magnesium before beginning treatment and every 3 days during therapy; hypocalcemia may occur

Patient/family education

• Teach patient to report sore throat, fever, fatigue; could indicate superinfection

• Advise patient not to drink alcohol or take aspirin, since gastric bleeding may occur

• Teach patient to make position changes slowly to prevent orthostatic hypotension

• Advise patient to maintain adequate fluid intake

Evaluation

Positive therapeutic outcome

• Decreased signs and symptoms of protozoan infections

• Decreased signs and symptoms of *P. jiroveci* pneumonia in HIV infections

---

⚠ Nurse Alert   ✴ Key NCLEX® Drug

> ⚠ **HIGH ALERT**

pentazocine (Rx)

(pen-taz′oh-seen)
Talwin, Talwin NX
Func. class.: Opiate analgesic
Chem. class.: Synthetic benzomorphan
(agonist/antagonist)
Pregnancy category C
Controlled substance schedule IV

ACTION: Inhibits ascending pain pathways in limbic system, thalamus, midbrain, hypothalamus by binding to opiate receptor sites, altering pain perception and response

Therapeutic outcome: Relief of pain

USES: Moderate to severe pain

CONTRAINDICATIONS:
Hypersensitivity to this product or sulfites, addiction (opioid)

Precautions: Pregnancy **C**, breastfeeding, child <18 yr, addictive personality, increased ICP, MI (acute), severe heart disease, respiratory depression, renal/hepatic disease, seizure disorder, head trauma, bowel impaction, geriatric patients

DOSAGE AND ROUTES
Adult: IV/IM/SUBCUT 30 mg q3-4hr prn, max 360 mg/day

Labor
Adult: IM 30 mg as a single dose; **IV** 20 mg q2-3hr when contractions are regular, max 2-3 times

Renal dose
Adult: CCr 10-50 ml/min reduce dose by 25%; CCr <10 ml/min reduce dose by 50%

Available forms: Inj 30 mg/ml

Implementation
• Give by inj (IM, **IV**), only when resuscitative equipment available; give slowly to prevent rigidity
• Store in light-resistant area at room temperature

PO route
• Tabs made in the United States contain naloxone 0.5 mg to prevent abuse if the PO preparation is used **IV**

IM/SUBCUT route
• Give IM inj deeply in large muscle mass; rotate inj sites; repeated SUBCUT inj may cause necrosis

Direct IV route
• Give after diluting 5 mg/ml of sterile water for inj; give 5 mg or less over 1 min

Syringe compatibilities: Atropine, benzquinamide, butorphanol, chlorproMAZINE, cimetidine, dimenhyDRINATE, diphenhydrAMINE, droperidol, fentaNYL, HYDROmorphone, hydrOXYzine, meperidine, metoclopramide, morphine, perphenazine, prochlorperazine, promazine, promethazine, propiomazine, ranitidine, scopolamine

Syringe incompatibilities: Glycopyrrolate, heparin, PENTobarbital, other barbiturates

Y-site compatibilities: Heparin, hydrocortisone, potassium chloride, vit B/C

Y-site incompatibilities: Nafcillin

Additive incompatibilities: Aminophylline, amobarbital, PENTobarbital, PHENobarbital, secobarbital, sodium bicarbonate

ADVERSE EFFECTS
CNS: *Drowsiness, dizziness, confusion, headache, sedation, euphoria, hallucinations,* dreaming, insomnia, light-headedness
CV: Palpitations, bradycardia, change in B/P, tachycardia, increased B/P (high doses), hypotension, syncope, flushing
EENT: Tinnitus, blurred vision, miosis, diplopia
GI: *Nausea,* vomiting, anorexia, constipation, cramps, dry mouth
GU: Urinary retention, increased urinary output, dysuria
HEMA: **Eosinophilia, decreased WBC**
INTEG: *Rash,* urticaria, bruising, flushing, diaphoresis, pruritus, severe irritation at inj sites, **Stevens-Johnson syndrome**
RESP: **Respiratory depression**

Pharmacokinetics

Absorption	Well absorbed (PO, SUBCUT, IM); completely absorbed (**IV**)
Distribution	Widely distributed; crosses placenta
Metabolism	Liver, extensively
Excretion	Kidneys, small amounts (unchanged)
Half-life	2-3 hr

P

Pharmacodynamics

	PO	SUB-CUT/ IM	IV
Onset	15-30 min	15-30 min	Rapid
Peak	1-3 hr	1-2 hr	15 min
Duration	3 hr	2-4 hr	1 hr

INTERACTIONS
Individual drugs
Alcohol: increased effects

Drug classifications
Antipsychotics, CNS depressants, sedative-hypnotics, skeletal muscle relaxants: increased effects

MAOIs: use cautiously; results are unpredictable

Opiates: decreased effects

Drug/lab test
Increased: amylase

NURSING CONSIDERATIONS
Assessment
• **Assess pain:** location, intensity, type of pain before, after treatment
• Assess bowel status: constipation; may need stimulant laxative/stool softener
• Monitor VS after parenteral route; note muscle rigidity, product history, liver, kidney function tests, respiratory dysfunction: respiratory depression, character, rate, rhythm; notify prescriber if respirations are <10/min
• Monitor CNS changes: dizziness, drowsiness, hallucinations, euphoria, LOC, pupil reaction
• **Monitor allergic reactions:** rash, urticaria
• Assess for withdrawal symptoms in opiate-dependent patients

Patient/family education
• Teach patient to report any symptoms of CNS changes, allergic reactions
• Advise patients to avoid CNS depressants: alcohol, sedative-hypnotics for at least 24 hr after taking this product
• Discuss with patient that dizziness, drowsiness, and confusion are common; to avoid getting up without assistance
• Discuss in detail all aspects of the product
• Instruct patient to change position slowly to prevent orthostatic hypotension
• Teach patient to turn, cough, breathe deeply after surgery to prevent atelectasis
• Teach patient to avoid operating machinery if drowsiness occurs

Evaluation
Positive therapeutic outcome
• Relief of pain

TREATMENT OF OVERDOSE:
Naloxone (Narcan) 0.2-0.8 mg IV, O$_2$, IV fluids, vasopressors

pentoxifylline (Rx)
(pen-tox-if'i-lin)
Trental
Func. class.: Hemorheologic agent
Chem. class.: Dimethylxanthine derivative
Pregnancy category C

ACTION: Decreases blood viscosity, stimulates prostacyclin formation, increases blood flow by increasing flexibility of RBCs; decreases RBC hyperaggregation; reduces platelet aggregation, decreases fibrinogen concentration

Therapeutic outcome: Decreased claudication and improved blood flow

USES: Intermittent claudication related to chronic occlusive vascular disease

Unlabeled uses: Diabetic neuropathies, sickle cell anemia

CONTRAINDICATIONS:
Hypersensitivity to this product or xanthines, retinal/cerebral hemorrhage

Precautions: Pregnancy **C**, breastfeeding, children, angina pectoris, impaired renal function, recent surgery, peptic ulcer, cardiac/hepatic disease, bleeding disorders

DOSAGE AND ROUTES
Adult: PO 400 mg tid with meals, may decrease to bid if side effects occur, must be taken for ≥8 wk for maximal effect

Available forms: Cont rel tabs 400 mg; ext rel tabs 400 mg

Implementation
• Do not break, crush, or chew cont rel or ext rel tab
• Give with meals to prevent GI upset

ADVERSE EFFECTS
CNS: *Headache,* anxiety, *tremors,* confusion, *dizziness*
GI: *Dyspepsia, nausea, vomiting*

Pharmacokinetics

Absorption	Well absorbed
Distribution	Unknown
Metabolism	Liver, degradation
Excretion	Kidneys
Half-life	½-1 hr

Pharmacodynamics

Onset	Unknown
Peak	2-4 hr
Duration	Unknown

INTERACTIONS

Individual drugs

Abciximab, clopidogrel, eptifibatide, ticlopidine, tirofiban, warfarin: increased bleeding risk

Cimetidine, ciprofloxacin: increased pentoxifyl-line level

Theophylline: increased theophylline level

Drug classifications

Antihypertensives, nitrates: increased hypotension

Thrombin inhibitors: increased bleeding risk

NURSING CONSIDERATIONS

Assessment

• Monitor B/P, respirations in patient taking antihypertensives

• Assess for intermittent claudication baseline, during treatment

• Monitor blood tests: pro-time, Hgb, Hct in patients at risk for hemorrhage

Patient/family education

• Teach patient that therapeutic response may take 2-4 wk

• Instruct patient to observe feet for arterial insufficiency

• Instruct patient to use cotton socks, well-fitted shoes; not to go barefoot

• Advise patient to watch for bleeding, bruises, petechiae, epistaxis

• Advise that there are many drug, herb interactions

Evaluation

Positive therapeutic outcome

• Decreased pain, cramping

• Increased ambulation

perampanel
(per-am′pa-nel)
Fycompa
Func. class.: Anticonvulsant
Pregnancy category C

ACTION: A noncompetitive AMPA-selective receptor antagonist; inhibits calcium influx

Therapeutic outcome: Decreased seizure activity

USES: Partial-onset seizures with/without secondary generalization

CONTRAINDICATIONS:
Hypersensitivity

Precautions: Pregnancy (C), breastfeeding, children <12 yr, geriatric patients, abrupt discontinuation, depression, liver disease, kidney disease, substance abuse, suicidal ideation, driving or operating machinery

> **BLACK BOX WARNING:** Bipolar disorder, psychosis, schizophrenia

DOSAGE AND ROUTES
Adult/adolescent/child <12 yr receiving enzyme-inducing AEDs: PO 4 mg/day at bedtime, increase dosage every wk by 2 mg/day to 4-12 mg/day at bedtime

Adult/adolescent/child ≥12 yr not receiving AEDs: PO 2 mg/day at bedtime, increase dosage every wk by 2 mg/day up to 4-8 mg/day at bedtime

Available forms: Tabs 2, 4, 6, 8, 10, 12 mg

Implementation
• Store at room temperature away from light

ADVERSE EFFECTS
CNS: Drowsiness, confusion, memory impairment, dizziness, fatigue, anxiety, ataxia, agitation, emotional lability, euphoria, hostility, lethargy, memory impairment, paranoia, paresthesias, **suicidal ideation,** vertigo, depression
CV: Peripheral edema
EENT: Blurred vision, diplopia
GI: Constipation, nausea, vomiting, weight gain
MS: Myalgia, arthralgia
SYST: Infection

Pharmacokinetics	
Absorption	Unknown
Distribution	Protein binding 95%–96%, antagonist of the AMPA receptor
Metabolism	Unknown
Excretion	Unknown

Pharmacodynamics	
Onset	Unknown
Peak	Unknown
Duration	Unknown

INTERACTIONS

Individual drugs
Alcohol: Increased CNS depression

Drug classifications
CYP3A4 inducers: Increased perampanel effect

Benzodiazepines, sedatives, antihistamines, all other CNS depressants: Increased CNS depression

Oral/implant contraceptives with levonorgestrel/estrogen: Decreased contraception

CYP3A4 inhibitors: Decreased perampanel effect

Drug/herb
St. John's wort: Decreased perampanel effect

NURSING CONSIDERATIONS

Assessment
• Seizures: Assess for aura, location, duration, activity at onset; institute seizure precautions: padded side rails; move objects that might harm patient

> **BLACK BOX WARNING:** Bipolar disorder, psychosis, schizophrenia: Assess for hostility, aggression, anger; homicidal ideation can occur

⚠ **Suicidal ideation: assess for suicidal thoughts/behaviors as early as 1 wk and any time during treatment**
• Mental status: Assess mood, sensorium, affect, behavioral changes, suicidal thoughts/behaviors; if mental status changes: notify prescriber

⚠ **Abrupt discontinuation: can increase seizures**

Patient/family education
• Advise patient to avoid driving, other activities that require alertness because dizziness, drowsiness can occur
• Teach patient not to discontinue medication quickly after long-term use; to taper over 1 wk

because withdrawal-precipitated seizures can occur
• Advise patient to notify prescriber if pregnancy is planned or suspected; to avoid breastfeeding
• Inform patient to take once daily at bedtime

Evaluation
Positive therapeutic outcome
• Decreased seizure activity

---

perindopril (Rx)
(per-in'doe-pril)
Aceon, Coversye ✦
Func. class.: Antihypertensive
Chem. class.: Angiotensin-converting enzyme (ACE) inhibitor
Pregnancy category D

ACTION: Selectively suppresses renin-angiotensin-aldosterone system; inhibits ACE; prevents conversion of angiotensin I to angiotensin II, resulting in dilatation of arterial and venous vessels

Therapeutic outcome: Decreased B/P in hypertension

USES: Hypertension alone or in combination, MI prophylaxis

Unlabeled uses: MI

CONTRAINDICATIONS:
Hypersensitivity, history of angioedema

> **BLACK BOX WARNING:** Pregnancy **D**

Precautions: Breastfeeding, renal disease, hyperkalemia, hepatic failure, dehydration, bilateral renal artery stenosis, cough, severe CHF, aortic stenosis, African descent

DOSAGE AND ROUTES

Hypertension
Adult: PO 4 mg/day, may increase or decrease to desired response; range 4-8 mg/day may give in 2 divided doses or as a single dose; max 16 mg/day

Patients taking diuretics
Adult: PO 2-4 mg/day in 1-2 divided doses, range 4-8 mg/day

Stable CAD
Adult: PO 4 mg/day × 2 wk, then increase as tolerated to 8 mg/day

---

Renal dose
Adult: PO CCr 16-29 ml/min, 2 mg every other day; CCr 30-59 ml/min 2 mg/day; **CCr ≤15 ml/min 2 mg on dialysis days only**

Available forms: Tabs, scored 2, 4, 8 mg

Implementation
• Store in airtight container at 86° F (30° C) or less
• Severe hypotension may occur after 1st dose of this medication; decreased hypotension may be prevented by reducing or discontinuing diuretic therapy 3 days before beginning perindopril therapy
• Give by **IV** inf of 0.9% NaCl (as ordered) to expand fluid volume if severe hypotension occurs

ADVERSE EFFECTS
CNS: *Insomnia, dizziness,* paresthesias, *headache,* fatigue, anxiety, depression
CV: *Hypotension,* chest pain, tachycardia, dysrhythmias, syncope, **cardiac arrest**
EENT: *Tinnitus,* visual changes, sore throat, double vision, dry burning eyes
GI: Nausea, vomiting, colitis, cramps, diarrhea, constipation, flatulence, dry mouth, loss of taste, **liver failure**
GU: Proteinuria, renal failure, increased frequency of polyuria or oliguria
HEMA: Agranulocytosis, neutropenia, bone marrow suppression
INTEG: Rash, purpura, alopecia, hyperhidrosis
META: *Hyperkalemia*
RESP: Dyspnea, dry cough, crackles
SYST: Angioedema

Pharmacokinetics

Absorption	Well absorbed
Distribution	Unknown
Metabolism	Liver
Excretion	Kidneys
Half-life	Unknown

Pharmacodynamics
Unknown

INTERACTIONS
Individual drugs
Allopurinol, NSAIDs: increased hypersensitivity
Lithium: increased serum levels

Drug classifications
Angiotensin II receptor antagonists, antihypertensives, diuretics: increased hypotension

Antihypertensives, neuromuscular blocking agents: increased effects
Diuretics (potassium-sparing), potassium supplements, salt substitutes: hyperkalemia
NSAIDs: decreased effects
NSAIDs, salicylates: decreased antihypertensive effect

Drug/herb
Hawthorn: increased antihypertensive effect
Ephedra: decreased antihypertensive effect

Drug/lab test
Interference: glucose/insulin tolerance tests

NURSING CONSIDERATIONS
Assessment
• **Hypertension:** monitor B/P, orthostatic hypotension, syncope; if changes occur dosage change may be required
• Monitor blood studies: neutrophils, decreased platelets
• **CHF:** Check for edema in feet, legs daily
• Monitor renal studies: protein, BUN, creatinine; increased levels may indicate nephrotic syndrome and renal failure
• Monitor renal symptoms: polyuria, oliguria, frequency, dysuria
• Establish baselines in renal, liver function tests before therapy begins
• Check potassium levels throughout treatment, although hyperkalemia rarely occurs
• **Assess for allergic reactions:** rash, fever, pruritus, urticaria; product should be discontinued if antihistamines fail to help; angioedema: facial swelling, urticaria, product should be discontinued, may be more common in African-Americans

Patient/family education
• Advise patient not to discontinue product abruptly; advise patient to tell all persons associated with health care
• Teach patient not to use OTC products (cough, cold, allergy medications) unless directed by physician; serious side effects can occur; xanthines, such as coffee, tea, chocolate, cola can prevent action of product
• Instruct patient on the importance of complying with dosage schedule, even if feeling better; to continue with medical regimen to decrease B/P; exercise, cessation of smoking, decreasing stress, diet modifications
• Emphasize the need to rise slowly to sitting or standing position to minimize orthostatic hypotension; not to exercise in hot weather, which can cause increased hypotension

- Advise patient to notify prescriber of mouth sores, sore throat, fever, swelling of hands or feet, irregular heartbeat, chest pain, coughing, shortness of breath
- Caution patient to report excessive perspiration, dehydration, vomiting, diarrhea; may lead to fall in B/P
- Caution patient that product may cause dizziness, fainting, light-headedness; may occur during 1st few days of therapy; to avoid activities that may be hazardous
- Teach patient how to take B/P, normal readings for age-group
- Teach patient to report persistent, sustained cough
- Teach patient to avoid potassium supplements, salt substitutes

BLACK BOX WARNING: Notify prescriber if pregnancy is planned or suspected, pregnancy category **D**

Evaluation
Positive therapeutic outcome
- Decreased B/P in hypertension

TREATMENT OF OVERDOSE:
Lavage, **IV** atropine for bradycardia, **IV** theophylline for bronchospasm, digoxin, O₂; diuretic for cardiac failure, hemodialysis

pertuzumab
(per-too'zoo-mab)
Perjeta
Func. class.: Antineoplastic biologic response modifier
Chem. class.: Monoclonal antibody, antineoplastic
Pregnancy category D

ACTION: Blocks liquid-dependent action of human epidermal growth factor-2 (HER2), inhibiting signal pathways

Therapeutic outcome: Decreased size, spread of tumor

USES: First-line treatment of (HER2) positive metastatic breast cancer with trastuzumab and DOCEtaxel

CONTRAINDICATIONS:

BLACK BOX WARNING: Pregnancy **(D)**

Precautions: Breastfeeding, children, infants, neonates, cardiac arrhythmias, MI, cardiac disease, heart failure, hypertension, infusion-related reactions

DOSAGE AND ROUTES
Adult: IV 840 mg over 60 min, then after 3 wk 420 mg over 30–60 min every 3 wk; give with trastuzumab 8 mg/kg IV over 90 min, then after 3 wk 6 mg/kg over 30–90 min every 3 wk and DOCEtaxel 75 mg/m 2 IV every 3 wk; dosage may be escalated to 100 mg/m²

Available forms: Solution for inj 420 mg/14 ml

Implementation
- Visually inspect for particulate matter and discoloration
Dilution and preparation
- Withdraw the calculated dose from the vial and add to 250 ml 0.9% sodium chloride to PVC or non-PVC polyolefin infusion bag; do not dilute with dextrose 5% solution
- Dilute in normal saline only; do not mix or dilute with other drugs or dextrose solutions
- Mix the diluted solution by gentle inversion; do not shake

IV infusion
- Administer the diluted solution immediately
- Do not administer as an IV push or bolus
- Give the first dose of 840 mg over 60 min and subsequent 420-mg doses over 30–60 min
- If the diluted solution is not used immediately, store at 2°–8° C for up to 24 hr
Delayed or missed doses
- If time since previous dose is 6 wk, give 420 mg IV (do not wait for next scheduled dose)
- If time since previous dose is 6 wk, give 840 mg IV over 60 min, followed 3 wk later by 420 mg IV over 30–60 min repeated every 3 wk
- If DOCEtaxel is discontinued, this product and trastuzumab may continue

ADVERSE EFFECTS
CNS: Headache, fever, peripheral neuropathy, chills, fatigue, asthenia
CV: Heart failure
EENT: Lacrimation, stomatitis
GI: Nausea, vomiting, diarrhea, dysgeusia
HEMA: Anemia, neutropenia
MS: Myalgia
RESP: Upper respiratory infection
SYST: Anaphylaxis, infection, antibody formation

Pharmacokinetics

Absorption	Unknown
Distribution	Unknown
Metabolism	Unknown
Excretion	Unknown
Half-life	Median 18 days

Pharmacodynamics

Onset	Unknown
Peak	Unknown
Duration	Unknown

NURSING CONSIDERATIONS

Assessment

• **HER2 overexpression**: Testing should be done to identify HER2 overexpression before using this product

⚠ **Decreased left ventricular ejection fraction (LVEF)**: Can occur and is increased in those with a history of prior anthracycline use or radiotherapy to the chest; evaluate LVEF at baseline and every 3 mo; withhold therapy × 3 wk if LVEF is <40% or LVEF is 40%–45% with a 10% or greater absolute decrease from baseline; resume therapy if the LVEF is recovered to >45% or to 40%–45% with <10% absolute decrease at reassessment; if the LVEF has not improved or has declined further, consider permanently discontinuing pertuzumab and trastuzumab after a risk/benefit assessment

⚠ **Infusion-related reactions/hypersensitivity**: Assess anaphylactoid reaction, acute infusion reaction, cytokine-release syndrome 60 min after the first infusion, 30 min after other infusions; monitor for pyrexia, chills, fatigue, headache, asthenia, hypersensitivity, and vomiting; if a significant reaction occurs, slow or interrupt the infusion; permanent discontinuation may be needed in severe reactions

BLACK BOX WARNING: Pregnancy: Determine if pregnancy is planned or suspected; patients who become pregnant during therapy should report exposure to the Genentech Adverse Event line at 1-888-835-2555 and enroll in the MOTHER pregnancy registry at 1-800-690-6720

⚠ **Neutropenia**: Can occur, but occurs more commonly when trastuzumab is also used

• **Upper respiratory infection**: Monitor for dyspnea, shortness of breath, fever

Patient/family education

BLACK BOX WARNING: Counsel women of childbearing age on the need for contraception during and for 6 mo after therapy; advise patients who suspect pregnancy to contact their health care provider immediately; discontinue breastfeeding

Evaluation

Positive therapeutic outcome
• Decreased size, spread of tumor

⚠ HIGH ALERT

PHENobarbital (Rx)

(fee-noe-bar'bit-tal)
Func. class.: Anticonvulsant
Chem. class.: Barbiturate
Pregnancy category D
Controlled substance schedule IV

Do not confuse:

PHENobarbital/PENTobarbital

ACTION: Decreases impulse transmission, increases seizure threshold at cerebral cortex level

Therapeutic outcome: Sedation, anticonvulsant, improved energy

USES: All forms of epilepsy, status epilepticus, febrile seizures in children, sedation, insomnia

Unlabeled uses: Hyperbilirubinemia, chronic cholestasis

CONTRAINDICATIONS:

Pregnancy **D**, hypersensitivity to barbiturates, porphyria, hepatic/respiratory disease

Precautions: Anemia, renal disease, breastfeeding, geriatric

DOSAGE AND ROUTES

Seizures

Adult: PO 1-3 mg/kg/day in divided doses bid-tid or total dose at bedtime

Child 5-12 yr: PO 3-6 mg/kg/day in 1-2 divided doses

Child 1-5 yr: PO 6-8 mg/kg/day in 1-2 divided doses

Infant: PO 5-6 mg/kg/day in 1-2 divided doses

Neonate: PO 3-4 mg/kg/day as a single dose

Adverse effects: *italics* = common; **bold** = life-threatening

Status epilepticus

Adult: **IV** INF loading dose 15-18 mg/kg, then 10 mg/kg; run no faster than 50 mg/min; may give up to 30 mg/kg

Child: **IV** INF 5-10 mg/kg; may repeat q10-15min up to 20 mg/kg; run no faster than 50 mg/min

Sedation

Adult: PO 30-120 mg/day in 2-3 divided doses

Child: PO 3-5 mg/kg/day in 3 divided doses

Preoperative sedation

Adult: IM 100-200 mg 1-1½ hr before surgery

Child: PO/IM/**IV** 1-3 mg/kg 1-1½ hr before surgery

Available forms: Caps 15 mg; elix 20 mg/5 ml; tabs 15, 30, 32, 60, 65, 100 mg; inj 30, 60, 65, 130 mg/ml

Implementation

• Give medication after removal of cigarettes to prevent fires

• Give medication after trying conservative measures for insomnia

PO route

• Tab may be crushed and mixed with food if swallowing is difficult; also may be mixed with other fluids 30-60 min before bedtime for expected sleeplessness; on empty stomach for best absorption

• **Oral sol:** use undiluted or mixed with water or other fluids, use calibrated measuring device

IM route

• Give inj in deep muscle mass (gluteal) to minimize irritation to tissues

• Split inj of >5 ml into two, since irritation to tissues may occur

Direct IV route

• Use large vein to prevent extravasation; if extravasation occurs, use moist heat to the area and 5% procaine sol injected into area; give at 60 mg or less/min; titrate to patient's response

Y-site compatibilities: Doxapram, enalaprilat, fentaNYL, fosphenytoin, levofloxacin, meropenem, methadone, morphine, propofol, SUFentanil

Y-site incompatibilities: HYDROmorphone

ADVERSE EFFECTS

CNS: Paradoxical excitement (geriatric), drowsiness, lethargy, *hangover headache,* flushing, hallucinations, **coma, suicidal ideation**

EENT: Miosis, mydriasis

GI: Nausea, vomiting, diarrhea, constipation

HEMA: Agranulocytosis, megaloblastic anemia, thrombocytopenia, thrombophlebitis

INTEG: Rash, urticaria, **Stevens-Johnson syndrome, angioedema,** local pain, swelling, necrosis, scaling eczema

RESP: Respiratory depression

Pharmacokinetics

Absorption	Slow (70%-90%) (PO/IM/**IV**)
Distribution	Not known; crosses placenta
Metabolism	Liver (75%)
Excretion	Kidneys (25% unchanged)
Half-life	2-6 days

Pharmacodynamics

	PO	IM	IV
Onset	30-60 min	10-30 min	5 min
Peak	Unknown	Unknown	30 min
Duration	6-8 hr	4-6 hr	4-6 hr

INTERACTIONS

Individual drugs

Alcohol: increased CNS depression

Chloramphenicol, disulfiram: increased effects

Doxycycline, metroNIDAZOLE, quiNIDine, theophylline: decreased effectiveness

Furosemide: increased orthostatic hypotension

Valproic acid: increased sedation

Drug classifications

Anticoagulants, glucocorticoids, estrogens, hormonal contraceptives: decreased effectiveness

CNS depressants: increased effects

MAOIs, skeletal muscle relaxants (nondepolarizing), sulfonamides: increased effects

Drug/herb

Chamomile, eucalyptus, hops, kava, valerian: increased CNS depression

St. John's wort: decreased barbiturate effect

NURSING CONSIDERATIONS

Assessment

• Assess mental status: mood, sensorium, affect, memory (long, short), especially geriatric; if using as a hypnotic, assess sleep patterns during therapy; product suppresses REM sleep with dreaming

• Withdrawal insomnia may occur after short-term use; do not start using product again; insomnia improves in 1-3 nights; may experience increased dreaming

- Assess respiratory dysfunction: respiratory depression, character, rate, rhythm when using **IV**; hold product if respirations are <10/min or if pupils are dilated; also check VS q30min after parenteral route for 2 hr
- **Assess for barbiturate toxicity:** hypotension, pulmonary constriction, cold, clammy skin, cyanosis of lips, CNS depression, nausea, vomiting, hallucinations, delirium, weakness, coma, pupillary constriction; mild symptoms occur in 8-12 hr without product
- **Assess for pain** in postop patients; pain threshold is lowered in patients taking this medication
- **Assess for blood dyscrasias:** fever, sore throat, bruising, rash, jaundice, epistaxis (long-term treatment only); monitor CBC, serum creatinine, BUN
- **Assess seizure activity** including type, location, duration, character; provide seizure precaution
- ⚠ Teach patient to report suicidal thoughts/behavior immediately

Patient/family education
- Teach patient that hangover is common
- Instruct patient that product is indicated only for short-term treatment of insomnia and is probably ineffective after 2 wk
- Inform patient that physical dependency may result when used for extended time (45-90 days depending on dosage)
- Teach patient to avoid driving and other activities requiring alertness
- Caution patient to avoid alcohol ingestion and CNS depressants; serious CNS depression may result
- Instruct patient not to discontinue medication quickly after long-term use; may cause seizures; product should be tapered over 1 wk; take exactly as prescribed
- Emphasize the need to tell all prescribers that a barbiturate is being taken
- Teach the patient to make position changes slowly; orthostatic hypotension may occur
- Teach patient that response may take 4 days to 2 wk
- Instruct patient to notify prescriber immediately if bruising, bleeding occur, which may indicate blood dyscrasias

Evaluation
Positive therapeutic outcome
- Improved sleeping patterns
- Decreased seizure activity
- Sedative preoperatively

TREATMENT OF OVERDOSE:
Lavage, activated charcoal, warming blanket, VS, hemodialysis, alkalinize urine, give **IV** volume expanders, **IV** fluids

phentolamine (Rx)
(fen-tole′a-meen)
Func. class.: Antihypertensive
Chem. class.: α-Adrenergic blocker
Pregnancy category C

Do not confuse:
phentolamine/phentermine

ACTION:
α-Adrenergic blocker; binds to α-adrenergic receptors, dilating peripheral blood vessels, lowering peripheral resistance, lowering blood pressure

Therapeutic outcome: Decreased B/P, reversal of vasoconstriction (dermal necrosis)

USES:
Hypertension; pheochromocytoma; prevention, treatment of dermal necrosis after extravasation of norepinephrine, DOPamine, EPINEPHrine

Unlabeled uses: Impotence, hypertensive crisis due to MAOIs

CONTRAINDICATIONS:
Hypersensitivity, MI, coronary insufficiency, angina, hypotension

Precautions: Pregnancy **C**, breastfeeding, dysrhythmia, peptic ulcer disease

DOSAGE AND ROUTES
Treatment of hypertensive episodes in pheochromocytoma
Adult: **IV**/IM 5 mg; repeat if necessary
Child: **IV** 0.05-0.1 mg/kg; repeat if necessary, max 5 mg

Diagnosis of pheochromocytoma
Adult: **IV** 5 mg
Child: **IV** 0.05 mg/kg; if negative, repeat with 0.1 mg/kg **IV**

Treatment of necrosis
Adult: 5-10 mg/10 ml 0.9% NaCl injected into area of extravasation within 12 hr
Child: 0.1-0.2 mg/kg; max 5 mg

Prevention of dermal necrosis
Adult: **IV** 10 mg/L of norepinephrine-containing sol
Child: **IV** 0.1-0.2 mg/kg, max 5 mg

Adverse effects: *italics* = common; **bold** = life-threatening

Available forms: Inj 5 mg/ml

Implementation
• Give with vasopressor nearby

IV route
• Give by direct **IV** after diluting 5 mg/1 ml of sterile water for inj or 0.9% NaCl; give 5 mg or less/min
• Give by cont inf by further diluting 5-10 mg/500 ml of D_5W, titrate to patient response
• Add 10 mg/L to norepinephrine in **IV** sol for prevention of dermal necrosis

Syringe compatibilities: MethylPRED-NISolone, papaverine

Y-site compatibilities: Amiodarone

Additive compatibilities: DOBUTamine, verapamil

ADVERSE EFFECTS
CNS: *Dizziness,* flushing, weakness, **cerebrovascular spasm,** paresthesias, CVA
CV: *Hypotension,* **tachycardia,** *angina,* **dysrhythmias, MI**
EENT: Nasal congestion
GI: *Dry mouth, nausea, vomiting, diarrhea, abdominal pain*
INTEG: Pruritus, injection site pain
RESP: Nasal congestion

Pharmacokinetics

Absorption	Well absorbed (IM); completely absorbed (**IV**)
Distribution	Unknown
Metabolism	Unknown
Excretion	Kidneys, unchanged (10%)
Half-life	Unknown

Pharmacodynamics

	IM	IV
Onset	Unknown	Rapid
Peak	20 min	2 min
Duration	½-1 hr	½ hr

INTERACTIONS
Individual drugs
EPINEPHrine: increased effects of EPINEPHrine
Sildenafil, tadalafil: increased hypotension

Drug classifications
Antihypertensives: increased effects of antihypertensives

NURSING CONSIDERATIONS
Assessment
• Monitor B/P, orthostatic hypotension, syncope, pulse, ECG until stable

Patient/family education
• Caution patient not to discontinue product abruptly
• Teach patient not to use OTC products (cough, cold, allergy) unless directed by prescriber
• Teach patient the importance of complying with dosage schedule, even if feeling better
• Emphasize the need to rise slowly to sitting or standing position to minimize orthostatic hypotension
• Teach patient to notify prescriber of mouth sores, sore throat, fever, swelling of hands or feet, irregular heartbeat, chest pain
• Caution patient to report excessive perspiration, dehydration, vomiting, diarrhea; may lead to fall in B/P
• Caution patient that product may cause dizziness, fainting, light-headedness; may occur during 1st few days of therapy
• Teach patient how to take B/P, teach normal readings for age group

Evaluation
Positive therapeutic outcome
• Decreased B/P in hypertension
• Resolution of impotence
• Prevention of dermal necrosis

TREATMENT OF OVERDOSE:
Administer norepinephrine; discontinue product

phenylephrine (Rx)
(fen-ill-ef′rin)
Neo-Synephrine
Func. class.: Adrenergic, direct acting
Chem. class.: Direct sympathomimetic amine (α-agonist)
Pregnancy category C

ACTION: Powerful and selective receptor agonist causing contraction of blood vessels, vasoconstriction of eye arterioles; decreases eye engorgement by stimulation of α-adrenergic receptors

Therapeutic outcome: Increased B/P, decreased nasal congestion, decreased eye irritation

USES: Hypotension, paroxysmal supraventricular tachycardia, shock, B/P maintenance during spinal anesthesia, topical ocular vasoconstrictor in uveitis, open-angle glaucoma; preoperatively, diagnostic procedures, refraction without cycloplegia; nasal congestion

CONTRAINDICATIONS:

Hypersensitivity, closed-angle glaucoma, ventricular fibrillation, tachydysrhythmias, pheochromocytoma, severe hypertension

Precautions: Pregnancy **C,** breastfeeding, geriatric, hyperthyroidism, severe arteriosclerosis, arterial embolism, peripheral vascular disease, bradycardia, myocardial disease, partial heart block

> **BLACK BOX WARNING:** Cardiac disease, extravasation

DOSAGE AND ROUTES
Hypotension
Adult: SUBCUT/IM 2-5 mg; may repeat q10-15min if needed, do not exceed initial dose; IV 0.1-0.5 mg; may repeat q10-15min if needed, do not exceed initial dose
Child: IM/SUBCUT 0.1 mg/kg/dose q1-2hr prn

Supraventricular tachycardia
Adult: IV max 0.5 mg given rapidly, max single dose 1 mg

Shock
Adult: IV INF 10 mg/500 ml of D_5W given 100-180 mcg/min (if 20 gtt/ml device is used), then maintenance of 40-60 mcg/min (if 20 gtt/ml device is used); use inf pump
Child: IV BOL 5-20 mcg/kg/dose q10-15min; IV INF 0.1-0.5 mg/kg/min

Available forms: Inj 1% (10 mg/ml)

Implementation
IV route
• Give plasma expanders for hypovolemia
• Give **IV** after diluting 1 mg/9 ml of sterile water for inj; give dose over 30-60 sec; may be diluted 10 mg/500 ml of D_5W or 0.9% NaCl; titrate to patient's response; low normal B/P; check for extravasation; check site for infiltration; use inf pump
• Store reconstituted sol in refrigerator for no longer than 24 hr
• Do not use discolored sol

Y-site compatibilities: Famotidine, haloperidol, inamrinone, zidovudine

Additive compatibilities: Chloramphenicol, DOBUTamine, lidocaine, potassium chloride, sodium bicarbonate

ADVERSE EFFECTS
CNS: *Headache, dizziness, anxiety, tremor, insomnia*
CV: Reflex bradycardia, **dysrhythmias,** *hypertension,* **tachycardia,** palpitations, ectopic beats, angina
GI: *Nausea, vomiting*
INTEG: Necrosis, tissue sloughing with extravasation, **gangrene**
MISC: Anaphylaxis

Pharmacokinetics
Absorption	Well absorbed (IM); completely absorbed (**IV**); minimally absorbed (nasal, ophth)
Distribution	Unknown
Metabolism	Liver
Excretion	Unknown
Half-life	Unknown

Pharmacodynamics
	SUBCUT/IM	IV
Onset	15 min	Rapid
Peak	Unknown	Unknown
Duration	45-60 min	20-30 min

INTERACTIONS
Individual drugs
Digoxin: increased dysrhythmias

Drug classifications
α-Blockers: decreased phenylephrine action
Antidepressants (tricyclics), β-adrenergic blockers, H_1 antihistamines: increased pressor effect
General anesthetics: increased dysrhythmias
MAOIs: do not use within 2 wk, hypertensive crisis may result
Oxytocics: increased B/P

NURSING CONSIDERATIONS
Assessment
• Monitor I&O ratio; notify prescriber if output <30 ml/hr
• Monitor ECG during administration continuously; if B/P increases, product is decreased
• Monitor B/P and pulse q5min after parenteral route; CVP or PWP during inf if possible
• Assess for paresthesias and coldness of extremities; peripheral blood flow may decrease

Patient/family education
• Inform patient of reason for product administration and expected result

Adverse effects: *italics* = common; **bold** = life-threatening

• Advise patient to report pain at inf site immediately
• Instruct patient to report change in vision, blurring, loss of sight; breathing trouble, sweating, flushing

Evaluation
Positive therapeutic outcome
• Increased B/P with stabilization

phenylephrine nasal agent
See Appendix B

phenylephrine ophthalmic
See Appendix B

phenytoin (Rx)
(fen′i-toyn)
Dilantin, Dilantin Infatabs, Phenytek
Func. class.: Anticonvulsant/antidysrhythmic (class IB)
Chem. class.: Hydantoin
Pregnancy category D 🟊

ACTION: Inhibits spread of seizure activity in motor cortex by altering ion transport; increases AV conduction to decrease dysrhythmias

Therapeutic outcome: Decreased seizures, absence of dysrhythmias

USES: Generalized tonic-clonic seizures, status epilepticus, nonepileptic seizures associated with Reye's syndrome or after head trauma, complex/partial seizures

CONTRAINDICATIONS:
Pregnancy **D**, hypersensitivity, psychiatric condition, bradycardia, SA and AV block, Stokes-Adams syndrome

Precautions: Geriatric, allergies, renal/hepatic disease, petit mal seizures, hypotension, myocardial insufficiency, Asian patients positive for HLA-B 1502, hepatic failure, acute intermittent porphyria

BLACK BOX WARNING: IV use

DOSAGE AND ROUTES
Seizures
Adult: PO 15-20 mg/kg (EXT REL) in 3-4 divided doses given q2hr or 400 mg, then 300 mg q2hr × 2 doses, maintenance 4-7 mg/kg/day; max 600 mg/day; **IV** 15-20 mg/kg, max 25-50 mg/min then 100 mg q6-8hr

Child: PO 5 mg/kg/day in 2-3 divided doses, maintenance 4-8 mg/kg/day in 2-3 divided doses, max 300 mg/day; **IV** 15-20 mg/kg at 1-3 mg/kg/min

Status epilepticus
Adult: **IV** 15-20 mg/kg, max 25-50 mg/min; may give 100 mg q6-8hr thereafter
Child: **IV** 15-20 mg/kg, max in divided doses 1-3 mg/kg/min

Ventricular dysrhythmias
Adult: PO loading dose 1 g divided over 24 hr, then 500 mg/day × 2 days; **IV** 250 mg given over 5 min until dysrhythmias subside or 1 g is given, or 100 mg q15min until dysrhythmias subside or 1 g is given
Child: PO 3-8 mg/kg or 250 mg/m²/day as single dose or divided in 2 doses; **IV** 3-8 mg/kg given over several min, or 250 mg/m²/day as single dose or divided in 2 doses

Renal dose
Adult: Do not use loading dose if CCr <10 ml/min or hepatic failure

Available forms: Susp 25 mg/5 ml; chew tabs 50 mg; inj 50 mg/ml; ext rel caps 100, 200, 300 mg; prompt rel caps 100 mg

Implementation
PO route
• Do not interchange chewable product with caps, not equivalent; only ext rel caps are to be used for once-a-day dosing
• Give with meals to decrease GI upset
• Chew tab can be crushed or chewed; cap can be opened and mixed with foods or fluids; cap and tab are not interchangeable, only ext rel cap is to be used for once a day dosing
• Do not take antacids or antidiarrheals within 2-3 hr of taking phenytoin
• **Oral suspension:** shake well before each dose G tube/NG tube; dilute susp prior to administration; flush tube with 20 ml water after dose; hold tube feedings 1 hr before and 1 hr after dose
• Allow 7-10 days between dosage changes
• Divided PO doses with or after meals to decrease adverse effects
• 2 hr before or after antacid, enteral feeding
• Shake oral susp well; use measuring device for correct dose

Direct IV route

BLACK BOX WARNING: Give undiluted at ≤50 mg/min (adult) 1-3 mg/kg/min (neonates); 0.5-1 mg/kg/min

Intermittent IV INF route

BLACK BOX WARNING: Dilute dose in NS to ≤6.7 mg/ml, complete inf within 1 hr of preparation, use 0.22 or 0.55 micron in-line particulate final filter between **IV** catheter and tubing, flush the **IV** line or catheter with NS before and after use, give at ≤50 mg/min (adult), 0.5-1 mg/kg/min (child, infant, neonate)

Additive compatibilities: Bleomycin, verapamil

Y-site compatibilities: Esmolol, famotidine, fluconazole, foscarnet, tacrolimus

Y-site incompatibilities: Enalaprilat, potassium chloride, vit B/C

ADVERSE EFFECTS

CNS: Dizziness, insomnia, paresthesias, depression, **suicidal tendencies**, aggression, headache, confusion, slurred speech, peripheral neuropathy
CV: Hypotension, **ventricular fibrillation, bradycardia, cardiac arrest**
EENT: Nystagmus, diplopia, blurred vision
ENDO: Diabetes insipidus
GI: Nausea, vomiting, constipation, anorexia, weight loss, **hepatitis**, jaundice, gingival hyperplasia, abdominal pain
GU: Nephritis, urine discoloration, sexual dysfunction
HEMA: Agranulocytosis, leukopenia, aplastic anemia, thrombocytopenia, megaloblastic anemia
INTEG: Rash, **lupus erythematosus, Stevens-Johnson syndrome**, hirsutism, **toxic epidermal necrolysis**
SYST: Hypocalcemia, **purple glove syndrome (IV)**, exacerbation of myasthenia gravis

Pharmacokinetics

Absorption	Slowly absorbed from GI tract; erratic (IM)
Distribution	Crosses placenta, 90%-95% protein binding
Metabolism	Liver, extensively
Excretion	Kidneys, minimally; enters breast milk
Half-life	7-42 hr, dose dependent

Pharmacodynamics

	PO	PO-EXT REL	IM	IV
Onset	2-24 hr	2-24 hr	Erratic	1-2 hr
Peak	1½-3 hr	4-12 hr	Erratic	Unknown
Duration	6-12 hr	12-36 hr	12-24 hr	12-24 hr

INTERACTIONS
Individual drugs
Alcohol (chronic use), calcium (high dose), carBAMazepine, folic acid, rifampin: decreased effects of phenytoin
Chloramphenicol, cimetidine, cycloSERINE, disulfiram, alcohol, amiodarone, FLUoxetine, gabapentin, methylphenidate, felbamate, traZODone, diazepam, valproate: increased phenytoin effect

Drug classifications
Antacids, barbiturates: decreased effect of phenytoin
Antidepressants (tricyclics), benzodiazepines, sulfonamides, H₂ antagonists, azole antifungals, estrogens, succinimides, phenothiazines, salicylates: increased phenytoin level

Drug/food
Enteral tube feeding: may decrease absorption of oral product, do not use enteral feedings 2 hr before and after dose

Drug/lab test
Increased: glucose, alkaline phosphatase, BSP
Decreased: dexamethasone, metyrapone test serum, urinary steroids

NURSING CONSIDERATIONS
Assessment
• Assess product level: toxic level 30-50 mcg/ml; therapeutic level 7.5-20 mcg/ml, wait ≥1 wk to determine level
⚠ **Assess mental status: mood, sensorium, affect, memory (long, short), especially geriatric; suicidal thoughts/behaviors**
⚠ **Phenytoin hypersensitivity syndrome: assess 3-12 wk after start of treatment: rash, temp, lymphadenopathy; may cause hepatotoxicity, renal failure, rhabdomyolysis**
⚠ **Serious skin disorders: assess for beginning rash that may lead to Stevens-Johnson syndrome or toxic epidermal necrolysis;**

Adverse effects: *italics* = common; **bold** = life-threatening

phenytoin should not be used again, may occur more often in Asian patients with HLA-B 1502

⚠ **Purple glove syndrome: with IV use**

- Phenytoin level: toxic level 30-50 mcg/ml, therapeutic level: 7.5-20 mcg/ml, wait ≥1 wk to draw levels
- **Seizures:** assess for duration, type, intensity precipitating factors, obtain EEG periodically, monitor therapeutic level
- Blood studies: CBC, platelets q2wk until stabilized, then qmo × 12, then q3mo; discontinue product if neutrophils <1600/m³; renal function: albumin conc; folic acid levels, LFTs
- **Blood dyscrasias:** assess fever, sore throat, bruising, rash, jaundice, epistaxis (long-term treatment only)
- Assess renal studies: urinalysis, BUN, urine creatinine
- Monitor blood studies: RBC, Hct, Hgb, reticulocyte counts weekly for 4 wk then monthly; also check thyroid function tests, serum calcium
- Monitor ECG, B/P, respiratory function during IV loading dose; verify potency of IV access port prior to IV infusion
- Monitor EEG function and serum levels periodically
- Monitor liver function tests for renal failure: ALT, AST, bilirubin, creatinine
- Assess for signs of physical withdrawal if medication suddenly discontinued
- Assess eye problems: need for ophth exam before, during, after treatment (slit lamp, funduscopy, tonometry)
- **Monitor for toxicity:** bone marrow depression, nausea, vomiting, ataxia, diplopia, CV collapse, slurred speech, confusion

Patient/family education

- Teach patient to carry/wear emergency ID stating name, products taken, condition, prescriber's name and phone number
- Advise patient to avoid driving and other activities that require alertness until product response is known; dizziness, drowsiness can occur
- Advise patient to avoid alcohol ingestion and CNS depressants unless approved by prescriber; increased sedation may occur
- Teach patient not to discontinue medication quickly after long-term use; taper off over several wk
- Advise patient that urine may turn pink, red, or brown
- Caution patient to avoid antacids or antidiarrheals within 2-3 hr of taking phenytoin

- Instruct patient in proper oral hygiene to prevent gingival hyperplasia; to visit dentist routinely
- Teach patient to use nonhormonal contraception, to notify prescriber if pregnancy is planned or suspected, pregnancy **D**
- Teach patient to notify prescriber of unusual bleeding, bruising, petechiae (bleeding), clay-colored stools, abdominal pain, dark urine, yellowing of skin/eyes (hepatotoxicity); slurred speech, headache, drowsiness

⚠ **Teach patient to report suicidal thoughts/behaviors immediately**

Evaluation

Positive therapeutic outcome

- Decreased seizure activity
- Decreased dysrhythmias
- Relief of pain

physostigmine ophthalmic
See Appendix B

phytonadione (vit K₁) (Rx)
(fye-toe-na-dye′one)
Mephyton
Func. class.: Vitamin K₁, fat-soluble vitamin
Pregnancy category C

ACTION: Needed for adequate blood clotting (factors II, VII, IX, X)

Therapeutic outcome: Prevention of bleeding

USES: Vitamin K malabsorption, hypoprothrombinemia, prevention of hypoprothrombinemia caused by oral anticoagulants, prevention of hemorrhagic disease of the newborn

CONTRAINDICATIONS:
Hypersensitivity, severe hepatic disease, last few wk of pregnancy

Precautions: Pregnancy **C**, neonates, hepatic disease

> **BLACK BOX WARNING: IV** use

DOSAGE AND ROUTES
Hypoprothrombinemia caused by vitamin K malabsorption
Adult: PO/IM 2.5-25 mg; may repeat or increase to 50 mg
Child: PO 2.5-5 mg
Infant: PO/IM 2 mg

Prevention of hemorrhagic disease of the newborn

Neonate: IM 0.5-1 mg within 1 hr after birth; repeat in 2-3 wk if required

Hypoprothrombinemia caused by oral anticoagulants

Adult and child: PO/SUBCUT/IM 1-10 mg, may repeat 12-48 hr after PO dose or 6-8 hr after SUBCUT/IM dose, based on INR

Available forms: Tabs 5 mg; inj 10 mg/ml, 1 mg/0.5 ml

Implementation

Intermittent IV infusion route
• Give **IV** after diluting with D_5 NS 10 ml or more; give max 1 mg/min
• Give **IV** only when other routes not possible (deaths have occurred)
• Store in airtight, light-resistant container

Y-site compatibilities: Alfentanil, amikacin, aminophylline, ascorbic acid, atracurium, atropine, azaTHIOprine, aztreonam, bumetanide, buprenorphine, butorphanol, calcium chloride/gluconate, ceFAZolin, cefonicid, cefoperazone, cefotaxime, cefoTEtan, cefOXitin, cefTAZidime, ceftizoxime, cefTRIAXone, cefuroxime, chloramphenicol, chlorproMAZINE, cimetidine, clindamycin, cyanocobalamin, cycloSPORINE, dexamethasone, digoxin, diphenhydrAMINE, DOPamine, doxycycline, enalaprilat, ePHEDrine, EPINEPHrine, epoetin alfa, erythromycin, esmolol, famotidine, fentaNYL, fluconazole, folic acid, furosemide, ganciclovir, gentamicin, glycopyrrolate, heparin, hydrocortisone, imipenem-cilastatin, indomethacin, insulin, isoproterenol, ketorolac, labetalol, lidocaine, mannitol, meperidine, metaraminol, methoxamine, methyldopa, metoclopramide, metoprolol, metroNIDAZOLE, midazolam, morphine, multivitamins, nafcillin, nalbuphine, naloxone, nitroglycerin, nitroprusside, norepinephrine, ondansetron, oxacillin, oxytocin, papaverine, penicillin G potassium, pentamidine, pentazocine, PENTobarbital, PHENobarbital, phentolamine, phenylephrine, potassium chloride, procainamide, prochlorperazine, propranolol, pyridoxime, ranitidine, sodium bicarbonate, succinylcholine, SUFentanil, theophylline, thiamine, ticarcillin/clavulanate, tobramycin, tolazoline, trimethaphan, urokinase, vancomycin, vasopressin, verapamil, vitamin B with C

Y-site incompatibilities: Dantrolene, diazepam, diazoxide, magnesium sulfate, phenytoin, trimethoprim/sulfamethoxazole

ADVERSE EFFECTS

CNS: Headache, **brain damage** (large doses)
GI: Nausea, decreased liver function tests
HEMA: Hemolytic anemia, **hemoglobinuria, hyperbilirubinemia**
INTEG: Rash, urticaria
RESP: **Bronchospasm,** dyspnea, chest constriction, **respiratory arrest**

Pharmacokinetics

Absorption	Well absorbed (PO, IM, SUBCUT)
Distribution	Crosses placenta
Metabolism	Liver, rapidly
Excretion	Breast milk
Half-life	Unknown

Pharmacodynamics

	PO	SUBCUT/IM
Onset	6-12 hr	1-2 hr
Peak	Unknown	6 hr
Duration	Unknown	14 hr

INTERACTIONS

Individual drugs

Sucralfate, mineral oil: decreased action of phytonadione
Warfarin: decreased action of warfarin (large dose of this product)

Drug classifications

Oral anticoagulants: decreased anticoagulant effect
Bile acid sequestrants, antiinfectives, salicylates: decreased action of phytonadione

Drug/food

Olestra: decreased vit K levels

NURSING CONSIDERATIONS

Assessment

• Monitor pro-time during treatment (2-sec deviation from control time, bleeding time, and clotting time)
• Monitor for bleeding, INR pulse, and B/P
• Assess nutritional status: liver (beef), spinach, tomatoes, coffee, asparagus, broccoli, cabbage, lettuce, greens
• Assess for bleeding or bruising: hematuria, black tarry stools, hematemesis

Patient/family education

• Teach patient not to take other supplements unless directed by prescriber; to take this medication as directed
• Teach patient necessary foods high in vit K to be included in diet

• Advise patient to avoid IM inj, hard toothbrush, flossing; use electric razor until treatment is terminated
• Instruct patient to report symptoms of bleeding: bruising, nosebleeds, blood in urine, heavy menstruation, black tarry stools
• Caution patient not to use OTC medications unless approved by prescriber
• Stress the need for periodic lab tests to monitor coagulation levels
• Stress the need for patient to carry/wear emergency ID with condition, treatment, and medications taken

Evaluation

Positive therapeutic outcome
• Decreased bleeding tendencies
• Decreased pro-time
• Decreased clotting time

pilocarpine ophthalmic
See Appendix B

pimecrolimus topical
See Appendix B

pioglitazone (Rx)
(pie-oh-glye′ta-zone)
Actos
Func. class.: Antidiabetic, oral
Chem. class.: Thiazolidinedione
Pregnancy category C

ACTION: Specifically targets insulin resistance, an insulin sensitizer; regulates the transcription of a number of insulin-responsive genes

Therapeutic outcome: Decreased symptoms of diabetes mellitus

USES: Type 2 diabetes mellitus

CONTRAINDICATIONS:
Breastfeeding, children, hypersensitivity to thiazolidinediones, diabetic ketoacidosis

> **BLACK BOX WARNING:** NYHA Class III/IV heart failure

Precautions: Pregnancy C, thyroid/renal/hepatic disease, edema, geriatric patients with CV disease, polycystic ovary syndrome, bladder cancer, osteoporosis, pulmonary disease, secondary malignancy

DOSAGE AND ROUTES
Monotherapy
Adult: PO 15-30 mg/day, may increase to 45 mg/day; with strong CYP2C8 max 15 mg/day; those with NYHA class I/II heart failure max 15 mg/day

Combination therapy
Adult: PO 15-30 mg/day with a sulfonylurea, metformin, or insulin; decrease sulfonylurea dose if hypoglycemia occurs; decrease insulin dose by 10%-25% if hypoglycemia occurs or if plasma glucose is <100 mg/dl; max 45 mg/day

Hepatic dose
Do not use in active liver disease or if ALT >2.5 × ULN

Available forms: Tabs 15, 30, 45 mg

Implementation
• Convert from other oral hypoglycemic agents; change may be made with gradual dosage change; monitor serum glucose during conversion
• Give once a day without regard to meals
• Give tabs crushed and mixed with meal or fluids for patients with difficulty swallowing
• Store in airtight container in cool environment

ADVERSE EFFECTS
CNS: *Headache*
CV: **MI, heart failure, death** (geriatric patients)
ENDO: Hyper/hypoglycemia
MISC: *Myalgia, sinusitis, upper respiratory tract infection, pharyngitis,* **hepatotoxicity,** edema, weight gain, anemia, macular edema; **risk of bladder cancer (use >1 yr),** peripheral/pulmonary edema
MS: Fractures (females), **rhabdomyolysis,** myalgia

Pharmacokinetics	
Absorption	Unknown
Distribution	Protein binding >99%
Metabolism	Unknown
Excretion	Kidneys
Half-life	3-7 hr, terminal 16-24 hr

Pharmacodynamics	
Onset	Unknown
Peak	6-12 wk
Duration	Unknown

INTERACTIONS
Individual drugs
Atorvastatin: decreased effect of this product
Fluconazole, itraconazole, ketoconazole, miconazole, voriconazole: decreased pioglitazone effect

Drug classifications
CYP2C8 inducers: decreased pioglitazone effect
Oral contraceptives: decreased effect, use an alternative contraceptive method

Drug/herb
Garlic, green tea, horse chestnut: increased hypoglycemia

Drug/lab test
Increased: CPK, LFTs, HDL, cholesterol
Decreased: glucose, Hct/Hgb

NURSING CONSIDERATIONS
Assessment

> **BLACK BOX WARNING: Heart failure:** do not use in NYHA Class III/IV; excessive/rapid weight gain > 5 lb, dyspnea, edema; may need to be reduced or discontinued

• **Hypoglycemic reactions:** assess for hypoglycemic reactions (sweating, weakness, dizziness, anxiety, tremors, hunger), hyperglycemic reactions soon after meals (rare)
• **Bladder cancer: Avoid use in patients with history of bladder cancer; use of pioglitazone >1 yr has been correlated with an increase in bladder cancer;** may occur more often with insulin or other antidiabetics
• **Hepatic disease:** check LFTs periodically: AST, LDH; do not start treatment in active heart disease or if ALT >2.5× upper limit of normal; if treatment has already begun, follow closely with continuing ALT levels; if ALT increases to >3× upper limit of normal, recheck ALT as soon as possible, if ALT remains >3× upper limit of normal, discontinue
• Monitor FBS, glycosylated HbA1c, plasma lipids/lipoproteins, B/P, body weight during treatment
• Monitor CBC with differential prior to and during therapy, more necessary in those with anemia, Hct/Hgb (may be decreased in first few months of treatment)

Patient/family education
• Teach patient to self-monitor using a blood glucose meter
• Teach patient symptoms of hypo/hyperglycemia, what to do about each (rare)
• Advise patient that product must be continued on daily basis; explain consequence of discontinuing product abruptly
• Advise patient to avoid OTC medications or herbal preparations unless approved by prescriber; to report weight gain, edema
• Advise patient that diabetes is life-long illness; that this product is not a cure, only controls symptoms
⚠ **Instruct patient to notify prescriber if oral contraceptives are used, effect may be decreased**
• Teach patient not to use if breastfeeding
• Teach patient that lab work, eye exams will be needed periodically

Evaluation
Positive therapeutic outcome
• Decrease in polyuria, polydipsia, polyphagia; clear sensorium; absence of dizziness; stable gait; blood glucose, A1c improvement

---

piperacillin/tazobactam (Rx)
(pip′er-ah-sill′in/ta-zoe-bak′tam)
Zosyn
Func. class.: Broad-spectrum antiinfective
Chem. class.: Extended-spectrum penicillin
Pregnancy category B

ACTION: Interferes with cell wall replication of susceptible organisms; tazobactam is a β-lactamase inhibitor, protects piperacillin from enzymatic degradation

Therapeutic outcome: Bactericidal effects for piperacillin-resistant β-lactamase, *Escherichia coli, Staphylococcus aureus, Bacteroides fragilis, Bacteroides ovatus, Bacteroides thetaiotaomicron, Bacteroides vulgatus, Haemophilus influenzae*

USES: Moderate to severe infections: piperacillin-resistant, β-lactamase strains causing infections in respiratory tract, skin, skin structure, urinary tract, bone, and joint; gonorrhea, pneumonia, infections from penicillinase-producing staphylococci, streptococci

Unlabeled uses: Endocarditis

CONTRAINDICATIONS:
Hypersensitivity to penicillins; neonates, carbapenem allergy

Precautions: Pregnancy **B,** breastfeeding, CHF, seizures, hypersensitivity to cephalosporins, renal insufficiency in neonates, GI disease, electrolyte imbalances, biliary obstruction

---

Adverse effects: *italics* = common; **bold** = life-threatening

DOSAGE AND ROUTES

Nosocomial pneumonia
Adult: **IV** 4.5 g q6hr or 3.375 g q4hr with an aminoglycoside or antipseudomonal fluoroquinolone × 1-2 wk

Appendicitis/peritonitis
Child ≥40 kg (88 lb): **IV** 3.375 g q6hr × 7-10 days
Child ≥9 mo and <40 g: **IV** 100 mg (piperacillin)/kg q8hr × 7-10 days
Infant 2 mo to <9 mo: **IV** 80 mg (piperacillin) q8hr × 7-10 days

Renal dose
Adult: **IV** CCr 20-40 ml/min give 3.375 g q6hr (nosocomial pneumonia); give 2.25 g q6hr (all other indications); CCr <20 ml/min, give 2.25 g q6hr (nosocomial pneumonia); give 2.25 g q8hr (all other indications)

Available forms: Powder for inj 2 g piperacillin/0.25 g tazobactam, 3 g piperacillin/0.375 g tazobactam, 4 g piperacillin/0.5 g tazobactam, 36 g piperacillin/4.5 g tazobactam

Implementation
• Separate aminoglycoside from piperacillin to avoid inactivation
• Product after C&S is complete

Intermittent IV infusion route
• Reconstitute each 1 g of product/5 ml 0.9% NaCl for inj or sterile water for inj, dextrose 5%; shake well; further dilute in at least 50 ml compatible IV sol and run as int inf over at least 30 min

ADD-Vantage IV solution: reconstitution
• Reconstitute with 0.9% NaCl or D₅W in the appropriate flexible diluent container provided; for 500 mg vials, use at least a 100 ml diluent container and for 750 mg and 1 g vials, use only the 250 ml diluent container
• Remove the protective covers from the top of the vial and vial port. Remove vial cap (do not access with a syringe) and vial port cover. Screw the vial into the vial port until it will go no further to assure a seal. Once vial is sealed to the port, do not remove. To activate the contents of the vial, squeeze the bottom of the diluent container gently to inflate the portion of the container surrounding the end of the drug vial. With the other hand, push the drug vial down into the container telescoping walls of the container and grasp the inner cap of the vial through the walls of the container. Pull the inner cap from the drug vial. Verify the rubber stopper has been pulled out, allowing the drug and diluent to mix. Mix the container contents thoroughly

• *Storage after reconstitution:* The admixture solution may be stored for up to 24 hr at room temperature. Do not refrigerate or freeze after reconstitution
• Do not use in series connections with flexible containers

Pre-mixed Galaxy IV solution
• Thaw frozen containers at room temperature (20-25° C or 68-77° F) or under refrigeration (2-8° C or 36-46° F). Do not force thaw by immersion in water baths or by microwaving. Check for leaks by squeezing bag firmly
• Do not admix
• Contents of the solution may precipitate in the frozen state and should dissolve with little or no agitation once the solution has reached room temperature
• *Storage:* The thawed solution is stable for 24 hours at room temperature or for 14 days under refrigeration. Do not refreeze thawed product
• Do not use plastic containers in series connections as this could result in an embolism due to residual air being drawn from the primary container before administration of the fluid from the secondary container is complete

IV infusion
• Infuse IV over at least 30 min. Ambulatory intravenous infusion pumps can be used; the solution is stable for up to 12 hr at room temperature

Y-site compatibilities: Alfentanil, allopurinol, amifostine, amikacin, aminocaproic acid, aminophylline, amphotericin B lipid complex, amphotericin B liposome, anidulafungin, argatroban, atenolol, aztreonam, bivalirudin, bleomycin, bumetanide, buprenorphine, busulfan, butorphanol, calcium acetate/chloride/gluconate, CARBOplatin, carmustine, cefepime, chloramphenicol, cimetidine, clindamycin, cyclophosphamide, cycloSPORINE, cytarabine, DACTINomycin, DAPTOmycin, dexamethasone, dexrazoxane, diazepam, digoxin, diphenhydrAMINE, DOCEtaxel, DOPamine, doxacurium, enalaprilat, ePHEDrine, EPINEPHrine, eptifibatide, erythromycin, esmolol, etoposide, fenoldopam, fentaNYL, floxuridine, fluconazole, fludarabine, fluorouracil, foscarnet, fosphenytoin, furosemide, gallium, granisetron, heparin, hydrocortisone, HYDROmorphone, ifosfamide, isoproterenol, ketorolac, lansoprazole, lepirudin, leucovorin, lidocaine, linezolid, LORazepam, magnesium sulfate, mannitol, mechlorethamine, melphalan, meperidine, mesna, metaraminol, methotrexate, methylPREDNISolone, metoclopramide, metoprolol, metroNIDAZOLE, milrinone, morphine, naloxone, nitroglycerin, nitroprusside, norepinephrine, octreotide, ondansetron, oxytocin, PACLitaxel, palonosetron, pamidronate, pancuronium, PEMEtrexed, PENTobarbital, PHENobarbital, phentolamine, phenylephrine, plicamycin, potassium chloride/phosphates, procainamide, ranitidine, remifentanil, riTUXimab, sargramostim, sodium acetate/bicarbonate/phosphates, succinylcholine, SUFentanil, sulfamethoxazole-trimethoprim, tacrolimus, telavancin, teniposide, theophylline, thiotepa, tigecycline, tirofiban, trimethobenzamide, vasopressin, vinBLAStine, vinCRIStine, voriconazole, zidovudine, zoledronic acid

Y-site incompatibilities: Fluconazole, ondansetron, sargramostim, vinorelbine

ADVERSE EFFECTS

CNS: Headache, insomnia, dizziness, fever, lethargy, hallucinations, anxiety, depression, twitching, **seizures,** vertigo
CV: Cardiac toxicity, edema
GI: *Nausea, vomiting, diarrhea,* increased AST, ALT, abdominal pain, glossitis, constipation, **pseudomembranous colitis, pancreatitis**
GU: Oliguria, proteinuria, hematuria, *vaginitis, moniliasis,* **glomerulonephritis, renal failure**
HEMA: Anemia, increased bleeding time, **bone marrow depression, agranulocytosis,** hemolytic anemia
INTEG: Rash, pruritus, **exfoliative dermatitis**
META: Hypokalemia, hypernatremia
SYST: Serum sickness, anaphylaxis, Stevens-Johnson syndrome

Pharmacokinetics

Absorption	Well absorbed (80%)
Distribution	Widely distributed; crosses placenta
Metabolism	Not metabolized
Excretion	Kidneys, unchanged (90%); bile (10%); breast milk
Half-life	0.7-1.3 hr

Pharmacodynamics

Onset	Rapid
Peak	Inf end
Duration	Unknown

INTERACTIONS

Individual drugs

Aspirin, probenecid: increased piperacillin levels
Methotrexate: increased effect of methotrexate

Drug classifications

Aminoglycosides (**IV**): decreased piperacillin effect
Anticoagulants (oral): increased effect of anticoagulants
Contraceptives (oral): decreased contraceptive effectiveness
Neuromuscular blockers: increased effects
Tetracyclines: decreased antimicrobial effectiveness of piperacillin

Drug/lab test

Increased: eosinophilia, neutropenia, leucopenia, serum creatinine, PTT, AST, ALT, alkaline phosphatase, bilirubin, BUN, electrolytes
Decreased: Hct, Hgb, electrolytes
False positive: urine glucose, urine protein, Coombs' test

NURSING CONSIDERATIONS

Assessment

• Assess patient for previous sensitivity reaction to penicillins or other cephalosporins; cross-sensitivity between penicillins and cephalosporins is common
• Assess patient for signs and symptoms of infection, including characteristics of wounds, sputum, urine, stool, WBC > 10,000/mm³, fever; obtain information baseline, during treatment
• Obtain C&S before beginning product therapy to identify if correct treatment has been initiated
• **Assess for allergic reactions:** rash, urticaria, pruritus, chills, fever, joint pain; angioedema may occur a few days after therapy begins; epinephrine, resuscitation equipment should be available for anaphylactic reaction
A Identify urine output; if decreasing, notify prescriber (may indicate nephrotoxicity); also check for increased BUN, creatinine
• Monitor blood studies: AST, ALT, CBC, Hct, bilirubin, LDH, alkaline phosphatase, Coombs' test monthly if patient is on long-term therapy
• Monitor electrolytes: potassium, sodium, chloride monthly if patient is on long-term therapy
• **Pseudomembranous colitis:** asssess for diarrhea, abdominal pain, fever, fatigue, anorexia; possible anemia, elevated WBC and low serum albumin; stop product and usually give either vancomycin or **IV** metroNIDAZOLE
• Monitor for bleeding: ecchymosis, bleeding gums, hematuria, stool guaiac daily if on long-term therapy
• **Assess for overgrowth of infection:** perineal itching, fever, malaise, redness, pain, swelling, drainage, rash, diarrhea, change in cough, sputum

Adverse effects: *italics* = common; **bold** = life-threatening

Patient/family education
• Teach patient to report sore throat, bruising, bleeding, joint pain; may indicate **blood dyscrasias (rare)**
• Advise patient to contact prescriber if vaginal itching, loose foul-smelling stools, furry tongue occur; may indicate **superinfection**
• Advise patient to notify prescriber of diarrhea with blood or pus, which may indicate **pseudomembranous colitis**

Evaluation
Positive therapeutic outcome
• Absence of signs/symptoms of infection (WBC $<$10,000/mm^3, temp WNL, absence of red, draining wounds)
• Reported improvement in symptoms of infection

TREATMENT OF ANAPHYLAXIS: Withdraw product, maintain airway, administer EPINEPHrine, aminophylline, O_2, **IV** corticosteroids

---

pitavastatin (Rx)
(pit'a-va-stat'in)
Livalo
Func. class.: Antilipidemic
Chem. class.: HMG-CoA reductase inhibitor
Pregnancy category X

Do not confuse:
pitavastatin/pravastatin

ACTION: Inhibits HMG-CoA reductase enzyme, which reduces cholesterol synthesis, high doses lead to plaque regression

Therapeutic outcome: Decreased cholesterol levels and LDLs, increased HDLs

USES: As an adjunct in primary hypercholesterolemia (types Ia, Ib), dysbetalipoproteinemia, elevated triglyceride levels; prevention of cardiovascular disease by reduction of heart risk in those with mildly elevated cholesterol

CONTRAINDICATIONS:
Pregnancy **X**, breastfeeding, hypersensitivity, active liver disease, cholestasis

Precautions: Past liver disease, alcoholism, severe acute infections, trauma, severe metabolic disorders, electrolyte imbalance, seizures, surgery, organ transplant, endocrine disease, females, hypotension, renal disease

DOSAGE AND ROUTES
Adult: PO 2 mg/day, usual range 1-4, max 4 mg/day

Renal dose
Adult: PO CCr 30-60 ml/min 1 mg qd, max 2 mg qd; CCr $<$30 ml/min on hemodialysis 1 mg qd, max 2 mg qd; CCr $<$30 ml/min not on hemodialysis—not recommended

Available forms: Tabs 1, 2, 4 mg

Implementation
• Administer total daily dose at any time of day
• Store in cool environment in tight container protected from light

ADVERSE EFFECTS
CNS: Headache
GI: Constipation, diarrhea
INTEG: Rash, pruritus, alopecia
MS: Myalgia, **rhabdomyolysis**, arthralgia
RESP: Pharyngitis

Pharmacokinetics	
Absorption	Unknown
Distribution	Concentrations are lower in healthy African-Americans
Metabolism	Liver
Excretion	Urine, feces
Half-life	12 hr

Pharmacodynamics
Unknown

INTERACTIONS
Individual drugs
Clofibrate, cycloSPORINE, erythromycin, gemfibrozil, niacin: increased risk of rhabdomyolysis
Colestipol: decreased action of atorvastatin
Erythromycin: increased levels of atorvastatin

Drug classifications
Antifungals (azole): possible rhabdomyolysis

Drug/herb
Red yeast rice: increased pitavastatin effect

Drug/lab test
Increased: bilirubin, alkaline phosphatase, ALT, AST
Interference: thyroid function tests

NURSING CONSIDERATIONS
Assessment
• Assess nutrition: fat, protein, carbohydrates; nutritional analysis should be completed by dietitian before treatment

---

- **Rhabdomyolysis:** assess for muscle pain, tenderness; obtain CPK if these occur; product may need to be discontinued
- Monitor bowel pattern daily; diarrhea may be a problem
- Monitor triglycerides, cholesterol at baseline, throughout treatment; LDL and VLDL should be watched closely; if increased, product should be discontinued
- Monitor liver function studies q1-2mo during the first 1½ yr of treatment; AST, ALT, liver function tests may be increased
- Monitor renal studies in patients with compromised renal system: BUN, I&O ratio, creatinine
- Assess eyes via ophthalmic exam 1 mo after treatment begins, annually

Patient/family education
- Inform patient that compliance is needed for positive results to occur, not to double doses
- Teach patient that risk factors should be decreased: high-fat diet, smoking, alcohol consumption, absence of exercise
- Advise patient to notify prescriber if the GI symptoms of diarrhea, abdominal or epigastric pain, nausea, vomiting; chills, fever, sore throat; muscle pain, weakness occur
- Advise patient that treatment will take several years
- Advise patient that blood work will be necessary during treatment
- Advise patient not to take if pregnant, pregnancy **X**

Evaluation
Positive therapeutic outcome
- Decreased cholesterol levels, serum triglyceride
- Improved ratio of HDLs

plasma protein fraction (Rx)
Plasmanate
Func. class.: Hematological agent
Chem. class.: Plasma volume expander
Pregnancy category C

ACTION: Exerts similar oncotic pressure as human plasma, expands blood volume, shifts water from extravascular space to intravascular space

Therapeutic outcome: Shift of fluid from extravascular into intravascular space

USES: Hypovolemic shock, hypoproteinemia, ARDS, preoperative cardiopulmonary bypass, acute liver failure, nephrotic syndrome, cardiogenic shock

CONTRAINDICATIONS:
Hypersensitivity to this product or albumin, CHF, severe anemia, renal insufficiency, hyponatremia, cardiopulmonary bypass

Precautions: Pregnancy **C**, decreased salt intake, decreased cardiac reserve, lack of albumin deficiency, hepatic disease

DOSAGE AND ROUTES
Hypovolemia
Adult: IV INF 250-500 ml (12.5-25 g of protein), max 10 ml/min
Child: IV INF 10-30 ml/kg max 5-10 ml/min

Hypoproteinemia
Adult: IV INF 1000-1500 ml/day, max 8 ml/min

Available forms: Inj 5%

Implementation
- Give by **IV;** no dilution required; use inf pump, large-gauge needle (≥20-G); discard unused portion; inf slowly to prevent hypotension; give within 4 hr of opening
- Provide adequate hydration before administration
- Do not use sol that has been frozen
- Adjust rate to changes in B/P
- Store at room temp, max 86° F

Additive compatibilities:
Carbohydrate and electrolyte sol, whole blood, packed RBCs, chloramphenicol, tetracycline

Additive incompatibilities:
Protein hydrolysate sol, amino acid sol, alcohol, norepinephrine

ADVERSE EFFECTS
CNS: Fever, chills, headache, paresthesias, flushing
CV: Fluid overload, hypotension, erratic pulse
GI: Nausea, vomiting, increased salivation
INTEG: Rash, urticaria, cyanosis
RESP: Altered respirations, dyspnea, **pulmonary edema**

Pharmacokinetics
Absorption	Completely absorbed
Distribution	Intravascular space
Metabolism	Unknown
Excretion	Unknown
Half-life	Unknown

Pharmacodynamics

Onset	15-30 min
Peak	Unknown
Duration	Unknown

INTERACTIONS
Drug/lab test
False increase: alkaline phosphatase

NURSING CONSIDERATIONS
Assessment
• Monitor blood studies: Hct, Hgb; electrolytes, serum protein; if serum protein declines, dyspnea, hypoxemia can result
• Monitor B/P (decreased), pulse (erratic), respiration during inf; CVP, jugular vein distention, PWP (increases if overload occurs); SOB, anxiety, insomnia, expiratory crackles, frothy blood-tinged cough, cyanosis indicate pulmonary overload
• Monitor I&O ratio; urinary output may decrease
• Assess for allergy: fever, rash, itching, chills, flushing, urticaria, nausea, vomiting, or hypotension require discontinuation of inf; use new lot if therapy is reinstituted, premedicate with diphenhydrAMINE

Patient/family education
• Explain reason for and expected result of medication

Evaluation
Positive therapeutic outcome
• Increased B/P
• Decreased edema
• Increased serum albumin

---

plerixafor (Rx)
(pler-ix'a-fore)
Mozobil
Func. class.: Biological modifier
Chem. class.: Colony-stimulating factor
Pregnancy category D

ACTION: Competitively inhibits the binding of stromal-derived factors, allowing hematopoietic stem cells to mobilize into peripheral blood

Therapeutic outcome: Successful collection of stem cells

USES: For peripheral blood stem cell (PBSC) mobilization for collection and autologous transplant in non-Hodgkin's lymphoma, multiple myeloma; used with a granulocyte colony stimulating factor (G-CSF)

CONTRAINDICATIONS:
Pregnancy **D**, hypersensitivity, breastfeeding

Precautions: Children, renal disease, thrombocytopenia

DOSAGE AND ROUTES
Adult: SUBCUT 0.24 mg/kg qd about 11 hr before initiating apheresis; give up to 4 consecutive days; give filgrastim 10 mcg/kg SUBCUT qd each AM beginning 4 days before the 1st evening dose of plerixafor and on each day of apheresis; give filgrastim before procedure

Available forms: Inj 300 mcg/ml, 480 mcg/1.6 ml, 480 mcg/0.8 ml, 3000 mcg/0.5 ml

Implementation
SUBCUT route
• Each single-use vial contains 24 mg of plerixafor (1.2 ml of 20 mg/ml sol); the volume is calculated by multiplying 0.012 by the actual body wt (kg)
• Give 11 hr before apheresis
• Max 40 mg/day, or 27 mg/day in renal disease
• Store at room temperature

ADVERSE EFFECTS
CNS: Syncope, dizziness, fatigue, headache, insomnia, malaise, paresthesias
GI: *Nausea,* vomiting, diarrhea, abdominal pain, constipation
HEMA: Thrombocytopenia, leukocytosis
INTEG: Rash, skin irritation, pruritus, inj site reaction, erythema, urticaria
MS: Musculoskeletal pain
RESP: Dyspnea, hypoxia

Pharmacokinetics

Absorption	Unknown
Distribution	Protein binding 58%
Metabolism	Unknown
Excretion	70% kidney as parent drug
Half-life	Terminal 3-5 hr

Pharmacodynamics

Onset	30-60 min
Peak	6-9 hr mobilization
Duration	Unknown

INTERACTIONS
Individual drugs
Lithium: increased adverse reactions, increased leukocytosis, do not use concomitantly

---

NURSING CONSIDERATIONS

Assessment
- Monitor blood studies: CBC/differential
- Monitor B/P, respirations, pulse before, during therapy
- Assess for bone pain; give mild analgesics

Patient/family education
- Explain reason for use and expected results

Evaluation
Positive therapeutic outcome
- Collection of stem cells

---

posaconazole (Rx)
(poe'sa-kon'a-zole)
Noxafil, Posanol ✦
Func. class.: Antifungal, systemic
Chem. class.: Triazole derivative
Pregnancy category C

ACTION: Inhibits a portion of cell wall synthesis; alters cell membranes and inhibits several fungal enzymes

Therapeutic outcome: Decreased fever, malaise, rash; negative C&S for infecting organism

USES: Prevention of aspergillus, candida infection, oropharyngeal candidiasis in the immunocompromised, chemotherapy-induced neutropenia, mucocutaneous candidiasis

CONTRAINDICATIONS:
Hypersensitivity to this product or other systemic antifungal or azoles, fungal meningitis, onchomycosis or dermatomycosis in cardiac dysfunction, use with ergots, sirolimus, CYP3A4 substrates

Precautions: Pregnancy C, breastfeeding, children, hepatic/cardiac/renal disease

DOSAGE AND ROUTES
Adult/adolescent: PO 800 mg/day in 2-4 divided doses

Thrush
Adult: PO 100 mg bid × 1 day, then 100 mg/day × 13 days

Available forms: Oral susp 200 mg/5 ml

Implementation
PO route
- **Oral susp:** give after shaking well; use calibrated measuring device; take only with a full meal or liquid nutritional supplements such as Ensure; rinse measuring device after each use
- Store in a tight container in refrigerator; do not freeze

ADVERSE EFFECTS
CNS: *Headache, dizziness,* insomnia, fever, rigors, weakness, anxiety
CV: Hypo/hypertension, tachycardia, anemia, **QT prolongation, torsades de pointes**
GI: *Nausea, vomiting, anorexia, diarrhea,* cramps, abdominal pain, flatulence, **GI bleeding, hepatotoxicity**
GU: Gynecomastia, impotence, decreased libido
INTEG: *Pruritus,* fever, *rash,* **toxic epidermal necrolysis**
MISC: *Edema, fatigue,* malaise, hypokalemia, tinnitus, **rhabdomyolysis**

Pharmacokinetics

Absorption	Well absorbed, enhanced by food
Distribution	Protein binding 98%-99%
Metabolism	Liver
Excretion	Feces, 77% unchanged
Half-life	19-35 hr

Pharmacodynamics

Onset	Unknown
Peak	3-5 hr
Duration	Unknown

INTERACTIONS
Individual drugs
⚠ Atorvastatin, lovastatin: do not use concurrently
⚠ BusPIRone, busulfan, clarithromycin, cycloSPORINE, diazepam, digoxin, felodipine, indinavir, isradipine, midazolam, niCARdipine, NIFEdipine, niMODipine, phenytoin, quiNIDine, ritonavir, saquinavir, tacrolimus, warfarin: increased levels, toxicity
Haloperidol, chloroquine, droperidol, pentamidine; arsenic trioxide, levomethadyl: increased QT prolongation
Cimetidine, phenytoin: decreased posaconazole level
Didanosine, rifamycin: decreased posaconazole action
⚠ Dofetilide, pimozide, quiNIDine, halofantrine: life-threatening reactions, increased QT prolongation
Midazolam (oral), triazolam: increased sedation
QuiNIDine: increased tinnitus, hearing loss

Adverse effects: *italics* = common; **bold** = life-threatening

Drug classifications

Antacids, H_2-receptor antagonists, rifamycins: decreased posaconazole action

Class IA/III antidysrhythmics, some phenothiazines, beta agonists, local anesthetics, tricyclics, CYP3A4 inhibitors (amiodarone, clarithromycin, erythromycin, telithromycin, troleandomycin), CYP3A4 substrates (methadone, pimozide, QUEtiapine, quiNIDine, risperidone, ziprasidone): increased QT prolongation

⚠ **Ergots: life-threatening reactions, increased QT prolongation**

Other hepatotoxic products: increased hepatotoxicity

Calcium channel blockers, HMG-CoA reductase inhibitors, vinca alkaloids: increased levels, toxicity

Oral contraceptives: decreased effect, use other contraceptives

Oral hypoglycemics: increased severe hypoglycemia

Drug/food

Food: increased absorption

NURSING CONSIDERATIONS

Assessment

• **Rhabdomyolysis:** assess for muscle pain, increased CPK, weakness, swelling of affected muscles; if these occur and if confirmed by CPK, product should be discontinued

• **QT prolongation:** monitor ECG for QT prolongation, ejection fraction; assess for chest pain, palpitations, dyspnea

• Assess for type of infection; may begin treatment before obtaining results

• Assess for infection: temp, WBC, sputum, baseline, periodically, breakthrough infections may occur when used with fosamprenavir

• Monitor I&O ratio, potassium levels

• Monitor liver function tests (ALT, AST, bilirubin) if on long-term therapy

• Assess for allergic reaction: rash, photosensitivity, uricaria, dermatitis

⚠ **Assess for hepatotoxicity: nausea, vomiting, jaundice, clay-colored stools, fatigue**

Patient/family education

• Teach patient that long-term therapy may be needed to clear infection (1 wk-6 mo depending on infection)

• Advise patient to avoid hazardous activities if dizziness occurs

• Advise patient to take 2 hr before administration of other products that increase gastric pH (antacids, H_2-blockers, omeprazole, sucralfate, anticholinergics); to notify health care provider of all medications taken (many interactions)

• Teach the patient the importance of compliance with product regimen; to use alternative method of contraception

• Teach patient to notify prescriber of GI symptoms, signs of hepatic dysfunction (fatigue, nausea, anorexia, vomiting, dark urine, pale stools)

• Teach patient to take during meal or within 20 min of eating

Evaluation

Positive therapeutic outcome

• Decreased fever, malaise, rash, negative C&S for infecting organism

---

potassium acetate/ potassium bicarbonate (Rx, OTC)

K-Effervescent, Klor-Con EF, K-Vescent

potassium bicarbonate/ potassium chloride (Rx, OTC)

Neo-K ✦

potassium bicarbonate/ potassium citrate (Rx, OTC)

potassium chloride (Rx, OTC)

Epiklor, Klor-Con, K-Tab, Micro-K, Odan K-20 ✦

potassium gluconate (Rx, OTC)

Kaon, Kaylixir, K-G Elixir, Potassium-Rougier ✦

Func. class.: Electrolyte, mineral replacement

Chem. class.: Potassium

Pregnancy category C

ACTION: Needed for adequate transmission of nerve impulses and cardiac contraction, renal function, intracellular ion maintenance

Therapeutic outcome: Potassium level 3.0-5.0 mg/dl

USES: Prevention and treatment of hypokalemia

CONTRAINDICATIONS:
Renal disease (severe), severe hemolytic disease, Addison's disease, hyperkalemia, acute dehydration, extensive tissue breakdown

Precautions: Pregnancy **C**, cardiac disease, potassium-sparing diuretic therapy, systemic acidosis

DOSAGE AND ROUTES
Hypokalemia (prevention) (bicarbonate, chloride, gluconate)
Adult: PO 20 mEq/day in 1-2 divided doses
Child: PO 1-2 mEq/day in 1-2 divided doses

Hypokalemia, digoxin toxicity (acetate, chloride)
Adult: serum potassium conc > 2.5 mEq/L: **IV** max 10 mEq/l hr, with 24 hr dose max 200 mEq, initial dose of 20-40 mEq has been recommended; **PO** 40-100 mEq/day in 2-4 divided doses
Child: IV 0.25-0.5 mEq/g/dose, at 0.25-0.5 mEq/kg/hr; PO 2-5 mEq/day in divided doses

Available forms: Tabs for sol 6.5, 25 mEq; ext rel caps 8, 10 mEq; powder for sol 3.3, 5, 6.7, 10, 13.3 mEq/5 ml; tabs 2, 4, 5, 13.4 mEq; ext rel tabs 6.7, 8, 10 mEq; elix 6.7 mEq/5 ml; oral sol 2.375 mEq/5 ml; inj for prep of IV 1.5, 2, 2.4, 3, 3.2, 4.4, 4.7 mEq/ml

Implementation
PO route
• Do not break, crush, or chew ext rel tabs/caps or enteric-coated products
• Give with meal or after meal; take cap with full glass of liquid; dissolve effervescent tab, powder in 8 oz of cold water or juice; do not give IM, SUBCUT
• Store at room temperature

IV route
• Give through large-bore needle to decrease vein inflammation; check for extravasation; administer in large vein, avoiding scalp vein in child
• After diluting in large volume of IV sol give as an IV inf slowly to prevent toxicity; never give IV bol or IM

Potassium acetate

Additive compatibilities: Metoclopramide
• **Potassium chloride** must be diluted, concentrated potassium injections are fatal

Continuous IV infusion route
• Conc max 80 mEq/L for peripheral line, 120 mEq/L central line

• Dehydrated patients should receive 1 L of potassium-free hydration sol; then infuse 10 mEq/hr; in severe hypokalemia rate may be 40 mEq/hr

Y-site compatibilities: Acyclovir, aldesleukin, allopurinol, amifostine, aminophylline, amiodarone, ampicillin, atropine, aztreonam, betamethasone, calcium gluconate, cefmetazole, cephalothin, cephapirin, chlordiazePOXIDE, chlorproMAZINE, ciprofloxacin, cladribine, cyanocobalamin, dexamethasone, digoxin, diltiazem, diphenhydrAMINE, DOBUTamine, DOPamine, droperidol, edrophonium, enalaprilat, EPINEPHrine, esmolol, estrogens, ethacrynate, famotidine, fentaNYL, filgrastim, fludarabine, fluorouracil, furosemide, gallium, granisetron, heparin, hydrALAZINE, IDArubicin, indomethacin, inamrinone, regular insulin, isoproterenol, kanamycin, labetalol, lidocaine, LORazepam, magnesium sulfate, melphalan, meperidine, methicillin, methoxamine, methylergonovine, midazolam, minocycline, morphine, neostigmine, norepinephrine, ondansetron, oxacillin, oxytocin, PACLitaxel, penicillin G potassium, pentazocine, phytonadione, piperacillin/tazobactam, predniSOLONE, procainamide, prochlorperazine, propofol, propranolol, pyridostigmine, sargramostim, scopolamine, sodium bicarbonate, succinylcholine, tacrolimus, teniposide, theophylline, thiotepa, trimethaphan, trimethobenzamide, vinorelbine, zidovudine

Additive compatibilities: Aminophylline, amiodarone, atracurium, bretylium, calcium chloride, cefepime, cephalothin, cephapirin, chloramphenicol, cimetidine, ciprofloxacin, clindamycin, cloxacillin, corticotropin, cytarabine, dimenhyDRINATE, DOPamine, enalaprilat, erythromycin, floxacillin, fluconazole, furosemide, heparin, hydrocortisone, isoproterenol, lidocaine, metaraminol, methicillin, methyldopate, metoclopramide, mitoXANtrone, nafcillin, netilmicin, norepinephrine, oxacillin, penicillin G potassium or sodium, phenylephrine, piperacillin, ranitidine, sodium bicarbonate, thiopental, vancomycin, verapamil, vit B/C

Potassium chloride

Y-site compatibilities: Aldesleukin, amifostine, granisetron, LORazepam, midazolam, thiotepa

ADVERSE EFFECTS
CNS: Confusion
CV: Bradycardia, *cardiac depression,* **dysrhythmias, arrest, peaking T waves,**

lowered R and depressed RST, prolonged P–R interval, widened QRS complex
GI: *Nausea, vomiting, cramps,* pain, *diarrhea,* ulceration of small bowel
GU: Oliguria
INTEG: Cold extremities, rash

Pharmacokinetics

Absorption	Unknown
Distribution	Unknown
Metabolism	Unknown
Excretion	Kidneys, feces
Half-life	Unknown

Pharmacodynamics

	PO	IV
Onset	30 min	Immediate
Peak	Unknown	Unknown
Duration	Unknown	Unknown

INTERACTIONS
Drug classifications
Angiotensin-converting enzyme inhibitors, calcium, diuretics (potassium-sparing), magnesium, potassium phosphate, **IV,** other potassium products: increased hyperkalemia

NURSING CONSIDERATIONS
Assessment
• Assess ECG for peaking T-waves, lowered R, depressed RST, prolonged PR interval, widening QRS complex, hyperkalemia; product should be reduced or discontinued
• Monitor potassium level during treatment (3.5-5.0 mg/dl is normal level)
• Monitor hydration status, I&O ratio; watch for decreased urinary output; notify prescriber immediately; check urinary pH in patients receiving the product as a urinary acidifier
• Assess cardiac status: rate, rhythm, CVP, PWP, PAWP if being monitored directly

Patient/family education
• Teach patient to eat foods rich in potassium after medication is discontinued
• Advise patient to avoid OTC products: antacids, salt substitutes, analgesics, vit preparations, unless specifically directed by prescriber; avoid licorice in large amounts, may cause hypokalemia, sodium retention
• Advise patient to report hyperkalemia symptoms or continued hypokalemia symptoms
• Tell patient to take cap with full glass of liquid; to dissolve powder or tab completely in at least 120 ml of water or juice; not to crush, chew caps or tabs

• Emphasize importance of regular follow-up and periodic potassium levels

Evaluation
Positive therapeutic outcome
• Absence of fatigue, muscle weakness, and decreased thirst and urinary output, cardiac changes
• Potassium level normal

---

pramipexole (Rx)
(pra-mi-pex'ol)
Mirapex, Mirapex ER
Func. class.: Antiparkinsonian agent
Chem. class.: Dopamine receptor agonist, nonergot
Pregnancy category C

ACTION: Selective agonist for D_2 receptors (presynaptic/postsynaptic sites); binding at D_3 receptor contributes to antiparkinson effects

Therapeutic outcome: Decreased symptoms of Parkinson's disease (involuntary movements)

USES: Idiopathic Parkinson's disease, restless leg syndrome

CONTRAINDICATIONS:
Hypersensitivity

Precautions: Pregnancy **C**, renal/cardiac disease, MI with dysrhythmias, affective disorders, psychosis, preexisting dyskinesias, history of falling asleep during daily activities

DOSAGE AND ROUTES
Initial treatment
Adult: PO from a starting dose of 0.375 mg/day given in 3 divided doses, increase gradually by 0.125 mg/dose at 5-7–day intervals until total daily dose of 4.5 mg is reached; ER 0.375 mg qd, may increase up to 0.75 mg/day, then increments of 0.75 mg/day ≤5-7 days, max 4.5 mg/day

Restless leg syndrome
Adult: PO 0.125 mg 2-3 hr before bedtime, increase gradually, max 0.5 mg/day

Renal dose
Adult: PO CCr 35-59 ml/min 0.125 mg bid, may increase q5-7day to 1.5 mg bid; CCr 15-34 ml/min 0.125 mg/day, may increase q5-7day to 1.5 mg/day

Available forms: Tabs 0.125, 0.25, 0.5, 1, 1.5 mg; cap ER 0.375, 0.75, 1.5, 3.0, 4.5 mg

---

Implementation
- Adjust dosage to patient's response
- Give with meals to decrease GI upset

ADVERSE EFFECTS

CNS: *Agitation, insomnia,* psychosis, hallucinations, depression, dizziness, headache, confusion, amnesia, dream disorder, asthenia, dyskinesia, hypersomnolence, sudden sleep onset, impulse-control disorders

CV: *Orthostatic hypotension,* edema, syncope, tachycardia, increased B/P, heart rate

EENT: Blurred vision

ENDO: Antidiuretic hormone secretion (SIADH)

GI: *Nausea, anorexia,* constipation, dysphagia, dry mouth

GU: Impotence, urinary frequency

HEMA: Hemolytic anemia, leukopenia, agranulocytosis

INTEG: Pruritus

Pharmacokinetics

Absorption	Well absorbed
Distribution	Widely distributed
Metabolism	Liver, minimally
Excretion	Kidneys, unchanged
Half-life	8 hr; 12 hr in geriatric

Pharmacodynamics

Onset	Unknown
Peak	2 hr
Duration	Unknown

INTERACTIONS

Individual drugs
Cimetidine, diltiazem, levodopa, quiNIDine, ranitidine, triamterine, verapamil: increased pramipexole levels

Metoclopramide: decreased pramipexole levels

Drug classifications
Butyrophenones, DOPamine agonists, phenothiazines: decreased pramipexole effect

NURSING CONSIDERATIONS

Assessment
- Monitor B/P, ECG, respiration during initial treatment; hypo/hypertension should be reported
- Assess mental status: affect, mood, behavioral changes, depression; complete suicide assessment

- Assess for involuntary movements in parkinsonism: akinesia, tremors, staggering gait, muscle rigidity, drooling; these symptoms should improve with therapy

⚠ **Assess for sleep attacks: may fall asleep during activities, without warning; may need to discontinue medication**

Patient/family education
- Advise patient that therapeutic effects may take several wk to a few mo
- Caution patient to change positions slowly to prevent orthostatic hypotension
- Instruct patient to use product exactly as prescribed; if product is discontinued abruptly, parkinsonian crisis may occur; if treatment is to be discontinued, taper over 1 wk; avoid alcohol, OTC sleeping products
- Advise patient to notify prescriber if pregnancy is planned or suspected
- Teach patient to notify prescriber of impulse control disorders: shopping

Evaluation

Positive therapeutic outcome
- Decreased akathisia, other involuntary movements
- Improved mood

---

pramlintide (Rx)
(pram′lin-tide)

Symlin

Func. class.: Antidiabetic

Chem. class.: Synthetic human amylin analog

Pregnancy category C

ACTION: Modulates and slows stomach emptying, prevents postprandial rise in plasma glucagon, decreases appetite, leads to decreased caloric intake and weight loss

Therapeutic outcome: Decreased polyuria, polydipsia, polyphagia; improved A1c

USES: As an adjunct to insulin therapy with uncontrolled type 1 or type 2 diabetes mellitus

CONTRAINDICATIONS:
Hypersensitivity to this product or cresol, gastroparesis

> **BLACK BOX WARNING:** Hypoglycemia

Precautions: Pregnancy **C**, breastfeeding

DOSAGE AND ROUTES

Type 1 diabetes
Adult: SUBCUT prior to each meal (≥30 g carbohydrate), titrate up from 15 mcg to target dose of 60 mcg/dose, each dose titration should occur after no nausea for 3 days

Type 2 diabetes
Adult: SUBCUT 60 mcg prior to each meal (≥30 g CHO), titrate up to 120 mcg SUBCUT with each meal after no nausea for 3-7 days

Available forms: PEN 60, 120 (1000 mcg/ml sol for j-injection)

Implementation
• Pre-meal insulin should be decreased by 50% when starting and adjusted to therapeutic dose to prevent hypoglycemia

SUBCUT route
• Rotate inj sites, allow sol to warm to room temp before use
• Give immediately before mealtime or if 30 g of carbohydrates will be consumed
• Do not use if a meal is skipped
• Do not use if discolored; do not give in arm; absorption is variable
• Store at room temperature for up to 30 days; keep away from heat and sunlight; refrigerate all other supply

ADVERSE EFFECTS

CNS: *Headache,* fatigue, dizziness, confusion
EENT: Blurred vision
GI: *Nausea, vomiting, anorexia,* abdominal pain
INTEG: Inj site reactions, diaphoresis
META: Hypoglycemia
MS: Arthralgia
RESP: *Cough,* pharyngitis
SYST: *Systemic allergy*

Pharmacokinetics

Absorption	30%-40%
Distribution	Not bound to blood cells or albumin, 40% bound in plasma
Metabolism	Kidneys
Excretion	Unknown
Half-life	48 min

Pharmacodynamics

Onset	Unknown
Peak	20 min
Duration	3 hr

INTERACTIONS

Individual drugs
Acetaminophen: may increase effect of acetaminophen
Alcohol, disopyramide, insulin: increased hypoglycemia
Dextrothyroxine, niacin, triamterene: decreased hypoglycemia
Diphenoxylate, loperamide, octreotide: increased pramlintide action
Erythromycin, metoclopramide: do not use

Drug classifications
ACE inhibitors, anabolic steroids, androgens, corticosteroids, fibric acid derivatives: increased hypoglycemia
α-Glucosidase inhibitors, antimuscarinics, opiate agonist, tricyclics: increased pramlintide action
Estrogens, MAOIs, oral contraceptives, progestins, thiazide diuretics: decreased hypoglycemia
Phenothiazines: increased hyperglycemia

NURSING CONSIDERATIONS

Assessment
• Monitor fasting blood glucose, 2 hr postprandial (80-150 mg/dl, normal fasting level; 70-130 mg/dl, normal 2 hr level); A1c may also be drawn to identify treatment effectiveness; also monitor weight, appetite
• **Assess for hypoglycemic reaction** (sweating, weakness, dizziness, chills, confusion, headache, nausea, rapid weak pulse, fatigue, tachycardia, memory lapses, slurred speech, staggering gait, anxiety, tremors, hunger)
• **Assess for hyperglycemia:** acetone breath, polyuria, fatigue, polydipsia, flushed, dry skin, lethargy

Patient/family education
• Advise patient that product does not cure diabetes but controls symptoms
• Advise patient to carry emergency ID as diabetic
• Teach patient to recognize hypoglycemia reaction: headache, fatigue, weakness, fast pulse
• Teach patient the dosage, route, mixing instructions, if any diet restrictions, disease process
• Advise patient to carry a glucose source (candy or lump sugar, glucose tabs) to treat hypoglycemia
• Teach patient symptoms of ketoacidosis: nausea, thirst, polyuria, dry mouth, decreased B/P, dry, flushed skin, acetone breath, drowsiness, Kussmaul respirations

---

• Advise patient that a plan is necessary for diet, exercise; all food on diet should be eaten; exercise routine should not vary
• Teach patient about blood glucose testing; make sure patient is able to determine glucose level
• Advise patient to avoid OTC products unless directed by prescriber, avoid alcohol
• Advise patient not to operate machinery or drive until effect is known
• Teach patient how to use pen

Evaluation
Positive therapeutic outcome
• Decrease in polyuria, polydipsia, polyphagia, clear sensorium; improved A1c, blood glucose; absence of dizziness; stable gait

TREATMENT OF OVERDOSE:
Glucose 25 g **IV**, via dextrose 50% sol, 50 ml or glucagon 1 mg SUBCUT

pramoxine topical
See Appendix B

prasugrel (Rx)
(pra′soo-grel)
Effient
Func. class.: Platelet aggregation inhibitor
Chem. class.: ADP receptor antagonist
Pregnancy category B

ACTION: Inhibits ADP-induced platelet aggregation

Therapeutic outcome: Absence of MI, stroke

USES: Reducing the risk of stroke, MI, vascular death, peripheral arterial disease in high-risk patients

CONTRAINDICATIONS:
Hypersensitivity, stroke, TIA

> **BLACK BOX WARNING:** Active bleeding

Precautions: Pregnancy **B**, breastfeeding, children, hepatic disease, increased bleeding risk, neutropenia, agranulocytosis, renal disease, surgery, trauma, thrombotic thrombocytopenia purpura, Asian patients, weight <60 kg, CABG, geriatric
Abrupt discontinuation

DOSAGE AND ROUTES
Adult/geriatric <75 yr and ≥60 kg: PO 60 mg loading dose, then 10 mg qd with aspirin (75-325 mg/day)
Adult/geriatric <75 yr and <60 kg: PO 60 mg loading dose, then 5 mg qd
Geriatric >75 yr: Not recommended

Available forms: Tabs 5, 10 mg

Implementation
• Give with food to decrease gastric symptoms
• Do not break tablets
• Do not discontinue therapy abruptly

ADVERSE EFFECTS
CNS: Headache, dizziness
CV: Edema, atrial fibrillation, bradycardia, chest pain, hyper/hypotension
GI: Nausea, vomiting, diarrhea
HEMA: Epistaxis, **leukopenia, thrombocytopenia, neutropenia, anaphylaxis, angioedema, anemia**
INTEG: Rash, hypercholesterolemia
MISC: Fatigue, **intracranial hemorrhage, secondary malignancy, angioedema**
MS: Back pain

Pharmacokinetics
Absorption	Rapidly absorbed
Distribution	Unknown
Metabolism	Liver CYP3A4, CYP2B6
Excretion	Urine, feces
Half-life	7-8 hr

Pharmacodynamics
Onset	Unknown
Peak	30 min
Duration	Unknown

INTERACTIONS
Individual drugs
Abciximab, aspirin, eptifibatide, rifampin, tirofiban, ticlopidine, treprostinil: increased bleeding risk

Drug classifications
Anticoagulants, thrombolytics, NSAIDs, SSRIs: increased bleeding risk

NURSING CONSIDERATIONS
Assessment
⚠ Assess for thrombotic/thrombocytic purpura: fever, thrombocytopenia, neurolytic anemia
• Monitor hepatic studies: AST, ALT, bilirubin, creatinine (long-term therapy)

Adverse effects: *italics* = common; **bold** = life-threatening

• Monitor blood studies: CBC, differential, Hct, Hgb, PT, cholesterol (long-term therapy)

> **BLACK BOX WARNING: Bleeding:** may be fatal, decreased B/P in those who have had CABG may be the first indication; bleeding should be controlled while continuing product; may use transfusion; do not use within 1 wk of CABG; may use lower doses in those <60 kg

Patient/family education
• Advise that blood work will be necessary during treatment
• Teach to report any unusual bruising, bleeding to prescriber; that it may take longer to stop bleeding
• Advise to take with food or just after eating to minimize GI discomfort
• Advise to report diarrhea, skin rashes, subcutaneous bleeding, chills, fever, sore throat
• Teach to tell all health care providers that prasugrel is used; may be withheld before surgery

Evaluation
Positive therapeutic outcome
• Absence of stroke, MI

---

pravastatin (Rx)
(pra′va-sta-tin)
Pravachol
Func. class.: Antilipidemic
Pregnancy category X

Do not confuse:
Pravachol/Prevacid

ACTION: Inhibits biosynthesis of VLDL, LDL, which are responsible for cholesterol development, by inhibiting the enzyme HMG-CoA reductase

Therapeutic outcome: Decreasing cholesterol levels and LDL, increased HDL

USES: As an adjunct in primary hypercholesterolemia types IIa, IIb, III, IV, artherosclerosis; to reduce the risk of recurrent MI, primary/secondary CV events; reduce stroke, TIAs

CONTRAINDICATIONS:
Pregnancy **X,** breastfeeding, hypersensitivity, active liver disease

Precautions: Past liver disease, alcoholism, severe acute infections, trauma, severe metabolic disorders, electrolyte imbalances, renal disease

DOSAGE AND ROUTES
Adult: PO 40-80 mg/day at bedtime (range 20-80 mg/day), start at 10 mg/day if also on immunosuppressants
Adolescent 14-18 yr: PO 40 mg/day
Child 8-13 yr: PO 20 mg/day
Geriatric/renal/hepatic dose: PO 10 mg/day, initially

Renal dose
Adult: PO 10-20 mg daily at bedtime, increase at 4-wk intervals

Available forms: Tabs 10, 20, 40, 80 mg

Implementation
• Give at bedtime only; give 1 hr before or 2 hr after bile acid sequestrants
• Store in cool environment in airtight, light-resistant container

ADVERSE EFFECTS
CNS: Headache, dizziness, fatigue, confusion
CV: Chest pain
EENT: Lens opacities
GI: Nausea, constipation, diarrhea, flatus, abdominal pain, heartburn, **liver dysfunction, pancreatitis, hepatitis**
GU: **Renal failure (myoglobinuria)**
INTEG: Rash, pruritus
MS: Muscle cramps, myalgia, **myositis, rhabdomyolysis**
RESP: Common cold, rhinitis, cough

Pharmacokinetics
Absorption	Poorly absorbed, erratic
Distribution	Protein binding 80%
Metabolism	Liver, extensively
Excretion	Feces (70%-75%); kidneys, unchanged (20%); breast milk (minimal)
Half-life	2 hr

Pharmacodynamics
Onset	Unknown
Peak	1-1½ hr
Duration	Unknown

INTERACTIONS
Individual drugs
Clarithromycin, clofibrate, cycloSPORINE, erythromycin, gemfibrozil, itraconazole, niacin: increased risk for myopathy

Drug classifications
Bile acid sequestrants: decreased pravastatin bioavailability
Protease inhibitors: increased risk of myopathy

Drug/herb
St. John's wort: decreased effect
Red yeast rice: increased adverse reactions
Eucalyptus: increased hepatotoxicity

Drug/lab test
Increased: CPK, liver function tests
Altered: thyroid function tests

NURSING CONSIDERATIONS
Assessment
• Assess nutrition: fat, protein, carbohydrates; nutritional analysis should be completed by dietitian before treatment
• Monitor triglycerides, esterol, cholesterol at baseline, throughout treatment; LDL and HDL should be watched closely; if increased, product should be discontinued
⚠ **Rhabdomyolysis: assess for muscle tenderness, pain; obtain CPK; therapy should be discontinued**
• Monitor ophth status yearly

Patient/family education
• Inform patient that compliance is needed for positive results to occur; not to double doses or skip doses
• Teach patient that risk factors should be decreased: high-fat diet, smoking, alcohol consumption, absence of exercise
• Advise patient to notify prescriber of weakness, tenderness, or limited mobility, blurred vision, severe GI symptoms, dizziness, headache, muscle pain, fever
⚠ **Explain to patient that contraception is necessary, since product produces teratogenic effects, pregnancy X, not to breastfeed**
• Advise patient to use sunscreen, protective clothing to prevent burns
⚠ **Hepatic disease: Instruct patient to notify prescriber of lack of appetite, yellow sclera and skin, dark urine, abdominal pain, weakness**

Evaluation
Positive therapeutic outcome
• Decreased cholesterol, serum triglyceride levels and improved ratio with HDL

---

prazosin (Rx)
(pra′zoe-sin)
Minipress
Func. class.: Antihypertensive
Chem. class.: α_1-Adrenergic blocker, peripheral
Pregnancy category C

ACTION: Blocks α-mediated vasoconstriction of adrenergic receptors, inducing peripheral vasodilatation

Therapeutic outcome: Decreased B/P in hypertension; decreased cardiac preload, afterload

USES: Hypertension

Unlabeled uses: Benign prostatic hypertrophy to decrease urine outflow obstruction, posttraumatic stress disorder (PTSD), scorpion venom poisoning

CONTRAINDICATIONS:
Hypersensitivity

Precautions: Pregnancy **C,** breastfeeding, children, geriatric patients, prostate cancer, ocular surgery, orthostatic hypotension

DOSAGE AND ROUTES
Hypertension (unlabeled)
Adult: PO 1 mg bid or tid, increasing to 20 mg/day in divided doses if required, usual range 6-15 mg/day; max 1 mg initially, max 20-40 mg/day
Child: PO 5 mcg/kg q6hr; max 400 mcg/kg/day or 15 mg/day

Benign prostatic hyperplasia (unlabeled)
Adult: PO 2 mg bid

Available forms: Caps 1, 2, 5 mg

Implementation
• Severe hypotension may occur after first dose of this medication; hypotension may be prevented by reducing or discontinuing diuretic therapy 3 days before beginning prazosin therapy
• Give same time each day
• Store in airtight container at 86° F (30° C) or less
• Give without regard to meals
• Store at room temperature

Adverse effects: *italics* = common; **bold** = life-threatening

ADVERSE EFFECTS

CNS: *Dizziness, headache, drowsiness,* anxiety, depression, vertigo, *weakness,* fatigue, syncope

CV: *Palpitations, orthostatic hypotension,* tachycardia, edema, rebound hypertension

EENT: Blurred vision, epistaxis, tinnitus, dry mouth, red sclera

GI: *Nausea,* vomiting, diarrhea, constipation, abdominal pain, **pancreatitis**

GU: Urinary frequency, incontinence, impotence, priapism, water and sodium retention

Pharmacokinetics

Absorption	60%
Distribution	Widely distributed
Metabolism	Liver, extensively; protein binding 97%
Excretion	Kidneys, unchanged (10%); bile (90%)
Half-life	2-3 hr

Pharmacodynamics

Onset	2 hr
Peak	1-3 hr
Duration	6-12 hr

INTERACTIONS

Individual drugs
Alcohol, nitroglycerin: increased hypotension
CloNIDine: decreased antihypertensive effect

Drug classifications
Antihypertensives, β-adrenergic blockers, phosphodiesterase inhibitors (vardenafil, tadalafil, sildenafil), diuretics, MAOIs: increased hypotension
NSAIDs: decreased antihypertensive effect

Drug/herb
Hawthorn: increased antihypertensive effect

Drug/lab test
Increased: urinary norepinephrine, VMA

NURSING CONSIDERATIONS

Assessment
• **Hypertension/CHF:** Monitor B/P, orthostatic hypotension, syncope; check for edema in feet, legs daily; monitor I&O, weight daily; notify prescriber of changes
• Assess for allergic reactions: rash, fever, pruritus, urticaria; product should be discontinued if antihistamines fail to help
• Assess for orthostatic hypotension; tell patient to rise slowly from sitting or lying position

Patient/family education
• Instruct patient not to discontinue product abruptly; stress the importance of complying with dosage schedule, even if feeling better; if dose is missed, take as soon as remembered; take at same time each day
• Advise patient not to use OTC products (cough, cold, allergy) unless directed by prescriber; also to avoid large amounts of caffeine, alcohol
• Emphasize the need to rise slowly to sitting or standing position to minimize orthostatic hypotension
• Teach patient to notify prescriber of mouth sores, sore throat, fever, swelling of hands or feet, irregular heartbeat, chest pain
• Caution patient to report excessive perspiration, dehydration, vomiting, diarrhea; may lead to fall in B/P
• Caution patient that product may cause dizziness, fainting, light-headedness; may occur during 1st few days of therapy; to avoid hazardous activities
• Teach patient how to take B/P and normal readings for age group; instruct to take B/P q7day

Evaluation
Positive therapeutic outcome
• Decreased B/P in hypertension

TREATMENT OF OVERDOSE:
Administer volume expanders or vasopressors, discontinue product, place patient in supine position

prednisoLONE (Rx)
(pred-niss'oh-lone)
Flo-Pred, Millipred, Orapred, Orapred ODT, Prelone, Veripred
Func. class.: Corticosteroid, synthetic
Chem. class.: Intermediate-acting glucocorticoid
Pregnancy category C

Do not confuse:
prednisoLONE/predniSONE

ACTION: Decreases inflammation by suppressing migration of polymorphonuclear leukocytes, fibroblasts; reversal to increase capillary permeability and lysosomal stabilization

Therapeutic outcome: Decreased inflammation, decreased adrenal insufficiency

USES: Severe inflammation, immunosuppression, neoplasms, asthma

CONTRAINDICATIONS:
Hypersensitivity, fungal infections, varicella, viral infection

Precautions: Pregnancy C, breastfeeding, children, diabetes mellitus, glaucoma, osteoporosis, seizure disorders, ulcerative colitis, CHF, myasthenia gravis, thromboembolism, peptic ulcer disease, renal disease, Cushing syndrome, abrupt discontinuation, children, acute MI, GI ulcers, hypertension, hepatitis, psychosis

DOSAGE AND ROUTES

Primary (Addison's disease)/secondary adrenocortical insufficiency or for the treatment of congenital adrenal hyperplasia
Adult: PO 5-60 mg/day as a single dose or in divided doses
Adolescent/child/infant: PO 0.14-2 mg/kg or 4-60 mg/m^2/day in 3-4 divided doses

Nonsuppurative thyroiditis
Adult: PO 5-60 mg/day as a single dose or in divided doses
Adolescent/child/infant: PO 0.14-2 mg/kg or 4-60 mg/m^2/day in 3-4 divided doses

Management of symptomatic sarcoidosis; or treatment of hypercalcemia associated with sarcoidosis or with various cancers
Adult: PO 5-60 mg/day as a single dose or divided doses
Adolescent/child/infant: PO 0.14-2 mg/kg or 4-60 mg/m^2/day in 3-4 divided doses

Adjunct in rheumatic disorders (ankylosing spondylitis, gout with gouty arthritis, juvenile rheumatoid arthritis (JRA)/juvenile idiopathic arthritis (JIA), post-traumatic osteoarthritis psoriatic arthritis, rheumatoid arthritis) or acute episodes or exacerbation of nonrheumatic inflammation (acute and subacute bursitis, epicondylitis, and acute nonspecific tenosynovitis)
Adult: PO 5-60 mg/day as a single dose or in divided doses
Adolescent/child/infant: PO 0.14-2 mg/kg or 4-60 mg/m^2/day in 3-4 divided doses

Adjunct in carpal tunnel syndrome (unlabeled)
Adult: PO 20 mg/day × 2 wk, then 10 mg/day for an additional 2 wk relief

Maintenance therapy in selected cases of acute rheumatic carditis, systemic dermatomyositis (polymyositis), systemic lupus erythematosus (SLE); (unlabeled): temporal arteritis, Churg-Strauss syndrome, mixed connective tissue disease, polyarteritis nodosa, relapsing polychondritis, polymyalgia rheumatica, vasculitis, or Wegener's granulomatosis
Adult: PO 5-60 mg/day as a single dose or in divided doses
Adolescent/child/infant: PO 0.14-2 mg/kg or 4-60 mg/m^2/day given in 3-4 divided doses

Corticosteroid-responsive respiratory disorders (airway-obstructing hemangioma in infant) (unlabeled), aspiration pneumonitis, berylliosis, chronic obstructive pulmonary disease (COPD), laryngotracheobronchitis (croup), Loeffler's syndrome, noncardiogenic pulmonary edema (unlabeled)
Adult: PO 5-60 mg/day as a single dose or in divided doses
Adolescent/child/infant: PO 0.14-2 mg/kg or 4-60 mg/m^2/day in 3-4 divided doses

Asthma; bronchospasm prophylaxis (unlabeled)
Adult/adolescent: PO 40-80 mg/day in 1-2 divided doses until the peak expiratory flow (PEF) reaches 70% of predicted or personal best; total course of treatment is 3-10 days
Child: PO 1 mg/kg/day (up to 60 mg) in 2 divided doses until PEF reaches 70% of predicted or personal best; if a patient is given systemic corticosteroids, continue PO corticosteroids for a total course of 3-10 days; tapering is not necessary for courses <1 wk

Acute asthma exacerbation on an outpatient basis
Adult/adolescent: PO 40-60 mg/day as a single dose or in 2 divided doses for 3-10 days
Child 5-12 yr: PO 1-2 mg/kg/day (up to 60 mg) in 2 divided doses for 3-10 days
Infant/child ≤4 yr: PO 1-2 mg/kg/day (up to 30 mg) in 2 divided doses for 3-10 days

Long-term prevention of symptoms in severe persistent asthma

Adult, adolescent, and child ≥12 yr: PO 7.5-60 mg once daily in the morning or every other day

Infant and child ≤11 yr: PO 0.25-2 mg/kg PO daily given as a single dose each morning or every other day

Hematologic disorders with thrombocytopenia (immune thrombocytopenia/idiopathic thrombocytopenic purpura (ITP), or secondary thrombocytopenia)

Adult: PO 5-60 mg/day as a single dose or in divided doses

Adolescent/child: PO 0.14-2 mg/kg or 4-60 mg/m²/day in 3-4 divided doses

Available forms: Tabs 5 mg; oral sol 5 mg/5 ml, 10 mg/5 ml, 15 mg/5 ml, 25 mg/5 ml; syrup 5 mg/5 ml; oral dissolving tab 10, 15, 30 mg

Implementation

• **Oral sol:** use calibrated measuring devices
• **Orally disintegrating tabs:** place on tongue, allow to dissolve, swallow; or swallow whole; do not cut, split

ADVERSE EFFECTS

CNS: *Depression,* flushing, sweating, headache, mood changes

CV: *Hypertension,* **circulatory collapse, thrombophlebitis, embolism,** tachycardia

EENT: Fungal infections, increased intraocular pressure, blurred vision

GI: *Diarrhea, nausea, abdominal distention,* **GI hemorrhage,** increased appetite, **pancreatitis**

INTEG: Acne, poor wound healing, ecchymosis, petechiae

MS: Fractures, osteoporosis, weakness, arthralgia, myopathy, tendon rupture

Pharmacokinetics

Absorption	Well absorbed (PO, IM), completely absorbed (**IV**)
Distribution	Widely distributed, crosses placenta
Metabolism	Liver, extensively
Excretion	Kidney, breast milk
Half-life	2-4 hr

Pharmacodynamics

	PO	IM (phosphate)	IV	IA/IL
Onset	1 hr	Rapid	Rapid	Slow
Peak	2 hr	1 hr	Unknown	Unknown
Duration	1½ days	Unknown	Unknown	Up to 1 mo

INTERACTIONS

Individual drugs

Alcohol, amphotericin B, cycloSPORINE, digitalis, indomethacin, **NSAIDs:** increased side effects

Ambenonium, isoniazid, neostigmine, somatrem: decreased effects of each specific product

Cholestyramine, colestipol, ePHEDrine, phenytoin, rifampin, theophylline: decreased action of prednisoLONE

Indomethacin, ketoconazole: increased action of prednisoLONE

Drug classifications

Antibiotics (macrolide), contraceptives (oral), estrogens, salicylates: increased action of prednisoLONE

Anticholinesterases, anticoagulants, anticonvulsants, antidiabetics, salicylates, toxoids, vaccines: decreased effects of each specific product

Azole antifungals, cycloSPORINE: increased toxicity

Barbiturates: decreased action of prednisoLONE

CYP3A4 inducers: decreased prednisoLONE effect

CYP3A4 inhibitors: increased prednisoLONE effect

Diuretics, salicylates: increased side effects

Quinolones: increased tendon rupture

Drug/lab test

Increased: cholesterol, sodium, blood glucose, uric acid, calcium, urine glucose

Decreased: calcium, potassium, T_4, T_3, thyroid ^{131}I uptake test, urine 17-OHCS, 17-KS, PBI

False negative: skin allergy tests

NURSING CONSIDERATIONS

Assessment

• Monitor potassium, blood glucose, urine glucose while patient is on long-term therapy; hypokalemia and hyperglycemia may occur
• Monitor weight daily; notify prescriber of weekly gain >5 lb; monitor I&O ratio; be alert

for decreasing urinary output and increasing edema
• Monitor B/P q4hr, pulse; notify prescriber if chest pain occurs
• Monitor plasma cortisol levels during long-term therapy (normal level 138-635 nmol/L [SI units] when measured at 8 AM)
• Assess adrenal function periodically for hypothalamic-pituitary-adrenal axis suppression
• **Assess infection:** increased temp, WBC even after withdrawal of medication; product masks infection symptoms
• **Assess for potassium depletion:** paresthesias, fatigue, nausea, vomiting, depression, polyuria, dysrhythmias, weakness, edema, hypertension, cardiac symptoms
• **Adrenal insufficiency:** assess for nausea, vomiting, lethargy, restlessness, confusion
• Assess mental status: affect, mood, behavioral changes, aggression
• Monitor temp; if fever develops, product should be discontinued
• Assess for systemic absorption: increased temp, inflammation, irritation (topical)

Patient/family education
• Advise patient to carry/wear emergency ID as steroid user
• Advise patient to notify prescriber if therapeutic response decreases; dosage adjustment may be needed
• Caution patient not to discontinue abruptly; adrenal crisis can result; take exactly as prescribed
• Caution patient to avoid OTC products: salicylates, cough products with alcohol, cold preparations unless directed by prescriber
• Teach patient all aspects of product usage including cushingoid symptoms
• Teach patient symptoms of adrenal insufficiency: nausea, anorexia, fatigue, dizziness, dyspnea, weakness, joint pain
• Advise patient that long-term therapy may be needed to clear infection (1-2 mo depending on type of infection)

Evaluation
Positive therapeutic outcome
• Decreased inflammation

prednisoLONE ophthalmic
See Appendix B

predniSONE (Rx)
(pred'ni-sone)
Rayos, Winpreo ✦
Func. class.: Corticosteroid
Chem. class.: Intermediate-acting glucocorticoid
Pregnancy category C

Do not confuse:
predniSONE/methylPREDNISolone/ prednisoLONE/PriLOSEC

ACTION: Decreases inflammation by increasing capillary permeability and lysosomal stabilization, minimal mineralocorticoid activity

Therapeutic outcome: Decreased inflammation, decreased adrenal insufficiency

USES: Severe inflammation, neoplasms, multiple sclerosis, collagen disorders, dermatologic disorders

CONTRAINDICATIONS:
Hypersensitivity

Precautions: Pregnancy **C**, diabetes mellitus, glaucoma, osteoporosis, seizure disorders, ulcerative colitis, CHF, myasthenia gravis, renal disease, esophagitis, peptic ulcer, cataracts, coagulopathy, abrupt discontinuation, children, corticosteroid hypersensitivity, Cushing syndrome, thromboembolism, geriatrics, acute MI

DOSAGE AND ROUTES
Adult: PO 5-60 mg/day or divided bid-qid
Child: PO 0.05-2 mg/kg/day divided 1-4 ×/day

Nephrotic syndrome
Child: PO 2 mg/kg/day in divided doses until urine is protein-free for 3 consecutive days, then 1-1.5 mg/kg/day every other day × 4 wk

Multiple sclerosis
Adult: PO 200 mg/day × 1 wk, then 80 mg every other day × 1 mo

Asthma
Adult/adolescent: PO 40-80 mg/day in 1-2 divided doses until PEF is 70% of predicted or personal best
Child: PO 1 mg/kg (max 60 mg)/day in 2 divided doses until PEF is 70% of predicted or personal best

Available forms: Tabs 1, 2.5, 5, 10, 20, 50 mg; oral sol 5 mg/5 ml; syr 5 mg/5 ml; del rel tab 1, 2, 5 mg

P

Implementation
• Give with food or milk to decrease GI symptoms; use measuring device for liquid route
• For long-term use, alternative product therapy is recommended, to decrease adverse reactions
• **Del rel tab:** swallow whole, do not break, crush, or chew; give once daily

ADVERSE EFFECTS
CNS: Depression, flushing, sweating, headache, mood changes
CV: Hypertension, **thrombophlebitis, embolism,** tachycardia, fluid retention
EENT: Fungal infections, increased intraocular pressure, blurred vision
GI: Diarrhea, nausea, abdominal distention, **GI hemorrhage,** increased appetite, **pancreatitis**
INTEG: Acne, poor wound healing, ecchymosis, petechiae
META: Hyperglycemia
MS: Fractures, osteoporosis, weakness

Pharmacokinetics	
Absorption	Well absorbed
Distribution	Widely distributed, crosses placenta
Metabolism	Liver, extensively
Excretion	Kidney, breast milk
Half-life	3-4 hr

Pharmacodynamics	
Onset	Unknown
Peak	1-2 hr; del rel 6-6½ hr
Duration	1½ days

INTERACTIONS
Individual drugs
Alcohol, amphotericin B, cycloSPORINE, digoxin: increased side effects
Ambenonium, isoniazid, neostigmine, sometrem: decreased effects of each specific product
Cholestyramine, colestipol, phenytoin, rifampin, theophylline: decreased action of predniSONE
Ketoconazole: increased action of predniSONE
NSAIDs: increased side effects, increased action of predniSONE

Drug classifications
Anticholinesterases, anticoagulants, anticonvulsants, antidiabetics, toxoids, vaccines: decreased effects of each specific product
Antiinfectives (macrolide), contraceptives (oral), estrogens: increased action of predniSONE

Barbiturates: decreased action of predniSONE
CYP3A4 inducers: decreased predniSONE effect
CYP3A4 inhibitors: increased predniSONE effect
Diuretics: increased side effects
Quinolones: increased tendon rupture
Salicylates: increased side effects, increased action of predniSONE, decreased effects of salicylates

Drug/herb
Ephedra (ma huang): decreased predniSONE effect

Drug/lab test
Increased: cholesterol, sodium, blood glucose, uric acid, calcium, urine glucose
Decreased: calcium, potassium, T_4, T_3, thyroid ^{131}I uptake test, urine 17-OHCS, 17-KS, PBI
False negative: skin allergy tests

NURSING CONSIDERATIONS
Assessment
• **Adrenal insufficiency:** assess for nausea, vomiting, anorexia, confusion, hypotension, weight loss before and during treatment; HPA suppression may be precipitated by abrupt withdrawal
• Monitor potassium, blood glucose, urine glucose while on long-term therapy; hypokalemia and hyperglycemia may occur
• Monitor weight daily; notify prescriber of weekly gain >5 lb; monitor I&O ratio; be alert for decreasing urinary output and increasing edema
• Monitor B/P, pulse; notify prescriber if chest pain occurs
• Monitor plasma cortisol levels during long-term therapy (normal level 138-635 nmol/L when measured at 8 AM)
• Assess adrenal function periodically for hypothalamic-pituitary-adrenal axis suppression
• **Assess infection:** increased temp, WBC even after withdrawal of medication; product masks infection symptoms
• **Assess for potassium depletion:** paresthesias, fatigue, nausea, vomiting, depression, polyuria, dysrhythmias, weakness, edema, hypertension, cardiac symptoms
• Assess mental status: affect, mood, behavioral changes, aggression
• Monitor temp; if fever develops, product should be discontinued
• Assess for systemic absorption: increased temp, inflammation, irritation (topical)

Patient/family education
• Advise patient that emergency ID as corticosteroid user should be carried or worn

---

- Advise patient to notify prescriber if therapeutic response decreases; dosage adjustment may be needed

⚠ **Caution patient not to discontinue abruptly; adrenal crisis can result**

- Caution patient to avoid OTC products: salicylates, cough products with alcohol, cold preparations unless directed by prescriber
- Teach patient all aspects of product use including cushingoid symptoms
- Teach patient symptoms of adrenal insufficiency: nausea, anorexia, fatigue, dizziness, dyspnea, weakness, joint pain
- Advise patient that long-term therapy may be needed to clear infection (1-2 mo depending on type of infection)

⚠ **Teach patient to notify prescriber if pregnancy is planned or suspected; cleft palate, stillbirth, abortion reported**

Evaluation

Positive therapeutic outcome
- Decreased inflammation

---

pregabalin (Rx)
(pre-gab'a-lin)
Lyrica
Func. class.: Anticonvulsant
Pregnancy category C
Controlled substance schedule V

ACTION: Binds to high-voltage–gated calcium channels in CNS tissues; this may lead to anticonvulsant action, similar to the inhibitory neurotransmitter GABA; anxiolytic, analgesic, and antiepileptic properties

Therapeutic outcome: Decreased seizure activity, decreased neuropathic pain

USES: Neuropathic pain associated with spinal cord injury, diabetic peripheral neuropathy, partial-onset seizures, postherpetic neuralgia, fibromyalgia

Unlabeled uses: Moderate pain, social anxiety disorder

CONTRAINDICATIONS:
Hypersensitivity to this product or gabapentin, abrupt discontinuation

Precautions: Pregnancy **C,** breastfeeding, children <12 yr, geriatric, renal disease, PR interval prolongation, creatine kinase elevations, CHF (class III, IV), decreased platelets, drug abuse, dependence, glaucoma, myopathy, angioedema history, suicidal behavior

DOSAGE AND ROUTES
Diabetic peripheral neuropathic pain
Adult: PO/oral sol 50 mg tid, may increase to 300 mg/day (max) within 1 wk, adjust in renal disease

Partial onset seizures
Adult: PO/oral sol 75 mg bid or 50 mg tid; may increase to 600 mg/day (max)

Postherpetic neuralgia
Adult: PO/oral sol 150 mg/day in 2-3 doses, may increase to 300 mg/day in 2-3 divided doses, if higher dose is needed in 2-4 wk, may increase to 600 mg/day in 2-3 divided doses

Fibromyalgia, spinal cord injury/pain
Adult: PO/oral sol 75 mg bid, may increase to 150 mg bid within 1 wk and 225 mg bid after 1 wk

Renal dose
PO CCr 30-60 ml/min 75-300 mg/day in 2-3 divided doses; CCr 15-30 ml/min 25-150 mg/day in 1-2 divided doses, CCr <15 ml/min 25-75 mg/day in a single dose

Available forms: Caps 25, 50, 75, 100, 150, 200, 225, 300 mg; oral sol 20 mg/ml

Implementation
- Do not crush or chew caps; caps may be opened and contents put in applesauce or dissolved in juice
- Give without regard to meals
- Gradually withdraw over 7 days; abrupt withdrawal may precipitate seizures
- Store at room temperature away from heat and light
- Give hard candy, frequent rinsing of mouth, gum for dry mouth
- Provide assistance with ambulation during early part of treatment; dizziness occurs
- Provide seizure precautions: padded side rails; move objects that may harm patient
- Provide increased fluids, bulk in diet for constipation
- **Oral sol:** should be written in mg and calculated to mL

ADVERSE EFFECTS
CNS: Dizziness, fatigue, confusion, euphoria, incoordination, nervousness, neuropathy, tremor, vertigo, somnolence, ataxia, amnesia, abnormal thinking
EENT: Dry mouth, blurred vision, nystagmus, amblyopia, sinusitis

---

Adverse effects: *italics* = common; **bold** = life-threatening

GI: Constipation, flatulence, abdominal pain, weight gain, nausea, vomiting, increased appetite
GU: Gynecomastia
HEMA: Ecchymosis, **thrombocytopenia**
MS: Back pain, **rhabdomyolysis**, myopathy
MISC: Pruritus, orgasm/erectile dysfunction, peripheral edema, **angioedema, suicidal ideation**, drowsiness
RESP: Dyspnea

Pharmacokinetics

Absorption	Well absorbed
Distribution	Not bound to plasma proteins
Metabolism	Negligible
Excretion	90% unchanged, urine
Half-life	6 hr

Pharmacodynamics

Onset	Unknown
Peak	1.5 hr
Duration	Unknown

INTERACTIONS
Individual drugs
Alcohol: increased CNS depression

Drug classifications
Anxiolytics, barbiturates, general anesthetics, hypnotics, opiate agonists, phenothiazines, sedating H_1 blockers, sedatives, thiazolidinediones, tricyclics: increased CNS depression
Thiazolidinediones: increased weight gain/fluid retention; avoid use if possible

Drug/lab test
Increased: creatine kinase
Decreased: platelets

NURSING CONSIDERATIONS
Assessment
• Assess for seizures: aura, location, duration, activity at onset, use seizure precaution
• **Assess for pain:** location, duration, characteristics if using for diabetic neuropathy
• Monitor renal function tests: urinalysis, BUN, urine creatinine q3mo, creatine kinase; if markedly increased, discontinue
• Assess mental status: mood, sensorium, affect, behavioral changes, suicidal thoughts, behavior; if mental status changes, notify prescriber
⚠ **Angioedema/hypersensitivity:** monitor for blisters, hives, rash, dyspnea, wheezing; **angioedema;** if these occur discontinue:

cross-hypersensitivity with this product and gabapentin may occur
⚠ **Rhabdomyolysis and creatinine kinase elevations: monitor for muscle pain, tenderness, weakness accompanied by malaise or fever; product should be discontinued**
• Hemolytic anemia may be severe in Asian, Mediterranean individuals

Patient/family education
• Advise patient to carry emergency ID stating patient's name, products taken, condition, prescriber's name and phone number
• Advise patient to avoid driving, other activities that require alertness: dizziness, drowsiness may occur
• Teach patient not to discontinue medication quickly after long-term use, taper over ≥1 wk; withdrawal-precipitated seizures may occur, not to double doses if dose is missed, take if 2 hr or more before next dose
• Teach patient to notify prescriber if pregnancy is planned or suspected; avoid breastfeeding
• Teach patient to report muscle pain, tenderness, weakness, when accompanied by fever, malaise
• Advise patient to avoid alcohol, live virus vaccines

Evaluation
Positive therapeutic outcome
• Decreased seizure activity; decrease in neuropathic pain

TREATMENT OF OVERDOSE:
Lavage, VS, hemodialysis

primidone (Rx)
(pri'mi-done)
Mysoline, Sertan ✦
Func. class.: Anticonvulsant
Chem. class.: Barbiturate derivative
Pregnancy category D

ACTION: Raises seizure threshold by conversion of product to phenobarbital; decreases neuron firing

Therapeutic outcome: Reduction in seizure activity

USES: Generalized tonic-clonic (grand mal), complex

CONTRAINDICATIONS:
Pregnancy **D**, hypersensitivity to this product or barbiturates, porphyria, breastfeeding

Precautions: COPD, renal/hepatic disease, hyperactive children, suicidal ideation/behavior, hepatic encephalopathy, sleep apnea

DOSAGE AND ROUTES
Adult and child >8 yr: PO 125-250 mg at bedtime, increase by 125-250 mg/day q3-7day, usual dose 750-1500 mg/day in 3-4 divided doses, max 2 g/day in divided doses
Child <8 yr: PO 50-125 mg at bedtime, increase by 50-125 mg/day q3-7day, usual dose 10-25 mg/kg/day in 3-4 divided doses

Neonate: PO 12-20 mg/kg/day in 2-4 divided doses, start at lower dose and titrate

Renal dose
Adult: CCr 10-15 ml/min: increase interval between doses to 8-12 hr; CCr <10 ml/min: increase interval to 12-24 hr

Available forms: Tabs 50, 250 mg; susp 250 mg/5 ml ✤; chew tabs 125 mg ✤

Implementation
• May give with food to decrease gastric irritation
• May crush tab and mix with food or fluid

ADVERSE EFFECTS
CNS: *Stimulation, drowsiness,* irritability, fatigue, emotional disturbances, mood changes, paranoia, psychosis, ataxia, *vertigo,* **suicidal ideation**
EENT: Diplopia, nystagmus, edema of eyelids, blurred vision, miosis
GI: *Nausea, vomiting, anorexia,* **hepatitis**
GU: Impotence
HEMA: **Thrombocytopenia, leukopenia, neutropenia, eosinophilia, megaloblastic anemia,** decreased serum folate level, lymphadenopathy
INTEG: Rash, edema, alopecia, lupuslike syndrome
MS: Osteopenia
RESP: Respiratory depression (dose related)

Pharmacokinetics
Absorption	60%-80%
Distribution	Widely distributed, crosses placenta
Metabolism	Liver, converted to phenobarbital + PEMA
Excretion	Kidneys, breast milk
Half-life	3-12 hr

Pharmacodynamics
Onset	Unknown
Peak	4 hr
Duration	Unknown

INTERACTIONS
Individual drugs
Acebutolol, lamotrigine, metoprolol, propranolol: decreased effectiveness
Acetazolamide, carBAMazepine: decreased primidone levels
Alcohol, heparin, isoniazid, nicotinamide, phenytoin: increased primidone levels

Drug classifications
Antidepressants (tricyclic), oral contraceptives, phenothiazines: decreased effectiveness
CNS depressants, MAOIs: increased primidone levels
CYP3A4 inducers (barbiturates, carBAMazepine, efavirenz, nevirapine), phenytoins: decreased primidone effect
CYP3A4 inhibitors (aprepitant, antiretroviral protease inhibitors, delavirdine, fluconazole, imatinib, voriconazole): increased toxicity
Succinimides: decreased primidone levels

Drug/herb
Ginkgo: increased effect
Ginseng, santonica: decreased effect
Kava, St. John's wort, valerian: avoid use

NURSING CONSIDERATIONS
Assessment
• Assess mental status: mood, sensorium, affect, memory (long, short), especially geriatric; suicidal thoughts/behavior
• Assess for blood dyscrasias: fever, sore throat, bruising, rash, jaundice, epistaxis (long-term treatment only)
• **Assess seizure activity** including type, location, duration, and character; provide seizure precaution
• Assess renal function tests: urinalysis, BUN, urine creatinine
• Monitor blood studies: RBC, Hct, Hgb, reticulocyte counts weekly for 4 wk then monthly
• Monitor liver function tests: ALT, AST, bilirubin, creatinine
• Monitor product levels during initial treatment: therapeutic level 5-12 mcg/ml; CBC, LFTs should be done q6mo
• Assess for signs of physical withdrawal if medication is suddenly discontinued
• Assess eye problems: need for ophth exam before, during, after treatment (slit lamp, funduscopy, tonometry)

- Assess allergic reaction: red raised rash; if this occurs, product should be discontinued
- Monitor for toxicity: bone marrow depression, nausea, vomiting, ataxia, diplopia, CV collapse

Patient/family education
- Teach patient to carry/wear emergency ID stating name, products taken, condition, prescriber's name, phone number
- Advise patient to avoid driving and other activities that require alertness
- Caution patient to avoid alcohol and CNS depressants; increased sedation may occur
- Teach patient to report rash
- ⚠ Teach patient to report suicidal thoughts/behaviors immediately
- Teach patient not to discontinue medication quickly after long-term use; taper off over several wk

Evaluation
Positive therapeutic outcome
- Decreased seizure activity

---

procainamide (Rx)
(proe'kane-ah-mide)
Func. class.: Antidysrhythmic (class IA)
Chem. class.: Procaine HCl amide analog
Pregnancy category C

ACTION: Depresses excitability of cardiac muscle to electrical stimulation and slows conduction velocity in atrium, bundle of His, ventricle; increases refractory period

Therapeutic outcome: Prevention of dysrhythmias

USES: Life-threatening ventricular dysrhythmias, paroxysmal atrial tachycardia, PSVT, Wolff-Parkinson-White (WPW) syndrome

CONTRAINDICATIONS:
Hypersensitivity, severe heart block, torsades de pointes

BLACK BOX WARNING: Lupus erythematosis

Precautions: Pregnancy **C**, breastfeeding, children, renal/hepatic disease, CHF, respiratory depression, cytopenia, dysrhythmia associated with digoxin toxicity, myasthenia gravis, digoxin toxicity

BLACK BOX WARNING: Bone marrow failure, cardiac arrhythmias

DOSAGE AND ROUTES
Ventricular tachycardia during CPR
Adult: IV loading dose 20 mg/min; either ventricular tachycardia resolves or patient becomes hypotensive; the QRS complex is widened by 50% of original width or total is 17 mg/kg (1.2 g for a 70 kg patient); may give up to 50 mg/min in urgent situations; maintenance 1-4 mg/min CONT IV INF; IM 50 mg/kg/day in divided doses q3-6hr
Child: IV PALS 15 mg/kg over 30-60 min

Renal dose
Adult: **IV** CCr 35-59 ml/min give 70% of maintenance dose; CCr 15-34 ml/min give 40%-60% maintenance dose; CCr <15 ml/min individualized

Available forms: inj 100, 500 mg/ml

Implementation
IM route
- IM inj in deltoid; aspirate to avoid intravascular administration, use only when unable to use IV

Direct IV route
- Dilute each 100 mg/10 ml of 0.9% NaCl, give at max 50 mg/min
Intermittent INF route
- Dilute 0.2-1 g/50-500 ml of D$_5$W (2-4 mg/ml) give over 30-60 min at max 25-50 mg/min, use inf pump

Y-site compatibilities: Alfentanil, amikacin, aminocaproic acid, aminophylline, amiodarone, amphotericin B lipid complex, amphotericin B liposome, anidulafungin, ascorbic acid, atenolol, atracurium, atropine, aztreonam, benztropine, bivalirudin, bleomycin, bumetanide, buprenorphine, butorphanol, calcium chloride/gluconate, caspofungin, ceFAZolin, cefmetazole, cefonicid, cefoperazone, cefotaxime, cefoTEtan, cefOXitin, cefTAZidime, cefTRIAXone, cefuroxime, cephalothin, chlorproMAZINE, cimetidine, cisatracurium, CISplatin, clindamycin, cyanocobalamin, cyclophosphamide, cycloSPORINE, cytarabine, DACTINomycin, DAPTOmycin, dexamethasone, digoxin, diphenhydrAMINE, DOBUTamine, DOCEtaxel, DOPamine, doxacurium, DOXOrubicin, doxycycline, enalaprilat, ePHEDrine, EPINEPHrine, epirubicin, epoetin alfa, eptifibatide, ertapenem, erythromycin, esmolol, etoposide, etoposide phosphate, famotidine, fenoldopam, fentaNYL, fluconazole, fludarabine, fluorouracil, folic acid, furosemide, gatifloxacin, gemcitabine, gentamicin, glycopyrrolate, granisetron, heparin, hydrocortisone, HYDROmorphone, IDArubicin, ifosfamide,

---

⚠ Nurse Alert   ✳ Key NCLEX® Drug

indomethacin, insulin (regular), irinotecan, isoproterenol, ketorolac, labetalol, lidocaine, linezolid, LORazepam, magnesium sulfate, mannitol, mechlorethamine, meperidine, metaraminol, methicillin, methotrexate, methoxamine, methyldopa, methylPREDNISolone, metoclopramide, metoprolol, mezlocillin, miconazole, midazolam, mitoXANtrone, morphine, moxalactam, multiple vitamins, mycophenolate, nafcillin, nalbuphine, naloxone, netilmicin, nitroglycerin, nitroprusside, norepinephrine, octreotide, ondansetron, oxacillin, oxaliplatin, oxytocin, PACLitaxel, palonosetron, pamidronate, pancuronium, pantoprazole, papaverine, PEMEtrexed, penicillin G potassium/sodium, pentamidine, pentazocine, PENTobarbital, PHENobarbital, phenylephrine, phytonadione, piperacillin, piperacillin-tazobactam, polymyxin B, potassium chloride, prochlorperazine, promethazine, propranolol, protamine, pyridoxine, quiNIDine, quinupristin-dalfopristin, ranitidine, remifentanil, ritodrine, rocuronium, sodium bicarbonate, succinylcholine, SUFentanil, tacrolimus, teniposide, theophylline, thiamine, thiotepa, ticarcillin, ticarcillin-clavulanate, tigecycline, tirofiban, tobramycin, tolazoline, trimetaphan, urokinase, vancomycin, vasopressin, vecuronium, verapamil, vinCRIStine, vinorelbine, vitamin B complex/C, voriconazole, zoledronic acid

Y-site incompatibilities: Milrinone

ADVERSE EFFECTS
CNS: *Headache, dizziness,* confusion, psychosis, restlessness, irritability, weakness, depression
CV: *Hypotension,* **heart block, cardiovascular collapse, arrest, torsades de pointes**
GI: Nausea, vomiting, anorexia, diarrhea, hepatomegaly, pain, bitter taste
HEMA: Systemic lupus erythematosus syndrome, **agranulocytosis, thrombocytopenia, neutropenia, hemolytic anemia**
INTEG: Rash, urticaria, edema, swelling (rare), pruritus, flushing, **angioedema**
SYST: SLE

Pharmacokinetics

Absorption	Well absorbed
Distribution	Rapidly distributed, protein binding 15%
Metabolism	Liver
Excretion	Kidneys, unchanged (50%-70%)
Half-life	2½-4½ hr; increased in renal disease

Pharmacodynamics

	IV
Onset	Rapid
Peak	½-1 hr
Duration	3-4 hr

INTERACTIONS
Individual drugs
Cimetidine, quiNIDine, ranitidine, trimethoprim: increased procainamide effect
Thioridazine: increased toxicity

Drug classifications
Antidysrhythmics, quinolones: increased toxicity
β-Adrenergic blockers: increased procainamide effects
Neuromuscular blockers: increased neuromuscular blocking effect

Drug/lab test
Increased: ALT, AST, alkaline phosphatase, LDH, bilirubin

NURSING CONSIDERATIONS
Assessment
• Assess for oxygenation or perfusion deficit: decreased B/P, chest pain, dizziness, loss of consciousness
• Assess respiratory status: auscultate lung fields for bibasilar crackles in patients with advanced CHF
• Monitor I&O ratio; electrolytes: potassium, sodium, chloride; watch for decreasing urinary output, possible retention
• Monitor liver function tests: AST, ALT, bilirubin, alkaline phosphatase

> **BLACK BOX WARNING: Cardiac dysrhythmias:** Monitor ECG continuously to determine product effectiveness; measure PR, QRS, QT intervals; check for PVCs, other dysrhythmias; check B/P continuously for hypo/hypertension; for rebound hypertension after 1-2 hr; prolonged PR/QT intervals, QRS complex; if QT or QRS increases by 50% or more, withhold next dose, notify prescriber

• Monitor ANA titer; during long-term treatment, watch for lupuslike symptoms
• Monitor for dehydration or hypovolemia
⚠ Monitor for CNS symptoms: confusion, seizures, psychosis, numbness, depression, involuntary movements; if these occur, product should be discontinued

BLACK BOX WARNING: Bone marrow suppression: CBC q2wk × 3 mo; leukocyte, neutrophil, platelet counts may be decreased, treatment may need to be discontinued

- Monitor blood levels (therapeutic level 4-10 mcg/ml), ANA titer or *N*-acetylprocainamide levels 10-20 mcg/ml; notify prescriber of abnormal results; assess for toxicity: confusion, drowsiness, nausea, vomiting, tachydysrhythmias, oliguria
- Assess cardiac rate, respiration: rate, rhythm, character, chest pain, ventricular tachycardia, supraventricular tachycardia or fibrillation

Patient/family education
- Advise patient to report side effects immediately to prescriber; to take exactly as prescribed; if dose is missed take when remembered if within 3-4 hr of next dose, do not double doses
- Caution patient that dark glasses may be needed for photophobia; to use sunscreen or stay out of sun to prevent burns; avoid temperature extremes; impairment of heat-regulating mechanism can occur
- Advise patient to complete follow-up appointment with prescriber, including pulmonary function tests, chest x-ray
- Instruct patient that dry mouth may be relieved by frequent sips of water, hard candy, sugarless gum
- Caution patient to make position changes from lying to standing slowly to prevent orthostatic hypotension

BLACK BOX WARNING: Advise prescriber immediately if lupuslike symptoms (joint pain, butterfly rash, fever, chills, dyspnea), leukopenia symptoms (sore mouth, gums, throat), or thrombocytopenia symptoms (bleeding, bruising) occur

- Teach patient how to take pulse and when to report to prescriber

Evaluation
Positive therapeutic outcome
- Decreased PVCs, ventricular tachycardia

TREATMENT OF OVERDOSE:
O_2, artificial ventilation, ECG, administer DOPamine for circulatory depression, diazepam or thiopental for seizures, isoproterenol

procarbazine (Rx)
(proe-kar'ba-zeen)
Matulane
Func. class.: Antineoplastic, alkylating agent
Chem. class.: Hydrazine derivative
Pregnancy category D

ACTION: Inhibits DNA, RNA, protein synthesis; has multiple sites of action; a nonvesicant

Therapeutic outcome: Prevention of rapidly growing malignant cells

USES: Lymphoma, Hodgkin's disease, cancers resistant to other therapy

Unlabeled uses: Brain, lung malignancies, other lymphomas, multiple myeloma, malignant melanoma, polycythemia vera

CONTRAINDICATIONS:
Pregnancy **D**, breastfeeding, hypersensitivity, thrombocytopenia, bone marrow depression

Precautions: Cardiac/renal/hepatic disease, radiation therapy, seizure disorder, anemia, bipolar disorder, Parkinson's disease

BLACK BOX WARNING: Requires a specialized care setting and an experienced clinician

DOSAGE AND ROUTES
Adult: PO 2-4 mg/kg/day for first wk; maintain dosage of 4-6 mg/kg/day until platelets and WBC fall; after recovery, 1-2 mg/kg/day
Child: PO 50 mg/m²/day for 7 days, then 100 mg/m² until desired response, leukopenia, or thrombocytopenia occurs; 50 mg/m²/day is maintenance after bone marrow recovery

Available forms: Caps 50 mg

Implementation
- Give with foods, fluids for GI upset; open cap and give with food/fluids for swallowing difficulty; administer as directed

ADVERSE EFFECTS
CNS: Headache, dizziness, **seizures,** insomnia, hallucinations, confusion, **coma,** pain, chills, fever, sweating, paresthesias, peripheral neuropathy
EENT: Retinal hemorrhage, nystagmus, photophobia, diplopia, dry eyes
GI: *Nausea, vomiting,* anorexia, diarrhea, constipation, dry mouth, stomatitis, elevated hepatic enzymes

GU: Azoospermia, cessation of menses
HEMA: Thrombocytopenia, anemia, leukopenia, myelosuppression, bleeding tendencies, purpura, petechiae, epistaxis, hemolysis
INTEG: *Rash,* pruritus, dermatitis, alopecia, herpes, hyperpigmentation
MS: Arthralgias, myalgias
RESP: Cough, pneumonitis, hemoptysis
SYST: Secondary malignancy

Pharmacokinetics

Absorption	Well absorbed
Distribution	Widely distributed, crosses blood-brain barrier
Metabolism	Liver
Excretion	Kidneys
Half-life	1 hr

Pharmacodynamics

Unknown

INTERACTIONS
Individual drugs
Alcohol: increased CNS depression
Caffeine, guanethidine, levodopa, methyldopa, reserpine: increased hypertension
Meperidine: hypotension; do not use together

Drug classifications
Anticoagulants, NSAIDs, platelet inhibitors, thrombolytics: increased bleeding risk
Antidepressants (tricyclics), MAOIs, SSRIs, SNRIs: confusion, seizures, hypertension
Antihistamines, barbiturates, hypotensive agents, opiates, phenothiazines: increased CNS depression
Sympathomimetics: disulfiram-like reaction, life-threatening hypertensive crisis

Drug/food
Tyramine-containing foods: increased disulfiram-like reaction, hypertensive crisis

NURSING CONSIDERATIONS
Assessment
⚠ **Bone marrow suppression: monitor CBC, differential, platelet count weekly; withhold product if WBC is <4000/mm³ or platelet count is <75,000/mm³; notify prescriber of results if WBC <20,000/mm³, platelets <150,000/mm³**

• Monitor pulmonary function tests, chest x-ray films before, during therapy; chest film should be obtained q2wk during treatment; check for dyspnea, crackles, unproductive cough, chest pain, tachypnea

• **Hepatic/renal disease:** can cause accumulation of drug, increased toxicity; monitor renal function tests: BUN, serum uric acid, urine CCr before, during therapy; I&O ratio; report fall in urine output of 30 ml/hr; check for decreased hyperuricemia; monitor hepatic studies before, during therapy: bilirubin, AST, ALT, ALK phos, LDH, PRN or qmo

> **BLACK BOX WARNING:** To be used only in a specialized care setting with emergency equipment

> **BLACK BOX WARNING:** To be given only by an experienced clinician knowledgeable in cytotoxic products

• Monitor for cold, fever, sore throat (may indicate beginning of infection); identify edema in feet, joint and stomach pain, shaking; prescriber should be notified

• **Assess for bleeding:** hematuria, guaiac, bruising or petechiae, mucosa or orifices; no rectal temp

• Assess for tyramine-containing foods in the diet; hypertensive crisis can occur

Patient/family education
• Teach patient to avoid use of products containing aspirin or NSAIDs, razors, commercial mouthwash, since bleeding may occur; to report symptoms of bleeding (hematuria, tarry stools)

• Caution patient to report signs of anemia (fatigue, headache, irritability, faintness, shortness of breath); CNS changes, diarrhea

• Advise patient to report any changes in breathing or coughing even several mo after treatment; to avoid crowds and persons with respiratory tract or other infections

• Inform patient hair loss is common; discuss the use of wigs or hairpieces

• Caution patient not to have any vaccinations without the advice of the prescriber; serious reactions can occur

• Advise patient that contraception is needed during treatment and for several mo after the completion of therapy; may cause infertility; avoid breastfeeding

• Teach patient to avoid sunlight, UV exposure; wear sunscreen or protective clothing

Evaluation
Positive therapeutic outcome
• Absence of swelling at night
• Increased appetite, increased weight
• Decreasing malignancy

prochlorperazine (Rx)

(proe-klor-pair'a-zeen)

Compro

Func. class.: Antiemetic/antipsychotic

Chem. class.: Phenothiazine, piperazine derivative

Pregnancy category C

Do not confuse:
prochlorperazine/chlorproMAZINE

ACTION: Decreases DOPamine neurotransmission by increasing DOPamine turnover through blockade of the D_2 somatodendritic autoreceptor in the meso-limbic system

Therapeutic outcome: Decreased nausea, vomiting, decreased signs and symptoms of psychosis

USES: Nausea, vomiting, psychosis

CONTRAINDICATIONS:

Hypersensitivity to phenothiazines, coma, infants/neonates/child <2 yr or <20 lb, surgery

Precautions: Pregnancy **C**, breastfeeding, geriatric, seizure, encephalopathy, glaucoma, hepatic disease, Parkinson's disease, BPH

> **BLACK BOX WARNING:** Increased mortality in elderly patients with dementia-related psychosis

DOSAGE AND ROUTES

Postoperative nausea/vomiting

Adult: IM 5-10 mg 1-2 hr before anesthesia; may repeat in 30 min; **IV** 5-10 mg 15-30 min before anesthesia; **IV** INF 20 mg/L D₅W or 0.9% NaCl 15-30 min before anesthesia, max 40 mg/day

Severe nausea/vomiting

Adult: PO 5-10 mg tid-qid; SUS REL 15 mg/day in AM or 10 mg q12hr; RECT 25 mg/bid; IM 5-10 mg; may repeat q3-4hr prn, max 40 mg/day

Child 18-39 kg: PO 2.5 mg tid or 5 mg bid; IM 0.132 mg/kg, q3-4hr prn, max 15 mg/day

Child 14-17 kg: PO/RECT 2.5 mg bid-tid; IM 0.132 mg/kg, q3-4hr prn, max 10 mg/day

Child 9-13 kg: PO/RECT 2.5 mg daily-bid; IM 0.132 mg/kg, q3-4hr prn, max 7.5 mg/day

Antipsychotic

Adult and child ≥12 yr: PO 5-10 mg tid-qid; may increase q2-3day, max 150 mg/day; IM 10-20 mg q2-4hr up to 4 doses, then 10-20 mg q4-6hr, max 200 mg/day; RECT 10 mg tid-qid, may increase by 5-10 mg q2-3day as needed

Child 2-12 yr: PO 2.5 mg bid-tid; IM 0.132 mg/kg, change to oral ASAP

Antianxiety

Adult and child ≥12 yr: PO 5 mg tid-qid, max 20 mg/day or >12 wk; IM 5-10 mg q3-4hr, max 40 mg/day; **IV** 2.5-10 mg; max 40 mg/day

Child 2-12 yr: IM 0.132 mg/kg, change to oral ASAP

Available forms: Syr 5 mg/ml; inj 5 mg/ml; tabs 5, 10, 25 mg; sus rel caps 10, 15 mg; supp 2.5, 5, 25 mg

Implementation

IM route

• Inject slowly in deep muscle mass; do not give SUBCUT; aspirate to avoid **IV** administration; do not administer sol with a precipitate; have patient lie down afterward for at least 30 min

Direct IV route

• No dilution needed, inject directly in a vein ≤5 mg/min, do not give as bolus

Intermittent IV infusion route

• May dilute 20 mg/L NaCl and give as inf 15-30 min prior to anesthesia induction

Syringe compatibilities: Atropine, butorphanol, chlorproMAZINE, cimetidine, diamorphine, diphenhydrAMINE, droperidol, fentanyl, glycopyrrolate, hydrOXYzine, meperidine, metoclopramide, nalbuphine, pentazocine, perphenazine, promazine, promethazine, ranitidine, scopolamine, SUFentanil

Syringe incompatibilities: DimenhyDRINATE, midazolam, PENTobarbital, thiopental

Y-site compatibilities: Amsacrine, calcium gluconate, CISplatin, cladribine, cyclophosphamide, cytarabine, DOXOrubicin, fluconazole, granisetron, heparin, hydrocortisone, melphalan, methotrexate, ondansetron, PACLitaxel, potassium chloride, propofol, sargramostim, SUFentanil, teniposide, thiotepa, vinorelbine, vit B/C

Y-site incompatibilities: Foscarnet

ADVERSE EFFECTS

CNS: Tardive dyskinesia, *euphoria*, **depression, EPS,** restlessness, tremor, dizziness, **neuroleptic malignant syndrome,** drowsiness, headache

CV: Circulatory failure, **tachycardia,** hypotension, ECG changes

EENT: Blurred vision

GI: Nausea, vomiting, anorexia, dry mouth, diarrhea, constipation, weight loss, metallic taste, cramps
HEMA: Agranulocytosis
MISC: Impotence
RESP: Respiratory depression

Pharmacokinetics

Absorption	Variably absorbed (PO); well absorbed (IM)
Distribution	Widely distributed, high concentration in CNS, crosses placenta
Metabolism	Liver, extensively; GI mucosa
Excretion	Kidneys, breast milk
Half-life	Unknown

Pharmacodynamics

	PO	PO-SUS REL	RECT	IM	IV
Onset	½ hr	Unkn	1 hr	10-20 min	4-5 min
Peak	Unkn	Unkn	Unkn	Unkn	Unkn
Duration	3-4 hr	10-12 hr	3-4 hr	4-6 hr; children: 12 hr	3-4 hr

INTERACTIONS
Individual drugs
Lithium: decreased prochlorperazine effect

Drug classifications
Antacids, barbiturates: decreased prochlorperazine effect
Anticholinergics, antidepressants, antiparkinson products: increased anticholinergic effects
SSRIs, SNRIs: increased serotonin syndrome, increased neuroleptic malignant syndrome
CNS depressants: increased CNS depression

Drug/herb
Betel palm, kava: increased EPS
Dong quai: avoid use

Drug/lab test
Increased: liver function tests, cardiac enzymes, cholesterol, blood glucose, prolactin, bilirubin, PBI, ^{131}I, alkaline phosphatase, leukocytes, granulocytes, platelets
Decreased: hormones (blood and urine)
False positive: pregnancy tests, urine bilirubin

False negative: urinary steroids, 17-OHCS, pregnancy tests

NURSING CONSIDERATIONS
Assessment
• Assess mental status: orientation, mood, behavior, presence and type of hallucinations before initial administration and monthly; this product should significantly reduce psychotic behavior
• Check for swallowing of PO medication; check for hoarding or giving of medication to other patients
• Monitor I&O ratio; palpate bladder if low urinary output occurs, especially in geriatric; urinalysis recommended before, during prolonged therapy
⚠ Monitor bilirubin, CBC, liver function tests monthly; blood dyscrasias, hepatotoxicity may occur
• Assess affect, orientation, LOC, reflexes, gait, coordination, sleep pattern disturbances
• Monitor B/P with patient sitting, standing, and lying; take pulse and respirations q4hr during initial treatment; establish baseline before starting treatment; report drops of 30 mm Hg; obtain baseline ECG, Q-wave and T-wave changes
• Check for dizziness, faintness, palpitations, tachycardia on rising; severe orthostatic hypotension is common
⚠ Identify neuroleptic malignant syndrome: hyperpyrexia, muscle rigidity, increased CPK, altered mental status, seizures, fever, tachycardia, dyspnea, fatigue, loss of bladder control; notify prescriber immediately; product should be discontinued
• Assess for EPS including akathisia (inability to sit still, no pattern to movements), tardive dyskinesia (bizarre movements of the jaw, mouth, tongue, extremities), pseudoparkinsonism (ragged tremors, pill rolling, shuffling gait); an antiparkinsonism product should be prescribed
• Assess for constipation, urinary retention daily; if these occur, increase bulk, water in diet

Patient/family education
• Teach patient to use good oral hygiene; frequent rinsing of mouth, sugarless gum for dry mouth since oral candidiasis may occur
• Caution patient to avoid hazardous activities until product response is determined; dizziness, blurred vision may occur
• Inform patient that orthostatic hypotension occurs often and to rise from sitting or lying position gradually; to remain lying down after IM inj for at least 30 min; tell patient to avoid hot tubs, hot showers, tub baths, since hypotension

may occur; tell patient that in hot weather heat stroke may occur; take extra precautions to stay cool

• Advise patient to avoid abrupt withdrawal of this product, or EPS may result; product should be withdrawn slowly

• Teach patient to avoid OTC preparations (cough, hay fever, cold) unless approved by prescriber, since serious product interactions may occur; avoid use with alcohol, CNS depressants; increased drowsiness may occur; avoid activities requiring mental alertness

• Instruct patient to avoid sun or use sunscreen, sunglasses, and protective clothing to prevent burns

• Advise patient to take antacids 2 hr before or after taking this product

• Advise patient to report sore throat, malaise, fever, bleeding, mouth sores; if these occur, CBC should be done and product discontinued

• Teach patient not to double or skip doses

• Inform patient that urine may turn pink to reddish brown

• Instruct patient to report dark urine, clay-colored stools, bleeding, bruising, rash, blurred vision

• Advise patient that suppositories may contain coconut/palm oil

Evaluation

Positive therapeutic outcome

• Relief of nausea and vomiting

• Decrease in emotional excitement, hallucinations, delusions, paranoia

• Reorganization of patterns of thought, speech

TREATMENT OF OVERDOSE:

Lavage if orally ingested; provide airway; *do not induce vomiting or use EPINEPHrine*

---

progesterone (Rx)

(proe-jess′ter-one)
Crinone, Endometrin, First-Progesterone, Prochieve, Prometrium
Func. class.: Progestogen
Chem. class.: Progesterone derivative
Pregnancy category D

ACTION: Inhibits secretion of pituitary gonadotropins, which prevents follicular maturation, ovulation; stimulates growth of mammary tissue; antineoplastic action against endometrial cancer

Therapeutic outcome: Decreased abnormal uterine bleeding, absence of amenorrhea

USES: Contraception, amenorrhea, premenstrual syndrome, abnormal uterine bleeding, endometrial hyperplasia prevention, assisted reproductive technology (ART) gel

Unlabeled uses: Corpus luteum insufficiency

CONTRAINDICATIONS:

Pregnancy **B**, thromboembolic disorders, reproductive cancer, genital bleeding (abnormal, undiagnosed), cerebral hemorrhage, ectopic pregnancy, PID, STDs, thrombophlebitis, hypersensitivity to this product, peanuts, or peanut oil

BLACK BOX WARNING: Breast cancer

Precautions: Breastfeeding, hypertension, asthma, blood dyscrasias, gallbladder disease, CHF, diabetes mellitus, bone disease, depression, migraine headache, seizure disorders, renal/hepatic disease, family history of breast or reproductive tract cancer

BLACK BOX WARNING: Cardiac disease, dementia

DOSAGE AND ROUTES

Infertility
Adult: Vag 90 mg/day (micronized gel); 100 mg 2-3 times/day, starting day after oocyte retrieval and up to 10 wk total

Amenorrhea/functional uterine bleeding
Adult: IM 5-10 mg/day × 6-8 doses

Endometrial hyperplasia prevention
Adult: PO 200 mg/day × 12 days

Assisted reproductive technology
Adult: GEL 90 mg (8%) vaginally daily, for supplementation; 90 mg (8%) vaginally bid for replacement; if pregnancy occurs, continue × 10-12 wk

Corpus luteum insufficiency (unlabeled)
Adult: VAG insert 90-100 mg bid-tid starting at oocyte retrieval and continuing up to 10-12 wk of gestation

Available forms: Caps 100, 200 mg; inj 50 mg/ml; powder micronized; vag gel 4%, 8%; vag insert 100 mg; supp 25, 100, 200, 500 mg, compounding kit 25, 50, 100, 200, 400 mg

---

Implementation
PO route
• Do not crush, break, chew caps, give one dose in AM
• With food or milk to decrease GI symptoms
• Start progesterone 14 days after estrogen dose, if given concomitantly
Vaginal route
• Wait at least 6 hr after any vaginal treatment before using vaginal gel
IM route
• Store in dark area
• Give titrated dose; use lowest effective dosage; give oil sol deep in large muscle mass; rotate sites; use after warming to dissolve crystals
• Check for particulate matter and discoloration prior to injecting

ADVERSE EFFECTS
CNS: *Dizziness, headache*, migraines, depression, *fatigue*, mood swings, dementia, drowsiness
CV: Hypotension, **thrombophlebitis**, edema, **thromboembolism, stroke, pulmonary embolism, MI**
EENT: Diplopia, retinal thrombosis
GI: *Nausea*, vomiting, anorexia, cramps, increased weight, **cholestatic jaundice**, *constipation*, abdominal pain
GU: Amenorrhea, cervical erosion, breakthrough bleeding, dysmenorrhea, vaginal candidiasis, nocturia, breast changes, *gynecomastia, testicular atrophy, impotence*, endometriosis, **spontaneous abortion**, breast pain, ectopic pregnancy
INTEG: Rash, urticaria, acne, hirsutism, alopecia, oily skin, seborrhea, purpura, melasma
META: Hyperglycemia
SYST: Angioedema, anaphylaxis

Pharmacokinetics

Absorption	Unknown
Distribution	Unknown
Metabolism	Unknown
Excretion	Breast milk
Half-life	Unknown

Pharmacodynamics

	IM	RECT	VAG
Onset	Unknown	Unknown	Unknown
Peak	Unknown	Unknown	Unknown
Duration	24 hr	24 hr	24 hr

INTERACTIONS
Drug classifications
Barbiturates, phenytoins: decreased progesterone effect
CYP3A4 inhibitors (cimetidine, clarithromycin, danazol, diltiazem, erythromycin, fluconazole, itraconazole, ketoconazole, troleandomycin, verapamil, voriconazole): increased progesterone effect

Drug/lab test
Increased: alkaline phosphatase, nitrogen (urine), pregnanediol, amino acids, factors VII, VIII, IX, X
Decreased: GTT, HDL

NURSING CONSIDERATIONS
Assessment
• Monitor B/P at beginning of treatment and periodically; check weight daily; notify prescriber of weekly weight gain >5 lb
• Monitor I&O ratio: be alert for decreasing urinary output, increasing edema, hypertension
• Assess liver function tests: ALT, AST, bilirubin periodically during long-term therapy
• Assess edema, hypertension, cardiac symptoms, jaundice
• Assess mental status: affect, mood, behavioral changes, depression
• Assess for hypercalcemia
• Assess cervical cytology
• Conduct breast exam

Patient/family education
• Teach patient to avoid activities requiring mental alertness until effects are realized; can cause dizziness
• Teach patient to report breast lumps, vaginal bleeding, edema, jaundice, dark urine, clay-colored stools, dyspnea, headache, blurred vision, abdominal pain, numbness or stiffness in legs, chest pain
• Teach patient to report suspected pregnancy
• Teach patient to avoid gel with other vaginal products; if to be used together, to separate by 6 hr; for vaginal route, teach patient proper insertion technique

Evaluation
Positive therapeutic outcome
• Decreased abnormal uterine bleeding
• Absence of amenorrhea
• Prevented pregnancy

promethazine (Rx)

(proe-meth'a-zeen)
Phenadoz, Phenergan, Promethagan
Func. class.: Antihistamine, H₁-receptor antagonist; antiemetic; sedative/hypnotic
Chem. class.: Phenothiazine derivative
Pregnancy category C

Do not confuse:
Phenergan/Theragran

ACTION: Acts on blood vessels, GI, respiratory system by competing with histamine for H₁-receptor site; decreases allergic response by blocking histamine

Therapeutic outcome: Absence of allergy symptoms and rhinitis, absence of nausea/vomiting, sedation

USES: Motion sickness, rhinitis, allergy symptoms, sedation, nausea, preoperative and postoperative sedation

CONTRAINDICATIONS: Hypersensitivity to H₁-receptor antagonist, agranulocytosis, bone marrow suppression, breastfeeding, coma, jaundice, Reye's syndrome

> **BLACK BOX WARNING:** Infants, intraarterial/SUBCUT use, neonates, children, extravasation

Precautions: Pregnancy **C**, renal/cardiac/hepatic disease, asthma, seizure disorder, prostatic hypertrophy, bladder obstruction, glaucoma, COPD, GI obstruction, ileus, CNS depression, diabetes, sleep apnea, urinary retention

> **BLACK BOX WARNING: IV** use

DOSAGE AND ROUTES
Nausea/vomiting
Adult: PO/IM/IV/RECT 12.5-25 mg; q4-6hr prn
Child >2 yr: PO/IM/IV/RECT 0.25-0.5 mg/kg q4-6hr prn

Motion sickness
Adult: PO 25 mg bid; give 30-60 min before departure and q8-12hr prn
Child >2 yr: PO/IM/RECT 12.5-25 mg bid; give 30-60 min before departure and q8-12hr prn

Allergy/rhinitis (unlabeled)
Adult: PO 12.5 mg qid, or 25 mg at bedtime
Child ≥2 yr: PO 6.25-12.5 mg tid or 25 mg at bedtime

Sedation
Adult: PO/IM 25-50 mg at bedtime
Child ≥2 yr: PO/IM/RECT 12.5-25 mg at bedtime

Sedation (preoperative/postoperative)
Adult: PO/IM/IV 25-50 mg
Child ≥2 yr: PO/IM/IV 0.5-1.1 mg/kg

Available forms: Tabs 12.5, 25, 50 mg; supp 12.5, 25, 50 mg; inj 25, 50 mg/ml

Implementation
PO route
• With meals for GI symptoms; absorption may slightly decrease
• When used for motion sickness, 30 min-1 hr before travel
IM route
• IM inj in deep in large muscle; rotate site

> **Direct IV route**
>
> **BLACK BOX WARNING:** Check for extravasation: burning, pain, swelling at **IV** site, can cause tissue necrosis

• Do not use if precipitate is present
• Rapid administration may cause transient decrease in B/P
• After diluting each 25-50 mg/9 ml of NaCl for inj; give 25 mg or less/2 min

Syringe compatibilities: Butorphanol, chlorproMAZINE, cimetidine, dihydroergotamine, diphenhydrAMINE, droperidol, fentaNYL, glycopyrrolate, HYDROmorphone, hydrOXYzine, meperidine, metoclopramide, midazolam, pentazocine, perphenazine, prochlorperazine, promazine, ranitidine, scopolamine

Y-site compatibilities: Alfentanil, amifostine, amikacin, aminocaproic acid, amsacrine, anidulafungin, ascorbic acid, atenolol, atracurium, atropine, aztreonam, benztropine, bivalirudin, bleomycin, bumetanide, buprenorphine, butorphanol, calcium chloride/gluconate, CARBOplatin, caspofungin, chlorproMAZINE, cimetidine, ciprofloxacin, cisatracurium, CISplatin, cladribine, codeine, cyanocobalamin, cyclophosphamide, cycloSPORINE, cytarabine, DACTINomycin, DAPTOmycin, dexmedetomidine, digoxin, diltiazem, diphenhydrAMINE, DOBUTamine, DOCEtaxel, DOPamine, doxacurium, DOXOrubicin, doxycycline, enalaprilat, ePHEDrine, EPINEPHrine, epirubicin, epoetin, eptifibatide, erythromycin, esmolol, etoposide, famotidine, fenoldopam, fentaNYL, filgrastim, fluconazole, fludarabine, gemcitabine, gentamicin, glycopyrrolate, granisetron, HYDROmorphone, hydrOXYzine, IDArubicin, ifosfamide, insulin (regular), irinotecan, isoproterenol, labetalol, levofloxacin, lidocaine, linezolid, LORazepam, LR, magnesium sulfate, mannitol, mechlorethamine, melphalan, meperidine, metaraminol, methoxamine, methyldopa, metoclopramide, metoprolol, metroNIDAZOLE, miconazole, midazolam, milrinone, mitoXANtrone, morphine, mycophenolate, nalbuphine, naloxone, netilmicin, nitroglycerin, norepinephrine, octreotide, ondansetron, oxaliplatin, oxytocin, PACLitaxel, palonosetron, pamidronate, pancuronium, PEMEtrexed, pentamidine, pentazocine, phenylephrine, polymyxin B, procainamide, prochlorperazine, propranolol, protamine, pyridoxine, quiNIDine, quinupristin-dalfopristin, ranitidine, remifentanil, Ringer's, ritodrine, riTUXimab, rocuronium, sargramostim, sodium acetate, succinylcholine, SUFentanil, tacrolimus, teniposide, theophylline, thiamine, thiotepa, tigecycline, tirofiban, TNA, tobramycin, tolazoline, trastuzumab, trimetaphan, vancomycin, vasopressin, vecuronium, verapamil, vinCRIStine, vinorelbine, voriconazole

ADVERSE EFFECTS
CNS: *Dizziness, drowsiness,* poor coordination, fatigue, anxiety, euphoria, confusion, paresthesia, neuritis, EPS, **neuroleptic malignant syndrome**
CV: Hyper/hypotension, palpitations, tachycardia
EENT: Blurred vision, dilated pupils, tinnitus, nasal stuffiness, dry nose, throat, mouth, photosensitivity
GI: *Constipation,* dry mouth, nausea, vomiting, anorexia, diarrhea
GU: *Retention,* dysuria, frequency
HEMA: Thrombocytopenia, agranulocytosis, hemolytic anemia
INTEG: Rash, urticaria, photosensitivity
RESP: Increased thick secretions, wheezing, chest tightness, **apnea in pediatric patients**

Pharmacokinetics
Absorption	Well absorbed (PO, IM); erratically absorbed (RECT)
Distribution	Widely distributed; crosses the blood-brain barrier, placenta
Metabolism	Liver
Excretion	Kidneys, breast milk
Half-life	Unknown

Pharmacodynamics
	PO/IM/RECT	IV
Onset	20 min	3-5 min
Peak	Unknown	Unknown
Duration	4-12 hr	4-6 hr

INTERACTIONS
Individual drugs
Alcohol: increased CNS depression
Heparin: decreased oral anticoagulants effect

Drug classifications
Antidepressants (tricyclics), barbiturates, CNS depressants, opiates, sedative/hypnotics: increased CNS depression
MAOIs: increased promethazine effect

Drug/lab test
False negative: skin allergy tests (discontinue antihistamines 3 days before testing)
False positive: urine pregnancy test
Interference: blood grouping (ABO), GTT

NURSING CONSIDERATIONS
Assessment

BLACK BOX WARNING: Not to be used in children <2 yr: fatal respiratory depression may occur; use cautiously in children >2 yr: seizures, paradoxical CNS stimulation may occur

• **Neuroleptic malignant syndrome:** assess for fever, confusion, diaphoresis, rigid muscles, elevated CPK, encephalopathy, discontinue product, notify prescriber
• Assess respiratory status: rate, rhythm, increase in bronchial secretions, wheezing, chest tightness; provide fluids to 2 L/day to decrease secretion thickness
• Monitor I&O ratio: be alert for urinary retention, frequency, dysuria, especially geriatric; product should be discontinued if these occur
• Monitor CBC during long-term therapy; blood dyscrasias may occur but are rare
• Monitor cardiac status: VS, palpitations, increased pulse, hypo/hypertension

Patient/family education
• Inform patient that a false-negative result may occur with skin testing; these procedures should not be scheduled until 3 days after discontinuing use
• Advise patient to take 30 min before departure to prevent motion sickness
• Caution patient to avoid hazardous activities, activities requiring alertness, since dizziness may

occur; instruct patient to request assistance with ambulation
• Advise patient to avoid alcohol, other depressants; serious CNS depression may occur
• Teach patient all aspects of product use; to notify prescriber if confusion, sedation, hypotension, jaundice, fever occur; to avoid driving and other hazardous activity if drowsiness occurs
• Advise patient to take 1 hr before or 2 hr after meals to facilitate absorption
• Caution patient not to exceed recommended dosage; dysrhythmias may occur
• Inform patient hard candy, gum, frequent rinsing of mouth may be used for dryness
• Advise that product may reduce sweating (heat stroke)

Evaluation
Positive therapeutic outcome
• Absence of motion sickness
• Absence of nausea, vomiting

propafenone (Rx)
(pro-paff'e-nown)
Rythmol, Rythmol SR
Func. class.: Antidysrhythmic (Class IC)
Pregnancy category C

ACTION: Slows conduction velocity; reduces membrane responsiveness; inhibits automaticity; increases ratio of effective refractory period to action potential duration; β-blocking activity

Therapeutic outcome: Absence of arrhythmias

USES: Atrial fibrillation (single dose), sustained ventricular tachycardia, paroxysmal supraventricular tachycardia (PSVT) prophylaxis, supraventricular dysrhythmias

CONTRAINDICATIONS:
2nd-, 3rd-degree AV block, right bundle branch block, cardiogenic shock, hypersensitivity, bradycardia, uncontrolled CHF, sick sinus syndrome, marked hypotension, bronchospastic disorders, electrolyte imbalance, Brugada syndrome

Precautions: Pregnancy **C**, breastfeeding, children, geriatric, CHF, hypo/hyperkalemia, nonallergic bronchospasm, renal/hepatic disease, hematologic disorders, myasthenia gravis, COPD

BLACK BOX WARNING: Recent MI, cardiac arrhythmias, QT prolongation, torsades de pointes

DOSAGE AND ROUTES
PSVT
Adult: PO 150 mg q8hr; allow a 3-4 day interval before increasing dose, max 900 mg/day

Atrial fibrillation
Adult: PO 450 or 600 mg as a single dose; SR 225 mg q12hr, may increase to 325 mg q12hr, max 425 mg q12hr

Available forms: Tabs 150, 225, 300 mg, SR cap 225, 325, 425 mg

Implementation
• Begin treatment in hospital
• Remove other antiarrhythmics before starting propafenone
• Adjust dosage q3-4day, no sooner

ADVERSE EFFECTS
CNS: Headache, dizziness, abnormal dreams, syncope, confusion, **seizures,** insomnia, tremor, anxiety, fatigue
CV: Supraventricular dysrhythmia, ventricular dysrhythmia, bradycardia, prodysrhythmia, palpitations, AV block, intraventricular conduction delay, AV dissociation, hypotension, chest pain, asystole
EENT: Blurred vision, altered taste, tinnitus
GI: *Nausea, vomiting,* constipation, dyspepsia, cholestasis, abnormal hepatic studies, dry mouth, diarrhea, anorexia
HEMA: Leukopenia, agranulocytosis, granulocytopenia, thrombocytopenia, anemia, bruising
INTEG: Rash
RESP: Dyspnea

Pharmacokinetics	
Absorption	Well absorbed
Distribution	Widely, crosses placenta
Metabolism	Rapid, liver, CYP1A2, CYP2D6, CYP3A4
Excretion	Kidneys
Half-life	2-32 hr, poor metabolizers 10-32 hr

Pharmacodynamics (antiarrhythmic)	
Onset	Hours to several days
Peak	4-5 days
Duration	Several hr

INTERACTIONS
Individual products
Arsenic trioxide, chloroquine, clarithromycin, droperidol, erythromycin, haloperidol, levomethadyl, methadone, pentamidine, chlorproMAZINE, mesoridazine, thioridazine: increased QT prolongation

Cimetidine, quiNIDine, rifampin: decreased propafenone effect

CycloSPORINE, digoxin: increased serum levels

Metropolol, propranolol: increased β-blocker effect

Warfarin: increased anticoagulation

Drug classifications
Local anesthetics: increased CNS effects

CYP1A2, CYP2D6, CYP3A4 inhibitors (protease inhibitors, quiNINE, PARoxetine, saquinavir, erythromycin, azole antifungals, sertraline, tricyclics): increased propafenone effects

Drug/food
Grapefruit juice: increased propafenone effect

Drug/herb
St. John's wort: decreased propafenone effect

Drug/lab test
Increased: CPK

NURSING CONSIDERATIONS
Assessment
• Monitor GI status: bowel pattern, number of stools

> **BLACK BOX WARNING:** Assess cardiac status: rate, rhythm, quality; ECG or Holter monitor prior to, during therapy; watch for PR, QT prolongation

• Monitor chest x-ray film, pulmonary function test during treatment
• Monitor I&O ratio; check for decreasing output; daily weight
• Monitor B/P for fluctuations

> **BLACK BOX WARNING:** Assess lung fields; bilateral crackles, dyspnea, peripheral edema, weight gain, jugular venous distention may occur in CHF patient

⚠ Assess toxicity: fine tremors, dizziness, hypotension, drowsiness, abnormal heart rate

Patient/family education
• Advise patient to avoid hazardous activities until response is known

• Advise patient to report fever, chills, sore throat, bleeding, shortness of breath, chest pain, palpitations, blurred vision
• Advise patient to take medication with food
• Advise patient to carry emergency ID identifying medication and prescriber
• Instruct patient not to use with grapefruit juice or St. John's wort

Evaluation
Positive therapeutic outcome
• Absence of dysrhythmias

TREATMENT OF OVERDOSE:
O_2, artificial ventilation, defibrillation ECG; administer DOPamine for circulatory depression, diazepam or thiopental for seizures, isoproterenol

proparacaine ophthalmic
See Appendix B

> ⚠ **HIGH ALERT**

propofol (Rx)
(pro′poh-fole)
Diprivan, Fresenius, Propoven
Func. class.: General anesthetic
Pregnancy category B

ACTION: Produces dose-dependent CNS depression by activation of GABA receptor

Therapeutic outcome: Induction of anesthesia

USES: Induction or maintenance of anesthesia as part of balanced anesthetic technique; sedation in mechanically ventilated patients

CONTRAINDICATIONS:
Hypersensitivity to product or soybean oil, egg, benzyl alcohol (some products)

Precautions: Pregnancy **B,** breastfeeding, children, geriatric, respiratory depression, severe respiratory disorders, cardiac dysrhythmias, labor and delivery, renal disease, hyperlipidemia

DOSAGE AND ROUTES
Anesthesia
Adult <55 yr and ASA I/II IV (Diprivan or generic): IV 40 mg q10sec until induction onset; maintenance: 100-200 mcg/kg/min or **IV BOL** 20-50 mg prn, allow 3-5 min between

P

adjustments; Fresenius Propoven 1% **IV** 20-40 q10sec until induction then 3-6 mg/kg/hr
Child ≥3 yr or ASA I or II: IV Induction: 2.5-3.5 mg/kg over 20-30 sec when not premedicated or lightly premedicated
Child 2 mo-16 yr maintenance: IV 125-300 mcg/kg/min, lower dose for ASA III or IV

ICU sedation

Adult: IV 5 mcg/kg/min over 5 min; may increase by 5-10 mcg/kg/min over 5-10 min until desired response (Diprivan or generic): 0.3-4 mg/kg/hr, max 4 mg/kg/hr (Fresenius Propoven)

Available forms: Inj 10 mg/ml in 20 ml ampule, 50 ml, 100 ml vials

Implementation

IV route
• Shake well before use; dilution is not necessary but if diluted, use only D₅W to ≥2 mg/ml; give over 3-5 min, titrate to needed level of sedation; use only glass containers when mixing, not stable in plastic; use aseptic technique when transferring from original container
• Fresenius Propoven 1%: Dilution is not necessary but if diluted use only D₅W or NS to ≥2 mg/ml (max dilution max 1 part Fresenius Propoven/4 parts D₅W or NS), do not admix, lidocaine can be used to reduce pain at site
• May be given by cont inf; give by inf pump
• Only with resuscitative equipment available, only by qualified persons trained in anesthesia

Y-site compatibilities: Acyclovir, alfentanil, aminophylline, ampicillin, aztreonam, bumetanide, buprenorphine, butorphanol, calcium gluconate, CARBOplatin, ceFAZolin, cefoperazone, cefotaxime, cefoTEtan, cefOXitin, ceftizoxime, cefTRIAXone, cefuroxime, chlorproMAZINE, cimetidine, CISplatin, clindamycin, cyclophosphamide, cycloSPORINE, cytarabine, dexamethasone, diphenhydrAMINE, DOBUTamine, DOPamine, doxycycline, droperidol, enalaprilat, ePHEDrine, EPINEPHrine, esmolol, famotidine, fentaNYL, fluconazole, fluorouracil, furosemide, ganciclovir, glycopyrrolate, granisetron, haloperidol, heparin, hydrocortisone, HYDROmorphone, hydrOXYzine, ifosfamide, imipenem/cilastatin, inamrinone, regular insulin, isoproterenol, ketamine, labetalol, levorphanol, lidocaine, LORazepam, magnesium sulfate, mannitol, meperidine, mezlocillin, miconazole, morphine, nafcillin, nalbuphine, naloxone, nitroglycerin, norepinephrine, ofloxacin, PACLitaxel, PENTobarbital, PHENobarbital, piperacillin, potassium chloride, prochlorperazine, propranolol, ranitidine, scopolamine, sodium bicarbonate, sodium nitroprusside, succinylcholine, SUFentanil, thiopental, ticarcillin, ticarcillin/clavulanate, vecuronium, verapamil

Solution compatibilities: (If given together via Y-site) D₅W, D₅LR, LR, D₅/0.45% NaCl, D₅/0.2% NaCl

ADVERSE EFFECTS

CNS: Involuntary movement, headache, jerking, fever, dizziness, shivering, tremor, confusion, somnolence, paresthesia, agitation, abnormal dreams, euphoria, fatigue, **increased ICP, impaired cerebral flow, seizures**
CV: *Bradycardia, hypotension,* hypertension, PVC, PAC, tachycardia, abnormal ECG, ST segment depression, **asystole, bradydysrhythmias**
EENT: Blurred vision, tinnitus, eye pain, strange taste, diplopia
GI: *Nausea, vomiting, abdominal cramping,* dry mouth, swallowing, hypersalivation, **pancreatitis**
GU: Urine retention, green urine, cloudy urine, oliguria
INTEG: *Flushing, phlebitis, hives, burning/stinging at inj site,* rash, pain of extremities
MS: Myalgia
RESP: Apnea, *cough, hiccups,* dyspnea, hypoventilation, sneezing, wheezing, tachypnea, hypoxia, respiratory acidosis
SYST: Propofol infusion syndrome

Pharmacokinetics

Absorption	Completely absorbed
Distribution	Rapid
Metabolism	Liver, conjugation to active metabolites; 95%-99% protein binding
Excretion	Urine
Half-life	3-12 hr

Pharmacodynamics

Onset	15-30 sec
Peak	Unknown
Duration	Unknown

INTERACTIONS

Individual drugs
Alcohol: increased CNS depression

Drug classifications
Antipsychotics, CNS depressants (sedativehypnotics, opioid analgesics), inhalational anesthetics, skeletal muscle relaxants: increased CNS depression
MAOIs: do not use within 10 days

Drug/herb
St. John's wort: increased propofol effect

NURSING CONSIDERATIONS
Assessment
• Assess inj site: phlebitis, burning, stinging
⚠ Monitor ECG for changes: PVC, PAC, ST segment changes; monitor VS
• Assess CNS changes: movement, jerking, tremors, dizziness, LOC, pupil reaction
• Assess allergic reactions: hives
⚠ Assess respiratory dysfunction: respiratory depression, character, rate, rhythm; notify prescriber if respirations are <10/min
⚠ Propofol infusion syndrome: assess for rhabdomyolysis, renal failure, hyperkalemia, metabolic acidosis, cardiac dysrhythmias, heart failure, usually between 35 and 93 hr after inf began, at >5 mg/kg/hr for >58 hr

Patient/family education
• Teach patient that this medication will cause dizziness, drowsiness, sedation; to avoid hazardous activities until drug effect wears off

Evaluation
Positive therapeutic outcome
• Induction of anesthesia

TREATMENT OF OVERDOSE:
Discontinue product; administer vasopressor agents or anticholinergics, artificial ventilation

propranolol (Rx)
(proe-pran′oh-lole)
Inderal, Inderal LA, InnoPran XL
Func. class.: Antihypertensive, antianginal, antidysrhythmic (class III)
Chem. class.: β-Adrenergic blocker
Pregnancy category C

Do not confuse:
Inderal/Toradol/Inderide/Adderall/Imuran, propranolol/Pravachol

ACTION: Nonselective β-blocker with negative inotropic, chronotropic, dromotropic properties

Therapeutic outcome: Decreased B/P, heart rate

USES: Chronic stable angina pectoris, hypertension, supraventricular dysrhythmias, migraine prophylaxis, pheochromocytoma, cyanotic spells related to hypertrophic subaortic stenosis, essential tremor, acute MI

Unlabeled uses: Prevention of variceal bleeding caused by portal hypertension, akathisia induced by antipsychotics, lithium-induced tremor

CONTRAINDICATIONS:
Hypersensitivity to this product, cardiogenic shock, AV heart block, bronchospastic disease, sinus bradycardia, bronchospasm, asthma

Precautions: Pregnancy **C,** breastfeeding, children, diabetes mellitus, renal/hepatic disease, hyperthyroidism, COPD, myasthenia gravis, peripheral vascular disease, hypotension, cardiac failure, Raynaud's disease, sick sinus syndrome, vasospastic angina, smoking, Wolff-Parkinson-White syndrome, thyrotoxicosis

> **BLACK BOX WARNING:** Abrupt discontinuation

DOSAGE AND ROUTES
Dysrhythmias
Adult: PO 10-30 mg tid-qid; **IV** BOL 1-3 mg given 1 mg/min; may repeat in 2 min; may repeat q4hr thereafter
Child: PO 1 mg/kg/day divided in 2 doses, **IV** 0.01-0.1 mg/kg over 5 min

Hypertension
Adult: PO 40 mg bid or 80 mg/day (EXT REL) initially; usual dosage 120-240 mg/day bid-tid or 120-160 mg/day (EXT REL)
Child: PO 0.5-1 mg/kg/day divided q6-12hr

Angina
Adult: PO 10-20 mg bid-qid, increase at 3-7 day intervals up to 160-320 mg/day, or 80 mg/day, increase at 3-7 day intervals up to 160-320 mg/day

MI prophylaxis
Adult: PO 180-240 mg/day tid-qid starting 5 days to 2 wk after MI

Pheochromocytoma
Adult: PO 60 mg/day × 3 days preoperatively in divided doses or 30 mg/day in divided doses (inoperable tumor)

Migraine
Adult: PO 80 mg/day (EXT REL) or in divided doses; may increase to 160-240 mg/day in divided doses
Child: PO 0.6-1.5 mg/kg/day divided q8hr
Child ≤35 kg (unlabeled): PO 10-20 mg tid

P

Essential tremor

Adult: PO 40 mg bid; usual dosage 120 mg/day

Available forms: Ext rel caps 60, 80, 120, 160 mg; tabs 10, 20, 40, 60, 80, 90 mg; inj 1 mg/ml; oral sol 4 mg, 8 mg/ml

Implementation

PO route

• Do not break, crush, chew, or open ext rel cap
• Do not use ext rel cap for essential tremor, MI, cardiac dysrhythmias; do not use InnoPran XL in hypertropic subaortic stenosis, migraine, angina pectoris
• Ext rel caps should be taken daily; InnoPran XL should be taken at bedtime
• May mix oral sol with liquid or semisolid food; rinse container to get entire dose
• Give with 8 oz water with food; food enhances bioavailability
• Do not give with aluminum-containing antacid; may decrease GI absorption

Direct IV route

• IV undiluted or diluted 10 ml D$_5$W for inj; give 1 mg or less/min

Intermittent IV infusion route

• May be diluted in 50 ml NaCl and run 1 mg over 10-15 min

Y-site compatibilities: Acyclovir, alfentanil, alteplase, amikacin, aminocaproic acid, aminophylline, anidulafungin, ascorbic acid, atracurium, atropine, azaTHIOprine, aztreonam, benztropine, bivalirudin, bleomycin, bumetanide, buprenorphine, butorphanol, calcium chloride/gluconate, CARBOplatin, caspofungin, cefamandole, ceFAZolin, cefmetazole, cefonicid, cefoperazone, cefotaxime, cefoTEtan, cefOXitin, cefTAZidime, ceftizoxime, cefTRIAXone, cefuroxime, cephalothin, cephapirin, chloramphenicol, chlorproMAZINE, cimetidine, CISplatin, clindamycin, cyanocobalamin, cyclophosphamide, cycloSPORINE, cytarabine, DACTINomycin, DAPTOmycin, dexamethasone, digoxin, diltiazem, diphenhydrAMINE, DOBUTamine, DOCEtaxel, DOPamine, doxacurium, DOXOrubicin, doxycycline, enalaprilat, ePHEDrine, EPINEPHrine, epirubicin, epoetin alfa, eptifibatide, ertapenem, erythromycin, esmolol, etoposide, etoposide phosphate, famotidine, fenoldopam, fentaNYL, fluconazole, fludarabine, fluorouracil, folic acid, furosemide, ganciclovir, gatifloxacin, gemcitabine, gemtuzumab, gentamicin, glycopyrrolate, granisetron, heparin, hydrocortisone, HYDROmorphone, hydrOXYzine, IDArubicin, ifosfamide, imipenem-cilastatin, inamrinone, irinotecan, isoproterenol, ketorolac, labetalol, levofloxacin, lidocaine, linezolid, LORazepam, magnesium, mannitol, mechlorethamine, meperidine, metaraminol, methicillin, methotrexate, methoxamine, methyldopate, methylPREDNISolone, metoclopramide, metoprolol, metroNIDAZOLE, mezlocillin, miconazole, midazolam, milrinone, minocycline, mitoXANtrone, morphine, moxalactam, multiple vitamins, mycophenolate, nafcillin, nalbuphine, naloxone, nesiritide, netilmicin, nitroglycerin, nitroprusside, norepinephrine, octreotide, ondansetron, oxacillin, oxaliplatin, oxytocin, palonosetron, pamidronate, pancuronium, papaverine, PEMEtrexed, penicillin G potassium/sodium, pentamidine, pentazocine, PENTobarbital, PHENobarbital, phenylephrine, phytonadione, piperacillin, polymyxin B, potassium chloride, procainamide, prochlorperazine, promethazine, propofol, protamine, pyridoxine, quiNIDine, quinupristin-dalfopristin, ranitidine, ritodrine, rocuronium, sodium acetate/bicarbonate, succinylcholine, SUFentanil, tacrolimus, teniposide, theophylline, thiamine, thiotepa, ticarcillin, ticarcillin-clavulanate, tigecycline, tirofiban, tobramycin, tolazoline, trimetaphan, urokinase, vancomycin, vasopressin, vecuronium, verapamil, vinCRIStine, vinorelbine, vitamin B complex/C, voriconazole, zoledronic acid

ADVERSE EFFECTS

CNS: Depression, hallucinations, *dizziness, fatigue,* lethargy, paresthesia, bizarre dreams, disorientation

CV: Bradycardia, *hypotension,* **CHF,** palpitations, AV block, peripheral vascular insufficiency, vasodilatation, **pulmonary edema, dysrhythmias,** cold extremities

EENT: Sore throat, **laryngospasm,** blurred vision, dry eyes

GI: Nausea, vomiting, diarrhea, colitis, constipation, cramps, dry mouth, hepatomegaly, gastric pain, acute pancreatitis

GU: Impotence, decreased libido, UTIs

HEMA: Agranulocytosis, thrombocytopenia

INTEG: Rash, pruritus, fever, **Stevens-Johnson syndrome, toxic epidermal necrolysis**

META: Hyperglycemia, hypoglycemia

MISC: Facial swelling, weight change, Raynaud's phenomenon

MS: Joint pain, arthralgia, muscle cramps, pain

RESP: Dyspnea, respiratory dysfunction, **bronchospasm,** cough

---

Pharmacokinetics

Absorption	Well absorbed (PO); slowly absorbed (ext rel); completely absorbed (**IV**)
Distribution	Widely distributed, crosses blood-brain barrier, protein binding 90%
Metabolism	Liver, extensively
Excretion	Kidneys
Half-life	3-8 hr; ext rel 8-11 hr

Pharmacodynamics

	PO	PO-EXT REL	IV
Onset	½ hr	Unknown	Rapid
Peak	1-1½ hr	6 hr	1 min
Duration	6-12 hr	24 hr	2-4 hr

INTERACTIONS

Individual drugs
Cimetidine: increased β-blocking effect
Disopyramide: increased negative inotropic effects
Haloperidol, prazosin, quiNIDine: increased hypotension
Propafenone: increased propranolol levels
Smoking: decreased propranolol levels

Drug classifications
Barbiturates: decreased β-blocking effect
Calcium channel blockers, neuromuscular blockers: increased effects
Phenothiazines: increased toxicity

Drug/herb
Hawthorn: increased antihypertensive effect
Avoid use with feverfew, ma huang: decreased antihypertensive effect

Drug/lab test
Increased: serum potassium, serum uric acid, AST, ALT, alkaline phosphatase, LDH
Decreased: blood glucose
Interference: glaucoma testing

NURSING CONSIDERATIONS
Assessment
• Monitor B/P during beginning treatment, periodically thereafter; pulse q4hr; note rate, rhythm, quality; check apical/radial pulse before administration; notify prescriber of any significant changes (pulse <50 bpm or systolic B/P <90 mm Hg)

• Check for baselines in renal, liver function tests before therapy begins and periodically thereafter
• Assess for edema in feet, legs daily; monitor I&O, weight daily; check for jugular vein distention, crackles bilaterally; dyspnea (CHF)
• Monitor skin turgor, dryness of mucous membranes for hydration status, especially geriatric
• Assess for headache, light-headedness, decreased B/P; may indicate need for decreased dose; may aggravate symptoms of arterial insufficiency

Patient/family education
⚠ Teach patient not to discontinue product abruptly (life-threatening dysrhythmias, exacerbation of angina, MI); to take at same time of day either with or without food consistently; taper over at least a few wk
• Teach patient not to use OTC products containing α-adrenergic stimulants (such as nasal decongestants, cold preparations); to avoid alcohol, smoking and to limit sodium intake as prescribed; blood glucose (diabetes mellitus)
• Teach patient how to take pulse and B/P at home; advise when to notify prescriber
• Instruct patient to comply with weight control, dietary adjustments, modified exercise program
• Instruct patient to carry/wear emergency ID to identify product being taken, allergies; tell patient product controls symptoms but does not cure
• Caution patient to avoid hazardous activities if dizziness, drowsiness are present
• **Teach patient to report symptoms of CHF:** difficulty breathing, especially on exertion or when lying down, night cough, swelling of extremities or bradycardia, dizziness, confusion, depression, fever
• Advise patient that sensitivity to cold may occur
• Teach patient to monitor blood glucose; may mask symptoms of hypoglycemia
• Teach patient how to take pulse, B/P; withhold if <50 bpm or systolic B/P <90 mm Hg

Evaluation
Positive therapeutic outcome
• Decreased B/P in hypertension (after 1-2 wk)
• Decreased tremors
• Absence of dysrhythmias
• Decreased migraine headaches

TREATMENT OF OVERDOSE:
Lavage, **IV** atropine for bradycardia, **IV** theophylline for bronchospasm, digoxin, O$_2$, diuretic for cardiac failure, hemodialysis, **IV** glucose for

hyperglycemia, **IV** diazepam (or phenytoin) for seizures

propylhexadrine nasal
See Appendix B

propylthiouracil (Rx)
(proe-pill-thye-oh-yoor′a-sill)
Propyl-Thyracil ✚
Func. class.: Thyroid hormone antagonist (antithyroid)
Chem. class.: Thioamide
Pregnancy category D

ACTION: Blocks synthesis peripherally of T_3, T_4, inhibits organification of iodine

Therapeutic outcome: Decreased T_3, T_4 levels, hyperthyroid symptoms

USES: Preparation for thyroidectomy, thyrotoxic crisis, hyperthyroidism, thyroid storm

CONTRAINDICATIONS:
Pregnancy **D**, breastfeeding, hypersensitivity, agranulocytosis, hepatitis, jaundice

Precautions: Infection, bone marrow depression, hepatic disease, fever

> **BLACK BOX WARNING:** Hepatic disease

DOSAGE AND ROUTES
Thyrotoxic crisis
Adult and child: PO 200-400 mg q4h for 1st 24 hr

Preparation for thyroidectomy
Adult: PO 600-1200 mg/day
Child: PO 10 mg/kg/day in divided doses

Hyperthyroidism
Adult: PO 100 mg tid increasing to 300 mg q8hr if condition is severe; continue to euthyroid state, then 100 mg daily-tid
Child >6 yr: PO 50 mg/day divided doses q8hr, titrate based on TSH/free T_4 levels
Neonate (unlabeled): PO 10 mg/kg/day in divided doses

Available forms: Tabs 50 mg

Implementation
• Give with meals to decrease GI upset
• Give at same time each day to maintain product level
• Give lowest dosage that relieves symptoms
• Store in light-resistant container

• Increase fluids to 3-4 L/day, unless contraindicated

ADVERSE EFFECTS
CNS: *Drowsiness, headache, vertigo, fever,* paresthesias, neuritis
GI: *Nausea, diarrhea, vomiting,* jaundice, **hepatitis,** loss of taste, **liver failure, death**
GU: Nephritis
HEMA: **Agranulocytosis, leukopenia, thrombocytopenia, hypothrombinemia, lymphadenopathy,** bleeding, vasculitis, periarteritis
INTEG: *Rash, urticaria, pruritus, alopecia, hyperpigmentation,* lupus-like syndrome
MS: Myalgia, arthralgia, nocturnal muscle cramps, osteoporosis

Pharmacokinetics
Absorption	Rapidly absorbed
Distribution	Crosses placenta, concentration in thyroid gland
Metabolism	Liver
Excretion	Urine, bile, breast milk
Half-life	1-2 hr

Pharmacodynamics
Onset	30-40 min
Peak	Unknown
Duration	2-4 hr

INTERACTIONS
Individual drugs
Heparin: decreased anticoagulant effect
Lithium: increased antithyroid effect
Potassium/sodium iodide: increased effects
Radiation: increased bone marrow depression

Drug classifications
Anticoagulants (oral): decreased anticoagulant effect
Antineoplastics: increased bone marrow depression
Phenothiazines: increased agranulocytosis

Drug/lab test
Increased: pro-time, AST, ALT, alkaline phosphatase

NURSING CONSIDERATIONS
Assessment
• Monitor pulse, B/P, temp; I&O ratio; check for edema (puffy hands, feet, periorbits); indicates hypothyroidism
• Check weight daily with same clothing, scale, time of day

• Hyperthyroidism: weight loss, nervousness, insomnia, fever, diaphoresis, tremors
• Hypothyroidism: constipation, dry skin, weakness, headache
• Monitor T_3, T_4, which are increased; check serum TSH, which is decreased; assess free thyroxine index, which is increased if dosage is too low; discontinue product 3-4 wk before radioactive iodine uptake test
⚠ **Blood dyscrasias: Monitor CBC with differential; leukopenia, thrombocytopenia, agranulocytosis**
⚠ **Overdose: Assess for peripheral edema, heat intolerance, diaphoresis, palpitations, dysrhythmias, severe tachycardia, increased temp, delirium, CNS irritability**
⚠ **Hypersensitivity: Assess for rash, enlarged cervical lymph nodes; product may have to be discontinued**
• **Hypoprothrombinemia:** assess for bleeding, petechiae, ecchymosis
• **Bone marrow depression:** assess for sore throat, fever, fatigue

---

BLACK BOX WARNING: Hepatotoxicity: monitor LFTs before and during treatment; jaundice, nausea, vomiting, abdominal pain, anorexia, diarrhea, fatigue

---

• Monitor clinical response: after 3 wk should include increased weight, decreased pulse, decreased T_4

Patient/family education
• Advise patient to abstain from breastfeeding after delivery; product appears in breast milk
• Teach patient to take pulse daily and to keep graph of weight, pulse, mood
• Advise patient to report redness, swelling, sore throat, mouth lesions, which indicate blood dyscrasias
• Caution patient to avoid OTC products that contain iodine; that seafood, other iodine-containing foods may be restricted by prescriber
• Caution patient not to discontinue this medication abruptly; thyroid crisis may occur; stress patient compliance
• Teach patient that response may take several mo if thyroid is large
• Teach patient symptoms/signs of overdose: periorbital edema, cold intolerance, mental depression; notify prescriber at once
• Teach patient symptoms of inadequate dose: tachycardia, diarrhea, fever, irritability; prescriber should be notified to adjust dosage
• Teach patient to take medication exactly as prescribed, not to skip or double doses; missed doses should be taken when remembered up to 1 hr before next dose
• Instruct patient to carry/wear emergency identification indicating medication taken and condition being treated

Evaluation
Positive therapeutic outcome
• Weight gain
• Decreased pulse
• Decreased T_4
• Decreased B/P

---

protamine (Rx)
(proe′ta-meen)
Func. class.: Heparin antagonist
Chem. class.: Low-molecular-weight protein
Pregnancy category C

ACTION: Binds heparin, making it ineffective

Therapeutic outcome: Prevention of heparin overdose

USES: Heparin overdose; neutralizes heparin in procedures, hemorrhage

CONTRAINDICATION: Hypersensitivity

Precautions: Pregnancy **C,** breastfeeding, fish allergy, diabetes, previous exposure to protamine, insulins, heparin rebound or bleeding

DOSAGE AND ROUTES
Heparin overdose
Adult and child: **IV** 1 mg of protamine/100 units of heparin given; administer slowly over 1-3 min; max 50 mg/10 min

Enoxaparin overdose
Adult: IV 1 mg of protamine/1 mg enoxaparin

Dalteparin/tinzaparin overdose
Adult: IV 1 mg of protamine/100 anti-Xa unit

Available forms: Inj 10 mg/ml

Implementation
Direct IV route
• After reconstituting 50 mg/5 ml sterile bacteriostatic water for inj, shake; give 20 mg or less over 1-3 min

Y-site compatibilities: Alfentanil, amikacin, aminophylline, ascorbic acid, atracurium, atropine, azaTHIOprine, aztreonam, benztropine, bumetanide, buprenorphine, butorphanol, calcium chloride/gluconate, ceftazidime, chlorproMAZINE, cimetidine, clindamycin, cyanocobalamin, cycloSPORINE, digoxin, diphenhydrAMINE, DOBUTamine, DOPamine, doxycycline, enalaprilat, ePHEDrine, EPINEPHrine, epoetin alfa, erythromycin, esmolol, famotidine, fentaNYL, fluconazole, ganciclovir, gentamicin, glycopyrrolate, hydrOXYzine, imipenemcilastatin, inamrinone, iohexol, iopamidol, iothalamate, isoproterenol, labetalol, lidocaine, magnesium, mannitol, meperidine, metaraminol, methoxamine, methyldopate, metoclopramide, metoprolol, miconazole, midazolam, minocycline, morphine, multiple vitamins, nalbuphine, naloxone, netilmicin, nitroglycerin, nitroprusside, norepinephrine, ondansetron, oxytocin, papaverine, pentazocine, phenylephrine, polymyxin B, potassium chloride, procainamide, prochlorperazine, promethazine, propranolol, pyridoxine, quiNIDine, ranitidine, Ringer's, ritodrine, sodium bicarbonate, succinylcholine, SUFentanil, theophylline, thiamine, tobramycin, tolazoline, trimetaphan, urokinase, vancomycin, vasopressin, verapamil

ADVERSE EFFECTS

CNS: Lassitude, flushing
CV: Hypotension, bradycardia, **circulatory collapse,** capillary leak
GI: Nausea, vomiting, anorexia
HEMA: Bleeding
INTEG: *Rash,* dermatitis, urticaria
RESP: Dyspnea, **pulmonary edema, severe respiratory distress, bronchospasm**
SYST: Anaphylaxis, angioedema

Pharmacokinetics

Absorption	Completely absorbed
Distribution	Unknown
Metabolism	Unknown
Excretion	Unknown
Half-life	Unknown

Pharmacodynamics

Onset	5 min
Peak	Unknown
Duration	2 hr

NURSING CONSIDERATIONS

Assessment

• Monitor blood studies (Hct, platelets, occult blood stools) q3mo
• Monitor coagulation tests (aPTT, ACT) 15 min after dose, then in several hr

• Monitor VS, B/P, pulse q30min, plus 3 hr after dose
⚠ **Assess for hypersensitivity: skin rash, urticaria, dermatitis, cough, wheezing, have emergency equipment nearby; men who have had a vasectomy may be more prone to hypersensitivity**
⚠ **Assess for allergy to salmon; use with caution in these patients**

Patient/family education

• Explain reason for medication and expected results; not to take if allergic to fish
• Caution patient to avoid contact activities that may result in bleeding

Evaluation

Positive therapeutic outcome
• Reversal of heparin overdose

pseudoephedrine (OTC)

(soo-doe-e-fed'rin)
Elix Sure Cold, Eltor ✦, Nasofed, Sudafed, Sudafed 24 hour, Sudogest
Func. class.: Adrenergic
Chem. class.: Substituted phenylethylamine
Pregnancy category C

ACTION: Primary activity through α-adrenergic effects on respiratory mucosal membranes reducing congestion, hyperemia, edema; minimal bronchodilatation secondary to β-adrenergic effects

Therapeutic outcome: Decreased nasal congestion, swelling

USES: Nasal decongestant, otitis media adjunct, adjunct with antihistamines

CONTRAINDICATIONS:

Hypersensitivity to sympathomimetics, closedangle glaucoma

Precautions: Pregnancy **C,** breastfeeding, cardiac disorders, hyperthyroidism, diabetes mellitus, prostatic hypertrophy, hypertension

DOSAGE AND ROUTES

Adult and child >12 yr: PO 60 mg q6hr; EXT REL 120 mg q12hr or 240 mg q24hr
Geriatric: PO 30-60 mg q6hr prn
Child 6-12 yr: PO 30 mg q6hr, max 120 mg/day
Child 2-6 yr: PO 15 mg q6hr, max 60 mg/day

Available forms: Ext rel caps 120, 240 mg; oral sol 15 mg, 30 mg/5 ml; drops 7.5

⚠ Nurse Alert   ⭐ Key NCLEX® Drug

mg/0.8 ml; tabs 30, 60 mg; caps 60 mg; ext rel tabs 120, 240 mg

Implementation
• Swallow tab and ext rel cap whole; do not break, crush, or chew
• Avoid taking at or near bedtime if insomnia occurs
• Store at room temperature

ADVERSE EFFECTS
CNS: *Tremors, anxiety,* stimulation, insomnia, headache, dizziness, hallucinations, **seizures** (geriatric)
CV: Palpitations, tachycardia, hypertension, chest pain, **dysrhythmias, CV collapse**
EENT: Dry nose, irritation of nose and throat
GI: *Anorexia, nausea, vomiting,* dry mouth, ischemic colitis
GU: Dysuria

Pharmacokinetics

Absorption	Well absorbed
Distribution	Enters CSF, crosses placenta
Metabolism	Liver, partially
Excretion	Kidneys, unchanged (75%); breast milk
Half-life	7 hr

Pharmacodynamics

	PO	PO-EXT REL
Onset	15-30 min	1 hr
Peak	Unknown	Unknown
Duration	4-6 hr	12 hr

INTERACTIONS
Drug classifications
Antidepressants (tricyclics), MAOIs: hypertensive crisis, do not use together
Urinary acidifiers: decreased effect of pseudoephedrine
Urinary alkalizers, adrenergics, β-blockers, phenothiazines, tricyclics: increased effect of pseudoephedrine

NURSING CONSIDERATIONS
Assessment
• Assess for CNS side effects in the geriatric: excitation, seizures, hallucinations
• Monitor for nasal congestion; auscultate lung sounds; check for tenacious bronchial secretions; children with otitis media should be assessed for eustachian tube congestion
• Monitor B/P and pulse throughout treatment

Patient/family education
• Teach patient reason for product administration and expected results
• Instruct patient not to use continuously, or more than recommended dose; rebound congestion may occur
• Advise patient to check with prescriber before using other products, as product interactions may occur
• Advise patient to avoid taking near bedtime; stimulation can occur
• Caution patient not to use if stimulation, restlessness, tremors occur
• Notify parents of possible excessive agitation in children
⚠ **Advise patient to notify prescriber of anxiety, slow or fast heart rate, dyspnea, seizures**
• Ext rel: do not divide, crush, chew, or dissolve
• Do not use within 14 days of MAOIs

Evaluation
Positive therapeutic outcome
• Decreased nasal congestion

pseudoephedrine nasal agent
See Appendix B

psyllium (OTC)
(sill'i-um)
Hydrocil, Leader Fiber Laxative, Metamucil, Natural Fiber, Natural Vegetable Fiber, Reguloid, Wal-Mucil
Func. class.: Laxative, bulk-forming
Chem. class.: Psyllium colloid
Pregnancy category C

ACTION: Bulk-forming laxative

Therapeutic outcome: Decreased constipation, decreased diarrhea in colitis

USES: Chronic constipation, ulcerative colitis, irritable bowel syndrome

CONTRAINDICATIONS:
Hypersensitivity, intestinal obstruction, abdominal pain, nausea/vomiting, fecal impaction

Precautions: Pregnancy **C**

DOSAGE AND ROUTES
Adult: PO 1-2 tsp in 8 oz of water bid or tid, then 8 oz of water; or 1 premeasured packet in 8 oz of water bid or tid, then 8 oz of water
Child >6 yr: 1 tsp in 4 oz of water at bedtime

P

Available forms: Chew pieces 1.7, 3.4 g/piece; powder effervescent 3.4, 3.7 g/packet; powder 3.3, 3.4, 3.5, 4.94 g/tsp; wafers 3.4 g/wafer

Implementation

- Give alone for better absorption; give after mixing with water immediately before use; administer with 8 oz of water or juice followed by another 8 oz of fluid
- Administer in AM or PM (oral dose)
- Shake susp well

ADVERSE EFFECTS

GI: *Nausea, vomiting, anorexia, diarrhea,* cramps, intestinal/esophageal blockage

Pharmacokinetics

Absorption	None
Distribution	None
Metabolism	Unknown
Excretion	Feces
Half-life	Unknown

Pharmacodynamics

Onset	12-24 hr
Peak	2-4 days
Duration	Unknown

INTERACTIONS

Drug classifications

Cardiac glycosides, oral anticoagulants, salicylates: decreased absorption of each specific product

Drug/herb

Flax, senna: increased laxative

NURSING CONSIDERATIONS

Assessment

- Monitor blood, urine electrolytes if used often by patient; check I&O ratio to identify fluid loss
- Assess for cramping, rectal bleeding, nausea, vomiting; if these symptoms occur, product should be discontinued; identify cause of constipation; identify whether fluids, bulk, or exercise is missing from lifestyle
- Assess stool for color, consistency, amount, presence of flatulence

Patient/family education

- Discuss with patient that adequate fluid consumption is necessary
- Teach patient that normal bowel movements do not always occur daily
- Caution patient not to use in presence of abdominal pain, nausea, vomiting; tell patient to notify prescriber if constipation is unrelieved or if symptoms of electrolyte imbalance occur (muscle cramps, pain, weakness, dizziness, excessive thirst)
- Teach patient not to use laxatives for long-term therapy; bowel tone will be lost and will decrease
- Teach patient not to take at bedtime as a laxative; may interfere with sleep; also problems with lipid pneumonia
- Teach patient not to use with food or vitamin preparations; delays digestion and absorption of fat-soluble vitamins

Evaluation

Positive therapeutic outcome

- Decreased constipation in 12-24 hr

---

pyridostigmine (Rx)

(peer-id-oh-stig′meen)
Mestinon, Mestinon Timespan, Regonol
Func. class.: Cholinergic, anticholinesterase
Chem. class.: Tertiary amine carbamate
Pregnancy category C

ACTION: Inhibits destruction of acetylcholine, which increases concentration at sites where acetylcholine is released; this facilitates transmission of impulses across myoneural junction

Therapeutic outcome: Decreased action of nondepolarizing muscle relaxant; increased muscle strength in myasthenia gravis

USES: Nondepolarizing muscle relaxant antagonist, myasthenia gravis, pretreatment in nerve gas exposure (military only)

CONTRAINDICATIONS:

Bradycardia, hypotension, obstruction of intestine, renal system, bromide, benzyl alcohol sensitivity, cholinesterase inhibitor toxicity

Precautions: Pregnancy **C**, seizure disorders, bronchial asthma, coronary occlusion, hyperthyroidism, dysrhythmias, peptic ulcer, megacolon, poor GI motility

DOSAGE AND ROUTES

Myasthenia gravis

Adult: PO 600 mg/day in 5-6 divided doses, max 1.5 g/day; IM/IV 2 mg or 1/30 of PO dose;

SUS REL 180-540 mg/day or bid at intervals of at least 6 hr
Child: PO 7 mg/kg/day in 5-6 divided doses; IM/IV 0.05-0.15 mg/kg/dose

Nondepolarizing neuromuscular blocker antagonist
Adult: 0.6-1.2 mg **IV** atropine, then 0.1-0.25 mg/kg/dose
Child: IV 0.1-0.25 mg/kg/dose

Nerve gas exposure prophylaxis (military)
Adult: PO 30 mg q8hr if threat of exposure to Soman gas is anticipated, start several hours before exposure and discontinue upon exposure; after this product is discontinued, give antidotes (atropine, pralidoxime)

Available forms: Tabs 60 mg; ext rel tabs 180 mg; syr 60 mg/5 ml; inj 5 mg/ml

Implementation
• Only with atropine sulfate available for cholinergic crisis
• Only after all other cholinergics have been discontinued
• Increased doses for tolerance, as ordered
• Larger doses after exercise or fatigue, as ordered
• Do not break, crush, or chew sus rel tabs
PO route
• On empty stomach for better absorption

IV route
• Undiluted (5 mg/ml), give through Y-tube or 3-way stopcock, give 0.5 mg or less/min (myasthenia gravis); 5 mg/min (reversal of nondepolarizing neuromuscular blockers)

Syringe compatibilities: Glycopyrrolate

Y-site compatibilities: Heparin, hydrocortisone, potassium chloride, vit B/C
• Storage at room temperature

ADVERSE EFFECTS
CNS: Dizziness, headache, sweating, weakness, **seizures,** uncoordination, paralysis, drowsiness, LOC
CV: Tachycardia, dysrhythmias, bradycardia, AV block, hypotension, ECG changes, **cardiac arrest,** syncope
EENT: Miosis, blurred vision, lacrimation, vision changes
GI: *Nausea, diarrhea, vomiting, cramps, increased salivary and gastric secretions, peristalsis*
GU: Frequency, incontinence, urgency
INTEG: Rash, urticaria, flushing

RESP: Respiratory depression, bronchospasm, constriction, laryngospasm, respiratory arrest
SYST: Cholinergic crisis

Pharmacokinetics
Absorption	Poorly absorbed (PO)
Distribution	Widely distributed, crosses placenta
Metabolism	Liver, plasma cholinesterase
Excretion	Kidneys
Half-life	2 hr (**IV**); 4 hr (PO)

Pharmacodynamics
	PO	PO-EXT REL	IM/IV
Onset	20-30 min	½-1 hr	2-15 min
Peak	Unknown	Unknown	Unknown
Duration	3-6 hr	3-6 hr	2-4 hr

INTERACTIONS
Individual drugs
Atropine, gallamine, metocurine, pancuronium, tubocurarine: decreased action
Succinylcholine: increased action of pyridostigmine
Magnesium, mecamylamine, polymyxin, procainamide, quiNIDine: decreased action of pyridostigmine

Drug classifications
Aminoglycosides, anesthetics, antidysrhythmics, corticosteroids, quinolones: decreased action of pyridostigmine

NURSING CONSIDERATIONS
Assessment
• **Myasthenia gravis:** assess for fatigue, ptosis, diplopia, difficulty swallowing, SOB, hand/gait before and after product, improvement should be seen after 1 hr
• Monitor I&O ratio; check for urinary retention or incontinence
⚠ **Toxicity: assess for bradycardia, hypotension, bronchospasm, headache, dizziness, seizures, respiratory depression; product should be discontinued if toxicity occurs**
• Monitor VS, respiration; increased B/P during test and at baseline
• Monitor diabetic patient carefully, since this product lowers blood glucose

Patient/family education
• Advise patient to carry/wear emergency ID specifying myasthenia gravis, products taken

---

Adverse effects: *italics* = common; **bold** = life-threatening

Evaluation
Positive therapeutic outcome
• Increased muscle strength, hand grasp, improved gait, absence of labored breathing (if severe); reversal of nondepolarizing neuromuscular blockers; prevention of nerve gas toxicity

TREATMENT OF OVERDOSE:
Discontinue product, atropine 1-4 mg **IV**

---

pyridoxine (vitamin B$_6$) (OTC, Rx)
(peer-i-dox'een)
Equaline Vitamin B$_6$, Neuro-K, Walgreens Finest B-6, Walgreens Gold Seal Vitamin B$_6$
Func. class.: Vitamin B$_6$, water soluble
Pregnancy category A

ACTION: Needed for fat, protein, carbohydrate metabolism; enhances glycogen release from liver and muscle tissue; needed as coenzyme for metabolic transformations of a variety of amino acids

Therapeutic outcome: Absence of vit B$_6$ deficiency

USES: Vitamin B$_6$ deficiency associated with the following: inborn errors of metabolism, seizures, isoniazid therapy, oral contraceptives, alcoholism, polyneuritis

Unlabeled uses: Palmar-plantar erythrodysesthesia syndrome

CONTRAINDICATION:
Hypersensitivity

Precautions: Pregnancy **A**, breastfeeding, children, Parkinson's disease, patients taking levodopa should avoid supplemental vitamins with >5 mg pyridoxine

DOSAGE AND ROUTES
RDA
Adult: PO (male) 1.7-2 mg; (female) 1.4-1.6 mg
Child 9-13 yr: PO 1 mg/day
Child 4-8 yr: PO 0.6 mg/day
Child 1-3 yr: PO 0.5 mg/day
Infant 7-12 mo: PO 0.3 mg/day

Vitamin B$_6$ deficiency
Adult: PO 5-25 mg/day × 3 wk
Child: PO 10 mg until desired response

Pyridoxine deficiency neuritis/seizure (not drug induced)
Adult: PO without neuritis 2.5-10 mg/day, after corrected 2-5 mg/day; with neuritis 100-200 mg/day × 3 wk, then 2-5 mg/day
Child: PO without neuritis 5-25 mg/day × 3 wk, then 1.5-2.5 mg/day in a multivitamin; with neuritis 10-50 mg/day × 3 wk, then 1-2 mg/day
Neonate with seizures: IM/IV 50-100 mg as a single dose

Deficiency caused by isoniazid, cycloSERINE, hydrALAZINE, penicillamine
Adult: PO 100-300 mg/day
Child: PO 10-50 mg/day

Prevention of deficiency caused by isoniazid, cycloSERINE, hydrALAZINE, penicillamine
Adult: PO 25-100 mg/day
Child: PO 1.2 mg/kg/day

Palmar-plantar erythrodysesthesia syndrome (unlabeled)
Adult: PO 50-150 mg/day

Available forms: Tabs 10, 25, 50, 100 mg; ext rel tabs 100 mg; inj 100 mg/ml; ext rel caps 150 mg

Implementation
PO route
• Swallow ext rel cap and ext rel tabs whole; do not break, crush, or chew
IM route
• Rotate sites to avoid pain; burning or stinging at site may occur; give by Z-track to minimize pain
• Store in airtight, light-resistant container

IV route
• Give **IV** undiluted or added to most **IV** sol; give 50 mg or less/1 min if undiluted

Syringe compatibilities: Doxapram

Additive incompatibilities: Erythromycin, iron salts, kanamycin, riboflavin, streptomycin

ADVERSE EFFECTS
CNS: Paresthesia, flushing, warmth, lethargy (rare with normal renal function)
INTEG: Pain at inj site

Pharmacokinetics

Absorption	Well absorbed (PO)
Distribution	Stored in liver, muscle, brain; crosses placenta
Metabolism	Unknown
Excretion	Kidneys, unchanged (not used)
Half-life	Unknown

Pharmacodynamics

Unknown

INTERACTIONS
Individual drugs
Chloramphenicol, cycloSERINE, hydrALAZINE, isoniazid, penicillamine: decreased effects of pyridoxine
Levodopa: decreased effects of levodopa

Drug classifications
Contraceptives (oral), immunosuppressants: decreased effects of pyridoxine

NURSING CONSIDERATIONS
Assessment
• Monitor pyridoxine levels throughout treatment
• Assess nutritional status: yeast, liver, legumes, bananas, green vegetables, whole grains
• Assess for pyridoxine (B$_6$) deficiency: nausea, vomiting, dermatitis, cheilosis, seizures, irritability, dermatitis before, during treatment
• Assess neurological status: paresthesia, lethargy
• Monitor blood tests: Hct, Hgb

Patient/family education
• Teach patient to avoid other vitamin supplements unless directed by prescriber
• Advise patient to increase meat, bananas, potatoes, lima beans, whole grain cereals in diet which are high in vit B$_6$
• Caution patient not to increase dosage, since serious reactions may occur

Evaluation
Positive therapeutic outcome
• Absence of nausea, vomiting, anorexia, skin lesions, glossitis, stomatitis, edema, seizures, restlessness, paresthesia

pyrimethamine (Rx)
(peer-i-meth′a-meen)
Daraprim
Func. class.: Antimalarial, antiprotozoal
Chem. class.: Folic acid antagonist
Pregnancy category C

ACTION: Inhibits folic acid metabolism in parasite; prevents transmission by stopping growth of fertilized gametes

Therapeutic outcome: Prevention of malaria

USES: Malaria prophylaxis, antiprotozoal action against *Plasmodium vivax, Pneumocystis jiroveci*

CONTRAINDICATIONS:
Hypersensitivity, chloroquine-resistant malaria, megaloblastic anemia caused by folate deficiency

Precautions: Pregnancy **C,** breastfeeding, geriatric patients, blood dyscrasias, seizure disorder, glucose-6-phosphate dehydrogenase (G6PD) disease, renal/hepatic disease

DOSAGE AND ROUTES
Prophylaxis of malaria
• Begin 2 wk before entering endemic area and continue for 6-10 wk after return
Adult and child >10 yr: PO 25 mg qwk
Child 4-10 yr: PO 12.5 mg qwk
Child <4 yr: PO 6.25 mg qwk

Malaria treatment
Adult/adolescent/child >10 yr: PO 25 mg/day × 2 days with sulfonamide
Child 4-10 yr: 25 mg/day × 2 days

Toxoplasmosis
Adult: PO 50-75 mg, then reduce by about 50% for 4-5 wk, with 1-4 g sulfADIAZINE × 1-3 wk, then reduce by 50% for 4-5 wk
Child: PO 1 mg/kg/day in 2 divided doses or 2 mg/kg/day × 3 days, then 1 mg/kg/day or divided twice daily × 4 wk, max 25 mg/day

Toxoplasmosis in AIDS patients
Adult: PO 100-200 mg/day × 1-2 days, then 50-100 mg/day × 3-6 wk, then 25-50 mg/day for life (given with clindamycin or sulfADIAZINE)

Available forms: Tabs 25 mg; combo tabs 500 mg sulfadoxine/25 mg pyrimethamine

P

Implementation
PO route
• Give leucovorin IM 3-9 mg/day × 3 days if folic acid deficiency occurs
• Give before or after meals at same time each day to maintain product level, decrease GI symptoms
• **Extemporaneous susp:** tabs may be crushed and mixed with 25 ml distilled water, sucrose-containing sol (1 mg/ml), shake well, stable for 5-7 days at room temp if mixed with sucrose-containing sol
• Store in tight, light-resistant container

ADVERSE EFFECTS
CNS: Stimulation, irritability, **seizures**, tremors, ataxia, fatigue, fever
CV: Dysrhythmias
GI: *Nausea, vomiting, cramps, anorexia,* diarrhea, atrophic glossitis, gastritis
HEMA: **Thrombocytopenia, leukopenia, pancytopenia, megaloblastic anemia,** decreased folic acid, **agranulocytosis**
INTEG: Skin eruptions, photosensitivity, **Stevens-Johnson syndrome**
RESP: **Respiratory failure**

Pharmacokinetics

Absorption	Well absorbed
Distribution	Widely distributed; crosses placenta
Metabolism	Liver, extensively
Excretion	Kidneys, unchanged (30%); breast milk
Half-life	4 days

Pharmacodynamics

Onset	Unknown
Peak	2 hr
Duration	Unknown

INTERACTIONS
Individual drugs
Folic acid: increased synergistic action
Radiation: increased bone marrow suppression
Zidovudine: increased risk of megaloblastic anemia, agranulocytosis, thrombocytopenia

Drug classifications
Bone marrow depressants, folate antagonists: increased bone marrow suppression

NURSING CONSIDERATIONS
Assessment
• **Serious skin disorders:** assess for **Stevens-Johnson syndrome** (swelling of face, lips, throat, fever)
• Monitor folic acid level; megaloblastic anemia occurs
⚠ Blood dyscrasias: assess blood studies, CBC, platelets; twice weekly if dosage is increased
⚠ Toxicity: assess for vomiting, anorexia, seizure, blood dyscrasia, glossitis; product should be discontinued immediately

Patient/family education
• Instruct patient that compliance with dosage schedule, duration is necessary; that scheduled appointments must be kept or relapse may occur
• Teach patient to report vision problems, fever, fatigue, bruising, bleeding, sore throat; may indicate **blood dyscrasias**
• Teach patient to report immediately skin rash; stop use

Evaluation
Positive therapeutic outcome
• Decreased symptoms of toxoplasmosis
• Decreased symptoms of *Pneumocystis jiroveci* pneumonia
• Decreased symptoms of malaria

TREATMENT OF OVERDOSE:
Gastric lavage, short-acting barbiturate, leucovorin, respiratory support if needed

QUEtiapine (Rx)

(kwe-tie′a-peen)

Seroquel, Seroquel XR

Func. class.: Antipsychotic

Chem. class.: Dibenzodiazepine

Pregnancy category C

ACTION: Functions as an antagonist at multiple neurotransmitter receptors in the brain including 5-HT_{1A}, 5-HT_2, DOPamine D_1, D_2, H_1, adrenergic α_1, α_2 receptors

Therapeutic outcome: Decreased hallucinations and disorganized thought

USES: Bipolar disorder, bipolar I disorder, depression, mania, schizophrenia

CONTRAINDICATIONS:

Hypersensitivity, breastfeeding

Precautions: Pregnancy **C**, geriatric, long-term use, seizures, hepatic disease, breast cancer, QT prolongation, CV disease, Parkinson's, brain tumor, hematological disease, torsades de pointes, cataracts, dehydration

> **BLACK BOX WARNING:** Children, suicide, dementia

DOSAGE AND ROUTES

Bipolar I disorder

Adult: PO (monotherapy or as adjunct to lithium or divalproex) 50 mg bid on day 1, 100 mg on day 2 in 2 divided doses as tolerated to 400 mg on day 4; range 400-800 mg/day

Psychotic disorders

Adult: PO 25 mg bid, titrate upward; XR: 300 mg/day in PM, range 400-800 mg/day

Depressive disorder (inadequate response to antidepressants alone)

Adult: PO EXT REL 50 mg/day in the PM on day 1, 2; on day 3 give 150 mg in the PM

Geriatric: PO EXT REL 50 mg; may increase by 50 mg/day based on response

Available forms: Tabs 25, 50, 100, 200, 300, 400 mg; ext rel tab 50, 150, 200, 300, 400 mg

Implementation

- Give reduced dosage in geriatric patients
- Give anticholinergic agent on order from prescriber to be used for EPS
- Avoid use of CNS depressants
- Give **immediate release** without regard to meals
- Give **extended release** without food or with light meal, swallow whole, do not split, crush, chew
- Supervise ambulation until patient is stabilized on medication; do not involve in strenuous exercise program because fainting is possible; patient should not stand still for a long time
- Sips of water, sugarless candy, gum for dry mouth
- Store in airtight, light-resistant container

ADVERSE EFFECTS

CNS: EPS, pseudoparkinsonism, akathisia, dystonia, tardive dyskinesia, drowsiness, insomnia, agitation, anxiety, *headache*, **seizures**, **neuroleptic malignant syndrome**, dizziness, dystonia, restless legs syndrome

CV: Orthostatic hypotension, **tachycardia**, QT prolongation, CV disease, Parkinson's disease, cardiomyopathy, myocarditis

ENDO: SIADH, hyperglycemia

GI: Nausea, anorexia, constipation, abdominal pain, dry mouth

HEMA: Leukopenia, **agranulocytosis**

INTEG: Rash

META: Hyponatremia

MISC: Asthenia, back pain, fever, ear pain

MS: **Rhabdomyolysis**

RESP: Rhinitis

SYST: **Stevens-Johnson syndrome**, **anaphylaxis**

Pharmacokinetics

Absorption	Rapidly absorbed
Distribution	Widely distributed
Metabolism	Liver, extensively; inhibits P450 CYP3A4 enzyme system; 83% protein binding
Excretion	Urine, feces
Half-life	≥ 6 hr

Pharmacodynamics

Onset	Unknown
Peak	1.5 hr
Duration	Up to 12 hr

INTERACTIONS

Individual drugs

Alcohol: increased CNS depression

CarBAMazepine, phenytoin, rifampin, thioridazine: increased QUEtiapine clearance

Chloroquine, clarithromycin, droperidol, erythromycin, haloperidol, methadone, pentamidine: increased QT prolongation

Cimetidine: decreased QUEtiapine clearance

Erythromycin: increased effects of erythromycin

Fluconazole, itraconazole, ketoconazole: increased action of QUEtiapine

Levodopa: decreased effect of levodopa

Lithium: increased neurotoxicity

LORazepam: decreased effect of LORazepam

Drug classifications

Analgesics (opioid), antihistamines, sedatives-hypnotics: increased CNS depression

Antihypertensives: increased hypotension

Barbiturates, glucocorticoids: increased clearance of quetiapine, decreased quetiapine effect

β-agonists, class IA/III antidysrhythmics, local anesthetics, phenothiazines (some), tricyclics: increased QT prolongation

DOPamine agonists: decreased effects of DOPamine agonists

NURSING CONSIDERATIONS
Assessment
• Assess CV status: QT prolongation, tachycardia, orthostatic B/P

> **BLACK BOX WARNING:** Mental status before initial administration, AIMS assessment; affect, orientation, LOC, reflexes, gait, coordination, sleep pattern disturbances; suicidal thoughts/behavior (child/young adult); dementia (geriatric patients)

• **Suicide:** restrict amount of product given, usually suicidal thoughts, behavior occur early in treatment and in children/adolescents/young adults

• Check that patient swallows all PO medication; check for hoarding or giving of medication to other patients

• Obtain baselines in blood glucose, liver function tests, neurologic status, ophthalmologic exam, cholesterol profile, weight

• Monitor B/P with patient in sitting, standing, and lying positions; take pulse and respirations q4hr during initial treatment; establish baseline before starting treatment; report drops of 30 mm Hg; obtain baseline ECG and monitor Q- and T-wave changes

• Check for dizziness, faintness, palpitations, tachycardia on rising; severe orthostatic hypotension is common

⚠ **Identify for neuroleptic malignant syndrome: hyperpyrexia, muscle rigidity, increased CPK, altered mental status, seizures, tachycardia, diaphoresis, hyper/hypotension, fatigue; product should be discontinued and prescriber notified immediately**

• **Assess for EPS** including akathisia (inability to sit still, no pattern to movements), tardive dyskinesia (bizarre movements of the jaw, mouth, tongue, extremities), pseudoparkinsonism (rigidity, tremors, pill rolling, shuffling gait); an antiparkinson product should be prescribed

Patient/family education
• Teach patient to use good oral hygiene; frequent rinsing of mouth, sugarless gum for dry mouth

• Caution patient to avoid hazardous activities until product response is determined; dizziness, blurred vision may occur

• Inform patient that orthostatic hypotension occurs often; patient should rise from sitting or lying position gradually; avoid hot tubs, hot showers, and tub baths because hypotension may occur; inform patient that heat stroke may occur in hot weather, to take extra precautions to stay cool

• Advise patient to avoid abrupt withdrawal of this product or EPS may result; product should be withdrawn slowly

• Teach patient to avoid OTC preparations (cough, hayfever, cold) unless approved by prescriber; serious product interactions may occur; avoid use with alcohol, CNS depressants because increased drowsiness may occur

• Advise patient to take medication only as prescribed

• Advise patient that follow-up is necessary including LFTs, blood glucose, neurologic/ophthalmic function, cholesterol profile, weight

• If drowsiness occurs, avoid hazardous activities such as driving

• Advise patient to notify prescriber if pregnancy is planned, suspected; do not breastfeed

• **Advise patient to notify prescriber immediately of fever, difficulty breathing, fatigue, sore throat, rash, bleeding**

• **Suicide: thoughts, behavior, primarily in children/adolescents/young adults**

Evaluation
Positive therapeutic outcome
• Decrease in emotional excitement, hallucinations, delusions, paranoia

• Reorganization of patterns of thought, speech

TREATMENT OF OVERDOSE:
Lavage, provide airway

⚠ Nurse Alert   ⭐ Key NCLEX® Drug

quinapril (Rx)

(kwin'a-pril)

Accupril

Func. class.: Antihypertensive

Chem. class.: Angiotensin-converting enzyme (ACE) inhibitor

Pregnancy category D (2nd/3rd trimester)

Pregnancy category C (1st trimester)

Do not confuse:

Accupril/Aciphex

ACTION: Selectively suppresses renin-angiotensin-aldosterone system; inhibits ACE, prevents conversion of angiotensin I to angiotensin II; results in dilatation of arterial, venous vessels

Therapeutic outcome: Decreased B/P in hypertension

USES: Hypertension, alone or in combination with thiazide diuretics, systolic CHF

CONTRAINDICATIONS:

Children, hypersensitivity to ACE inhibitors, angioedema

> **BLACK BOX WARNING:** Pregnancy D (2nd/3rd trimester)

Precautions: Breastfeeding, geriatric, impaired renal/liver function, dialysis patients, hypovolemia, blood dyscrasias, bilateral renal stenosis, cough, pregnancy C 1st trimester, hyperkalemia, aortic stenosis, African descent

DOSAGE AND ROUTES

Hypertension

Adult: PO 10-20 mg/day initially, then 20-80 mg/day divided bid or daily (monotherapy), start at 2.5 mg/day (with diuretics)

Geriatric: PO 10 mg/day, titrate to desired response (monotherapy), start at 2.5 mg/day (with diuretics)

Congestive heart failure

Adult: PO 5 mg bid, may increase qwk until 20-40 mg/day in 2 divided doses

Renal dose

Adult: PO CCr 61-89 ml/min start or 10 mg/day (hypertension), 5 mg bid (heart failure); CCr 30-60 ml/min 5 mg/day initially; CCr 10-29 ml/min 2.5 mg/day initially

Available forms: Tabs 5, 10, 20, 40 mg

Implementation

- Tabs may be crushed if necessary, without regard to food
- Store in airtight container at 86° F (30° C) or less
- Severe hypotension may occur after 1st dose of this medication; may be prevented by reducing or discontinuing diuretic therapy 3 days before beginning quinapril therapy

ADVERSE EFFECTS

CNS: Headache, dizziness, fatigue, somnolence, depression, malaise, nervousness, vertigo, syncope

CV: Hypotension, postural hypotension, syncope, palpitations, *angina pectoris,* **MI, tachycardia,** vasodilatation, chest pain

GI: Nausea, diarrhea, constipation, vomiting, gastritis, **GI hemorrhage,** dry mouth

GU: Increased BUN, creatinine, decreased libido, impotence

INTEG: **Angioedema,** rash, sweating, photosensitivity, pruritus

META: Hyperkalemia

MISC: Back pain, amblyopia

MS: Myalgia

RESP: Cough, pharyngitis, dyspnea

Pharmacokinetics

Absorption	≥60%
Distribution	Protein binding 97%, crosses placenta
Metabolism	Liver (active metabolites quinaprilat)
Excretion	Metabolites urine (60%), feces (37%)
Half-life	2 hr

Pharmacodynamics

Onset	½-1 hr
Peak	1-2 hr
Duration	24 hr

INTERACTIONS

Individual drugs

Alcohol: increased hypotension (large amounts)

Lithium: increased toxicity

HydrALAZINE, prazosin: use caution

Tetracycline: decreased absorption of tetracycline

Drug classifications

Adrenergic blockers, antihypertensives, diuretics, ganglionic blockers, nitrates, phenothiazines: increased hypotension

Diuretics (potassium sparing), potassium supplements, sympathomimetics, ACE/angiotensin II receptor antagonists, vasodilators: use caution

NSAIDs: decreased hypotensive effect of quinapril

Drug/lab test
Increased: Potassium, creatinine, BUN, LFTs

NURSING CONSIDERATIONS
Assessment
• **Collagen vascular disease:** monitor blood studies: neutrophils, decreased platelets; WBC with differential baseline, periodically q3mo; if neutrophils <1000/mm³ discontinue treatment
• **Hypertension:** monitor B/P, check for orthostatic hypotension, syncope; if changes occur, dosage change may be required
• Monitor renal function tests (protein, BUN, creatinine) and periodically liver function tests, uric acid; glucose may be elevated; watch for increased levels that may indicate nephrotic syndrome and renal failure; monitor renal symptoms: polyuria, oliguria, frequency, dysuria
• Check potassium levels throughout treatment, although hyperkalemia rarely occurs
• **CHF:** check for edema in feet, legs daily, weight daily
• **Allergic reactions:** assess for allergic reactions: rash, fever, pruritus, urticaria; product should be discontinued if antihistamines fail to help

> **BLACK BOX WARNING:** Assess for pregnancy; pregnancy **D**, 2nd/3rd trimester; if pregnancy is suspected, discontinue product

Patient/family education
• Advise patient not to discontinue product abruptly; advise patient to tell all persons associated with care
• Teach patient not to use OTC products (cough, cold, allergy) unless directed by physician; serious side effects can occur; avoid high-fat meal at time of dose
• Inform patient that xanthines such as coffee, tea, chocolate, cola can prevent action of product
• Caution patient on the importance of complying with dosage schedule, even if feeling better; to continue with medical regimen to decrease B/P: exercise, cessation of smoking, decreasing stress, diet modifications
• Emphasize the need to rise slowly to sitting or standing position to minimize orthostatic hypotension; not to exercise in hot weather or increased hypotension can occur

• Teach patient to notify prescriber of mouth sores, sore throat, fever, swelling of hands or feet, irregular heartbeat, chest pain, coughing, shortness of breath
• Caution patient to report excessive perspiration, dehydration, vomiting, diarrhea; may lead to fall in B/P, maintain adequate hydration
• Caution patient that product may cause dizziness, fainting, light-headedness; may occur during 1st few days of therapy; to avoid activities that may be hazardous
• Teach patient how to take B/P, and normal readings for age group
• Teach patient product may cause skin rash or impaired taste perception

> **BLACK BOX WARNING:** Pregnancy **D**, 2nd/3rd trimester, to report if pregnancy is planned or suspected, do not breastfeed

Evaluation
Positive therapeutic outcome
• Decreased B/P in hypertension

TREATMENT OF OVERDOSE:
0.9% NaCl **IV** inf, hemodialysis

quiNIDine gluconate (Rx)
(kwin'i-deen)
quiNIDine sulfate (Rx)
Func. class.: Antidysrhythmic (class IA)
Chem. class.: QuiNINE dextro isomer
Pregnancy category C

Do not confuse:
quiNIDine/quiNINE

ACTION: Prolongs action potential duration and effective refractory period, thus decreasing myocardial excitability; anticholinergic properties

Therapeutic outcome: Treatment of dysrhythmias

USES: Wolff-Parkinson-White syndrome, PVST, atrial fibrillation, flutter; paroxysmal atrial tachycardia, ventricular tachycardia, malaria (**IV** quiNIDine gluconate)

Unlabeled uses: Singultus (hiccups)

CONTRAINDICATIONS:
Hypersensitivity or idiosyncratic response, digoxin toxicity, blood dyscrasias, myasthenia gravis, AV block

Precautions: Pregnancy **C**, breastfeeding, children, geriatric, renal/hepatic disease, potas-

---

sium imbalance, CHF, respiratory depression, bradycardia, hypotension, syncope

> **BLACK BOX WARNING:** Cardiac arrhythmias, MI

DOSAGE AND ROUTES

QuiNIDine sulfate

Atrial fibrillation/flutter/PVST/WPW

Adult: PO 200 mg q6-8hr × 5-8 doses; may increase daily until sinus rhythm is restored; max 4 g/day given only after digitalization; maintenance 200-300 mg tid-qid or 300-600 mg q8-12hr (EXT REL)

Hiccups (unlabeled)

Adult: PO 200 mg qid

QuiNIDine gluconate

Adult: PO 324-648 mg q8-12hr (EXT REL); IM 600 mg, then 400 mg q2hr; **IV** give 16 mg/min

Available forms: Gluconate: ext rel tabs 324, 330 mg; inj gluconate 80 mg/ml; **sulfate:** tabs 200, 300 mg; ext rel tabs 300 mg

Implementation

- Give AV node blocker (digoxin) before starting quiNIDine to avoid increased ventricular rate

PO route

- Do not break, crush, or chew ext rel tab
- Give on an empty stomach with a full glass of water; may be given with meals if GI irritation occurs, absorption will be decreased
- Ext rel forms are not interchangeable
- Tab may be crushed and mixed with fluid or foods for patients with swallowing difficulties

IM route

- Give IM injection in deltoid, aspirate to avoid intravascular administration

Intermittent IV infusion route

- Give after diluting 800 mg/50 ml or more D_5W (16 mg/ml); give max 0.25 mg/kg/min, quiNIDine is absorbed by PVC tubing, minimize length; use inf pump

Y-site compatibilities: Alfentanil, amikacin, anidulafungin, ascorbic acid, atenolol, atracurium, atropine, benztropine, bleomycin, bumetanide, buprenorphine, butorphanol, calcium gluconate, caspofungin, chlorproMAZINE, cimetidine, CISplatin, cyanocobalamin, cycloSPORINE, DACTINomycin, digoxin, diltiazem, diphenhydrAMINE, DOBUTamine, DOCEtaxel, DOPamine, doxycycline, enalaprilat, ePHEDrine, EPINEPHrine, epoetin alfa, erythromycin, esmolol, etoposide, famotidine, fenoldopam, fentaNYL, fluconazole, fludarabine, gatifloxacin, gemcitabine, gentamicin, glycopyrrolate, granisetron, HYDROmorphone, IDArubicin, imipenem-cilastatin, irinotecan, isoproterenol, labetalol, lidocaine, linezolid, LORazepam, magnesium sulfate, mannitol, mechlorethamine, meperidine, metaraminol, methoxamine, methyldopate, metoclopramide, metoprolol, metroNIDAZOLE, miconazole, milrinone, mitoXANtrone, morphine, multiple vitamins, mycophenolate, nalbuphine, naloxone, nesiritide, netilmicin, nitroglycerin, norepinephrine, octreotide, ondansetron, oxaliplatin, PACLitaxel, palonosetron, pamidronate, pancuronium, papaverine, pentamidine, pentazocine, phenylephrine, phytonadione, polymyxin B, potassium chloride, procainamide, prochlorperazine, promethazine, propranolol, protamine, pyridoxine, ranitidine, ritodrine, succinylcholine, SUFentanil, tacrolimus, teniposide, theophylline, thiamine, thiotepa, tirofiban, tobramycin, tolazoline, trimetaphan, urokinase, vancomycin, vasopressin, verapamil, vinorelbine, voriconazole, zoledronic acid

ADVERSE EFFECTS

CNS: *Headache, dizziness,* involuntary movement, confusion, psychosis, restlessness, irritability, syncope, excitement, depression, ataxia

CV: Hypotension, *bradycardia, PVCs,* **heart block, cardiovascular collapse, arrest, torsades de pointes,** widening QRS complex, **ventricular tachycardia**

EENT: Cinchonism: tinnitus, blurred vision, hearing loss, mydriasis, disturbed color vision

GI: Nausea, vomiting, anorexia, *diarrhea,* **hepatotoxicity,** abdominal pain

HEMA: Thrombocytopenia, hemolytic anemia, agranulocytosis, hypoprothrombinemia

INTEG: Rash, urticaria, **angioedema,** swelling, photosensitivity, flushing with severe pruritus

RESP: Dyspnea, **respiratory depression**

Pharmacokinetics

Absorption	Well absorbed (PO, IM), slowly absorbed (sus rel)
Distribution	Widely distributed, crosses placenta, protein binding 80%-90%
Metabolism	Liver
Excretion	Kidney unchanged, 10%-50% breast milk
Half-life	6-7 hr (prolonged in geriatrics, cirrhosis, CHF)

Adverse effects: *italics* = common; **bold** = life-threatening

Pharmacodynamics

	PO (SULFATE)	PO EXT REL	PO (GLUCONATE)	IM	IV
Onset	½ hr	Unknown	Unknown	½ hr	5 min
Peak	1-6 hr	4 hr	4 hr	½-1½ hr	Unknown
Duration	6-8 hr	8-12 hr	6-8 hr	6-8 hr	6-8 hr

INTERACTIONS
Individual drugs
Amiodarone, cimetidine, NIFEdipine: increased quiNIDine level

Digoxin: increased digoxin level

NIFEdipine, sodium bicarbonate, verapamil: increased quiNIDine effect

Phenytoin, rifampin, sucralfate: decreased effects of quiNIDine

Propranolol: increased effect of propranolol

Reserpine: increased cardiac depression

Warfarin: increased levels of warfarin

Drug classifications
Antacids, carbonic anhydrase inhibitors, hydroxide suspensions: increased effects of quiNIDine

Anticholinergic blockers: increased vagolytic effects

Anticoagulants (oral): increased levels of anticoagulant

Antidepressants (tricyclics): increased effect of antidepressant

Antidysrhythmics: increased cardiac depression

Barbiturates, cholinergics: decreased effects of quiNIDine

Neuromuscular blockers: increased neuromuscular blocking

Phenothiazines: increased cardiac depression

Drug/herb
Hawthorn: increased quiNIDine effect

Drug/food
Grapefruit juice: decreased absorption, decreased metabolism

Drug/lab test
Increased: CPK

Interference: triamterene therapy interferes with quiNIDine test levels

NURSING CONSIDERATIONS
Assessment
• Monitor ECG continuously to determine product effectiveness, measure PR, QRS, QT intervals, check for PVCs, other dysrhythmias; monitor B/P continuously for hypo/hypertension; for rebound hypertension after 1-2 hr; check for dehydration or hypovolemia

• Monitor blood levels (therapeutic level 2-7 mcg/ml)

• **Cinchonism:** assess for tinnitus, headache, nausea, dizziness, fever, vertigo, tremor, may lead to hearing loss

• Monitor I&O ratio, electrolytes (potassium, sodium, chloride); check weight daily; check for signs of CHF or pulmonary toxicity: dyspnea, fatigue, cough, fever, chest pain; if these occur, product should be discontinued

• Monitor liver function tests: AST, ALT, bilirubin, alkaline phosphatase

• Assess for CNS symptoms: confusion, psychosis, numbness, depression, involuntary movements; if these occur, product should be discontinued

• Monitor cardiac rate, respiration: rate, rhythm, character, chest pain; watch for ventricular tachycardia, supraventricular tachycardia, or fibrillation that indicates toxicity

Patient/family education
• Instruct patient to report adverse effects immediately to prescriber

• Caution patient that sunglasses may be needed for photophobia; to use sunscreen, protective clothing, or stay out of sun to prevent burns

• Instruct patient to complete follow-up appointments with health care provider including pulmonary function tests, chest x-ray, ophth and otoscopic exams

• Advise patients to report signs of cinchonism, diarrhea, anorexia, decreased B/P

• Avoid grapefruit

Evaluation
Positive therapeutic outcome
• Resolution of dysrhythmias

---

quiNINE (OTC, Rx)
(kwye′nine)
Apo-Quinine ✿, Qualaquin
Func. class.: Antimalarial
Chem. class.: Cinchona tree alkaloid
Pregnancy category C

ACTION: Inhibits parasite replications, transcription of DNA to RNA by forming complexes with DNA of parasite

---

Therapeutic outcome: Reduction/death of *Plasmodium falciparum*; decreased leg cramps

USES: *P. falciparum,* malaria

CONTRAINDICATIONS:
Hypersensitivity, G6PD deficiency, retinal field changes, myasthenia gravis

Precautions: Pregnancy **C,** blood dyscrasias, breastfeeding, severe GI/hepatic disease, neurologic disease, psoriasis, cardiac dysrhythmias, tinnitus, hypoglycemia

> **BLACK BOX WARNING:** Nocturnal leg cramps

DOSAGE AND ROUTES
Malaria
Adult: PO 648 mg q8hr × 3 days or 7 days in SE Asia, given with tetracycline 250 mg q5hr × 7 days or clindamycin 900 mg q8hr × 7 days or doxycycline 100 mg q12hr × 7 days
Child: PO 25 mg/kg/day divided q8hr for 3-7 days in conjunction with another agent

Available forms: Tabs 324 mg

Implementation
• Give before or after meals at same time each day to maintain level
• Store in airtight, light-resistant container

ADVERSE EFFECTS
CNS: Headache, stimulation, fatigue, irritability, **seizures,** bad dreams, dizziness, fever, confusion, anxiety
CV: Angina, dysrhythmias, tachycardia, hypotension, **acute circulatory failure**
EENT: *Blurred vision, corneal changes, retinal changes, difficulty focusing,* tinnitus, vertigo, deafness, photophobia, diplopia, night blindness
ENDO: Hypoglycemia
GI: *Nausea, vomiting, anorexia,* diarrhea, epigastric pain
GU: Renal tubular damage, **anuria**
HEMA: **Thrombocytopenia, purpura, hypothrombinemia, hemolysis**
INTEG: Pruritus, pigmentary changes, skin eruptions, lichen planus–like eruptions, flushing, facial edema, sweating
MISC: **Hemolytic uremic syndrome**
RESP: Dyspnea

Pharmacokinetics

Absorption	Rapidly absorbed, 80%
Distribution	Crosses placenta, excreted breast milk, protein binding 70%-90% in malaria
Metabolism	Liver, extensively 80%
Excretion	Urine, 20% unchanged
Half-life	8-12 hr, increases in malaria

Pharmacodynamics

Onset	Unknown
Peak	1-3 hr
Duration	8 hr

INTERACTIONS
Individual products
AcetaZOLAMIDE, sodium bicarbonate: increased toxicity
Digoxin, digitoxin: increased levels
QuiNIDine: increased QT prolongation
Rifampin: increased treatment failure

Drug classifications
CYP2D6 substrates (amoxapine, atomoxetine, carvedilol, metoprolol, propranolol, timolol, encainide, flecainide, mexiletine, cloZAPine, codeine, cyclobenzaprine, fenfluramine, darifenacin, dexfenfluramine, dextromethorphan, donepezil, FLUoxetine, galantamine, haloperidol, HYDROcodone, maprotiline, meperidine, methadone, methamphetamine, oxyCODONE, PARoxetine, risperidone, fluPHENAZine, perphenazine, thioridazine, traMADol, traZODone, venlafaxine, zolpidem): increased levels
Antacids (magnesium or aluminum salts): decreased absorption of quiNINE
Anticoagulants: increased levels of anticoagulants
CYP3A4 inhibitors (clarithromycin, cycloSPORINE, diltiazem, etravirine, azole antifungals, lapatinib, mifepristone, protease inhibitors): increased quiNINE levels
Neuromuscular blockers: increased effect of neuromuscular blockers
Tricyclics: increased levels of tricyclics

Drug/lab test
Increased: 17-ks
Interference: 17-ohcs

Drug/herb
St. John's wort: decreased quiNINE level

Adverse effects: *italics* = common; **bold** = life-threatening

NURSING CONSIDERATIONS
Assessment
• Monitor B/P, pulse; watch for hypotension, tachycardia
• Assess liver studies qwk: ALT, AST, bilirubin
• Assess blood tests, CBC, since blood dyscrasias occur
• **Assess for cinchonism:** nausea, blurred vision, tinnitus, headache, difficulty focusing; quiNIDine levels >10 mcg/ml
• Assess for symptoms of malaria and improvement
• Assess frequency/duration of nocturnal leg cramps

Patient/family education
• Advise patient to avoid OTC preparations: cold preparations, tonic water
• Advise patient to take only as prescribed
• Teach patient visual changes may occur, to avoid driving or hazardous activities until response is known
• Teach patient to stop product and call prescriber if difficulty breathing, ringing in the ears, or allergic reaction occurs
• Teach patient to use insect repellant, protective clothing if in area with mosquitoes

Evaluation
Positive therapeutic outcome
• Decreased symptoms of malaria

rabeprazole (Rx)

(rab-ee-pray′zole)

Aciphex, Dariet ✦

Func. class.: Proton pump inhibitor

Chem. class.: Benzimidazole

Pregnancy category C

Do not confuse:

Aciphex/Aricept/Accupril

ACTION: Suppresses gastric secretion by inhibiting hydrogen/potassium ATPase enzyme system in the gastric parietal cell; characterized as a gastric acid pump inhibitor, since it blocks the final step of acid production

Therapeutic outcome: Absence of duodenal ulcers; decreased gastroesophageal reflux

USES: Gastroesophageal reflux disease (GERD), severe erosive esophagitis, poorly responsive systemic GERD, pathologic hypersecretory conditions (Zollinger-Ellison syndrome, systemic mastocytosis, multiple endocrine adenomas); treatment of duodenal ulcers with or without antiinfectives for *Helicobacter pylori;* daytime, nighttime heartburn

CONTRAINDICATIONS:

Hypersensitivity to this product or proton pump inhibitors (PPIs)

Precautions: Pregnancy **C**, breastfeeding, children, Asian patients, diarrhea, geriatric patients, gastric cancer, hepatic/GI disease, IBS, osteoporosis, pseudomembranous colitis, ulcerative colitis, vit B$_{12}$ deficiency

DOSAGE AND ROUTES

Healing of duodenal ulcers

Adult: PO 20 mg/day × ≤4 wk, to be taken after breakfast

Erosive esophagitis/GERD

Adult: PO 20 mg/day × 4-8 wk

Adolescent and child ≥12 yr: PO 20 mg/day up to 8 wk

Pathologic hypersecretory conditions

Adult: PO 60 mg/day; may increase to 120 mg in 2 divided doses

Available forms: Del rel tabs 20 mg

Implementation

PO route

- Do not break, crush, or chew del rel tab
- Give after breakfast daily with a full glass of water, without regard to food

ADVERSE EFFECTS

CNS: *Headache, dizziness, asthenia*

CV: Chest pain, angina, tachycardia, bradycardia, palpitations, peripheral edema

EENT: Tinnitus, taste perversion

GI: *Diarrhea, abdominal pain, vomiting, nausea, constipation, flatulence, acid regurgitation,* abdominal swelling, anorexia, irritable colon, esophageal candidiasis, dry mouth, **pseudomembranous colitis**

GU: UTI, frequency, increased creatinine, **proteinuria, hematuria,** testicular pain, glycosuria

HEMA: Pancytopenia, thrombocytopenia, neutropenia, leukocytosis, anemia

INTEG: Rash, dry skin, urticaria, pruritus, alopecia

META: Hypoglycemia, increased hepatic enzymes, weight gain

MISC: *Back pain,* fever, fatigue, malaise, **Stevens-Johnson syndrome**

RESP: *Upper respiratory tract infections, cough,* epistaxis, **pneumonia**

Pharmacokinetics

Absorption	Unknown
Distribution	Protein binding 96.3%
Metabolism	Liver, extensively by CYP2C19
Excretion	Kidneys, feces, metabolites
Half-life	1-2 hr

Pharmacodynamics

Unknown

INTERACTIONS

Individual drugs

Digoxin, nelfinavir/omeprazole: increased levels

Ketoconazole, itraconazole, iron salts, atazanavir/ritonavir, ampicillin: decreased levels

Calcium carbonate, sucralfate, vitamin B$_{12}$: decreased rabeprazole levels

Clarithromycin, phenytoin: increased levels of rabeprazole

Warfarin, clopidogrel: increased bleeding risk

Drug classifications

Benzodiazepines, antacids, other proton pump inhibitors, H$_2$ blockers: increased levels of rabeprazole

R

Adverse effects: *italics* = common; **bold** = life-threatening

Drug/herb
St. John's wort: decreased levels of rabeprazole

Drug/lab test
Decreased: magnesium

NURSING CONSIDERATIONS

Assessment
• Assess GI system: bowel sounds q8hr, abdomen for pain and swelling, anorexia

⚠ **Pseudomembranous colitis: may occur with most antibiotic therapy; assess for watery diarrhea, abdominal pain, fever**

• **Vitamin B$_{12}$ deficiency/cyanocobalamin/ hypomagnesemia:** may occur after 3-12 mo of treatment; use magnesium, Vit B$_{12}$, cyanocobalamin supplement, if severe, discontinuing of product may be needed

• Monitor hepatic enzymes: AST, ALT, increased alkaline phosphatase during treatment

• **Serious skin reactions:** assess for Stevens-Johnson syndrome

• **Blood dyscrasias (rare):** CBC with differential before and periodically during treatment

• Obtain susceptibility testing if *H. pylori* treatment is ineffective; another antiinfective may be needed

Patient/family education
• Advise patient to report severe diarrhea; product may have to be discontinued

• Advise patient to notify prescriber if pregnancy is planned or suspected

• Teach patient to report diarrhea, black, tarry stools, product may need to be discontinued

• Inform diabetic patient that hypoglycemia can occur

• Caution patient to avoid driving and other hazardous activities until response to product is known

• Caution patient to avoid alcohol, salicylates, NSAIDs; may cause GI irritation

• Advise patient to wear sunscreen, protective clothing to prevent burns

Evaluation
Positive therapeutic outcome
• Absence of epigastric pain, swelling, fullness; decreased symptoms of GERD after 4-8 wk

---

raloxifene (Rx)
(ral-ox'ih-feen)
Evista
Func. class.: Bone resorption inhibitor
Chem. class.: Hormone modifier, selective estrogen receptor modulator (SERM)
Pregnancy category X

ACTION: Tissue-selective estrogen agonist/ antagonist; agonist activity in bone and lipid metabolism, antagonistic activity on breast and uterus, reduces resorption of bone and decreases bone turnover

Therapeutic outcome: Absence or decrease of osteoporosis in postmenopausal women

USES: Prevention, treatment of osteoporosis in postmenopausal women, breast cancer prophylaxis in postmenopausal women with osteoporosis or in postmenopausal women at high risk for developing the disease

CONTRAINDICATIONS:
Pregnancy **X,** breastfeeding, hypersensitivity

> **BLACK BOX WARNING:** Women with active or history of venous thromboembolic events

Precautions: Hepatic/CV disease, cervical/ uterine cancer, elevated triglycerides, pulmonary embolism

> **BLACK BOX WARNING:** Stroke

DOSAGE AND ROUTES
Hormone replacement
Adult: PO 60 mg/day, max 60 mg/day

Available forms: Tabs 60 mg

Implementation
• Administer without regard to meals
• Add calcium supplement, vit D if lacking

ADVERSE EFFECTS
CNS: Insomnia
CV: Hot flashes, peripheral edema, **thromboembolism, stroke**
EENT: Retinal vein occlusion (rare)
GI: *Nausea,* vomiting, diarrhea, dyspepsia
GU: Vaginitis, leukorrhea, *hot flashes,* cystitis, vaginal bleeding
INTEG: Rash, sweating
META: Weight gain, peripheral edema

MS: Arthralgia, myalgia, *leg cramps,* arthritis

RESP: Sinusitis, pharyngitis, increased cough, pneumonia, laryngitis, rhinitis, bronchitis, **pulmonary embolism,** flulike symptoms

Pharmacokinetics

Absorption	Unknown
Distribution	Highly protein bound
Metabolism	Unknown
Excretion	Feces, breast milk
Half-life	28-32 hr (elimination)

Pharmacodynamics

Unknown

INTERACTIONS

Individual drugs

Ampicillin, cholestyramine: decreased action of raloxifene

Desiccated thyroid, levothyroxine, liotrix: decreased action

Drug classifications

Anticoagulants: decreased action of anticoagulants

Highly protein-bound products, systemic estrogens: administer cautiously

Drug/food

Soy: decreased effect of raloxifene

Drug/lab test

Increased: apolipoprotein, corticosteroid-binding globulin, thyroxine-binding globulin (TBG)

Decreased: lipoprotein, LDL cholesterol, total cholesterol, calcium, total protein, albumin

NURSING CONSIDERATIONS

Assessment

> **BLACK BOX WARNING:** For history of stroke, TIA, thrombosis, atrial fibrillation, hypertension, smoking; venous thrombosis may occur; avoid prolonged sitting, discontinue 3 days before surgery or other immobilization

• Obtain bone density test baseline, periodically throughout treatment; bone-specific alkaline phosphatase; osteocalcin, collagen breakdown

• Monitor B/P q4hr, watch for increase caused by H_2O and sodium retention

Patient/family education

> **BLACK BOX WARNING:** Teach patients to discontinue product 72 hr before prolonged bedrest

• Advise patient to avoid maintaining one position for long periods

• Advise patient to take calcium supplements, vit D if intake is inadequate

• Advise patient to increase exercise using weights

• Advise patient to stop smoking and to decrease alcohol consumption

• Inform patient that this product does not help control hot flashes

• Instruct patient to report fever, acute migraine, insomnia, emotional distress, UTI, or vaginal itching

> **BLACK BOX WARNING:** Teach patient to report swelling, warmth, or pain in calves

Evaluation

Positive therapeutic outcome

• Prevention, treatment of osteoporosis

---

raltegravir (Rx)

(ral-teg'ra-vir)

Isentress

Func. class.: Antiretroviral

Chem. class.: HIV integrase strand transfer inhibitor (ISTIs)

Pregnancy category C

ACTION: Inhibits catalytic activity of HIV integrase, which is an HIV-encoded enzyme needed for replication

Therapeutic outcome: Improvement in CD4, T-cell counts

USES: HIV in combination with other antiretrovirals

CONTRAINDICATIONS:

Hypersensitivity, breastfeeding

Precautions: Pregnancy **C,** children, geriatric, hepatic disease, immune reconstitution syndrome, hepatitis, antimicrobial resistance, lactase deficiency

DOSAGE AND ROUTES

Adult and adolescent ≥16 yr: PO 400 mg bid, if using with rifampin give 800 mg bid, max 800 mg/day with or without food

Available forms: Tabs 400 mg

Implementation
- Do not break, crush, or chew tabs
- May give without regard to meals, with 8 oz of water
- Store at room temperature

ADVERSE EFFECTS
CNS: *Fatigue*, fever, *dizziness*, *headache*, asthenia, **suicidal ideation**
CV: MI
GI: *Nausea*, vomiting, diarrhea, abdominal pain, gastritis, **hepatitis**
GU: Oliguria, proteinuria, hematuria, glomerulonephritis, acute renal failure, renal tubular necrosis
HEMA: Anemia, neutropenia
INTEG: Rash, urticaria, pruritus, pain or phlebitis at IV site, unusual sweating, alopecia
META: Hyperamylasia, hyperglycemia
MS: Myopathy, **rhabdomyolysis**
SYST: Immune reconstitution syndrome

Pharmacokinetics

Absorption	Max 3 hr if taken on empty stomach
Distribution	Unknown
Metabolism	Liver by uridine diphosphate glucuronosyltransferase (UGT A1A enzyme system)
Excretion	51% feces, 32% urine
Half-life	Terminal 9 hr

Pharmacodynamics

Unknown

INTERACTIONS
Individual drugs
Rifampin, efavirenz, tenofovir, tipranavir/ritonavir: decreased raltegravir levels

Drug classifications
Fibric acid derivatives, HMG-CoA reductase inhibitors: increased rhabdomyolysis, myopathy, elevated CPK
H$_2$ blockers, protein pump inhibitors, UGT1A1 inhibitors (atazanavir): increased raltegravir effect

Drug/lab test
Increased: total/HDL/LDL cholesterol

NURSING CONSIDERATIONS
Assessment
- **Rhabdomyolysis:** Assess for calf pain, increased CPK; product should be discontinued

- **HIV infection:** monitor CD4, T-cell count, plasma HIV RNA, viral load; resistance testing prior to therapy and at treatment failure
- **A Suicidal thoughts, behavior: monitor for depression, more comon in those with mental illness**
- **A Immune reconstitution syndrome: usually during initial phase of treatment, may give antiinfective before starting**
- Monitor total HDL/LDL cholesterol baseline and periodically; all may be elevated
- Assess skin eruptions: rash, urticaria, itching

Patient/family education
- Teach patient to take as prescribed; if dose is missed, take as soon as remembered up to 1 hr before next dose; do not double dose, do not share with others
- Teach patient that sexual partners need to be told that patient has HIV
- Advise patient that product does not cure infection, just controls symptoms, does not prevent infecting others
- **A Teach patient to report sore throat, fever, fatigue (may indicate superinfection)**
- Advise patient that product must be taken in equal intervals 2×/day to maintain blood levels for duration of therapy
- Advise patient to notify prescriber immediately of suicidal thoughts, behavior
- Advise patient to notify prescriber if pregnancy is planned or suspected, avoid breastfeeding

Evaluation
Positive therapeutic outcome
- Improvement in CD4, T-cell counts

---

ramelteon (Rx)
(rah-mel′tee-on)
Rozerem
Func. class.: Sedative-hypnotic, antianxiety
Chem. class.: Melatonin receptor agonist
Pregnancy category C

ACTION: Binds selectively to melatonin receptors (MT$_1$, MT$_2$); thought to be involved in circadian rhythm and the normal sleep-wake cycle

Therapeutic outcome: Ability to fall asleep easily and decrease early-morning awakenings

USES: Insomnia (difficulty with sleep onset)

CONTRAINDICATIONS:
Breastfeeding, infants, children, hypersensitivity

Precautions: Pregnancy **C**, hepatic disease, alcoholism, seizure disorder, sleep apnea, suicidal ideation, angioedema, depression, sleep-related behavior (sleepwalking), schizophrenia, bipolar disorder, alcohol intoxication, hepatic encephalopathy, aortic stenosis

DOSAGE AND ROUTES
Adult: PO 8 mg within 30 min of bedtime

Hepatic dose
Do not use in severe hepatic disease; use with caution in mild to moderate hepatic disease

Available forms: Tabs 8 mg

Implementation
• Give within 30 min of bedtime for sleeplessness, give on empty stomach for fast onset
• Store in tight container in cool environment
• Do not break tabs, swallow whole

ADVERSE EFFECTS
CNS: Dizziness, somnolence, fatigue, headache, insomnia, depression, complex sleep-related reactions: sleep driving, sleep eating, **suicidal thoughts/behavior,** syncope
GI: Nausea, diarrhea, dysgeusia, vomiting
MISC: Myalgia, arthralgia, decreased blood cortisol, influenza, upper respiratory tract infection
SYST: Severe allergic reactions, angio-edema

Pharmacokinetics

Absorption	Rapidly absorbed
Distribution	Protein binding 82%
Metabolism	Rapid first-pass metabolism, liver
Excretion	84% urine, 4% feces
Half-life	2-5 hr

Pharmacodynamics

Onset	Unknown
Peak	0.75 hr
Duration	Unknown

INTERACTIONS
Individual drugs
Alcohol, ciprofloxacin, fluconazole, fluvox-aMINE, ketoconazole: increased ramelteon effect, toxicity
Rifampin: decreased effect of ramelteon

Drug classifications
Antiretroviral protease inhibitors: possible toxicity
Anxiolytics, azole antifungals, barbiturates, CYP1A2 inhibitors, hypnotics, sedatives: increased ramelteon effect, toxicity
Potassium-sparing diuretics, potassium supplement, angiotensin II receptor agonists: increased hyperkalemia

Drug/food
High-fat/heavy meal: prolonged absorption, sleep onset reduced

NURSING CONSIDERATIONS
Assessment
• **Sleep characteristics:** assess type of sleep problem: falling asleep, staying asleep; complex sleep disorders (sleep walking/driving/eating) after taking product
• Assess mental status: mood, sensorium, affect, memory (long, short)

Patient/family education
• Advise patient to avoid driving or other activities requiring alertness until product is stabilized; drowsiness may continue the next day
• Advise patient to avoid alcohol ingestion or CNS depressants
• Teach patient alternative measures to improve sleep: reading, exercise several hr before bedtime, warm bath, warm milk, TV, self-hypnosis, deep breathing
• Teach patient to report if pregnancy is planned or suspected (C), avoid breastfeeding
• Advise patient to take immediately before going to bed
• Advise patient not to ingest a high-fat/heavy meal before taking
• Teach patient to report cessation of menses, galactorrhea (women), decreased libido, infertility, worsening of insomnia, behavioral changes, suicidal thoughts/behavior
• Med guide should be given to patient and reviewed

Evaluation
Positive therapeutic outcome
• Ability to sleep at night, decreased amount of early-morning awakening

R

ramipril (Rx)
(ra-mi′pril)
Altace
Func. class.: Antihypertensive
Chem. class.: Angiotensin-converting enzyme (ACE) inhibitor
Pregnancy category D

Do not confuse:
ramipril/enalapril, Altace/alteplase

ACTION: Selectively suppresses renin-angiotensin-aldosterone system; inhibits ACE; prevents conversion of angiotensin I to angiotensin II; results in dilatation of arterial, venous vessels

Therapeutic outcome: Decreased B/P in hypertension

USES: Hypertension, alone or in combination with thiazide diuretics; CHF (after MI), reduction in risk of MI, stroke, death from CV disorders

CONTRAINDICATIONS:
Breastfeeding, children, hypersensitivity to ACE inhibitors, history of ACE inhibitor–induced angioedema

BLACK BOX WARNING: Pregnancy **D** (2nd/3rd trimesters)

Precautions: Impaired renal/liver function, dialysis patients, hypovolemia, blood dyscrasias, COPD, CHF, asthma, geriatric, renal artery stenosis, cough, African descent

DOSAGE AND ROUTES
Hypertension
Adult: PO 2.5 mg/day initially, then 2.5-20 mg/day divided bid or daily

CHF/Post MI
Adult: PO 1.25-2.5 mg bid, may increase to 5 mg bid

Reduction in risk of MI, stroke, death
Adult: PO 2.5 mg/day × 7 days, then 5 mg/day × 21 days, then may increase to 10 mg/day

Renal impairment
Adult: PO CCr <40 ml/min; reduce by 50%, titrate upward to max 5 mg/day

Available forms: Caps 1.25, 2.5, 5, 10 mg

Implementation
• Caps may be opened and added to food, mixture is stable for 24 hr at room temperature, 48 hr refrigerated
• Store in airtight container at 86° F (30° C) or less

ADVERSE EFFECTS
CNS: *Headache, dizziness,* anxiety, insomnia, paresthesia, fatigue, depression, malaise, vertigo
CV: *Hypotension,* chest pain, palpitations, angina, syncope, **dysrhythmia, heart failure, MI**
EENT: Hearing loss
GI: Nausea, constipation, vomiting, dyspepsia, dysphagia, anorexia, diarrhea, abdominal pain, **hepatitis, hepatic failure, pancreatitis, hepatic necrosis**
GU: Proteinuria, increased BUN, creatinine, impotence
HEMA: Decreased Hct, Hgb, **eosinophilia, leukopenia, pancytopenia, thrombocytopenia, agranulocytosis (rare)**
INTEG: Rash, sweating, photosensitivity, pruritus
META: *Hyperkalemia,* hyperglycemia
MISC: **Angioedema, toxic epidermal necrolysis, anaphylaxis, Stevens-Johnson syndrome**
MS: Arthralgia, arthritis, myalgia
RESP: Cough, dyspnea

Pharmacokinetics
Absorption	Well absorbed
Distribution	Not known, crosses placenta
Metabolism	Liver, extensively; protein binding 73%
Excretion	Urine
Half-life	Ramipril (5 hr), ramiprilat (24 hr)

Pharmacodynamics
Onset	½-1 hr
Peak	6-8 hr
Duration	24-72 hr

INTERACTIONS
Individual drugs
Alcohol: increased hypotension (large amounts)
Lithium: increased serum levels
HydrALAZINE, prazocin: increased toxicity
Indomethacin: decreased antihypertensive effect

Drug classifications

Adrenergic blockers, antihypertensives, diuretics, ganglionic blockers, nitrates: increased hypotension

Antacids: decreased absorption

Diuretics (potassium sparing), potassium supplements, sympathomimetics, vasodilators: increased toxicity

NSAIDs, salicylates: decreased antihypertensive effect

Drug/food

Potassium salt substitutes: increased hyperkalemia, avoid use

Drug/herb

Hawthorn: increased antihypertensive effect
Ephedra: decreased antihypertensive effect

Drug/lab test

Increased: LFTs, BUN, creatinine, glucose, potassium

Decreased: RBC, Hgb, platelets

NURSING CONSIDERATIONS

Assessment

• Monitor blood tests: neutrophils, decreased platelets; WBC with differential baseline, periodically q3mo; if neutrophils are <1000/mm³, discontinue treatment

• **Hypertension:** Monitor B/P baseline and regularly, check for orthostatic hypotension, syncope; if changes occur, dosage may need to be changed

• **Renal disease:** Monitor renal function tests: protein, BUN, creatinine, potassium, sodium; watch for increased levels that may indicate nephrotic syndrome and renal failure; monitor renal symptoms: polyuria, oliguria, frequency, dysuria; establish baselines in renal, liver function tests before therapy begins and monitor periodically; liver function tests, uric acid, and glucose may be increased

• Check potassium levels throughout treatment, hyperkalemia occurs

• **CHF:** check for edema in feet, legs daily, weight daily

• **Allergic reactions:** angioedema, **Stevens-Johnson syndrome;** rash, fever, pruritus, urticaria; product should be discontinued if antihistamines fail to help

• Monitor electrolytes baseline and periodically, potassium may be increased

Patient/family education

• Caution patient not to discontinue product abruptly; advise patient to tell all persons associated with care

• Teach patient not to use OTC products (cough, cold, allergy) unless directed by physician; serious side effects can occur; xanthines such as coffee, tea, chocolate, cola can prevent action of product

• Instruct patient on the importance of complying with dosage schedule, even if feeling better; to continue with medical regimen to decrease B/P: exercise, cessation of smoking, decreasing stress, diet modifications

• Emphasize the need to rise slowly to sitting or standing position to minimize orthostatic hypotension; not to exercise in hot weather because increased hypotension can occur

• Teach patient to notify prescriber of mouth sores, sore throat, fever, swelling of hands or feet, irregular heartbeat, chest pain, coughing, shortness of breath

• Caution patient to report excessive perspiration, dehydration, vomiting, diarrhea; may lead to fall in B/P, maintain hydration

• Caution patient that product may cause dizziness, fainting, light-headedness; may occur during 1st few days of therapy; to avoid activities that may be hazardous

• Teach patient how to take B/P, and normal readings for age group

> **BLACK BOX WARNING:** Inform prescriber if pregnancy is planned or suspected, pregnancy **D,** do not breastfeed

Evaluation

Positive therapeutic outcome

• Decreased B/P in hypertension

TREATMENT OF OVERDOSE:

0.9% NaCl **IV** inf, hemodialysis

ranibizumab (Rx)

(ran-ih-biz′oo-mab)
Lucentis
Func. class.: Ophthalmic
Chem. class.: Selective vascular endothelial growth factor antagonist
Pregnancy category C

ACTION: Binds to receptor-binding site of active forms of vascular endothelial growth factor A (VEGF-A) that causes angiogenesis and cell proliferation

Therapeutic outcome: Prevention of increasing neovascular macular degeneration

USES: Macular degeneration (neovascular) (wet), macular edema after retinal vein occlusion (RVO)

CONTRAINDICATIONS:
Hypersensitivity, ocular infections

Precautions: Pregnancy **C**, breastfeeding, children, retinal detachment, increased intraocular pressure

DOSAGE AND ROUTES
Adult: Intravitreal 0.3 mg (0.05 ml) q28 days

Available forms: Sol for inj 0.5 mg/0.05 ml

Implementation
• Given by ophthalmologist via intravitreal injection using adequate anesthesia; use 19-gauge filter
• Store in refrigerator; do not freeze
• Protect from light

ADVERSE EFFECTS
CNS: Dizziness, headache
EENT: Blepharitis, cataract, conjunctival hemorrhage/hyperemia, detachment of the retinal pigment epithelium, dryness/irritation/pain in the eye, visual impairment, vitreous floaters, ocular infection
GI: Constipation, nausea
MISC: Hypertension, UTI, **thromboembolism, non-ocular bleeding**
RESP: Bronchitis, cough, sinusitis, URI

Pharmacokinetics

Absorption	Minimal
Distribution	None
Metabolism	None
Excretion	None
Half-life	Elimination 9 days

Pharmacodynamics

Unknown

INTERACTIONS
Individual drugs
Verteporfin photodynamic therapy (PDT): increased severe inflammation

NURSING CONSIDERATIONS
Assessment
• Assess for eye changes: redness, sensitivity to light, vision change, intraocular pressure change; report to ophthalmologist immediately

Patient/family education
• Teach patient that if eye becomes red, sensitive to light, or painful or if there is a change in vision, seek immediate care from ophthalmologist
• Teach patient reason for treatment, expected results

Evaluation
Positive therapeutic outcome
• Prevention of increasing neovascular macular degeneration

ranitidine (Rx)
(ra-nit′i-deen)
Equaline Heartburn Relief, Nu-Ranit ✿, Top Care Heartburn Relief, Wal-Zan, Zantac, Zantac-C ✿, Zantac EFFER-dose
ranitidine bismuth citrate
Tritec
Func. class.: H₂ histamine receptor antagonist
Pregnancy category B

Do not confuse:
ranitidine/amantadine/rimantadine,
Zantac/Xanax/Zofran/ZyrTEC

ACTION: Inhibits histamine at H₂ receptor site in the gastric parietal cells, which inhibits gastric acid secretion

Therapeutic outcome: Healing of duodenal ulcers or gastric ulcers; prevention of duodenal ulcers; decreased symptoms of gastroesophageal reflux disease (GERD), Zollinger-Ellison syndrome, or heartburn

USES: Short-term treatment of duodenal and gastric ulcers and maintenance; management of GERD, Zollinger-Ellison syndrome, active duodenal ulcers with *Helicobacter pylori* in combination with clarithromycin, hypersecretory conditions, stress ulcers, erosive esophagitis (maintenance), systemic mastocytosis, multiple endocrine adenoma syndrome, heartburn

Unlabeled uses: Prevention of aspiration pneumonitis, upper GI bleeding

CONTRAINDICATIONS:
Hypersensitivity

Precautions: Pregnancy **B**, breastfeeding, child <12 yr, renal/hepatic disease

---

DOSAGE AND ROUTES
Ranitidine

Erosive esophagitis
Adult: PO 150 mg qid for up to 12 wk
Child ≥1 mo: PO 5-10 mg/kg/day in 2-3 divided doses

Duodenal ulcer
Adult: PO 150 mg bid or 300 mg/day after PM meal or at bedtime, maintenance 150 mg at bedtime
Infant and child: PO 2-4 mg/kg bid, max 300 mg/day

Zollinger-Ellison syndrome
Adult: PO 150 mg bid, may increase if needed

Gastric ulcer
Adult: PO 150 mg bid × 6 wk, then 150 mg at bedtime
Infant/child: PO 2-4 mg/kg bid, max 300 mg/day

GERD
Adult: PO 150 mg bid

Renal dose
Adult: CCr <50 ml/min give 50% of dose or extend dosing interval

Ranitidine bismuth citrate
Adult: PO 400 mg bid × 4 wk with clarithromycin 500 mg tid × first 2 wk

Available forms: Ranitidine: tabs 75, 150, 300 mg; caps 150, 300 mg; syr 15 mg/ml; sol for inj 25 mg/ml; effervescent tabs 25 mg; ranitidine bismuth citrate: tabs 400 mg

Implementation
• Store at room temp
PO route
• May be given with or without meals; **EFFER-dose tab:** dissolves 25 mg/5 ml or more, give after dissolved; do not chew, swallow whole, or dissolve on tongue
• Give antacids 1 hr before or 1 hr after this product
IM route
• No dilution needed; inject in large muscle mass, aspirate

IV direct route
• Dilute to max 2.5 mg/ml (50 mg/20 ml) using 0.9% NaCl (nonpreserved) or D₅W, give dose over ≥5 min (max 4 mg/ml)
Intermittent IV INF route
• Dilute to max 0.5 mg/ml with D₅W, 0.9% NaCl, give over 15-20 min (5-7 ml/min); premixed ready-to-use bags as 1 mg/ml (50 mg/50 ml), inf over 15-20 min

Continuous 24 hr IV INF route
• **Adult:** dilute 150 mg/250 ml of D₅W or 0.9% NaCl, run over 24 hr (6.25 mg/hr or as directed); use inf device and use within 48 hr; *Zollinger-Ellison:* dilute in D₅W or 0.9% NaCl, max concentration 2.5 mg/ml, use inf device

Y-site compatibilities: Acyclovir, aldesleukin, alemtuzumab, alfentanil, allopurinol, amifostine, amikacin, aminophylline, amphotericin B liposome, amsacrine, anikinra, anidulafungin, ascorbic acid, atracurium, atropine, aztreonam, bivalirudin, bumetanide, buprenorphine, butorphanol, calcium chloride/gluconate, CARBOplatin, ceFAZolin, cefepime, cefonicid, cefoperazone, cefotaxime, cefoTEtan, cefOXitin, cefTAZidime, ceftizoxime, cefTRIAXone, cefuroxime, chloramphenicol, chlorproMAZINE, cimetidine, ciprofloxacin, cisatracurium, CISplatin, clindamycin, cyanocobalamin, cyclophosphamide, cycloSPORINE, cytarabine, DACTINomycin, DAPTOmycin, dexamethasone, dexmedetomidine, digoxin, diltiazem, DOBUTamine, DOCEtaxel, DOPamine, doripenem, doxacurium, doxapram, DOXOrubicin, DOXOrubicin liposome, doxycycline, enalaprilat, ePHEDrine, EPINEPHrine, epirubicin, epoetin alfa, ertapenem, erythromycin, esmolol, etoposide, etoposide phosphate, famotidine, fenoldopam, fentaNYL, filgrastim, fluconazole, fludarabine, fluorouracil, folic acid, foscarnet, furosemide, ganciclovir, gemcitabine, gentamicin, glycopyrrolate, granisetron, heparin, hydrocortisone, HYDROmorphone, IDArubicin, ifosfamide, imipenem/cilastatin, inamrinone, indomethacin, isoproterenol, ketorolac, labetalol, levofloxacin, lidocaine, linezolid, LORazepam, magnesium sulfate, mannitol, mechlorethamine, melphalan, meperidine, metaraminol, methotrexate, methoxamine, methyldopate, methylPREDNISolone, metoclopramide, metoprolol, metroNIDAZOLE, midazolam, milrinone, mitoXANtrone, morphine, nalbuphine, naloxone, nesiritide, niCARdipine, nitroglycerin, nitroprusside, norepinephrine, octreotide, ondansetron, oxacillin, oxaliplatin, oxytocin, PACLitaxel, palonosetron, pancuronium, papaverine, PEMEtrexed, penicillin G, pentamidine, pentazocine, PENTobarbital, PHENobarbital, phentolamine, phenylephrine, phytonadione, piperacillin/tazobactam, potassium chloride, procainamide, prochlorperazine, promethazine, propofol, propranolol, protamine, pyridoxime, remifentanil, riTUXimab, rocuronium, sargramostim, sodium acetate/bicarbonate, succinylcholine, SUFentanil, tacrolimus, teniposide, theophylline, thiamine, thiopental, thiotepa, ticarcillin/clavulanate,

Adverse effects: *italics* = common; **bold** = life-threatening

R

tigecycline, tirofiban, tobramycin, tolazoline, trastuzumab, trimetaphan, urokinase, vancomycin, vecuronium, vinCRIStine, vinorelbine, warfarin, zidovudine, zoledronic acid

Y-site incompatibilities: Amphotericin B cholesteryl, caspofungin, diazepam, diazoxide, insulin, pantoprazole, phenytoin, quinupristin/dalfopristin, trimethoprim/sulfamethoxazole

ADVERSE EFFECTS
CNS: Headache, sleeplessness, dizziness, confusion, agitation, depression; hallucinations (geriatric)
CV: Tachycardia, bradycardia, premature ventricular contractions
EENT: Blurred vision, increased ocular pressure
GI: Constipation, abdominal pain, diarrhea, nausea, vomiting, **hepatotoxicity**
GU: Impotence, **acute interstitial nephritis (rare)**
INTEG: Urticaria, rash, fever
RESP: Pneumonia
SYST: Anaphylaxis (rare)

Pharmacokinetics

Absorption	Well absorbed (PO, IM), completely absorbed (**IV**)
Distribution	Widely distributed, crosses placenta
Metabolism	Liver (30%)
Excretion	Kidneys unchanged (70%)
Half-life	2-3 hr, increased renal disease

Pharmacodynamics

	PO	IM/IV
Onset	Unknown	Unknown
Peak	2-3 hr	15 min
Duration	8-12 hr	8-12 hr

INTERACTIONS
Individual drugs
Adefovir, pramipexole, procainamide, trospium, triazolam, memantine, saquinavir: increased effect of each product
Diazepam, metoclopramide: decreased absorption of ranitidine
Ketoconazole: decreased effect of ketoconazole
NIFEdipine, ext rel products: increased GI obstruction risk
Procainamide: increased absorption, toxicity

Drug classifications
Anticholinergics, antacids: decreased ranitidine absorption
Anticoagulants, sulfonylureas: increased absorption, toxicity
Benzodiazepines, calcium channel blockers: increased effect of each product
Cephalosporins: decreased effects of cephalosporins
Iron salts: decreased effects of iron salts

Drug/lab test
Increased: AST, creatinine, ALT
False positive: urine protein (multistix)

NURSING CONSIDERATIONS
Assessment
• **GI complaints:** assess patient with ulcers or suspected ulcers: epigastric or abdominal pain, hematemesis, occult blood in stools, blood in gastric aspirate before, throughout treatment
• Monitor I&O ratio, BUN, creatinine, CBC with differential monthly

Patient/family education
• Caution patient that gynecomastia, impotence may occur and are reversible after treatment is discontinued
• Advise patient to avoid driving, other hazardous activities until stabilized on this medication; drowsiness or dizziness may occur
• Inform patient that smoking decreases the effectiveness of the product; that smoking cessation should be considered
• Instruct patient that product must be continued for prescribed time to be effective and taken exactly as prescribed; doses should not be doubled; a missed dose should be taken when remembered up to 1 hr before next dose
• Advise patient to report bruising, fatigue, malaise; blood dyscrasias may occur
• Inform patient to report diarrhea, black tarry stools, sore throat, rash, dizziness, confusion, or delirium to prescriber immediately
• Teach patient to take once-daily dose before bedtime

Evaluation
Positive therapeutic outcome
• Decreased pain in abdomen, heartburn
• Healing of ulcers
• Absence of gastroesophageal reflux

ranolazine (Rx)

(ruh-no'luh-zeen)

Ranexa

Func. class.: Antianginal

Pregnancy category C

ACTION: Antianginal, antiischemic; unknown, may work by inhibiting portal fatty-acid oxidation

Therapeutic outcome: Decreased anginal pain and number of episodes

USES: Chronic stable angina pectoris; use in those that have not responded to other treatment options; should be used in combination with other antianginals such as amlodipine, β-blockers, or nitrates

CONTRAINDICATIONS:

Preexisting QT prolongation, hepatic disease (Child-Pugh class A, B, C), hypersensitivity, hypokalemia, renal failure, torsades de pointes, ventricular dysrhythmia, ventricular tachycardia, hepatic cirrhosis

Precautions: Pregnancy C, breastfeeding, children, geriatric, renal disease, hypotension, females at risk for torsades de pointes

DOSAGE AND ROUTES

Adult: PO 500 mg bid and increased to 1000 mg bid based on response; max 1000 mg bid

Available forms: Ext rel tabs 500, 1000 mg

Implementation

• **Ext rel tabs:** Do not break, crush, or chew tabs; give products as prescribed; do not double or skip dose

• Give bid, without regard to meals

• Do not use with grapefruit juice

ADVERSE EFFECTS

CNS: *Headache, dizziness,* hallucinations

CV: Palpitations, **QT prolongation,** orthostatic hypotension

EENT: Tinnitus

GI: Nausea, vomiting, constipation, dry mouth

MISC: Peripheral edema

RESP: Dyspnea

Absorption	Varied absorption
Distribution	Protein binding 62%
Metabolism	Liver, extensively by CYP3A, CYP2D6 (lesser)
Excretion	Urine 75%, feces 25%
Half-life	7 hr

Onset	Unknown
Peak	2-5 hr
Duration	Unknown

INTERACTIONS

Individual drugs

Haloperidol, chloroquine, droperidol, pentamidine, arsenic trioxide, levomethadyl; CYP3A4 substrates (methadone, pimozide, QUEtiapine, quiNIDine, risperidone, ziprasidone): increased QT prolongation

Digoxin, simvastatin: increased action of digoxin, simvastatin

Diltiazem, dofetilide, ketoconazole, PARoxetine, quiNIDine, sotalol, thioridazine, verapamil, ziprasidone: increased ranolazine action

Drug classifications

Anti-retroviral protease inhibitors: increased ranolazine absorption, toxicity

Class IA/III antidysrhythmics, some phenothiazines, β-agonists, local anesthetics, tricyclics; CYP3A4 inhibitors (amiodarone, clarithromycin, erythromycin, telithromycin, troleandomycin); CYP3A4 substrates (methadone, pimozide, QUEtiapine, quiNIDine, risperidone, ziprasidone): increased QT prolongation

Macrolide antibiotics, protease inhibitors: increased ranolazine action

Macrolides (clarithromycin, erythromycin, troleandomycin): increased QTc interval

Drug/food

Do not use with grapefruit or grapefruit juice

NURSING CONSIDERATIONS

Assessment

• Assess cardiac status: B/P, pulse, respiration, ECG; watch for prolongation of QT

• **QT prolongation:** ECG for QT prolongation, ejection fraction; assess for chest pain, palpitations, dyspnea

• **Angina:** characteristics of pain (intensity, location, duration, alleviating/precipitating factors)

R

Patient/family education
• Teach patient to avoid hazardous activities until stabilized on product, dizziness is no longer a problem
• Advise patient to avoid OTC drugs, grapefruit juice, drugs prolonging QTc (quiNIDine, dofetilide, sotalol, erythromycin, thioridazine, ziprasidone or protease inhibitors, diltiazem, ketoconazole, macrolide antibiotics, verapamil) unless directed by prescriber
• Advise patient to comply in all areas of medical regimen
• Teach patient to notify all health care providers of this product use
• Teach patient not to chew or crush, and to avoid grapefruit juice
• Advise patient to notify prescriber of palpitations, dizziness, fainting, edema, dyspnea
• For acute angina take other products prescribed; this product doesn't decrease acute attack

Evaluation
Positive therapeutic outcome
• Decreased anginal pain and number of episodes

rasagiline (Rx)
(ra-sa′ji-leen)
Azilect
Func. class.: Antiparkinson agent
Chem. class.: MAOI, type B
Pregnancy category C

ACTION: Inhibits MAO type B at recommended doses; may increase DOPamine levels

Therapeutic outcome: Improved symptoms in those with Parkinson's disease

USES: Idiopathic Parkinson's disease monotherapy or with levodopa

CONTRAINDICATIONS:
Breastfeeding, hypersensitivity to this product or MAOIs, pheochromocytoma

Precautions: Pregnancy **C**, children, psychiatric disorders, severe hepatic disorders

DOSAGE AND ROUTES
Monotherapy
Adult: PO 1 mg/day

Adjunctive therapy
Adult: PO 0.5 mg/day, may be increased to 1 mg/day; change of levodopa dose in adjunct therapy; reduced levodopa dose may be needed

Hepatic dose
Adult: PO 0.5 mg in mild hepatic disease

Concomitant ciprofloxacin, other CYP1A2 inhibitors
Adult: PO 0.5 mg; plasma concentrations of rasagiline may double

Available forms: Tabs 0.5, 1 mg

Implementation
• Give with meals to prevent nausea; continuing therapy usually reduces or eliminates nausea; do not give with foods/liquids containing large amounts of tyramine
• Give reduced dose of carbidopa/levodopa cautiously
⚠ Renal failure: in dialysis, increase dose slowly

ADVERSE EFFECTS
CNS: Drowsiness, hallucinations, depression, headache, malaise, paresthesia, vertigo, syncope
CV: Angina, **hypertensive crisis** (ingestion of tyramine products), orthostatic hypotension
GI: *Nausea,* diarrhea, dry mouth, dyspepsia
GU: Impotence, decreased libido
HEMA: Leukopenia
INTEG: Alopecia, **skin cancers**
MISC: Conjunctivitis, fever, flu syndrome, neck pain, allergic reaction, alopecia
MS: Arthralgia, arthritis, dyskinesia, falls
RESP: Rhinitis

Pharmacokinetics

Absorption	Well absorbed
Distribution	Protein binding >88%-94%
Metabolism	Liver, CYP1A2
Excretion	Kidneys
Half-life	Unknown

Pharmacodynamics

Unknown

INTERACTIONS
Individual drugs
Ciprofloxacin: increased levels of rasagiline up to twofold
⚠ Meperidine: do not give; serious reaction including coma and death may occur

---

Drug classifications
⚠ **Analgesics, sympathomimetics: do not give; serious reaction including coma and death may occur**
⚠ **Antidepressants (tricyclics, SSRIs, SNRIs, mirtazapine, cyclobenzaprine): increased severe CNS toxicity**
CYP1A2 inhibitors (atazanavir, mexiletine, taurine): increased levels of rasagiline up to twofold
⚠ **MAOIs: increased hypertensive crisis**

Drug/herb
⚠ **St. John's wort, yohimbe: do not give**

Drug/food
Do not use with food/liquids that contain large amounts of tyramine

Drug/lab test
Increased: LFTs
Decreased: WBCs

NURSING CONSIDERATIONS
Assessment
• **Assess for Parkinson's symptoms:** tremor, ataxia, muscle weakness and rigidity; baseline, periodically; assess for increased dyskinesia and postural hypotension if used in combination with levodopa
• Assess mental status: hallucinations, confusion, notify prescriber
• **Assess for hypertensive crisis:** severe headache, blurred vision, seizures, chest pain, difficulty thinking, nausea/vomiting, signs of stroke; any unexplained severe headache should be considered to be hypertensive crisis
• **Assess for melanomas** frequently, perform periodic skin exams by a dermatologist
• Monitor cardiac status: B/P, ECG; periodically during beginning treatment
• **Tyramine products:** assess for foods, other medications, may lead to hypertensive crisis (tachycardia, bradycardia, chest pain, nausea, vomiting, sweating, dilated pupils)

Patient/family education
• Advise patient to change position slowly to prevent orthostatic hypotension
• Instruct patient to avoid hazardous activities until stabilized; dizziness can occur
• Advise patient to rinse mouth frequently, use sugarless gum to alleviate dry mouth
• Teach patient to take as prescribed, not to miss dose or double doses; take missed dose as soon as remembered if several hours before next dose
• Teach patient to prevent hypertensive crisis by avoiding tyramine foods >150 mg

• Teach patient to report signs of hypertensive crisis
• Teach patient to avoid CNS depressants, alcohol

Evaluation
Positive therapeutic outcome
• Improved symptoms in those with Parkinson's disease (decreasing tremors, ataxia, muscle weakness/rigidity)

---

rasburicase (Rx)
(rass-burr′i-case)
Elitek, Fasturtec ✦
Func. class.: Enzyme
Chem. class.: Recombinant urate-oxidase enzyme
Pregnancy category C

ACTION: Catalyzes enzymatic oxidation of uric acid into an inactive and a soluble metabolite (allantoin)

Therapeutic outcome: Decreased uric acid levels

USES: To reduce uric acid levels in children with leukemia, lymphoma, solid tumor malignancies who are receiving chemotherapy

CONTRAINDICATIONS:
Hypersensitivity

> **BLACK BOX WARNING:** G6PD deficiency (Mediterranean, African descent), hemolytic reactions, or methemoglobinemia reactions to this product

Precautions: Pregnancy **C**, breastfeeding, children <2 yr, anemia

> **BLACK BOX WARNING:** Acute bronchospasm, angina, angioedema, patients of African or Mediterranean ancestry, hypotension, urticaria

DOSAGE AND ROUTES
Adult/adolescent/child/infant: IV INF 0.2 mg/kg as a single daily dose given as **IV** INF over ½ hr × 5 days

Available forms: Powder for inj 1.5, 7.5 mg/vial

Implementation
Intermittent IV INF route
• Reconstitute with diluent provided, add 1 ml of diluent/vial, swirl, withdraw amount needed

---

Adverse effects: *italics* = common; **bold** = life-threatening

and mix with 0.9% NaCl to final volume of 50 ml, use within 24 hr, give over 30 min, do not use filter, use different line, if not possible flush with ≥15 ml of NaCl before and after use
• Chemotherapy is started 4-24 hr after 1st dose

ADVERSE EFFECTS
CNS: *Headache*, fever
CV: Chest pain, hypotension
GI: *Nausea, vomiting, anorexia, diarrhea, abdominal pain, constipation, dyspepsia, mucositis*
HEMA: Neutropenia with fever, hemolysis, methemoglobinemia
INTEG: *Rash*
MISC: Edema
RESP: Bronchospasm, wheezing, dyspnea
SYST: Anaphylaxis, hemolysis, methemoglobinemia, sepsis

Pharmacokinetics

Absorption	Unknown
Distribution	Unknown
Metabolism	Unknown
Excretion	Unknown
Half-life	Elimination 16-21 hr

Pharmacodynamics

Unknown

INTERACTIONS
Individual drugs
Allopurinol: increased toxicity

NURSING CONSIDERATIONS
Assessment
• Monitor blood studies: BUN, serum uric acid, urine CCr, electrolytes, CBC with differential before, during therapy
• Monitor temp q4hr; fever may indicate beginning infection; no rectal temp
• **Assess for anaphylaxis** (dyspnea, urticaria, flushing, wheezing, swelling of lips, tongue, throat); have emergency equipment nearby
• **Assess for G6PD deficiency, hemolytic reactions, methemoglobinemia;** these patients should not be given this agent, screen patients who are higher risk for these disorders
• Assess GI symptoms: frequency of stools, cramping; if severe diarrhea occurs, fluid and electrolytes may need to be given

Patient/family education
• Advise of reason for therapy, expected results
• Advise to report trouble breathing, jaundice, chest pain

Evaluation
Positive therapeutic outcome
• Decreased uric acid levels in children when antineoplastics causing high uric acid levels are used

regorafenib
(re′goe-raf′e-nib)
Stivarga
Func. class.: Antineoplastic biologic response modifier; multikinase inhibitor
Chem. class.: Signal transduction inhibitor (STI)
Pregnancy category D

ACTION: Inhibits tyrosine kinase in patients with colorectal cancer

Therapeutic outcome: Decrease in spread or size of tumor

USES: Metastatic colorectal cancer in those who have received fluoropyrimidine, oxaliplatin, irinotecan-based chemotherapy, an anti-VEGF therapy; and an anti-EGFR therapy if *KRAS* wild type

CONTRAINDICATIONS:
Pregnancy (D)

Precautions: Breastfeeding, children, geriatric patients, cardiac/renal/hepatic/dental disease, fistula, GI bleeding or perforation, bone marrow suppression, infection, wound dehiscence, thrombocytopenia, neutropenia, immunosuppression

> **BLACK BOX WARNING:** Hepatic disease

DOSAGE AND ROUTES
Adult: PO 160 mg/day with a low-fat breakfast × 21 days of a 28-day cycle, cycles may be repeated

Available forms: Tabs 40 mg

Implementation
• Store at 77°F (25°C)
• Give at the same time each day with a low-fat breakfast that contains less than 30% fat such as 2 slices of white toast with 1 TBSP of low-fat margarine and 1 TBSP of jelly, and 8 oz of skim milk; or 1 cup of cereal, 8 oz of skim milk, 1 slice of toast with jam, apple juice, and 1 cup of coffee or tea
• Swallow tablets whole
• If a dose is missed, take as soon as possible that day; do not take 2 doses on the same day

---

Hand–foot skin reaction:
Reduce to 120 mg (grade 2 palmar–plantar erythrodysesthesia); hold if grade 2 toxicity does not improve in 7 days or recurs; hold for 7 days in grade 3 toxicity; reduce to 80 mg for recurrent grade 2 toxicity; discontinue if 80 mg is not tolerated

Hypertension:
Hold in grade 2 hypertension

Other severe toxicity (except hepatotoxicity)
Hold until toxicity resolves in grade 3 or 4 toxicity; consider the risk/benefits of continuing therapy in grade 4 toxicity, reduce dosage to 120 mg; if grade 3 or 4 toxicity recurs, hold until toxicity resolves, then reduce to 80 mg; discontinue in those who do not tolerate 80-mg dose

Hepatic dose

Baseline mild (Child-Pugh class A) or moderate (Child-Pugh class B): No change; baseline severe hepatic impairment (Child-Pugh class C): use not recommended

AST/ALT elevations during therapy:
For grade 3 AST/AST level elevations, hold dose; if therapy is continued, reduce to 120 mg after levels recover; discontinue in those with AST/ALT $> 20 \times$ ULN; AST/ALT $> 3 \times$ ULN and bilirubin $> 2 \times$ ULN; recurrence of AST/ALT $> 5 \times$ ULN despite a reduction to 120 mg

ADVERSE EFFECTS

CNS: Headache, tremor
CV: Hypertensive crisis, MI
EENT: Blurred vision, conjunctivitis
GI: Hepatotoxicity, GI hemorrhage, diarrhea, GI perforation, xerostomia
HEMA: Neutropenia, thrombocytopenia, bleeding
INTEG: Rash, alopecia
META: Hypokalemia
MISC: Fatigue, decreased weight, hand–foot syndrome, hypothyroidism

Pharmacokinetics

Absorption	Unknown
Distribution	Protein binding 99%
Metabolism	by CYP3A4, UGT1A0
Half-life	14–58 hr

Pharmacodynamics

Onset	Unknown
Peak	Unknown
Duration	Unknown

INTERACTIONS

Individual drugs

Simvastatin: Increased plasma concentrations of simvastatin
Warfarin: Increased plasma concentration of warfarin; avoid use; use low-molecular-weight anticoagulants instead

Drug classifications

CYP3A4 inhibitors (ketoconazole, itraconazole, erythromycin, clarithromycin): Increase: regorafenib concentrations
Calcium-channel blockers, ergots: Increased plasma concentrations of each product
CYP3A4 inducers (dexamethasone, phenytoin, carBAMazepine, rifampin, PHENobarbital): Decrease: regorafenib concentrations

Drug/food

Grapefruit juice; avoid use while taking product: Increased regorafenib effect

Drug/herb

St. John's wort: Decreased imatinib concentration

NURSING CONSIDERATIONS

Assessment

> **BLACK BOX WARNING:** Hepatic disease: fatal hepatotoxicity can occur; obtain LFTs baseline and at least every 2 wk × 2 mo, then monthly

⚠ **Fatal bleeding:** From GI, respiratory, GU tracts; permanently discontinue in those with severe bleeding
⚠ **Palmar–plantar erythrodysesthesia (hand–foot syndrome):** More common in those previously treated; reddening swelling, numbness, desquamation on palms, soles
⚠ **GI perforation/fistula:** Discontinue if this occurs, assess for pain in epigastric area, dyspepsia, flatulence, fever, chills
⚠ **Hypertension/hypertensive crisis:** Hypertension usually occurs in the first cycle in those with preexisting hypertension, do not start treatment until B/P is controlled; monitor B/P every wk × 6 wk, then at start of each cycle or more often if needed, temporarily or permanently discontinue for severe uncontrolled hypertension

Patient/family education

• Teach patient to report adverse reactions immediately: bleeding, rash
• Teach patient the reason for treatment, expected results

R

• Advise patient that effect on male fertility is unknown

Evaluation
Positive therapeutic outcome
• Decrease in spread or size of tumor

> **⚠ HIGH ALERT**

remifentanil (Rx)
(re-me-fin′ta-nill)
Ultiva
Func. class.: Opiate agonist analgesic
Chem. class.: μ-Opioid agonist
Pregnancy category C
Controlled substance schedule II

ACTION: Inhibits ascending pain pathways in limbic system, thalamus, midbrain, hypothalamus

Therapeutic outcome: Maintenance of anesthesia

USES: In combination with other products in general anesthesia to provide analgesia

CONTRAINDICATIONS:
Hypersensitivity

Precautions: Pregnancy **C**, breastfeeding, geriatric, increased ICP, acute MI, severe heart disease, GI/renal/hepatic disease, asthma, respiratory conditions, seizure disorders, bradyarrhythmias, child <12 yr

DOSAGE AND ROUTES
Adult: Induction **IV** 0.5-1 mcg/kg/min with a hypnotic or volatile agent; maintenance with isoflurane (0.4-1.5 MAC) or propofol (100-200 mcg/kg/min); CONT INF 0.25-0.4 mcg/kg/min
Child 1-12 yr: CONT **IV** INF 0.25 mcg/kg/min with isoflurane
Full-term neonate and infant up to 2 mo: CONT **IV** INF 0.4 mcg/kg/min with nitrous oxide

Available forms: Powder for inj, lyophilized 1, 2, 5 mg

Implementation
• Add 1 ml diluent/remifentanil
• Shake well; further dilute to a final concentration of 20, 25, 50 or 250 mcg/mg
• Interruption of inf results in rapid reversal (no residual opioid effect within 5-10 min)
• Store in light-resistant area at room temperature

Direct IV route
• Use only during maintenance of general anesthesia; inject into tubing close to venous cannula, give in nonintubated patients over 30-60 sec
CONT IV INF route
• Use infusion device, max 16 hr, do not use same tubing as blood, do not admix

Y-site compatibilities: Acyclovir, alfentanil, amikacin, aminophylline, ampicillin, ampicillin/sulbactam, aztreonam, bretylium, bumetanide, buprenorphine, butorphanol, calcium gluconate, ceFAZolin, cefepime, cefotaxime, cefoTEtan, cefOXitin, cefTAZidime, ceftizoxime, cefTRIAXone, cefuroxime, cimetidine, ciprofloxacin, cisatracurium, clindamycin, dexamethasone, digoxin, diltiazem, diphenhydrAMINE, DOBUTamine, DOPamine, doxacurium, doxycycline, droperidol, enalaprilat, EPINEPHrine, esmolol, famotidine, fentaNYL, fluconazole, furosemide, ganciclovir, gatifloxicin, gentamicin, haloperidol, heparin, hydrocortisone sodium succinate, HYDROmorphone, hydrOXYzine, imipenem/cilastatin, inamrinone, isoproterenol, ketorolac, lidocaine, LORazepam, magnesium sulfate, mannitol, meperidine, methylprednisoLONE sodium succinate, metoclopramide, metroNIDAZOLE, mezlocillin, midazolam, morphine, nalbuphine, nitroglycerin, norepinephrine, ondansetron, phenylephrine, pipericillin, potassium chloride, procainamide, prochlorperazine, promethazine, ranitidine, trimethroprim, SUFentanil, theophylline, thiopental, ticarcillin/clavulate, tobramycin, vancomycin, zidovudine

Solution compatibilities: D₅, 0.45% NaCl, LR, D₅LR, 0.9% NaCl

ADVERSE EFFECTS
CNS: Drowsiness, *dizziness,* confusion, *headache,* sedation, euphoria, delirium, agitation, anxiety
CV: Palpitations, **bradycardia**, change in B/P; facial flushing, syncope, **asystole**
EENT: Tinnitus, blurred vision, miosis, diplopia
GI: *Nausea, vomiting,* anorexia, constipation, cramps, dry mouth
GU: Urinary retention, dysuria
INTEG: Rash, urticaria, bruising, flushing, diaphoresis, pruritus
MS: Rigidity
RESP: **Respiratory depression, apnea**

Pharmacokinetics

Absorption	Complete
Distribution	70% protein binding
Metabolism	Unknown
Excretion	Urine
Half-life	Terminal 3-10 min

Pharmacodynamics

Onset	1-3 min
Peak	Unknown
Duration	Unknown

INTERACTIONS

Individual drugs
Alcohol: increased respiratory depression, hypotension, profound sedation

Drug classifications
Antihistamines, CNS depressants, phenothiazines, MAOIs, sedative/hypnotics: increased respiratory depression, hypotension, profound sedation

Drug/herb
Kava: increased CNS depression

NURSING CONSIDERATIONS

Assessment
• Monitor I&O ratio, check for decreasing output; may indicate urinary retention, especially in geriatric
• Assess CNS changes: dizziness, drowsiness, hallucinations, euphoria, LOC pupil reaction
• Assess allergic reactions: rash, urticaria
• **Assess respiratory dysfunction:** respiratory depression, character, rate, rhythm; notify prescriber if respirations are <12/min; CV status, bradycardia, syncope
• Monitor GI status: nausea, vomiting, anorexia, constipation
• Use pain scoring to determine pain perception

Patient/family education
• Advise patient to call for assistance when ambulating or smoking; drowsiness, dizziness may occur
• Advise patient to make position changes slowly to prevent orthostatic hypotension

Evaluation

Positive therapeutic outcome
• Maintenance of anesthesia

repaglinide (Rx)
(re-pag′lih-nide)
Gluco Norm ✤, **Prandin**
Func. class.: Antidiabetic
Chem. class.: Meglitinides
Pregnancy category C

ACTION: Causes functioning β-cells in pancreas to release insulin, leading to drop in blood glucose levels; closes ATP-dependent potassium channels in the β-cell membrane; this leads to opening of calcium channels; increased calcium influx induces insulin secretion

Therapeutic outcome: Blood glucose controlled

USES: Type 2 diabetes mellitus

CONTRAINDICATIONS:
Hypersensitivity to meglitinides, diabetic ketoacidosis, type 1 diabetes

Precautions: Pregnancy **C**, breastfeeding, children, geriatric, cardiac disease, severe renal/hepatic disease, thyroid disease, severe hypoglycemic reactions

DOSAGE AND ROUTES
Adult: PO 1-2 mg with each meal, max 16 mg/day, adjust at weekly intervals; oral hypoglycemic-naïve patients or those with A1c <8% should start with 0.5 mg with each meal

Renal/hepatic dose
Adult: PO CCr 20-39 ml/min: 0.5 mg/day; titrate upward cautiously

Available forms: Tabs 0.5, 1, 2 mg

Implementation
• 15 min before meals: 2, 3, or 4 ×/day preprandially
• Skip dose if meal is skipped; add dose if meal is added
• Store in airtight container at room temperature

ADVERSE EFFECTS
CNS: *Headache, weakness,* paresthesia
CV: Angina
EENT: Sinusitis, tinnitus
ENDO: **Hypoglycemia**
GI: Nausea, vomiting, diarrhea, constipation, dyspepsia, **pancreatitis**
HEMA: **Hemolytic anemia, leukopenia**
INTEG: Rash, allergic reactions
MISC: Chest pain, UTI, allergy

R

Adverse effects: *italics* = common; **bold** = life-threatening

MS: Back pains, arthralgia
RESP: URI, sinusitis, rhinitis, bronchitis

Pharmacokinetics

Absorption	Complete
Distribution	98% protein binding, crosses placenta
Metabolism	Liver by CYP3A4
Excretion	Urine/feces
Half-life	1 hr

Pharmacodynamics

Onset	30 min
Peak	1 hr
Duration	<4 hr

INTERACTIONS
Individual drugs
CarBAMazepine, rifampin: increased repaglinide metabolism

Chloramphenicol, deferasirox, fenofibrate, gemfibrozil, probenecid, simvastatin: increased effect of repaglinide

Erythromycin, ketoconazole, miconazole: decreased repaglinide metabolism

Gemfibrozil, **isophane insulin (NPH)**: Do not use together

Isoniazid, phenobarbital, phenytoin, rifampin: decreased action of repaglinide

Levonorgestrel/ethinyl estradol: increase in both

Drug classifications
Antifungals, CYP3A4 inhibitors, macrolides: decreased repaglinide metabolism

Barbiturates, CYP3A4 inducers: increased repaglinide metabolism

β-Adrenergic blockers, coumarins, MAOIs, NSAIDs, salicylates, sulfonamides: increased repaglinide effect

Calcium channel blockers, contraceptives (oral), corticosteroids, diuretics (thiazide), estrogens, phenothiazines, sympathomimetics, thyroid preparations: decreased repaglinide effect

CYP3A4, OATP1B1, CYP2C9 inhibitors: increased repaglinide effect

Drug/herb
Chromium, garlic, horse chestnut: increased antidiabetic effect

Drug/food
Decreased: repaglinide level; give before meals
Grapefruit juice: decreased repaglinide metabolism

Drug/lab test
Increased/decreased: glucose

NURSING CONSIDERATIONS
Assessment
• Assess for hypoglycemic or hyperglycemic reaction, which can occur soon after meals; dizziness, weakness, headache, tremor, anxiety, tachycardia, hunger, sweating, abdominal pain, monitor A1c, fasting, postprandial glucose during treatment

Patient/family education
• Teach patient technique of blood glucose monitoring using blood glucose meter
• Teach patient the symptoms of hypoglycemia and hyperglycemia, what to do about each
• Teach patient that product must be continued on daily basis; explain consequence of discontinuing product abruptly
• Advise patient to avoid OTC medications unless ordered by prescriber
• Advise patient that diabetes is a lifelong illness; product will not cure disease
• Advise patient to eat all food included in diet plan to prevent hypoglycemia; that if a meal is omitted, dose should be omitted; to have glucagon emergency kit available; to take repaglinide 15-30 min before meals 2, 3, or 4×/day
• Instruct patient to carry/wear emergency ID for emergency purposes

Evaluation
Positive therapeutic outcome
• Decrease in polyuria, polydipsia, polyphagia; clear sensorium; absence of dizziness; stable gait; blood glucose, A1c improvement

retapamulin topical
See Appendix B

retinoic acid
See tretinoin

Rh$_o$ (D) immune globulin, standard dose IM
BayRho-D, HyperRHO SD, Rho Gam Ultra Filtered Plus
Rh$_o$ (D) immune globulin microdose IM
MICRhoGAM Ultra Filtered Plus
Rh$_o$ (D) immune globulin IV
Rhophylac, WinRho SDF
Func. class.: Immune globulins
Pregnancy category C

ACTION: Suppresses immune nonsensitized Rh$_o$ (D or D^u)-negative patients who are exposed to Rh$_o$ (D or D^u)-positive blood

Therapeutic outcome: Absence of Rh factor and transfusion error

USES: Prevention of isoimmunization in Rh-negative women exposed to Rh-positive blood given after abortions, miscarriages, amniocentesis, chronic idiopathic thrombocytopenic purpura (Rhophylac)

CONTRAINDICATIONS:
Previous immunization with this product, Rh$_o$ (D)-positive/D^u-positive patient

> **BLACK BOX WARNING:** Hemolysis

Precautions: Pregnancy **C**

> **BLACK BOX WARNING:** Requires a specialized setting

DOSAGE AND ROUTES
To reduce risk of Rh isoimmunization antepartum/suppression of Rh isoimmunization postpartum following delivery of full-term infant
Adult and adolescent ≥16 yr: IM (BayRho-D [HyperRHO SD] [full dose only]) 300 mcg (1500 international units) at 28 wk gestation, repeat within 72 hr of delivery of confirmed Rho(D)-positive infant; a dose is not needed after delivery, if delivery is within 3 wk of last dose and no fetal maternal hemorrhage of >15 ml of RBC; IM (RhoGam only) 300 mcg (1500 international units) at 26-28 wk gestation, repeat within 72 hr even if status of Rho is unknown or if 72 hr have passed; IM/**IV** (WinRho SDF only) 300 mcg (1500 international units) at 28 wk gestation; if given earlier in pregnancy, give at 12-wk intervals during pregnancy, a 120-mcg (600 international units) dose; IM/**IV** should be given as soon as possible and preferably within 72 hr of delivery of a confirmed Rho(D)-positive infant, and even if status is unknown give up to 28 days after delivery

Known or suspected massive feto-maternal hemorrhage (>15 ml of fetal RBC or >30 ml of fetal whole blood)
Adult and adolescent ≥16 yr: IM (BayRho-D [HyperRHO SD] [full dose only]) 300 mcg (1500 international units) per every 15 ml of fetal blood cells or 30 ml of whole blood, multiple syringes may be injected IM at the same time in different sites, give within 72 hr of exposure, repeat dose within 72 hr of delivery; IM (RhoGAM only) 300 mcg (1500 international

units) for every 15 ml of fetal blood cells or 30 ml of whole blood, give total dose within 72 hr of exposure; IM/**IV** (WinRho SDF only) if large fetomaternal hemorrhage is suspected, give **IV** 9 mcg (45 international units) or IM 12 mcg (60 international units) for every ml of fetal whole blood, give **IV** 600 mcg (3000 international units) q8hr or IM 1200 mcg (6000 international units) q12hr until total dose is given, total dose should be given within 72 hr of exposure

Threatened abortion at any stage of pregnancy
Adult and adolescent ≥16 yr: IM (BayRho-D [HyperRHO SD] [full dose only]) 300 mcg (1500 international units) as soon as possible; if given 13-18 wk gestation, give another 300 mcg (1500 international units) at 26-28 wk gestation; repeat dose within 72 hr of delivery; IM (RhoGam only) 300 mcg (1500 international units) as soon as possible and within 72 hr; IM/**IV** (Rhophylac only) 300 mcg (1500 international units) as soon as possible and within 72 hr; IM/**IV** (WinRho SDF only) 300 mcg (1500 international units) as soon as possible and within 72 hr, repeat dose at 12-wk intervals during pregnancy and 120 mcg (600 international units) as soon as possible after delivery and within 72 hr

Following spontaneous abortion, induced termination of pregnancy, or ectopic pregnancy that occurs ≤12 wk gestation
Adult and adolescent ≥16 yr: IM (BayRho-D Minidose, HYperRHO Minidose, MICRORhoGAM only) 50 mcg (250 international units) as soon as possible, give within 3 hr of spontaneous or surgical removal, if possible within 72 hr

Following spontaneous abortion, induced termination of pregnancy, or ruptured tubal pregnancy that occurs ≥13 wk
Adult and adolescent ≥16 yr: IM(BayRho-D full dose [HyperRHO SD full dose] RhoGAM only) 300 mcg (1500 international units) as soon as possible and within 72 hr of event

Following spontaneous abortion, induced termination of pregnancy, aminocentesis, chorionic villus sampling, abdominal trauma, ruptured tubal pregnancy, or percutaneous umbilical cord sampling up to 34 wk gestation
Adult and adolescent ≥16 wk: IM/**IV** (WinRho SDF only) 300 mcg (1500 international units) within 72 hr, repeat at 12-wk intervals

R

during pregnancy, give 120 mcg (600 international units) as soon as possible and preferably within 72 hr of delivery

Available forms: BayRho-D sol for inj 300 mcg/ml (HyperRHO SD solution for injection); MICRhoGAM Ultra Filtered Plus Solution for inj 50 mcg/ml; RhoGam Ultra Filtered Plus Solution for inj 50 mcg; Rhophylac Pre-Filled Syringes Solution for inj 300 mcg/2 ml; WinRho SDF Liquid for inj; WinRho powder for inj

Implementation
- BayRho-D is being changed to HyperRHO SD
- BayRho-D (HyperRHO SD), MICRhoGAM, RhoGAM are given by IM only; do not give **IV**
- WinRho SDF and Rhophylac may be given IM or **IV**
- Inspect for particulate matter; do not use if particulate matter is present
- Reconstitution/dilution: no reconstitution or dilution is needed for BayRho-D (HyperRHO SD), Rhophylac, MICRoGAM, RhoGAM, or the liquid formulation of WinRho SDF
- WinRho SDF powder for **IV** use: if giving **IV**, reconstitute 600 international units or 1500 international units immediately before use with 2.5 ml of sterile diluent; reconstitute 5000 international units with 8.5 ml sterile diluent; add diluent to vial slowly down the wall of the vial; gently swirl until powder is dissolved; do not shake
- WinRho SDF powder for IM use: **IV** giving IM, reconstitute 600 international units or 1500 international units immediately before use with 1.25 ml of sterile diluent; 5000 international units with 8.5 ml of sterile diluent; add diluent to the vial slowly down the wall of the vial; gently swirl until powder is dissolved; do not shake

IM route
- Use aseptic technique, observe for 20 min after administration
- Bring Rhophylac to room temperature before using
- Inject into the deltoid muscle of upper arm or anterolateral portion of the upper thigh; do not inject into gluteal muscle
- If dose calculated will need multiple vials or syringes, use different sites at the same time

IV route
- Use aseptic technique
- WinRhoSDF: remove entire contents of vial to obtain calculated dose; if partial vial contents are required for dosage calculation, withdraw the entire vial contents to ensure correct calculation; inf correct calculated dose over 3-5 min; do not inf with other fluids or products

- Rhophylac: bring to room temperature; inf by slow **IV**; observe for 20 min

ADVERSE EFFECTS
CNS: Lethargy
CV: Hypo/hypertension
INTEG: Irritation at inj site, fever
MISC: Infection, **ARDS, anaphylaxis, pulmonary edema, DIC**
MS: Myalgia

Pharmacokinetics

Absorption	Well absorbed
Distribution	Unknown
Metabolism	Unknown
Excretion	Unknown
Half-life	Unknown

Pharmacodynamics

Onset	Rapid
Peak	Unknown
Duration	Unknown

INTERACTIONS
Drug classifications
Live virus vaccines (measles, mumps, rubella): decreased antibody response to vaccine

NURSING CONSIDERATIONS
Assessment
- Assess for allergies, reactions to immunizations; previous immunization with this product
- **Intravascular hemolysis:** assess for back pain, chills, hemoglobinuria, renal insufficiency; usually when WinRho SDF is given in those with immune thrombocytopenia purpura
- Obtain type and cross-match of mother's blood and of neonate's cord blood; neonate must be Rh₀(D)-positive, mother must be Rh₀(D)-negative and (Dᵘ)-negative, medication should be given if there is a doubt

Patient/family education
- Teach patient how product works; that product must be given after subsequent deliveries if subsequent babies are Rh-positive
- **Intravascular hemolysis:** Teach patient to report immediately: shaking, fever, chills, dark urine, swelling of hand or feet, back pain, SOB

Evaluation
Positive therapeutic outcome
- Prevention of Rh₀(D) sensitization in transfusion error
- Prevention of erythroblastosis fetalis in subsequent Rh₀(D)-positive neonates

---

ribavirin (Rx)
(rye-ba-vye′rin)
Virazole
Func. class.: Synthetic antiviral
Chem. class.: Tricyclic amine
Pregnancy category X

ACTION: Prevents replication of DNA and RNA synthesis

Therapeutic outcome: Resolution of severe lower respiratory tract infections

USES: Severe lower respiratory tract infections in infants and children

Unlabeled uses: Influenza A or B (early)

CONTRAINDICATIONS:
Pregnancy **X**, breastfeeding, children <1 yr, hypersensitivity

Precautions: Epilepsy, renal/hepatic disease

DOSAGE AND ROUTES
Infant and young child: INH 20 mg/ml × 12-18 hr/day × 3-7 days

Available forms: Powder for reconstitution for aerosol 6 g/vial

Implementation
• Give by the Viratek small particle aerosol generator (SPAG-2), do not use other inhalation equipment
• May be given by an oxygen hood for infants, or a face mask may be attached to the SPAG-2
• Reconstitute 6 g of sterile water for inj or inh, place sol in the Erlenmeyer flask and dilute further to 20 mg/ml

ADVERSE EFFECTS
CNS: Dizziness, faintness
CV: Hypotension, cardiac arrest
EENT: Eye irritation, conjunctivitis, blurred vision, photosensitivity
INTEG: Rash

Pharmacokinetics

Absorption	Inhalation (systemic)
Distribution	To respiratory tract
Metabolism	Liver
Excretion	Respiratory tract
Half-life	9½ hr

Pharmacodynamics

Onset	Unknown
Peak	Inhalation's end
Duration	Unknown

INTERACTIONS
Individual products
Zidovudine: decreased antiviral action, increased toxicity

Drug classification
Cardiac glycosides: increased toxicity

NURSING CONSIDERATIONS
Assessment
• Assess allergies before initiation of treatment, reaction of each medication; list allergies on chart in bright red letters
• Monitor respiratory status: rate, character, wheezing, tightness in chest
• Obtain C&S test results before starting treatment

Patient/family education
• Teach patient and parents aspects of product therapy

Evaluation
Positive therapeutic outcome
• Absence of respiratory syncytial virus

riboflavin (vitamin B₂) (OTC)
(rye′bo-flay-vin)
Func. class.: Vitamin B₂, water soluble
Pregnancy category A

ACTION: Needed for respiratory reactions (catalyzes proteins) and for normal vision

Therapeutic outcome: Prevention or treatment of riboflavin deficiency

USES: Vitamin B₂ deficiency or polyneuritis; cheilosis adjunct with thiamine

Precautions: Pregnancy A

DOSAGE AND ROUTES
Deficiency
Adult: PO 5-30 mg/day
Child ≥12 yr: PO 3-10 mg/day, then 0.6 mg/1000 cal ingested

RDA
Adult: PO (Males) 1.3 mg; (females) 1.1 mg

Adverse effects: *italics* = common; **bold** = life-threatening

Available forms: Tabs 5, 10, 25, 50, 100, 250 mg

Implementation
- Give with food for better absorption
- Store in airtight, light-resistant container

ADVERSE EFFECTS
GU: Yellow discoloration of urine (large doses)

Pharmacokinetics

Absorption	Well absorbed (by active transport)
Distribution	60% protein bound, widely distributed, crosses placenta
Metabolism	Unknown
Excretion	Kidneys (unchanged), excess amounts
Half-life	1-1½ hr

Pharmacodynamics

Unknown

INTERACTIONS
Individual drugs
Alcohol, probenecid: increased riboflavin need
Tetracycline: decreased action of tetracycline

Drug classifications
Antidepressants (tricyclics), phenothiazines: increased riboflavin need

Drug/lab test
False increase: urinary catecholamines

NURSING CONSIDERATIONS
Assessment
- Assess patient's nutritional status: liver, eggs, dairy products, yeast, whole grain, green vegetables
- Assess for vit B_2 deficiency: photophobia, cheilosis, stomatitis, ocular swelling

Patient/family education
- Inform patient that urine may turn bright yellow
- Instruct patient about needed addition of foods that are rich in riboflavin

Evaluation
Positive therapeutic outcome
- Absence of headache, GI problems, cheilosis, skin lesions, depression, burning itchy eyes, anemia

rifabutin (Rx)
(riff'a-byoo-tin)
Mycobutin
Func. class.: Antimycobacterial
Chem. class.: Rifamycin S derivative
Pregnancy category B

Do not confuse:
rifabutin/rifampin/rifapentine

ACTION: Inhibits DNA-dependent RNA polymerase in susceptible strains

Therapeutic outcome: Antimycobacterial death of *Escherichia coli, Bacillus subtilis;* mechanism of action against *Mycobacterium avium* unknown

USES: Prevention of *M. avium* complex (MAC) in patients with advanced HIV infection

Unlabeled uses: *Helicobacter pylori* that has not responded to other treatment

CONTRAINDICATIONS:
Hypersensitivity, active TB, WBC <1000/mm³, platelets <50,000/mm³

Precautions: Pregnancy **B**, breastfeeding, children, hepatic disease, blood dyscrasias

DOSAGE AND ROUTES
Adult: PO 300 mg/day (may take as 150 mg bid); max 600 mg/day

Renal dose
Adult: PO CCr <30 ml/min reduce dose by 50%

Available forms: Caps 150 mg

Implementation
- Give with meals to decrease GI symptoms; better to take on empty stomach 1 hr before or 2 hr after meals; high-fat food slows absorption, may take in 2 divided doses, may open capsule and mix with applesauce if unable to swallow whole
- Give antiemetic if vomiting occurs

ADVERSE EFFECTS
CNS: *Headache,* fatigue, anxiety, confusion, insomnia
GI: *Nausea, vomiting, anorexia, diarrhea,* heartburn, **hepatitis,** discolored saliva, **pseudomembranous colitis**
GU: Discolored urine
HEMA: Hemolytic anemia, eosinophilia, thrombocytopenia, leukopenia
INTEG: *Rash*

MISC: Flulike syndrome, shortness of breath, chest pressure
MS: Asthenia, arthralgia, myalgia

Pharmacokinetics

Absorption	Well absorbed
Distribution	Widely distributed
Metabolism	Liver
Excretion	Kidney
Half-life	45 hr

Pharmacodynamics

Onset	Unknown
Peak	2-3 hr
Duration	Unknown

INTERACTIONS
Individual drugs
Amprenavir, busPIRone, clofibrate, cycloSPO-RINE, dapsone, delavirdine, disopyramide, doxycycline, efavirenz, fluconazole, indinavir, ketoconazole, losartan, nelfinavir, nevirapine, phenytoin, quiNIDine, saquinavir, theophylline, zidovudine, zolpidem: decreased action of each specific product
Ritonavir: increased rifabutin level

Drug classifications
Anticoagulants, antidepressants (tricyclics), barbiturates, β-blockers, contraceptives (oral), corticosteroids, estrogens, sulfonylureas: decreased action of each specific product

Drug/food
High-fat foods: decreased absorption

Drug/lab test
Interference: folate level, vit B_{12}, BSP, gallbladder tests

NURSING CONSIDERATIONS
Assessment
• **Assess for active TB:** chest x-ray, sputum culture, blood culture, biopsy of lymph nodes, obtain PPD test; product should be given only for MAC and never for TB
• Monitor CBC for neutropenia, thrombocytopenia, eosinophilia
• **Pseudomembranous colitis:** assess for diarrhea, abdominal pain, fever, fatigue, anorexia; possible anemia, elevated WBC and low serum albumin; stop product and usually give either vancomycin or IV metroNIDAZOLE

Patient/family education
• Caution patient that compliance with dosage schedule and duration is necessary

• Instruct patient that scheduled appointments must be kept or relapse may occur
• Instruct patient to notify prescriber if hepatitis, neutropenia, or thrombocytopenia occurs: sore throat, fever, bleeding, bruising, yellow sclera, anorexia, nausea, vomiting, fatigue, weakness; myositis: muscle or bone pain
• Advise patient that urine, feces, saliva, sputum, sweat, tears may be colored red-orange; soft contact lenses may become permanently stained
• Caution patients using oral contraceptives to use a nonhormonal method of birth control because rifabutin may decrease efficiency of oral contraceptives; to notify prescriber if pregnancy is planned or suspected

Evaluation
Positive therapeutic outcome
• Decreased symptoms of *M. avium* in patients with HIV

rifampin (Rx)
(rif'am-pin)
Rifadin, Rofact ♣
Func. class.: Antitubercular
Chem. class.: Rifamycin B derivative
Pregnancy category C

Do not confuse:
rifampin/rifabutin

ACTION: Inhibits DNA-dependent polymerase, decreases tubercle bacilli replication

Therapeutic outcome: Bactericidal against the following organisms: mycobacteria, *Staphylococcus aureus*, *Haemophilus influenzae*, *Neisseria meningitidis*, *Legionella pneumophila*

USES: Pulmonary TB, meningococcal carriers (prevention)

CONTRAINDICATIONS:
Hypersensitivity to this product or rifamycins, active *Neisseria meningitidis* infection

Precautions: Pregnancy **C**, breastfeeding, children <5 yr, hepatic disease, blood dyscrasias

DOSAGE AND ROUTES
Tuberculosis
Adult: PO/IV max 600 mg/day as single dose 1 hr before or 2 hr after meals, or 10 mg/kg/day 2-3 ×/wk

Child >5 yr: PO/IV 10-20 mg/kg/day as single dose 1 hr before or 2 hr after meals, max 600 mg/day, with other antitubercular products
6-mo regimen: 2-mo treatment of isoniazid, rifampin, pyrazinamide, and possibly streptomycin or ethambutol; then rifampin and isoniazid × 4 mo
9-mo regimen: Rifampin and isoniazid supplemented with pyrazinamide or streptomycin or ethambutol

Meningococcal carriers
Adult: PO/IV 600 mg bid × 2 days, max 600 mg/dose
Child >5 yr: PO/IV 10-20 mg/kg bid × 2 days, max 600 mg/dose
Infant 3 mo-1 yr: PO 5 mg/kg bid for 2 days

Available forms: Caps 150, 300 mg; powder for inj 600 mg/vial

Implementation
• Do not give IM or SUBCUT
PO route
• On empty stomach, 1 hr before or 2 hr after meals with a full glass of water; give with other products for TB
• Antiemetic if vomiting occurs
• Capsules may be opened and mixed with applesauce or gelatin

Intermittent IV INF route
• After diluting each 600 mg/10 ml of sterile water for inj (60 mg/ml), swirl, withdraw dose, and dilute in 100 ml or 500 ml of D_5W given as an inf over 3 hr, or if diluted in 100 ml, give over ½ hr; do not admix with other sol or medications

Y-site compatibilities: Amiodarone, bumetanide, midazolam, pantoprazole, vancomycin

ADVERSE EFFECTS
CNS: Headache, fatigue, anxiety, drowsiness, confusion
EENT: Visual disturbances
GI: *Nausea, vomiting, anorexia, diarrhea,* **pseudomembranous colitis,** *heartburn,* sore mouth and tongue, **pancreatitis,** elevated liver function tests
GU: **Hematuria, acute renal failure, hemoglobinuria**
HEMA: **Hemolytic anemia, eosinophilia, thrombocytopenia, leukopenia**
INTEG: Rash, pruritus, urticaria
MISC: Flulike syndrome, menstrual disturbances, edema, SOB, **Stevens-Johnson syndrome, toxic epidermal necrolysis, angioedema, anaphylaxis**
MS: Ataxia, weakness

⚠ Nurse Alert   ✳ Key NCLEX® Drug

Pharmacokinetics
Absorption	Well absorbed (PO), completely absorbed (**IV**)
Distribution	Widely distributed, crosses placenta
Metabolism	Liver—extensively
Excretion	Feces
Half-life	3 hr

Pharmacodynamics
	PO	IV
Onset	Rapid	Rapid
Peak	2-3 hr	Inf end
Duration	Unknown	Unknown

INTERACTIONS
Individual drugs
Acetaminophen, alcohol, chloramphenicol, clofibrate, cycloSPORINE, dapsone, digoxin, diltiazem, doxycycline, haloperidol, NIFEdipine, phenytoin, theophylline, verapamil, zidovudine: decreased effect of specific product
Isoniazid: increased hepatotoxicity

Drug classifications
Anticoagulants, antidiabetics, barbiturates, benzodiazepines, β-blockers, contraceptives (oral), glucocorticoids, hormones, imidazole antifungals: decreased effect of each product
Protease inhibitors: do not use together

Drug/lab test
Increased: LFTs
Decreased: Hgb
Interference: folate level, vit B_{12}

NURSING CONSIDERATIONS
Assessment
• Monitor liver function tests qmo: ALT, AST, bilirubin, decreased appetite, jaundice, dark urine, fatigue
• Monitor renal status: before, qmo: BUN, creatinine, output, specific gravity, urinalysis
• **Pseudomembranous colitis:** assess for diarrhea, abdominal pain, fever, fatigue, anorexia; possible anemia, elevated WBC and low serum albumin; stop product and usually give either vancomycin or IV metroNIDAZOLE
• Monitor mental status often: affect, mood, behavioral changes; psychosis may occur
• **Infection:** assess sputum culture, lung sounds
• C&S should be performed before beginning treatment, during, and after therapy is completed

- **Serious skin reactions:** assess for fever, sore throat, fatigue, ulcers, lesions in mouth, lips, rash; can be fatal

Patient/family education
- Instruct patient that compliance with dosage schedule, duration is necessary
- Instruct patient that scheduled appointments must be kept or relapse may occur
- Instruct patient to notify prescriber if hepatitis, neutropenia, or thrombocytopenia occurs: sore throat, fever, bleeding, bruising, yellow sclera, anorexia, nausea, vomiting, fatigue, weakness, diarrhea with pus, mucus, blood
- Advise patient that urine, feces, saliva, sputum, sweat, tears may be colored red-orange; soft contact lenses may be permanently stained
- Caution patients using oral contraceptives to use a nonhormonal method of birth control because rifabutin may decrease the efficiency of oral contraceptives, to notify prescriber if pregnancy is planned or suspected
- Advise patient to avoid alcohol; hepatotoxicity may occur

Evaluation
Positive therapeutic outcome
- Decreased symptoms of TB

---

rifaximin (Rx)
(rif-ax′i-min)
Xifaxan
Func. class.: Misc. antiinfective
Chem. class.: Analog of rifampin
Pregnancy category C

Do not confuse:
rifaximin/rifampin

ACTION: Binds to bacterial DNA dependent RNA polymerase, thereby inhibiting bacterial RNA synthesis

Therapeutic outcome: Bacterial action against *E. coli*

USES: Traveler's diarrhea in those ≥12 yr old, caused by *E. coli,* hepatic encephalopathy, irritable bowel syndrome

CONTRAINDICATIONS:
Hypersensitivity to this product or rifamycins, diarrhea with fever, blood in stool

Precautions: Pregnancy C, breastfeeding, children, geriatric patients

DOSAGE AND ROUTES
Traveler's diarrhea
Adult and child ≥12 yr: PO 200 mg tid × 3 days without regard to meals

Hepatic encephalopathy
Adult: PO 550 mg bid

Available forms: Tabs 200, 550 mg

Implementation
- May be administered without regard to food

ADVERSE EFFECTS
CNS: Abnormal dreams, dizziness, insomnia, *headache,* fatigue, depression
CV: Hypotension, chest pain, peripheral edema, ascites
GI: *Abdominal pain, constipation, defecation urgency, flatulence, nausea, rectal tenesmus,* vomiting, ascites, **pseudomembranous colitis**
GU: Proteinuria, polyuria, increased urinary frequency
MISC: *Pyrexia,* motion sickness, tinnitus, rash, photosensitivity, **exfoliative dermatitis**
MS: Arthralgia, muscle pain, myalgia
RESP: Dyspnea, cough, pharyngitis

Pharmacokinetics
Absorption	Low, systemic
Distribution	Unknown
Metabolism	Induces CYP3A4
Excretion	Feces
Half-life	6 hr

Pharmacodynamics
Onset	Unknown
Peak	1-4 hr
Duration	Unknown

INTERACTIONS
Individual drugs
Afatinib: increased effect of afatinib

Drug/lab test
Increased: LFTs, potassium
Decreased: blood glucose, sodium

NURSING CONSIDERATIONS
Assessment
- Assess for GI symptoms: amount and character of diarrhea, abdominal pain, nausea, vomiting; do not use in those with blood in stool, increased temperature with diarrhea
- ⚠ Assess for overgrowth of infection and pseudomembranous colitis

---

Adverse effects: *italics* = common; **bold** = life-threatening

Patient/family education
• Instruct patient to discontinue rifaximin and notify prescriber if diarrhea persists for more than 24-48 hr, if diarrhea worsens, or if blood is in stools and fever is present
• Advise patient to avoid hazardous activities if dizziness occurs
• Teach patient to take without regard to food
• Teach patient to take as directed, to consume all of the product prescribed

Evaluation
Positive therapeutic outcome
• Absence of infection

---

rilpivirine
(ril-pi-vir′ine)
Edurant
Func. class.: Antiretroviral
Chem. class.: Non-nucleoside transcriptase inhibitors (NNTIs)

ACTION: Inhibits HIV-1 reverse transcriptase; unlike nucleoside reverse transcriptase inhibitors (NRTIs), it does not compete for binding nor does it require phosphorylation to be active. Binds directly to a site on reverse transcriptase; causing disruption of the enzyme's active site thereby blocking RNA-dependent and DNA-dependent DNA polymerase activities

USES: HIV in combination with other antiretrovirals

CONTRAINDICATIONS:
Hypersensitivity

Precautions: Pregnancy category **B**, breast-feeding, immune reconstitution syndrome, antimicrobial resistance, pancreatitis, depression, suicidal ideation, neonates, infants, children, adolescents <18 yr, QT prolongation, torsades de pointes, hyperlipidemia, hypertriglyceridemia, hypercholesterolemia

DOSAGE AND ROUTES
Treatment of antiretroviral treatment-naive adults with human immunodeficiency virus (HIV) in combination with other antiretroviral agents
Adult: PO 25 mg/day with a meal; give in combination with other antiretroviral agents. In antiretroviral-treatment–naive adults, rilpivirine is used as an alternative to efavirenz in NNRTI-based treatment regimens. Potential rilpivirine-based treatment regimens combine rilpivirine with either tenofovir plus emtricitabine or

lamiVUDine, or abacavir plus emtricitabine or lamiVUDine, or zidovudine plus emtricitabine or lamiVUDine

Available forms: Tab 25 mg
Implementation
• Store at room temperature away from heat and moisture

ADVERSE EFFECTS
CNS: Depressed mood, dizziness, drowsiness, dysphoria, fatigue, headache, major depression, mood alteration, negative thoughts, **suicide attempts**
GI: Abdominal pain, cholecystitis, cholelithiasis, decreased appetite, diarrhea, elevated hepatic enzymes, hyperbilirubinemia, hypercholesterolemia, nausea, vomiting
GU: Glomerulonephritis membranous/glomerulonephritis mesangioproliferative

Pharmacokinetics

Absorption	Increased effect 40% (food), decreased effect 50% (high protein drink)
Distribution	Protein binding (99.7%) to albumin
Metabolism	Via oxidation CYP3A system
Excretion	Feces 25% excreted unchanged (85%); urine (6.1%)
Half-life	Terminal elimination 50 hr

Pharmacodynamics

Onset	Unknown
Peak	4-5 hr
Duration	Unknown

INTERACTIONS
Individual drugs
Aminoglutethimide, bexarotene, bosentan, efavirenz, flutamide, griseofulvin, metyrapone, modafinil, nafcillin, nevirapine, pioglitazone, primidone, ritonavir, topiramate: Decreased rilpivirine effect, treatment failure
Abarelix, alfuzosin, amiodarone, amoxapine, apomorphine, artemether, asenapine, chloroquine, ciprofloxacin, citalopram, cloZAPine, cyclobenzaprine, dasatinib, dolasetron, dronedarone, droperidol, eribulin, flecainide, fluconazole, gatifloxacin, gemifloxacin, haloperidol, iloperidone, lapatinib, levofloxacin, lopinavir, lumefantrine, maprotiline, mefloquinem, moxifloxacin, nilotinib, norfloxacin, octreotide, ofloxacin, OLANZapine, ondansetron, paliperidone, palonosetron, pentami-

---

dine, posconazole, QUEtiapine, ranolazine, saquinavir: Increased QT prolongation
Fluconazole, voriconazole: Increased rilpivirine adverse reactions, fungal infections

Drug classifications

CYP3A4 inducers (phenytoin, fosphenytoin, barbiturates, OXcarbazepine, carBAMazepine, rifabutin, rifampin, rifapentine, dexamethasone), proton pump inhibitors (PPIs): Decreased rilpivirine effect, treatment failure

H_2 receptor antagonists (cimetidine, famotidine, nizatidine, ranitidine): Decreased rilpivirine effect, treatment failure; give 12 hr before or 4 hr after rilpivirine

Antacids: Decreased rilpivirine effect; use 2 hr or more before, or 4 hr after rilpivirine

CYP3A4 inhibitors (aldesleukin, amiodarone, aprepitant, atazanavir, basiliximab, boceprevir, bromocriptine, chloramphenicol, clarithromycin, conivaptan, daloprisitin, danazol, darunavir, dasatinib, delavirdine, diltiazem, dronedarone, efavirenz, erythromycin, ethinyl estradiol, fluconazole, FLUoxetine, fluvoxaMINE, fosamprenavir, fosaprepitant, IL-2, imatinib, indinavir, isoniazid, itraconazole, ketoconazole, lanreotide, lapatinib, miconazole, nefazodone, nelfinavir, niCARdipine, octreotide, posaconazole, quiNINE, ranolazine, rifaximin, tamoxifen, telaprevir, telithromycin, tipranavir, troleandomycin, verapamil, voriconazole, zafirlukast): Increased rilpivirine effect

Class IA/III antidysrhytmics, some phenothiazines, beta agonists, local anesthetics, tricyclics, CYP3A4 inhibitors (amiodarone, arsenic trioxide, clarithromycin, erythromycin, levomethadyl, telithromycin, troleandomycin); CYP3A4 substrates (methadone, pimozide, QUEtiapine, quiNIDine, risperidone, ziprasidone), halogenated anesthetics: Increased QT prolongation

Drug/food

Increased adverse reactions: grapefruit juice

NURSING CONSIDERATIONS

Assessment

• **HIV:** Assess symptoms of HIV, including opportunistic infections before and during treatment; some may be life-threatening; monitor plasma HIV RNA, CD4+, CD8+ cell counts, serum β-2 microglobulin, serum ICD+24 antigen levels; treatment failures occur more frequently in those with baseline HIV-1 RNA concs >100,000 copies/ml than in patients with concs <100,000 copies/ml; monitor serum cholesterol, lipid panel

• Antiretroviral drug resistance testing is recommended before initiation of therapy in antiretroviral treatment-naive patients

• For adults and adolescents, initiation of antiretroviral therapy is recommended in any patient with a history of an AIDS-defining infection; with a CD4 ≤500/mm³; who is pregnant; who has HIV-associated nephropathy; or who is being treated for hepatitis B (HBV) infection

⚠ **Suicidal thoughts/behaviors:** Assess frequently for suicidal ideation; report any increase in depressive symptoms

• Hepatic disease: monitor for elevated hepatic enzymes (>2.5 × ULN); grade 3 and 4 may be higher in patients co-infected with hepatitis B or C

Patient/family education

• Teach patient that product is not a cure but controls symptoms

• Teach patient that product must be taken in combination with other prescribed products

Evaluation

Positive therapeutic outcome

• Control of HIV-related symptoms

---

riluzole (Rx)

(ri-loo′zole)

Rilutek

Func. class.: Amyotropic lateral sclerosis (ALS) agent

Chem. class.: Benzathiazole

Pregnancy category C

ACTION: Unknown; may act by inhibiting glutamate, interfering with binding of amino acid receptors, inactivation of voltage-dependent sodium channels

Therapeutic outcome: Decreased symptoms of ALS

USES: ALS

CONTRAINDICATIONS: Hypersensitivity

Precautions: Pregnancy **C**, breastfeeding, children, geriatric, neutropenia, renal/hepatic disease, cigarette smoking, febrile illness, pneumonia

DOSAGE AND ROUTES

Adult: PO 50 mg q12hr; take 1 hr before or 2 hr after meals

Available forms: Tabs 50 mg

Implementation
• Give 1 hr before or 2 hr after meals; a high-fat meal decreases absorption
• Store in tight, dry container

ADVERSE EFFECTS
CNS: Hypertonia, depression, dizziness, insomnia, somnolence, vertigo, paresthesia
CV: Hypertension, tachycardia, phlebitis, palpitation, postural hypertension
GI: Nausea, vomiting, dyspepsia, anorexia, diarrhea, flatulence, stomatitis, dry mouth, increased liver function tests, jaundice, abdominal pain
GU: UTI, dysuria
HEMA: Neutropenia
INTEG: Pruritus, eczema, alopecia, **exfoliative dermatitis**
MS: Arthralgia
RESP: Decreased lung function; rhinitis, increased cough, pneumonia

Pharmacokinetics

Absorption	Well
Distribution	Unknown
Metabolism	Liver, extensively
Excretion	Urine, feces
Half-life	Unknown

Pharmacodynamics

Unknown

INTERACTIONS
Individual drugs
Allopurinol, leflunomide, methotrexate, methyldopa, sulfasalazine, tacrine: increased hepatic injury
Amitriptyline, caffeine, theophylline: decreased elimination of riluzole
CarBAMazepine: increased liver function tests
Cigarette smoke, omeprazole, rifampin: increased elimination of riluzole

Drug classifications
Barbiturates: increased liver function tests
Quinolones: decreased elimination of riluzole

Drug/food
Charcoal-broiled foods: increased elimination of riluzole
High-fat meal: decreased absorption

NURSING CONSIDERATIONS
Assessment
• Assess for clinical improvement in neurologic function

• Monitor liver function tests: AST, ALT, bilirubin, GGT, baseline and qmo × 3 mo, then q3mo
• Assess for neutropenia (neutrophils <500/mm^3)

Patient/family education
• Advise to report febrile illness, may indicate neutropenia; cardiac/respiratory changes
• Teach reason for product and expected results

Evaluation
Positive therapeutic outcome
• Decreasing symptoms of ALS

rimantadine (Rx)
(ri-man'ti-deen)
Flumadine
Func. class.: Synthetic antiviral
Chem. class.: Tricyclic amine
Pregnancy category C

Do not confuse:
rimantadine/amantadine/ranitidine

ACTION: Prevents uncoating of nucleic acid in viral cell, preventing penetration of virus to host; causes release of DOPamine from neurons

Therapeutic outcome: Prevention of influenza type A

USES: Prophylaxis or treatment of influenza type A

CONTRAINDICATIONS:
Hypersensitivity to products of adamantine class (this product, amantadine)

Precautions: Pregnancy **C**, breastfeeding, children <1 yr, epilepsy, renal/hepatic disease

DOSAGE AND ROUTES
Influenza type A prophylaxis
Adult and child >10 yr: PO 100 mg bid
Child 1-10 yr: PO 5 mg/kg/day, max 150 mg

Treatment
Adult: PO 100 mg bid; start treatment at onset of symptoms, continue for at least 1 wk
Geriatric: PO 100 mg/day

Renal/hepatic dose
Adult: PO ≤10 ml/min 100 mg qd

Available forms: Tabs 100 mg; syr 50 mg/5 ml

Implementation
- Give before exposure to influenza; continue for 10 days after contact
- Give at least 4 hr before bedtime to prevent insomnia
- Administer after meals for better absorption, to decrease GI symptoms; cap may be opened and mixed with food for easy swallowing
- Give in divided doses to prevent CNS disturbances: headache, dizziness, fatigue, drowsiness
- Store in airtight, dry container
- Give with full glass of water

ADVERSE EFFECTS
CNS: *Headache, dizziness,* fatigue, depression, hallucinations, tremors, **seizures,** insomnia, poor concentration, asthenia, gait abnormalities, anxiety, confusion
CV: Pallor, palpitations, edema
EENT: Tinnitus, taste abnormality, eye pain
GI: *Nausea, vomiting,* constipation, *dry mouth, anorexia, abdominal pain, diarrhea,* dyspepsia
INTEG: Rash

Pharmacokinetics
Absorption	Minimally absorbed (PO)
Distribution	Widely distributed, crosses placenta, CSF concentration 50% plasma
Metabolism	Liver
Excretion	95% unchanged—kidneys
Half-life	13-65 hr, increased in renal disease

Pharmacodynamics
	PO
Onset	Unknown
Peak	1½-2½ hr
Duration	Unknown

INTERACTIONS
Individual drugs
Acetaminophen, aspirin, intranasal influenza vaccine: decreased peak concentration of rimantadine
Cimetidine: increased rimantadine concentration

NURSING CONSIDERATIONS
Assessment
- **Assess for seizures;** if seizures occur, product should be discontinued
- Monitor respiratory status: rate, character, wheezing, tightness in chest

Patient/family education
- Instruct patient about aspects of product therapy: need to report dyspnea, dizziness, poor concentration, behavioral changes
- Advise patient to avoid hazardous activities if dizziness occurs
- Caution patient to consult prescriber before taking OTC medications, alcohol; serious product interactions may result

Evaluation
Positive therapeutic outcome
- Absence of fever, malaise, cough, dyspnea

---

risedronate (Rx)
(rih-sed′roh-nate)
Actonel, Atelvia
Func. class.: Bone resorption inhibitor
Chem. class.: Bisphosphonate
Pregnancy category C

Do not confuse:
Actonel/Actos

ACTION: Inhibits bone resorption; absorbs calcium phosphate crystal in bone and may directly block dissolution of hydroxyapatite crystals of bone

Therapeutic outcome: Increased bone mass, activity without fractures

USES: Paget's disease; prevention, treatment of osteoporosis in postmenopausal women; glucocorticoid-induced osteoporosis; osteoporosis in men

CONTRAINDICATIONS:
Hypersensitivity to bisphosphonates, inability to stand or sit upright for ≥30 min, esophageal stricture, achalasia, hypocalcemia

Precautions: Pregnancy C, breastfeeding, children, renal disease, active upper GI disorders, dental disease, hyperparathyroidism, infection, vitamin D deficiency, coagulopathy, chemotherapy, asthma

DOSAGE AND ROUTES
Paget's disease
Adult: PO 30 mg/day × 2 mo; give calcium and vit D if dietary intake is lacking; if relapse occurs, retreatment is advised

R

Treatment/prevention of post-menopausal osteoporosis
Adult: PO 5 mg/day or 35 mg qwk or 75 mg/day × 2 consecutive days 2 × mo or 150 mg qmo

Glucocorticoid osteoporosis
Adult: PO 5 mg/day

Osteoporosis in men
Adult: PO 35 mg qwk

Renal dose
Adult: PO CCr <30 mg/min, avoid use

Available forms: Tabs 5, 30, 35, 75, 150 mg; tab gastro-resistant, weekly 35 mg; tab, weekly 35 mg

Implementation
• Give PO for 2 mo to be effective in Paget's disease
• Give with a full glass of water; patient should be in upright position
• Administer supplemental calcium and vit D in Paget's disease
• Give daily ≥30 min before meals
• Store in cool environment out of direct sunlight

ADVERSE EFFECTS
CNS: Dizziness, headache, depression
CV: Chest pain, hypertension, **atrial fibrillation**
GI: *Abdominal pain,* diarrhea, *nausea,* constipation, esophagitis
MS: *Severe muscle/joint/bone pain,* **osteonecrosis of the jaw,** fractures
MISC: Rash, UTI, pharyngitis, hypocalcemia, hypophosphatemia, increased PTH
SYST: Angioedema

Pharmacokinetics

Absorption	Unknown
Distribution	To bones (50%)
Metabolism	Unknown
Excretion	Kidneys
Half-life	Terminal 220 hr

Pharmacodynamics

Unknown

INTERACTIONS
Drug classifications
Aluminum, antacids, calcium, iron, magnesium salts: decreased absorption of risedronate
NSAIDs, salicylates: increased GI irritation

Drug/food
Food: decreased bioavailability; take ½ hr before food or drinks other than water

Drug/lab test
Decreased: calcium

NURSING CONSIDERATIONS
Assessment
• **Paget's disease:** assess for headache, bone pain, increased head circumference
• **Osteoporosis:** in men or postmenopausal women; bone density study prior to and periodically during treatment
• **Hypocalcemia:** assess for paresthesia, twitching, laryngospasm, Chvostek's/Trousseau's signs
⚠ **Serious skin reactions: assess for angioedema**
⚠ **Assess for atrial fibrillation**
• Monitor phosphate, alkaline phosphatase, calcium; creatinine, BUN (renal disease)
• **Hypercalcemia:** assess for paresthesia, twitching, laryngospasm, Chvostek's/Trousseau's signs
⚠ **Assess dental health, cover with antiinfectives prior to dental extraction**

Patient/family education
• Advise patient to sit upright for ½ hr after dose to prevent irritation
• Instruct patient to comply with dietary restrictions, maintain good oral hygiene
• Advise patient to notify prescriber if pregnancy is planned or suspected

Evaluation
Positive therapeutic outcome
• Increased bone mass, absence of fractures

---

risperiDONE (Rx)
(res-pare′a-done)
Risperdal, Risperdal Consta, Risperdal M-TAB
Func. class.: Antipsychotic
Chem. class.: Benzisoxazole derivative
Pregnancy category C

Do not confuse:
Risperdal/reserpine

ACTION: Unknown; may be mediated through both DOPamine type 2 (D_2) and serotonin type 2 (5-HT_2) antagonism

Therapeutic outcome: Decreased hallucinations and disorganized thought

---

USES: Irritability associated with autism, bipolar disorder, mania, schizophrenia

CONTRAINDICATIONS:

Hypersensitivity, seizure

Precautions: Pregnancy **C**, children, geriatric, cardiac/renal/hepatic disease, breast cancer, Parkinson's disease, CNS depression, brain tumor, dehydration, diabetes, hematologic disease, seizure disorders, breastfeeding, abrupt discontinuation, suicidal ideation, phenylketonuria

> **BLACK BOX WARNING:** Increased mortality in elderly patients with dementia-related psychosis

DOSAGE AND ROUTES

Adult: PO 2 mg/day as a single dose or 2 divided doses, adjust dose at intervals of ≥24 hr and 1-2 mg/day as tolerated to 4-8 mg/day; IM establish dosing with PO prior to IM 25 mg q2wk, may increase to max 50 mg q2wk

Adolescent: PO 0.5 mg/day in AM or PM, adjust dose at intervals of ≥24 hr and 0.5-1 mg/day as tolerated to 3 mg/day

Geriatric: PO 0.5 mg daily-bid, increase by 1 mg qwk; IM 25 mg q2wk

Hepatic dose/renal dose

Adult: PO 0.5 mg, increase by 0.5 mg bid, then increase to 1.5 mg bid at intervals ≥1 wk

Available forms: Tabs 0.25, 0.5, 1, 2, 3, 4 mg; oral sol 1 mg/ml; orally disintegrating tabs 0.25, 0.5, 1, 2, 3, 4 mg; long-acting inj kit (Risperdal Consta) 12.5, 25, 37.5, 50 mg

Implementation

PO route

- Reduced dosage in geriatric patients
- Anticholinergic agent on order from prescriber, to be used for EPS
- Avoid use with CNS depressants
- Conventional tabs: give without regard to meals
- *Oral disintegrating tab* (Risperdal M-Tab): do not open blister pack until ready to use; tear 1 of the 4 units apart at perforation; bend corner where indicated; peel back foil; do not push tab through foil; remove from pack and place on tongue; tab disintegrates in seconds and can be swallowed with or without liquids, do not split or chew
- *Oral solution:* may dilute 3-4 oz of a beverage, measure dose using calibrated pipette, not compatible with tea, cola; compatible with water, coffee, orange juice, low-fat milk

IM route

- Only suspend in the diluent provided and with the supplied needle; do not substitute any components of the dose pack including the SmartSite Needle-Free Vial Access Device or Needle-Pro device; prior to admixing, remove the dose pack from the refrigerator and allow to come to room temperature for about 30 minutes prior to reconstitution
- Remove the plastic colored cap from the vial without removing the grey rubber stopper. Wipe top of the grey stopper with an alcohol wipe and allow to dry
- Peel back the blister pouch and remove the Vial Access Device by holding between the white luer cap and the skirt. Do not touch the spike tip at any time
- Place the vial on a hard surface and hold the base. Orient the Vial Access Device vertically over the vial so that the spike tip is at the center of the vial's rubber stopper
- With a straight downward push, press the spike tip of the Vial Access Device through the center of the vial's rubber stopper until the device securely snaps onto the vial top. Improper placement of the Vial Access Device on the vial could result in leakage of the diluent upon transfer
- Hold the base of the vial and swab the syringe connection point (blue circle) of the Vial Access Device with an alcohol wipe and allow to dry prior to attaching the syringe
- During syringe assembly steps, avoid overtightening, or syringe component parts may loosen from the syringe body
- To open the syringe, hold syringe only by the white collar and snap off the smooth white cap. Do not twist or cut off the white cap. Remove white cap together with the rubber tip cap inside
- While holding the white collar of the syringe, insert and press the syringe tip into the blue circle of the Vial Access Device and twist in a clockwise motion to secure the connection of the syringe to the Vial Access Device. Hold the skirt of the Vial Access Device during attachment to prevent it from spinning. Keep the syringe and the Vial Access Device aligned
- Inject the entire contents of the syringe containing the diluent into the vial
- Shake the vial vigorously for a minimum of 10 seconds while holding the plunger rod down with the thumb. Mixing is complete when the suspension appears uniform, thick, and milky colored, and all the powder is dispersed in liquid. The microspheres will be visible in liquid, but no dry microspheres remain

R

Adverse effects: *italics* = common; **bold** = life-threatening

• Invert the vial completely and slowly withdraw the entire content of the suspension from the vial into the syringe. Tear the section of the vial label at the perforation and apply the detached label to the syringe for identification purposes

• While holding the white collar of the syringe, unscrew the syringe from the Vial Access Device, then discard both the vial and the Vial Access Device appropriately

• Select the appropriate color-coded needle provided with the kit. Two distinct needles are provided. The needle with the yellow colored hub and print is for injection into the gluteal muscle (2-inch needle) and the needle with the green colored hub and print is for deltoid muscles (1-inch needle). They are not interchangeable; do not use the needle intended for gluteal injection for deltoid injection, and vice versa

• Peel the blister pouch of the Needle-Pro safety device open halfway. Grasp the transparent needle sheath using the plastic peel pouch. To prevent contamination, do not touch the orange Needle-Pro safety device's luer connector. While holding the white collar of the syringe, attach the luer connection of the orange Needle-Pro safety device to the syringe with an easy clockwise twisting motion

• While holding the white collar of the syringe, grasp the transparent needle sheath and seat the needle firmly on the orange Needle-Pro safety device with a push and a clockwise twist. Seating the needle will secure the connection between the needle and the orange Needle-Pro safety device

• While holding the white collar of the syringe, pull the transparent needle sheath straight away from the needle. Do not twist the sheath since this may loosen the luer connection

• Re-suspension will be necessary prior to administration, since settling will occur after reconstitution. Re-suspend the microspheres in the syringe by shaking vigorously

• May refer to the Instructions for Use section of the product labeling for detailed visual aids that accompany the written instructions

Administration

• **Only for IM; do not give IV**

• Re-suspension will be necessary prior to administration, since settling will occur after reconstitution. Re-suspend the microspheres in the syringe by shaking vigorously

• Remove any air bubbles by tapping the syringe and slowly depressing the plunger with the needle in an upright position

• Inject the entire contents of the syringe into the upper outer quadrant of the gluteal area or the deltoid muscle of the arm; inject immediately after reconstitution to avoid settling. Gluteal injections should be alternated between the two buttocks

• After the injection is complete, press the needle into the orange Needle-Pro safety device by gently pressing the orange Needle-Pro safety device against a flat surface with one hand. As the orange Needle-Pro safety device is pressed, the needle will firmly engage into the orange Needle-Pro safety device

• Visually confirm full engagement of the needle into the Needle-Pro safety device, then appropriately discard both the used and unused needle provided in the dose pack

• Do not store the vial after reconstitution or the suspension may settle

• Do not combine 2 different dosage strengths of Risperdal Consta in a single administration

• The dose pack device is for single use only. Do not re-process for subsequent re-use because the integrity of the device may be compromised leading to a deterioration in performance

• *Stability after reconstitution:* Once in suspension, the product may remain at room temperature but must be used within 6 hr. Always re-suspend prior to administration if not used immediately

• When switching from oral to inj, give oral dose with first inj and continue for 3 wk, then discontinue

ADVERSE EFFECTS

CNS: *EPS (pseudoparkinsonism, akathisia, dystonia, tardive dyskinesia), drowsiness, insomnia, agitation, anxiety, headache,* **neuroleptic malignant syndrome,** dizziness, **seizures, suicidal ideation,** head titubation (shaking)

CV: Orthostatic hypotension, **tachycardia, heart failure, sudden death (geriatric),** AV block

EENT: Blurred vision, tinnitus

GI: *Nausea,* vomiting, *anorexia, constipation,* jaundice, weight gain

GU: Hyperprolactinemia, gynecomastia, dysuria

HEMA: Neutropenia, granulocytopenia

MS: Rhabdomyolysis

MISC: Renal artery disease; weight gain, hyperprolactinemia (child)

RESP: Rhinitis, sinusitis, upper respiratory infection, cough

Pharmacokinetics

Absorption	Unknown
Distribution	Unknown
Metabolism	Liver, extensively
Excretion	Urine 90%
Half-life	3-24 hr

Pharmacodynamics

Onset	Unknown
Peak	1-2 hr
Duration	Up to 12 hr

INTERACTIONS

Individual drugs
Alcohol: increased sedation

⚠ **Chloroquine, clarithromycin, droperidol, erythromycin, haloperidol, methadone, pentamidine, thioridazine, ziprasidone: increased QT prolongation**

CarBAMazepine: increased risperiDONE excretion

⚠ **Furosemide: increased risk of death in dementia-related psychosis**

Levodopa: decreased levodopa effect

⚠ **TraMADol: increased seizures**

⚠ **Valproic acid, verapamil: increased risperidone levels**

Drug classifications
Acetylcholinesterase inhibitors, CYP2D6 inhibitors, SSRIs: increased risperiDONE levels

Antipsychotics: increased EPS

⚠ **β-agonists, class IA/III antidysrhythmics, local anesthetics, some phenothiazines, tricyclics: increased QT prolongation**

CNS depressants: increased sedation

CYP2D6 inducers (carBAMazepine, barbiturates, phenytoin, rifampin): decreased risperiDONE action

CYP2D6 inhibitors (selective serotonin reuptake inhibitors): serotonin syndrome, neuroleptic malignant syndrome

Drug/herb
Echinacea: decreased risperiDONE effect

Drug/lab test
Increased: prolactin levels, blood glucose, lipids

NURSING CONSIDERATIONS

Assessment
• **Suicidal thoughts, behaviors** often occur when depression is lessened; assess mental status: orientation, mood, behavior, presence and type of hallucinations before initial administration, monthly; this product should significantly reduce psychotic behavior

• Monitor bilirubin, CBC, liver function tests monthly

• Assess affect, orientation, LOC, reflexes, gait, coordination, sleep pattern disturbances

• **QT prolongation:** Monitor B/P with patient in sitting, standing, and lying positions; take pulse and respirations q4hr during initial treatment; establish baseline before starting treatment; report drops of 30 mm Hg; obtain baseline ECG and monitor Q- and T-wave changes

• Check for dizziness, faintness, palpitations, tachycardia on rising; severe orthostatic hypotension is common

⚠ **Assess for neuroleptic malignant syndrome: hyperpyrexia, muscle rigidity, increased CPK, altered mental status; product should be discontinued**

• EPS: Assess for akathisia (inability to sit still, no pattern to movements), tardive dyskinesia (bizarre movements of the jaw, mouth, tongue, extremities), pseudoparkinsonism (rigidity, tremors, pill rolling, shuffling gait); an antiparkinsonian product should be prescribed

• Assess for constipation, urinary retention daily; if these occur, increase bulk, water in diet

• Assess for weight gain, hyperglycemia, metabolic changes in diabetes, increased lipids

Patient/family education
• Teach patient to use good oral hygiene; frequent rinsing of mouth, sugarless gum for dry mouth

• Caution patient to avoid hazardous activities until product response is determined; dizziness, blurred vision may occur

• Inform patient that orthostatic hypotension occurs often; patient should rise from sitting or lying position gradually and remain lying down for at least 30 min after IM inj

• Instruct patient to avoid hot tubs, hot showers, tub baths; hypotension may occur

• Inform patient that heat stroke may occur in hot weather and to take extra precautions to stay cool

• Advise patient to avoid abrupt withdrawal of this product, or EPS may result; product should be withdrawn slowly

• Teach patient to avoid OTC preparations (cough, hay fever, cold) unless approved by prescriber; serious product interactions may occur; avoid use with alcohol, CNS depressants because increased drowsiness may occur

• Advise patient to use contraception, to inform prescriber if pregnancy is planned or suspected

⚠ **Teach patient to notify provider of suicidal thoughts/behaviors**

R

Evaluation
Positive therapeutic outcome
- Decrease in emotional excitement, hallucinations, delusions, paranoia
- Reorganization of patterns of thought, speech

TREATMENT OF OVERDOSE:
Lavage, provide airway

---

ritonavir (Rx)
(ri-toe′na-veer)
Norvir
Func. class.: Antiretroviral
Chem. class.: Protease inhibitor
Pregnancy category B

Do not confuse:
ritonavir/retrovir

ACTION: Inhibits HIV-1 protease and prevents maturation of the infectious virus

Therapeutic outcome: Improvement of HIV-1 infection

USES: HIV-1 in combination with at least 2 other antiretrovirals

CONTRAINDICATIONS:
Hypersensitivity

BLACK BOX WARNING: Coadministration with other drugs

Precautions: Pregnancy **B**, breastfeeding, children, liver disease, pancreatitis, diabetes, hemophilia, AV block, hypercholesterolemia, immune reconstitution syndrome, neonates, cardiomyopathy, immune reconstitution syndrome

DOSAGE AND ROUTES
Adult/adolescent >16 yr: PO 600 mg bid; if nausea occurs, begin dose at ½ and gradually increase, max 1200 mg/day
Adolescent ≤16 yr/child/infant: PO 400 mg/m² bid up to 1200 mg/day; may start lower and escalate

Available forms: Caps 100 mg; oral sol 80 mg/ml, tab 100 mg

Implementation
- Oral sol: Shake oral sol well, use calibrated measuring device
- Store caps in refrigerator
- Mix liquid formulation with chocolate milk or liquid nutritional supplement to improve taste

- When switching from cap to tab, more GI symptoms may occur that will lessen over time
- Use dosage titration to minimize side effects

ADVERSE EFFECTS
CNS: *Paresthesia*, headache, **seizures,** dizziness, insomnia, fever, asthenia, **intracranial bleeding**
CV: **QT, PR interval prolongation**
GI: *Diarrhea*, buccal mucosa ulceration, *abdominal pain, nausea, taste perversion,* dry mouth, *vomiting, anorexia*
INTEG: Rash
MISC: Asthenia, **angioedema, anaphylaxis, Stevens-Johnson syndrome,** increased lipids, lipodystrophy, **toxic epidermal necrolysis**
MS: Pain, **rhabdomyolysis,** myalgia

Pharmacokinetics
Absorption	Well
Distribution	Unknown
Metabolism	98% protein binding, liver
Excretion	Unknown
Half-life	3-5 hr

Pharmacodynamics
Onset	Unknown
Peak	2-4 hr
Duration	Unknown

INTERACTIONS
Individual drugs

BLACK BOX WARNING: Amiodarone, astemizole, buPROPion, cisapride, cloZAPine, desipramine, encainide, ergotamine, flecainide, meperidine, midazolam, pimozide, piroxicam, propafenone, propoxyphene, quiNIDine, ranolazine, saquinavir, terfenadine, triazolam, zolpidem: toxicity, do not use together

---

Atovaquone, divalproex, ethinyl estradiol, lamoTRIgine, phenytoin, sulfamethoxazole, theophylline, voriconazole, zidovudine: decreased levels of each drug
Bosentan: increased levels of bosentan
Clarithromycin: increased level of both products
ddI: increased levels of both products
Fluconazole: increased ritonavir level
Haloperidol, chloroquine, droperidol, pentamidine, arsenic trioxide, levomethadyl: increased QT prolongation
Nevirapine, phenytoin: decreased ritonavir levels

Drug classifications
Anticoagulants: decreased levels of anticoagulants

Azole antifungals, benzodiazepines, HMG-CoA reductase inhibitors, interleukins: toxicity, do not use together

Barbiturates, rifamycins: decreased ritonavir level

> **BLACK BOX WARNING:** Class IA/III antidys-rhythmics, some phenothiazines, β-agonists, local anesthetics, tricyclics, CYP3A4 inhibitors (amiodarone, clarithromycin, erythromycin, telithromycin, troleandomycin), CYP3A4 substrates (dasatinib, methadone, pimozide, QUEtiapine, quiNIDine, risperidone, ziprasi-done): increased QT prolongation

CYP2D6 inhibitors: toxicity, do not use together

Drug/herb
Red yeast rice: avoid use
St. John's wort: decreased ritonavir levels, avoid concurrent use

Drug/lab test
Increased: ALT, GGT, AST, CK, cholesterol, triglycerides, uric acid
Decreased: Hct, RBC, Hgb, neutrophils, WBC

NURSING CONSIDERATIONS
Assessment
• **QT prolongation:** ECG for QT prolongation, ejection fraction; assess for chest pain, palpitations, dyspnea
• **Rhabdomyolysis:** muscle pain, increased CPK, weakness, swelling of affected muscles; if these occur and if confirmed by CPK, product should be discontinued
⚠ **Immune reconstitution syndrome: may occur with combination therapy, may develop inflammatory response with opportunistic infection (MAC, Graves disease, Guillain-Barré syndrome, TB, PCP), may occur during initial treatment or months afterward**
• Assess signs of infection, anemia
• Monitor viral load and CD4, blood glucose, plasma HIV RNA, serum cholesterol, lipid profile baseline, throughout therapy
• Resistance testing prior to starting therapy and after treatment failure
• Assess liver function tests: ALT, AST; in those with hepatic disease, monitor q3mo
• Monitor C&S before product therapy; product may be taken as soon as culture is done; repeat C&S after treatment; determine the presence of other STDs
• Assess bowel pattern before, during treatment; if severe abdominal pain with bleeding occurs, product should be discontinued; monitor hydration

• **Serious skin disorders: Stevens-Johnson syndrome,** angioedema; anaphylaxis, toxic epidermal necrolysis

Patient/family education
• Teach patient to take as prescribed; if dose is missed, take as soon as remembered up to 1 hr before next dose; do not double dose
• Teach patient that product must be taken in equal intervals around the clock to maintain blood levels for duration of therapy
• Teach patient that product is not a cure for HIV; opportunistic infections may continue to be acquired, and others may continue to contract HIV from the patient
• Advise patient not to use St. John's wort, that it decreases this product's effect
• Inform that redistribution of body fat or accumulation of body fat may occur

Evaluation
Positive therapeutic outcome
• Decreasing symptoms of HIV
• Improving viral load and CD4 cell counts

---

riTUXimab (Rx)
(rih-tuks'ih-mab)
Rituxan
Func. class.: Antineoplastic—miscellaneous; DMARD
Chem. class.: Murine/human monoclonal antibody
Pregnancy category C

ACTION: Directed against the CD20 antigen that is found on malignant B lymphocytes; CD20 regulates a portion of cell cycle initiation/differentiation

Therapeutic outcome: Decreased tumor size, prevention of spread of cancer

USES: Non-Hodgkin's lymphoma (CD20 positive, B-cell), bulky disease (tumors >10 cm), rheumatoid arthritis, Wegener's granulomatosis, microscopic polyangitis

CONTRAINDICATIONS:
Hypersensitivity, murine proteins

Precautions: Pregnancy **C**, breastfeeding, children, geriatric, cardiac/renal/pulmonary conditions

> **BLACK BOX WARNING:** Exfoliative dermatitis, infusion-related reactions, progressive multifocal leukoencephalopathy

DOSAGE AND ROUTES

Relapsed or refractory low-grade or follicular, CD20 positive, B-cell non-Hodgkin's lymphoma (NHL)
Adult: IV 375 mg/m² qwk × 4 doses, may retreat with 4 more doses of 375 mg/m² qwk

First-line treatment of follicular, CD20-positive, B-cell non-Hodgkin's lymphoma (NHL), in combination with chemotherapy
Adult: IV 375 mg/m² on day 1 of each cycle for up to 8; may be given with cyclophosphamide IV 750 mg/m² on day 1, vinCRIStine IV 1.4 mg/m² (max of 2 mg) on day 1, and predniSONE 40 mg/m²/day PO on days 1-5

Single-agent maintenance therapy in patients with follicular, CD20-positive, B-cell non-Hodgkin's lymphoma (NHL) (complete or partial response following first-line treatment with riTUXimab in combination with chemotherapy)
Adult: IV 375 mg/m² IV q8wk × 12 doses as maintenance therapy starting 8 wk after the completion of induction chemotherapy with 8 doses of riTUXimab with 6-8 cycles of cyclophosphamide, vinCRIStine, and predniSONE 4-6 cycles of cyclophosphamide, DOXOrubicin, vinCRIStine, and predniSONE

As a component of the Zevalin (ibritumomab tiuxetan) regimen
Adult: IV; as a required component of the ibritumomab regimen; riTUXimab 250 mg/m² given within 4 hr prior to the administration of Yttrium-90 ibritumomab that may occur on day 7, 8, or 9

First-line treatment of diffuse large B-cell, CD20-positive non-Hodgkin's lymphoma (NHL), in combination with CHOP or other anthracycline-based chemotherapy regimen
Adult 18-59 yr: IV 375 mg/m² on day 1 of each cycle for up to 8 infusions

As single-agent maintenance therapy in patients with low-grade, CD20-positive, B-cell non-Hodgkin's lymphoma (NHL) with nonprogressing disease (stable disease or better) following first-line treatment with cyclophosphamide, vinCRIStine, and predniSONE (CVP)
Adult: IV 375 mg/m² qwk × 4 wk repeated q6mo × 2 years (total of 16 doses) as maintenance therapy starting 4 wk after the completion of first-line chemotherapy with 6 to 8 cycles of cyclophosphamide, vinCRIStine, and predniSONE (CVP)

Available forms: Inj 10 mg/ml (100 mg/10 ml, 500 mg/50 ml)

Implementation

Intermittent IV infusion route
- Hold antihypertensive 2 hr before administration
- Administer after diluting to a final conc of 1-4 mg/ml; use 0.9% NaCl, D₅W, gently invert bag to mix; do not mix with other products
- Increase fluid intake to 2-3 L/day to prevent dehydration, unless contraindicated
- Store vials at 36° F-40° F; protect vials from direct sunlight; inf sol is stable at 36° F-46° F for 24 hr and at room temp for another 12 hr

Y-site compatibilities: Acyclovir, amifostine, amikacin, aminophylline, ampicillin, ampicillin/sulbactam, aztreonam, bleomycin, bumetanide, buprenorphine, busulfan, butorphanol, calcium gluconate, CARBOplatin, carmustine, ceFAZolin, cefoperazone, cefotaxime, cefoTEtan, cefOXitin, cefTAZidime, ceftizoxime, cefTRIAXone, cefuroxime, chlorproMAZINE, cimetidine, CISplatin, clindamycin, cyclophosphamide, cytarabine, DACTINomycin, DAUNOrubicin hydrochloride, dexamethasone, dexrazoxane, digoxin, diphenhydrAMINE, DOBUTamine, DOCEtaxel, DOPamine, DOXOrubicin liposome, doxycycline, droperidol, enalaprilat, etoposide phosphate, famotidine, fentaNYL, filgrastim, floxuridine, fluconazole, fludarabine, fluorouracil, ganciclovir, gemcitabine, gentamicin, granisetron, haloperidol, heparin, hydrocortisone, HYDROmorphone, IDArubicin, ifosfamide, imipenem/cilastatin, irinotecan, leucovorin, levorphanol, LORazepam, magnesium sulfate, mannitol, meperidine, mesna, methotrexate, methylPREDNISolone, metoclopramide, metroNIDAZOLE, mitoMYcin, mitoXANtrone, morphine, nalbuphine, netilmicin, PACLitaxel, pentamidine, piperacillin/tazobactam, plicamycin, potassium chloride, prochlorperazine, promethazine, ranitidine, sargramostim, streptozocin, teniposide, theophylline, thiotepa, ticarcillin/clavulanate, tobramycin, trimethoprim/sulfamethoxazole, trimethobenzamide, vinBLAStine, vinCRIStine, vinorelbine, zidovudine

Y-site incompatibilities: Aldesleukin, amphotericin B colloidal, ciprofloxacin, cycloSPORINE, DAUNOrubicin liposome, DOXOrubicin hydrochloride, furosemide, levofloxacin,

minocycline, ondansetron, quinupristin/
dalfopristin, sodium bicarbonate, topotecan,
vancomycin

Additive incompatibilities: Do not
admix with other products

ADVERSE EFFECTS

CNS: Life-threatening brain infection (pro-
gressive multifocal leukoencephalopathy)
CV: Cardiac dysrhythmias, heart failure,
MI, superventricular tachycardia, hypertension, angina
GI: *Nausea, vomiting, anorexia,* GI obstruc-
tion/perforation
GU: Renal failure
HEMA: Leukopenia, neutropenia, thrombocytopenia, anemia
INTEG: *Irritation at inj site, rash,* fatal
mucocutaneous infections (rare)
MISC: *Fever,* chills, asthenia, *headache,*
angioedema, hypotension, myalgia, bronchospasm, ARDs
SYST: Stevens-Johnson syndrome,
exfoliative dermatitis, toxic epidermal
necrolysis, tumor lysis syndrome

Pharmacokinetics

Absorption	Unknown
Distribution	Binds to CD20 sites on lymphoma cells
Metabolism	Unknown
Excretion	Unknown
Half-life	60-174 hr

Pharmacodynamics

Unknown

INTERACTIONS

Individual drugs
CISplatin: increased nephrotoxicity—avoid
concurrent use; if used, monitor renal status

Drug classifications
Anticoagulants, NSAIDs: increased bleeding risk
Antihypertensives: increased hypotension,
separate by 12 hr

NURSING CONSIDERATIONS

Assessment

> **BLACK BOX WARNING:** Assess for signs
> of fatal inf reaction: hypoxia, pulmonary
> infiltrates, ARDS, MI, ventricular fibrillation,
> cardiogenic shock; most fatal inf reactions
> occur with first inf, discontinue product

> **BLACK BOX WARNING:** Assess for signs of
> severe mucocutaneous reactions: Stevens-
> Johnson syndrome, lichenoid dermatitis, toxic
> epidermal lysis; signs occur 1-13 wk after
> product was given, discontinue treatment
> immediately

> **BLACK BOX WARNING:** Assess for tumor
> lysis syndrome: acute renal failure requiring
> hemodialysis, hyperkalemia, hypocalcemia, hy-
> peruricemia, hyperphosphatasemia; allopurinol
> and adequate hydration may be needed

> **BLACK BOX WARNING: Multifocal leuko-
> encephalopathy:** confusion, dizziness,
> lethargy, hemiparesis, monitor periodically

• Monitor CBC, differential, platelet count
weekly; withhold product if WBC is <3500/
mm^3 or platelet count <100,000/mm^3; notify
prescriber of these results; product should be
discontinued
• Monitor ECG, serum creatinine/BUN, electrolytes, uric acid
• Assess GI symptoms: frequency of stools,
abdominal pain, perforation/obstruction may
occur
⚠ Infection: assess for fever, increased
temperature, flulike symptoms in those with
WG and MPA, in those using DMARDs

Patient/family education
• Advise patient to report to prescriber possible
infection (cough, fever, chills, sore throat),
renal issues (painful urination, back/side pain),
bleeding (gums, stools, bruising, urine, emesis,
fatigue)
• Advise to avoid OTC products
⚠ Teach to use contraception during and
up to 12 mo after therapy
• Avoid use with vaccines, toxoids

Evaluation
Positive therapeutic outcome
• Prevention of increasing cancer progression

rivaroxaban
(ri-va-rox′a-ban)
Xarelto
Func. class.: Anticoagulant
Chem. class.: Factor Xa inhibitor
Pregnancy category C

ACTION: A novel, oral anticoagulant that
selectively and potently inhibits coagulation
factor Xa

Therapeutic outcome: Prevention of DVT, stroke, and systemic embolism

USES: For deep venous thrombosis (DVT) prophylaxis, pulmonary embolism (PE), in patients undergoing knee or hip replacement surgery; for stroke prophylaxis and systemic embolism prophylaxis in patients with nonvalvular atrial fibrillation

CONTRAINDICATIONS:
Severe hypersensitivity

Precautions: Moderate or severe hepatic disease (Child-Pugh Class B or C), hepatic disease associated with coagulopathy, creatinine clearance <30 ml/min for use as DVT prophylaxis and <15 ml/min for stroke and systemic embolism prophylaxis in nonvalvular atrial fibrillation, dental procedures, neonates, infants, children, adolescents, pregnancy category C, aneurysm, diabetes retinopathy, breastfeeding, diverticulitis, endocarditis, geriatrics, GI bleeding, hypertension, obstetric delivery, peptic ulcer disease, stroke, surgery

DOSAGE AND ROUTES
Deep venous thrombosis (DVT) prophylaxis, which may lead to pulmonary embolism (PE) (knee or hip replacement surgery)
Administer the initial dose at least 6–10 hr after surgery once hemostasis has been established
Adult: PO 10 mg daily for 12 days after knee replacement surgery or for 35 days after hip replacement

Stroke prophylaxis and systemic embolism prophylaxis (nonvalvular atrial fibrillation)
Adult: PO 20 mg daily with the evening meal (CrCl > 50 ml/min); **converting from warfarin to rivaroxaban:** discontinue warfarin and start rivaroxaban when INR is <3; **converting from another anticoagulant other than warfarin to rivaroxaban:** start rivaroxaban 0-2 hr before the next scheduled evening administration of anticoagulant (omit that dose of anticoagulant); for continuous infusion of unfractionated heparin, stop the infusion and initiate rivaroxaban simultaneously; **converting from rivaroxaban to another anticoagulant with rapid onset (not warfarin):** Discontinue rivaroxaban and give the first dose of the other anticoagulant (oral or parenteral) at the time that the next dose of rivaroxaban would have been administered

Renal dose
Adult: PO (nonvalvular atrial fibrillation) CCr 15-50 ml/min, 15 mg/day; CCr <15 ml/min, avoid use; (treatment/prophylaxis of DVT/pulmonary embolism) CCr <30 ml/min, avoid use

Hepatic dose
Adult: PO Child-Pugh class B or C: avoid use

Available forms: Tab 10, 15, 20, 50 mg

Implementation
• **For DVT prophylaxis:** give daily without regard to food, give initial dose ≥6-10 hr after surgery when hemostasis has been established
• For stroke/systemic embolism prophylaxis: give daily with evening meal
• If dose is not given at correct time, give as soon as possible on the same day
• Unless pathological bleeding occurs, do not discontinue rivaroxaban in the absence of alternative
• Store at room temperature
• 15, 20 mg tablets should be taken with food, for those unable to swallow whole, 15 mg and 20 mg tablets may be crushed, mixed with applesauce, immediately following administration, instruct to eat, crushed tablets are stable in applesauce for up to 4 hr
• 10 mg tablet can be taken without regard to food
Nasogastric (NG) tube or gastric feeding tube
• Confirm gastric placement of tube
• Crush 15 mg or 20 mg tablet, suspend in 50 ml of water, and administer via NG or gastric feeding tube
• To minimize reduced absorption, avoid administration distal to the stomach
• Enteral feeding should immediately follow administration of a crushed dose
• Crushed tablets are stable in water for up to 4 hours
Missed doses
• Patients receiving 15 mg twice daily should take their missed dose immediately to ensure intake of 30 mg per day. Two 15-mg tablets may be taken at once followed by the regular 15 mg twice daily dose the next day
• For patients receiving once daily dosing, take the missed dose as soon as it is remembered

ADVERSE EFFECTS
GI: Cholestasis, **cytolytic hepatitis**, hyperbilirubinemia, increased hepatic enzymes, jaundice, nausea

HEMA: Adrenal bleeding, bleeding, cerebral hemorrhage, epidural hematoma, GI bleeding, hemiparesis, intracranial bleeding, retinal hemorrhage, retroperitoneal hemorrhage, subdural hematoma, thrombocytopenia
INTEG: Anaphylactic reaction, anaphylactic shock, blister, hypersensitivity, pruritus
SYST: Stevens-Johnson syndrome

BLACK BOX WARNING: Active bleeding

BLACK BOX WARNING: Abrupt discontinuation, epidermal/spinal anesthesia

---

Pharmacokinetics

Absorption	80%-100%
Distribution	Protein binding (92%-95%)
Metabolism	Oxidative degradation
Excretion	Urine (66%), feces (17%)
Half-life	5-9 hr; geriatric: 11-13 hr

Pharmacodynamics

Onset	Unknown
Peak	2-4 hrs
Duration	Unknown

INTERACTIONS

Individual drugs

Clarithromycin, conivaptan, erythromycin, itraconazole, ketoconazole, lopinavir/ritonavir, nicardipine: increased rivaroxaban effect, possible bleeding

CarBAMazepine, phenytoin, rifampin, ritonavir: decreased rivaroxaban effect

Amiodarone, azithromycin, darunavir, diltiazem, dronedarone, felodipine, fluconazole, lapatinib, mifepristone, nelfinavir, pantoprazole, posaconazole, quiNIDine, ranolazine, saquinavir, tamoxifen, telithromycin, verapamil: increased rivaroxaban effect in renal impairment

Drug classifications

NSAIDs, other anticoagulants, platelet inhibitors, salicylates, thrombolytics: increased rivaroxaban effect, possible bleeding

Drug/herb

St. John's wort: decreased rivaroxaban effect

Drug/food

Grapefruit juice: increased rivaroxaban effect in renal disease
Food: decreased rivaroxaban effect

NURSING CONSIDERATIONS
Assessment

BLACK BOX WARNING: Bleeding: Monitor for bleeding, including bleeding during dental procedures, easy bruising, blood in urine, stools, emesis, sputum, epistaxis; there is no specific antidote

---

BLACK BOX WARNING: Abrupt discontinuation: Avoid the abrupt discontinuation unless an alternative anticoagulant is used in those with atrial fibrillation; discontinuing puts patients at increased risk for thrombotic events; if this product must be discontinued for reasons other than pathological bleeding, consider administering another anticoagulant

---

• **Pregnancy/breastfeeding:** pregnancy category C; identify if pregnancy is suspected or planned; pregnancy-related hemorrhage may occur, and anticoagulation cannot be monitored with standard laboratory testing; breastfeeding should be discontinued prior to use of this product

---

BLACK BOX WARNING: Epidural/spinal anesthesia: Epidural or spinal hematomas that may result in long-term/permanent paralysis may occur in patients who have received anticoagulants and are receiving neuraxial anesthesia or undergoing spinal puncture. The epidural catheter should not be removed <18 hr after the last dose of rivaroxaban; do not administer the next rivaroxaban dose <6 hr after the catheter removal; delay rivaroxaban administration for 24 hr if traumatic puncture occurs. Monitor for neuro changes

---

• **Hepatic/Renal disease:** Increase in effect of this product in hepatic disease (Child-Pugh Class B or C), hepatic disease with coagulopathy; renal failure/severe renal impairment (creatinine clearance <30 ml/min in DVT prophylaxis and <15 ml/min for stroke/systemic embolism prophylaxis in nonvalvular atrial fibrillation); product should be discontinued in acute renal failure; reduce dose in those with atrial fibrillation and CrCl 15-50 ml/min; monitor renal function periodically (creatinine clearance, BUN)

Patient/family education

• Advise patient to report if pregnancy is planned or suspected, not to breastfeed
• Teach patient to report bleeding (bruising, blood in urine, stools, sputum, emesis, heavy

---

menstrual flow) and to use soft toothbrush, electric shaver
• Advise patient to inform all health care providers of use
• Advise patient to avoid abrupt discontinuation without another blood thinner
• Instruct patients, especially those with dental disease, in proper oral hygiene, including caution in use of regular toothbrushes, dental floss, and toothpicks.

Evaluation
Positive therapeutic outcome
• Prevention of DVT, stroke and systemic embolism

---

rivastigmine (Rx)
(riv-as-tig′mine)
Exelon, Exelon Patch
Func. class.: Anti-Alzheimer's agent
Chem. class.: Cholinesterase inhibitor
Pregnancy category B

ACTION: Potent selective inhibitor of brain acetylcholinesterase (AChE) and butycholinerase (BChE)

Therapeutic outcome: Decreased signs and symptoms of Alzheimer's dementia

USES: Mild to severe Alzheimer's dementia, mild to moderate Parkinson's disease dementia (PDD)

CONTRAINDICATIONS:
Hypersensitivity to this product, other carbamates

Precautions: Pregnancy **B,** breastfeeding, children, renal/hepatic/respiratory disease, seizure disorder, asthma, urinary obstruction, peptic ulcer, increased intracranial pressure, surgery, GI bleeding, jaundice

DOSAGE AND ROUTES
Adult: PO 1.5 mg bid with food for 4 wk or more, may increase to 3 mg bid after 4 wk or more; may increase to 4.5 mg bid and thereafter 6 mg bid, max 12 mg/day; transdermal apply 4.6 mg/24 hr after 4 wk or more, may increase to 9.5 mg/24 hr; max 13.3 mg/24 hr; for those using 6-12 mg/day PO and switching to transdermal use one 9.5 mg/24 hr; for those using <6 mg/day PO and switching to transdermal use one 4.6 mg/24 hr

Available forms: Caps 1.5, 3, 4.5, 6 mg; sol 2 mg/ml; transdermal patch 4.6, 9.5 mg/24 hr

Implementation
• Give with meals; take with AM and PM meal even though absorption may be decreased
• Provide assistance with ambulation during beginning therapy
• Discontinue treatment for several doses and restart at same or next lower dosage level if adverse reactions cause intolerance
• If treatment is interrupted for longer than several days treatment should be initiated with the lowest daily dose and titrated as indicated above

Transdermal route
• Apply to clean, hairless, dry skin; not in an area that clothing will rub; rotate sites daily; remove liner; apply firmly; may be used during water activities; avoid saunas, avoid excess sunlight or external heat, each 5 cm^2 patch contains 9 mg base, rate of 4.6 mg/24 hr, each 10 cm^2 patch is 18 mg base, rate of 9.5 mg/24 hr

ADVERSE EFFECTS
CNS: *Tremors, confusion, insomnia,* psychosis, hallucination, depression, dizziness, headache, anxiety, somnolence, fatigue, syncope, EPS, exacerbation of Parkinson's disease
CV: QT prolongation, AV block, cardiac arrest, MI, angina, palpitations
GI: *Nausea, vomiting, anorexia, abdominal distress, flatulence,* diarrhea, constipation, dyspepsia, colitis, eructation, fecal incontinence, **GI bleeding/obstruction,** GERD, gastritis, **pancreatitis**
MISC: UTI, asthenia, increased sweating, hypertension, flulike symptoms, weight change

Pharmacokinetics	
Absorption	Rapidly, completely absorbed
Distribution	40% protein binding
Metabolism	To decarbamylated metabolite
Excretion	Kidney—metabolites, clearance lowered in geriatric, hepatic disease, increased nicotine use
Half-life	1½ hr

Pharmacodynamics	
Onset	Unknown
Peak	1 hr
Duration	Unknown

INTERACTIONS
Individual drugs
Nicotine: increased metabolism, decreased blood level of rivastigmine
Drug classifications
Anticholinergics, phenothiazines, sedating H_1 blockers, tricyclics: decreased rivastigmine effect

Cholinergic agonists, other cholinesterase inhibitors: increased synergistic effect

NSAIDs: increased GI effects

NURSING CONSIDERATIONS
Assessment
• Monitor liver function tests: AST, ALT, alkaline phosphatase, LDH, bilirubin, CBC
• Assess for severe GI effects: nausea, vomiting, anorexia, weight loss
• Monitor B/P, respiration during initial treatment; hypo/hypertension should be reported
• **Cognitive/mental status:** affect, mood, behavioral changes, depression; complete suicide assessment

Patient/family education
• Teach patient procedure for giving **oral sol**; use instruction sheet provided; teach application of **transdermal** product, to fold in half and discard, not to get in eyes, to wash hands after application, to not use heating pad, sauna, tanning bed
• Teach patient to notify prescriber of severe GI effects, do not discontinue abruptly
• Teach patient that product may cause dizziness, anorexia, weight loss

Evaluation
Positive therapeutic outcome
• Increased coherence, decreased symptoms of Alzheimer's disease, improved mood

rizatriptan (Rx)
(rye-zah-trip′tan)
Maxalt, Maxalt-MLT
Func. class.: Migraine agent
Chem. class.: 5-HT$_1$-like receptor agonist
Pregnancy category C

ACTION: Binds selectively to the vascular 5-HT$_{1B/1D}$ receptor subtype, exerts antimigraine effect; causes vasoconstriction in cranial arteries

Therapeutic outcome: After treatment, relief of migraine

USES: Acute treatment of migraine

CONTRAINDICATIONS:
Angina pectoris, history of MI, documented silent ischemia, Prinzmetal's angina, ischemic heart disease, concurrent ergotamine-containing preparations, uncontrolled hypertension, hypersensitivity, basilar or hemiplegic migraine

Precautions: Pregnancy C, breastfeeding, children, postmenopausal women, men >40 yr, geriatric, risk factors for CAD, hypercholesterolemia, obesity, diabetes, impaired renal/hepatic function

DOSAGE AND ROUTES
Adult: PO 5-10 mg single dose, redosing separate by 2 hr or more; max 30 mg/24 hr, use 5 mg in patient on propanolol; max 15 mg/24 hr

Available forms: Tabs (Maxalt) 5, 10 mg; orally disintegrating tabs (Maxalt-MLT) 5, 10 mg

Implementation
• Provide quiet, calm environment with decreased stimulation for noise, bright light, excessive talking
• Do not open blister pack until ready to use, put orally disintegrating tab on tongue to dissolve; swallow with saliva

ADVERSE EFFECTS
CNS: *Dizziness,* drowsiness, *headache, fatigue,* warm/cold sensation, flushing
CV: MI, ventricular fibrillation, ventricular tachycardia, coronary artery vasospasm, peripheral vascular ischemia, ECG changes
ENDO: Hot flashes, mild increase in growth hormone
GI: *Nausea,* dry mouth, diarrhea, abdominal pain, ischemic colitis
RESP: Chest tightness, pressure, dyspnea

Pharmacokinetics
Absorption	Unknown
Distribution	Unknown
Metabolism	Liver (metabolite)
Excretion	Urine/feces
Half-life	2-3 hr

Pharmacodynamics
Onset	10 min-2 hr
Peak	Unknown
Duration	Unknown

R

Adverse effects: *italics* = common; **bold** = life-threatening

INTERACTIONS
Individual drugs
Cimetidine, isocarboxazide, pargyline, phenelzine, propranolol, trancyclomine: increased rizatriptan action

Ergot: increased vasospastic effects

Sibutramine: increased levels of sibutramine

Drug classifications
Contraceptives (oral), MAOIs, MAOIs (nonselective types A and B): increased rizatriptan action

Ergot derivatives, 5-HT$_1$ receptor agonists: increased vasospastic effects

Selective serotonin reuptake inhibitors: increased weakness, hyperreflexia, incoordination

Drug/herb
St. John's wort: serotonin syndrome

NURSING CONSIDERATIONS
Assessment
• Assess for stress level, activity, recreation, coping mechanisms
• Assess neurologic status: LOC, blurring vision, nausea, vomiting, tingling in extremities preceding headache
• **Ingestion of tyramine-containing foods:** Monitor for pickled products, beer, wine, aged cheese, food additives, preservatives, colorings, artificial sweeteners, chocolate, caffeine, which may precipitate these types of headaches

Patient/family education
• **Teach patient use of orally disintegrating tab:** instruct patient not to open blister until use, to peel blister open with dry hands, to place tab on tongue, where it will dissolve, and to swallow with saliva (contains phenylalanine)
• Advise patient to report any side effects to prescriber
• Advise patient to use alternative contraception while taking product if oral contraceptives are being used
• Teach patient that product does not prevent or reduce number of migraines, main action is abortive, if first dose does not relieve pain, do not use more, notify prescriber

Evaluation
Positive therapeutic outcome
• Decrease in frequency, severity of headache

---

roflumilast
(roe-flue'mi-last)
Daliresp
Func. class.: Respiratory anti-inflammatory agent
Chem. class.: Phosphodiesterase-4 (PDE4) inhibitor
Pregnancy category C

ACTION: Roflumilast and the active metabolite (roflumilast N-oxide), selectively inhibit phosphodiesterase-4 (PDE4); not a bronchodilator; instead, inhibition of the PDE4 enzyme blocks the hydrolyses and inactivation of cyclic adenosine monophosphate (cAMP), resulting in intracellular cAMP accumulation; decreases inflammatory activity, PDE4 inhibition may affect migration and actions of pro-inflammatory cells (neutrophils, other leukocytes, T-lymphocytes, monocytes, macrophages, fibroblasts)

Therapeutic outcome: Decreasing exacerbations in COPD

USES: For the prevention of COPD exacerbations in those with severe chronic obstructive pulmonary disease (COPD) associated with chronic bronchitis and a history of exacerbations

CONTRAINDICATIONS:
Moderate to severe hepatic disease (Child-Pugh B or C)

Precautions: Pregnancy category C, breastfeeding, neonates, infants, children, and adolescents, acute bronchospasm, anxiety, insomnia, depression, and/or suicidal ideation or behavior

DOSAGE AND ROUTES
Adult: PO 500 mcg/day

Available forms: Tab 500 mcg

Implementation
PO route
• Give without regard to meals
• Store at room temperature

ADVERSE EFFECTS
CNS: Anxiety, depression, dizziness, headache, insomnia, suicidal ideation, tremor
EENT: Rhinitis, sinusitis
GI: Abdominal pain, anorexia, diarrhea, dyspepsia, gastritis, nausea, vomiting, weight loss
GU: Urinary tract infection

MS: Back pain, muscle cramps/spasm
SYST: Infections, influenza

Pharmacokinetics

Absorption	80%
Distribution	Protein binding 99%
Metabolism	Exclusively by CYP3A4, CYP1A2
Excretion	Unknown
Half-life	17 hr (parent); 30 hr (metabolite)

Pharmacodynamics

Onset	Unknown
Peak	1 hr (parent drug); 8 hrs (metabolite)
Duration	Unknown

INTERACTIONS

Drug classifications

CYP3A4 inducers (alcohol, barbiturates, bexarotene, bosentan, carBAMazepine, dexamethasone, erythromycin, etravirine, fluvoxaMINE, ketoconazole, metyrapone, modafinil, nevirapine, OXcarbazepine, PHENobarbital, phenytoin, rifabutin, rifampin, ritonavir: decreased roflumilast effect

CYP3A4/CYP1A2 inhibitors (cimetidine, dalfopristin, delavirdine, enoxacin, indinavir, isoniazid, itraconazole, quinupristin, tipranavir): increased roflumilast effect

Oral contraceptives (gestodene and ethinyl estradiol): increased roflumilast effect

Fosamprenavir: altered effect

Drug/herb

St. John's wort: decreased roflumilast effect

NURSING CONSIDERATIONS

Assessment

• Monitor lung sounds and respiratory function baseline and periodically thereafter
• Assess behavioral changes including mood, depression and suicidal thoughts/behaviors
• Monitor liver function tests baseline and periodically thereafter; if increases in liver function studies occur, product should be discontinued
• Monitor weight baseline and periodically, as weight loss is common

Patient/family education

• Advise patient to take product as directed, do not skip or double doses, take missed doses as soon as remembered unless almost time for next dose

• Teach patient not to use OTC or other products without prescriber approval; not to discontinue other respiratory products unless approved by prescriber
• Advise patient not to be used for acute bronchospasm, but may be continued during acute asthma attacks
• **Suicidal thoughts/behaviors: Instruct patient to notify prescriber of worsening depression or suicidal thoughts/behaviors**

Evaluation

Positive therapeutic outcome

• Decreasing exacerbations in COPD

romiPLOStim (Rx)

(roe-mi-ploe′stim)
Nplate
Func. class.: Hematopoietin
Chem. class.: Thrombopoietin receptor agonist
Pregnancy category C

ACTION: A thrombopoietin-like fusion protein produced by DNA recombinant technology

Therapeutic outcome: Increase in platelet counts, absence of bleeding

USES: Chronic idiopathic thrombocytopenic purpura in patients who have had an insufficient response to corticosteroids, immunoglobulins, or splenectomy

CONTRAINDICATIONS:

Hypersensitivity to this product or mannitol

Precautions: Pregnancy **C**, breastfeeding, malignancies, bleeding, bone marrow suppression, children

DOSAGE AND ROUTES

Thrombocytopenia in chronic idiopathic thrombocytopenic purpura (ITP) with insufficient response to corticosteroids, immunoglobulins, splenectomy

Adult: SUBCUT; initial dose is 1 mcg/kg SC qwk (based on actual body weight). Increase the weekly dose by 1 mcg/kg until the patient achieves a platelet count $\geq$50,000/mm^3; do not exceed a maximum weekly dose of 10 mcg/kg; use the lowest dose needed to achieve and maintain a platelet count $\geq$50,000/mm^3; monitor CBC, including platelet counts, qwk until a stable platelet count is achieved;

R

Adverse effects: *italics* = common; **bold** = life-threatening

platelets ≥50,000/mm³ ≥4 wk without dose adjustment; then, monitor the CBC, including platelet counts, monthly. Once a stable dose is achieved, if the platelet count falls to <50,000/mm³, increase the dose by 1 mcg/kg/wk. If the platelet count increases to >200,000/mm³ for 2 consecutive wk, reduce dose by 1 mcg/kg; if the platelet count is >400,000/mm³, temporarily stop romiplostim, and continue to monitor the platelet count weekly; once the platelets are <200,000/mm³, restart, but reduce the previous dose by 1 mcg/kg/wk. RomiPLOStim may be administered concomitantly with other medical ITP therapies. If platelet counts exceed 50,000/mm³, other medical ITP therapies may be reduced or discontinued. Discontinue romiPLOStim if the platelet count does not increase to avoid important bleeding after 4 wk of therapy at max dose of 10 mcg/kg

Available forms: Inj vials 250, 500 mcg

Implementation
• Store vials in refrigerator, do not freeze; protect from light; diluted sol is stable refrigerated or at room temperature for 24 hrs
SUBCUT route
• Use 0.01 ml graduations syringe
• Discard any unused portion in vial; do not pool unused portions from vials
• Dilute 250 mcg/0.72 preservative-free sterile water for inj; 500 mcg/1.2 preservative-free sterile water for inj; final concentration 500 mcg/ml
• Gently swirl until dissolved; do not shake
• Do not use if discolored or if particulate matter is present
• Inj into outer aspect of upper arm or abdomen except for 2 inches around navel or front aspect of middle thigh; do not use areas that are bruised, scratched, or scarred
• Rotate inj sites

ADVERSE EFFECTS
CNS: *Dizziness, insomnia, headache,* fatigue
GI: Abdominal pain, dyspepsia, diarrhea
HEMA: Thromboembolism, thrombosis, bleeding, myelofibrosis, erythromelalgia
MS: Myalgia
SYST: Secondary malignancy, antibody formation

Pharmacokinetics

Absorption	Unknown
Distribution	Unknown
Metabolism	Unknown
Excretion	Unknown
Half-life	Terminal 1-34 days

Pharmacodynamics

Onset	Unknown
Peak	7-50 hr
Duration	Unknown

INTERACTIONS
Drug classifications
Anticoagulants, NSAIDs, platelet inhibitors, thrombolytics, salicylates: possible risk of bleeding

NURSING CONSIDERATIONS
Assessment
⚠ Bone marrow suppression: If cytopenias occur, product should be discontinued; may use a bone marrow biopsy and straining for fibrosis
• **Thromboembolic disease:** Do not use to normalize patients, use only in those with thrombocytopenia in ITP, maintain platelets ≥50,000/mm³
• Assess blood studies: CBC during treatment weekly and for 2 wks after discontinuing

Patient/family education
• Instruct patient to report bleeding, to avoid hazardous activities that may cause bleeding
• Inform the patient the reason for product and expected results
• Advise patient to report a missed dose to prescriber due to increased risk of bleeding
• Teach patient that lab tests will be done qwk and dose may be changed; if dose is not changed lab will be checked qmo; after drug is discontinued, labs will be checked qwk × 2 wk
• Teach patient to advise prescriber if spleen has been removed: bleeding or clotting problems
⚠ Teach patient to notify prescriber if pregnancy is planned or suspected, pregnancy (C); if pregnancy occurs, call registry 1-877-675-2831

Evaluation
Positive therapeutic outcome
• Increase in platelet counts, absence of bleeding

---

rOPINIRole (Rx)
(roe-pin'e-role)
Requip, Requip XL
Func. class.: Antiparkinsonian agent
Chem. class.: Dopamine-receptor agonist, nonergot
Pregnancy category C

Do not confuse:
rOPINIRole/risperiDONE

ACTION: Selective agonist for DOPamine D_2 receptors (presynaptic/postsynaptic sites); binding at D_3 receptor contributes to antiparkinson effects

Therapeutic outcome: Decreased symptoms of Parkinson's disease (involuntary movements)

USES: Parkinsonism, restless legs syndrome

CONTRAINDICATIONS:
Hypersensitivity

Precautions: Pregnancy **C**, cardiac/renal/hepatic disease, dysrhythmias, affective disorders, psychosis

DOSAGE AND ROUTES
Parkinson's disease
Adult: **PO** (regular release) Initially, 0.25 mg PO tid × first wk; gradually titrate at weekly intervals; wk 2: give 0.5 mg tid; wk 3: 0.75 mg tid; wk 4; titrate to 1 mg tid; after wk 4, may increase by 1.5 mg/day wk, max 9 mg/day total dose, and then by 3 mg/day qwk, max 24 mg/day; PO (ext rel) Initially, 2 mg/day × 1-2 wk, may increase by mg/day at intervals ≥1 wk based upon response; max 24 mg/day. If significant interruption of therapy occurs, retitration may be necessary

For conversion from immediate-release to ext rel tablets
Oral dosage (ext rel tablets):
Adults currently on 0.75-2.25 mg/day: Give 2 mg/day ext rel
Adults currently on 3-4.5 mg/day: Give 4 mg/day ext rel
Adults currently on 6 mg/day: Give 6 mg/day ext rel
Adults currently on 7.5-9 mg/day: Give 8 mg/day ext rel
Adults currently on 12 mg/day: Give 12 mg/day ext rel
Adults currently on 15-18 mg/day: Give 16 mg/day ext rel
Adults currently on 21 mg/day: Give 20 mg/day ext rel
Adults currently on 24 mg/day: Give 24 mg/day ext rel

For the treatment of restless legs syndrome (RLS)
Adult: PO (reg rel) Initially, 0.25 mg/day, give 1-3 hr before bedtime; days 3-7, may increase to 0.5 mg/day; at the beginning of wk 2 (day 8) the dose may be increased to 1 mg/day × 1 wk; weeks 3-6, dose may be titrated up by 0.5 mg/wk (from 1.5-3 mg over the 5-wk period), as needed to achieve desired effect; wk 7, may increase dose to 4 mg/day; dose is titrated based on clinical response; give all doses 1-3 hr before bedtime

Available forms: Tabs 0.25, 0.5, 1, 2, 3, 4, 5 mg; ext rel tab 2, 4, 8, 12 mg

Implementation
• Give product until NPO before surgery
• Adjust dosage to patient's response
• Give with meals to decrease GI upset
• Test for diabetes mellitus, acromegaly if patient is receiving long-term therapy

ADVERSE EFFECTS
CNS: Dystonia, *agitation, insomnia,* dizziness, psychosis, hallucinations, depression, somnolence, **sleep attacks,** impulse-control disorders
CV: *Orthostatic hypotension,* hypotension, syncope, palpitations, **tachycardia,** hypertension
EENT: Blurred vision
GI: *Nausea, vomiting, anorexia, dry mouth,* constipation, dyspepsia, flatulence
GU: Impotence, urinary frequency
HEMA: **Hemolytic anemia, leukopenia, agranulocytosis**
INTEG: Rash, sweating
RESP: Pharyngitis, rhinitis, sinusitis, bronchitis, dyspnea

Pharmacokinetics	
Absorption	Well absorbed
Distribution	Widely distributed
Metabolism	Liver, extensively by the liver by CYP450 CYP1A2 enzyme system
Excretion	Kidneys
Half-life	6 hr

Pharmacodynamics

Unknown

INTERACTIONS
Individual drugs
Cimetidine, ciprofloxacin, digoxin, diltiazem, enoxacin, erythromycin, fluvoxamine, levodopa, mexiletine, norfloxacin, tacrine, theophylline: increased effect of rOPINIRole
Metoclopramide: decreased rOPINIRole effect

Drug classifications
Butyrophenones, phenothiazines, thioxanthenes: decreased ropinirole effect

NURSING CONSIDERATIONS
Assessment
• Monitor B/P, respiration during initial treatment; hypotension or hypertension should be reported
• Assess mental status: affect, mood, behavioral changes, depression; complete suicide assessment
• **Parkinsonism:** assess for akinesia, tremors, staggering gait, muscle rigidity, drooling; these symptoms should improve with therapy
⚠ **Sleep attacks: assess for drowsiness, falling asleep without warning even during hazardous activities**

Patient/family education
• Teach patient to notify prescriber if pregnancy is planned or suspected, pregnancy (C)
• Teach patient to take with food to prevent nausea
• Teach patient to report hallucinations, confusion (usually in geriatrics)
• Advise patient that therapeutic effects may take several wk to a few mo
• Caution patient to change positions slowly to prevent orthostatic hypotension
• Instruct patient to use product exactly as prescribed; if product is discontinued abruptly, parkinsonian crisis may occur
• Teach patient that drowsiness, sleeping attacks may occur, to avoid driving or other hazardous activities until response is known
• Teach patient to avoid alcohol and CNS depressants (cough and cold products)
• Teach patient to notify prescriber of unusual urges

Evaluation
Positive therapeutic outcome
• Decreased akathisia, other involuntary movements
• Increased mood

---

ropivacaine (Rx)
(roe-pi'va-kane)
Naropin
Func. class.: Local anesthetic
Chem. class.: Amide
Pregnancy category B

ACTION: Competes with calcium for sites in nerve membrane that control sodium transport across cell membrane; decreases rise of depolarization phase of action potential

Therapeutic outcome: Maintenance of local anesthesia

USES: Peripheral nerve block, caudal anesthesia, central neural block, vaginal, epidural, spinal block

CONTRAINDICATIONS:
Children <12 yr, geriatric, hypersensitivity to amide local anesthetics, severe liver disease, severe hypotension, complete heart block

Precautions: Pregnancy **B**, severe product allergies, hyperthyroidism, CV, hepatic/neurologic disease

DOSAGE AND ROUTES
Lumbar epidural block for C-section
Adult: 20-30 ml of 0.5% SOL, or 15-20 ml of 0.75% SOL

Thoracic epidural
Adult: 5-15 ml of 0.5%-0.75% SOL

Major nerve block
Adult: 35-50 ml of 0.5% SOL or 10-40 ml of 0.75% SOL

Labor pain epidural
Adult: 10-20 ml of 0.2% SOL, then 6-14 ml/hr

Postoperative (lumbar/thoracic epidural)
Adult: 6-14 ml/hr of 0.2% SOL

Infiltration/minor nerve block
Adult: 1-100 ml of 0.2% SOL or 1-40 ml of 0.5% SOL

Available forms: Inj 2, 5, 7.5 mg/ml

Implementation
• Give only with resuscitative equipment nearby
• Give only products without preservatives for epidural or caudal anesthesia
• Use new sol; discard unused portions

ADVERSE EFFECTS
CNS: Anxiety, restlessness, **seizures, loss of consciousness,** drowsiness, disorientation, tremors, shivering, paresthesia
CV: Myocardial depression, cardiac arrest, dysrhythmias, bradycardia, *hypo*/hypertension, **fetal bradycardia**
EENT: Blurred vision, tinnitus, pupil constriction
ENDO: Hypokalemia
GI: Nausea, vomiting
GU: Urinary retention
INTEG: Rash, urticaria, allergic reactions, edema, burning, skin discoloration at injection site, tissue necrosis

---

RESP: Status asthmaticus, respiratory arrest, anaphylaxis

Pharmacokinetics

Absorption	Complete
Distribution	Unknown
Metabolism	Liver
Excretion	Kidneys
Half-life	Unknown

Pharmacodynamics

Onset	2-8 min
Peak	Unknown
Duration	3 hr, varies with inj site

INTERACTIONS
Individual drugs
Amiodarone, cimetidine, ciprofloxacin, fluvox-aMINE, imipramine, theophylline: increased effect

Chloroprocaine: decreased action of ropivacaine

Enflurane, EPINEPHrine, halothane: increased dysrhythmias

Drug classifications
Antidepressants (tricyclics), MAOIs, phenothi-azines: increased hypertension

Azole antifungals: increased effect

NURSING CONSIDERATIONS
Assessment
• Assess B/P, pulse, respiration during treatment
• Assess fetal heart tones during labor
• Assess allergic reactions: rash, urticaria, itching
• Assess cardiac status: ECG for dysrhythmias, pulse, B/P during anesthesia

Evaluation
Positive therapeutic outcome
• Anesthesia necessary for procedure

TREATMENT OF OVERDOSE:
Airway, O₂, vasopressor, **IV** fluids, anticonvulsants for seizures

---

rosiglitazone (Rx)
(rose-i-glye′ta-zone)
Avandia
Func. class.: Antidiabetic, oral
Chem. class.: Thiazolidinedione
Pregnancy category C

ACTION: Improves insulin resistance by hepatic glucose metabolism, insulin receptor kinase activity, insulin receptor phosphorylation

Therapeutic outcome: Decreased symptoms of diabetes mellitus

USES: Stable type 2 diabetes mellitus alone or in combination with sulfonylureas, metformin, or insulin

CONTRAINDICATIONS:
Breastfeeding, children, hypersensitivity to thia-zolidinediones, diabetic ketoacidosis, jaundice, type 1 diabetes

> **BLACK BOX WARNING:** NYHA III or IV acute heart failure, heart failure

Precautions: Pregnancy C, geriatric, thy-roid/renal/hepatic disease, heart failure, NYHA class I, II

> **BLACK BOX WARNING:** MI

DOSAGE AND ROUTES
Adult: PO 4 mg/day or in 2 divided doses, may increase to 8 mg/day or in 2 divided doses after 12 wk; may be added to metformin, sulfonyl-ureas at the adult dose

Available forms: Tabs 2, 4, 8 mg

Implementation
• Convert from other oral hypoglycemic agents if needed; change may be made without gradual dosage change; monitor blood glucose during conversion
• Give tabs crushed and mixed with meal or fluids for patients with difficulty swallowing
PO route
• Give once or in 2 divided doses without regard to food
• Store in airtight container in cool environment
• **Available only through the REMS Program 1-800-Avandia**

ADVERSE EFFECTS
CNS: Fatigue, *headache*
CV: CHF, MI, death (geriatric patients)
ENDO: Hyper/hypoglycemia
GI: Weight gain, **hepatotoxicity,** increased total cholesterol, LDL, HDL, decreased free fatty acids
MISC: Accidental injury, upper respiratory tract infection, sinusitis, anemia, back pain, diarrhea, edema, bone fractures (female), pulmonary/macular/peripheral edema
SYST: Anaphylaxis, Stevens-Johnson syndrome, lactic acidosis

Adverse effects: *italics* = common; **bold** = life-threatening

R

Pharmacokinetics

Absorption	Unknown
Distribution	Protein binding 99.8%
Metabolism	Unknown
Excretion	Urine, feces, breast milk
Half-life	Elimination 3-4 hr

Pharmacodynamics

Onset	Unknown
Peak	6-12 wk
Duration	Unknown

INTERACTIONS

Individual drugs
FluvoxaMINE, gemfibrozil, ketoconazole: increased hypoglycemia; monitor glucose
Insulin: avoid concurrent use

Drug classifications
CYP2C5 inducers/inhibitors: may increase/decrease effect
Nitrates: avoid concurrent use

Drug/herb
Horse chestnut: increased antidiabetic effect

Drug/lab test
Increased: ALT, HDL, LDL, total cholesterol, blood glucose
Decreased: Hgb/Hct

NURSING CONSIDERATIONS

Assessment

> **BLACK BOX WARNING:** Use in NYHA III or IV acute heart failure is contraindicated; any deterioration in any cardiac status, discontinue product

> **BLACK BOX WARNING: CHF/MI:** assess for dyspnea, edema, weight gain ≥5 lb, jugular vein distention; may need to change or discontinue; do not use in acute coronary syndrome

• **Lactic acidosis:** assess for dyspnea, abdominal pain, muscle pain; notify prescriber immediately
• Assess for hypoglycemic reactions (sweating, weakness, dizziness, anxiety, tremors, hunger), hyperglycemic reactions soon after meals
• **Assess for systemic reactions:** anaphylaxis, Stevens-Johnson syndrome
• **Hepatotoxicity:** check liver function tests periodically; AST, FBS, ALT (if ALT is >2.5 × ULN, do not use), HbA$_{2c}$, plasma lipids, lipoproteins, B/P, body weight during treatment

Patient/family education
• Teach patient that in order to use product, provider/patient must be enrolled in the Avandia-Rosiglitazone Access Program
• Teach patient to monitor capillary blood glucose test, that periodic liver function tests are mandatory; to report edema, weight gain
• Teach patient symptoms of hypo/hyperglycemia, what to do about each
• Advise patient that product must be continued on daily basis; explain consequence of discontinuing product abruptly
• Advise patient to avoid OTC medications, nitrates, insulin, or herbal preparations unless approved by prescriber
• Advise patient that diabetes is lifelong illness; that this product is not a cure, only controls symptoms
• Advise patient that all food included in diet plan must be eaten to prevent hypoglycemia
• Advise patient to carry/wear emergency ID and glucagon emergency kit for emergencies
• Instruct patient to notify prescriber if oral contraceptives are used
• Teach patient not to use if breastfeeding; may be secreted in breast milk
• **Hepatotoxicity:** advise patient to report nausea, vomiting, abdominal pain, fatigue, anorexia, dark urine, jaundice
• Teach patient that 2 wk is needed to see a reduction in blood glucose, 2-3 mo to see full effect

Evaluation
Positive therapeutic outcome
• Decrease in polyuria, polydipsia, polyphagia; clear sensorium; absence of dizziness; stable gait; blood glucose, A1c improvement

---

rosuvastatin (Rx)
(roe-soo′va-sta-tin)
Crestor
Func. class.: Antilipemic
Chem. class.: HMG-CoA reductase inhibitor
Pregnancy category X

ACTION: Inhibits HMG-CoA reductase, which reduces cholesterol synthesis

Therapeutic outcome: Decreasing cholesterol levels

USES: As an adjunct in primary hypercholesterolemia (types IIa, IIb), mixed dyslipidemia elevated serum triglycerides, homozygous/heterozygous familial hypercholesterolemia (FH),

---

slowing of atherosclerosis, CV disease prophylaxis, MI, stroke prophylaxis (normal LDL)

CONTRAINDICATIONS:
Pregnancy **X**, breastfeeding, hypersensitivity, active liver disease

Precautions: Children <10 yr, geriatric, past liver disease, alcoholism, severe acute infections, trauma, hypotension, uncontrolled seizure disorders, severe metabolic disorders, electrolyte imbalances, severe renal impairment, hypothyroidism, Asian patients

DOSAGE AND ROUTES
Patient should first be placed on a cholesterol-lowering diet

Hypercholesterolemia
Adult: PO 5-40 mg/day; initial dose 10 mg/day, reanalyze lipid levels at 2-4 wk and adjust dosage accordingly

Homozygous FH
Adult: PO 20 mg/day, max 40 mg; Asian patients 5 mg/day

Dose in patients taking cycloSPO-RINE/gemfibrozil/lopinavir/ritonavir/atazanavir
Adult: 5 mg/day, max 10 mg/day

Heterozygous familial hypercholesterolemia
Females ≥1 yr post-menarche and ≥10 yr and males ≥10 yr: PO 5-20 mg/day individualized

Asian patients/predisposition for myopathy
Adult: PO 5 mg/day

Atherosclerosis slowing
Adult: PO 10 mg/day (for those not taking cycloSPORINE or gemfibrozil)

Renal/hepatic dose
Adult: PO CCr <30 ml/min 5 mg daily; max 10 mg daily; avoid use in hepatic disease

Available forms: Tabs 5, 10, 20, 40 mg

Implementation
• May be taken at any time of day, with or without food
• Store in cool environment in airtight, light-resistant container

ADVERSE EFFECTS
CNS: *Headache, dizziness,* insomnia, paresthesia, confusion

GI: *Nausea, constipation, abdominal pain, flatus, diarrhea, dyspepsia, heartburn,* **kidney failure, liver dysfunction,** vomiting
HEMA: Thrombocytopenia, hemolytic anemia, leukopenia
INTEG: *Rash, pruritus*
MS: *Asthenia, muscle cramps, arthritis, arthralgia, myalgia,* **myositis, rhabdomyolysis,** leg, shoulder, or localized pain
RESP: Rhinitis, sinusitis, *pharyngitis,* increased cough

Pharmacokinetics

Absorption	Unknown
Distribution	88% protein bound, crosses placenta
Metabolism	Minimal liver metabolism (about 10%)
Excretion	Primarily in feces (90%)
Half-life	19 hr

Pharmacodynamics

Onset	Unknown
Peak	3-5 hr
Duration	Unknown

INTERACTIONS
Individual drugs
Alcohol: increased hepatotoxicity
Clofibrate, cycloSPORINE, gemfibrozil, niacin: increased myalgia, myositis
Warfarin: increased bleeding

Drug classifications
Antifungals (azole), anti-retroviral protease inhibitors, fibric acid derivatives: increased myalgia, myositis
Bile acid sequestrants: increased effects

Drug/herb
St. John's wort: decreased rosuvastatin effect

Drug/lab test
Increased: CPK, liver function tests

NURSING CONSIDERATIONS
Assessment
• Assess diet: obtain diet history including fat, cholesterol in diet
• Monitor fasting cholesterol, LDL, HDL, triglycerides periodically during treatment
• Liver function: monitor liver function tests q1-2mo during the first 1½ yr of treatment; AST, ALT, liver function tests may increase
• Monitor renal function in patients with compromised renal system: BUN, creatinine, I&O ratio

R

• Obtain ophthalmic exam before, 1 mo after treatment begins, annually; lens opacities may occur

⚠ **Rhabdomyolysis: Assess for muscle pain, tenderness, obtain CPK; if these occur, product may need to be discontinued; for Asian ancestry: increased blood levels, rhabdomyolysis**

Patient/family education

• Advise to report suspected pregnancy, to use contraception while taking this product, pregnancy category **X**, not to breastfeed
• Advise that blood work and ophthalmic exam will be necessary during treatment
• Teach to report blurred vision, severe GI symptoms, dizziness, headache, muscle pain, weakness
• Teach that previously prescribed regimen will continue: low-cholesterol diet, exercise program, smoking cessation; liver injury (jaundice, anorexia, abdominal pain)

Evaluation

Positive therapeutic outcome
• Cholesterol at desired level after 8 wk

---

rufinamide (Rx)
(roo-fin′a-mide)
Banzel
Func. class.: Anticonvulsant
Chem. class.: Triazole derivative
Pregnancy category C

ACTION: May act through action at sodium channels; exact action is unknown

Therapeutic outcome: Decrease in severity of seizures

USES: Lennox-Gastaut syndrome

CONTRAINDICATIONS:
Hypersensitivity, familial short QT syndrome

Precautions: Pregnancy **C**, breastfeeding, renal/hepatic disease, geriatric patients, child <16 yr, depression, dialysis, hazardous activities, suicidal ideation

DOSAGE AND ROUTES
Adult: PO 400-800 mg/day divided bid, increase by 400-800 mg/day q2day to 3200 mg/day
Child ≥4 yr: PO 10 mg/kg/day divided equally bid; increase by 10 mg/kg/day every other day to 45 mg/kg/day or 3200 mg/day, whichever is less

Available forms: Tabs 200, 400 mg; oral susp 40 mg/ml

Implementation
• **PO tabs:** Give with food, may give whole, crushed, or halved
• **Oral susp:** Shake well before use, use provided adapter and calibrated oral dosing syringe, insert adapter firmly in neck of bottle before use and keep in place for the duration of bottle use, insert dosing syringe into the adapter and withdraw dose from inverted bottle, replace cap after each use, use within 90 days of opening, give with food

ADVERSE EFFECTS

CNS: Dizziness, ataxia, drowsiness, fever, seizures, tremor, fatigue, headache, gait disturbance
EENT: Diplopia, blurred vision, nystagmus
GI: Nausea, hepatitis, vomiting
HEMA: Anemia, leukopenia, neutropenia, thrombocytopenia, lymphadenopathy
INTEG: Rash, urticaria
MISC: Edema, hematuria, influenzae, nephrolithiasis

Pharmacokinetics

Absorption	Unknown
Distribution	Unknown
Metabolism	Liver
Excretion	Kidneys
Half-life	Terminal 6-10 hr

Pharmacodynamics

Onset	Unknown
Peak	4-6 hr
Duration	Unknown

INTERACTIONS

Individual drugs
CarBAMazepine, PHENobarbital, phenytoin, primidone: decreased effect of rufinamide
Valproate: increased rufinamide effect

Drug classifications
Hormonal contraceptives: decreased effect

Drug/lab test
Increased: LFTs

NURSING CONSIDERATIONS

Assessment
• **Seizures:** Assess for duration, type, intensity precipitating factors

---

⚠ Assess mental status: mood, sensorium, affect, memory (long, short), increased suicidal thoughts/actions

Patient/family education
• Caution patient not to discontinue product abruptly; seizures may occur
• Advise patient to avoid hazardous activities until stabilized on product
• Instruct patient to carry emergency ID stating product use
• Instruct patient to notify prescriber if pregnancy is planned or suspected, to use alternative form of contraception; hormonal contraceptives may be decreased
• Inform patient to take adequate fluids

Evaluation
Positive therapeutic outcome
• Decrease in severity of seizures

R

Adverse effects: *italics* = common; **bold** = life-threatening

salicylic acid topical
See Appendix B

salmeterol (Rx)
(sal-met′er-ole)
Serevent, Serevent Diskus
Func. class.: Adrenergic β$_2$ agonist,
bronchodilator
Pregnancy category C

ACTION: Causes bronchodilatation by
action on β$_2$ (pulmonary) receptors by increasing levels of cyclic AMP, which relaxes smooth
muscle; with very little effect on heart rate,
maintains improvement in FEV from 3 to 12 hr;
prevents nocturnal asthma symptoms

Therapeutic outcome: Ease of breathing

USES: Prevention of exercise-induced
asthma, bronchospasm, COPD

CONTRAINDICATIONS:
Hypersensitivity to sympathomimetics, tachydysrhythmias, severe cardiac disease, monotherapy
treatment of asthma

Precautions: Pregnancy **C,** breastfeeding,
cardiac disorders, hyperthyroidism, diabetes
mellitus, hypertension, prostatic hypertrophy,
closed-angle glaucoma, seizures, acute asthma,
as a substitute for corticosteroids, QT prolongation

> **BLACK BOX WARNING:** Asthma-related
> death, children <4 yr

DOSAGE AND ROUTES
Adult/child ≥4 yr: INH 50 mcg (one inhalation as dry powder); exercise-induced bronchospasm: 50 mcg (2 INH) ½-1 hr prior to exercise

Available forms: Inhalation powder 50
mcg/blister

Implementation
• Shake aerosol container, ask patient to
exhale, then place mouthpiece in mouth, inhale
slowly, hold breath, remove, exhale slowly; allow
at least 1 min between inhalations
• Use this medication before other medications
and allow at least 1 min between each
• Use spacing device for pediatric/geriatric
patients
• Store in foil pouch; do not expose to temp
>86° F (30° C); discard 6 wk after removal
from foil pouch

• Use 1 hr prior to exercise for exercise-
induced bronchospasm prevention

ADVERSE EFFECTS
CNS: *Tremors, anxiety,* insomnia, headache,
dizziness, fever
CV: Palpitations, **tachycardia**, angina, hypo/
hypertension, **dysrhythmias**
EENT: Dry nose, irritation of nose and throat
GI: Heartburn, nausea, vomiting, abdominal
pain
MS: Muscle cramps
RESP: Bronchospasm, cough

Pharmacokinetics
Unknown

Pharmacodynamics
Onset	5-15 min
Peak	4 hr
Duration	12 hr

INTERACTIONS
Drug classifications
Antidepressants (tricyclics): increased salme-
terol action
β-Adrenergic blockers: block therapeutic effect
Bronchodilators, aerosol: increased action of
bronchodilator
CYP3A4 inhibitors (itraconazole, ketoconazole,
nelfinavir, nefazodone, saquinavir): increased
CV effects
MAOIs: increased action of salmeterol

Drug/herb
Betel palm, butterbur, coffee, cola nut, figwort,
fumitory, guarana, hawthorn, lily of the valley,
motherwort, plantain, tea (black, green),
yerba maté: increased stimulation

NURSING CONSIDERATIONS
Assessment
• **Respiratory function:** assess vital capacity,
FEV, ABGs, lung sounds, heart rate, rhythm
(baseline)
• **Paradoxical bronchospasm:** monitor for
dyspnea, wheezing, chest tightness

> **BLACK BOX WARNING:** Children should not
> use this product as monotherapy for asthma;
> use only with persistent asthma in those
> that are not well-controlled with a long-term
> asthma product

Patient/family education
• Caution patient not to use OTC medications
because extra stimulation may occur

• Instruct patient to use this medication before other medications and to allow at least 1 min between each, to prevent overstimulation

• Teach patient how to use inhaler; to avoid getting aerosol in eyes; blurring may result; to wash inhaler in warm water daily and dry; to avoid smoking, smoke-filled rooms, and persons with respiratory infections; review package insert with patient

• Instruct patient on administration of dose, not to use more than prescribed; serious side effects may occur

• Teach patient not to use for exercise-induced bronchospasm, never exhale into diskus, hold level, keep mouthpiece dry

• Teach patient not to use for treatment of acute exacerbation, a fast-acting β-blocker should be used instead

• Teach patient to report immediately dyspnea after use, if 1 canister or more is used in 2 mo time

Evaluation

Positive therapeutic outcome
• Absence of dyspnea, wheezing
• Improved airway exchange
• Improved ABGs

TREATMENT OF OVERDOSE:
Administer a β$_2$-adrenergic blocker

sargramostim (Rx)
(sar-gram′oh-stim)
Leukine, rhu GM-CSF
Func. class.: Biological modifier: cytokine
Chem. class.: Granulocyte-macrophage colony-stimulating factor (GM-CSF)
Pregnancy category C

Do not confuse:
Leukine/leucovorin/Leukeran

ACTION: Stimulates proliferation and differentiation of hematopoietic progenitor cells (granulocyte, macrophage)

Therapeutic outcome: WBC and differential recovery

USES: Acceleration of myeloid recovery in patients with non-Hodgkin's lymphoma, acute lymphoblastic leukemia, acute myelogenous leukemia, autologous bone marrow transplantation in Hodgkin's disease; bone marrow transplantation failure or engraftment delay; mobilization and transplant of peripheral blood progenitor cells (PBPCs)

Unlabeled uses: Aplastic anemia, Crohn's disease, ganciclovir- or zidovudine-induced neutropenia

CONTRAINDICATIONS:
Hypersensitivity to GM-CSF, benzyl alcohol, yeast products; excessive leukemic myeloid blast in the bone marrow or peripheral blood, neonates

Precautions: Pregnancy **C**, breastfeeding, children, renal/hepatic/lung/cardiac disease, pleural/pericardial effusions, peripheral edema, leukocytosis, mannitol hypersensitivity, hepatic/renal disease

DOSAGE AND ROUTES
Myeloid reconstitution after autologous bone marrow transplantation
Adult: IV 250 mcg/m²/day × 3 wk; give over 2 hr, begin 2-4 hr after bone marrow INF, and not less than 24 hr after last dose of antineoplastics and 12 hr after last dose of radiotherapy, bone marrow transplantation failure, or engraftment delay

Acceleration of myeloid recovery
Adult: IV 250 mcg/m²/day × 14 days; give over 2 hr; may repeat in 7 days, may repeat 500 mcg/m²/day × 14 days after another 7 days if no improvement

Mobilization of PBPCs
Adult: IV/SUBCUT 250 mcg/m²/day during collection of PBPCs

After PBPC transplantation
Adult: IV/SUBCUT 250 mcg/m²/day until ANC >1500/mm³ × 3 days

Available forms: Powder for inj lyophilized 250 mcg; solution for injection 500 mcg/ml

Implementation
• Store in refrigerator; do not freeze
SUBCUT route
• No further dilution of reconstituted sol is needed; take care not to inject intradermally

Intermittent IV infusion route
• After reconstituting with 1 ml sterile water for inj without preservative; do not reenter vial; discard unused portion; direct reconstitution sol at side of vial; rotate contents, do not shake
• Dilute in 0.9% NaCl inj to prepare IV inf; if final concentration is <10 mcg/ml, add human albumin to make a final concentration of 0.1% to NaCl before adding sargramostim to prevent adsorption; for a final concentration of

0.1% albumin, add 1 mg human albumin/1 ml 0.9% NaCl inj run over 2 hr **(bone marrow transplant or failure of graft)**; over 4 hr **(chemotherapy for AML)**; over 24 hr as cont inf **(PBPCs)**; give within 6 hr after reconstitution

Y-site compatibilities: Amikacin, aminophylline, aztreonam, bleomycin, butorphanol, calcium gluconate, CARBOplatin, carmustine, ceFAZolin, cefepime, cefotaxime, cefoTEtan, ceftizoxime, cefTRIAXone, cefuroxime, cimetidine, CISplatin, clindamycin, cyclophosphamide, cycloSPORINE, cytarabine, dacarbazine, DACTINomycin, dexamethasone, diphenhydrAMINE, DOPamine, DOXOrubicin, doxycycline, droperidol, etoposide, famotidine, fentaNYL, floxuridine, fluconazole, fluorouracil, furosemide, gentamicin, granisetron, heparin, IDArubicin, ifosfamide, immune globulin, magnesium sulfate, mannitol, mechlorethamine, meperidine, mesna, methotrexate, metoclopramide, metroNIDAZOLE, minocycline, mitoXANtrone, netilmicin, pentostatin, piperacillin/tazobactam, potassium chloride, prochlorperazine, promethazine, ranitidine, teniposide, ticarcillin, ticarcillin-clavulanate, trimethoprim-sulfamethoxazole, vinBLAStine, vinCRIStine, zidovudine

Y-site incompatibilities: Acyclovir, ampicillin, ampicillin/sulbactam, cefonicid, cefoperazone, cefTAZidime, chlorproMAZINE, ganciclovir, haloperidol, hydrocortisone, HYDROmorphone, hydrOXYzine, IDArubicin, imipenem/cilastatin, LORazepam, methylPREDNISolone sodium succinate, mitoMYcin, morphine, nalbuphine, ondansetron, piperacillin, sodium bicarbonate, tobramycin

ADVERSE EFFECTS
CNS: Fever, malaise, CNS disorder, weakness, chills, dizziness, syncope, headache
CV: **Transient supraventricular tachycardia**, peripheral edema, **pericardial effusion**, hypotension, tachycardia
GI: Nausea, vomiting, diarrhea, anorexia, **GI hemorrhage**, stomatitis, **liver damage**, hyperbilirubinemia
GU: Urinary tract disorder, abnormal kidney function
HEMA: Blood dyscrasias, **hemorrhage**
INTEG: Alopecia, rash, peripheral edema
MS: Bone pain, myalgia
RESP: Dyspnea

Pharmacokinetics
Absorption	Completely absorbed
Distribution	Unknown
Metabolism	Unknown
Excretion	Unknown
Half-life	Elimination **IV** 60 min; SUBCUT 2-3 hr

Pharmacodynamics
Onset	Rapid
Peak	2 hr
Duration	Unknown

INTERACTIONS
Individual drugs
Lithium: increased myeloproliferation

Drug classifications
Antineoplastics or radiation, separate by ≥24 hr
Corticosteroids: increased myeloproliferation

Drug/lab test
Increased: bilirubin, BUN, creatinine, eosinophils, LFTs, leukocytes

NURSING CONSIDERATIONS
Assessment
• Monitor blood studies: CBC, differential count before treatment and twice weekly; leukocytosis may occur (WBC >50,000 cells/mm³, ANC >20,000 cells/mm³), platelets; if ANC >20,000/mm³ or 10,000/mm³ after nadir has occurred or platelets >500,000/mm³, reduce dose by ½ or discontinue; if blast cells occur, discontinue
• Monitor renal/liver function tests before treatment: BUN, creatinine, urinalysis; AST, ALT, alkaline phosphatase; monitoring is needed twice a week in renal/hepatic disease
⚠ **Gasping syndrome in neonates: assess for, due to benzyl alcohol hypersensitivity**
• Assess for **hypersensitivity reactions**/rashes and local inj site reactions; usually transient
• Assess for increased fluid retention in cardiac disease, body weight, hydration status, pulmonary function
• Constitutional symptoms: asthenia, chills, fever, headache, malaise
• Assess for myalgia, arthralgia in legs, feet; use analgesics, antipyretics

Patient/family education
• Teach patient reason for medication and expected results
• Advise patient to notify nurse or prescriber of dyspnea
• Review all aspects of product use

⚠ Nurse Alert　　　★ Key NCLEX® Drug

Evaluation
Positive therapeutic outcome
- WBC and differential recovery
- Absence of infection

saxagliptin (Rx)
(sax-a-glip'tin)
Onglyza
Func. class.: Antidiabetic, oral
Chem. class.: Dipeptidyl-peptidase-4
(DPP-4) inhibitor
Pregnancy category C

Do not confuse:
saxagliptin/sitaGLIPtin

ACTION: Slows the inactivation of incretin hormones, improves glucose homeostasis, improves glucose-dependent insulin synthesis, lowers glucagon secretions and slows gastric emptying time

Therapeutic outcome: Decrease in polyuria, polydipsia, polyphagia; clear sensorium; absence of dizziness; stable gait; blood glucose at normal level

USES: Type 2 diabetes mellitus as monotherapy or in combination with other antidiabetic agents

CONTRAINDICATIONS:
Hypersensitivity, angioedema

Precautions: Pregnancy **B**, geriatric, GI obstruction, thyroid disease, surgery, renal/hepatic disease, trauma, diabetic ketoacidosis (DKA), type 1 diabetes mellitus

DOSAGE AND ROUTES
Adult: PO 2.5-5 mg; may use with other antidiabetic agents (metformin, pioglitazone, rosiglitazone), if used with insulin, a lower dose is needed; max 2.5 mg with strong 3A415 inhibitors

Renal dose
Adult: PO CCr ≤50 ml/min 2.5 mg/day

Available forms: Tabs 2.5; 5 mg

Implementation
PO route
- May be taken with or without food
- Conversion from other antidiabetic agents; change may be made with gradual dosage change
- Store in tight container at room temperature

ADVERSE EFFECTS
CNS: *Headache*
ENDO: Hypoglycemia (renal impairment)
GI: *Nausea, vomiting,* abdominal pain, pancreatitis
INTEG: Urticaria, **angioedema,** anaphylaxis
MISC: Lymphopenia, peripheral edema

Pharmacokinetics
Absorption	Rapidly
Distribution	Unknown
Metabolism	Unknown
Excretion	Kidneys 24% unchanged
Half-life	Terminal 2.5 hr, 3.1 hr metabolite

Pharmacodynamics
Onset	Unknown
Peak	1-4 hr
Duration	24 hr

INTERACTIONS
Individual drugs
Aripiprazole, cloZAPine, fosphenytoin, OLANZapine, phenytoin, QUEtiapine, risperiDONE, ziprasidone: decreased antidiabetic effect
Cimetidine, disopyramide: increased saxagliptin level
Cimetidine, FLUoxetine: increased hypoglycemia
Digoxin: increased levels of digoxin

Drug classifications
ACE inhibitors, estrogens, oral contraceptives, phenothiazines, progestins, protease inhibitors, sympathomimetics, thiazide diuretics: decreased antidiabetic effect
Androgens, β-blockers, corticosteroids, fibric acid derivatives, insulins, MAOIs, salicylates: increased hypoglycemia

Drug/herb
Garlic, horse chestnut: increased antidiabetic effect

Drug/lab test
Decreased: lymphocytes, glucose

NURSING CONSIDERATIONS
Assessment
- **Hypoglycemic reactions** (sweating, weakness, dizziness, anxiety, tremors, hunger); monitor blood glucose (BG) as needed
- Monitor CBC (baseline, q3mo) during treatment; check liver function tests periodically, AST, LDH, renal studies: BUN, creatinine during treatment; glycosylated hemoglobin HbA1c

S

Adverse effects: *italics* = common; **bold** = life-threatening

Patient/family education
• Teach patient to use regular self-monitoring of blood glucose using blood glucose meter
• Teach patient the symptoms of hypo/hyperglycemia; what to do about each
• Teach patient that product must be continued on daily basis; explain consequence of discontinuing product abruptly
• Advise patient to avoid OTC medications, alcohol, digoxin, exenatide, insulins, nateglinide, repaglinide, and other products that lower blood sugar, unless approved by prescriber
• Teach patient that diabetes is a lifelong illness; that this product is not a cure, only controls symptoms
• Teach patient that all food included in diet plan must be eaten to prevent hypo/hyperglycemia
• Teach patient to carry emergency ID
• Teach patient to take product without regard to food
• Teach patient to notify prescriber when surgery, trauma, or stress occurs, as dose may need to be adjusted

Evaluation
Positive therapeutic outcome
• Decrease in polyuria, polydipsia, polyphagia; clear sensorium; absence of dizziness; stable gait; blood glucose at normal level

scopolamine (Rx)
(skoe-pol′a-meen)
Maldemar, Scopace, Transderm-Scop
Func. class.: Cholinergic blocker
Chem. class.: Belladonna alkaloid
Pregnancy category C

ACTION: Inhibits acetylcholine at receptor sites in autonomic nervous system, which controls secretions, free acids in stomach; blocks central muscarinic receptors, which decreases involuntary movements

Therapeutic outcome: Absence of vomiting, secretions (preoperatively), involuntary movements

USES: Reduction of secretions before surgery, production of amnesia, prevention of motion sickness, Parkinson's symptoms

Unlabeled uses: Drooling (TD)

CONTRAINDICATIONS:
Hypersensitivity, closed-angle glaucoma, myasthenia gravis, GI/GU obstruction, hypersensitivity to belladonna, barbiturates

Precautions: Pregnancy **C**, breastfeeding, children, geriatric, prostatic hypertrophy, CHF, hypertension, dysrhythmias, gastric ulcer, renal/hepatic disease, hiatal hernia, GERD, ulcerative colitis, hyperthyroidism

DOSAGE AND ROUTES
Prevention of motion sickness
Adult: Transdermal 1 patch placed behind ear 4 hr before travel, reapply q3day

Parkinson's symptoms
Adult: PO 0.4-0.8 mg q8hr

Preoperatively
Adult: IM/IV/SUBCUT 0.32-0.65 mg; TD apply 1 patch PM before surgery or 1 hr before C-section

Nausea and vomiting
Adult: SUBCUT 0.6-1 mg
Child: SUBCUT 0.006 mg/kg; max 0.3 mg/dose

Drooling (unlabeled)
Adult: Transdermal 1.5 mg patch q3day

Available forms: Patch 1.5 mg delivered in 72 hr; 0.4 mg/ml

Implementation
Transdermal route
• Instruct patient to wash, dry hands before and after applying to surface behind ear; to change patch q72hr; to apply at least 4 hr before traveling
• Store at room temperature in light-resistant container

IM/SUBCUT/IV route
• Administer parenteral dose with patient recumbent to prevent postural hypotension
Direct IV route
• Give by direct **IV** after diluting with sterile water; give slowly

Syringe compatibilities: Atropine, benzquinamide, butorphanol, chlorproMAZINE, cimetidine, dimenhyDRINATE, diphenhydrAMINE, droperidol, fentaNYL, glycopyrrolate, HYDROmorphone, hydrOXYzine, meperidine, metoclopramide, midazolam, morphine, nalbuphine, pentazocine, PENTobarbital, perphenazine, prochlorperazine, promazine, promethazine, ranitidine, SUFentanil, thiopental

Y-site compatibilities: Heparin, hydrocortisone, potassium chloride, propofol, SUFentanil, vit B/C

ADVERSE EFFECTS

CNS: Confusion, anxiety, restlessness, irritability, delusions, headache, fatigue, hallucinations, sedation, depression, incoherence, dizziness, excitement, delirium, flushing, weakness; transdermal: memory disturbances

CV: Palpitations, **tachycardia**, postural hypotension, paradoxical bradycardia

EENT: Transdermal: blurred vision, photophobia, dilated pupils, difficulty swallowing, mydriasis, cycloplegia

GI: *Dryness of mouth, constipation,* nausea, vomiting, abdominal distress, **paralytic ileus**

GU: Hesitancy, retention, difficult urination (patch)

INTEG: Urticaria, dry skin

MISC: Suppression of breastfeeding, nasal congestion, decreased sweating

Pharmacokinetics

Absorption	Well absorbed (IM, SUBCUT, TD)
Distribution	Crosses placenta, blood-brain barrier
Metabolism	Liver
Excretion	Unknown
Half-life	8 hr

Pharmacodynamics

	SUBCUT/IM	IV	TRANSDERMAL
Onset	30-45 min	10-15 min	4-5 hr
Peak	1 hr	1 hr	Unknown
Duration	6 hr	4 hr	72 hr

INTERACTIONS

Individual drugs
Alcohol: increased anticholinergic effect

Drug classifications
Antidepressants (tricyclics), antihistamines, opioids, phenothiazines: increased anticholinergic effect

NURSING CONSIDERATIONS

Assessment
• Monitor I&O ratio; retention commonly causes decreased urinary output
• **Parkinsonism, EPS:** assess for shuffling gait, muscle rigidity, involuntary movements; affect, mood, CNS depression, worsening of mental symptoms during early therapy
• Assess for urinary hesitancy, retention; palpate bladder if retention occurs
• Assess for constipation; increase fluids, bulk, exercise if this occurs
• Assess for tolerance over long-term therapy; dose may have to be increased or changed

Patient/family education
• Tell patient to avoid hazardous activities, activities requiring alertness; dizziness may occur
• Instruct patient to read labels of all OTC medications; if any scopolamine is found in product, avoid use
• Inform patient that blurred vision will decrease with repeated use of ophthalmic product
• Caution patient not to discontinue this product abruptly; to taper off over 1 wk

Transdermal route
• Apply with clean, dry hands; wash, dry hands before and after applying to surface behind ear, press patch firmly
• Teach patient to avoid hazardous activities, activities requiring alertness; dizziness may occur
• Teach patient to change patch q72hr
• Advise patient to discontinue use if blurred vision, severe dizziness, drowsiness occurs; another type of antiemetic may be used or the patch rotated to the other ear
• Advise patient to keep medication out of children's reach
• Caution patient to report change in vision, blurring or loss of sight, trouble breathing, inhibition of sweating, flushing

Evaluation
Positive therapeutic outcome
• Decreased secretions
• Absence of motion sickness

S

scopolamine ophthalmic
See Appendix B

selegiline (Rx)
(se-le′ji-leen)
Eldepryl, Emsam, Zelapar
Func. class.: Antiparkinson agent
Chem. class.: MAOI, type B
Pregnancy category C

Do not confuse:
Eldepryl/enalapril

ACTION: Increased dopaminergic activity by inhibition of MAO type B activity; not fully understood

Therapeutic outcome: Decreased symptoms of Parkinson's disease

USES: Adjunct management of Parkinson's disease in patients being treated with levodopa/carbidopa who have responded poorly to therapy, depression (transdermal)

Unlabeled use: Alzheimer's disease, depression

CONTRAINDICATIONS:
Children/adolescents (suicide/hypertensive crisis), hypersensitivity, breastfeeding

Precautions: Pregnancy **C**

DOSAGE AND ROUTES
Adult: PO 10 mg/day in divided doses, 5 mg at breakfast and lunch with levodopa/carbidopa; after 2-3 days begin to reduce the dose of levodopa/carbidopa 10%-30%; **oral disintegrating tab** 1.25 mg (1 tab) initially, then 2.5 (2 tabs) dissolved on tongue daily before breakfast × 6 wk or more; max 2.5 mg/day; **transdermal** 6 mg/24 hr initially, increase by 3 mg/24 hr at ≥2 wk, up to 12 mg/24 hr if needed

Alzheimer's disease (unlabeled)
Adult: PO 5 mg bid AM, PM

Available forms: Tabs 5 mg, caps 5 mg; oral disintegrating tabs 1.25 mg; transdermal 6 mg/24 hr (20 mg/20 cm²), 9 mg/24 hr (30 mg/30 cm²), 12 mg/24 hr (40 mg/40 cm²)

Implementation
- Do not use in children due to risk for hypertensive crisis
- Adjust dosage to patient's response
- Give with meals; limit protein taken with product
- Give at doses <10 mg/day because of risks associated with nonselective inhibition of MAO
- **Oral disintegrating tab:** peel back foil, place tab on tongue, allow to dissolve, swallow with saliva

Transdermal route
- Apply to dry, intact skin on upper torso/thigh or outer surface of upper arm q12hr

ADVERSE EFFECTS
CNS: Increased tremors, chorea, restlessness, blepharospasm, increased bradykinesia, grimacing, tardive dyskinesia, dystonic symptoms, involuntary movements, increased apraxia, hallucinations, dizziness, mood changes, nightmares, delusions, lethargy, apathy, overstimulation, sleep disturbances, headache, migraine, numbness, muscle cramps, confusion, anxiety, tiredness, vertigo, personality change, back/leg pain, **suicide in children/adolescents, suicidal ideation in adults**

CV: Orthostatic hypotension, hypertension, **dysrhythmia,** palpitations; angina pectoris, hypotension, tachycardia, edema, sinus bradycardia, syncope, **hypertensive crisis (children)**

EENT: Diplopia, dry mouth, blurred vision, tinnitus

GI: *Nausea,* vomiting, constipation, weight loss, anorexia, diarrhea, heartburn, rectal bleeding, poor appetite, dysphagia, xerostomia

GU: Slow urination, nocturia, prostatic hypertrophy, hesitation, retention, frequency, sexual dysfunction

INTEG: Increased sweating, alopecia, hematoma, rash, photosensitivity, facial hair

RESP: Asthma, shortness of breath

Pharmacokinetics

Absorption	Well absorbed
Distribution	Widely distributed
Metabolism	Rapidly, liver
Excretion	Metabolites *N*-desmethyl-deprenyl, amphetamine, methamphetamine
Half-life	10 hr; oral disintegrating tab 1.3 hr

Pharmacodynamics

Onset	Unknown
Peak	½-2 hr
Duration	Unknown

INTERACTIONS
Individual drugs
Dextromethorphan: increased unusual behavior, psychosis

FLUoxetine, fluvoxaMINE, PARoxetine, sertraline: increased serotonin syndrome (confusion, seizures, fever, hypertension, agitation) discontinue 5 wk before selegiline

Levodopa/carbidopa: increased side effects

⚠ **Meperidine: do not use, fatal reaction**

Drug classifications
⚠ **Antidepressants (tricyclics), opioids (especially meperidine): do not use, fatal reaction**

Antihypertensives: increased hypotension

Drug/lab test
Decreased: VMA

False positive: urine ketones, urine glucose

False negative: urine glucose (glucose oxidase)

False increase: uric acid, urine protein

Patient/family education
• Teach patient that therapeutic effects may take 1 wk or longer
• Instruct patient to notify prescriber if pregnant or planning to become pregnant or breastfeed, pregnancy (C)
• Instruct patient to use caution in driving or other activities requiring alertness because of drowsiness, dizziness, blurred vision; to avoid rising quickly from sitting to standing, especially geriatric
• Advise patient to avoid alcohol ingestion, other CNS depressants
⚠ Teach patient not to discontinue medication quickly after long-term use: may cause nausea, headache, malaise
• Caution patient to wear sunscreen or large hat because photosensitivity can occur
• Teach patient to increase fluids, bulk in diet if constipation, urinary retention occur, especially geriatric
• Instruct patient to take gum, hard sugarless candy, or frequent sips of water for dry mouth
• Teach patient that medication may be taken without regard to food
• **Serotonin syndrome:** teach patient to report agitation, nausea, vomiting, diarrhea, twitching, sweating, shivering to prescriber immediately

> **BLACK BOX WARNING:** Teach patient that suicidal thoughts/behavior may occur (children/adolescents)

Evaluation
Positive therapeutic outcome
• Decrease in depression, OCD
• Absence of suicidal thoughts

TREATMENT OF OVERDOSE:
ECG monitoring, induce emesis, lavage, activated charcoal, administer anticonvulsant

sildenafil (Rx)
(sil-den′a-fill)
Revatio, Viagra
Func. class.: Erectile agent; antihypertensive, peripheral vasodilator
Chem. class.: Selective inhibitor of cyclic GMP-PDE5
Pregnancy category B   ✳

Do not confuse:
Viagra/Allegra

ACTION: Enhances the effect of nitric oxide (NO) by inhibiting phosphodiesterase type 5 (PDE5), which is necessary for degrading cyclic GMP in the corpus cavernosum

Therapeutic outcome: Ability to achieve and maintain erection

USES: Treatment of erectile dysfunction, pulmonary hypertension; improvement in exercise ability

Unlabeled uses: Sexual dysfunction (women)

CONTRAINDICATIONS:
Hypersensitivity to this product or nitrates

Precautions: Pregnancy **B**, anatomical penile deformities, sickle cell anemia, leukemia, multiple myeloma, retinitis pigmentosa, bleeding disorders, active peptic ulceration, CV/renal/hepatic disease, multidrug antihypertensive regimens, geriatric patients

DOSAGE AND ROUTES
Erectile dysfunction (Viagra only)
Adult male <65 yr: PO 50 mg 1 hr before sexual activity; may be increased to 100 mg or decreased to 25 mg; max once/day
Adult ≥65 yr (male): PO 25 mg prn about 1 hr before sexual activity

Renal/hepatic dose
Adult: PO (Child-Pugh A, B) 25 mg, take 1 hr before sexual activity, do not use more than 1 ×/day; CCr <30 ml/min 25 mg starting dose

Pulmonary hypertension (Revatio only)
Adult: PO 20 mg tid, take 4-6 hr apart; **IV** BOL 10 mg tid

Available forms: Tabs 20, 25, 50, 100 mg, sol for inj 10 mg/12.5 ml

Implementation
• **Erectile dysfunction:** give approximately 1 hr before sexual activity, do not use more than once a day, give on empty stomach for better absorption
• Tab may be split
• **Pulmonary hypertension:** Give 3×/day, 4-6 hr apart

ADVERSE EFFECTS
CNS: *Headache, flushing, dizziness,* transient global amnesia, **seizures**
CV: MI, sudden death, CV collapse, TIAs, ventricular dysrhythmias, CV hemorrhage

S

MISC: *Dyspepsia, nasal congestion, UTI, abnormal vision, diarrhea, rash,* **NAION (nonarteritic ischemic optic neuropathy),** hearing loss, priapism, **sickle cell crisis**

Pharmacokinetics

Absorption	Rapidly, bioavailability (40%)
Distribution	Unknown
Metabolism	Liver (active metabolites)
Excretion	Feces, urine
Half-life	4 hr

Pharmacodynamics

Onset	Unknown
Peak	½-1½ hr
Duration	Unknown

INTERACTIONS
Individual drugs
Alcohol, amLODIPine: decreased B/P

Bosentan, rifampin, carBAMazepine, dexamethasone, phenytoin, nevirapine, rifabutin, troglitazone: decreased sildenafil levels

Cimetidine, erythromycin, itraconazole, ketoconazole, tacrolimus: increased sildenafil levels

Drug classifications
Antacids, barbiturates, CYP450 inducers: decreased sildenafil levels

Antiretroviral protease inhibitors: increased sildenafil levels

α-Blockers, angiotensin II receptor blockers: decreased B/P

⚠ Nitrates: fatal fall in B/P; do not use together

Drug/food
Grapefruit: increased product effect

High-fat meal: decreased absorption

NURSING CONSIDERATIONS
Assessment
⚠ **Phosphodiesterase type 5 inhibitors with lopinavir/ritonavir (Kaletra):** assess for hypotension, visual changes, prolonged erection, syncope; give only 25 mg q48hr and monitor for adverse reactions

⚠ **Identify organic nitrates that should not be used with this product**

⚠ **Assess for any severe loss of vision while taking this or any similar products; these products should not be used if vision loss has occurred**

• **Assess for MI, sudden death, CV collapse:** Those with an MI within 6 mo, resting hypotension <90/50, resting hypertension >170/100, fluid depletion should use this product cautiously, may occur right after sexual activity to days afterward

• **Sickle cell crisis (vasoocclusive crisis):** when used for pulmonary hypertension, may require hospitalization

Patient/family education
• Teach patient that product does not protect against STDs, including HIV

• Teach patient that product absorption is reduced with a high-fat meal

• Teach patient that product should not be used with nitrates in any form

• Teach patient that tab may be split

• Teach patient to notify prescriber immediately and stop taking product if vision loss occurs

• Do not use more often than 100 mg in 24 hr

⚠ **Teach patient to notify prescriber immediately and to stop taking product if vision/hearing loss occurs or erection lasts >4 hr**

Evaluation
Positive therapeutic outcome
• Ability to achieve and maintain an erection

---

silodosin (Rx)
(si-lo'do-seen)
Rapaflo
Func. class.: Selective α₁-adrenergic blocker, BPH agent
Chem. class.: Sulfamoylphenethylamine derivative
Pregnancy category B

ACTION: Binds preferentially to α_{1A}-adrenoceptor subtype located mainly in the prostate

Therapeutic outcome: Decreased symptoms of benign prostatic hyperplasia

USES: Symptoms of benign prostatic hyperplasia (BPH)

CONTRAINDICATIONS:
Hypersensitivity, renal failure, hepatic disease

Precautions: Pregnancy **B**, breastfeeding, children, renal/hepatic disease, females, hypotension, ocular surgery, orthostatic hypotension, prostate cancer, syncope, geriatric patients

---

DOSAGE AND ROUTES
Adult: PO 8 mg/day with a meal; max 8 mg/day

Renal dose
Adult: PO CCr 30-49 ml/min 4 mg/day; CCr <30 ml/min not recommended

Available forms: Tabs 8 mg

Implementation
• Give with meal at same time of day
• Store at room temperature; protect from light and moisture

ADVERSE EFFECTS
CNS: *Dizziness, headache,* asthenia, insomnia, syncope
CV: Orthostatic hypotension
EENT: Nasal congestion, rhinorrhea, sinusitis
GI: Diarrhea, abdominal pain, jaundice
GU: Abnormal ejaculation, priapism, urinary incontinence
HEMA: Purpura

Pharmacokinetics	
Absorption	Decreased with high-fat/high-calorie meal
Distribution	Extensive protein binding 97%
Metabolism	Liver
Excretion	Urine
Half-life	24 hr (metabolite)

Pharmacodynamics

Unknown

INTERACTIONS
Drug classifications
CYP3A4 inhibitors (clarithromycin, itraconazole, ritonavir, anti-retroviral protease inhibitors, aprepitant, chloramphenicol, conivaptan, dalfopristin, danazol, delavirdine, efavirenz, fosaprepitant, fluconazole, fluvoxaMINE, imatinib, isoniazid, mifepristone, nefazodone, tamoxifen, telithromycin, troleandomycin, voriconazole, zileuton, zafirlukast): increased silodosin effect

Drug/food
Grapefruit juice: increased silodosin effect

Drug/lab test
Increased: LFTs

NURSING CONSIDERATIONS
Assessment
• **Prostatic hyperplasia:** assess for change in urinary patterns, baseline and throughout

treatment, testing for prostate cancer prior to administration is recommended
• Monitor BUN, uric acid, urodynamic studies (urinary flow rates, residual volume)
• Assess I&O ratios, weight daily, edema, report weight gain or edema
• B/P, monitor for orthostatic hypotension

Patient/family education
• Caution patient not to drive or operate machinery until effect is known
• Advise patient not to use with grapefruit juice
• Teach patient to take with same meal each day

Evaluation
Positive therapeutic outcome
• Decreased symptoms of benign prostatic hyperplasia

silver nitrate 1% ophthalmic
See Appendix B

silver nitrate sulfacetamide sodium ophthalmic
See Appendix B

silver sulfADIAZINE topical
See Appendix B

simethicone (Rx, OTC)
(si-meth′i-kone)
Barriere ✤, Equaline Extra Strength Gas Relief, Gas Relief ✤, Gas-Relief, Gas-X, Good Sense Ultra Strength Gas Relief, Mylanta Gas, Mylanta Gas Relief, Mylicon, Ovol ✤, Phazyme, Top Care Gas Relief Extra Strength, Walgreens Gas Relief
Func. class.: Antiflatulent
Pregnancy category C

Do not confuse:
Mylicon/Mylanta Gas

ACTION: Disperses, prevents gas pockets in GI system; lowers surface tension of gas bubbles

Therapeutic outcome: Belching or flatus

USES: Flatulence

Unlabeled uses: Dyspepsia

CONTRAINDICATIONS:
Hypersensitivity, GI obstruction/perforation

Precautions: Pregnancy **C**, abdominal pain, fistula, hiatal hernia

DOSAGE AND ROUTES
Adult and child >12 yr: PO 40-125 mg after meals and at bedtime prn, max 500 mg/day
Child 2-12 yr: PO 40 mg after meals and at bedtime prn, max 240 mg/day
Child <2 yr: PO 20 mg qid prn

Available forms: Chew tabs 40, 150, 166 mg; tabs 60, 80, 95, 125 mg; drops 20 mg/0.3 ml, 95 mg/1.425 ml; caps 95, 180 mg; caps, soft gel 125, 180 mg; oral dissolving film 62.5 mg

Implementation
• Give after meals and at bedtime
• Shake susp well before administering
• Chew tab should be chewed and not swallowed whole

ADVERSE EFFECTS
GI: Belching, rectal flatus, diarrhea

Pharmacokinetics	
Absorption	None
Distribution	None
Metabolism	None
Excretion	None
Half-life	Unknown

Pharmacodynamics	
Onset	Rapid
Peak	Unknown
Duration	3 hr

NURSING CONSIDERATIONS
Assessment
• Identify the reason for excess gas production: decreased bowel sounds, recent surgery, other GI conditions

Patient/family education
• Caution patient that tab must be chewed; to shake susp well before pouring

Evaluation
Positive therapeutic outcome
• Absence of flatulence

simvastatin (Rx)
(sim-va-stat'in)
Zocor
Func. class.: Antilipidemic
Chem. class.: HMG-CoA reductase inhibitor
Pregnancy category X

Do not confuse:
Zocor/Cozaar/Zoloft

ACTION: Inhibits HMG-CoA reductase enzyme, which reduces cholesterol synthesis; this enzyme is needed for cholesterol production

Therapeutic outcome: Decreasing cholesterol levels and LDLs, increased HDLs

USES: As an adjunct in primary hypercholesterolemia (types IIa, IIb), isolated hypertriglyceridemia (Frederickson type IV) and type III hyperlipoproteinemia, CAD, heterozygous familial hypercholesterolemia; MI/stroke prophylaxis

CONTRAINDICATIONS:
Pregnancy **X**, breastfeeding, hypersensitivity, active liver disease

Precautions: Past liver disease, alcoholism, severe acute infections, trauma, severe metabolic disorders, electrolyte imbalances, Chinese patients

DOSAGE AND ROUTES
Adult: PO 20-40 mg/day in PM initially, usual range 5-40 mg/day daily in PM max, 40 mg/day for most patients; max 80 mg/day (for patients taking 80 mg/day chronically without myopathy); dosage adjustments may be made at 4-wk intervals or more; those taking verapamil and amiodarone max 20 mg/day, max <80 mg for Chinese patients taking lipid-modifying niacin doses

With diltiazem/verapamil
Adult: PO 5-10 mg q PM, max 10 mg/day with amiodarone/amLODIPine/ranolazine
Adult: PO 5-20 mg q PM, max 20 mg/day
Child and adolescent ≥10 yr including girls ≥1 yr postmenarche: PO 10 mg q PM, range 10-40 mg/day

With amiodarone, amLODIPine, ranolazine
Adult: PO 5-20 mg/day in evening, max 20 mg/day

⚠ Nurse Alert   ✴ Key NCLEX® Drug

Heterozygous familial hypercholesterolemia

Adolescent 10-17 yr: PO 10 mg daily, max 40 mg daily

Available forms: Tabs 5, 10, 20, 40, 80 mg

Implementation
• Give 30 min before AM and PM meals
• Store in cool environment in tight container protected from light

ADVERSE EFFECTS

CNS: Headache, cognitive impairment
GI: Nausea, constipation, diarrhea, dyspepsia, flatus, abdominal pain, **liver dysfunction, pancreatitis,** hyperglycemia
INTEG: Rash, pruritus
MS: Muscle cramps, myalgia, **myositis, rhabdomyolysis,** myopathy
RESP: Upper respiratory tract infection

Pharmacokinetics	
Absorption	85%
Distribution	Unknown
Metabolism	Liver—extensively
Excretion	70% feces, 20% kidneys
Half-life	3 hr

Pharmacodynamics
Unknown

INTERACTIONS

Individual drugs
Clarithromycin, clofibrate, cycloSPORINE, erythromycin, gemfibrozil, itraconazole, ketoconazole, niacin, danazol, delavirdine, nefazodone, verapamil, diltiazem, amiodarone, azole antifungals, telithromycin: increased myalgia, myositis, rhabdomyolysis
CycloSPORINE, gemfibrozil: do not use with simvastatin
Digoxin: increased digoxin levels
Warfarin: increased risk of bleeding

Drug classifications
Macrolide antiinfectives, protease inhibitors: increased myalgia, myositis, rhabdomyolysis

Drug/herb
Red yeast rice: increased simvastatin effect
St. John's wort: decreased effect

Drug/lab test
Increased: CPK, liver function tests

NURSING CONSIDERATIONS

Assessment
• Assess nutrition: fat, protein, carbohydrates; nutritional analysis should be completed by dietitian before treatment is initiated
⚠ **Rhabdomyolysis: assess for increase tenderness, increased CPK levels 10× ULN; therapy should be discontinued, more likely in those receiving >80 mg/day, first year of treatment, those ≥65 yr, females**
• Monitor bowel pattern daily; diarrhea may be a problem
• Monitor triglycerides, cholesterol baseline, throughout treatment; LDL, HDL, triglycerides and cholesterol should be watched closely at 6-8 wk and q6mo; if increased, product should be discontinued

Patient/family education
• Inform patient that compliance is needed for positive results to occur, not to double doses
• Advise patient to lower risk factors: high-fat diet, smoking, alcohol consumption, absence of exercise
• Advise patient to notify prescriber of planned or suspected pregnancy **X**

Evaluation
Positive therapeutic outcome
• Decreased cholesterol levels, serum triglycerides and improved ratio with HDLs

sirolimus (Rx)
(seer-roe′li-mus)
Rapamune
Func. class.: Immunosuppressant
Chem. class.: Macrolide
Pregnancy category C

S

ACTION: Produces immunosuppression by inhibiting T-lymphocyte activation and proliferation

Therapeutic outcome: Prevention of rejection in organ transplant

USES: Organ transplants: to prevent rejection, recommended use is with cycloSPORINE and corticosteroids

CONTRAINDICATIONS:
Breastfeeding, hypersensitivity to this product or to components of the product

Precautions: Pregnancy **C,** children <13 yr, severe cardiac/renal/hepatic disease, diabetes mellitus, hyperkalemia, hyperuricemia, hypertension, interstitial lung disease, hyperlipidemia

---

Adverse effects: *italics* = common; **bold** = life-threatening

---

BLACK BOX WARNING: Lymphomas, infection, other malignancies

DOSAGE AND ROUTES
Adult/adolescent ≥40 kg: PO 2 mg daily with 6 mg loading dose
Child >13 yr <40 kg (88 lb): PO 1 mg/m²/day, 3 mg/m²/loading dose

Hepatic dose
Adult and child ≥13 yr <40 kg: PO reduce by 33% in maintenance dose (mild to moderate hepatic impairment); reduce by 50% in maintenance dose (severe hepatic impairment)

Available forms: Oral sol 1 mg/ml; tabs 0.5, 1, 2 mg

Implementation
• Administer prophylaxis for *Pneumocystis jiroveci* pneumonia for 1 yr after transplantation; prophylaxis for cytomegalovirus (CMV) is recommended for 90 days after transplantation in those at increased risk for CMV
• Use amber oral dose syringe and withdraw amount of oral sol needed from the bottle, empty correct dose into plastic/glass container holding 60 ml of water/orange juice, stir vigorously and have patient drink at once, refill container with additional 120 ml of water/orange juice, stir vigorously, and have patient drink at once; if using a pouch squeeze entire contents into container and follow preceding directions
• Give all medications PO if possible; avoid IM inj because bleeding may occur
• Give for 3 days before transplant surgery; patients should be placed in protective isolation, give at same time of day, give 4 hr after cycloSPORINE oral sol or caps, do not use with grapefruit juice
• Store protected from light; refrigerate; stable for 24 months

ADVERSE EFFECTS
CNS: *Tremors, headache, insomnia,* paresthesia, chills, fever
CV: Hypo/hypertension, **atrial fibrillation, CHF,** palpitations, **tachycardia,** peripheral edema, **thrombosis**
EENT: Blurred vision, photophobia
GI: Nausea, vomiting, diarrhea, constipation, **hepatotoxicity**
GU: UTI, **albuminuria, hematuria, proteinuria, renal failure,** nephrotic syndrome
HEMA: Anemia, **thrombocytopenia purpura, leukopenia,** pancytopenia
INTEG: *Rash, acne,* photosensitivity

META: Increased creatinine, edema, hypercholesterolemia, *hyperlipemia,* hypophosphatemia, weight gain, hyperglycemia, hypo/hyperkalemia, hyperuricemia, hypomagnesemia, hypertriglyceridemia
MS: Arthralgia
RESP: Pleural effusion, atelectasis, *dyspnea,* pneumonitis, pulmonary embolism/fibrosis
SYST: Lymphoma, exfoliative dermatitis

Pharmacokinetics
Absorption	Rapidly absorbed
Distribution	92% protein binding
Metabolism	Liver; extensively by CYP3A4 enzyme system
Excretion	Unknown
Half-life	57-63 hr

Pharmacodynamics
Onset	Unknown
Peak	1 hr single dose, 2 hr multiple dosing
Duration	Unknown

INTERACTIONS
Individual drugs
Bromocriptine, cimetidine, cycloSPORINE, danazol, erythromycin, metoclopramide: increased blood level
CarBAMazepine, PHENobarbital, phenytoin, rifamycin, rifapentine: decreased blood levels

Drug classifications
ACE inhibitors, angiotensin II receptor antagonists, cephalosporins, iodine-containing radiopaque contrast media, neuromuscular blockers, NSAIDs, penicillins, salicylates, thrombolytics: increased angioedema
Antifungal agents, calcium channel blockers, HIV protease inhibitors: increased blood levels
Live virus vaccines: decreased effect of vaccines

Drug/herb
St. John's wort: decreased sirolimus effect

Drug/food
Food: alters bioavailability, use consistently with or without food
Grapefruit juice: do not use with grapefruit juice

Drug/lab test
Increased: LFTs, alk phos, lipids, triglycerides, total cholesterol, BUN, creatinine, LDH, phosphate
Decreased: platelets, sodium

⚠ Nurse Alert   ✴ Key NCLEX® Drug

Increased or decreased: magnesium, glucose, calcium

NURSING CONSIDERATIONS
Assessment
⚠ **Wound dehiscence and anastomotic disruption:** assess wound, vascular, airway, ureteral, biliary, inhibition of growth factors; do not combine with corticosteroids
⚠ **Anaphylaxis, angioedema, exfoliative dermatitis:** assess for, more common when given with ACE inhibitors; do not use if a hypersensitivity reaction occurs
• **Bone marrow depression:** Hgb, WBC, platelets monthly during treatment; if leukocytes are <3000/mm³ or platelets <100,000/mm³, product should be discontinued or reduced; decreased Hgb level
• Monitor blood levels in those who may have altered metabolism, trough levels ≥15 ng/ml are associated with increased adverse reactions
• **Pulmonary fibrosis, pulmonary effusion, pneumonitis:** assess for dyspnea, cough, hypoxia; some fatal cases have occurred
• Monitor lipid profile: cholesterol, triglycerides; a lipid-lowering agent may be needed

> **BLACK BOX WARNING:** Creatinine/BUN, CBC, serum potassium

• Assess for infection and development of lymphoma
• Only those experienced in immunosuppressant therapy and organ transplantation should use this product; use only in renal transplant
• **High risk:** those with Banff grade 3 acute rejection or vascular rejection prior to cycloSPORINE withdrawal, dialysis dependent, creatinine >4.5 mg/dl, African descent, re-transplant, multiorgan transplant, high panel of reactive antibodies
• **Hepatotoxicity:** alk phos, AST, ALT, amylase, bilirubin: dark urine, jaundice, itching, light-colored stools; product should be discontinued

Patient/family education
• Instruct patient to report fever, rash, severe diarrhea, chills, sore throat, fatigue because serious infections may occur; clay-colored stools, cramping may indicate hepatotoxicity
• Caution patient to avoid crowds or persons with known infections to reduce risk of infection
• Teach patient to use contraception before, during, and 12 wk after product has been discontinued, avoid breastfeeding
• Teach patient to use sunscreen, protective clothing to prevent burns

• Teach patient that lifelong use is required to prevent rejection
• Teach patient that continuing follow-up exams and blood work will be required
• Teach patient not to get on skin
• Teach patient how to use product
• Teach patient to take at same time, consistently, with or without regard to food
• Teach patient to take 4 hr after cycloSPORINE

Evaluation
Positive therapeutic outcome
• Absence of graft rejection

---

sitaGLIPtin (Rx)
(sit-a-glip'tin)
Januvia
Func. class.: Antidiabetic, oral
Chem. class.: Dipeptidyl-peptidase-4 inhibitor (DPP-4 inhibitor)
Pregnancy category B

ACTION: Slows the inactivation of incretin hormones; improves glucose homeostasis, improves glucose-dependent insulin secretion, lowers glucagon secretions and slows gastric emptying time

Therapeutic outcome: Decrease in polyuria, polydipsia, polyphagia; clear sensorium; absence of dizziness; stable gait; blood glucose at normal level

USES: Type 2 diabetes mellitus as monotherapy or in combination with other antidiabetic agents

CONTRAINDICATIONS:
Angioedema, diabetic ketoacidosis (DKA)

Precautions: Pregnancy **B**, geriatric, hypersensitivity, GI obstruction, thyroid disease, surgery, renal/hepatic disease, trauma, breastfeeding, pancreatitis, hypercortisolism, hyperglycemia, hyperthyroidism, hypoglycemia, ileus, pituitary insufficiency, surgery, type 1 diabetes mellitus, adrenal insufficiency, burns, diabetic ketoacidosis

DOSAGE AND ROUTES
Adult: PO 100 mg/day; may use with other antidiabetic agents (metformin, pioglitazone, rosiglitazone) other than insulin

Renal dose
Adult: PO CCr 30-50 ml/min 50 mg qd; CCr <30 ml/min 25 mg qd

S

Available forms: Tabs 25, 50, 100 mg

Implementation

- May be taken with or without food
- Conversion from other antidiabetic agents; change may be made with gradual dosage change
- Store in tight container at room temperature
- Do not split, crush, chew, swallow whole

ADVERSE EFFECTS

CNS: *Headache*
ENDO: Hypoglycemia
GI: *Nausea, vomiting,* abdominal pain, diarrhea, **pancreatitis,** constipation
GU: Acute renal failure
MISC: Peripheral edema
SYST: Anaphylaxis, Stevens-Johnson syndrome, angioedema

Pharmacokinetics

Absorption	Rapidly
Distribution	Unknown
Metabolism	Unknown
Excretion	Kidneys, 79% unchanged
Half-life	Terminal 12.4 hr

Pharmacodynamics

Onset	Unknown
Peak	1-4 hr
Duration	Unknown

INTERACTIONS

Individual drugs

ARIPiprazole, cloZAPine, fosphenytoin, OLANZapine, phenytoin, QUEtiapine, risperiDONE, ziprasidone: decreased antidiabetic effect
Cimetidine, disopyramide: increased sitaGLIPtin level
Cimetidine, FLUoxetine: increased hypoglycemia
Digoxin: increased levels of digoxin

Drug classifications

ACE inhibitors, estrogens, oral contraceptives, progestins, phenothiazines, protease inhibitors, sympathomimetics, thiazide diuretics: decreased antidiabetic effect
Androgens, β-blockers, corticosteroids, fibric acid derivatives, insulins, MAOIs, salicylates, sulfonylureas: increased hypoglycemia

Drug/herb

Garlic, green tea, horse chestnut: increased antidiabetic effect

Drug/lab test

Increased: creatinine, LFTs

NURSING CONSIDERATIONS

Assessment

- **Hypoglycemic reactions:** assess for sweating, weakness, dizziness, anxiety, tremors, hunger, hyperglycemic reactions soon after meals
- Monitor CBC (baseline, q3mo) during treatment; check liver function tests periodically, AST, LDH, renal studies: BUN, creatinine during treatment; Hgb A1c
- Monitor blood glucose (BG) as needed
- **Serious skin reactions:** assess for swelling of face, mouth, lips, dyspnea, wheezing
- **Pancreatitis:** assess for severe abdominal pain, nausea, vomiting; discontinue product
- **Renal studies:** monitor BUN, creatinine during treatment, especially in geriatrics or those with renal disease
- Monitor hemoglobin A1c; monitor blood glucose as needed

Patient/family education

- Teach patient to use regular self-monitoring of blood glucose using blood glucose meter
- Teach patient the symptoms of hypo/hyperglycemia, what to do about each
- Teach patient that product must be continued on daily basis; explain consequence of discontinuing product abruptly
- Teach patient to notify prescriber if pregnancy is planned or suspected; to continue health regimen (diet, exercise)
- Advise patient to avoid OTC medications, alcohol, digoxin, exenatide, insulins, nateglinide, repaglinide, and other products that lower blood sugar, unless approved by prescriber
- Teach patient that diabetes is a lifelong illness; that this product is not a cure, only controls symptoms
- Teach patient that all food included in diet plan must be eaten to prevent hypo/hyperglycemia
- Teach patient to carry emergency ID
- Teach patient to notify prescriber immediately of hypersensitivity reactions (rash, swelling of face, trouble breathing)

Evaluation

Positive therapeutic outcome

- Decrease in polyuria, polydipsia, polyphagia; clear sensorium; absence of dizziness; stable gait, blood glucose, A1c improvement

sodium bicarbonate (Rx, OTC)

baking soda, Brosch-Neut, Citrocarbonate, Neut, Sellymin ✤

Func. class.: Alkalinizer; antacid
Chem. class.: NaHCO₃

Pregnancy category C

ACTION: Orally neutralizes gastric acid, which forms water, NaCl, CO_2; increases plasma bicarbonate, which buffers H^+ ion concentration; reverses acidosis **IV**

Therapeutic outcome: Correction of acidosis, gastric acid neutralization

USES: Acidosis (metabolic), cardiac arrest, alkalinization (systemic/urinary); antacid (PO); salicylate poisoning

CONTRAINDICATIONS:

Respiratory/metabolic alkalosis, hypochloremia, hypocalcemia

Precautions: Pregnancy **C**, CHF, cirrhosis, toxemia, renal disease, hypertension, hypokalemia, breastfeeding, hypernatremia, Bartter's syndrome, Cushing's syndrome, hyperaldosteronism, children

DOSAGE AND ROUTES

Acidosis, metabolic (not associated with cardiac arrest)

Adult and child: IV INF 2-5 mEq/kg over 4-8 hr depending on CO_2, pH, ABGs

Cardiac arrest

Adult and child: IV BOL 1 mEq/kg of 7.5% or 8.4% SOL, then 0.5 mEq/kg q5-10min, then doses based on ABGs

Infant: IV 1 mEq/kg over several min (use only the 0.5 mEq/ml [4.2%] sol for inj)

Alkalinization of urine

Adult: PO 325 mg-2 g qid or 48 mEq/kg (4 g), then 12-24 mEq q4hr

Child: PO 84-840 mg/kg/day (1-10 mEq/kg), in divided doses q4-6hr

Antacid

Adult: PO 300 mg-2 g chewed, taken with water daily-qid

Available forms: Tabs 300, 325, 600, 650 mg; inj 4.2%, 5%, 7.5%, 8.4%

Implementation

PO route

• Antacid tab must be chewed and taken with 8 oz of water
• Dissolve effervescent tab in water
• May be used to neutralize gastric acid in peptic ulcer disease, given 1 and 3 hr after meals and at bedtime

Direct IV route

• Use in cardiac emergencies, use ampules or prefilled syringes only, give by rapid bolus dose, flush with 0.9% NaCl before and after use

Continuous IV infusion route

• Prepared sol or diluted in an equal amount of any dextrose/saline combination; administer 2-5 mEq/kg over 4-8 hr, max 50 mEq/hr; slower rate in children

Y-site compatibilities: Acyclovir, amifostine, asparaginase, aztreonam, bivalirudin, bumetanide, cefepime, cefmetazole, cefTRIAXone, chloramphenicol, cyclophosphamide, cytarabine, DAUNOrubicin, dexamethasone, DOXOrubicin, etoposide, famotidine, fentaNYL, filgrastim, fluconazole, fludarabine, furosemide, gallium nitrate, gemcitabine, gentamicin, granisetron, heparin, hydrocortisone sodium succinate, ifosfamide, indomethacin, insulin, ketorolac, labetalol, levofloxacin, lidocaine, linezolid, LORazepam, magnesium sulfate, melphalan, mesna, meperidine, methylPREDNISolone, metoclopramide, metoprolol, metroNIDAZOLE, milrinone, morphine, nafcillin, nitroglycerin, nitroprusside, PACLitaxel, palonosetron, pantoprazole, PEMEtrexed, penicillin G potassium, phenylephrine, phytonadione, piperacillin/tazobactam, potassium chloride, procainamide, propofol, propranolol, protamine, ranitidine, remifentanil, tacrolimus, teniposide, thiotepa, ticarcillin/clavulanate, tirofiban, tobramycin, tolazoline, vasopressin, vitamin B complex with C, voriconazole

Y-site incompatibilities: Allopurinol, amiodarone, amphotericin B, amphotericin B cholesteryl sulfate complex, ampicillin, anidulafungin, calcium chloride, calicum gluconate, caspofungin, cefotaxime, cefOXitin, cefuroxime, diazepam, diphenhydrAMINE, DOBUTamine, DOXOrubicin liposome, doxycycline, EPINEPHrine, fenoldopam, ganciclovir, haloperidol, hydrOXYzine, IDArubicin, imipenem/cilastatin, inamrinone, isoproterenol, lansoprazole, leucovorin, midazolam, nalbuphine, norepinephrine, ondansetron, phenytoin, prochlorperazine, promethazine, quinupristin/dalfopristin,

S

Adverse effects: *italics* = common; **bold** = life-threatening

sargramostim, trimethoprim/sulfamethoxazole, verapamil, vinCRIStine, vinorelbine

ADVERSE EFFECTS

CNS: Irritability, headache, confusion, stimulation, tremors, *twitching, hyperreflexia,* **tetany,** weakness, **seizures** caused by alkalosis
CV: Irregular pulse, **cardiac arrest,** water retention, edema, weight gain
GI: Flatulence, *belching, distention*
GU: Calculi
META: *Alkalosis*
MS: Muscular twitching, tetany, irritability

Pharmacokinetics

Absorption	Unknown
Distribution	Widely distributed—extracellular fluids
Metabolism	Unknown
Excretion	Kidneys
Half-life	Unknown

Pharmacodynamics

	PO	IV
Onset	2 min	Rapid
Peak	½ hr	Rapid
Duration	1-3 hr	Unknown

INTERACTIONS

Individual drugs

ChlorproPAMIDE, lithium: decreased effect of each specific product
Flecainide, mecamylamine, pseudoephedrine, quiNIDine, quiNINE: increased effects of each specific product

Drug classifications

Amphetamines, anorexiants, sympathomimetics: increased effects of each specific product
Barbiturates: decreased effects of barbiturates
Benzodiazepines: decreased effects of each specific product
Corticosteroids: increased sodium; decreased potassium, decreased effects of corticosteroids
Ketoconazoles: decreased effects of ketoconazoles
Salicylates: decreased effect of salicylates

Drug/herb

Oak bark: decreased action of sodium bicarbonate

Drug/lab test

Increased: sodium, lactate
Decreased: potassium

NURSING CONSIDERATIONS

Assessment

• Assess respiratory and pulse rate, rhythm, depth, lung sounds; notify prescriber of abnormalities
• Assess for CO_2 in GI tract; may lead to perforation if ulcer is severe
• **Fluid balance** (I&O ratio, weight daily, edema); notify prescriber of fluid overload, assess for edema, crackles, SOB
• Monitor electrolytes, blood pH, PO_2, HCO_3 during beginning treatment; ABGs frequently during emergencies
• Monitor extravasation with **IV** administration (tissue sloughing, ulceration, and necrosis)
• **Alkalosis:** irritability, confusion, twitching, hyperreflexia, stimulation, slow respirations, cyanosis, irregular pulse
• **Milk-alkali syndrome:** confusion, headache, nausea, vomiting, anorexia, urinary stones, hypercalcemia

Patient/family education

• Instruct patient to chew antacid tab and drink 8 oz of water; not to take antacid with milk because milk-alkali syndrome may result; not to use antacid for more than 2 wk
• Advise patient to notify prescriber if indigestion is accompanied by chest pain; trouble breathing; diarrhea; dark, tarry stools; vomit that looks like coffee grounds; swelling of feet/ankles
• Teach patient about sodium-restricted diet; to avoid use of baking soda for indigestion

Evaluation

Positive therapeutic outcome
• ABGs, electrolytes, blood pH, HCO_3 normal levels
• Decreased gastric pain

sodium biphosphate/ sodium phosphate (OTC)

Fleet Enema, Phospho-soda
Func. class.: Laxative, saline
Pregnancy category C

ACTION: Increases water absorption in the small intestine by osmotic action; laxative effect occurs by increased peristalsis and water retention

Therapeutic outcome: Absence of constipation

USES: Constipation, bowel or rectal preparation for surgery, examination

---

CONTRAINDICATIONS:

Hypersensitivity, rectal fissures, abdominal pain, nausea/vomiting, appendicitis, acute surgical abdomen, ulcerated hemorrhoids, Na-restricted diets, renal failure, hyperphosphatemia, hypocalcemia, hypokalemia, hypernatremia, Addison's disease, CHF, ascites, bowel perforation, megacolon, imperforate anus

> **BLACK BOX WARNING:** GI obstruction, renal failure

Precautions: Pregnancy **C**

> **BLACK BOX WARNING:** Colitis, elderly, hypovolemia, renal disease

DOSAGE AND ROUTES

Adult: PO 20-30 ml (Phospho-soda)
Child: PO 5-15 ml (Phospho-soda)
Adult and child >12 yr: RECT enema (118 ml)
Child 2-12 yr: RECT ½ enema (59 ml)

Available forms: Enema 7 g/phosphate and 19 g/biphosphate/118 ml; oral sol 18 g phosphate/48 g biphosphate/100 ml

Implementation
PO route
- Give on empty stomach
- Mix oral sol in cold water
- Take alone for better absorption; do not take within 1 hr of other products

ADVERSE EFFECTS

CV: **Dysrhythmias, cardiac arrest,** hypotension, widening QRS complex
GI: *Nausea, cramps,* diarrhea
META: Electrolyte, fluid imbalances

Pharmacokinetics

Absorption	Up to 20% (rec)
Distribution	Unknown
Metabolism	Unknown
Excretion	Kidneys
Half-life	Unknown

Pharmacodynamics

	PO	Rect
Onset	½-3 hr	5 min
Peak	Unknown	Unknown
Duration	Unknown	Unknown

NURSING CONSIDERATIONS
Assessment
- Assess stools: color, amount, consistency
- Assess for bowel pattern, bowel sounds (frequency, intensity), flatulence, distention, increased temp, dietary patterns (fluid, bulk), exercise
- Assess for cramping, rectal bleeding, nausea, vomiting; if these symptoms occur, product should be discontinued

Patient/family education
- Advise patient not to use laxatives or enema for long-term therapy; bowel tone will be lost
- Teach patient that normal bowel movements do not always occur daily
- Caution patient not to use in presence of abdominal pain, nausea, vomiting
- Caution patient to notify prescriber if constipation is unrelieved or if symptoms of electrolyte imbalance occur: muscle cramps, pain, weakness, dizziness, excessive thirst
- Instruct patient to maintain adequate fluid consumption to help prevent constipation

Evaluation
Positive therapeutic outcome
- Decrease in constipation

sodium polystyrene sulfonate (Rx)
(po-lee-stye'reen)
Kayexalate, Kionex, SPS
Func. class.: Potassium-removing resin
Chem. class.: Cation exchange resin
Pregnancy category C

ACTION: Removes potassium by exchanging sodium for potassium in body; occurs primarily in large intestine

Therapeutic outcome: Potassium levels within accepted range

USES: Hyperkalemia in conjunction with other measures

CONTRAINDICATIONS:
Hypersensitivity to saccharin or parabens that may be in some products; GI obstruction, neonate (reduced gut motility)

Precautions: Pregnancy **C**, geriatric, renal failure, CHF, severe edema, severe hypertension, sodium restriction, constipation, GI bleeding, hypocalcemia

DOSAGE AND ROUTES
Adult: PO 15 g daily-qid; RECT enema 30-50 q1-2hr initially prn, then q6hr prn
Child (unlabeled): PO 1 g/kg q6hr prn; RECT 1 g/kg q2-6hr prn

Available forms: Powder for susp 453.6 g, 454 g; oral susp 15 g/60 ml

Implementation
PO route
• Powdered resin: Each dose of the sodium polystyrene sulfonate powdered resin is usually given orally as a suspension in water or in a syrup. Usually, the amount of fluid ranges 20-100 ml, depending on the dose, or 3-4 ml per g of resin. Suspensions should be freshly prepared and not stored for longer than 24 hr. The suspension may also be introduced into the stomach via a tube or the powdered resin may be mixed with the patient's food; the powder should not be mixed with foods or liquids that contain a large amount of potassium (bananas or orange juice)

Rectal route
• Precede retention enema with a cleansing enema; instruct patient to lie down on left side with lower leg extended and the upper leg flexed for support or place the patient in the knee-chest position. Gently insert a soft, large (French 28) rubber tube into the rectum for a distance of about 20 cm; the tip should be well into the sigmoid colon. Tape the tube in place. Suspend the sodium polystyrene sulfonate powdered resin in 100 ml of an aqueous vehicle (water or sorbitol) which has been warmed to body temperature and introduce through the tube by gravity. The particles should be kept suspended by stirring the suspension during administration. Alternatively, 120-180 ml of a commercially available suspension may be administered as a retention enema after the suspension has been warmed to body temperature. Following administration, flush the tube with 50-100 ml of fluid and clamp the tube and leave in place. The suspension should be retained in the colon for at least 30-60 min or for several hours, if possible
• After several hours have passed, administer a cleansing enema using a nonsodium containing solution at body temperature. Up to 2 quarts of fluid may be necessary. Drain fluid through a Y-tube connection. Observe the drainage if sorbitol was used

ADVERSE EFFECTS
GI: *Constipation,* anorexia, nausea, vomiting, diarrhea (sorbitol), *fecal impaction,* gastric irritation
META: Hypocalcemia, hypokalemia, hypomagnesemia, sodium retention

Pharmacokinetics
Absorption	None
Distribution	None
Metabolism	None
Excretion	Feces
Half-life	Unknown

Pharmacodynamics
	PO	Rect
Onset	2-12 hr	2-12 hr
Peak	Unknown	Unknown
Duration	6-24 hr	4-6 hr

INTERACTIONS
Individual drugs
Sorbitol: increased colonic necrosis, do not use concurrently
Lithium: decreased effect of lithium

Drug classifications
Diuretics (loop), cardiac glycosides: increased hypokalemia
Magnesium/calcium antacids: increased metabolic acidosis
Thyroid hormones: decreased effect of thyroid hormones

NURSING CONSIDERATIONS
Assessment
• Assess bowel function daily: amount of stool, color, characteristics
• Assess for hypotension: confusion, irritability, muscular pain, weakness
• Hyperkalemia: assess for confusion, dyspnea, weakness, dysrhythmias
• Monitor electrolytes: potassium, sodium, calcium, magnesium; I&O ratio, weight daily
• Monitor ECG for spiked T-waves, depressed ST segments, prolonged QT interval, and widening QRS complex
• Monitor I&O ratio, weight daily, crackles, dyspnea, jugular vein distention, edema
• Monitor for digoxin toxicity (nausea, vomiting, blurred vision, anorexia, dysrhythmia) in those receiving digoxin

Patient/family education
• Explain reason for medication and expected results

- Teach patient to avoid laxatives, antacids, electrolyte-based products unless approved by prescriber
- Teach patient to use a low-potassium diet, provide sample diet

Evaluation
Positive therapeutic outcome
- Potassium level 3.5-5 mg/dl

---

solifenacin (Rx)
(sol-i-fen′a-sin)
VESIcare
Func. class.: Urinary antispasmodic, anticholinergic
Chem. class.: Antimuscarinic receptor antagonist
Pregnancy category C

ACTION: Relaxes smooth muscles in urinary tract by inhibiting acetylcholine at postganglionic sites

Therapeutic outcome: Decreased dysuria, frequency, nocturia, incontinence

USES: Overactive bladder (urinary frequency, urgency, incontinence)

CONTRAINDICATIONS:
Hypersensitivity, uncontrolled closed-angle glaucoma, urinary retention, gastric retention

Precautions: Pregnancy **C**, breastfeeding, children, geriatric patients, renal/hepatic disease, controlled closed-angle glaucoma, bladder outflow obstruction, GI obstruction, decreased GI motility, history of QT prolongation

DOSAGE AND ROUTES
Adult: PO 5 mg/day, max 10 mg/day

Renal/hepatic dose
Adult: PO CCr <30 ml/min 5 mg/day; Child-Pugh B max 5 mg/day

Available forms: Tabs 5, 10 mg

Implementation
PO route
- Without regard to meals
- Swallow product whole with water, liquid

ADVERSE EFFECTS
CNS: Anxiety, paresthesia, fatigue, *dizziness,* headache, confusion, delirium, depression, drowsiness, fatigue

CV: Chest pain, hypertension, **QTc prolongation, peripheral edema,** palpitations, sinus tachycardia
EENT: *Vision abnormalities, xerophthalmia,* nasal dryness
GI: *Nausea, vomiting, anorexia,* abdominal pain, *constipation,* dry mouth, dyspepsia
GU: Dysuria, urinary retention, frequency, UTI
INTEG: Rash, pruritus, **angioedema,** exfoliative dermatitis, erythema multiforme
MISC: Hyperthermia
RESP: Bronchitis, cough, pharyngitis, URI

Pharmacokinetics

Absorption	Rapid (90%)
Distribution	98% protein bound
Metabolism	Extensively metabolized by CYP3A4
Excretion	Excreted in urine (69%)/feces (22%)
Half-life	Terminal half-life 45-68 hr

Pharmacodynamics

Unknown

INTERACTIONS
Drug classifications
Azoles, macrolides, fluoroquinolones, class IA, III antidysrhythmics: increased QT prolongation

Benzodiazepines, hypnotics, opioids, sedatives: increased CNS depression

CYP3A4 inducers (carBAMazepine, nevirapine, phenobarbitol, phenytoin): decreased effects of solifenacin

CYP3A4 inhibitors (clarithromycin, diclofenac, doxycycline, erythromycin, isoniazid, ketoconazole, nefazodone, propofol, protease inhibitors, verapamil): increased action of solifenacin, max dose 5 mg

Drug/herb
St. John's wort: decreased effects

Drug/food
Grapefruit juice: increased effect

Drug/lab test
Increased: LFTs

NURSING CONSIDERATIONS
Assessment
- **Urinary patterns:** assess for distention, nocturia, frequency, urgency, incontinence
- **Allergic reactions:** assess for rash; if this occurs, product should be discontinued

S

• **Cardiac patients:** monitor ECG for QT prolongation, avoid products that can increase QT prolongation
• **Angioedema:** assess for swelling of face, lips, tongue, larynx

Patient/family education
• Caution patient to avoid hazardous activities; dizziness may occur
• Advise patient that constipation, blurred vision may occur, to notify prescriber if abdominal pain with constipation occurs
• Instruct patient to call prescriber if severe abdominal pain or constipation lasts for 3 or more days
• Advise patient that heat prostration may occur if used in a hot environment, sweating is decreased
• Teach patient to take without regard to food
• Teach patient to swallow tab whole, do not crush, chew

Evaluation
Positive therapeutic outcome
• Urinary status: decreased dysuria, frequency, nocturia, incontinence

---

somatropin (Rx)
(soe-ma-troe′pin)
Genotropin, Humatrope, Norditropin, Norditropin Flexpro, Nutropin, Nutropin AQ, Omnitrope, Saizen, Serostim, Tev-Tropin, Zorbtive
Func. class.: Pituitary hormone
Chem. class.: Growth hormone
Pregnancy category C

Do not confuse:
somatropin/somatrem/SUMAtriptan

ACTION: Stimulates growth; similar to natural growth hormone—both preparations are developed by recombinant DNA technique

Therapeutic outcome: Increase in height as a result of skeletal growth in pituitary growth hormone deficiency

USES: Pituitary growth hormone deficiency (hypopituitary dwarfism), children with human growth hormone deficiency, AIDS wasting syndrome, cachexia, adults with somatropin deficiency syndrome (SDS), short stature in Noonan syndrome, SHOX deficiencies; Turner's syndrome, Prader-Willi syndrome

CONTRAINDICATIONS:
Hypersensitivity to benzyl alcohol, creosol, glycerin hypersensitivity (for medications that contain these products), closed epiphyses, acute respiratory failure, Prader-Willi syndrome with obesity, trauma

Precautions: Pregnancy **C**, breastfeeding, newborns, geriatric, diabetes mellitus, hypothyroidism, intracranial lesions, prolonged treatment in adults, scoliosis, sleep apnea, chemotherapy, respiratory disease

DOSAGE AND ROUTES
Genotropin
Child: SUBCUT 0.16-0.24 mg/kg/wk, divided into 6 or 7 daily inj, give in abdomen, thigh, buttocks
Adult: SUBCUT 0.4-0.8 mg/kg/wk divided in 6-7 daily doses

Humatrope
Child: SUBCUT/IM 0.006 mg/kg divided into equal doses either on 3 alternate days or 6 ×/wk, max 0.3 mg/kg/wk
Adult: IM 0.018 units/kg/day, max 0.0125 units/kg/day

Growth hormone deficiency

Nutropin/Nutropin AQ
Child: SUBCUT 0.3 mg/kg/wk

Serostim
Adult: SUBCUT at bedtime >55 kg 6 mg, 45-55 kg 5 mg, 35-45 kg 4 mg

Norditropin
Child: SUBCUT 0.024-0.034 mg/kg 6-7 ×/wk

Accretropin
Child: SUBCUT 0.18-0.3 mg/kg/wk divided into 6 or 7 equal daily inj

Replacement of GH in GH deficiency
Adult: SUBCUT (Saizen) 0.005 mg/kg/day; may increase after 4 wk to max 0.01 mg/kg/day

Available forms: Powder for inj (lyophilized) 1.5 mg (4 international units/ml), 4 mg (12 international units/vial), 5 mg (13 international units/vial), 5 mg (15 international units/vial), rDNA origin, 5.8 mg (15 international units/ml), 6 mg (18 international units/ml), 8 mg (24 international units/vial), 10 mg (26 international units/vial), inj 10 mg (30 international units/vial); 5, 10, 15 mg/1.5 ml

---

Implementation

- Store in refrigerator for <1 mo; if reconstituted, <1 wk; do not use discolored or cloudy sol
- Give IM or subcut, do not use IV
- Discontinue therapy if final height is achieved or epiphyseal fusion occurs
- Visually inspect parenteral products for particulate matter and discoloration

Accretropin

- No reconstitution needed, prior to use, swirl the contents of the vial with a gentle rotary motion; do not shake, the solution should be clear, store unopened vials refrigerated, do not freeze, protect from light. Once opened, the vial may be stored refrigerated ≤14 days

Genotropin

- This product is supplied as a powder, filled in a two-chamber cartridge with the active substance in the front chamber and the diluent in the rear chamber. The product is available in a 5 mg cartridge (green tip) and a 12 mg cartridge (purple tip). The 5 and 12 mg cartridges can be used with the Genotropin Pen or the Genotropin Mixer. Genotropin is also available, in various doses ranging from 0.2 mg to 2 mg, in single use, auto-mix devices called Genotropin Miniquicks
- *Cartridges:* Store cartridges refrigerated prior to reconstitution, do not freeze; protect from light. A reconstitution device supplied by the manufacturer is used to mix the powder and the diluent. After the powder and diluent are mixed, gently tip the cartridge upside down a few times until completely dissolved. DO NOT SHAKE; this may cause denaturation of the protein. If the solution is cloudy, do not use. Following reconstitution, the 5 mg cartridge will contain a 5 mg/ml solution and the 12 mg cartridge will contain a 12 mg/ml solution; both the 5 mg and 12 mg cartridges contain overfill. The cartridges contain diluent with preservative (m-cresol) and may be stored refrigerated ≤28 days after reconstitution. Do not use the 5 mg and 12 mg cartridges in patients with m-cresol hypersensitivity
- *Genotropin Miniquicks:* After dispensing, but prior to reconstitution, store at or 77 degrees ≤3 mo. A reconstitution device supplied by the manufacturer is used to mix the powder and diluent. Ten different strengths are available that each deliver a fixed volume of 0.25 ml. This product contains a diluent with no preservative, refrigerate after reconstitution and use within 24 hr. Use the reconstituted solution only once and discard any remaining solution

Humatrope

- Prior to reconstitution, store refrigerated
- *Vials:* Reconstitute each 5-mg vial with 1.5-5 ml of the supplied diluent (contains m-cresol as a preservative) or Bacteriostatic Water for Injection (contains benzoyl alcohol as a preservative); sterile water for injection can be used for patients with a hypersensitivity to both m-cresol and benzoyl alcohol. Direct the liquid against the glass vial wall. Swirl vial with a gentle rotary motion until contents are dissolved completely. Do not shake. If the solution is cloudy, do not use. Small, colorless particles may be present after refrigeration; this is not unusual for solutions containing proteins. Vials reconstituted with the diluent or bacteriostatic water are stable for 14 days when stored refrigerated; for vials reconstituted with sterile water, use the vial only once and discard the unused portion; if not used immediately, refrigerate and use within 24 hr; avoid freezing reconstituted solutions
- *Cartridges:* Reconstitute cartridges using ONLY the supplied diluent syringe; the cartridges are designed for use only with the Humatrope injection device. Once reconstituted, the cartridges are stable for up to 28 days when stored refrigerated. Store the injection device without the needle attached; avoid freezing reconstituted solutions

Norditropin

- Do not use reconstituted solution if cloudy or contains particulate matter
- Prior to use, store refrigerated
- Reconstitution of the cartridges is not required. The cartridge is intended for use only with the NordiPen injector; a prefilled, disposable pen, NordiFlex Pen injector, is also available. Each cartridge size (5 mg, 10 mg, or 15 mg per 1.5 ml cartridge) has a color-coded corresponding pen, which is graduated to deliver an appropriate dose based on the solution concentration; NordiPen and NordiFlex Pen allow for administration of a minimum 0.25-mg dose to a maximum 4.5-mg dose, depending on cartridge concentrations. Follow directions provided in Pen injector instruction booklet
- After a cartridge has been inserted into the NordiPen injector or once a NordiFlex pen is in use, the pen should be stored refrigerated and used within 4 wk. Alternatively, the 5-mg and 10-mg cartridges may be stored in the pen at room temperatures, no higher than 77° F, for up to 3 wk. NovoFine needles are recommended for administration. Wipe the stopper of the pen cartridge with rubbing alcohol

Nutropin
- Prior to reconstitution, store refrigerated
- Reconstitute each 5-mg vial with 1-5 ml bacteriostatic water for injection (benzyl alcohol preserved) and each 10-mg vial with 1-10 ml of bacteriostatic water for injection (benzyl alcohol preserved). If using for newborns, reconstitute with sterile water for injection. Direct the liquid against the glass vial wall. Swirl vial with a gentle rotary motion until contents are dissolved completely. Do not shake. If the solution is cloudy after reconstitution or refrigeration, do not use. Small, colorless particles may be present after refrigeration; this is not unusual for solutions containing proteins
- Solutions reconstituted with bacteriostatic water for injection are stable for 14 days refrigerated
- Solutions reconstituted with sterile water for injection should be used immediately and only once; discard any unused portions. Avoid freezing reconstituted solutions

Nutropin AQ
- Does not require reconstitution. Solution should be clear. Small, colorless particles may be present after refrigeration; this is not unusual for solutions containing proteins. Allow vial or pen cartridge to come to room temperature and gently swirl. If solution is cloudy, do not use
- *Vials:* Before needle insertion, wipe the vial septum with rubbing alcohol or antiseptic solution to prevent contamination by microorganisms that may be introduced by repeated needle insertions. Administer using sterile, disposable syringes and needles. Use syringes with small enough volume that the prescribed dose can be drawn from the vial with reasonable accuracy
- *Pen cartridge:* Two strengths are available: 10 mg and 20 mg; intended for use only with Nutropin AQ Pen. Each pen and cartridge are color coded to ensure accurate placement of the 10-mg or 20-mg cartridge into the appropriate pen. Do not use the 20-mg cartridge in the pen intended for the 10-mg cartridge, and vice versa. Wipe septum of pen cartridge with rubbing alcohol or antiseptic solution to prevent contamination by microorganisms that may be introduced by repeated needle insertions. Administer using sterile, disposable needles. Follow the directions provided in the Nutropin AQ Pen Instructions for Use. The Nutropin AQ 10 pen allows for administration of a minimum 0.1-mg dose to a maximum 4-mg dose, in 0.1-mg increments. The Nutropin AQ 20 pen allows for administration of a minimum 0.2-mg dose to a maximum 8-mg dose, in 0.2-mg increments

- *Prefilled device:* A prefilled multi-dose, dial-a-dose device is available in 3 strengths. Administer using disposable needles. Follow the directions provided in the Nutropin AQ NuSpin Instructions for Use. The Nutropin AQ Nuspin 5 allows for administration of a minimum dose of 0.05 mg to a maximum dose of 1.75 mg, in increments of 0.05 mg. The Nutropin AQ Nuspin 10 allows for administration of a minimum dose of 0.1 mg to a maximum dose of 3.5 mg, in increments of 0.1 mg. The Nutropin AQ Nuspin 20 allows for administration of a minimum dose of 0.2 mg to a maximum dose of 7 mg, in increments of 0.2 mg
- After initial use, vials, cartridges, and prefilled devices are stable for 28 days refrigerated; avoid freezing. Vials, cartridges, and prefilled devices are light sensitive; protect from light

Omnitrope
- Prior to reconstitution, store vials refrigerated. Store in the carton; Omnitrope is sensitive to light
- *Vials:* Reconstitute the vial with diluent provided using a sterile, disposable syringe. Swirl the vial gently, but do not shake. If the solution is cloudy after reconstitution, the contents must not be injected. After reconstitution, the 1.5-mg vial may be refrigerated ≤24 hr. The 1.5-mg vial does not contain a preservative and should only be used once; discard any remaining solution. The 5.8-mg vial diluent contains benzoyl alcohol as a preservative. After reconstitution, the contents must be used within 3 wk. After the first injection, store the 5.8-mg vial in the carton, to protect from light, in the refrigerator; avoid freezing
- *Omnitrope Pen 5 cartridge:* Each 5-mg cartridge must be inserted into the Omnitrope Pen 5 delivery system. Follow the directions provided in the Omnitrope Instructions for Use. The cartridge contains benzyl alcohol as a preservative. Once initially used, store refrigerated ≤28 days, protect from light, avoid freezing
- *Omnitrope Pen 10 cartridge:* Each 10-mg cartridge must be inserted into the Omnitrope Pen 10 delivery system. Follow the directions provided in the Omnitrope Instructions for Use. Once initially used, store refrigerated ≤28 days, protect from light, avoid freezing

Saizen
- Prior to reconstitution, store at room temperature
- *Vials:* Reconstitute each 5 mg vial with 1-3 ml bacteriostatic water for injection; reconstitute each 8.8-mg vial with 2-3 ml bacteriostatic water for injection (benzyl alcohol preserved).

In patients with hypersensitivity to benzyl alcohol, the vials can be mixed with sterile water for injection. Direct the liquid against the glass vial wall. Swirl vial with a gentle rotary motion until contents are dissolved completely. Do not shake. The solution should be clear; if it is cloudy immediately after reconstitution or refrigeration, do not use. Small, colorless particles may be present after refrigeration; this is not unusual for solutions containing proteins. After reconstitution, store vials mixed with bacteriostatic water for injection refrigerated and use within 14 days. For vials mixed with sterile water for injection, the solution should be used immediately, and any unused portion should be discarded. Avoid freezing

• *Cartridges:* Available in 4-mg and 8.8-mg click.easy cartridges for use in a compatible injection device. A reconstitution device supplied by the manufacturer is used to mix the Saizen with accompanying diluent containing metacresol. Cartridges reconstituted with the diluent containing metacresol are stable under refrigeration for up to 21 days. Avoid freezing

Serostim
• Prior to reconstitution, store vials and diluent at room temperature (15-30° C / 59-86° F).
• *Vials:* Reconstitute the 5-mg or 6-mg vials with 0.5-1 ml of supplied diluent (sterile water for injection). Reconstitute the 4-mg vial with 0.5-1 ml of bacteriostatic water for injection (benzyl alcohol preserved) and the 8.8-mg vial with 1-2 ml of bacteriostatic water for injection (benzyl alcohol preserved). Direct the liquid against the glass vial wall. Swirl vial with a gentle rotary motion until contents are dissolved completely. Do not shake. The solution should be clear; if it is cloudy immediately after reconstitution or refrigeration, do not use. Small, colorless particles may be present after refrigeration; this is not unusual for solutions containing proteins. If reconstituted with sterile water for injection, use within 24 hr. If reconstituted with bacteriostatic water for injection (benzyl alcohol preserved), the solution is stable for up to 14 days under refrigeration (2-8° C or 36-46° F). Avoid freezing

• *Cartridges:* Available in 8.8-mg click.easy cartridges for use in a compatible injection device. A reconstitution device is supplied by the manufacturer and is used to mix the Serostim with accompanying diluent containing metacresol. After reconstitution, cartridges are stable under refrigeration for up to 21 days. Avoid freezing

Serostim LQ
• Prior to use, store refrigerated
• Available in 6-mg single-use cartridges that do not require reconstitution. Administer using sterile, disposable syringes and needles
• Bring to room temperature prior to use. Discard single-use cartridge after use, even if some drug remains. Discard cartridges after the expiration date stated on the product. Do not freeze. Protect from light

Tev-Tropin
• Prior to reconstitution, store refrigerated
• Reconstitute each 5-mg vial with 1-5 ml bacteriostatic 0.9% sodium chloride (benzyl alcohol preserved) for injection. Direct the liquid against the glass vial wall. Swirl vial with a gentle rotary motion until contents are dissolved completely. Do not shake. The solution should be clear; if it is cloudy immediately after reconstitution, do not inject. Small, colorless particles may be present after refrigeration; this is not unusual for solutions containing proteins. When administering to newborns, reconstitute with sterile normal saline for injection that is unpreserved
• Solution reconstituted with bacteriostatic 0.9% sodium chloride is stable for 14 days when stored refrigerated. Solution reconstituted with sterile normal saline should be used only once, with any remaining solution discarded. Avoid freezing

Valtropin
• Prior to dispensing, store vials and diluent refrigerated. After dispensing to patients, may be stored at or below 77° F for up to 3 months
• Reconstitute each 5-mg vial with the entire contents of the accompanying diluent, which contains metacresol as a preservative. If patients are allergic to metacresol, sterile water for injection can be used. Direct the liquid against the glass vial wall. Swirl vial with a gentle rotary motion until contents are dissolved completely. Do not shake. The solution should be clear; if it is cloudy or contains particulate matter immediately after reconstitution or after refrigeration, do not inject. The final concentration of the reconstituted solution is 3.33 mg/ml
• After reconstituted with the provided diluent, solutions can be stored refrigerated for up to 14 days. After reconstituted with sterile water for injection, use only one dose of Valtropin per vial and discard the unused portion if not used immediately

Zorbtive
• Unreconstituted vials of drug and diluent may be stored at room temperature until expiration date

• Reconstitute each vial of 4 mg, 5 mg, or 6 mg with 0.5-1 ml sterile water for injection, USP. Reconstitute each 8.8 mg with 1-2 ml bacteriostatic water for injection (0.9% benzyl alcohol preserved); in newborns or patients with a benzyl alcohol hypersensitivity, sterile water for injection can be used. Review manufacturer's labeling for expected concentrations. Direct the liquid against the glass vial wall. Swirl vial with a gentle rotary motion until contents are dissolved completely. Do not shake. The solution should be clear; if it is cloudy after reconstitution or refrigeration, do not use. Small, colorless particles may be present after refrigeration; this is not unusual for solutions containing proteins

• After reconstitution with sterile water for injection, use the solution immediately and discard any unused portion. When using bacteriostatic water for injection, reconstituted solutions are stable for up to 14 days refrigerated. Avoid freezing vials of drug or diluent, or reconstituted vials

IM route

• Inject deeply into a large muscle; aspirate prior to injection; rotate injection sites daily

Subcut route

• Volumes >1 ml of reconstituted solution is not recommended; do not inject intradermally

• Allow refrigerated solutions to come to room temperature prior to injection

• Subcutaneous injections may be given in the thigh, buttocks, or abdomen; rotate injection sites daily

ADVERSE EFFECTS

CNS: Headache, growth of intracranial tumor, fever, aggressive behavior
ENDO: *Hyperglycemia, ketosis, hypothyroidism*
GI: Nausea, vomiting
GU: *Hypercalciuria*
INTEG: Rash, urticaria, pain, inflammation at inj site; hematoma
MS: Tissue swelling, joint and muscle pain
SYST: Antibodies to growth hormone

Pharmacokinetics

Absorption	Well absorbed (SUBCUT/IM)
Distribution	Unknown
Metabolism	Unknown
Excretion	Unknown
Half-life	15-60 min

Pharmacodynamics

	IM/SUBCUT (growth)
Onset	Unknown
Peak	Unknown
Duration	7 days

INTERACTIONS

Drug classifications

Androgens, thyroid hormones: increased epiphyseal closure
Glucocorticosteroids: decreased growth
Insulins, antidiabetics: decreased antidiabetic effect, adjust dosage

Drug/lab test

Increased: glucose, urine glucose
Decreased: glucose thyroid hormones

NURSING CONSIDERATIONS

Assessment

• Assess for signs/symptoms of diabetes

• Identify growth hormone antibodies if patient fails to respond to therapy

• Monitor thyroid function tests: T_3, T_4, T_7, TSH to identify hypothyroidism, thyroid hormone replacement may be needed

• Assess for allergic reaction: rash, itching, fever, nausea, wheezing

• Assess for hypercalciuria: urinary stones; groin, flank pain; nausea, vomiting, frequency, hematuria, chills

• Monitor growth rate, bone age of child at intervals during treatment

• **Respiratory infection:** in those with Prader-Willi syndrome, may have sleep apnea, upper airway obstruction; discontinue if obstruction occurs

• Rapid growth: assess for slipped capital femoral epiphysis; may also occur in endocrine disorders

• Monitor ophthalmologic status baseline and periodically, intracranial hypertension may occur

• Identify creosol or benzyl alcohol hypersensitivity before use

Patient/family education

• Explain reason for medication and expected results; that treatment may continue for yr

• Advise patient that routine follow-up is needed to monitor growth rate

• Instruct parents on procedure for medication preparation and inj use; request demonstration, return demonstration; provide written instructions

---

- Teach patient to maintain growth record, report knee, hip pain or limping
- Advise patient treatment is very expensive

Evaluation
Positive therapeutic outcome
- Growth in children until epiphyseal plates close

---

sotalol (Rx)
(soe-ta′lole)
Betapace, Betapace AF, Sorine
Func. class.: Antidysrhythmic, group III
Chem. class.: Nonselective β-blocker
Pregnancy category B

ACTION: Blockade of $β_1$- and $β_2$-receptors leads to antidysrhythmic effect, prolongs action potential in myocardial fibers without affecting conduction, prolongs QT interval, no effect on QRS duration

Therapeutic outcome: Decreased B/P, heart rate, AV conduction

USES: Life-threatening ventricular dysrhythmias; Betapace AF: to maintain sinus rhythm in symptomatic atrial fibrillation/flutter

CONTRAINDICATIONS:
Hypersensitivity to β-blockers, cardiogenic shock, heart block (2nd or 3rd degree), sinus bradycardia, CHF, bronchial asthma, CCr <40 ml/min

> **BLACK BOX WARNING:** Congenital or acquired long QT syndrome, hypokalemia

Precautions: Pregnancy B, breastfeeding, major surgery, diabetes mellitus, renal/thyroid disease, COPD, well-compensated heart failure, CAD, nonallergic bronchospasm, electrolyte disturbances, bradycardia, peripheral vascular disease

> **BLACK BOX WARNING:** Cardiac dysrhythmias, torsades de pointes, ventricular dysrhythmias, ventricular fibrillation

DOSAGE AND ROUTES
Adult: PO initial 80 mg bid, may increase to total of 240-320 mg/day, each dosage increase is made after ≥3 days and QTc interval <550 msecs
Child >2 yr with normal renal function (unlabeled): PO 30 mg/m² tid, adjust dosage gradually after ≥36 hr to max 60 mg/m² tid

Renal dose
Adult: PO CCr 30-60 ml/min q24hr; CCr 10-29 ml/min q36-48hr; CCr <10 ml/min individualize dose

Life-threatening ventricular dysrhythmias
Adult: with CCr 40-60 ml/min **IV** 75 mg over 5 hr/day, monitor QTc at end of each infusion during initiation and titration; 80 mg PO = 75 mg **IV**; 120 mg PO = 112.5 mg **IV**; 160 mg PO = 150 mg **IV**

Betapace AF
Adult: PO initial 80 mg bid, titrate upward to 120 mg bid during initial hospitalization, monitor OTC interval for 2-4 hr after each dose

Renal dose (Betapace AF)
Adult: CCr >60 ml/min q12hr; CCr 40-60 ml/min q24hr; CCr <40 ml/min do not use

Available forms: Tabs 80, 120, 160, 240 mg; (Betapace AF) 80, 120, 160 mg; inj 150 mg/10 ml (15 mg/ml)

Implementation
PO route
- Given before meals, at bedtime, tab may be crushed or swallowed whole; give with food to prevent GI upset; reduce dosage in renal dysfunction
- **Betapace and Betapace AF are not interchangeable**
- Store in dry area at room temp; do not freeze

IV route
- Dilute to a volume of either 120 ml or 300 ml with D_5W, LR
- **75-mg dose:** withdraw 6 ml sotalol inj (90 mg), add 114 ml dilute to make 120 ml (0.75% mg/ml); or withdraw 6 ml sotalol inj (90 mg), add 294 ml, dilute to make 300 ml (0.3 mg/ml)
- **112.5-mg dose:** withdraw 9 ml sotalol inj, (135 ml), add 111 ml, dilute to 120 ml (1.125 mg/ml); or withdraw 9 ml sotalol (135 mg) and add 291 ml dilute to 300 ml (0.45 mg/ml)
- **150-mg dose:** withdraw 12 ml sotalol (180 mg), add 108 ml to 120 ml (1.5 mg/ml); or withdraw 12 ml of sotalol (180 mg), add 288 ml to 300 ml (0.6 mg/ml)
- Use inf pump and infuse 100 or 250 ml over 5 hr at a constant rate

ADVERSE EFFECTS
CNS: Dizziness, mental changes, drowsiness, fatigue, headache, catatonia, depression, anxiety, nightmares, paresthesia, lethargy, insomnia, decreased concentration

S

Adverse effects: *italics* = common; **bold** = life-threatening

CV: Orthostatic hypotension, bradycardia, **CHF,** chest pain, **ventricular dysrhythmias, prolonged QT,** AV block, peripheral vascular insufficiency, palpitations, **prodysrhythmia, torsades de pointes; Betapace AF:** life-threatening ventricular dysrhythmias
EENT: Tinnitus, visual changes, sore throat, double vision, dry, burning eyes
GI: Nausea, vomiting, diarrhea, dry mouth, flatulence, constipation, anorexia, indigestion
GU: Impotence, dysuria, ejaculatory failure, urinary retention
HEMA: Agranulocytosis, thrombocytopenic purpura (rare), thrombocytopenia, leukopenia
INTEG: Rash, alopecia, urticaria, pruritus, fever, diaphoresis
MISC: Facial swelling, decreased exercise tolerance, weight change, Raynaud's disease
MS: Joint pain, arthralgia, muscle cramps, pain
RESP: Bronchospasm, dyspnea, wheezing, nasal stuffiness, pharyngitis

Pharmacokinetics

Absorption	Variable (30%)
Distribution	Crosses placenta, minimal penetration in CNS
Metabolism	Liver, protein binding 0%
Excretion	70% unchanged—kidneys
Half-life	10-24 hr, increased in renal disease

Pharmacodynamics

Onset	Several hr
Peak	Unknown
Duration	Unknown

INTERACTIONS
Individual drugs

> **BLACK BOX WARNING:** Haloperidol, chloroquine, droperidol, pentamidine; arsenic trioxide, levomethadyl: increased QT prolongation

Insulin: increased hypoglycemia
Lidocaine: increased effects of lidocaine
Nitroglycerin: increased hypotension
Theophylline: decreased bronchodilating effects of theophylline

Drug classifications

Antihypertensives, diuretics: increased hypotension
β_2-Agonists: decreased bronchodilating effects
Class IA/III antidysrhythmics, some phenothiazines, β-agonists, local anesthetics, tricyclics, CYP3A4 inhibitors (amiodarone, clarithromycin, erythromycin, telithromycin, troleandomycin), CYP3A4 substrates (methadone, pimozide, QUEtiapine, quiNIDine, risperiDONE, ziprasidone): increased QT prolongation
Sulfonylureas: decreased hypoglycemic effects
Sympathomimetics: decreased β-blocker effects

Drug/herb

Hawthorn: do not use concurrently

Drug/lab test

False: increased urinary catecholamines
Interference: glucose, insulin tolerance tests

NURSING CONSIDERATIONS
Assessment

> **BLACK BOX WARNING: QT syndrome:** Monitor B/P during beginning treatment, periodically thereafter; pulse q4hr; note rate, rhythm, quality: apical/radial pulse before administration; notify prescriber of any significant changes (pulse <50 bpm); monitor ECG continuously (Betapace AF); use QT interval to determine patient eligibility; baseline QT must be ≤450 msec, if ≥500 msec, frequency or dosage must be decreased or drug must be discontinued

> **BLACK BOX WARNING:** Requires a specialized care setting: for a minimum of at least 3 days on maintenance dose with continuous ECG monitoring, creatinine clearance, calculate before dosing

> **BLACK BOX WARNING:** Cardiogenic shock, acute pulmonary edema: do not use, as effect can further depress cardiac output

• Check for baselines in renal function tests, before therapy begins
• Assess for edema in feet, legs daily, monitor I&O ratio, daily weight; check for jugular vein distention, crackles, bilaterally, dyspnea (CHF)
⚠ Abrupt discontinuation: do not discontinue abruptly; taper over 1-2 wk
• Dose should be adjusted slowly, with at least 3 days between changes; monitor ECG for QT interval
• Monitor electrolytes (hypokalemia, hypomagnesemia); may increase dysrhythmias

Patient/family education

• Teach patient not to discontinue product abruptly, taper over 2 wk; may cause precipitate angina if stopped abruptly

---

• Teach patient not to use OTC products containing α-adrenergic stimulants (such as nasal decongestants, cold preparations); to avoid alcohol and smoking and to limit sodium intake as prescribed

• Teach patient how to take pulse and B/P at home, advise when to notify prescriber

• Instruct patient to comply with weight control, dietary adjustments, modified exercise program

• Caution patient to carry/wear emergency ID to identify product being taken, allergies

• Inform patient that product controls symptoms but does not cure

• Caution patient to avoid hazardous activities if dizziness, drowsiness are present

• Teach patient to report symptoms of **CHF**: difficulty breathing, especially on exertion or when lying down; night cough; swelling of extremities; bradycardia; dizziness; confusion; depression; fever

• Teach patient to take product as prescribed, not to double or skip doses; take any missed doses as soon as remembered if at least 4 hr until next dose

• Teach patient that hospitalization will be required for ≥3 days

Evaluation
Positive therapeutic outcome
• Absence of dysrhythmias

TREATMENT OF OVERDOSE:
Lavage; **IV** atropine for bradycardia; **IV** theophylline for bronchospasm; digoxin, O₂, diuretic for cardiac failure; hemodialysis; **IV** glucose for hyperglycemia; **IV** diazepam (or phenytoin) for seizures

spironolactone (Rx)
(speer'on-oh-lak'tone)
Aldactone, Novo-Spiroton ✦
Func. class.: Potassium-sparing diuretic
Chem. class.: Aldosterone antagonist
Pregnancy category D

Do not confuse:
Aldactone/Aldactazide

ACTION: Competes with aldosterone at receptor sites in the distal tubule in the renal system, resulting in excretion of sodium chloride, water, retention of potassium, phosphate

Therapeutic outcome: Diuretic and antihypertensive effect while retaining potassium; lowered aldosterone levels

USES: Edema of CHF, hypertension, diuretic-induced hypokalemia, primary hyperaldosteronism (diagnosis, short-term treatment, long-term treatment), edema of nephrotic syndrome, cirrhosis of the liver with ascites

Unlabeled uses: CHF, hirsutism in women

CONTRAINDICATIONS:
Pregnancy **D**, hypersensitivity, anuria, severe renal disease, hyperkalemia

Precautions: Breastfeeding, dehydration, renal/hepatic disease, electrolyte imbalances, metabolic acidosis, gynecomastia

> **BLACK BOX WARNING:** Secondary malignancy

DOSAGE AND ROUTES
Edema/hypertension
Adult: PO 25-200 mg/day in 1-2 divided doses

CHF
Adult: PO 12.5-25 mg/day, max 50 mg/day

Edema
Child: PO 1.5-3.3 mg/kg/day in single or divided doses

Hypertension
Child (unlabeled): PO 1.5-3.3 mg/kg in divided doses

Hypokalemia
Adult: PO 25-100 mg/day; if PO, potassium supplements must not be used

Primary hyperaldosteronism diagnosis
Adult: PO 400 mg/day × 4 days or 4 wk depending on the test, then 100-400 mg/day maintenance

Edema (nephrotic syndrome, CHF, hepatic disease)
Adult: PO 100 mg/day given as a single dose or in divided doses, titrate to response
Child: PO 1.5-3.3 mg/kg/day or 60 mg/m²/day given once daily or in 2-4 divided doses

Renal dose
Adult: PO CCr 10-50 ml/min; give dose q12-24hr; CCr <10 ml/min, avoid use

Polycystic ovary syndrome/hirsutism in women (unlabeled)
Adult: PO 50-200 mg in 1-2 divided doses

Available forms: Tabs 25, 50, 100 mg

S

Implementation
- Give in AM to avoid interference with sleep
- Give with food if nausea occurs; absorption may be increased; take at same time each day
- Effect may take 2 wk

ADVERSE EFFECTS
CNS: Headache, confusion, drowsiness, lethargy, ataxia
ELECT: Hyperchloremic metabolic acidosis, **hyperkalemia,** hyponatremia
ENDO: Impotence, gynecomastia, irregular menses, amenorrhea, postmenopausal bleeding, hirsutism, deepening voice, breast pain
GI: Diarrhea, cramps, **bleeding,** gastritis, vomiting, anorexia, nausea, **hepatocellular toxicity**
HEMA: Agranulocytosis
INTEG: *Rash, pruritus,* urticaria

Pharmacokinetics

Absorption	GI tract; well absorbed
Distribution	Crosses placenta
Metabolism	Liver to canrenone (active metabolite)
Excretion	Renal; breast milk
Half-life	12-24 hr (canrenone)

Pharmacodynamics

Onset	24-48 hr
Peak	48-72 hr
Duration	Unknown

INTERACTIONS
Individual drugs
Aspirin: decreased action of spironolactone
Cholestyramine: increased hyperchloremic acidosis in cirrhosis
Digoxin: increased digoxin action
Lithium: increased action, toxicity

Drug classifications
ACE inhibitors, diuretics (potassium-sparing), potassium products, salt substitute: increased hyperkalemia
Anticoagulants: decreased effects of anticoagulants, monitor INR/PT
Antihypertensives: increased action
NSAIDs: decreased effect of spironolactone

Drug/food
Potassium-rich foods, potassium salt substitutes: increased hyperkalemia

Drug/herb
Ephedra: decreased antihypertensive effect
Hawthorn, horse chestnut: increased hypotension
St. John's wort: severe photosensitivity

Drug/lab test
Increased: BUN, potassium
Decreased: sodium, magnesium
Interference: 17-OHCS, 17-KS, radioimmunoassay, digoxin assay

NURSING CONSIDERATIONS
Assessment
- **Hypokalemia:** assess for polyuria, polydipsia, dysrhythmias including a U wave on ECG
- **Hyperkalemia:** assess for weakness, fatigue, dyspnea, dysrhythmias, confusion
- Assess fluid volume status: I&O ratios and record, count or weigh diapers as appropriate, weight, distended red veins, crackles in lung, color, quality, and specific gravity of urine, skin turgor, adequacy of pulses, moist mucous membranes, bilateral lung sounds, peripheral pitting edema; dehydration symptoms of decreasing output, thirst, hypotension, dry mouth and mucous membranes should be reported
- Monitor electrolytes: potassium, sodium, calcium, magnesium; also include BUN, ABGs, uric acid, CBC, blood glucose

Patient/family education
- Teach patient to take medication early in day to prevent nocturia
- Instruct patient to take with food or milk if GI symptoms of nausea and anorexia occur
- Teach patient to maintain a record of weight on a weekly basis and notify prescriber of weight loss of >5 lb
- Caution patient that this product causes an increase in potassium levels, that foods high in potassium should be avoided: oranges, bananas, salt substitutes, dried apricots, dates; avoid potassium salt substitutes; refer to dietitian for assistance planning
- Teach patient to take in AM, to prevent sleeplessness
- Teach patient to avoid hazardous activities until reaction is known
- Teach patient to notify prescriber if pregnancy is planned or suspected, pregnancy (C), do not breastfeed
- Teach patient not to use alcohol or any OTC medications without prescriber's approval; serious product reactions may occur
- Emphasize the need to contact prescriber immediately if muscle cramps, weakness, nausea, dizziness, or numbness occur
- Teach patient to take own B/P and pulse and record
- Teach patient to notify prescriber of cramps, diarrhea, lethargy, thirst, headache, skin rash,

---

menstrual abnormalities, deepening voice, breast enlargement

• Advise patient that dizziness and confusion may occur; avoid driving or other hazardous activities if alertness is decreased

• Teach patient to continue taking medication even if feeling better; this product controls symptoms but does not cure the condition

• Advise patient with hypertension to continue other treatment (exercise, weight loss, relaxation techniques, cessation of smoking)

Evaluation

Positive therapeutic outcome

• Prevention of hypokalemia (diuretic use)
• Decreased edema
• Decreased B/P
• Decreased aldosterone levels
• Increased diuresis

TREATMENT OF OVERDOSE:

• Lavage if taken orally, monitor electrolytes
• Administer sodium bicarbonate
• Monitor hydration, CV, renal status

---

stavudine d4t (Rx)

(sta'vu-deen)
Zerit
Func. class.: Antiretroviral
Chem. class.: Nucleoside reverse transcriptase inhibitor (NRTI)
Pregnancy category C

ACTION: Prevents replication of HIV-1 by inhibition of reverse transcriptase; causes DNA chain termination

Therapeutic outcome: Decreasing diarrhea, fatigue, night sweats; increased body weight

USES: Treatment of HIV-1; used in combination with other antiretrovirals

CONTRAINDICATIONS:

Hypersensitivity to this product or zidovudine, didanosine, zalcitabine; severe peripheral neuropathy

> **BLACK BOX WARNING:** Lactic acidosis

Precautions: Breastfeeding, advanced HIV infections, bone marrow suppression, renal, peripheral neuropathy, osteoporosis, obesity

> **BLACK BOX WARNING:** Pregnancy **C**, hepatic disease, pancreatitis

DOSAGE AND ROUTES

Adult >60 kg: PO 40 mg q12hr
Adult <60 kg: PO 30 mg q12hr
Child <30 kg: PO 1 mg/kg q12hr
Child ≥30 kg ≤60 kg: PO 30 mg q12hr
Child >60 kg: PO 40 mg q12hr

Renal dose

Adult >60 kg: CCr 26-50 ml/min 20 mg q12hr; CCr 10-25 ml/min 20 mg q24hr
Adult <60 kg: CCr 26-50 ml/min 15 mg q12hr; CCr 10-25 ml/min 15 mg q24hr

Available forms: Caps 15, 20, 30, 40 mg; oral powder for sol 1 mg/ml

Implementation

• Give with or without meals; absorption does not appear to be lowered when taken with food
• Give product q4hr around the clock, even during night
• Shake susp well before using
• Use after hemodialysis

ADVERSE EFFECTS

CNS: *Peripheral neuropathy,* insomnia, anxiety, depression, dizziness, confusion, *headache,* chills/fever, malaise, neuropathy
CV: Chest pain, vasodilatation, hypertension
EENT: Conjunctivitis, abnormal vision
GI: Hepatotoxicity, *diarrhea, nausea, vomiting,* anorexia, dyspepsia, constipation, stomatitis, **pancreatitis**
HEMA: Bone marrow suppression, leukopenia, macrocytosis
INTEG: *Rash,* sweating, pruritus, benign neoplasms
MISC: Lactic acidosis, asthenia, lipodystrophy
MS: Myalgia, arthralgia
RESP: Dyspnea, pneumonia, asthma

Pharmacokinetics

Absorption	Rapidly absorbed, 82% bioavailability
Distribution	Cerebrospinal fluid
Metabolism	Unknown
Excretion	Kidneys, breast milk
Half-life	Elimination: 1-1.6 hr

Pharmacodynamics

Onset	Unknown
Peak	1 hr
Duration	Unknown

S

INTERACTIONS
Individual drugs
Chloramphenicol, dapsone, didanosine, ethambutol, hydrALAZINE, lithium, phenytoin, vinCRIStine, zalcitabine: increased peripheral neuropathy

Methadone, zidovudine: decreased stavudine effect

Probenecid: increased stavudine levels

Drug classifications
Myelosuppressants: increased myelosuppression

NURSING CONSIDERATIONS
Assessment

> **BLACK BOX WARNING:** Assess for lactic acidosis and severe hepatomegaly with steatosis; death may result

- Monitor viral load and CD4 counts, plasma HIV RNA baseline, throughout treatment
- Monitor for peripheral neuropathy: tingling, pain in extremities; if these occur, discontinue product
- **Monitor for pancreatitis:** severe upper abdominal pain, weakness, fatigue, dyspnea, nausea, vomiting throughout treatment; if these occur, discontinue product
- Monitor blood tests: WBC, differential, RBC, Hct, Hgb, platelets, serum amylase, lipase
- Monitor renal function tests: urinalysis, protein, blood, serum creatinine
- Obtain C&S before product therapy; product may be taken as soon as culture is performed; repeat C&S after therapy
- Monitor bowel pattern before, during treatment
- Monitor fluid overload; product requires large volume to stay in sol
- Assess for weakness, tremors, confusion, dizziness, psychosis; if these occur, product may have to be decreased or discontinued

Patient/family education
- Teach patient signs of peripheral neuropathy: burning, weakness, pain, pricking feeling in the extremities
- Caution patient that this product should not be given with antineoplastics
- Inform patient that GI complaints and insomnia resolve after 3-4 wk of treatment
- Inform patient that product is not a cure for AIDS but controls symptoms
- Advise patient to call prescriber if sore throat, swollen lymph nodes, malaise, fever occur; may indicate presence of other infections
- Caution patient that even with product administration, virus is still infective and may be passed on to others
- Caution patient that follow-up visits must be continued because serious toxicity may occur; blood counts must be done q2wk
- Teach patient that product must be taken q4hr around the clock even during night
- Caution patient that serious product interactions with other medications may occur, check with prescriber first if taking chloramphenicol, dapsone, cisplatin, didanosine, ethambutol, lithium, antifungals

> **BLACK BOX WARNING:** Teach patient to notify prescriber if pregnancy is planned or suspected, fatal lactic acidosis may occur, pregnancy (C), avoid breastfeeding

- Inform patient that other products may be necessary to prevent other infections
- Inform patient that product may cause fainting or dizziness

Evaluation
Positive therapeutic outcome
- Decreased symptoms of HIV infection

⚠ HIGH ALERT

succinylcholine (Rx)
(suk-sin-ill-koe′leen)
Anectine, Quelicin
Func. class.: Neuromuscular blocker (depolarizing—ultra short)
Pregnancy category C

ACTION: Inhibits transmission of nerve impulses by binding with cholinergic receptor sites, antagonizing action of acetylcholine; causes release of histamine

Therapeutic outcome: Paralysis of skeletal muscles

USES: Facilitation of endotracheal intubation, skeletal muscle relaxation during orthopedic manipulations

CONTRAINDICATIONS:
Hypersensitivity, malignant hyperthermia, trauma

Precautions: Pregnancy **C**, breastfeeding, geriatric or debilitated patients, severe burns, fractures (fasciculation may increase damage), electrolyte imbalances, dehydration, neuro-

---

muscular disease, respiratory disease, collagen diseases, glaucoma, eye surgery, renal/hepatic/cardiac disease

> **BLACK BOX WARNING:** Hyperkalemia, myopathy, rhabdomyolysis, children <2 yr

DOSAGE AND ROUTES

Adult: **IV** 0.3-1.1 mg/kg, max 150 mg, maintenance 0.04-0.07 mg/kg q5-10min as needed; CONT **IV** INF dilute to concentration of 1-2 mg/ml in D₅W or NS 10-100 mcg/kg/min

Child: **IV** initially 1-2 mg/kg; CONT **IV** INF not recommended

Available forms: Inj 20, 50, 100 mg/ml; powder for inj 100, 500 mg/vial, 1 g/vial

Implementation

• Store in refrigerator, powder at room temp; close tightly

• Give IV or IM; only experienced clinicians familiar with the use of neuromuscular blocking drugs should administer or supervise the use of this product

• Visually inspect parenteral products for particulate matter and discoloration prior to use

• Monitor heart rate and mechanical ventilator status during use

Rapid IV injection route

• Due to tachyphylaxis and prolonged apnea, this method is not recommended for prolonged procedures. Rapid IV injection of succinylcholine may result in profound bradycardia or asystole in pediatric patients; as with adults, the risk increases with repeated doses. Pretreatment with atropine may be needed

• No dilution of injection solution necessary

• Inject rapidly IV over 10-30 seconds

Continuous IV infusion route

• Not recommended for infants and children due to risk of malignant hyperthermia

• This route is preferred for long surgical procedures due to possible tachyphylaxis and prolonged apnea associated with administration of repeated fractional doses

• Dilute succinylcholine to a concentration of 1-2 mg/ml with D₅W, D₅NS, NS, or 1/6 M sodium lactate injection. One g of the powder for injection or 20 ml of a 50-mg/ml solution may be added to 1 L or 500 ml of diluent to give solutions containing 1 or 2 mg/ml, respectively. Alternatively, 500 mg of the powder for injection or 10 ml of a 50 mg/ml solution may be added to 500 ml or 250 ml of diluent to give solutions containing 1 or 2 mg/ml, respectively

• Infuse IV at a rate of 2.5 mg/min (range = 0.5-10 mg/min); adjust rate based on patient response and requirements

IM route

• Recommended for infants and other patients in whom a suitable vein is not accessible

• Inject into a large muscle, preferably high into the deltoid muscle. Aspirate prior to injection

Syringe compatibilities: Heparin

Y-site compatibilities: Etomidate, heparin, potassium chloride, propofol, vit B/C

Additive compatibilities: Amikacin, cephapirin, isoproterenol, meperidine, methyldopate, morphine, norepinephrine, scopolamine

Additive incompatibilities: Barbiturates, nafcillin, sodium bicarbonate

ADVERSE EFFECTS

CV: Bradycardia, tachycardia; increased, decreased B/P, **sinus arrest, dysrhythmias,** edema

EENT: Increased secretions, increased intraocular pressure

HEMA: Myoglobulinemia

INTEG: Rash, flushing, pruritus, urticaria

MS: Weakness, muscle pain, fasciculation, prolonged relaxation, myalgia, **rhabdomyolysis**

RESP: Prolonged apnea, bronchospasm, cyanosis, respiratory depression, wheezing, dyspnea

SYST: Anaphylaxis, angioedema

Pharmacokinetics

Absorption	Well absorbed (IM)
Distribution	Widely distributed, crosses placenta
Metabolism	Plasma (90%)
Excretion	Hydrolyzed in blood, excreted in urine (active/inactive metabolites)
Half-life	Unknown

Pharmacodynamics

	IM	IV
Onset	2-3 min	1 min
Peak	Unknown	2-3 min
Duration	10-30 min	6-10 min

S

INTERACTIONS
Individual products
Clindamycin, enflurane, isoflurane, lincomycin, lithium, oxytocin, procainamide, quiNIDine: increased neuromuscular blockade
Theophylline: increased dysrhythmias

Drug classifications
Aminoglycosides, anesthetics (local), antibiotics (polymyxin), β-adrenergic blockers, cardiac glycosides, magnesium salts, opioids, thiazides: increased neuromuscular blockade

Drug/herb
Melatonin: blocks succinylcholine

NURSING CONSIDERATIONS
Assessment
• Assess for electrolyte imbalances (potassium, magnesium); may lead to increased action of this product
• Monitor VS (B/P, pulse, respirations, airway) until fully recovered; rate, depth, pattern of respirations, strength of hand grip
• Monitor I&O ratio; check for urinary retention, frequency, hesitancy
• **Recovery:** assess for decreased paralysis of face, diaphragm, leg, arm, rest of body
• **Allergic reactions:** assess for rash, fever, respiratory distress, pruritus; product should be discontinued if these occur
• **Myopathy, rhabdomyolysis:** in pediatric patients (rare)

Patient/family education
• Explain reason for medication and expected results
• Provide reassurance if communication is difficult during recovery from neuromuscular blockade; postoperative stiffness is normal, soon subsides

Evaluation
Positive therapeutic outcome
• Paralysis of jaw, eyelid, head, neck, rest of body

TREATMENT OF OVERDOSE:
Edrophonium or neostigmine, atropine, monitor VS; may require mechanical ventilation

---

sucralfate (Rx)
(soo-kral´fate)
Carafate, Sulcrate ✚
Func. class.: Protectant; antiulcer
Chem. class.: Aluminum hydroxide/sulfated sucrose
Pregnancy category B

Do not confuse:
Carafate/Cafergot

ACTION: Forms a complex that adheres to ulcer site, adsorbs pepsin

Therapeutic outcome: Healing of ulcers

USES: Duodenal ulcer, oral mucositis, stomatitis after radiation of head and neck

Unlabeled uses: Gastric ulcers, gastroesophageal reflux

CONTRAINDICATIONS:
Hypersensitivity

Precautions: Pregnancy **B,** breastfeeding, children, renal failure, hypoglycemia (diabetics)

DOSAGE AND ROUTES
Duodenal ulcers
Adult: PO 1 g qid 1 hr before meals and at bedtime
Child: PO 40-80 mg/kg/day divided

Available forms: Tabs 1 g; oral susp 1 g/10 ml

Implementation
• Do not break, crush, or chew tabs
• Give on empty stomach 1 hr before meals and at bedtime
• Avoid antacids ½ hr before or 1 hr after taking this product
• Store at room temperature

ADVERSE EFFECTS
CNS: Drowsiness, dizziness
ENDO: Hyperglycemia (diabetes mellitus)
GI: *Dry mouth, constipation,* nausea, gastric pain, vomiting, bezoar (critically ill patients)
INTEG: Urticaria, rash, pruritus

Pharmacokinetics	
Absorption	Minimally absorbed
Distribution	Unknown
Metabolism	Not metabolized
Excretion	Feces (90%)
Half-life	6-20 hr

Pharmacodynamics

Onset	½ hr
Peak	Unknown
Duration	6 hr

INTERACTIONS
Individual drugs
Cimetidine, ranitidine: decreased absorption of sucralfate

Digoxin, ketoconazole, phenytoin, tetracycline, theophylline: decreased action of each specific product

Drug classifications
Antacids: decreased absorption of sucralfate

Fat-soluble vitamins: decreased action of fat-soluble vitamins

Fluoroquinolones: decreased absorption

NURSING CONSIDERATIONS
Assessment
• **GI symptoms:** assess for abdominal pain, blood in stools
• **Hypoglycemia:** may occur in those with diabetes mellitus, monitor blood glucose carefully

Patient/family education
• Instruct patient to take medication on empty stomach
• Caution patient to take full course of therapy, not to use >8 wk, to avoid smoking
• Caution patient to avoid antacids within ½ hr of product or 1 hr after this product
• Advise patient to increase fluids, bulk, exercise to lessen constipation

Evaluation
Positive therapeutic outcome
• Absence of pain or GI complaints

---

sulfamethoxazole/ trimethoprim (cotrimoxazole) (Rx)
(sul-fa-meth-ox′a-zole/trye-meth′oh-prim [ko-trye-mox′a-zole])
Bacter-Aid DS, Bactrim DS, Novo-Trimel ♣, Nu-Cotrimox ♣, Septra, Septra DS, SMZ/TMP, Sultrex
Func. class.: Antiinfective
Chem. class.: Sulfonamide—miscellaneous
Pregnancy category C

ACTION: Sulfamethoxazole (SMZ) interferes with bacterial biosynthesis of proteins by competitive antagonism of PABA when adequate levels are maintained; trimethoprim (TMP) blocks synthesis of tetrahydrofolic acid; combination blocks two consecutive steps in bacterial synthesis of essential nucleic acids, protein

Therapeutic outcome: Absence of infection, based on C&S

USES: UTI, otitis media, acute and chronic prostatitis, shigellosis, chancroid, traveler's diarrhea, *Enterobacter, Escherichia coli, Haemophilus influenzae* (beta-lactamase negative), *Haemophilus influenzae* (beta-lactamase positive), *Klebsiella, Morganella morganii, Pneumocystis carinii, Pneumocystis jiroveci, Proteus mirabilis, Proteus, Shigella flexneri, Shigella sonnei, Streptococcus* pneumonia; **may also be effective for** *Acinetobacter baumannii, Actinomadura madurae, Actinomadura pelletieri, Bordetella pertussis, Burkholderia pseudomallei, Cyclospora cayetanensis, Haemophilus ducreyi, Isospora belli, Klebsiella granulomatis, Legionella micdadei, Legionella pneumophila, Listeria monocytogenes, Moraxella catarrhalis, Neisseria gonorrhoeae, Nocardia asteroides, Nocardia brasiliensis, Nocardia otitidiscaviarum, Pediculus capitis, Plasmodium falciparum, Providencia, Salmonella, Serratia, Shigella, Staphylococcus aureus* (MRSA), *Staphylococcus aureus* (MSSA), *Staphylococcus epidermidis, Stenotrophomonas maltophilia, Streptococcus pyogenes* (group A beta-hemolytic streptococci), *Streptomyces somaliensis, Toxoplasma gondii, Vibrio cholerae, Viridans* streptococci, *Yersinia enterocolitica*

CONTRAINDICATIONS:
Pregnancy at term, breastfeeding, infants <2 mo, hypersensitivity to trimethoprim or sulfonamides, megaloblastic anemia, CCr <15 ml/min

Precautions: Pregnancy **C**, infants, geriatric, renal disease, G6PD deficiency, impaired renal/hepatic function, possible folate deficiency, severe allergy, bronchial asthma, UV exposure, porphyria, hyperkalemia, hypothyroidism

DOSAGE AND ROUTES
Based on TMP content

UTI
Adult: PO 160 mg TMP q12hr × 10-14 days
Child: PO 8 mg/kg TMP daily in 2 divided doses q12hr (treatment); 2 mg/kg/day (prophylaxis)

S

Otitis media
Child: PO 8 mg/kg TMP daily in 2 divided doses q12hr × 10 days

Chronic bronchitis
Adult: PO 160 mg TMP q12hr × 10-14 days

Pneumocystis jiroveci pneumonitis
Adult and child: PO 15-20 mg/kg TMP daily in 4 divided doses q6hr × 14-21 days; **IV** 15-20 mg/kg/day (based on TMP) in 3-4 divided doses for up to 14 days

Renal dose
Dosage reduction necessary in moderate to severe renal impairment (CCr <30 ml/min)

Available forms: Tabs 80 mg TMP/400 mg SMZ, 160 mg TMP/800 mg SMZ; susp 200 mg-40 mg/5 ml, 800 mg-160 mg/20 ml; **IV** 16 mg/80 mg/ml

Implementation
• Give with full glass of water to maintain adequate hydration; increase fluids to 2 L/day to decrease crystallization in kidneys
• Give medication after C&S; repeat C&S after full course of medication
• Store in airtight, light-resistant container at room temp
• Give without regard to meals

Intermittent IV infusion route
• Dilute 5 ml ampule/100-125 ml of D₅W, stable for 6 hr, give over ½ hr, do not refrigerate, if using Septra ADD-Vantage vials dilute each 10-ml vial in ADD-Vantage diluent containers containing 250 ml of D₅W, infuse over 60-90 min, change site q48-72hr

Y-site compatibilities: Acyclovir, aldesleukin, allopurinol, amifostine, atracurium, aztreonam, cefepime, cyclophosphamide, diltiazem, enalaprilat, esmolol, filgrastim, fludarabine, gallium, granisetron, HYDROmorphone, labetalol, LORazepam, magnesium sulfate, melphalan, meperidine, morphine, pancuronium, perphenazine, piperacillin/tazobactam, sargramostim, tacrolimus, teniposide, thiotepa, vecuronium, zidovudine

Y-site incompatibilities: Alfentanil, amikacin, aminophylline, amphotericin B colloidal, ampicillin, ampicillin/sulbactam, ascorbic acid, atropine, azaTHIOprine, benztropine, bumetanide, buprenorphine, butorphanol, calcium chloride/gluconate, caspofungin, ceFAZolin, cefotaxime, cefOXitin, cefTAZidime, cefTRIAXone, chloramphenicol, chlorproMAZINE, cimetidine, clindamycin, codeine, cyanocobalamin, cycloSPORINE, dantrolene, dexamethasone, diazepam, diazoxide, digoxin, diphenhydrAMINE, DOBUTamine, DOPamine, DOXOrubicin, doxycycline, ePHEDrine, EPINEPHrine, epirubicin, epoetin alfa, erythromycin, famotidine, fentaNYL, fluconazole, folic acid, furosemide, ganciclovir, gentamicin, glycopyrrolate, haloperidol, heparin, hydrALAZINE, hydrocortisone, hydrOXYzine, IDArubicin, imipenem/cilastatin, inamrinone, indomethacin, insulin, isoproterenol, ketorolac, lidocaine, mannitol, mechlorethamine, metaraminol, methoxamine, methyldopate, methylPREDNISolone, metoclopramide, metoprolol, metroNIDAZOLE, midazolam, multi-vitamins, nafcillin, nalbuphine, naloxone, nitroglycerin, nitroprusside, norepinephrine, ondansetron, oxacillin, oxytocin, papaverine, penicillin G, pentamidine, pentazocine, PENTobarbital, PHENobarbital, phentolamine, phenylephrine, phenytoin, phytonadione, potassium chloride, procainamide, prochlorperazine, promethazine, propranolol, protamine, quinupristin/dalfopristin, ranitidine, sodium bicarbonate, succinylcholine, SUFentanil, thiamine, ticarcillin/clavulanate, tobramycin, tolazoline, trimetaphan, urokinase, vancomycin, verapamil, vinorelbine

ADVERSE EFFECTS
CNS: Headache, insomnia, hallucinations, depression, vertigo, fatigue, anxiety, seizures, product fever, chills, **aseptic meningitis**
CV: Allergic myocarditis
EENT: Tinnitus
GI: *Nausea, vomiting, abdominal pain,* stomatitis, **hepatitis,** glossitis, pancreatitis, diarrhea, **enterocolitis,** anorexia, **pseudomembranous colitis**
GU: Renal failure, toxic nephrosis; increased BUN, creatinine; crystalluria
HEMA: Leukopenia, neutropenia, thrombocytopenia, agranulocytosis, hemolytic anemia, hypoprothrombinemia, HenochSchölein purpura, methemoglobinemia, eosinophilia I
INTEG: Rash, dermatitis, urticaria, erythema, photosensitivity, pain, inflammation at injection site, **toxic epidermal necrolysis, erythema multiforme**
RESP: Cough, shortness of breath
SYST: Anaphylaxis, systemic lupus erythematosus, Stevens-Johnson syndrome

Pharmacokinetics

Absorption	Rapid
Distribution	Breast milk, crosses placenta, 68% protein bound
Metabolism	Liver
Excretion	Kidneys
Half-life	8-13 hr

Pharmacodynamics

Onset	Unknown
Peak	1-4 hr
Duration	Unknown

INTERACTIONS

Individual drugs

CycloSPORINE: decreased response
Dofetilide: increased levels of dofetilide
Methenamine: increased crystalluria
Methotrexate: increased bone marrow depression
Phenytoin: decreased hepatic clearance of phenytoin

Drug classifications

Anticoagulants (oral): increased anticoagulant effect
CYP2C9, CYP3A4 inducers: decreased hepatic clearance
Diuretics (potassium-sparing), potassium supplements: increased potassium levels
Diuretics (thiazide): increased thrombocytopenia
Sulfonylureas: increased hypoglycemic response

Drug/lab test

Increased: creatinine, bilirubin
Decreased: Hgb, platelets

NURSING CONSIDERATIONS

Assessment

• Monitor I&O ratio; note color, character, pH of urine if product administered for UTI; output should be 800 ml less than intake; if urine is highly acidic, alkalization may be needed
• Monitor renal function tests: BUN, creatinine, urinalysis (long-term therapy)
• Assess type of infection; obtain C&S before starting therapy
• Assess blood dyscrasias, skin rash, fever, sore throat, bruising, bleeding, fatigue, joint pain
• Assess allergic reaction: rash, dermatitis, urticaria, pruritus, dyspnea, bronchospasm, AIDS patients are more susceptible

Patient family education

• Teach patient to take each oral dose with full glass of water to prevent crystalluria; drink 8-10 glasses of water/day
• Teach patient to complete full course of treatment to prevent superinfection
• Teach patient to avoid sunlight or use sunscreen to prevent burns
• Teach patient to avoid OTC medications (aspirin, vit C) unless directed by prescriber
• If diabetic, teach patient to use Clinistix or Tes-Tape
• Teach patient to use alternative contraceptive measures; decreased effectiveness of oral contraceptives may result
• Teach patient to notify prescriber if skin rash, sore throat, fever, mouth sores, unusual bruising, bleeding occur

Evaluation

Positive therapeutic outcome

• Absence of pain, fever, C&S negative

sulfaSALAzine (Rx)

(sul-fa-sal′a-zeen)
Azulfidine, Azulfidine EN-tabs, Salazopyrin ✦
Func. class.: GI Antiinflammatory, antirheumatic (DMARD)
Chem. class.: GI Sulfonamide
Pregnancy category B

Do not confuse:

sulfaSALAzine/sulfiSOXAZOLE

ACTION: Proproduct to deliver sulfapyridine and 5-aminosalicylic acid to colon; antinflammatory in connective tissue

Therapeutic outcome: Treatment of ulcerative colitis, rheumatoid arthritis

USES: Ulcerative colitis, rheumatoid arthritis, juvenile rheumatoid arthritis (Azulfidine EN-tabs)

Unlabeled uses: Crohn's disease

CONTRAINDICATIONS:

Pregnancy at term, children <2 yr, hypersensitivity to sulfonamides or salicylates, intestinal, urinary obstruction, porphyria

Precautions: Pregnancy **B**, breastfeeding, impaired renal/hepatic function, severe allergy, bronchial asthma, megaloblastic anemia

S

DOSAGE AND ROUTES
Bowel disease
Adult: PO 3-4 g/day in divided doses; maintenance 2 g/day in divided doses q6hr
Child ≥6 yr: PO 40-60 mg/kg/day in 4-6 divided doses, then 30 mg/kg/day in 4 doses, max 2 g/day

Rheumatoid arthritis
Adult: PO 0.5-1 g/day, then increase daily dose by 500 mg qwk to 2 g/day in 2-3 divided doses

Juvenile rheumatoid arthritis
Child ≥6 yr: PO 30-50 mg/kg/24 hr, divided into 2 doses

Renal dose
Adult: PO CCr 10-30 ml/min give bid; CCr <10 ml/min give daily

Available forms: Tabs 500 mg; oral susp 250 mg/5 ml; del rel tabs 500 mg

Implementation
• Give with full glass of water to maintain adequate hydration; increase fluids to 2 L/day to decrease crystallization in kidneys; contact lenses, urine, skin may be yellow-orange
• Give total daily dose in evenly spaced doses and after meals to help minimize GI intolerance
• Give at bedtime
• Store in airtight, light-resistant container at room temperature

ADVERSE EFFECTS
CNS: Headache, confusion, insomnia, hallucinations, depression, vertigo, fatigue, anxiety, **seizures,** product fever, chills
CV: Allergic myocarditis
GI: *Nausea, vomiting, abdominal pain,* stomatitis, **hepatitis,** glossitis, **pancreatitis,** diarrhea
GU: Renal failure, toxic nephrosis, increased BUN, creatinine, crystalluria
HEMA: Leukopenia, neutropenia, thrombocytopenia, agranulocytosis, hemolytic anemia
INTEG: Rash, dermatitis, urticaria, **Stevens-Johnson syndrome,** erythema, photosensitivity
SYST: Anaphylaxis

Absorption	Partially absorbed
Distribution	Crosses placenta
Metabolism	Liver
Excretion	Kidneys, breast milk
Half-life	6 hr

Onset	1 hr
Peak	1½-6 hr
Duration	6-12 hr

INTERACTIONS
Individual drugs
AzaTHIOprine, mercaptopurine: increased leucopenia risk
CycloSPORINE: decreased effect of cycloSPORINE
Digoxin: decreased digoxin effect
Folic acid: decreased folic acid effect
Methotrexate: decreased renal excretion

Drug classifications
Anticoagulants (oral): increased anticoagulant effect
Hypoglycemics (oral): increased hypoglycemic response

Drug/food
Iron, folic acid will be poorly absorbed

Drug/lab test
False positive: urinary glucose test

NURSING CONSIDERATIONS
Assessment
• Monitor I&O ratio; note color, amount, character, pH of urine if product administered for UTIs; output should be 800 ml less than intake; if urine is highly acidic, alkalization may be needed
• Monitor kidney function tests: BUN, creatinine, urinalysis if on long-term therapy
⚠ **Blood dyscrasias: assess for rash, fever, sore throat, bruising, bleeding, fatigue, joint pain; monitor CBC before and q3mo**
⚠ **Allergic reaction: assess for rash, dermatitis, urticaria, pruritus, dyspnea, bronchospasm**
• **Ulcerative colitis, proctitis, other inflammatory bowel disease:** monitor character, amount, consistency of stools, abdominal pain, cramping, blood, mucus
• **Rheumatoid arthritis:** assess mobility, joint swelling, pain, activities of daily living

Patient/family education
• Advise patient to take each oral dose with full glass of water to prevent crystalluria
• Teach patient to avoid sunlight or to use sunscreen to prevent burns
• Teach patient to avoid OTC medication (aspirin, vit C) unless directed by prescriber

• Advise patient to notify prescriber if skin rash, sore throat, fever, mouth sores, unusual bruising, bleeding occur

• Advise patient to use rectal susp at bedtime and retain all night

Evaluation

Positive therapeutic outcome

• Absence of fever, mucus in stools or pain in joints

SUMAtriptan (Rx)

(soo-ma-trip′tan)

ALSUMA Auto-injector, Imitrex, Sumavel Dose Pro, Zecuity

Func. class.: Antimigraine agent

Chem. class.: 5-HT$_1$ receptor agonist

Pregnancy category C

Do not confuse:

SUMAtriptan/somatropin

ACTION: Binds selectively to the vascular 5-HT$_1$ receptor subtype and exerts antimigraine effect; causes vasoconstriction in cranial arteries

Therapeutic outcome: Absence of migraines

USES: Acute treatment of migraine with or without aura and cluster headache

CONTRAINDICATIONS:

Angina pectoris, history of MI, documented silent ischemia, Prinzmetal's angina, ischemic heart disease, **IV** use, concurrent ergotamine-containing preparations, uncontrolled hypertension, hypersensitivity, basilar or hemiplegic migraine

Precautions: Pregnancy **C**, breastfeeding, children <18 yr, postmenopausal women, men >40 yr, geriatric, risk factors for CAD, hypercholesterolemia, obesity, diabetes, impaired renal/hepatic function, overuse

DOSAGE AND ROUTES

Adult: SUBCUT 6 mg or less, may repeat in 1 hr, max 12 mg/24 hr; PO 25 mg with fluids if no relief in 2 hr, give another dose, max 200 mg/day; NASAL 1 dose of 5, 10, or 20 mg in one nostril, may repeat in 2 hr, max 40 mg/24 hr, 1 puff each nostril q2hr; TD 1 patch (6.5 mg/4 hr); after application push activation button

Hepatic dose

Adult: PO 25 mg, if no response after 2 hr, give up to 50 mg

Available forms: Inj 4, 6 mg/0.5 ml; tabs 25, 50, 100 mg; nasal spray 5 mg/100 mcl-units dose spray device 20 mg/100 mcl-units; transdermal patch 6.5 mg/4 hr

Implementation

PO route

• Swallow tab whole; do not break, crush, or chew

• Take with fluids as soon as symptoms appear; may take a second dose >4 hr, max 200 mg/24 hr

SUBCUT route

• Give by SUBCUT route only, avoid IM or **IV** administration, use only for actual migraine attack

• Give 1st dose supervised by medical staff in those with CAD or those at risk for CAD

Nasal route

• Spray once in 1 nostril, may repeat if headache returns, do not repeat if pain continues after 1st dose

Transdermal route

• Do not cut; apply to dry, intact skin of upper arm or thigh; do not use over scars, tattoos, cuts, scratches, burns, abrasions

• Apply another patch if headache is not relieved ≥2 hr after 1st patch; push activation button within 15 min of applying or patch will not work; do not bathe, shower, swim; may be taped with medical tape if needed

• Do not use with MRI

• Remove slowly, cleanse with soap and water, may cause redness

• Dispose of after folding in half

ADVERSE EFFECTS

CNS: *Tingling, hot sensation, burning, feeling of pressure, tightness, numbness, dizziness, sedation,* headache, anxiety, fatigue, cold sensation

CV: *Flushing,* **MI,** hypo/hypertension

EENT: Throat, mouth, nasal discomfort, vision changes

GI: Abdominal discomfort

INTEG: *Inj site reaction,* sweating

MS: *Weakness, neck stiffness,* myalgia

RESP: Chest tightness, pressure

Pharmacokinetics

Absorption	Well absorbed (SUBCUT)
Distribution	10%-20% plasma protein binding
Metabolism	Liver (metabolite)
Excretion	Urine, feces
Half-life	2 hr

Adverse effects: *italics* = common; **bold** = life-threatening

Pharmacodynamics

	SUBCUT
Onset	10-20 min
Peak	10 min-2 hr
Duration	Up to 24 hr (pain relief)

INTERACTIONS
Individual drugs
Ergotamine: increased risk of vasospastic reaction

Drug classifications
Ergot derivatives: extended vasospastic effects
MAOIs, SSRIs, SNRIs, serotonin-receptor agonists: increased SUMAtriptan levels

Drug/herb
SAM-e, St. John's wort: serotonin syndrome

NURSING CONSIDERATIONS
Assessment
• **Serotonin syndrome:** assess for delirium, coma, agitation, diaphoresis, hypertension, fever, tremors, may resemble neuroleptic malignant syndrome (in patients taking SSRIs, SNRIs)
• Assess for tingling, hot sensation, burning, feeling of pressure, numbness, flushing, inj site reaction
• Assess B/P; signs/symptoms of coronary vasospasm
• Monitor stress level, activity, reaction, coping mechanisms of patient
• Assess neurologic status: LOC, blurring vision, nausea, vomiting, tingling in extremities preceding headache
• Assess for ingestion of tyramine-containing foods (pickled products, beer, wine, aged cheese), food additives, preservatives, colorings, artificial sweeteners, chocolate, caffeine, which may precipitate these types of headaches

Patient/family education
• Caution patient not to take more than 2 doses/day or 12 mg/day; allow at least 1 hr between doses
• Caution patient to avoid driving or hazardous activities if dizziness or drowsiness occurs
• Teach patient to report chest tightness, heat, flushing, drowsiness, dizziness, fatigue, sudden severe abdominal pain or any allergic reactions that occur to prescriber immediately
• Inform patient to report any side effects to prescriber
• Caution patient to use contraception when taking product, to notify prescriber if pregnancy is suspected or planned

• **Nasal spray:** one spray in one nostril, may repeat if headache returns, do not repeat if pain continues after 1st dose

Evaluation
Positive therapeutic outcome
• Decrease in frequency, severity of headache

SUNItinib (Rx)
(soo-nit'in-ib)
Sutent
Func. class.: Antineoplastic—miscellaneous
Chem. class.: Protein-tyrosine kinase inhibitor
Pregnancy category D

ACTION: Inhibits multiple receptor tyrosine kinases (RTKs), some are responsible for tumor growth

Therapeutic outcome: Decrease in size of tumor

USES: Gastrointestinal stromal tumors (GIST) after disease progression or intolerance to imatinib; advanced renal carcinoma, pancreatic neuroendocrine tumors (pNET) in those with unresectable locally advanced/metastatic disease

CONTRAINDICATIONS: Pregnancy **D**, breastfeeding, hypersensitivity

Precautions: Children, geriatric, active infections, QT prolongation, torsades de pointes, stroke, heart failure

> **BLACK BOX WARNING:** Hepatic disease

DOSAGE AND ROUTES
Gastrointestinal stromal tumors (GIST)/renal cell cancer
Adult: PO 50 mg/day × 4 wk, then 2 wk off; may increase or decrease dose by 12.5 mg; if administered with CYP3A4 inducers, give 87.5 mg/day; if given with CYP3A4 inhibitors give 37.5 mg/day

Pancreatic neuroendocrine (pNET)
Adult: PO 37.5 mg/day continuously, increase or decrease by 12.5 mg based on tolerance, avoid potent CYP3A4 inhibitors/inducers, if used with CYP3A4 inhibitor decrease sunitinib dose to a minimum of 25 mg/day; if used with CYP3A4 inducer increase sunitinib to a max of 62.5 mg/day

---

Available forms: Caps 12.5, 25, 50 mg

Implementation
- Give with meal and large glass of water to decrease GI symptoms
- Give nutritious diet with iron, vitamin supplement, low fiber, few dairy products
- Store at 25°C (77°F)

ADVERSE EFFECTS
CNS: **CNS hemorrhage**, headache, dizziness, insomnia, **seizures**, fatigue
CV: Hypertension, **left ventricular dysfunction; QT prolongation, cardiotoxicity, thrombotic microangiopathy, torsades de pointes**
ENDO: Hyper/hypothyroidism
GI: *Nausea,* **hepatotoxicity,** vomiting, dyspepsia, *anorexia, abdominal pain,* altered taste, *constipation,* stomatitis, mucositis, **pancreatitis,** diarrhea, **GI bleeding/perforation**
GU: **Nephrotic syndrome**
HEMA: **Neutropenia, thrombocytopenia, hemolytic anemia, leukopenia**
INTEG: *Rash, yellow skin discoloration,* depigmentation of hair or skin, alopecia
MS: Pain, arthralgia, myalgia, myopathy, **rhabdomyolysis**
RESP: Cough, dyspnea, pulmonary embolism
SYST: **Bleeding,** electrolyte abnormalities, hand-foot syndrome, **serious infection**

Pharmacokinetics

Absorption	Unknown
Distribution	Protein binding 95%
Metabolism	By CYP3A4
Excretion	Feces, small amount in urine
Half-life	Terminal 40-60 hr (sunitinib); active metabolite 80-110 hr

Pharmacodynamics

Onset	Unknown
Peak	6-12 hr
Duration	Unknown

INTERACTIONS
Individual drugs
Acetaminophen: increased hepatotoxicity
Bevacizumab: microangiopathic hemolytic anemia; avoid concurrent use
Dexamethasone, carBAMazepine, PHENobarbital, phenytoin, rifampin: decreased SUNItinib concentrations

Haloperidol, chloroquine, droperidol, pentamidine, arsenic trioxide, levomethadyl: increased QT prolongation
Simvastatin: increased plasma concentrations
Warfarin: increased plasma concentration; avoid use with warfarin, use low-molecular-weight anticoagulants instead

Drug classifications
Calcium channel blockers: increased plasma concentrations
Class IA/III antidysrhythmics, some phenothiazines, β-agonists, local anesthetics, tricyclics, CYP3A4 inhibitors (amiodarone, clarithromycin, erythromycin, telithromycin, troleandomycin), CYP3A4 substrates (methadone, pimozide, QUEtiapine, quiNIDine, risperidone, ziprasidone): increased QT prolongation

Drug/herb
St. John's wort: decreased sunitinib concentration

Drug/food
Grapefruit juice: increased plasma concentrations

NURSING CONSIDERATIONS
Assessment
- Monitor ANC and platelets; if ANC $<1 \times 10^9$/L and/or platelets $<50 \times 10^9$/L, stop until ANC $>1.5 \times 10^9$/L and platelets $>75 \times 10^9$/L; if ANC $<0.5 \times 10^9$/L and/or platelets $<10 \times 10^9$/L, reduce dose by 200 mg; if cytopenia continues, reduce dose by another 100 mg; if cytopenia continues for 4 wk, stop product until ANC $\geq 1 \times 10^9$/L
- Assess CV status: hypertension, QT prolongation can occur; monitor left ventricular ejection fraction (LVEF) (MUGA) baseline periodically, ECG, B/P
- Assess for **renal toxicity:** if bilirubin $>3 \times$ IULN, withhold sunitinib until bilirubin levels return to $<1.5 \times$ IULN; electrolytes
- **Hepatotoxicity:** monitor liver function tests, before treatment and qmo; if liver transaminases $>5 \times$ IULN, withhold sunitinib until transaminase levels return to $<2.5 \times$ IULN
- Assess for **CHF:** adrenal insufficiency in those experiencing trauma
- Assess for bleeding: epistaxis rectal, gingival, upper GI, genital, wound bleeding; tumor-related hemorrhage may occur rapidly

Patient/family education
- Advise patient to report adverse reactions immediately: shortness of breath, bleeding

• Teach patient reason for treatment, expected result
• Teach patient that many adverse reactions may occur: high B/P, bleeding, mouth swelling, taste change, skin discoloration, depigmentation of hair/skin
• Teach patient to avoid persons with known upper respiratory infections; immunosuppression is common
• Teach to avoid grapefruit juice

• Teach patient to report if pregnancy is planned or suspected, pregnancy **D**

Evaluation

Positive therapeutic outcome
• Decrease in size of tumor

suprofen ophthalmic
See Appendix B

tacrolimus (PO, IV) (Rx)

(tak-row'lim-us)

Prograf

tacrolimus (topical) (Rx)

Protopic

Func. class.: Immunosuppressant

Chem. class.: Macrolide

Pregnancy category C

ACTION: Produces immunosuppression by inhibiting lymphocytes (T)

Therapeutic outcome: Prevention of rejection in organ transplant

USES: Organ transplants, to prevent rejection; **topical:** atopic dermatitis

Unlabeled uses: Severe recalcitrant psoriasis

CONTRAINDICATIONS:

Hypersensitivity to this product or to some kinds of castor oil, long-term use (topical), child <2 yr (topical)

Precautions: Pregnancy **C,** breastfeeding, children <12 yr, severe renal/hepatic disease, diabetes mellitus, hyperkalemia, hyperuricemia, lymphomas, hypertension, acute bronchospasm, African descent, heart failure, seizures, QT prolongation

> **BLACK BOX WARNING:** Children <12 yr, lymphomas, infection, neoplastic disease, neonates, infants; requires a specialized setting and an experienced clinician

DOSAGE AND ROUTES

Kidney transplant rejection prophylaxis

Adult: **IV** 0.03-0.05 mg/kg/day as cont INF, give no sooner than 6 hr after transplantation

Liver transplant rejection prophylaxis

Adult: **PO** 0.10-0.15 mg/kg/day in 2 divided doses q12h, give no sooner than 6 hr after transplantation; **IV** 0.03-0.05 mg/kg/day as a cont INF, give no sooner than 6 hr after transplantation

Heart transplant rejection prophylaxis

Adult: **PO** 0.075 mg/kg/day in 2 divided doses q12h, give no sooner than 6 hr after transplantation; **IV** 0.01 mg/kg/day as a cont INF, give no sooner than 6 hr after transplantation

Atopic dermatitis

Adult: **TOP** use 0.03% or 0.1% ointment, apply bid × 7 day after clearing of signs

Child 2-5 yr: **TOP** 0.03% ointment, apply bid × 7 day after clearing of signs

Available forms: Inj **IV** 5 mg/ml; caps 0.5, 1, 5 mg; ointment 0.03%, 0.1%

Implementation

PO route

• Give on empty stomach, food decreases absorption

• Give for several days before transplant surgery; patients should be placed in protective isolation

• Apply thin layers to affected skin only, rub in gently

• Use on small area of skin

• **Topical ointment has risk of developing cancer; use only when other options have failed**

Continuous IV infusion route

• Give after diluting in 0.9% NaCl or D₅W to a concentration of 0.004-0.02 mg/ml as a cont inf

Y-site compatibilities: Alemtuzumab, alfentanil, amifostine, amikacin, aminophylline, amiodarone, amphotericin B colloidal, amphotericin B liposome, anidulafungin, atracurium, aztreonam, benztropine, bivalirudin, bleomycin, bumetanide, buprenorphine, busulfan, butorphanol, calcium acetate/chloride/gluconate, CARBOplatin, carmustine, caspofungin, ceFAZolin, cefoperazone, cefotaxime, cefoTEtan, cefOXitin, cefTAZidime, ceftizoxime, cefTRIAXone, cefuroxime, chloramphenicol, chlorproMAZINE, cimetidine, ciprofloxacin, cisatracurium, CISplatin, clindamycin, cyclophosphamide, cycloSPORINE, cytarabine, DACTINomycin, DAPTOmycin, dexamethasone, dexmedetomidine, dexrazoxane, digoxin, diltiazem, diphenhydrAMINE, DOBUTamine, DOCEtaxel, dolasetron, DOPamine, doripenem, doxacurium, DOXOrubicin hydrochloride, doxycycline, droperidol, enalaprilat, ePHEDrine, EPINEPHrine, epirubicin, ertapenem, erythromycin, esmolol, etoposide, etoposide phosphate, famotidine, fenoldopam, fentaNYL, fluconazole, fludarabine, foscarnet, fosphenytoin, gemcitabine, gentamicin, glycopyrrolate, granisetron, haloperidol, heparin, hydrALAZINE, hydrocortisone, HYDROmorphone, IDArubicin, ifosfamide, imipenem/cilastatin, inamrinone, insulin, isoproterenol, ketorolac, labetalol, leucovorin, levofloxacin, levorphanol, lidocaine, linezolid, LORazepam, magnesium sulfate, mannitol, mechlorethamine, meperidine, meropenem, mesna, metaraminol,

methotrexate, methyldopa, methylPREDNISolone, metoclopramide, metoprolol, metroNI-
DAZOLE, micafungin, midazolam, milrinone,
mitoMYcin, mitoXANtrone, mivacurium,
morphine, multivitamins, nafcillin, nalbuphine,
naloxone, nesiritide, niCARdipine, nitroglycerin,
nitroprusside, norepinephrine, octreotide,
ondansetron, oxacillin, oxaliplatin, oxytocin,
PACLitaxel, palonosetron, pancuronium, PEME-
trexed, penicillin G, pentamidine, pentazocine,
perphenazine, phentolamine, phenylephrine,
piperacillin/tazobactam, potassium chloride/
phosphates, procainamide, prochlorperazine,
promethazine, propranolol, quinupristin/dal-
fopristin, ranitidine, remifentanil, rocuronium,
sodium acetate/bicarbonate/phosphates, streptozocin, succinylcholine, SUFentanil, teniposide,
theophylline, thiotepa, ticarcillin/clavulanate,
tigecycline, tirofiban, tobramycin, tolazoline,
trimethobenzamide, vancomycin, vasopressin,
vecuronium, verapamil, vinCRIStine, vinorelbine, voriconazole, zidovudine, zoledronic acid

Y-site incompatibilities: Acyclovir, allopurinol, azaTHIOprine, cefepime, dantrolene,
diazepam, diazoxide, espmeprazole, folic
acid, ganciclovir, iron sucrose, levothyroxine,
omeprazole, phenytoin, thiopental

ADVERSE EFFECTS

CNS: *Tremors, headache,* insomnia, paresthesia, chills, fever, **seizures,** posterior reversible
encephalopathy syndrome, BK-virus-associated
nephropathy
CV: Hypertension, myocardial hypertrophy,
prolonged QTc, cardiomyopathy
EENT: Blurred vision, photophobia
GI: Nausea, vomiting, diarrhea, constipation,
GI bleeding
GU: Urinary tract infections, **albuminuria,
hematuria, proteinuria, renal failure, hemo-
lytic uremic syndrome**
HEMA: Anemia, **leukocytosis, thrombocy-
topenia, purpura**
INTEG: Rash, flushing, itching, alopecia
META: Hirsutism, hyperglycemia, hyperurice-
mia, hypo/hyperkalemia, hypomagnesemia
MS: Back pain, muscle spasms
RESP: **Pleural effusion, atelectasis,**
dyspnea, **interstitial lung disease**
SYST: **Anaphylaxis,** infection, malignancy

Absorption	Erractically absorbed (PO), completely absorbed (**IV**)
Distribution	Crosses placenta, 75% protein binding
Metabolism	Liver to metabolite
Excretion	Kidney—minimal; breast milk, bile
Half-life	10 hr

Pharmacodynamics

	PO	IV
Onset	Unknown	Unknown
Peak	1-4 hr	Unknown
Duration	12 hr	12 hr

INTERACTIONS
Individual drugs
CarBAMazepine, PHENobarbital, phenytoin,
rifamycin: decreased blood levels
Cimetidine, danazol, erythromycin, mycopheno-
late, mofetil: increased blood levels
CISplatin, cycloSPORINE: increased toxicity
Haloperidol, chloroquine, droperidol, pent-
amidine, arsenic trioxide, levomethadyl;
CYP3A4 substrates (methadone, pimozide,
QUEtiapine, quiNIDine, risperiDONE, zipra-
sidone): increased QT prolongation; do not
use together
Ibuprofen: increased oliguria

Drug classifications
Aminoglycosides: increased toxicity
Antifungals, calcium channel blockers: increased blood levels
Class IA/III antidysrhythmics, some phenothiazines, β-agonists, local anesthetics, tricyclics,
CYP3A4 inhibitors (amiodarone, clarithromycin, erythromycin, telithromycin, troleandomycin), CYP3A4 substrates (methadone, pimozide, QUEtiapine, quiNIDine, risperiDONE,
ziprasidone): increased QT prolongation
Live virus vaccines: decreased effect of vaccines

Drug/herb
Astragalus, echinacea, melatonin: decreased
immunosuppression
Ginseng, St. John's wort: decreased effect

Drug/food
Decreased absorption of food
Grapefruit juice: increased effect of tacrolimus

Drug/lab test
Increased: glucose, BUN, creatinine
Decreased: magnesium, Hgb, platelets
Increased or decreased: LFTs, potassium

⚠ Nurse Alert   **✳ Key NCLEX® Drug**

NURSING CONSIDERATIONS
Assessment
• Monitor blood studies: Hgb, WBC, platelets during treatment monthly; if WBC is <3000/mm³ or platelet count <100,000/mm³, product should be discontinued or reduced; decreased Hgb level may indicate bone marrow suppression

• **QT prolongation:** ECG for QT prolongation, ejection fraction; assess for chest pain, palpitations, dyspnea

• Monitor liver function tests: alkaline phosphatase, AST, ALT, amylase, bilirubin, and for hepatotoxicity: dark urine, jaundice, itching, light-colored stools; product should be discontinued

• Monitor serum creatinine/BUN, serum electrolytes, lipid profile, serum tacrolimus concentration

⚠ Assess for anaphylaxis: rash, pruritus, wheezing, laryngeal edema; stop inf, initiate emergency procedures

Patient/family education

> **BLACK BOX WARNING:** Advise patient to report if pregnancy is planned or suspected

> **BLACK BOX WARNING:** Advise patient to report symptoms of lymphoma

• Instruct patient to report fever, rash, severe diarrhea, chills, sore throat, fatigue because serious infections may occur; clay-colored stools, cramping may indicate hepatotoxicity, signs of diabetes mellitus

• Caution patient to avoid crowds or persons with known infections to reduce risk of infection, to avoid eating raw shellfish

Evaluation
Positive therapeutic outcome
• Absence of graft rejection
• Immunosuppression in autoimmune disorders

---

tadalafil (Rx)
(tah-dal′a-fil)
Adcirca, Cialis
Func. class.: Impotence agent
Chem. class.: Phosphodiesterase type 5 inhibitor
Pregnancy category B

ACTION: Inhibits phosphodiesterase type 5 (PDE5); enhances erectile function by increasing the amount of cyclic GMP, which causes smooth muscle relaxation and increased blood flow into the corpus cavernosum; improves erectile function for up to 36 hr

Therapeutic outcome: Erection

USES: Treatment of erectile dysfunction; pulmonary arterial hypertension (PAH) (Adcirca only), benign prostatic hyperplasia (BPH) with or without erectile dysfunction

CONTRAINDICATIONS:
Newborns, women, children, hypersensitivity, patients taking organic nitrates regularly or intermittently, patients taking any α-adrenergic antagonist other than 0.4 mg once-daily tamsulosin

Precautions: Pregnancy **B,** although not indicated for women, anatomic penile deformities, sickle cell anemia, leukemia, multiple myeloma, CV/renal/hepatic disease, bleeding disorders, active peptic ulcer, prolonged erection

DOSAGE AND ROUTES
Erectile dysfunction
Adult: PO (Cialis) CCr 51-80 ml/min erectile dysfunction no adjustment; 20 mg/day initially, pulmonary hypertension; 10 mg, taken prior to sexual activity, dose may be reduced to 5 mg or increased to a max of 20 mg; usual max dosing frequency is once per day; once-daily dosing 2.5 mg/day at same time each day

BPH
Adult: PO 5 mg bid at the same time every day

Renal dose
Adult: PO CCr 31-50 ml/min 5 mg/day, max 10 mg q48hr; CCr <30 ml/min, max 5 mg q72hr

Hepatic dose
Adult: PO Child-Pugh class A, B, max 10 mg/day or 20 mg/day (pulmonary hypertension) max 40 mg/day; Child-Pugh class C, not recommended

Concomitant medications
Ketoconazole, itraconazole, ritonavir, max 10 mg q72hr

Pulmonary hypertension
Adult: PO **(Adcirca only)** 40 mg qd; **Adult taking ritonavir:** PO 20 mg qd initially, then increase to 40 mg qd as tolerated

Available forms: Tabs 2.5, 5, 10, 20 mg; tab 20 mg (Adcirca)

T

Adverse effects: *italics* = common; **bold** = life-threatening

Implementation
• **Sexual dysfunction:** give before sexual activity; do not use more than once a day
• **Pulmonary hypertension:** give Adcirca without regard to meals
• **Product should not be used with nitrates in any form**

ADVERSE EFFECTS
CNS: *Headache, flushing, dizziness,* seizures, transient global amnesia
CV: **MI,** hypotension, **QT prolongation**
INTEG: **Stevens-Johnson syndrome, exfoliative dermatitis,** urticaria
MISC: Back pain/myalgia, *dyspepsia, nasal congestion, UTI,* blurred vision, changes in color vision, *diarrhea,* pruritus, priapism, **nonarteritic ischemic optic neuropathy (NAION),** hearing loss

Pharmacokinetics

Absorption	Rapid; rate and extent of absorption of tadalafil are not influenced by food
Distribution	94% protein bound
Metabolism	Liver
Excretion	Excreted primarily as metabolites, feces, urine; plasma concentration 61% in feces, 36% in urine
Half-life	17.5 hr

Pharmacodynamics

Onset	Rapid
Peak	6 hr
Duration	Unknown

INTERACTIONS
Individual drugs
Alcohol, amlodipine, enalapril: decreased B/P
Bosentan: decreased effects of tadalafil
Itraconazole, ketoconazole, ritonavir: increased levels (although not studied, may also include other HIV protease inhibitors)

Drug classifications
⚠ **Do not use with nitrates because of unsafe drop in B/P that could result in heart attack or stroke**
α-blockers, angiotensin II receptor blockers: decreased B/P
Antacids: decreased effects of tadalafil

Drug/food
Grapefruit: increased tadalafil effect

NURSING CONSIDERATIONS
Assessment
• **Cialis:** assess for underlying cause of erectile dysfunction prior to treatment; organic nitrates that should not be used with this product; assess for severe loss of vision
• **Adcirca:** monitor hemodynamic parameters baseline and periodically

Patient/family education
• Teach patient to take 1 hr before sexual activity
• Teach patient not to drink large amounts of alcohol
• Advise that product does not protect against STDs, including HIV
• Instruct to tell physician if patient has a bleeding problem
• Advise that product should not be used with nitrates in any form
• Advise that product has no effect in the absence of sexual stimulation
• Instruct to seek medical help if an erection lasts more than 4 hr or if chest pain occurs
• Advise to tell physician of all medicines, vitamins, and herbs patient is taking, especially α-blockers, erythromycin, indinavir, itraconazole, ketoconazole, nitrates, ritonavir
• **Advise that tadalafil is contraindicated for use with α-blockers except 0.4 mg/ daily tamsulosin**

Evaluation
Positive therapeutic outcome
• Sustainable erection
• Improvement in exercise ability (pulmonary hypertension)

---

tamoxifen (Rx)
(ta-mox′i-fen)
Apo-Tamox ✦, Nolvadex, Tamofen ✦
Func. class.: Antineoplastic
Chem. class.: Antiestrogen
Pregnancy category D   ✴

ACTION: Inhibits cell division by binding to cytoplasmic estrogen receptors; resembles normal cell complex but inhibits DNA synthesis and estrogen response of target tissue

Therapeutic outcome: Prevention of rapidly growing malignant cells

USES: Advanced breast carcinoma that has not responded to other therapy in estrogen receptor–positive patients (usually postmenopausal), prevention of breast cancer, after breast

---

surgery/radiation in ductal carcinoma in situ (DCIS)

Unlabeled uses: Mastalgia, pain/size of gynecomastia, ovulation stimulation, malignant carcinoid tumor, carcinoid syndrome, meta-plastic melanoma, desmoid tumors, McCune-Albright syndrome (female pediatric patients)

CONTRAINDICATIONS:
Pregnancy **D**, breastfeeding, hypersensitivity

> **BLACK BOX WARNING:** Thromboembolic disease

Precautions: Leukopenia, thrombocytopenia, cataracts, women of childbearing age

> **BLACK BOX WARNING:** Endometrial cancer, stroke

DOSAGE AND ROUTES
Breast cancer
Adult: PO 20-40 mg/day × 5 yr, doses >20 mg/day divide AM/PM

High risk for breast cancer
Adult: PO 20 mg/day × 5 yr

Ductal carcinoma in situ
Adult: PO 20 mg/day × 5 yr

McCune-Albright syndrome (unlabeled)
Child 2-10 yr (girls): PO 20 mg/day for up to 1 yr

Available forms: Tabs 10, 20 mg

Implementation
• Do not break, crush, or chew tabs
• Give with food or fluids for GI upset; repeat dose may be needed if vomiting occurs
• Store in light-resistant container at room temperature

ADVERSE EFFECTS
CNS: *Hot flashes, headache, lightheadedness,* depression, mood changes
CV: Chest pain, stroke, fluid retention, flushing
EENT: Ocular lesions, cataracts, retinopathy, corneal opacity, blurred vision (high doses)
GI: *Nausea, vomiting,* altered taste (anorexia)
GU: Vaginal bleeding, pruritus vulvae, uterine malignancies, *altered menses, amenorrhea*
HEMA: **Thrombocytopenia, leukopenia,** deep vein thrombosis
INTEG: *Rash,* alopecia
META: Hypercalcemia
RESP: **Pulmonary embolism**

Pharmacokinetics
Absorption	Adequately absorbed
Distribution	Unknown
Metabolism	Liver—extensively
Excretion	Feces—slowly, small amounts (kidneys)
Half-life	1 wk

Pharmacodynamics
Onset	Unknown
Peak	4-7 hr
Duration	Unknown

INTERACTIONS
Individual drugs
Aminoglutethimide, rifamycin: decreased tamoxifen levels
Bromocriptine: increased tamoxifen level
Letrozole: decreased levels of letrozole
PARoxetine: increased risk for death from breast cancer
Radiation: increased myelosuppression

Drug classifications
Anticoagulants: increased risk of bleeding
Cytotoxics: increased thromboembolic action
CYP2D6 inhibitors (antidepressants): decreased tamoxifen effect
CYP3A4 inducers (barbiturates, bosentan, carBAMazepine, efavirenz, phenytoin, nevirapine, rifabutin, rifampin): decreased tamoxifen effect
CYP3A4 inhibitors (aprepitant, antiretroviral protease inhibitors, clarithromycin, danazol, delavirdine, diltiazem, erythromycin, fluconazole, FLUoxetine, fluvoxaMINE, imatinib, ketoconazole, mibefradil, nefazodone, telithromycin, voriconazole): increased toxicity

Drug/herb
Black cohosh, dong quai, St. John's wort: avoid use

Drug/lab test
Increased: serum calcium, T_4, AST, ALT, cholesterol, triglycerides

NURSING CONSIDERATIONS
Assessment
• Monitor CBC, differential, platelet count weekly; withhold product if WBC is <4000/mm³ or platelet count is <75,000/mm³; notify prescriber of results; monitor calcium levels (hypercalcemia is common); breast exam, mammogram, pregnancy test, bone mineral

Adverse effects: *italics* = common; **bold** = life-threatening

density, LFTs, serum calcium, serum lipid profile, periodic eye exams (cataracts, retinopathy)
⚠ **Assess for tumor flare: increase in bone, tumor pain during beginning treatment; give analgesics as ordered to decrease pain**
• **Assess for bleeding:** hematuria, guaiac, bruising or petechiae, mucosa or orifices q8hr, no rectal temp

> **BLACK BOX WARNING: Assess for uterine malignancies:** symptoms of stroke, PE that may occur in women with DCIS and women at high risk for breast cancer

Patient/family education
• Teach patient to use nonhormonal contraception during treatment and for 2 months after discontinuing treatment
• Teach patient to notify prescriber of stroke: blurred vision, headache, weakness on one side of the body; pulmonary embolism: chest pain, fainting sweating, difficulty breathing
• Instruct patient to report any complaints, side effects to prescriber; if dose is missed, do not double next dose; that use may be 5 yr
• Advise patient that vaginal bleeding, pruritus, hot flashes can occur and are reversible after discontinuing treatment
• Instruct patient to report immediately decreased visual acuity, which may be irreversible; stress need for routine eye exams
• Inform patient about who should be told about tamoxifen therapy
• Advise patient to report vaginal bleeding immediately; that tumor flare (increase in size or tumor, increased bone pain) may occur and will subside rapidly; may take analgesics for pain; that premenopausal women must use mechanical birth control method because ovulation may be induced (teratogenic product)
• **Tumor flare:** Advise patient that increase in size of tumor, increased bone pain may occur and will subside rapidly; may take analgesics for pain
• Teach patient that hair loss may occur during treatment; a wig or hairpiece may make patient feel better; new hair may be different in color, texture
• Advise patient to increase fluids to 2 L/day unless contraindicated

Evaluation
Positive therapeutic outcome
• Decreased spread of malignant cells in breast cancer

tamsulosin (Rx)
(tam-sue-lo'sen)
Flomax
Func. class.: Selective α-adrenergic blocker, BPH agent
Chem. class.: Sulfamoyl phenethylamine derivative
Pregnancy category B

Do not confuse:
Flomax/Fosamax/Volmax

ACTION: Binds preferentially to α IA-adrenoceptor subtype located mainly in the prostate

Therapeutic outcome: Decreased symptoms of benign prostatic hyperplasia (BPH)

USES: Symptoms of BPH

CONTRAINDICATIONS:
Hypersensitivity

Precautions: Pregnancy **B**, breastfeeding, children, hepatic disease, CAD, severe renal disease, prostate cancer; cataract surgery (floppy iris syndrome)

DOSAGE AND ROUTES
Adult: PO 0.4 mg/day, increasing to 0.8 mg/day if required

Hepatic dose (moderate impairment)
Adult: PO reg rel 50 mg q8hr, titrate; ext rel 50 mg q24hr, titrate, max 100 mg q24hr; avoid use in severe impairment

Available forms: Caps 0.4 mg

Implementation
• Swallow caps whole; do not break, crush, or chew
• Store in airtight container at 86° F (30° C) or less
• Give without regard to food, but may be given with food to prevent GI symptoms; ½ hr after same meal each day
• If treatment is interrupted for several days, restart at lowest dose (0.4 mg/day)

ADVERSE EFFECTS
CNS: *Dizziness, headache,* asthenia, insomnia
CV: Chest pain, orthostatic hypotension
EENT: Amblyopia, floppy iris syndrome
GI: Nausea, diarrhea, dysgeusia

GU: Decreased libido, abnormal ejaculation, priapism
MS: Back pain
RESP: Rhinitis, pharyngitis, cough
SYST: Angioedema

Pharmacokinetics

Absorption	Well absorbed
Distribution	Not known; 98% plasma protein bound
Metabolism	Liver, extensively
Excretion	Kidneys
Half-life	9-15 hr

Pharmacodynamics

Unknown

INTERACTIONS
Individual drugs
Cimetidine: increased toxicity
Doxazosin, prazosin, terazosin, vardenafil: do not use together

Drug classifications
α-blockers: do not use together

Drug/food
Decreased: absorption with food

NURSING CONSIDERATIONS
Assessment
• Monitor CBC with differential and liver function tests; B/P and heart rate
• Monitor urodynamic studies/urinary flow rates, residual volume
• **Assess for BPH:** change in urinary patterns, baseline, throughout treatment; monitor I&O ratios, weight daily, edema, report weight gain or edema
• **Orthostatic hypotension:** monitor B/P standing, sitting

Patient/family education
• Teach patient not to discontinue product abruptly; emphasize the importance of complying with dosage schedule, even if feeling better; if dose is missed take as soon as remembered; take at same time each day
• Teach patient not to use OTC products (cough, cold, allergy) unless directed by prescriber; also to avoid large amounts of caffeine
• Caution patient that product may cause dizziness, may occur during 1st few days of therapy; to avoid hazardous activities
• Teach patient to take ½ hr before same meal each day

• Teach patient about priapism (rare)
• Advise patient not to crush, break, chew caps

Evaluation
Positive therapeutic outcome
• Decreased symptoms of BPH

tapentadol (Rx)
(ta-pen′ta-dol)
Nucynta, Nucynta ER
Func. class.: Analgesic, miscellaneous
Chem. class.: μ-Opioid receptor agonist
Pregnancy category C
Controlled substance schedule II

ACTION: Centrally acting synthetic analgesic; μ-opioid agonist activity is thought to result in analgesia; inhibits norepinephrine uptake

Therapeutic outcome: Relief of pain

USES: Moderate to severe pain

CONTRAINDICATIONS:
Hypersensitivity, asthma, ileus

> **BLACK BOX WARNING:** Respiratory depression

Precautions: Pregnancy **C,** breastfeeding, children <18 yr, increased intracranial pressure, MI (acute), severe heart disease, respiratory depression, renal/hepatic disease, GI obstruction, ulcerative colitis, sleep apnea, seizure disorder

> **BLACK BOX WARNING:** Accidental exposure, avoid ethanol, substance abuse

DOSAGE AND ROUTES
Adult: PO 50-100 mg q4-6hr; may give second dose 1 hr or more after 1st dose; max 700 mg on day 1, 600 mg/day thereafter; ext rel 50 mg q12hr (opioid-naive), titrate to 100-250 mg q12hr, max 250 mg q12hr

Available forms: Tab 50, 75, 100 mg; tabs, ext rel 50, 100, 150, 200, 250 mg

Implementation
• Give with antiemetic if nausea, vomiting occur
• Give when pain is beginning to return; determine dosing interval by response
• Store in light-resistant area at room temperature
• Provide assistance with ambulation
• Provide safety measures: night-light, call bell within easy reach

- Not to crush, chew, break, or use with alcohol: ext rel product
- Preferred analgesic in those with altered cytochrome P450 or mild hepatic disease, mild to moderate renal disease

ADVERSE EFFECTS

CNS: *Drowsiness, dizziness, confusion, headache, euphoria,* hallucinations, restlessness, syncope, anxiety, flushing, psychological dependence, insomnia, lethargy, tremor, **seizures**
CV: Palpitations, bradycardia, hypo/hypertension, orthostatic hypotension, sinus tachycardia
GI: *Nausea, vomiting, anorexia, constipation, cramps,* gastritis, dyspepsia, biliary spasms
GU: Urinary retention/frequency
INTEG: *Rash,* urticaria, diaphoresis, pruritus
RESP: Respiratory depression, cough
SYST: Anaphylaxis, infection, serotonin syndrome

Pharmacokinetics	
Absorption	32%
Distribution	Protein binding 20%
Metabolism	Liver, extensively
Excretion	Urine 99%
Half-life	Terminal 4 hr

Pharmacodynamics	
Onset	Unknown
Peak	Unknown
Duration	Unknown

INTERACTIONS
Individual drugs
Alcohol: increased effects with other CNS depressants

Drug classifications
Antipsychotics, opioids, sedatives/hypnotics, skeletal muscle relaxants: increased effects with other CNS depressants
MAOIs: increased toxicity
Serotonin-receptor agonists, SSRIs, SNRIs, tricyclics: increased serotonin syndrome

Drug/herb
Kava, St. John's wort, valerian: increased sedative effect

NURSING CONSIDERATIONS
Assessment
- Monitor I&O ratio; check for decreasing output; may indicate urinary retention

- Assess CNS changes: dizziness, drowsiness, hallucinations, euphoria, LOC, pupil reaction
- Assess for allergic reactions: rash, urticaria, anaphylaxis
- **Serotonin syndrome:** Assess for increased heart rate, shivering, sweating, dilated pupils, tremors, high B/P, hyperthermia, headache, confusion; if these occur, stop product, administer a serotonin antagonist if needed

> **BLACK BOX WARNING: Assess for respiratory dysfunction:** respiratory depression, character, rate, rhythm; notify prescriber if respirations are <10/min; also B/P, pulse

- **Assess for pain:** intensity, location, type, characteristics; need for pain medication by pain/sedation scoring; physical dependence

Patient/family education
- Teach patient to report any symptoms of CNS changes, allergic reactions
- Advise that physical dependency may result from extended use
- Inform that withdrawal symptoms may occur: nausea, vomiting, cramps, fever, faintness, anorexia
- Teach to avoid CNS depressants, alcohol
- Advise to avoid driving, operating machinery if drowsiness occurs

Evaluation
Positive therapeutic outcome
- Decrease in pain

tazobactam
See piperacillin/tazobactam

tbo-filgrastim
(fil-gras′tim)
Neutrophil
Func. class.: Biologic modifier
Chem. class.: Short-acting granulocyte colony-stimulating factor (G-CSF)
Pregnancy category C

ACTION: Stimulates proliferation and differentiation of neutrophils by binding to G-CSF receptors

Therapeutic outcome: Absence of severe neutropenia in cancer

USES: Chemotherapy-induced neutropenia prophylaxis to reduce the duration of severe neutropenia in nonmyeloid malignancies

CONTRAINDICATIONS:
Hypersensitivity

Precautions: Pregnancy (C), breastfeeding, children, sickle cell disease, chemotherapy, neoplastic disease

DOSAGE AND ROUTES
Adult: SUBCUT 5 mcg/kg/day

Available forms: Solution for injection 300 mcg/0.5 ml, 480 mcg/0.8 ml

Implementation
SUBCUT route
• Visually inspect for particulate matter and discoloration before use, the solution should be clear; do not shake
• Injection sites include the front of the middle thighs, the upper outer areas of the buttocks, the upper back portion of the upper arms, or the abdomen except for the 2 inches around the navel; vary sites daily
• After removing the needle shield, expel unneeded volume based on the needed dose, discard unused portions
• Inject SUBCUT, avoiding any area that is tender, red, bruised, or hard or that has stretch marks or scars; push the plunger as far as it will go, because injection of the entire contents is necessary to activate the needle guard
• Remove needle from skin while keeping plunger depressed; slowly let the plunger go to allow the empty syringe to move inside the device and guard the needle

ADVERSE EFFECTS
CNS: Fever, headache
GI: Nausea, vomiting, diarrhea, anorexia, abdominal pain
HEMA: Excessive leukocytosis
INTEG: Alopecia
RESP: Acute respiratory distress syndrome (ARDS)
SYST: Anaphylaxis, angioedema, sickle cell crisis, splenic rupture

Pharmacokinetics

Absorption	Unknown
Distribution	Unknown
Metabolism	Unknown
Excretion	Unknown
Half-life	3.2–3.8 hr

Pharmacodynamics

Onset	Unknown
Peak	Unknown
Duration	Unknown

INTERACTIONS
Individual drugs
Lithium: increased adverse reactions—do not use this product concomitantly with lithium

Drug classifications
Antineoplastics: Increased adverse reactions—do not use this product concomitantly with antineoplastics

NURSING CONSIDERATIONS
Assessment
• Blood studies: obtain CBC, platelet count before treatment and twice weekly; neutrophil counts may be increased for 2 days after therapy
• Obtain B/P, respirations, pulse before and during therapy
• Assess for bone pain; give mild analgesics with chemotherapy

Patient/family education
• Teach patient about the technique for self-administration: dose, side effects, disposal of containers and needles; provide instruction sheet

Evaluation
Positive therapeutic outcome
• Absence of severe neutropenia in cancer

telaprevir
(tel-a′pre-vir)
Incivek
Func. class.: Antiviral, antihepatitis agent
Chem. class.: NS3/4A protease inhibitor
Pregnancy category B (alone); X (combination therapy)

ACTION: Prevents hepatitis C viral (HCV) replication by blocking the proteolytic activity of HCV NS3/4A serine protease; hepatitis C virus NS3/4A serine protease is an enzyme responsible for the conversion of HCV-encoded polyproteins to mature/functioning viral proteins. These proteins (NS4A, NS4B, NS5A, NS5B), are needed for viral replication.

Therapeutic outcome: Decreasing hepatitis C viral infection

USES: Chronic hepatitis C

CONTRAINDICATIONS:
Pregnancy **X** in combination, male partners of women who are pregnant

Precautions: Breastfeeding, anemia, neutropenia, thrombocytopenia, HIV, hepatitis B,

Adverse effects: *italics* = common; **bold** = life-threatening

decompensated hepatic disease, in liver or other organ transplants, neonates, infants, children, adolescents <18 years of age

> **BLACK BOX WARNING:** Serious rash

DOSAGE AND ROUTES
For the treatment of chronic hepatitis C infection (genotype 1) in adults with compensated liver disease

In patients without cirrhosis who are previously untreated or have relapsed after treatment with interferon and ribavirin therapy:

Adult: PO 750 mg tid (q7-9hr) with peginterferon alfa and ribavirin; duration is determined by the patient's HCV RNA level at treatment wk 4, 12. If the HCV RNA is undetectable at wk 4, 12, give the three-drug regimen for 12 wk, then give an additional 12 wk of only peginterferon alfa and ribavirin (24 wk total); if the HCV RNA is detectable but ≤1000 international units/ml at wk 4, or 12, give the three-drug regimen for 12 wk, then an additional 36 wk of only peginterferon alfa and ribavirin (48 wk total)

Those without cirrhosis who are previously partial or null responders to interferon and ribavirin therapy/or those with cirrhosis

Adult: PO 750 mg tid (q7-9hr) with peginterferon alfa and ribavirin; give the three drug regimen for 12 wk, then another 36 wk (48 wk total) of only peginterferon alfa and ribavirin

Available forms: Tab 375 mg

Implementation
• Only use in combination with peginterferon alfa and ribavirin; never give as monotherapy
• Discontinue in hepatitis C virus (HCV) RNA concentrations ≥1000 international units/ml at wk 4 or 12 or a confirmed detectable HCV RNA concentration at wk 24
• Any contraindication to peginterferon alfa or ribavirin also applies to this product. See ribavirin monograph for additional information regarding contraindications and warnings associated with these products
• Give with food, not low-fat
• Store tabs at room temperature

ADVERSE EFFECTS
CNS: Fatigue
GI: Anorectal discomfort, diarrhea, dysgeusia, hemorrhoids, hyperbilirubinemia, nausea, pruritus ani, rectal burning, vomiting

HEMA: Anemia, decreased Hgb, leukopenia, lymphopenia, neutropenia, thrombocytopenia
INTEG: Drug reaction with eosinophilia and systemic symptoms (DRESS), pruritus, rash, Stevens-Johnson Syndrome (SJS); severe rashes (bullous rash, skin ulcerations, and vesicular rash)
META: Increased uric acid

Pharmacokinetics
Absorption	Unknown
Distribution	59%-76% protein binding
Metabolism	Liver
Excretion	82% (feces)
Half-life	9-11 hr

Pharmacodynamics
Onset	Unknown
Peak	4-5 hrs
Duration	Unknown

INTERACTIONS
Individual drugs
Acetaminophen, alfentanil, aliskiren, almotriptan, alosetron, ALPRAZolam, aminophylline, amiodarone, amitriptyline, amLODIPine, ARIPiprazole, astemizole, atorvastatin, atorvastin, bepridil, boceprevir, bosentan, budesonide, bupivacaine, buprenorphine, busPIRone, carvedilol, cevimeline, chloroquine, cilostazol, cinacalcet, citalopram, clarithromycin, clomiPRAMINE, clonazePAM, clopidogrel, cloZAPine, colchicine, cyclobenzaprine, cycloSPORINE, dapsone, DAUNOrubicin, desipramine, desloratadine, dexamethasone, dexlansoprazole, dextromethorphan, diazepam, diclofenac, digoxin, diltiazem, disopyramide, disulfiram, DOCEtaxel, dolasetron, donepezil, DOXOrubicin, droperidol, dutasteride, ebastine, eletriptan, eplerenone, erlotinib, erythromycin, estazolam, eszopiclone, ethosuximide, etoposide, exemestane, felodipine, fentaNYL, fexofenadine, finasteride, flecainide, flunitrazepam, flurazepam, galantamine, gefitinib, glyburide, granisetron, halofantrine, haloperidol, HYDROcodone, ifosfamide, imipramine, indinavir, isradipine, irinotecan, itraconazole, ivermectin, ixabepilone, ketoconazole, lansoprazole, lidocaine, loperamide, loratadine, losartan, maraviroc, mefloquine, meloxicam, mirtazapine, mitoMYcin, montelukast, morphine, nateglinide, niCARdipine, NIFEdipine, nisoldipine, nortriptyline, omeprazole, ondansetron, oxybutynin, oxyCODONE, PACLitaxel, palonosetron,

paricalcitol, plicamycin, posaconazole, prasugrel, praziquantel, propafenone, quazepam, QUEtiapine, quinacrine, quiNIDine, ramelteon, repaglinide, rifabutin, risperiDONE, ropivacaine, salmeterol, selegiline, sertraline, sibutramine, silodosin, sirolimus, sitaxsentan, solifenacin, SUFentanil, SUNItinib, tacrolimus, telithromycin, teniposide, terfenadine, testosterone, theophylline, tiagabine, tinidazole, tolterodine, tolvaptan, traMADol, traZODone, vardenafil, venlafaxine, verapamil, vinBLAStine, vinCRIStine, voriconazole, warfarin, and others: use cautiously; may need to reduce dose: increased effect, adverse reactions of each product

Alfuzosin, cisapride, ezetimibe, lovastatin, niacin with simvastatin and boceprevir, pimozide, simvastatin; oral midazolam, triazolam; sildenafil, tadalafil (pulmonary arterial hypertension): do not use concurrently; increased; life-threatening reactions of each product

Atazanavir, efavirenz, lopinavir with ritonavir, ritonavir: possible treatment failure

Drosperinone: increased hyperkalemia

Ethinyl estradiol: Decreased estrogen levels

Methadone: decreased effect of methadone

Drug classifications

CYP3A4 inhibitors (carBAMazepine, PHENobarbital, phenytoin, rifampin): decreased telaprevir effect

Ergots (dihydroergotamine, ergotamine, ergonovine, methylergonovine): do not use concurrently; increased; life-threatening reactions of each product

Phosphodiesterase type 5 (PDE5) inhibitors (for erectile dysfunction), systemic corticosteroids: use cautiously; may need to reduce dose: increased effect, adverse reactions of each product

Drug/herb

Do not use with St. John's wort

NURSING CONSIDERATIONS

Assessment

• **Pregnancy:** Pregnancy (**X**) combination therapy; obtain a pregnancy test prior to, monthly during, and for 6 months after treatment is completed; those who are not willing to practice strict contraception should not receive treatment with these products; report any cases of prenatal ribavirin exposure to the Ribavirin Pregnancy registry at (800) 593-2214

• **Anemia:** Monitor hemoglobin prior to, at treatment wks 4, 8, and 12, and as needed. If Hgb is less than 10 g/dl, decrease ribavirin dosage; if Hgb is less than 8.5 g/dl, discontinuation of therapy is recommended; telaprevir dosage should not be altered based on adverse reactions; Anemia may be managed through ribavirin dose modifications; never alter the dose of telaprevir. If anemia persists despite a reduction in ribavirin dose, consider discontinuing telaprevir. If management of anemia requires permanent discontinuation of ribavirin, treatment with telaprevir must also be permanently discontinued. Once telaprevir has been discontinued, it must not be restarted; monitor CBC with differential at treatment wks 4, 8, 12, and at other treatment points as needed

> **BLACK BOX WARNING: Serious rash:** Assess for toxic epidermal necrolysis, Stevens-Johnson syndrome, eosinophilia, fever, mucosal skin erosion, mucosal ulceration, target lesions; if serious skin reaction occurs, immediately discontinue all components of the three-drug regimen and refer the patient for urgent medical care

• Thyroid function tests, LFTs, serum bilirubin/creatinine, BUN, bilirubin, serum electrolytes, serum uric acid, baseline and periodically during treatment

Patient/family education

• Instruct patient to use two forms of effective contraception (intrauterine devices and barrier methods) during treatment and for 6 months after treatment (pregnancy **X**), avoid breast feeding

• If a serious skin reaction occurs, patients should be instructed to seek urgent medical care and all components of the triple-drug regimen must be discontinued immediately

Evaluation

Positive therapeutic outcome

• Decreasing hepatitis C viral infection

---

telavancin (Rx)

(tel-a-van'sin)

Vibativ

Func. class.: Antiinfective—miscellaneous

Chem. class.: Lipoglycopeptide

Pregnancy category C

ACTION: Inhibits bacterial cell wall synthesis, disrupts cell membrane integrity, blocks glycopeptides

Therapeutic outcome: Negative culture

USES: Skin/skin structure infections caused by *Enterococcus faecalis, E. faecium, Staphylococcus aureus* (MSRA), *S. aureus* (MSSA), *S. epidermidis, S. haemolyticus, Streptococcus agalactiae* (group B), *S. dysgalactiae, S. pyogenes* (group A beta tremolytic), *S. anginosus, S. intermedius, S. constellates,* nosocomial pneumonia caused by susceptible gram-positive bacteria

Unlabeled uses: Bacteremia

CONTRAINDICATIONS:
Hypersensitivity

Precautions: Breastfeeding, geriatric patients, renal disease, antimicrobial resistance, children, diabetes mellitus, diarrhea, GI disease, heart failure, hypertension, pseudomembranous colitis, QT prolongation, vancomycin hypersensitivity

> **BLACK BOX WARNING:** Pregnancy **C,** females

DOSAGE AND ROUTES
Skin/skin structure infections
Adult: IV INF 10 mg/kg over 60 min q24hr × 7-14 days

Nosocomial pneumonia
Adult: IV INF 10 mg/kg q24hr × 7-21 days

Renal dose
Adult: IV CCr 30-50 ml/min 7.5 mg/kg q24hr; CCr 10-29 ml/min 10 mg/kg q48hr

Available forms: Lyophilized powder for inj 250, 750 mg

Implementation
• Use only for susceptible organisms to prevent drug-resistant bacteria
• Give antihistamine if red man syndrome occurs: decreased B/P, flushing of neck, face
• Store in refrigerator
• Have EPINEPHrine, suction, tracheostomy set, endotracheal intubation equipment on unit; anaphylaxis may occur
• Give adequate intake of fluids (2 L/day) to prevent nephrotoxicity
• Avoid IM, subcut use

Intermittent IV infusion route
• Administer after reconstituting with 15 ml D₅W sterile water for inj; 0.9% NaCl (15 mg/ml) 250 mg vial; add 45 ml to 750 mg vial (15 mg/ml) for dose of 150-800 mg; further dilute with 100-250 ml of compatible sol; for dose <150 mg or 800 mg, further dilute to a conc of 0.6-8 mg/ml with compatible sol; give over 60 min, **avoid rapid IV, may cause red man syndrome;** reconstituted or diluted solution is stable for 4 hr at room temperature, 7 hr refrigerated

Y-site compatibilities: Amphotericin B lipid complex (Abelcet), ampicillin-sulbactam, azithromycin, calcium gluconate, caspofungin, cefepime, cefTAZidime, cefTRIAXone, ciprofloxacin, dexamethasone, diltiazem, DOBUTamine, DOPamine, doripenem, doxycycline, ertapenem, famotidine, fluconazole, gentamicin, hydrocortisone, labetalol, magnesium sulfate, mannitol, meropenem, metoclopramide, milrinone, norepinephrine, ondansetron, pantoprazole, phenylephrine, piperacillin-tazobactam, potassium chloride/phosphates, ranitidine, sodium bicarbonate, sodium phosphates, tigecycline, tobramycin, vasopressin

ADVERSE EFFECTS
CNS: Anxiety, chills, flushing, headache, insomnia, dizziness
CV: QT prolongation, irregular heartbeat
EENT: Hearing loss
GI: Nausea, vomiting, **pseudomembranous colitis,** abdominal pain, constipation, diarrhea, metallic/soapy taste
GU: Nephrotoxicity, *increased BUN, creatinine,* renal failure, foamy urine
HEMA: Leukopenia, eosinophilia, anemia, thrombocytopenia
INTEG: Chills, fever, rash, thrombophlebitis at inj site, urticaria, pruritus, necrosis (red man syndrome)
SYST: Anaphylaxis, superinfection

Pharmacokinetics

Absorption	Unknown
Distribution	Unknown, protein binding 90%
Metabolism	Unknown, hepatic metabolism
Excretion	Urine 76%
Half-life	8-9 hr

Pharmacodynamics

Onset	Rapid
Peak	Unknown
Duration	Unknown

INTERACTIONS
Individual drugs
Adefovir, amphotericin B, bacitracin, cidofovir, CISplatin, colistin, cycloSPORINE, foscarnet, ganciclovir, IV pentamine

---

⚠ Nurse Alert   ✴ Key NCLEX® Drug

acyclovir, pamidronate, polymyxin, strep-tozotocin, tacrolimus, zoledronic acid: increased toxicity, **nephrotoxicity**
Chloroquine, clarithromycin, dronedarone, droperidol, erythromycin, grepafloxacin, haloperidol, levomethadyl, methadone, pimozide, ziprasidone: increased QT prolongation

Drug classifications
Aminoglycosides, cephalosporins, nondepolarizing muscle relaxants: increased toxicity, nephrotoxicity
Class IA, III antidysrhythmics, some phenothiazines: increased QT prolongation

Drug/lab test
False increase: INR, PT, PTT

NURSING CONSIDERATIONS
Assessment
• Monitor I&O ratio; report hematuria, oliguria; nephrotoxicity may occur
• Monitor C&S throughout treatment
• Assess auditory function during, after treatment, hearing loss, ringing, roaring in ears; product should be discontinued

> **BLACK BOX WARNING:** Obtain a pregnancy test before use; if a woman has taken this product during pregnancy, the national registry should be notified at 866-658-4228

• Monitor B/P during administration; sudden drop may indicate red man syndrome; also flushing, pruritus, rash
• Assess respiratory status: rate, character, wheezing, tightness in chest
• Assess allergies before treatment, reaction of each medication

Patient/family education
• Teach all aspects of product therapy; culture may be taken after completed course of medication
• Advise to report sore throat, fever, fatigue; could indicate superinfection; diarrhea (pseudomembranous colitis); hearing loss
• Teach patient to use contraception while taking this product; do not breastfeed; **to notify prescriber if pregnancy is planned or suspected**

Evaluation
Positive therapeutic outcome
• Negative culture

telbivudine (Rx)
(tel-bi'vyoo-deen)
Sebivo ✦, Tyzeka
Func. class.: Antiretroviral
Chem. class.: Nucleoside reverse transcriptase inhibitor (NRTI)
Pregnancy category B

ACTION: Inhibits replication of HBV DNA polymerase, which inhibits HBV replication

Therapeutic outcome: Decreased hepatitis B serology

USES: Treatment of chronic hepatitis B

CONTRAINDICATIONS:
Hypersensitivity, breastfeeding

Precautions: Pregnancy **B,** children, severe renal disease, anemia, organ transplant, dialysis, HIV, obesity, alcoholism; hispanic or African descent (safety not established)

> **BLACK BOX WARNING:** Impaired hepatic function, lactic acidosis

DOSAGE AND ROUTES
Adult and adolescent >16 yr: PO 600 mg/day; max 600 mg/day

Renal dose
Adult: PO CCr 30-49 ml/min 600 mg tab q48hr or 400 mg oral sol/day; CCr <30 ml/min (not requiring dialysis) 600 mg tab q72hr or 200 mg oral sol/day

Available forms: Tabs 600 mg

Implementation
• Give with or without food with a full glass of water
• Store at room temperature

ADVERSE EFFECTS
CNS: *Fever, headache, malaise,* weakness, *dizziness, insomnia*
EENT: Taste change, hearing loss, photophobia
GI: *Nausea, vomiting, diarrhea, anorexia,* abdominal pain, hepatomegaly
INTEG: *Rash*
MISC: Lactic acidosis
MS: Myalgia, arthralgia, muscle cramps
RESP: Cough

T

Adverse effects: *italics* = common; **bold** = life-threatening

Pharmacokinetics

Absorption	Unknown
Distribution	Steady state 5-7 days, protein binding 3.3%
Metabolism	Unknown
Excretion	Kidneys, unchanged
Half-life	Terminal 40-49 hr

Pharmacodynamics

Onset	Unknown
Peak	1-4 hr
Duration	Unknown

INTERACTIONS
Individual drugs
CycloSPORINE, erythromycin, hydrochloroquine, niacin, penicillamine, zidovudine, ZDV: increased myopathy risk

Do not use with pegylated interferon alfa-2a

Drug classifications
Any agent altering renal function: altered telbivudine levels

Azole antifungals, corticosteroids, fibric acid derivatives, HMG-CoA reductase inhibitors: increased myopathy risk

NURSING CONSIDERATIONS
Assessment

BLACK BOX WARNING: Monitor liver function tests, hepatitis B serology, creatine kinase, periodically; monitor HBV DNA after 24 wk, if viral suppression is incomplete (≥300 copies/ml) start alternate therapy, monitor HBV DNA q6mo

BLACK BOX WARNING: Lactic acidosis, severe hepatomegaly with steatosis: obtain baseline LFTs, if elevated, discontinue treatment; discontinue even if LFTs are normal but lactic acidosis, hepatomegaly are present, may be fatal

Patient/family education
• Advise patient that GI complaints and insomnia may resolve after 3-4 wk of treatment
• Teach patient that product does not cure hepatitis B and does not stop the spread to others
• Teach patient that follow-up visits must be continued
• Teach patient that serious product interactions may occur if OTC products are ingested; check with prescriber before taking

• Advise patient that product may cause dizziness; avoid hazardous activities until response is known
• Teach patient to report symptoms of cough, difficulty sleeping or excessive headache, muscle pain/weakness

Evaluation
Positive therapeutic outcome
• Decreased hepatitis B serology

telmisartan (Rx)
(tel-mih-sar'tan)
Micardis
Func. class.: Antihypertensive
Chem. class.: Angiotensin II receptor (type AT₁)
**Pregnancy category C (1st trimester)
D (2nd/3rd trimesters)**

ACTION: Blocks the vasoconstrictor and aldosterone-secreting effects of angiotensin II; selectively blocks the binding of angiotensin II to the AT₁ receptor found in tissues

Therapeutic outcome: Decreased B/P

USES: Hypertension, alone or in combination; stroke, MI prophylaxis (>55 yr) in those unable to take ACE inhibitors

Unlabeled uses: Heart failure, proteinuria in diabetic nephropathy

CONTRAINDICATIONS:
Hypersensitivity

BLACK BOX WARNING: Pregnancy **D** (2nd/3rd trimesters)

Precautions: Pregnancy **C** (1st trimester), breastfeeding, children, geriatric, hypersensitivity to angiotensin-converting enzyme (ACE) inhibitors, renal/hepatic disease, renal artery stenosis, dialysis, CHF, hyperkalemia, hypotension, hypovolemia, African descent

DOSAGE AND ROUTES
Adult: PO 40 mg/day; range 20-80 mg/day

Stroke, MI prophylaxis
Adult >55 yr: PO 80 mg/day

Available forms: Tabs 20, 40, 80 mg

Implementation
• Give without regard to meals
• Give increased dose to African American, hispanic patients, B/P response may be reduced

---

• Do not remove from blister pack until ready to use

ADVERSE EFFECTS

CNS: Dizziness, insomnia, *anxiety,* headache, fatigue, syncope
GI: *Diarrhea,* dyspepsia, *anorexia, vomiting*
META: Hyperkalemia
MS: *Myalgia, pain*
RESP: *Cough, upper respiratory tract infection,* sinusitis, pharyngitis
SYST: Angioedema

Pharmacokinetics

Absorption	Unknown
Distribution	Highly protein bound
Metabolism	Liver, extensively
Excretion	Urine/feces
Half-life	Terminal 24 hr

Pharmacodynamics

Onset	3-hr
Peak	0.5-1 hr
Duration	Unknown

INTERACTIONS

Individual drugs
Digoxin: increased digoxin peak, trough concentrations

Drug classifications
ACE inhibitors, potassium-sparing diuretics, potassium salt substitutes: increased hyperkalemia
Antihypertensives, diuretics, NSAIDs: increased antihypertensive action
NSAIDs, salicylates: decreased antihypertensive effect

Drug/lab test
Increased: LFTs

NURSING CONSIDERATIONS

Assessment
• Monitor B/P, pulse q4hr; note rate, rhythm, quality; if severe hypotension occurs, place in supine position and give **IV** NS
• Monitor baselines in renal, electrolytes, liver function tests before therapy begins
• Assess edema in feet, legs daily
• Assess skin turgor, dryness of mucous membranes for hydration status
• Overdose: dizziness, bradycardia or tachycardia

Patient/family education
• Instruct patient to comply with dosage schedule, even if feeling better
• Advise patient to notify prescriber of mouth sores, fever, swelling of hands or feet, irregular heartbeat, chest pain
• Teach patient that excessive perspiration, dehydration, vomiting, diarrhea may lead to fall in blood pressure; consult prescriber if these occur
• Teach patient not to stop medication abruptly

> **BLACK BOX WARNING:** Teach patient that product may cause dizziness, fainting; lightheadedness may occur; to avoid hazardous activities until response is known; to rise slowly from sitting to prevent drop in B/P

> **BLACK BOX WARNING:** Advise patient to use contraception while taking this product, pregnancy category **D**, 2nd/3rd trimester

• Teach patient to notify prescriber of all prescriptions, OTC preparations, and supplements taken

Evaluation
Positive therapeutic outcome
• Decreased B/P

temazepam (Rx)

(tem-az′a-pam)
Restoril
Func. class.: Sedative-hypnotic
Chem. class.: Benzodiazepine, short-intermediate acting
Pregnancy category X
Controlled substance schedule IV (USA), schedule F (Canada)

Do not confuse:
temazepam/flurazepam

ACTION: Produces CNS depression at limbic, thalamic, hypothalamic levels of the CNS; may be mediated by neurotransmitter γ-aminobutyric acid (GABA); results are sedation, hypnosis, skeletal muscle relaxation, anticonvulsant activity, anxiolytic action

Therapeutic outcome: Decreased insomnia

USES: Insomnia (short-term treatment, generally 7-10 days)

CONTRAINDICATIONS:

Pregnancy **X,** breastfeeding, hypersensitivity to benzodiazepines

Precautions: Children <15 yr, geriatric, anemia, pulmonary/renal/hepatic disease, suicidal patients, product abuse, psychosis, acute closed-angle glaucoma, seizure disorders, angioedema, sleep-related behavior (sleep walking), COPD, dementia, myasthenia gravis, intermittent porphyria

DOSAGE AND ROUTES

Adult: PO 7.5-30 mg at bedtime
Geriatric: PO 7.5 mg at bedtime

Available forms: Caps 7.5, 15, 22.5, 30 mg

Implementation

• Give with food or milk to decrease GI symptoms; if patient is unable to swallow medication whole, tab may be crushed and mixed with foods or fluids
• Give sugarless gum, hard candy, frequent sips of water for dry mouth
• Store in tight container in cool environment

ADVERSE EFFECTS

CNS: *Lethargy, drowsiness, daytime sedation,* dizziness, confusion, light-headedness, headache, anxiety, irritability, complex sleep-related reactions (sleep driving, sleep eating), fatigue
CV: Chest pain, pulse changes, hypotension
EENT: Blurred vision
GI: Nausea, vomiting, diarrhea, heartburn, abdominal pain, constipation, anorexia
SYST: Severe allergic reactions

Pharmacokinetics

Absorption	Well absorbed
Distribution	Widely distributed, crosses placenta, crosses blood-brain barrier
Metabolism	Liver
Excretion	Kidneys, breast milk
Half-life	10-20 hr

Pharmacodynamics

Onset	½ hr
Peak	1-2 hr
Duration	6-8 hr

INTERACTIONS

Individual drugs

Alcohol: increased actions of both products
Cimetidine, disulfiram: increased effect of each specific product
Probenecid: increased effect of temazepam
Rifampin: decreased action of rifampin
Theophylline: decreased effects of theophylline

Drug classifications

Antacids: decreased effect of antacids
Contraceptives (oral): increased effect
CNS depressants: increased action of both products

Drug/herb

Chamomile, skullcap, valerian: increased CNS depression

Drug/food

Caffeine: decreased temazepam effect

Drug/lab test

Increased: AST/ALT
Decreased: radioactive iodine uptake
False increase: 17-OHCS

NURSING CONSIDERATIONS

Assessment

• Assess mental status: mood, sensorium, anxiety, affect, sleeping pattern (baseline, periodically), drowsiness, dizziness, especially geriatric; physical dependency, withdrawal symptoms: anxiety, panic attacks, agitation, orientation, headache, nausea, vomiting, muscle pain, weakness; indications of increasing tolerance and abuse

Patient/family education

• Inform patient that product may be taken with food, and that tab may be crushed or swallowed whole
• Advise patient not to use for everyday stress or longer than 3 mo unless directed by prescriber; not to take more than prescribed amount; may be habit forming; not to double or skip doses
• Caution patient to avoid OTC preparations unless approved by prescriber; alcohol and CNS depressants will increase CNS depression
• Advise patient to avoid driving, activities that require alertness, drowsiness may occur; to avoid alcohol ingestion or other psychotropic medications; to rise slowly or fainting may occur, especially in geriatric; that drowsiness may worsen at beginning of treatment
• Caution patient not to discontinue medication abruptly after long-term use; withdrawal symptoms include vomiting, cramping, tremors, seizures
• Advise patient to use contraception while taking this product, to notify prescriber if pregnancy is planned or suspected, pregnancy **X**
• Advise patient that complex sleep-related behavior may occur (sleep driving/eating)

⚠ Nurse Alert   ✹ Key NCLEX® Drug

- Teach patient to limit to 7-10 days continuous use

Evaluation
Positive therapeutic outcome
- Decreased anxiety, restlessness, sleeplessness (short-term treatment only)

TREATMENT OF OVERDOSE:
Lavage, VS, supportive care

---

temozolomide (Rx)
(tem-oo-zole′oo-mide)
Temodar
Func. class.: Antineoplastic alkylating agents
Chem. class.: Imidazotetrazine derivative
Pregnancy category D

ACTION: A proproduct that undergoes conversion to 5-(3-methyl-1-triazeno) imidazole-4-carboxamide (MTIC); MTIC action prevents DNA transcription

Therapeutic outcome: Prevention of rapidly growing malignant cells

USES: Anaplastic astrocytoma with relapse, glioblastoma multiforme, malignant glioma

Unlabeled uses: Metastatic melanoma

CONTRAINDICATIONS:
Pregnancy **D**, breastfeeding, hypersensitivity to this product, carbazine, or gelatin

Precautions: Radiation therapy, renal/hepatic disease, bone marrow suppression, infection, geriatric, myelosuppression

DOSAGE AND ROUTES
Anaplastic astrocytoma
Adult: PO adjust dose based on nadir neutrophil and platelet counts 150 mg/m^2/day × 5 days during 28-day cycle

Glioblastoma multiforme
Adult: PO/IV 75 mg/m^2/day × 42 days with focal radiotherapy, then maintenance of 6 cycles

Malignant glioma
Adult: 150 mg/m^2/day over 90 min day 1-5, q28day; may increase to 200 mg/m^2/day on day 1-5, q28day if hematologic parameters permit

Available forms: Caps 5, 20, 100, 140, 180, 250 mg; powder for inj 100 mg

Implementation
PO route
- Give fluids **IV** or PO before chemotherapy to hydrate patient
- Give antiemetic 30-60 min before giving product to prevent vomiting, and prn; antibiotics for prophylaxis of infection
- Capsules should not be opened; if accidentally damaged, do not allow contact with skin, or inhale; take caps one at a time with 8 oz of water at the same time of day; use cytotic handling procedure
- Give on empty stomach at bedtime to prevent nausea/vomiting
- Store in light-resistant container in a dry area

IV route
- Bring vial to room temperature, discard if cloudy
- Inject 41 ml sterile water for inj into vial (2.5 mg/ml)
- Gently swirl, do not shake
Intermittent IV infusion route
- Withdraw up to 40 ml from each vial to make total dose and transfer to empty 250 ml PVC inf bag, flush before and after inf
- Run over 90 min
- Use reconstituted sol within 14 hr including inf time
- Do not admix

ADVERSE EFFECTS
CNS: Seizures, *hemiparesis, dizziness, poor coordination, amnesia, insomnia, paresthesia, somnolence, paresis, ataxia, anxiety, dysphagia, depression, confusion*
GI: *Nausea, anorexia, vomiting,* abdominal pain, constipation
GU: *Urinary incontinence, UTI, frequency*
HEMA: **Thrombocytopenia, leukopenia,** anemia, **myelosuppression, neutropenia**
INTEG: *Rash, pruritus*
MISC: *Headache, fatigue, asthenia, fever, edema, back pain, weight increase, diplopia*
RESP: *Upper respiratory tract infection, pharyngitis, sinusitis, coughing*
SYST: **Anaphylaxis, secondary malignancy**

Pharmacokinetics
Absorption	Rapid, complete
Distribution	Crosses blood-brain barrier
Metabolism	To MTIC and metabolite
Excretion	Urine, feces
Half-life	1.8 hr

Pharmacodynamics

Onset	Unknown
Peak	1 hr
Duration	Unknown

INTERACTIONS
Individual drugs
Digoxin: decreased action of digoxin

Filgrastim, G-CSF, pegfilgrastim, sargramostim: do not use within 24 hr of these products

Radiation: increased toxicity, bone marrow suppression

Drug classifications
Anticoagulants, NSAIDs, platelet inhibitors, thrombolytics: increased bleeding risk

Antineoplastics: increased bone marrow suppression

Live virus vaccines, toxoids: increased adverse reactions, decreased antibody reaction

Drug/food
Decreased drug absorption

Drug/lab test
Decreased: Hgb, platelets, WBC, neutrophils

NURSING CONSIDERATIONS
Assessment
• Assess symptoms indicating severe allergic reaction: rash, pruritus, urticaria, purpuric skin lesions, itching, flushing; product should be discontinued

• Assess tumor response during treatment

• Obtain CBC on day 22 (21 days after 1st dose), CBC weekly until recovery if ANC is <1.5 × 10⁹/L and platelets <100 × 10⁹/L, do not administer to patients that do not tolerate 100 mg/m²; myelosuppression usually occurs late in the treatment cycle

• Assess for seizures, mental status throughout treatment

• Monitor renal function studies: BUN, creatinine, urine CCr before, during therapy; I&O ratio; report fall in urine output to <30 ml/hr

• Monitor temp q4hr (may indicate beginning of infection)

• Monitor liver function tests before, during therapy (bilirubin, AST, ALT, LDH) as needed or monthly; note jaundice of skin or sclera, dark urine, clay-colored stools, itchy skin, abdominal pain, fever, diarrhea; hepatotoxicity can be serious and fatal

• Assess for bleeding: hematuria, stool guaiac, bruising or petechiae, mucosa or orifices; check for inflammation of mucosa, breaks in skin

Patient/family education
• Teach patient to avoid use of products containing aspirin or NSAIDs, razors, commercial mouthwash, since bleeding may occur; to report symptoms of bleeding (hematuria, tarry stools)

• Instruct patient to report signs of anemia (fatigue, headache, irritability, faintness, shortness of breath)

• Caution patient not to have any vaccinations without the advice of prescriber; serious reactions can occur

• Advise patient contraception is needed during treatment and for several months after completion of therapy; product has teratogenic properties, pregnancy **D**, not to breastfeed

Evaluation
Positive therapeutic outcome
• Prevention of rapid division of malignant cells

temsirolimus (Rx)
(tem-sir-oh′li-mus)

Torisel

Func. class.: Biological response modifier

Chem. class.: Kinase inhibitor, mTOR antagonist

Pregnancy category D

ACTION: Inhibits mammalian target of rapamycin (mTOR), a protein kinase

Therapeutic outcome: Decreased time of progression of renal cell carcinoma

USES: Renal cell carcinoma

CONTRAINDICATIONS:
Pregnancy **D**, breastfeeding, hypersensitivity to this product or to sirolimus, polysorbate 80

Precautions: Children <13 yr, females, severe pulmonary/renal/hepatic disease (bilirubin >1-1.5 × ULN or AST > ULN, but bilirubin ≤ULN), diabetes mellitus, hyperkalemia, hyperuricemia, hypertension, bone marrow suppression, hypertriglyceridemia/hyperlipidemia, surgery, brain tumor

DOSAGE AND ROUTES
Adult: IV 25 mg over 30-60 min qwk; treat until disease progression or severe toxicity occurs

Hepatic dose
Adult: IV (mild impairment) (bilirubin >1-1.5 × ULN or AST > ULN but bilirubin ≤ ULN)

Available forms: 25 mg/ml sol for inj kit

Implementation

• Premedicate with 25-50 mg diphenhydrAMINE **IV** 30 min before dose; if reaction occurs, stop for ½-1 hr; may resume at slower rate

• Use in-line filter ≤5 micrometers and inf pump; inf over 30-60 min; complete inf within 6 hr

• Dilute product with 1.8 ml of provided diluent; the result is 3 ml (10 mg/ml); invert to mix well; withdraw the required amount and inject rapidly into 250 ml of 0.9% NaCl; do not use PVC infusion bags/sets

• Protect from light during preparation; use only glass

ADVERSE EFFECTS

CNS: *Headache*, seizures
CV: Hypertension, **thrombophlebitis**
ENDO: Hypertriglyceridemia, hyperlipidemia, hyperglycemia
GI: Nausea, vomiting, diarrhea, constipation, **bowel perforation**
GU: UTIs, **albuminuria, hematuria, proteinuria, renal failure,** mucositis
HEMA: Anemia, leukopenia, thrombocytopenia
INTEG: *Rash*, pruritus
META: Metabolic acidosis, hyperglycemia, hyperlipidemia
RESP: Interstitial lung disease
SYST: Lymphoma

Pharmacokinetics

Absorption	Rapidly absorbed
Distribution	Unknown
Metabolism	Extensively via liver by CYP3A4
Excretion	Eliminated via feces
Half-life	Unknown

Pharmacodynamics

Onset	Unknown
Peak	0.5-2 hr
Duration	Unknown

INTERACTIONS

Individual drugs

Bromocriptine, cimetidine, clarithromycin, cycloSPORINE, danazol, erythromycin, metoclopramide: increased blood levels
CarBAMazepine, dexamethasone, PHENobarbital, phenytoin, rifamycin, rifapentine: decreased blood levels
SUNItinib: increased toxicity

Drug classifications

Antifungals, benzodiazepines, calcium channel blockers, CYP3A4 inhibitors, HIV protease inhibitors, HMG-CoA reductase inhibitors: increased blood levels
CYP3A4 inducers: decreased blood levels
Vaccines: decreased effect of vaccines; avoid with vaccines

Drug/herb

Astragalus, echinacea, melatonin: decreased immunosuppression
Ginseng, maitake, mistletoe: increased effect
St. John's wort: may decrease the effect of sirolimus

Drug/food

Alters bioavailability; use consistently with or without food; do not use with grapefruit juice

NURSING CONSIDERATIONS

Assessment

• Assess cardiac status: B/P, heart rate
• Assess for interstitial lung disease
• Assess for hypersensitive reactions: anaphylaxis
• Monitor lipid profile: cholesterol, triglycerides, a lipid-lowering agent may be needed; blood glucose
⚠ **Assess for infection and development of lymphoma**
⚠ **Monitor blood tests: Hgb, WBC, platelets during treatment qmo**
• Monitor renal function tests: BUN, creatinine, phosphate potassium; proteinuria, hematuria, albuminemia may indicate renal failure
• **Hepatic disease:** monitor liver function test baseline and periodically

Patient/family education

• Advise patient to report fever, rash, severe diarrhea, chills, sore throat, fatigue; serious infections may occur; clay-colored stools, cramping (hepatotoxicity)
• Advise patient to avoid crowds, persons with known infections to reduce risk of infection
• Teach patient to use contraception before, during, and 12 wk after product has been discontinued; avoid breastfeeding; men should also use reliable contraception during and 12 wk after cessation of product, pregnancy **D**
• Advise to report excessive thirst, urinary frequency, new or worsening breathing problems, blood in stool, abdominal pain

Evaluation

Positive therapeutic outcome

• Decreased time of progression of renal cell carcinoma

tenecteplase (TNK-tPA) (Rx)

(ten-ek´ta-place)

TNKase

Func. class.: Thrombolytic

Chem. class.: Tissue plasminogen activator

Pregnancy category C

ACTION: Activates conversion of plasminogen to plasmin (fibrinolysin): plasmin breaks down clots (fibrin), fibrinogen, factors V, VII; occlusion of venous access lines

Therapeutic outcome: Resolution of MI

USES: Acute MI, coronary artery thrombosis

CONTRAINDICATIONS:

Hypersensitivity, arteriovenous malformation, aneurysm, active bleeding, intracranial, intraspinal surgery or trauma within 2 mo, CNS neoplasms, severe hypertension, severe renal disease, hepatic disease, history of CVA, increased ICP, stroke

Precautions: Pregnancy **C**, breastfeeding, children, geriatric, arterial emboli from left side of heart, hypocoagulation, subacute bacterial endocarditis, rheumatic valvular disease, cerebral embolism/thrombosis/hemorrhage, intraarterial diagnostic procedure or surgery (10 days), recent major surgery, dysrhythmias, hypertension

DOSAGE AND ROUTES

Total dose, max 50 mg, based on patient's weight

Adult <60 kg: **IV** BOL 30 mg, give over 5 sec

Adult 60-70 kg: **IV** BOL 35 mg, give over 5 sec

Adult 70-80 kg: **IV** BOL 40 mg, give over 5 sec

Adult 80-90 kg: **IV** BOL 45 mg, give over 5 sec

Adult ≥90 kg: **IV** BOL 50 mg, give over 5 sec, max 50 mg total dose

Available forms: Powder for inj, lyophilized 50 mg

Implementation

Intermittent IV infusion route

• Give as soon as thrombi are identified; not useful for thrombi >1 wk old

• Administer cryoprecipitate or fresh frozen plasma if bleeding occurs

• Give heparin after fibrinogen level >100 mg/dl; heparin inf to increase PTT to 1.5-2 × baseline for 3-7 days; **IV** heparin with loading dose is recommended

• Aseptically withdraw 10 ml of sterile water for inj from diluent vial, use red cannula syringe-filling device, inject all contents of syringe into product vial, direct into powder, swirl, withdraw correct dose, discard any unused sol; stand the shield with dose vertically on flat surface and passively recap the red cannula; remove entire shield assembly by twisting counterclockwise; give by **IV** bol

• **IV** therapy: use upper extremity vessel that is accessible to manual compression

• Provide bed rest during entire course of treatment

• Avoid venous or arterial puncture, inj, rectal temp, any invasive treatment

• Treat fever with acetaminophen or aspirin

• Apply pressure for 30 sec to minor bleeding sites; inform prescriber if this does not attain hemostasis; apply pressure dressing

ADVERSE EFFECTS

CV: Dysrhythmias, hypotension, pulmonary edema, **pulmonary embolism, cardiogenic shock, cardiac arrest, heart failure, myocardial reinfarction, myocardial rupture, tamponade, pericarditis, pericardial effusion, thrombosis, CVA**

HEMA: Decreased Hct, **bleeding**

INTEG: Rash, urticaria, phlebitis at **IV** inf site, itching, flushing

SYST: GI, GU, intracranial, **retroperitoneal bleeding, surface bleeding, anaphylaxis**

Pharmacokinetics

Absorption	Unknown
Distribution	Unknown
Metabolism	Liver
Excretion	Unknown
Half-life	20-24 min

Pharmacodynamics

Onset	Immediate
Peak	Unknown
Duration	Unknown

INTERACTIONS

Individual drugs

Aspirin, cefamandole, cefoperazone, cefoTEtan, clopidogrel, dipyridamole, indomethacin, phenylbutazone, ticlopidine: increased bleeding potential

Drug classifications
Anticoagulants, antithrombolytics, glycoprotein IIb, IIIa inhibitors, NSAIDs, SNRIs, SSRIs: increased bleeding

Drug/herb
Anise, basil, dong quai, fenugreek, feverfew, garlic, ginger, ginkgo, ginseng, green tea, horse chestnut: increased risk of bleeding

Drug/lab test
Increased: INR, PT, PTT

NURSING CONSIDERATIONS
Assessment
• **Assess for allergy:** fever, rash, itching, chills; mild reaction may be treated with antihistamines

⚠ **Assess for bleeding during 1st hr of treatment; hematuria, hematemesis, bleeding from mucous membranes, epistaxis, ecchymosis; may require transfusion (rare), continue to assess for bleeding for 24 hr**

• Monitor blood tests (Hct, platelets, PTT, protime, TT, aPTT) before starting therapy; protime or aPTT must be less than 2 × control before starting therapy; PTT or pro-time q3-4hr during treatment

⚠ **Cholesterol embolism: assess for blue-toe syndrome, renal failure, MI, cerebral/spinal cord/bowel/retinal infarction, hypertension; can be fatal**

• Assess for hypersensitive reactions: fever, rash, dyspnea; product should be discontinued
• Monitor VS, B/P, pulse, respirations, neurologic signs, temp at least q4hr; temp >104° F (40° C) indicates internal bleeding; systolic pressure increase >25 mm Hg should be reported to prescriber

⚠ **Assess for neurologic changes that may indicate intracranial bleeding**

⚠ **Assess for retroperitoneal bleeding: back pain, leg weakness, diminished pulses**

Patient/family education
• Teach patient to notify prescriber immediately of severe headache
• Advise patient to notify prescriber of bleeding, hypersensitivity, fast, slow, or uneven heart rate, feeling of fainting, blood in urine/stools, nose bleeds
• Teach patient about proper dental care to avoid bleeding

Evaluation
Positive therapeutic outcome
• Resolution of myocardial infarction

tenofovir (Rx)
(ten-oh-foh′veer)
Viread
Func. class.: Antiretroviral
Chem. class.: Nucleoside reverse transcriptase inhibitor (NRTI)
Pregnancy category B

ACTION: Inhibits replication of HIV-1 virus by competing with the natural substrate and then incorporating into cellular DNA by viral reverse transcriptase, thereby terminating cellular DNA chain

Therapeutic outcome: Improved symptoms of HIV-1 infection

USES: HIV-1 infection with at least 2 other antiretrovirals, hepatitis B

CONTRAINDICATIONS:
Hypersensitivity

> **BLACK BOX WARNING:** Lactic acidosis

Precautions: Pregnancy **B**, breastfeeding, children, geriatric, renal disease, hepatic insufficiency, CCr <60 ml/min, osteoporosis, immune reconstitution syndrome

> **BLACK BOX WARNING:** Hepatic disease, hepatitis

DOSAGE AND ROUTES
Adult: PO 300 mg with meal; if used with didanosine, give tenofovir 2 hr before or 1 hr after didanosine

Renal dose
Adult: PO CCr 30-49 ml/min 300 mg q48hr; CCr 10-29 ml/min 300 mg q72-96hr; CCr <10 ml/min not recommended
Child ≥2 yr: PO 8 mg/kg/day approximate; ≥35 kg 300 mg/day; 28-34 kg 250 mg/day; 22-27 kg 200 mg/day; 17-21 kg 150 mg/day

Available forms: Tabs 150, 200, 250, 300 mg; oral powder 40 mg/scoop

Implementation
• Administer PO without regard to meals
• Store at 25° C (77° F)
• Give product 2 hr before or 1 hr after taking didanosine (if used)
• Oral powder: use scoop provided, mix powder into 2-4 oz (¼-½ cup) of applesauce or yogurt, do not mix with liquid; product is bitter; use immediately after mixing, clean scoop

T

Adverse effects: *italics* = common; **bold** = life-threatening

ADVERSE EFFECTS
CNS: *Headache,* asthenia
GI: *Nausea, vomiting, diarrhea,* anorexia, *flatulence, abdominal pain,* pancreatitis
GU: Renal failure, renal tubular acidosis/necrosis, Fanconi syndrome
HEMA: Neutropenia, osteopenia
INTEG: *Rash,* angioedema
META: Lactic acidosis, hypokalemia, hypophosphatemia
MS: *Myopathy,* rhabdomyolysis
SYST: Lipodystrophy

Pharmacokinetics

Absorption	Rapidly absorbed
Distribution	Extravascular space; bound to serum plasma <0.7%, to serum proteins <7.2%
Metabolism	Unknown
Excretion	Urine, unchanged (70%-80%)
Half-life	Terminal 17 hr

Pharmacodynamics

Onset	Unknown
Peak	1-2 hr
Duration	Unknown

INTERACTIONS
Individual drugs
Acyclovir, cidofovir, ganciclovir, valacyclovir, valganciclovir: increased level of tenofovir
Didanosine: increased level of didanosine when coadministered with tenofovir

Drug classifications
Increased: levels of tenofovir with any product that decreases renal function

NURSING CONSIDERATIONS
Assessment
• Monitor viral load, CD4+ T cell count, plasma HIV RNA, serum creatinine/BUN/phosphate
• Resistance testing at start of therapy and at treatment failure
• Assess liver function tests: AST, ALT, bilirubin; amylase, lipase, triglycerides periodically during treatment
• Assess for bone, renal toxicity: if bone abnormalities are suspected, obtain tests: serum phosphorus, creatinine
• **Lactic acidosis, severe hepatomegaly with steatosis: Obtain baseline LFTs, if el-** evated discontinue treatment; discontinue even if LFTs are normal but lactic acidosis, hepatomegaly are present, may be fatal

Patient/family education
• Instruct patient to take this product 2 hr before or 1 hr after taking didanosine (if used)
• Instruct patient to take product with meal
• Advise patients that GI complaints resolve after 3-4 wk of treatment
• Caution patient not to breastfeed while taking this product
• Inform patient that product must be taken daily even if patient feels better
• Advise patient to continue follow-up visits since serious toxicity may occur; blood counts must be done q2wk
• Inform patient that product controls symptoms but is not a cure for HIV; patient is still infectious, may pass HIV virus on to others
• Advise patient that other products may be necessary to prevent other infections
• Advise patient that changes in body fat distribution may occur
⚠ **Lactic acidosis: teach patient symptoms of lactic acidosis, to notify prescriber**

Evaluation
Positive therapeutic outcome
• Decrease in signs/symptoms of HIV

---

terazosin (Rx)
(ter-ay'zoe-sin)
Func. class.: Antihypertensive
Chem. class.: α-Adrenergic blocker (peripherally acting)
Pregnancy category C

ACTION: Peripheral blood vessels are dilated, peripheral resistance is lowered; reduction in blood pressure results from α-adrenergic receptors being blocked

Therapeutic outcome: Decreased B/P in hypertension, decreased symptoms of benign prostatic hyperplasia (BPH)

USES: Hypertension, as a single agent or in combination with diuretics or β-blockers, BPH

CONTRAINDICATIONS:
Hypersensitivity

Precautions: Pregnancy **C,** breastfeeding, children, prostate cancer, renal disease, syncope

---

DOSAGE AND ROUTES

Hypertension

Adult: PO 1 mg at bedtime, may increase dosage slowly to desired response; max 20 mg/day divided q12hr

Benign prostatic hyperplasia

Adult: PO 1 mg at bedtime, gradually increase up to 5-10 mg, max 20 mg divided q12hr

Available forms: Caps 1, 2, 5, 10 mg

Implementation

• May be used in combination with other antihypertensives
• Give at same time each day
• May be given with food to prevent GI symptoms
• Store in airtight container at 86° F (30° C) or less
• If treatment is interrupted for several days, restart with initial dose
• Give without regard to food
• Feeding tube: place cap in 60 ml of warm tap water, stir until liquid spills from ruptured shell (5 min), stir until cap dissolves, draw solution into oral syringe, give through feeding tube, flush with water

ADVERSE EFFECTS

CNS: *Dizziness, headache, drowsiness,* anxiety, depression, vertigo, weakness, fatigue, syncope
CV: *Palpitations, orthostatic hypotension,* tachycardia, *edema,* rebound hypertension
EENT: Blurred vision, epistaxis, tinnitus, dry mouth, red sclera, nasal congestion, sinusitis
GI: *Nausea,* vomiting, diarrhea, constipation, abdominal pain
GU: Urinary frequency, incontinence, impotence, priapism
RESP: Dyspnea, cough, pharyngitis

Pharmacokinetics

Absorption	Well absorbed
Distribution	Not known
Metabolism	Liver (50%)
Excretion	Kidneys unchanged (10%), feces unchanged (20%)
Half-life	9-12 hr

Pharmacodynamics

Onset	15 min
Peak	2-3 hr
Duration	24 hr

INTERACTIONS

Individual drugs

Alcohol, nitroglycerin, verapamil: increased hypotensive effects, not to drink alcohol

Drug classifications

Antihypertensives (other): increased hypotension
β-Blockers: increased hypotensive effects
Estrogens, NSAIDs, salicylates, sympathomimetics: decreased antihypertensive effect

Drug/herb

Hawthorn: increased antihypertensive effect
Ephedra: decreased antihypertensive effect

NURSING CONSIDERATIONS

Assessment

• **Hypertension:** monitor B/P, orthostatic hypotension, syncope; check for edema in feet, legs daily; I&O ratio; weight daily; notify prescriber of changes
• **Benign prostatic hyperplasia (BPH):** assess urinary patterns (hesitancy, frequency, change in stream, dribbling, dysuria, urgency)

Patient/family education

• Caution patient not to discontinue product abruptly; the importance of complying with dosage schedule, even if feeling better; if dose is missed take as soon as remembered; take medication at same time each day
• Teach patient not to use OTC products (cough, cold, allergy) unless directed by prescriber; to avoid large amounts of caffeine
• Emphasize the need to rise slowly to sitting or standing position to minimize orthostatic hypotension
• Teach patient to notify prescriber of mouth sores, sore throat, fever, swelling of hands or feet, irregular heartbeat, chest pain
• Caution patient to report excessive perspiration, dehydration, vomiting, diarrhea; may lead to fall in B/P
• Caution patient that product may cause dizziness, fainting, light-headedness; may occur during 1st few days of therapy; to avoid hazardous activities
• **Hypertension:** teach patient how to take B/P and normal readings for age group; to take B/P q7day; to continue with regimen including diet and exercise

Evaluation

Positive therapeutic outcome

• Decreased B/P in hypertension
• Decreased symptoms of BPH

T

Adverse effects: *italics* = common; **bold** = life-threatening

TREATMENT OF OVERDOSE:
Administer volume expanders or vasopressors; discontinue product; place patient in supine position

terbinafine (Rx)
(ter-bin'a-feen)
Lamisil
Func. class.: Antifungal, systemic
Chem. class.: Synthetic allylamine derivative
Pregnancy category B

Do not confuse:
LamISIL/LaMICtal/lamoTRIgine

ACTION: Interferes with cell membrane permeability in fungi such as *Trichophyton rubrum, Trichophyton mentagrophytes, Trichophyton tonsurans, Epidermophyton floccosum, Microsporum canis, Microsporum audouinii, Microsporum gypseum, Candida,* broad-spectrum antifungal

Therapeutic outcome: Resolution of fungal infection

USES: Onychomycosis of the toenail or fingernail due to dermatophytes, tinea capitis/corporis/cruris/pedis/versicolor

Unlabeled uses: Cutaneous candidiasis, tinea versicolor

CONTRAINDICATIONS:
Hypersensitivity

Precautions: Pregnancy **B**, breastfeeding, children, chronic/active renal/hepatic disease GFR ≤50 mg/min, immunosuppression

DOSAGE AND ROUTES
Adult: PO 250 mg/day × 6 wk (fingernail); × 12 wk (toenail)

Available forms: Tabs 250 mg; oral granules 125, 187.5 mg

Implementation
• **PO:** give without regard to food
• **Granules:** take with food, sprinkle packet contents on pudding or non-acidic soft food, swallow without chewing, do not use fruit-based foods
• Store at 25° C (77° F), protect from light

ADVERSE EFFECTS
CNS: Depression
EENT: Tinnitus, hearing impairment
GI: Diarrhea, dyspepsia, abdominal pain, nausea, hepatitis
HEMA: Neutropenia
INTEG: Rash, pruritus, urticaria, **Stevens-Johnson syndrome,** photosensitivity
MISC: Headache, hepatic enzyme changes, taste, visual/olfactory disturbance

Pharmacokinetics

Absorption	80%
Distribution	Extensive, most to hair, scalp, nails; excreted in breast milk; protein binding 99%
Metabolism	Liver, extensively
Excretion	Unknown
Half-life	22 days or longer

Pharmacodynamics

Onset	Up to 1 wk
Peak	Several days-weeks
Duration	Several weeks

INTERACTIONS
Individual drugs
Atomoxetine: decreased metabolism of atomoxetine
Cimetidine: increased effect
CycloSPORINE: increased cycloSPORINE clearance
Dextromethorphan: increased levels
Rifampin: increased terbinafine clearance

Drug/herb
Cola nut, guarana, yerba maté, tea (black, green), coffee: side effects

Drug/lab test
Increased: LFTs

NURSING CONSIDERATIONS
Assessment
• Assess hepatic studies (ALT, AST) before beginning treatment; do not use in presence of hepatic disease
• Monitor CBC in treatment >6 wk
• Assess for continuing infection

Patient/family education
• Teach patient to notify prescriber of nausea, vomiting, fatigue, jaundice, dark urine, clay-colored stool, RUQ pain, that may indicate hepatic dysfunction
• Teach patient to avoid using OTC medication unless approved by prescriber
• Teach patient that treatment may take 10 wk (toenail), 4 wk (fingernail)

⚠ Nurse Alert   ✳ Key NCLEX® Drug

Evaluation
Positive therapeutic outcome
• Decrease in size, number of lesions

terbinafine topical
See Appendix B

terbutaline (Rx)
(ter-byoo'ta-leen)
Bricanye ✦
Func. class.: Selective β₂-agonist; bronchodilator
Chem. class.: Catecholamine
Pregnancy category B

Do not confuse:
terbutaline/TOLBUTamide/terbinafine

ACTION: Relaxes bronchial smooth muscle by direct action on β₂-adrenergic receptors through accumulation of cyclic AMP at β-adrenergic receptor sites; results are bronchodilatation, diuresis, and CNS and cardiac stimulation; relaxes uterine smooth muscle

Therapeutic outcome: Bronchodilatation with ease of breathing

USES: Bronchospasm

Unlabeled uses: Premature labor

CONTRAINDICATIONS:
Hypersensitivity to sympathomimetics; closed-angle glaucoma, tachydysrhythmias

Precautions: Pregnancy **B**, breastfeeding, geriatric, cardiac disorders, hyperthyroidism, diabetes mellitus, prostatic hypertension, hypertension, seizure disorder

> **BLACK BOX WARNING:** Labor

DOSAGE AND ROUTES
Bronchospasm
Adult and child >12 yr: PO 2.5-5 mg q8hr; SUBCUT 0.25 mg q15-30min, max 0.5 mg in 4 hr
Adolescent ≤15 yr and child ≥12 yr: PO 2.5 mg tid, max 7.5 mg/day

Renal dose
Adult: PO CCr 10-50 ml/min 50% of dose; CCr <10 ml/min avoid use

Severe renal failure
Adult: PO avoid if GFR <10 ml/min

Tocolytic (preterm labor) (unlabeled)
Adult: SUBCUT 0.25 mg q20min to 6 hr, hold if pulse >120 bpm

Available forms: Tabs 2.5, 5 mg; inj 1 mg/ml

Implementation
• Use this medication before other medications and allow 5 min between each to prevent overstimulation
PO route
• Give PO with meals to decrease gastric irritation; tab may be crushed and mixed with food or fluid
SUBCUT route
• May give by SUBCUT route; do not give by IM route
Aerosol route
• Give after shaking; ask patient to exhale, place mouthpiece in mouth, then inhale slowly; hold breath, remove, exhale slowly; allow at least 1 min between inhalations
• Store in light-resistant container, do not expose to temperatures over 86° F (30° C)

IV route
• Give at 5 mcg q10min until contractions are stopped; use inf pump for correct dose; after ½-1 hr with no contraction decrease dose by 5 mcg; switch to PO dose when possible

Y-site compatibilities: Regular insulin

ADVERSE EFFECTS
CNS: Tremors, anxiety, insomnia, headache, dizziness, stimulation
CV: Palpitations, tachycardia, hypertension, dysrhythmias, **cardiac arrest, QT prolongation**
GI: Nausea, vomiting
META: Hypokalemia, hyperglycemia
RESP: Paradoxical bronchospasm, dyspnea

Pharmacokinetics

Absorption	Well absorbed (SUBCUT), partially absorbed (PO)
Distribution	Unknown
Metabolism	Liver, partially
Excretion	Unknown
Half-life	PO 3-4 hr, subcut 5-7 hr

Adverse effects: *italics* = common; **bold** = life-threatening

Pharmacodynamics

	PO	INH	SUB-CUT	IV
Onset	½ hr	5-15 min	10-15 min	Rapid
Peak	1-2 hr	1-2 hr	½-1 hr	Unknown
Duration	4-8 hr	4-6 hr	1½-4 hr	Unknown

INTERACTIONS

Individual drugs
Arsenic trioxide, chloroquine, droperidol, haloperidol, levomethadyl, pentamidine: increased QT prolongation

Drug classifications
Beta agonists, class IA/III antidysrhythmics, CYP3A4 inhibitors (amiodarone, clarithromycin, erythromycin, telithromycin, troleandomycin), CYP3A4 substrates (methadone, pimozide, QUEtiapine, quiNIDine, risperiDONE, ziprasidone), local anesthetics, some phenothiazines, tricyclics: increased QT prolongation

β-Adrenergic blockers: do not use together, block therapeutic effect

MAOIs: increased chance of hypertensive crisis

Sympathomimetics: increased effects of both products

Drug/herb
Green tea (large amounts), guarana: increased effect

NURSING CONSIDERATIONS

Assessment
• Monitor respiratory function: vital capacity, FEV, ABGs, lung sounds, heart rate, rhythm (baseline)
• Determine that patient has not received theophylline therapy before giving dose; assess client's ability to self-medicate
• Monitor for evidence of allergic reactions; withhold dose and notify prescriber
• **Assess for paradoxical bronchospasm:** dyspnea, wheezing; keep emergency resuscitative equipment nearby

> **BLACK BOX WARNING:** Assess for labor: maternal heart rate, B/P, contractions, fetal heart rate; can inhibit uterine contractions, labor; monitor for hypoglycemia

Patient/family education
• Advise patient not to use OTC medications; extra stimulation may occur; to use this medication before other medications and allow at least 5 min between each to prevent overstimulation
• Teach patient how to use inhaler; to avoid getting aerosol in eyes because blurring may result; to wash inhaler in warm water daily and dry; to avoid smoking, smoke-filled rooms, persons with respiratory infections; review package insert with patient
• Teach patient that paradoxical bronchospasm may occur; to stop product immediately and notify prescriber; to limit caffeine products such as chocolate, coffee, tea, and colas
• Instruct patient on administration of dose, not to use more than prescribed; serious side effects may occur; if taking PO regularly and dose is missed, take when remembered; space other doses on new time schedule

Evaluation
Positive therapeutic outcome
• Absence of dyspnea, wheezing after 1 hr
• Improved airway exchange
• Improved ABGs

TREATMENT OF OVERDOSE:
Administer a β₂-adrenergic blocker

terconazole vaginal antifungal
See Appendix B

teriflunomide
(ter′i-floo′noe-mide)
Aubagio
Func. class.: Multiple sclerosis agent
Chem. class.: Pyrimidine synthesis inhibitor
Pregnancy category X

ACTION: Antiproliferative effects including peripheral T- and B-lymphocytes, might reduce inflammatory demyelination

Therapeutic outcome: Decreased symptoms of MS

USES: Reduction of the frequency of relapses or remitting MS

CONTRAINDICATIONS:
Hypersensitivity

> **BLACK BOX WARNING:** Pregnancy: X

Precautions: Breastfeeding, alcoholism, diabetes mellitus, eosinophilic pneumonia,

---

🅐 Nurse Alert   🌟 Key NCLEX® Drug

hepatitis, jaundice, male-mediated teratogenicity, pneumonitis, pulmonary disease/fibrosis, sarcoidosis, TB, vaccination

> **BLACK BOX WARNING:** Hepatic disease

DOSAGE AND ROUTES
Adult: PO 7 or 14 mg/day

Available forms: Tabs 7, 14 mg

Implementation
PO route
May be taken without regard to food

ADVERSE EFFECTS
CNS: Anxiety, headache
CV: Palpitations, hypertension, **MI**
EENT: Blurred vision, conjunctivitis, sinusitis
GI: Nausea, vomiting, diarrhea, cystitis
HEMA: Leukopenia, lymphopenia, neutropenia
INTEG: Acne vulgaris, alopecia, pruritus
META: Weight loss
MISC: Infection, cystitis

Pharmacokinetics

Absorption	Unknown
Distribution	Protein binding >99%
Metabolism	Unknown
Excretion	Unknown
Half-life	Median 18–19 days, peak 1–4 hr

INTERACTIONS
Individual drugs
Do not use with leflunomide
CycloSPORINE, eltrombopag, gefitinib: increased teriflunomide effect
Methotrexate: increased hepatotoxicity
Zidovudine: increased hematologic toxicity
Repaglinide, pioglitazone, rosiglitazone, PACLitaxel, naproxen, topotecan, bosentan, furosemide: increased effect of each agent
Warfarin, alosetron, DULoxetine, theophylline, tiZANidine, quiNINE, tamoxifen, bendamustine, rasagiline, rOPINIRole, selegiline, propafenone, mexiletine, lidocaine, anagrelide, cloZAPine, cinacalcet, caffeine: decreased effect of each agent, monitor closely
Cholestyramine, activated charcoal: decreased effect of teriflunomide

Drug classifications
Do not use with live virus vaccines
HMG-CoA reductase inhibitors: Increase: hepatotoxicity

Oral contraceptives: increased effect of oral contraceptives

NURSING CONSIDERATIONS
Assessment
• CNS symptoms: assess for anxiety, confusion, vertigo
• GI status: assess for diarrhea, vomiting, abdominal pain
• Cardiac status: assess for tachycardia, palpitations, vasodilation, chest pain

Patient/family education
• Teach patient that blurred vision can occur
• Advise patient to notify prescriber if pregnancy is planned or suspected
• Inform patient not to change dosing or stop taking without advice of prescriber

Evaluation
Positive therapeutic outcome
• Decreased symptoms of MS

teriparatide (Rx)
(tah-ree-par'ah-tide)
Forteo
Func. class.: Parathyroid hormone (rDNA)
Chem. class.: Teriparatide
Pregnancy category C

ACTION: Contains human recombinant parathyroid hormone, which stimulates new bone growth

Therapeutic outcome: Calcium levels at 9-10 mg/dl, decreased symptoms of hypocalcemia, hypoparathyroidism

USES: Postmenopausal women with osteoporosis, men with primary or hypogonadal osteoporosis who are at high risk for fracture, glucocorticoid-induced osteoporosis

CONTRAINDICATIONS:
Hypersensitivity, increased baseline risk of osteosarcoma (Paget's disease, open epiphyses, previous bone radiation), bone metastases, history of skeletal malignancies, other metabolic bone diseases, preexisting hypercalcemia

Precautions: Pregnancy C, breastfeeding, children, urolithiasis, hypotension, use >2 yr

> **BLACK BOX WARNING:** Secondary malignancy

T

DOSAGE AND ROUTES
Adult: SUBCUT 20 mcg/day up to 2 yr (osteoporosis); use for years/lifetime is recommended (glucocorticoid-induced osteoporosis)

Available forms: Prefilled pen delivery device (delivers 20 mcg/day)

Implementation
• Store refrigerated; do not freeze
SUBCUT route
• Give by SUBCUT only, rotate inj sites
• Protect from freezing, light; refrigerate pen

ADVERSE EFFECTS
CNS: Dizziness, headache, insomnia, depression, vertigo
CV: Hypertension, angina, syncope
GI: Nausea, diarrhea, dyspepsia, vomiting, constipation
INTEG: Rash, sweating
MISC: Pain, asthenia, hyperuricemia
MS: Arthralgia, leg cramps, back/leg pain, weakness, **osteosarcoma (rare)**
RESP: Rhinitis, cough, pharyngitis, pneumonia, dyspnea

Pharmacokinetics

Absorption	Extensively, rapidly
Distribution	Unknown
Metabolism	Liver
Excretion	Kidneys
Half-life	Unknown

Pharmacodynamics

Onset	Rapid
Peak	½ hr
Duration	3 hr

INTERACTIONS
Individual drug
Digoxin: increased digoxin toxicity

Drug/lab test
Increased: calcium, uric acid, urinary calcium
Decreased: magnesium, phosphorus

NURSING CONSIDERATIONS
Assessment
• **Secondary malignancy:** osteosarcoma depends on length of treatment, those at higher risk for osteosarcoma should not use this product
• Monitor uric acid, chloride, magnesium, electrolytes, urine pH, vit D, phosphate for normal serum levels; serum calcium may be transiently increased after dosing (max at 4-6 hr after dose)
• Assess for bone pain, headache, fatigue, changes in LOC, leg cramps
• Monitor for signs of persistent hypercalcemia: nausea, vomiting, constipation, lethargy, muscle weakness
• Assess nutritional status: diet for sources of vit D (milk, some seafood), calcium (dairy products, dark green vegetables), phosphates (dairy products)

Patient/family education
• Advise patient of the symptoms of hypercalcemia
• Teach about foods rich in calcium
• Teach how to use delivery device, dispose of needles, not to share pen with others, use at same time of day
• Advise to sit or lie down if dizziness or fast heartbeat occurs after the first few doses
• Pen may be used for 28 days

Evaluation
Positive therapeutic outcome
• Increased bone mineral density

tesamorelin
(tes-a-moe-rel′in)
Egrifta
Func. class.: Pituitary hormone, growth hormone modifiers
Pregnancy category X

ACTION: Binds to growth hormone releasing factor receptors on the pituitary somatotroph cells; binding stimulates the production, release of endogenous growth hormone (GH)

Therapeutic outcome: Decreasing lipodystrophy in HIV patients

USES: Treatment of excess abdominal fat in HIV-infected patients with lipodystrophy

CONTRAINDICATIONS:
Hypersensitivity to this product or mannitol, neoplastic disease, pregnancy **X,** disruption of the hypothalamic-pituitary axis (hypothalamic-pituitary-adrenal [HPA] suppression) resulting from hypophysectomy, hypopituitarism, pituitary tumor/surgery, radiation therapy of the head, head trauma, IV/IM administration

Precautions: Breastfeeding, CABG, diabetes, diabetic retinopathy, edema, geriatrics, children, infants, adolescents

---

⚠ Nurse Alert   ✳ Key NCLEX® Drug

DOSAGE AND ROUTES
Adult: SUBCUT 2 mg/day

Available forms: Powder for injection
1 mg

Implementation
SUBCUT route
• Visually inspect parenteral products for
particulate matter and discoloration before use
whenever solution and container permit
• To reconstitute, inject 2.1 ml sterile water for
injection into the 2-mg vial; use the syringe with
the needle already attached. To avoid foaming,
push the plunger in slowly with the needle at
a slight angle so the sterile water goes down
the inside wall of the vial; with the needle and
syringe attached to the vial, keep the vial upright
and gently roll the vial for 30 sec until mixed; do
not shake; withdraw 2.1 ml of the reconstituted
solution
• Take the syringe out of the vial, place the
needle cap on its side against a clean, flat surface; do not touch needle; hold syringe and slide
the needle into cap; *push the cap all the way or
until it snaps shut; do not touch cap until it
covers the needle completely*
• Remove needle and insert a ½″ 27-G safety injection needle onto the syringe; use immediately;
throw away any unused product or used sterile
water for injection
• Solution should be clear; do not use if discolored, cloudy, or has particles, but slight foaming
is acceptable
• Inject subcut into abdomen; avoid scar tissues, bruises, or the navel; rotate injection sites
in the abdomen; slowly push plunger down until
all solution has been injected
• After removing the injection from the skin, flip
back the needle shield until it snaps, covering
the injection needle completely; keep pressing
until you hear a click; that means the injection
needle is protected
• Use a piece of sterile gauze to rub the
injection site clean; if there is bleeding, apply
pressure to the injection site with gauze for 30
seconds; if bleeding continues, apply a bandage
to the site
• Properly dispose of used syringe, needles,
vial, and sterile water for injection bottle in a
sharps container

ADVERSE EFFECTS
CNS: Depression, flushing, headache,
hypoesthesia, insomnia, night sweats, peripheral
neuropathy paresthesias, spasms

CV: Chest pain, edema, hypertension, palpita-
tions, peripheral edema
GI: Diarrhea, dyspepsia, nausea, upper ab-
dominal pain, vomiting
INTEG: Flushing, injection site reactions,
pruritus, rash, urticaria
MS: Arthralgia, carpal tunnel syndrome, joint
swelling, myalgias, stiffness
RESP: *Upper respiratory tract infection*
SYST: Secondary malignancy

Pharmacokinetics

Absorption	Unknown
Distribution	Unknown
Metabolism	Unknown
Excretion	Unknown
Half-life	26 and 38 mins in healthy and HIV-infected patients, respectively, peak 0.15 hrs

Pharmacodynamics

Onset	Unknown
Peak	0.15 hrs
Duration	Unknown

INTERACTIONS
Individual drugs
Cortisone, predniSONE, simvastatin, ritonavir:
decreased effect of each specific product

NURSING CONSIDERATIONS
Assessment
• Lipsodystrophy: Assess for sunken cheeks;
thinning arms and legs; fat accumulation in the
abdomen, jaws, and back of neck; after treatment these should lessen
• Monitor glycosylated hemoglobin A1c
(HbA1c), serum IGF-1 concentrations, ophthalmologic exam

Patient/family education
• Explain reason for product and expected
result
⚠ **Teach patient to use contraception
(Pregnancy X)**

Evaluation
Positive therapeutic outcome
• Decreasing lipodystrophy in HIV patients

T

testosterone (Rx)
(tess-toss′te-rone)
testosterone enanthate (Rx)
Delatestryl
testosterone cypionate (Rx)
Depo-Testosterone
testosterone pellets (Rx)
Testopel
testosterone transdermal (Rx)
Androderm
testosterone gel (Rx)
AndroGel Fortesta, Testim
testosterone buccal (Rx)
Striant
testosterone topical solution (Rx)
Axiron

Func. class.: Androgenic anabolic steroid
Chem. class.: Halogenated testosterone derivative
Pregnancy category X
Controlled substance schedule III

ACTION: Increases weight by building body tissue; increases potassium, phosphorus, chloride, nitrogen levels; increases bone development; responsible for maintenance of secondary sex characteristics (male)

Therapeutic outcome: Increased hormone levels in eunuchoidism, decreased tumor growth in female breast cancer, onset of male puberty

USES: Female breast cancer, hypogonadism, eunuchoidism, male climacteric, oligospermia, impotence, vulvar dystrophies, low testosterone levels, delayed male puberty (inj)

CONTRAINDICATIONS:
Pregnancy **X**, breastfeeding, severe renal/cardiac/hepatic disease, hypersensitivity, genital bleeding (rare), male breast/prostate cancer

Precautions: Diabetes mellitus, CV disease, MI, urinary tract disorders, prostate cancer, hypercalcemia

BLACK BOX WARNING: Children, accidental exposure

DOSAGE AND ROUTES
Replacement
Adult: **IM** (enanthate or cypionate) 50-400 mg q2-4wk; transdermal (Testoderm) 4-6 mg applied q24hr; (Androderm, AndroGel) 5 mg applied q24hr; once daily (gel); topical sol (Axiron) 60 mg (2 pump activations) each AM; BUCCAL 1 buccal system (30 mg) to the gum region q12hr before meals/PM
Adult (male) and child: SUBCUT (pellets) 150-450 mg (2-6 pellets) inserted q3-6mo

Breast cancer
Adult: IM 50-100 mg 3 ×/wk (propionate) or 200-400 mg q2-4wk (cypionate or enanthate)

Delayed male puberty
Child >12 yr: IM up to 100 mg/mo for up to 6 mo

Available forms: **Enanthate:** inj 200 mg/ml; **cypionate:** inj 100, 200 mg/ml; pellets 75 mg; **transdermal** 2, 4 mg/24 hr; **gel** 1%, 1.62%, 10 mg/actuation; **buccal system** 30 mg; **topical solution** 30 mg/actuation

Implementation
• Administer diet with increased calories, protein; decreased sodium if edema occurs
• Administer supportive product if anemia occurs
• Give titrated dose; use lowest effective dose
• Give IM inj deep into upper outer quadrant of gluteal muscle; route can be painful
Transdermal route
• Apply Testoderm to skin of scrotum, Androderm to skin of back, upper arms, thighs, abdomen; area must be clean and dry, free of hair
Gel route
• Products are not interchangeable, dosage and administration for AndroGel 1% differs from AndroGel 1.62%
• Apply daily to clean dry area on shoulders, upper arms, or abdomen; women, children should not touch gel or treated skin
Buccal system route
• Do not chew or swallow buccal system
• Rotate sites; place above incisor tooth on either side of mouth
• Open packet; place rounded side of surface against gum and hold firmly in place with finger over lip for 30 sec; if product falls off, replace with new system; discard in trash can away from children or pets
Topical solution
• Using the provided applicator, apply the solution to clean, dry, intact skin of the axilla, preferably at the same time each morning. Do

not apply to any other part of the body. Allow the solution to dry completely before dressing. If an antiperspirant or deodorant is used, apply at least 2 min before applying the solution. The pump must be primed before the first use by fully depressing the pump mechanism 3 times and discarding any solution that is released during the priming. To dispense the solution, position the nozzle over the applicator cup and carefully depress the pump once fully; the cup should be filled with no more than 1 pump actuation (30 mg). With the applicator upright, place it up into the axilla and wipe steadily down and up into the axilla. Do not use fingers or hand to rub the solution. If multiple applications are necessary for the required dose, alternate application between the left and right axilla. When repeat application to the same axilla is necessary, allow the solution to dry completely before the next application. After use, rinse the applicator under running water and pat dry with tissue. Wash hands with soap and water

• Following application, allow the site to dry a few minutes before putting on clothing

• Direct contact of the medicated skin with the skin of another person can result in the transfer of residual testosterone and absorption by the other person. To reduce accidental transfer, the patient should cover the application site(s) with clothing (e.g., a T-shirt) after the solution has dried. The application site should be washed with soap and water prior to any skin-to-skin contact regardless of the length of time since application. In the case of direct contact, the other person should wash the area of contact with soap and water as soon as possible

• Patients should be advised that the topical solution is flammable; therefore, fire, flame, and smoking should be avoided during use

• Advise patients to avoid swimming or washing the application site until 2 hr following application of solution

ADVERSE EFFECTS

CNS: Dizziness, headache, fatigue, tremors, paresthesias, flushing, sweating, anxiety, lability, insomnia, carpal tunnel syndrome
CV: Increased B/P
EENT: Conjunctival edema, nasal congestion
ENDO: Abnormal GTT
GI: Nausea, vomiting, constipation, weight gain, **cholestatic jaundice**
GU: Hematuria, amenorrhea, vaginitis, decreased libido, decreased breast size, clitoral hypertrophy, testicular atrophy, gynecomastia, enlarged prostate

HEMA: Polycythemia
INTEG: Rash, acneiform lesions, oily hair and skin, flushing, sweating, acne vulgaris, alopecia, hirsutism
MS: Cramps, spasms

Pharmacokinetics

Absorption	Well but slowly absorbed
Distribution	Crosses placenta
Metabolism	Liver
Excretion	Kidneys, breast milk
Half-life	8 days (cypionate)
	10-100 min (base)

Pharmacodynamics

	IM (base)	IM (cypionate)	IM (enanthate)	IM (propionate)
Onset	Unknown	Unknown	Unknown	Unknown
Peak	Unknown	Unknown	Unknown	Unknown
Duration	1-3 days	2-4 wk	2-4 wk	1-3 days

INTERACTIONS
Individual drugs
ACTH, buPROPion: increased edema
Insulin: decreased glucose levels may alter need for insulin
Oxyphenbutazone: increased effects of oxyphenbutazone

Drug classifications
Adrenal steroids: increased edema
Anticoagulants: increased pro-time
Antidiabetics, oral: decreased need for oral antidiabetics

Drug/lab test
Increased: serum cholesterol, blood glucose, urine glucose
Decreased: serum Ca, serum K, T_4, T_3, thyroid ^{131}I uptake test, urine 17-OHCS, 17-KS, PBI

NURSING CONSIDERATIONS
Assessment
• Monitor patient's weight daily; notify prescriber if weekly weight gain is >5 lb; assess I&O ratio; be alert for decreasing urinary output, increasing edema
• Monitor B/P q4hr, Hgb/Hct
• Assess growth rate, bone age in adolescent because growth rate may be uneven (linear/bone growth) if used for extended periods

T

Adverse effects: *italics* = common; **bold** = life-threatening

- Monitor electrolytes: potassium, sodium, chloride, calcium; cholesterol
- Monitor liver function tests: ALT, AST, bilirubin
- Assess edema, hypertension, cardiac symptoms, jaundice
- Assess mental status: affect, mood, behavioral changes, aggression
- **Assess signs of masculinization** in female: increased libido, deepening of voice, decreased breast tissue, enlarged clitoris, menstrual irregularities; male: gynecomastia, impotence, testicular atrophy
- **Assess hypercalcemia:** lethargy, polyuria, polydipsia, nausea, vomiting, constipation; product may have to be decreased
- **Assess hypoglycemia** in diabetics because oral antidiabetic action is increased

Patient/family education
- Inform patient that product needs to be combined with complete health plan: diet, rest, exercise
- Caution patient to notify prescriber if therapeutic response decreases; not to discontinue this medication abruptly
- Inform women patients to report menstrual irregularities; about changes in sex characteristics
- Discuss that 1-3 mo course is necessary for response in breast cancer
- Inform patient about application of transdermal patches: Testoderm to skin of scrotum, Androderm to skin of back, upper arms, thighs, abdomen; area must be dry and free of hair; may be reapplied after bathing, swimming
- Teach about changes in sex characteristics: priapism, gynecomastia, increased libido

Evaluation
Positive therapeutic outcome
- Decrease size of tumor in breast cancer
- Increased androgen levels

tetracaine ophthalmic
See Appendix B

tetracaine topical
See Appendix B

tetracycline (Rx)
(tet-ra-sye′kleen)
Apo-Tetra ❖, Nu-Tetra ❖
Func. class.: Antiinfective—broad-spectrum
Chem. class.: Tetracycline
Pregnancy category D

ACTION: Inhibits protein synthesis and phosphorylation in microorganisms; bacteriostatic

Therapeutic outcome: Bactericidal action against susceptible organisms: gram-positive pathogens *Bacillus anthracis, Clostridium perfringens, Clostridium tetani, Listeria monocytogenes, Nocardia, Propionibacterium acnes, Actinomyces israelii;* gram-negative pathogens *Haemophilus influenzae, Legionella pneumophila, Yersinia enterocolitica, Yersinia pestis, Neisseria gonorrhoeae, Neisseria meningitidis*

USES: Syphilis, *Chlamydia trachomatis,* gonorrhea, lymphogranuloma venereum, uncommon gram-positive, gram-negative organisms, rickettsial infections

CONTRAINDICATIONS:
Pregnancy **D**, breastfeeding, children <8 yr, hypersensitivity to tetracyclines

Precautions: Renal/hepatic disease, UV exposure

DOSAGE AND ROUTES
Susceptible gram-positive/gram-negative infections
Adult: PO 250-500 mg q6hr
Child >8 yr: PO 25-50 mg/kg/day in divided doses q6hr

Chlamydia trachomatis
Adult: PO 500 mg qid × 7 days

Syphilis
Adult and adolescent: PO 500 mg qid × 2 wk; if syphilis duration >1 yr, must treat 30 days

Brucellosis
Adult: PO 500 mg qid × 3 wk with 1 g of streptomycin IM 2 ×/day × 1 wk, and 1 ×/day the 2nd wk

Urethral, endocervical, rectal infections *(C. trachomatis)*
Adult: PO 500 mg qid × 7 days

Acne
Adult and adolescent: PO 250 mg q6hr, then 125-500 mg/day or every other day

Renal dose
Adult: PO CCr 51-90 ml/min give dose q8-12hr, CCr 10-50 ml/min give dose q12-24hr, CCr <10 ml/min give dose q24hr

Available forms: Caps 250, 500 mg

Implementation
PO route
• Give around the clock to maintain proper blood levels; give with food to increase absorption of product; do not give within 3 hr of other agents; product interactions may occur; take on an empty stomach (1 hr before or 2 hr after meals)
• Give with 8 oz of water
• Shake liquid preparation well before giving; use calibrated device for proper dosing
• Store in tight, light-resistant container at room temp

ADVERSE EFFECTS
CNS: Fever, headache, paresthesia
CV: Pericarditis
EENT: Dysphagia, glossitis, decreased calcification (permanent discoloration) of deciduous teeth, oral candidiasis, oral ulcers
GI: *Nausea,* abdominal pain, *vomiting, diarrhea,* anorexia, enterocolitis, **hepatotoxicity,** flatulence, abdominal cramps, epigastric burning, stomatitis, hepatitis, **pseudomembranous colitis**
GU: *Increased BUN,* azotemia, **acute renal failure**
HEMA: Eosinophilia, neutropenia, thrombocytopenia, leukocytosis, hemolytic anemia
INTEG: *Rash, urticaria, photosensitivity, increased pigmentation,* exfoliative dermatitis, pruritus, **angioedema, Stevens-Johnson syndrome**
MISC: Increased intracranial pressure, candidiasis

Pharmacokinetics

Absorption	60%-80% (PO), lower (IM)
Distribution	Widely distributed, some in CSF; crosses placenta
Metabolism	Not metabolized
Excretion	Unchanged—kidneys
Half-life	6-10 hr

Pharmacodynamics

Onset	1-2 hr
Peak	2-3 hr
Duration	Unknown

INTERACTIONS
Individual drugs
Cimetidine, NaHCO₃: decreased tetracycline effect
Digoxin: increased digoxin effect
Iron: forms chelates, decreased absorption
Methoxyflurane: fatal nephrotoxicity
Warfarin: increased warfarin effect

Drug classifications
Alkali products, antacids: decreased tetracycline effect
Penicillins: decreased penicillin effect

Drug/herb
Dong quai: increased photosensitivity

Drug/food
Decreased: absorption with dairy products; forms insoluble chelate

Drug/lab test
Increased: BUN, LFTs

NURSING CONSIDERATIONS
Assessment
⚠ Serious skin reactions: angioedema, Stevens-Johnson syndrome, exfoliative dermatitis, report immediately after stopping product
• Assess patient for previous sensitivity reaction
• Assess patient for signs and symptoms of infection including characteristics of wounds, sputum, urine, stool, WBC >10,000/mm³, temp; obtain baseline information before, during treatment
• Complete C&S testing before beginning product therapy to identify if correct treatment has been initiated
• **Assess for allergic reactions:** rash, urticaria, pruritus, chills, fever, joint pain; angioedema may occur a few days after therapy begins; EPINEPHrine, resuscitation equipment should be available for anaphylactic reaction
• Identify urine output; if decreasing, notify prescriber (may indicate nephrotoxicity); increased BUN, creatinine
• **Pseudomembranous colitis:** assess for diarrhea, abdominal pain, fever, fatigue, anorexia; possible anemia, elevated WBC and low serum albumin; stop product and usually give either vancomycin or IV metroNIDAZOLE

T

Adverse effects: *italics* = common; **bold** = life-threatening

• Assess for superinfection: perineal itching, fever, malaise, redness, pain, swelling, drainage, rash, diarrhea, change in cough, sputum if on prolonged therapy

Patient/family education
• Teach patient to report sore throat, bruising, bleeding, joint pain; may indicate blood dyscrasias (rare)
• Advise patient to use sunscreen when outdoors to decrease photosensitivity reaction
• Advise patient to contact prescriber if vaginal itching, loose foul-smelling stools, furry tongue occur; may indicate superinfection; report itching, rash, pruritus, urticaria
• Teach patient to take 1 hr before bedtime to prevent esophageal ulceration
• Instruct patient to take all medication prescribed for the length of time ordered; product must be taken around the clock to maintain blood levels; do not give medication to others
• Teach patient to notify prescriber immediately of diarrhea with pus, mucus, fever, abdominal pain
• Teach patient to notify prescriber if pregnancy is planned or suspected, pregnancy **D**
⚠ Teach patient not to use outdated products, as Fanconi syndrome (nephrotoxicity) may occur

Evaluation
Positive therapeutic outcome
• Absence of signs/symptoms of infection (WBC <10,000/mm³, temp WNL, absence of red, draining wounds)
• Reported improvement in symptoms of infection, resolution of infection, prevention of malaria

---

tetrahydrozoline nasal agent
See Appendix B

tetrahydrozoline ophthalmic
See Appendix B

theophylline (Rx)
(thee-off′i-lin)
Elixophyllin, Theo-24, Theochron, Uniphyl
Func. class.: Spasmolytic, bronchodilator
Chem. class.: Xanthine, ethylenediamine
Pregnancy category C

ACTION: Relaxes smooth muscle of respiratory system by blocking phosphodiester-

ase, which increases cyclic AMP, exact action unknown

Therapeutic outcome: Ability to breathe without difficulty

USES: Bronchial asthma, bronchospasm of COPD, chronic bronchitis, emphysema

CONTRAINDICATIONS:
Hypersensitivity to xanthines, tachydysrhythmias

Precautions: Pregnancy **C**, children, geriatric, CHF, cor pulmonale, hepatic disease, active peptic ulcer disease, diabetes mellitus, hyperthyroidism, hypertension, seizure disorder

DOSAGE AND ROUTES
Acute exacerbations of reversible airway obstructions
Adult: PO/IV 5 mg/kg loading dose over 20-30 min

COPD, chronic bronchitis
Adult: IV 0.4 mg/kg/hr in nonsmokers or 0.7 mg/kg/hr in smokers
Adult, child >45 kg: Maintenance PO (regular release) 10 mg/kg/day, in divided doses q1-8hr; after 3 days increase dosage to 400 mg in divided doses q6-8hr; after 3 more days increase to 600 mg in divided doses q6-8hr; max 800 mg/day

Apnea of prematurity
Neonate: IV 4 mg/kg over 20-30 min, then maintenance IV/PO neonate ≥24 days 1.5 mg/kg q12h

Available forms: Cap, ext rel 100, 200, 300, 400 mg; tab ext rel 100, 200, 400, 450, 600 mg; elixir 80 mg/15 ml; sol for inj 250 mg/10 ml, 500 mg/20 ml

Implementation
PO route
• Do not crush or chew time release products
• Contents of bead-filled cap may be sprinkled over food for children's use
• Give PO with 8 oz water; to decrease GI symptoms; avoid food, absorption may be affected
• Store diluted sol for 24 hr if refrigerated

IV route
• Give loading dose over 20-30 min; max 20-25 mg/min; do not give by rapid IV; use only by cont inf

Y-site compatibilities: Acyclovir, ampicillin, aztreonam, ceFAZolin, cefoTEtan, cefTAZidime, cefTRIAXone, cimetidine, clindamycin, dexamethasone, diltiazem, DOBUTamine, DO-

---

Pamine, doxycycline, erythromycin, famotidine, fluconazole, gentamicin, haloperidol, heparin, hydrocortisone, lidocaine, methyldopa, methylPREDNISolone, metroNIDAZOLE, midazolam, nafcillin, nitroglycerin, nitroprusside, penicillin G potassium, piperacillin, potassium chloride, ranitidine, ticarcillin, ticarcillin/clavulanate, tobramycin, vancomycin

ADVERSE EFFECTS

CNS: *Anxiety, restlessness, insomnia, dizziness, seizures,* headache, light-headedness, muscle twitching, tremors
CV: *Palpitations, sinus tachycardia,* hypotension, **dysrhythmias,** fluid retention with tachycardia
ENDO: Hyperglycemia
GI: *Nausea, vomiting, anorexia,* diarrhea, bitter taste, dyspepsia, gastric distress
INTEG: Flushing, urticaria
MISC: SIADH, urinary frequency
RESP: Increased rate, tachypnea

Pharmacokinetics

Absorption	Well absorbed (PO), slowly absorbed (ext rel)
Distribution	Crosses placenta, widely distributed
Metabolism	Liver
Excretion	Kidneys, breast milk
Half-life	6.5-10.5 hr; increased in liver disease, CHF, geriatric

Pharmacodynamics

	PO	PO–TIME REL	IV
Onset	Rapid	Slow	Immediate
Peak	1 hr	4-8 hr	Inf end
Duration	6 hr	12-24 hr	6-8 hr

INTERACTIONS
Individual drugs
CarBAMazepine: decreased theophylline level
Cimetidine, disulfiram, erythromycin, fluvoxaMINE, influenza vaccine, mexiletine, propranolol: increased theophylline action
Lithium: decreased effect of lithium
PHENobarbital, phenytoin, rifampin: decreased theophylline

Drug classifications
Anticoagulants: increased anticoagulant level
β-Adrenergic blockers: cardiotoxicity

Contraceptives (oral), corticosteroids, fluoroquinolones, interferons: increased theophylline action
Smoking: decreased theophylline level

Drug/herb
Coffee, cola nut, guarana, ma huang (ephedra), tea (black, green), yerba maté: increased toxicity
St. John's wort: decreased theophylline level

NURSING CONSIDERATIONS
Assessment
• Monitor theophylline blood levels (therapeutic level is 5-15 mcg/ml); toxicity may occur with small increase above 15 mcg/ml
• Monitor I&O; diuresis occurs; dehydration may result in children or geriatric
• Assess for signs of toxicity: irritability, insomnia, restlessness, tremors, nausea, vomiting
• Monitor respiratory rate, rhythm, depth; auscultate lung fields bilaterally; notify prescriber of abnormalities
• Assess for allergic reactions: rash, urticaria; if these occur, product should be discontinued

Patient/family education
• Advise patient to check OTC medications, current prescription medications for ePHEDrine, which increases stimulation, and to avoid alcohol, caffeine
• Caution patient to avoid hazardous activities; dizziness may occur
• Inform patient that if GI upset occurs, to take product with 8 oz of water; avoid food; absorption may be decreased
• Advise patient to notify prescriber of toxicity: nausea, vomiting, anxiety, insomnia, seizures
• Advise patient to notify prescriber of change in smoking habit; dosage may have to be changed

Evaluation
Positive therapeutic outcome
• Ability to breathe more easily

thiamine (vitamin B$_1$) (PO, OTC; IV, IM, Rx)
Betaxin ✦, **Betalin S, Biamine, Revitonus, Thiamilate**
Func. class.: Vitamin B$_1$
Chem. class.: Water soluble
Pregnancy category A

Do not confuse:
thiamine/Tenormin

T

ACTION: Needed for pyruvate metabolism, carbohydrate metabolism

Therapeutic outcome: Prevention and treatment of thiamine deficiency

USES: Vit B$_1$ deficiency or polyneuritis, cheilosis adjunct with thiamine beriberi, Wernicke-Korsakoff syndrome, pellagra, metabolic disorders, alcoholism

CONTRAINDICATIONS:
Hypersensitivity

Precautions: Pregnancy **A**

DOSAGE AND ROUTES
RDA
Adult: PO (Male) 1.2-1.5 mg; (female) 1.1 mg; (pregnancy) 1.4 mg; (breastfeeding) 1.4 mg
Child 9-13 yr: PO 0.9 mg
Child 4-8 yr: PO 0.6 mg
Child 1-3 yr: PO 0.5 mg
Infant 6 mo-1 yr: PO 0.3 mg
Neonate and infant to 6 mo: PO 0.3 mg

Beriberi
Adult: PO 5-30 mg qd or given in 3 divided doses × 1 month; IM/IV 5-30 mg qd or in 3 doses, then convert to PO
Child/infant: PO 10-50 mg qd × 2 wk, then 5-10 mg qd × 1 mo; IV/IM 10-25 mg/day × 2 wk, then 5-10 mg qd × 1 mo

Available forms: Tabs 50, 100, 250, 500 mg; inj 100 mg/ml; enteric-coated tabs 20 mg

Implementation
IM route
• Give by IM inj; rotate sites if pain and inflammation occur; do not mix with alkaline sol; Z-track to minimize pain
• Application of cold compress may decrease pain
• Store in airtight, light-resistant container

Direct IV route
• **IV** undiluted given over 5 min
Continuous IV infusion route
• Dilute in compatible **IV** sol

Syringe compatibilities: Doxapram

Y-site compatibilities: Famotidine

ADVERSE EFFECTS
CNS: Weakness, restlessness
CV: Collapse, pulmonary edema, hypotension
EENT: Tightness of throat

GI: Hemorrhage, *nausea, diarrhea*
INTEG: Angioneurotic edema, cyanosis, sweating, warmth
SYST: Anaphylaxis

Pharmacokinetics
Absorption	Well absorbed (PO, IM), completely absorbed (**IV**)
Distribution	Widely distributed
Metabolism	Liver
Excretion	Kidneys (unchanged—excess amounts)
Half-life	Unknown

Pharmacodynamics
Unknown

NURSING CONSIDERATIONS
Assessment
• **Anaphylaxis (IV only):** assess for swelling of face, eyes, lips, throat, wheezing
• **Thiamine deficiency:** assess for anorexia, weakness, pain, depression, confusion, blurred vision, tachycardia
• Assess nutritional status: yeast, beef, liver, whole or enriched grains, legumes

Patient/family education
• Teach patient necessary foods to be included in diet: yeast, beef, liver, legumes, whole grains

Evaluation
Positive therapeutic outcome
• Absence of nausea, vomiting, anorexia, insomnia, tachycardia, paresthesias, depression, muscle weakness

thioridazine (Rx)
(thye-or-rid′a-zeen)
Func. class.: Antipsychotic (typical)
Chem. class.: Phenothiazine, piperidine
Pregnancy category C

Do not confuse:
thioridazine/thiothixene/thorazine

ACTION: Depresses cerebral cortex, hypothalamus, limbic system, which control activity, aggression; blocks neurotransmission produced by dopamine at synapse; exhibits strong α-adrenergic, anticholinergic blocking action; mechanism for antipsychotic effects is unclear

Therapeutic outcome: Decreased signs and symptoms of psychosis

USES: Psychotic disorders, schizophrenia, behavioral problems in children, anxiety, major depressive disorders, organic brain syndrome

CONTRAINDICATIONS:
Children <2 yr, hypersensitivity, coma, CNS depression

> **BLACK BOX WARNING:** QT prolongation, cardiac dysrhythmias

Precautions: Pregnancy C, breastfeeding, seizure disorders, hypertension, hepatic/pulmonary disease, renal failure, BPH, glaucoma, phenothiazine hypersensitivity, suicidal ideation, smoking, Reye's syndrome, Parkinson's disease

> **BLACK BOX WARNING:** Cardiac disease, dementia, AV block, bundle branch block, torsades de pointes

DOSAGE AND ROUTES
Psychosis
Adult: PO 25-100 mg tid, max dose 800 mg/day; dose is gradually increased to desired response, then reduced to minimum maintenance

Depression/behavioral problems/organic brain syndrome
Adult: PO 25 tid, range from 10 mg bid-qid to 50 mg tid-qid; max 800 mg/day for short period
Geriatric: PO 10-25 mg daily-bid, increase 4-7 days by 10-25 mg to desired dose, max 300 mg/day for short period
Child 2-12 yr: PO 0.5-3 mg/kg/day in divided doses, max 3 mg/kg/day

Available forms: Tabs 10, 25, 50, 100 mg

Implementation
• Decrease dosage in geriatric because metabolism is slowed
• Administer PO with full glass of water, milk; or give with food to decrease GI upset
• Give antacids 2 hr before or after this product
• Store in airtight, light-resistant container, oral sol in amber bottle

ADVERSE EFFECTS
CNS: *EPS (pseudoparkinsonism, akathisia, dystonia, tardive dyskinesia)*, **seizures,** *headache*, confusion, **neuroleptic malignant syndrome, dizziness,** drowsiness
CV: Orthostatic hypotension, **cardiac arrest,** ECG changes, **tachycardia, QT prolongation, torsades de pointes**
EENT: Blurred vision, glaucoma, dry eyes

GI: *Dry mouth, nausea, vomiting, anorexia, constipation,* diarrhea, jaundice, weight gain
GU: Urinary retention, urinary frequency, enuresis, impotence, amenorrhea, gynecomastia, ejaculation dysfunction, priapism
HEMA: Anemia, **leukopenia, leukocytosis, agranulocytosis**
INTEG: *Rash*, photosensitivity, dermatitis
RESP: **Laryngospasm,** dyspnea, **respiratory depression**

Pharmacokinetics

Absorption	Variably absorbed (tab)
Distribution	Widely distributed, high concentrations in CNS, crosses placenta, protein binding 91%-99%
Metabolism	Liver, extensively; GI mucosa
Excretion	Kidneys, breast milk
Half-life	26-36 hr

Pharmacodynamics

Onset	Erratic
Peak	2-4 hr
Duration	8-12 hr

INTERACTIONS
Individual drugs
Alcohol: oversedation
Aluminum hydroxide, magnesium hydroxide: decreased absorption

> **BLACK BOX WARNING:** Haloperidol, chloroquine, droperidol, pentamidine, arsenic trioxide, levomethadyl: increased QT prolongation

Lithium: decreased thioridazine levels

Drug classifications
Anesthetics (barbiturate), CNS depressants: oversedation
Antacids: decreased absorption
Anticholinergics: increased anticholinergic effects
Antiparkinson agents: decreased effect of these agents
Barbiturates: decreased thioridazine effect
Centrally acting antihypertensives: decreased antihypertensive effect

T

BLACK BOX WARNING: Class IA/III antidys-rhythmics, some phenothiazines, β-agonists, local anesthetics, tricyclics, CYP3A4 inhibitors (amiodarone, clarithromycin, erythromycin, telithromycin, troleandomycin); CYP3A4 substrates (methadone, pimozide, QUEtiap-ine, quiNIDine, risperiDONE, ziprasidone): increased QT prolongation; CYP2D6 inhibitors

Drug/lab test
Increased: liver function tests, prolactin, bilirubin, alk phos
Decreased: Hct/Hgb, platelets, granulocytes, leukocytes, neutrocytes, eosinophils

NURSING CONSIDERATIONS
Assessment
• Assess mental status: orientation, mood, behavior, presence of hallucinations, and type before initial administration and monthly; this product should significantly reduce psychotic behavior
• Check for swallowing of PO medication; check for hoarding or giving of medication to other patients
• Monitor I&O ratio; palpate bladder if low urinary output occurs, especially in geriatric; urinalysis recommended before, during prolonged therapy
• Monitor bilirubin, CBC, liver function tests monthly
• Assess affect, orientation, LOC, reflexes, gait, coordination, sleep pattern disturbances
• Monitor B/P sitting, standing, and lying, take pulse and respirations q4hr during initial treatment; establish baseline before starting treatment; report drops of 30 mm Hg; obtain baseline ECG, monitor Q- and T-wave changes
• Check for dizziness, faintness, palpitations, tachycardia on rising; severe orthostatic hypotension is common
• **QT prolongation:** monitor ECG for QT prolongation, ejection fraction; assess for chest pain, palpitations, dyspnea
⚠ **Neuroleptic malignant syndrome: assess for hyperpyrexia, muscle rigidity, increased CPK, altered mental status, dyspnea, fatigue; product should be discontinued**
• **EPS** including akathisia (inability to sit still, no pattern to movements), tardive dyskinesia (bizarre movements of the jaw, mouth, tongue, extremities), pseudoparkinsonism (ragged tremors, pill rolling, shuffling gate); an antiparkinsonian product should be prescribed

• Assess for constipation, urinary retention daily; if these occur, increase bulk, water in diet

Patient/family education
• Teach patient to use good oral hygiene; frequent rinsing of mouth, sugarless gum for dry mouth
• Advise patient to avoid hazardous activities until product response is determined; dizziness, blurred vision are common
• Inform patient that orthostatic hypotension occurs often and to rise from sitting or lying position gradually; to avoid hot tubs, hot showers, tub baths because hypotension may occur
• Instruct patient that in hot weather, heat stroke may occur; take extra precautions to stay cool
• Caution patient to avoid abrupt withdrawal of this product, or EPS may result; product should be withdrawn slowly
• Teach patient to avoid OTC preparations (cough, hay fever, cold) unless approved by prescriber; serious product interactions may occur; avoid use with alcohol, CNS depressants; increased drowsiness may occur
• Advise patient to use sunglasses and sunscreen to prevent burns
• Teach patient about EPS and necessity for meticulous oral hygiene because oral candidiasis may occur
• Advise patient to take antacids 2 hr before or after this product
• Instruct patient to report sore throat, malaise, fever, bleeding, mouth sores; if these occur, CBC should be performed and product discontinued; may cause vision impairment, report to prescriber
• Advise patient that urine may be discolored

Evaluation
Positive therapeutic outcome
• Decrease in emotional excitement, hallucinations, delusions, paranoia
• Reorganization of patterns of thought, speech

TREATMENT OF OVERDOSE:
Lavage if orally ingested; provide airway; *do not induce vomiting or use EPINEPHrine*, CV monitoring, continuous ECG

thyroid USP (desiccated) (Rx)

(thye′roid)

Armour Thyroid, Bio-Throid, Nature Thyroid, NP Thyroid

Func. class.: Thyroid hormone

Chem. class.: Active thyroid hormone in natural state and ratio

Pregnancy category A

ACTION: Increases metabolic rate; increases cardiac output, O_2 consumption, body temp, blood volume, growth, development at cellular level

Therapeutic outcome: Correction of lack of thyroid hormone

USES: Hypothyroidism, cretinism (juvenile hypothyroidism), myxedema

CONTRAINDICATIONS:

Adrenal insufficiency, MI, thyrotoxicosis, porcine protein hypersensitivity

BLACK BOX WARNING: Obesity treatment

Precautions: Pregnancy **A,** breastfeeding, geriatric, angina pectoris, hypertension, ischemia, cardiac disease

DOSAGE AND ROUTES

Hypothyroidism

Adult: PO 60-65 mg/day, increased by 30 mg qmo until desired response; maintenance dose 65-120 mg/day

Geriatric: PO 7.5-15 mg/day, increase dose q6-8wk until desired response

Cretinism/juvenile hypothyroidism

Child: PO 15 mg/day, then 30 mg/day after 2 wk, then 60 mg/day after another 2 wk; maintenance dose 60-180 mg/day

Myxedema

Adult: PO 15 mg/day, double dose q2wk, maintenance 60-180 mg/day

Available forms: Tabs 16, 32, 60, 65, 98, 130, 195, 260, 325 mg; enteric-coated tabs 32, 65, 130 mg; sugar-coated tabs 32, 65, 130, 195 mg; caps 65, 130, 195, 325 mg

Implementation

• Give in AM if possible as a single dose to decrease sleeplessness; at same time each day to maintain product level

• Do not give with food because absorption will be decreased

• Give only for hormone imbalances; not to be used for obesity, male infertility, menstrual conditions, lethargy; give lowest dose that relieves symptoms; lower dosage in the geriatric and in cardiac diseases

• Store in airtight, light-resistant container

• Wean patient off medication 4 wk before RAIU test

ADVERSE EFFECTS

CNS: *Insomnia, tremors,* headache, **thyroid storm**

CV: *Tachycardia, palpitations, angina,* **dysrhythmias,** hypertension, **cardiac arrest**

GI: Nausea, diarrhea, increased or decreased appetite, cramps

MISC: Menstrual irregularities, weight loss, sweating, heat intolerance, fever

Pharmacokinetics

Absorption	Well absorbed
Distribution	Widely distributed, does not cross placenta
Metabolism	Liver, tissues
Excretion	Feces via bile, breast milk
Half-life	T_3, 2 days; T_4, 1 wk

Pharmacodynamics

Onset	1 hr
Peak	12-48 hr
Duration	Unknown

INTERACTIONS

Individual drugs

Aluminum, calcium, magnesium: decreased thyroid absorption

Drug classifications

Anticoagulants, oral: increased effects of anticoagulants

Antidepressants (tricyclic): increased antidepressant (tricylics) effect

Bile acid sequestrants: decreased thyroid absorption

Catecholamines: increased effects of catecholamines

Estrogens: decreased thyroid hormone effect

Sympathomimetics: increased effects of sympathomimetics

Drug/lab test
Increased: CPK, LDH, AST, PBI, blood glucose
Decreased: thyroid function tests

NURSING CONSIDERATIONS
Assessment

> **BLACK BOX WARNING: Obesity treatment:** use can lead to serious or life-threatening toxicity

- Identify if the patient is taking anticoagulants, antidiabetic agents; document on chart
- Take B/P, pulse before each dose; monitor I&O ratio and weight every day in same clothing, using same scale, at same time of day
- Monitor height, weight, psychomotor development, growth rate if given to a child
- Monitor T_3, T_4, FTIs, which are decreased; radioimmunoassay of TSH, which is increased; radioactive iodine uptake (RAIU), which is increased if patient's dose of medication is too low
- Monitor pro-time; patient may require decreased dosage of anticoagulant; check for bleeding, bruising
- **Hyperthyroidism:** assess for increased nervousness, excitability, irritability, which may indicate that dose of medication is too high, usually after 1-3 wk of treatment
- **Hypothyroidism:** lethargy, cold intolerance, weight gain, constipation, muscle cramps, may indicate dosage is too low
- Assess cardiac status: angina, palpitation, chest pain, change in VS; the geriatric patient may have undetected cardiac problems; baseline ECG should be completed before treatment

Patient/family education
- Teach patient that product is not a cure but controls symptoms and that treatment is long-term, that strong odor is normal
- Instruct patient to report excitability, irritability, anxiety, sweating, heat intolerance, chest pain, palpitations, which indicate overdose
- Advise patient not to switch brands unless approved by prescriber; bioavailability may differ; do not take with food; absorption will be decreased
- Teach patient that product might be discontinued after giving birth; thyroid panel will be evaluated after 1-2 mo
- Teach patient that hyperthyroid child will show almost immediate behavior/personality change; that hair loss will occur in child and is temporary

- Caution patient that product is not to be taken to reduce weight
- Caution patient to avoid OTC preparations containing iodine; read labels; other medications should not be used unless approved by prescriber
- Teach patient to avoid iodine-containing food: iodized salt, soybeans, tofu, turnips, certain kinds of seafood and bread

Evaluation
Positive therapeutic outcome
- Absence of depression
- Weight loss, increased diuresis, pulse, appetite
- Absence of constipation, peripheral edema, cold intolerance, pale, cool dry skin, brittle nails, alopecia, coarse hair, menorrhagia, night blindness, paresthesias, syncope, stupor, coma, rosy cheeks
- Improved levels of T_3, T_4 by laboratory tests
- Child: Age-appropriate weight, height, and psychomotor development

TREATMENT OF OVERDOSE:
Withhold dose for up to 1 wk; acute overdose—gastric lavage or induce emesis, then activated charcoal; provide supportive treatment to control symptoms

tiaGABine (Rx)
(tie-ah-ga′been)
Gabitril
Func. class.: Anticonvulsant
Pregnancy category C

Do not confuse:
tiaGABine/tiZANidine

ACTION: Inhibits reuptake and metabolism of GABA; may increase seizure threshold, structurally similar to GABA; tiaGABine binding sites in neocortex, hippocampus

USES: Adjunct treatment of partial seizures in adults and children ≥12 yr

CONTRAINDICATIONS:
Hypersensitivity

Precautions: Pregnancy **C,** breastfeeding, child <12 yr, geriatric, renal/hepatic disease, suicidal ideation/behavior, status epilepticus, mania, bipolar disorder, abrupt discontinuation, depression

---

DOSAGE AND ROUTES

When not given with a CYP3A4 enzyme, effect of tiagabine is doubled; lower dosages are indicated

Adult: PO (those on an enzyme-inducing antiepileptic) 4 mg/day in divided doses, may increase by 4-8 mg qwk until desired response, max 56 mg/day

Child 12-18 yr: PO 4 mg/day, may increase by 4 mg at beginning of wk 2, may increase by 4-8 mg qwk until desired response, max 32 mg/day

Hepatic dose

Adult: PO reduce dose or increase dosing interval

Available forms: Tabs 2, 4, 12, 16 mg

Implementation

• Store at room temperature away from heat and light
• Provide assistance with ambulation during early part of treatment; dizziness occurs
• Provide seizure precautions: padded side rails; move objects that may harm patient

ADVERSE EFFECTS

CNS: *Dizziness, anxiety,* somnolence, ataxia, confusion, *asthenia,* unsteady gait, depression, **suicidal ideation,** seizures, tremor, hostility, EEG changes
CV: Vasodilatation, tachycardia, hypertension
ENDO: Goiter, hypothyroidism
GI: Nausea, diarrhea, vomiting, increased appetite
INTEG: Pruritus, rash, **Stevens-Johnson syndrome,** alopecia, hyperhidrosis
MS: Myalgia
RESP: Pharyngitis, coughing

Pharmacokinetics	
Absorption	>95%
Distribution	Protein binding 96%
Metabolism	Liver
Excretion	Kidneys
Half-life	7-9 hr

Pharmacodynamics	
Onset	Unknown
Peak	45 min
Duration	Unknown

INTERACTIONS

Individual drugs

CarBAMazepine, PHENobarbital, phenytoin, primidone: decreased effect of these products
Sevelamer: decreased tiagabine effect

Valproate: lower dose of tiaGABine may be required

Drug classifications

Alcohol, CNS depressants: increased CNS depression

Drug/food

High-fat meal: decreased rate of absorption

NURSING CONSIDERATIONS

Assessment

• Monitor renal function tests: urinalysis, BUN, urine creatinine q3mo
• Monitor liver function tests: ALT, AST, bilirubin
• Assess description of seizures: location, duration, presence of aura; assess for weakness
⚠ **Withdraw gradually to prevent seizures**
⚠ **May cause status epilepticus and unexplained death**
⚠ **Assess mental status: mood, sensorium, affect, behavioral changes, suicidal thoughts; if mental status changes, notify prescriber, increased affect and hypnomania may be present**

Patient/family education

• Advise patient to carry/wear emergency ID stating patient's name, products taken, condition, prescriber's name and phone number
• Advise patient to avoid driving, other activities that require alertness
• Teach patient not to discontinue medication quickly after long-term use
• Teach patient to notify prescriber if pregnancy is planned or suspected, avoid breastfeeding
⚠ **Teach patient to report suicidal thoughts, behaviors immediately**

Evaluation

Positive therapeutic outcome

• Decreased seizure activity; document on patient's chart

TREATMENT OF OVERDOSE:

Lavage, VS

ticagrelor

(tye-ka′gre-lor)
Brilinta
Func. class.: Platelet inhibitor
Chem. class.: ADP receptor antagonist
Pregnancy category C

ACTION: Reversibly binds to the platelet receptor, preventing platelet activation

Therapeutic outcome: Prevention of thromboembolism

USES: Arterial thromboembolism prophylaxis in acute coronary syndrome (ACS) (unstable angina, acute MI), including in patients undergoing percutaneous coronary intervention (PCI)

CONTRAINDICATIONS:
Hypersensitivity, severe hepatic disease, bleeding

Precautions: Abrupt discontinuation, breastfeeding, children, infants, neonates, GI bleeding, hepatic disease, pregnancy C

DOSAGE AND ROUTES
Adult: PO Loading dose 180 mg with aspirin (usually 325 mg PO); then, give 90 mg bid with aspirin 75-100 mg/day, do not give maintenance doses of aspirin >100 mg/day

Available forms: Tab 90 mg

Implementation
PO route
- May be taken without regard to food
- Store at room temperature, in original container in dry place
- Discontinue 5-7 days before surgery
- Ensure entire dose is given by flushing mortar, syringe, NG tube with 2 additional 50 ml of water

ADVERSE EFFECTS
CNS: Dizziness, fatigue, headache
CV: Atrial fibrillation, bradyarrhythmias, chest pain, hypertension, hypotension, syncope, ventricular pauses
GI: Diarrhea, nausea
HEMA: Fatal bleeding
MISC: Back pain, gynecomastia, hyperuricemia
RESP: Cough, dyspnea

BLACK BOX WARNING: Bleeding, intracranial bleeding

BLACK BOX WARNING: Coronary artery bypass graft (CABG) surgery

Pharmacokinetics
Absorption	36%
Distribution	Protein binding >99%
Metabolism	By CYP3A4
Excretion	26% (urine)
Half-life	7 hr; 9 hr metabolite

Pharmacodynamics
Onset	Unknown
Peak	1.5 hr (product), 2.5 hrs (metabolite)
Duration	≥8 hrs

INTERACTIONS
Individual drugs
Simvastatin, lovastatin: increased effect
Digoxin: change in effect

Drug classifications
Anticoagulants, NSAIDs, platelet inhibitors: increased bleeding risk
CYP3A4 inducers (carBAMazepine, dexamethasone, PHENobarbital, phenytoin, rifampin): decreased ticagrelor action
CYP3A4 inhibitors (atazanavir, clarithromycin, dalfopristin, delavirdine, indinavir, isoniazid, itraconazole, ketoconazole, lopinavir, nefazodone, nelfinavir, quinupristin, ritonavir, saquinavir, telithromycin, tipranavir, voriconazole): increased bleeding risk

Drug/lab
Serum creatinine: increased

NURSING CONSIDERATIONS
Assessment
- Thromboembolism: Monitor CBC differential with platelet count baseline and periodically during treatment

BLACK BOX WARNING: Assess for bleeding that may occur when aspirin is combined with this product, some bleeding can be fatal

- Abrupt discontinuation: Do not discontinue abruptly, may increase risk for MI, stent thrombosis, death

Patient/family education
- Teach patient to take only as prescribed, do not skip or double doses, if a dose is missed, take next dose at scheduled time
- Advise patient to notify prescriber of chills, fever, bruising, bleeding
- Teach patient not to use any Rx, OTC products, herbs without approval of prescriber; products with aspirin, NSAIDs may cause bleeding
- Instruct patient to notify all health care providers of product use
- Advise patient that product can be taken without regard to meals
- Teach patient it may take longer for bleeding to stop

Evaluation
Positive therapeutic outcome
- Prevention of thromboembolism

---

ticarcillin/clavulanate (Rx)
(tye-kar-sill′in)
Timentin
Func. class.: Extended-spectrum penicillin, beta lactamase inhibitor
Chem. class.: Antiinfective—broad-spectrum
Pregnancy category B

ACTION: Interferes with cell wall replication of susceptible organisms; osmotically unstable cell wall swells, bursts from osmotic pressure; clavulanate inhibits β-lactamase and protects against enzymatic degradation of ticarcillin

Therapeutic outcome: Resolution of infection

USES: Respiratory, soft tissue, urinary tract infections; bacterial septicemia; effective for gram-positive cocci *(Staphylococcus aureus, Streptococcus faecalis, Streptococcus pneumoniae)*, gram-negative cocci *(Neisseria gonorrhoeae)*, gram-positive bacilli *(Clostridium perfringens, Clostridium tetani)*, gram-negative bacilli *(Bacteroides, Fusobacterium nucleatum, Escherichia coli, Proteus mirabilis, Salmonella, Morganella morganii, Proteus rettgeri, Enterobacter, Pseudomonas aeruginosa, Serratia, Peptococcus, Peptostreptococcus, Eubacterium)*

CONTRAINDICATIONS:
Hypersensitivity to penicillins; neonates

Precautions: Pregnancy **B,** hypersensitivity to cephalosporins, renal disease

DOSAGE AND ROUTES
Systemic/urinary tract infections, moderate/severe infections
Adult ≥60 kg: **IV** INF 3.1 g q4-6hr
Adult <60 kg: **IV** INF 200-300 mg/kg/day q4-6hr
Child >60 kg: **IV** INF 3.1 g q4hr
Child <60 kg: **IV** INF 300 mg/kg/day q4hr
Full-term neonate/infant <3 mo (unlabeled):
IV 50 mg/kg q4hr

Mild/moderate infections
Child ≥60 kg: **IV** INF 3.1 g q6hr
Child <60 kg: **IV** INF 200 mg/kg/day q6hr
Full-term neonate/infant <3 mo (unlabeled):
IV 50 mg/kg q6hr

Renal dose
Adult: **IV** INF loading dose 3.1 g; CCr 60 ml/min 3.1 g q4hr; CCr 30-60 ml/min 2 g q4hr; CCr 10-30 ml/min 2 g q8hr; CCr <10 ml/min 2 g q12hr; CCr <10 ml/min with hepatic dysfunction 2 g q24hr

Available forms: Inj IM, **IV** 3 g ticarcillin and 0.1 g clavulanate; **IV** inf 3 g ticarcillin and 0.1 g clavulanate; powder for inj 3 g ticarcillin, 0.1 g clavulanate

Implementation
- Give product after C&S has been completed, give ≥q1hr before bactericidal antiinfectives, change IV site q48hr
- Have adrenalin, suction, tracheostomy set, endotracheal intubation equipment available
- Obtain scratch test results to assess allergy after securing order from prescriber; usually done when penicillin is only product of choice
- Store at room temperature, reconstituted sol for 12-24 hr or 3-7 days refrigerated

Intermittent IV infusion route
- Give **IV** after diluting 3.1 g or less/13 ml of sterile water or 0.9% NaCl (200 mg/ml), shake; may further dilute in 50-100 ml or more 0.9% NaCl, D₅W, or LR and run over ½ hr

Y-site compatibilities: Allopurinol, amifostine, amikacin, anidulafungin, atropine, aztreonam, bivalirudin, bumetanide, ceFAZolin, cefepime, cefotaxime, cefOXitin, cefTAZidime, ceftizoxime, cefTRIAXone, cefuroxime, chloramphenicol, cimetidine, clindamycin, cyclophosphamide, cycloSPORINE, dexamethasone, dexmedetomidine, digoxin, diltiazem, diphenhydrAMINE, DOCEtaxel, DOPamine, DOXOrubicin liposome, doxycycline, enalaprilat, EPINEPHrine, esmolol, etoposide phosphate, famotidine, fenoldopam, filgrastim, fluconazole, furosemide, gemcitabine, gentamicin, granisetron, heparin, hydrocortisone, HYDROmorphone, imipenem/cilastatin, insulin, isoproterenol, labetalol, levofloxacin, lidocaine, linezolid, LORazepam, melphalan, meperidine, methylPREDNISolone, metoclopramide, metoprolol, metroNIDAZOLE, milrinone, morphine, nitroglycerin, nitroprusside, norepinephrine, ondansetron, palonosetron, pantoprazole, PEMEtrexed, penicillin G potassium, perphenazine, phenylephrine, procainamide, propofol, propranolol, ranitidine,

---

Adverse effects: *italics* = common; **bold** = life-threatening

remifentanil, sargramostim, sodium bicarbonate, tacrolimus, teniposide, theophylline, thiotepa, tirofiban, tobramycin, vasopressin, verapamil, vinorelbine, voriconazole

Y-site incompatibilities: Acyclovir, amphotericin B cholesteryl sulfate, azithromycin, caspofungin, diazepam, DOBUTamine, drotrecogin, erythromycin, ganciclovir, haloperidol, hydrOXYzine, lansoprazole, phenytoin, promethazine, protamine, quinupristin/dalfopristin, trimethoprim/sulfamethoxazole

ADVERSE EFFECTS

CNS: Anxiety, **coma, seizures,** confusion, drowsiness
GI: *Nausea, vomiting, diarrhea,* increased AST, ALT, abdominal pain, glossitis, colitis, **pseudomembranous colitis,** hepatotoxicity
HEMA: Anemia, increased bleeding time, **bone marrow depression, granulocytopenia**
INTEG: Rash, urticaria, **toxic epidermal necrolysis,** pain at injection site
META: Hypokalemia, hypernatremia
SYST: Anaphylaxis, Stevens-Johnson syndrome, overgrowth of organisms

Pharmacokinetics	
Absorption	Completely absorbed (**IV**)
Distribution	Widely distributed, crosses blood-brain barrier
Metabolism	Liver
Excretion	Kidneys
Half-life	64-68 min

Pharmacodynamics	
	IV
Onset	Unknown
Peak	30-45 min
Duration	4 hr

INTERACTIONS
Individual drugs
Chloramphenicol: decreased antimicrobial effect of ticarcillin
Heparin: increased effect of heparin
Methotrexate: increased methotrexate level
Probenecid, sulfinpyrazone: increased ticarcillin concentration

Drug classifications
Aminoglycosides (**IV**): decreased antimicrobial effect of ticarcillin
Anticoagulants: increased bleeding
Contraceptives (oral): decreased effect of oral contraceptives

Erythromycins: decreased absorption
Macrolides, sulfonamides, tetracyclines: decreased ticarcillin effect

Drug/lab test
Increased: LFTs, sodium, eosinophils, INR, bleeding time, uric acid, bilirubin, BUN, creatinine, alk phos, LDH
Decreased: Hgb, potassium, platelets, WBC, granulocytes
False positive: urine glucose, urine protein, Coombs' test

NURSING CONSIDERATIONS
Assessment
• Infection: WBC, wound, temperature, sputum, urine, baseline and periodically
• **Pseudomembranous colitis:** assess for diarrhea, abdominal pain, fever, fatigue, anorexia; possible anemia, elevated WBC, low serum albumin; stop product and usually give either vancomycin or IV metroNIDAZOLE
• Monitor liver function tests: AST, ALT
• Monitor blood tests: WBC, RBC, Hgb, Hct, bleeding time, platelets, baseline and periodically
• Monitor renal function tests; sodium, potassium
• Assess bowel pattern before, during treatment
• Assess skin eruptions after administration of penicillin to 1 wk after discontinuing product
⚠ **Assess for anaphylaxis: wheezing, rash, laryngeal edema; have emergency equipment nearby**
• **Serious skin reactions:** Stevens-Johnson syndrome, toxic epidermal necrolysis

Patient/family education
• Advise patient that C&S may be performed after completed course of medication
• Instruct patient to report sore throat, fever, fatigue (may indicate superinfection)
• Advise patient to carry/wear emergency ID if allergic to penicillins
• Advise patient to use alternative birth control methods instead of hormonal
• Advise patient to report persistent diarrhea with blood, pus, mucus, or fever

Evaluation
Positive therapeutic outcome
• Absence of fever, purulent drainage, redness, inflammation

TREATMENT OF OVERDOSE:
Withdraw product, maintain airway, administer EPINEPHrine, aminophylline, O₂, **IV** corticosteroids for anaphylaxis

---

⚠ Nurse Alert ⬙ Key NCLEX® Drug

ticlopidine (Rx)

(tye-cloe'pi-deen)
Func. class.: Platelet aggregation inhibitor
Chem. class.: Thienopyridine compound
Pregnancy category B

ACTION: Irreversible inhibition of platelet aggregation through antagonism of ADP

Therapeutic outcome: Decreased stroke by decreasing platelet aggregation

USES: Reducing the risk of stroke in high-risk patients

Unlabeled uses: Intermittent claudication, chronic arterial occlusion, subarachnoid hemorrhage, uremic patients with AV shunts/fistulas, open heart surgery, coronary artery bypass grafts, primary glomerulonephritis, diabetic neuropathy

CONTRAINDICATIONS:
Hypersensitivity, severe liver disease, active bleeding, coagulopathy

> **BLACK BOX WARNING:** Agranulocytosis, neutropenia, thrombocytopenia, thrombotic thrombocytopenic purpura (TTP)

Precautions: Pregnancy **B**, breastfeeding, children, geriatric, past liver disease, renal disease, increased bleeding risk, peptic ulcer disease, surgery

> **BLACK BOX WARNING:** Anemia, hematological disease

DOSAGE AND ROUTES
Adult: PO 250 mg bid with food

Available forms: Tabs 250 mg

Implementation
• Give with food or after eating to decrease GI effects; may use methylPREDNISolone **IV** 20 mg to provide normal bleeding time in 2 hr

ADVERSE EFFECTS
CNS: Dizziness, headache, weakness
EENT: Tinnitus, epistaxis
GI: Nausea, vomiting, diarrhea, GI discomfort, **cholestatic jaundice, hepatitis,** increased cholesterol LDL, VLDL, triglycerides
GU: Hematuria
HEMA: **Bleeding (epistaxis, hematuria, conjunctival hemorrhage, GI bleeding),**
agranulocytosis, neutropenia, thrombocytopenia, thrombotic thrombocytopenic purpura
INTEG: Rash, pruritus
META: Hypercholesterolemia, hypertriglyceridemia

Pharmacokinetics

Absorption	Well absorbed
Distribution	Unknown
Metabolism	Liver, extensively; 98% protein binding
Excretion	Kidneys, unchanged product
Half-life	Increased with repeat dosing; 4-5 days (multiple doses)

Pharmacodynamics

Onset	Unknown
Peak	1-3 hr
Duration	Unknown

INTERACTIONS
Individual drugs
Abciximab, aspirin, eptifibatide, tirofiban: increased bleeding tendencies
Ambrisenten, fosphenytoin, phenytoin, theophylline: increased levels of each specific drug
Cimetidine: increased effects of ticlopidine
CycloSPORINE: decreased plasma levels of cycloSPORINE
Digoxin: decreased plasma levels of digoxin

Drug classifications
Antacids: decreased plasma levels of ticlopidine
Anticoagulants, NSAIDs, salicylates, SSRIs, thrombin inhibitors, thrombolytics: increased bleeding risk
CYP2C19, CYP2DC substrates: increased levels of each specific drug

Drug/herb
Ginger, ginkgo, garlic, feverfew, horse chestnut, green tea: increased bleeding risk

NURSING CONSIDERATIONS
Assessment
• Monitor liver function tests: AST, ALT, bilirubin, creatinine if patient is on long-term therapy (4 mo or more)

T

BLACK BOX WARNING: Blood dyscrasias, bone marrow depression, do not use in those with a history of these conditions; monitor blood tests: CBC, Hct, Hgb, pro-time if patient is on long-term therapy; CBC q2wk × 3 mo therapy; thrombocytopenia, neutropenia may occur

---

• Monitor bleeding time baseline and throughout therapy, levels may be 2-5 × normal limit

Patient/family education
• Advise patient that blood studies are necessary during treatment
• Advise patient to report any unusual bleeding to prescriber
• Instruct patient to take with food or just after eating to minimize GI discomfort, not to double missed dose
• Caution patient to report side effects such as diarrhea, skin rashes, subcutaneous bleeding, signs of cholestasis (yellow skin and sclera, dark urine, light-colored stools)
• Advise patient that product should be discontinued 10-14 days before surgery
• Advise there are many drug and herb interactions; to avoid all OTC products unless approved by prescriber

Evaluation
Positive therapeutic outcome
• Absence of stroke

---

tigecycline (Rx)
(tye-ge-sye′kleen)
Tygacil
Func. class.: Broad-spectrum antiinfective
Chem. class.: Glycylcyclines
Pregnancy category D

ACTION: Inhibits protein synthesis and phosphorylation in microorganisms; bacteriostatic, structurally similar to the tetracyclines

Therapeutic outcome: Resolution of infection

USES: Complicated skin/skin structure infections: *Escherichia coli, Enterococcus faecalis* (vancomycin-susceptible only), *Staphylococcus aureus, Streptococcus agalactiae, S. anginosus* group, *S. pyogenes, Bacteroides fragilis;* complicated intraabdominal infections (*Citrobacter freundii*), *Enterobacter cloacae, Escherichia coli, Klebsiella oxytoca, K. pneumoniae, E. faecalis* (vancomycin-susceptible only), *S. aureus* (methicillin-susceptible only),

S. anginosus group, *B. fragilis, Bacteroides thetaiotaomicron, B. uniformis, B. vulgatus, Clostridium perfringens, Peptostreptococcus micros,* community-acquired pneumonia

CONTRAINDICATIONS:
Pregnancy **D**, breastfeeding, children <18 yr, hypersensitivity to tigecycline

Precautions: Renal/hepatic disease, hypersensitivity to tetracyclines, ventricular-associated hospital-acquired pneumonias

DOSAGE AND ROUTES
Adult: IV 100 mg, then 50 mg q12hr, **IV INF** is given over 30 min to 60 min q12hr; given for 5-14 days depending on infection

Hepatic dose (Child-Pugh C)
Adult: IV 100 mg, then 25 mg q12hr

Available forms: Powder for inj, lyophilized 50 mg

Implementation
• Tigecycline allergy test before using, obtain C&S, do not begin treatment before results

Intermittent IV infusion route
• Reconstitute each vial with 5.3 ml of 0.9% NaCl, or D₅W (10 mg/ml); swirl to dissolve; immediately withdraw 5 ml of the reconstituted sol and add to a 100-ml **IV** bag for inf (1 mg/ml); may be yellow or orange, if not, sol should be discarded; do not give if particulate matter is present, use a dedicated IV line or Y-site, flush with NS before and after use, give over ½ hr
• Store in tight, light-resistant container at room temperature, diluted sol at room temp for up to 24 hr, 6 hr in vial, and remaining time in IV bag, 48 hr refrigerated

Y-site compatibilities: Acyclovir, alfentanil, allopurinol, amifostine, amikacin, aminocaproic acid, aminophylline, amphotericin B liposome, ampicillin, ampicillin/sulbactam, argatroban, azithromycin, aztreonam, bivalirudin, bumetanide, buprenorphine, butorphanol, calcium chloride/gluconate, CARBOplatin, carmustine, caspofungin, ceFAZolin, cefepime, cefotaxime, cefoTEtan, cefOXitin, cefTAZidime, ceftizoxime, cefTRIAXone, cefuroxime, cimetidine, ciprofloxacin, cisatracurium, CISplatin, clindamycin, cyclophosphamide, cycloSPORINE, cytarabine, dacarbazine, DACTINomycin, DAPTOmycin, DAUNOrubicin hydrochloride, dexamethasone, dexmedetomidine, dexrazoxane, digoxin, diltiazem, diphenhydrAMINE, DOBUTamine, DOCEtaxel, dolasetron, DOPamine, doripenem, DOXOrubicin hydrochloride, DOXOrubicin

---

liposome, droperidol, enalaprilat, EPINEPHrine, eptifibatide, ertapenem, erythromycin, esmolol, etoposide, etoposide phosphate, famotidine, fenoldopam, fentaNYL, fluconazole, fludarabine, fluorouracil, foscarnet, fosphenytoin, furosemide, ganciclovir, gemcitabine, gentamicin, glycopyrrolate, granisetron, haloperidol, heparin, hydrocortisone, HYDROmorphone, ifosfamide, imipenem/cilastatin, insulin, irinotecan, isoproterenol, ketorolac, labetalol, lansoprazole, lepirudin, leucovorin, levofloxacin, lidocaine, linezolid, LORazepam, magnesium sulfate, mannitol, mechlorethamine, melphalan, meperidine, meropenem, mesna, methohexital, methotrexate, methyldopa, metoclopramide, metoprolol, metroNIDAZOLE, midazolam, milrinone, mitoMYcin, mitoXANtrone, morphine, moxifloxacin, mycophenolate, nafcillin, nalbuphine, naloxone, nesiritide, nitroglycerin, nitroprusside, norepinephrine, octreotide, ondansetron, oxaliplatin, oxytocin, PACLitaxel, palonosetron, pamidronate, pancuronium, pantoprazole, PEMEtrexed, pentamidine, pentazocine, PENTobarbital, PHENobarbital, phenylephrine, piperacillin/tazobactam, potassium acetate/chloride/phosphate, procainamide, prochlorperazine, promethazine, propofol, propranolol, ranitidine, remifentanil, rocuronium, sodium acetate/bicarbonate/phosphate, streptozocin, succinylcholine, SUFentanil, tacrolimus, teniposide, theophylline, thiopental, thiotepa, ticarcillin/clavulanate, tirofiban, tobramycin, topotecan, trimethoprim/sulfamethoxazole, vancomycin, vasopressin, vecuronium, vinBLAStine, vinCRIStine, vinorelbine, zidovudine, zoledronic acid

Y-site incompatibilities: Amiodarone, amphotericin B colloidal, bleomycin, chloramphenicol, chlorproMAZINE, dantrolene, DAUNOrubicin liposome, diazepam, epirubicin, hydrALAZINE, IDArubicin, niCARdipine, phenytoin, quinapristin/dalfopristin, verapamil

ADVERSE EFFECTS
CNS: Headache, dizziness, insomnia
CV: Hypo/hypertension, phlebitis
EENT: Tooth discoloration
GI: *Nausea, vomiting, diarrhea,* anorexia, constipation, dyspepsia, **hepatotoxicity, hepatic failure, pseudomembranous colitis**
HEMA: **Anemia, leukocytosis, thrombocytopenia**
INTEG: *Rash,* pruritus, sweating, photosensitivity
META: Increased ALT, AST, BUN, lactic acid, alkaline phosphatase, amylase, hyperglycemia, hypokalemia, hypoproteinemia, bilirubinemia

MISC: Back pain, fever, abnormal healing, abdominal pain, abscess, asthenia, infection, pain, peripheral edema, local reactions
RESP: Cough, dyspnea
SYST: **Anaphylaxis**

Pharmacokinetics

Absorption	Unknown
Distribution	Protein binding 71%-89%
Metabolism	Not extensively
Excretion	22% unchanged, urine; primarily biliarily excreted
Half-life	Terminal 42 hr

Pharmacodynamics
Unknown

INTERACTIONS
Individual drugs
Warfarin: increased effect of tigecycline

Drug classifications
Oral contraceptives: decreased effect of tigecycline

Drug/lab test
Increased: amylase, LFTs, alk phos, BUN, creatinine, LDH, WBC, INR, PTT, PT
Decreased: potassium, calcium, sodium, Hgb/Hct, platelets

NURSING CONSIDERATIONS
Assessment
• **Pseudomembranous colitis:** assess for diarrhea, abdominal pain, fever, fatigue, anorexia; possible anemia, elevated WBC, low serum albumin; stop product and usually give either vancomycin or IV metroNIDAZOLE
• Assess for signs of anemia: Hct, Hgb, fatigue
• Monitor blood tests: PT, CBC, AST, ALT, BUN creatinine
• **Assess for allergic reactions:** rash, itching, pruritus, angioedema
⚠ **Serious allergic skin reactions: assess for Stevens-Johnson syndrome, anaphylaxis**
• Assess for nausea, vomiting, diarrhea; administer antiemetic, antacids as ordered
• **Assess for overgrowth of infection:** fever, malaise, redness, pain, swelling, drainage, perineal itching, diarrhea, changes in cough or sputum
⚠ **Toxicity: assess for pseudotumor cerebri, photosensitivity, anti-anabolic actions (azotemia, BUN, hypophosphatemia, metabolic acidosis): tigecycline is structurally similar to tetracycline**

T

⚠ Assess for pancreatitis, hyperamylasemia: may be fatal; if these occur, discontinue; improvement usually occurs after product is discontinued

Patient/family education
• Teach patient to avoid sun exposure; sunscreen does not seem to decrease photosensitivity
• Teach patient to avoid pregnancy while taking this product; fetal harm may occur; to avoid breastfeeding
• Teach patient to report burning, pain at inj site

Evaluation
Positive therapeutic outcome
• Decreased temp, absence of lesions, negative C&S

---

timolol (Rx)
(tye'moe-lole)
Apo-Timol ✦, Novo-Timol ✦
Func. class.: Antihypertensive; antiglaucoma
Chem. class.: Nonselective β-blocker
Pregnancy category C   ✴

ACTION: Competitively blocks stimulation of β-adrenergic receptor within vascular smooth muscle (decreases rate of SA node discharge, increases recovery time), slows conduction of AV node, decreases heart rate, which decreases O_2 consumption in myocardium; also decreases renin-aldosterone-angiotensin system; at high doses inhibits $β_2$ receptors in bronchial system

Therapeutic outcome: Decreased B/P, decreased arrhythmias, absence of death from MI, decreased aqueous humor in the eye, absence of migraine headaches

USES: Mild to moderate hypertension, migraine prophylaxis, to decrease mortality following MI

Unlabeled uses: Tremors, angina pectoris

CONTRAINDICATIONS:
Hypersensitivity to β-blockers, cardiogenic shock, heart block (2nd or 3rd degree), sinus bradycardia, CHF, cardiac failure, severe COPD, asthma

Precautions: Pregnancy **C,** breastfeeding, major surgery, diabetes mellitus, thyroid/renal/hepatic disease, COPD, well-compensated heart failure, nonallergic bronchospasm, peripheral vascular disease

> **BLACK BOX WARNING:** Abrupt discontinuation

DOSAGE AND ROUTES
Hypertension
Adult: PO 10 mg bid, or 20 mg/day, may increase by 10 mg q7day, max 60 mg/day
Geriatric: PO Initiate dose cautiously

Myocardial infarction
Adult: 10 mg bid beginning 1-4 wk after MI for ≥2 yr

Glaucoma
Adult: Ophth 1 gtt daily or bid
Child: Ophth 1 gtt daily or bid (0.25% SOL only)

Migraine headache prevention
Adult: PO 10 mg bid, or 20 mg/day; may increase to 30 mg/day, 20 mg in AM, 10 mg in PM; discontinue if not effective after 8 wk

Available forms: Tabs 5, 10, 20 mg

Implementation
• Given before meals, at bedtime; tab may be crushed or swallowed whole; give with food to prevent GI upset; reduce dosage in renal dysfunction
• Store at room temp; do not freeze

ADVERSE EFFECTS
CNS: *Insomnia, dizziness,* hallucinations, anxiety, fatigue, depression, headache
CV: Hypotension, bradycardia, **CHF,** edema, chest pain, claudication, angina, AV block, ventricular dysrhythmias
EENT: *Vision changes,* sore throat, *double vision,* dry burning eyes
GI: *Nausea,* vomiting, **ischemic colitis,** diarrhea, *abdominal pain,* **mesenteric arterial thrombosis,** flatulence, constipation
GU: Impotence, urinary frequency
HEMA: Agranulocytosis, thrombocytopenia, purpura
INTEG: Rash, alopecia, pruritus, fever
META: Hypoglycemia
MUSC: *Joint pain, muscle pain*
RESP: Bronchospasm, dyspnea, cough, crackles, nasal stuffiness

---

Pharmacokinetics

Absorption	Well absorbed (PO), minimally absorbed (ophth)
Distribution	Protein binding <10%
Metabolism	Liver, extensively
Excretion	Breast milk
Half-life	3 hr

Pharmacodynamics

	PO
Onset	Unknown
Peak	2-4 hr
Duration	12-24 hr

INTERACTIONS

Individual drugs

Alcohol: increased hypotension, bradycardia (large amounts)

HydrALAZINE, methyldopa, prazosin, reserpine: increased hypotension, bradycardia

Insulin: decreased hypoglycemia

Thyroid hormones: decreased antihypertensive effect

Drug classifications

Anticholinergics, nitrates: increased hypotension, increased bradycardia

β_2-Adrenergic agonists: increased β-blocking effect

Calcium channel blockers: increased effects of calcium channel blockers

NSAIDs, salicylates, sympathomimetics: decreased antihypertensive effect

Sulfonylureas: decreased hypoglycemic effect

Theophyllines: decreased bronchodilatation

Drug/lab test

Increased: renal, liver function tests, uric acid

Interference: glucose, insulin tolerance test

NURSING CONSIDERATIONS

Assessment

BLACK BOX WARNING: Abrupt discontinuation: may result in myocardial ischemia, MI, severe hypotension, ventricular dysrhythmias in those with preexisting cardiovascular disease

• Assess for headaches: location, severity, duration, frequency baseline, throughout treatment

• Monitor B/P during beginning treatment, periodically thereafter; pulse q4hr; note rate, rhythm, quality: apical/radial pulse before administration; notify prescriber of any significant changes (pulse <50 bpm)

• Check baselines in renal, liver function tests before therapy begins

• Assess for edema in feet, legs daily, monitor I&O ratio, daily weight; check for jugular vein distention, crackles bilaterally, dyspnea (CHF)

• Monitor skin turgor, dryness of mucous membranes for hydration status, especially geriatric

Patient/family education

BLACK BOX WARNING: Teach patient not to discontinue product abruptly; taper over 2 wk; may cause precipitate angina if stopped abruptly

• Advise patient not to use OTC products containing α-adrenergic stimulants (nasal decongestants, cold preparations); to avoid alcohol, smoking; to limit sodium intake as prescribed

• Teach patient how to take pulse and B/P at home; advise patient when to notify prescriber

• Instruct patient to comply with weight control, dietary adjustments, modified exercise program

• Advise patient to carry/wear emergency ID to identify product being taken, any allergies; tell patient product controls symptoms but does not cure

• Caution patient to avoid hazardous activities if dizziness, drowsiness are present

• Teach patient to report symptoms of CHF; difficult breathing, especially on exertion or when lying down; night cough; swelling of extremities or bradycardia; dizziness; confusion; depression; fever

• Teach patient to take product as prescribed, not to double dose, skip doses; take any missed doses as soon as remembered if at least 4 hr until next dose

• Product masks hypoglycemia; monitor blood sugar

Evaluation

Positive therapeutic outcome

• Decreased B/P in hypertension (after 1-2 wk)
• Absence of dysrhythmias

TREATMENT OF OVERDOSE:

Lavage, IV atropine for bradycardia, IV theophylline for bronchospasm, digoxin, O_2, diuretic for cardiac failure, hemodialysis, IV glucose for hyperglycemia, IV diazepam (or phenytoin) for seizures

timolol ophthalmic
See Appendix B

tinidazole (Rx)
(tye-ni′da-zole)
Tindamax
Func. class.: Antiprotozoal
Chem. class.: Nitroimidazole derivative
Pregnancy category C

ACTION: Interferes with DNA/RNA synthesis in protozoa

Therapeutic outcome: Decrease in infection

USES: Amebiasis, giardiasis, trichomoniasis

CONTRAINDICATIONS:
Breastfeeding, hypersensitivity to this product or nitroimidazole derivative, pregnancy

Precautions: Pregnancy **C**, children, geriatric, hepatic disease, CNS depression, blood dyscrasias, candidiasis, seizures, viral infection, alcoholism

> **BLACK BOX WARNING:** Secondary malignancy

DOSAGE AND ROUTES
Intestinal amebiasis
Adult: PO 2 g/day × 3 days
Adolescent/child ≥3 yr: PO 50 mg/kg/day × 3 days, max 2 g/day

Amebic involvement (liver)
Adult: PO 2 g/day × 3-5 days
Child ≥3 yr: PO 50 mg/kg/day × 3-5 days, max 2 g

Giardiasis
Adult: PO 2 g as a single dose
Child ≥3 yr: PO 50 mg/kg as a single dose, max 2 g

Trichomoniasis
Adult: PO 2 g as a single dose

Bacterial vaginosis
Adult (not pregnant): PO 2 g/day × 2 days with food or 1 g/day × 5 days with food

Available forms: Tabs 250, 500 mg

Implementation
• Administer to those >3 yr old
• Give with food; tabs can be crushed and mixed with artificial cherry syrup

ADVERSE EFFECTS
CNS: *Dizziness, headache,* **seizures,** *peripheral neuropathy,* malaise, fatigue

GI: *Nausea, vomiting,* anorexia, increased AST and ALT, constipation, abdominal pain, indigestion, altered taste
HEMA: Leukopenia, neutropenia
INTEG: Pruritus, urticaria, *rash,* oral candidiasis
SYST: Angioedema, cramping

Pharmacokinetics

Absorption	Unknown
Distribution	Crosses blood-brain barrier
Metabolism	Extensively in the liver
Excretion	Unchanged (20%-25%) in urine, (12%) feces
Half-life	12-14 hr

Pharmacodynamics

Unknown

INTERACTIONS
Individual drugs
Do not use within 2 wk of taking disulfiram
Cholestyramine, oxytetracycline: decreased action of tinidazole
CycloSPORINE, fluorouracil, lithium, tacrolimus: increased action

Drug classifications
Anticoagulants, hydantoins: increased action
CYP3A4 inducers (phenobarbital, phenytoin, rifampin): decreased action of tinidazole
CYP3A4 inhibitors (cimetidine, ketoconazole): increased action of tinidazole

Drug/herb
St. John's wort: increased or decreased tinidazole level

Drug/lab test
Increase: triglycerides, LDH, AST/ALT, glucose
Decrease: WBCs

NURSING CONSIDERATIONS
Assessment
• Giardiasis: obtain 3 stool samples several days apart beginning q3-4wk after treatment
• **Assess for amebic liver abscess:** monitor CBC, ESR, amebic gel diffusion test, ultrasound, total and differential leukocyte count
• Assess for signs of infection, anemia
• Assess bowel pattern before, during treatment

> **BLACK BOX WARNING: Secondary malignancy:** Avoid unnecessary use

Patient/family education
• Instruct patient to take with food to increase plasma concentrations, minimize epigastric

---

⚠ Nurse Alert   ✳ Key NCLEX® Drug

distress and other GI effects; not to use alcoholic beverages during or for 3 days afterward
• Advise patient that in cases of trichomoniasis, both partners should be treated at the same time
• Teach patient to avoid alcohol, may cause disulfiram reaction
• Teach patient to avoid doing hazardous activities until reaction is known
• Teach patient that product causes taste change
• Teach patient not to use OTC, Rx or herbal products unless approved by prescriber

Evaluation
Positive therapeutic outcome
• Decrease in infection as evidenced by negative culture

⚠ HIGH ALERT

tinzaparin (Rx)
(tin-zay-par′in)
Innohep
Func. class.: Anticoagulant
Chem. class.: Unfractionated porcine heparin
Pregnancy category C

ACTION: Inhibits the effect of factor Xa, thrombin IIa

Therapeutic outcome: Resolution of DVT

USES: Treatment of DVT, pulmonary emboli after abdominal, knee, hip surgery or knee, hip replacement, cerebral thromboembolism, thrombosis prophylaxis

Unlabeled uses: DVT prophylaxis

CONTRAINDICATIONS:
Hypersensitivity to this product, heparin, pork or benzyl alcohol, sulfites; hemophilia, leukemia with bleeding, peptic ulcer disease, thrombocytopenic purpura, heparin-induced thrombocytopenia

Precautions: Pregnancy C, breastfeeding, children, geriatric, alcoholism, severe renal/hepatic disease, blood dyscrasias, severe uncontrolled hypertension, subacute bacterial endocarditis, acute nephritis, elderly >70 yr (renal disease with DVT/PE)

BLACK BOX WARNING: Spinal/epidural anesthesia, lumbar puncture

DOSAGE AND ROUTES
Treatment of deep vein thrombosis
Adult: SUBCUT 175 anti-Xa international units/kg daily ≥6 days and until adequate anticoagulation with warfarin (INR ≥2 for 2 consecutive days)
Adolescent/child 10-16 yr: SUBCUT 275 anti-Xa international units/kg/day, adjust dose to maintain anti-Xa 0.5-1 international units/ml drawn 4 hr after inj
Child 5-10 yr: SUBCUT 200 anti-Xa international units/kg/day, adjust dose to maintain anti-Xa of 0.5-1 international units drawn 4 hr after injection

Prophylaxis of DVT/thromboembolism/PE (unlabeled)
Adult: 3500 anti-Xa units (50 anti-Xa units/kg) daily beginning 1-2 hr before surgery and continued for 5-10 days

Prophylaxis of deep vein thrombosis in orthopedic procedures (unlabeled)
Adult: 75 anti-Xa units/kg/day started 12-24 hr after surgery

Available forms: Inj 20,000 international units/ml

Implementation
• Give only after screening patient for bleeding disorders
• Give SUBCUT only; do not give IM/IV
• Give for 6 days and until warfarin has been given to result in adequate coagulation
• Give SUBCUT to recumbent patient; rotate inj sites (left/right anterolateral, left/right posterolateral abdominal wall)
• Insert whole length of needle into skin fold held with thumb and forefinger
⚠ Use only this product when ordered; not interchangeable with heparin (unfractionated) or LMWHs
• Give at same time each day to maintain steady blood levels
• Do not massage area or aspirate when giving SUBCUT inj
• Alternate injection sites
• For excessive bruising at injection site, may use ice at site before subcut injection
• Do not mix with other products or inf fluids
• Store at 77° F (25° C); do not freeze

ADVERSE EFFECTS
CNS: Fever, confusion, dizziness, insomnia
CV: Angina, dysrhythmias, peripheral edema, tachycardia, hypo/hypertension

GI: Nausea, constipation, flatulence, dyspepsia, **hepatitis**
GU: UTI, hematuria, urinary retention, dysuria
HEMA: Hemorrhage, **anemia, thrombocytopenia,** bleeding
INTEG: Ecchymosis, inj site reaction
MISC: Headache, chest pain, hypersensitivity
SYST: Stevens-Johnson syndrome

Pharmacokinetics

Absorption	Unknown
Distribution	Unknown
Metabolism	Unknown
Excretion	Unknown
Half-life	3-4 hr

Pharmacodynamics

Onset	Unknown
Peak	4 hr (max antithrombin activity)
Duration	Unknown

INTERACTIONS

Individual drug
Clopidogrel, ticlopidine: increased tinzaparin action

Drug classifications
Anticoagulants (oral), NSAIDs, platelet inhibitors, salicylates, thrombolytics: increased tinzaparin action

Drug/herb
Feverfew, garlic, ginger, ginkgo, horse chestnut, green tea: increased bleeding risk

NURSING CONSIDERATIONS

Assessment

> **BLACK BOX WARNING:** Spinal/epidermal anesthesia, lumbar puncture: monitor neurological impairment; if impairment occurs, urgent treatment is needed

• Monitor blood tests (Hct, platelets, occult blood in stools), anti-Xa; thrombocytopenia may occur
• **Assess for bleeding** gums, petechiae, ecchymosis, black tarry stools, hematuria

Patient/family education
• Instruct patient to report any signs of bleeding: gums, under skin, urine, stools

Evaluation

Positive therapeutic outcome
• Resolution of deep vein thrombosis

TREATMENT OF OVERDOSE:
Protamine 1 mg/100 anti-Xa international units of tinzaparin

tioconazole vaginal antifungal
See Appendix B

tiotropium (Rx)
(ty-oh'tro-pee-um)
Spiriva, HandiHaler
Func. class.: Anticholinergic, bronchodilator
Chem. class.: Synthetic quaternary ammonium compound
Pregnancy category C

Do not confuse:
Spiriva/Inspra

ACTION: Inhibits interaction of acetylcholine at receptor sites on the bronchial smooth muscle, resulting in decreased cGMP and bronchodilatation

Therapeutic outcome: Improved breathing

USES: COPD, for long-term treatment, once daily maintenance of bronchospasm, associated with COPD including chronic bronchitis and emphysema

CONTRAINDICATIONS:
Hypersensitivity to this product, atropine, or its derivatives

Precautions: Pregnancy **C**, breastfeeding, children, geriatric, closed-angle glaucoma, prostatic hypertrophy, bladder neck obstruction, renal disease

DOSAGE AND ROUTES
Adult: INH content of 1 cap/day (18 mcg) using HandiHaler inhalation device

Available forms: Powder for inhalation 18 mcg in blister packs containing 6 caps with inhaler; 30 caps with inhaler

Implementation
Inhalation route
• **Caps are for INH only; do not swallow**
• Immediately before administration, peel back foil until cap is visible (until "stop" line); open dust cap of HandiHaler by pulling upward, then open mouthpiece

---

• Place cap in center chamber; firmly close mouthpiece until it clicks, leaving dust cap open
• Hold HandiHaler with mouthpiece upward; press button in once, completely, and release; this allows medication to be released
• Breathe out completely; do not breathe into mouthpiece at any time
• Raise device to mouth and close lips tightly around mouthpiece
• With head upright, breathe in slowly/deeply, but allowing the cap to vibrate; breathe until lungs fill; hold breath and remove mouthpiece; resume normal breathing
• Repeat
• Remove used capsule and discard; close the mouthpiece and dust cap; store

ADVERSE EFFECTS

CNS: Depression, paresthesia
CV: Chest pain, increased heart rate
EENT: Dry mouth, blurred vision, glaucoma
GI: *Vomiting,* abdominal pain, constipation, dyspepsia
GU: Urinary difficulty, urinary retention, UTI
INTEG: Rash, **angioedema**
MISC: Candidiasis, flu-like syndrome, herpes zoster, infections, angina pectoris
MS: Arthritis, myalgic leg/skeletal pain
RESP: *Cough, worsening of symptoms,* sinusitis, URI, epistaxis, pharyngitis

Pharmacokinetics

Absorption	Unknown
Distribution	Does not cross blood-brain barrier
Metabolism	Very little metabolized in the liver
Excretion	Excreted in urine, 72% protein binding
Half-life	5-6 days in animals

Pharmacodynamics

Unknown

INTERACTIONS

Drug classifications
Anticholinergics: avoid use with other anticholinergics

Drug/lab test
Increased: cholesterol, glucose

NURSING CONSIDERATIONS

Assessment
• For tolerance over long-term therapy; dose may have to be increased or changed

• **Respiratory status:** assess for dyspnea, rate, breath sounds before and during treatment; pulmonary function tests baseline and periodically; upper respiratory infection, cough, sinusitis

Patient/family education
• Teach patient how to use HandiHaler
• Teach patient signs of closed-angle glaucoma (eye pain, blurred vision, visual halos)
• Advise patient that product is used for long-term maintenance, not for immediate relief of breathing problems
• Caution patient to avoid getting the powder in the eyes; may cause blurred vision and pupil dilatation
• Teach patient to report immediately blurred vision, eye pain, halos
• Teach patient to keep caps in sealed blisters before use, store at room temperature

Evaluation
Positive therapeutic outcome
• Ability to breathe easier

---

tipranavir (Rx)
(ti-pran´a-veer)
Aptivus
Func. class.: Antiretroviral
Chem. class.: Protease inhibitor
Pregnancy category C

ACTION: Inhibits HIV protease; this prevents the maturation of virus

Therapeutic outcome: Prevention of worsening of HIV

USES: HIV in combination with other antiretrovirals

CONTRAINDICATIONS:
Hypersensitivity

BLACK BOX WARNING: Hepatic disease (Child-Pugh B to C)

Precautions: Pregnancy **C**, breastfeeding, children, renal disease, history of renal stones, sulfa allergy, hemophilia, diabetes mellitus, pancreatitis, alcoholism, immune reconstitution syndrome, surgery, trauma, infection

BLACK BOX WARNING: Intracranial bleeding, hepatitis

Adverse effects: *italics* = common; **bold** = life-threatening

DOSAGE AND ROUTES

Reduce dosage in mild or moderate hepatic impairment and ketoconazole coadministration
Adult: PO 500 mg coadministered with ritonavir 200 mg bid with food
Adolescent and child ≥2 yr: PO 14 mg/kg given with ritonavir 6 mg/kg bid or 375 mg/m² given with ritonavir 150 mg/m² bid; max 500 mg with ritonavir 200 mg bid

Available forms: Caps 250 mg; oral sol 100 mg/ml

Implementation

• Swallow cap whole; do not break, crush, or chew
• Store caps in refrigerator before use; after opening, store at room temp; use within 60 days
• Give after meals
• Give in equal intervals around the clock to maintain blood levels

ADVERSE EFFECTS

CNS: *Headache, insomnia,* dizziness, somnolence, fatigue, *fever,* **intracranial bleeding**
GI: *Diarrhea, abdominal pain, nausea, vomiting,* anorexia, dry mouth, **hepatitis B or C, fatalities when given with ritonavir, pancreatitis**
GU: Nephrolithiasis
INTEG: *Rash,* urticaria, lipodystrophy, serious rash
MS: Pain
OTHER: Asthenia, **insulin-resistant hyperglycemia,** *hyperlipidemia,* **ketoacidosis**

Pharmacokinetics

Absorption	Unknown
Distribution	Protein binding, 99.9%, steady state 7-10 days
Metabolism	CYP3A4
Excretion	80% feces
Half-life	Terminal 6 hr

Pharmacodynamics

Onset	Unknown
Peak	3 hr
Duration	Unknown

INTERACTIONS

Individual drugs

⚠ **Amiodarone, astemizole, cisapride, flecainide, midazolam, pimozide, propafenone, quiNIDine, rifabutin, rifampin, terfenadine, triazolam: life-threatening dysrhythmias**
Clarithromycin, zidovudine: increased levels of both products

Delavirdine, itraconazole, ketoconazole: increased tipranavir levels
Efavirenz, fluconazole, nevirapine: decreased tipranavir levels
Lovastatin, simvastatin: increased myopathy, rhabdomyolysis

Drug classifications

⚠ **Ergots: life-threatening dysrhythmias**
Oral contraceptives: increased levels of tipranavir
Rifamycins: decreased tipranavir levels

Drug/herb

St. John's wort: decreased tipranavir levels; avoid concurrent use

Drug/food

Grapefruit juice, high-fat, high-protein foods: decreased tipranavir absorption

Drug/lab test

Increased: AST, ALT, cholesterol, blood glucose, amylase, lipase, triglycerides

NURSING CONSIDERATIONS

Assessment

• Assess for signs of infection, anemia, the presence of other STDs

> **BLACK BOX WARNING:** Assess for hepatic studies: ALT, AST; total bilirubin, amylase, all may be elevated, discontinue in those with hepatic insufficiency or hepatitis or AST/ALT 10× upper limit or AST/ALT 5-10× ULN and total bilirubin 2.5× ULN

• **HIV:** Monitor viral load, CD4, plasma HIV RNA, serum cholesterol/triglycerides during treatment
• Monitor bowel pattern before, during treatment; if severe abdominal pain with bleeding occurs, product should be discontinued; monitor hydration
• **Immune reconstitution syndrome:** has been reported with combination antiretroviral therapy; patients may develop pain (MAC, CMV, PcP, TB) and autoimmune disease months after treatment
• **Intercranial bleeding:** more common in those with trauma or surgery, or those taking antiplatelets or anticoagulants
• Cushingoid symptoms: assess for buffalo hump, facial/peripheral wasting, breast enlargement, central obesity
• **Serious rash:** if a serious rash occurs, product should be discontinued
• Assess for allergies before treatment, reaction of each medication; place allergies on chart

Patient/family education
• Teach patient to take as prescribed; if dose is missed, take as soon as remembered up to 1 hr before next dose; do not double dose
• Teach patient that product must be taken in equal intervals around the clock to maintain blood levels for duration of therapy
⚠ Advise that hyperglycemia may occur; watch for increased thirst, weight loss, hunger, dry, itchy skin; notify prescriber
• Advise patient that product does not cure AIDS, only controls symptoms; not to donate blood

Evaluation
Positive therapeutic outcome
• Prevention of viral replication

⚠ HIGH ALERT

tirofiban (Rx)
(tie-roh-fee′ban)
Aggrastat
Func. class.: Antiplatelet
Chem. class.: Glycoprotein IIb/IIIa inhibitor
Pregnancy category B

ACTION: Antagonist of platelet glycoprotein (GP) IIb/IIIa receptor that leads to binding of fibrinogen and von Willebrand's factor, which inhibits platelet aggregation

Therapeutic outcome: Decreased platelet count

USES: Acute coronary syndrome in combination with heparin

CONTRAINDICATIONS:
Hypersensitivity, active internal bleeding, stroke, major surgery, severe trauma within 30 days, intracranial neoplasm, aneurysm, hemorrhage, acute pericarditis, platelets <100,000/mm³, history of thrombocytopenia, coagulopathy, systolic B/P >180 mm Hg or diastolic B/P >110 mm Hg

Precautions: Pregnancy **B**, breastfeeding, children, geriatric, renal disease, bleeding tendencies, hypertension, platelets <150,000/mm³

DOSAGE AND ROUTES
Adult: **IV** 0.4 mcg/kg/min × 30 min, then 0.1 mcg/kg/min for 12-24 hr after angioplasty or atherectomy

Renal dose
Adult: **IV** CCr <30 ml/min 0.2 mcg/kg/min × 30 min, then 0.05 mcg/kg/min, during angiography and for up to 12-24 hr after angioplasty

Available forms: Inj 50 ml vials; inj premixed bag 50 mcg/ml in 100, 250 ml

Implementation
• Dilute inj: withdraw and discard 100 ml from a 500-ml bag of sterile 0.9% NaCl or D₅ and replace this vol with 100 ml of tirofiban inj from two vials
• Tirofiban inj for sol is premixed in containers of 500 ml 0.9% NaCl (50 mg/ml), give over 30 min
• Minimize other arterial/venous punctures, IM inj, catheter use, intubation to reduce bleeding risks

Y-site compatibilities: Acyclovir, alfentanil, allopurinol, amifostine, amikacin, aminocaproic acid, aminophylline, amiodarone, ampicillin, ampicillin/sulbactam, anidulafungin, argatroban, arsenic trioxide, atracurium, atropine, azithromycin, aztreonam, bivalirudin, bleomycin, bumetanide, buprenorphine, butorphanol, calcium chloride/gluconate, capreomycin, CARBOplatin, carmustine, caspofungin, ceFAZolin, cefepime, cefotaxime, cefoTEtan, cefOXitin, cefTAZidime, ceftizoxime, cefTRIAXone, cefuroxime, chloramphenicol, chlorproMAZINE, cimetidine, ciprofloxacin, cisatracurium, CISplatin, clindamycin, cyclophosphamide, cycloSPORINE, cytarabine, DACTINomycin, DAPTOmycin, dexamethasone, dexmedetomidine, dexrazoxane, digoxin, diltiazem, diphenhydrAMINE, DOBUTamine, DOCEtaxel, dolasetron, DOPamine, doxacurium, DOXOrubicin, DOXOrubicin liposome, doxycycline, droperidol, enalaprilat, ePHEDrine, EPINEPHrine, epirubicin, eptifibatide, ertapenem, erythromycin, esmolol, etoposide, etoposide phosphate, famotidine, fenoldopam, fentaNYL, fluconazole, fludarabine, fluorouracil, foscarnet, fosphenytoin, furosemide, ganciclovir, gemcitabine, gentamicin, glycopyrrolate, granisetron, haloperidol, heparin, hydrALAZINE, hydrocortisone, HYDROmorphone, IDArubicin, ifosfamide, imipenem/cilastatin, insulin, irinotecan, isoproterenol, ketorolac, labetalol, leucovorin, lidocaine, linezolid, LORazepam, magnesium sulfate, mannitol, mechlorethamine, melphalan, meperidine, meropenem, mesna, methylhexital, methotrexate, methyldopate, methylPREDNISolone, metoclopramide, metoprolol, metroNIDAZOLE, midazolam, milrinone, mitoXANtrone, morphine, mycophenolate, nafcillin, nalbuphine,

T

naloxone, nesiritide, niCARdipine, nitroglycerin, nitroprusside, norepinephrine, octreotide, ondansetron, oxaliplatin, oxytocin, PACLitaxel, palonosetron, pamidronate, pancuronium, pantoprazole, PEMEtrexed, PENTobarbital, PHENobarbital, phentolamine, phenylephrine, piperacillin/tazobactam, potassium acetate/chloride/phosphates, procainamide, prochlorperazine, promethazine, propranolol, quinupristin/dalfopristin, ranitidine, remifentanil, rocuronium, sodium acetate/bicarbonate, streptozocin, succinylcholine, SUFentanil, tacrolimus, teniposide, theophylline, thiopental, thiotepa, ticarcillin/clavulanate, tigecycline, tobramycin, topotecan, vancomycin, vasopressin, vecuronium, verapamil, vinBLAStine, vinCRIStine, vinorelbine, voriconazole, zidovudine, zoledronic acid

Y-site incompatibilities: Amphotericin B colloidal, amphotericin B liposome, dantrolene, diazepam, phenytoin

ADVERSE EFFECTS
CNS: Dizziness, headache
CV: Bradycardia, hypotension
GI: Nausea, vomiting
HEMA: Bleeding, **thrombocytopenia**
INTEG: *Rash*
MISC: Dissection, edema, pain in legs/pelvis, sweating
SYST: Anaphylaxis

Pharmacokinetics

Absorption	Unknown
Distribution	Plasma clearance 20%-25%
Metabolism	Liver
Excretion	Urine/feces
Half-life	2 hr

Pharmacodynamics

Unknown

INTERACTIONS
Individual drugs
Abciximab, aspirin, cefamandole, cefoperazone, cefoTEtan, clopidogrel, dipyridamole, eptifibatide, heparin, ticlopidine, valproic acid: increased bleeding risk

Drug classifications
Heparins, NSAIDs, SNRIs, SSRIs, thrombin inhibitors: increased bleeding risk

NURSING CONSIDERATIONS
Assessment
• **Bleeding:** Monitor platelet counts, Hct, Hgb before treatment, within 6 hr of loading dose

and at least daily thereafter; watch for bleeding from puncture sites, catheters, or in stools, urine
• **Multiple sclerosis, spinal cord injury:** assess muscle spasms, dizziness, drowsiness, difficulty moving, coordination, balance

Patient/family education
• Advise patient that it is necessary to quit smoking to prevent excessive vasoconstriction
• Teach signs/symptoms of bleeding, low platelets
• Advise that there are many drug and herb interactions

Evaluation
Positive therapeutic outcome
• Treatment of acute coronary syndrome

---

tiZANidine (Rx)
(tye-za'na-deen)
Zanaflex
Func. class.: Skeletal muscle relaxant, central acting
Chem. class.: Imidazole
Pregnancy category C

Do not confuse:
tiZANidine/tiaGABine

ACTION: Increases presynaptic inhibition of motor neurons and reduces spasticity by α_2-adrenergic agonism

Therapeutic outcome: Decreased pain/spasticity in multiple sclerosis

USES: Acute/intermittent management of increased muscle tone associated with spasticity, symptoms of MS

CONTRAINDICATIONS:
Hypersensitivity

Precautions: Pregnancy **C**, breastfeeding, children, geriatric, renal/hepatic disease, hypotension

DOSAGE AND ROUTES
Adult: PO 8 mg q6-8hr; max 36 mg/24 hr

Renal dose
Adult: PO CCr <25 ml/min, start with lower dosage

Available forms: Tabs 2, 4 mg; caps 2, 4, 6 mg

Implementation
- Give with meals for GI symptoms
- Store in airtight container at room temperature
- Give consistently either with or without food; food may affect absorption
- Titrate dose carefully

ADVERSE EFFECTS
CNS: *Dizziness,* somnolence, speech disorder, dyskinesia, nervousness, hallucination, psychosis
CV: Hypotension, bradycardia
GI: *Constipation, vomiting, dry mouth,* increased ALT, abnormal liver function tests
GU: Urinary frequency
OTHER: Blurred vision, pharyngitis, rhinitis, tremor, rash, muscle weakness

Pharmacokinetics

Absorption	Completely absorbed
Distribution	Widely distributed
Metabolism	Liver, extensively
Excretion	Kidneys, feces
Half-life	2½ hr

Pharmacodynamics

Onset	Unknown
Peak	1-2 hr
Duration	3-6 hr

INTERACTIONS
Individual drugs
Acyclovir, alcohol, amiodarone, ciprofloxacin, enoxacin, famotidine, fluvoxaMINE, norfloxacin, propafenone, tacrine, verapamil, zileuton: increased tizanidine levels; avoid concurrent use
Rasagiline: increased effect of rasagiline

Drug classifications
Antihypertensive: increased hypotension
CNS depressants: increased CNS depression

Drug/herb
Kava, St. John's wort: increased CNS depression

Drug/lab test
Increased: AST, alkaline phosphatase, ALT, serum glucose

NURSING CONSIDERATIONS
Assessment
- Assess for muscle spasticity baseline and throughout treatment
- Monitor B/P, heart rate

- Perform neurologic exam in spasticity: deep tendon reflexes, muscle tone, clonus, sensory function
- Monitor renal/liver function tests, electrolytes, CBC with differential during long-term treatment
- Assess for allergic reactions: rash, fever, respiratory distress; severe weakness, numbness in extremities
- Assess CNS depression: dizziness, drowsiness, psychiatric symptoms
- Check dosage, because individual titration is required

Patient/family education
- Advise patient not to discontinue medication quickly; spasticity will occur; product should be tapered off over 1-2 wk
- Advise patient not to take with alcohol, other CNS depressants; take as directed; if dose is missed, take as soon as remembered, unless it is almost time for next dose
- Caution patient to avoid altering activities while taking this product; to avoid hazardous activities if drowsiness or dizziness occurs; to rise from sitting or lying slowly to prevent fainting
- Teach patient to use gum, frequent sips of water for dry mouth
- Advise patient to avoid using OTC medications (cough preparations, antihistamines) unless directed by prescriber
- Notify prescriber if fainting, hallucinations, dark urine, stomach pain, yellowing of skin/eyes occurs
- Advise patient to rise slowly from lying or sitting to upright position to prevent orthostatic hypotension

Evaluation
Positive therapeutic outcome
- Decreased pain, spasticity

tobramycin (Rx)
(toe-bra-mye'sin)
TOBI, TOBI Podhaler
Func. class.: Antiinfective
Chem. class.: Aminoglycoside
Pregnancy category D

ACTION: Interferes with protein synthesis in bacterial cell by binding to ribosomal subunit, causing inaccurate peptide sequence to form in protein chain, causing bacterial death

Therapeutic outcome: Bactericidal effects for the following organisms: *Pseudomonas aeruginosa, Enterobacter, Escherichia coli,*

Providencia, Citrobacter, Staphylococcus, Proteus, Klebsiella, Serratia

USES: Severe systemic infections of CNS, respiratory, GI, urinary tract, bone, skin, soft tissues, cystic fibrosis (nebulizer), *Acinetobacter calcoaceticus, Citrobacter, Enterobacter, Enterococcus, Escherichia coli, Haemophilus aegyptius, Haemophilus influenzae* (beta-lactamase negative), *Haemophilus influenzae* (beta-lactamase positive), *Klebsiella, Moraxella lacunata, Morganella morganii, Neisseria, Proteus mirabilis, Proteus vulgaris, Providencia, Pseudomonas aeruginosa, Serratia, Staphylococcus aureus* (MSSA), *Staphylococcus epidermidis, Staphylococcus, Streptococcus;* **may also be used for the following:** *Acinetobacter, Aeromonas, Bacillus anthracis, Salmonella, Shigella*

CONTRAINDICATIONS:
Hypersensitivity to aminoglycosides

BLACK BOX WARNING: Pregnancy **D,** severe renal disease

Precautions: Breastfeeding, geriatric, neonates, mild renal disease, myasthenia gravis, Parkinson's disease

BLACK BOX WARNING: Hearing deficits, neuromuscular disease

DOSAGE AND ROUTES
Adult: IM/IV 3 mg/kg/day in divided doses q8hr; may give up to 6 mg/kg/day in divided doses q8-12hr; once-daily dosing (pulse dosing) (unlabeled) **IV** 5-7 mg/kg; dosing intervals are determined using a nomogram and are based on random levels drawn 8-12 hr after first dose
Child: IM/IV 6-7.5 mg/kg/day in 3-4 equal divided doses
Child ≥6 yr: NEB 300 mg bid in repeating cycles of 28 days on/28 days off; give inh over 10-15 min using a hand-held PARI LC PLUS reusable nebulizer with a DeVilbiss Pulmo-Aid compressor
Neonate <1 wk: IM/IV ≤4 mg/kg/day divided q12hr
Conventional dosing: Multiply the serum creatinine (mg/100 ml) by 6 to determine the dosing; to decrease the dose, divide the standard dose by the serum creatinine (mg/100 ml) to determine the lower recommended dose

Interval adjustment of extended-interval dosing of 5 or 7 mg/kg (unlabeled): Adjust doses based on serum concentrations and organism MIC; CCr 40-59 ml/min: 5 or 7 mg/kg **IV** q36hr; CCr 20-39 ml/min: 5 or 7 mg/kg **IV** q48hr; CCr <20 ml/min: 5 or 7 mg/kg **IV** once, then follow serial levels to determine time of next dose (serum concentration <1 mcg/ml)
Dose adjustment of extended dosing of 5 mg/kg (unlabeled): Adjust doses based on serum concentrations and organism MIC; CCr >80 ml/min: no dosage adjustment is needed; CCr 60-79 ml/min: 4 mg/kg **IV** q24hr; CCr 50 ml/min: 3.5 mg/kg **IV** q24hr CrCl 40 ml/min: 2.5 mg/kg **IV** q24hr; CrCl <30 ml/min: Use traditional dosing

Cystic fibrosis with *Pseudomonas aeruginosa*
Adult/adolescent/child: IV 2.5-3.3 mg/kg q8hr, neb 300 mg via inhalation bid × 28 days, then 28 days after

Available forms: Inj 10, 40 mg/ml; powder for inj 1.2 g; neb sol 300 mg/5 ml; powder for inh 28 mg

Implementation
IM route
• Give inj deeply in large muscle mass, aspirate
• Draw peak 1 hr after dose, trough right before next dose; absorption erratic
Nebulizer route
• The solution for nebulization is for inhalation only; use over 10-15 min
Inhalation route (TOBI Podhaler)
• Use with Podhaler device, do not swallow caps, use device for 7 days then discard
• Keep caps in blister pack until ready to use, administer other inhaled products or chest physiotherapy before
• While holding base of Podhaler device, unscrew lid, stand upright, unscrew mouthpiece; while holding body, tear blister card in half lengthwise along precut lines; peel back foil, place cap in chamber at top of device, reattach mouthpiece, and tighten; with mouthpiece pointed down, press blue button down with thumb, release; exhale completely, place mouth over mouthpiece, close lips, inhale with single breath, hold 5 sec, and exhale normally away from device; after a few normal breaths, repeat, unscrew mouthpiece, and remove cap: cap should be empty; repeat process 3 more times (total 4 caps); after use reattach mouthpiece and wipe with clean, dry cloth

---

⚠ Nurse Alert   ✴ Key NCLEX® Drug

Intermittent IV infusion route
- Visually inspect solution; do not use if discolored or if particulate is present
- ADD-Vantage vials are for IV only and only for exactly 60 or 80 mg
- Give **IV** diluted in 50-100 ml of 0.9% NaCl, $D_{10}W$, D_5/0.9% NaCl, 0.9% NaCl, Ringer's, LR, D_5W (adult), inf over 20-60 min, volume for pediatric patients needs and should be sufficient to allow for 20-60 min infusion
- Flush after inf with D_5W, 0.9% NaCl
- Separate aminoglycosides and penicillins by ≥1 hr

Syringe compatibilities: Doxapram

Syringe incompatibilities: Cefamandole, clindamycin, heparin, sargramostim

Y-site compatibilities: Acyclovir, aldesleukin, alfentanil, alprostadil, amifostine, aminophylline, amiodarone, amsacrine, anidulafungin, ascorbic acid, atracurium, atropine, aztreonam, bivalirudin, bretylium, bumetanide, buprenorphine, butorphanol, calcium chloride/gluconate, CARBOplatin, caspofungin, chloramphenicol, cimetidine, ciprofloxacin, cisatracurium, CISplatin, clindamycin, cyanocobalamin, cyclophosphamide, cycloSPORINE, cytarabine, DACTINomycin, DAPTOmycin, dexmedetomidine, digoxin, diltiazem, diphenhydrAMINE, DOBUTamine, DOCEtaxel, DOPamine, doripenem, doxacurium, DOXOrubicin hydrochloride, DOXOrubicin liposome, doxycycline, enalaprilat, ePHEDrine, EPINEPHrine, epirubicin, epoetin alfa, ertapenem, esmolol, etoposide, etoposide phosphate, famotidine, fenoldopam, fentaNYL, filgrastim, fluconazole, fludarabine, fluorouracil, foscarnet, furosemide, gemcitabine, gentamicin, glycopyrrolate, granisetron, HYDROmorphone, ifosfamide, imipenem/cilastatin, isoproterenol, ketorolac, labetalol, levofloxacin, lidocaine, linezolid, LORazepam, magnesium sulfate, mannitol, mechlorethamine, melphalan, meperidine, metaraminol, methicillin, methotrexate, methoxamine, methyldopate, methylPREDNISolone, metoclopramide, metoprolol, metroNIDAZOLE, miconazole, midazolam, milrinone, minocycline, mitoXANtrone, morphine, moxalactam, multiple vitamins, nafcillin, nalbuphine, naloxone, niCARdipine, nitroglycerin, nitroprusside, norepinephrine, octreotide, ondansetron, oxaliplatin, oxytocin, PACLitaxel, palonosetron, pantoprazole, papaverine, penicillin G, pentazocine, perphenazine, PHENobarbital, phentolamine, phenylephrine, phytonadione, potassium chloride, procainamide, prochlorperazine, promethazine, propranolol, protamine, pyridoxime, quinupristin/dalfopristin, ranitidine, remifentanil, riTUXimab, rocuronium, sodium acetate/bicarbonate, succinylcholine, SUFentanil, tacrolimus, teniposide, theophylline, thiamine, thiotepa, ticarcillin/clavulanate, tigecycline, tirofiban, tolazoline, trastuzumab, trimetaphan, urokinase, vancomycin, vasopressin, vecuronium, verapamil, vinCRIStine, vinorelbine, voriconazole, zidovudine

Y-site incompatibilities: Allopurinol, amphotericin B cholesteryl, amphotericin B colloidal, amphotericin B liposome, azaTHIOprine, azithromycin, ceFAZolin, cefoperazone, cefoTEtan, cefTRIAXone, dantrolene, dexamethasone, diazepam, diazoxide, drotrecogin, folic acid, ganciclovir, heparin, indomethacin, oxacillin, PEMEtrexed, pentamidine, PENTobarbital, phenytoin, piperacillin/tazobactam, propofol, sargramostim, trimethoprim/sulfamethoxazole

ADVERSE EFFECTS
CNS: Confusion, depression, numbness, tremors, **seizures,** muscle twitching, **neurotoxicity,** dizziness, vertigo
CV: Hypo/hypertension, palpitations
EENT: *Ototoxicity,* deafness, visual disturbances, tinnitus
GI: *Nausea, vomiting, anorexia,* increased ALT, AST, bilirubin, hepatomegaly, **hepatic necrosis,** splenomegaly
GU: Oliguria, hematuria, renal damage, azotemia, renal failure, nephrotoxicity
HEMA: Agranulocytosis, thrombocytopenia, leukopenia, eosinophilia, anemia
INTEG: *Rash,* burning, urticaria, dermatitis, alopecia

Pharmacokinetics

Absorption	Well absorbed (IM), completely absorbed (**IV**)
Distribution	Widely distributed in extracellular fluids
Metabolism	Minimal liver
Excretion	Mostly unchanged (>90%) kidneys
Half-life	2-3 hr, increased in renal disease, neonates

Pharmacodynamics

	IM	IV	OPHTH
Onset	Rapid	Rapid	Rapid
Peak	1 hr	Inf end	Unknown
Duration	Unknown	Unknown	Unknown

INTERACTIONS
Individual drugs
Acyclovir, amphotericin B, bacitracin, cidofovir, CISplatin, ethacrynic acid, furosemide, mannitol, methoxyflurane, polymyxin, vancomycin: increased ototoxicity, neurotoxicity, nephrotoxicity

Drug classifications
Aminoglycosides, cephalosporins, penicillins: increased otoxicity, neurotoxicity, nephrotoxicity

NURSING CONSIDERATIONS
Assessment
• Assess patient for previous sensitivity reaction
Systemic route
• Assess patient for signs and symptoms of infection including characteristics of wounds, sputum, urine, stool, WBC >10,000/mm³, temp baseline, during treatment
• Complete C&S testing before beginning product therapy to identify if correct treatment has been initiated
• Assess for allergic reactions: rash, urticaria, pruritus, chills, fever, joint pain

> **BLACK BOX WARNING: Renal disease:** Identify urine output; if decreasing, notify prescriber (may indicate nephrotoxicity); also, obtain BUN, creatinine, urine CCr (<80 ml/min) values; urinalysis daily for proteinuria, cells, casts; report sudden change in urine output

• Monitor blood studies: AST, ALT, CBC, Hct, bilirubin, LDH, alkaline phosphatase, Coombs' test monthly if patient is on long-term therapy
• Monitor electrolytes: potassium, sodium, chloride, magnesium monthly if patient is on long-term therapy
• Monitor for bleeding: ecchymosis, bleeding gums, hematuria, stool guaiac daily if patient is on long-term therapy
• **Assess for overgrowth of infection:** perineal itching, fever, malaise, redness, pain, swelling, drainage, rash, diarrhea, change in cough, sputum
• Obtain weight before treatment; calculation of dosage is usually based on ideal body weight but may be calculated on actual body weight
• Monitor VS during inf, watch for hypotension, change in pulse
• Assess **IV** site for thrombophlebitis including pain, redness, swelling q30min; change site if needed; apply warm compresses to discontinued site

• Obtain serum peak, drawn at 30-60 min after **IV** inf or 60 min after IM inj, trough level drawn just before next dose; peak 4-12 mcg/ml, trough 1-2 mcg/ml

> **BLACK BOX WARNING:** Monitor for deafness by audiometric testing, ringing, roaring in ears, vertigo; assess hearing before, during, after treatment

Patient/family education
• Teach patient to report sore throat, bruising, bleeding, joint pain; may indicate blood dyscrasias (rare)
• Advise patient to contact prescriber if vaginal itching, loose foul-smelling stools, furry tongue occur; may indicate superinfection

> **BLACK BOX WARNING:** Advise patient to notify prescriber if pregnancy is planned or suspected, pregnancy **D**

• Advise patient to notify prescriber of diarrhea with blood or pus; may indicate pseudomembranous colitis

Nebulizer route
• Advise patient to use multiple therapies first, then tobramycin

Evaluation
Positive therapeutic outcome
• Absence of signs/symptoms of infection (WBC <10,000/mm³, temp WNL, absence of red, draining wounds)
• Reported improvement in symptoms of infection

TREATMENT OF OVERDOSE:
Withdraw product, hemodialysis, exchange transfusion in the newborn, monitor serum levels of product, may give ticarcillin or carbenicillin

tobramycin ophthalmic
See Appendix B

tocilizumab (Rx)
(toe′si-liz′oo-mab)
Actemra
Func. class.: DMARDs (Disease modifying anti-rheumatoid drugs)/tumor necrosis factor (TNF) modifier
Pregnancy category C

ACTION: Interleukin- 6 (IL-6) receptor inhibiting monoclonal antibody

---

Therapeutic outcome: Ability to move more easily with less pain

USES: Rheumatoid arthritis, active systemic juvenile idiopathic arthritis

CONTRAINDICATIONS:
Hypersensitivity

Precautions: Breastfeeding, pregnancy **C,** risk for GI perforation, active hepatic disease, severe neutropenia/thrombocytopenia, demyelinating disorders

> **BLACK BOX WARNING:** Invasive fungal infection, active TB

DOSAGE AND ROUTES
Adult: **IV** 4 mg/kg over 1 hr q4wk, may increase to 8 mg/kg q4wk based on clinical response, max dose 800 mg/inf; do not initiate if ANC is >2000 and platelets are <100,000.

Juvenile idiopathic arthritis
Child ≥2 yr/adolescent ≥30 kg: **IV** 8 mg/kg over 1 hr q2wk
Child ≥2 yr/adolescent <30 kg: **IV** 12 mg/kg over 1 hr

Available forms: Sol for inj 80 mg/4 ml, 200 mg/10 ml, 400 mg/20 ml

Implementation
Intermittent IV route
• Visually inspect for particulate matter and discoloration before administration whenever solution and container permit, colorless to pale yellow liquid
• From a 100-ml infusion bag or bottle, withdraw a volume of 0.9% NaCl for inj equal to the volume of the tocilizumab solution required for the patient's dose
• Slowly add tocilizumab from each vial into the infusion bag or bottle. Gently invert the bag to avoid foaming. Fully diluted solutions are compatible with polypropylene, polyethylene, and polyvinyl chloride infusion bags and polypropylene, polyethylene, and glass infusion bottles
• The fully diluted sol for inf may be stored refrigerated or at room temp for up to 24 hours and should be protected from light. Do not use unused product remaining in vials; no preservatives
• Allow the fully diluted solution to reach room temp before infusing
• Give over 60 min with an infusion set. Do not administer as an **IV** push or bolus

• Do not infuse concomitantly in the same intravenous line with other drugs

ADVERSE EFFECTS
CNS: Headache, dizziness
CV: Hypertension
GI: **Perforation,** abdominal pain, gastritis, mouth ulcerations
HEMA: **Neutropenia, thrombocytopenia**
INTEG: Rash, infusion reactions
RESP: Upper respiratory infections, nasopharyngitis, bronchitis
SYST: **Serious infections, anaphylaxis,** infusion-related reactions, anti-tocilizumab antibody formation

Pharmacokinetics

Absorption	Unknown
Distribution	Unknown
Metabolism	Unknown
Excretion	Unknown
Half-life	~6 days with a single dose and ~11 days with multiple (steady state) doses

Pharmacodynamics
Unknown

INTERACTIONS
Individual drugs
CycloSPORINE, theophylline, warfarin: decreased product level

Drug classifications
CYP3A4 substrates (hormonal contraceptives, omeprazole, atorvastatin, simvastatin): decreased levels of these products
Live virus vaccines: Do not use together
TNF modifiers, DMARDs, immunosuppressives: avoid use due to increased risk of infection

NURSING CONSIDERATIONS
Assessment
• **Rheumatoid arthritis:** assess ROM, pain, stiffness baseline q1-2wk
• Monitor blood studies: CBC with differential, LFTs, platelet count, serum lipid profile, baseline and periodically
• Assess for infection before and periodically, obtain TB screening before beginning treatment

Patient/family education
• Teach patient that this treatment must continue unless safety or effectiveness is an issue; reason for use and expected result

T

> **BLACK BOX WARNING:** Advise patient to
> avoid use of live vaccines, bring immunizations
> up to date before treatment

• Instruct patient to report signs/symptoms
of infection (including TB and Hepatitis B),
invasive fungal infections, discontinue if infection occurs during administration; may use
antituberculosis therapy prior to tocilizumab in
past history of latent or active TB when adequate
course of treatment cannot be confirmed and
those with a negative TB with risk factors for
infections
• Teach patient to notify prescriber if pregnancy
is planned or suspected, pregnancy (C); do not
use if breastfeeding

Evaluation
Positive therapeutic outcome
• Ability to move more easily with less pain

---

tofacitinib
(toe´fa-sye´ti-nib)
Xeljanz
Func. class.: antirheumatic agent (disease
modifying), immunomodulator/biologic
DMARD
Chem. class.: Janus kinase inhibitor
Pregnancy category: C

ACTION: Affects the signaling pathway of
Janus kinase

Therapeutic outcome: Decreased
inflammation, pain in joints, decreased joint
destruction

USES: Rheumatoid arthritis (moderately to
severely active) in those who have taken methotrexate with inadequate response or intolerance

CONTRAINDICATIONS:
Hypersensitivity

Precautions: Pregnancy (C), breastfeeding,
neonates, infants, children, geriatric patients,
neoplastic disease, ulcerative colitis, neutropenia, peptic ulcer disease, active infections, risk
of lymphomas/leukemias, TB, posttransplant
lymphoproliferative disorder (PTLD), kidney
disease, diabetes mellitus, HIV, hypercholesterolemia

> **BLACK BOX WARNING:** Infection, secondary
> malignancy

DOSAGE AND ROUTES
Adult: PO 5 mg/day with or without methotrexate or other nonbiologic DMARDs

Available forms: Tabs 5 mg

Implementation
PO route
Give without regard to food

ADVERSE EFFECTS
CNS: Headache, paresthesias, insomnia,
fatigue
CV: Hypertension
GI: Abdominal pain, nausea, **liver damage,**
dyspepsia, vomiting, diarrhea, gastritis, **GI
perforation, steatosis**
**HEMA: Anemia, lymphocytosis, lympho-
penia, neutropenia**
INTEG: Rash, pruritus
**MISC: Increased cancer risk, risk of infec-
tion (TB, invasive fungal infections, other
opportunistic infections), may be fatal,
posttransplant lymphoproliferative disorder
(PTLD)**

Pharmacokinetics

Absorption	Bioavailability 70%
Distribution	Protein binding 40% (albumin)
Metabolism	Mediated by CYP3A4
Excretion	Unknown
Half-life	3 hr

Pharmacodynamics

Onset	Unknown
Peak	0.5–1 hr
Duration	Unknown

INTERACTIONS
Drug classifications
Do not use with TNF modifiers, vaccines, potent
    immunosuppressants, other biologic DMARDS
CYP3A4 inhibitors (amprenavir, boceprevir,
    delavirdine, ketoconazole, indinavir, itracon-
    azole, dalfopristin/quinupristin, ritonavir, tip-
    ranavir, fluconazole, isoniazid, miconazole):
    increased tofacinib effect
CYP3A4 inducers (rifampin, rifapentine, rifabu-
    tin, primidone, phenytoin, PHENobarbital,
    nevirapine, nafcillin, modafinil, griseofulvin,
    etravirine, efavirenz, barbiturates, bexarotene,
    bosentan, carBAMazepine, enzalutamide,
    dexamethasone): decreased tofacinib effect

Drug/lab test
Increase: LFTs, cholesterol
Decrease: neutrophils, lymphocytes, Hct, Hgb

NURSING CONSIDERATIONS
Assessment
• Monitor lipid profile, Hct/Hgb WBC, LFTs
• RA: assess for pain, stiffness, ROM, swelling of joints before, during treatment

> **BLACK BOX WARNING:** Active infection, including localized infection: evaluate and test patients for latent or active TB before use; treat with antimycobacterials before use of product; this product increases the risk of serious illness including fatal infections (pulmonary or extrapulmonary TB; invasive fungal infections; and bacterial, viral, and opportunistic infections); during and after use, monitor for infection including TB in those who tested negative for latent TB before use; if a serious infection develops, interrupt receipt until the infection is controlled

> **BLACK BOX WARNING:** Secondary malignancy: lymphoma and other malignancies have been noted with product use

⚠ **Epstein–Barr virus–associated post transplant lymphoproliferative disorder (PTLD):** in kidney transplant patients when used with this product and immunosuppressives
• **Liver disease:** not recommended in severe liver disease, impairment; dose modification is needed with moderate liver impairment, monitor LFTs
⚠ **GI perforation:** assess in those with diverticulitis, peptic ulcer disease, or ulcerative colitis
⚠ **Immunosuppression:** obtain neutrophil and lymphocyte counts before use, do not start the product in lymphocyte count < 500 cells/mm^3 or < ANC 1000 cells/mm^3; for ANC >1000 cells/ mm^3, monitor neutrophil counts after 4-8 wk and every 3 mo thereafter; lymphocyte count > 500 cells/ mm^3, monitor lymphocyte counts every 3 mo
⚠ **Anemia:** determine Hgb, do not start in Hgb 9 g/dl; in Hgb 9 g/dl, monitor Hgb after 4-8 wk and every 3 mo thereafter
⚠ **Pregnancy (C)/breastfeeding:** use during pregnancy only if the potential benefit justifies the potential risk to the fetus; if pregnancy occurs, enrollment in the pregnancy registry is encouraged by calling 1–877–311–8972; discontinue product or breastfeeding, serious adverse reactions can occur in nursing infants

> **BLACK BOX WARNING:** Neoplastic disease (lymphomas/leukemias)

Patient/family education
• Teach patient not to have vaccines while taking this product
• Advise patient not to take any live virus vaccines during treatment
• Inform patient to report signs of infection, allergic reaction
⚠ **Pregnancy C:** teach patient to report if pregnancy is planned or suspected, do not breastfeed

Evaluation
Positive therapeutic outcome
• Decreased inflammation, pain in joints, decreased joint destruction

tolcapone (Rx)
(toll′cah-pone)
Tasmar
Func. class.: Antiparkinson agent
Chem. class.: Catecholamine inhibitor (COMT)
Pregnancy category C

ACTION: Selective, reversible inhibitor of catecholamine; used as adjunct to levodopa/carbidopa therapy

Therapeutic outcome: Increased ability to move and speak

USES: Parkinsonism

CONTRAINDICATIONS:
Hypersensitivity, rhabdomyolysis

> **BLACK BOX WARNING:** Hepatic disease

Precautions: Pregnancy **C**, breastfeeding, cardiac/renal disease, hypertension, asthma, history of rhabdomyolysis

DOSAGE AND ROUTES
Adult: PO 100-200 mg tid, with levodopa/carbidopa therapy; max 600 mg/day; discontinue if no benefit in 3 wk

Available forms: Tabs 100, 200 mg

Implementation
• Administer tid with levodopa/carbidopa therapy

Adverse effects: *italics* = common; **bold** = life-threatening

• Provide assistance with ambulation during beginning therapy
• Give without regard to food

ADVERSE EFFECTS

CNS: Dystonia, dyskinesia, dreaming, *fatigue, headache, confusion,* psychosis, hallucination, dizziness, sleep disorders
CV: *Orthostatic hypotension,* chest pain, hypotension
EENT: Cataract, eye inflammation
GI: *Nausea, vomiting, abdominal distress,* diarrhea, constipation, **fatal liver failure,** elevated liver function tests
GU: UTI, urine discoloration, uterine tumor, micturition disorder, hematuria
HEMA: **Hemolytic anemia, leukopenia, agranulocytosis**
INTEG: Sweating, alopecia
MS: **Rhabdomyolysis**

Pharmacokinetics

Absorption	Rapidly absorbed
Distribution	Protein binding 99%
Metabolism	Liver, extensively
Excretion	Urine (60%), feces (40%)
Half-life	2-3 hr

Pharmacodynamics

Onset	Unknown
Peak	2 hr
Duration	Unknown

INTERACTIONS

Individual drugs
Apomorphine, DOBUTamine, isoproterenol, α-methyldopa: may influence pharmacokinetics

Drug classifications
CNS depressants: increased CNS depression
MAOIs: decreased normal catecholamine metabolism; MAO-B inhibitor may be used

NURSING CONSIDERATIONS

Assessment
• **Hepatic disease:** monitor liver function tests: AST, ALT, alkaline phosphatase, LDH, bilirubin, CBC
• Assess involuntary movements in parkinsonism: akinesia, tremors, staggering gait, muscle rigidity, drooling
• Monitor B/P, respiration during initial treatment; hypo/hypertension should be reported
• Monitor mental status: affect, mood, behavioral changes

Patient/family education
• Advise patient to change positions slowly to prevent orthostatic hypotension
• Advise patient that urine, sweat may change color
• Teach patient to notify prescriber if pregnancy is planned or suspected, pregnancy (C)
• Teach patient that CNS changes may occur, hallucinations, involuntary movement
• Teach patient to avoid hazardous activities until reaction is known, dizziness occurs
• Advise patient that nausea and diarrhea are common

> **BLACK BOX WARNING:** Advise patient to report signs of hepatic injury: clay-colored stools, jaundice, fatigue, appetite loss, lethargy, fatigue, itching, right upper abdominal pain

• Teach patient to report nausea, vomiting, anorexia
• May be taken without regard to food

Evaluation
Positive therapeutic outcome
• Decrease in akathisia, improved mood

tolnaftate topical
See Appendix B

tolterodine (Rx)
(tol-tehr'oh-deen)
Detrol, Detrol LA
Func. class.: Overactive bladder product
Chem. class.: Muscarinic receptor antagonist
Pregnancy category C

ACTION: Relaxes smooth muscles in urinary tract by inhibiting acetylcholine at postganglionic sites

Therapeutic outcome: Decreased symptoms of overactive bladder

USES: Overactive bladder (frequency, urgency), urinary incontinence

CONTRAINDICATIONS:
Hypersensitivity, uncontrolled closed-angle glaucoma, urinary retention, gastric retention

Precautions: Pregnancy **C**, breastfeeding, children, renal/hepatic disease, controlled closed-angle glaucoma, bladder obstruction, QT prolongation, decreased GI motility

---

⚠ Nurse Alert   ✴ Key NCLEX® Drug

DOSAGE AND ROUTES
Adult and geriatric: PO 2 mg bid, may decrease to 1 mg bid; EXT REL 4 mg/day, may decrease to 2 mg if needed, max 4 mg/day

Hepatic disease
Adult: PO 1 mg bid (50% dose) or EXT REL 2 mg/day

Renal dose
Adult: PO CCr ≤30 ml/min reduce by 50%

Available forms: Tabs 1, 2 mg; ext rel caps 2, 4 mg

Implementation
• Swallow whole; give with liquids

ADVERSE EFFECTS
CNS: *Anxiety,* paresthesia, fatigue, *dizziness,* headache, increasing dementia, memory impairment
CV: Chest pain, hypertension, **QT prolongation**
EENT: Vision abnormalities, xerophthalmia
GI: *Nausea, vomiting, anorexia,* abdominal pain, constipation, dry mouth, dyspepsia
GU: Dysuria, retention, frequency, UTI
INTEG: Rash, pruritus
RESP: Bronchitis, cough, pharyngitis, upper respiratory tract infection
SYST: **Angioedema, Stevens-Johnson syndrome**

Pharmacokinetics

Absorption	Rapidly absorbed
Distribution	Highly protein bound
Metabolism	Liver, extensively by CYP2D6, a portion of the population may be poor metabolizers
Excretion	Urine/feces
Half-life	Unknown

Pharmacodynamics
Unknown

INTERACTIONS
Individual drugs
Chloroquine, clarithromycin, droperidol, erythromycin, grepafloxacin, halofantrine, haloperidol, methadone, pentamidine: increased QT prolongation
Festerodine: do not use in those with known hypersensitivity

Drug classifications
Antibiotics (macrolide), antifungal agents, antiretroviral protease inhibitors: increased action of tolterodine

Antimuscarinics: increased anticholinergic effect
β-agonists, class IA/III antidysrhythmics, local anesthetics, some phenothiazines, tricyclics: increased QT prolongation
Diuretics: increased urinary frequency

Drug/food
Increased: bioavailability of tolterodine

Drug/lab test
Increased: LFTs, bilirubin

NURSING CONSIDERATIONS
Assessment
• **Assess urinary patterns:** distention, nocturia, frequency, urgency, incontinence
• **Serious skin disorders:** assess for angioedema, Stevens-Johnson syndrome; assess allergic reactions: rash; if this occurs, product should be discontinued
• **QT prolongation:** ECG for QT prolongation, ejection fraction; assess for chest pain, palpitations, dyspnea

> **BLACK BOX WARNING:** Fatal hepatic injury: increased LFTs, bilirubin during first 18 mo of therapy in those with autosomal dominant polycystic kidney disease; assess for fatigue, anorexia, right upper abdominal pain, dark urine, jaundice; if these occur, discontinue product and do not restart if cause is liver injury

Patient/family education
• Advise patient to avoid hazardous activities; dizziness may occur
• Advise patient not to drink liquids before bedtime
• Teach patient importance of bladder maintenance
• Teach patient to take with liquids; swallow whole

Evaluation
Positive therapeutic outcome
• Decreased urinary frequency, urgency

---

tolvaptan (Rx)
(tole-vap′tan)
Samsca
Func. class.: Antihypertensive
Chem. class.: Vasopressin receptor antagonist, V2
Pregnancy category C

ACTION: Arginine vasopressin (AVP) antagonist with affinity for V_2 receptors; level of

Adverse effects: *italics* = common; **bold** = life-threatening

circulating AVP in circulating blood is critical for regulation of water, electrolyte balance and is usually elevated in euvolemic/hypervolemic hyponatremia

Therapeutic outcome: Normal serum sodium level

USES: Hypervolemic/euvolemic hyponatremia in heart failure, cirrhosis, SIADH

CONTRAINDICATIONS:
Hypersensitivity, hypovolemia, anuria

Precautions: Pregnancy **C,** breastfeeding, children, dehydration, geriatric patients, hyperkalemia, autosomal dominant PKD

> **BLACK BOX WARNING:** Alcoholism, malnutrition, hepatic disease

DOSAGE AND ROUTES
Adult: PO 15 mg qd; after 24 hr, may increase to 30 mg qd; max 60 mg/day for ≤30 days

Available forms: Tab 15, 30 mg

Implementation
- Give PO with or without food
- Avoid fluid restriction the first 24 hr
- Initiate in hospital setting

ADVERSE EFFECTS
CNS: Fever, dizziness
CV: Ventricular fibrillation, DIC, stroke, thrombosis
GI: *Nausea,* vomiting, *constipation,* colitis, hepatic injury
GU: Polyuria
HEMA: Bleeding
META: *Dehydration, hyperglycemia,* hyperkalemia, hypernatremia
MS: Rhabdomyolysis
RESP: Respiratory depression, pulmonary embolism

Pharmacokinetics

Absorption	Unknown
Distribution	Protein binding 99%
Metabolism	CYP3A4
Excretion	Unknown
Half-life	Terminal 12 hr

Pharmacodynamics

Onset	Unknown
Peak	2-4 hr
Duration	Unknown

INTERACTIONS
Drug classifications
CYP3A4 inducers (carBAMazepine, dexamethasone, etravirine, flutamide, griseofulvin, metyrapone, modafinil, nafcillin, nevirapine, OXcarbazepine, phenytoin, rifampin, rifabutin, rifapentine, topiramate): decreased concentrations of tolvaptan
CYP3A4 inhibitors (efavirenz, fosamprenavir, quiNINE), P-gp inhibitors (azithromycin, cycloSPORINE, mefloquine, palperidone, propafenone, quiNIDine, testosterone): increased concentrations of tolvaptan

Drug/herb
St. John's wort: decreased tolvaptan effect

Drug/food
Grapefruit juice: do not use together

NURSING CONSIDERATIONS
Assessment
- Assess renal, hepatic function
- Monitor frequent sodium volume status; overly rapid correction of sodium concentration (>12 mEq/L per 24 hr) may result in osmotic demyelination syndrome; may occur in alcoholism, severe malnutrition, advanced liver disease, SIADH
- Assess CV status: ventricular fibrillation, hypertension, monitor B/P, pulse
- Monitor electrolytes (sodium, potassium)

Patient/family education
- Teach patient to avoid pregnancy, breastfeeding while taking this product
- Advise of administration procedure and expected result
- Teach patient to report difficulty swallowing or speaking, seizures, dizziness, drowsiness: embolism may be the cause
- Teach patient to drink fluid in response to thirst
- Teach patient to not use grapefruit juice

Evaluation
Positive therapeutic outcome
- Correction of serum sodium levels

---

topiramate (Rx)
(toh-pire′a-mate)
Topamax, Topamax Sprinkle, Topiragen
Func. class.: Anticonvulsant— miscellaneous
Chem. class.: Monosaccharide derivative
Pregnancy category D

ACTION: Increased GABA activity; may prevent seizure spread as opposed to an elevation of seizure threshold

Therapeutic outcome: Absence of seizures

USES: Partial seizures in adults and children 2-16 yr old; tonic-clonic seizures; seizures in Lennox-Gastaut syndrome, migraine prophylaxis

Unlabeled uses: Infantile spasms, bulimia nervosa

CONTRAINDICATIONS:
Hypersensitivity, metabolic acidosis, pregnancy **D**

Precautions: Breastfeeding, children, renal/hepatic disease, acute myopia, secondary closed-angle glaucoma, behavioral disorders, COPD, dialysis, encephalopathy, status asthmaticus, status epilepticus, surgery, paresthesias, maculopathy, nephrolithiasis

DOSAGE AND ROUTES
Adjunctive therapy
Adult/adolescent/child ≥ 10 yr: PO 25-50 mg/day initially, titrate by 25-50 mg/wk, up to 200-400 mg/day in 2 divided doses
Child 2-9 yr: PO week 1 25 mg q PM, then 25 mg bid if tolerated (week 2), then increase by 25-50 mg/day each week as tolerated over 5-7 wk titration period, maintenance given in 2 divided doses; <11 kg minimum 150 mg/day, max 250 mg/day; 12-22 kg minimum 200 mg/day, max 300 mg/day; 23-31 kg minimum 200 mg, max 350 mg/day, 32-38 kg minimum 250 mg/kg, max 350 mg/day; >38 kg minimum 250 mg/day, max 400 mg/day

Migraine prophylaxis
Adult: PO 25 mg/day initially, increase by 25 mg/day qwk up to 100 mg/day in 2 divided doses

Renal dose
Adult: PO CCr <70 ml/min ½ dose

Available forms: Tabs 25, 50, 100, 200 mg; sprinkle caps 15, 25 mg

Implementation
- Do not break, crush, or chew tabs; very bitter
- May take without regard to meals
- Sprinkle cap can be given whole or opened and sprinkled on soft food; do not chew, drink water after sprinkle
- Store at room temp away from heat, light

ADVERSE EFFECTS
CNS: Dizziness, fatigue, cognitive disorder, *insomnia,* anxiety, depression, paresthesia, motor retardation, **suicidal ideation,** memory loss, tremor, poor balance, ataxia
CV: Flushing, chest pain
EENT: Diplopia, vision abnormality
GI: *Diarrhea, anorexia,* nausea, dyspepsia, abdominal pain, constipation, dry mouth, **pancreatitis**
GU: Breast pain, dysmenorrhea, menstrual disorder
INTEG: Rash, alopecia
MISC: Weight loss, **leukopenia,** metabolic acidosis, increased body temperature, **unexplained death (epilepsy)**
RESP: Upper respiratory tract infection, pharyngitis, sinusitis

Pharmacokinetics
Absorption	Well absorbed
Distribution	Crosses placenta, plasma protein binding (9%-17%), steady state 4 days
Metabolism	Unknown
Excretion	Kidneys unchanged 55%-97%
Half-life	19-25 hr

Pharmacodynamics
Onset	Unknown
Peak	2-4 hr
Duration	Unknown

INTERACTIONS
Individual drugs
Alcohol: increased CNS depression
Amitriptyline: increased effect of amitriptyline
CarBAMazepine, phenytoin, probenecid: decreased levels of topiramate
Digoxin: decreased levels of digoxin
Estrogen: decreased levels of estrogen
Hydrochlorothiazide, lamoTRIgine, metformin: increased topiramate levels
Lithium: decreased levels of lithium

RisperiDONE: decreased levels of risperidone
Valproic acid: decreased levels of both products

Drug classifications

Carbonic anhydrase inhibitors: increased kidney
stone formation
CNS depressants: increased CNS depression
Oral contraceptives: decreased level of oral
contraceptives

NURSING CONSIDERATIONS

Assessment

• **Bipolar disorder:** assess mood, behavior
⚠ **Assess mental status: mood, sensorium,
affect, memory (long, short), especially in
geriatric; suicidal thoughts/behavior**
• Assess for blood dyscrasias: fever, sore throat,
bruising, rash, jaundice, epistaxis (long-term
treatment only)
• **Assess seizure activity** including type, location, duration, and character; provide seizure
precaution
• Monitor CBC during long-term therapy; serum
bicarbonate
• Assess body weight and evidence of cognitive
disorder

Patient/family education

• Teach patient to carry/wear emergency ID
stating name, products taken, condition, prescriber's name and phone number
• Advise patient to avoid driving, other activities
that require alertness
• Teach patient not to discontinue medication
abruptly after long-term use
• Advise patient to use nonhormonal contraceptive; effect of oral contraceptives is decreased,
pregnancy **D**
• Teach patient to drink plenty of fluids to
prevent kidney stones
• Teach patient that increased dietary intake
might be necessary, weight loss may occur

Evaluation

Positive therapeutic outcome
• Decreased seizure activity

TREATMENT OF OVERDOSE:

Lavage, VS

⚠ **HIGH ALERT**

topotecan (Rx)

(to-poe′ti-kan)
Hycamtin
Func. class: Antineoplastic natural; topo-
isomerase inhibitor
Chem. class.: Camptothecin analog
Pregnancy category D

ACTION: Antitumor product with topoisomerase I–inhibitory activity; topoisomerase
I relieves torsional strain in DNA by causing
single-strand breaks; causes double-strand DNA
damage

Therapeutic outcome: Decreased tumor
size

USES: Metastatic ovarian cancer after failure of traditional chemotherapy, relapsed small
cell lung cancer, cervical cancer

CONTRAINDICATIONS:

Pregnancy **D**, breastfeeding, hypersensitivity,
severe bone marrow depression

BLACK BOX WARNING: Neutropenia

Precautions: Children, renal disease, gelatin
hypersensitivity

DOSAGE AND ROUTES

**Metastatic carcinoma of the ovary
after failure of first or subsequent
chemotherapy; SCLC-sensitive
disease after failure of first-line
therapy**
Adult: IV INF 1.5 mg/m^2 over 30 min/day ×
5 days starting on day 1 of a 21-day course ×
4 courses; may be reduced to 0.25 mg/m^2 for
subsequent courses if severe neutropenia occurs

**Relapsed small-cell lung cancer
(SCLC) in those with a prior complete or partial response, 45 days
from end of first-line treatment**
Adult: PO 2.3 mg/m^2/day on days 1-5 of a
21-day course

Renal dose
Adult: IV CCr 20-39 ml/min 0.75 mg/m^2/day
× 5 days on day 1 of a 21-day course

Available forms: Lyophilized powder for
inj 4 mg; cap 0.25, 1 mg

Implementation
- Provide increased fluid intake to 2-3 L/day to prevent dehydration, unless contraindicated
- Change **IV** site q48hr
- Store caps in refrigerator; IV INF unopened at room temperature; protect both from light

Intermittent IV infusion route
- Visually inspect for particulate matter and discoloration prior to use
- Reconstitute each 4-mg vial with 4 ml sterile water for injection; use immediately, no preservative
- Withdraw the appropriate volume of the reconstituted solution; dilute further in 0.9% NaCl or D₅W prior to administration
- The reconstituted solution is yellow or yellow-green
- Topotecan injection diluted for infusion is stable at room temperature with normal light for 24 hr
- Infuse over 30 min

ADVERSE EFFECTS
CNS: Arthralgia, *asthenia, headache,* myalgia, *pain,* weakness
GI: *Abdominal pain, constipation,* diarrhea, obstruction, *nausea,* stomatitis, *vomiting,* increased ALT, AST, anorexia
HEMA: Neutropenia, leukopenia, thrombocytopenia, anemia, sepsis
INTEG: *Total alopecia*
RESP: Dyspnea, cough, interstitial lung disease

Pharmacokinetics

Absorption	Rapidly, completely absorbed
Distribution	7%-35% protein binding
Metabolism	Liver
Excretion	Urine, feces to metabolites
Half-life	2.8 hr

Pharmacodynamics
Unknown

INTERACTIONS
Individual drugs
CISplatin: increased myelosuppression
Itraconazole, mefloquine, niCARdipine, quiNIDine, RU-486, tamoxifen, testosterone, verapamil: avoid giving together

Drug classifications
Anticoagulants, NSAIDs, platelet inhibitors, thrombolytics: increased bleeding risk

P-glycoprotein, breast cancer resistance protein inhibitors (amiodarone, clarithromycin, diltiazem, erythromycin, indinavir vaccines, toxoids: avoid using together

Drug/food
Grapefruit juice: avoid use

NURSING CONSIDERATIONS
Assessment
- Monitor liver function tests: AST, ALT, alkaline phosphatase, which may be elevated; creatinine, BUN

BLACK BOX WARNING: Monitor CBC, differential, platelet count weekly; withhold product if WBC is <3500/mm³ or platelet count is <100,000/mm³; notify prescriber of these results; product should be discontinued

- Assess buccal cavity for dryness, sores or ulceration, white patches, oral pain, bleeding, dysphagia
- **Interstitial lung disease (ILD):** assess for fever, cough, dyspnea, hypoxia, may be fatal

Patient/family education
- Advise patient to avoid foods with citric acid or hot flavor or rough texture if stomatitis is present; to drink adequate fluids
- Advise patient that total alopecia may occur; hair grows back but may be different in color and texture
- Advise patient to report stomatitis; any bleeding, white spots, ulcerations in mouth; tell patient to examine mouth daily; report symptoms

BLACK BOX WARNING: Teach patient to report signs of anemia; fatigue, headache, faintness, shortness of breath, irritability

- Teach patient to rinse mouth tid-qid with water, club soda; brush teeth bid-tid with soft brush or cotton-tipped applicator for stomatitis; use unwaxed dental floss
- Teach patient to use effective contraception during treatment and up to 6 mo after, pregnancy (D), avoid breastfeeding
- Advise patient to avoid OTC products without approval of prescriber
- Advise to avoid driving or other activities requiring alertness
- Advise to avoid vaccines, toxoids

Evaluation
Positive therapeutic outcome
- Decreased tumor size, spread of malignancy

Adverse effects: *italics* = common; **bold** = life-threatening

toremifene (Rx)

(tor-em'ih-feen)

Fareston

Func. class.: Antineoplastic

Chem. class.: Antiestrogen hormone

Pregnancy category D

ACTION: Inhibits cell division by binding to cytoplasmic estrogen receptors; resembles normal cell complex but inhibits DNA synthesis and estrogen response of target tissue

Therapeutic outcome: Prevention of rapidly growing malignant cells

USES: Advanced breast carcinoma that has not responded to other therapy in estrogen-receptor-positive patients (usually postmenopausal)

CONTRAINDICATIONS:

Pregnancy **D**, hypersensitivity, history of thromboembolism

> **BLACK BOX WARNING:** QT prolongation

Precautions: Breastfeeding, children, cataracts, leukopenia, thrombocytopenia, hypercalcemia, hepatic disease, endometrial hyperplasia

DOSAGE AND ROUTES

Adult: PO 60 mg/day

Available forms: Tabs 60 mg

Implementation

• Do not break, crush, or chew tabs

• Give with food or fluids to decrease GI upset; repeat dose may be needed if vomiting occurs

• Store in light-resistant container at room temperature

ADVERSE EFFECTS

CNS: *Hot flashes, headache, light-headedness,* depression

CV: Chest pain, **CHF, MI, PE,** chest pain, angina

EENT: Ocular lesions, retinopathy, corneal opacity, blurred vision (high doses)

GI: *Nausea, vomiting,* altered taste (anorexia)

GU: Vaginal bleeding, pruritus vulvae

HEMA: **Thrombocytopenia, leukopenia, thrombosis**

INTEG: *Rash,* alopecia, sweating

META: Hypercalcemia

RESP: **Pulmonary embolism**

Pharmacokinetics

Absorption	Adequately absorbed
Distribution	99% protein binding
Metabolism	Liver, extensively
Excretion	Feces, slowly, small amounts (kidneys)
Half-life	Terminal 5-6 days

Pharmacodynamics

Onset	Unknown
Peak	3 hr
Duration	Unknown

INTERACTIONS

Individual drugs

Warfarin: increased warfarin effect

> **BLACK BOX WARNING:** Haloperidol, chloroquine, droperidol, pentamidine, arsenic trioxide, levomethadyl: increased QT prolongation

Drug classifications

> **BLACK BOX WARNING:** Class IA/III antidysrhythmics, some phenothiazines, β-agonists, local anesthetics, tricyclics, pentamidine; CYP3A4 inhibitors (amiodarone, clarithromycin, erythromycin, telithromycin, troleandomycin); CYP3A4 substrates (methadone, pimozide, QUEtiapine, quiNIDine, risperidone, ziprasidone): increased QT prolongation

CYP3A4 inducers (barbiturates, bosentan, carBAMazepine, efavirenz, phenytoins, nevirapine, rifabutin, rifampin): decreased toremifene effect

CYP3A4 inhibitors (aprepitant, antiretroviral protease inhibitors, clarithromycin, danazol, delivirdine, diltiazem, erythromycin, fluconazole, FLUoxetine, fluvoxaMINE, imatinib, ketoconazole, mibefradil, nefazodone, telithromycin, voriconazole): increased toxicity

Drug/herb

St. John's wort: avoid use

Drug/lab test

Increased: serum Ca

NURSING CONSIDERATIONS

Assessment

• Monitor CBC, differential, platelet count weekly; withhold product if WBC is <4000/mm^3 or platelet count is <75,000/mm^3; notify prescriber of results; monitor calcium levels

---

(hypercalcemia is common), LFTs, serum calcium
• **Assess for tumor flare:** increase in bone, tumor pain during beginning treatment; give analgesics as ordered to decrease pain
• Assess for bleeding: hematuria, guaiac, bruising or petechiae, mucosa or orifices q8hr, no rectal temp
• **QT prolongation:** ECG for QT prolongation, ejection fraction; assess for chest pain, palpitations, dyspnea

> **BLACK BOX WARNING: Allergic reactions:** assess for rash, pruritus, urticaria, purpuric skin lesions, itching, flushing

Patient/family education
• Advise patient that vaginal bleeding, pruritus, hot flashes can occur and are reversible after discontinuing treatment
• Instruct patient to report immediately decreased visual acuity, which may be irreversible; stress need for routine eye exams
• Inform patient about who should be told about toremifene therapy
• Advise patient to report vaginal bleeding immediately; that tumor flare (increase in size of tumor, increased bone pain) may occur and will subside rapidly; may take analgesics for pain; that premenopausal women must use mechanical birth control method because ovulation may be induced (teratogenic product), pregnancy (D)
• Caution patient to use sunscreen and protective clothing to prevent burns because photosensitivity is common
• Teach patient that hair loss may occur during treatment; a wig or hairpiece may make patient feel better; new hair may be different in color, texture
• Inform patient rash or lesions are temporary and may become large during beginning therapy

Evaluation
Positive therapeutic outcome
• Decreased spread of malignant cells in breast cancer

---

traMADol (Rx)
(trah′mah-dol)
ConZip, Ryzolt, Ultram, Ultram ER, Zytram ✦
Func. class.: Analgesic, miscellaneous
Pregnancy category C

Do not confuse:
traMADol/Toradol

ACTION: Binds to μ-opioid receptors and inhibits reuptake of norepinephrine, serotonin

Therapeutic outcome: Relief of pain

USES: Management of moderate to severe pain, chronic pain, headache, osteoarthritis

CONTRAINDICATIONS:
Hypersensitivity, acute intoxication with any CNS depressant, alcohol, asthma, respiratory depression

Precautions: Pregnancy C, breastfeeding, children, geriatric, seizure disorder, renal/hepatic disease, respiratory depression, head trauma, increased ICP, acute abdominal condition, product abuse, depression, suicidal ideation

DOSAGE AND ROUTES
Mild to moderate pain
Adult: PO 25 mg qd, titrate by 25 mg ≥3 days to 100 mg/day (25 mg qid), then may increase by 50 mg ≥3 days to 200 mg (50 mg qid), then 50-100 mg q4-6hr, max 400 mg/day; use caution in elderly
Geriatric >75 yr: PO <300 mg/day in divided dose

Hepatic dose
Adult: PO 50 mg q12hr

Renal dose
Adult (Child-Pugh C): PO CCr <30 ml/min q12hr, max 200 mg/day; do not use ext rel tabs

Moderate to severe chronic pain
Adult: PO-ER (Ultram ER) 100 mg daily, titrate upward q5day by 100 mg, max 300 mg/day; (Ryzolt) 100 mg, titrate upward q2-3day in 100-mg increments; max 300 mg/day; products are not interchangeable

Available forms: Tabs 50 mg; ext rel tab 100, 200, 300 mg; orally disintegrating tab 50 mg; ext rel caps 100, 200, 300 mg

Implementation
• Do not break, crush, or chew ext rel product
• Give with antiemetic for nausea, vomiting
• Administer when pain is beginning to return; determine dosage interval by patient response
• **Ext rel** products (Ryzolt/Ultram ER) are not interchangeable
• Store in cool environment, protect from sunlight
• Give with or without food; ext rel: always give with food, or always give on empty stomach

---

ADVERSE EFFECTS
CNS: Dizziness, CNS stimulation, somnolence, headache, anxiety, confusion, euphoria, **seizures,** hallucinations, sedation, **neuroleptic malignant syndrome–like reactions**
CV: Vasodilatation, orthostatic hypotension, tachycardia, hypertension, abnormal ECG
EENT: Visual disturbances
GI: Nausea, constipation, vomiting, dry mouth, diarrhea, abdominal pain, anorexia, flatulence, GI bleeding
GU: Urinary retention/frequency, menopausal symptoms, dysuria, menstrual disorder
INTEG: Pruritus, rash, urticaria, vesicles, flushing
SYST: Anaphylaxis, Stevens-Johnson syndrome, toxic epidermal necrolysis, serotonin syndrome

Pharmacokinetics

Absorption	Rapidly, almost completely absorbed
Distribution	Steady state 2 days
Metabolism	Extensively in liver, may cross blood-brain barrier
Excretion	Unchanged product 30% in urine, protein binding 20%
Half-life	Unknown

Pharmacodynamics

Unknown

INTERACTIONS
Individual drugs
Alcohol: increased CNS depression
CarBAMazepine: decreased tramadol level

Drug classifications
CYP3A4 inducers (barbiturates, bosentan, carBAMazepine, efavirenz, nevirapine, phenytoin, rifabutin, rifampin): decreased tramadol effect
CYP3A4 inhibitors (aprepitant, antiretroviral protease inhibitors, clarithromycin, danazol, delavirdine, diltiazem, erythromycin, fluconazole, FLUoxetine, fluvoxaMINE, imatinib, ketoconazole, mibefradil, nefazodone, telithromycin, voriconazole): increased traMADol levels
MAOIs: inhibition of norepinephrine and serotonin reuptake; use together with caution
Opiates, sedative/hypnotics: increased CNS depression
SSRIs, SNRIs, serotonin-receptor agonists: increased serotonin syndrome

Drug/herb
Chamomile, hops, kava, skullcap, valerian: increased CNS depression
St. John's wort: avoid use

Drug/lab test
Increased: creatinine, liver enzymes
Decreased: Hgb

NURSING CONSIDERATIONS
Assessment
• **Pain:** assess location, type, character; give before pain becomes extreme
• Assess for increased side effects in renal/hepatic disease
• **Respiratory depression:** withhold if respirations <12/min
• Monitor I&O ratio: check for decreasing output; may indicate urinary retention
• Assess need for product
• Assess for constipation and bowel pattern; increase fluids, bulk in diet
⚠ **Hypersensitivity: usually after beginning treatment**
• Monitor CNS changes: dizziness, drowsiness, hallucinations, euphoria, LOC, pupil reaction
• Determine allergic reactions: rash, urticaria
• **Serotonin syndrome, neuroleptic malignant syndrome:** assess for increased heart rate, shivering, sweating, dilated pupils, tremors, high B/P, hyperthermia, headache, confusion; if these occur, stop product, administer a serotonin antagonist if needed

Patient/family education
• Teach patient to report any symptoms of CNS changes, allergic reactions
• Teach patient that drowsiness, dizziness, and confusion may occur; to call for assistance
• Instruct patient to make position changes slowly; orthostatic hypotension may occur
• Tell patient to avoid OTC medication and alcohol unless approved by prescriber
• Instruct patient not to discontinue abruptly, taper

Evaluation
Positive therapeutic outcome
• Decreased pain

⚠ Nurse Alert   ✳ Key NCLEX® Drug

trandolapril (Rx)

(tran-doe′la-prill)

Mavik

Func. class.: Antihypertensive

Chem. class.: Angiotensin-converting enzyme (ACE) inhibitor

Pregnancy category D (2nd/3rd trimester), C (1st trimester)

ACTION: Selectively suppresses renin-angiotensin-aldosterone system; inhibits ACE; prevents conversion of angiotensin I to angiotensin II, resulting in dilatation of arterial and venous vessels and lowered B/P

Therapeutic outcome: Decreased B/P in hypertension

USES: Hypertension alone or in combination, heart failure, after MI, LV dysfunction after MI

CONTRAINDICATIONS:

Breastfeeding, hypersensitivity, history of angioedema

> **BLACK BOX WARNING:** Pregnancy **D** (2nd/3rd trimester), pregnancy **C** (1st trimester)

Precautions: Geriatric, hyperkalemia, hepatic disease, bilateral renal stenosis, after kidney transplant, aortal/mitral valve stenosis, cirrhosis, severe renal disease, untreated CHF, autoimmune diseases, cough

DOSAGE AND ROUTES

Hypertension

Adult: PO 1 mg/day, 2 mg/day in African Americans, make dosage adjustment ≥1 wk; up to 8 mg/day

Heart failure (after MI/left ventricular dysfunction)

Adult: PO 1 mg/day, titrate upward to 4 mg/day if tolerated, 2-4 yr

Renal dose/hepatic dose

Adult: PO CCr <30 ml/min or hepatic disease 0.5 mg/day

Available forms: Tabs 1, 2, 4 mg

Implementation

• Store in airtight container at ≤77° F (≤25° C) or less
• Give without regard to food
• Space antacids by 2 hr after dose

ADVERSE EFFECTS

CNS: *Dizziness,* paresthesias, headache, *syncope,* fatigue, drowsiness, depression, sleep disturbances, anxiety, syncope

CV: *Hypotension,* **MI,** palpitations, angina, TIAs, **stroke,** bradycardia, dysrhythmias

GI: Nausea, vomiting, cramps, diarrhea, constipation, **pancreatitis,** *dyspepsia*

GU: Proteinuria, renal failure

HEMA: Agranulocytosis, neutropenia, leukopenia, anemia

INTEG: Rash, purpura, pruritus, **angioedema**

MISC: Hyperkalemia, hyponatremia, impotence, *myalgia,* **angioedema,** muscle cramps, asthenia, hypocalcemia, gout

RESP: Dyspnea, cough

Pharmacokinetics

Absorption	40%-60%
Distribution	Unknown
Metabolism	Liver
Excretion	Kidneys (33%), feces (66%)
Half-life	0.6-1.1 hr, 16-24 hr

Pharmacodynamics

Onset	½ hr
Peak	4-10 hr
Duration	>8 days

INTERACTIONS

Individual drugs

Levodopa, lithium, reserpine: increased effect of each specific product

Drug classifications

Antacids, NSAIDs, salicylates: decreased effect of trandolapril

Antihypertensives, diuretics: increased severe hypotension

Barbiturates, ergots, hypoglycemics, neuromuscular blocking agents: increased effects of each specific product

Diuretics (potassium-sparing): increased potassium levels

Phenothiazines: increased antihypertensive effects

Potassium supplements: increased potassium levels

Salt substitutes: increased potassium levels

Drug/lab test

Increased: potassium, LFTs, BUN, creatinine

Decreased: sodium, WBC

T

Adverse effects: *italics* = common; **bold** = life-threatening

NURSING CONSIDERATIONS
Assessment
• Monitor blood tests: neutrophils, decreased platelets
• Monitor B/P, orthostatic hypotension, syncope; if changes occur dosage change may be required
• Monitor renal studies: protein, BUN, creatinine; increased levels may indicate nephrotic syndrome and renal failure
• Monitor renal symptoms: polyuria, oliguria, frequency, dysuria
• Establish baselines in renal, liver function tests before therapy begins
• Check potassium levels throughout treatment, although hyperkalemia rarely occurs
• Check for edema in feet, legs daily
• Assess for allergic reactions: rash, fever, pruritus, urticaria; product should be discontinued if antihistamines fail to help
⚠ **Hepatotoxicity (rare): assess for increased LFTs, jaundice, fulminating hepatic necrosis; if jaundice occurs, discontinue product**
• Angioedema: of the face, edema of the extremities, mucus membranes, may need to discontinue
⚠ **Hyperkalemia: monitor electrolytes, check potassium**

Patient/family education
• Advise patient not to discontinue product abruptly; advise patient to tell all persons associated with health care
• Teach patient not to use OTC products (cough, cold, allergy) unless directed by physician; serious side effects can occur; xanthines, such as coffee, tea, chocolate, cola, can prevent action of product
• Instruct patient on the importance of complying with dosage schedule, even if feeling better; to continue with medical regimen to decrease B/P: exercise, cessation of smoking, decreasing stress, diet modifications
• Emphasize the need to rise slowly to sitting or standing position to minimize orthostatic hypotension; not to exercise in hot weather, which can cause increased hypotension
• Advise patient to notify prescriber of mouth sores, sore throat, fever, swelling of hands or feet, irregular heartbeat, chest pain, coughing, shortness of breath
• Caution patient to report excessive perspiration, dehydration, vomiting, diarrhea; may lead to fall in B/P
• Caution patient that product may cause dizziness, fainting, light-headedness; may occur during 1st few days of therapy; to avoid activities that may be hazardous
• Teach patient how to take B/P and normal readings for age group

> **BLACK BOX WARNING:** Teach patient to notify prescriber if pregnancy is suspected or planned, pregnancy **D**

Evaluation
Positive therapeutic outcome
• Decreased B/P in hypertension

TREATMENT OF OVERDOSE:
Lavage, **IV** atropine for bradycardia, **IV** theophylline for bronchospasm, digoxin, O_2, diuretic for cardiac failure, hemodialysis

---

⚠ **HIGH ALERT**

trastuzumab (Rx)
(tras-tuz'uh-mab)
Herceptin
Func. class.: Antineoplastic—miscellaneous
Chem. class.: Humanized monoclonal antibody
Pregnancy category D

ACTION: DNA-derived monoclonal antibody selectively binds to extracellular portion of human epidermal growth factor receptor 2 (HER2); it inhibits proliferation of cancer cells

Therapeutic outcome: Decreasing symptoms of breast cancer

USES: Metastatic breast cancer with overexpression of HER2, early breast cancer (adjuvant, neoadjuvant), gastric cancer; previously untreated HER2 overexpressing metastatic gastric or gastroesophageal junction adenocarcinoma with CISplatin, 5-fluorouracil or capecitabine

CONTRAINDICATIONS:
Pregnancy **D**, hypersensitivity to this product, Chinese hamster ovary cell protein

Precautions: Breastfeeding, children, geriatric, pulmonary disease, anemia, leukopenia

> **BLACK BOX WARNING:** Cardiac disease, respiratory distress syndrome, respiratory insufficiency, infusion-related reactions, cardiomyopathy

---

DOSAGE AND ROUTES
Breast cancer
Several regimens may be used
Adult: **IV** 4 mg/kg given over 90 min, then maintenance 2 mg/kg given over 30 min; do not give as **IV** PUSH or BOL; may be given in combination with other antineoplastics

Gastric cancer
Adult: **IV** 8 mg/kg over 90 min on day 1, then 6 mg/kg over 30-90 min q21days from day 22, give with CISplatin 80 mg/m^2 on day 1 plus 5-fluorouracil 800 mg/m^2 CONT INF on days 1-5 or capecitabine 1000 mg/m^2 bid on days 1-14, repeat cycle q3wk

Available forms: Lyophilized powder 440 mg

Implementation
• Give acetaminophen as ordered to alleviate fever and headache
• Increase fluid intake to 2-3 L/day

Intermittent IV infusion route
• Administer after reconstituting vial with 20 ml of bacteriostatic water for inj, 1.1% benzyl alcohol preserved (supplied) to yield 21 mg/ml, mark date on vial 28 days from reconstitution date; if patient is allergic to benzyl alcohol, reconstitute with sterile water for inj; use immediately; inf over 90 min; q3wk give 8 mg/kg loading dose over 90 min; subsequent doses 6 mg/kg may be given over 30-60 min
• Do not mix or dilute with other products or dextrose sol

ADVERSE EFFECTS
CNS: *Dizziness, numbness, paresthesias,* depression, *insomnia,* neuropathy, peripheral neuritis
CV: **Tachycardia, CHF**
GI: Nausea, vomiting, *anorexia, diarrhea,* abdominal pain, **hepatotoxicity,** dysgeusia
HEMA: *Anemia,* leukopenia
INTEG: *Rash,* acne, herpes simplex
META: Edema, peripheral edema
MISC: *Flulike symptoms; fever, headache, chills*
MS: Arthralgia, *bone pain*
RESP: *Cough, dyspnea, pharyngitis, rhinitis,* sinusitis, **pneumonia, pulmonary edema/fibrosis,** acute respiratory distress syndrome (ARDS)
SYST: **Anaphylaxis, angioedema**

Pharmacokinetics
Absorption	Unknown
Distribution	Unknown
Metabolism	Unknown
Excretion	Unknown
Half-life	1-32 days

Pharmacodynamics
Unknown

INTERACTIONS
Individual drugs
Cyclophosphamide: increased cardiomyopathy risk; avoid use
Warfarin: increased bleeding risk

Drug classifications
Anthracyclines: increased cardiomyopathy risk
Vaccines/toxoids: decreased immune response

NURSING CONSIDERATIONS
Assessment
• Monitor CBC, HER2 overexpression
• Assess for symptoms of infection; may be masked by product
• Assess CNS reaction: LOC, mental status, dizziness, confusion

> **BLACK BOX WARNING: CHF** and other cardiac symptoms: assess for dyspnea, coughing, gallop; obtain a full cardiac workup including ECG, echocardiogram, multigated angiogram

• Hypersensitivity reactions, anaphylaxis

> **BLACK BOX WARNING: Potentially fatal infusion reactions:** assess for fever, chills, nausea, vomiting, pain, headache, dizziness, hypotension; discontinue product

• **Pulmonary toxicity:** assess for dyspnea, interstitial pneumonitis, pulmonary hypertension, ARDS; can occur after infusion reaction, those with lung disease may have more severe toxicity

Patient/family education
• Advise patient to take acetaminophen for fever
• Teach patient to avoid hazardous tasks, since confusion, dizziness may occur
• Teach patient to report signs of infection: sore throat, fever, diarrhea, vomiting
• Inform patient that emotional lability is common; instruct patient to notify prescriber if severe or incapacitating
• Advise patient to use contraception while taking this product, pregnancy **D**; avoid breastfeeding

BLACK BOX WARNING: Teach patient to report pain at infusion site

Evaluation
Positive therapeutic outcome
• Decrease in size of tumors

travoprost ophthalmic
See Appendix B

traZODone (Rx)
(tray'zoe-done)
Oletpro
Func. class.: Antidepressant—miscellaneous
Chem. class.: Triazolopyridine
Pregnancy category C

ACTION: Selectively inhibits serotonin, norepinephrine uptake by brain, potentiates behavioral changes

Therapeutic outcome: Decreased symptoms of depression after 2-3 wk

USES: Depression

CONTRAINDICATIONS:
Hypersensitivity to tricyclics

Precautions: Pregnancy C, suicidal patients, severe depression, increased intraocular pressure, closed-angle glaucoma, urinary retention, cardiac/hepatic disease, hyperthyroidism, electroshock therapy, elective surgery, bleeding, abrupt discontinuation, bipolar disorder, breastfeeding, dehydration, hyponatremia, hypovolemia, recovery phase of MI, seizure disorders, prostatic hypertrophy, family history of long QT

BLACK BOX WARNING: Suicidal ideation in children/adolescents

DOSAGE AND ROUTES
Depression
Adult: PO 150 mg/day in divided doses; may increase by 50 mg/day q3-4day, max 400 mg/day (outpatient), 600 mg/day (inpatient); EXT REL 150 mg/day in the evening, may increase gradually by 75 mg/day at 3 day intervals, max 375 mg/day
Geriatric: PO 25-50 at bedtime, increase by 25-50 mg q3-7day to desired dose, usual 75-150 mg/day

Child 6-18 yr (unlabeled): PO 1.5-2 mg/kg/day in divided doses, may increase q3-4day up to 6 mg/kg/day or 400 mg/day in divided doses, whichever is less

Available forms: Tabs 50, 100, 150, 300 mg; ext rel tabs 150, 300 mg

Implementation
• Give with food or milk for GI symptoms; crush if patient is unable to swallow medication whole
• Give dose at bedtime if oversedation occurs during day; may take entire dose at bedtime; geriatric may not tolerate once/day dosing
• Store in tight, light-resistant container at room temp; do not freeze

ADVERSE EFFECTS
CNS: *Dizziness, drowsiness,* confusion, headache, anxiety, tremors, stimulation, weakness, insomnia, nightmares, EPS (geriatric), increase in psychiatric symptoms, **suicide in children/adolescents**
CV: *Orthostatic hypotension, ECG changes, tachycardia,* **hypertension,** palpitations
EENT: *Blurred vision,* tinnitus, mydriasis
GI: *Diarrhea, dry mouth,* nausea, vomiting, **paralytic ileus,** increased appetite, cramps, epigastric distress, jaundice, **hepatitis,** stomatitis, constipation
GU: *Retention,* **acute renal failure, priapism**
HEMA: **Agranulocytosis, thrombocytopenia, eosinophilia, leukopenia**
INTEG: Rash, urticaria, sweating, pruritus, photosensitivity

Pharmacokinetics
Absorption	Well absorbed
Distribution	Widely distributed
Metabolism	Liver, extensively
Excretion	Kidneys, minimally unchanged
Half-life	4½-7½ hr

Pharmacodynamics
Onset	Unknown
Peak	1 hr without food, 2 hr with food
Duration	Unknown

INTERACTIONS
Individual drugs
Alcohol, carBAMazepine, digoxin, phenytoin: increased effect of each product
FLUoxetine, nefazodone: increased levels, increased toxicity, serotonin syndrome

---

Guanethidine, cloNIDine: decreased effects of each product

Warfarin: increased or decreased effects of warfarin

Drug classifications

Barbiturates, benzodiazepines, CNS depressants: increased effects

CYP3A4, 2D6 inhibitors (phenothiazenes, protease inhibitors, azole antifungals): increased effects of trazodone

MAOIs: increased hyperpyretic crisis, seizures, hypertensive episode, do not use within 14 days

SNRIs, SSRIs: increased toxicity, serotonin syndrome

Sympathomimetics (direct-acting): increased sympathomimetic effects

Sympathomimetics (indirect-acting): decreased effects

Drug/herb

Hops, kava, lavender, valerian: increased CNS depression

SAM-e, St. John's wort: increased serotonin syndrome

Drug/lab test

Increased: LFTs

Decreased: Hgb

NURSING CONSIDERATIONS

Assessment

• Monitor B/P (lying, standing), pulse q4hr; if systolic B/P drops 20 mm Hg hold product, notify prescriber; take vital signs q4hr in patients with CV disease

• Monitor blood tests: CBC, leukocytes, differential

• Monitor liver function tests: AST, ALT, bilirubin

• Check weight qwk; appetite may increase with product

• Assess ECG for flattening of T wave, bundle branch block, AV block, dysrhythmias in cardiac patients

• Assess for EPS primarily in geriatric: rigidity, dystonia, akathisia

> **BLACK BOX WARNING:** Assess mental status: mood, sensorium, affect, suicidal tendencies in children/adolescents; increase in psychiatric symptoms: depression, panic, not approved for children

• Monitor urinary retention, constipation; constipation is more likely to occur in children or geriatric

• **Withdrawal symptoms:** assess for headache, nausea, vomiting, muscle pain, weakness; do not usually occur unless product was discontinued abruptly

• Identify alcohol consumption; if alcohol is consumed, hold dose until AM

• **Serotonin syndrome, neuroleptic malignant syndrome:** assess for increased heart rate, shivering, sweating, dilated pupils, tremors, high B/P, hyperthermia, headache, confusion; if these occur, stop product, administer a serotonin antagonist if needed

Patient/family education

• Teach patient that therapeutic effects may take 2-3 wk

• Teach patient to use caution in driving or other activities requiring alertness because of drowsiness, dizziness, blurred vision; to avoid rising quickly from sitting to standing, especially geriatric

• Teach patient not to crush, chew ext rel product

• Caution patient to avoid alcohol ingestion, other CNS depressants

• Teach patient not to discontinue medication quickly after long-term use: may cause nausea, headache, malaise

• Advise patient to wear sunscreen or large hat because photosensitivity occurs

• Teach patient to increase fluids, bulk in diet if constipation, urinary retention occur, especially geriatric

• Advise patient to take gum, hard sugarless candy, or frequent sips of water for dry mouth

• Advise patient to rise slowly to prevent dizziness

> **BLACK BOX WARNING:** Teach family to watch for suicidal ideation or tendencies, usually in children/adolescents

• Teach patient to notify prescriber if pregnancy is planned or suspected, pregnancy (C), avoid breastfeeding

Evaluation

Positive therapeutic outcome

• Decrease in depression

• Absence of suicidal thoughts

TREATMENT OF OVERDOSE:

ECG monitoring, induce emesis, lavage, activated charcoal, administer anticonvulsant

treprostinil (Rx)

(treh-prah'stin-ill)

Remodulin, Tyvaso

Func. class.: Antihypertensive vasodilator

Chem. class.: Tricyclic benzidine prostacy-clin analog

Pregnancy category B

ACTION: Direct vasodilatation of pulmonary, systemic arterial vascular beds, inhibition of platelet aggregation

Therapeutic outcome: Decreased pulmonary arterial hypertension (PAH)

USES: PAH, NYHA class II through IV

CONTRAINDICATIONS:

Hypersensitivity to this product or other prostacyclin analogs

Precautions: Pregnancy **B**, breastfeeding, children, geriatric, past hepatic disease, renal/thromboembolic disease, abrupt discontinuation, **IV** administration

DOSAGE AND ROUTES

Pulmonary arterial hypertension (WHO group 1)

Adult: SUBCUT INF 1.25 ng/kg/min by cont INF, may reduce to 0.625 ng if not tolerated; may increase by 1.25 ng/kg/min qwk for first 4 wk, then 2.5 ng/kg/min qwk for remainder of INF; oral INH 3 breaths via Tyvaso INH system qid

Hepatic dose

Adult: SUBCUT INF 0.625 ng/kg ideal body weight/min and increase cautiously

Available forms: Inj 1, 2.5, 5, 10 mg/ml; neb sol 1.74 mg/2.9 ml

Implementation

SUBCUT INF route

• By continuous subcut infusion

• No dilution required

CONT IV INF route

• By surgically placed CV catheter using an ambulatory inf pump

• The IV pump, product, and patient education can be obtained from Priority Healthcare in the United States

• Must be diluted with sterile water for inj or 0.9% NaCl

• Calculate the concentration using this formula: diluted conc = [dose (ng/kg/min) × weight (kg) × 0.00006]/inf rate (ml/hr)

• Sudden decreased doses or abrupt withdrawal may worsen pulmonary atrial hypertension symptoms

Oral inhalation route

• Avoid skin or eyes, do not take orally; use Tyvaso Inhalation System only

• Patient should have a backup Optineb-ir device to avoid interruptions

• Follow instructions for use and cleaning

• Do not mix with other medications in Optineb-ir device

• Twist off cap and squeeze total contents into medicine cup, volume is sufficient for 4 treatments

ADVERSE EFFECTS

CNS: Dizziness, headache, syncope

CV: Vasodilatation, *hypotension, edema,* right ventricular heart failure

GI: Nausea, *diarrhea*

INTEG: *Rash,* pruritus

OTHER: Jaw pain, cough, throat irritation

SYST: Infusion site reactions, inf site pain, increased risk of infection

Pharmacokinetics

Absorption	Unknown
Distribution	Unknown
Metabolism	Liver, 90% protein binding
Excretion	Urine, feces
Half-life	2-4 hr, terminal

Pharmacodynamics

Unknown

INTERACTIONS

Individual drug

Aspirin: increased risk of bleeding

Drug classifications

Anticoagulants, NSAIDs, SSRIs, thrombin inhibitors: increased risk of bleeding

Antihypertensives, β-blockers, calcium channel blockers, diuretics, MAOIs, vasodilators: increased hypotension

NURSING CONSIDERATIONS

Assessment

• **Hypertension:** monitor B/P baseline and periodically

• Monitor liver function tests: AST, ALT, bilirubin, creatinine (long-term therapy)

⚠ **Monitor blood tests: CBC; CBC q2wk × 3 mo, Hct, Hgb, pro-time (long-term therapy), ABGs**

⚠ Monitor bleed time baseline and throughout; levels may be 2-5 × normal limit

Patient/family education
- Teach patient that blood work will be necessary during treatment
- Teach patient to report side effects such as diarrhea, skin rashes
- Teach patient that therapy will be needed for prolonged periods of time, sometimes years
- Advise patient that aseptic technique must be used in preparing and administering to prevent infection
- Teach that there are many drug and herb interactions
- Teach signs/symptoms of bleeding: blood in urine, stools
- Teach patient to avoid abrupt discontinuation
- Teach patient how to use inhaled solution and how to care for equipment

Evaluation
Positive therapeutic outcome
- Decreased pulmonary arterial hypertension

---

tretinoin (vitamin A acid, retinoic acid) (Rx)
(tret´i-noyn)
Avita, Renova, Retin-A, Retin-A Micro, Stieva-A ✦

Func. class.: Vitamin A acid/acne product, antineoplastic—miscellaneous
Chem. class.: Tretinoin derivative
Pregnancy category C (TOPICAL), D (PO)

ACTION: (Topical) Decreases cohesiveness of follicular epithelium, decreases microcomedone formation; (PO) induces maturation of acute promyelocytic leukemia, exact action is unknown

Therapeutic outcome: Decreased signs/symptoms of leukemia

USES: (Topical) Acne vulgaris (grades 1-3); (PO) acute promylocytic leukemia, facial wrinkles, photoaging

Unlabeled uses: Acne rosacea, actinic keratosis, ichthyosis, Kaposi's sarcoma, keloids, keratosis follicularis, melasma

CONTRAINDICATIONS:
Hypersensitivity to retinoids or sensitivity to parabens

> **BLACK BOX WARNING:** Pregnancy **D** (PO)

Precautions: Pregnancy **C** (topical), breast-feeding, eczema, sunburn, sun exposure

> **BLACK BOX WARNING:** Rapid-evolving leukocytosis, respiratory compromise, acute promyelocytic leukemia differentiation syndrome

DOSAGE AND ROUTES
Adult and child: TOP cleanse area, apply 0.025%-0.1% cream or 0.05% liquid at bedtime; cover lightly

Promyelocytic leukemia
Adult: PO 45 mg/m²/day given as 2 evenly divided doses until remission; discontinue treatment 30 days after remission or after 90 days of treatment, whichever is first

Available forms: Topical cream 0.01%, 0.02%, 0.025%, 0.05%, 0.1%; topical gel 0.025%, 0.04%, 0.05%, 0.1%; topical liquid 0.05%; caps 10 mg

Implementation
Topical route
- Apply using gloves or cotton, once daily before bedtime; cover area lightly using gauze
- Store at room temperature
- Wash hands after application
- Apply only to affected areas

ADVERSE EFFECTS
PO route
CNS: Headache, fever, sweating, fatigue
CV: Cardiac dysrhythmias, pericardial effusion
GI: Nausea, vomiting, **hemorrhage,** abdominal pain, diarrhea, constipation, dyspepsia, distention, **hepatitis**
META: Hypercholesterolemia, hypertriglyceridemia
RESP: Pneumonia, upper respiratory tract disease

Topical route
INTEG: Rash, stinging, warmth, redness, erythema, blistering, crusting, peeling, contact dermatitis, hypo/hyperpigmentation, dry skin, pruritus, scaly skin, retinoic acid syndrome (RAS)

Pharmacokinetics

Absorption	Small amounts
Distribution	Unknown
Metabolism	Unknown
Excretion	Kidneys
Half-life	Unknown

Pharmacodynamics

Unknown

INTERACTIONS
Individual drugs
Aminocaproic acid, aprotinin, tranexamic acid: increased thrombotic complications

Benzoyl peroxide, resorcinol, salicylic acid (topical), sulfur: increased peeling

Ketoconazole: increased plasma concentrations of tretinoin (oral)

Drug classifications
Alcohol, astringents, cleansers with drying effect, medicated, abrasive soaps: use with caution (topical)

Diuretics (thiazide), phenothiazines, quinolones, retinoids, sulfonamides, sulfonylureas: increased photosensitivity

Tetracyclines: increased ICP, risk of pseudotumor cerebri; do not use together

Drug/lab test
Increased: AST, ALT

NURSING CONSIDERATIONS
Assessment
Topical route
• Assess part of body involved, including time involved, what helps or aggravates condition, cysts, dryness, itching; lesions may become worse at beginning of treatment

PO route
• Monitor hepatic function, coagulation, hematologic parameters, also cholesterol, triglycerides

Patient/family education
Topical route
• Instruct patient to avoid application on normal skin, to avoid getting cream in eyes, nose, other mucous membranes
• Advise patient to avoid sunlight, sunlamps or to use protective clothing or sunscreen to prevent burns
• Advise patient that treatment may cause warmth, stinging; dryness, peeling will occur
• Inform patient that cosmetics may be used over product; not to use shaving lotions
• Inform patient that rash may occur during first 1-3 wk of therapy
• Caution patient that product does not cure condition, only relieves symptoms; that therapeutic results may be seen in 2-3 wk but may not be optimal until after 6 wk

PO route

> **BLACK BOX WARNING:** Advise patient to report to prescriber if pregnancy is planned or suspected, pregnancy **D** (PO)

Evaluation
Positive therapeutic outcome
• Decrease in size and number of lesions

tretinoin topical
See Appendix B

triamcinolone (Rx)
(trye-am-sin'oh-lone)
Aristospan, Kenalog-10, Kenalog-40, Tac-3, Tac-40, Triesence
Func. class.: Corticosteroid, synthetic; antiinflammatory
Chem. class.: Glucocorticoid, intermediate-acting
Pregnancy category C

ACTION: Decreases inflammation by suppressing migration of polymorphonuclear leukocytes, fibroblasts, reversal of increased capillary permeability and lysosomal stabilization

Therapeutic outcome: Decreased inflammation, normal immune response

USES: Severe inflammation, immunosuppression, neoplasms, asthma (steroid dependent), collagen, respiratory, dermatologic disorders, rheumatic disorders

CONTRAINDICATIONS:
Hypersensitivity, neonatal prematurity, epidural/intrathecal administration (triamcinolone acetonide injections [Kenalog]), systemic fungal infections

Precautions: Pregnancy **C,** breastfeeding, diabetes mellitus, glaucoma, osteoporosis, seizure disorders, ulcerative colitis, CHF, myasthenia gravis, renal disease, esophagitis, peptic ulcer, acne, cataracts, coagulopathy, head trauma, children <2 yr, psychosis, idiopathic thrombocytopenia, acute glomerulonephritis, amebiasis, fungal infections, nonasthmatic bronchial disease, AIDS, TB, adrenal insufficiency, acute bronchospasm, acne rosacea, Cushing's syndrome, acute MI, thromboembolism

DOSAGE AND ROUTES

Adult: IM 40 mg qwk (acetonide), 5-48 mg into neoplasms (acetonide), 2-40 mg into joint or soft tissue (hexacetonide), 0.5 mg/sq in of affected intralesional skin (hexacetonide), 2-20 mg into joint or soft tissue (hexacetonide)

Severe/incapacitating allergic conditions such as asthma

Adult: IM (Trivaris) 60 mg, titrate; usual range 40-80 mg

Child: IM (Trivaris) 0.11-1.6 mg/kg/day (3.2-48 mg/m²/day) given in 3-4 divided doses

Available forms: Inj 3, 10, 40 mg/ml acetonide; inj 5, 20 mg/ml hexacetonide; inh 100 mcg/spray

Implementation
PO route
• Give with food or milk to decrease GI symptoms; tablet may be crushed
IM route
• Give IM inj deeply in large muscle mass; rotate sites; avoid deltoid; use 21-G needle
• Avoid SUBCUT administration, may damage tissue
Inhalation route
• Use spacer device for geriatric
• Give inh with water to decrease possibility of fungal infections; titrated dose, use lowest effective dose
• Give after cleaning aerosol top daily with warm water, dry thoroughly
• Store in cool environment; do not puncture or incinerate container
Topical route
• Apply only to affected areas; do not get in eyes
• Apply medication, then cover with occlusive dressing (only if prescribed), seal to normal skin, change q12hr; systemic absorption may occur
• Apply only to dermatoses; do not use on weeping, denuded, or infected areas
• Cleanse skin before applying product
• Continue treatment for a few days after area has cleared
• Store at room temperature
Nasal route
• Have patient clear nasal passages before administration; use decongestant if needed; shake inhaler, invert, tilt head backward, insert nozzle into nostril, away from septum; hold other nostril closed and depress activator, inhale through nose, exhale through mouth

ADVERSE EFFECTS

CNS: *Depression,* headache, mood changes
CV: *Hypertension,* **circulatory collapse, embolism,** tachycardia, edema
EENT: Fungal infections, increased intraocular pressure, blurred vision
GI: *Diarrhea, nausea, abdominal distention,* **GI hemorrhage,** *increased appetite,* **pancreatitis**
HEMA: **Thrombocytopenia**
INTEG: Acne, poor wound healing, ecchymosis, petechiae
MS: Fractures, osteoporosis, weakness

Pharmacokinetics

Absorption	Well absorbed (PO, IM)
Distribution	Crosses placenta, widely distributed
Metabolism	Liver, extensively
Excretion	Kidney, breast milk
Half-life	2-5 hr, adrenal suppression 3-4 days

Pharmacodynamics

	PO	IM	TOPICAL	INH	INTRANASAL
Onset	Unknown	Unknown	Min to hr	1-2 wk	Unknown
Peak	1-2 hr	1-2 hr	Hr to days	Unknown	2-3 wk
Duration	3 days	Unknown	Hr to days	Unknown	Unknown

INTERACTIONS
Individual drugs
Alcohol, amphotericin B, cycloSPORINE, digoxin, indomethacin, quinolones: increased side effects

Ambenonium, isoniazid, neostigmine, somatrem: decreased effects of each specific product

Cholestyramine, colestipol, ePHEDrine, phenytoin, rifampin, theophylline: decreased action of triamcinolone

Indomethacin, ketoconazole: increased action of triamcinolone

Drug classifications
Anticholinesterases, anticoagulants, anticonvulsants, antidiabetics, salicylates: decreased effects of each specific product

Antidiabetic agents: increased need for antidiabetic agents

Antiinfectives (macrolide), carBAMazepine, contraceptives (oral), estrogens, salicylates: increased action of triamcinolone

Barbiturates: decreased action of triamcinolone

Diuretics, salicylates: increased side effects

Toxoids, vaccines: decreased effects of toxoids, vaccines

Drug/herb
Aloe, cascara sagrada, senna: increased hypokalemia

Drug/lab test
Increased: cholesterol, sodium, blood glucose, uric acid, calcium, urine glucose

Decreased: calcium, potassium, T_4, T_3, thyroid ^{131}I uptake test, urine 17-OHCS, 17-KS

False negative: skin allergy tests

NURSING CONSIDERATIONS
Assessment
• Monitor potassium, blood glucose, urine glucose while on long-term therapy; hypokalemia and hyperglycemia

• Monitor weight daily; notify prescriber of weekly gain >5 lb; I&O ratio; be alert for decreasing urinary output and increasing edema

• Monitor B/P q4hr, pulse; notify prescriber if chest pain occurs

• Monitor plasma cortisol levels during long-term therapy (normal level 138-635 nmol/L [SI units] when measured at 8 AM); adrenal function periodically for hypothalamic-pituitary-adrenal axis suppression

• Assess for infection: increased temp, WBC even after withdrawal of medication; product masks infection symptoms

• Assess for potassium depletion: paresthesias, fatigue, nausea, vomiting, depression, polyuria, dysrhythmias, weakness

• Assess mental status: affect, mood, behavioral changes, aggression

• Assess nasal passages during long-term treatment for changes in mucus (nasal)

• Monitor temp; if fever develops, product should be discontinued

• Assess for systemic absorption: increased temp, inflammation, irritation (topical)

Patient/family education
• Advise patient that emergency ID as corticosteroid user should be carried/worn; not to discontinue abruptly, taper dose

• Instruct patient to notify prescriber if therapeutic response decreases; dosage adjustment may be needed

• Caution patient to avoid OTC products: salicylates, alcohol in cough products, cold preparations unless directed by prescriber; to avoid live vaccines

• Advise patient on all aspects of product use including cushingoid symptoms

• Teach patient symptoms of adrenal insufficiency: nausea, anorexia, fatigue, dizziness, dyspnea, weakness, joint pain

• Teach patient that long-term therapy may be needed to clear infection (1-2 mo depending on type of infection)

Inhalation route
• Teach patient proper administration technique; to wash inhaler with warm water and dry after each use

• Teach patient all aspects of product use including cushingoid symptoms

Topical route
• Instruct patient to avoid sunlight on affected area; burns may occur

Nasal route
• Instruct patient to clear nasal passages if sneezing attack occurs, repeat dose

• Advise patient to continue using product even if mild nasal bleeding occurs; is usually transient

• Teach patient method of instillation after providing written instruction from manufacturer

Evaluation
Positive therapeutic outcome
• Decrease in runny nose (nasal)

• Decreased dyspnea, wheezing, dry crackles on auscultation (inh)

• Ease of respirations, decreased inflammation

• Absence of severe itching, patches on skin, flaking (topical)

triamcinolone nasal agent
See Appendix B

triamcinolone ophthalmic
See Appendix B

triamcinolone topical
See Appendix B

triazolam (Rx)
(trye-az'oh-lam)
**Apo-Triazo ✢, Gen-Triazolam ✢,
Halcion**
Func. class.: Sedative-hypnotic, antianxiety
Chem. class.: Benzodiazepine, short acting
Pregnancy category X
**Controlled substance schedule IV
(USA), targeted (CDSA IV) (Canada)**

Do not confuse:
Halcion/Haldol/halcinonide

ACTION: Produces CNS depression at limbic, thalamic, hypothalamic levels of CNS; may be mediated by neurotransmitter; γ-aminobutyric acid (GABA); results are sedation, hypnosis, skeletal muscle relaxation, anticonvulsant activity, anxiolytic action

Therapeutic outcome: Decreased anxiety, insomnia

USES: Insomnia (short-term), sedative/hypnotic

CONTRAINDICATIONS:
Pregnancy **X**, breastfeeding, hypersensitivity to benzodiazepines

Precautions: Children <15 yr, geriatric, anemia, renal/hepatic disease, suicidal individuals, product abuse, psychosis, acute closed-angle glaucoma, seizure disorders, angioedema, respiratory disease, depression, sleep-related behaviors (sleep walking), intermittent porphyria, myasthenia gravis, Parkinson's disease

DOSAGE AND ROUTES
Adult: PO 0.125-0.5 mg at bedtime, max 0.5 mg/day
Geriatric: PO 0.0625-0.125 mg at bedtime, max 0.25 mg/day

Available forms: Tabs 0.125, 0.25 mg

Implementation
• Give with food or milk to decrease GI symptoms; if patient is unable to swallow medication whole, tab may be crushed and mixed with food or fluid
• Give sugarless gum, hard candy, frequent sips of water for dry mouth

ADVERSE EFFECTS
CNS: *Headache, lethargy, drowsiness, daytime sedation,* dizziness, confusion, light-headedness, anxiety, irritability, amnesia, poor coordination, complex sleep-related reactions (sleep driving, sleep eating)
CV: Chest pain, pulse changes, ECG changes
GI: Nausea, vomiting, diarrhea, heartburn, abdominal pain, constipation, **hepatic injury**
SYST: Severe allergic reactions

Pharmacokinetics

Absorption	Well absorbed
Distribution	Widely distributed, crosses placenta, crosses blood-brain barrier
Metabolism	Liver
Excretion	Kidneys, breast milk
Half-life	1.5-5.5 hr

Pharmacodynamics

Onset	15-30 min
Peak	Unknown
Duration	6-8 hr

INTERACTIONS
Individual drugs
Alcohol: increased action of both products
Cimetidine, clarithromycin, disulfiram, erythromycin, isoniazid, probenecid: increased effects; do not use concurrently
Rifampin: decreased action of rifampin
Theophylline: decreased effects of theophylline

Drug classifications
Antacids: decreased effects of antacids
Antiinfectives (clarithromycin): increased effects
CNS depressants: increased effects of both products
Contraceptives (oral): increased effects; do not use concurrently
CYP3A4 inhibitors, protease inhibitors: increased triazolam levels
Smoking: decreased hypnotic effects

Drug/food
Grapefruit may increase action, avoid concurrent use

Drug/herb
Chamomile, hops, kava, lavender, valerian:
increased CNS depression

Drug/lab test
Increased: AST, ALT, serum bilirubin
Decreased: radioactive iodine uptake
False increase: 17-OHCS

NURSING CONSIDERATIONS
Assessment
• Assess patient's mental status: mood,
sensorium, anxiety, affect, sleeping pattern,
drowsiness, dizziness, especially geriatric; physical dependency, withdrawal symptoms: anxiety,
panic attacks, agitation, seizures, headache,
nausea, vomiting, muscle pain, weakness;
suicidal tendencies; for indications of increasing
tolerance and abuse
• Monitor patient's B/P (lying, standing), pulse;
if systolic B/P drops 20 mm Hg, hold product,
notify prescriber
• Monitor blood tests: CBC during long-term
therapy; blood dyscrasias have occurred rarely;
decreased hematocrit, neutropenia may occur
• Monitor liver function tests: AST, ALT, bilirubin, creatinine LDH, alkaline phosphatase
• Monitor I&O ratio; indicate renal dysfunction

Patient/family education
• Advise patient that product may be taken with
food or fluids, and tab may be crushed or swallowed whole
• Caution patient not to use for everyday
stress or longer than 3 mo unless directed by
prescriber; not to take more than prescribed
amount; may be habit forming; not to double
doses or skip doses
• Instruct patient to avoid OTC preparations
unless approved by prescriber; alcohol and CNS
depressants will increase CNS depression
• Caution patient to avoid driving, activities
that require alertness because drowsiness may
occur; to avoid alcohol ingestion or other psychotropic medications; to rise slowly or fainting
may occur, especially geriatric; that drowsiness
may worsen at beginning of treatment
• Teach patient to use reliable contraception,
pregnancy **X**
• Teach patient that complex sleep-related
behaviors (sleep eating/driving) may occur
• Advise patient not to discontinue medication abruptly after long-term use; withdrawal
symptoms include vomiting, cramping, tremors,
seizures; decrease dosage by 50% q2nights until
0.125 mg for 2 nights, then stop

Evaluation
Positive therapeutic outcome
• Decreased anxiety, restlessness, sleeplessness
(short-term treatment only)

TREATMENT OF OVERDOSE:
Lavage, VS, supportive care

trifluridine ophthalmic
See Appendix B

trimethobenzamide (Rx)
(trye-meth-oh-ben'za-mide)
Tigan
Func. class.: Antiemetic, anticholinergic
Chem. class.: Ethanolamine derivative
Pregnancy category C

ACTION: Acts centrally by blocking
chemoreceptor trigger zone, which in turn acts
on vomiting center

Therapeutic outcome: Absence of
nausea and vomiting

USES: Nausea, vomiting, prevention of
postoperative vomiting

CONTRAINDICATIONS:
Children (parenterally), hypersensitivity to
opioids, shock

Precautions: Pregnancy **C**, children,
geriatric, cardiac dysrhythmias, acute febrile illness, encephalitis, gastroenteritis, dehydration,
electrolyte imbalances, Reye's syndrome

DOSAGE AND ROUTES
Postoperative vomiting
Adult: IM 200 mg followed by a second dose
1 hr later

Nausea/vomiting
Adult: PO 300 mg tid-qid; IM 200 mg tid-qid

Renal dose
Adult: IM CCr 15-30 ml/min give 50% of dose

Available forms: Caps 300 mg; inj 100
mg/ml

Implementation
PO route
• Cap may be swallowed whole or opened and
mixed with food or fluids
IM route
• Administer IM inj in large muscle mass;
aspirate to avoid **IV** administration

- Patient should remain lying down for 30 min after IM inj

Syringe compatibilities: Glycopyrrolate, HYDROmorphone, midazolam, nalbuphine

ADVERSE EFFECTS
CNS: *Drowsiness,* headache, dizziness, confusion, *vertigo,* EPS, disorientation, **coma, seizures,** depression
CV: Hyper/hypotension, palpitations, **cardiac dysrhythmias**
EENT: Dry mouth, blurred vision, photosensitivity
GI: Nausea, diarrhea, vomiting, difficulty swallowing
INTEG: Rash, urticaria, fever, chills, flushing, hyperpyrexia

Pharmacokinetics
Absorption	Unknown
Distribution	Unknown
Metabolism	Liver, extensively
Excretion	Kidneys
Half-life	Unknown

Pharmacodynamics
	PO	IM	RECT
Onset	20-40 min	15 min	10-40 min
Peak	Unknown	Unknown	Unknown
Duration	3-4 hr	2-3 hr	3-4 hr

INTERACTIONS
Individual drugs
Alcohol: increased effect

Drug classifications
CNS depressants: increased effect

NURSING CONSIDERATIONS
Assessment
- Monitor VS, B/P; check patients with cardiac disease more often
- Assess for signs of toxicity of other products or masking of symptoms of disease: brain tumor, intestinal obstructions
- Observe for drowsiness, dizziness
- Assess for nausea, vomiting before and after treatment

Patient/family education
- Teach patient to use good oral hygiene; frequent rinsing of mouth, sugarless gum for dry mouth
- Caution patient to avoid hazardous activities until product response is determined; drowsiness may occur
- Inform patient that orthostatic hypotension occurs often and to rise from sitting or lying position gradually; avoid hot tubs, hot showers, and tub baths because hypotension may occur
- Advise patient to remain lying down after IM inj for at least 30 min
- Inform patient that in hot weather, heat stroke may occur; take extra precautions to stay cool
- Teach patient to avoid OTC preparations (cough, hay fever, cold) unless approved by prescriber, serious product interactions may occur; avoid use with alcohol, CNS depressants, increased drowsiness may occur
- Teach patient about EPS
- Instruct patient to report sore throat, malaise, fever, bleeding, mouth sores; if these occur, CBC should be performed and product discontinued

Evaluation
Positive therapeutic outcome
- Decreased nausea, vomiting

triptorelin (Rx)
(trip-toe′rel-in)
Trelstar, Trelstar Depot, Trelstar LA
Func. class.: Gonadotropin-releasing hormone antagonist
Chem. class.: Synthetic decapeptide analog of LHRH
Pregnancy category X

ACTION: Inhibitor of pituitary gonadotropin secretion; initially increases LH and FSH, with increases in testosterone, reduction in sex steroid levels

Therapeutic outcome: Decreased signs/symptoms of advanced prostate cancer

USES: Advanced prostate cancer

CONTRAINDICATIONS:
Pregnancy **X**, breastfeeding, hypersensitivity to this product or other LHRH agonists or LHRH

Precautions: Metastatic vertebral lesions, urinary tract obstruction, spinal cord compression, renal disease

DOSAGE AND ROUTES
Adult: IM 3.75 mg q4wk; 11.25 mg q12wk, 22.5 mg q24wk

Available forms: Microgranules, depot inj 3.75 mg, 11.25 mg

Implementation
• Give IM using implant, inserted by qualified person
• Use syringe with 20-G needle, withdraw 2 ml of sterile water for inj, inject into vial, shake well, withdraw vial contents, inject immediately

ADVERSE EFFECTS
CNS: Headache, insomnia, dizziness, lability, fatigue
CV: *Hypertension,* peripheral edema
ENDO: Gynecomastia, breast tenderness, hot flashes
GI: Nausea, vomiting, diarrhea
GU: Impotence, urinary retention, UTI
INTEG: Rash, pain on injection, pruritus, hypersensitivity
MISC: Anaphylaxis, angioedema
MS: Osteoneuralgia

Pharmacokinetics	
Absorption	Unknown
Distribution	Unknown
Metabolism	CYP450
Excretion	Liver, kidneys
Half-life	3 hr

Pharmacodynamics
Unknown

INTERACTIONS
Drug/lab test
Increased: alk phos, estradiol, FSH, LH, testosterone levels
Decreased: testosterone levels, progesterone

NURSING CONSIDERATIONS
Assessment
• **Assess for severe hypersensitivity:** discontinue product and give antihistamines, have emergency equipment nearby
• Monitor I&O ratios; palpate bladder for distention in urinary obstruction
• Monitor for relief of bone pain (back pain)
• Assess levels of testosterone and PSA

Patient/family education
• Teach patient that gynecomastia may occur but will decrease after treatment is discontinued
• Advise patient to report allergic reaction immediately
• Teach patient that disease flare may occur at beginning of therapy

Evaluation
Positive therapeutic outcome
• More normal levels of PSA, acid phosphatase, alkaline phosphatase, testosterone level of <25 ng/dl, tumor response

tropicamide ophthalmic
See Appendix B

trospium (Rx)
(trose'pee-um)
Sanctura, Sanctura XR
Func. class.: Anticholinergic, overactive bladder product, urinary antispasmodic
Chem. class.: Muscarinic receptor antagonist
Pregnancy category C

ACTION: Relaxes smooth muscles in bladder by inhibiting acetylcholine effect on muscarinic receptors

Therapeutic outcome: Absence of bladder distention, nocturia, frequency, urgency, incontinence

USES: Overactive bladder (urinary frequency, urgency)

CONTRAINDICATIONS:
Hypersensitivity, uncontrolled closed-angle glaucoma, urinary retention, gastric retention, myasthenia gravis

Precautions: Pregnancy **C**, breastfeeding, children, renal/hepatic disease, controlled closed-angle glaucoma, ulcerative colitis, intestinal atony, bladder outflow obstruction

DOSAGE AND ROUTES
Adult: PO 20 mg bid, give 5 ml ≥1 hr prior to meals or on empty stomach ER 60 mg qAM

Renal dose
Adult: PO CCr < 30 ml/min 20 mg/day at bedtime
Geriatric ≥75 yr: PO titrate down to 20 mg/day based on response and tolerance

Available forms: Tabs 20 mg caps ER 60 mg

Implementation
• Take 1 hr before meals or on empty stomach

ADVERSE EFFECTS
CNS: Fatigue, dizziness, headache
CV: Tachycardia

EENT: Dry eyes, vision abnormalities
GI: Flatulence, abdominal pain, *constipation, dry mouth,* dyspepsia
GU: Urinary retention, UTI
INTEG: Dry skin, **angioedema**
MISC: **Heat stroke,** fever

Pharmacokinetics

Absorption	Rapidly absorbed (10%)
Distribution	Protein bound (50%-85%)
Metabolism	Not fully understood in humans; extensively metabolized
Excretion	Urine (6%), feces (85%); excreted in urine by active tubular secretion
Half-life	Unknown

Pharmacodynamics

Unknown

INTERACTIONS
Individual drugs
Alcohol: increased drowsiness
MetFORMIN, procainamide, quiNIDine, ranitidine, tenofovir, triamterene, vancomycin: increased or decreased action of trospium

Drug classifications
CNS depressants: increased drowsiness
Products excreted by active renal secretion (aMILoride, digoxin, morphine): increased or decreased action of trospium

Drug/food
High-fat meal: decreased absorption

NURSING CONSIDERATIONS
Assessment
• **Assess urinary patterns:** distention, nocturia, frequency, urgency, incontinence, voiding patterns

Patient/family education
• Advise patient to avoid hazardous activities; dizziness may occur
• Caution patient that alcohol may increase drowsiness
• Inform patient about anticholinergic effects that may occur
• Teach patient to avoid all other products unless approved by prescriber

Evaluation
Positive therapeutic outcome
• Correction of urinary status: absence of dysuria, frequency, nocturia, incontinence

uliprista (Rx)

(ue'li-pris'tal)

Ella

Func. class.: Progesterone agonist/
antagonist-abortifacient

Pregnancy category X

ACTION: Binds to the progesterone receptor and prevents progesterone from occupying the receptor, postpones follicular rupture when taken immediately prior to ovulation

Therapeutic outcome: Absence of pregnancy

USES: Emergency contraception

CONTRAINDICATIONS:

Pregnancy **X,** children/infants/neonates, postmenopausal females

Precautions: History of ectopic pregnancy, HIV

DOSAGE AND ROUTES

Adult/adolescent females: PO 30 mg (1 tab) as soon as possible within 120 hr (5 days) of unprotected intercourse or a known or suspected contraceptive failure

Available forms: Tab 30 mg

Implementation

• Administer without regard to food
• Store at room temperature, protect from light

ADVERSE EFFECTS

CNS: Dizziness, headache, fatigue
GI: Nausea, vomiting, abdominal pain
GU: Dysmenorrhea, breakthrough bleeding
INTEG: Acne vulgaris

Pharmacokinetics

Absorption	Unknown
Distribution	Protein binding >94%
Metabolism	Metabolized by CYP3A4
Excretion	Unknown
Half-life	Terminal half-life 27-38 hrs

Pharmacodynamics

Onset	Unknown
Peak	1 hr
Duration	Unknown

INTERACTIONS

Individual drugs

Bosentan, carBAMazepine, felbamate, griseofulvin, OXcarbazepine, phenytoin, rifampin, St. John's wort, topiramate, bexarotene, dexamethasone, etravirine, flutamide, metyrapone, modafinil, nafcillin, nevirapine, pioglitazone, rifabutin, itraconazole, ketoconazole: decreased effect of ulipristal

Aldesleukin, IL-2, amiodarone, atazanavir, basiliximab, chloramphenicol, cimetidine, clarithromycin, dalfopristin, danazol, darunavir, delavirdine, diltiazem, dronedarone, erythromycin, fluconazole, FLUoxetine, fluvoxaMINE, imatinib, isoniazid, lapatinib, nefazodone, nelfinavir, niCARdipine, octreotide, pantoprazole, quinupristin, ranolazine, saquinavir, tamoxifen, telithromycin, tipranavir, verapamil, voriconazole, zafirlukast: increased ulipristal effect and adverse reactions

Aprepitant, fosaprepitant, efavirenz, fosamprenavir, quiNINE, ritonavir: increased or decreased ulipristal effect

Drug classifications

Regular hormonal contraceptive methods: decreased contraceptive action

CYP3A4 inducers, barbiturates: decreased effect of ulipristal

CYP3A4 inhibitors: increased ulipristal effect and adverse reactions

Drug/herb

St. John's wort: decreased effect of ulipristal

NURSING CONSIDERATIONS

Assessment

• **Assess need for emergency contraception,** pregnancy planned or suspected, obtain pregnancy test before use (pregnancy **X**)
• Assess medications taken, many drug interactions may occur

Patient/family education

• Instruct patient that if vomiting occurs within 3 hours of taking the tablet, consider repeating the dose
• Advise patient to report to provider any side effects
• Explain reason for medication and expected results
• Advise patient to avoid use in breastfeeding

Evaluation

Positive therapeutic outcome
• Absence of pregnancy

undecylenic acid topical

See Appendix B

unoprostone ophthalmic

See Appendix B

---

valacyclovir (Rx)

(val-a-sye′kloh-vir)

Valtrex

Func. class.: Antiviral

Chem. class.: Synthetic acyclic purine nucleoside analog

Pregnancy category B

Do not confuse:

valacyclovir/valganciclovir, **Valtrex**/Valcyte

ACTION: Interferes with DNA synthesis by conversion to acyclovir, causing decreased viral replication, time of lesional healing

Therapeutic outcome: Absence of itching, painful lesions; crusting and healing of lesions

USES: Treatment or suppression of herpes zoster (shingles), recurrent genital herpes, herpes labialis (cold sores), varicella, varicella-zoster

Unlabeled uses: Prevention of CMV infection in advanced HIV, posttransplant patients, Bell's palsy, herpes simplex virus prophylaxis

CONTRAINDICATIONS:

Hypersensitivity to this product, acyclovir, valganciclovir

Precautions: Pregnancy **B**, breastfeeding, geriatric, renal/hepatic disease, electrolyte imbalance, dehydration, hypersensitivity to penciclovir, famciclovir, ganciclovir, varicella

DOSAGE AND ROUTES

Genital herpes (suppressive initial)

Adult: PO 1 g bid × 10 days initially

Genital herpes (recurrent episodes)

Adult: PO 500 mg bid × 3 days

Genital herpes (suppressive therapy)

Adult: PO 1 g/day with normal immune function; 500 mg/day for those with ≤9 recurrences/yr; 500 mg bid in HIV-infected patients with CD4 ≥100

Reduction of transmission

Adult: PO 500 mg/day for source partner

Herpes zoster (shingles)

Adult: PO 1 g tid × 1 wk

Herpes labialis

Adult: PO 2 g bid × 1 day at first sign of lesions

Varicella (chickenpox) in immunocompetent patients

Adolescent and child ≥2 yr: PO 20 mg/kg/dose tid × 5 days, max 3 g/day; start at first sign, preferably within 24 hr of rash

Renal dose

Adult: PO CCr 30-49 ml/min 1g q12hr (herpes zoster); 1 g q12hr × 1 day (herpes labialis); CCr 10-29 ml/min 1 g q24hr (genital herpes/herpes zoster); 500 mg q24hr (recurrent genital herpes); CCr <10 ml/min 500 mg q24hr (genital herpes/herpes zoster), 500 mg q24hr (recurrent genital herpes)

Available forms: Tabs 500, 1000 mg

Implementation

• Give within 72 hr of outbreak (herpes zoster); as soon as possible (herpes labialis, genital herpes)

• Give orally before infection occurs

• Store at room temp; protect from light, moisture

ADVERSE EFFECTS

CNS: Tremors, lethargy, *dizziness, headache, weakness,* depression

ENDO: *Dysmenorrhea*

GI: *Nausea, vomiting, diarrhea, abdominal pain, constipation,* increased AST

HEMA: Thrombocytopenic purpura, hemolytic uremic syndrome

INTEG: *Rash*

Pharmacokinetics	
Absorption	Unknown
Distribution	Crosses placenta, enters breast milk, protein binding 13.5%-17.9%
Metabolism	Converts to acyclovir
Excretion	Urine, as acyclovir
Half-life	2½-3½ hr

Pharmacodynamics
Unknown

INTERACTIONS

Individual drugs

Cimetidine, probenecid: increased blood levels of valacyclovir (only if renal disease is significant)

Drug/lab test

Increased: LFTs, creatinine

Decreased: WBC, platelets

NURSING CONSIDERATIONS
Assessment
• **Assess for signs of infection;** characteristics of lesions; therapy should be started at first sign of herpes and is most effective within 72 hr of outbreak
• Assess C&S before product therapy; product may be given as soon as culture is performed; repeat C&S after treatment; determine the presence of other STDs
• Assess bowel pattern before, during treatment
• Assess for skin eruptions: rash
• Assess allergies before treatment, reaction of each medication
⚠ Assess for thrombocytopenic purpura, hemolytic uremic syndrome, may be fatal

Patient/family education
• Advise patient to take as prescribed; if dose is missed, take as soon as remembered up to 2 hr before next dose; do not double dose
• Instruct patient to take product orally before infection occurs; product should be taken when itching or pain occurs, usually before eruptions
• Inform patient that partners need to be told that patient has herpes; they can become infected; condoms must be worn to prevent reinfections
• Tell patient that product does not cure infection, just controls symptoms and does not prevent infection to others

Evaluation
Positive therapeutic outcome
• Absence of itching, painful lesions; crusting and healed lesions

---

valganciclovir (Rx)
(val-gan-sy′kloh-veer)
Valcyte
Func. class.: Antiviral
Chem. class.: Synthetic nucleoside
Pregnancy category C

Do not confuse:
valganciclovir/valacyclovir, **Valcyte**/Valtrex

ACTION: Valganciclovir is metabolized to ganciclovir; inhibits replication of human CMV in vivo and in vitro by selectively inhibiting viral DNA synthesis

Therapeutic outcome: Decreased proliferation of virus responsible for CMV retinitis

USES: Cytomegalovirus (CMV) retinitis in immunocompromised persons, including those with AIDS, after indirect ophthalmoscopy confirms diagnosis; prevention of CMV in transplantation; prevention of CMV in patients at risk going through transplant (kidney, heart, pancreas)

CONTRAINDICATIONS:
Breastfeeding, hypersensitivity to ganciclovir or valacyclovir, absolute neutrophil count <500/mm^3, platelet count <25,000/mm^3, hemodialysis, liver transplant

Precautions: Pregnancy **C**, children, geriatric, renal function impairment, hypersensitivity to acyclovir, penciclovir, famciclovir

> **BLACK BOX WARNING:** Preexisting cytopenias, secondary malignancy, infertility, anemia

DOSAGE AND ROUTES
Treatment of CMV
Adult: PO induction 900 mg bid × 21 days with food; maintenance 900 mg/day with food

Transplant (CMV prophylaxis)
Adult/adolescent >16 yr: PO 900 mg/day with food starting within 10 days before transplantation until 100 days after transplantation
Infant ≥4 mo/child/adolescent ≤16 yr: PO give within 10 days of heart/kidney transplant; calculate dose as 7 × BSA × CCr and give a single daily dose

Renal dose
CCr ≥60 ml/min same dosage as above; CCr 40-59 ml/min 450 mg bid × 21 days, then 450 mg/day; CCr 25-39 ml/min 450 mg/day × 21 days, then 450 mg q2day; CCr 10-24 ml/min 450 mg q2day, then 450 mg 2 ×/week

Available forms: Tabs 450 mg; powder for oral sol 50 mg/ml

Implementation
PO tab
• Give with food for better absorption, avoid getting on skin, do not break tab
Oral SOL
• Measure 9 ml of purified water in graduated cylinder, shake bottle to loosen powder, add ½ liquid, shake well, add remaining water, shake, remove child-resistant cap and push bottle adapter into neck of bottle, close with cap, give using the dispenser provided
• Store liquid in refrigerator; do not freeze; throw away any unused portion after 49 days

ADVERSE EFFECTS
CNS: *Fever,* chills, **coma,** *confusion,* abnormal thoughts, dizziness, bizarre dreams,

---

⚠ Nurse Alert   ✹ Key NCLEX® Drug

headache, psychosis, tremors, somnolence, *paresthesia, weakness,* **seizures,** insomnia
EENT: Retinal detachment in CMV retinitis
GI: *Abnormal liver function tests, nausea, vomiting, anorexia, diarrhea, abdominal pain,* **hemorrhage**
GU: **Hematuria,** increased creatinine, BUN
HEMA: **Granulocytopenia, thrombocytopenia, irreversible neutropenia, anemia,** eosinophilia
INTEG: *Rash,* alopecia, *pruritus,* urticaria, pain at inj site, phlebitis, **Stevens-Johnson syndrome**
MISC: Local and systemic infections and sepsis

Pharmacokinetics

Absorption	Well absorbed from GI tract
Distribution	Plasma protein binding unknown; crosses blood-brain barrier, CSF
Metabolism	Rapidly metabolized in intestinal wall and liver to ganciclovir
Excretion	Kidneys (ganciclovir)
Half-life	3-4½ hr

Pharmacodynamics

Onset	Unknown
Peak	1-3 hr
Duration	Unknown

INTERACTIONS
Individual drugs
Adriamycin, amphotericin B, cycloSPORINE, dapsone, DOXOrubicin, flucytosine, pentamidine, trimethoprim/sulfamethoxazole, vinBLAStine, vinCRIStine: increased toxicity
Didanosine: increased effect; monitor for adverse effects, toxicity
Imipenem/cilastatin: increased seizures
Mycophenolate: increased effect of both drugs
Probenecid: decreased renal clearance of valganciclovir
Radiation, zidovudine: severe granulocytopenia; do not coadminister

Drug classifications
Antineoplastics, immunosuppressants: increased severe granulocytopenia; do not coadminister
Nucleoside analogs, other: increased toxicity

Drug/food
Absorption: increased with high-fat meal

Drug/lab test
Increased: creatinine
Decreased: RBC/WBC, Hct/Hgb

NURSING CONSIDERATIONS
Assessment

> **BLACK BOX WARNING:** Assess for leukopenia/neutropenia/thrombocytopenia: WBCs, platelets q2day during 2 ×/day dosing and then qwk

- Assess serum creatinine or CCr ≥q2wk
- Assess for CMV retinitis by ophthalmoscopy before beginning treatment and q2wk
- Obtain culture for CMV

Patient/family education
- Inform patient that product does not cure condition, that regular ophthalmologic and blood tests are necessary
- Caution patient that major toxicities may necessitate discontinuing product
⚠ Caution patient to use contraception during treatment and that infertility may occur; men should use barrier contraception for 90 days after treatment
- Instruct patient to take with food
⚠ Instruct patient to report seizures, dizziness; to avoid hazardous activities
- Caution patient to use sunscreen to prevent burns

Evaluation
Positive therapeutic outcome
- Decreased symptoms of CMV

TREATMENT OF OVERDOSE:
Maintain adequate hydration; dialysis may help reduce serum concentrations; consider use of hematopoietic growth factors

---

valproate (Rx)
(val-proh′ate)
Depacon
valproic acid (Rx)
Depakene, Stavzor
divalproex sodium (Rx)
Depakote, Depakote ER, Epival ✦
Func. class.: Anticonvulsant, vascular headache suppressant
Chem. class.: Carboxylic acid derivative
Pregnancy category D

ACTION: Increases levels of γ-aminobutyric acid (GABA) in the brain, which decreases seizure activity

Adverse effects: *italics* = common; **bold** = life-threatening

Therapeutic outcome: Decreased symptoms of epilepsy, bipolar disorder

USES: Simple (petit mal), complex (petit mal), absence, mixed seizures, manic episode associated with bipolar disorder, prophylaxis of migraine, adjunct in schizophrenia, tardive dyskinesia, aggression in children with ADHD, organic brain syndrome, tonic-clonic (grand mal)/myoclonic seizures

Unlabeled uses: Rectal for seizures (valproic acid)

CONTRAINDICATIONS:
Hypersensitivity, urea cycle disorders

> **BLACK BOX WARNING:** Pregnancy **D,** hepatic disease, pancreatitis

Precautions: Breastfeeding, geriatric

> **BLACK BOX WARNING:** Children <2 yr

DOSAGE AND ROUTES
Epilepsy
Adult and child: PO 10-15 mg/kg/day divided in 2-3 doses, may increase by 5-10 mg/kg/day qwk, max 60 mg/kg/day in 2-3 divided doses; **IV** ≤20 mg/min over 1 hr

Mania (divalproex sodium)
Adult: PO 750 mg/day in divided doses, max 60 mg/kg/day or 3000 mg/day

Mania (valproic acid: Stavzor)
Adult: DEL REL cap 750 mg/day in divided doses

Migraine (divalproex sodium)
Adult: PO 250 mg bid, may increase to 1000 mg/day; or 500 mg (Depakote ER) daily × 7 days, then 1000 mg/day

Available forms: Valproic acid: caps 250 mg; syr 250 mg/5 ml del rel cap (Stavzor) 125 mg; divalproex: del rel tabs 125, 250, 500 mg; ext rel tabs 250, 500 mg; sprinkle caps 125 mg; valproate: inj 100 mg/ml

Implementation
• Swallow tabs and caps whole; do not break, crush, or chew
• Sprinkle cap contents on food
• Give elixir alone; do not dilute with carbonated beverage; do not give syrup to patients on sodium restriction
• Give with food or milk to decrease GI symptoms

IV route
• Dilute dose with ≥50 ml D₅W, NS, LR
• Run over 60 min (20 mg/min)

ADVERSE EFFECTS
CNS: *Sedation, drowsiness,* dizziness, headache, incoordination, depression, hallucinations, behavioral changes, tremors, aggression, weakness, **coma, suicidal ideation**
CV: Hypotension/hypertension, chest pain, palpitations, peripheral edema
EENT: Visual disturbances, taste perversion
GI: *Nausea, vomiting, constipation, diarrhea, dyspepsia,* anorexia, cramps, **hepatic failure, pancreatitis, toxic hepatitis,** stomatitis, weight gain, dry mouth
GU: Enuresis, irregular menses
HEMA: **Thrombocytopenia, leukopenia, lymphocytosis,** increased pro-time, bruising, epistaxis, **pancytopenia**
INTEG: *Rash,* alopecia, photosensitivity, dry skin
META: Hyperammonemia, SIADH
RESP: Dyspnea

Pharmacokinetics	
Absorption	Unknown
Distribution	Breast milk, crosses placenta, widely distributed, protein binding 90%
Metabolism	Liver
Excretion	Kidneys
Half-life	6-16 hr

Pharmacodynamics	
Onset	15-30 min
Peak	1-4 hr
Duration	4-6 hr

INTERACTIONS
Individual drugs
Abciximab, cefoperazone, cefoTEtan, eptifibatide, heparin, tirofiban: increased bleeding risk
Alcohol: increased CNS depression
Cimetidine: decreased metabolism of valproic acid
ChlorproMAZINE, erythromycin, felbamate: increased valproic acid level
Phenytoin: increased action of phenytoin
Warfarin: increased bleeding

Drug classifications
Antidepressants (tricyclics), barbiturates: increased action

Antihistamines, barbiturates, MAOIs, opioids,
    sedative/hypnotics: increased CNS depression
Tricyclics: decreased seizure threshold

Drug/lab test
Increased: LFTs, bleeding time, ammonia
Decreased: sodium
False positive: ketones, urine
Interference: thyroid function tests

NURSING CONSIDERATIONS
Assessment
• Monitor blood tests: Hct, Hgb, RBC, serum
folate, ammonia, platelets, pro-time, PTT, vit D if
on long-term therapy
• Monitor liver function tests: AST, ALT, bilirubin, creatinine, failure
• Monitor blood levels: therapeutic level 50-125
mcg/ml
• **Assess seizure disorder:** location, aura,
activity, duration; seizure precautions should be
in place
⚠ **Assess bipolar disorder: mood, activity, sleeping, eating, behavior; suicidal
thoughts/behaviors**
⚠ **Hyperammonemic encephalopathy: can
be fatal in those with urea cycle disorders
(UCD); lethargy, confusion, coma, CV, respiratory changes; discontinue**
• **Assess migraines:** frequency, intensity
• Overdose symptoms: heart block, coma

> **BLACK BOX WARNING:** Assess for pancreati-
> tis, may be fatal

Patient/family education
• Teach patient that physical dependency may
result from extended use
⚠ **Instruct patient to report immediately
suicidal thoughts/behaviors**
• Instruct patient to avoid driving, other activities that require alertness
⚠ **Advise patient not to discontinue medication quickly after long-term use; seizures
may result**
⚠ **Advise patient to report visual disturbances, rash, diarrhea, light-colored stools,
jaundice, protracted vomiting to prescriber**
⚠ **Advise patient to use contraception
while taking this product, pregnancy D**
• Instruct patient to drink plenty of fluids

Evaluation
Positive therapeutic outcome
• Decreased seizures

---

valsartan (Rx)
(val-zar′tan)
Diovan
Func. class.: Antihypertensive
Chem. class.: Angiotensin II receptor
antagonist (type AT_1)
Pregnancy category D

Do not confuse:
Diovan/Dioval

ACTION: Blocks the vasoconstrictor and
aldosterone-secreting effects of angiotensin II;
selectively blocks the binding of angiotensin II to
the AT_1 receptor found in tissues

Therapeutic outcome: Decreased B/P

USES: Hypertension, alone or in combination, in patients >6 yr; CHF, after MI with left
ventricular dysfunction/failure in stable patients

CONTRAINDICATIONS:
Hypersensitivity, severe hepatic disease, bilateral
renal artery stenosis

> **BLACK BOX WARNING:** Pregnancy **D** 2nd/3rd
> trimester

Precautions: Breastfeeding, children,
geriatric, CHF, hypertrophic cardiomyopathy,
aortic/mitral valve stenosis, CAD, angioedema,
renal/hepatic disease, hypersensitivity to ACE
inhibitors, hyperkalemia, hypovolemia, African
descent

DOSAGE AND ROUTES
Adult: PO 80 or 160 mg/day alone or in
combination with other antihypertensives, may
increase to 320 mg CHF
Geriatric: PO Adjust based on clinical response; may start with lower dose
Child/adolescent 6-16 yr: PO 1.3 mg/kg/day,
max 40 mg/day

CHF
Adult: PO 40 mg bid, up to 60 mg bid

Post MI
Adult: PO 20 mg bid as early as 12 hr after MI,
may be titrated within 7 days to 40 mg bid, then
titrate to maintenance of 160 mg bid

Available forms: Tabs 80, 160, 320 mg

Implementation
• Administer without regard to meals

V

Adverse effects: *italics* = common; **bold** = life-threatening

ADVERSE EFFECTS

CNS: *Dizziness, insomnia,* drowsiness, vertigo, headache, fatigue
CV: Angina pectoris, 2nd-degree AV block, **cerebrovascular accident,** hypotension, **MI, dysrhythmias**
EENT: Conjunctivitis
GI: Diarrhea, abdominal pain, nausea, **hepatotoxicity**
GU: Impotence, **nephrotoxicity, renal failure**
HEMA: *Anemia,* neutropenia
META: Hyperkalemia
MISC: Vasculitis, angioedema
MS: Cramps, myalgia, pain, stiffness
RESP: *Cough*

Pharmacokinetics

Absorption	Well absorbed
Distribution	Bound to plasma proteins
Metabolism	Extensive
Excretion	Feces, urine, breast milk
Half-life	9 hr

Pharmacodynamics

Onset	Up to 2 hr
Peak	2-4 hr
Duration	24 hr

INTERACTIONS

Individual drugs

Aliskiren: do not use concurrently
Gemfibrozil, rifampin, ritonavir, telithromycin: increased valsartan levels
Lithium: increased effects of lithium

Drug classifications

Diuretics (potassium-sparing, potassium supplements, ACE inhibitors): increased hyperkalemia
NSAIDs, salicylates: decreased antihypertensive effects

Drug/herb

Ephedra, ma huang: decreased antihypertensive effect
Hawthorn: increased antihypertensive effect

Drug/food

Decreased AUC by 40%
Salt substitutes with potassium: increased hyperkalemia

NURSING CONSIDERATIONS

Assessment

• Assess B/P (lying, sitting, standing), pulse q4hr; note rate, rhythm, quality periodically

• Monitor electrolytes: potassium, sodium, chloride; total CO_2
• Assess for angioedema: facial swelling, shortness of breath
• Obtain baselines in renal, liver function tests before therapy begins
• Assess blood tests: BUN, creatinine, before treatment
• Monitor for edema in feet, legs daily
• Assess for skin turgor, dryness of mucous membranes for hydration status; correct volume depletion before initiating therapy
• Overdose symptoms: bradycardia or tachycardia, circulatory collapse

Patient/family education

• Teach patient not to take this product if breastfeeding or pregnant, or have had an allergic reaction to this product
• If a dose is missed, instruct patient to take as soon as possible, unless it is within an hour before next dose
• Advise patient to comply with dosage schedule, even if feeling better
• Teach patient to notify prescriber of fever, swelling of hands or feet, irregular heartbeat, chest pain, persistent cough
• Advise patient excessive perspiration, dehydration, diarrhea may lead to fall in blood pressure; consult prescriber if these occur
• Inform patient that product may cause dizziness, fainting; light-headedness may occur, maintain hydration
• Instruct patient to avoid potassium supplements and foods, salt substitutes
• Caution patient to rise slowly to sitting or standing position to minimize orthostatic hypotension; how to take B/P

> **BLACK BOX WARNING:** Teach patient not to take this medication if pregnant (D) or breastfeeding

Evaluation

Positive therapeutic outcome
• Decreased B/P

vancomycin
(van-koe-mye′sin)
Vancocin
Func. class.: Antiinfective—miscellaneous
Chem. class.: Tricyclic glycopeptide
Pregnancy category B

ACTION: Inhibits bacterial cell wall synthesis, blocks glycopeptides

Therapeutic outcome: Bactericidal for the following organisms: staphylococci, streptococci, *Corynebacterium, Clostridium*

USES: *Actinomyces* sp., *Bacillus* sp., *Clostridium difficile, Clostridium* sp., *Enterococcus faecalis, Enterococcus faecium, Enterococcus* sp., *Lactobacillus* sp., *Listeria monocytogenes, Staphylococcus aureus* (MRSA), *Staphylococcus aureus* (MSSA), *Staphylococcus epidermidis, Staphylococcus* sp., *Streptococcus agalactiae* (group B streptococci), *Streptococcus bovis, Streptococcus pneumoniae, Streptococcus pyogenes* (group A beta-hemolytic streptococci), *Viridans streptococci;* may be effective against *Corynebacterium jeikeium, Corynebacterium* sp.; pseudomembranous colitis, staphylococcal enterocolitis, group A β-hemolytic streptococci, endocarditis prophylaxis for dental procedures, bacteremia, join/bone infections, osteomyelitis, pneumonia, septicemia

Unlabeled uses: Bacterial infection prophylaxis, brain abscess, endocarditis prophylaxis, meningitis, orthopedic device–related infection, peritonitis, surgical infection prophylaxis, vancomycin desensitization, ventriculitis

CONTRAINDICATIONS:
Hypersensitivity, previous hearing loss

Precautions: Pregnancy **B** (PO); **C** (IV), breastfeeding, neonates, geriatric, renal disease

DOSAGE AND ROUTES
Serious staphylococcal infections
Adult: **IV** 500 mg (7.5 mg/kg) q6-8hr or 1 g (15 mg/kg) q12hr
Child: **IV** 40-60 mg/kg/day divided q6-8hr
Neonate: **IV** 15 mg/kg initially followed by 10 mg/kg q8-24hr

Pseudomembranous/ staphylococcal enterocolitis
Adult: PO 125 mg qid × 10-14 days
Child: PO (unlabeled) 40 mg/kg/day divided q6hr × 7-10 days, max 2 g/day

Endocarditis prophylaxis for dental procedure
Adult: **IV** 2 g divided
Child: **IV** 20 mg/kg over 1 hr; 1 hr before procedure

Renal dose
Adult: **IV** 15-20 mg/kg loading dose in seriously ill; individualize all other doses

Available forms: Cap 125, 250 mg; powder for inj **IV** 500, 750 mg; vials 1, 5, 10 g; dextrose sol for inj 500 mg/100 ml, 750 mg/150 ml, 1 g/200 ml

Implementation
• Give antihistamine if red man syndrome occurs: decreased B/P, flushing of neck, face; stop or slow infusion
• Give dose based on serum conc
• Give in equal intervals around the clock to maintain blood levels
• Store at room temp for up to 2 wk after reconstitution
• Have adrenaline, suction, tracheostomy set, endotracheal intubation equipment on unit; anaphylaxis may occur
• Provide adequate intake of fluids (2 L) to prevent nephrotoxicity
PO route
• Give without regard to food, swallow whole

Intermittent IV INF route
• Give after reconstitution with 10 ml of sterile water for inj (500 mg/10 ml); further dilution is needed for **IV**, 500 mg/100 ml of 0.9% NaCl, D₅W given as intermittent inf over 1 hr; decrease rate of inf if red man syndrome occurs
Continuous IV INF route (unlabeled)
• Reconstitute, then may inf 1-2 g in volume to give over 24 hr if intermittent **IV** route cannot be used

Y-site compatibilities: Acetylcysteine, acyclovir, alatrofloxacin, aldesleukin, alemtuzumab, alfentanil, allopurinol, alprostadil, amifostine, amikacin, amino acids injection, aminocaproic acid, amiodarone, amoxicillin-clavulanate, amsacrine, anidulafungin, argatroban, ascorbic acid injection, atenolol, atracurium, atropine, azithromycin, benztropine, bleomycin, bretylium, bumetanide, buprenorphine, butorphanol, calcium chloride/gluconate, CARBOplatin, carmustine, caspofungin, cefpirome, chlorproMAZINE, cimetidine, ciprofloxacin, cisatracurium, CISplatin, clarithromycin, clindamycin, codeine, cyanocobalamin, cyclophosphamide, cycloSPORINE, cytarabine, DACTINomycin, DAUNOrubicin liposome, dexamethasone, dexmedetomidine, dexrazoxane, digoxin, diltiazem, diphenhydrAMINE, DOBUTamine, DOCEtaxel, dolasetron, DOPamine, doripenem, doxacurium, doxapram, DOXOrubicin, DOXOrubicin liposomal, doxycycline, enalaprilat, ePHEDrine, EPINEPHrine, epirubicin, eptifibatide, ertapenem, erythromycin, esmolol, etoposide, etoposide phosphate, famotidine, fenoldopam, fentaNYL, filgrastim, fluconazole, fludarabine, folic acid (as

Adverse effects: *italics* = common; **bold** = life-threatening

sodium salt), gallium, gemcitabine, gentamicin, glycopyrrolate, granisetron, HYDROmorphone, hydrOXYzine, ifosfamide, insulin, regular, irinotecan, isoproterenol, isosorbide, ketamine, labetalol, lactated Ringer's injection, lepirudin, levofloxacin, lidocaine, linezolid, LORazepam, magnesium sulfate, mannitol, mechlorethamine, melphalan, meperidine, meropenem, metaraminol, methyldopate, metoclopramide, metoprolol, metroNIDAZOLE, midazolam, milrinone, minocycline, mitoXANtrone, morphine, multiple vitamins injection, mycophenolate, nalbuphine, naloxone, nesiritide, netilmicin, niCARdipine, nitroglycerin, nitroprusside, norepinephrine, octreotide, ofloxacin, ondansetron, oxacillin, oxaliplatin, oxytocin, PACLitaxel (solvent/surfactant), palonosetron, pamidronate, pancuronium, papaverine, PEMEtrexed, penicillin G potassium/sodium, pentamidine, pentazocine, PENTobarbital, perphenazine, PHENobarbital, phentolamine, phenylephrine, phytonadione, piritramide, polymyxin B, potassium acetate/chloride, procainamide, prochlorperazine, promethazine, propranolol, protamine, pyridoxine, quiNIDine, ranitidine, remifentanil, rifampin, Ringer's injection, riTUXimab, sodium acetate/bicarbonate/citrate, succinylcholine, SUFentanil, tacrolimus, teniposide, thiamine, thiotepa, tigecycline, tirofiban, TNA (3-in-1), tobramycin, tolazoline, TPN (2-in-1), trastuzumab, urapidil, vasopressin, vecuronium, verapamil, vinBLAStine, vinCRIStine, vinorelbine, voriconazole, zidovudine, zoledronic acid

Additive compatibilities: Amikacin, atracurium, calcium gluconate, cefepime, cimetidine, corticotropin, dimenhyDRINATE, hydrocortisone, meropenem, ofloxacin, potassium chloride, ranitidine, verapamil, vit B/C

ADVERSE EFFECTS
CNS: Headache
CV: Cardiac arrest, vascular collapse (rare), hypotension, peripheral edema
EENT: *Ototoxicity, permanent deafness,* tinnitus, nystagmus
GI: Nausea, pseudomembranous colitis
GU: Nephrotoxicity: increased BUN, creatinine, albumin, fatal uremia
HEMA: Leukopenia, eosinophilia, neutropenia
INTEG: Chills, fever, rash, thrombophlebitis at inj site, urticaria, pruritus, necrosis (red man syndrome), skin/subcutaneous tissue disorders
MS: Back pain
RESP: Wheezing, dyspnea
SYST: Anaphylaxis, superinfection

Pharmacokinetics

Absorption	Poorly absorbed (PO), completely absorbed (**IV**)
Distribution	Widely distributed, crosses placenta
Metabolism	Liver
Excretion	PO, feces; **IV**, kidneys
Half-life	4-8 hr

Pharmacodynamics

	IV
Onset	Immediate
Peak	Inf end
Duration	Unknown

INTERACTIONS
Individual drugs
Acyclovir, adefovir, amphotericin B, capreomycin, CISplatin, colistin, cycloSPORINE, foscarnet, ganciclovir, methotrexate, pamidronate, IV pentamidine, polymyxin B, streptozocin, tacrolimus, zoledronic acid: increased ototoxicity or nephrotoxicity
Cholestyramine, colestipol, cidofovir: do not use concurrently
MetFORMIN: increased lactic acidosis

Drug classifications
Aminoglycosides, cephalosporins, NSAIDs: increased ototoxicity or nephrotoxicity
Nodepolarizing muscle relaxants: increased neuromuscular effects

Drug/lab test
Increased: BUN/creatinine, eosinophils
Decreased: WBC

NURSING CONSIDERATIONS
Assessment
• **Assess for infection:** WBC, urine, stools, sputum, wound characteristics, throughout treatment
• Monitor I&O ratio, BUN, creatinine; report hematuria, oliguria because nephrotoxicity may occur
• Monitor blood tests: WBC; serum levels; peak 1 hr after 1-hr inf 25-40 mg/L; trough before next dose 5-10 mg/L, especially in renal disease
• Obtain C&S before product therapy; product may be given as soon as culture is performed
• Assess auditory function during, after treatment; hearing loss, ringing, roaring in ears; product should be discontinued
• Monitor B/P during administration; sudden drop may indicate red man syndrome
• Assess for signs of infection

- Red man syndrome: flushing of neck, face, upper body, arms, back; may lead to anaphylaxis, slow IV infusion to >1 hr

Patient/family education

- Teach patient aspects of product therapy: need to complete entire course of medication to ensure organism death (7-10 days); culture may be performed after completed course of medication
- Advise patient to report sore throat, fever, fatigue; could indicate superinfection
- Instruct patient that product must be taken in equal intervals around the clock to maintain blood levels

Evaluation

Positive therapeutic outcome

- Absence of fever, sore throat
- Negative culture after treatment

---

vardenafil (Rx)

(var-den'a-fil)
Levitra, Staxyn
Func. class.: Impotence agent
Chem. class.: Phosphodiesterase type 5 inhibitor
Pregnancy category B

ACTION: Inhibits phosphodiesterase type 5 (PDE5); enhances erectile function by increasing the amount of cyclic GMP, which causes smooth muscle relaxation and increased blood flow into the corpus cavernosum

Therapeutic outcome: Erection

USES: Treatment of erectile dysfunction

CONTRAINDICATIONS:

Hypersensitivity, coadministration of α-blockers or nitrates, renal failure, congenital or acquired QT prolongation

Precautions: Pregnancy **B**; not indicated for women, children, or newborns; hepatic impairment; retinitis pigmentosa; cardiovascular disease; anatomic penile deformities; sickle cell anemia; leukemia; multiple myeloma; bleeding disorders; active peptic ulceration; renal disease

DOSAGE AND ROUTES

Adult: PO 10 mg, taken 1 hr before sexual activity, dose may be reduced to 5 mg or increased to a max of 20 mg; max dosing frequency is once/day; orally disintegrating tab 10 mg 60 min before sexual activity; do not use with potent CYP3A4 inhibitors

Geriatric >65 yr: PO 5 mg initially, titrate as needed/tolerated

Hepatic dose (Child-Pugh B)
Adult: PO 5 mg, max 10 mg

Concomitant medications

Ritonavir, max 2.5 mg q72hr; for indinavir, ketoconazole 400 mg/day and itraconazole 400 mg/day, max 2.5 mg/day; for ketoconazole 200 mg/day, itraconazole 200 mg/day and erythromycin, max 5 mg/day

Available forms: Tabs 2.5, 5, 10, 20 mg; orally disintegrating tab 10 mg

Implementation

- Take approximately 1 hr before sexual activity; do not use more than once a day
- Orally disintegrating tabs are not interchangeable with film-coated tabs
- **Orally disintegrating tab:** place on tongue, allow to dissolve, do not use water

ADVERSE EFFECTS

CNS: *Headache, flushing, dizziness, insomnia,* **seizures,** transient global amnesia
CV: Hypertension, **MI, CV collapse,** chest pain
EENT: Conjunctivitis, tinnitus, photophobia, diminished vision, glaucoma, hearing loss
GU: Abnormal ejaculation, priapism
MISC: Rash, GERD, GGTP increased, **NAION (nonarteritic ischemic optic neuropathy),** dyspepsia
MS: Myalgia, arthralgia, neck pain
RESP: Rhinitis, sinusitis, dyspnea, pharyngitis, epistaxis

Pharmacokinetics

Absorption	Rapid; reduced absorption with high-fat meal
Distribution	Bioavailability 15%; protein binding 95%
Metabolism	Liver
Excretion	Primarily in feces (91%-95%)
Half-life	4-5 hr

Pharmacodynamics

Onset	20 min
Peak	½-1½ hr
Duration	<5 hr

INTERACTIONS

Individual drugs

Alcohol, amLODIPine, metoprolol, NIFEdipine: increased hypotension, do not use concurrently

---

Adverse effects: *italics* = common; **bold** = life-threatening

Cimetidine, erythromycin, itraconazole, ketoconazole: increased levels
Clarithromycin, droperidol, procainamide,
quiNIDine: serious dysrhythmias; do not use
concurrently

Drug classifications
⚠ Do not use with nitrates because of
unsafe decrease in B/P that could result in
heart attack or stroke
α-Blockers, protease inhibitors: increased
hypotension; do not use concurrently
Angiotensin II receptor blockers: increased
hypotension; do not use concurrently
Antidysrhythmics class Ia, III, quinolones: serious dysrhythmias; do not use together
Antiretroviral protease inhibitors: increased
vardenafil levels

Drug/food
High-fat meal: decreased absorption

Drug/lab test
Increase: CK

NURSING CONSIDERATIONS
Assessment
• Assess for use of organic nitrates that should
not be used with this product
• Assess for severe loss of vision while taking
this or any similar products; these products
should not be used if vision loss has occurred

Patient/family education
• Advise that product does not protect against
STDs, including HIV
• Teach that product absorption is reduced with
a high-fat meal
⚠ Instruct that product should not be used
with nitrates in any form
• Inform that product has no effect in the
absence of sexual stimulation
• Teach that patient should seek immediate
medical attention if erection lasts for more than
4 hr
• Advise to inform physician of all medications
being taken
• Teach patient to notify prescriber immediately
and stop taking product if vision loss occurs

Evaluation
Positive therapeutic outcome
• Sustainable erection

varenicline (Rx)
(var-e-ni′kleen)
Champix ✦, **Chantix**
Func. class.: Smoking cessation agent
Pregnancy category C

ACTION: Partial agonist for nicotine
receptors; partially activates receptors to help
curb cravings; occupies receptors to prevent
nicotine binding

Therapeutic outcome: Smoking cessation

USES: Smoking deterrent

CONTRAINDICATIONS:
Hypersensitivity, eating disorders

Precautions: Pregnancy **C**, breastfeeding,
children <18 yr, geriatric, renal disease, recent
MI, angioedema

> **BLACK BOX WARNING:** Bipolar disorder,
> depression, schizophrenia, suicidal ideation

DOSAGE AND ROUTES
Smoking cessation
Adult: PO therapy should begin 1 week prior
to smoking stop date (i.e., take product plus
tobacco for 7 days); titrate for 1 wk, days 1
through 3, 0.5 mg/day; days 4 through 7, 0.5 mg
bid; day 8 through end of treatment 1 mg bid;
treatment is 12 wk and may repeat for another
12 wk

Renal dose
Adult: PO CCr ≤50 ml/min, titrate to max 0.5
mg bid

Available forms: Tabs 0.5, 1 mg, Chantix
continuing month PAK; Chantix starting month
PAK

Implementation
• Do not break, crush, or chew tabs
• Give increased fluids, bulk in diet if constipa-
tion occurs
• Give with a full glass of water after eating
• Give sugarless gum, hard candy, or frequent
sips of water for dry mouth

ADVERSE EFFECTS
CNS: Headache, agitation, dizziness, insomnia,
abnormal dreams, fatigue, malaise, behavior
changes, depression, **suicidal ideation, suicide,** amnesia, hallucinations, hostility, mania,
psychosis, tremor

CV: **Dysrhythmias,** hypertension, palpitations, **tachycardia,** angina, hypotension, **MI**
EENT: *Blurred vision,* tinnitus
GI: *Nausea, vomiting,* anorexia, *dry mouth,* increased/decreased appetite, *constipation,* flatulence, GERD
GU: Erectile dysfunction, urinary frequency, menstrual irregularities
INTEG: Rash, pruritus, **angioedema, Stevens-Johnson syndrome**
MISC: Weight loss or gain
RESP: Dyspnea, rhinorrhea

Pharmacokinetics

Absorption	Unknown
Distribution	Steady state 4 days
Metabolism	Minimal
Excretion	Urine 92%, unchanged
Half-life	Elimination 24 hr

Pharmacodynamics

Unknown

NURSING CONSIDERATIONS
Assessment
• **Assess smoking history:** motivation for smoking cessation, years used, amount each day
• Assess for renal function in geriatric
• Assess for smoking cessation after 12 wk; if progress has not been made, product may be used for an additional 12 wk
• Assess mental status: mood, sensorium, affect

Patient/family education
• Teach patient that treatment for smoking cessation lasts 12 wk and another 12 wk may be required
• Teach patient to use caution in driving, other activities requiring alertness; blurred vision may occur
• Advise patient to set a date to quit smoking and initiate treatment 1 wk prior to that date
• Teach patient how to titrate product
• Advise patient not to use with nicotine patches unless directed by prescriber; may increase B/P
• Advise patient to notify prescriber if pregnancy is suspected or planned
• Teach patient common side effects to be expected

> **BLACK BOX WARNING:** Instruct patient to notify prescriber immediately of change in thought/behavior (suicidal ideation, hostility, depression); stop product

Evaluation
Positive therapeutic outcome
• Smoking cessation

vasopressin (Rx)
(vay-soe-press′in)
Pitressin, Pressyn ✦
Func. class.: Pituitary hormone
Chem. class.: Lysine vasopressin
Pregnancy category C

ACTION: Promotes reabsorption of water by action on renal tubular epithelium; causes vasoconstriction on muscles in the GI system

Therapeutic outcome: Increased osmolality, decreased urine output in diabetes insipidus

USES: Diabetes insipidus (nonnephrogenic/nonpsychogenic), abdominal distention postoperatively, bleeding esophageal varices

CONTRAINDICATIONS:
Hypersensitivity, chronic nephritis

Precautions: Pregnancy **C,** breastfeeding, CAD, asthma, renal/vascular disease, migraines, seizures

DOSAGE AND ROUTES
Diabetes insipidus
Adult: IM/SUBCUT 5-10 units bid-qid prn; CONT **IV** INF 0.0005 units/kg/hr, (0.05 milliunit/kg/hr), double dose q30min as needed
Child: IM/SUBCUT 2.5-10 units bid-qid prn; IM/SUBCUT 1.25-2.5 units q2-3day (Pitressin Tannate) for chronic therapy

Abdominal distention
Adult: IM 5 units, then q3-4hr, increasing to 10 units if needed (aqueous)

Available forms: Sol for inj 20 units/ml, 10 units/0.5 ml

Implementation
IM/SUBCUT route
• May be given IM/SUBCUT for diagnosis of diabetes insipidus
• Give patient 16 oz water at administration to prevent nausea, vomiting, cramping

ADVERSE EFFECTS
CNS: Drowsiness, headache, lethargy, flushing, vertigo
CV: Increased B/P, dysrhythmias, chest pain, **cardiac arrest, shock, MI**

V

EENT: Nasal irritation, congestion, rhinitis
GI: Nausea, heartburn, cramps, vomiting, flatus
GU: Vulval pain, uterine cramping
MISC: Tremor, sweating, vertigo, urticaria, bronchial constriction

Pharmacokinetics

Absorption	Erratically absorbed (IM)
Distribution	Widely distributed extracellular fluid
Metabolism	Liver, rapidly
Excretion	Kidneys, unchanged
Half-life	10-20 min

Pharmacodynamics

	IM	IV
Onset	1 hr	Unknown
Peak	Unknown	Unknown
Duration	3-8 hr	3-8 hr

INTERACTIONS
Individual drugs
CarBAMazepine, chlorproPAMIDE, clofibrate, fludrocortisone, urea: decreased antidiuretic effect
Demeclocycline, lithium: increased antidiuretic effect

Drug classifications
Tricyclics: increased antidiuretic effect

NURSING CONSIDERATIONS
Assessment
• Assess intranasal use: nausea, congestion, cramps, headache; usually decreased with decreased dose
• Monitor pulse, B/P when giving product **IV** or SUBCUT
• Monitor I&O ratio, weight daily, fluid/electrolyte balance; check for edema in extremities; if water retention is severe, diuretic may be prescribed; **check for water intoxication: lethargy, behavioral changes, disorientation, neuromuscular excitability**
• Small doses may precipitate coronary adverse effects; keep emergency equipment nearby

Patient/family education
• Teach patient technique for nasal instillation: to insert tube into nasal cavity to instill product
• Caution patient to avoid OTC products for cough, hay fever because these preparations may contain epinephrine, decrease product response; do not use with alcohol
• Advise patient to carry/wear emergency ID specifying therapy, disease process (diabetes insipidus)
• Teach patient to measure/record I&O
• Teach patient to avoid alcohol, all OTC medications unless approved by prescriber

Evaluation
Positive therapeutic outcome
• Absence of severe thirst
• Decreased urine output, osmolality

vemurafenib
(vem-ue-raf'e-nib)
Zelboraf
Func. class.: Biologic response modifiers; signal transduction inhibitors (STIs)
Pregnancy category D

ACTION: Inhibitor of some mutated forms of BRAF serine threonine kinase, thereby blocking cellular proliferation in melanoma cells with the mutation. It also inhibits other kinases including CRAF, ARAF, wild-type BRAF, SRMA, ACK1, MAP4H5, and FGR. It is a potent adenosine triphosphate-competitive inhibitor of RAFs with a modest preference for mutant BRAF and CRAF as compared with wild-type BRAF.

Therapeutic outcome: Decreased spread of malignancy

USES: Unresectable or metastatic malignant melanoma with V600E mutation of the BRAF gene

CONTRAINDICATIONS:
Hypersensitivity

Precautions: Pregnancy D, breastfeeding, children, infants, neonates, hepatic disease, QT prolongation, secondary malignancy, torsades de pointes, hypokalemia, hypomagnesium, sunlight exposure

DOSAGE AND ROUTES
Adult: PO 960 mg (4 tabs) bid about q12h

Dose adjustments for toxicity due to symptomatic adverse reactions or QTc prolongation for Grade 1 or tolerable Grade 2 adverse events: No dosage change

For Intolerable Grade 2 or Grade 3 adverse events (1st episode):
Interrupt treatment until toxicity resolves to grade ≤1; when resuming, reduce dosage to 720 mg (3 tabs) bid

---

For Intolerable Grade 2 or Grade 3 adverse events (2nd episode):
Interrupt treatment until toxicity resolves to grade ≤1; when resuming, reduce dose to 480 mg (2 tabs) bid

For Intolerable Grade 2 or Grade 3 adverse events (3rd episode)
Discontinue treatment permanently

For Grade 4 adverse events (1st episode):
Discontinue permanently or interrupt until toxicity resolves to grade ≤1; when resuming, reduce dose to 480 mg (2 tablets) bid

For Grade 4 adverse events (2nd episode):
Discontinue permanently

Available forms: Tab 240 mg

Implementation
• Continue until disease progresses or unacceptable toxicity occurs
• Missed doses can be taken up to 4 hr before the next dose is due; take about 12 hr apart; take without regard to meals
• Swallow whole with a full glass of water; do not crush or chew
• Store at room temperature in original container

ADVERSE EFFECTS
CNS: Asthenia, fatigue, fever, dizziness, headache, muscle paralysis, peripheral neuropathy
CV: Atrial fibrillation, hypotension, peripheral edema, QT prolongation
EENT: Blurred vision, iritis, photophobia, uveitis
GI: Constipation, decreased appetite, diarrhea, dysgeusia, nausea, vomiting, weight loss
INTEG: Actinic keratosis, alopecia, hyperkeratosis, maculopapular rash, palmar-plantar erythrodysesthesia (hand and foot syndrome), papular rash, photosensitivity, pruritus, xerosis/dry skin
MS: Arthralgia, arthritis, back pain, extremity pain, musculoskeletal pain, myalgias
RESP: Cough
SYST: Anaphylaxis, secondary malignancy

Pharmacokinetics

Absorption	Unknown
Distribution	Protein binding 99%
Metabolism	Unknown
Excretion	94% feces
Half-life	30-120 hr

Pharmacodynamics

Onset	Unknown
Peak	Unknown
Duration	Unknown

INTERACTIONS
Individual drugs
Abarelix, alfuzosin, amoxapine, apomorphine, arsenic trioxide, asenapine, chloroquine, ciprofloxacin, citalopram, clarithromycin, cloZAPine, cyclobenzaprine, dasatinib, dolasetron, dronedarone, droperidol, eribulin, erythromycin, ezogabine, flecainide, fluconazole, gatifloxacin, gemifloxacin, grepafloxacin, halofantrine, haloperidol, iloperidone, indacaterol, lapatinib, levofloxacin, levomethadyl, lopinavir/ritonavir, magnesium sulfate, maprotiline, mefloquine, methadone, moxifloxacin, nilotinib, norfloxacin, octreotide, ofloxacin, OLANZapine, ondansetron, paliperidone, palonosetron, pentamidine, pimozide, posaconazole, potassium sulfate, probucol, propafenone, QUEtiapine, quiNIDine, ranolazine, rilpivirine, risperiDONE, saquinavir, sodium, sparfloxacin, SUNItinib, tacrolimus, telavancin, telithromycin, tetrabenazine, troleandomycin, vardenafil, vemurafenib, venlafaxine, vorinostat, ziprasidone: increased QT prolongation, torsades de pointes

Drug classifications
Beta-agonists, Class IA antiarrhythmics (disopyramide, procainamide, quiNIDine), Class III antiarrhythmics (amiodarone, dofetilide, ibutilide, sotalol), halogenated anesthetics, local anesthetics, certain phenothiazines (chlorproMAZINE, fluPHENAZine, mesoridazine, perphenazine, prochlorperazine, thioridazine and trifluoperazine), tricyclic antidepressants: increased QT prolongation, torsades de pointes
CYP3A4 inducers (alcohol, barbiturates, bexarotene, carBAMazepine, erythromycin, etravirine, fluvoxaMINE, ketoconazole, metyrapone, modafinil, nevirapine, OXcarbazepine, phenytoin, rifabutin, rifampin, ritonavir): decreased vemurafenib effect
CYP3A4/CYP1A2 inhibitors (cimetidine, dalfopristin, delavirdine, enoxacin, indinavir, isoniazid, itraconazole, quinupristin, tipranavir): increased vemurafenib effect

Drug/lab test
Alkaline phosphatase, bilirubin, LFTs, serum creatinine: increase

Adverse effects: *italics* = common; **bold** = life-threatening

NURSING CONSIDERATIONS
Assessment
• **Hepatic disease:** Liver function test (LFT) abnormalities, altered bilirubin levels, may occur during treatment; monitor LFTs and bilirubin levels prior to treatment, then monthly; more frequent testing is needed in those presenting with grade 2 or greater toxicities; Laboratory alterations should be managed with dose reduction, treatment interruption, or discontinuation
• **QT prolongation:** has been reported with the use of crizotinib; therefore, crizotinib should be avoided in patients with QT prolongation; Monitor ECG and electrolytes in those with congestive heart failure, bradycardia, electrolyte imbalance (hypokalemia, hypomagnesemia), or in those who are taking concomitant medications known to prolong the QT interval; treatment interruption, dosage adjustment, treatment discontinuation may be needed in those who develop QT prolongation
• **Pregnancy/breastfeeding:** Identify if pregnancy is planned or suspected, pregnancy category D, avoid breastfeeding
• Serum electrolytes

Patient/family education
• Decreased spread of malignancy

venlafaxine (Rx)
(ven-la-fax′een)
Effexor, Effexor XR
Func. class.: Second-generation SNRI antidepressant—miscellaneous
Pregnancy category C

ACTION: Potent inhibitor of neuronal serotonin and norepinephrine uptake, weak inhibitor of dopamine; no muscarinic, histaminergic, or α-adrenergic receptors in vitro

Therapeutic outcome: Relief of depression

USES: Prevention/treatment of major depression, to treat depression at end of life; long-term treatment of generalized anxiety disorder, panic disorder, social anxiety disorder (Effexor XR only)

CONTRAINDICATIONS:
Hypersensitivity

Precautions: Pregnancy **C,** breastfeeding, geriatric, mania, recent MI, cardiac/renal/hepatic disease, seizure disorder, hypertension, eosinophilic pneumonia, desvenlafaxine hypersensitivity

BLACK BOX WARNING: Children, suicidal ideation, bipolar disorder, interstitial lung disease

DOSAGE AND ROUTES
Depression
Adult: PO 75 mg/day in 2 or 3 divided doses; taken with food, may be increased to 150 mg/day; if needed may be further increased to 225 mg/day; increments of 75 mg/day should be made at intervals of no less than 4 days; some hospitalized patients may require up to 375 mg/day in 3 divided doses; EXT REL 37.5-75 mg PO daily, max 225 mg/day; give Effexor XR daily

Anxiety disorders
Adult: PO 75 mg/day or 37.5 mg/day × 4-7 days initially, max 225 mg/day

Hepatic dose
Adult: PO moderate impairment 50% of dose

Renal dose
Adult: PO CCr 10-70 ml/min reduce dose by 25%-50%; CCr <10 ml/min reduce by 50%

Hot flashes (unlabeled)
Adult (male, prostate cancer): PO 12.5 mg bid × 4 wk
Adult female: PO 37.5-75 mg/day

Available forms: Tabs scored (Effexor) 25, 37.5, 50, 75, 100 mg; ext rel caps (Effexor XR) 37.5, 75, 150, 225 mg

Implementation
• Give with food or milk for GI symptoms
• Crush if patient is unable to swallow medication whole
• Store at room temperature; do not freeze

ADVERSE EFFECTS
CNS: *Emotional lability, dizziness, weakness,* apathy, ataxia, headache, tremors, hypertonia, euphoria, hallucinations, hostility, insomnia, anxiety, **suicidal ideation in children/adolescents, seizures,** neuroleptic malignant syndrome–like reaction
CV: Angina pectoris, extrasystoles, postural hypotension, syncope, thrombophlebitis, hypertension, tachycardia, change in QTc interval, increased cholesterol
EENT: *Abnormal vision,* taste, *ear pain*
GI: *Dysphagia, eructation,* colitis, gastritis, gingivitis, *constipation,* stomatitis, stomach and mouth ulceration, nausea, anorexia, dry mouth

GU: *Anorgasmia,* abnormal ejaculation, urinary frequency, decreased libido, impotence, menstrual changes
HEMA: Thrombocytopenia, leukocytosis, leukopenia, **abnormal bleeding**
INTEG: Ecchymosis, acne, alopecia, brittle nails, dry skin, photosensitivity, sweating, **angioedema (ext rel), Stevens-Johnson syndrome**
META: *Peripheral edema, weight loss,* edema, glycosuria, hyperlipemia, hypokalemia
MS: Arthritis, bone pain, tenosynovitis, arthralgia
RESP: *Bronchitis, dyspnea,* cough
SYST: **Neonatal abstinence syndrome**

Pharmacokinetics

Absorption	Well absorbed
Distribution	Widely distributed, 27% protein binding
Metabolism	Liver, extensively
Excretion	Kidneys, 87%
Half-life	5 hr, 11 hr (active metabolite)

Pharmacodynamics

Unknown

INTERACTIONS
Individual drugs
Alcohol: increased CNS depression
Cimetidine: increased venlafaxine effect
CloZAPine, desipramine, haloperidol, warfarin: increased levels of these products
Cyproheptadine: decreased venlafaxine effect
Indinavir: decreased effect of indinavir
Linezolid, methylene blue, sibutramine, SUMAtriptan, traMADol, traZODone, tryptophan: increased serotonin syndrome

Drug classifications
Antihistamines, opioids, sedative-hypnotics: increased CNS depression
MAOIs: hyperthermia, rigidity, rapid fluctuations of vital signs, mental status changes, neuroleptic malignant syndrome
Salicylates, NSAIDs, platelet inhibitors, anticoagulants: increased bleeding risk
SSRIs, SNRIs, serotonin-receptor agonists: increased serotonin syndrome

Drug/herb
Kava, valerian: increased CNS depression
St. John's wort: serotonin syndrome

Drug/lab test
Increased: alkaline phosphatase, bilirubin, AST, ALT, BUN, creatinine, serum cholesterol, CPK, LDH
False positive: amphetamines, phencyclidine

NURSING CONSIDERATIONS
Assessment
• Monitor B/P (lying, standing), pulse q4hr; if systolic B/P drops 20 mm Hg hold product, notify prescriber; take vital signs q4hr in patients with CV disease
• Monitor blood tests: CBC, leukocytes, differential, cardiac enzymes if patient is receiving long-term therapy
• Monitor liver function tests: AST, ALT, bilirubin
• Check weight qwk; weight loss or gain; appetite may increase, peripheral edema may occur

BLACK BOX WARNING: Assess mental status: mood, sensorium, affect; increase in psychiatric symptoms: depression, panic; for suicidal ideation in children/adolescents

• Monitor urinary retention, constipation; constipation is more likely to occur in children or geriatric
• **Assess for withdrawal symptoms:** headache, nausea, vomiting, muscle pain, weakness; do not usually occur unless product was discontinued abruptly
• Identify alcohol consumption; if alcohol is consumed, hold dose
• **Serotonin syndrome, neuroleptic malignant syndrome:** assess for increased heart rate, shivering, sweating, dilated pupils, tremors, high B/P, hyperthermia, headache, confusion; if these occur, stop product, administer a serotonin antagonist if needed; usually worse if given with linezolid, methylene blue, tryptophan

Patient/family education
• Advise patient to notify prescriber of rash, hives, or allergic reactions
• Teach patient that therapeutic effects may take 2-3 wk
• Teach patient to use caution in driving or other activities requiring alertness because of drowsiness, dizziness, blurred vision; to avoid rising quickly from sitting to standing, especially geriatric
• Teach patient to avoid alcohol ingestion, other CNS depressants
⚠ Advise patient to avoid pregnancy, breastfeeding while taking this product, birth defects have occurred when used in the 3rd trimester

Adverse effects: *italics* = common; **bold** = life-threatening

⚠ Teach patient that worsening of symptoms, suicidal thoughts/behavior may occur in children, young adults

Evaluation
Positive therapeutic outcome
• Decreased depression, anxiety; sense of well-being
• Absence of suicidal thoughts

TREATMENT OF OVERDOSE:
ECG monitoring, induce emesis, lavage, activated charcoal, administer anticonvulsant

---

verapamil (Rx)
(ver-ap′a-mil)
Apo-Verap, Calan, Calan SR, Covera-HS ✦, Isoptin, Isoptin SR, Nu-Verap ✦, Verelan, Verelan PM
Func. class.: Calcium-channel blocker; antihypertensive; antianginal, antidys-rhythmic (Class IV)
Chem. class.: Diphenylalkylamine
Pregnancy category C

ACTION: Inhibits calcium ion influx across cell membrane during cardiac depolarization; produces relaxation of coronary vascular smooth muscle, peripheral vascular smooth muscle; dilates coronary vascular arteries; decreases SA/AV node conduction; dilates peripheral arteries

Therapeutic outcome: Decreased angina pectoris, dysrhythmias, B/P

USES: Chronic stable vasospastic, unstable angina; dysrhythmias, hypertension, supraventricular tachycardia, atrial flutter or fibrillation

Unlabeled uses: Prevention of migraine headaches, claudication, mania

CONTRAINDICATIONS:
Sick sinus syndrome, 2nd- or 3rd-degree heart block, hypotension <90 mm Hg systolic, cardiogenic shock, severe CHF, Lown-Ganong-Levine syndrome, Wolff-Parkinson-White syndrome

Precautions: Pregnancy **C**, breastfeeding, children, geriatric, CHF, hypotension, hepatic injury, renal disease, concomitant β-blocker therapy

DOSAGE AND ROUTES
Angina
Adult: PO 80-120 mg tid, increase qwk, max 480 mg/day

Dysrhythmias
Adult: PO 240-320 mg/day in 3-4 divided doses in digitalized patients
Adult: IV BOL 5-10 mg (0.075-0.15 mg/kg) over 2 min, may repeat 10 mg (0.15 mg/kg) ½ hr after first dose
Child 1-15 yr: IV BOL 0.1-0.3 mg/kg over >2 min, repeat in 30 min, max 5 mg in a single dose
Child 0-1 yr: IV BOL 0.1-0.2 mg/kg over ≥2 min, may repeat after 30 min

Hypertension
Adult: PO 80 mg tid, may titrate upward; EXT REL 120-240 mg/day as a single dose, may increase to 240-480 mg/day

Hepatic dose/geriatric/compromised ventricular function
Adult: PO 40 mg tid initially, increase as tolerated

Available forms: Tabs 40, 80, 120 mg; ext rel tabs 120, 180, 240 mg; inj 2.5 mg/ml in ampules, syringes, vials; ext rel caps 100, 200, 240, 300 mg

Implementation
PO route
• **Regular release:** give without regard to food
• **Extended release:** do not crush or chew ext rel products
• Cap may be opened and contents sprinkled on food; do not dissolve, chew cap
• Give once a day before meals at bedtime; sus rel give with food to decrease GI symptoms

Direct IV route
• Give by direct **IV** undiluted (Y-site, 3-way stopcock) over at least 2 min, or 3 min geriatric; discard unused sol; to prevent serious hypotension, patient should be recumbent for 1 hr or more, with continuous ECG and B/P monitoring
• **Do not use IV with IV β-blockers, may cause AV nodal blockade**

Y-site compatibilities: Alfentanil, amikacin, argatroban, ascorbic acid, atracurium, atropine, aztreonam, bivalirudin, bumetanide, buprenorphine, butorphanol, calcium chloride/gluconate, CARBOplatin, caspofungin, ceFAZolin, cefonicid, cefotaxime, cefoTEtan, cefOXitin, ceftizoxime, cefTRIAXone, cefuroxime, chlorproMAZINE, cimetidine, ciprofloxacin, clindamycin, cyanocobalamin, cyclophosphamide, cycloSPORINE, cytarabine, DACTINomycin, DAPTOmycin, dexamethasone, dexmedetomidine, digoxin, diltiazem, diphenhydrAMINE, DOBUTamine, DOCEtaxel, DOPamine, doxacurium, DOXOrubicin hydrochloride, doxycycline, enalaprilat, ePHEDrine, EPINEPHrine, epirubicin, epoetin alfa, eptifibatide, erythromycin, esmolol, etoposide, etoposide phosphate, famotidine, fenoldopam, fentaNYL, fluconazole, fludarabine, gemcitabine, gentamicin, glycopyrrolate, granisetron, heparin, hydrALAZINE, hydrocortisone, HYDROmorphone, ifosfamide, imipenem/cilastatin, inamrinone, insulin, isoproterenol, ketorolac, labetalol, levofloxacin, lidocaine, linezolid, LORazepam, magnesium sulfate, mannitol, mechlorethamine, meperidine, metaraminol, methotrexate, methoxamine, methyldopate, methylPREDNISolone, metoclopramide, metoprolol, metroNIDAZOLE, miconazole, midazolam, milrinone, mitoXANtrone, morphine, multivitamins, nalbuphine, naloxone, nesiritide, nitroglycerin, nitroprusside, norepinephrine, octreotide, ondansetron, oxaliplatin, oxytocin, PACLitaxel, palonosetron, papaverine, PEMEtrexed, penicillin G, pentamidine, pentazocine, phentolamine, phenylephrine, phytonadione, piperacillin/tazobactam, potassium chloride, procainamide, prochlorperazine, promethazine, propranolol, protamine, pyridoxine, quinupristin/dalfopristin, ranitidine, rocuronium, sodium acetate, succinylcholine, SUFentanil, tacrolimus, teniposide, theophylline, thiamine, ticarcillin/clavulanate, tirofiban, tobramycin, tolazoline, trimethaphan, urokinase, vancomycin, vasopressin, vecuronium, vinCRIStine, vinorelbine, voriconazole

Y-site incompatibilities: Acyclovir, albumin, aminophylline, amphotericin B cholesteryl, amphotericin B colloidal, amphotericin B liposome, ampicillin, ampicillin/sulbactam, azaTHIOprine, cefoperazone, cefTAZidime, chloramphenicol, dantrolene, diazepam, diazoxide, ertapenem, fluorouracil, folic acid, furosemide, ganciclovir, indomethacin, pantoprazole, PENTobarbital, PHENobarbital, phenytoin, piperacillin/tazobactam, propofol, sodium bicarbonate, thiotepa, tigecycline, trimethoprim/sulfamethoxazole

ADVERSE EFFECTS
CNS: *Headache, drowsiness,* dizziness, anxiety, depression, weakness, asthenia, fatigue, insomnia, confusion, light-headedness

CV: *Edema,* **CHF,** bradycardia, hypotension, palpitations, AV block, **dysrhythmias**
GI: *Nausea,* diarrhea, gastric upset, *constipation,* elevated liver function tests
GU: Impotence, nocturia, polyuria, gynecomastia
HEMA: Bruising, petechiae, bleeding
INTEG: Rash, bruising
MISC: Gingival hyperplasia
SYST: Stevens-Johnson syndrome

Pharmacokinetics

Absorption	Well absorbed (PO)
Distribution	Not known
Metabolism	Liver, extensively
Excretion	Kidneys (70%)
Half-life	Biphasic 4 min, 3-7 hr

Pharmacodynamics

	PO	PO-EXT REL	IV
Onset	1-2 hr	Unknown	1-5 min
Peak	½-1½ hr	5-7 hr	3-5 min
Duration	3-7 hr	24 hr	2 hr

INTERACTIONS
Individual drugs
CarBAMazepine, cycloSPORINE, digoxin, theophylline: increased levels of each specific product
Cimetidine, clarithromycin, erythromycin: increased effect of verapamil
FentaNYL, prazosin, quiNIDine: increased hypotension
Lithium: decreased lithium levels

Drug classifications
Antihypertensive, β-adrenergic blockers, nitrates: increased effects of verapamil, monitor for CV effects
Nondepolarizing muscle relaxants: increased effect
NSAIDs: decreased antihypertensive effect

Drug/herb
Ephedra (ma huang): increased hypertension
Ginseng, ginkgo: increased verapamil effect
St. John's wort: decreased verapamil effect

Drug/food
Grapefruit juice: increased hypotension

Drug/lab test
Increased: alkaline phosphatase, AST, ALT, BUN, creatinine, serum cholesterol

V

NURSING CONSIDERATIONS
Assessment
• **CHF:** Assess fluid volume status: I&O ratio and record; weight; distended red veins; crackles in lung; color; quality, specific gravity of urine; skin turgor; adequacy of pulses; moist mucous membranes; bilateral lung sounds; peripheral pitting edema; dehydration symptoms of decreasing output, thirst, hypotension, dry mouth, and mucous membranes should be reported
• Monitor B/P and pulse, pulmonary capillary wedge pressure (PCWP), central venous pressure, index, often during inf; notify prescriber if <50 bpm, systolic B/P <90 mm Hg
• Monitor ALT, AST, bilirubin daily; if these are elevated, hepatotoxicity is suspected
• Monitor platelets; if <150,000/mm³, product is usually discontinued and another product started
• Assess for extravasation; change site q48hr
• **Monitor cardiac status:** B/P, pulse, respiration, ECG
• Monitor renal/hepatic function tests during long-term treatment, serum potassium, periodically

Patient/family education
• Advise patient to increase fluids/fiber to counteract constipation
• Caution patient to avoid hazardous activities until stabilized on product and dizziness is no longer a problem
• Teach patient how to take pulse, B/P before taking product; to keep record or graph
• Instruct patient to limit caffeine consumption; to avoid alcohol, grapefruit, and OTC products unless directed by prescriber
• Advise patient to comply with medical regimen: diet, exercise, stress reduction, product therapy; to notify prescriber of irregular heartbeat, shortness of breath, swelling of feet and hands, pronounced dizziness, constipation, nausea, hypotension, **IV** calcium
• Teach patient to use as directed even if feeling better; may be taken with other CV products (nitrates, β-blockers)
• Caution patient not to discontinue abruptly; chest pain may occur
• Advise to report chest pain, palpitations, irregular heart beats, swelling of extremities, skin irritation, rash, tremors, weakness
• Instruct patient to notify prescriber if pregnancy is planned; may breastfeed (American Academy of Pediatrics)
• Inform patient that cap (Covera-HS ✦) may appear in stool

Evaluation
Positive therapeutic outcome
• Decreased anginal pain
• Decreased dysrhythmias
• Decreased B/P

TREATMENT OF OVERDOSE:
Defibrillation, atropine for AV block, vasopressor for hypotension, **IV** calcium

vidarabine ophthalmic
See Appendix B

vigabatrin (Rx)
(vye-ga′ba-trin)
Sabril
Func. class.: Anticonvulsant
Chem. class.: GABA transaminase inhibitor
Pregnancy category C

ACTION: May inhibit reuptake and metabolism of GABA, may increase seizure threshold; structurally similar to GABA

Therapeutic outcome: Prevention of seizure activity

USES: Adjunct treatment of partial seizures in adults and children ≥12 yr, infantile spasm

CONTRAINDICATIONS:
Hypersensitivity to this product

Precautions: Pregnancy **C**, breastfeeding, children <2 yr, geriatric patients, renal/hepatic disease, suicidal ideation/behavior, abrupt discontinuation

> **BLACK BOX WARNING:** Visual disturbance

DOSAGE AND ROUTES
Partial seizures
Adult: PO 500 mg bid, titrate in 500-mg increments at weekly intervals, up to 1.5 g bid

Infantile spasm
Infant >1 mo, child ≤2 yr: PO 50 mg/kg/day in 2 divided doses titrate in 25-50 mg/kg/day increments q3days, max 150 mg/kg/day

Renal dose
Adult: PO CCr 50-80 ml/min, reduce dosage by 25%; PO CCr 30-50 ml/min, reduce dosage by 50%; PO CCr 10-30 ml/min, reduce dosage by 75%

Available forms: Powder for oral sol 500 mg; tablet 500 mg

Implementation
PO route (tab)
- Give without regard to meals

PO route (oral solution)
- Reconstitute immediately before using
- Empty contents of appropriate number of packets into a clean cup
- For each packet, dissolve 10 ml of water, conc. 50 mg/ml; do not use other liquids
- Stir until dissolved; solution should be clear
- Use calibrated oral syringe to measure correct dosage
- Discard any unused solution

ADVERSE EFFECTS

CNS: Headache, memory impairment, *dizziness*, irritability, lethargy, **malignant hyperthermia**, insomnia, **suicidal ideation**
CV: Edema
EENT: **Vision impairment**
GI: Nausea, vomiting, diarrhea, increased appetite, abdominal pain, GI bleeding, hemorrhoids, weight gain, constipation
GU: Impotence, dysmenorrhea
HEMA: Anemia
INTEG: Pruritus, rash
RESP: Coughing, **respiratory depression, pulmonary embolism**

Pharmacokinetics

Absorption	>95%
Distribution	Widely; no protein binding
Metabolism	Not metabolized
Excretion	Urine 80% parent drug, slowed in renal disease
Half-life	7.5 hr

Pharmacodynamics

Onset	Unknown
Peak	2 hr
Duration	Unknown

INTERACTIONS
Individual drugs
AzaTHIOprine, chloroquine, deferoxamine, ethambutol, hydroxychloroquine, interferons, loxapine, mecasermin, rh-IGF-1, pentostatin, tamoxifen, thiothixene: increased serious ophthalmic effects (glaucoma, retinopathy); avoid concurrent use

Drug classifications
CNS depressants: increased CNS depression
Corticosteroids, phenothiazines, phosphodiesterase inhibitors: increased serious ophthalmic effects (glaucoma, retinopathy)

Drug/lab test
Decreased: ALT/AST

NURSING CONSIDERATIONS
Assessment
⚠ **Visual impairment: prescribers must be registered with the SHARE program due to risk of permanent vision loss; if no clinical response in 2-4 wk in pediatric patients or 3 mo in adults, provide vision assessment; assess again after ≤4 wk, at least q3mo, and 3-6 mo after stopping product**
- Monitor renal studies: urinalysis, BUN, urine creatinine q3mo in those with renal disease
- Monitor hepatic studies: ALT, AST, bilirubin
- Assess description of seizures: location, duration, presence of aura
- Assess mental status: mood, sensorium, affect, behavioral changes; if mental status changes, notify prescriber

Perform/provide
- Store at room temperature
- Provide assistance with ambulation during early part of treatment; dizziness occurs
- Provide seizure precautions: padded side rails; move objects that may harm patient

Patient/family education
- Teach patient to carry emergency ID stating patient's name, products taken, condition, prescriber's name and phone number
- Advise patient to avoid driving, other activities that require alertness
- Inform patient not to discontinue medication quickly after long-term use
- Instruct patient to notify prescriber if pregnancy is planned or suspected
⚠ **Instruct patient to report suicidal thoughts/behaviors immediately**
⚠ **Instruct patient to avoid alcohol; drowsiness, dizziness may occur**

Evaluation
Positive therapeutic outcome
- Decreased seizure activity; document on patient's chart

V

vilazodone (Rx)

(vil-az'oh-done)
Viibryd
Func. class.: Antidepressant, miscellaneous

Pregnancy category C

ACTION: A novel antidepressant unrelated to other antidepressants, enhances serotoninergic action by a dual mechanism

Therapeutic outcome: Remission of depressive symptoms

USES: Major depression

CONTRAINDICATIONS:

Concomitant use of MAOIs or within 14 days after discontinuing an MAOI or within 14 days after discontinuing vilazodone

Precautions: Abrupt discontinuation, bipolar disorder, bleeding, operating machinery, ECT, geriatrics, hepatic disease, hyponatremia, hypovolemia, infants, labor, pregnancy **C**, substance abuse, history of seizures, serotonin syndrome, neuroleptic malignant syndrome, use with serotonin precursors (e.g., tryptophan) or serotonergic drugs, suicidal ideation and worsening depression or behavior

> **BLACK BOX WARNING:** Child, suicidal ideation

DOSAGE AND ROUTES

Adult: PO 10 mg ×7 days, then 20 mg ×7 days, then 40 mg/day; if taking a potent CYP3A4 inhibitor, the max is 20 mg/day

Available forms: Tabs 10, 20, 40 mg

Implementation
• Administer with food to increase absorption
• Store at room temperature, away from moisture, heat
• Do not use within 2 wk of MAOIs

ADVERSE EFFECTS

CNS: Restlessness, dizziness, drowsiness, fatigue, mania, insomnia, migraine, **neuroleptic malignant-like syndrome,** paresthesias, **seizures, suicidal ideation,** tremor, night sweats, dream disorders
CV: Palpitations, ventricular extrasystole
EENT: Cataracts, blurred vision

GI: *Nausea,* vomiting, flatulence, *diarrhea, xerostomia,* altered taste, gastroenteritis, increased appetite
GU: Decreased libido, ejaculation disorder, increased frequency of urination, sexual dysfunction
HEMA: Bleeding, decreased platelets
INTEG: Sweating
MS: Arthralgia
SYST: Neonatal abstinence syndrome, withdrawal, **serotonin syndrome**

Pharmacokinetics

Absorption	Unknown
Distribution	Protein binding 96-99%
Metabolism	Metabolized by the liver by CYP 3A4 (major) and CYP2C19 and CYP2D (minor) and non-CYP pathways
Excretion	Unknown
Half-life	25 hr

Pharmacodynamics

Onset	Unknown
Peak	4-5 hr
Duration	Unknown

INTERACTIONS
Individual drugs
Selegline, busPIRone, dextromethorphan, fenfluramine, dexfluramine, lithium, meperidine, fentaNYL, methylphenidate, dexmethylphenidate, metoclopramide, mirtazapine, nefazodone, pentazocine, phenothiazines, haloperidol, loxapine, thiothixene, molidone: increased serotonin syndrome

Drug classifications
MAO inhibitors: do not use within 2 wk of SSRIs, SNRIs, serotonin receptor agonists, ergots, amphetamines: increased serotonin syndrome
Anticoagulants, NSAIDs, platelet inhibitors, salicylates, thrombolytics: increased bleeding
CYP3A4 inducers: decreased vilazodone effect
CYP3A4 inhibitors (clarithromycin, dronedarone, efavirenz, erythromycin, ketoconazole and others): increased vilazodone levels

Drug/herb
St. John's wort: increased serotonin syndrome

Drug/food
Grapefruit juice: avoid use

Drug/lab test
Decreased: sodium

NURSING CONSIDERATIONS
Assessment
• Assess mental status: orientation, mood behavior initially and periodically.

BLACK BOX WARNING: Initiate suicide precautions if indicated

• Assess for history of seizures, mania
• Monitor renal, hepatic status: hyponatremia
⚠ **Abrupt discontinuation: do not discontinue abruptly; taper, monitor for symptoms of withdrawal; if intolerable, resume previous dose and decrease more slowly**
⚠ **Serotonin syndrome/neuroleptic malignant syndrome: nausea, vomiting, sedation, sweating, facial flushing, high B/P; discontinue product**

Patient/family education
• Teach patient to take as directed, do not double doses
• Advise patient to avoid abrupt discontinuation unless approved by prescriber
• Instruct patient not to drive or operate machinery until effects are known
• Instruct patient not to use other products unless approved by prescriber
• Advise patient to contact prescriber if allergic reactions, personality changes (aggression, anxiety, anger, hostility), extreme sleepiness or drowsiness, confusion, nervousness, restlessness, clumsiness, numbness, tingling or burning pain in hands, arms, legs or feet, tremors, or having unusual behavior or thoughts about self-harm
• Instruct patient to notify prescriber if pregnancy is planned or suspected; avoid breastfeeding

Evaluation
Positive therapeutic outcome
• Remission of depressive symptoms

⚠ HIGH ALERT

vinBLAStine (VLB) (Rx)
(vin-blast′een)
Velbe ✿
Func. class.: Antineoplastic
Chem. class.: Vinca rosea alkaloid
Pregnancy category D

Do not confuse:
vinBLAStine/vinCRIStine/vinorelbine

ACTION: Inhibits mitotic activity, arrests cell cycle at metaphase; inhibits RNA synthesis, blocks cellular use of glutamic acid needed for purine synthesis; a vesicant

Therapeutic outcome: Prevention of rapid growth of malignant cells; immunosuppression

USES: Breast, testicular cancer; lymphomas; neuroblastoma; Hodgkin's, non-Hodgkin's lymphomas; mycosis fungoides; histiocytosis; Kaposi's sarcoma, Langerhan's cell histiocytosis

CONTRAINDICATIONS:
Pregnancy **D**, breastfeeding, infants, hypersensitivity, leukopenia, granulocytopenia, bone marrow suppression, infection

BLACK BOX WARNING: Intrathecal use

Precautions: Renal/hepatic disease, tumor lysis syndrome

BLACK BOX WARNING: Extravasation

DOSAGE AND ROUTES
Breast cancer
Adult: IV 4.5 mg/m^2 on day 1 of every 21 days in combination with DOXOrubicin and thiotepa

Hodgkin's disease
Adult: IV 6 mg/m^2 on days 1 and 15 q28 days with DOXOrubicin (ABVD)
Child: IV 2.5-6 mg/m^2/day once q 1-2 wk × 3-6 wks; max weekly dose 12.5 mg/m^2

Available forms: Inj powder 10 mg for 10 ml **IV** inj; sol for inj 1 mg/ml

Implementation
IV inj route
• Administer **IV** after diluting 10 mg/10 ml NaCl; give through Y-tube or 3-way stopcock or directly over 1 min
Intermittent IV INF route
• Further dilute in 50-100 ml of NS, inf over 15-30 min
• Give by intermittent inf
• Sol should be prepared by qualified personnel only under controlled conditions
• Use Luer-Lok tubing to prevent leakage; do not let sol come in contact with skin; if contact occurs, wash well with soap and water

BLACK BOX WARNING: Give hyaluronidase 150 units/ml in 1 ml of NaCl, warm compress for extravasation for vesicant activity treatment

---

✿ Canada only   Adverse effects: *italics* = common; **bold** = life-threatening

> **BLACK BOX WARNING:** Do not administer intrathecally: fatal

Syringe compatibilities: Bleomycin, CISplatin, cyclophosphamide, droperidol, fluorouracil, leucovorin, methotrexate, metoclopramide, mitomycin, vinCRIStine

Y-site compatibilities: Allopurinol, amifostine, aztreonam, bleomycin, CISplatin, cyclophosphamide, DOXOrubicin, droperidol, filgrastim, fludarabine, fluorouracil, granisetron, heparin, leucovorin, melphalan, methotrexate, metoclopramide, mitomycin, ondansetron, PACLitaxel, piperacillin/tazobactam, sargramostim, teniposide, thiotepa, vinCRIStine, vinorelbine

Y-site incompatibilities: Furosemide

Additive compatibilities: Bleomycin

ADVERSE EFFECTS
CNS: Paresthesias, peripheral neuropathy, depression, headache, **seizures**, malaise
CV: Tachycardia, orthostatic hypotension, hypertension
GI: *Nausea, vomiting,* ileus, *anorexia, stomatitis, constipation,* abdominal pain, GI and rectal bleeding, **hepatotoxicity,** pharyngitis
GU: Urinary retention, **renal failure,** hyperuricemia
HEMA: **Thrombocytopenia, leukopenia, myelosuppression,** agranulocytosis, granulocytosis, aplastic anemia, neutropenia, pancytopenia
INTEG: *Rash, alopecia,* photosensitivity, **extravasation, tissue necrosis**
META: SIADH
SYST: Tumor lysis syndrome (TLS)
RESP: Fibrosis, pulmonary infiltrate, bronchospasm

Pharmacokinetics

Absorption	Complete bioavailability
Distribution	Crosses blood-brain barrier slightly
Metabolism	Liver—active antineoplastic
Excretion	Biliary, kidneys
Half-life	Triphasic <5 min, 50-155 min, 23-85 hr

Pharmacodynamics
Unknown

INTERACTIONS
Individual drugs
Bleomycin: increased synergism
Methotrexate: increased methotrexate action
MitoMYcin: increased bronchospasm
Phenytoin: decreased phenytoin level
Radiation: increased toxicity, bone marrow suppression; do not use together

Drug classifications
Anticoagulants, antiplatelets, NSAIDs, thrombolytics: increased bleeding risk
Antineoplastics: increased toxicity, bone marrow suppression
CYP3A4 inducers (barbiturates, bosentan, carBAMazepine, efavirenz, phenytoin, nevirapine, rifabutin, rifampin): decreased vinBLAStine effect
CYP3A4 inhibitors (aprepitant, antiretroviral protease inhibitors, clarithromycin, danazol, delavirdine, diltiazem, erythromycin, fluconazole, FLUoxetine, fluvoxaMINE, imatinib, ketoconazole, mebefradil, nefazodone, telithromycin, voriconazole): increased toxicity
Live virus vaccines: increased adverse reactions

Drug/herb
St. John's wort: avoid use

Drug/lab test
Increased: uric acid, bilirubin
Decreased: Hgb, platelets, WBC

NURSING CONSIDERATIONS
Assessment
• Monitor B/P (baseline and q15min) during administration
• Monitor CBC, differential, platelet count weekly; withhold product if WBC is $<2000/$mm^3 or platelet count is $<75,000/$mm^3; notify prescriber of results; recovery will take 3 wk; RBC, Hct, Hgb may be decreased; nadir occurs on days 4-10, and continues for another 1-2 wk
⚠ **Tumor lysis syndrome: monitor for hyperkalemia, hyperphosphatemia, hyperuricemia; usually occurs with leukemia, lymphoma; alkalinization of the urine; allopurinol should be used to prevent urate nephropathy; monitor electrolytes and renal function (BUN, uric acid, urine CCR)**
• Monitor renal function tests: BUN, serum uric acid, urine CCr before, during therapy; I&O ratio; report fall in urine output of 30 ml/hr; for decreased hyperuricemia
⚠ **Bronchospasm: can be life threatening; usually occurs when giving mitoMYcin**

- Monitor for cold, fever, sore throat (may indicate beginning of infection); notify prescriber if these occur
- Assess for bleeding: hematuria, guaiac, bruising or petechiae, mucosa or orifices q8hr, no rectal temp; avoid IM inj; use pressure to venipuncture sites
- Identify nutritional status: an antiemetic may need to be prescribed
- Assess for gout, joint pain, swelling, increased uric acid; allopurinol or other treatment may be used
- Assess for symptoms indicating severe allergic reactions: rash, pruritus, urticaria, itching, flushing, bronchospasm, hypotension; EPINEPHrine and resuscitative equipment should be nearby
- Hepatitis: transient hepatitis may occur with continuous IV

Patient/family education

- Teach patient to avoid use of products containing aspirin or NSAIDs, razors, commercial mouthwash because bleeding may occur; to report symptoms of bleeding (hematuria, tarry stools)
- Instruct patient to report signs of anemia, (fatigue, headache, irritability, faintness, shortness of breath)
- Caution patient to report any changes in breathing or coughing even several mo after treatment; avoid breastfeeding; may cause male infertility
- Advise patient that contraception will be necessary during treatment; teratogenesis may occur
- Advise patient to use sunscreen, wear protective clothing and sunglasses
- Inform patient that hair may be lost during treatment; a wig or hairpiece may make patient feel better; new hair will be different in color, texture
- Advise patient to avoid vaccinations during treatment; serious reactions may occur
- Teach patient to report signs/symptoms of infection: fever, chills, sore throat; patient should avoid crowds and persons with known infections
- **Pregnancy:** teach patient to notify prescriber if pregnancy is planned or suspected, pregnancy D, avoid breastfeeding, may cause male infertility
⚠ **Instruct patient to avoid persons with known infections**
⚠ **Infection: instruct patient to report sore throat, flulike symptoms**

Evaluation
Positive therapeutic outcome
- Decreased spread of malignant cells

⚠ HIGH ALERT

vinCRIStine (VCR) (Rx)
(vin-kris′teen)
Vincasar PFS
Func. class.: Antineoplastic—miscellaneous
Chem. class.: Vinca alkaloid
Pregnancy category D

Do not confuse:
vinCRIStine/vinBLAStine/vinorelbine

ACTION: Inhibits mitotic activity, arrests cell cycle at metaphase; inhibits RNA synthesis, blocks cellular use of glutamic acid needed for purine synthesis; a vesicant

Therapeutic outcome: Prevention of rapid growth of malignant cells, immunosuppression

USES: Lymphomas, neuroblastomas, Hodgkin's disease, acute lymphoblastic and other leukemias, rhabdomyosarcoma, Wilms' tumor, non-Hodgkin's lymphoma, malignant glioma, soft-tissue sarcoma

CONTRAINDICATIONS:
Pregnancy **D**, breastfeeding, infants, hypersensitivity, radiation therapy

> **BLACK BOX WARNING:** Intrathecal use

Precautions: Renal/hepatic disease, hypertension, neuromuscular disease

> **BLACK BOX WARNING:** Extravasation

V

DOSAGE AND ROUTES
Adult: IV 0.4-1.4 mg/m^2/wk, max 2 mg
Child >10 kg: IV 1-2 mg/m^2/wk, max 2 mg

Available forms: Inj 1 mg/ml; powder for inj 5 mg/vial

Implementation

> **BLACK BOX WARNING:** Do not give intrathecally: fatal

- Administer **IV** after diluting with diluent provided or 1 mg/10 ml of sterile water or 0.9%

Adverse effects: *italics* = common; **bold** = life-threatening

NaCl; give through Y-tube or 3-way stopcock or directly over 1 min; do not use 5-mg vial for single doses

> **BLACK BOX WARNING:** Hyaluronidase 150 units/ml in 1 ml of NaCl; apply warm compress for extravasation

Syringe compatibilities: Bleomycin, CISplatin, cyclophosphamide, doxapram, DOXOrubicin, droperidol, fluorouracil, heparin, leucovorin, methotrexate, metoclopramide, mitoMYcin, ondansetron, vinCRIStine

Syringe incompatibilities: Furosemide

Y-site compatibilities: Allopurinol, amifostine, aztreonam, bleomycin, CISplatin, cladribine, cyclophosphamide, DOXOrubicin, droperidol, filgrastim, fludarabine, fluorouracil, granisetron, heparin, leucovorin, methotrexate, metoclopramide, mitoMYcin, ondansetron, PACLitaxel, sargramostim, teniposide, thiotepa, vinCRIStine, vinorelbine

Y-site incompatibilities: Furosemide

ADVERSE EFFECTS
CNS: *Decreased reflexes, numbness, weakness, motor difficulties,* CNS depression, cranial nerve paralysis, **seizures,** peripheral neuropathy
CV: Orthostatic hypotension
EENT: *Diplopia*
GI: *Nausea, vomiting, anorexia, stomatitis, constipation,* **paralytic ileus, abdominal pain, hepatotoxicity**
GU: Renal tubular obstruction
HEMA: **Thrombocytopenia, leukopenia, myelosuppression, anemia**
INTEG: *Alopecia,* extravasation
SYST: Tumor lysis syndrome (TLS)

Pharmacokinetics

Absorption	Complete bioavailability
Distribution	Rapidly, widely distributed; crosses blood-brain barrier
Metabolism	Liver
Excretion	Biliary, in feces, crosses placenta
Half-life	Triphasic <5 min, 50-155 min, 23-85 hr

Pharmacodynamics

Onset	Unknown
Peak	Unknown
Duration	1 wk

INTERACTIONS
Individual drugs
Digoxin: decreased digoxin level
MitoMYcin-C: increased acute pulmonary reactions
Radiation: increased toxicity, bone marrow suppression; do not use together

Drug classifications
CYP3A4 inducers (barbiturates, bosentan, carBAMazepine, efavirenz, phenytoins, nevirapine, rifabutin, rifampin): decreased vinCRIStine effect
CYP3A4 inhibitors (aprepitant, antiretroviral protease inhibitors, clarithromycin, danazol, delavirdine, diltiazem, erythromycin, fluconazole, FLUoxetine, fluvoxaMINE, imatinib, ketoconazole, mibefradil, nefazodone, telithromycin, voriconazole): increased toxicity
Peripheral nervous system products: increased neurotoxicity
Vaccines/toxoids: decreased immune response

Drug/herb
St. John's wort: avoid use

Drug/lab test
Increased: uric acid
Decreased: Hgb, WBC, platelets, sodium

NURSING CONSIDERATIONS
Assessment
• Monitor CBC, differential, platelet count weekly; withhold product if WBC is <4000/mm^3 or platelet count is <75,000/mm^3; notify prescriber of results; platelets may increase or decrease
• Assess neurologic status: paresthesia, weakness, cranial nerve palsies, orthostatic hypotension, lethargy, agitation, psychosis; notify prescriber
• **Bronchospasm:** more common with mitoMYcin
• Identify for increased uric acid levels, joint pain in extremities; increase fluid intake to 2-3 L/day unless contraindicated
⚠ **Tumor lysis syndrome: hyperkalemia, hyperphosphatemia, hyperuricemia, hypocalcemia; more common in leukemia, lymphoma, use alkalinization of urine with allopurinol, monitor electrolytes, renal function (BUN, urine, CCR, uric acid)**

Patient/family education
• Teach patient to avoid use of products containing aspirin or NSAIDs, razors, commercial mouthwash because bleeding may occur; to report symptoms of bleeding (hematuria, tarry stools)

⚠ Nurse Alert   ✦ Key NCLEX® Drug

• Instruct patient to report signs of anemia (fatigue, headache, irritability, faintness, shortness of breath)
• Caution patient to report any changes in breathing or coughing, even several mo after treatment
⚠ **Pregnancy: instruct patient to notify prescriber if pregnancy is planned or suspected**
• Advise patient that contraception will be necessary during and 2 mo after treatment; may be teratogenic, pregnancy **D**, avoid breastfeeding
• Inform patient that hair may be lost during treatment; a wig or hairpiece may make patient feel better; new hair will be different in color, texture
• Advise patient to avoid vaccinations during treatment; serious reactions may occur
• Teach patient to report signs/symptoms of infection: fever, chills, sore throat; patient should avoid crowds or persons with known infections
• Advise patient to increase fluids, bulk in diet, exercise to prevent constipation
⚠ **Infection: instruct patient to report sore throat, fever, flulike symptoms; avoid persons with known infection**

Evaluation
Positive therapeutic outcome
• Decreased spread of malignancies

⚠ HIGH ALERT

vinorelbine (Rx)
(vi-nor′el-bine)
Navelbine
Func. class.: Antineoplastic—miscellaneous
Chem. class.: Semisynthetic vinca alkaloid
Pregnancy category D

ACTION: Inhibits mitotic spindle activity, arrests cell cycle at metaphase; inhibits RNA synthesis, blocks cellular use of glutamic acid needed for purine synthesis; a vesicant

Therapeutic outcome: Decreased spread of malignancy

USES: Unresectable, advanced non–small-cell lung cancer (NSCLC) stage IV; may be used alone or in combination with cisplatin for stage III or IV NSCLC

CONTRAINDICATIONS:
Pregnancy **D**, breastfeeding, hypersensitivity, infants, granulocyte count <1000 cells/mm^3 pretreatment

---

BLACK BOX WARNING: Severe neutropenia, intrathecal use

Precautions: Children, geriatric, hepatic/pulmonary/neurologic/renal disease, bone marrow suppression

BLACK BOX WARNING: Extravasation

DOSAGE AND ROUTES
Adult: **IV** 30 mg/m^2 qwk

ANC: 1000-1499, give 50% dose; <1000 hold dose; $<1000 \times 3$ wk, discontinue

Hepatic dose
Adult: **IV** total bilirubin 2.1-3 mg/dl 15 mg/m^2 qwk; total bilirubin ≥3 mg/dl 7.5 mg/m^2/day

Available forms: Inj 10 mg/ml

Implementation

BLACK BOX WARNING: Do not give intrathecally: fatal

BLACK BOX WARNING: Hyaluronidase 150 units/ml in 1 ml of 0.9% NaCl, warm compress for extravasation for vesicant activity treatment

• Antacid before oral agent; give product after evening meal before bedtime
• Antiemetic 30-60 min before giving product and prn to prevent vomiting
Intermittent IV infusion route
• Dilute to 0.5-2 mg/ml with 0.9% NaCl, 0.45% NaCl, D$_5$W, D$_5$/0.45% NaCl, LR, Ringer's; give over 6-10 min into Y-site or central line; flush line
Continuous IV infusion route
• Give 40 mg/m^2 q3wk after **IV** bol of 8 mg/m^2; may be given in combination with DOXOrubicin, fluorouracil, cisplatin

Y-site compatibilities: Amikacin, aztreonam, bleomycin, buprenorphine, butorphanol, calcium gluconate, CARBOplatin, cefotaxime, CISplatin, cimetidine, clindamycin, dexamethasone, enalaprilat, etoposide, famotidine, filgrastim, fluconazole, fludarabine, gentamicin, hydrocortisone, LORazepam, meperidine, morphine, netilmicin, ondansetron, plicamycin, streptozocin, teniposide, ticarcillin, tobramycin, vancomycin, vinBLAStine, vinCRIStine, zidovudine

ADVERSE EFFECTS
CNS: Paresthesias, peripheral neuropathy, depression, headache, **seizures,** weakness, jaw pain, asthenia

V

CV: Chest pain
GI: *Nausea, vomiting,* ileus, *anorexia, stomatitis,* constipation, abdominal pain, *diarrhea,* **hepatotoxicity, GI obstruction/perforation**
HEMA: Neutropenia, anemia, thrombocytopenia, granulocytopenia
INTEG: *Rash, alopecia,* photosensitivity, inj site reaction, necrosis
META: Syndrome of inappropriate diuretic hormone
MS: Myalgia
RESP: Shortness of breath, **dyspnea, pulmonary edema, acute bronchospasm, acute respiratory distress syndrome (ARDS)**

Pharmacokinetics

Absorption	Poor bioavailability ($<$50%)
Distribution	Highly bound to platelets, lymphocytes
Metabolism	Liver, to metabolite
Excretion	Bile
Half-life	43 hr

Pharmacodynamics

Onset	Unknown
Peak	1-2 hr
Duration	Unknown

INTERACTIONS

Drug classifications
NSAIDs, anticoagulants: increased bleeding risk
CYP3A4 inhibitors (antiretroviral protease inhibitors, aprepitant, clarithromycin, danazol, delavirdine, diltiazem, erythromycin, fluconazole, FLUoxetine, fluvoxaMINE, imatinib, ketoconazole, mibefradil, nefazodone, telithromycin, voriconazole): increased toxicity
CYP3A4 inducers (barbiturates, bosentan, carBAMazepine, efavirenz, phenytoins, nevirapine, rifabutin, rifampin): decreased vinorelbine effect

Drug/herb
St. John's wort: avoid use

Drug/lab test
Increased: LFTs, bilirubin
Decreased: Hgb, WBC, platelets

NURSING CONSIDERATIONS

Assessment
• Monitor B/P (baseline and q15min) during administration

BLACK BOX WARNING: Monitor CBC, differential, platelet count before each dose; withhold product if WBC is $<$4000/mm^3 or platelet count is $<$75,000/mm^3; notify prescriber of results; recovery will take 3 wk; liver function tests: AST, ALT, bilirubin, LDH

⚠ **Bronchospasm: more common with mitoMYcin; also dyspnea, wheezing; may be treated with oxygen, bronchodilators, corticosteroids, especially if there is underlying pulmonary disease**
• Assess for dyspnea, crackles, unproductive cough, chest pain, tachypnea
• Monitor renal function tests: BUN, serum uric acid, urine CCr before, during therapy, I&O ratio; report fall in urine output of 30 ml/hr; for decreased hyperuricemia
• Monitor for cold, fever, sore throat (may indicate beginning **infection**); notify prescriber if these occur; effects of alopecia on body image
• **Assess for bleeding:** hematuria, guaiac, bruising or petechiae, mucosa or orifices q8hr: no rectal temp; avoid IM inj; use pressure on venipuncture sites
• **Assess for symptoms indicating severe allergic reactions:** rash, pruritus, urticaria, itching, flushing, bronchospasm, hypotension; epinephrine and resuscitative equipment should be nearby
• Assess neurologic status: numbness, pain, tingling, loss of Achilles reflex, weakness, palsies

Patient/family education
• Teach patient to use liquid diet: cola, gelatin; dry toast or crackers may be added if patient is not nauseated or vomiting
• Advise patient to rinse mouth 3-4 ✕/day with water and brush teeth 2-3 ✕/day with soft brush or cotton-tipped applicators for stomatitis; use unwaxed dental floss
• Advise patient to avoid crowds, people with infections, vaccinations
• **Pregnancy:** notify prescriber if pregnancy is planned or suspected; advise patient to use effective contraception during and for $\geq$2 mo after product is discontinued; pregnancy **D,** avoid breastfeeding
• Teach patient hair may be lost but will grow back; new hair may be different texture, color
⚠ **Infection: report sore throat, fever, flulike symptoms**

Evaluation
Positive therapeutic outcome
• Decreased spread of malignant cells

---

vismodegib

(vis'moe-deg'ib)
Erivedge
Func. class.: Antineoplastic biologic response modifier
Chem. class.: Signal transduction inhibitor (STI)
Pregnancy category: D

ACTION: A hedgehog (Hh) signaling pathway inhibitor

Therapeutic outcome: Decreased spread of tumor

USES: Patients who have metastatic basal cell carcinoma, locally advanced, that has recurred after surgery and who are not candidates for surgery/radiation

CONTRAINDICATIONS:

Hypersensitivity, breastfeeding

> **BLACK BOX WARNING:** Intrauterine fetal death, male-mediated teratogenicity, pregnancy **(D)**

Precautions: Children, blood donation

DOSAGE AND ROUTES

Adult: **PO** 150 mg/day

Available forms: Cap 150 mg

Implementation
• Give without regard to food
• To be swallowed whole, do not open or crush caps
• If a dose is missed, do not take additional dose, take at usual time
• Store at 77°F (25°C)

ADVERSE EFFECTS

GI: Nausea, vomiting, dysgeusia
GU: Amenorrhea, azotemia
INTEG: Alopecia
META: Hyponatremia
MISC: Fatigue, decreased weight
MS: Arthralgia

Pharmacokinetics

Absorption	Unknown
Distribution	Protein binding >99%
Metabolism	Unknown
Excretion	Unknown
Half-life	Elimination 4 days

Pharmacodynamics

Onset	Unknown
Peak	Unknown
Duration	Unknown

INTERACTIONS

Drug classifications

Pgp inhibitors (amiodarone, clarithromycin, cycloSPORINE, diltiazem, erythromycin, indinavir, itraconazole, ketoconazole, nelfinavir, niCARdipine, propafenone, quiNIDine, ritonavir, saquinavir, tacrolimus, tamoxifen, verapamil); CYP2C19 substrates (amitriptyline, clomiPRAMINE, imipramine, citalopram, diazepam, phenytoin, PHENobarbital, lansoprazole, omeprazole, pantoprazole, RABEprazole, esomeprazole, clopidogrel, proguanil, propranolol, carisoprodol, chloramphenicol, cyclophosphamide, indomethacin, nelfinavir, nilutamide, progesterone, teniposide, warfarin): Increased effect of each product

NURSING CONSIDERATIONS

Assessment

> **BLACK BOX WARNING:** Pregnancy **D:** Verify pregnancy status of all women within 7 days before starting therapy; effective contraception is needed during and for 7 mo after treatment; men receiving this product should use condoms with spermicide (even after vasectomy) during sexual intercourse with female partners and for 2 mo after the last dose; report exposure during pregnancy to the Genentech Adverse Event Line

Patient/family education

> **BLACK BOX WARNING:** Pregnancy **D:** Teach patient to notify their provider immediately if pregnancy is suspected (or in a female partner for male patients); effective contraception is needed during and for 7 mo after treatment; men receiving this product should use condoms with spermicide (even after vasectomy) during sexual intercourse with female partners and for 2 mo after the last dose; if product is used during pregnancy or if the patient becomes pregnant during use, the woman (or female partner for male patients) should be apprised of the potential hazard to the fetus; encourage exposed women (either directly or through seminal fluid) to participate in the ERIVEDGE pregnancy pharmacovigilance program

• Teach patient about reason for treatment, expected Results

V

Adverse effects: *italics* = common; **bold** = life-threatening

Evaluation
Positive therapeutic outcome
• Decreased spread of tumor

---

vitamin A (PO, OTC; IM, Rx)
Aquasol A, Del-Vi-A, Vitamin A
Func. class.: Vitamin, fat-soluble
Chem. class.: Retinol
Pregnancy category C (PO); X (parenteral)

ACTION: Needed for normal bone and tooth development, visual dark adaptation, skin disease, mucosa tissue repair; assists in production of adrenal steroids, cholesterol, RNA

Therapeutic outcome: Prevention, absence of vit A deficiency

USES: Vit A deficiency

CONTRAINDICATIONS:
Pregnancy **X** (parenteral), hypersensitivity to vit A, malabsorption syndrome (PO), hypervitaminosis A, parenteral, **IV** administration

Precautions: Pregnancy **C** (PO), breastfeeding, impaired renal function, children, hepatic disease, infants, alcoholism, hepatitis

DOSAGE AND ROUTES
Adult and child >8 yr: PO 100,000-500,000 international units/day × 3 days, then 50,000 international units/day × 2 wk; dose based on severity of deficiency; maintenance 10,000-20,000 international units for 2 mo
Child 1-8 yr: IM 5000-15,000 international units/day × 10 days
Infant <1 yr: IM 5000-15,000 international units × 10 days

Maintenance
Child 4-8 yr: IM 15,000 international units/day × 2 mo
Child <4 yr: IM 10,000 international units/day × 2 mo

Available forms: Caps 10,000, 25,000, 50,000 international units; drops 5000 international units; inj 50,000 international units/ml; tabs 10,000, 25,000, 50,000 international units

Implementation
PO route
• Give with food (PO) for better absorption; do not give **IV** because anaphylaxis may occur, IM only

• Oral preparations are not indicated for vit A deficiency in those with malabsorption syndrome
• Store in airtight, light-resistant container
IM route
• Give deep in large muscle mass; do not use deltoid muscle for administration of >1 ml

ADVERSE EFFECTS
CNS: Headache, increased ICP, intracranial hypertension, lethargy, malaise
EENT: Gingivitis, papilledema, exophthalmos, inflammation of tongue and lips
GI: Nausea, vomiting, anorexia, abdominal pain, *jaundice*
INTEG: Drying of skin, pruritus, increased pigmentation, night sweats, alopecia
META: Hypomenorrhea, hypercalcemia
MS: Arthralgia, retarded growth, hard areas on bone

Pharmacokinetics
Absorption	Rapidly absorbed
Distribution	Stored in liver, kidneys, lungs
Metabolism	Liver
Excretion	Breast milk
Half-life	Unknown

Pharmacodynamics
Unknown

INTERACTIONS
Individual drugs
Cholestyramine, colestipol, mineral oil: decreased absorption of vit A

Drug classifications
Contraceptives (oral), corticosteroids: increased levels of vit A

Drug/lab test
False increase: bilirubin, serum cholesterol

NURSING CONSIDERATIONS
Assessment
• Assess nutritional status: increase intake of yellow and dark green vegetables, yellow/orange fruits, vit A–fortified foods, liver, egg yolks
• Assess vit A deficiency: decreased growth; night blindness; dry, brittle nails; hair loss; urinary stones; increased infection; hyperkeratosis of skin; drying of cornea
• Identify vit A deficiency by plasma vit A, carotene level

• Assess for chronic vit A toxicity: increased calcium, BUN, glucose, cholesterol, triglyceride level

Patient/family education
• Instruct patient that if dose is missed, it should be omitted
• Inform patient that ophth exams may be required periodically throughout therapy
• Instruct patient not to use mineral oil while taking this product because absorption will be decreased
• Advise patient to notify prescriber of nausea, vomiting, lip cracking, loss of hair, headache
• Caution patient not to take more than the prescribed amount

Evaluation
Positive therapeutic outcome
• Increase in growth rate, weight
• Absence of dry skin and mucous membranes, night blindness

TREATMENT OF OVERDOSE:
Discontinue product

vitamin A acid
See tretinoin

vitamin B₁
See thiamine

vitamin B₁₂ (cyano-cobalamin) (PO, OTC; IM/SUBCUT, Rx)
(sye-an-oh-koe-bal'a-min)
Alphamin, Anacobin ✦, Bedoz ✦, Cobex, Cobolin-M Crystamine, Crysti-1000, Cyanabin ✦, Cyanoject, Cyomin, Ener-B, Hydrobexan, Hydro Cobex, Hydro-Crysti-12
Func. class.: Vitamin B₁₂, water-soluble vitamin

vitamin B₁₂a (hydroxoco-balamin) (vit B₁₂) (Rx)
(hye-drox'o-ko-bal'a-min)
Hydro Cobex, Hydroxycobal, LA-12, Nascobal, Neuroforter, Rubesol-1000, Rubramin PC, Shovite, Vibral LA, Vibral, Vitamin B₁₂
Pregnancy category A

ACTION: Needed for adequate nerve functioning, protein and carbohydrate metabolism, normal growth, RBC development and cell reproduction

Therapeutic outcome: Prevention, correction of vit B₁₂ deficiency

USES: Vit B₁₂ deficiency; pernicious anemia; vit B₁₂ malabsorption syndrome; Schilling test; increased requirements with pregnancy, thyrotoxicosis, hemolytic anemia, hemorrhage, renal and hepatic disease

CONTRAINDICATIONS:
Hypersensitivity, optic nerve atrophy

Precautions: Pregnancy **A**, breastfeeding, children

DOSAGE AND ROUTES
Cyanocobalamin
Adult: PO up to 1000 mcg/day; SUBCUT/IM 30-100 mcg/day × 1 wk, then 100-200 mcg/mo

Shilling test
Adult and child: IM 1000 mcg in 1 dose
Child: PO up to 1000 mcg/day; SUBCUT/IM 30-50 mcg/day × 2 wk, then 100 mcg/mo; NASAL 500 mcg qwk

Hydroxocobalamin
Adult: SUBCUT/IM 30-50 mcg/day × 5-10 days, then 100-200 mcg/mo
Child: SUBCUT/IM 30-50 mcg/day × 5-10 days, then 30-50 mcg/mo

Available forms: Cyanocobalamin: tabs 25, 50, 100, 250, 500, 1000, 5000 mcg; ext rel tabs 100, 200, 500, 1000 mcg; lozenges: 100, 250, 500 mcg; nasal gel 500 mcg/spray; inj 100, 1000 mcg/ml; hydroxocobalamin: inj 1000 mcg/ml

Implementation
PO route
• Give with fruit juice to disguise taste; administer immediately after mixing
• Give with meals if possible for better absorption; large doses should not be used because most is excreted
IM route
• Give by IM inj for pernicious anemia for life unless contraindicated
IV route
• May be mixed with TPN sol, but **IV** route is not recommended

Y-site compatibilities: Heparin, hydrocortisone sodium succinate, potassium chloride

Solution compatibilities: Dextrose/Ringer's or LR's combinations, dextrose/saline combinations, D_5W, $D_{10}W$, 0.45% NaCl, Ringer's or LR's sol, ascorbic acid

ADVERSE EFFECTS

CNS: Flushing, optic nerve atrophy
CV: CHF, peripheral vascular thrombosis, **pulmonary edema**
GI: *Diarrhea*
INTEG: Itching, rash, pain at inj site
META: Hypokalemia
SYST: Anaphylactic shock

Pharmacokinetics

Absorption	Well absorbed (IM, SUBCUT)
Distribution	Crosses placenta
Metabolism	Stored in liver, kidney, stomach
Excretion	50%-90% (urine), breast milk
Half-life	Unknown

Pharmacodynamics

Unknown

INTERACTIONS

Individual drugs

Aminosalicylic acid, chloramphenicol, cimetidine, colchicine: decreased absorption
PredniSONE: increased absorption

Drug classifications

Aminoglycosides, anticonvulsants, potassium products: decreased absorption

Drug/herb

Goldenseal: decreased vit B_{12} absorption

Drug/lab test

False positive: intrinsic factor

NURSING CONSIDERATIONS

Assessment

• Assess for deficiency: anorexia, dyspepsia on exertion, palpitations, paresthesias, psychosis, visual disturbances, pallor, red inflamed tongue, neuropathy, edema of legs
• Monitor potassium levels during beginning treatment in patients with megaloblastic anemia
• Monitor CBC for increase in reticulocyte count during 1st wk of therapy, then increase in RBC and hemoglobin; folic acid levels, vit B_{12} levels
• Assess nutritional status: egg yolks, fish, organ meats, dairy products, clams, oysters, which are good sources of vit B_{12}
• Monitor for pulmonary edema or worsening of CHF in cardiac patients

Patient/family education

• Instruct patient that treatment must continue for life if diagnosed as having pernicious anemia
• Advise patient to eat well-balanced diet from the food pyramid and comply with dietary recommendation
• Caution patient not to exceed the RDA of vit B_{12} because adverse reactions may occur

Evaluation

Positive therapeutic outcome

• Decreased anorexia, dyspnea on exertion, palpitations, paresthesias, psychosis, visual disturbances, edema of legs
• Prevention or correction of vit B_{12} deficiency

TREATMENT OF OVERDOSE:

Discontinue products

vitamin D (cholecalciferol, vitamin D_3 or ergocalciferol, vitamin D_2) (Rx, OTC)
Calciferol, Delta-D, Drisdol, Radiostol ✦, Radiostol Forte ✦, vitamin D, vitamin D_3
Func. class.: Vitamin D
Chem. class.: Fat-soluble vitamin
Pregnancy category C

Do not confuse:

Calciferol/calcitriol

ACTION: Needed for regulation of calcium, phosphate levels; normal bone development; parathyroid activity; neuromuscular functioning

Therapeutic outcome: Prevention of rickets, osteomalacia, normal calcium/phosphate levels

USES: Vit D deficiency, rickets, renal osteodystrophy, hypoparathyroidism, hypophosphatemia, psoriasis, rheumatoid arthritis

CONTRAINDICATIONS:

Hypersensitivity, hypercalcemia, renal dysfunction, hyperphosphatemia

Precautions: Pregnancy **C,** CV disease, renal calculi

DOSAGE AND ROUTES

Deficiency

Adult: PO/IM 12,000 international units/day, then increased to 500,000 international units/day

---

Child: PO/IM 1500-5000 international units/day × 2-4 wk, may repeat after 2 wk or 600,000 international units as single dose

Hypoparathyroidism
Adult and child: PO/IM 200,000 international units given with 4 g calcium tab

Available forms: Tabs 400, 1000, 50,000 international units; caps 25,000, 50,000 international units; oral sol 8000 international units/ml; inj 500,000 international units/ml, 500,000 international units/5 ml

Implementation
PO route
• PO may be increased q4wk depending on blood level
• Store in airtight, light-resistant container at room temperature
IM route
• Give inj deeply in large muscle mass, administer slowly, aspirate to avoid **IV** administration, rotate inj site

ADVERSE EFFECTS
CNS: Fatigue, weakness, drowsiness, **seizures,** headache, psychosis
CV: Hypertension, dysrhythmias
GI: Nausea, vomiting, anorexia, cramps, diarrhea, constipation, metallic taste, dry mouth
GU: Polyuria, nocturia, **hematuria, albuminuria, renal failure,** decreased libido
INTEG: Pruritus, photophobia
MS: Decreased bone growth, early joint pain, early muscle pain

Pharmacokinetics
Absorption	Well absorbed
Distribution	Stored in liver
Metabolism	Liver, sun
Excretion	Bile, kidney
Half-life	12-22 hr

Pharmacodynamics
	PO	IM
Onset	Unknown	Unknown
Peak	4 hr	Unknown
Duration	15-20 days	Unknown

INTERACTIONS
Individual drugs
Cholestyramine, colestipol, PHENobarbital, phenytoin: decreased effects of vit D
Verapamil: increased toxicity

Drug classifications
Antacids, diuretics (thiazide): increased toxicity

NURSING CONSIDERATIONS
Assessment
• Monitor BUN, urinary calcium, AST, ALT, cholesterol, creatinine, uric acid, chloride, magnesium, electrolytes, urine pH, phosphate—may increase; calcium should be kept at 9-10 mg/dl; vit D at 50-135 international units/dl, phosphate at 70 mg/dl; alkaline phosphatase may be decreased
• Monitor for increased blood level; toxic reactions may occur rapidly
• Assess for dry mouth, metallic taste, polyuria, bone pain, muscle weakness, headache, fatigue, tinnitus, change in LOC, irregular pulse, dysrhythmias, increased respirations, anorexia, nausea, vomiting, cramps, diarrhea, constipation; may indicate hypercalcemia
• Assess renal status: decreased urinary output (oliguria, anuria), edema in extremities, weight gain ≥5 lb, periorbital edema
• Assess nutritional status, diet for sources of vit D (milk, cod, halibut, salmon, sardines, egg yolk), calcium (dairy products, dark green vegetables), phosphates (dairy products)

Patient/family education
• Advise patient to omit dose if missed; to avoid vitamin supplements unless directed by prescriber
• Inform patient of necessary foods to be included in diet
• Advise patient to keep appointments for evaluation because therapeutic and toxic levels are narrow
• Instruct patient to report weakness, lethargy, headache, anorexia, loss of weight; to report nausea, vomiting, abdominal cramps, diarrhea, constipation, excessive thirst, polyuria, muscle and bone pain
• Caution patient to decrease intake of antacids and laxatives containing magnesium

Evaluation
Positive therapeutic outcome
• Calcium levels 9-10 ml/dl
• Decreasing symptoms of bone disease

vitamin E (OTC)
Aquasol E
Func. class.: Vitamin E
Chem. class.: Fat-soluble vitamin
Pregnancy category A

ACTION: Needed for digestion and metabolism of polyunsaturated fats, decreases platelet aggregation, decreases blood clot formation,

Adverse effects: *italics* = common; **bold** = life-threatening

promotes normal growth and development of muscle tissue, prostaglandin synthesis

Therapeutic outcome: Prevention and treatment of vit E deficiency

USES: Vit E deficiency, impaired fat absorption, hemolytic anemia in premature neonates, prevention of retrolental fibroplasia, sickle cell anemia, supplement in malabsorption syndrome

CONTRAINDICATIONS:
IV use in infants

Precautions: Pregnancy **A**, anemia, breastfeeding, hypothrombinemia

DOSAGE AND ROUTES
Deficiency
Adult: PO 60-75 international units/day
Child: PO 1 international unit/kg (malabsorption)

Prevention of deficiency
Adult: PO 30 international units/day
Infant: PO 5 international units/day

Topical route
Adult and child: TOP apply to affected areas as needed

Available forms: Caps 100, 200, 400, 500, 600, 1000 international units; tabs 100, 200, 400 international units; drops 50 mg/ml; chew tabs 400 units; ointment, cream, lotion, oil

Implementation
PO route
• Chew chewable tabs well
• Sol may be dropped in mouth or mixed with food
• Store in airtight, light-resistant container
Topical route
• Apply topical to moisturize dry skin

ADVERSE EFFECTS
CNS: Headache, fatigue
CV: Increased risk of thrombophlebitis
EENT: Blurred vision
GI: Nausea, cramps, diarrhea
GU: Gonadal dysfunction
INTEG: Sterile abscess, contact dermatitis
META: Altered metabolism of hormones (thyroid, pituitary, adrenal), altered immunity
MS: Weakness

Pharmacokinetics
Absorption	20%-80% (PO)
Distribution	Widely distributed, stored in fat
Metabolism	Liver
Excretion	Bile
Half-life	Unknown

Pharmacodynamics
Unknown

INTERACTIONS
Individual drugs
Cholestyramine, colestipol, mineral oil, sucralfate: decreased absorption

Drug classification
Anticoagulants (oral): increased action of anticoagulants

NURSING CONSIDERATIONS
Assessment
• Assess nutritional status: intake of wheat germ, dark green leafy vegetables, nuts, eggs, liver, vegetable oils, dairy products, cereals
• Assess for vit E deficiency (usually in neonates): irritability, restlessness, hemolytic anemia

Patient/family education
• Inform patient necessary foods to be included in diet high in vit E
• Instruct patient to omit if dose is missed
• Instruct patient to avoid vit supplements unless directed by prescriber because overdose may occur

Evaluation
Positive therapeutic outcome
• Absence of hemolytic anemia
• Adequate vit E levels
• Improvement in skin lesions
• Decrease in edema

voriconazole (Rx)
(vohr-i-kahn′a-zol)
Vfend
Func. class.: Antifungal
Pregnancy category D

Do not confuse:
Vfend/Venofer

ACTION: Inhibits fungal CYP 450-mediation demethylation, needed for biosynthesis, causing leakage from cell membrane

Therapeutic outcome: Decreasing signs, symptoms of infection

USES: Invasive aspergillosis, serious fungal infections (*Candida* sp., *Scedosporium apiospermum, Fusarium* sp.), *Monosportum, Apiospermum*

CONTRAINDICATIONS:
Pregnancy **D**, breastfeeding, children, hypersensitivity, severe bone marrow depression, severe hepatic disease

Precautions: Renal disease (**IV**); Asian/African descent, cardiomyopathy, cholestasis, chemotherapy, lactase deficiency, visual disturbances, renal failure, pancreatitis, QT prolongation, hypokalemia, ventricular dysrhythmias, torsades de pointes

DOSAGE AND ROUTES
Esophageal candidiasis
Adult/geriatric/child ≥12 yr: PO ≥**40 kg** 200 mg q12hr; <**40 kg** 100 mg q12hr
Adult/geriatric/child ≥12 yr: IV loading dose 6 mg/kg q12hr × 2 dose, then 3-4 mg/kg q12hr; may switch to oral dosing

Candidemia of the skin, kidney, bladder wall, abdomen (non-neutropenic patients)
Adult/child ≥12 yr: IV loading dose 6 mg/kg q12hr × 24 hr, then 3-4 mg/kg q12hr × ≥14 days and ≥7 days after resolution of symptoms; PO after loading dose >**40 kg** 200 mg q12hr × ≥14 days and ≥7 days after resolution of symptoms; <**40 kg** 100 mg q12hr × ≥14 days and ≥7 days after resolution of symptoms

Invasive aspergillosis
Adult/adolescent: IV 6 mg/kg q12hr (loading dose) then 4 mg/kg q12hr, may reduce to 3 mg/kg q12hr if intolerable
Child ≥12 yr: IV 6 mg/kg q12hr, then 4 mg/kg q12hr

Renal dose
Adult: PO CCr <50 ml/min, use only orally

Hepatic dose
Adult: PO 6 mg/kg q12hr × 2 doses, then 2 mg/kg q12hr or 100 mg q12hr if ≥40 kg; 50 mg q12hr if <40 kg

Available forms: Tabs 50, 200 mg; powder for inj, lyophilized 200 mg voriconazole, powder for oral susp 45 g (40 mg/ml after reconstitution)

Implementation
• Give 1 hr before or after meals
• Store at room temperature (powder, tabs)

Intermittent IV infusion route
• Give product only after C&S confirms organism, product needed to treat condition; make sure product is used in life-threatening infections
• Reconstitute powder with 19 ml water for inj to 10 mg/ml, shake until dissolved; infuse over 1-2 hr at a conc of 5 mg/ml or less; do not admix with other products, 4.2% sodium bicarbonate inf

Y-site compatibilities: Acyclovir, alfentanil, allopurinol, amifostine, amikacin, aminocaproic acid, aminophylline, amiodarone, amphotericin B liposome, ampicillin, ampicillin/sulbactam, anidulafungin, azithromycin, aztreonam, bivalirudin, bleomycin, bumetanide, buprenorphine, butorphanol, calcium acetate/chloride/gluconate, CARBOplatin, carmustine, caspofungin, ceFAZolin, cefotaxime, cefoTEtan, cefOXitin, cefTAZidime, ceftizoxime, cefTRIAXone, chloramphenicol, chlorproMAZINE, cimetidine, ciprofloxacin, cisatracurium, CISplatin, clindamycin, cyclophosphamide, cytarabine, dacarbazine, DACTINomycin, DAPTOmycin, DAUNOrubicin, dexamethasone, dexmedetomidine, dexrazoxane, digoxin, diltiazem, diphenhydrAMINE, DOBUTamine, DOCEtaxel, dolasetron, DOPamine, doripenem, doxacurium, doxycycline, droperidol, enalaprilat, ePHEDrine, EPINEPHrine, epirubicin, ertapenem, erythromycin, esmolol, etoposide, etoposide phosphate, famotidine, fenoldopam, fentaNYL, fluconazole, fludarabine, fluorouracil, foscarnet, fosphenytoin, furosemide, ganciclovir, gemcitabine, gentamicin, glycopyrrolate, granisetron, haloperidol, heparin, hydrALAZINE, hydrocortisone, ifosfamide, imipenem/cilastatin, inamrinone, insulin, irinotecan, isoproterenol, ketorolac, labetalol, leucovorin, levofloxacin, lidocaine, linezolid, LORazepam, magnesium sulfate, mannitol, mechlorethamine, melphalan, meperidine, meropenem, mesna, metaraminol, methohexital, methotrexate, methyldopate, methylPREDNISolone, metoclopramide, metoprolol, metroNIDAZOLE, midazolam, milrinone, mitoMYcin, morphine, nafcillin, nalbuphine, naloxone, niCARdipine, nitroglycerin, norepinephrine, octreotide, ondansetron, oxaliplatin, oxytocin, PACLitaxel, palonosetron, pancuronium, pentamidine, pentazocine, PENTobarbital, PHENobarbital, phentolamine, phenylephrine, piperacillin/tazobactam, potassium chloride/

Adverse effects: *italics* = common; **bold** = life-threatening

phosphates, procainamide, promethazine, propranolol, quinupristin/dalfopristin, remifentanil, rocuronium, sodium acetate/bicarbonate/phosphates, streptozocin, succinylcholine, SUFentanil, tacrolimus, teniposide, theophylline, thiotepa, ticarcillin/clavulanate, tirofiban, tobramycin, topotecan, trimethobenzamide, trimethoprim/sulfamethoxazole, vancomycin, vasopressin, vecuronium, verapamil, vinBLAStine, vinCRIStine, vinorelbine, zidovudine

Y-site incompatibilities: Amphotericin B colloidal, busulfan, cefepime, cyclopSPORINE, dantrolene, diazepam, DOXOrubicin, IDArubicin, mitoXANtrone, nitroprusside, pantoprazole, phenytoin, thiopental

ADVERSE EFFECTS
CNS: *Headache,* paresthesias, peripheral neuropathy, *hallucinations,* psychosis, EPS, depression, Guillain-Barré syndrome, insomnia, **suicidal ideation,** dizziness, fever
CV: **Tachycardia,** hyper/hypotension, vasodilatation, **atrial dysrhythmias, atrial fibrillation, AV block, bradycardia, CHF, MI, QT prolongation, torsades de pointes,** peripheral edema
EENT: Blurred vision, eye hemorrhage, *visual disturbances*
GI: *Nausea, vomiting, anorexia, diarrhea,* cramps, **hemorrhagic gastroenteritis, acute liver failure, hepatitis, intestinal perforation, pancreatitis**
GU: *Hypokalemia,* azotemia, **renal tubular necrosis, permanent renal impairment, anuria, oliguria**
HEMA: Anemia, **eosinophilia,** hypomagnesemia, **thrombocytopenia, leukopenia, pancytopenia**
INTEG: *Burning, irritation,* pain, necrosis at inj site with extravasation, dermatitis, *rash,* photosensitivity
MISC: Respiratory disorder
SYST: Stevens-Johnson syndrome, toxic epidermal necrolysis, sepsis, melanoma (photosensitivity reaction)

Pharmacokinetics
Absorption	Unknown
Distribution	Unknown
Metabolism	CYP3A4/CYP2C9
Excretion	Via hepatic metabolism
Half-life	Elimination 6 hr (dose dependent)

Pharmacodynamics
Onset	Unknown
Peak	1-2 hr
Duration	Unknown

INTERACTIONS
Individual drugs
CISplatin, cycloSPORINE, polymyxin B, vancomycin: increased nephrotoxicity

CycloSPORINE, phenytoin, pimozide, prednisoLONE, quiNIDine, rifabutin, sirolimus, tacrolimus, warfarin: increased effects of each specific product

Digoxin: increased hypokalemia

Haloperidol, chloroquine, droperidol, pentamidine; arsenic trioxide, levomethadyl: increased QT prolongation

Drug classifications
Aminoglycosides: increased nephrotoxicity

Benzodiazepines, calcium channel blockers, ergots, HMG-CoA reductase inhibitors, nonnucleoside reverse transcriptase inhibitors, protease inhibitors, proton pump inhibitors, sulfonylureas, vinca alkaloids: increased effects of each specific product

Class IA/III antidysrhythmics, some phenothiazines, beta agonists, local anesthetics, tricyclics, CYP3A4 inhibitors (amiodarone, clarithromycin, erythromycin, telithromycin, troleandomycin); CYP3A4 substrates (methadone, pimozide, QUEtiapine, quiNIDine, risperiDONE, ziprasidone): increased QT prolongation

Corticosteroids, diuretics (thiazide), skeletal muscle relaxants: increased hypokalemia

Drug/herb
St. John's wort: do not use together

Drug/food
High-fat foods: avoid use with high-fat meals, take 1 hr before or after a meal

Drug/lab test
Increased: AST/ALT, alkaline phosphatase, creatinine, bilirubin
Decreased: Hgb/Hct, platelets, WBC

NURSING CONSIDERATIONS
Assessment
• Monitor VS q15-30min during first inf; note changes in pulse, B/P
• Monitor I&O ratio; watch for decreasing urinary output, change in specific gravity; discontinue product to prevent permanent damage to renal tubules

---

• Monitor blood tests: CBC, K, Na, Ca, Mg q2wk; BUN, creatinine weekly
• Monitor weight weekly; if weight increases >2 lb/wk, edema is present; renal damage should be considered
⚠ **Assess for renal toxicity: increasing BUN, serum creatinine; if BUN is >40 mg/dl or if serum creatinine >3 mg/dl, product may be discontinued or dosage reduced**
⚠ **Assess for hepatotoxicity: increasing AST, ALT, alkaline phosphatase, bilirubin, baseline and periodically**
• **Assess for allergic reaction:** dermatitis, rash; product should be discontinued, antihistamines (mild reaction) or epinephrine (severe reaction) administered
• **Assess for hypokalemia:** anorexia, drowsiness, weakness, decreased reflexes, dizziness, increased urinary output, increased thirst, paresthesias
• **Assess for ototoxicity:** tinnitus (ringing, roaring in ears), vertigo, loss of hearing (rare)

• **QT prolongation:** ECG for QT prolongation, ejection fraction; assess for chest pain, palpitations, dyspnea

Patient/family education
• Teach that long-term therapy may be needed to clear infection (2 wk-3 mo depending on type of infection)
• Advise patient to notify prescriber of bleeding, bruising, or soft tissue swelling
• Teach to take 1 hr before or after meal (PO)
• Advise patient not to drive at night because of vision changes
• Advise to avoid strong, direct sunlight
• Advise women of childbearing age to use effective contraceptive

Evaluation
Positive therapeutic outcome
• Decreased fever, malaise, rash, negative C&S for infecting organism

> **⚠ HIGH ALERT**

warfarin (Rx)
(war'far-in)
Coumadin, Jantoven
Func. class.: Anticoagulant
Pregnancy category X

Do not confuse:
Coumadin/Cardura/Compazine

ACTION: Interferes with blood clotting by indirect means; depresses hepatic synthesis of vit K–dependent coagulation factors (II, VII, IX, X)

Therapeutic outcome: Prevention of clotting

USES: Antiphospholipid antibody syndrome, arterial thromboembolism prophylaxis, deep vein thrombosis, MI prophylaxis, post MI, stroke prophylaxis, thrombosis prophylaxis

CONTRAINDICATIONS:
Pregnancy **X,** breastfeeding, hypersensitivity, hemophilia, leukemia with bleeding, peptic ulcer disease, thrombocytopenic purpura, hepatic disease (severe), malignant hypertension, subacute bacterial endocarditis, acute nephritis, blood dyscrasias, preeclampsia, eclampsia, hemorrhagic tendencies, surgery of CNS, eye, traumatic surgery with large open surface, bleeding tendencies of GI/GU/respiratory, stroke, aneurysms, pericardial effusion, spinal puncture, major regional/lumbar block anesthesia

> **BLACK BOX WARNING:** Bleeding

Precautions: Alcoholism, geriatric, CHF, debilitated patients, trauma, indwelling catheters, severe hypertension, active infections, protein C deficiency, polycythemia vera, vasculitis, severe diabetes, Asian patients (CYP2C9, protein C,S deficiency)

DOSAGE AND ROUTES
Adult: PO/IV 2.5-10 mg/day × 3 days, then titrated to INR/pro-time
Adolescent/child/infant: PO/IV 0.2 mg/kg/day titrated to INR

Available forms: Tabs 1, 2, 2.5, 3, 4, 5, 6, 7.5, 10 mg; 5.4 mg powder for inj

Implementation
PO route
• Warfarin is usually given with **IV** heparin for 3 or more days, warfarin blood level may take several days

Direct IV route
• Reconstitute with 2.7 ml of sterile water for inj; do not use solution that is discolored or has particulates
• Give over 1-2 min into peripheral vein

Y-site compatibilities: CeFAZolin, cefTRIAXone, DOPamine, heparin, lidocaine, morphine, nitroglycerin, potassium chloride, ranitidine

ADVERSE EFFECTS
CNS: *Fever,* dizziness, fatigue, headache, lethargy
CV: Angina, chest pain, edema, hypotension, syncope
GI: *Diarrhea,* nausea, vomiting, anorexia, stomatitis, cramps, **hepatitis,** cholestatic jaundice
GU: Hematuria
HEMA: Hemorrhage, agranulocytosis, leukopenia, eosinophilia, ecchymosis, anemia, petechiae
INTEG: *Rash,* dermatitis, urticaria, alopecia, pruritus
MISC: Epistaxis, hemoptysis, mouth ulcers, taste disturbances, priapism, dyspnea
MS: Bone fractures
SYST: Anaphylaxis, coma, cholesterol, microembolisms, **exfoliative dermatitis, purple toe syndrome**

Pharmacokinetics

Absorption	Well absorbed (PO), completely absorbed
Distribution	Crosses placenta, 99% plasma protein binding
Metabolism	Liver
Excretion	Kidney, feces (active, inactive metabolites)
Half-life	Effective ½-2½ days

Pharmacodynamics

	PO
Onset	12-24 hr
Peak	½-4 days
Duration	3-5 days

INTERACTIONS
Individual drugs

Allopurinol, amiodarone, chloral hydrate, chloramphenicol, cimetidine, clofibrate, clotrimoxazole, dextrothyroxine, diflunisal, disulfiram, erythromycin, furosemide, glucagon, heparin, indomethacin, isoniazid, mefenamic acid, metroNIDAZOLE, mifepristone, phenylbutazone, quiNIDine, RU-486, sulfinpyrazone, sulindac, thyroid: increased warfarin action

Aprepitant, azoTHIOprine, bosentan, carBAMazepine, dicloxicillin, ethchlorvynol, factor IX/VIIa, griseofulvin, nafcillin, phenytoin, rifampin, sucralfate, sulfaSALAzine, thyroid, vitamin K: decreased warfarin action

Phenytoin: increased toxicity

Drug classifications

Antidepressants (tricyclic), ethacrynic acids, HMG-CoA reductase inhibitors, NSAIDs, oxyphenbutazones, COX-2 selective inhibitors, penicillins, quinolones, salicylates, selective serotonin reuptake inhibitors, steroids, sulfonamides, thrombolytics: increased warfarin action

Barbiturates, bile acid sequestrants, contraceptives (oral), estrogens: decreased warfarin action

Sulfonylureas (oral): increased toxicity

Drug/herb

Angelica, anise, basil, chamomile, chondroitin, dong quai, evening primrose, feverfew, garlic, ginger, ginkgo, ginseng, horse chestnut, kava, licorice, melatonin, red yeast rice, saw palmetto: increased risk of bleeding

Coenzyme Q10, St. John's wort: decreased anticoagulant effect

Drug/food

Vit K foods: decreased warfarin action

Drug/lab test

Increased: T_3 uptake, liver function tests
Decreased: uric acid

NURSING CONSIDERATIONS
Assessment

BLACK BOX WARNING: Monitor blood studies (Hct, PT, platelets, occult blood in stools) q3mo; INR: in hospital daily after 2nd or 3rd dose; once in therapeutic range for 2 consecutive days, monitor 2-3× wk for 1-2 wk, then less frequently depending on stability of INR results; *Outpatient:* monitor every few days until stable dose, then periodically thereafter depending on stability of INR results, usually at least monthly

BLACK BOX WARNING: Assess for bleeding gums, petechiae, ecchymosis, black tarry stools, hematuria; fatal hemorrhage can occur

• Monitor B/P, watch for increasing signs of hypertension
• Assess for fever, skin rash, urticaria
• Assess for needed dosage change q1-2wk

Patient/family education
• Caution patient to avoid OTC preparations unless directed by prescriber; may cause serious product interactions
• Advise patient that product may be withheld during active bleeding (menstruation), depending on condition
• Advise patient to use soft-bristle toothbrush to avoid bleeding gums, avoid contact sports, use electric razor, avoid IM inj
• Instruct patient to carry/wear emergency ID identifying product taken
• Advise patient to report any signs of bleeding: gums, under skin, urine, stools
• Teach patient to read food labels; limited intake of vit K foods (green leafy vegetables) is necessary to maintain consistent prothrombin levels

Evaluation
Positive therapeutic outcome
• Decrease of deep vein thrombosis
• Pro-time (1.3-2.0 × control)

W

xylometazoline nasal agent
See Appendix B

zafirlukast (Rx)

(za-feer′loo-cast)

Accolate

Func. class.: Bronchodilator

Chem. class.: Leukotriene receptor antagonist

Pregnancy category B

ACTION: Antagonizes the contractile action of leukotrienes (LTC_4, LTD_4, LTE_4) in airway smooth muscle; inhibits bronchoconstriction caused by antigens

Therapeutic outcome: Ability to breathe more easily

USES: Prophylaxis and treatment of chronic asthma in adults/children >5 yr

CONTRAINDICATIONS:

Hypersensitivity, hepatic encephalopathy

Precautions: Pregnancy **B**, breastfeeding, children, geriatric, hepatic disease, Churg-Strauss syndrome, acute bronchospasm

DOSAGE AND ROUTES

Adult and child ≥12 yr: PO 20 mg bid

Child 5-11 yr: PO 10 mg bid

Available forms: Tabs 10, 20 mg

Implementation

• Give PO 1 hr before or 2 hr after meals; absorption may be decreased if given with food

ADVERSE EFFECTS

CNS: Headache, dizziness, **suicidal ideation,** fever, insomnia

GI: Nausea, diarrhea, abdominal pain, vomiting, dyspepsia, **hepatic failure, hepatitis**

HEMA: Agranulocytosis

MISC: Infections, pain, asthenia, myalgia, fever, increased ALT, urticaria, rash, **angioedema**

Pharmacokinetics

Absorption	Rapidly absorbed
Distribution	Unknown
Metabolism	Extensively by CYP2C9, CYP3A4 enzyme systems, protein binding (99%)
Excretion	Feces
Half-life	10 hr

Pharmacodynamics

Onset	Unknown
Peak	3 hr
Duration	Unknown

INTERACTIONS

Individual drugs

Aspirin: increased plasma levels of zafirlukast

Erythromycin, theophylline: decreased plasma levels of zafirlukast

Warfarin: increased pro-time

Drug/food

Decreased: bioavailability of zafirlukast

NURSING CONSIDERATIONS

Assessment

• Assess respiratory rate, rhythm, depth; auscultate lung fields bilaterally; notify prescriber of abnormalities; not to be used for acute bronchospasm in acute asthma

• **Churg-Strauss syndrome (rare):** assess adults carefully (eosinophilia, vasculitic rash, worsening pulmonary symptoms, cardiac complications, neuropathy), may be caused by reducing oral corticosteroids

• **Hepatic disease:** Monitor liver function tests

• Assess for renal/pancreatic/visual function

Patient/family education

• Advise patient to check OTC medications, current prescription medications that may increase stimulation

• Advise patient to avoid hazardous activities; dizziness may occur

• Advise patient that if GI upset occurs, to take product with 8 oz of water; avoid food if possible; absorption may be decreased

• Advise to take even if symptom-free

• Advise patient to notify prescriber of nausea, vomiting, diarrhea, abdominal pain, fatigue, jaundice, anorexia, flulike symptoms (hepatic dysfunction)

• Advise patient not to use for acute asthma episodes, or to use while breastfeeding

• Advise patient to avoid: driving at night (blurred vision); direct sunlight (photosensitivity); taking <1 hr before or after a meal

Evaluation

Positive therapeutic outcome

• Ability to breathe more easily

Z

zaleplon (Rx)

(zal'eh-plon)
Sonata
Func. class.: Hypnotic, non-barbiturate
Chem. class.: Pyrazolopyrimidine
Pregnancy category C
Controlled substance schedule IV

ACTION: Binds selectively to ω-1 receptor of the γ-aminobutyric acid type A (GABA$_A$) receptor complex; results are sedation, hypnosis, skeletal muscle relaxation, anticonvulsant activity, anxiolytic action

Therapeutic outcome: Ability to sleep

USES: Insomnia (short-term treatment)

CONTRAINDICATIONS:
Hypersensitivity, severe hepatic disease

Precautions: Pregnancy **C**, breastfeeding, children <15 yr, geriatric, renal/hepatic disease, psychosis, angioedema, respiratory disease, depression, sleep-related behavior (sleep walking)

DOSAGE AND ROUTES
Adult: PO 10 mg at bedtime; may increase dosage to 20 mg at bedtime if needed; 5 mg may be used in low-weight persons
Geriatric: PO 5 mg at bedtime; may increase if needed

Available forms: Caps 5, 10 mg

Implementation
• Give ½-1 hr before bedtime for sleeplessness; give on empty stomach
• Store in tight container in cool environment

ADVERSE EFFECTS
CNS: *Drowsiness,* amnesia, depersonalization, hallucinations, hyperesthesia, paresthesia, somnolence, tremor, vertigo, dizziness, anxiety, *lethargy, daytime sedation,* confusion, complex sleep-related reactions (sleep driving, sleep eating)
CV: Chest pain, peripheral edema
EENT: Vision changes, ear/eye pain, hyperacusis, parosmia
GI: Nausea, anorexia, colitis, dyspepsia, dry mouth, constipation, abdominal pain
MISC: Asthenia, fever, headache, myalgia, dysmenorrhea
MS: Myalgia, back pain, arthritis
RESP: Bronchitis
SYST: Severe allergic reactions

Pharmacokinetics

Absorption	Rapidly absorbed
Distribution	Extravascular tissues, crosses blood-brain barrier; crosses placenta
Metabolism	Extensively, liver to inactive metabolites
Excretion	Kidneys
Half-life	1 hr

Pharmacodynamics

Onset	Rapid
Peak	1 hr
Duration	3-4 hr

INTERACTIONS
Individual drugs
Cimetidine: increased action of zaleplon

Drug classifications
CYP3A4 inhibitors/inducers: increased or decreased zaleplon levels

Drug/herb
Chamomile, hops, kava, valerian: increased CNS depression

Drug/food
High-fat/heavy meal: prolonged absorption, sleep onset reduced

NURSING CONSIDERATIONS
Assessment
• **Sleep disorders:** assess for type of sleep problem, falling asleep, staying asleep; monitor for complex sleep disorders
• Assess for previous product dependence or tolerance; if product dependent or tolerant, amount of medication should be restricted
• Monitor patient's mental status: mood, sensorium, affect, sleeping patterns, drowsiness, dizziness, suicidal tendencies, excessive sedation, impaired coordination

Patient/family education
• Inform patient that product is for short-term use only
• Teach patient to take immediately before going to bed
• Advise patient that product may cause memory problems, dependence (if used for longer periods of time), changes in behavior/thinking, complex sleep-related behavior (sleep eating/driving)
• Advise patient not to ingest a high-fat/heavy meal before taking

---

⚠ Nurse Alert　　　✦ Key NCLEX® Drug

• Advise patient to avoid OTC preparations unless approved by a physician, to avoid alcohol ingestion or other psychotropic medications unless prescribed by a health care provider, that 1-2 wk of therapy may be required before therapeutic effects occur

• Caution patient to avoid driving, activities requiring alertness; drowsiness may occur; until medication response is known, tell patient that drowsiness may worsen at beginning of treatment

• Instruct patient not to discontinue medication abruptly after long-term use

Evaluation

Positive therapeutic outcome

• Decreased sleeplessness

---

zanamivir (Rx)

(zan-a-mee′veer)

Relenza

Func. class.: Antiviral

Chem. class.: Neuramidase inhibitor

Pregnancy category C

ACTION: Inhibits neuramidase enzyme needed for influenza virus replication

Therapeutic outcome: Decreased symptoms of influenza types A and B for those who have been symptomatic for no more than 2 days

USES: Treatment of influenza types A and B for those who have been symptomatic for no more than 2 days

Unlabeled uses: Prophylaxis against influenza A and B infections; swine flu (H1N1)

CONTRAINDICATIONS:

Hypersensitivity

Precautions: Pregnancy **C**, breastfeeding, children <7 yr, geriatric, respiratory disease, angioedema, milk protein hypersensitivity, Reye's syndrome

DOSAGE AND ROUTES

Adult and child >7 yr: INH 2 inh (two 5-mg blisters) q12hr × 5 days, on the 1st day 2 doses should be taken with at least 2 hr between doses

H1N1 (swine flu) (unlabeled)

Adult/adolescent/child ≥7 yr: INH 2 inh bid × 5 days

Available forms: Blisters of powder for inhalation 5 mg

Implementation

• Give before exposure to influenza; continue for 5 days after contact

• Store in airtight, dry container

ADVERSE EFFECTS

CNS: *Headache, dizziness,* fatigue, **seizures,** self-injury, delirium (child)

EENT: Ear, nose, throat infections

GI: *Nausea, vomiting, diarrhea*

RESP: Nasal symptoms, cough, sinusitis, bronchitis, **bronchospasm**

SYST: Angioedema

Pharmacokinetics	
Absorption	4%-17% absorbed
Distribution	<10% protein binding
Metabolism	Not metabolized
Excretion	Kidneys unchanged
Half-life	2½-5 hr

Pharmacodynamics
Unknown

INTERACTIONS

Individual drugs

Intranasal influenza vaccine: decreased effect; separate by ≥48 hr, do not restart antiviral drugs for ≥2 wk

NURSING CONSIDERATIONS

Assessment

• Assess for symptoms of influenza A: increased temp, malaise, aches and pains

• Assess for skin eruptions, photosensitivity after administration of product

• Monitor respiratory status: rate, character, wheezing, tightness in chest

• Assess for allergies before initiation of treatment, reaction of each medication

Patient/family education

• Give patient "Patient's instructions for use" and review all points before using delivery system

• Teach patient to avoid hazardous activities if dizziness occurs

• Teach patient to use for the entire 5 days

• Inform patient that this product does not reduce transmission risk of influenza to others

• Advise patients with asthma or COPD to carry a fast-acting inhaled bronchodilator since bronchospasm may occur; to use scheduled inhaled bronchodilators before using this product

---

Evaluation
Positive therapeutic outcome
• Absence of fever, malaise, cough, dyspnea in influenza A

---

zidovudine (Rx)

(zye-doe'vue-deen)
Apo-Zidovudine ✚, **Novo-AZT** ✚,
Retrovir
Func. class.: Antiretroviral
Chem. class.: Nucleoside reverse transcriptase inhibitor (NRTI)
Pregnancy category C

Do not confuse:
Retrovir/ritonavir

ACTION: Inhibits replication of HIV-1 by incorporating into cellular DNA by viral reverse transcriptase, thereby terminating the cellular DNA chain

Therapeutic outcome: Decreased symptoms of HIV-1 infection

USES: Used in combination with at least 2 other antiretrovirals for HIV-1 infection

CONTRAINDICATIONS:
Hypersensitivity

Precautions: Pregnancy **C**, breastfeeding, children, granulocyte count <1000/mm³ or Hgb <9.5 g/dl, severe renal disease, obesity

> **BLACK BOX WARNING:** Impaired hepatic function, anemia, lactic acidosis, myopathy, neutropenia

DOSAGE AND ROUTES
HIV infections with other antiretrovirals
Adult: PO (tabs, caps, syrup) 600 mg/day in divided doses, either 200 mg tid or 300 mg bid in combination with other antiretrovirals; **IV** 1-mg/kg q4hr, initiate PO as soon as possible, up to 1000 mg
Adolescent/child ≥30 kg: PO (tabs/caps/syrup) 300 mg bid or 200 mg tid
Child 25 kg to <30 kg: PO (tabs/caps) 500 mg/day divided bid
Child 19 kg to <25 kg: PO (tabs/caps) 400 mg/day divided bid
Child/infant ≥4 wk and 13 kg to <19 kg: PO (tabs/caps) 300 mg/day divided bid

Child/infant ≥4 wk and 7 kg to <13 kg: PO (tabs/caps) 200 mg/day divided bid
Child/infant ≥4 wk and 5 kg to <7 kg: PO (tabs/caps) 150 mg/day divided bid
Infant ≥4 wk, child/adolescent ≥9 kg and <30 kg: PO (syrup) 18 mg/kg/day divided bid or tid
Infant ≥4 wk and 4 kg to <9 kg: PO (syrup) 24 mg/kg/day divided bid or tid

Perinatal transmission prophylaxis
Full-term neonate: PO (syrup) 2 mg/kg or **IV** 1.5 mg/kg q6hr starting 12 hr after birth; continue up to 6 wk of age

Prevention of maternal-fetal HIV transmission
Neonate ≥34 wk: PO 2 mg/kg/dose q6hr × 6 wk beginning 8-12 hr after birth; **IV** 1.5 mg/kg/dose over 30 min q6hr until able to take PO
Maternal (>14 wk gestation): PO 100 mg 5 ×/day until start of labor, then during labor/delivery **IV** 2 mg/kg over 1 hr followed by **IV** INF 1 mg/kg/hr until umbilical cord is clamped

Prevention of HIV after needlestick
Adult: PO 200 mg tid plus lamiVUDine 150 mg bid, plus a protease inhibitor for high-risk exposure; begin within 2 hr of exposure

Available forms: Caps 100 mg; tabs 300 mg; inj 10 mg/ml; oral syr 50 mg/5 ml

Implementation
PO route
• Give on empty stomach
• Do not take dapsone at same time as didanosine
• Store in cool environment; protect from light

Intermittent IV infusion route
• Give after diluting with D₅W; give over 1 hr (<4 mg/ml), do not give by direct **IV**
• Protect unopened product from light; use diluted solutions within 24 hr if stored at room temperature, 48 hr if refrigerated

Y-site compatibilities: Acyclovir, allopurinol, amikacin, amphotericin B, aztreonam, ceftazidime, cefTRIAXone, cimetidine, clindamycin, dexamethasone, DOBUTamine, DOPamine, erythromycin, fluconazole, fludarabine, gentamicin, heparin, imipenem/cilastatin, LORazepam, metoclopramide, morphine, nafcillin, ondansetron, oxacillin, pentamidine, phenylephrine, piperacillin, potassium chloride, ranitidine, sargramostim, tobramycin, trimethoprim/sulfamethoxazole, vancomycin

---

Additive incompatibilities: Blood products or protein solutions

ADVERSE EFFECTS

CNS: *Fever, headache, malaise,* diaphoresis, *dizziness, insomnia,* paresthesia, somnolence, chills, tremor, twitching, anxiety, confusion, depression, lability, vertigo, loss of mental acuity, **seizures,** malaise
EENT: Taste change, hearing loss, photophobia
GI: *Nausea, vomiting, diarrhea,* anorexia, cramps, *dyspepsia, constipation,* dysphagia, *flatulence,* rectal bleeding, mouth ulcer, abdominal pain, hepatomegaly
GU: Dysuria, polyuria, frequency, hesitancy
HEMA: **Granulocytopenia, anemia**
INTEG: *Rash,* acne, pruritus, urticaria
MS: Myalgia, arthralgia, muscle spasm
RESP: Dyspnea
SYST: **Lactic acidosis**

Pharmacokinetics

Absorption	Well absorbed (PO), completely absorbed (**IV**)
Distribution	Widely distributed—crosses placenta, CSF, protein binding 38%
Metabolism	Liver, mostly
Excretion	Kidneys
Half-life	Terminal ½-3 hr

Pharmacodynamics

	PO	IV
Onset	Unknown	Rapid
Peak	½-1½ hr	Inf end
Duration	Unknown	Unknown

INTERACTIONS

Individual drugs
DOXOrubicin, ribavarin, staduvine: avoid concurrent use
Ganciclovir, radiation, SMZ/TMP, valganciclovir: increased bone marrow suppression
Methadone: increased zidovudine level

Drug classifications
Antineoplastics: increased bone marrow suppression
Interferons, NRTIs: decreased zidovudine levels

Drug/lab test
Increased: LFTs
Decreased: platelets

NURSING CONSIDERATIONS

Assessment
• **Assess for peripheral neuropathy:** tingling or pain in hands and feet, distal numbness; if these occur, product may be decreased or discontinued
• **Assess for pancreatitis:** abdominal pain, nausea, vomiting, elevated liver enzymes; product should be discontinued because condition can be fatal
• Assess children by dilated retinal examination q6mo to rule out retinal depigmentation

> **BLACK BOX WARNING:** Monitor CBC, differential, platelet count qmo; withhold product if WBC is <4000/mm³ or platelet count is <75,000/mm³; notify prescriber of results; monitor viral load, CD4 counts, LFTs, plasma HIV RNA, serum creatinine/BUN baseline, throughout treatment

• **Lactic acidosis, severe hepatomegaly with steatosis:** obtain baseline LFTs; if elevated, discontinue treatment; discontinue even if LFTs are normal but lactic acidosis, hepatomegaly are present: may be fatal

Patient/family education
• Caution patient to take on empty stomach; to use exactly as prescribed
• Advise patient to report signs of infection: increased temp, sore throat, flulike symptoms; to avoid crowds and those with known infections
• Instruct patient to report signs of anemia: fatigue, headache, faintness, shortness of breath, irritability
• Advise patient to report bleeding; avoid use of razors or commercial mouthwash
• Inform patient that hair may be lost during therapy (rare); a wig or hairpiece may make patient feel better
• Caution patient to avoid OTC products or other medications without approval of prescriber
• Caution patient not to have any sexual contact without use of a condom; needles should not be shared; blood from infected individual should not come in contact with another's mucous membranes

Evaluation
Positive therapeutic outcome
• Decreased infection; decreased symptoms of HIV infection, decreased viral load, increased CD4 counts

Z

zinc (PO, OTC; IV, Rx)
(zink sul'fate)
Orazinc, PMS Egozinc ✦, Verazinc, Zinca-Pak, Zincate, Zinc 15, Zinc-220
Func. class.: Trace element; nutritional supplement
Pregnancy category C, parenteral

ACTION: Needed for adequate healing, bone and joint development, (23% zinc)

Therapeutic outcome: Replacement of zinc

USES: Prevention of zinc deficiency, adjunct to vit A therapy

Unlabeled uses: Wound healing

Precautions: Pregnancy **C** (parenteral), breastfeeding, hypocupremia, neonatal prematurity, neonates, renal disease

DOSAGE AND ROUTES
Dietary supplement (elemental zinc)
Adult/adolescent pregnant females: PO 11-13 mg/day

Nutritional supplement (IV)
Adult: IV 2.5-4 mg/day, may increase by 2 mg/day if needed
Child 1-5 yr: IV 50 mcg/kg/day
Adult and lactating female: PO 12-14 mg/day × 12 mo
Adult and adolescent male ≥14 yr: PO 11 mg/day
Adult female ≥19 yr: PO 8 mg/day
Adolescent female ≥14 yr: PO 9 mg/day
Child 9-13 yr: PO 8 mg/day
Child 4-8 yr: PO 5 mg/day
Child 1-3 yr: PO 3 mg/day
Infant 7-12 mo: PO 3 mg/day
Infant birth to 6 mo: PO 2 mg/day (adequate intake)

Wound healing
Adult: PO 50 mg tid until healed (elemental iron)

Available forms: Tabs 66, 110 mg; caps 220 mg; inj 1, 5 mg/ml

Implementation
PO route
• Give with meals to decrease gastric upset; restrict dairy products, caffeine, which decrease absorption

IV route
• Part of TPN

ADVERSE EFFECTS
GI: Nausea, vomiting, cramps, heartburn, ulcer formation
OVERDOSE: Diarrhea, rash, dehydration, restlessness

Pharmacokinetics

Absorption	Poorly absorbed (PO), completely absorbed (**IV**)
Distribution	Widely distributed
Metabolism	Liver
Excretion	90% (feces), 10% (kidneys)
Half-life	Unknown

Pharmacodynamics
Unknown

INTERACTIONS
Drug classifications
Fluoroquinolones, tetracyclines: decreased absorption

Drug/food
Caffeine, dairy products: decreased absorption of PO zinc

NURSING CONSIDERATIONS
Assessment
• Zinc deficiency: poor wound healing, absence of taste, smell, slowing growth
• Alkaline phosphatase, HDL monthly in long-term therapy
• Monitor zinc levels during treatment

Patient/family education
• Inform patient that element must be taken for 3 mo to be effective
• Advise patient to report immediately nausea, diarrhea, rash, severe vomiting, restlessness, abdominal pain, tarry stools

Evaluation
Positive therapeutic outcome
• Absence of zinc deficiency
• Improved wound healing

ziprasidone (Rx)

(zi-praz'ih-dohn)
Geodon, Zeldox ✦
Func. class.: Antipsychotic/neuroleptic
Chem. class.: Benzisoxazole derivative
Pregnancy category C

ACTION: Unknown; may be mediated through both dopamine type 2 (D_2) and serotonin type 2 (5-HT_2) antagonism

Therapeutic outcome: Decreased signs/symptoms of psychosis

USES: Schizophrenia, acute agitation, acute psychosis, bipolar disorder, mania, psychotic depression, agitation

CONTRAINDICATIONS:

Hypersensitivity, breastfeeding

Precautions: Pregnancy C, children, geriatric, renal/cardiac/hepatic disease, breast cancer, diabetes, AV block, CNS depression, seizure disorders, abrupt discontinuation, agranulocytosis, ambient temperature increase, suicidal ideation, torsades de pointes, strenuous exercise

BLACK BOX WARNING: Increased mortality in elderly patients with dementia-related psychosis

DOSAGE AND ROUTES

Schizophrenia

Adult: PO 20 mg bid with food, adjust dosage every 2 days upward to max of 80 mg bid; IM 10-20 mg; may give 10 mg q2hr, doses of 20 mg may be given q4hr, max 40 mg/day (acute episodes); switch to PO as soon as possible

Bipolar disorder

Adult: PO 40 mg bid with food, on day 2 increase to 60 or 80 mg bid, then adjust to response; maintenance as adjunct to lithium/valproate 40-80 mg bid

Available forms: Tabs 20, 40, 60, 80 mg; inj 20 mg/ml single-dose vials

Implementation

- Give reduced dosage in geriatric
- Give antiparkinsonian agent on order from prescriber, to be used for EPS
- Provide decreased stimulus by dimming lights, avoiding loud noises
- Store in tight, light-resistant container
- Provide supervised ambulation until patient is stabilized on medication; do not involve in strenuous exercise program because fainting is possible; patient should not stand still for a long time

PO route
- Take cap whole and with food
- Food increases absorption
- Store in airtight, light-resistant container

IM route
- Add 1.2 ml sterile water for inj to vial, shake vigorously until product is dissolved; give deeply in large muscle; do not mix with other drugs in same syringe

ADVERSE EFFECTS

CNS: *EPS (pseudoparkinsonism, akathisia, dystonia, tardive dyskinesia), drowsiness, insomnia, agitation, anxiety, headache,* **seizures, neuroleptic malignant syndrome,** dizziness, tremor, facial droop

CV: Orthostatic hypotension, **tachycardia, prolonged QT/QTc, sudden death, heart failure (geriatric), torsades de pointes**

EENT: Blurred vision, diplopia

ENDO: Metabolic changes, hyperprolactinemia (rare)

GI: *Nausea,* vomiting, *anorexia, constipation,* jaundice, weight gain, diarrhea, dry mouth, abdominal pain

GU: Enuresis, urinary incontinence, gynecomastia, impotence, priapism

MS: Decreased bone density

RESP: Rhinitis, dyspnea, infection, cough

Pharmacokinetics

Absorption	Unknown
Distribution	Protein binding 99%
Metabolism	Liver, extensively to metabolite
Excretion	Unknown
Half-life	Terminal 7 hr

Pharmacodynamics

Onset	Unknown
Peak	PO 6-8 hr; IM 60 min
Duration	Unknown

INTERACTIONS

Individual drugs

Alcohol: increased sedation

Chloroquine, clarithromycin, droperidol, erythromycin, grepafloxacin, haloperidol, methadone, moxifloxacin, pentamidine: increased QT prolongation

CarBAMazepine, phenytoin, rifampin: increased excretion of ziprasidone

---

✦ Canada only

Z

Ketoconazole: increased ziprasidone level
Lithium: increased EPS, possible neurotoxicity

Drug classifications
Antihypertensives: increased hypotension
Antipsychotics: increased EPS
β-agonists, class IA/III antidysrhythmics, local anesthetics, phenothiazines (some), tricyclics: increased QT prolongation
Barbiturates: increased excretion of ziprasidone
CNS depressants: increased sedation
SSRIs, SNRIs: increased serotonin syndrome, increased neuroleptic malignant syndrome

NURSING CONSIDERATIONS
Assessment

> **BLACK BOX WARNING:** Assess geriatric with dementia closely; heart failure, sudden death have occurred

• Assess mental status before initial administration, AIMS assessment
• Monitor bilirubin, CBC, liver function tests, fasting blood glucose, cholesterol profile; potassium, magnesium when taken with loop/thiazide diuretics qmo
• Monitor urinalysis before, during prolonged therapy
• Monitor B/P standing and lying; also pulse, respirations; take these q4hr during initial treatment; establish baseline before starting treatment; report drops of 30 mm Hg; watch for ECG changes; **QT prolongation may occur**
• Assess dizziness, faintness, palpitations, tachycardia on rising
• **Assess EPS,** including akathisia (inability to sit still, no pattern to movements), tardive dyskinesia (bizarre movements of the jaw, mouth, tongue, extremities), pseudoparkinsonism (rigidity, tremors, pill rolling, shuffling gait)
⚠ **Assess for neuroleptic malignant syndrome: hyperthermia, increased CPK, altered mental status, muscle rigidity**
• Assess constipation, urinary retention daily; if these occur, increase bulk and water in diet

Patient/family education
• Advise patient that orthostatic hypotension may occur and to rise from sitting or lying position gradually; avoid hot tubs, hot showers, tub baths because hypotension may occur
• Advise patient to avoid abrupt withdrawal of this product; EPS may result; product should be withdrawn slowly
• Advise patient to avoid OTC preparations (cough, hay fever, cold) unless approved by prescriber, since serious product interactions may occur; avoid use with alcohol, CNS depressants; increased drowsiness may occur
• Teach patient to avoid hazardous activities if drowsy or dizzy
• Advise patient to increase fluids to prevent constipation
• Teach patient to use sips of water, candy, gum for dry mouth
• Teach patient to report impaired vision, tremors, muscle twitching
• Teach patient that in hot weather, heat stroke may occur; take extra precautions to stay cool

Evaluation
Positive therapeutic outcome
• Decrease in emotional excitement, hallucinations, delusions, paranoia; reorganization of patterns of thought, speech

TREATMENT OF OVERDOSE:
Lavage if orally ingested; provide airway; *do not induce vomiting*

ziv-aflibercept
(ziv-a-flih′ber-sept)
Zaltrap
Func. class.: Antineoplastic biologic response modifier
Chem. class.: Signal transduction inhibitor (STI)
Pregnancy category: C

ACTION: An angiogenesis inhibitor, a fusion protein that binds to vascular endothelial growth factors (VEGF-A, VEGF-B) and placental growth factor 1 and 2

Therapeutic outcome: Decrease in spread or size of tumor

USES: Metastatic colorectal cancer that is resistant or has progressed after an oxaliplatin-containing regimen in combination with 5-fluorouracil, leucovorin, irinotecan (FOLFIRI)

CONTRAINDICATIONS:
Hypersensitivity

Precautions: Infertility, male-mediated teratogenicity, encephalopathy, hypertension, dental work, breastfeeding, children, neonates, geriatric patients, infection, neutropenia, pregnancy (C)

> **BLACK BOX WARNING:** Bleeding, GI bleeding/perforation, intracranial bleeding, surgery

DOSAGE AND ROUTES

Adult: IV 4 mg/kg over 1 hr on day 1 every 2 wk in combination with the FOLFIRI regimen (irinotecan 180 mg/m^2 over 90 min on day 1 with dl-racemic leucovorin 400 mg/m^2 over 2 hr) (infused at the same time, in same Y-line; then on day 1 by 5-fluorouracil 400 mg/m^2 as a bolus, then 2400 mg/m^2 as a 46-hr cont IV inf)

Available forms: Solution for injection 100 mg/4 ml; 200 mg/8 ml

Implementation
• Give before FOLFIRI chemotherapy; visually inspect for particulate matter and discoloration before use

Dilution and preparation
• Withdraw the calculated dose, add to 0.9% sodium chloride or dextrose 5% solution to 0.6–8 mg/mL; use polyvinyl chloride (PVC) infusion bags containing bis (2-ethylhexyl) phthalate (DHEP) or polyolefin infusion bags; do not re-enter the vial after first puncture; discard any unused portion; do not mix or combine with other drugs in the same infusion bag; the diluted solution may be stored refrigerated for ≤4 hr; discard any unused portion in the infusion bag

IV infusion
• Give diluted solution over 1 hr using a 0.2 micrometer polyethersulfone filter; do not use nylon or polyvinylidene fluoride (PVDF) filters; do not give IV push or bolus; do not mix or combine with other drugs in the same IV line; give using an infusion set made of one of the following: PVC containing DEHP, DEHP-free PVC containing trioctyl-trimellitate (TOTM), polypropylene, polyethylene-lined PVC, or polyurethane

Dosage adjustments for recurrent or severe hypertension
Hold until B/P is controlled and then permanently reduce dose to 2 mg/kg; discontinue in hypertensive crisis or hypertensive encephalopathy

Dosage adjustments for proteinuria (2 g/24 hr)
Hold until proteinuria is <2 g/24 hr; if proteinuria recurs, hold therapy until proteinuria is <2 g/24 hr, then reduce to 2 mg/kg; discontinue in nephrotic syndrome or thrombotic microangiopathy

ADVERSE EFFECTS

CNS: *Intracranial bleeding*, headache, dizziness
CV: **Hypertensive crisis**, hypertension, stroke

GI: Nausea, hepatotoxicity, dyspepsia, **GI hemorrhage**, abdominal pain, **GI perforation**
GU: Proteinuria, hematuria
HEMA: **Neutropenia, leukopenia**
INTEG: Rash, pruritus, alopecia, hypersensitivity
MISC: Fatigue, epistaxis, night sweats, decreased weight, flulike symptoms, infection
RESP: Dyspnea, **pulmonary embolism**

Pharmacokinetics

Absorption	Unknown
Distribution	Unknown
Metabolism	Unknown
Excretion	Unknown
Half-life	Elimination 6 days

Pharmacodynamics

Onset	Unknown
Peak	Unknown
Duration	Unknown

NURSING CONSIDERATIONS

Assessment
⚠ **Severe bleeding: Assess for GI bleeding, intracranial bleeding, and pulmonary hemorrhage/hemoptysis; may be fatal; monitor patients for signs and symptoms of bleeding**
⚠ **GI perforation: some cases are fatal; monitor patients for signs and symptoms of GI perforation; discontinue therapy if GI perforation develops**
• **Poor wound healing:** hold ≥4 wk before elective surgery; after major surgery, do not restart for ≥4 wk and until the surgical wound is entirely healed
⚠ **Severe hypertension/hypertensive crisis: usually occurs within the first 2 cycles (grade 3 or 4 hypertension); monitor B/P every 2 wk or more often if needed; treatment with antihypertensives may be needed; product may need to be discontinued**
⚠ **Severe proteinuria/nephrotic syndrome/ thrombotic microangiopathy (TMA): monitor urine protein by dipstick analysis and urinary protein–to–creatinine ratio (UPCR); obtain a 24-hr urine collection for a UPCR >1; for proteinuria of <2 g/24 hr, temporarily hold doses until proteinuria is <2 g/24 hr; if proteinuria recurs, hold doses until proteinuria is <2 g/24 hr, then permanently reduce; discontinue in nephrotic syndrome or TMA**
⚠ **Febrile neutropenia, neutropenic infection/sepsis: monitor CBC with differential**

at baseline and before each cycle, hold FOLFIRI until the neutrophil count is ≥1.5 × 10⁹/L

⚠ Geriatric toxicity: assess for diarrhea, dizziness, asthenia, weight loss, and dehydration that can indicate toxicity

⚠ Pregnancy C/Breastfeeding: highly effective contraception during treatment and up to 3 mo after the last dose is needed for all patients of reproductive potential because infertility and male-mediated teratogenicity can occur; infertility can occur but is reversible within 18 wk after stopping product: do not breastfeed

Patient/family education

⚠ Pregnancy C/breastfeeding: teach that highly effective contraception should be used during treatment and up to 3 mo after the last dose in all patients of reproductive potential, infertility and male-mediated teratogenicity is reversible within 18 wk after stopping product; do not breastfeed
• Teach patient about reason for treatment, expected results

⚠ Notify prescriber immediately of bleeding, severe abdominal pain, poor wound healing

Evaluation

Positive therapeutic outcome
• Decrease in spread of size of tumor

---

zoledronic acid (Rx)
(zoh'leh-drah'nick ass'id)
Reclast, Zometa
Func. class.: Bone-resorption inhibitor
Chem. class.: Bisphosphonate
Pregnancy category D

ACTION: Inhibits normal and abnormal bone resorption; potent inhibitor of osteoclastic bone resorption; inhibits osteoclastic activity, reduces bone resorption and inhibits skeletal calcium release caused by stimulating factors released by tumors; reduction of abnormal bone resorption is responsible for therapeutic effect in hypercalcemia; may directly block dissolution of hydroxyapatite bone crystals

Therapeutic outcome: Serum calcium at normal level

USES: Moderate to severe hypercalcemia associated with malignancy; multiple myeloma; bone metastases from solid tumors (used with

antineoplastics), active Paget's disease, osteoporosis, glucocorticoid-induced osteoporosis, osteoporosis prophylaxis in postmenopausal women

CONTRAINDICATIONS:
Pregnancy **D**, breastfeeding, hypocalcemia, hypersensitivity to this product or bisphosphonates

Precautions: Children, geriatric, renal dysfunction, asthmatic patients, asthma, acute bronchospasm, anemia, chemotherapy, coagulopathy, dehydration, dental disease, diabetes mellitus, renal disease, electrolyte imbalance, hypertension, hypovolemia, phosphate hypersensitivity, infection, multiple myeloma

DOSAGE AND ROUTES
Hypercalcemia of malignancy
Adult: IV INF 4 mg, given as a single INF over ≥15 min, may re-treat with 4 mg if serum calcium does not return to normal within 1 wk

Multiple myeloma/metastatic bone lesions
Adult: IV INF 4 mg, given over 15 min q3-4wk

Osteoporosis
Adult: IV 5 mg over 15 min or more q12mo

Active Paget's disease
Adult: IV INF 5 mg over ≥15 min

Osteoporosis prophylaxis (Reclast), postmenopausal women
Adult: IV INF 5 mg every other yr

Osteoporosis prophylaxis (Reclast) taking systemic glucocorticoids
Adult: IV 5 mg qyr

Early breast cancer (unlabeled)
Adult: IV 4 mg q6mo with goserelin 3.6 mg subcut qmo and tamoxifen 20 mg/day or anastrozole 1 mg/day for 3 yr

Available forms: Sol for inj 4 mg/5 ml (Zometa); inj 5 mg/100 ml (Reclast)

Implementation
• Give acetaminophen before and for 72 hr after to decrease pain
• Sol reconstituted with sterile water may be stored under refrigeration for up to 24 hr **IV**
• Administer in separate IV line from all other products
Zometa
• Administer after reconstituting by adding 5 ml of sterile water for inj to each vial, then add up to ≥100 ml of sterile 0.9% NaCl, D₅W, run over ≥15 min

---

Reclast
• No further dilution required; inf over ≥15 min at constant rate; max 5 mg

ADVERSE EFFECTS
CNS: Dizziness, headache, anxiety, confusion, insomnia, agitation
CV: Hypotension, leg edema, **atrial fibrillation**, chest pain
GI: Abdominal pain, anorexia, constipation, nausea, diarrhea, vomiting, taste change
GU: UTI, possible reduced renal function, **renal damage**
META: Anemia, hypokalemia, hypomagnesemia, hypophosphatemia, hypocalcemia, increased serum creatinine
MISC: *Fever, chills, flulike symptoms*
MS: Severe bone pain, *arthralgias, myalgias*, osteonecrosis of the jaw

Pharmacokinetics

Absorption	Rapidly cleared from circulation
Distribution	Taken up mainly by bones; plasma protein binding ~22%
Metabolism	Not metabolized
Excretion	Kidneys (~50% eliminated in urine within 24 hr)
Half-life	Terminal 167 hr

Pharmacodynamics

Onset	Unknown
Peak	15 min
Duration	Max effect 7 days

INTERACTIONS
Individual drugs
Calcium, vitamin D: decreased zoledronic acid effect
Digoxin: hypomagnesemia, hypokalemia

Drug classifications
Aminoglycosides, NSAIDs, radiopaque contrast agents: increased neurotoxicity
Aminoglycosides, loop diuretics: decreased serum calcium
Infusion solutions (calcium-containing): do not mix with calcium-containing inf sol such as lactated Ringer's sol

Drug/lab test
Increased: creatinine
Decreased: calcium, phosphorus, magnesium, potassium, Hct/Hgb, RBC, platelets, WBC

NURSING CONSIDERATIONS
Assessment
• Assess renal function tests and calcium, phosphate, magnesium, potassium, creatinine; if creatinine is elevated hold treatment
• **Assess for hypocalcemia:** paresthesia, twitching, laryngospasm; Chvostek's/Trousseau's signs
• Assess dental status; cover with antiinfectives for dental extraction
• Assess for atrial fibrillation

Patient/family education
• Instruct patient to report hypercalcemic relapse: nausea, vomiting, bone pain, thirst
• Advise patient to continue with dietary recommendations including calcium and vit D; take a multiple vitamin daily, 500 mg of calcium, 400 international units vit D in multiple myeloma
• Teach patient if nausea/vomiting occur, eat small meals, use lozenges or chewing gum
• Advise patient if bone pain occurs, notify prescriber to obtain analgesic
• Advise patient to avoid pregnancy
• Instruct patient to continue good oral hygiene

Evaluation
Positive therapeutic outcome
• Calcium levels decreased to normal

TREATMENT OF OVERDOSE:
Correct clinically relevant reductions in serum calcium by administering **IV** calcium gluconate; in serum phosphorus, with potassium or sodium phosphate; in serum magnesium, with magnesium sulfate

ZOLMitriptan (Rx)
(zole-mih-trip′tan)
Zomig, Zomig-ZMT
Func. class.: Migraine agent, abortive
Chem. class.: 5HT$_{1B}$/5HT$_{1D}$ receptor agonist (triptan)
Pregnancy category C

ACTION: Binds selectively to the vascular serotonin type 1 (5HT$_{1B}$/5HT$_{1D}$) receptor subtype, exerts antimigraine effect; causes vasoconstriction in cranial arteries

Therapeutic outcome: Decreased severity, frequency of headache

USES: Acute treatment of migraine with or without aura

Z

Adverse effects: *italics* = common; **bold** = life-threatening

CONTRAINDICATIONS:

Angina pectoris, history of MI, documented silent ischemia, ischemic heart disease, uncontrolled hypertension, hypersensitivity, basilar or hemiplegic migraine, risk of CV events

Precautions: Pregnancy **C,** breastfeeding, children, postmenopausal women, men >40 yr, geriatric, risk factors for CAD, hypercholesterolemia, obesity, diabetes, impaired renal/hepatic function

DOSAGE AND ROUTES:

Adult: PO start at 2.5 mg or lower (tab may be broken), may repeat after 2 hr, max 10 mg/24 hr; NASAL 1 spray in 1 nostril at onset of migraine, repeat in 2 hr if no relief

Available forms: Tabs 2.5, 5 mg; orally disintegrating tabs 2.5, 5 mg; nasal spray 5 mg

Implementation

• Give with fluids as soon as symptoms of migraine occur
• Provide quiet, calm environment with decreased stimulation for noise, bright light, excessive talking

Orally disintegrating tablet

• Give orally disintegrating tablet after opening; do not crush or chew, allow to dissolve on tongue

ADVERSE EFFECTS

CNS: *Tingling, hot sensation, burning, feeling of pressure, tightness, numbness, dizziness, sedation*
CV: Palpitations, chest pain
GI: Abdominal discomfort, nausea, dry mouth, dyspepsia, dysphagia
MISC: Odd taste (spray)
MS: *Weakness, neck stiffness,* myalgia
RESP: Chest tightness, pressure

Pharmacokinetics	
Absorption	Unknown
Distribution	25% plasma protein binding
Metabolism	Liver
Excretion	Urine, feces
Half-life	3-3½ hr

Pharmacodynamics	
Onset	Unknown
Peak	Unknown
Duration	2-3½ hr

INTERACTIONS

Individual drugs

Cimetidine: increased half-life of ZOLMitriptan
Ergot: increased vasospastic effects
FLUoxetine, fluvoxaMINE, PARoxetine, sertraline: increased weakness, hyperreflexia, incoordination
Sibutramine: increased ZOLMitriptan levels

Drug classifications

Contraceptives (oral): increased half-life of ZOLMitriptan
Ergot derivatives: increased vasospastic effects
MAOIs: do not use within 2 wk
Selective serotonin reuptake inhibitors: increased weakness, hyperreflexia, incoordination

Drug/herb

SAM-e, St. John's wort: serotonin syndrome

Drug/lab test

Increased: alkaline phosphatase

NURSING CONSIDERATIONS

Assessment

• Assess for tingling, hot sensation, burning, feeling of pressure, numbness, flushing
• Assess neurologic status: LOC, blurring vision, nausea, vomiting, tingling in extremities preceding headache
• Monitor ingestion of tyramine foods (pickled products, beer, wine, aged cheese), food additives, preservatives, colorings, artifical sweeteners, chocolate, caffeine, which may precipitate these types of headaches
• **Assess for serotonin syndrome** if also taking an SSRI

Patient/family education

• Teach patient to report any side effects to prescriber
• Advise patient to use contraception while taking product
• Teach patient to report pain, rash, swelling of face
• Instruct patient not to double doses; if second dose is needed, wait at least 2 hr

Evaluation

Positive therapeutic outcome

• Decrease in frequency, severity of headache

---

zolpidem (Rx)

(zole-pi'dem)

Ambien, Ambien CR, Edluar, Zolpimist

Func. class.: Sedative-hypnotic

Chem. class.: Nonbenzodiazepine of imidazopyridine class

Pregnancy category C

Controlled substance schedule IV

ACTION: Produces CNS depression at limbic, thalamic, hypothalamic levels of CNS; may be mediated by neurotransmitter γ-aminobutyric acid (GABA); results are sedation, hypnosis, skeletal muscle relaxation, anticonvulsant activity, anxiolytic action

Therapeutic outcome: Ability to sleep, sedation

USES: Insomnia, short-term treatment; insomnia with difficulty of sleep onset/maintenance (ext rel)

CONTRAINDICATIONS:

Hypersensitivity to benzodiazepines

Precautions: Pregnancy **C**, breastfeeding, children <18 yr, geriatric, anemia, renal/hepatic disease, suicidal individuals, product abuse, psychosis, seizure disorders, angioedema, depression, respiratory disease, sleep apnea, sleep-related behavior (sleep walking), myasthenia gravis, pulmonary disease, next-morning impairments; females (lower dose needed)

DOSAGE AND ROUTES

Adult: PO 10 mg at bedtime × 7-10 days only; total dose max 10 mg; EXT REL 12.5 mg immediately before bedtime, may be useful for up to 24 wk in people 18-64 yr with primary insomnia; oral spray (Zolpimist) 10 mg (2 sprays) immediately before bedtime, max 10 mg/day; SL (Edluar) 10 mg just before bedtime

Geriatric: PO 5 mg at bedtime; EXT REL 6.25 mg

Available forms: Tabs 5, 10 mg; ext rel tabs 6.25, 12.5 mg; SL 1.75, 3.5, 5, 10 mg; oral spray 5 mg/spray

Implementation

PO route

• Do not break, crush, or chew ext rel product or orally disintegrating tab

• Give ½-1 hr before bedtime for sleeplessness; give several hr before patient is to rise (to avoid hangover)

• Give with food or fluids; tab may be crushed or swallowed whole

• Do not use spray with or after a meal

• Store in airtight container in cool environment

ADVERSE EFFECTS

CNS: Headache, lethargy, drowsiness, daytime sedation, dizziness, confusion, light-headedness, anxiety, irritability, amnesia, poor coordination, complex sleep-related reactions (sleep driving, sleep eating), depression, somnolence, **suicidal ideation**, abnormal thinking/behavioral changes

CV: Chest pain, palpitation

GI: Nausea, vomiting, diarrhea, heartburn, abdominal pain, constipation

HEMA: Leukopenia, granulocytopenia (rare)

MISC: Myalgia

SYST: Severe allergic reactions, angioedema, anaphylaxis

Pharmacokinetics

Absorption	Rapidly absorbed
Distribution	Unknown
Metabolism	Liver—inactive metabolite
Excretion	Kidneys, breast milk
Half-life	2½ hr, increased in geriatric

Pharmacodynamics

Onset	PO up to 1.5 mg

INTERACTIONS

Individual drugs

Alcohol: increased action of both products

Drug classifications

CNS depressants: increased action of both products

CYP3A4 inhibitors/inducers: increased or decreased zolpidem levels

NURSING CONSIDERATIONS

Assessment

• Assess mental status: mood, sensorium, anxiety, affect, sleeping pattern, drowsiness, dizziness, especially geriatric; physical dependency, withdrawal symptoms: anxiety, panic attacks, agitation, seizures, headache, nausea, vomiting, muscle pain, weakness; suicidal tendencies; for indications of increasing tolerance and abuse

• Monitor B/P (lying, standing), pulse; if systolic B/P drops 20 mm Hg, hold product, notify prescriber

• Monitor I&O ratio for renal dysfunction

Z

Patient/family education
- Advise patient that complex sleep-related behavior may occur (sleep driving/eating)
- Instruct patient that product may be taken with food or fluids, next-morning impairment may occur
- Caution patient not to use for everyday stress or longer than 3 mo unless directed by prescriber; not to take more than prescribed amount; may be habit forming; not to double or skip doses
- Caution patient to avoid OTC preparations unless approved by prescriber; alcohol and CNS depressants will increase CNS depression
- Advise patient to avoid driving, activities that require alertness, because drowsiness may occur; to avoid alcohol ingestion or other psychotropic medications; to rise slowly or fainting may occur, especially geriatric; that drowsiness may worsen at beginning of treatment
- Instruct patient not to discontinue medication abruptly after long-term use; withdrawal symptoms include vomiting, cramping, tremors, seizures
- Teach patient use of orally disintegrating tabs: place on tongue, allow to dissolve before swallowing
- Teach patient not to crush, chew, break ext rel tabs
- Teach patient to prime spray pump before using

Evaluation
Positive therapeutic outcome
- Ability to sleep at night
- Decreased amount of early-morning awakening if taking product for insomnia

TREATMENT OF OVERDOSE:
Lavage, VS, supportive care

---

zonisamide (Rx)
(zone-is'a-mide)
Zonegran
Func. class.: Anticonvulsant
Chem. class.: Sulfonamides
Pregnancy category C

ACTION: May act through sodium and calcium channels, but exact action is unknown; serotoninergic action

Therapeutic outcome: Decreased seizures

USES: Epilepsy, adjunctive therapy of partial seizures

CONTRAINDICATIONS:
Hypersensitivity to this product or sulfonamides

Precautions: Pregnancy **C**, breastfeeding, children <16 yr, geriatric, allergies, renal/hepatic disease, psychiatric condition, hepatic failure

DOSAGE AND ROUTES
Adults and child >16 yr: PO 100 mg/day, may increase after 2 wk to 200 mg/day, may increase q2wk, max dose 600 mg/day

Available forms: Caps 25, 50, 100 mg

Implementation
- Give without regard to food, swallow whole

ADVERSE EFFECTS
CNS: Dizziness, insomnia, paresthesias, depression, fatigue, headache, confusion, somnolence, agitation, irritability, speech disturbance, **suicidal ideation, seizures, status epilepticus**
EENT: Diplopia, verbal difficulty, speech abnormalities, taste perversion, amblyopia, pharyngitis, rhinitis, tinnitus, nystagmus
GI: Nausea, constipation, anorexia, weight loss, diarrhea, dyspepsia, dry mouth, abdominal pain
GU: Kidney stones
HEMA: Aplastic anemia, granulocytopenia (rare), ecchymosis
INTEG: Rash
MISC: Flulike symptoms
SYST: Stevens-Johnson syndrome, metabolic acidosis

Pharmacokinetics
Absorption	Unknown
Distribution	Protein binding 40%
Metabolism	Liver
Excretion	Kidneys
Half-life	In RBCs 105 hr

Pharmacodynamics
Onset	Unknown
Peak	2-6 hr
Duration	Unknown

INTERACTIONS
Individual drugs
Alcohol: increased CNS depression

Drug classifications
CarBAMazepine, PHENobarbital, phenytoin: decreased half-life of zonisamide
CYP3A4 inducers, inhibitors: altered product levels

Drug/herb

St. John's wort: increased effect of zonisamide

Drug/food

Grapefruit: do not use together

Drug/lab test

Increased: BUN, creatinine

NURSING CONSIDERATIONS

Assessment

• Assess for seizures: duration, type, intensity, precipitating factors
• Renal function: albumin conc, BUN, urinalysis, creatinine; serum bicarbonate baseline, periodically
⚠ Assess mental status: mood, sensorium, affect, memory (long, short); suicidal thoughts/behavior
⚠ Stevens-Johnson syndrome, aplastic anemia, fulminant hepatic necrosis; may cause death; monitor for rashes and hypersensitive reactions
• Assess for rash, hypersensitivity reaction
• Obtain bicarbonate before treatment/periodically; metabolic acidosis may occur in child

Patient/family education

• Advise patient not to discontinue product abruptly; seizures may occur
• Advise patient to avoid hazardous activities until stabilized on product
• Advise patient to carry/wear emergency ID stating product use
• Teach patient not to use grapefruit juice
• Teach patient to notify prescriber of sore throat, fever, easy bruising
⚠ Teach patient to notify prescriber of rash immediately; to notify prescriber of back pain, abdominal pain, blood in urine; to increase fluid intake to reduce risk of kidney stones
⚠ Teach patient to report suicidal thoughts, behaviors immediately

Evaluation

Positive therapeutic outcome
• Decrease in severity of seizures

Adverse effects: *italics* = common; **bold** = life-threatening

Alpha-adrenergic Blockers

ACTION: α-Adrenergic blockers bind to α-adrenergic receptors, causing dilatation of peripheral blood vessels and lower peripheral resistance resulting in decreased blood pressure.

USES: α-Adrenergic blockers are used for benign prostatic hyperplasia, pheochromocytoma, prevention of tissue necrosis, and sloughing associated with extravasation of IV vasopressors.

CONTRAINDICATIONS:
Hypersensitive reactions may occur, and allergies should be identified before these products are given. Patients with myocardial infarction, coronary insufficiency, angina, or other evidence of coronary artery disease should not use these products.

IMPLEMENTATION
PO route
• Start with low dose, gradually increasing to prevent side effects
• Give with food or milk for GI symptoms

ADVERSE EFFECTS: The most common side effects are hypotension, tachycardia, nasal stuffiness, nausea, vomiting, and diarrhea.

PHARMACOKINETICS: Onset, peak, and duration vary among products.

INTERACTIONS: Vasoconstrictive and hypertensive effects of EPINEPHrine are antagonized by α-adrenergic blockers.

NURSING CONSIDERATIONS
Assessment
• Monitor electrolytes: potassium, sodium chloride, carbon dioxide
• Monitor weight daily, I&O
• Monitor B/P with patient lying, standing before starting treatment, q4hr thereafter
• Assess for nausea, vomiting, diarrhea
• Assess for skin turgor, dryness of mucous membranes for hydration status

Patient/family education
• Caution patient to avoid alcoholic beverages
• Advise patient to report dizziness, palpitations, fainting
• Instruct patient to change position slowly or fainting may occur

• Teach patient to take product exactly as prescribed; to avoid all OTC products (cough, cold, allergy) unless directed by prescriber

Evaluation
Positive therapeutic outcome
• Decreased B/P
• Increased peripheral pulses

Generic Names
α 1 blockers:
silodosin

Anesthetics—general/local

ACTION: Anesthetics (general) act on the CNS to produce tranquilization and sleep before invasive procedures. Anesthetics (local) inhibit conduction of nerve impulses from sensory nerves.

USES: General anesthetics are used to premedicate for surgery, and for induction and maintenance in general anesthesia. For local anesthetics, refer to individual product listing for indications.

CONTRAINDICATIONS:
Persons with CVA, increased ICP, severe hypertension, and cardiac decompensation should not use these products since severe adverse reactions can occur.

Precautions: Anesthetics (general) should be used with caution in the geriatric, children <2 yr, and those with cardiovascular disease (hypotension, bradydysrhythmias), renal/hepatic disease, and Parkinson's disease. The precaution for anesthetics (local) is pregnancy.

IMPLEMENTATION
• Give anticholinergic preoperatively to decrease secretions
• Administer only with resuscitative equipment nearby
• Provide quiet environment for recovery to decrease psychotic symptoms

ADVERSE EFFECTS: The most common side effects are dystonia, akathisia, flexion of arms, fine tremors, drowsiness, restlessness, and hypotension. Also common are chills, respiratory depression, and laryngospasm.

PHARMACOKINETICS: Onset, peak, and duration vary widely among products.

Most products are metabolized in the liver and excreted in urine.

INTERACTIONS: AOIs, tricyclics, and phenothiazines may cause severe hypo/hypertension when used with local anesthetics. CNS depressants will potentiate general and local anesthetics.

NURSING CONSIDERATIONS
Assessment
• Monitor VS q10min during **IV** administration, q30min after IM dose
Evaluation
Positive therapeutic outcome
• Maintenance of anesthesia
• Decreased pain

Generic Names
General anesthetics:
droperidol (high alert), **fentaNYL** (high alert), fentaNYL/droperidol, fentaNYL transdermal, fospropofol, midazolam, **propofol** (high alert)

Local anesthetics:
lidocaine, parenteral (high alert), penicillin G procaine, ropivacaine

Antacids

ACTION: Antacids are basic compounds that neutralize gastric acidity and decrease the rate of gastric emptying. Products are divided into those containing aluminum, magnesium, calcium, or a combination of these.

USES: Antacids decrease hyperacidity in conditions such as peptic ulcer disease, reflux esophagitis, gastritis, or hiatal hernia.

CONTRAINDICATIONS:
Sensitivity to aluminum or magnesium products may cause hypersensitive reactions. Aluminum products should not be used by persons sensitive to aluminum. Magnesium products should not be used by persons sensitive to magnesium. Check for sensitivity before administering.

Precautions: Magnesium products should be given cautiously to patients with renal insufficiency, and during pregnancy and breastfeeding. Sodium content of antacids may be significant. Use with caution for patients with hypertension, or CHF or those on a low-sodium diet.

IMPLEMENTATION
• Advise patient not to take other products within 1-2 hr of antacid administration, since antacids may impair absorption of other products
• Give all products with an 8-oz glass of water to ensure absorption in the stomach
• Give another antacid if constipation occurs with aluminum products

ADVERSE EFFECTS: The most common side effect caused by aluminum-containing antacids is constipation, which may lead to fecal impaction and bowel obstruction. Diarrhea occurs often when magnesium products are given. Alkalosis may occur when systemic products are used. Constipation occurs more frequently than laxation with calcium carbonate. The release of CO_2 from carbonate-containing antacids causes belching, abdominal distention, and flatulence. Sodium bicarbonate may act as a systemic antacid and produce systemic electrolyte disturbances and alkalosis. Calcium carbonate and sodium bicarbonate may cause rebound hyperacidity and milk-alkali syndrome. Alkaluria may occur when products are used on a long-term basis, particularly in persons with abnormal renal function.

PHARMACOKINETICS: Duration is 20-40 min. If ingested 1 hr after meals, acidity is reduced for at least 3hr.

INTERACTIONS: Products whose effects may be increased by some antacids include quiNIDine, amphetamines, pseudoephedrine, levodopa, valproic acid, and dicumarol. Products whose effects may be decreased by some antacids include cimetidine, corticosteroids, ranitidine, iron salts, phenothiazines, phenytoin, digoxin, tetracyclines, ketoconazole, salicylates, and isoniazid.

NURSING CONSIDERATIONS
Assessment
• Assess for aggravating and alleviating factors of epigastric pain or hyperacidity; identify the location, duration, and characteristics of epigastric pain
• Assess GI symptoms, including constipation, diarrhea, abdominal pain; if severe abdominal pain with fever occurs, these products should not be given
• Assess renal symptoms, including increasing urinary pH, electrolytes

Evaluation
Positive therapeutic outcome
- Absence of epigastric pain
- Decreased acidity

Generic Names
aluminum hydroxide, bismuth subsalicylate, calcium carbonate, magaldrate, magnesium oxide, sodium bicarbonate

Anti-Alzheimer Agents

ACTION: Anti-Alzheimer agents improve cognitive functioning by increasing acetylcholine and inhibiting cholinesterase in the CNS. They do not cure the condition, but improve symptoms.

USES: Anti-Alzheimer agents are used for the treatment of Alzheimer's symptoms.

CONTRAINDICATIONS:
Persons with hypersensitivity reactions should not use these products.

Precautions: Anti-Alzheimer agents should be used cautiously in pregnancy **(C)**, breastfeeding, sick sinus syndrome, GI bleeding, bladder obstruction, and seizures.

IMPLEMENTATION
- Give lowest possible dose for therapeutic result; adjust dose to response
- Provide assistance with ambulation during beginning therapy if dizziness, ataxia occur

ADVERSE EFFECTS: The most common side effects are nausea, vomiting, diarrhea, dry mouth, insomnia, dizziness, urinary frequency, incontinence, and rash. The most serious side effects are seizures and dysrhythmias.

PHARMACOKINETICS: Onset, peak, and duration vary widely among products. Most products are metabolized in the liver and excreted by the kidneys.

INTERACTIONS: Increased synergistic reactions may occur with succinylcholine, cholinesterase inhibitors, and cholingeric agonists. There may be a decrease in the action of anticholinergics, and there may be additive effects when used with cholinergic agents.

NURSING CONSIDERATIONS
Assessment
- B/P, hypo/hypertension
- Mental status: affect, mood, behavioral changes, depression, confusion
- GI status: nausea, vomiting, anorexia, diarrhea
- GU status: urinary frequency, incontinence

Patient/family education
- Instruct patient to report side effects, adverse reactions to healthcare provider
- Advise patient to use exactly as prescribed, at regular intervals
- Caution patient not to increase or abruptly decrease dose; serious consequences may result
- Inform patient that product is not a cure, but relieves symptoms

Evaluation
Positive therapeutic outcome
- Decrease in confusion
- Improved mood

Generic Names
donepezil, memantine, rivastigmine

Antianginals

ACTION: Antianginals are divided into the nitrates, calcium channel blockers, and β-adrenergic blockers. The nitrates dilate coronary arteries, causing decreased preload, and dilate systemic arteries, causing decreased afterload. Calcium channel blockers dilate coronary arteries and decrease SA/AV node conduction. β-Adrenergic blockers decrease heart rate so that myocardial O_2 use is decreased. Dipyridamole selectively dilates coronary arteries to increase coronary blood flow.

USES: Antianginals are used in chronic stable angina pectoris, unstable angina, and vasospastic angina. Some (i.e., calcium channel blockers and β-blockers) may be used as dysrhythmics and in hypertension.

CONTRAINDICATIONS:
Persons with known hypersensitivity, increased ICP, or cerebral hemorrhage should not use some of these products.

Precautions: Antianginals should be used with caution in pregnancy, breastfeeding, children, postural hypotension, renal disease, and hepatic injury.

IMPLEMENTATION
- Store protected from light, moisture; place in cool environment

ADVERSE EFFECTS:
The most common side effects are postural hypotension, headache, flushing, dizziness, nausea, edema, and drowsiness. Also common are rash, dysrhythmias, and fatigue.

PHARMACOKINETICS:
Onset, peak, and duration vary widely among coronary products. Most products are metabolized in the liver and excreted in urine.

INTERACTIONS:
Interactions vary widely among products. Check individual monographs for specific information.

NURSING CONSIDERATIONS
Assessment
- Monitor orthostatic B/P, pulse
- Assess for pain: duration, time started, activity being performed, character
- Assess for tolerance if taken over long period
- Assess for headache, light-headedness, decreased B/P; may indicate a need for decreased dosage

Patient/family education
- Instruct patient to keep tabs in original container
- Instruct patient not to use OTC products unless directed by prescriber
- Advise patient to report bradycardia, dizziness, confusion, depression, fever
- Teach patient to take pulse at home; advise when to notify prescriber
- Advise patient to avoid alcohol, smoking, sodium intake
- Advise patient to comply with weight control, dietary adjustments, modified exercise program
- Teach patient to carry/wear emergency ID to identify product being taken, allergies
- Caution patient to make position changes slowly to prevent fainting

Evaluation
Positive therapeutic outcome
- Decrease, prevention of anginal pain

Generic Names
Nitrates:
isosorbide, nitroglycerin

β-Adrenergic blockers:
atenolol, dipyridamole, metoprolol, nadolol, propranolol

Calcium channel blockers:
amLODIPine, **diltiazem** (high alert), niCARdipine, NIFEdipine, verapamil

Miscellaneous:
ranolazine

Antianxiety Agents

ACTION:
Benzodiazepines potentiate the action of GABA, including any other inhibitory transmitters in the CNS, resulting in decreased anxiety. Most agents cause a decrease in CNS excitability.

USES:
Anxiety is relieved in conditions such as generalized anxiety disorder and phobic disorders. Benzodiazepines are also used for acute alcohol withdrawal to prevent delirium tremens, and some products are used for relaxation before surgery.

CONTRAINDICATIONS:
These products are contraindicated in hypersensitivity, acute closed-angle glaucoma, breastfeeding (diazepam), children <6 mo, and hepatic disease (clonazePAM).

Precautions: Antianxiety agents should be used cautiously in geriatric or debilitated patients. Usually smaller doses are needed since metabolism is slowed. Persons with renal/hepatic disease may show delayed excretion. ClonazePAM may increase the incidence of seizures.

IMPLEMENTATION
- Give with food or milk for GI symptoms; may give crushed if patient is unable to swallow whole (tabs only, no controlled or sustained-release products)

ADVERSE EFFECTS:
The most common side effects are dizziness, drowsiness, blurred vision, and orthostatic hypotension. Most adverse reactions are mediated through the CNS. There is potential for abuse and physical dependence with some products.

PHARMACOKINETICS:
Most of these agents are metabolized by the liver and excreted via the kidneys.

INTERACTIONS: Increased CNS depression may occur when given with other CNS depressants. These products should be used together cautiously. Alcohol should not be used, as fatal reactions have occurred. The serum concentration and toxicity may be increased when used with benzodiazepines.

NURSING CONSIDERATIONS

Assessment

• Assess B/P (lying and standing), pulse; if systolic B/P drops 20 mm Hg, hold product and notify prescriber; orthostatic hypotension can be severe

• Monitor renal/hepatic function tests: AST, ALT, bilirubin, creatinine, LDH, alkaline phosphatase

• Monitor physical dependency and withdrawal with some products, including headache, nausea, vomiting, muscle pain, and weakness after long-term use

Patient/family education

• Inform patient that product should not be used for everyday stress or long-term use; not to take more than prescribed amount since product is habit forming

• Caution patient to avoid driving and activities that require alertness since drowsiness and dizziness may occur

• Instruct patient to abstain from alcohol, other psychotropic medications unless directed by prescriber

• Caution patient not to discontinue abruptly; after extended periods, withdrawal symptoms may occur

Evaluation

Positive therapeutic outcome

• Decreased anxiety
• Increased relaxation

Generic Names

Benzodiazepines:
ALPRAZolam, chlordiazePOXIDE, clonazePAM, diazepam, LORazepam, midazolam, triazolam

Miscellaneous:
busPIRone, doxepin, hydrOXYzine, PARoxetine, venlafaxine

Antiasthmatics

ACTION: Bronchodilators are divided into anticholinergics, α/β-adrenergic agonists, β-adrenergic agonists, and phosphodiesterase inhibitors. Also included in antiasthmatic agents are corticosteroids, leukotriene antagonists, mast cell stabilizers, and monoclonal antibodies. Anticholinergics act by inhibiting interaction of acetylcholine at receptor sites on bronchial smooth muscle. α/β-Adrenergic agonists act by relaxing bronchial smooth muscle and increasing diameter of nasal passages. β-Adrenergic agonists act by action on β_2-receptors, which relaxes bronchial smooth muscle. Phosphodiesterase inhibitors act by blocking phosphodiesterase and increasing cAMP, which mediates smooth muscle relaxation in the respiratory system. Corticosteroids act by decreasing inflammation in the bronchial system. Leukotriene receptor antagonists decrease leukotrienes, and mast cell stabilizers decrease histamine; both act to decrease bronchospasm.

USES: Antiasthmatics are used for bronchial asthma; bronchospasm associated with bronchitis, emphysema, or other obstructive pulmonary diseases; Cheyne-Stokes respirations; and prevention of exercise-induced asthma. Some products are used for rhinitis and other allergic reactions.

CONTRAINDICATIONS:
Persons with hypersensitivity, closed-angle glaucoma, tachydysrhythmias, and severe cardiac disease should not use some of these products.

Precautions: Antiasthmatics should be used with caution in pregnancy, breastfeeding, hyperthyroidism, hypertension, prostatic hypertrophy, and seizure disorders.

IMPLEMENTATION

• Give inhaled product after shaking; exhale, place mouthpiece in mouth, inhale slowly, hold breath, remove, exhale slowly

• Give PO product with meals to decrease gastric irritation

• Store inhaled product in light-resistant container; do not expose to temperatures >86° F (30° C)

• Give gum, small sips of water for dry mouth

ADVERSE EFFECTS: The most common side effects are tremors, anxiety, nausea, vomiting and irritation in the throat. The most serious adverse reactions are bronchospasm and dyspnea.

PHARMACOKINETICS: Onset, peak, and duration vary widely among products. Most products are metabolized by the liver and excreted in urine.

INTERACTIONS: Interactions vary widely among products. Check individual monographs for specific information.

NURSING CONSIDERATIONS
Assessment
- Monitor respiratory function: vital capacity, forced expiratory volume, ABGs, lung sounds, heart rate and rhythm, aggravating and alleviating factors

Patient/family education
- Caution patient to avoid hazardous activities; drowsiness or dizziness may occur with some products
- Instruct patient to obtain bloodwork as required; some products require blood levels to be drawn
- Advise patient to avoid all OTC medications unless approved by provider
- Instruct patient to report side effects, including insomnia, heart palpitations, light-headedness; these side effects may occur with some products

Evaluation
Positive therapeutic outcome
- Decreased severity and number of asthma attacks
- Absence of dyspnea, wheezing

Generic Names
Bronchodilators:
albuterol, arformoterol, **atropine** (high alert), formoterol, ipratropium, levalbuterol, terbutaline, theophylline, tiotropium

Adrenergics:
EPINEPHrine (high alert)

Corticosteroids:
beclomethasone, betamethasone, budesonide, cortisone, dexamethasone, flunisolide, fluticasone, hydrocortisone, methylPREDNISolone, predniSONE, triamcinolone

Leukotriene antagonists:
zafirlukast

Monoclonal antibodies:
omalizumab

Anticholinergics

ACTION: Anticholinergics inhibit the muscarinic actions of acetylcholine at receptor sites in the autonomic nervous system. Anticholinergics are also known as antimuscarinic products.

USES: Anticholinergics are used for a variety of conditions: decreasing involuntary movements in parkinsonism (benztropine, trihexyphenidyl); bradydysrhythmias (atropine); nausea and vomiting (scopolamine); and as cycloplegic mydriatics (atropine, hematropine, scopalamine, cyclopentolate, tropicamide). Gastrointestinal anticholinergics are used to decrease motility (smooth muscle tone) in the GI, biliary, and urinary tracts and for their ability to decrease gastric secretions (propantheline, glycopyrrolate).

CONTRAINDICATIONS:
Persons with closed-angle glaucoma, myasthenia gravis, or GI/GU obstruction should not use some of these products.

Precautions: Anticholinergics should be used with caution in pregnant, breastfeeding, or geriatric patients, or in those with prostatic hypertrophy, CHF, or hypertension. Use with caution in the presence of high environmental temperature.

IMPLEMENTATION
PO route
- Give with or after meals to prevent GI upset; may give with fluids other than water
- Store at room temperature
- Give hard candy, frequent drinks, sugarless gum to relieve dry mouth

IM/IV route
- Give parenteral dose with patient recumbent to prevent postural hypotension
- Give parenteral dose slowly; keep in bed for at least 1 hr after dose; monitor VS
- Give after checking dose carefully; even slight overdose could lead to toxicity

ADVERSE EFFECTS: The most common side effects are dry mouth, constipation, urinary retention, urinary hesitancy, headache, and dizziness. Also common is paralytic ileus.

PHARMACOKINETICS: Onset, peak, and duration vary widely among products. Most products are metabolized in the liver and excreted in urine.

INTERACTIONS: Increased anticholinergic effects may occur when used with MAOIs, tricyclics, and amantadine. Anticholinergics may cause a decreased effect of phenothiazines and levodopa.

NURSING CONSIDERATIONS
Assessment
• Assess I&O ratio; retention commonly causes decreased urinary output
• Assess for urinary hesitancy, retention; palpate bladder if retention occurs
• Assess for constipation; increase fluids, bulk, exercise if this occurs
• Identify tolerance over long-term therapy; dosage may need to be increased or changed
• Assess mental status: affect, mood, CNS depression, worsening of mental symptoms during early therapy

Patient/family education
• Caution patient to avoid driving and other hazardous activities; drowsiness may occur
• Advise patient to avoid OTC medication: cough, cold preparations with alcohol, antihistamines unless directed by prescriber

Evaluation
Positive therapeutic outcome
• Decreased secretions
• Absence of nausea and vomiting

Generic Names
atropine (high alert), benztropine, glycopyrrolate, hyoscyamine, scopolamine (transdermal), solifenacin

Anticoagulants

ACTION: Anticoagulants interfere with blood clotting by preventing clot formation.

USES: Anticoagulants are used for DVT, pulmonary emboli, myocardial infarction, open heart surgery, disseminated intravascular clotting syndrome, atrial fibrillation with embolization, and in transfusion and dialysis.

CONTRAINDICATIONS:
Persons with hemophilia and related disorders, leukemia with bleeding, peptic ulcer disease, thrombocytopenic purpura, blood dyscrasias, acute nephritis, and subacute bacterial endocarditis should not use these products.

Precautions: Anticoagulants should be used with caution in pregnancy, geriatric, and alcoholism.

IMPLEMENTATION
• Store in tight container (PO dose)
SUBCUT route
• Give at same time each day to maintain steady blood levels

• Do not massage area or aspirate when giving SUBCUT inj; give in abdomen between pelvic bones; rotate sites; do not pull back on plunger, leave in for 10 sec; apply gentle pressure for 1 min
• Do not change needles
• Avoid all IM inj that may cause bleeding

ADVERSE EFFECTS: The most serious adverse reactions are hemorrhage, agranulocytosis, leukopenia, eosinophilia, and thrombocytopenia, depending on the specific product. The most common side effects are diarrhea, rash, and fever.

PHARMACOKINETICS: Onset, peak, and duration vary widely among products. Most products are metabolized in the liver and excreted in urine.

INTERACTIONS: Salicylates, steroids, and nonsteroidal antiinflammatories will potentiate the action of anticoagulants. Anticoagulants may cause serious effects. Check individual monographs for specific information.

NURSING CONSIDERATIONS
Assessment
• Monitor blood tests (Hct, platelets, occult blood in stools) q3mo
• Monitor PTT, which should be 1½-2 × control, PPT; daily, APTT, ACT, INR
• Monitor B/P; watch for increasing signs of hypertension
• Monitor for bleeding gums, petechiae, ecchymosis, black tarry stools, hematuria
• Monitor for fever, skin rash, urticaria
• Monitor for needed dosage change q1-2wk

Patient/family education
• Advise patient to avoid OTC preparations that may cause serious product interactions unless directed by prescriber
• Inform patient that product may be held during active bleeding (menstruation), depending on condition
• Caution patient to use soft-bristle toothbrush to prevent bleeding gums; avoid contact sports; use electric razor
• Instruct patient to carry/wear emergency ID identifying product taken
• Instruct patient to report any signs of bleeding: gums, under skin, urine, stools

Evaluation
Positive therapeutic outcome
• Decrease of DVT

Generic Names

argatroban, dabigatran, **dalteparin** (high alert), **enoxaparin** (high alert), fondaparinux, **heparin** (high alert), **lepirudin** (high alert), **tinzaparin** (high alert), **warfarin** (high alert)

Anticonvulsants

ACTION: Anticonvulsants are divided into the barbiturates, benzodiazepines, hydantoins, succinimides, and miscellaneous products. Barbiturates and benzodiazepines are discussed in separate sections. Hydantoins act by inhibiting the spread of seizure activity in the motor cortex. Succinimides act by inhibiting spike and wave formation; they also decrease amplitude, frequency, duration, and spread of discharge in seizures.

USES: Hydantoins are used in generalized tonic-clonic seizures, status epilepticus, and psychomotor seizures. Succinimides are used for absence (or petit mal) seizures. Barbiturates are used in generalized tonic-clonic and cortical focal seizures.

CONTRAINDICATIONS:

Hypersensitive reactions may occur, and allergies should be identified before these products are given.

Precautions: Persons with renal/hepatic disease should be watched closely.

IMPLEMENTATION
PO route

• Give with food, milk to decrease GI symptoms
• Provide good oral hygiene as it is important for patients taking hydantoins

ADVERSE EFFECTS: Bone marrow

depression is the most life-threatening adverse reaction associated with hydantoins or succinimides. The most common side effects are GI symptoms. Other common side effects for hydantoins are gingival hyperplasia and CNS effects such as nystagmus, ataxia, slurred speech, and confusion.

PHARMACOKINETICS: Onset,

peak, and duration vary widely among products. Most products are metabolized in the liver and excreted in urine, bile, and feces.

INTERACTIONS: Hydantoins cause

decreased effects of estrogens, and oral contraceptives.

NURSING CONSIDERATIONS
Assessment

• Monitor renal function tests, including BUN, creatinine, serum uric acid, urine CCr before, during therapy
• Monitor blood tests: RBC, Hct, Hgb, reticulocyte counts weekly for 4 wk then monthly
• Monitor hepatic function tests: AST, ALT, bilirubin, creatinine
• Assess mental status, including mood, sensorium, affect, behavioral changes; if mental status changes, notify prescriber
• Assess for eye problems, including need for ophth examinations before, during, and after treatment (slit lamp, fundoscopy, tonometry)
• Assess for allergic reaction, including red, raised rash; if this occurs, product should be discontinued
• Assess for blood dyscrasias, including fever, sore throat, bruising, rash, jaundice
• Monitor toxicity, including bone marrow depression, nausea, vomiting, ataxia, diplopia, cardiovascular collapse, Stevens-Johnson syndrome

Patient/family education

• Advise patient to carry/wear emergency ID stating products taken, condition, prescriber's name, phone number
• Advise patient to avoid driving, other activities that require alertness

Evaluation
Positive therapeutic outcome

• Decreased seizure activity; document on patient's chart

Generic Names

Succinimides:
ethosuximide

Hydantoins:
fosphenytoin, phenytoin

Miscellaneous:
acetaZOLAMIDE, carBAMazepine, clonazePAM, diazepam, eslicarbazepine, ezogabine, gabapentin, lacosamide, lamoTRIgine, **magnesium sulfate** (high alert), rufinamide, tiaGABine, topiramate, valproate/valproic acid/divalproex sodium, vigabatrin, zonisamide

Barbiturates:
PHENobarbital (high alert), primidone, **thiopental** (high alert)

Antidepressants

ACTION: Antidepressants are divided into the tricyclics, MAOIs, and miscellaneous antidepressants (SSRIs). The tricyclics work by blocking reuptake of norepinephrine and serotonin into nerve endings and increasing action of norepinephrine and serotonin in nerve cells. MAOIs act by increasing concentrations of endogenous epinephrine, norepinephrine, serotonin, and dopamine in storage sites in the CNS by inhibition of MAO; increased concentration reduces depression.

USES: Antidepressants are used for depression and, in some cases, enuresis in children.

CONTRAINDICATIONS:
The contraindications for antidepressants are seizure disorders, prostatic hypertrophy, and severe renal/hepatic/cardiac disease depending on the type of medication.

Precautions: Antidepressants should be used cautiously in pregnant, geriatric, and suicidal patients; severe depression; schizophrenia; hyperactivity; and diabetes mellitus.

IMPLEMENTATION
PO route
• Give increased fluids, bulk in diet if constipation, urinary retention occur
• Give with food or milk for GI symptoms
• Give gum, hard candy, or frequent sips of water for dry mouth
• Store in airtight container at room temperature; do not refreeze
• Provide assistance with ambulation during beginning therapy since drowsiness/dizziness occurs

ADVERSE EFFECTS: The most serious adverse reactions are paralytic ileus, acute renal failure, hypertension, and hypertensive crisis, depending on the specific product. Common side effects are dizziness, drowsiness, diarrhea, dry mouth, urinary retention, and orthostatic hypotension.

PHARMACOKINETICS: Onset, peak, and duration vary widely among products. Most products are metabolized in the liver and excreted in urine.

INTERACTIONS: Interactions vary widely among products. Check individual monographs for specific information.

NURSING CONSIDERATIONS
Assessment
• Monitor B/P (lying, standing), pulse q4hr; if systolic B/P drops 20 mm Hg, hold product, notify prescriber; take VS q4hr in patients with CV disease
• Monitor blood tests: CBC, leukocytes, differential, cardiac enzymes if patient is receiving long-term therapy
• Monitor hepatic function tests: AST, ALT, bilirubin, creatinine
• Monitor weight weekly; appetite may increase with product
• Monitor for EPS primarily in geriatric: rigidity, dystonia, akathisia
• Assess mental status: mood, sensorium, affect, suicidal tendencies, increase in psychiatric symptoms (depression, panic)
• Check for urinary retention, constipation; constipation is more likely to occur in children, geriatric patients
• Assess for withdrawal symptoms: headache, nausea, vomiting, muscle pain, weakness; do not usually occur unless product was discontinued abruptly
• Identify alcohol consumption; if alcohol is consumed, hold dose until AM

Patient/family education
• Teach patient that therapeutic effects may take 2-3 wk
• Advise patient to use caution in driving or other activities requiring alertness because of drowsiness, dizziness, blurred vision
• Caution patient to avoid alcohol ingestion, other CNS depressants
• Instruct patient not to discontinue medication quickly after long-term use; may cause nausea, headache, malaise
• Instruct patient to wear sunscreen or large hat, since photosensitivity may occur

Evaluation
Positive therapeutic outcome
• Decreased depression

Generic Names
Tetracyclics:
mirtazapine

Tricyclics:
amitriptyline, clomiPRAMINE, desipramine, doxepin, imipramine, nortriptyline

Miscellaneous:
buPROPion, DULoxetine, levomilnacipran, traZODone, venlafaxine, vortioxetine

SSRIs:
citalopram, escitalopram, FLUoxetine, PARoxetine, sertraline

Antidiabetics

ACTION: Antidiabetics are divided into the insulins that decrease blood glucose, phosphate, and potassium and increase blood pyruvate and lactate and oral antidiabetics that cause functioning β-cells in the pancreas to release insulin and improve the effect of endogenous and exogenous insulin.

USES: Insulins are used for ketoacidosis and diabetes mellitus types 1 and 2; oral antidiabetics are used for diabetes mellitus type 2.

CONTRAINDICATIONS:
Hypersensitive reactions may occur, and allergies should be identified before these products are given. Oral antidiabetics should not be used in juvenile or brittle diabetes, diabetic ketoacidosis, or severe renal/hepatic disease.

Precautions: Oral antidiabetics should be used with caution in pregnancy, breastfeeding, geriatric, cardiac disease, and in the presence of alcohol.

IMPLEMENTATION
PO route
• Give oral antidiabetic 30 min before meals
SUBCUT route
• Give insulin after warming to room temperature by rotating in palms to prevent lipodystrophy from injecting cold insulin
• Give human insulin to those allergic to beef or pork
• Rotate inj sites when giving insulin; use abdomen, upper back, thighs, upper arm, buttocks; keep a record of sites

ADVERSE EFFECTS: The most common side effect of insulin and oral antidiabetics is hypoglycemia. Other adverse reactions for oral antidiabetics include blood dyscrasias, hepatotoxicity, and, rarely, cholestatic jaundice. Adverse reactions for insulin products include allergic responses and, more rarely, anaphylaxis.

PHARMACOKINETICS: Onset, peak, and duration vary widely among products. Oral antidiabetics are metabolized in the liver, with metabolites excreted in urine, bile, and feces.

INTERACTIONS: Interactions vary widely among products. Check individual monographs for specific information.

NURSING CONSIDERATIONS
Assessment
• Monitor blood, urine glucose levels during treatment to determine diabetes control (oral products)
• Monitor fasting blood glucose, 2 hr PP (60-100 mg/dl normal fasting level) (70-130 mg/dl—normal 2-hr level)
• Assess for hypoglycemic reaction that can occur during peak time

Patient/family education
• Advise patient to avoid alcohol and salicylates except on advice of prescriber
• Teach patient symptoms of ketoacidosis: nausea, thirst, polyuria, dry mouth, decreased B/P, dry, flushed skin, acetone breath, drowsiness, Kussmaul respirations
• Teach patient symptoms of hypoglycemia: headache, tremors, fatigue, weakness; that candy or sugar should be carried to treat hypoglycemia
• Advise patient to test urine for glucose/ketones tid if this product is replacing insulin
• Advise patient to continue weight control, dietary restrictions, exercise, hygiene

Evaluation
Positive therapeutic outcome
• Decrease in polyuria, polydipsia, polyphagia
• Clear sensorium
• Absence of dizziness
• Stable gait

Generic Names
canagliflozin, dapagliflozin, empagliflozin, glipiZIDE, glyBURIDE, **insulin aspart** (high alert), **insulin detemir** (high alert), **insulin glargine** (high alert), **insulin glulisine** (high alert), **insulin lispro** (high alert), **insulin, regular** (high alert), **insulin, regular concentrated** (high alert), insulin, zinc suspension (Lente), insulin, zinc suspension extended (Ultralente), liraglutide, linagliptin, metformin, miglitol, pioglitazone, repaglinide, rosiglitazone, saxagliptin, sitaGLIPtin

Antidiarrheals

ACTION: Antidiarrheals work by various actions including direct action on intestinal muscles to decrease GI peristalsis or by inhibiting prostaglandin synthesis responsible for

Adverse effects: *italics* = common; **bold** = life-threatening

GI hypermotility, acting on mucosal receptors responsible for peristalsis, or decreasing water content of stools.

USES: Antidiarrheals are used for diarrhea of undetermined causes.

CONTRAINDICATIONS:
The contraindications are persons with severe ulcerative colitis, and pseudomembranous colitis with some products.

Precautions: Antidiarrheals should be used with caution in pregnancy, breastfeeding, children, geriatric patients, dehydration.

IMPLEMENTATION
PO route
• Give for 48 hr only

ADVERSE EFFECTS: The most serious adverse reactions of some products are paralytic ileus, toxic megacolon, and angioneurotic edema. The most common side effects are constipation, nausea, dry mouth, and abdominal pain.

PHARMACOKINETICS: Onset, peak, and duration vary widely among products. Most products are metabolized in the liver and excreted in urine.

INTERACTIONS: Interactions vary widely among products. Check individual monographs for specific information.

NURSING CONSIDERATIONS
Assessment
• Monitor electrolytes (potassium, sodium, chloride) if on long-term therapy
• Monitor bowel pattern before; for rebound constipation after termination of medication
• Assess response after 48 hr; if no response, product should be discontinued
• Identify dehydration in children

Patient/family education
• Advise patient to avoid OTC products
• Caution patient not to exceed recommended dose

Evaluation
Positive therapeutic outcome
• Decreased diarrhea

Generic Names
bismuth subsalicylate, kaolin/pectin, loperamide

Antidysrhythmics

ACTION: Antidysrhythmics are divided into four classes and miscellaneous antidysrhythmics:
• Class I increases the duration of action potential and the effective refractory period and reduces disparity in the refractory period between a normal and infarcted myocardium; further subclasses include Ia, Ib, Ic
• Class II decreases the rate of SA node discharge, increases recovery time, slows conduction through the AV node, and decreases heart rate, which decreases O_2 consumption in the myocardium
• Class III increases the duration of action potential and the effective refractory period
• Class IV inhibits calcium ion influx across the cell membrane during cardiac depolarization; decreases SA node discharge, decreases conduction velocity through the AV node
• Miscellaneous antidysrhythmics include those such as adenosine, which slows conduction through the AV node, and digoxin, which decreases conduction velocity and prolongs the effective refractory period in the AV node

USES: Antidysrhythmics are used for PVCs, tachycardia, hypertension, atrial fibrillation, and angina pectoris.

CONTRAINDICATIONS:
Contraindications vary widely among products.

Precautions: Precautions vary widely among products.

ADVERSE EFFECTS: Side effects and adverse reactions vary widely among products.

PHARMACOKINETICS: Onset, peak, and duration vary widely among products.

INTERACTIONS: Interactions vary widely among products. Check individual monographs for specific information.

NURSING CONSIDERATIONS
Assessment
• Monitor ECG continuously to determine product effectiveness, PVCs, or other dysrhythmias
• Assess for dehydration or hypovolemia
• Monitor B/P continuously for hypo/hypertension
• Monitor I&O ratio

- Monitor serum potassium
- Assess for edema in feet and legs daily

Patient/family education

- Advise patient to comply with dosage schedule, even if patient is feeling better
- Instruct patient to report bradycardia, dizziness, confusion, depression, fever

Evaluation

Positive therapeutic outcome

- Decrease in B/P in hypertension
- Decreased B/P, edema, moist crackles in CHF

Generic Names

Class Ia:
disopyramide, procainamide, quiNIDine

Class Ib:
lidocaine, parenteral (high alert), phenytoin

Class Ic:
flecainide, propafenone

Class II:
acebutolol, esmolol, propranolol, sotalol

Class III:
amiodarone (high alert), **dronedarone** (high alert), **ibutilide** (high alert)

Class IV:
verapamil

Miscellaneous:
adenosine (high alert), **atropine** (high alert), **digoxin** (high alert)

Antiemetics

ACTION: The antiemetics are divided into the 5-HT$_3$ receptor antagonists, the phenothiazines, and the miscellaneous products. The 5-HT$_3$ receptor antagonists work by blocking serotonin peripherally, centrally, and in the small intestine. The phenothiazines act by blocking the chemoreceptor trigger zone in the brain. The miscellaneous products work by either decreasing motion sickness or delaying gastric emptying.

USES: Antiemetics are used to prevent nausea and vomiting due to cancer chemotherapy, radiotherapy, and surgery (5-HT$_3$ receptor antagonists); some of the miscellaneous products (antihistamines) work by decreasing motion sickness. Most other products are used for many types of nausea and vomiting.

CONTRAINDICATIONS:
Persons developing hypersensitive reactions should not use these products.

Precautions: Antiemetics should be used cautiously in pregnancy, breastfeeding, hepatic disease, and some GI disorders.

IMPLEMENTATION

- Give prophylactically, before nausea and vomiting occur, in cancer chemotherapy
- Store at room temperature vial/ampules, oral products

ADVERSE EFFECTS: The most common side effects are headache, dizziness, fatigue, and diarrhea.

PHARMACOKINETICS: Onset, peak, and duration vary widely among products. Most products are metabolized by the liver and excreted by the kidneys.

INTERACTIONS: Interactions vary widely among products. Check individual monographs for specific information. Other CNS depressants increase CNS depression.

NURSING CONSIDERATIONS

Assessment

- Assess reason for nausea, vomiting; absence of nausea and vomiting after giving product
- Monitor hypersensitivity reactions: rash, bronchospasm with some products

Patient/family education

- Caution patient to avoid hazardous activities if dizziness occurs; ask for assistance if hospitalized
- Instruct patient to rise slowly to prevent orthostatic hypotension
- Teach patient all aspects of product usage
- Teach patient conservative methods to control nausea and vomiting such as sips of water or other fluids and dry crackers

Evaluation

Positive therapeutic outcome

- Absence or decreasing nausea and vomiting after use

Generic Names

5-HT$_3$ antagonists:
dolasetron, granisetron, ondansetron, palono-setron

Phenothiazines:
chlorproMAZINE, prochlorperazine, promethazine

Miscellaneous:
aprepitant, meclizine, metoclopramide, scopolamine, trimethobenzamide

Antifungals (systemic)

ACTION: Antifungals act by increasing cell membrane permeability in susceptible organisms by binding sterols and decreasing potassium, sodium, and nutrients in the cell.

USES: Antifungals are used for infections of histoplasmosis, blastomycosis, coccidioidomycosis, cryptococcosis, aspergillosis, phycomycosis, candidiasis, sporotrichosis causing severe meningitis, septicemia, and skin infections.

CONTRAINDICATIONS:
Persons with severe bone marrow depression or hypersensitivity should not use these products.

Precautions: Antifungals should be used with caution in renal/hepatic disease and pregnancy.

IMPLEMENTATION
IV route
• Give by **IV** using in-line filter (mean pore diameter >1 μm) using distal veins; check for extravasation, necrosis q8hr
• Give product only after C&S confirms organism, make sure product is used in life-threatening infections
• Provide protection from light during infusion; cover with foil
• Give symptomatic treatment as ordered for adverse reactions: aspirin, antihistamines, antiemetics, antispasmodics
• Store protected from moisture and light; diluted sol is stable for 24 hr

ADVERSE EFFECTS: The most serious adverse reactions include renal tubular acidosis, permanent renal impairment, anuria, oliguria, hemorrhagic gastroenteritis, acute liver failure, and blood dyscrasias. Some common side effects include hypokalemia, nausea, vomiting, anorexia, headache, fever, and chills.

PHARMACOKINETICS: Onset, peak, and duration vary widely among products. Most products are metabolized in the liver and excreted in urine.

INTERACTIONS: Interactions vary widely among products. Check individual monographs for specific information.

NURSING CONSIDERATIONS
Assessment
• Monitor VS q15-30min during first infusion; note changes in pulse,B/P
• Monitor I&O ratio; watch for decreasing urinary output, change in specific gravity; discontinue product to prevent permanent damage to renal tubules
• Monitor blood tests; CBC, potassium, sodium, calcium, magnesium q2wk
• Monitor weight weekly; if weight increases over 2 lb/wk, edema is present; renal damage should be considered
• Assess for renal toxicity: increasing BUN, if >40 mg/dl or if serum creatinine >3 mg/dl; product may be discontinued or dosage reduced
• Assess for hepatotoxicity: increasing AST, ALT, alkaline phosphatase, bilirubin
• Assess for allergic reaction: dermatitis, rash; product should be discontinued; antihistamines (mild reaction) or epINEPHrine (severe reaction) administered
• Assess for hypokalemia: anorexia, drowsiness, weakness, decreased reflexes, dizziness, increased urinary output, increased thirst, paresthesias
• Assess for ototoxicity: tinnitus (ringing, roaring in ears), vertigo, loss of hearing (rare)

Patient/family education
• Teach patient that long-term therapy may be needed to clear infection (2 wk-3 mo depending on type of infection)

Evaluation
Positive therapeutic outcome
• Decreased fever, malaise, rash
• Negative C&S for infecting organism

Generic Names
amphotericin B, anidulafungin, fluconazole, itraconazole, ketoconazole, micafungin, nystatin, posaconazole, voriconazole

Antihistamines

ACTION: Antihistamines compete with histamines for H_1 receptor sites. They antagonize in varying degrees most of the pharmacologic effects of histamines.

USES: Antihistamines are used to control the symptoms of allergies, rhinitis, and pruritus.

CONTRAINDICATIONS:
Hypersensitivity to H_1-receptor antagonists occurs rarely. Patients with acute asthma and lower respiratory tract disease should not use these products since thick secretions may result. Other contraindications include closed-angle glaucoma, bladder neck obstruction, stenosing peptic ulcer, symptomatic prostatic hypertrophy, breastfeeding, and in the newborn.

Precautions: Antihistamines must be used cautiously in conjunction with intraocular pressure since they increase intraocular pressure. Caution should also be used in pregnancy, breastfeeding, and geriatric patients and patients with renal/cardiac disease, hypertension, and seizure disorders.

ADVERSE EFFECTS:
Most products cause drowsiness; however, loratadine and fexofenadine produce little, if any, drowsiness. Other common side effects are headache and thickening of bronchial secretions. Serious blood dyscrasias may occur, but are rare. Urinary retention, GI effects occur with many of these products.

PHARMACOKINETICS:
Onset varies from 20-60 min, with duration lasting 4-24 hr. In general, pharmacokinetics vary widely among products.

INTERACTIONS:
Barbiturates, opioids, hypnotics, tricyclics, and alcohol can increase CNS depression when taken with antihistamines.

NURSING CONSIDERATIONS
Assessment
- Check I&O ratio; be alert for urinary retention, frequency, dysuria; product should be discontinued if these occur
- Assess for blood dyscrasias: thrombocytopenia, agranulocytosis (rare)
- Assess for respiratory status, including rate, rhythm, increase in bronchial secretions, wheezing, chest tightness
- Assess for cardiac status, including palpitations, increased pulse, hypotension
- Assess CBC during long-term therapy, since hemolytic anemia, although rare, may occur
- Administer with food or milk to decrease GI symptoms; absorption may be decreased slightly
- Administer whole (sus rel tab)
- Provide hard candy, gum, frequent rinsing of mouth for dryness

Patient/family education
- Advise patient to notify prescriber if confusion, sedation, hypotension occur
- Caution patient to avoid driving and other hazardous activity if drowsiness occurs
- Instruct patient to avoid concurrent use of alcohol and other CNS depressants
- Inform patient to discontinue a few days before skin testing

Evaluation
Positive therapeutic outcome
- Absence of allergy symptoms, itching

Generic Names
brompheniramine, budesonide, cetirizine, chlorpheniramine, cyproheptadine, desloratadine, diphenhydrAMINE, fexofenadine, levocetirizine, loratadine, promethazine

Antihypertensives

ACTION: Antihypertensives are divided into angiotensin converting enzyme (ACE) inhibitors, β-adrenergic blockers, calcium channel blockers, centrally acting adrenergics, diuretics, peripherally acting antiadrenergics, and vasodilators. β-Blockers, calcium channel blockers, and diuretics are discussed in separate sections. ACE inhibitors selectively suppress conversion of renin-angiotensin I to angiotensin II; dilatation of arterial and venous vessels occurs. Centrally acting adrenergics act by inhibiting the sympathetic vasomotor center in the CNS, which reduces impulses in the sympathetic nervous system; blood pressure, pulse rate, and cardiac output decrease. Peripherally acting antiadrenergics inhibit sympathetic vasoconstriction by inhibiting release of norepinephrine and/or depleting norepinephrine stores in adrenergic nerve endings. Vasodilators act on arteriolar smooth muscle by producing direct relaxation or vasodilatation; a reduction in blood pressure, with concomitant increases in heart rate and cardiac output, occurs.

USES: Antihypertensives are used for hypertension and for heart failure not responsive to conventional therapy. Some products are used in hypertensive crisis, angina, and for some cardiac dysrhythmias.

CONTRAINDICATIONS:
Hypersensitive reactions may occur, and allergies should be identified before these products

are given. Antihypertensives should not be used in children or in patients with heart block.

Precautions: Antihypertensives should be used with caution in geriatric and dialysis patients, and in the presence of hypovolemia, leukemia, and electrolyte imbalances.

IMPLEMENTATION
• Place patient in supine or Trendelenburg position for severe hypotension

ADVERSE EFFECTS: The most
common side effects are marked hypotension, bradycardia, tachycardia, headache, nausea, and vomiting. Side effects and adverse reactions may vary widely between classes and specific products.

PHARMACOKINETICS: Onset,
peak, and duration vary widely among products. Most products are metabolized in the liver, with metabolites excreted in urine, bile, and feces.

INTERACTIONS: Interactions vary
widely among products. Check individual monographs for specific information.

NURSING CONSIDERATIONS
Assessment
• Monitor blood tests: neutrophil; decreased platelets occur with many of the products
• Monitor renal function tests: protein, BUN, creatinine; watch for increased levels, which may indicate nephrotic syndrome; obtain baselines in renal/hepatic function tests before beginning treatment
• Assess for edema in feet and legs daily
• Identify allergic reaction, including rash, fever, pruritus, urticaria: product should be discontinued if antihistamines fail to help
• Identify symptoms of CHF: edema, dyspnea, wet crackles, B/P
• Assess for renal symptoms: polyuria, oliguria, frequency

Patient/family education
• Instruct patient to comply with dosage schedule, even if feeling better
• Advise patient to rise slowly to sitting or standing position to minimize orthostatic hypotension

Evaluation
Positive therapeutic outcome
• Decrease in B/P in hypertension
• Decreased B/P, edema, moist crackles in CHF

Generic Names
Angiotensin-converting enzyme inhibitors:
benazepril, enalapril, fosinopril, lisinopril, quinapril, ramipril, trandolapril

Angiotensin II receptor blockers:
azilsartan, candesartan, eprosartan, irbesartan, losartan, olmesartan, telmisartan, valsartan

Centrally acting adrenergics:
cloNIDine, guanfacine, methyldopa

Peripherally acting antiadrenergics:
doxazosin, prazosin, reserpine

Vasodilators:
ambrisentan, fenoldopam, hydrALAZINE, macitentan, minoxidil, **nitroprusside** (high alert)

Antiadrenergic: Combined α/β-blocker:
labetalol

Direct renin inhibitors:
aliskiren

Antiinfectives

ACTION: Antiinfectives are divided into
several groups, which include but are not limited to penicillins, cephalosporins, aminoglycosides, sulfonamides, tetracyclines, monobactam, erythromycins, and quinolones. These products inhibit the growth and replication of susceptible bacterial organisms.

USES: Antiinfectives are used for infections
of susceptible organisms. These products are effective against bacterial, rickettsial, and spirochete infections.

CONTRAINDICATIONS:
Hypersensitive reactions may occur, and allergies should be identified before these products are given. Cross-sensitivity can occur between products of different classes (penicillins or cephalosporins). Often persons allergic to penicillins are also allergic to cephalosporins.

Precautions: Antiinfectives should be used with caution in persons with renal/hepatic disease.

IMPLEMENTATION
• Give for 10-14 days to ensure organism death, prevention of superinfection
• Give after C&S completed; product may be taken as soon as culture is obtained

---

ADVERSE EFFECTS: The most common side effects are nausea, vomiting, and diarrhea. Adverse reactions include bone marrow depression and anaphylaxis.

PHARMACOKINETICS: Onset, peak, and duration vary widely among products. Most products are metabolized in the liver. Metabolites are excreted in urine, bile, and feces.

INTERACTIONS: Interactions vary widely among products. Check individual monographs for specific information.

NURSING CONSIDERATIONS
Assessment
• Assess for nephrotoxicity: increased BUN, creatinine
• Monitor blood tests: AST, ALT, CBC, Hct, bilirubin; test monthly if patient is on long-term therapy
• Monitor bowel pattern daily; if severe diarrhea occurs, product should be discontinued
• Monitor urine output; if decreasing, notify prescriber; may indicate nephrotoxicity
• Assess for allergic reaction: rash, fever, pruritus, urticaria; product should be discontinued
• Assess for bleeding: ecchymosis, bleeding gums, hematuria, stool guaiac daily
• Assess for overgrowth of infection: perineal itching, fever, malaise, redness, pain, swelling, drainage, rash, diarrhea, change in cough, sputum

Patient/family education
• Teach patient to comply with dosage schedule, even if feeling better
• Advise patient to report sore throat, bruising, bleeding, joint pain; may indicate blood dyscrasias (rare)

Evaluation
Positive therapeutic outcome
• Absence of fever, fatigue, malaise, draining wounds

Generic Names
Aminoglycosides:
amikacin, azithromycin, clarithromycin, gentamicin, neomycin, streptomycin, tobramycin

Cephalosporins:
cefaclor, cefadroxil, ceFAZolin, cefdinir, cefditoren, cefepime, cefixime, cefotaxime, cefprozil, ceftibuten, cefuroxime, cephalexin, cephradine

Fluoroquinolones:
ciprofloxacin, gemifloxacin, levofloxacin, norfloxacin, ofloxacin

Ketolides:
telithromycin

Miscellaneous:
adefovir, dalbavancin, daptomycin, doripenem, ertapenem, fidaxomicin, meropenem, oritavancin, peginterferon alfa-2a, telavancin, vancomycin

Penicillins:
amoxicillin/clavulanate, ampicillin/sulbactam, imipenem/cilastatin, nafcillin, penicillin G benzathine, penicillin G, penicillin G procaine, penicillin V, piperacillin/tazobactam, ticarcillin, ticarcillin/clavulanate

Sulfonamides:
sulfaSALAzine

Tetracyclines:
doxycycline, minocycline, tetracycline

Antilipidemics

ACTION: Antilipidemics are divided into three categories or subclassifications; HMG-CoA reductase inhibitors (statins), bile acid sequestrants, and miscellaneous products. The HMG-CoA reductase inhibitors work by reduction of an enzyme that is responsible for the beginning step in cholesterol production. Bile acid sequestrants work by binding cholesterol in the GI system. The miscellaneous products work by various actions.

USES: Primary hypercholesterolemia in individuals as an adjunct with other lifestyle changes.

CONTRAINDICATIONS: Persons breastfeeding (some products) or those with hypersensitivity to any product or severe hepatic disease should not take these products. Antilipidemics are identified as pregnancy category **X** on some products.

Precautions: Some products are identified as pregnancy category **C.**

IMPLEMENTATION
• Give as directed by health care provider; times will vary with medication used
• Provide protection from sunlight and heat

ADVERSE EFFECTS: The most common side effects are headache, dizziness, fatigue, insomnia, peripheral edema, dysrhythmias, sinusitis, pharyngitis, abdominal pain, diarrhea, constipation, flatulence, and back pain.

PHARMACOKINETICS: Pharmacokinetics and pharmacodynamics vary with each product.

INTERACTIONS: Interactions vary widely among products. Check individual monographs for specific information.

NURSING CONSIDERATIONS

Assessment
• Obtain a diet and lifestyle history, including exercise, smoking, alcohol, and stress-related activities

Patient/family education
• Teach patient all aspects of medication use
• Instruct patient to combine medication with lifestyle changes, including low-cholesterol diet, decreasing LDL in diet; avoid smoking, alcohol, and sedentary daily routine

Evaluation
Positive therapeutic outcome
• Decrease in triglycerides and LDL cholesterol levels

Generic Names

HMG-CoA reductase inhibitors:
atorvastatin, fluvastatin, lovastatin, pitavastatin, pravastatin, simvastatin

Bile acid sequestrants:
cholestyramine, colesevelam

Miscellaneous:
ezetimibe, fenofibrate, fenofibric acid, gemfibrozil, mipomersen, niacin, niacinamide

Antineoplastics

ACTION: Antineoplastics are divided into alkylating agents, antimetabolites, antibiotic agents, hormonal agents, and miscellaneous agents. Alkylating agents act by cross-linking strands of DNA. Antimetabolites act by inhibiting DNA synthesis. Antibiotic agents act by inhibiting RNA synthesis and by delaying or inhibiting mitosis. Hormones alter the effect of androgens, luteinizing hormone, follicle-stimulating hormone, or estrogen by changing the hormonal environment.

USES: Antineoplastics vary widely among products and classes of products. They are used to treat leukemia, Hodgkin's disease, lymphomas, and other tumors throughout the body.

CONTRAINDICATIONS: Hypersensitive reactions may occur, and allergies should be identified before these products are given. Also, persons with severe renal/hepatic disease should not use these products unless the benefits outweigh the risks.

Precautions: Persons with bleeding, severe bone marrow depression, or renal/hepatic disease should be watched closely.

IMPLEMENTATION
• Check **IV** site for irritation; phlebitis
• Have epINEPHrine available for hypersensitivity reaction
• Give antibiotics for prophylaxis of infection
• Provide strict medical asepsis, protective isolation if WBC levels are low
• Provide comprehensive oral hygiene, using careful technique and soft-bristle brush

ADVERSE EFFECTS: Most products cause thrombocytopenia, leukopenia, and anemia. If these reactions occur, the product may need to be stopped until the problem is corrected. Other side effects include nausea, vomiting, glossitis, and hair loss. Some products also cause hepatotoxicity, nephrotoxicity, and cardiotoxicity.

PHARMACOKINETICS: Onset, peak, and duration vary widely among products. Most products cross the placenta and are excreted in breast milk and in urine.

INTERACTIONS: Toxicity may occur when used with other antineoplastics or radiation.

NURSING CONSIDERATIONS

Assessment
• Monitor CBC, differential, platelet count weekly; withhold product if WBC is <4000 or platelet count is <75,000; notify prescriber of results
• Monitor renal function tests: BUN, creatinine, serum uric acid, and urine creatinine clearance before, during therapy
• Monitor I&O ratio; report fall in urine output of 30 ml/hr
• Monitor temp q4hr (may indicate beginning infection)

• Monitor hepatic function tests before, during therapy (bilirubin, AST, ALT, LDH) monthly or as needed
• Assess for bleeding, including hematuria, guaiac, bruising or petechiae, mucosa, or orifices q8hr; obtain prescription for viscous lidocaine (Xylocaine)
• Identify jaundice of skin, sclera, dark urine, clay-colored stools, itchy skin, abdominal pain, fever, diarrhea
• Assess for edema in feet, joint pain, stomach pain, shaking
• Assess for inflammation of mucosa, breaks in skin

Patient/family education
• Advise patient to report signs of infection, including increased temp, sore throat, malaise
• Instruct patient to report signs of anemia, including fatigue, headache, faintness, shortness of breath, irritability
• Instruct patient to report bleeding and to avoid use of razors and commercial mouthwash

Evaluation
Positive therapeutic outcome
• Decreased tumor size

Generic Names
Alkylating agents:
bendamustine, **busulfan** (high alert), **CARBOplatin** (high alert), **carmustine** (high alert), chlorambucil, **CISplatin** (high alert), **cyclophosphamide** (high alert), **dacarbazine** (high alert), **melphalan** (high alert), oxaliplatin

Antimetabolites:
capecitabine, **cytarabine** (high alert), decitabine, **etoposide** (high alert), **fluorouracil** (high alert), mercaptopurine, **methotrexate** (high alert), PEMEtrexed

Antibiotic agents:
bleomycin (high alert), **DACTINomycin** (high alert), **DAUNOrubicin** (high alert), **DOXOrubicin** (high alert), **mitoMYcin** (high alert), **mitoXANtrone** (high alert)

Hormonal agents:
flutamide, fulvestrant, goserelin, **irinotecan** (high alert), **leuprolide** (high alert), megestrol, tamoxifen, **topotecan** (high alert)

Miscellaneous agents:
ado-trastuzumab, afatinib, alemtuzumab, anastrozole, azacitidine, belinostat, bortezomib, brentuximab, cabazitaxel, cetuximab, crizotinib, dabrafenib, dasatinib, eribulin, erlotinib, gemcitabine, ibritumomab, ibrutinib, idelalisib, imatinib, interferon alfa-2a, interferon alfa-2b, ipilimumab, irinotecan, ixabepilone, lapatinib, nilotinib, olaparib, palbociclib, panitumumab, pembrolizumab, pomalidomide, procarbazine, ranibizumab, riTUXimab, sipuleucel-T, trametinib, vemurafenib, **vinBLAStine** (high alert), **vinCRIStine** (high alert), **vinorelbine** (high alert)

Antiparkinsonian Agents

ACTION: Antiparkinsonian agents are divided into cholinergics, dopamine agonists, and monoamine oxidase type B inhibitors. Cholinergics work by blocking or competing at central acetylcholine receptors. Dopamine agonists work by decarboxylation to dopamine or by activation of dopamine receptors. Monoamine oxidase type B inhibitors increase dopamine activity by inhibiting MAO type B activity.

USES: Antiparkinson agents are used alone or in combination for patients with Parkinson's disease.

CONTRAINDICATIONS:
Persons with hypersensitivity, closed-angle glaucoma, and undiagnosed skin lesions should not use these products.

Precautions: Antiparkinsonian agents should be used with caution in pregnancy, breastfeeding, children, renal/cardiac/hepatic disease, and affective disorder.

IMPLEMENTATION
• Give product up until NPO before surgery
• Adjust dosage depending on patient response
• Give with meals; limit protein taken with product
• Give only after MAOIs have been discontinued for 2 wk
• Assist with ambulation during beginning therapy if needed
• Test for diabetes mellitus and acromegaly if on long-term therapy

ADVERSE EFFECTS: Side effects and adverse reactions vary widely among products. The most common side effects include involuntary movements, headache, numbness, insomnia, nightmares, nausea, vomiting, dry mouth, and orthostatic hypotension.

PHARMACOKINETICS: Onset, peak, and duration vary widely among products. Most products are metabolized in the liver and excreted in urine.

INTERACTIONS: Interactions vary widely among products. Check individual monographs for specific information.

NURSING CONSIDERATIONS
Assessment
• Monitor B/P, respiration
• Assess mental status: affect, behavioral changes, depression, complete suicide assessment

Patient/family education
• Advise patient to change positions slowly to prevent orthostatic hypotension
• Instruct patient to report side effects: twitching, eye spasm; indicate overdose
• Advise patient to use product exactly as prescribed; if product is discontinued abruptly, parkinsonian crisis may occur

Evaluation
Positive therapeutic outcome
• Decrease in akathisia
• Improvement in mood

Generic Names
amantadine, benztropine, bromocriptine, carbidopa-levodopa, pramipexole, rasagiline, selegiline, tolcapone

Antiplatelets

ACTION: The antiplatelets are divided into the platelet aggregation inhibitors, platelet adhesion inhibitors, and the glycoprotein IIb, IIIa inhibitors. The platelet aggregation inhibitors work by action on thrombin; the platelet adhesion inhibitors work by inhibition of phosphodiesterase; and the glycoprotein IIb, IIIa inhibitors work by preventing fibrin from binding to glycoprotein IIb, IIIa receptors.

USES: Antiplatelets are used to prevent myocardial infarction and stroke; other products are used for coronary syndromes.

CONTRAINDICATIONS:
Persons developing hypersensitive reactions should not use these products.

Precautions: Antiplatelets should be used cautiously in pregnancy, breastfeeding, and bleeding disorders.

IMPLEMENTATION
• Give with heparin or other aspirin (some products)
• Store at room temperature vial/ampules, oral products

ADVERSE EFFECTS: The most common side effects are headache, dizziness, bleeding, and diarrhea.

PHARMACOKINETICS: Onset, peak, and duration vary widely among products. Most products are metabolized by the liver and excreted by the kidneys.

INTERACTIONS: Interactions vary widely among products. Check individual monographs for specific information.

NURSING CONSIDERATIONS
Assessment
• Assess reason for use of these products
• Monitor hypersensitivity reactions with some products
• Monitor bleeding from orifices, stool urine
• Monitor blood tests: platelets, Hgb, Hct, PT/APTT, and INR

Patient/family education
• Caution patient to avoid hazardous activities if drowsiness, dizziness occurs; ask for assistance if hospitalized
• Teach patient all aspects of product usage

Evaluation
Positive therapeutic outcome
• Absence of MI, stroke, or other coronary syndromes

Generic Names
Platelet aggregation inhibitors:
cilostazol, clopidogrel, ticagrelol, ticlopidine

Platelet adhesion inhibitors:
dipyridamole

Glycoprotein IIb, IIIa inhibitors:
eptifibatide (high alert), **tirofiban** (high alert)

Antipsychotics

ACTION: Antipsychotics/neuroleptics are divided into several subgroups: phenothiazines, thioxanthenes, butyrophenones, dibenzoxazepines, dibenzodiazepines, and indolones and other heterocyclic compounds. Although chemically different, these subgroups share many pharmacologic and clinical properties. All antipsychotics work to block postsynaptic DOPamine receptors in the brain that are responsible for psychotic behavior, including hallucinations, delusions, and paranoia.

USES: Antipsychotic behavior is decreased in conditions such as schizophrenia, paranoia, and mania. These agents are also effective for severe anxiety, intractable hiccups, nausea, vomiting, behavioral problems in children, and for relaxation before surgery.

CONTRAINDICATIONS:

Persons with liver damage, severe hypertension or coronary disease, cerebral arteriosclerosis, blood dyscrasias, bone marrow depression, parkinsonism, severe depression, or closed-angle glaucoma; children <12 yr; persons withdrawing from alcohol or barbiturates should not use antipsychotics until these conditions are corrected.

Precautions: Caution must be used when antipsychotics are given to geriatric patients, since metabolism is slowed and adverse reactions can occur rapidly. Renal/hepatic disease may cause poor metabolism and excretion of the product. Seizure threshold is decreased with these products; increases in the dose of anticonvulsants may be required. Persons with diabetes mellitus, prostatic hypertrophy, chronic respiratory disease, and peptic ulcer disease should be monitored closely.

IMPLEMENTATION

• Give antiparkinsonian agent if extrapyramidal symptoms occur
• Administer liquid conc mixed in glass of juice or cola since taste is unpleasant; avoid contact with skin when preparing liquid conc or parenteral medications
• Supervise ambulation until stabilized on medication; do not involve in strenuous exercise program, since fainting is possible; patient should not stand still for long periods
• Increase fluids to prevent constipation
• Give sips of water, candy, gum for dry mouth
• Patient should remain lying down for at least 30 min after IM inj

ADVERSE EFFECTS: The most common side effects include extrapyramidal symptoms such as pseudoparkinsonism, akathisia, dystonia, and tardive dyskinesia, which may be controlled by use of antiparkinsonian agents.

Serious adverse reactions such as hypotension, agranulocytosis, cardiac arrest, and laryngospasm have occurred. Other common side effects include dry mouth and photosensitivity.

PHARMACOKINETICS: Onset, peak, and duration vary widely with different products and routes. Products are metabolized by the liver, are excreted in urine as metabolites, are highly bound to plasma proteins, cross the placenta, and enter breast milk. Half-life can be extended over 3 days.

INTERACTIONS: Because other CNS depressants can cause oversedation, these combinations should be used carefully. Anticholinergics may decrease the therapeutic actions of phenothiazines and also cause increased anticholinergic effects.

NURSING CONSIDERATIONS
Assessment
• Monitor bilirubin, CBC, hepatic function tests monthly, since these products are metabolized in the liver and excreted in urine
• Monitor I&O ratio: palpate bladder if low urinary output occurs, since urinary retention occurs with many of these products
• Assess affect, orientation, LOC, reflexes, gait, coordination, sleep pattern disturbances
• Assess dizziness, faintness, palpitations, tachycardia on rising
• Check B/P with patient lying and standing; wide fluctuations between lying and standing B/P may require dosage or product change, since orthostatic hypotension is occurring
• Assess for EPS, including akathisia, tardive dyskinesia, pseudoparkinsonism

Patient/family education
• Advise patient to rise from sitting or lying position gradually, since fainting may occur
• Caution patient to avoid hot tubs, hot showers, or tub baths, since hypotension may occur
• Advise patient to wear sunscreen or protective clothing to prevent burns
• Advise patient to take extra precautions during hot weather to stay cool; heat stroke can occur
• Caution patient to avoid driving and other activities requiring alertness until response to medication is known
• Inform patient that drowsiness or impaired mental/motor activity is evident the first 2 wk, but tends to decrease over time

Evaluation
Positive therapeutic outcome
- Decrease in excitement, hallucinations, delusions, paranoia
- Reorganization of thought patterns, speech

Generic Names
Phenothiazines:
chlorproMAZINE, fluPHENAZine

Butyrophenone:
haloperidol

Miscellaneous:
ARIPiprazole, asenapine, iloperidone, loxapine, OLANZapine, paliperidone, QUEtiapine, risperiDONE, ziprasidone

Antipyretics

ACTION: The antipyretics act on the CNS to control fever and also inhibit prostaglandin production.

USES: Antipyretics are used to decrease fever.

CONTRAINDICATIONS:
Persons developing hypersensitive reactions should not use these products.

Precautions: Antipyretics should be used cautiously in pregnancy, breastfeeding, geriatric patients, hepatic disease, and those with certain GI disorders.

IMPLEMENTATION
- Give around the clock to keep fever reduced
- Store at room temperature

ADVERSE EFFECTS: The most common side effects are nausea, vomiting, and rash.

PHARMACOKINETICS: Onset, peak, and duration vary widely among products. Most products are metabolized by the liver and excreted by the kidneys.

INTERACTIONS: Interactions vary widely among products. Check individual monographs for specific information.

NURSING CONSIDERATIONS
Assessment
- Monitor temp frequently
- Assess reason for use and expected outcome

- Monitor hypersensitivity reactions: rash, bronchospasm with some products

Patient/family education
- Teach patient all aspects of product usage

Evaluation
Positive therapeutic outcome
- Absence or decreasing fever after use

Generic Names
acetaminophen, aspirin, choline/magnesium salicylates, ibuprofen, ketoprofen, magnesium salicylate, naproxen, salsalate

Antiretrovirals

ACTION: Antiretrovirals act by blocking DNA synthesis.

USES: Antiretrovirals are used in HIV infections, chronic hepatitis C to slow the progression of the disease.

CONTRAINDICATIONS:
Persons with hypersensitivity should not use these products.

Precautions: Antiretrovirals should be used cautiously in pregnancy, breastfeeding, and renal/hepatic disease. Protease inhibitors should be used cautiously in diabetes.

IMPLEMENTATION
- Give in equal intervals around the clock
- Store at room temperature

ADVERSE EFFECTS: The most common side effects are nausea, vomiting, anorexia, headache, and diarrhea. The most serious adverse reactions are nephrotoxicity and blood dyscrasias.

PHARMACOKINETICS: Onset, peak, and duration vary widely among products. Most products are metabolized by the liver and excreted by the kidneys.

INTERACTIONS: Interactions vary widely among products. Check individual monographs for specific information.

NURSING CONSIDERATIONS
Assessment
- Monitor for signs of HIV infection: increased CD4 counts, decreased viral load; signs of chronic hepatitis C

⚠ Nurse Alert   ✦ Key NCLEX® Drug

- Monitor patients with compromised renal system; since product is excreted slowly in poor renal system function, toxicity may occur rapidly

Patient/family education
- Instruct patient to report sore throat, fever, fatigue; may indicate superinfection
- Caution patient that product does not cure condition or prevent infecting others, but controls symptoms
- Instruct patient that product must be taken around the clock, in equal intervals to maintain blood levels for duration of therapy
- Instruct patient to notify prescriber of side effects such as bruising, bleeding, fatigue, malaise; may indicate blood dyscrasias

Evaluation
Positive therapeutic outcome
- Decreased viral load
- Increased CD4 count
- Improvement in the symptoms of HIV/AIDS

Generic Names
Nonnucleoside reverse transcriptase inhibitors:
delavirdine, efavirenz, etravirine, nevirapine, rilpivirine

Nucleoside reverse transcriptase inhibitors:
abacavir, didanosine, emtricitabine, lamiVUDine, stavudine d4t, tenofovir, zidovudine

Protease inhibitors:
atazanavir, boceprevir, fosamprenavir, indinavir, nelfinavir, ritonavir, saquinavir, telaprevir, tipranavir

Fusion inhibitors:
enfuvirtide

Miscellaneous:
dolutegravir, raltegravir

Antituberculars

ACTION: Antituberculars act by inhibiting RNA or DNA, or interfering with lipid and protein synthesis, thereby decreasing tubercle bacilli replication.

USES: Antituberculars are used for pulmonary tuberculosis.

CONTRAINDICATIONS:
Persons with severe renal disease or hypersensitivity should not use these products.

Precautions: Antituberculars should be used with caution in pregnancy, breastfeeding, and hepatic disease.

IMPLEMENTATION
- Give some of these agents on empty stomach, 1 hr before meals (only for isoniazid and rifampin) or 2hr after meals
- Give antiemetic if vomiting occurs
- Give after C&S is completed; monthly to detect resistance

ADVERSE EFFECTS: Adverse effects vary widely among products. Most products can cause nausea, vomiting, anorexia, and rash. Serious adverse reactions include renal failure, nephrotoxicity, ototoxicity, and hepatic necrosis.

PHARMACOKINETICS: Onset, peak, and duration vary widely among products. Most products are metabolized in the liver and excreted in urine.

INTERACTIONS: Interactions vary widely among products. Check individual monographs for specific information.

NURSING CONSIDERATIONS
Assessment
- Assess for signs of anemia: Hct, Hgb, fatigue
- Monitor hepatic function tests weekly: ALT, AST, bilirubin
- Monitor renal status before treatment and monthly thereafter: BUN, creatinine, output, specific gravity, urinalysis
- Monitor hepatic status: decreased appetite, jaundice, dark urine, fatigue

Patient/family education
- Teach patient that compliance with dosage schedule, duration is necessary
- Teach patient that scheduled appointments must be kept; relapse may occur
- Advise patient to avoid alcohol while taking product
- Advise patient to report flulike symptoms: excessive fatigue, anorexia, vomiting, sore throat; unusual bleeding, yellowish discoloration of skin/eyes

Evaluation
Positive therapeutic outcome
- Decreased symptoms of TB
- Negative culture

Adverse effects: *italics* = common; **bold** = life-threatening

Generic Names
ethambutol, isoniazid, pyrazinamide, rifabutin, rifampin, streptomycin

Antitussives/Expectorants

ACTION: Antitussives suppress the cough reflex by direct action on the cough center in the medulla. Expectorants act by liquefying and reducing the viscosity of thick, tenacious secretions.

USES: Antitussives/expectorants are used to treat cough occurring in pneumonia, bronchitis, TB, cystic fibrosis, and emphysema; as an adjunct in atelectasis (expectorants); and for nonproductive cough (antitussives).

CONTRAINDICATIONS:
Some products are contraindicated in pregnancy, breastfeeding, and hypothyroidism

Precautions: Some products should be used cautiously with asthma and in geriatric and debilitated patients.

IMPLEMENTATION
• Give decreased dosage to geriatric patients; their metabolism may be slowed
• Increase fluids to liquefy secretions
• Humidify patient's room

ADVERSE EFFECTS: The most common side effects are drowsiness, dizziness, and nausea.

PHARMACOKINETICS: Onset, peak, and duration vary widely among products. Some products are metabolized in the liver and excreted in urine.

INTERACTIONS: Interactions vary widely among products. Check individual monographs for specific information.

NURSING CONSIDERATIONS
Assessment
• Assess cough: type, frequency, character including sputum

Patient/family education
• Advise patient to avoid driving and other hazardous activities until stabilized on this medication
• Caution patient to avoid smoking, smoke-filled rooms, perfumes, dust, environmental pollutants, cleaners that increase cough

Evaluation
Positive therapeutic outcome
• Absence of cough

Generic Names
acetylcysteine, codeine, dextromethorphan, diphenhydrAMINE, guaiFENesin, HYDROcodone

Antivirals

ACTION: Antivirals act by interfering with DNA synthesis that is needed for viral replication.

USES: Antivirals are used for mucocutaneous herpes simplex virus, herpes genitalis (HSV-1, HSV-2), varicella infections, herpes zoster, and herpes simplex encephalitis.

CONTRAINDICATIONS:
Persons with hypersensitivity or immunosuppressed individuals should not use these products.

Precautions: Antivirals should be used cautiously in pregnancy, breastfeeding, and renal/hepatic disease.

IMPLEMENTATION
• Give increased fluids to 3 L/day to decrease crystalluria when given **IV**
• Store at room temperature for up to 12 hr after reconstitution

ADVERSE EFFECTS: The most common side effects are nausea, vomiting, anorexia, headache, and diarrhea. The most serious adverse reactions are nephrotoxicity and blood dyscrasias.

PHARMACOKINETICS: Onset, peak, and duration vary widely among products. Most products are metabolized by the liver and excreted by the kidneys.

INTERACTIONS: Interactions vary widely among products. Check individual monographs for specific information.

NURSING CONSIDERATIONS
Assessment
• Monitor for signs of infection, anemia
• Monitor patients with a compromised renal system; since product is excreted slowly in poor renal system function, toxicity may occur rapidly

---

⚠ Nurse Alert   ✴ Key NCLEX® Drug

• Monitor renal function tests: urinalysis, BUN, serum creatinine or decreased CCr may indicate nephrotoxicity; I&O ratio; report hematuria, oliguria, fatigue, weakness; check for protein in the urine during treatment
• Assess C&S before treatment; agent may be given as soon as culture is taken; repeat C&S after treatment
• Monitor bowel pattern before, during treatment; if severe abdominal pain with bleeding occurs, agent should be discontinued
• Monitor skin reactions: rash, urticaria, itching
• Monitor hepatic function tests: AST, ALT
• Monitor blood tests: WBC, RBC, Hct, Hgb, bleeding time; blood dyscrasias

Patient/family education

• Instruct patient to report sore throat, fever, fatigue; may indicate superinfection
• Caution patient that product does not prevent infecting others or cure condition but controls symptoms
• Instruct patient that product must be taken around the clock in equal intervals to maintain blood levels for duration of therapy
• Instruct patient to notify prescriber of side effects such as bruising, bleeding, fatigue, malaise; may indicate blood dyscrasias

Evaluation

Positive therapeutic outcome

• Absence or control of infection

Generic Names

acyclovir, amantadine, cidofovir, docosanol, entecavir, famciclovir, foscarnet, ganciclovir, lamiVUDine, maraviroc, oseltamivir, penciclovir, rapivab, ribavirin, simeprevir, sofosbuvir, valacyclovir, valganciclovir, zanamivir

β-Adrenergic Blockers

ACTION: β-Blockers are divided into selective and nonselective blockers. Selective β-blockers competitively block stimulation of β_1-receptors in cardiac smooth muscle; these products produce chronotropic and inotropic effects. Nonselective blockers produce a fall in blood pressure without reflex tachycardia or reduction in heart rate through a mixture of β-blocking effects; elevated plasma renins are reduced.

USES: β-Blockers are used for hypertension, ventricular dysrhythmias, and prophylaxis of angina pectoris.

CONTRAINDICATIONS:

Hypersensitive reactions may occur, and allergies should be identified before these products are given. β-Adrenergic blockers should not be used in heart block, CHF, or cardiogenic shock.

Precautions: β-Blockers should be used with caution in pregnant and geriatric patients or in renal/thyroid disease, COPD, CAD, diabetes mellitus, and asthma.

IMPLEMENTATION

• Give PO before meals and at bedtime; tab may be crushed or swallowed whole
• Give reduced dosage in renal dysfunction

ADVERSE EFFECTS: The most common side effects are orthostatic hypotension, bradycardia, diarrhea, nausea, and vomiting. Serious adverse reactions include blood dyscrasias, bronchospasm, and CHF.

PHARMACOKINETICS: Onset, peak, and duration vary widely among products. Most products are metabolized in the liver, with metabolites excreted in urine, bile, and feces.

INTERACTIONS: Interactions vary widely among products. Check individual monographs for specific information.

NURSING CONSIDERATIONS

Assessment

• Monitor renal function tests: protein, BUN, creatinine; watch for increased levels that may indicate nephrotic syndrome; obtain baselines in renal/hepatic function tests before beginning treatment
• Monitor I&O ratio, weight daily
• Monitor B/P during beginning of treatment and periodically thereafter, pulse q4hr; note rate, rhythm, quality
• Monitor apical/radial pulse before administration; notify prescriber of significant changes
• Check for edema in feet and legs daily

Patient/family education

• Instruct patient to comply with dosage schedule, even if feeling better
• Caution patient to rise slowly to sitting or standing position to minimize orthostatic hypotension
• Advise patient to report bradycardia, dizziness, confusion, depression, fever
• Teach patient to take pulse at home; advise when to notify prescriber

- Instruct patient to comply with weight control, dietary adjustment, modified exercise program
- Advise patient to wear support hose to minimize effects of orthostatic hypotension
- Advise patient not to discontinue product abruptly; taper over 2 wk; may precipitate angina

Evaluation
Positive therapeutic outcome
- Decrease in B/P in hypertension
- Decreased B/P, edema, moist crackles inCHF

Generic Names

Selective β1-receptor blockers:
acebutolol, atenolol, esmolol, metoprolol, nebibolol

β2-receptor blocker:
indacaterol

Nonselective β1 and β2-blockers:
carteolol, nadolol, propranolol, timolol

Combined α1, β1, and β2-receptor blocker:
labetalol

Bone Resorption Inhibitors

ACTION: Bone resorption inhibitors are divided into the biphosphonates and the selective estrogen receptor modulators. The biphosphonates act by absorbing calcium phosphate crystals in bone and may directly block dissolution of hydroxyapatite crystals of bone, inhibiting normal and abnormal bone resorption and mineralization. Selective estrogen receptor modulators act by reducing resorption of bone and decreasing bone turnover, mediated through estrogen receptor binding.

USES: Bone resorption inhibitors are used for prevention and treatment of osteoporosis in postmenopausal women, treatment of Paget's disease, and treatment of osteoporosis in men.

CONTRAINDICATIONS:
Persons developing hypersensitive reactions or those with hypocalcemia should not use these products.

Precautions: Bone resorption inhibitors should be used cautiously in pregnancy, breastfeeding, the geriatric patient, renal/hepatic disease, and some GI disorders.

IMPLEMENTATION
- Give for 6 months or more in Paget's disease
- Store at room temperature

ADVERSE EFFECTS: The most common side effects are nausea, vomiting, headache, bone pain, and rash.

PHARMACOKINETICS: Onset, peak, and duration vary widely among products. Most products are taken up by the bones and excreted by the kidneys.

INTERACTIONS: Interactions vary widely among products. Check individual monographs for specific information.

NURSING CONSIDERATIONS
Assessment
- Assess reason for use and expected outcome
- Monitor bone density test; hormonal status (women) before starting treatment and thereafter
- Monitor hypercalcemia: paresthesia, twitching, laryngospasm; Chvostek's, Trousseau's signs

Patient/family education
- Instruct patient to remain upright for at least 30 min after taking to prevent esophageal irritation
- Teach patient all aspects of product usage
- Instruct patient to use weight-bearing exercise to increase bone density

Evaluation
Positive therapeutic outcome
- Increase in bone mass
- Absence of fractures

Generic Names

Bisphosphonates:
alendronate, etidronate, ibandronate, pamidronate, risedronate

Selective estrogen receptor modulator:
raloxifene

Monoclonal antibody:
denosumab

Calcium Channel Blockers

ACTION: Calcium channel blockers inhibit calcium ion influx across the cell membrane in cardiac and vascular smooth muscle. This action produces relaxation of coronary vascular smooth muscle, dilates coronary arteries, slows

---

SA/AV node conduction, and dilates peripheral arteries.

USES: Calcium channel blockers are used for chronic stable angina pectoris, vasospastic angina, dysrhythmias, hypertension, and unstable angina.

CONTRAINDICATIONS:
Persons with 2nd- or 3rd-degree heart block, sick sinus syndrome, hypotension of <90 mm Hg systolic, Wolff-Parkinson-White syndrome, or cardiogenic shock should not use these products, since worsening of those conditions may occur.

Precautions: CHF may worsen since edema may be increased. Hypotension may worsen, since B/P is decreased. Patients with renal/hepatic disease should use these products cautiously since they are metabolized in the liver and excreted by the kidneys.

IMPLEMENTATION
• Give PO before meals and at bedtime

ADVERSE EFFECTS: The most common side effects are dysrhythmias and edema. Also common are headache, fatigue, drowsiness, and flushing.

PHARMACOKINETICS: Onset, peak, and duration vary widely with route of administration. Products are metabolized by the liver and excreted in the urine primarily as metabolites.

INTERACTIONS: Increased levels of digoxin and theophylline may occur when used with these products. Increased effects of β-blockers and antihypertensives may occur with calcium channel blockers.

NURSING CONSIDERATIONS
Assessment
• Monitor cardiac system: B/P, pulse, respirations, ECG intervals (PR, QRS, QT)

Patient/family education
• Teach patient how to take pulse before taking product; patient should record or graph pulses to identify changes
• Advise patient to avoid hazardous activities until stabilized on this product since dizziness occurs frequently
• Inform patient of the need for compliance to all areas of medical regimen, including diet, exercise, stress reduction, and product therapy

Evaluation
Positive therapeutic outcome
• Decreased anginal pain
• Decreased B/P, dysrhythmias

Generic Names
amLODIPine, clevidipine, **diltiazem** (high alert), felodipine, isradipine, niCARdipine, NIFEdipine, verapamil

Cardiac Glycosides

ACTION: Cardiac glycosides act by inhibiting sodium and potassium ATPase and then making more calcium available to activate contracted proteins. Cardiac contractility and cardiac output are increased.

USES: Cardiac glycosides are used for CHF, atrial fibrillation, atrial flutter, atrial tachycardia, and rapid digitalization in these disorders.

CONTRAINDICATIONS:
Hypersensitive reactions may occur, and allergies should be identified before these products are given. Also, persons with ventricular tachycardia, ventricular fibrillation, and carotid sinus syndrome should not use these products.

Precautions: Persons with acute MI and those who have or may develop serum potassium, calcium, or magnesium imbalances should use these products cautiously. Also, geriatric patients and those with AV block, severe respiratory disease, hypothyroidism, or renal/hepatic disease should exercise caution when these products are prescribed.

IMPLEMENTATION
• Give potassium supplements if ordered for potassium levels <3

ADVERSE EFFECTS: The most common side effects are cardiac disturbances, headache, hypotension, and GI symptoms. Also common are blurred vision and yellow-green halos.

PHARMACOKINETICS: Onset, peak, and duration vary widely with the route of administration. Digitoxin is inactivated by the liver, and inactive metabolites are excreted in urine. Digoxin is excreted in urine mainly as the parent product and metabolites.

INTERACTIONS: Toxicity may occur when used with diuretics, succinylcholine, quinidine, and thioamines. Increased blood levels may occur with propantheline bromide, spironolactone, quinidine, verapamil, amino-glycosides (PO), amiodarone, anticholinergics, and quinine. Diuretics may increase toxicity.

NURSING CONSIDERATIONS
Assessment
• Montior cardiac system: B/P, pulse, respirations, and increased urine output
• Monitor apical pulse for 1 min before giving product; if pulse <60, take again in 1 hr; if <60 notify prescriber
• Monitor electrolytes: potassium, sodium, chloride, calcium, magnesium; renal function tests, including BUN and creatinine; and blood tests, including AST, ALT, bilirubin
• Monitor I&O ratio, daily weights
• Monitor therapeutic product levels

Patient/family education
• Teach patient how to take pulse before taking product; patient should record or graph pulse to identify changes
• Advise patient to avoid hazardous activities until stabilized on this product since dizziness occurs frequently
• Inform patient of the need for compliance to all areas of medical regimen, including diet, exercise, stress reduction, product therapy

Evaluation
Positive therapeutic outcome
• Decreased weight, edema, pulse, respiration
• Increased urine output

Generic Names
digoxin (high alert)

Cholinergics

ACTION: Cholinergics act by preventing destruction of acetylcholine, which increases concentration at sites where acetylcholine is released. This exaggerates the effects of acetylcholine and facilitates transmission of impulses across the myoneural junction. Cholinergics may also act by stimulating receptors for acetylcholine.

USES: Cholinergics are used for myasthenia gravis, as antagonists of nondepolarizing neuromuscular blockade, postoperative bladder distention and urinary distention, postoperative ileus.

CONTRAINDICATIONS: Persons with obstruction of the intestine or renal system should not use these products.

Precautions: Caution should be used in patients with bradycardia, hypotension, seizure disorders, bronchial asthma, coronary occlusion, and hyperthyroidism, and in breastfeeding and children.

IMPLEMENTATION
• Give only with atropine sulfate available for cholinergic crisis
• Give only after all other cholinergics have been discontinued
• Give increased dosages if tolerance occurs
• Give larger doses after exercise or fatigue
• Give on empty stomach for better absorption
• Store at room temperature

ADVERSE EFFECTS: The most serious adverse reactions are respiratory depression, bronchospasm, constriction, laryngospasm, respiratory arrest, convulsions, and paralysis. The most common side effects are nausea, diarrhea, and vomiting.

PHARMACOKINETICS: Onset, peak, and duration vary widely among products. Most products are metabolized in the liver and excreted in urine.

INTERACTIONS: Interactions vary widely among products. Check individual monographs for specific information.

NURSING CONSIDERATIONS
Assessment
• Monitor VS, respiration q8hr
• Monitor I&O ratio; check for urinary retention or incontinence
• Assess for bradycardia, hypotension, bronchospasm, headache, dizziness, seizures, respiratory depression; product should be discontinued if toxicity occurs

Patient/family education
• Inform patient that product is not a cure; it only relieves symptoms (myasthenia gravis)
• Advise patient to carry/wear emergency ID specifying myasthenia gravis, products taken

Evaluation
Positive therapeutic outcome
• Increased muscle strength, hand grasp
• Improved muscle gait
• Absence of labored breathing (if severe)

Generic Names
bethanechol, physostigmine, pyridostigmine

Cholinergic Blockers

ACTION: Cholinergic blockers inhibit or block acetylcholine at receptor sites in the autonomic nervous system.

USES: Many cholinergic blockers are used to decrease secretions before surgery, to reverse neuromuscular blockade, and to decrease motility of the GI, biliary, and urinary tracts. Other products are used for parkinsonian symptoms, including dystonia associated with neuroleptic products.

CONTRAINDICATIONS:
Hypersensitivity can occur, and allergies should be identified before administering these products. Persons with GI and GU obstruction should not use these products, since constipation and urinary retention may occur. They are also contraindicated in closed-angle glaucoma and myasthenia gravis.

Precautions: Caution must be used when these products are given to the geriatric patient, since metabolism is slowed. Also, persons with tachycardia or prostatic hypertrophy should use these products with caution.

IMPLEMENTATION
• Give with food or milk to decrease GI symptoms
• Give parenteral dose with patient recumbent to prevent postural hypotension; give dose slowly, monitoring VS
• Give hard candy, gum, frequent rinsing of mouth for dryness

ADVERSE EFFECTS: The most
common side effects are dryness of the mouth and constipation, which can be prevented by frequent rinsing of the mouth and increasing water and bulk in the diet.

PHARMACOKINETICS: Onset, peak, and duration vary with route.

INTERACTIONS: Increase in anticholinergic effect occurs when used with opioids, barbiturates, antihistamines, MAOIs, phenothiazines, amantadine.

NURSING CONSIDERATIONS
Assessment
• Assess I&O ratio; be alert for urinary retention, frequency, dysuria; product should be discontinued if these occur
• Assess urinary hesitancy, retention; palpate bladder if retention occurs
• Assess constipation; increase fluids, bulk, exercise
• Assess for tolerance over long-term therapy; dosage may need to be changed
• Assess mental status: affect, mood, CNS depression, worsening of mental symptoms during early therapy

Patient/family education
• Caution patient to avoid driving and other hazardous activities if drowsiness occurs
• Advise patient to avoid concurrent use of cough, cold preparations with alcohol, antihistamines unless directed by prescriber
• Caution patient to use with caution in hot weather, since medication may increase susceptibility to heat stroke

Evaluation
Positive therapeutic outcome
• Absence of cramps
• Absence of EPS

Generic Names
atropine (high alert), benztropine, glycopyrrolate, scopolamine

Corticosteroids

ACTION: Corticosteroids are divided into glucocorticoids and mineralocorticoids. Glucocorticoids decrease inflammation by the suppression of migration of polymorphonuclear leukocytes, fibroblasts, increased capillary permeability, and lysosomal stabilization. They also have varied metabolic effects and modify the body's immune responses to many different stimuli. Mineralocorticoids act by increasing resorption of sodium by increasing hydrogen and potassium excretion in the distal tubule.

USES: Glucocorticoids are used to decrease inflammation and for immunosuppression. In addition, some products may be given for allergy, adrenal insufficiency, or cerebral edema. Mineralocorticoids are given for adrenal insufficiency or adrenogenital syndrome.

CONTRAINDICATIONS:

Hypersensitivity may occur and should be identified before administering. Since these products mask infection, they should not be used in systemic fungal infections or amebiasis. Mothers taking pharmacologic doses of corticosteroids should not breastfeed.

Precautions: Caution must be used when these products are prescribed for diabetic patients since hyperglycemia may occur. Also, patients with glaucoma, seizure disorders, peptic ulcer, impaired renal function, CHF, hypertension, ulcerative colitis, or myasthenia gravis should be monitored closely if corticosteroids are given. Use with caution during pregnancy, in children, and in the geriatric patient.

IMPLEMENTATION

• Give with food or milk to decrease GI symptoms
• Give single daily or alternate-day doses in the morning before 9 AM (for replacement therapy)

ADVERSE EFFECTS:

The most common side effects include change in behavior, including insomnia and euphoria; GI irritation, including peptic ulcer; metabolic reactions, including hypokalemia, hyperglycemia, and carbohydrate intolerance; and sodium and fluid retention. Most adverse reactions are dose dependent.

PHARMACOKINETICS:

For oral preparations the onset of action occurs between 1-2 hr, and duration can be up to 2 days, with a half-life of 2-4 days. Pharmacokinetics vary widely among products. These products cross the placenta and appear in breast milk.

INTERACTIONS:

Decreased corticosteroid effect may occur with barbiturates, rifampin, and phenytoin; corticosteroid dosage may need to be increased. There is a possibility of GI bleeding when used with salicylates and indomethacin. Steroids may reduce salicylate levels. When using with digoxin, glycosides, potassium-depleting diuretics, and amphotericin, serum potassium levels should be monitored.

NURSING CONSIDERATIONS

Assessment

• Monitor potassium, blood glucose, urine glucose while on long-term therapy; hypokalemia and hyperglycemia are common

• Monitor weight daily; notify prescriber if weekly gain of >5 lb since these products alter fluid and electrolyte balance
• Assess for potassium depletion: paresthesias, fatigue, nausea, vomiting, depression, polyuria, dysrhythmias, weakness
• Assess for mental status: affect, mood, behavioral changes, aggression; if severe personality changes occur, including depression, product may need to be tapered and then discontinued
• Monitor I&O ratio; be alert for decreasing urinary output and increasing edema
• Monitor plasma cortisol levels during long-term therapy (normal level is 138-635 nmol/L when drawn at 8 AM)
• Assess for infection: increased temp, WBC, even after withdrawal of medication; product masks symptoms of infection
• Assess for adrenal insufficiency: nausea, anorexia, fatigue, dizziness, dyspnea, weakness, joint pain

Patient/family education

• Advise patient that emergency ID as steroid user should be carried/worn
• Advise patient not to discontinue this medication abruptly; adrenal crisis can result
• Teach patient all aspects of product use, including cushingoid symptoms
• Instruct patient to take with meals or a snack
• Teach patient to avoid exposure to chickenpox or measles if taking immunosuppressives

Evaluation

Positive therapeutic outcome
• Decreased inflammation

Generic Names

Glucocorticoids:
beclomethasone, betamethasone, cortisone, dexamethasone, hydrocortisone, hydrocortisone sodium succinate, methylPREDNISolone, predniSOLONE, predniSONE, triamcinolone

Diuretics

ACTION:

Diuretics are divided into subgroups: thiazides and thiazide-like diuretics, loop diuretics, carbonic anhydrase inhibitors, osmotic diuretics, and potassium-sparing diuretics. Each one of these subgroups differs in its mechanism of action. Thiazides and thiazide-like diuretics increase excretion of water and sodium by inhibiting resorption in the early distal tubule. Loop diuretics inhibit resorption of sodium and chloride in the thick ascending limb

---

of the loop of Henle. Carbonic anhydrase inhibitors increase sodium excretion by decreasing sodium-hydrogen ion exchange throughout the renal tubule. Carbonic anhydrase inhibitors also decrease secretion of aqueous humor in the eye and thus decrease intraocular pressure. Osmotic diuretics increase the osmotic pressure of glomerular filtrate, thus decreasing net absorption of sodium. The potassium-sparing diuretics interfere with sodium resorption at the distal tubule, thus decreasing potassium excretion.

USES: Blood pressure is reduced in hypertension; edema is reduced in CHF; intraocular pressure is decreased in glaucoma.

CONTRAINDICATIONS:
Persons with electrolyte imbalances (sodium, chloride, potassium), dehydration, or anuria should not be given these products until the problem is corrected.

Precautions: Caution must be used when diuretics are given to the geriatric patient, since electrolyte disturbances and dehydration can occur rapidly. Renal/hepatic disorders may cause poor metabolism and excretion of the product.

IMPLEMENTATION
• Give in AM to avoid interference with sleep if using product as a diuretic
• Give potassium replacement if potassium is less than 3 mg/dl

ADVERSE EFFECTS: Hypokalemia, hyperuricemia, and hyperglycemia occur most frequently with thiazide diuretics. Aplastic anemia, blood dyscrasias, volume depletion, and dehydration may occur when thiazide-like diuretics, loop diuretics, or carbonic anhydrase inhibitors are given. Side effects and adverse reactions vary widely for the miscellaneous products.

PHARMACOKINETICS: Onset, peak, and duration vary widely among the different subgroups of these products.

INTERACTIONS: Cholestyramine and colestipol decrease the absorption of thiazide diuretics. Concurrent use of thiazides with diazoxide may increase hyperuricemia, hyperglycemia, and antihypertensive effects of thiazides. Ototoxicity may occur when loop diuretics are used with aminoglycosides. Thiazide and loop diuretics may increase therapeutic and toxic effects of lithium.

NURSING CONSIDERATIONS
Assessment
• Monitor weight, I&O ratio daily to determine fluid loss; check skin turgor for dehydration
• Monitor electrolytes: potassium, sodium, chloride: include BUN, blood glucose, CBC, serum creatinine, blood pH, ABGs, uric acid, calcium; electrolyte imbalances may occur quickly
• Monitor B/P with patient lying, standing; postural hypotension may occur since fluid loss occurs from intravascular spaces first
• Assess for signs of metabolic alkalosis, including drowsiness and restlessness
• Assess for signs of hypokalemia with some products: postural hypotension, malaise, fatigue, tachycardia, leg cramps, weakness

Patient/family education
• Teach patient to take product early in the day (diuretic) to prevent nocturia

Evaluation
Positive therapeutic outcome
• Improvement in edema of feet, legs, sacral area daily if medication is being used in CHF
• Improvement in B/P if medication is being used as a diuretic
• Improvement in intraocular pressure if medication is being used to decrease aqueous humor in the eye

Generic Names
Thiazides:
chlorothiazide, hydrochlorothiazide

Thiazide-like:
chlorthalidone, indapamide, metolazone

Loop:
bumetanide, furosemide

Carbonic anhydrase inhibitors:
acetaZOLAMIDE

Potassium-sparing:
aMILoride, spironolactone

Osmotic:
mannitol, urea

Histamine H₂ Antagonists

ACTION: Histamine H₂ antagonists act by inhibiting histamine at H₂ receptor site in parietal cells, which inhibits gastric acid secretion.

USES: Histamine H₂ antagonists are used for short-term treatment of duodenal and gastric

Adverse effects: *italics* = common; **bold** = life-threatening

ulcers and maintenance therapy for duodenal ulcer and for gastroesophageal reflux disease.

CONTRAINDICATIONS:
Persons with hypersensitivity should not use these products.

Precautions: Caution should be used in pregnancy, breastfeeding, children <16 yr, organic brain syndrome, and renal/hepatic disease.

IMPLEMENTATION
• Give with meals for prolonged product effect
• Give antacids 1 hr before or 1 hr after cimetidine
• Give **IV** slowly; bradycardia may occur; give over 30 min
• Store diluted sol at room temperature for up to 48 hr

ADVERSE EFFECTS: The most
serious adverse reactions are agranulocytosis, thrombocytopenia, neutropenia, aplastic anemia, and exfoliative dermatitis. The most common side effects are confusion (not with rantidine), headache, and diarrhea.

PHARMACOKINETICS: Onset,
peak, and duration vary widely among products. Most products are metabolized in the liver and excreted in urine.

INTERACTIONS: Antacids interfere
with absorption of histamine H_2 antagonists. Check individual monographs for specific information.

NURSING CONSIDERATIONS
Assessment
• Monitor gastric pH (>5 should be maintained)
• Monitor I&O ratio, BUN, creatinine

Patient/family education
• Advise patient that gynecomastia, impotence may occur but is reversible
• Caution patient to avoid driving and other hazardous activities until patient is stabilized on this medication
• Caution patient to avoid black pepper, caffeine, alcohol, harsh spices, extremes in temperature of food
• Caution patient to avoid OTC preparations: aspirin, cough, cold preparations
• Inform patient that product must be continued for prescribed time to be effective

• Advise patient to report bruising, fatigue, malaise; blood dyscrasias may occur

Evaluation
Positive therapeutic outcome
• Decreased pain in abdomen

Generic Names
cimetidine, famotidine, ranitidine

Immunosuppressants

ACTION: Immunosuppressants produce
immunosuppression by inhibiting T lymphocytes.

USES: Most immunosuppressants are used
for organ transplants to prevent rejection.

CONTRAINDICATIONS:
Products are contraindicated in hypersensitivity.

Precautions: Caution should be used in pregnancy and severe renal/hepatic disease.

IMPLEMENTATION
• Give for several days before transplant surgery
• Give with meals for GI upset or place product in chocolate milk
• Give with oral antifungal for *Candida* infections

ADVERSE EFFECTS: The most
serious adverse reactions are albuminuria, hematuria, proteinuria, renal failure, and hepatotoxicity. The most common side effects are oral *Candida* infection, gum hyperplasia, tremors, and headache. The most serious adverse reactions for azathioprine are hematologic (leukopenia and thrombocytopenia) and GI (nausea and vomiting). There is a risk of secondary infection.

PHARMACOKINETICS: Onset,
peak, and duration vary widely among products. Most products are metabolized in the liver and excreted in urine.

INTERACTIONS: Interactions vary
widely among products. Check individual monographs for specific information.

NURSING CONSIDERATIONS
Assessment
• Monitor renal function tests: BUN, creatinine at least monthly during treatment, 3 mo after treatment

---

• Monitor hepatic function tests: alkaline phosphatase, AST, ALT, bilirubin
• Monitor product blood levels during treatment
• Assess for hepatotoxicity: dark urine, jaundice, itching, light-colored stools; product should be discontinued

Patient/family education
• Advise patient to report fever, chills, sore throat, fatigue since serious infections may occur
• Caution patient to use contraceptive measures during treatment and for 12 wk after ending therapy

Evaluation
Positive therapeutic outcome
• Absence of rejection

Generic Names
azaTHIOprine, basiliximab (high alert), cycloSPORINE, everolimus, muromonab-CD3, sirolimus, tacrolimus, vedolizumab

---

Laxatives

ACTION: Laxatives are divided into bulk products, lubricants, osmotics, saline laxative stimulants, and stool softeners. Bulks work by absorbing water and expanding to increase moisture content and bulk in the stool. Lubricants increase water retention in the stool, causing reabsorption of water in the bowel. Saline draws water into the intestinal lumen. Osmotics increase distention and promote peristalsis. Stimulants act by increasing peristalsis by direct effect on the intestine. Stool softeners reduce surface tension of liquid in the bowel.

USES: Laxatives are used as a preparation for bowel or rectal examination, for constipation, or as stool softeners.

CONTRAINDICATIONS:
Persons with GI obstruction, perforation, gastric retention, toxic colitis, megacolon, abdominal pain, nausea, vomiting, and fecal impaction should not use these products.

Precautions: Caution should be used in rectal bleeding, large hemorrhoids, and anal excoriation.

IMPLEMENTATION
• Give alone only with water for better absorption; do not take within 1 hr of antacids, milk, or cimetidine

• Swallow tab whole; do not break, crush, or chew

ADVERSE EFFECTS: The most common side effects are nausea, abdominal cramps, and diarrhea.

PHARMACOKINETICS: Onset, peak, and duration vary among products.

INTERACTIONS: Interactions vary widely among products. Check individual monographs for specific information.

NURSING CONSIDERATIONS
Assessment
• Monitor blood, urine electrolytes if product is used often by patient
• Monitor I&O ratio to identify fluid loss
• Determine cause of constipation; identify whether fluids, bulk, or exercise is missing from lifestyle
• Assess for cramping, rectal bleeding, nausea, vomiting; if these symptoms occur, product should be discontinued

Patient/family education
• Caution patient not to use laxatives for long-term therapy; bowel tone will be lost; that normal bowel movements do not always occur daily
• Caution patient not to use in presence of abdominal pain, nausea, vomiting
• Advise patient to notify prescriber of abdominal pain, nausea, vomiting
• Advise patient to notify prescriber if constipation is unrelieved or if symptoms of electrolyte imbalance occur: muscle cramps, pain, weakness, dizziness

Evaluation
Positive therapeutic outcome
• Decrease in constipation

Generic Names
Bulk laxative:
psyllium

Osmotic agent:
lactulose

Saline laxatives:
magnesium salts, sodium biphosphate/sodium phosphate

Stimulants:
bisacodyl, senna

Stool softener:
docusate

Adverse effects: *italics* = common; **bold** = life-threatening

Neuromuscular Blocking Agents

ACTION: Neuromuscular blocking agents are divided into depolarizing and nondepolarizing blockers. They act by inhibiting transmission of nerve impulses by binding with cholinergic receptor sites.

USES: Neuromuscular blocking agents are used to facilitate endotracheal intubation and skeletal muscle relaxation during mechanical ventilation, surgery, or general anesthesia.

CONTRAINDICATIONS: Persons who are hypersensitive should not be given this product.

Precautions: Caution should be used in pregnancy, breastfeeding, children <2 yr, thyroid disease, collagen disease, cardiac disease, electrolyte imbalances, dehydration, neuromuscular disease (myasthenia gravis), and respiratory disease.

IMPLEMENTATION
• Administer using nerve stimulator by anesthesiologist to determine neuromuscular blockade
• Administer anticholinesterase to reverse neuromuscular blockade
• Give **IV** undiluted over 1-2 min (only by qualified person, usually an anesthesiologist)
• Store in light-resistant, cool area
• Reassure patient if communication is difficult during recovery from neuromuscular blockade

ADVERSE EFFECTS: The most serious adverse reactions are prolonged apnea, bronchospasm, cyanosis, respiratory depression, and malignant hyperthermia. The most common side effects are bradycardia and decreased motility.

PHARMACOKINETICS: Onset, peak, and duration vary widely among products. Most products are metabolized in the liver and excreted in urine.

INTERACTIONS: Aminoglycosides potentiate neuromuscular blockade. Check individual monographs for specific information.

NURSING CONSIDERATIONS
Assessment
• Monitor for electrolyte imbalances (potassium, magnesium); may lead to increased action of this product
• Monitor VS (B/P, pulse, respirations, airway) q15min until fully recovered; rate, depth, pattern of respirations, strength of hand grip
• Monitor I&O ratio; check for urinary retention, frequency, hesitancy
• Assess for recovery: decreased paralysis of face, diaphragm, leg, arm, rest of body
• Assess for allergic reactions: rash, fever, respiratory distress, pruritus; product should be discontinued

Evaluation
Positive therapeutic outcome
• Paralysis of jaw, eyelid, head, neck, rest of body

Generic Names
pancuronium (high alert), **succinylcholine** (high alert), **vecuronium** (high alert)

Nonsteroidal Antiinflammatories

ACTION: Nonsteroidal antiinflammatories decrease prostaglandin synthesis by inhibiting an enzyme needed for biosynthesis.

USES: Nonsteroidal antiinflammatories are used to treat mild to moderate pain, osteoarthritis, rheumatoid arthritis, and dysmenorrhea.

CONTRAINDICATIONS: Persons with hypersensitivity, asthma, or severe renal/hepatic disease should not use these products.

Precautions: Caution should be used in pregnancy, breastfeeding, children, geriatric patients, bleeding/GI/cardiac disorders, and hypersensitivity to other antiinflammatory agents.

IMPLEMENTATION
• Give with food to decrease GI symptoms; however, best to take on empty stomach to facilitate absorption
• Store at room temperature

ADVERSE EFFECTS: The most serious adverse reactions are nephrotoxicity (dysuria, hematuria, oliguria, azotemia), blood dyscrasias, and cholestatic hepatitis. The most common side effects are nausea, abdominal pain, anorexia, dizziness, and drowsiness.

PHARMACOKINETICS: Onset, peak, and duration vary widely among products.

Most products are metabolized in the liver and excreted in urine.

INTERACTIONS: Interactions vary widely among products. Check individual monographs for specific information.

NURSING CONSIDERATIONS
Assessment
• Monitor renal, hepatic, blood tests: BUN, creatinine, AST, ALT, Hgb, before treatment, periodically thereafter
• Monitor audiometric, ophth examination before, during, and after treatment.
• Check for eye, ear problems: blurred vision, tinnitus; may indicate toxicity

Patient/family education
• Advise patient to report blurred vision, ringing, roaring in ears; may indicate toxicity
• Caution patient to avoid driving, other hazardous activities if dizziness, drowsiness occurs, especially in geriatric patients
• Advise patient to report change in urine pattern, increased weight, edema, increased pain in joints, fever, blood in urine; indicate nephrotoxicity
• Inform patient that therapeutic effects may take up to 1 mo to occur

Evaluation
Positive therapeutic outcome
• Decreased pain, stiffness in joints
• Decreased swelling in joints
• Ability to move more easily

Generic Names
celecoxib, diclofenac, etodolac, ibuprofen, indomethacin, ketoprofen, ketorolac, nabumetone, naproxen, piroxicam, sulindac

Opioid Analgesics

ACTION: These agents depress pain impulse transmission at the spinal cord level by interacting with opioid receptors. Products are divided into opiates and nonopiates.

USES: Most opioid analgesics are used to control moderate to severe pain and are used before and after surgery.

CONTRAINDICATIONS:
Hypersensitive reactions occur frequently. Check for sensitivity before administering. These products should not be used if opioid addiction is suspected.

Precautions: Caution must be used when these products are given to persons with an addictive personality, since the possibility of addiction is so great. Also, persons with increased ICP may experience an even greater increase in ICP. Persons with severe heart disease, renal/hepatic disease, respiratory conditions, and seizure disorders should be monitored closely for worsening condition.

IMPLEMENTATION
• Give with antiemetic if nausea or vomiting occurs
• Give when pain is beginning to return; determine dosage interval by patient response
• Provide assistance with ambulation; patient should not be ambulating during product peak

ADVERSE EFFECTS: GI symptoms, including nausea, vomiting, anorexia, constipation, and cramps are the most common side effects. Other common side effects include lightheadedness, dizziness, and sedation. Serious adverse reactions such as respiratory depression, respiratory arrest, circulatory depression, and increased ICP may result but are less common and usually dose dependent.

PHARMACOKINETICS: Onset of action is immediate by **IV** route and rapid by IM and PO routes. Peak occurs from 1-2 hr, depending on route, with a duration of 2-8 hr. These agents cross the placenta and appear in breast milk.

INTERACTIONS: Barbiturates, other opioids, hypnotics, antipsychotics, or alcohol can increase CNS depression when taken with opioids.

NURSING CONSIDERATIONS
Assessment
• Monitor I&O ratio; be alert for urinary retention, frequency, dysuria; product should be discontinued if these occur
• Assess for respiratory dysfunction: respiratory depression, rate, rhythm, character; notify prescriber if respirations are <12/min
• Assess for CNS changes: dizziness, drowsiness, hallucinations, euphoria, LOC, pupil reaction
• Assess for allergic reactions: rash, urticaria
• Assess for need for pain medication, use pain scoring

Patient/family education
- Advise patient to report any symptoms of CNS changes, allergic reactions, or shortness of breath
- Caution patient that physical dependency may result when used for extended periods
- Teach patient that withdrawal symptoms may occur, including nausea, vomiting, cramps, fever, faintness, anorexia
- Advise patient to avoid alcohol and other CNS depressants

Evaluation
Positive therapeutic outcome
- Decrease in pain

Generic Names
buprenorphine, butorphanol, codeine, **fentaNYL** (high alert), **fentaNYL** transdermal, **HYDROmorphone** (high alert), **meperidine** (high alert), **methadone** (high alert), **morphine** (high alert), nalbuphine, **oxyCODONE** (high alert), **oxymorphone** (high alert), **pentazocine** (high alert), **remifentanil** (high alert)

Salicylates

ACTION: Salicylates have analgesic, antipyretic, and antiinflammatory effects. The analgesic and antiinflammatory activities may be mediated through the inhibition of prostaglandin synthesis. Antipyretic action results from inhibition of the hypothalamic heat-regulating center.

USES: The primary uses of salicylates are relief of mild to moderate pain and fever and ininflammatory conditions such as arthritis, thromboembolic disorders, and rheumatic fever.

CONTRAINDICATIONS: Hypersensitivity to salicylates is common. Check for sensitivity before administering. Persons with bleeding disorders, GI bleeding, and vit K deficiency should not use these products since salicylates increase pro-time. Children should not use these products since salicylates have been associated with Reye's syndrome.

Precautions: Caution is needed when salicylates are given to patients with anemia, renal/hepatic disease, and Hodgkin's disease. Caution should also be exercised in pregnancy and breastfeeding.

IMPLEMENTATION
- Give with food or milk to decrease gastric irritation; give 30 min before or 1 hr after meals with a full glass of water

ADVERSE EFFECTS: The most common side effects are GI symptoms and rash. Serious blood dyscrasias and hepatotoxicity may result when used for long periods at high doses. Tinnitus or impaired hearing may indicate that blood salicylate levels are reaching or exceeding the upper limit of the therapeutic range.

PHARMACOKINETICS: Onset of action occurs in 15-30 min, with a peak of 1-2 hr and a duration up to 6 hr. These products are metabolized by the liver and excreted by the kidneys.

INTERACTIONS: Increased effects of anticoagulants, insulin, methotrexate, heparin, valproic acid, and oral sulfonylureas may occur when used with salicylates. Aspirin may decrease serum concentrations of nonsteroidal antiinflammatory agents.

NURSING CONSIDERATIONS
Assessment
- Monitor renal/hepatic function tests: AST, ALT, bilirubin, creatinine, LDH, alkaline phosphatase, BUN if patient is on long-term therapy since these products are metabolized and excreted by the liver and kidney
- Monitor blood tests: CBC, Hct, Hgb, and pro-time if patient is on long-term therapy, since these products increase the possibility of bleeding and blood dyscrasias
- Assess for hepatotoxicity: dark urine, clay-colored stools, jaundiced skin and sclera, itching, abdominal pain, fever, diarrhea, which may occur with long-term use
- Assess for ototoxicity: tinnitus, ringing, roaring in ears; audiometric testing is needed before and after long-term therapy

Patient/family education
- Advise patient that blood sugar levels should be monitored closely if patient is diabetic
- Caution patient not to exceed recommended dosage; acute poisoning may result
- Inform patient that therapeutic response takes 2 wk in arthritis
- Caution patient to avoid use of alcohol since GI bleeding may result
- Advise patient to notify prescriber if ringing in the ears or persistent GI pain occurs

- Advise patient to take with full glass of water to reduce risk of lodging in esophagus

Evaluation
Positive therapeutic outcome
- Decreased pain, fever

Generic Names
aspirin, magnesium salicylate, salsalate

Sedatives/Hypnotics

ACTION: The sedatives/hypnotics depress the CNS; some products at the cerebral cortex, others inhibit transmitters in the CNS.

USES: Sedatives/hypnotics are used for the treatment of sleep disorders, seizures, muscle spasms, and alcohol withdrawal.

CONTRAINDICATIONS:
Persons with hypersensitivity reactions should not use these products.

Precautions: Sedatives/hypnotics should be used cautiously in pregnancy (**C**) and breastfeeding.

IMPLEMENTATION
- Give lowest possible dose for therapeutic result; adjust dose to response
- Provide assistance with ambulation during beginning therapy if dizziness, ataxia occur

ADVERSE EFFECTS: The most common side effects are nausea and drowsiness. The most serious side effects are Stevens-Johnson syndrome, blood dyscrasias, and risk of dependency.

PHARMACOKINETICS: Onset, peak, and duration vary widely among products. Most products are metabolized in the liver and excreted by the kidneys.

INTERACTIONS: Increased CNS depression may occur with other CNS depressants such as alcohol, opiates, antipsychotics, and antidepressants.

NURSING CONSIDERATIONS
Assessment
- Monitor mental status: affect, mood, behavioral changes, depression, confusion; seizure activity

Patient/family education
- Inform patient that these products should only be used for short-term insomnia
- Caution patient not to drive or engage in other hazardous activities while taking these products
- Instruct patient to avoid breastfeeding while taking these products
- Instruct patient to avoid alcohol or other CNS depressants as drowsiness will increase
- Teach patient that some of the products take two nights to be effective
- Advise patient to report side effects, adverse reactions to health care provider
- Instruct patient to use exactly as prescribed, at regular intervals

Evaluation
Positive therapeutic outcome
- Ability to sleep throughout the night
- Absence or decreasing seizure activity

Generic Names
Barbiturates:
PHENobarbital (high alert)

Benzodiazepines:
chlordiazePOXIDE, clorazepate, diazepam, flurazepam, LORazepam, midazolam, oxazepam, temazepam, triazolam

Miscellaneous products:
chloral hydrate, dexmedetomidine, **droperidol** (high alert), eszopiclone, hydrOXYzine, promethazine, ramelteon, suvorexant, tasimelton, zaleplon, zolpidem

Skeletal Muscle Relaxants

ACTION: Most skeletal muscle relaxants inhibit synaptic responses in the CNS by stimulating receptors and decreasing neurotransmission, decreasing pain and spasticity.

USES: Skeletal muscle relaxants are used for musculoskeletal disorders with pain or spasticity related to spinal cord injuries.

CONTRAINDICATIONS:
Persons with hypersensitivity should not use these products.

Precautions: Skeletal muscle relaxants should be used cautiously in pregnancy (**C**), breastfeeding, the geriatric patient, peptic ulcer, renal/hepatic disease, stroke, seizure disorder, and diabetes.

IMPLEMENTATION
• Give when pain is beginning to return, not after pain is severe
• Store in dry area, away from heat and sunlight

ADVERSE EFFECTS:
The most common side effects are dizziness, weakness, fatigue, drowsiness, and headache. Some products can cause seizures, cardiovascular collapse, and severe CNS depression.

PHARMACOKINETICS:
Pharmacokinetics vary widely among products. Check individual monographs for specific information.

INTERACTIONS:
CNS depressants used with skeletal muscle relaxants may lead to increased CNS depression.

NURSING CONSIDERATIONS
Assessment
• Monitor pain: character, location, duration, alleviating/aggravating factors

Patient/family education
• Advise patient not to use with other CNS depressant unless prescriber approved
• Inform patient that many products require 1-2 mo of treatment for full effect
• Caution patient to avoid hazardous activities until response to medication is known
• Caution patient that most products should not be discontinued quickly, but tapered over 1-2 wk

Evaluation
Positive therapeutic outcome
• Decrease in pain or spasticity

Generic Names
Centrally acting:
baclofen, carisoprodol, cyclobenzaprine, diazepam, methocarbamol

Direct-acting:
dantrolene

Thrombolytics

ACTION: Thrombolytics activate conversion of plasminogen to plasmin (fibrinolysin). Plasmin is able to break down clots (fibrin).

USES: Thrombolytics are used to treat DVT, PE, arterial thrombosis, arterial embolism, arteriovenous cannula occlusion, lysis of coronary artery thrombi after MI, and acute evolving transmural MI.

CONTRAINDICATIONS:
Persons with hypersensitivity, active bleeding, intraspinal surgery, neoplasms of the CNS, ulcerative colitis/enteritis, severe hypertension, renal/hepatic disease, hypocoagulation, COPD, subacute bacterial endocarditis, rheumatic valvular disease, cerebral embolism/thrombosis/hemorrhage, intra-arterial diagnostic procedure or surgery (10 days), and recent major surgery should not use these products.

Precautions: Caution should be used in arterial emboli from left side of heart and pregnancy.

IMPLEMENTATION
• Administer as soon as thrombi identified; not useful for thrombi over 1wk old
• Administer cryoprecipitate or fresh, frozen plasma if bleeding occurs
• Give loading dose at beginning of therapy; may require increased loading doses
• Give heparin after fibrinogen level is over 100 mg/dl; heparin INF to increase PTT to 1.5-2 × baseline for 3-7 days
• About 10% of patients have high streptococcal antibody titers requiring increased loading doses
• Give **IV** therapy using 0.8-μm filter
• Store reconstituted sol in refrigerator; discard after 24 hr
• Provide bed rest during entire course of treatment

ADVERSE EFFECTS:
Serious adverse reactions include GI, GU, intracranial, and retroperitoneal bleeding and anaphylaxis. The most common side effects are decreased Hct, urticaria, headache, and nausea.

PHARMACOKINETICS:
Onset, peak, and duration vary widely among products. Most products are metabolized in the liver and excreted in urine.

INTERACTIONS:
Interactions vary widely among products. Check individual monographs for specific information.

NURSING CONSIDERATIONS
Assessment
• Monitor VS, B/P, pulse, respirations, neurologic signs, temp at least q4hr (increased temp is an indicator of internal bleeding), cardiac

rhythm following intracoronary administration; systolic pressure increase of >25 mm Hg should be reported to prescriber
• Assess for neurologic changes that may indicate intracranial bleeding
• Assess retroperitoneal bleeding: back pain, leg weakness, diminished pulses
• Assess for allergy: fever, rash, itching, chills; mild reaction may be treated with antihistamines
• Assess for bleeding during 1st hr of treatment: hematuria, hematemesis, bleeding from mucous membranes, epistaxis, ecchymosis
• Monitor blood tests (Hct, platelets, PTT, PT, TT, APTT) before starting therapy; PT or APTT must be less than 2 times control before starting therapy; TT or PT q3-4hr during treatment

Patient/family education
• Teach patient to avoid venous or arterial puncture, injection, rectal temp
• Teach patient to treat fever with acetaminophen or aspirin
• Teach patient to apply pressure for 30 sec to minor bleeding sites; inform prescriber if this does not attain hemostasis; apply pressure dressing

Evaluation
Positive therapeutic outcome
• Resolution of thrombosis, embolism

Generic Names
alteplase (high alert), drotrecogin alfa, **tenecteplase** (high alert), **urokinase** (high alert)

Thyroid Hormones

ACTION: Thyroid hormones increase metabolic rates, resulting in increased cardiac output, O_2 consumption, body temp, blood volume, growth, development at cellular level, respiratory rate, and enzyme system activity.

USES: Thyroid hormones are used for thyroid replacement.

CONTRAINDICATIONS:
Persons with adrenal insufficiency, myocardial infarction, or thyrotoxicosis should not use these products.

Precautions: Caution should be used in pregnancy (A) and breastfeeding. Geriatric patients and those with angina pectoris, hypertension, ischemia, cardiac disease, or diabetes mellitus or insipidus should be watched closely when using these products.

IMPLEMENTATION
• Give at same time each day to maintain product level
• Give only for hormone imbalances; not to be used for obesity, male infertility, menstrual conditions, lethargy
• Remove medication 4 wk before RAIU test

ADVERSE EFFECTS: The most
common side effects include insomnia, tremors, tachycardia, palpitations, angina, dysrhythmias, weight loss, and changes in appetite. Serious adverse reactions include thyroid storm.

PHARMACOKINETICS: Pharmaco-
kinetics vary widely among products. Check individual monographs for specific information.

INTERACTIONS
• Impaired absorption of thyroid products may occur when administered with cholestyramine, iron products (separate by 4-5 hr).
• Increased effects of anticoagulants, sympathomimetics, tricyclics, catecholamines may occur.
• Decreased effects of digoxin, glycosides, insulin, hypoglycemics may occur.
• Decreased effects of thyroid products may occur with estrogens.

NURSING CONSIDERATIONS
Assessment
• Monitor B/P, pulse before each dose
• Monitor I&O ratio
• Monitor weight daily in same clothing, using same scale, at same time of day
• Monitor height, growth rate if given to a child
• Monitor T_3, T_4, which are decreased; radioimmunoassay of TSH, which is increased; ratio uptake, which is decreased if patient is on too low a dosage of medication
• Assess for increased nervousness, excitability, irritability; may indicate too high a dosage of medication, usually after 1-3 wk of treatment
• Assess for cardiac status: angina, palpitation, chest pain, change in VS

Patient/family education
• Advise patient/family that hair loss will occur in children and is temporary
• Advise patient to report excitability, irritability, anxiety; indicates overdose
• Caution patient not to switch brands unless directed by prescriber
• Caution family that hypothyroid children will show almost immediate behavior/personality change

Adverse effects: *italics* = common; **bold** = life-threatening

• Advise patient that treatment product is not to be taken to reduce weight
• Advise patient to avoid OTC preparations with iodine; read labels; to avoid iodine-containing foods: iodized salt, soybeans, tofu, turnips, some seafood, some bread

Evaluation
Positive therapeutic outcome
• Absence of depression
• Increased weight loss, diuresis, pulse, appetite
• Absence of constipation, peripheral edema, cold intolerance, pale, cool, dry skin, brittle nails, alopecia, coarse hair, menorrhagia, night blindness, paresthesias, syncope, stupor, coma, rosy cheeks

Generic Names
levothyroxine, liothyronine (T_3), liotrix, thyroid USP

Vasodilators

ACTION: Vasodilators act in various ways. Check individual monographs for specific action.

USES: Vasodilators are used to treat intermittent claudication, arteriosclerosis obliterans, vasospasm and muscular ischemia, ischemic cerebral vascular disease, hypertension, and angina.

CONTRAINDICATIONS:
Some products are contraindicated in acute MI, paroxysmal tachycardia, and thyrotoxicosis.

Precautions: Caution should be used in uncompensated heart disease or peptic ulcer disease.

IMPLEMENTATION
• Give with meals to reduce GI symptoms
• Store in tight container at room temperature

ADVERSE EFFECTS: The most common side effects are headache, nausea, hypotension, hypertension, and ECG changes.

PHARMACOKINETICS: Onset, peak, and duration vary widely among products. Most products are metabolized in the liver and excreted in urine.

INTERACTIONS: Interactions vary widely among products. Check individual monographs for specific information.

NURSING CONSIDERATIONS
Assessment
• Assess bleeding time in individuals with bleeding disorders
• Assess cardiac status: B/P, pulse, rate, rhythm, character; watch for increasing pulse

Patient/family education
• Inform patient that medication is not cure, may need to be taken continuously
• Advise patient that it is necessary to quit smoking to prevent excessive vasoconstriction
• Advise patient that improvement may be sudden, but usually occurs gradually over several weeks
• Instruct patient to report headache, weakness, increased pulse, since product may need to be decreased or discontinued
• Instruct patient to avoid hazardous activities until stabilized on medication; dizziness may occur

Evaluation
Positive therapeutic outcome
• Ability to walk without pain
• Increased temp in extremities
• Increased pulse volume

Generic Names
amyl nitrite, bosentan, dipyridamole, hydrALA-ZINE, minoxidil, nesiritide

Vitamins

ACTION: The action of vitamins varies widely among products and classes. Check individual monographs for specific action.

USES: Vitamins are used to correct and prevent vitamin deficiencies.

CONTRAINDICATIONS:
Hypersensitive reactions may occur, and allergies should be identified before these products are given.

IMPLEMENTATION
• Give PO with food for better absorption
• Store in tight, light-resistant container

ADVERSE EFFECTS: There is an absence of side effects or adverse reactions with the water-soluble vitamins (C, B). However, fat-soluble vitamins (A, D, E, K) may accumulate in the body and cause adverse reactions (refer to individual monographs).

PHARMACOKINETICS: Onset,
peak, and duration vary widely among products. Check individual monographs for specific information.

NURSING CONSIDERATIONS
Patient/family education
• Advise patient not to take more than prescribed amount

Evaluation
Positive therapeutic outcome
• Absence of vitamin deficiency

Generic Names
Fat-soluble:
phytonadione (vitamin K_1), vitamin A, vitamin D, vitamin E

Water-soluble:
ascorbic acid (C), cyanocobalamin (B_{12}), pyridoxine (B_6), riboflavin (B_2), thiamine (B_1)

Miscellaneous:
multivitamins

Appendix A

Selected New Drugs

ado-trastuzumab
(a'doe-tras-tooz'ue-mab)
Kadcyla
Func. class.: Antineoplastic-biologic response modifier
Chem. class.: Signal transduction inhibitor (STI), humanized anti-HER2 antibody
Pregnancy category D

ACTION: Humanized anti-HER2 monoclonal antibody that is linked to DM1, a small molecule microtubular inhibitor. Once the antibody is bound to the HER2 receptor, the complex is internalized and the DM1 is released to bind with tubulin to lead to apoptosis

Therapeutic outcome: Decrease in size of tumors

USES: Breast cancer, metastatic with over-expression of HER2, in patients who previously received trastuzumab and a taxane separately or in combination

CONTRAINDICATIONS:
Hypersensitivity to this product, Chinese hamster ovary cell protein, pregnancy **(D)**

Precautions: Breastfeeding, children, acute bronchospasm, anticoagulants, Asian patients, asthma, cardiomyopathy/CHF, COPD, extravasation, fever, hepatitis, human anti-human antibody, hypotension, neuropathy, hepatotoxicity, interstitial lung disease/pneumonitis; pulmonary disease, thrombocytopenia

DOSAGE AND ROUTES
Adult: **IV** 3.6 mg/kg over 30-90 min q3wk; give first infusion over 90 min; if tolerated, give over 30 min

Dosage adjustments for toxicities
Hepatotoxicity
AST/ALT >5 to ≤20× ULN: withhold, resume treatment at a reduced dose when AST/ALT is ≤5× ULN
• First dose reduction: reduce the dose to 3 mg/kg

• Second dose reduction: reduce the dose to 2.4 mg/kg
• Requirement for further dose reduction: discontinue
AST/ALT >20× ULN: discontinue
Total bilirubin >3 to ≤10× ULN: withhold; resume treatment at a reduced dose when total bilirubin recovers to ≤1.5
• First dose reduction: reduce the dose to 3 mg/kg
• Second dose reduction: reduce the dose to 2.4 mg/kg
• Requirement for further dose reduction: discontinue treatment
Total bilirubin >10× ULN: permanently discontinue
• Permanently discontinue treatment in patients with AST/ALT > 3× ULN and total bilirubin > 2× ULN
• Permanently discontinue treatment in patients diagnosed with nodular regenerative hyperplasia (NRH)
• Left ventricular ejection fraction (LVEF) 40%-45% and decrease is <10% points from baseline: continue treatment; repeat LVEF assessment within 3 wk
• LVEF 40%-45% and decrease is ≥10% points from baseline: withhold; repeat LVEF assessment within 3 wk; if LVEF remains ≥10% points from baseline, discontinue
• LVEF < 40%: withhold; repeat LVEF assessment within 3 wk; if LVEF remains <40%, discontinue
• Symptomatic congestive heart failure (CHF): discontinue

Thrombocytopenia
Platelet count 25,000/mm³ to <50,000/mm³: withhold; resume treatment at same dose when platelet count recovers to ≥75,000/mm³
Platelet count <25,000/mm³: withhold; resume treatment at a reduced dose when platelet count recovers to ≥75,000/mm³
• First dose reduction: reduce the dose to 3 mg/kg
• Second dose reduction: reduce the dose to 2.4 mg/kg
• Requirement for further dose reduction: discontinue

Adverse effects: *italics* = common; **bold** = life-threatening

Pulmonary toxicity
• Permanently discontinue in patients diagnosed with interstitial lung disease or pneumonitis

Peripheral neuropathy
• Withhold in patients experiencing grade 3 or 4 peripheral neuropathy; resume treatment upon resolution to ≤ grade 2

Available forms: Lyophilized powder 100, 160 mg

Implementation

IV route
• Visually inspect for particulate matter and discoloration prior to use
• Give as (IV) infusion with a 0.22-micron in-line filterl do not administer as an IV push or bolus
• Use cytotoxic handling procedures; do not mix with, or administer as an infusion with, other IV products

Reconstitution
• Slowly inject 5 ml of sterile water for injection into each 100 mg vial, or 8 ml of sterile water for injection into each 160 mg vial, to yield a single-use solution of 20 mg/ml
• Direct the stream of sterile water toward the wall of the vial and not directly at the cake or powder
• Gently swirl the vial to aid in dissolution; do not shake
• After reconstitution, withdraw desired amount from the vial and dilute immediately in 250 ml of 0.9% sodium chloride; do not use dextrose 5% solution; gently invert the bag to mix the solution in order to avoid foaming
• The reconstituted single-use product does not contain a preservative. Use the diluted solution immediately or store at 2-8°C (36-46°F) for up to 24 hr after reconstitution; discard any unused drug after 24 hr. Do not freeze.

IV infusion
• Closely monitor for possible subcutaneous infiltration during drug administration
• First infusion: Give over 90 min. The infusion rate should be slowed or interrupted if the patient develops an infusion-related reaction. Patients should be observed for at least 90 min following the initial dose for fever, chills, or other infusion-related reactions. Permanently discontinue for life-threatening infusion-related reactions.
• Subsequent infusions: Administer over 30 min if prior infusions were well tolerated. The infusion rate should be slowed or interrupted if the patient develops an infusion-related reaction.

Patients should be observed for at least 30 min after the infusion. Permanently discontinue for life-threatening infusion-related reactions

ADVERSE EFFECTS

CNS: Dizziness, insomnia, neuropathy, chills, fatigue, fever, flushing, headache, neuropathy
CV: Heart failure, tachycardia
EENT: Blurred vision, conjunctivitis, stomatitis
GI: Diarrhea, nausea, vomiting, abdominal pain, constipation, dyspepsia, hepatotoxicity
HEMA: Anemia, bleeding, thrombocytopenia
INTEG: Rash
MISC: Elevated LFTs, hand-foot syndrome
MS: Arthralgia
RESP: Cough, dyspnea, bronchospasm, pneumonitis, interstitial lung disease
SYST: Anaphylaxis

Pharmacokinetics

Absorption	Unknown
Distribution	93% Protein binding
Metabolism	Liver
Excretion	Unknown
Half-life	Unknown

Pharmacodynamics

Onset	Unknown
Peak	Unknown
Duration	Unknown

INTERACTIONS

Drug classifications
Anticoagulants, 5% dextrose, strong CYP3A4 inhibitors, platelets: avoid concurrent use
Do not give with other IV products

NURSING CONSIDERATIONS

Assessment
• Monitor liver function tests; pregnancy test;
• Monitor CBC, HER2 overexpression

BLACK BOX WARNING: CHF, other cardiac symptoms: assess for dyspnea, coughing; gallop; obtain full cardiac workup including ECG, echo, MUGA

• Monitor for symptoms of infection; may be masked by product
• CNS reaction: monitor LOC, mental status, dizziness, confusion

BLACK BOX WARNING: Monitor hypersensitive reactions, anaphylaxis

• Infusion reactions that may be fatal: monitor fever, chills, nausea, vomiting, pain, headache, dizziness, hypotension; discontinue product
• Pulmonary toxicity: monitor dyspnea, interstitial pneumonitis, pulmonary hypertension, ARDs: can occur after infusion reaction; those with lung disease may have more severe toxicity

BLACK BOX WARNING: Hepatic disease: may be fatal

Patient/family education
• Teach patient to take acetaminophen for fever
• Teach patient to avoid hazardous tasks because confusion, dizziness may occur
• Teach patient to report signs of infection: sore throat, fever, diarrhea, vomiting, bleeding, decreased heart function/SOB with exertion, neuropathy, liver toxicity
• Teach patient that emotional lability is common: to notify prescriber if severe or incapacitating
• Teach patient to use contraception while taking this product; and for additional 6 months after discontinuing this drug; pregnancy (D); to avoid breastfeeding
• Teach patient to report pain at infusion site

Evaluation
Positive therapeutic outcome
• Decrease in size of tumors

afatinib
(a-fat′i-nib)
Gilotrif
Func. class.: Antineoplastic biologic response modifiers
Chem. class.: Signal transduction inhibitors (STIs), epidermal growth factor receptor tyrosine kinase inhibitor
Pregnancy category D

Do not confuse:
afatinib/afinitor/axitinib

ACTION: Selective inhibitor of EGFR (ErbB1), HER2 (ErbB2), and HER4 (ErbB4); irreversible, covalent binding of intracellular tyrosine kinase inhibiting (and causing regression in) tumor growth by decreasing EGFR signal transduction, cell cycle arrest, and inhibition of angiogenesis.

Therapeutic outcome: Decrease in progression of disease

USES: Treatment of non-small cell lung cancer whose tumors have epidermal growth factor receptor Exon 19 deletions or 21 substitution mutations

CONTRAINDICATIONS:
Pregnancy **(D)**, hypersensitivity

Precautions: Contact lenses, dehydration, inflammation, keratitis, ocular disease, pneumonitis, pulmonary disease, renal disease, respiratory distress syndrome, serious rash, skin disease, diarrhea, hepatic disease, ocular disease

DOSAGE AND ROUTES
Adult: PO 40 mg/day

Dosage adjustments for toxicities
Hepatotoxicity
AST/ALT >5 to ≤20× ULN: withhold; resume at a reduced dose when AST/ALT is ≤5× ULN:
• First dose reduction: reduce the dose to 3 mg/kg
• Second dose reduction: reduce the dose to 2.4 mg/kg
• Requirement for further dose reduction: discontinue
AST/ALT >20× ULN: discontinue
Total bilirubin >3 to ≤10× ULN: withhold; resume treatment at a reduced dose when total bilirubin recovers to ≤1.5:
• First dose reduction: reduce the dose to 3 mg/kg
• Second dose reduction: reduce the dose to 2.4 mg/kg
• Requirement for further dose reduction: discontinue treatment
Total bilirubin >10× ULN: permanently discontinue
• Permanently discontinue treatment in patients with AST/ALT >3× ULN and total bilirubin >2× ULN
• Permanently discontinue treatment in patients diagnosed with nodular regenerative hyperplasia (NRH)
Left ventricular ejection fraction *(LVEF) 40%-45% and decrease is <10% points from baseline:* continue treatment. Repeat LVEF assessment within 3 wk.
LVEF 40%-45% and decrease is ≥10% points from baseline: withhold; repeat LVEF assessment within 3 wk; if LVEF remains ≥10% points from baseline, discontinue
LVEF <40%: withhold; repeat LVEF assessment within 3 wk; if LVEF remains <40%, discontinue

---

Symptomatic congestive heart failure (CHF): discontinue

Thrombocytopenia
Platelet count 25,000/mm³ to <50,000/mm³: withhold; resume treatment at same dose when platelet count recovers to ≥75,000 /mm³.
Platelet count <25,000/mm³: withhold; resume treatment at a reduced dose when platelet count recovers to ≥75,000/mm³.
• First dose reduction: reduce the dose to 3 mg/kg.
• Second dose reduction: reduce the dose to 2.4 mg/kg.
• Requirement for further dose reduction: discontinue

Pulmonary toxicity
• Permanently discontinue in patients diagnosed with interstitial lung disease or pneumonitis

Peripheral neuropathy
• Withhold in patients experiencing grade 3 or 4 peripheral neuropathy. Resume treatment upon resolution to ≤ grade 2

Available forms: Tabs 20, 30, 40 mg

Implementation
PO route
• Give on empty stomach 1 hr before, 2 hr after food
• Give at same time of day
• Do not take a missed dose if within 12 hr of next dose

ADVERSE EFFECTS
CNS: Fatigue, fever
CV: Heart failure
EENT: Blurred vision, conjunctivitis
GI: Diarrhea, nausea, vomiting, stomatitis, decreased appetite
HEMA: Anemia, neutropenia, leukopenia, epistaxis
INTEG: Rash, pruritus, acne vulgaris, photosensitivity, nail bed infections
MISC: Elevated LFTs, infection, hand foot syndrome, dehydration, renal failure, cystitis, hypokalemia
MS: Arthralgia
RESP: Cough, dyspnea, acute respiratory distress syndrome, interstitial lung disease, pneumonitis

Absorption	Unknown
Distribution	95% protein binding; time to steady state is approx. 8 days
Metabolism	Unknown
Excretion	Primarily excreted as unchanged drug in feces
Half-life	37 hr

Pharmacodynamics

Onset	Unknown
Peak	2-5 hr
Duration	Unknown

INTERACTIONS
Drug classifications
P-gp inhibitors: increased afatinib effect

Drug/food
Grapefruit juice: increased afatinib effect; avoid use while taking product

Drug/herb
St. John's wort: increased afatinib concentrations

NURSING CONSIDERATIONS
Assessment

BLACK BOX WARNING: Myelosuppression: anemia, neutropenia; obtain a CBC weekly × 1 mo, then monthly as needed; LFTs every mo × 3 mo, then as clinically indicated, hepatic failure may occur

Patient/family education
• Teach patient to report adverse reactions immediately, bleeding
• Teach patient about reason for treatment, expected results
• Teach patient to use effective contraception during treatment and up to 30 days after discontinuing treatment
• Teach patient to treat skin rash with topicals and oral antibiotics; use loperamide for diarrhea; if any side effect is severe or is persistent, contact prescriber
• Teach patient that complicated dosing changes may occur based on toxicity or drug-drug interaction
• Teach patient to take on empty stomach (at least 1 hr before or 2 hr after meal); do not take missed dose within 12 hr of next scheduled dose

Evaluation
Positive therapeutic outcome
• Decrease in progression of disease

---

canagliflozin
(kan′a-gli-floe′zin)
Invokana
Func. class.: Oral antidiabetic
Chem. class.: SGLT-2 inhibitor
Pregnancy category B

ACTION: Blocks reabsorption by the kidney, increases glucose excretion, lowers blood glucose concentrations

Therapeutic outcome: Improved signs/symptoms of diabetes mellitus (decreased polyuria, polydipsia, polyphagia; clear sensorium; absence of dizziness; stable gait)

USES: Type 2 diabetes mellitus, with diet and exercise

CONTRAINDICATIONS:
Dialysis, renal failure, hypersensitivity, breastfeeding, diabetic ketoacidosis

Precautions: Pregnancy (B), children, renal/hepatic disease, hypothyroidism, hyperglycemia, hypotension, pituitary insufficiency, type 1 diabetes mellitus, malnutrition, fever, dehydration, adrenal insufficiency, geriatrics

DOSAGE AND ROUTES
Renal dose
Adult: **PO** eGFR 45-59 ml/min/1.73 m², max 100 mg/day; <45 ml/min/1.73 m², do not use

Available forms: Tabs 100, 300 mg

Implementation
PO route
• Once daily with first meal of the day

ADVERSE EFFECTS
CNS: *Dizziness, fatigue*
GI: Abdominal pain, pancreatitis, constipation, nausea
GU: Candidiasis, urinary frequency, polydipsia, polyuria
INTEG: Photosensitivity, rash, pruritus
META: Hypercholesterolemia, lipidemia, hypoglycemia, hyperkalemia, hypermagnesemia, hyperphosphatemia
MISC: Bone fractures

Pharmacokinetics
Absorption	Unknown
Distribution	99% protein binding
Metabolism	By UGT1A9, UGT2B4
Excretion	33% in urine
Half-life	Unknown

Pharmacodynamics
Onset	Unknown
Peak	Unknown
Duration	Unknown

INTERACTIONS
Individual drugs
Baclofen, cycloSPORINE, estrogen, isoniazid, tacrolimus: decreased effect, hyperglycemia
Gatifloxacin: do not use concurrently
Lithium: increased or decreased glycemic control

Drug classifications
ACE inhibitors, angiotensin II receptor antagonists, β-blockers, bile acid sequestrants, fibric acid derivatives, insulin, MAOIs, salicylates, sulfonylureas: increased hypoglycemia
Atypical antipsychotics, carbonic anhydrase inhibitors, corticosteroids, digestive enzymes, intestinal absorbents, loop diuretics, oral contraceptives, phenothiazines, progestins, protease inhibitors, sympathomimetics, thiazide diuretics: decreased effect, hyperglycemia

NURSING CONSIDERATIONS
Assessment
• Assess for hypoglycemia (weakness, hunger, dizziness, tremors, anxiety, tachycardia, sweating), hyperglycemia; even though product does not cause hypoglycemia, if patient is on sulfonylureas or insulin, hypoglycemia may be additive; if hypoglycemia occurs, treat with dextrose, or, if severe, with IV glucagon
• Monitor for stress, surgery, or other trauma that may require a change in dose
• A1c q3mo, monitor serum glucose; 1 hr PP throughout treatment; serum cholesterol, serum creatinine/BUN, serum electrolytes

Patient/family education
• Teach patient the symptoms of hypoglycemia/hyperglycemia, what to do about each
• Instruct patient that medication must be taken as prescribed; explain consequences of discontinuing medication abruptly; that insulin may need to be used for stress, including trauma, fever, surgery

---

• Instruct patient to avoid OTC medications and herbal supplements unless approved by health care provider

• Instruct patient that diabetes is a lifelong illness; that the diet and exercise regimen must be followed; that this product is not a cure

• Instruct patient to carry emergency ID and glucose source; to avoid sugar, because sugar is blocked by acarbose

• Teach patient that blood glucose monitoring is required to assess product effect

• Teach patient that GI side effects may occur

Evaluation: Therapeutic response: improved signs/symptoms of diabetes mellitus (decreased polyuria, polydipsia, polyphagia; clear sensorium, absence of dizziness, stable gait

crofelemer
(kroe-fel′e-mer)
Fulyzaq
Func. class.: Antidiarrheal
Chem. class.: Red sap of *Croton lechleri* plant
Pregnancy category C

ACTION: Blocks chloride channel and high volume water loss in diarrhea

Therapeutic outcome: Decreasing diarrhea

USES: Noninfectious diarrhea in those with HIV/AIDS using antiretrovirals

CONTRAINDICATIONS:
Hypersensitivity

Precautions: Pregnancy (C), breastfeeding, black patients, children/ adolescents, GI disease, infection, malabsorption syndrome, pancreatitis

DOSAGE AND ROUTES
Adult: PO 125 mg bid

Available forms: Del rel tabs 125 mg

Implementation
PO route
• Do not break, crush, or chew
• Give without regard to meals

ADVERSE EFFECTS
CNS: Dizziness, depression
GI: Nausea, constipation, abdominal pain, anorexia, flatulence, hyperbilirubinemia
INTEG: Acne vulgaris, contact dermatitis
MISC: Arthralgia, cough, increased urinary frequency

Pharmacokinetics
Absorption	Unknown
Distribution	Unknown
Metabolism	Unknown
Excretion	Unknown
Half-life	Unknown

Pharmacodynamics
Onset	Unknown
Peak	Unknown
Duration	Unknown

INTERACTIONS
Individual drugs
Alosetron: increased serious constipation, bowel obstruction

Drug classifications
Antimuscarinics, opiate agonists: increased constipation

NURSING CONSIDERATIONS
Assessment
• Stools: volume, color, characteristic frequency; bowel pattern before protein rebound constipation
• Electrolytes (K, Na, Cl), hydration status
• Monitor effect in black patients; may be less effective

Patient/family education
• Instruct patient to avoid OTC products unless directed by prescriber
• Instruct patient not to operate machinery if drowsiness occurs

Evaluation
Positive therapeutic outcome:
• Decreased diarrhea

dabrafenib
(da-braf′e-nib)
Tafinlar
Func. class.: Antineoplastic
Chem. class.: Signal transduction inhibitor, kinase inhibitor
Pregnancy category D

ACTION: Inhibits kinase, inhibitor against mutated forms of BRAF kinases in melanoma cells

Therapeutic outcome: Decrease in melanoma progression

USES: Unresectable or metastatic BRAD V600E-mutated malignant melanoma

---

⚠ Nurse Alert   ✴ Key NCLEX® Drug

CONTRAINDICATIONS:
Pregnancy **D**, hypersensitivity

Precautions: Breastfeeding, children, infection, dehydration, diabetes mellitus, fever, G6PD deficiency, hemolytic anemia, hyperglycemia, hypotension, infertility, iritis, renal failure, secondary malignancy

DOSAGE AND ROUTES
Adult: **PO** 150 mg q12hr until disease progression, avoid strong CYP3A4/CYP2C8 inhibitors or inducers

Available forms: Caps 50, 75 mg

Implementation
PO route
• Swallow whole
• If dose is missed, take within 6 hr of missed dose, if >6 hr have passed, skip dose
• Space doses q12hr
• Take at least 1 hr before or 2 hr after a meal

ADVERSE EFFECTS
CNS: Headache, fever
GI: Pancreatitis
INTEG: Rash, alopecia
MISC: Arthralgia, back pain, hand/foot syndrome, hyperglycemia, hypophosphatemia, hyponatremia, myalgia, secondary malignancy

Pharmacokinetics	
Absorption	Unknown
Distribution	Protein binding 99.7%
Metabolism	Unknown
Excretion	71% (feces), 23% (urine)
Half-life	8 hr (dabrafenib), 10 hr, 21-22 hr metabolites

Pharmacodynamics	
Onset	Unknown
Peak	Unknown
Duration	Unknown

INTERACTIONS
Drug classifications
Antacids, CYP3A4 inducers (dexamethasome, phenytoin, carBAMazepine, rifampin, PHENobarbital), proton-pump inhibitors: decreased dabrafenib concentrations
CYP3A4 inhibitors (ketoconazole, itraconazole, erythromycin, clarithromycin): altered dabrafenib concentrations

Drug/food
Grapefruit juice: increased dabrafenib effect; avoid use while taking product

Drug/herb
St. John's wort: decreased dabrafenib concentrations

NURSING CONSIDERATIONS
Assessment
• Toxicity: Assess for fever, grade 2, 3

Patient/family education
• Instruct patient to report adverse reactions immediately
• Teach patient about reason for treatment, expected results
• Instruct patient to use effective contraception during treatment and for 30 days after discontinuing treatment, Pregnancy **D**

Evaluation
Positive therapeutic outcome
• Decrease in melanoma progression

---

dapagliflozin
(dap′a-gli-floe′zin)
Farxiga
Func. class.: Oral antidiabetic
Chem. class.: SGLT-2 inhibitor
Pregnancy category C

ACTION: Blocks reabsorption of glucose by the kidneys, increases glucose excretion, lowers blood glucose concentrations

Therapeutic outcome: Improved signs/symptoms of diabetes mellitus (decreased polyuria, polydipsia, polyphagia; clear sensorium, absence of dizziness, stable gait); HbA1c WNL

USES: Type 2 diabetes mellitus, with diet and exercise

CONTRAINDICATIONS:
Dialysis, renal failure, hypersensitivity, breastfeeding, diabetic ketoacidosis

Precautions: Pregnancy C, children, renal/hepatic disease, hypothyroidism, hyperglycemia, hypotension, bladder cancer, hypercholesterolemia, pituitary insufficiency, type 1 diabetes mellitus, malnutrition, fever, dehydration, adrenal insufficiency, geriatrics, genital fungal infections, hypoglycemia

DOSAGE AND ROUTES
Adult: **PO** 5 mg in AM; may increase to 10 mg/day if needed

---

Adverse effects: *italics* = common; **bold** = life-threatening

Renal dose
Adult: PO eGFR $\geq$60 ml/min/1.73m^2, no change; eGFR<60 ml/min, do not use

Available forms: Tabs 5, 10 mg

Implementation
PO route
• Give once/day in AM without regard to food

ADVERSE EFFECTS
CNS: Dizziness, fatigue
GI: Abdominal pain, pancreatitis, constipation, nausea
GU: Cystitis, candidiasis, urinary frequency, polydipsia, polyuria, increased serum creatinine, renal impairment/failure, infections
META: Hypercholesterolemia, lipidemia, hypoglycemia, hyperkalemia, hypomagnesemia, hypophosphatemia/hyperphosphatemia
MISC: Bone fractures, hypotension, dehydration, orthostatic hypotension, hypersensitivity, new bladder cancer; increased hematocrit

Pharmacokinetics	
Absorption	Unknown
Distribution	91% protein binding
Metabolism	Primarily metabolized by O-glucuronidation by UGT1A9; minor CYP3A4
Excretion	Urine
Half-life	12.9 hr

Pharmacodynamics	
Onset	Unknown
Peak	Less than 2 hr
Duration	Unknown

INTERACTIONS
Individual drugs:
Baclofen, cycloSPORINE, isoniazid, tacrolimus: decreased effect, hyperglycemia
Bortezomib, lithium: increased or decreased glycemic control
Gatifloxacin: do not use concurrently

Drug classifications
Androgens, quinolones: increased or decreased glycemic control
ACE inhibitors, angiotensin II receptor antagonists, bile acid sequestrates, β-blockers, fibric acid derivatives, insulins, MAOIs, salicylates, sulfonylureas: increased hypoglycemia
Atypical antipsychotics, carbonic anhydrase inhibitors, corticosteroids, digestive enzymes, estrogen, intestinal absorbents, loop diuretics, oral contraceptives, phenothiazines, progestins, protease inhibitors, sympathomimetics, thiazide diuretics: decrease effect, hyperglycemia

NURSING CONSIDERATIONS
Assessment
• Hypoglycemia (assess hunger, dizziness, tremors, anxiety, tachycardia, sweating, weakness), hyperglycemia; even though product does not cause hyperglycemia, if patient is on sulfonylureas or insulin, hypoglycemia may be additive; if hypoglycemia occurs, treat with dextrose, or, if severe, with IV glucagon; HbA1c; lipid panel; renal function tests; volume status; blood pressure;

Patient/family education
• Teach patient the symptoms of hypoglycemia and hyperglycemia, what to do about each
• Instruct patient that medication must be taken as prescribed; explain consequences of discontinuing medication abruptly; that insulin may need to be used for stress, including trauma, fever, surgery
• Instruct patient to avoid OTC medications and herbal supplements unless approved by health care provider
• Instruct patient that diabetes is a lifelong illness; that the diet and exercise regimen must be followed; that this product is not a cure
• Instruct patient to carry emergency ID and glucose source
• Instruct patient that blood glucose monitoring is required to assess product effect
• Instruct patient that GI side effects may occur
• Instruct patient that there is a risk of renal impairment, dehydration, and new bladder cancer

Evaluation
Positive therapeutic outcome
• Improved signs/symptoms of diabetes mellitus (decreased polyuria, polydipsia, polyphagia); clear sensorium, absence of dizziness, stable gait; HbA1c WNL

dolegravir
(dole-oo-teg'ra-vir)
Tivicity
Func. class.: Antiretroviral
Chem. class.: HIV integrase strand transfer inhibitor (ISTIs)
Pregnancy category C

ACTION: Inhibits catalytic activity of HIV integrase, which is an HIV-encoded enzyme needed for replication

Therapeutic outcome: Improvement in cell counts, T-cell counts

USES: HIV in combination with other retrovirals

CONTRAINDICATIONS:
Breastfeeding, hypersensitivity

Precautions: Pregnancy C, children, geriatric patients, hepatic disease, immune reconstitution syndrome, hepatitis, antimicrobial resistance, lactase deficiency

DOSAGE AND ROUTES
Adult and child >12 yr and ≥40 kg (treatment-naïve or treatment-experienced but integrase strand transfer inhibitor–naïve) PO 50 mg/day; if given with efavires, fosanprenavir/ritonavir, tipranavir/ritonavir or rifampin give 50 mg bid

Available forms: Tabs 50 mg

Implementation
• May give without regard to meals, with 8 oz of water
• Store at room temperature
• Give 2 hr before or 6 hr after cation-containing antacids or laxatives, sucralfate, oral iron, oral calcium, or buffered products

ADVERSE EFFECTS
CNS: Fatigue, fever, dizziness, headache, asthenia, suicidal ideation
CV: MI
GI: Nausea, vomiting, diarrhea, abdominal pain, asthenia, gastritis, hepatitis
INTEG: Rash, pruritis, urticarial
META: Hyperglycemia
SYST: Immune reconstitution syndrome

Pharmacokinetics

Absorption	Unknown
Distribution	Steady state 5 days, 98% protein binding
Metabolism	Liver
Excretion	Feces 53%, urine 31%
Half-life	Terminal 14 hr

Pharmacodynamics

Onset	Unknown
Peak	Peak 2-3 hr
Duration	Unknown

INTERACTIONS
Individual drugs
Efavirenz, rifampin tenofovir, tipranavir/ritonavir: decreased levels of each product

Drug classifications
Antacids, buffered products, laxatives/sucralfate, oral iron products, oral calcium products, buffered products: decreased effect of dolutegravir

Drug/herb
St. John's wort: avoid concurrent use

NURSING CONSIDERATIONS
Assessment
• HIV infection: monitor CD4, T-cell count, plasma HIV RNA, viral load; resistance testing before treatment, at treatment failure
• Perform drug resistance testing prior to use in treatment naïve patients
• Immune reconstitution syndrome RED, usually during initial phase of treatment, may be anti-infective before starting
• Monitor total/HDL/LDL cholesterol baseline and periodically, all may be elected

Patient/family education
• Teach patient to take as prescribed; if dose missed to take as soon as remembered up to 1 hr before next dose; not to double dose; not to share with others
• Teach patient that sexual partners need to be told that patient has HIV; that product does not cure infection, just controls symptoms, does not prevent infecting others
• Teach patient to report sore throat, fever, fatigue (may indicate superinfection)
• Teach patient to notify prescriber if pregnancy is planned, or suspected; to avoid breastfeeding and to continue follow up exams, and work

Evaluation
Positive therapeutic outcome
• Improvement in cell counts, T-cell counts

---

eslicarbazepine
(es'lye-kar-bay'ze-peen)
Aptiom
Func. class.: Anticonvulsant, misc
Chem class.: Voltage-gated sodium channel (VGSC) blocker
Pregnancy category C

ACTION: Exact mechanism unknown; a voltage-gated sodium-channel blocker inhibits repetitive neuronal firing

Adverse effects: *italics* = common; **bold** = life-threatening

USES: Partial seizures, adjunctive treatment

CONTRAINDICATIONS:
Hypersensitivity to this product or OXcarbazepine

Precautions: Breastfeeding, abrupt discontinuation, depression, driving/operating machinery, ethanol intoxication, hepatic disease, renal disease, hyponatremia, suicidal ideation, pregnancy **C**

DOSAGE AND ROUTES
Adult: PO 400 mg/day, after 1 wk increase to 800 mg/day, max 1200 mg/day

Renal dose
Adult: PO CCr <50 ml/min, 200 mg/day, after 2 wk increase to 400 mg/day, max 600 mg/day

Available forms: Tab 200, 400, 600, 800 mg

Implementation
- May be taken without regard to food
- May be crushed or swallowed whole

ADVERSE EFFECTS
CNS: Drowsiness, dizziness, amnesia, depression, insomnia, lethargy, memory impairment, confusion, fatigue, headache, speech disturbance, suicidal thoughts/behaviors, tremor
CV: Hypertension, peripheral edema
EENT: Blurred vision, nystagmus, diplopia
GI: Nausea, constipation, diarrhea, hypercholesterolemia/hypertriglyceride, vomiting, hepatotoxicity
GU: Cystitis
INTEG: Rash, Stevens-Johnson syndrome, toxic epidermal necrolysis, anaphylaxis, angioedema
META: Hyponatremia
RESP: Cough

Pharmacokinetics	
Absorption	Unknown
Distribution	Unknown
Metabolism	Liver
Excretion	Urine, feces
Half-life	Terminal 13-20 hr

Pharmacodynamics	
Onset	Unknown
Peak	1-4 hr
Duration	Unknown

INTERACTIONS
Individual drugs
Bedaquiline, boceprevir, bosutinib, carbozantinib, cobicistant, elvitegravir, emtricitubine, crizotinib, cycloSPORINE, dronederone, erlotinib, fosamprenavir, galantamine, gefitinib, HYDROcodone, maraviroc, oxyCODONE, paliperidone, perm panel, pimozide, praziquantel, QUEtiapine, ranolazine, rilpivirine: decreased effects of these agents
CYP1A2, CYP2C19 substrates: decreased eslicarbamazepine effect

Drug classifications
CYP3A inducers: decreased effect of these agents

NURSING CONSIDERATIONS
Assessment
- Seizures: character, location, duration, intensity, frequency, presents of aura
- Hepatic studies: ALT, AST, bilirubin; sodium

> **BLACK BOX WARNING** Mental status: mood, sensorium, affect, behavioral changes, suicidal thoughts/behaviors; if mental status changes, notify prescriber

- Eye problems: need for ophthalmic examinations before, during, after treatment (slit lamp, funduscopy, tonometry)
- Allergic reaction: purpura, red, raised rash; if these occur; product should be discontinued

Patient/family education
- Instruct patient to carry emergency ID stating patient's name, products taken, condition, prescriber's name and phone number
- Instruct patient too avoid driving, other activities that require alertness, usually for the first 3 days of treatment
- Instruct patient not to discontinue medication quickly after long-term use
- Instruct patient to notify prescriber if pregnancy is planned or suspected, pregnancy **C**, avoid breastfeeding
- Instruct patient to report signs of decreased renal function, dizziness, increased cholesterol, ocular toxicity, suicidal ideation, skin rashes
- Teach patient to take with or without food; tablet can be crushed

Evaluation
Positive therapeutic outcome
- Decreased seizure activity; document on patients chart

⚠ Nurse Alert   ✳ Key NCLEX® Drug

ibrutinib

(eye-broo'ti-nib)

Imbruvica

Func. class.: Antineoplastic-biologic response modifier

Chem. class.: Signal transduction inhibitor (STI)

Pregnancy category D

ACTION: Irreversible inhibitor of Bruton's tyrosine kinases in B cells responsible for tumor growth

Therapeutic outcome: Decrease in progression of disease

USES: Recurrent mantle cell lymphoma in patients who have received at least 1 prior treatment

CONTRAINDICATIONS:

Pregnancy (D), breastfeeding, hypersensitivity

Precautions: Children, geriatric patients, active infections, anticoagulant therapy, bleeding, hepatic/renal disease, neutropenia, surgery

DOSAGE AND ROUTES

Adult: PO 560 mg (4×140 mg caps)/day

Dosage adjustment for ≥ grade 3 non-hematologic, ≥ grade 3 neutropenia with infection or fever, or grade 4 hematologic toxicities

Interrupt therapy; resume upon recovery to grade 1 or baseline as indicated below:

• **First occurrence:** resume dosing at original dose (daily dose = 560 mg/day);
• **Second occurrence:** reduce dose by 1 capsule (daily dose = 420 mg/day);
• **Third occurrence:** reduce dose by 2 capsules (daily dose = 280 mg/day);
• **Fourth occurrence:** discontinue

Available forms: Caps 140 mg

Implementation

• Give at same time of day with water; if dose is missed, take as soon as possible on same day; do not double
• Do not open, break, chew cap

ADVERSE EFFECTS

CNS: Fatigue, fever

CV: Hypertension, atrial fibrillation, peripheral edema

EENT: Sinusitis

GI: Nausea, vomiting, dyspepsia, anorexia, abdominal pain, constipation, stomatitis, diarrhea, GI bleeding

GU: Increased serum creatinine, UTI

HEMA: Neutropenia, thrombocytopenia, anemia, bleeding, epistaxis, transient lymphocytosis

INTEG: Rash, skin infections

MS: Pain, arthralgia, muscle cramps

RESP: Cough, dyspnea

SYST: Secondary malignancy, infection

Pharmacokinetics

Absorption	Unknown
Distribution	Protein binding 97.3%
Metabolism	By CYP3A4/CYP2D6
Excretion	Primarily in feces, small amount in urine
Half-life	Terminal 4-8 hr

Pharmacodynamics

Onset	Unknown
Peak	1-2 hr
Duration	Unknown

INTERACTIONS

Drug classifications

Moderate or strong CYP3A4 inducers: decreased ibrutinib effect; avoid concurrent use

Moderate or strong CYP3A4 inhibitors: increased ibrutinib effect; avoid concurrent use

Drug/food

Grapefruit juice: increased plasma concentrations

Drug/herb

St. John's wort: decreased SUNItinib concentration

NURSING CONSIDERATIONS

Assessment

• **Bleeding:** bruising, grade 3 or higher bleeding events may occur
• Monitor hepatic/renal function, signs/symptoms of infection

Patient/family education

• Instruct patient-to report adverse reactions immediately: SOB, bleeding
• Teach patient about reason for treatment, expected result
• Teach patient that many adverse reactions may occur: high B/P, bleeding, mouth swelling
• Teach patient to avoid persons with known upper respiratory infections; that immunosuppression is common

---

Adverse effects: *italics* = common; **bold** = life-threatening

- Teach patient to avoid grapefruit juice or medications, herbs; there are many interactions
- Teach patient to report if pregnancy is planned or suspected, pregnancy (D)
- Teach patient to report bleeding, severe infections, renal toxicity (maintain hydration), development of second malignancies, diarrhea (contact physician if it persists)
- Teach patient to take with water (avoid food because increases drug levels) at same time each day; do not open, break, or chew

Evaluation
Positive therapeutic outcome
- Decrease in progression of disease

---

levomilnacipran
(lee′voe-mil-na′si-pran)
Fetzima
Chem. class.: Antidepressant
Func. class.: Serotonin
Pregnancy category C

ACTION: May pootentiate serotonergic, andrenergic activity in the CNS; is a potent inhibitor of adrenal serotonin and norepinephrine reuptake

Therapeutic outcome: Decreased depression

USES: Major depressive disorder in adults

CONTRAINDICATIONS:
Alcohol intoxication, alcoholism, closed angle glaucoma, hepatic disease, hepatitis, jaundice, hypersensitivity

Precautions: Pregnancy C, breastfeeding, geriatric patients, mania, hypertension, renal/cardiac disease, seizures, increased intraocular pressure, anorexia,, bleeding, dehydration, diabetes, hypotension, hypovolemia, orthostatic hypotension, abrupt product withdrawal

> **BLACK BOX WARNING:** Children, suicidal ideation

DOSAGE AND ROUTES
Adult: PO 20 mg/day × 2 days, then 40 mg/day, may increase in increments of 40 mg at intervals of at least 2 days, max 120 mg/day; max 80 mg/day (Strong CYP3A4 inhibitors therapy)

Renal dose
Adult: PO CCr 30-59 ml/min, max 80 mg/day; 15-29 ml/min, max 40 mg/day; <15 ml/min, avoid use

Available forms: Ext rel caps 20, 40, 80, 120 mg

Implementation
- Swallow cap whole; do not break, crush, or chew; do not sprinkle on food or mix with liquid
- Give without regard to food
- Give at the same time of day

ADVERSE EFFECTS
CNS: Dizziness, agitation, hallucinations, seizures, drowsiness, mania, migraine, paresthesias, serotonin syndrome, suicidal ideation, syncope
CV: Hypertension, palpitations, dysrhythmia, sinus tachycardia
EENT: Teeth grinding, blurred vision
GI: Constipation, diarrhea, nausea, vomiting, anorexia, dry mouth, abdominal pain
GU: Urinary retention
SYST: Serotonin syndrome, **Stevens-Johnson syndrome**

Pharmacokinetics	
Absorption	Unknown
Distribution	22% protein binding
Metabolism	By CYP2D6 in the liver
Excretion	Unknown
Half-life	12 hr

Pharmacodynamics	
Onset	Unknown
Peak	6-8 hr
Duration	Unknown

INTERACTIONS
Individual drugs
Linezolid, methylene blue IV: do not use concurrently

Drug classifications
Anticoagulants, antiplatelets, NSAIDs, salicylates: increased bleeding risk
CYP34A Inhibitors: increased levomilnacipran effect
MAOIs: Coadministration contraindicated within 14 days of MAOI
SSRIs, serotonin receptor agonists, SNRIs: increased serotonin syndrome

NURSING CONSIDERATIONS
Assessment
- Serotonin syndrome: assess for nausea/vomiting, dizziness, facial flush, shivering, sweating

---

• Monitor B/P lying, standing; pulse q4hr; if systolic B/P drops 20 mm Hg, hold product, notify prescriber; take VS q4hr in patients with CV disease
• Hepatic studies: monitor AST ALT, bilirubin
• Withdrawal symptoms: assess for headache, nausea, vomiting, muscle pain, weakness; not common unless product is discontinued abruptly

Patient/family education
• Teach patient signs and symptoms of bleeding (GI bleeding, nosebleed, ecchymoses, bruising)
• Instruct patient to use caution when driving and in other activities requiring alertness because of drowsiness and blurred vision
• Instruct patient to avoid alcohol ingestion, MAOIs, other CNS depressants
• Instruct patient not to discontinue medication quickly after long-term use; may cause headache, malaise; taper

• Teach patient to notify prescriber if pregnancy is planned or suspected, or if breastfeeding
• Teach patient improvement may occur in 4-8 wk or up to 12 wk (geriatric patients)

Evaluation
Positive therapeutic outcome
• Decreased depression

macitentan
(ma'si-ten'tan)
Opsumit
Func. class.: Antihypertensive
Chem class.: Vasodilator/endothelin receptor antagonist
Pregnancy category X

ACTION: Prevents the binding of ET-1, to ETA and ETB receptors on human pulmonary arterial smooth muscle

USES: Pulmonary arterial hypertension; WHO Group 1 to delay disease progression

CONTRAINDICATIONS:
Breastfeeding, hypersensitivity, (pregnancy category X)

Precautions: Anemia, hepatic disease, pulmonary edema

DOSAGE AND ROUTES
Adult: **PO** 10 mg/day

Available forms: Tabs 10 mg

Implementation
• Do not break, crush, chew tabs; take without regard to food; if a dose is missed, then take when remembered (do not take more than 1 tab/day)
• Do not discontinue abruptly

ADVERSE EFFECTS
CNS: Headache
GI: Hepatotoxicity
GU: Decreased sperm counts
HEMA: Anemia
RESP: Pharyngitis, pulmonary edema, bronchitis

Pharmacokinetics
Absorption	Rapid
Distribution	Unknown
Metabolism	By CYP3A4, CYP2C19
Excretion	Unknown
Half-life	Terminal: 15 hr; effective: 9 hr

Pharmacodynamics
Onset	Unknown
Peak	2 hr
Duration	Unknown

INTERACTIONS
Drug classifications
CYP3A4 inhibitors: increased macitentan effect

Drug/herb
St. John's wort, ephedra (ma huang): require macitentan dosage change

NURSING CONSIDERATIONS
Assessment
• **Pulmonary status:** improvement in breathing, ability to exercise; pulmonary edema that may indicate veno-occlusive disease
• Blood studies: CBC with differential; Hct, Hgb may be decreased
• Liver function tests: AST, ALT. bilirubin

BLACK BOX WARNING: Assess pregnancy status before giving this product; pregnancy category X

Patient/family education
• Teach patient the importance of complying with dosage schedule even if feeling better
• Instruct patient to notify prescriber if pregnancy is planned or suspected (if pregnant, product will need to be discontinued; pregnancy test done monthly); to use 2 contraception methods while taking this product
• Instruct patient not to use OTC products including herbs, supplements, unless approved by prescriber
• Instruct patient to report to prescriber immediately: dizziness, faintness, chest pain, palpitations, uneven or rapid heart rate, headache, edema, weight gain
• Instruct patient not to split, crush, or chew tabs; if a dose is missed, take as soon as remembered (do not more than 1 tab per day); there are many drug interactions
• Teach patient the signs and symptoms of hepatotoxicity

Evaluation
Positive therapeutic outcome
• Decrease in B/P, decreased shortness of breath

mipomersen
(mye′poe-mer-sen)
Kynamro
Func. class.: Antilipemic
Chem. class.: Antisense oligonucleotide
Pregnancy category B

ACTION: Inhibits synthesis of the principal apoliprotein of LDL, VLDL, binds to messenger ribonucleic acid (mRNA)

Therapeutic outcome: Decreasing LDL, total cholesterol, apolipoprotein B, non-high density lipoprotein cholesterol

USES: Reduction of LDL, total cholesterol, apolipoprotein B, non–high-density lipoprotein cholesterol (homozygous familial hypercholesterolemia)

CONTRAINDICATIONS:

BLACK BOX WARNING: Hepatic disease

Precautions: Pregnancy (B), breastfeeding, dialysis, alcohol ingestion, geriatrics, proteinuria, renal disease, low-density lipoprotein apheresis

DOSAGE AND ROUTES
Homozygous familial hypercholesterolemia
Adult: Subcut 200 mg qwk

Renal/hepatic dose
Adult: Do not use in severe renal, hepatic disease

Dose adjustments for elevated transaminases during treatment
• ALT or AST ≥ 3× and < 5× ULN: confirm elevation with a repeat test within 1 wk. If confirmed, withhold product, obtain other tests if not already obtained (total bilirubin, alkaline phosphatase, INR) to identify the probable cause. If resuming product after transaminases resolve to <3× ULN, consider monitoring liver-related tests more frequently
• ALT or AST ≥ 5× ULN: withhold, obtain additional liver-related tests if not already obtained (total bilirubin, alkaline phosphatase, INR) and identify the probable cause. If resuming product after transaminases resolve to < 3× ULN, monitor liver-related tests more frequently

Available forms: Sol for injection 200 mg/ml

Implementation
• Give on the same day each wk; if a dose is missed, give ≥3 days from the next weekly dose
• Monitor ALT, AST, alkaline phosphatase, and total bilirubin prior to start of therapy; monitor lipid levels ≥q3-4 mo for the first year.
• Monitor LDL-C level after 6 mo

ADVERSE EFFECTS
CNS: Fatigue, headache, fever
CV: Hypertension, palpitations
GI: Abdominal pain, vomiting
GU: Glomerulonephritis, proteinuria
MS: Musculoskeletal pain
SYST: Angioedema

Pharmacokinetics	
Absorption	Unknown
Distribution	Protein binding >90%
Metabolism	Unknown
Excretion	Unknown
Half-life	1-2 mo

Onset	Unknown
Peak	Unknown
Duration	Unknown

INTERACTIONS
Individual drugs
Acetaminophen, methotrexate, tamoxifen, tetra-cyclines, tamoxifen: increased hepatotoxicity risk

NURSING CONSIDERATIONS
Assessment
• Determine if the LDL-C reduction achieved is sufficient to warrant the potential risk of liver toxicity
• Assess geriatric patients: increased risk for hypertension, peripheral edema, hepatic steatosis
• Hypercholesterolemia: diet history: fat content, lipid levels (triglycerides, LDL, HDL, cholesterol); LFTs at baseline, periodically during treatment

Patient/family education
• Teach patient/family that compliance is needed
• Instruct patient to decrease risk factors: high fat diet, smoking, alcohol consumption, absence of exercise
• Instruct patient to notify prescriber if pregnancy is suspected or planned or if breastfeeding
• Instruct patient to notify prescriber of dietary/herbal supplements

Evaluation
Positive therapeutic outcome
• Decreasing LDL, total cholesterol, apolipoprotein B, non-high density lipoprotein cholesterol

obinutuzumab
(oh′bi-nue-tooz′ue-mab)
Gazyva
Func. class.: Antineoplastic
Chem. class.: Biologic response modifier
Pregnancy category C

ACTION: A recombinant, human monoclonal antibody that binds to the gastric B-lymphocyte-associated antibody, action is indirect, possible through T-cell-mediated anti-tumor responses

Therapeutic outcome: Decreased disease progression

USES: Chronic lymphocytic leukemia

CONTRAINDICATIONS:
Hypersensitivity

Precautions: Pregnancy C, breastfeeding, cardiac disease, Children, human antichimeric antibody (HACA) human antimurine antibody (HAMA), infection, infusion-related reactions, neutropenia, pulmonary disease, thrombocytopenia, tumor lysis syndrome, vaccination

> **BLACK BOX WARNING:** Hepatitis, progressive multifocal leukoencephalopathy

DOSAGE AND ROUTES
Adult: **IV Cycle 1** 100 mg over 4 hr (day 1); then 900 mg (0 mg/hr, increased by 50 mg/hr q30min, to max 400 mg/hr) (day 2); then 1000 mg (100 mg/hr, increased by 100 mg/hr q30min to max 400 mg/hr) (day 8, day 115); **Cycle 2-6** 1000 mg (100 mg/hr increased by 100 mg/hr q30min to max 400 mg/hr (day 1 repeat q28 days)

Available forms: Sol for inj 1000 mg/40 ml

Implementation
IV intermittent infusion route
• Due to the risk of hypotension, consider withholding antihypertensive medications for 12 hr before, during, and for the 1st hr after use until BP is stable
• Give antimicrobial prophylaxis to neutropenic patients throughout treatment; consider antiviral and antifungal prophylaxis as needed
• **Premedication for cycle 1, days 1 and 2:** acetaminophen 650-1000 mg, and diphenhydrAMINE 50 mg at least 30 min prior to infusion, dexamethasone 20 mg IV or methylPREDNISolone 80 mg IV at least 1 hr before infusion
• **Premedication for cycle 1, days 8 and 15 and cycles 2-6, day 1:** acetaminophen 650-1000 mg at least 30 min prior to the infusion; those with any infusion-related reaction with the previous infusion should also receive diphenhydrAMINE 50 mg at least 30 min before the infusion; if the patient had a grade 3 infusion-related reaction with the previous dose or has a lymphocyte count $> 25 \times 10^9$/L, additionally administer dexamethasone 20 mg IV or methylPREDNISolone 80 mg IV at least 1 hr before infusion
• Use in a facility to adequately monitor and treat infusion reactions

• Visually inspect parenteral products for particulate matter and discoloration prior to use
• Prepare all doses in 0.9% NaCl; do not admix; use a final concentration of 0.4-4 mg/mL; give as an IV infusion only

Reconstitution

Cycle 1, day 1 and 2
• Withdraw 4 mL (100 mg) from the vial and dilute into 100 mL 0.9% NaCL; use on day 1; mix by gentle inversion; do not shake, use immediately
• Withdraw the remaining 36 mL (900 mg) and dilute into 250 mL 0.9% NaCl for use on day 2; mix by gentle inversion; do not shake

Cycle 1, day 8 and 15; cycles 2-6
• Withdraw 40 mL (1000 mg) from the vial and dilute into 250 mL 0.9% NaCl mix by gentle inversion; do not shake.
• Storage following reconstitution: Store at 2-8°C (36-46°F) for up to 24 hr. Do not freeze. Allow to come to room temperature before administration, use a dedicated line
• **Day 1 (100-mg dose):** Give at an initial rate of 25 mg/hr over 4 hr. Do not increase the infusion rate.
• **Day 2 (900-mg dose):** Give at an initial rate of 50 mg/hr × 30 min; if no hypersensitivity or infusion-related events occur, increase the infusion rate by 50 mg/hr q30min to a max rate of 400 mg/hr. If a grade 1-2 infusion-related reaction occurs, the infusion should be temporarily interrupted or the rate reduced. The infusion may be resumed or continued at a reduced rate upon improvement of the patient's symptoms; if the reaction does not recur, the rate may be increased as appropriate for the current cycle and dose. If a grade 3 hypersensitivity or infusion-related event develops, the infusion should be temporarily interrupted. Upon improvement of the patient's symptoms, the infusion can be resumed at half the rate being used at the time that the reaction occurred; if the reaction does not recur, the rate may be increased as appropriate for the current cycle and dose. If a grade 4 hypersensitivity or infusion-related event develops, discontinue the infusion and do not resume.
• **Subsequent infusions (1000-mg dose):** Give at an initial rate of 100 mg/hr for 30 min; if no hypersensitivity or infusion-related events occur, increase the infusion rate by 100 mg/hr q30min to a max rate of 400 mg/hr; if a grade 1-2 infusion-related reaction occurs, the infusion should be temporarily interrupted or the rate reduced. The infusion may be resumed or continued at a reduced rate upon improve-

ment of the patient's symptoms; if the reaction does not recur, the rate may be increased as appropriate for the current cycle and dose. If a grade 3 hypersensitivity or infusion-related event develops, the infusion should be temporarily interrupted. Upon improvement of the patient's symptoms, the infusion can be resumed at half the rate being used at the time that the reaction occurred; if the reaction does not recur, the rate may be increased as appropriate for the current cycle and dose. If a grade 4 hypersensitivity or infusion-related event develops, discontinue the infusion and do not resume

ADVERSE EFFECTS
CNS: Headache, fever, chills, flushing
CV: Cardiac arrest, MI, sinus tachycardia, hypertension
GI: Constipation, decreased appetite, diarrhea, hepatitis/hepatic failure nausea, vomiting
HEMA: Neutropenia, thrombocytopenia, lymphopenia, leukopenia
META: Lower potassium/sodium/calcium, aluminum, higher potassium/uric acid
RESP: Wheezing, dyspnea
SYST: Tumor lysis syndrome

Pharmacokinetics

Absorption	Unknown
Distribution	Unknown
Metabolism	Unknown
Excretion	Unknown
Half-life	Terminal half-life 28.4 days

Pharmacodynamics

Onset	Unknown
Peak	Unknown
Duration	Unknown

NURSING CONSIDERATIONS
Assessment

BLACK BOX WARNING: Hepatitis B: reactivation of HBV in those who are HBsAg positive, HBsAg negative and core antibody anti-HBc positive; may result in fulminant hepatitis, hepatic failure and death

BLACK BOX WARNING: Progressive multifocal leukoencephalopathy (PML): Notify prescriber any new or worsening neurological signs/symptoms (ataxia, visual changes, confusion)

⚠ Tumor lysis syndrome: Can occur within 24 hr of 1st infusion, those with high tumor burden or lymphocyte count >25×10⁹/L are at increased risk; monitor serum creatinine, potassium, calcium, uric acid, phosphate closely

> **BLACK BOX WARNING:** Severe/life-threatening infusion reactions: 2/3 of patients have a reaction to 1st dose; consider withholding antihypertensives for 12 hr prior to, during, and after 1st hr of infusion

Patient/family education
• Teach patient about the reason for treatment and expected results

Evaluation
Positive therapeutic outcome
• Decreased disease progression

pomalidomide
(pom-a-lid′o-mide)
Pomalyst
Func. class.: TNF modifier
Chem. class.: Antineoplastic, biologic response modifier, hormone
Pregnancy category X

ACTION: Inhibits growth of tumor cells and induces apoptosis; can be used in those resistant to lenalidomide

Therapeutic outcome: Decreased growth of tumor cells

USES: Multiple myeloma in those who have received ≥2 treatments including lenalidomide and bortezomib, and in whom disease has progressed within 60 days of completion of the treatment

CONTRAINDICATIONS:
Breastfeeding, hypersensitivity

> **BLACK BOX WARNING:** Pregnancy (X)

Precautions: Children, geriatric patients, accidental exposure, bone marrow suppression, uterine bleeding, dental disease, fungal/viral infections, smoking

> **BLACK BOX WARNING:** Thrombocytopenia

DOSAGE AND ROUTES
Adult: PO 4 mg on days 1-21

Hepatic/renal dose
Adult: PO bilirubin >2 mg/dl and AST/ALT >3× ULN or CCr >3 mg/dl, do not use

Available forms: Tabs 1, 2, 3, 4 mg
Implementation
• With or without dexamethasone; may use dexamethasone 40 mg on days 1, 8, 15, 22 of each cycle; if age >75 yr, decrease dexamethasone to 20 mg/dose

ADVERSE EFFECTS
CNS: Dizziness, fatigue, fever, headache, peripheral neuropathy
CV: Chest pain
GI: Constipation, diarrhea, nausea/vomiting
HEMA: Leukopenia, neutropenia, thrombocytopenia
META: Hypokalemia
MS: Arthralgia, back pain
RESP: Cough, dyspnea, **pulmonary embolism**, epistaxis
SYST: Secondary malignancy

Pharmacokinetics
Absorption	Unknown
Distribution	12%-44% protein binding
Metabolism	Unknown
Excretion	Unknown
Half-life	Unknown

Pharmacodynamics
Onset	Unknown
Peak	Unknown
Duration	Unknown

INTERACTIONS
Drug classifications
CYP3A4 inducers (rifampin, rifapentine, rifabutin, primadone, phenytoin, PHENobarbital, nevirapine, nafacillin, modafinil, griseofulvin, etravirine, efavirenz, barbiturates, bexarotene, bosentan, carBAMazepine, enzalutamide, dexamethasone): decreased pomalidomide effect; avoid concurrent use
CYP3A4 inhibitors (amprenavir, bocenavir, delavirdine, ketoconazole, indinavir, itraconazole, dalfopristin/quinupristin, ritonavir, tipranavir, fluconazole, isoniazid, miconazole); P-gb inhibitors: increased pomalidomide effect; avoid concurrent use

NURSING CONSIDERATIONS
Assessment

> **BLACK BOX WARNING:** Blood studies: monitor Hct, Hgb; thrombolytic disease may occur

BLACK BOX WARNING: Monitor for pregnancy before treatment, pregnancy X

Patient/family education
• Instruct patient to avoid driving or hazardous activity during beginning of treatment

BLACK BOX WARNING: Advise patient to use adequate contraception, pregnancy (X)

Evaluation
Positive therapeutic outcome
• Decreased growth of tumor cells

riociguat
(rye′oh-sig′ue-at)
Adempas
Func. class.: Antihypertensive/vasodilator
Chem. class.: Guanylate cyclase stimulator
Pregnancy category X

ACTION: Guanylate cyclase stimulator; also a vasoconstrictor

Therapeutic outcome: Decrease in B/P; decreased shortness of breath

USES: WHO group I pulmonary arterial hypertension and WHO Group IV persistent/recurrent chronic thromboembolic pulmonary hypertension

CONTRAINDICATIONS:
Breastfeeding, hypersensitivity

BLACK BOX WARNING: Pregnancy (X)

Precautions: Hypotension, hypovolemia, pulmonary edema, smoking

DOSAGE AND ROUTES
1 mg tid, may start at 0.5 mg tid if needed; if systolic B/P remains >95 mmHg, increase by 0.5 mg tid; increase no sooner than 2 wk, max 2.5 mg tid

Renal/hepatic dose
Adult: Not recommended in CCr <15ml/min or Child Pugh C

Available forms: Tabs 0.5, 1, 1.5, 2, 2.5 mg

Implementation
• Give tid without regard to food
• Do not discontinue abruptly

• If dose is missed, take at next scheduled dose; if stopped for ≥3 days, begin with initial dose

ADVERSE EFFECTS
CNS: Dizziness
CV: Hypotension, peripheral edema, palpitations
EENT: Sinusitis, rhinitis
GI: Constipation, gastritis, gastroesophageal reflux, nausea, vomiting
GU: Decreased sperm counts
HEMA: Anemia, bleeding, nosebleeds
RESP: Pulmonary edema

Pharmacokinetics
Absorption	Unknown
Distribution	95% protein binding
Metabolism	By P-gb, CYP1A1, CYP3A4, CYP#A, CYP2C8, CYP2J2
Excretion	Unknown
Half-life	Terminal 15 hr

Pharmacodynamics
Onset	Unknown
Peak	1.5 hr
Duration	Unknown

INTERACTIONS
Drug classifications
CYP3A4 inhibitors (amprenavir, aprepitant, atazanavir, clarithromycin, conivaptan, cyclo-SPORINE, dalfopristin, danazol, darunavir, erythromycin, estradiol, imatinib, itraconazole, ketoconazole, nefazodone, nelfinavir, propoxyphene, quinupristin, ritonavir, RU-486, saquinavir, tamoxifen, telithromycin, troleandomycin, zafirlukast): increased riociguat effect
Nitrates, nitric oxide donors, phosphodiesterase-5 inhibitors: do not use concurrently
Tobacco smoking: decreased riociguat effect

Drug/Herbs
St. John's wort, ephedra (ma huang): require dosage change

NURSING CONSIDERATIONS
Assessment
• Pulmonary status: assess for improvement in breathing, ability to exercise; pulmonary edema may indicate veno-occlusive disease

BLACK BOX WARNING: Assess pregnancy status before giving this product; pregnancy category X

Patient/family education
• Teach patient the importance of complying with dosage schedule even if feeling better

> **BLACK BOX WARNING:** Teach patient to notify if pregnancy is planned or suspected (if pregnant, product will need to be discontinued, pregnancy test done monthly); to use 2 contraception methods while taking this product

• Instruct patient not to use OTC products including herbs, supplements, unless approved by prescriber

Evaluation
Positive therapeutic outcome
• Decrease in B/P; decreased shortness of breath

---

simeprevir
(sim-e′pre-vir)
Olysio
Func. class.: Antiviral, anti-hepatitis agent
Pregnancy category X

ACTION: Prevents formation of mature viral proteins by inhibiting hepatitis C viral (HCV) replication by blocking proteolytic activity of the hepatitis C virus NS3/4A protease

Therapeutic outcome: Decreased symptoms of chronic hepatitis C

USES: Chronic hepatitis C infection, hepatitis, (HCV, genotype 1) in adults with compensated liver disease

CONTRAINDICATIONS:
Hypersensitivity, male-mediated teratogenicity, pregnancy (X) in combination

Precautions: Pregnancy C,(alone), breastfeeding, Asian patients, liver transplant, UV exposure, hepatic disease, serious rash, children

DOSAGE AND ROUTES
Adult: **PO** 150 mg/day with food with peginterferon alfa and ribavirin × 12 wk

Available forms: Cap 150 mg

Implementation
• Give by mouth with food, swallow whole
• Do not use monotherapy; if peginterferon alfa or ribavirin are discontinued, discontinue simeprevir and do not restart
• Obtain NS3 Q80K polymorphism test before starting treatment

• Treatment-naïve/prior relapse: after initial 3-drug treatment, give another 12 wk with peginterferon alfa and ribavirin × another 12 wk; if HCV RNA concentrations ≥25 interstitial units/ml, discontinue all 3 drugs
• Prior nonresponders (partial/null): after initial 3-drug treatment give an additional 36 wk of peginterferon alfa and ribavirin; monitor HCV RNA at wk 4, 12, 24; if ≥25 interstitial units/ml, discontinue products

ADVERSE EFFECTS
EENT: Blurred vision, conjunctivitis
GI: Hyperbilirubinemia, nausea
INTEG: exfoliative dermatitis, pruritus, photosensitivity, vasculitis
MISC: Rash, dyspnea

Pharmacokinetics
Absorption	Unknown
Distribution	99.9 % protein binding
Metabolism	Primarily by CYP3A4, also a mild inhibitor of intestinal CYP3A4 and CYP1A2
Excretion	91% feces
Half-life	40 hr

Pharmacodynamics
Onset	Unknown
Peak	Unknown
Duration	Unknown

INTERACTIONS
Individual drugs
Bromocriptone, chloramphenicol, cimetidine, dalfopristin/quinupristin, danazol, erythromycin, FLUoxetine, isoniazid, lanreotide, octreotide, zafirlukast: increased simeprevir effect

Drug classifications
CYP3A4 inhibitors: increased effects of these agents

NURSING CONSIDERATIONS
Assessment
• Allergic reaction: assess for rash, pruritus, exfoliative dermatitis
• Asian patients: levels may be 3-fold to 4-fold higher
⚠ **Pregnancy: if planned or suspected; if pregnant call the Pregnancy Registry 800-258-4263, pregnancy X in combination**
• Liver function tests; Monitor HCV, RNA concentrations at weeks 4, 12 and 24 and at end of treatment
• Pregnancy tests

Adverse effects: *italics* = common; **bold** = life-threatening

Patient/family education

• Teach patient that optimal duration of treatment is unknown, that product is not a cure, that transmission may still occur
• Teach patient to avoid use with other medications unless approved by prescriber
• Teach patient to use protective clothing, sunscreen; photosensitivity may occur and can be severe
• Teach patient not to stop abruptly unless directed; worsening of hepatitis may occur

⚠ **Teach patient to notify prescriber if pregnancy is planned or suspected, avoid breastfeeding; use 2 reliable forms of contraception, do not try to conceive for at least 6 mo after discontinuation of this drug combination**

• Teach patient to use cautiously in sulfonamide allergy; do not take the drug as single agent; must use as combination therapy

Evaluation

Positive therapeutic outcome
• Decreased symptoms of chronic hepatitis C

---

sofosbuvir
(soe-fos'bue-vir)
Sovaldi
Func. class.: Antiviral, antihepatitis agent
Chem. class.: Adenosine monophosphate analog
Pregnancy category B

ACTION: Inhibits hepatitis C virus RNA polymerase by incorporating the polymerase into the viral RNA, also acts as a chain terminator

Therapeutic outcome: Decreased symptoms of chronic hepatitis C

USES: Chronic hepatitis C (genotypes 1, 2, 3, 4) with compensated liver disease

CONTRAINDICATIONS:
Hypersensitivity, pregnancy (X) in combination; male-mediated teratogenicity

Precautions: Pregnancy (B) breastfeeding, children, hepatic/renal disease

DOSAGE AND ROUTES

Genotype 1, 4
Adult: PO 400 mg/day with peginterferon alfa and ribavirin × 12 wk; may consider use for genotype 1 with ribavirin × 24 wk

Genotype 2
Adult: PO 400 mg/day with ribavirin × 12 wk

Genotype 3
Adult: PO 400 mg/day with ribavirin × 24 wk

Available forms: Tabs 400 mg

Implementation
• Give by mouth without regard to food
• Do not use as monotherapy

ADVERSE EFFECTS
CNS: Headache, chills, weakness, fatigue, fever, insomnia
GI: Diarrhea, hyperbilirubinemia
MISC: Rash, pruritus, neutropenia, anemia, myalgia

Pharmacokinetics

Absorption	Unknown
Distribution	61%-65% protein
Metabolism	Unknown
Excretion	By kidneys 80%
Half-life	0.4-27 hr

Pharmacodynamics

Onset	Unknown
Peak	½-2 hr
Duration	Unknown

INTERACTIONS
Individual drugs
OXcarbazepine, rifabutin, rifapentine, tipranavir: decreased sofosbuvir effect, avoid concurrent use

Drug classifications
P-glycoprotein (P-gp) inducers (carBAMazepine, PHENobarbital, phenytoin, rifampin): decreased sofosbuvir effect, avoid concurrent use

NURSING CONSIDERATIONS
Assessment
• Severe renal disease /eGFR <30 ml/min/1.73 m^2): monitor BUN, creatinine
• Monitor geriatric patients more carefully; may develop renal, cardiac symptoms more rapidly

⚠ **Pregnancy: if planned or suspected; if pregnant call the Pregnancy Registry 800-258-4263, obtain pregnancy test before starting treatment**

Patient/family education
• Teach patient that optimal duration of treatment is unknown, that product is not a cure, that transmission may still occur

---

• Instruct patient to avoid use with other medications unless approved by prescriber
• Instruct patient not to stop abruptly unless directed, worsening of hepatitis may occur
⚠ **Teach patient to notify prescriber if pregnancy is planned or suspected, use 2 forms of reliable contraception, avoid breastfeeding**

Evaluation
Positive therapeutic outcome
• Therapeutic response: decreased symptoms of chronic hepatitis C

---

teduglutide
(te'due-gloo'tide)
Gattex
Func. class.: GI disorder agent
Chem. class.: Recombinant glucagon-like peptide-2 analog
Pregnancy category B

ACTION: Increases intestinal, portal blood flow, inhibits gastric acid secretion, decreases gastric motility

Therapeutic outcome: Increased absorption of nutrients

USES: Short bowel syndrome in patients who are dependent on parenteral support

Precautions: Pregnancy C, breastfeeding, diarrhea, pancreatitis, renal disease, electrolyte imbalances, GI obstruction, heart failure, neoplastic disease, bilary tract disease, cardiac disease gastric cancer, GI disease

DOSAGE AND ROUTES
Adult: Subcut 0.05 mg/kg/day

Available forms: Powder for injection 5 mg

Implementation
Subcut route
• *Reconstitution:* Slowly inject the 0.5 ml of preservative-free sterile water for injection provided in the prefilled syringe into the vial ; allow to stand for 30 sec and gently roll the vial between your palms for 15 sec; do not shake; allow to stand 2 min; if undissolved powder is present, roll the vial again until all material is dissolved; if the product remains undissolved after the second attempt, do not use; discard unused portion; use within 3 hr after reconstitution

Subcut injection
• Calculate dose, withdraw into a syringe, and give; do not use IV, IM; if a dose is missed, it should be given as soon as possible on the same day; two doses should not be given on the same day; alternate sites

ADVERSE EFFECTS
CNS: Headache, fatigue
GI: Nausea, abdominal pain, cholecystitis, cholestasis, GI obstruction, pancreatitis, vomiting

Pharmacokinetics
Absorption	Unknown
Distribution	Unknown
Metabolism	Unknown
Excretion	Unknown
Half-life	2 hr; 1.3 hr (short bowel syndrome)

Pharmacodynamics
Onset	Unknown
Peak	Unknown
Duration	Unknown

INTERACTIONS
Individual drugs
Benzodiazepine, carBAMazepine, cycloSPORINE, digoxin, disopyramide, ethosuximide, flecainamide, lerothyromixe, lithium, phenytoin, procainamide, quiNIDine, sirolimus, tacrolimus, theophylline, valproic acid, warfarin: increased absorption of each of these products

NURSING CONSIDERATIONS
Assessment
• GI symptoms: nausea, abdominal pain
• Monitor alk phos, amylase, bilirubin, serum electrolytes, lipase—baseline and q6mo

Patient/family education
• Instruct patient to notify prescriber of GI symptoms

Evaluation
Positive therapeutic outcome
• Increased absorption of nutrients

Adverse effects: *italics* = common; **bold** = life-threatening

trametinib
(tra-me′ti-nib)
MeKinist
Func. class.: Antineoplastic biologic response modifier
Chem. class.: Signal transduction inhibitor (STI), tyrosine kinase inhibitor
Pregnancy category D

ACTION: Inhibits MEK-1, MEK-2 tyrosine kinase created in patients with malignant melanoma

Therapeutic outcome: Decrease in progression of disease

USES: Unresectable or metastatic BRAD V600E or BRAF V600K mutated malignant melanoma

CONTRAINDICATIONS: Pregnancy (D), hypersensitivity

Precautions: Breastfeeding, children, diarrhea, geriatric patients, hepatic disease, bone marrow suppression, infection, thrombocytopenia, neutropenia, immunosuppression

DOSAGE AND ROUTES
Adult: PO 2 mg/day, may be used in combination with dacarbazine or PACLitaxel in those with BRAF V600E

Management of treatment-related toxicity
Cutaneous toxicity
• *Grade 2 rash:* reduce dose by 0.5 mg (e.g., 2 mg/day to 1.5 mg/day) or discontinue in patients who are receiving trametinib 1 mg/day. In patients with an intolerable grade 2 rash that does not improve within 3 wk of a dosage reduction, withhold trametinib for up to 3 wk. If the rash is improved within 3 wk, resume therapy at a lower dose (reduce the previous dose by 0.5 mg). If the rash does not improve within 3 wk, permanently discontinue
• *Grade 3 or 4 rash:* withhold for up to 3 wk. If the rash is improved within 3 wk, resume at a lower dose (reduce the previous dose by 0.5 mg); discontinue in patients who are receiving trametinib 1 mg/day. If the rash does not improve within 3 wk, permanently discontinue
Cardiac toxicity
• Asymptomatic cardiac toxicity and an absolute decrease in LVEF of ≥10% from baseline and below institutional lower limits of normal (LLN)

from pretreatment value: withhold for up to 4 wk. If the LVEF is improved within 4 wk, resume at a lower dose (reduce the previous dose by 0.5 mg); discontinue in patients who are receiving 1 mg/day; if the LVEF does not improve to normal within 4 wk, permanently discontinue
• Symptomatic CHF or an absolute decrease in LVEF of >20% from baseline and below institutional LLN: permanently discontinue
Ocular toxicity
• *Grade 2 or 3 retinal pigment epithelial detachment (RPED)*: withhold for up to 3 wk. If the RPED improves to grade 1 or less within 3 wk, resume at a lower dose (reduce the previous dose by 0.5 mg); discontinue therapy in patients who are receiving 1 mg/day. If the RPED does not improve to at least grade 1 within 3 wk, permanently discontinue
• *Retinal vein occlusion*: permanently discontinue therapy
Pulmonary toxicity
• Interstitial lung disease/pneumonitis: permanently discontinue
Other toxicity
• *Grade 3 toxicity:* withhold for up to 3 wk. If the toxicity improves to grade 1 or less within 3 wk, resume at a lower dose (reduce the previous dose by 0.5 mg); discontinue in patients who are receiving 1 mg/day. If the toxicity does not improve to at least grade 1 within 3 wk, permanently discontinue
• *Grade 4 toxicity:* permanently discontinue

Available forms: Tabs 0.5, 2 mg

Implementation
• Give 1 hr before or 2 hr after a meal
• If dose is missed, take within 12 hr of missed dose; if >12 hr have passed, skip dose
• Follow cytotoxic handling procedures

ADVERSE EFFECTS
CNS: Dizziness
CV: Heart failure, hypertension, cardiomyopathy
EENT: Occular hemorrhage, retinal detachment, blurred vision
GI: Diarrhea, nausea, vomiting, abdominal pain, stomatitis
GU: Hematuria
INTEG: Rash, pruritus, acne, folliculitis, erythema
MISC: Elevated LFTs, hand-foot syndrome
MS: Rhabdomolysis
RESP: Cough, dyspnea, pleural effusion, pneumonitis, edema

Pharmacokinetics

Absorption	Unknown
Distribution	Protein binding 97.4%
Metabolism	Unknown
Excretion	In feces
Half-life	Unknown

Pharmacodynamics

Onset	Unknown
Peak	1.5 hr
Duration	Unknown

INTERACTIONS
None known

NURSING CONSIDERATIONS
Assessment
• Monitor LFTs every mo × 3 mo, then as clinically indicated

Patient/family education
• Teach patient to report adverse reactions immediately, bleeding
• Teach patient about reason for treatment, expected results
• Teach patient to use effective contraception during treatment and up to 30 days after discontinuing treatment

Evaluation
Positive therapeutic outcome
• Decrease in progression of disease

---

vortioxetine
(vor'tye-ox'e-teen)
Brintellix
Func. class.: Antidepressant
Chem. class.: Serotonin modulator
Pregnancy category C

ACTION: Reuptake inhibition at the serotonin transporter and agonist, or antagonist effects at serotonin receptors

Therapeutic outcome: Decreased depression

USES: Major depressive disorder in adults

CONTRAINDICATIONS:
Hypersensitivity, MAOI therapy

Precautions: Pregnancy C, breastfeeding, seizure disorder, hypersensitivity, bipolar disorder, hyponatremia, hypovolemia, children, suicidal ideation

DOSAGE AND ROUTES
Adult: PO 10 mg/day, may start with 5 mg/day initially, increase to 20 mg/day as tolerated, max 20 mg/day; poor metabolizers of CYP2D6 max 10 mg/day

Available forms: Tabs 5, 10, 20 mg

Implementation
• Give without regard to food

ADVERSE EFFECTS
CNS: Flushing, mania, serotonin syndrome, vertigo, dizziness, suicidal attempts
GI: Nausea, diarrhea, dyspnea, constipation, vomiting, flatulence
GU: Impotence
INTEG: Pruritus
SYST: Serotonin syndrome, neonatal abstinence syndrome

Pharmacokinetics

Absorption	Unknown
Distribution	Protein binding 98%
Metabolism	Unknown
Excretion	Urine (59%), feces (26%)
Half-life	Unknown

Pharmacodynamics

Onset	Unknown
Peak	Unknown
Duration	Unknown

INTERACTIONS
Individual drugs
CarBAMazepine: decreased vortioxetine levels
Lithium, traMADol, traZODone: increased serotonin syndrome

Drug classifications
Anticoagulants, antiplatelets, NSAIDs, salicylates, thrombolytics: increased bleeding risk
Barbiturates, sedative/hypnotics, other CNS depressants: increased CNS effects
Serotonin receptor agonists, SSRIs, MAOIs, SNRIs (venlafaxine, DULoxetine): increased serotonin syndrome
Tricyclics: increased effect of tricyclics; use cautiously

Drug/herb
St. John's wort: increased serotonin syndrome

NURSING CONSIDERATIONS
Assessment

> **BLACK BOX WARNING:** Mental status: assess mood, sensorium, affect, suicidal tendencies, increase in psychiatric symptoms, depression, panic

• Serotonin syndrome: monitor for increased heart rate, sweating, dilated pupils, tremors, twitching, hyperthermia, agitation
• Alcohol consumption: if alcohol is consumed, hold dose until AM
• Sexual dysfunction: assess for impotence

Patient/family education
• Teach patient that therapeutic effect may take several wk
• Teach patient to use caution when driving, performing other activities that require alertness, because of drowsiness, dizziness, blurred vision; to report signs, symptoms or bleeding

• Teach patient to avoid alcohol, other CNS depressants

> **BLACK BOX WARNING:** Teach patient that suicidal ideas, behaviors may occur in children or young adults

• Teach patient to notify prescriber if pregnant, planning to become pregnant, or breastfeeding, pregnancy C

> **BLACK BOX WARNING:** Teach patient about the effects of serotonin syndrome: nausea/vomiting, tremors; if symptoms occur, to discontinue immediately, notify prescriber

Evaluation
Positive therapeutic outcome
• Decreased depression

Appendix B

Ophthalmic, Nasal, Topical, and Otic Products

OPHTHALMIC PRODUCTS

α-ADRENERGIC BLOCKER
dapiprazole (Rx)
(da-pip'ra-zole)
Rev-Eyes

ANESTHETICS
lidocaine (Rx)
(lye'doe-kane)
Akten
proparacaine (Rx)
(proe-par'a-kane)
Alcaine, Diocaine ♣, Ophthaine, Ophthetic
tetracaine (Rx)
(tet'ra-kane)
Minims Tetracaine ♣, Pontocaine, Tetracaine

ANTIHISTAMINES
alcaftadine
(al-caf'tah-deen)
Lastacalf
azelastine (Rx)
(ay-zell'ah-steen)
Optivar
emedastine (Rx)
(ee-med'a-steen)
Emadine
epinastine (Rx)
(ep-een-as'teen)
Elestat
ketotifen (Rx, OTC)
(kee-toh-tif'en)
Zaditor
levocabastine (Rx)
(lee-voh-cab'ah-steen)
Livostin
olopatadine (Rx)
(oh-loh-pat'ah-deen)
Patanol

ANTIINFECTIVES
azithromycin (Rx)
(ay-zi-thro-my'sin)
AzaSite
besifloxacin (Rx)
(be'si-flox'a-sin)
Besivance
chloramphenicol (Rx)
(klor-am-fen'i-kole)
AK-Chlor, Chloramphenicol, Chloromycetin Ophthalmic, Chloroptic, Chloroptic S.O.P., Fenicol ♣, Isopto Fenical ♣, Pentamycin ♣
ciprofloxacin (Rx)
(sip-ro-floks'a-sin)
Ciloxan
erythromycin (Rx)
(er-ith-roe-mye'sin)
Erythromycin, Ilotycin
ganciclovir (Rx)
(gan-sye'kloe-vir)
Virgan
gatifloxacin (Rx)
(gat-ih-floks'ah-sin)
Zymar, Zymaxid
gentamicin (Rx)
(jen-ta-mye'sin)
Garamycin Ophthalmic, Genoptic Ophthalmic, Genoptic S.O.P., Gentacidin, Gentamicin Ophthalmic, Gentak
levofloxacin (Rx)
(lee-voh-flock'sah-sin)
Quixin
moxifloxacin (Rx)
(mox-i-flox'a-sin)
Vigamox
natamycin (Rx)
(nat-a-mye'sin)
Natacyn

norfloxacin (Rx)
(nor-floks'a-sin)
Chibroxin
ofloxacin (Rx)
(oh-floks'a-sin)
Ocuflox
silver nitrate 1% (Rx)
silver nitrate
sulfacetamide sodium (Rx)
(sul-fa-seet'a-mide)
AK-Sulf, Bleph-10, Bleph-10
S.O.P., Cetamide, Isopto Cetamide,
Ocusulf-10, Sodium Sulamyd, Sodium
Sulfacetamide, Storzsulf, Sulf-10,
Sulster
tobramycin (Rx)
(toe-bra-mye'sin)
AKTob, Defy, Tobrex
trifluridine (Rx)
(trye-floor'i-deen)
Viroptic
vidarabine (Rx)
(vye-dare'a-been)
Vira-A

β-ADRENERGIC BLOCKERS
betaxolol (Rx)
(beh-tax'oh-lole)
Betoptic, Betoptic S
carteolol (Rx)
(kar-tee'oh-lole)
Carteolol HCl, Ocupress
levobetaxolol (Rx)
(lee-voh-beh-tax'oh-lohl)
Betaxon
levobunolol (Rx)
(lee-voe-byoo'no-lole)
AK Beta, Betagen
metipranolol (Rx)
(met-ee-pran'oh-lole)
OptiPranolol
timolol (Rx)
(tym'moe-lole)
Apo-Timop ✦, Betimol, Timoptic,
Timoptic-XE

**CARBONIC ANHYDRASE
INHIBITORS**
brinzolamide (Rx)
(brin-zoh'la-mide)
Azopt
dorzolamide (Rx)
(dor-zol'a-mide)
Trusopt

**CHOLINERGICS
(Direct-acting)**
acetylcholine (Rx)
(ah-see-til-koe'leen)
Miochol-E
carbachol (Rx)
(kar'ba-kole)
**Carbastat, Carboptic, Isopto
Carbachol, Miostat**
pilocarpine (Rx)
(pye-loe-kar'peen)
**Adsorbocarpine, Akarpine, Isopto
Carpine, Ocu-Carpine, Ocusert Pilo-
20, Ocusert Pilo-40, Pilagan, Pilocar,
pilocarpine, Pilopine HS, Piloptic-1/2,
Piloptic-1, Piloptic-2, Piloptic-3,
Piloptic-4, Piloptic-6, Pilostat,
Pilopto-Carpine**

**CHOLINESTERASE
INHIBITORS**
demecarium (Rx)
(dem-e-kare'ee-um)
Humorsol
ecothiophate (Rx)
(ek-oh-thye'oh-fate)
Phospholine Iodide
isoflurophate (Rx)
(i-se'flur-e'fate)
Floropryl
physostigmine (Rx)
(fi-zoe-stig'meen)
Eserine Salicylate, Isopto Eserine

CORTICOSTEROIDS
dexamethasone (Rx)
(dex-a-meth'a-sone)
**AK-Dex, Decadron Phosphate,
Dexamethasone Ophthalmic
Suspension, Maxidex, Ozurdex**

fluocinolone (Rx)
(floo-oh-sin'oh-lone)
Retisert

fluorometholone (Rx)
(flure-oh-meth'oh-lone)
Flarex, Fluor-Op, FML, FML Forte, FML S.O.P.

loteprednol (Rx)
(loe-tee-pred-nole)
Alrex, Lotemax

medrysone (Rx)
(me'dri-sone)
HMS

prednisoLONE (Rx)
(pred-niss'oh-lone)
Econopred, Econopred Plus, AK-Pred, Inflamase Forte, Inflamase Mild, Pred-Forte

rimexolone (Rx)
(ri-mex'a-lone)
Vexol

triamcinolone (Rx)
(trye-am-sin'oh-lone)
Triesence

MYDRIATICS
atropine (Rx)
(a'troe-peen)
Atropine-1, Atropine Care, Atropine Sulfate Ophthalmic, Atropisol, Isopto Atropine

cyclopentolate (Rx)
(sye-kloe-pen'toe-late)
AK-Pentolate, Cyclogyl, Cyclopentolate HCl

homatropine (Rx)
(home-a'troe-peen)
Homatropine HBr, Isopto Homatropine, Minims Homatropine ♣

phenylephrine (OTC)
(fen-ill-ef'rin)
AK-Dilate, AK-Nefrin, Isopto Frin, Neo-Synephrine 2.5%, Neo-Synephrine 10%, phenylephrine HCl, 2.5% Mydfrin, Phenoptic Relief, Prefrin

scopolamine (Rx)
(skoe-pol'a-meen)
Isopto Hyoscine

tropicamide (Rx)
(troe-pik'a-mide)
Mydriacyl, Opticyl, Tropicacyl, Tropicamide

NONSTEROIDAL ANTIINFLAMMATORIES
bromfenac (Rx)
(brome'fen-ak)
Xibrom

diclofenac (Rx)
(dye-kloe'fen-ak)
Voltaren

flurbiprofen (Rx)
(flure-bi'pro-fen)
Ocufen

ketorolac (Rx)
(kee-toe'role-ak)
Acular, Acuvail

nepafenac (Rx)
(ne-pa-fen'ak)
Nevanac

suprofen (Rx)
(soo-proe'fen)
Profenal

SYMPATHOMIMETICS
apraclonidine (Rx)
(a-pra-klon'i-deen)
Iopidine

brimonidine (Rx)
(brem-on'i-dine)
Alphagan, Alphagan P

dipivefrin (Rx)
(dye-pi'vef-rin)
Propine, AKPro

epINEPHrine/epinephryl borate (Rx)
(ep-i-nef'rin)
Epifrin, Glaucon/Epinal, Eppy ♣

OPHTHALMIC DECONGESTANTS/ VASOCONSTRICTORS
lodoxamide
(loe-dox'ah-mide)
Alomide

---

naphazoline (Rx, OTC)
(naf-az'oh-leen)
20/20 Eye Drops, AK-Con, Albalon, Allerest Eye Drops, Allergy Drops, Clear Eyes, Clear Eyes ACR, Comfort Eye Drops, Degest 2, Maximum Strength Allergy Drops, Nafazair, naphazoline HCl, Naphcon, Naphcon Forte, Opcon, Vasoclear, Vasocon Regular

oxymetazoline (Rx)
(ox-i-met-ah-zoh'leen)
OcuClear, Visine L.R.

tetrahydrozoline (OTC)
(tet-ra-hye-dro'zoe-leen)
Collyrium Fresh, Eyesine, Geneye, Geneye Extra, Mallazine Eye Drops, Murine Plus, Optigene 3, tetrahydrozoline HCl, Tetrasine, Tetrasine Extra, Visine Moisturizing

MISCELLANEOUS OPHTHALMICS
bimatoprost (Rx)
(bih-mat'o-prost)
Latisse, Lumigan
latanoprost (Rx)
(la-tan'oh-prost)
Xalatan
travoprost (Rx)
(tra'voe-prost)
Travatan
unoprostone (Rx)
(yoo-noe-pros'tone)
Rescula

β-Adrenergic blockers
ACTION: Reduces production of aqueous humor by unknown mechanism

USES: Ocular hypertension, chronic open angle glaucoma

Anesthetics
ACTION: Decreases ion permeability by stabilizing neuronal membrane

USES: Cataract extraction, tonometry, gonioscopy, removal of foreign objects, corneal suture removal, glaucoma surgery (ophthalmic); pruritus, sunburn, toothache, sore throat, cold sores, oral pain, rectal pain and irritation, control of gagging (topical)

Antiinfectives
ACTION: Inhibits folic acid synthesis by preventing PABA use, which is necessary for bacterial growth

USES: Conjunctivitis, superficial eye infections, corneal ulcers, prophylaxis against infection after removal of foreign matter from the eye

Antiinflammatories
ACTION: Decreases inflammation, resulting in decreased pain, photophobia, hyperemia, cellular infiltration

USES: Inflammation of eye, eyelids, conjunctiva, cornea; uveitis, iridocyclitis, allergic conditions, burns, foreign bodies, postoperatively in cataract

Carbonic anhydrase inhibitor
ACTION: Converted to epINEPHrine, which decreases aqueous production and increases outflow

USES: Open angle glaucoma, ocular hypertension

Direct-acting miotic
ACTION: Acts directly on cholinergic receptor sites; induces miosis, spasm of accommodation, fall in intraocular pressure, caused by stimulation of ciliary, pupillary sphincter muscles, which leads to pulling away of iris from filtration angle, resulting in increased outflow of aqueous humor

USES: Primary glaucoma, early stages of wide angle glaucoma (less useful in advanced stages), chronic open angle glaucoma, acute closed angle glaucoma before emergency surgery; also neutralizes mydriatics used during eye exam; may be used alternately with mydriatics to break adhesions between iris and lens

CONTRAINDICATIONS:
Hypersensitivity

Precautions: Pregnancy, breastfeeding, children, aphakia, hypersensitivity to carbonic anhydrase inhibitors, sulfonamides, thiazide diuretics, ocular inhibitors, renal/hepatic insufficiency

Implementation
• Storage at room temperature away from light

ADVERSE EFFECTS
CNS: Headache
CV: Hypertension, tachycardia, dysrhythmias
EENT: Burning, stinging
GI: Bitter taste

NURSING CONSIDERATIONS
Assessment
• Monitor ophthalmic exams and intraocular pressure readings
• Monitor blood counts; renal/hepatic function tests and serum electrolytes during long-term treatment

Patient/family education
• Teach how to instill drops
• Advise patient that product may cause burning, itching, blurring, dryness of eye area

Evaluation
Positive therapeutic outcome
• Absence of increased intraocular pressure

NASAL AGENTS

NASAL ANTIHISTAMINES
olopatadine (Rx)
(oh-low-pat'uh-deen)
Patanase

NASAL DECONGESTANTS
azelastine (Rx)
(ay-zell'ah-steen)
Astelin, Astepro
desoxyephedrine (OTC)
(des-oxy-e-fed'rin)
Vicks Vapor Inhaler
ePHEDrine (OTC)
(e-fed'rin)
Pretz-D
EPINEPHrine (OTC)
(ep-i-neff'rin)
Adrenalin
naphazoline (OTC)
(naff-a-zoe'leen)
Privine

oxymetazoline (OTC)
(ox-i-met-az'oh-leen)
12 Hour Nasal, Afrin 12 Hour Original, Afrin 12-Hour Original Pump Mist, Afrin Severe Congestion with Menthol, Afrin Sinus with Vapornase, Afrin No-Drip 12-Hour, Afrin No-Drip 12-Hour Extra Moisturizing, Dristan, Duramist Plus, Duration, Genasal, Nafrine ✦, Neo-Synephrine 12 Hour, Nostrilla, oxymetazoline HCl, Nasal Relief, Nasal Decongestant Maximum Strength, Vicks Sinex 12 Hour Long-Acting, Vicks Sinex 12-Hour Ultra Fine Mist for Sinus Relief
phenylephrine (OTC)
(fen-ill-eff'rin)
Alconefrin 12, Children's Nostril, Neo-Synephrine, Sinex
propylhexadrine (OTC)
(proe-pil-hex'a-dreen)
Benzedrex Inhaler
pseudoephedrine (Rx, OTC)
(soo-doe-e-fed'rin)
Cenafed, Decofed, Dimetapp, Genaphed, Sudafed, Triaminic
tetrahydrozoline (OTC)
(tet-ra-hye-dro'zoe-leen)
Tyzine, Tyzine Pediatric
xylometazoline (OTC)
(zye-loh-meh-tazz'oh-leen)
Natru-vent, Otrivin, Otrivin Pediatric Nasal

NASAL STEROIDS
beclomethasone (Rx)
(be-kloe-meth'a-sone)
Beconase AQ Nasal, Beconase Inhalation, Vancenase AQ Nasal, Vancenase Pocket Inhaler
budesonide (Rx)
(byoo-des'oh-nide)
Rhinocort, Rhinocort Aqua
flunisolide (Rx)
(floo-niss'oh-lide)
Nasalide, Nasarel
fluticasone (Rx)
(floo-tic'a-son)
Flonase, Veramyst

---

triamcinolone (Rx)
(trye-am-sin'oh-lone)
Nasacort AQ

NONSTEROIDAL ANTIINFLAMMATORY
ketorolac (Rx)
(kee'toe-role-ak)
Sprix

ACTION: Produces vasoconstriction (rapid, long acting) of arterioles, thereby decreasing fluid exudation, mucosal engorgement by stimulation of α-adrenergic receptors in vascular smooth muscle

Therapeutic outcome: Absence of nasal congestion

USES: Nasal congestion

CONTRAINDICATIONS:
Hypersensitivity to sympathomimetic amines

Precautions: Pregnancy **C**, children <6 yr, geriatric, diabetes, CV disease, hypertension, hyperthyroidism, increased ICP, prostatic hypertrophy, glaucoma

DOSAGE AND ROUTES
Desoxyephedrine
Adult and child >6 yr: 1-2 INH in each nostril q2hr or less

EPHEDrine
Adult: Fill dropper to the level marked, then use in each nostril q4hr or less

EPINEPHrine
Adult and child >6 yr: Apply with swab, drops, spray prn

Naphazoline
Adult and child >6 yr: 1-2 drops/spray q6hr or less

Oxymetazoline
Adult and child >6 yr: INSTILL 2-3 gtt or sprays to each nostril bid
Child 2-6 yr: INSTILL 2-3 gtt or sprays 0.025 SOL bid, max 3 days

Phenylephrine
Adult and child >12 yr: 2-3 drops/spray (0.25-0.5) in each nostril q3-4hr or less; or 2-3 drops/spray (1%) in each nostril q4hr or less
Child 6-12 yr: 2-3 drops/spray (0.25%) in each nostril q3-4hr
Infant >6 mo: 1-2 drops (0.16%) in each nostril q3hr

Propylhexadrine
Adult and child >6 yr: 1-2 INH in each nostril q2hr or less

Tetrahydrozoline
Adult and child >6 yr: 2-4 drops (0.1%) q3-4hr prn or 3-4 sprays in each nostril q4hr prn
Child 2-6 yr: 2-3 drops (0.05%) in each nostril q4-6hr prn

Xylometazoline
Adult and child >12 yr: 2-3 drops/spray (0.1%) in each nostril q8-10hr
Child 2-12 yr: 2-3 drops (0.05%) in each nostril q8-10hr

Available forms: Nasal sol 0.025%, 0.05%

Implementation
• Have patient tilt head back, squeeze bulb to create a vacuum, and draw correct amount of sol into dropper; insert 2 gtt of sol into nostril; repeat in other nostril
• Store in light-resistant container; do not expose to high temperature or let sol come into contact with aluminum
• Give for <4 consecutive days
• Provide environmental humidification to decrease nasal congestion, dryness

ADVERSE EFFECTS
CNS: Anxiety, restlessness, tremors, weakness, insomnia, dizziness, fever, headache
EENT: Irritation, burning, sneezing, stinging, dryness, rebound congestion
GI: Nausea, vomiting, anorexia
INTEG: Contact dermatitis

NURSING CONSIDERATIONS
Assessment
• Assess for redness, swelling, pain in nasal passages before, during treatment
• Assess for systemic absorption; hypertension, tachycardia; notify prescriber; systemic absorption occurs at high doses or after prolonged use

Patient/family education
• Advise patient that stinging may occur for several applications; drying of mucosa may be decreased by environmental humidification
• Caution patient to notify prescriber if irregular pulse, insomnia, dizziness, or tremors occur
• Teach patient proper administration to avoid systemic absorption
• Advise patient to rinse dropper with very hot water to prevent contamination

Evaluation
Positive therapeutic outcome
• Decreased nasal congestion

TOPICAL GLUCOCORTICOIDS

betamethasone (Rx)
(bay-ta-meth'a-sone)
Alphatrex, Beben ✦,
Betacort ✦, Betatrex, Beta-Val,
Betnovate ✦, Celestoderm ✦,
Diprosone, Ectosone ✦, Luxiq,
Maxivate, Metaderm ✦, Psorion,
Valisone

betamethasone (augmented) (Rx)
(bay-ta-meth'a-sone)
Diprolene, Diprolene AF

clobetasol (Rx)
(kloe-bay'ta-sol)
Clobex, Cormax, Dermovate ✦,
Embeline E 0.05%, Temovate

desonide (Rx)
(dess'oh-nide)
Verdeso Foam

desoximetasone (Rx)
(dess-ox-i-met'a-sone)
Topicort, Topicort LP

dexamethasone (Rx)
(dex-a-meth'a-sone)
Aeroseb-Dex, Decaspray

fluocinolone (Rx)
(floo-oh-sin'oh-lone)
Derma-Smoothe/FS oil, Fluocin,
Licon, Lidemol ✦, Lidex, Lyderm ✦,
Topsyn ✦, Vasoderm

flurandrenolide (Rx)
(flure-an-dren'oh-lide)
Cordran, Cordran SP, Drenison 1/4 ✦,
Drenison Tape ✦

fluticasone (Rx)
(floo-tik'a-sone)
Cutivate

halcinonide (Rx)
(hal-sin'oh-nide)
Halog, Halog-E

hydrocortisone (Rx)
(hye-droe-kor'ti-sone)
Actiocort, Aeroseb-HC, Ala-Cort,
Allercort, Alphaderm, Anusol HC,
Bactine, Barriere-HC ✦, CaldeCORT
Anti-Itch, Carmol HC, Cetacort,
Cortacet ✦, Cortaid, Cortalo,
Cortate ✦, Cort-Dome, Cortef ✦,
Corticaine, Corticreme ✦, Cortifair,
Cortizone, Cortoderm ✦, Cortril,
Delcort, Dermacort, DemiCort,
Dermtex HC, Emo-Cort, Epifoam,
FoilleCort, Gly-Cort, Gynecort, Hi-
Cor, Hycort, Hyderm ✦, Hydro-Tex,
Hytone, Lacti-Care-HC, Lanacort,
Lemoderm, Locoid, Locoid Lotion, My
Cort, Novoehydrocort ✦, Nutracort
Pharm, Pharmacort, Pentacort,
Rederm, Rhulicort S-T Cort, Synacort,
Sarna HC ✦, Texa-Cort,
Unicort ✦, Westcort

triamcinolone (Rx)
(trye-am-sin'oh-lone)
Aristocort, Delta-Tritex, Flutex,
Kenac, Kenalog, Kenonel, Triaderm,
Trianide ✦, Triderm, Trymex

ACTION: Antipruritic, antiinflammatory

Therapeutic outcome: Decreased itching, inflammation

USES: Psoriasis, eczema, contact dermatitis, pruritus; usually reserved for severe dermatoses that have not responded to less potent formulation

CONTRAINDICATIONS:
Hypersensitivity, viral infections, fungal infections

Precautions: Pregnancy C

DOSAGE AND ROUTES
Adult and child: Apply to affected area

Implementation
- Apply only to affected areas; do not get in eyes
- Apply and leave site uncovered or lightly covered; occlusive dressing is not recommended—systemic absorption may occur
- Use only on dermatoses; do not use on weeping, denuded, or infected area
- Cleanse area before application of product

• Continue treatment for a few days after area has cleared
• Store at room temperature

ADVERSE EFFECTS
INTEG: *Acne, atrophy, epidermal thinning, purpura, striae*

NURSING CONSIDERATIONS
Assessment
• Monitor temp; if fever develops, product should be discontinued
• Monitor for systemic absorption, increased temp, inflammation, irritation

Patient/family education
• Teach patient to avoid sunlight on affected area; burns may occur
• Teach patient to limit treatment to 14 days

Evaluation
Positive therapeutic outcome
• Absence of severe itching, patches on skin, flaking

TOPICAL ANTIFUNGALS

clotrimazole (OTC)
(kloe-trye'ma-zole)
Canestew ✷, Clotrimaderm ✷, Clotrimazole, Cruex, Desenex, Lotrimin AF, Myclo ✷, Neozol ✷
econazole (OTC)
(ee-kon'a-zole)
Spectazole
ketoconazole (OTC)
(kee-toe-kon'a-zole)
Nizoral, Xolegel
miconazole (OTC)
(mye-kon'a-zole)
Absorbine Antifungal Foot Powder, Breeze Mist Antifungal, Fungoid Tincture, Lotrimin AF, Maximum Strength Desenex Antifungal, Micatin, Monistat-Derm, Ony-Clear, Tetterine, ZeaSob-AF
nystatin (OTC)
(nye-stat'in)
Mycostatin, Nodostine ✷, Nilstat, Nyoderm ✷, Nystex

selenium (OTC)
(see-leen'ee-um)
Exsel, Head and Shoulders Intensive Treatment, Selenium Sulfide, Selsun, Selsun Blue
terbinafine (OTC)
(ter-bin'a-feen)
Lamisil
tolnaftate (OTC)
(tole-naf'tate)
Absorbine Athlete's Foot Cream, Aftate for Athlete's Foot, Aftate for Jock Itch, Genaspor, Quinsana Plus, Tinactin, Ting, tolnaftate
undecylenic acid (OTC)
(un-deh-sih-len'ik)
Blis-To-Sol, Breeze Mist, Caldesene, Cruex, Decylenes, Desenex, Desenex Maximum Strength, Pedi-Pro, Phicon F, Protectol

ACTION: Interferes with fungal cell membrane permeability

Therapeutic outcome: Absence of itching and white patches of the skin

USES: Tinea cruris, tinea pedis, diaper rash, minor skin irritations; amphotericin B is used for *Candida* infections

CONTRAINDICATIONS:
Hypersensitivity

Precautions: Pregnancy **B,** breastfeeding, children

DOSAGE AND ROUTES
Massage into affected area, surrounding area daily or bid, continue for 7-14 days, max 4 wk

Implementation
• Apply to affected area, surrounding area; do not cover with occlusive dressings
• Store below 30° C (86° F)

ADVERSE EFFECTS
INTEG: Burning, stinging, dryness, itching, local irritation

NURSING CONSIDERATIONS
Assessment
• Assess skin for fungal infections: peeling, dryness, itching before, throughout treatment
• Assess for continuing infection; increased size, number of lesions

---

Patient/family education
- Instruct to apply with glove to prevent further infection; not to cover with occlusive dressings
- Teach patient that long-term therapy may be needed to clear infection (2 wk-6 mo depending on organism); compliance is needed even after feeling better
- Teach patient proper hygiene: hand-washing technique, nail care, use of concomitant top agents if prescribed
- Caution patient to avoid use of OTC creams, ointments, lotions unless directed by prescriber
- Instruct patient to use medical asepsis (hand washing) before, after each application; to change socks and shoes once a day during treatment of tinea pedis
- Advise patient to report to health care prescriber if infection persists or recurs; if blisters, burning, oozing, swelling occur
- Caution patient to avoid alcohol because nausea, vomiting, hypertension may occur
- Caution patient to use sunscreen or avoid direct sunlight to prevent photosensitivity
- Advise patient to notify prescriber of sore throat, fever, skin rash, which may indicate overgrowth of organisms

Evaluation
Positive therapeutic outcome
- Decrease in size, number of lesions

TOPICAL ANTIINFECTIVES

azelaic acid (Rx)
(a-zuh-lay'ic)
Azelex, Finacea
bacitracin (OTC)
(bass-i-tray'sin)
Bacitin ✤, Bacitracin
clindamycin (Rx)
(klin-da-my'sin)
Cleocin T, Clindets, Clindagel, ClindaMax
erythromycin (Rx, OTC)
(er-ith-roe-mye'sin)
A/T/S, Akne-Mycin, Eryderm, Erygel, Erythromycin, Staticin, T-Stat
gentamicin (Rx)
(jen-ta-mye'sin)
Gentamicin

---

mafenide (Rx)
(ma'fe-nide)
Sulfamylon
metronidazole (Rx)
(met-roh-nye'da-zole)
MetroGel, MetroCream, MetroLotion, Noritate
mupirocin (Rx)
(myoo-peer'oh-sin)
Bactroban
neomycin (OTC)
(nee-oh-mye'sin)
Neomycin Sulfate
nitrofurazone (Rx)
(nye-troe-fyoor'a-zone)
Furacin, Nitrofurazone
retapamulin (Rx)
(re-tap'a-mue'lin)
Altabax
salicylic acid (Rx)
(sal'i-sil'ik)
Salitop
silver sulfADIAZINE (Rx)
(sul-fa-dye'a-zeen)
Flamazine ✤, Silvadene, SSD, SSD AF, Thermazene
tretinoin (Rx)
(treh'tih-noyn)
Atralin

ACTION: Interferes with bacterial protein synthesis

Therapeutic outcome: Resolution of infection

USES: Skin infections, minor burns, wounds, skin grafts, primary pyodermas, otitis externa

CONTRAINDICATIONS: Hypersensitivity, large areas, burns, ulcerations

Precautions: Pregnancy **C**, breastfeeding, impaired renal function, external ear or perforated eardrum

Implementation
- Apply enough medication to cover lesions completely
- Apply after cleansing with soap, water before each application; dry well

---

Adverse effects: *italics* = common; **bold** = life-threatening

• Apply to less than 20% of body surface area when patient has impaired renal function
• Store at room temperature in dry place

ADVERSE EFFECTS
INTEG: Rash, urticaria, scaling, redness

NURSING CONSIDERATIONS
Assessment
• Assess for allergic reaction: burning, stinging, swelling, redness
• Assess for signs of nephrotoxicity or ototoxicity

Evaluation
Positive therapeutic outcome
• Decrease in size, number of lesions

TOPICAL ANTIVIRALS

acyclovir (Rx)
(ay-sye′kloe-ver)
Zovirax
penciclovir (Rx)
(pen-sye′kloe-ver)
Denavir

ACTION: Interferes with viral DNA replication

Therapeutic outcome: Resolution of infection

USES: Simple mucocutaneous herpes simplex, in immunocompromised clients with initial herpes genitalis

CONTRAINDICATIONS:
Hypersensitivity

Precautions: Pregnancy **C**, breastfeeding

Implementation
• Apply with finger cot or rubber glove to prevent further infection
• Apply enough medication to cover lesions completely
• Apply after cleansing with soap, water before each application; dry well
• Store at room temperature in dry place

ADVERSE EFFECTS
INTEG: Rash, urticaria, stinging, burning, pruritus, vulvitis

NURSING CONSIDERATIONS
Assessment
• Assess for allergic reaction: burning, stinging, swelling, redness, rash, vulvitis, pruritus
• Assess for signs of nephrotoxicity or ototoxicity

Patient/family education
• Teach patient not to use in eyes or when there is no evidence of infection
• Advise patient to apply with glove to prevent further infection
• Advise patient to avoid use of OTC creams, ointments, lotions unless directed by prescriber
• Advise patient to use medical asepsis (hand washing) before, after each application and avoid contact with eyes
• Advise patient to adhere strictly to prescribed regimen to maximize successful treatment outcome
• Advise patient to begin taking product when symptoms arise

Evaluation
Positive therapeutic outcome
• Decrease in size, number of lesions

TOPICAL ANESTHETICS

benzocaine (OTC)
(ben′zoe-kane)
Americaine Anesthetic, Anbesol Maximum Strength, Baby Anbesol, Biozene, Boil-Ease, Children's Chloraseptic, Dermoplast, Foille, Foille Plus, Hurricane, Lanacane, Medamint, Orabase, Oracin, Ora-Jel
dibucaine (OTC)
(dye′byoo-kane)
Dibucaine, Nupercainal
lidocaine (Rx, OTC)
(lye′doe-kane)
Anestacon, Burn-O-Jel, Dentipatch, Derma Flex, ELA-Max, Lidoderm, Numby Staff, Solarcaine Aloe Extra Burn Relief, Xylocaine, Xylocaine 10% Oral, Xylocaine Viscous, Zilactin-L
pramoxine (OTC)
(pra-mox′een)
Itch-X, PrameGel, Prax, Tronothane

tetracaine (OTC, Rx)
(tet´ra-cane)
Pontocaine, Viractin

ACTION: Inhibits conduction of nerve impulses from sensory nerves

Therapeutic outcome: Decreasing inflammation, itching, pain

USES: Oral irritation, sore throat, toothache, cold sore, canker sore, sunburn, minor cuts, insect bites, pain, itching

CONTRAINDICATIONS:
Hypersensitivity, infants <1 yr, application to large areas

Precautions: Pregnancy **C,** children <6 yr, sepsis, denuded skin

DOSAGE AND ROUTES
Adult and child: TOP apply qid as needed; RECT insert tid and after each BM

Implementation
• Store in tight, light-resistant container; do not freeze, puncture, or incinerate aerosol container

ADVERSE EFFECTS
INTEG: Rash, irritation, sensitization

NURSING CONSIDERATIONS
Assessment
• Assess pain: location, duration, characteristics before, after administration
• Assess for infection: redness, drainage, inflammation; this product should not be used until infection is treated

Patient/family education
• Teach patient to avoid contact with eyes
• Teach patient not to use for prolonged periods: use for <1 wk; if condition remains, prescriber should be contacted

Evaluation
Positive therapeutic outcome
• Decreased redness, swelling, pain

**TOPICAL
MISCELLANEOUS**

docosanol (OTC)
(doh-koh´sah-nohl)
Abreva
pimecrolimus (Rx)
(pim-eh-kroh-ly´mus)
Elidel

ACTION: Docosanol unknown; pimecrolimus may bind with macrophilin and inhibit calcium-dependent phosphatase

Therapeutic outcome: Decreased redness, swelling, pain

USES: Docosanol applied to fever blisters to promote more rapid healing; pimecrolimus used to treat mild to moderate atopic dermatitis in nonimmunocompromised patients ≥2 yr who are unresponsive to other treatment

CONTRAINDICATIONS:
Hypersensitivity

Precautions: Pregnancy **C,** breastfeeding, dermal infections

DOSAGE AND ROUTES
Docosanol
Adult: TOP rub into blisters 5 ×/day until healing occurs

Pimecrolimus
Adult and child ≥2 yr: TOP apply thin layer 2 ×/day and rub in; use as long as needed

Implementation
• Apply to skin, rub in gently

ADVERSE EFFECTS
Docosanol
NONE known

Pimecrolimus
INTEG: Burning

NURSING CONSIDERATIONS
Assessment
• Assess skin condition (color, pain, inflammation) before, after administration
• Assess for signs and symptoms of skin infections (redness, draining lesions); if present, avoid use of product (pimecrolimus)

Patient/family education
• Advise patient to avoid contact between medication and eyes
• Instruct patient to discontinue use of product when condition clears

Evaluation
Positive therapeutic outcome
• Decreased inflammation, redness

VAGINAL ANTIFUNGALS

butoconazole (OTC)
(byoo-toh-kone′ah-zole)
Femstat-3, Gynazol-1, Mycelex-3
clotrimazole (OTC)
(kloe-trye′ma-zole)
Canesten ✿, Clotriamazole, Gyne-Lotrimin 3, Gyne-Lotrimin 7, Mycelex 7, Myclo ✿
miconazole (OTC)
(mye-kon′a-zole)
Femizole-M, Monistat, Monistat 3, Monistat 7, Monistat Dual Pak, M-Zole 7 Dual Pack
nystatin (OTC)
(nye-stat′in)
Nystatin
terconazole (OTC)
(ter-kone′ah-zole)
Terazol 7, Tetrazol 3
tioconazole (OTC)
(tye-oh-kone′ah-zole)
Gyne-Trosyd ✿, Monistat 1, Vagistat-1

ACTION: Interferes with fungal DNA replication; binds sterols in fungal cell membranes, which increases permeability, leaking of nutrients

Therapeutic outcome: Fungistatic/fungicidal against susceptible organisms: *Candida* only

USES: Vaginal, vulval, vulvovaginal candidiasis (moniliasis)

CONTRAINDICATIONS:
Hypersensitivity

Precautions: Pregnancy, breastfeeding, children <2 yr

DOSAGE AND ROUTES
Butoconazole
Adult: VAG 5 g (1 applicator) at bedtime × 3-6 days

Clotrimazole
Adult: 100 mg (1 vag tab, 100 mg) at bedtime × 1 wk, or 200 mg (2 vag tab, 100 mg) at bedtime × 3 nights, or 500 mg (1 vag tab, 500 mg), or 5 g (1 applicator) at bedtime × 1-2 wk

Miconazole
Adult: 200 mg SUPP at bedtime × 3 days or 100 mg SUPP × 1 wk

Nystatin
Adult: 100,000 units/day × 2 wk

Terconazole
Adult: VAG 5 g (1 applicator) at bedtime × 7 days

Tioconazole
Adult: 1 applicator at bedtime × 1 wk

Implementation
Topical route
• Administer one full applicator every night high into the vagina
• Store at room temperature in dry place

ADVERSE EFFECTS
GU: Vulvovaginal burning, itching, pelvic cramps
INTEG: Rash, urticaria, stinging, burning
MISC: *Headache,* body pain

NURSING CONSIDERATIONS
Assessment
• Assess for allergic reaction: burning, stinging, itching, discharge, soreness

Patient/family education
• Instruct patient in asepsis (hand washing) before, after each application
• Teach patient to apply with applicator only; to avoid use of any other vaginal product unless directed by prescriber; sanitary napkin may prevent soiling of undergarments
• Instruct patient to abstain from sexual intercourse until treatment is completed; reinfection and irritation may occur
• Advise patient to notify prescriber if symptoms persist

Evaluation
Positive therapeutic outcome
• Decrease in itching or white discharge (vaginal)

OTIC ANTIINFECTIVES

boric acid (OTC)
(bor'ik as'id)
Auro-Dri, Dri/Ear, Ear Dry
chloramphenicol (Rx)
(klor-am-fen'i-kole)
Chloromycetin Otic
ciprofloxacin (Rx)
(sip'roe-flox'a-sin)
Cetraxel

ACTION: Inhibits protein synthesis in susceptible microorganisms

USES: Ear infection (external), short-term use

CONTRAINDICATIONS:
Hypersensitivity, perforated eardrum

Precautions: Pregnancy **C**

Implementation
• After removing impacted cerumen by irrigation
• After cleaning stopper with alcohol
• After restraining child if necessary
• After warming sol to body temp

ADVERSE EFFECTS
EENT: Itching, irritation in ear
INTEG: Rash, urticaria

NURSING CONSIDERATIONS
Assessment
• Assess for redness, swelling, fever, pain in ear, which indicates superinfection

Patient/family education
• Teach patient correct method of instillation using aseptic technique, including not touching dropper to ear
• Inform patient that dizziness may occur after instillation

Evaluation
Positive therapeutic outcome
• Decreased ear pain

Appendix C Vaccines and toxoids

GENERIC NAME	TRADE NAME	USES	DOSAGE AND ROUTES	CONTRAINDICATIONS
adenovirus vaccine		Prevention of adenovirus types 4/7	Adult ≤50 yr/adolescent ≥17 yr in the military PO 1 tab of each 4/7 as a single dose	Pregnancy
avian influenza A (H5N1) virus vaccine		Prophylaxis	Adult: IM 1 ml (90 mcg) 2 doses, 28 days apart	IV
anthrax vaccine	BioThrax	Pre-/postexposure prophylaxis	**Preexposure** Adult: SUBCUT 0.5 ml at 0, 2, 4 wk, then 0.5 ml at 6, 12, 18 mo **Postexposure** Adult: SUBCUT 0.5 ml 0, 2, 4 wk, with antibiotics	Hypersensitivity
BCG vaccine	TICE BCG	TB exposure	Adult and child >1 mo: 0.2–0.3 ml Child <1 mo: Reduce dose by 50% using 2 ml of sterile water after reconstituting	Hypersensitivity, hypogamma-globulinemia, positive TB test, burns
cholera vaccine	No trade name	Immunization for cholera outside the United States	Adult and child >10 yr: IM/SUBCUT 2× of 0.5 ml, 7-30 days before traveling to cholera areas Booster is used q6mo 0.5 ml prn	Hypersensitivity, acute febrile illness
diphtheria and tetanus toxoids, adsorbed	No trade name	Induces antitoxins to provide immunity to diphtheria and tetanus	Adult and child ≥7 yr: IM (adult strength) 0.5 ml q4-8wk × 2 doses, then 3rd dose 6-12 mo after 2nd dose, booster IM 0.5 ml q10yr Child 1-6 yr: IM (pediatric strength) 0.5 ml q4wk × 2 doses, booster 6-12 mo after 2nd dose Infant 6 wk-1 yr: IM (pediatric strength) 0.5 ml q4wk × 3 doses, booster 6-12 mo after 3rd dose	Hypersensitivity to mercury; thimerosal; immunocompromised patients; radiation; corticosteroids; acute illness
diphtheria and tetanus toxoids and whole-cell pertussis vaccine (DPT, DTP)	DTwP, Tr-Immunol	Prevention of diphtheria, tetanus, pertussis	Doses vary Check product information	Hypersensitivity, active infection, poliomyelitis outbreak, immunosuppression, febrile illness
diphtheria and tetanus toxoids and acellular pertussis vaccine	Adacel, Boostrix, Daptacel, Infanrix, Tripedia			
diphtheria, tetanus, pertussis, haemophilus, polio IPV	Pentacel	Immunity to diphtheria, tetanus, pertussis, haemophilus, polio	Infant >6 wk and child ≤5 yr: IM 0.5 ml at 2, 4, 6, and 15-18 mo	Hypersensitivity, polio outbreak, acute infection, immunosuppression
diphtheria, tetanus, pertussis, polio vaccine IPV	Kinrix	Immunity to diphtheria, tetanus, pertussis, polio vaccine IPV	Child: IM 0.5 ml	Hypersensitivity, polio outbreak, acute infection, immunosuppression

H1N1 influenza A (swine flu) virus vaccine	Influenza A (H1N1)	Immunity to H1N1	Adult <50 yr, adolescent, child ≥2 yr: Intranasal 1 dose (roughly 0.1 ml) into each nostril; child 2-9 repeat dose ≥4 wk later Adult, adolescent, child ≥3 yr: IM 0.5 ml as a single dose; child 3-9 yr repeat dose ≥4 wk later (Sanofi) (CSL); child 4-9 yr repeat dose ≥4 wk later (Novartis); infants ≥6 mo, child <36 mo: IM 0.25 ml, repeat in 4 wk (Sanofi) Adult: IM 0.5 ml as a single dose (GSK)	Hypersensitivity, febrile illness, active infection
haemophilus b conjugate vaccine, diphtheria CRM$_{197}$ protein conjugate (HbOC)	HibTITER	Polysaccharide immunization of children 2-6 yr against *H. influenzae* b, conjugate	**HibTITER (IM only)** Child: IM 0.5 ml Child 2-6 mo: 0.5 ml q2mo × 3 inj	
haemophilus b conjugate vaccine, meningococcal protein conjugate (PRP-OMP)	PedvaxHIB	Immunization of child 2, 4, 6 mo	Child 7-11 mo: Previously unvaccinated 0.5 ml q2mo inj Child 12-14 mo: Previously unvaccinated 0.5 ml × 1 inj **PedvaxHIB (IM only)** Child 2-14 mo: 0.5 ml × 2 inj at 2, 4 mo of age (6 mo dose not needed), then booster at 12-18 mo against invasive disease Child ≥15 mo: Previously unvaccinated 0.5 ml inj	
hepatitis A vaccine, inactivated	Havrix, VAQTA	Active immunization against hepatitis A virus	Adult: IM 1440 EL units (Havrix) or 50 units (VAQTA) as a single dose; booster dose is the same given at 6, 12 mo Child 2-18 yr: IM 720 EL units (Havrix) or 25 units (VAQTA) as a single dose, booster dose is the same given at 6, 12 mo	Hypersensitivity
hepatitis B vaccine, recombinant	Engerix-B, Recombivax HB	Immunization against all subtypes of hepatitis B virus	Varies widely	Hypersensitivity to this vaccine or yeast
herpes zoster virus vaccine	Zostavax	Prevention of herpes zoster	Adult ≥60 yr: SUBCUT 0.65 ml	<60 yr, child, infant, AIDS, IM/IV, leukemia, lymphoma, pregnancy
human papillomavirus recombinant vaccine, quadrivalent	Gardasil	Prevention of HPV types 6, 11, 16, 18, cervical cancer, genital warts, precancerous dysplasic lesions, anal cancer/anal intraepithelial neoplasia	Adult up to 26 yr and child >9 yr to 26 yr: IM give as 3 separate doses; 1st dose as elected; 2nd dose 2 mo after 1st dose; 3rd dose 6 mo after 1st dose	Child <9 yr, pregnancy, breastfeeding, geriatric, active disease, hypersensitivity

Continued

Appendix C Vaccines and toxoids—cont'd

GENERIC NAME	TRADE NAME	USES	DOSAGE AND ROUTES	CONTRAINDICATIONS
influenza virus vaccine	Afluria, FluMist, Fluogen, Flu-Shield, Fluviral*, Fluvirin, Fluzone, influenza virus vaccine, trivalent	Prevention of Russian, Chilean, Philippine influenza	Adult and child >12 yr: IM 0.5 ml in 1 dose Adult 18-64 yr: ID 0.1 ml as a single dose Child 3-12 yr: IM 0.5 ml, repeat in 1 mo (split) unless 1978-1985 vaccine was given; also given nasal Child 6 mo to 3 yr: IM 0.25 ml, repeat in 1 mo (split) unless 1978-1985 vaccine was given; also given nasal child ≤2 yr	Hypersensitivity; active infection, chicken egg allergy, Guillain-Barré syndrome, active neurologic disorders
Japanese encephalitis virus vaccine, inactivated	JE-VAX	Active immunity against Japanese encephalitis (JE)	Adult and child ≥3 yr: SUBCUT 1 ml, days 0, 7, 30; booster SUBCUT 1 ml 2 yr after last dose Child 1-3 yr: SUBCUT 0.5 ml, days 0, 7, 30; booster SUBCUT 0.5 ml 2 yr after last dose	Hypersensitivity to murine, thimerosal; allergic reactions to previous dose
Lyme disease vaccine (recombinant OspA)	LYMErix	Immunization against Lyme disease	Adult and adolescent 15-70 yr: IM 30 mcg in deltoid, repeat at 1, 12 mo after first dose	Hypersensitivity, antibiotic refractory Lyme arthritis
measles and rubella virus vaccine, live attenuated	M-R-Vax II	Immunity to measles and rubella by antibody production	Adult and child ≥15 mo: SUBCUT 0.5 ml (1000 units)	Hypersensitivity, immunocompromised patients, active untreated TB, cancer, blood dyscrasias, radiation, corticosteroids, pregnancy; allergic reactions to neomycin, eggs
measles, mumps, and rubella vaccine, live	M-M-R-II	Prevention of measles, mumps, rubella	Adult: SUBCUT 1 vial; 2 vials separated by 1 mo, in person born after 1957 Child >15 mo and adult: SUBCUT 0.5 ml	Hypersensitivity, blood dyscrasias, anemia, active infection, immunosuppression; egg, chicken allergy; pregnancy, febrile illness, neomycin allergy; neoplasms
measles, mumps, rubella, varicella	ProQuad	Immunity to measles, mumps, rubella, varicella	Child: SUBCUT 0.5 ml	Hypersensitivity to eggs, neomycin, cancer, radiation, corticosteroids, blood dyscrasias, active untreated TB
measles virus vaccine, live attenuated	Attenuvax	Immunity to measles by antibody production	Adult and child ≥15 mo: SUBCUT 0.5 ml (1000 units), 1 dose 15 mo, 2nd dose age 4-6 or 11-12	Hypersensitivity to eggs, neomycin; cancer, radiation, corticosteroids, pregnancy; immunocompromised patients, blood dyscrasias, active untreated TB
meningococcal diphtheria toxoid conjugate vaccine	Menomune, Menactra, Menveo	Prophylaxis to meningococcal meningitis/diphtheria	All doses are different; check product information	Latex hypersensitivity
meningococcal polysaccharide vaccine	Menomune-A/C/Y/W-135, Menactra	Prophylaxis to meningococcal meningitis	Adult and child >2 yr: SUBCUT 0.5 ml	Hypersensitivity to thimerosal, pregnancy, acute illness

mumps virus vaccine, live	Mumpsvax	Active immunity to mumps	Adult and child ≥1 yr: SUBCUT 0.5 ml (20,000 units)	Hypersensitivity to eggs, neomycin; cancer, radiation, corticosteroids, pregnancy, immunocompromised patients, blood dyscrasias, active untreated TB
plague vaccine	No trade name	Active immunity to *Yersinia pestis* plague	Adult: IM 1 ml, then 0.2 ml in 4-12 wk, then 0.2 ml 5-6 mo after 2nd dose; booster 0.1-0.2 ml q6mo when in plague area	Hypersensitivity to phenol, sulfites, formaldehyde, beef, soy, casein; pregnancy, coagulation disorders
pneumococcal 7-valent conjugate vaccine	Prevnar	Immunity against *Streptococcus pneumoniae*	Child: IM 0.5 ml ×3 doses (7-11 mo); ×2 doses (12-23 mo); ×1 dose >2-9 yr	Hypersensitivity to diphtheria toxoid or this product
pneumococcal vaccine, polyvalent	Pneumovax 23, Pnu-Imune 23	Pneumococcal immunization	Adult and child >2 yr: IM/SUBCUT 0.5 ml	Hypersensitivity, Hodgkin's disease, ARDS
poliovirus vaccine, live, oral, trivalent (TOPV), poliovirus vaccine (IPV)	Orimune, IPOL	Prevention of polio	Adult and child >2 yr: PO 0.5 ml, given q8wk ×2 doses, then 0.5 ml ½-1 yr after dose 2; Infant: PO 0.5 ml at 2, 4, 18 mo; booster at 4-6 yr; may also be given: IPV at 2, 4 mo, then TOPV at 12-18 mo, booster at 4-6 yr	Hypersensitivity, active infection, allergy to neomycin/streptomycin, immunosuppression, vomiting, diarrhea
rabies vaccine, adsorbed	No trade name	Active immunity to rabies	**Preexposure** Adult and child: IM 1 ml day 0, 7, 21, or 28 days (total 3 doses); booster IM 1 ml prn q2-5yr **Postexposure** Adult and child not vaccinated: IM 20 international units/kg of human rabies immune globulin (HRIG), give 5 total doses of 1-ml inj of rabies vaccine on days 0, 3, 7, 14, 28	Severe hypersensitivity to previous inj of vaccine, thimerosol
rabies vaccine, human diploid cell (HDCV)	Imovax Rabies, Imovax Rabies I.D.	Active immunity to rabies	**Preexposure** Adult and child: IM 1 ml day 0, 7, 21, or 28 (total 4 doses) **Postexposure** Adult and child: IM 1 ml on day 0, 3, 7, 14, 28 (total 5 doses)	No contraindications
rotovirus	RotaTeq, Rotarix	Prevents rotavirus	Infant: PO 3 doses given between 6 and 32 wk of age; 1st dose between 6-12 wk of age; 2nd and 3rd doses q4-10wk	Hypersensitivity to this product or latex, immunocompromised, blood products given within 6 wk, lymphatic disorders

*Canada only.

Continued

Appendix C Vaccines and toxoids—cont'd

GENERIC NAME	TRADE NAME	USES	DOSAGE AND ROUTES	CONTRAINDICATIONS
rubella and mumps virus vaccine, live	Biavax II	Immunity to rubella and mumps by antibody production	Adult and child ≥1 yr: SUBCUT 0.5 ml	Hypersensitivity to eggs, neomycin; cancer, radiation, corticosteroids, pregnancy; immuno-compromised patients, blood dyscrasias, active untreated TB
rubella virus vaccine, live attenuated (RA 27/3)	Meruvax II	Immunity to rubella by antibody production	Adult and child ≥1 yr: SUBCUT 0.5 ml (1000 units)	Hypersensitivity to eggs, neomycin; cancer, radiation, corticosteroids
smallpox vaccine	ACAM 2000, Dry Vax	Prevention of smallpox	See package insert	No contraindications
tetanus toxoid, adsorbed/tetanus toxoid	No trade name	Tetanus toxoid: Used for prophylactic treatment of wounds	Adult and child: IM 0.5 ml q4-6wk × 2 doses, then 0.5 ml 1 yr after dose 2 (adsorbed); SUBCUT/IM 0.5 ml q4-8wk × 3 doses, then 0.5 ml ¹⁄₂-1 yr after dose 3. booster dose 0.5 ml q10yr	Hypersensitivity, active infection, poliomyelitis outbreak, immunosuppression
typhoid vaccine, parenteral typhoid vaccine, oral	No trade name Vivotif Berna Vaccine	Active immunity to typhoid fever	Parenteral: PO 1 cap 1 hr before meals × 4 doses, booster q5yr Adult and child >10 yr: SUBCUT 0.5 ml, repeat in 4 wk, booster q3yr Child 6 mo-10 yr: SUBCUT 0.25 ml, repeat in 4 wk, booster q3yr	Parenteral: Systemic or allergic reaction, acute respiratory or other acute infection, intensive physical exercise in high temperatures Oral: Hypersensitivity, acute febrile illness, suppressive or antibiotic products
typhoid Vi polysaccharide vaccine	Typhim Vi	Active immunity to typhoid fever	Adult and child ≥2 yr: IM 0.5 ml as a single dose, reimmunize q2yr 0.5 ml IM, if needed	Hypersensitivity, chronic typhoid carriers
varicella virus vaccine	Varivax	Prevention of varicella-zoster (chickenpox)	Adult and child ≥13 yr: SUBCUT 0.5 ml, 2nd dose SUBCUT 0.5 ml 4-8 wk later	Hypersensitivity to neomycin; blood dyscrasias, immunosuppression, active untreated TB, acute illness, pregnancy, diseases of lymphatic system
yellow fever vaccine	YF-Vax	Active immunity to yellow fever	Adult and child ≥9 mo: SUBCUT 0.5 ml deeply; booster q10yr Child 6-9 mo: same as above if exposed	Hypersensitivity to egg or chicken embryo protein, pregnancy, child <6 mo, immunodeficiency
zoster vaccine, live	Zostavax	Herpes zoster prevention	Reconstitute immediately after removing from freezer; give SUBCUT as a single dose; inject total amount of single-dose vial	Immunosuppression; neomycin, gelatin allergy; children, TB, pregnancy (C)

Appendix D

Abbreviations and Pregnancy Categories

abd	abdomen	GPC	giant papillary conjunctivitis
ABG	arterial blood gas	gr	grain
ac	before meals	GTT	glucose tolerance test
ACE	angiotensin-converting enzyme	gtt	drops
ACT	activated clotting time	GU	genitourinary
ADA	American Diabetes Association	GVHD	graft-versus-host disease
ADH	antidiuretic hormone	H_2	histamine$_2$
ALT	alanine aminotransferase	hCG	human chorionic gonadotropin
ANA	antinuclear antibody	Hct	hematocrit
AP	anteroposterior	HDCV	human diploid cell rabies vaccine
APLA	antiphospholipid antibody syndrome	Hgb	hemoglobin
APTT	activated partial thromboplastin time	H&H	hematocrit and hemoglobin
ASA	acetylsalicylic acid, aspirin	5-HIAA	5-hydroxyindoleacetic acid
ASHD	arteriosclerotic heart disease	HIV	human immunodeficiency virus (AIDS)
AST	aspartate aminotransferase (SGOT)	H_2O	water
AV	atrioventricular	HOB	head of bed
bid	twice a day	HR	heart rate
BM	bowel movement	hr	hour
BMR	basal metabolic rate	IBD	inflammatory bowel disease
B/P	blood pressure	IC	intracardiac
BPH	benign prostatic hypertrophy	ICP	intracranial pressure
BPM	beats per minute	ID	intradermal
BS	blood sugar	IgG	immunoglobulin G
BUN	blood urea nitrogen	IM	intramuscular
C	Celsius (centigrade)	inf	infusion
CAD	coronary artery disease	INH	inhalation
cap	capsule	inj	injection
Cath	catheterization or catheterize	I&O	intake and output
CBC	complete blood cell count	IPPB	intermittent positive-pressure breathing
CHF	congestive heart failure	IT	intrathecal
CHo	carbohydrates	ITP	idiopathic thrombocytopenic purpura
cm	centimeter	IUD	intrauterine device
CNS	central nervous system	IV	intravenous
CO_2	carbon dioxide	IVP	intravenous pyelogram
cont	continuous	K	potassium
COPD	chronic obstructive pulmonary disease	kg	kilogram
CPAP	continuous positive airway pressure	L	liter
CPK	creatinine phosphokinase	lb	pound
CPR	cardiopulmonary resuscitation	LDH	lactic dehydrogenase
CCr	creatinine clearance	LE	lupus erythematosus
C&S	culture and sensitivity	LH	luteinizing hormone
C sect	cesarean section	LLQ	left lower quadrant
CSF	cerebrospinal fluid	LMP	last menstrual period
CTCL	cutaneous T-cell lymphoma	LOC	level of consciousness
CV	cardiovascular	LR	lactated Ringer's solution
CVA	cerebrovascular accident	LUQ	left upper quadrant
CVP	central venous pressure	M	meter
D&C	dilatation and curettage	m	minim
dir inf	direct infusion	m^2	square meter
dr	dram	MAOI	monoamine oxidase inhibitor
D_5W	5% glucose in distilled water	mcg	microgram
DVT	deep vein thrombosis	mEq	milliequivalent
ECG	electrocardiogram (EKG)	mg	milligram
EDTA	ethylenediamine tetraacetic acid	MI	myocardial infarction
EEG	electroencephalogram	min	minute
EENT	ear, eye, nose, and throat	ml	milliliter
EPS	extrapyramidal symptoms	mm	millimeter
ESR	erythrocyte sedimentation rate	mo	month
ext rel	extended release	Na	sodium
FBS	fasting blood sugar	neg	negative
FHT	fetal heart tones	NGU	nongonococcal urethritis
FSH	follicle-stimulating hormone	NHL	non-Hodgkin's lymphoma
g	gram	NPO	nothing by mouth (Lat. *nulla per os*)
GABA	γ-aminobutyric acid	NS	normal saline
GI	gastrointestinal	O_2	oxygen

OBS	organic brain syndrome	**RUQ**	right upper quadrant
OD	right eye	**Rx**	prescription
OR	operating room	**SARS**	severe acute respiratory syndrome
OS	left eye	**SCr**	serum creatinine
OTC	over-the-counter	**SIMV**	synchronous intermittent mandatory ventilation
OU	each eye	**SL**	sublingual
oz	ounce	**SLE**	systemic lupus erythematosus
p̄	after	**SOB**	shortness of breath
P56	Plasma-Lyte 56	**sol**	solution
PaCO₂	arterial carbon dioxide tension (pressure)	**sp gr**	specific gravity
PaO₂	arterial oxygen tension (pressure)	**ss**	one half
PAT	paroxysmal atrial tachycardia	**STD**	sexually transmitted disease
PBI	protein-bound iodine	**SUBCUT**	subcutaneous
pc	after meals	**supp**	suppository
PCI	percutaneous coronary intervention	**sus rel**	sustained release
PCWP	pulmonary capillary wedge pressure	**syr**	syrup
PEEP	positive end-expiratory pressure	**T&A**	tonsillectomy and adenoidectomy
PERRLA	pupils equal, round, react to light and accom- modation	**tab**	tablet
		tbsp	tablespoon
pH	hydrogen ion concentration	**TD**	transdermal
PO	by mouth	**temp**	temperature
postop	postoperative	**tid**	three times daily
PP	postprandial	**tinc**	tincture
PPHN	persistent pulmonary hypertension of the newborn	**TPN**	total parenteral nutrition
preop	preoperative	**TOP**	topical
prn	as required	**TSH**	thyroid-stimulating hormone
PT	prothrombin time	**tsp**	teaspoon
PTT	partial thromboplastin time	**TT**	thrombin time
PVC	premature ventricular contraction	**UA**	urinalysis
q	every	**UTI**	urinary tract infection
qAM	every morning	**UV**	ultraviolet
qhr	every hour	**vag**	vaginal
q2hr	every 2 hours	**VMA**	vanillylmandelic acid
q3hr	every 3 hours	**vol**	volume
q4hr	every 4 hours	**VS**	vital sign
q6hr	every 6 hours	**WBC**	white blood cell count
q12hr	every 12 hours	**wk**	week
qid	four times daily	**wt**	weight
qmo	every month	**yr**	year
qPM	every night	**>**	greater than
qs	sufficient quantity	**<**	less than
qt	quart	**=**	equal
qwk	every week	**°**	degree
R	right	**%**	percent
RAIU	radioactive iodine uptake	**α**	alpha
RBC	red blood count or cell	**γ**	gamma
RLQ	right lower quadrant	**β**	beta
ROM	range of motion		

- For a list of the Institute for Safe Medicine Practices (ISMP) error-prone abbreviations, symbols, and dose designations, please see http://www.ismp.org/tools/errorproneabbreviations.pdf.
- For frequently asked questions regarding the 2010 National Patient Safety Goals, please visit The Joint Commission website at http://www.jointcommission.org/PatientSafety/NationalPatientSafetyGoals.

FDA Pregnancy Categories

A No risk demonstrated to the fetus in any trimester

B No adverse effects in animals, no human studies available

C Only given after risks to the fetus are considered; animal studies have shown adverse reactions, no human studies available

D Definite fetal risks, may be given despite risks if needed in life-threatening conditions

X Absolute fetal abnormalities; not to be used any time during pregnancy

Note: **UK** = Unknown fetal risk (used in this text but not an official FDA pregnancy category).

Appendix E

Immunization Schedules

Recommended Childhood and Adolescent Immunization Schedule—United States, 2010
Immunization Schedule for Persons Aged 0-6 Years

Vaccine ▼ / Age ▶	Birth	1 month	2 months	4 months	6 months	12 months	15 months	18 months	19-23 months	2-3 years	4-6 years
Hepatitis B*	HepB	HepB				HepB					
Rotavirus*			Rota	Rota	Rota						
Diphtheria, Tetanus, Pertussis*			DTaP	DTaP	DTaP		DTaP				DTaP
Haemophilus Influenzae Type b*			Hib	Hib	Hib*	Hib					
Pneumococcal*			PCV	PCV	PCV	PCV				PPSV	
Inactivated Poliovirus*			IPV	IPV		IPV					IPV
Influenza*						Influenza (Yearly)					
Measles, Mumps, Rubella*						MMR					MMR
Varicella*						Varicella					Varicella
Hepatitis A*						HepA (2 doses)				HepA Series	
Meningococcal*										MCV	

Range of recommended ages

Certain high-risk groups

This schedule indicates the recommended ages for routine administration of currently licensed childhood vaccines, as of December 15, 2009, for children aged 0-6 years. Any dose not administered at the recommended age should be administered at any subsequent visit, when indicated and feasible. Additional vaccines may be licensed and recommended during the year. Licensed combination vaccines may be used whenever any components of the combination are indicated and other components of the vaccine are not contraindicated and if approved by the Food and Drug Administration for that dose of the series. **Providers should consult the respective Advisory Committee on Immunization Practices statement for detailed recommendations, including for high-risk conditions: http://www.cdc.gov/vaccines/pubs/ACIP-list.htm.** Clinically significant adverse events that follow immunization should be reported to the Vaccine Adverse Event Reporting System (VAERS). Guidance about how to obtain and complete a VAERS form is available at http://www.vaers.hhs.gov or by telephone, 800-822-7967.

*For complete information go to http://www.cdc.gov/vaccines/schedules/index

Immunization Schedule for Persons Aged 7-18 Years

Vaccine ▶ Age ▶	7-10 years	11-12 years	13-18 years
Tetanus, Diphtheria, Pertussis*		Tdap	Tdap
Human Papillomavirus*	*	HPV (3 doses)	HPV Series
Meningococcal*	MCV	MCV	MCV
Influenza*		Influenza (Yearly)	
Pneumococcal*		PPSV	
Hepatitis A*		HepA Series	
Hepatitis B*		HepB Series	
Inactivated Poliovirus*		IPV Series	
Measles, Mumps, Rubella*		MMR Series	
Varicella*		Varicella Series	

Legend:
- Range of recommended ages
- Catch-up immunization
- Certain high-risk groups

This schedule indicates the recommended ages for routine administration of currently licensed childhood vaccines, as of December 15, 2009, for children aged 7-18 years. Any dose not administered at the recommended age should be administered at any subsequent visit, when indicated and feasible. Additional vaccines may be licensed and recommended during the year. Licensed combination vaccines may be used whenever any components of the combination are indicated and other components of the vaccine are not contraindicated and if approved by the Food and Drug Administration for that dose of the series. **Providers should consult the respective Advisory Committee on Immunization Practices statement for detailed recommendations, including for high-risk conditions: http://www.cdc.gov/vaccines/pubs/ACIP-list.htm.** Clinically significant adverse events that follow immunization should be reported to the Vaccine Adverse Event Reporting System (VAERS). Guidance about how to obtain and complete a VAERS form is available at http://www.vaers.hhs.gov or by telephone, 800-822-7967.

*For complete information go to http://www.cdc.gov/nip/recs/child-schedule.htm#printable.

Appendix F

Standard Precautions

The following precautions are used in the care of all patients regardless of their diagnosis or disease. They are also applied when handling or cleaning equipment or supplies that are potentially contaminated.

1. Wear gloves any time that you may contact blood, any moist body fluid (except sweat), secretions, excretions, nonintact skin, or mucous membranes.
2. Remove your gloves, wash your hands, and reapply clean gloves if your gloves become soiled with infective material.
3. Even if you are wearing gloves, remove them, wash your hands, and apply clean gloves *immediately before* contact with mucous membranes or nonintact skin.
4. Wear a protective cover gown of waterproof material if your clothing is likely to have substantial contact with infective material or if splashing of body fluids is likely.
5. Wear a face shield or goggles to protect your eyes if splashing of secretions is likely.
6. Any time a face shield or goggles are worn, wear a surgical mask to protect the mucous membranes of your nose and mouth. A surgical mask may be worn during certain sterile procedures without protective eyewear. However, protective eyewear is *never* worn without a surgical mask.
7. Handle needles, razors, broken glass, and other sharp objects with care. Needles should never be recapped. All sharps should be disposed of in a puncture-resistant sharps container.
8. Wash your hands before and after each patient contact.
9. Wash your hands before you apply and after you remove gloves. Do not assume that hand washing is unnecessary because gloves were worn. Do not wash your hands with gloves on them.
10. Gloves are used for the care of one patient only, then discarded.
11. Follow your facility policy for disposal of gloves and other contaminated items. These items are generally not disposed of in open trash containers. Facilities have designated disposal sites for these biohazardous waste materials.
12. Use resuscitation barrier devices as an alternative to mouth-to-mouth resuscitation.
13. Linen should be handled in a manner that prevents contamination of the outside of the container. Linen from isolation rooms was previously double bagged. Double bagging is no longer recommended since all linen is handled as potentially infectious. Double bag linen only if the outside of the bag becomes contaminated during the bagging process.

Appendix G

Illustrated Mechanisms and Sites of Action

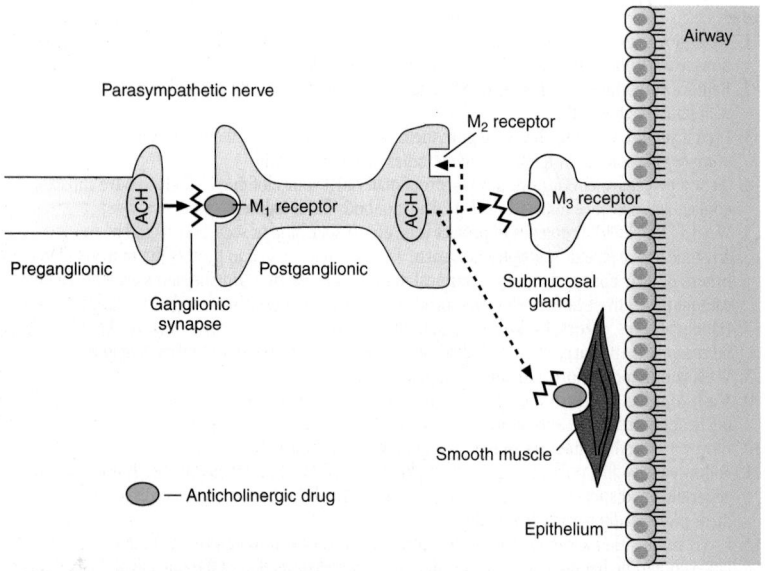

Fig. G-1 Sites and Mechanisms of Action: Anticholinergic Bronchodilators: Anticholinergic bronchodilators, such as ipratropium, work by blocking muscarinic-1 (M_1) receptors on postganglionic parasympathetic nerve endings and muscarinic-3 (M_3) receptors on the cell membranes of bronchial smooth muscles and submucosal glands. Normally, stimulation of the M_1 and M_3 receptors by acetylcholine (ACH) causes bronchoconstriction and mucus secretion from submucosal glands. Anticholinergic bronchodilators block these specific muscarinic receptors from the effects of acetylcholine, causing bronchial smooth muscle relaxation, bronchodilatation, and decreased mucus production. (From Gardenhire OS: *Rau's Respiratory Care Pharmacology,* ed 8, St. Louis, 2012, Mosby.)

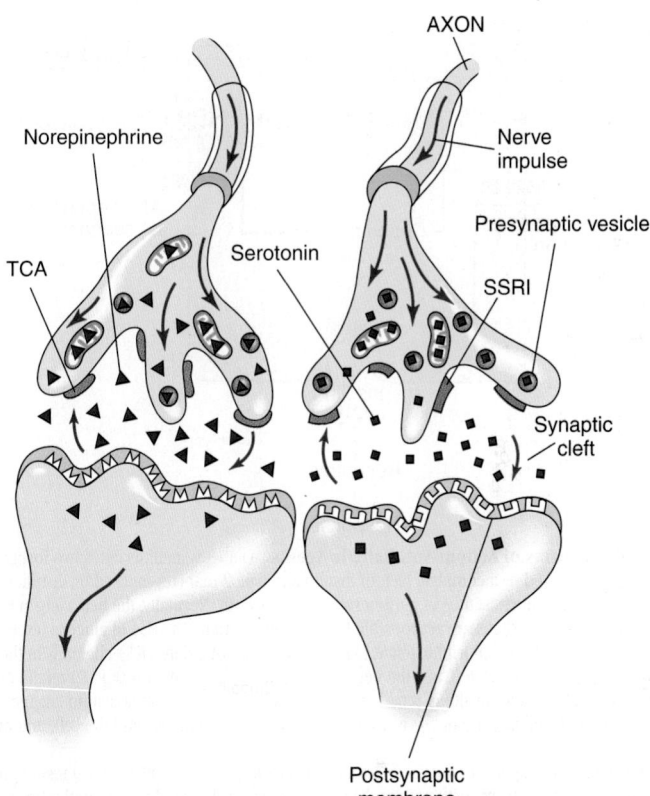

Fig. G-2 Mechanisms of Action: Antidepressants. Depression is thought to occur when levels of neurotransmitters, such as norepinephrine and serotonin, are reduced at postsynaptic receptor sites. These neurotransmitters affect a wide array of functions, including mood, obsessions, appetite, and anxiety. Antidepressants work by increasing the availability of these neurotransmitters at postsynaptic membranes and by enhancing and prolonging their effects. As a result, these agents improve mood, reduce anxiety, and minimize obsessions.

Antidepressants typically are classified as tricyclic antidepressants (TCAs), monoamine oxidase inhibitors (not shown), selective serotonin reuptake inhibitors (SSRIs), and atypical antidepressants (not shown). TCAs, such as amitriptyline and desipramine, primarily block norepinephrine reuptake at presynaptic membranes, thereby increasing the norepinephrine concentration at synapses and making more available at postsynaptic receptors.

SSRIs, such as fluoxetine and paroxetine, selectively inhibit serotonin uptake at presynaptic membranes. This action leads to increased serotonin availability at postsynaptic receptors. (From Gutierrez K: *Pharmacotherapeutics: Clinical Reasoning in Primary Care,* ed 2, Philadelphia, 2008, Saunders.)

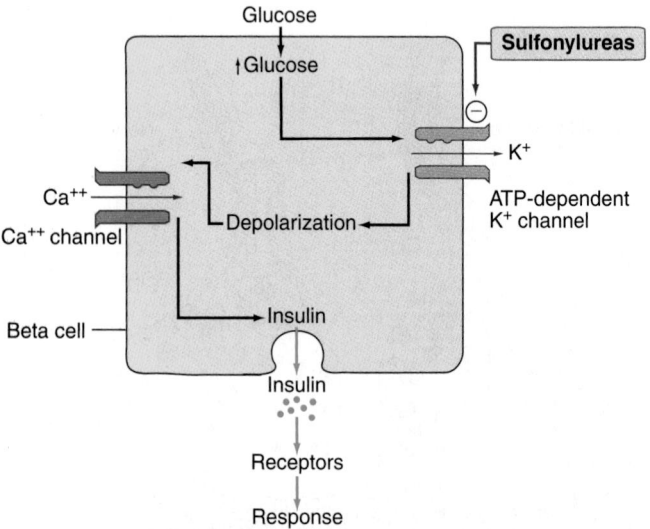

Fig. G-3 Mechanisms of Action: Antidiabetic Agents. Diabetes mellitus takes two forms: type 1 diabetes characterized by a complete lack of insulin and type 2 diabetes marked by insufficient insulin secretion, insulin resistance in peripheral tissues, or both. Normally, the beta cells in the pancreatic islets of Langerhans are responsible for secreting insulin. The rise of glucose levels in the beta cell triggers adenosine triphosphate (ATP)-dependent potassium (K$^+$) channels in the membranes of beta cells to close. Then the beta cells depolarize and calcium (Ca^{++}) enters the cell through Ca^{++} channel, and insulin is released from the cell. When circulating insulin engages with insulin receptors on cell membranes, it facilitates the movement of glucose into the cell, among other actions.

Type 1 diabetes is treated with the use of exogenous insulin, which mimics natural insulin in the body. Insulin takes many forms with varying degrees of onset, peak, and duration, including rapid, regular, intermediate, and long acting.

Type 2 diabetes is usually treated with oral agents. Sulfonylureas, such as glyburide, block ATP-dependent K$^+$ channels in the cell membranes of beta cells, ultimately resulting in the release of insulin. (From Taylor: *Mosby's Crash Course Pharmacology,* St. Louis, 1998, Mosby.)

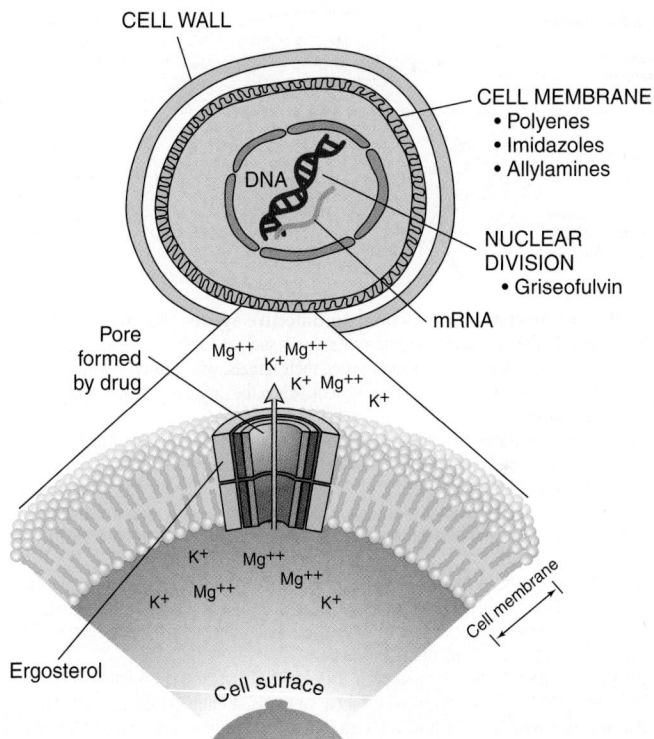

Fig. G-4 Sites and Mechanisms of Action: Antifungal Agents. Antifungal agents primarily affect fungi at one of two sites: the cell membrane or the cell nucleus. Most of these agents, such as polyene, imidazole, and allylamine antifungals, act on the fungal cell membrane. Polyene antifungals, such as amphotericin B, bind to ergosterol and increase cell membrane permeability. Imidazole antifungals, such as fluconazole and ketoconazole, interfere with ergosterol synthesis by inhibiting the cytochrome P_{450} enzyme system, altering the cell membrane, and inhibiting fungal growth. Allylamine antifungals, such as terbinafine, inhibit the enzyme squaline epoxidase, which disrupts ergosterol production—and cell membrane integrity. When cell membrane permeability increases, cellular components, including potassium (K^+) and magnesium (Mg^{++}), leak out. Loss of these cellular components leads to cell death.

Another antifungal agent, griseofulvin, directly affects the fungal nucleus, interfering with mitosis. By binding to structures in the mitotic spindle, it prevents cells from dividing, which eventually leads to their death. (From Gutierrez K: *Pharmacotherapeutics: Clinical Reasoning in Primary Care,* ed 2, Philadelphia, 2008, Saunders.)

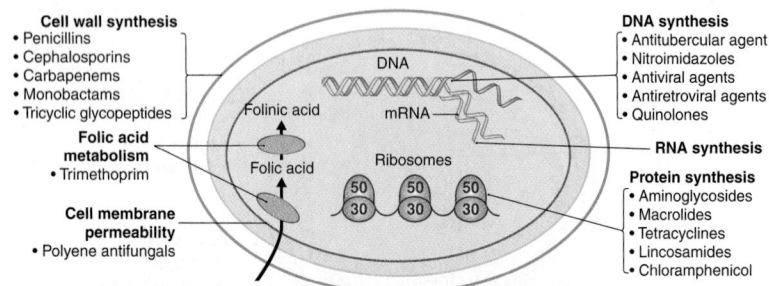

Fig. G-5 Sites and Mechanisms of Action: Antiinfective Agents. The goal of antiinfective therapy is to kill or inhibit the growth of microorganisms such as bacteria, viruses, and fungi. To achieve this goal, antiinfective agents must reach their targets, which usually occurs through absorption and distribution by the circulatory system. When the target is reached, a drug can kill or suppress microorganisms by:

• Inhibiting cell wall synthesis or activating enzymes that disrupt the cell wall, which leads to cellular weakening, lysis, and death. Penicillins (ampicillin), cephalosporins (cefazolin), carbapenems (imipenem), monobactams (aztreonam), and tricyclic glycopeptides (vancomycin) act in this way.

• Altering cell membrane permeability through direct action on the cell wall, which allows intracellular substances to leak out and destabilizes the cell. Polyene antifungals (amphotericin) work by this mechanism.

• Altering protein synthesis by binding to bacterial ribosomes (50/30) or affecting ribosomal function, which leads to cell death or slowed growth respectively. Aminoglycosides (gentamicin), macrolides (erythromycin), tetracyclines (doxycycline), lincosamides (clindamycin), and the miscellaneous antiinfective chloramphenicol use this action.

• Inhibiting DNA or RNA, including messenger RNA (mRNA), synthesis by binding to nucleic acids or interacting with enzymes required for their synthesis. Antitubercular agents (rifampin), nitroimidazoles (metronidazole), antiviral agents (acyclovir), antiretroviral agents (stavudine), and quinolones (ciprofloxacin) act like this.

• Inhibiting the metabolism of folic acid and folinic acid or other cellular components that are essential for bacterial cell growth. The miscellaneous antiinfective trimethoprim employs this mechanism of action. (From Page C et al: *Integrated Pharmacology,* ed 3, St. Louis, 2006, Mosby.)

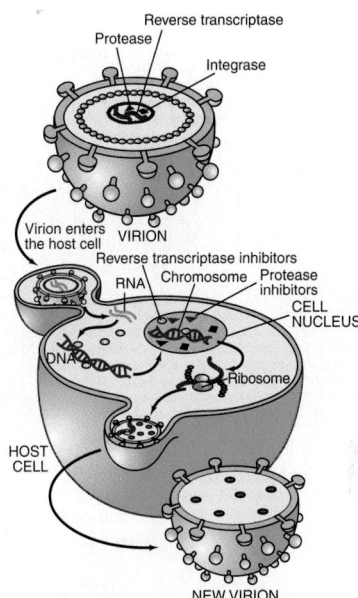

Fig. G-6 Mechanisms and Sites of Action: Antiretroviral Agents. When viruses reproduce, the infectious viral particle, or virion **(A)**, enters the host cell. The virion attaches to the cell's surface and then inserts itself into the host cell **(B)**. Once inside, the virion uncoats, and the enzyme reverse transcriptase makes two copies of the viral RNA: one copy is identical; the other is a mirror image. These two copies form double-stranded viral DNA that enters the host cell's nucleus, where it inserts itself into the host cell's DNA with the help of the enzyme integrase. Then viral DNA reprograms the host cell to produce additional viral RNA, which begins the process of forming new viruses. Specifically, messenger RNA (mRNA) instructs ribosomal RNA (rRNA) to produce a new chain of proteins and enzymes that are used to form new viruses. Protease cuts the chains, creating individual proteins. These combine with new RNA to create new virions, which bud and are released from the host cell **(C)**.

Antiretroviral agents target specific enzymes during viral reproduction. Nucleoside reverse transcriptase inhibitors, such as stavudine, interfere with the action of reverse transcriptase by mimicking naturally occurring nucleosides. Nucleotide reverse transcriptase inhibitors, such as tenofovir, block reverse transcriptase by competing with the natural substrate deoxyadenosine triphosphate and by causing DNA chain termination. Nonnucleoside reverse transcriptase inhibitors, such as delavirdine, work by directly binding to reverse transcriptase. As a result, no viral DNA is available to insert itself into the host cell's DNA. Protease inhibitors, such as indinavir, bind to and interfere with the action of protease; thus, the new chain of proteins formed by rRNA cannot be cut into individual proteins to make new viruses. (From Gutierrez K: *Pharmacotherapeutics: Clinical Reasoning in Primary Care,* ed 2, Philadelphia, 2008, Saunders.)

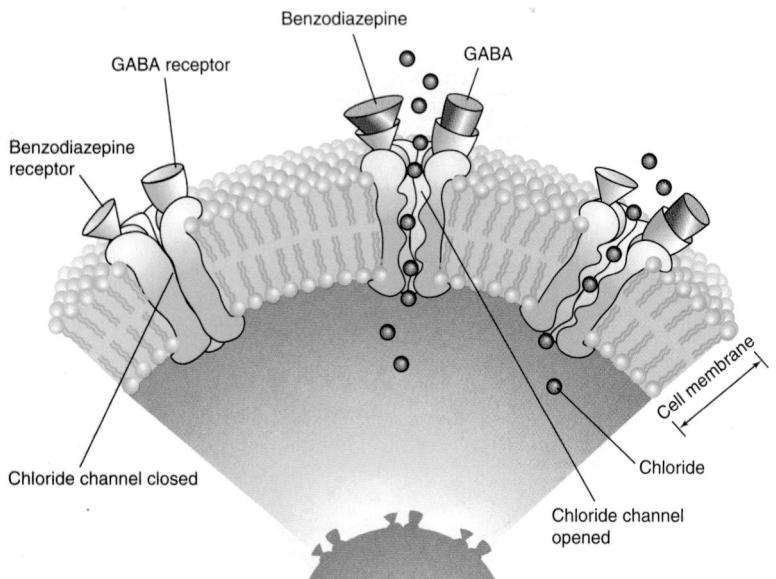

Fig. G-7 Mechanisms of Action: Benzodiazepines. Benzodiazepines reduce anxiety by stimulating the action of the inhibitory neurotransmitter, gamma-aminobutyric acid (GABA), in the limbic system. The limbic system plays an important role in the regulation of human behavior. Dysfunction of GABA neurotransmission in the limbic system may be linked to the development of certain anxiety disorders.

The limbic system contains a highly dense area of benzodiazepine receptors that may be linked to the antianxiety effects of benzodiazepines. These benzodiazepine receptors are located on the surface of neuronal cell membranes and are adjacent to GABA receptors. The binding of a benzodiazepine to its receptor enhances the affinity of a GABA receptor for GABA. In the absence of a benzodiazepine, the binding of GABA to its receptor causes the chloride channel in the cell membrane to open, which increases the influx of chloride into the cell. This influx of chloride results in hyperpolarization of the neuronal cell membrane and reduces the neuron's ability to fire, which is why GABA is considered an inhibitory neurotransmitter.

A benzodiazepine acts only in the presence of GABA. When it binds to a benzodiazepine receptor, it prolongs the time that the chloride channel remains open. This results in greater depression of neuronal function and a reduction in anxiety. (From Gutierrez K: *Pharmacotherapeutics: Clinical Reasoning in Primary Care,* ed 2, Philadelphia, 2008, Saunders.)

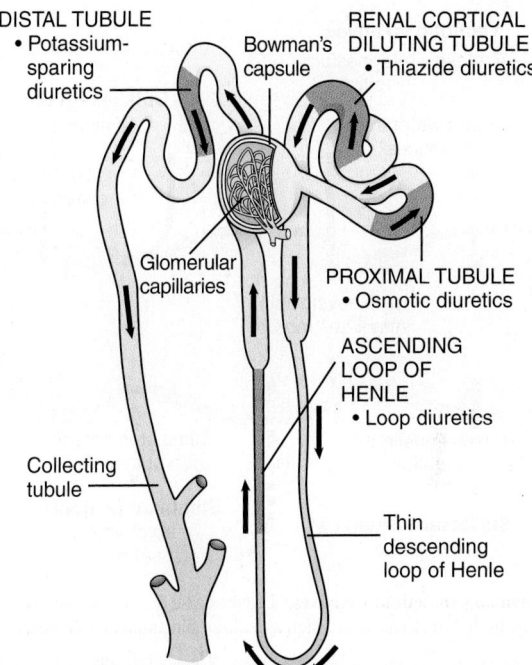

Fig. G-8 Sites of Action: Diuretics. Diuretics act primarily to increase water and sodium excretion by the kidneys, thereby increasing urine output. In the process, chloride, potassium, and other electrolytes may also be excreted. Most diuretics act by blocking sodium, water, and chloride reabsorption by peritubular capillaries in the nephrons. As a result, water and electrolytes remain in the convoluted tubules to be excreted as urine. The increased water and electrolyte excretion reduces blood volume—and ultimately blood pressure.

Diuretics belong to four major subclasses:

1. Thiazide diuretics, such as hydrochlorothiazide, act in the early portion of the distal convoluted tubule, called the cortical diluting segment. These drugs block sodium, chloride, and water reabsorption and promote their excretion along with potassium.

2. Loop diuretics, such as furosemide, act primarily in the thick ascending limb of the loop of Henle, blocking sodium, water, and chloride reabsorption. Then these substances are excreted along with potassium.

3. Potassium-sparing diuretics, such as spironolactone, act in the late portion of the distal convoluted tubule and collecting tubule. Here, they inhibit the action of aldosterone, leading to sodium excretion and potassium retention. Although triamterene and amiloride, two other potassium-sparing diuretics, act at the same site, they do not affect aldosterone. Instead, these drugs directly block the exchange of sodium and potassium, leading to decreased sodium reabsorption and decreased potassium excretion.

4. Osmotic diuretics, such as mannitol, work in the proximal convoluted tubule. As their name implies, these diuretics increase the osmotic pressure of the glomerular filtrate, inhibiting the passive reabsorption of water, sodium, and chloride. (From Gutierrez K: *Pharmacotherapeutics: Clinical Reasoning in Primary Care,* ed 2, Philadelphia, 2008, Saunders.)

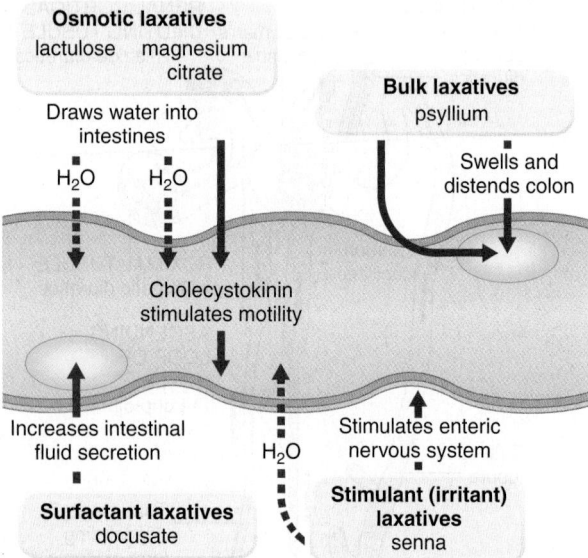

Fig. G-9 Mechanisms of Action: Laxatives. Laxatives ease or stimulate defecation. Typically, they are classified by their mechanism of action as bulk-forming, osmotic, stimulant, or surfactant laxatives.

Bulk-forming laxatives, such as psyllium, act in the small and large bowel. Because ingredients in these laxatives are undigestible, they remain within the stool and increase the fecal mass by drawing in water. These agents also enhance bacterial growth in the colon, further adding to the fecal mass.

Osmotic laxatives, such as lactulose, draw water into the intestinal lumen, causing the fecal mass to soften and swell. This osmotic action may be enhanced by the metabolism of colonic bacteria to lactate and other organic acids. These acids decrease colonic pH and increase colonic motility.

Stimulant (or irritant) laxatives, such as senna, act on the intestinal wall to increase water and electrolytes in the intestinal lumen. In addition, they directly irritate the colon, increasing motility.

Surfactant laxatives (or fecal softeners), such as docusate, reduce the surface tension of the stool, allowing water to enter it. These laxatives may also help to increase water and electrolyte excretion into the intestinal lumen, softening and increasing the fecal mass. (From Page C et al: *Integrated Pharmacology,* ed 3, St. Louis, 2006, Mosby.)

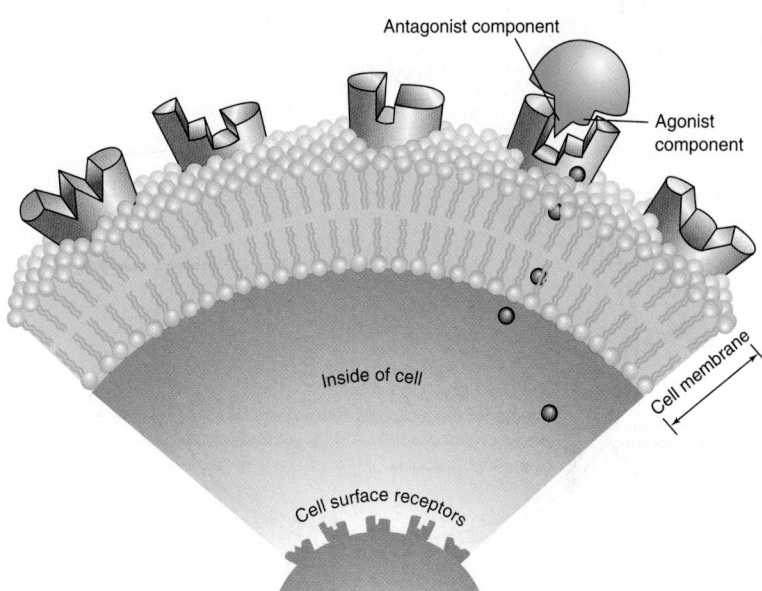

Fig. G-10 Mechanisms of Action: Narcotic Agonist-Antagonist Analgesics. Cell membranes have different types of opioid receptors, such as mu, kappa, and delta receptors. Opioid agonist-antagonists work by stimulating one type of receptor, while simultaneously blocking another type. As agonists, they work primarily by activating kappa receptors to produce analgesia and such other effects as CNS and respiratory depression, decreased GI motility, and euphoria. As antagonists, they compete with opioids at mu receptors, helping to reverse or block some of the other effects of agonists. (From Gutierrez K: *Pharmacotherapeutics: Clinical Reasoning in Primary Care,* ed 2, Philadelphia, 2008, Saunders.)

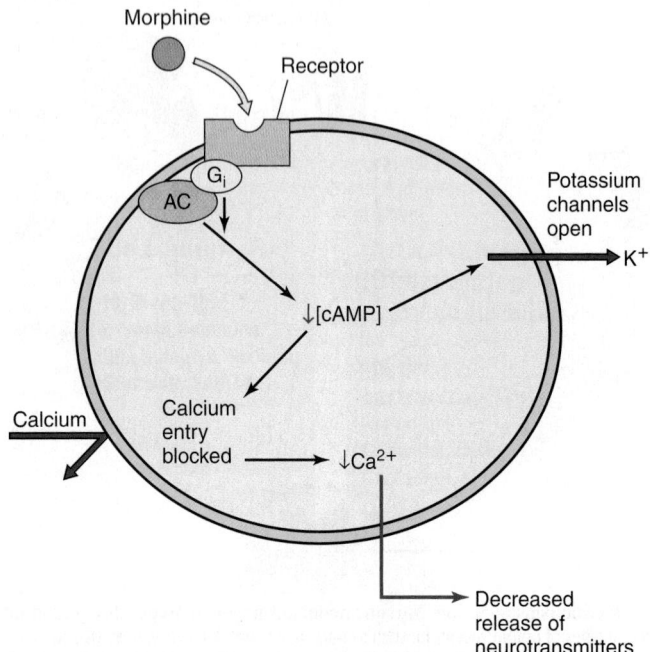

Fig. G-11 Mechanisms of Action: Narcotic Analgesics. Narcotic analgesics bind to three types of opioid receptors: mu, kappa, and delta receptors. They produce analgesia primarily by activating mu receptors. However, they also engage with and activate kappa and delta receptors, producing other effects, such as sedation and vasomotor stimulation.

When morphine or another narcotic analgesic binds to opioid receptors, activation occurs. The receptors send signals to the enzyme adenyl cyclase (AC) to slow activity by way of G proteins (G_i). Decreased adenyl cyclase activity causes reduced production of cyclic adenosine monophosphate (cAMP). A secondary messenger substance, cAMP is important for regulating cell membrane channels. A reduced cAMP level allows fewer potassium ions to leave the cell and blocks calcium ions from entering the cell. This ion imbalance—especially the reduced intracellular calcium level—ultimately decreases the release of neurotransmitters from the cell, thereby blocking or reducing pain impulse transmission. (From Minneman KP, Wecker L: *Brody's Human Pharmacology: Molecular to Clinical,* ed 4, St. Louis, 2005, Mosby.)

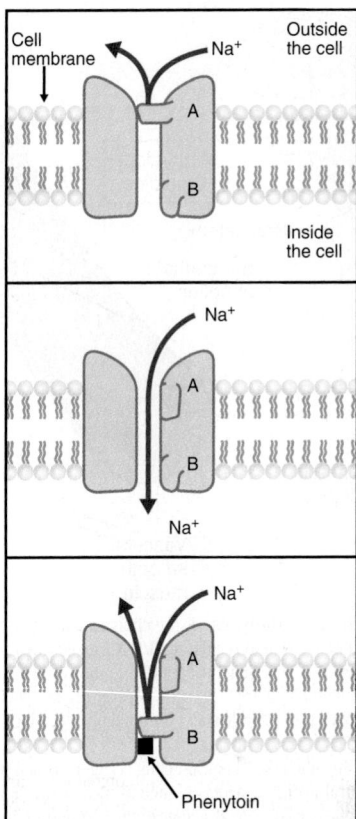

Fig. G-12 Mechanisms of Action: Phenytoin. Phenytoin, which is used to treat tonic-clonic seizures, acts in the motor cortex and brain stem, where the tonic phase of tonic-clonic seizures originates. By altering sodium transport across neuronal cell membranes, phenytoin stabilizes the cell membrane, reduces repetitive firing of the neurons, and halts or limits the spread of seizures. The first illustration shows a neuronal cell membrane in its resting state. The activation gate **(A)** of the sodium channel in the cell membrane is closed and blocks sodium (Na^+) from entering the cell. In the second illustration, a nerve impulse has caused depolarization and opening of the activation gate, allowing Na^+ to move into the cell. In the third illustration, depolarization continues and an inactivation gate **(B)** moves into the channel. This prevents Na^+ from moving into the cell. Phenytoin prolongs the inactivated state of the sodium channel by preventing reopening of the inactivation gate. By further preventing Na^+ from entering the cell, phenytoin slows impulse transmission, and thus slows the rate at which neurons fire. (From Minneman KP, Wecker L: *Brody's Human Pharmacology: Molecular to Clinical,* ed 4, St. Louis, 2005, Mosby.)

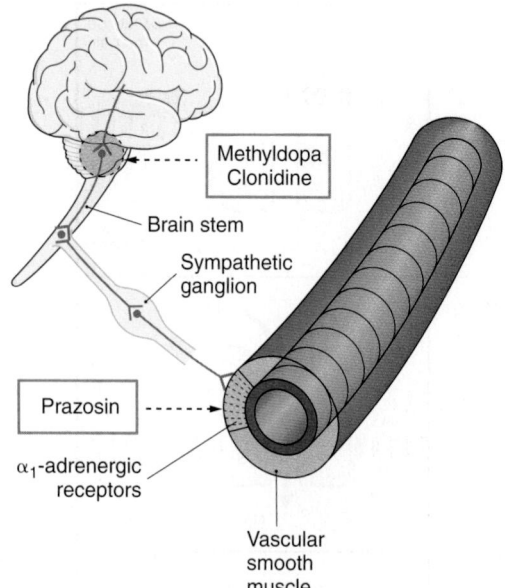

Fig. G-13 Sites of Action: Sympatholytics. Sympatholytics inhibit sympathetic nervous system (SNS) activity, which plays a major role in regulating B/P. Normally when the SNS is stimulated, nerve impulses travel from the cardiovascular center of the CNS to the sympathetic ganglia. From there, the impulses travel along postganglionic fibers to specific effector organs, such as the heart and blood vessels. SNS stimulation also triggers the release of norepinephrine, which acts primarily at alpha-adrenergic receptors.

Sympatholytics fall into two subclasses: central-acting α_2 agonists and peripheral-acting α_1-adrenergic antagonists. Central-acting α_2 agonists, such as methyldopa and clonidine, stimulate α_2-adrenergic receptors in the cardiovascular center of the CNS and reduce activity in the vasomotor center of the brain, interfering with sympathetic stimulation of the heart and blood vessels. This causes blood vessel dilatation and decreased cardiac output, which leads to reduced B/P.

Peripheral-acting α_1-adrenergic antagonists, such as prazosin, inhibit the stimulation of α_1-adrenergic receptors by norepinephrine in vascular smooth muscle, interfering with SNS-induced vasoconstriction. As a result, the blood vessels dilate, reducing peripheral vascular resistance and venous return to the heart. These effects, in turn, lead to decreased B/P. (From Prosser S, Worster B, Dewar K: *Applied Pharmacology for Nurses and Other Health Care Professionals,* St. Louis, 2000, Mosby.)

Appendix H

Photo Atlas of Drug Administration

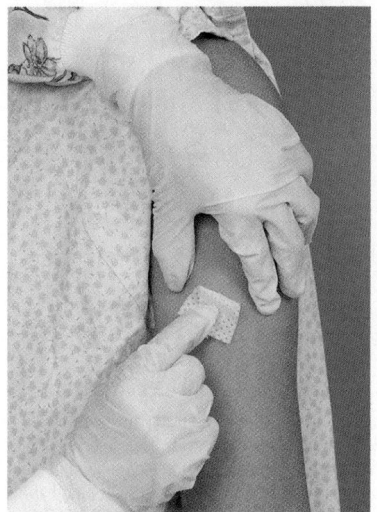

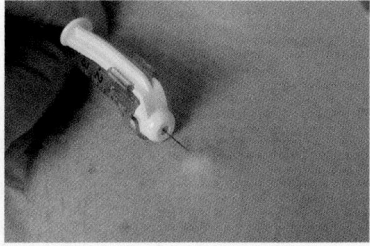

Fig. H-2 Intradermal Injection. For an intradermal injection, note formation of small bleb approximately 6 mm (¼ in) in diameter at injection site. (From Perry AG, Potter PA, and Elkin MK: *Nursing Interventions & Clinical Skills,* ed 5, St. Louis, 2012, Mosby.)

Fig. H-1 Administering an Injection. Cleanse site with antiseptic swab. Apply swab at center of site and rotate outward in circular direction for about 5 cm (2 in). (From Perry AG, Potter PA, and Elkin MK: *Nursing Interventions & Clinical Skills,* ed 5, St. Louis, 2012, Mosby.)

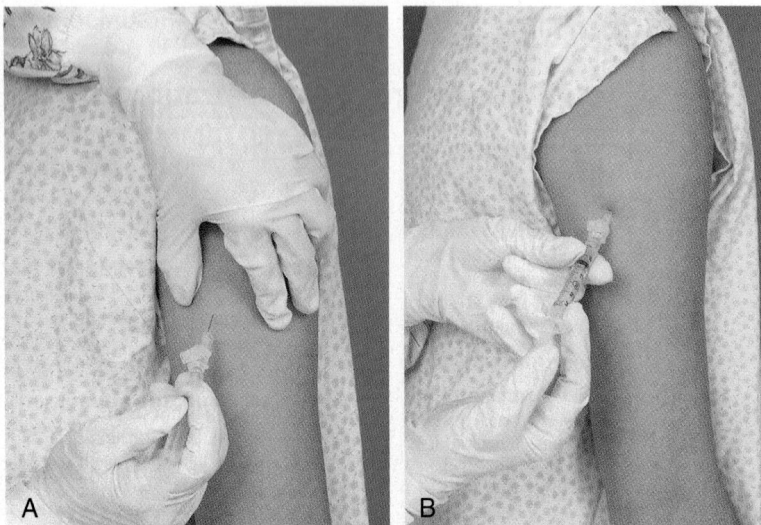

Fig. H-3 Subcutaneous Injection. A, For a subcutaneous injection, hold the syringe between the thumb and forefinger of the dominant hand as a dart, with the palm down. **B,** After injecting the needle at a 45- to 90-degree angle, grasp lower end of syringe barrel with nondominant hand to end of plunger. Avoid moving syringe while slowly pulling back on plunger to aspirate drug. If blood appears in syringe, remove needle, discard medication and syringe, and repeat procedure. *Exception:* Do not aspirate when giving heparin. (From Perry AG, Potter PA, and Elkin MK: *Nursing Interventions & Clinical Skills,* ed 5, St. Louis, 2012, Mosby.)

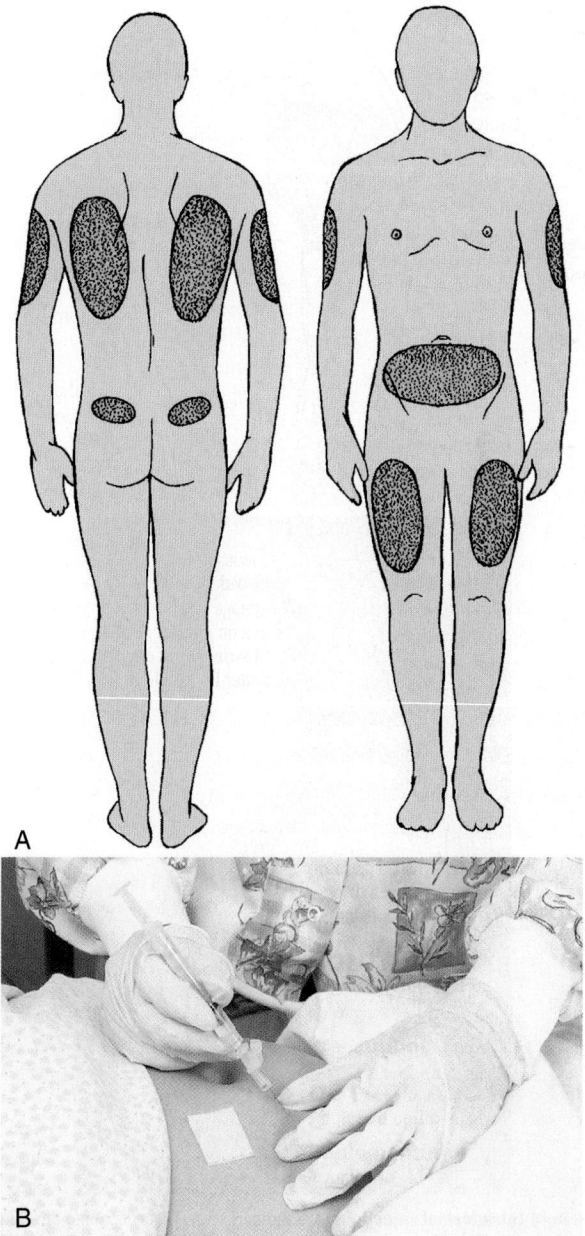

Fig. H-4 Subcutaneous Injection. A, Sites recommended for subcutaneous injections. **B,** Giving subcutaneous injection in the abdomen. (From Perry AG, Potter PA, and Elkin MK: *Nursing Interventions & Clinical Skills,* ed 5, St. Louis, 2012, Mosby.)

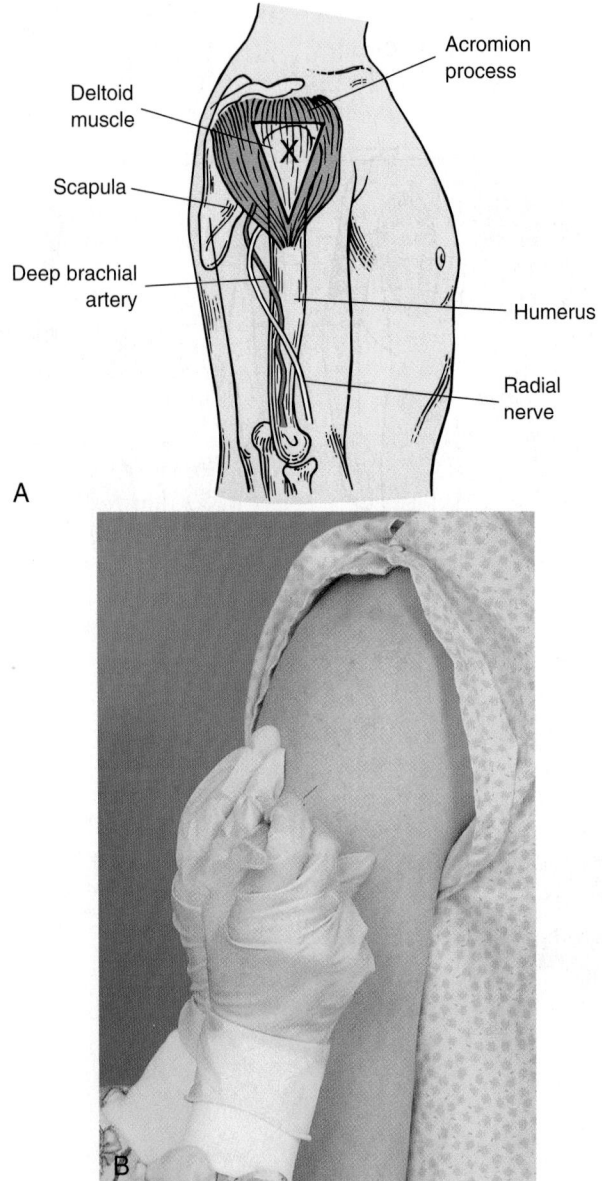

Fig. H-5 Deltoid Intradermal Injection. **A,** Landmarks for IM injection into the deltoid muscle. **B,** Giving IM injection in deltoid muscle. (From Perry AG, Potter PA, and Elkin MK: *Nursing Interventions & Clinical Skills,* ed 5, St. Louis, 2012, Mosby.)

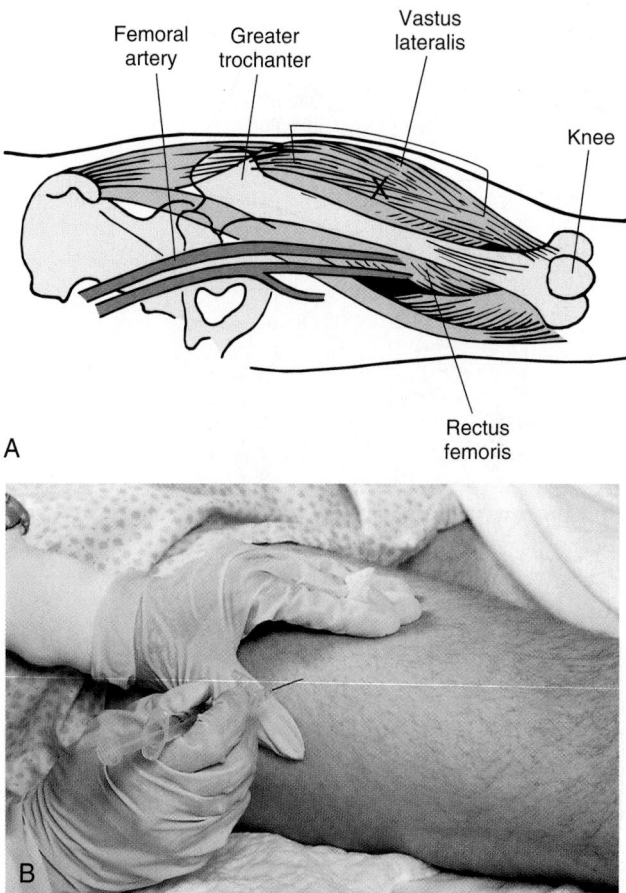

Fig. H-6 Vastus Lateralis Intramuscular Injection. A, Landmarks for IM injection in vastus lateralis. **B,** Giving IM injection in vastus lateralis site. (From Perry AG, Potter PA, and Elkin MK: *Nursing Interventions & Clinical Skills,* ed 5, St. Louis, 2012, Mosby.)

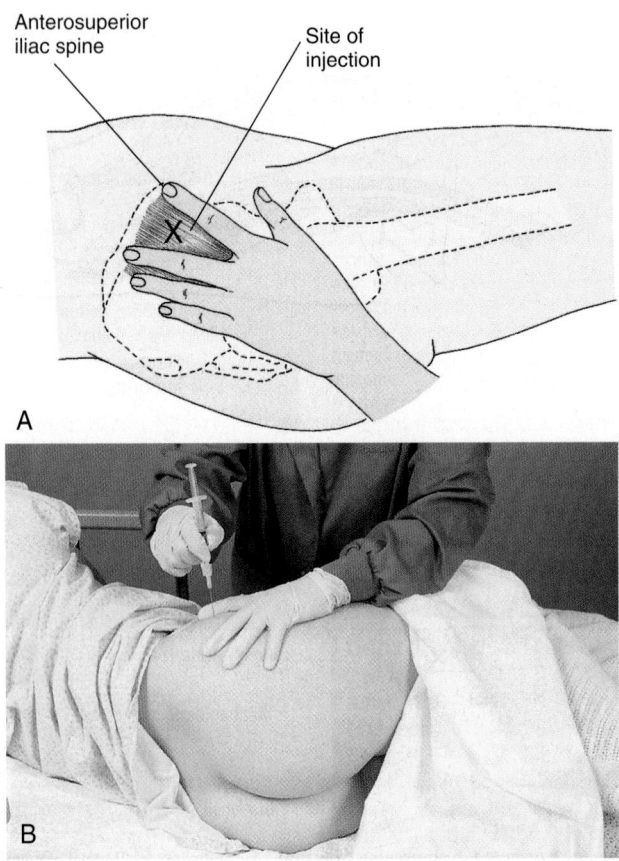

Fig. H-7 Ventrogluteal Intramuscular Injection. A, Anatomical view of ventrogluteal site. **B,** Giving IM injection into ventrogluteal muscle to avoid major nerves and blood vessels. (From Perry AG, Potter PA, and Elkin MK: *Nursing Interventions & Clinical Skills,* ed 5, St. Louis, 2012, Mosby.)

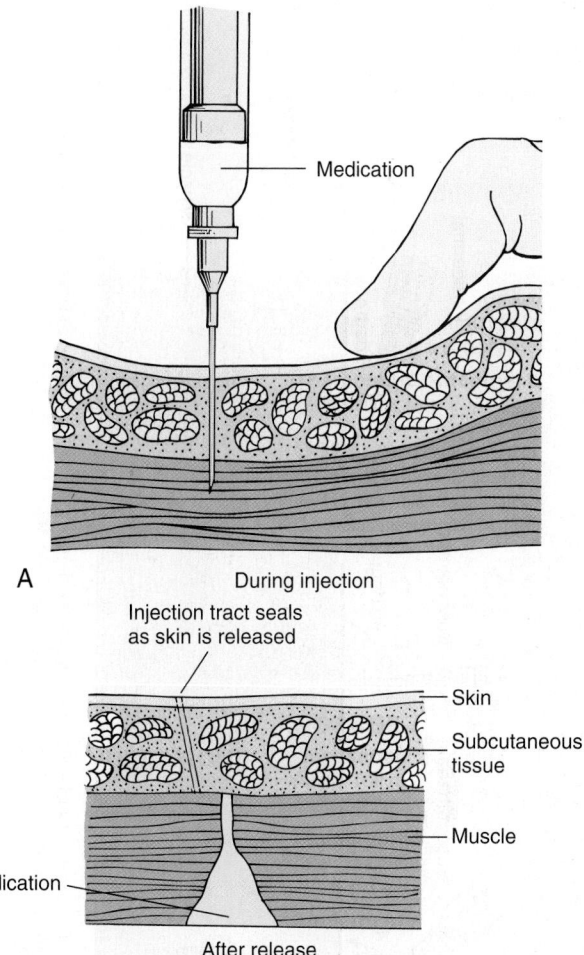

A   During injection

Fig. H-8 Z-Track Method of Injection. A, Pulling on overlying skin during IM injection moves tissues to prevent later tracking. **B,** The Z-track left after injection prevents the deposit of medication through sensitive tissue. (From Perry AG, Potter PA, and Elkin MK: *Nursing Interventions & Clinical Skills,* ed 5, St. Louis, 2012, Mosby.)

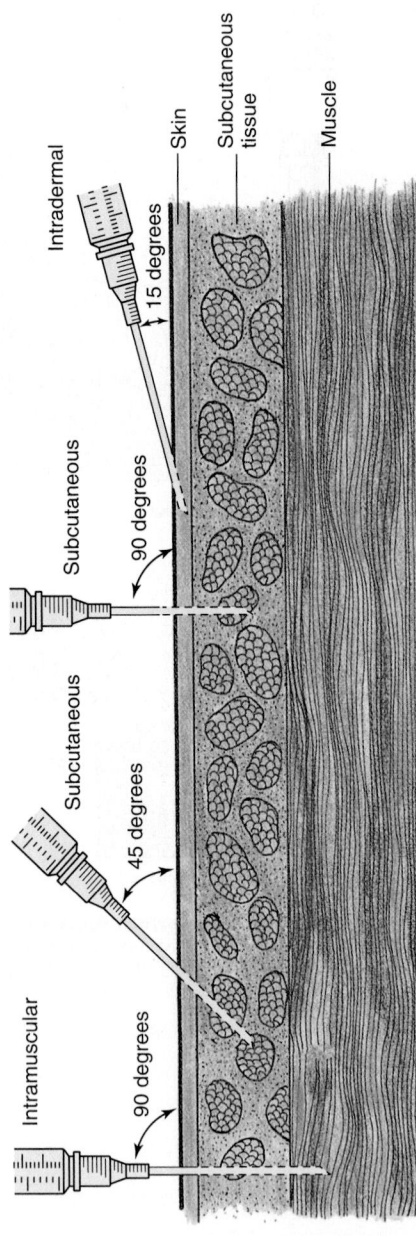

Fig. H-9 Comparison of Needle Angles. Comparison of angles of insertion for IM (90 degrees), SUBCUT (45 degrees and 90 degrees), and ID (15 degrees) injections. (From Potter PA, Perry AG: *Fundamentals of Nursing*, ed 7, St. Louis, 2009, Mosby.)

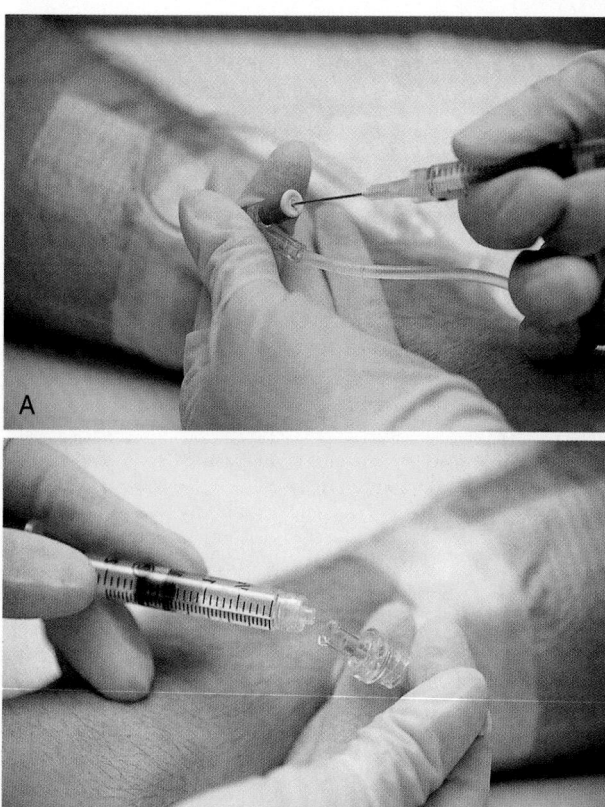

Fig. H-10 Administering Medication by IV Bolus (push). A, Needle system: Insert small-gauge needle of syringe containing prepared drug through center of injection port. **B,**Needleless system: Remove cap of needleless injection port. Connect tip of syringe directly. (From Potter PA, Perry AG: *Fundamentals of Nursing,* ed 6, St. Louis, 2005, Mosby.)

Continued

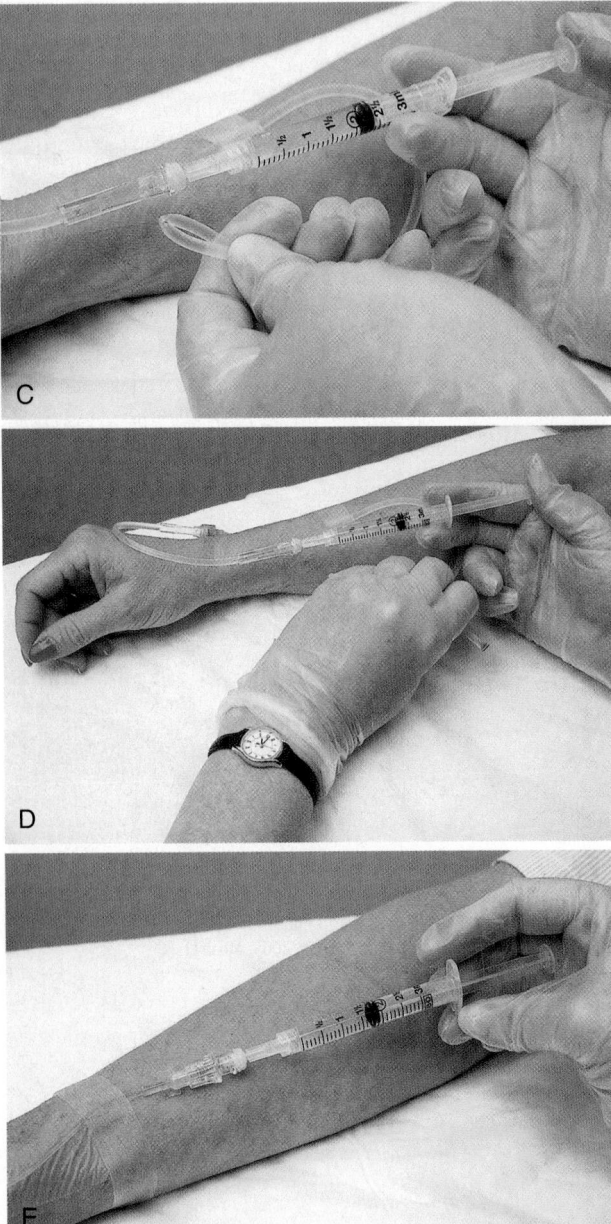

Fig. H-10, cont'd **C,** Occlude **IV** line by pinching tubing just above injection port. Pull back gently on syringe's plunger to aspirate blood return. **D,** After noting blood return, continue to occlude tubing and inject medication slowly over several minutes (read directions on drug package). Use watch to time administration. **E, IV** lock: Insert needle of syringe containing prepared drug through center of diaphragm. (From Potter PA, Perry AG: *Fundamentals of Nursing,* ed 6, St. Louis, 2005, Mosby.)

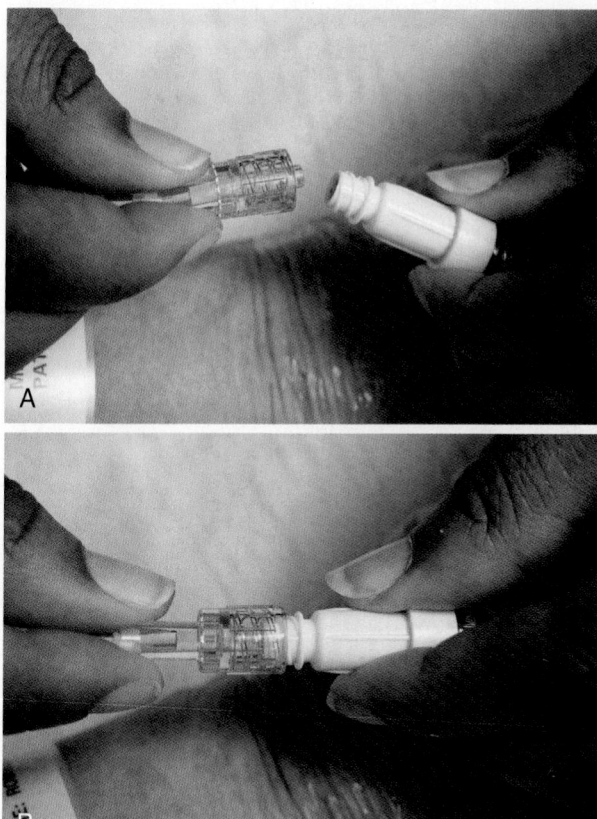

Fig. H-11 Administering IV Medication by Piggyback, Volume Administration Sets of Miniinfusors (Syringe Pump). Use needle-lock device to secure needle of secondary piggyback line through injection port of main line. (From Perry AG, Potter PA, and Elkin MK: *Nursing Interventions & Clinical Skills,* ed 5, St. Louis, 2012, Mosby.)

Index

Drug names listed with SEE EVOLVE are found on your Evolve Resources at http://elsevier.com/nursingdrugupdates/Skidmore/NDG.

Entries can be identified as follows: generic name, Trade Name, DRUG CATEGORY

Entries can be identified as follows: generic name, Trade Name, DRUG CATEGORY

Entries can be identified as follows: generic name, Trade Name, DRUG CATEGORY

M

Entries can be identified as follows: generic name, Trade Name, DRUG CATEGORY

Entries can be identified as follows: generic name, Trade Name, DRUG CATEGORY

Entries can be identified as follows: generic name, Trade Name, DRUG CATEGORY

Entries can be identified as follows: generic name, Trade Name, DRUG CATEGORY

- Does the patient have any allergies?
- Is the patient NPO?
- Is the patient taking any other medication and/or herbal supplements that may interact with this drug?
- Are there any vital signs that I need to check before administering the drug?
- Do I need to check any lab values (i.e., glucose)?
- Are there any other assessments that I need to make before giving this drug?

The 5 rights of medication administration

Always adhere to the 5 rights of medication administration when transcribing, preparing, administering, and documenting medications:

1. **Right patient:** Compare the patient's armband with the medication administration record. Compare the patient's name on the medication administration record (MAR) with that on the medication drawer or computerized equipment.
2. **Right drug:** Verify the correct medication by comparing the name on the label on the drug container with that written on the MAR.
3. **Right route:** Check the ordered route by reading the medication order, and verify the appropriateness of the route based on knowledge of the patient's condition.
4. **Right dose:** Always independently double-check dosages of medications with the pharmacy's calculations or with a second nurse. The nurse must also be aware of therapeutic dosages for each medication and question an order that is not within that range.
5. **Right time:** All medications should be administered within 30 minutes of the scheduled time. The medications must also be prepared to correlate appropriately with meal times and to avoid drug interactions.

Following appropriate drug administration, assess the patient for the expected therapeutic outcome and/or potential side effects.

RARELY USED

alemtuzumab

(al'em-tooz'ue-mab)
Lemtrada
Func. class.: Biologic response modifier

USES: Reserved for those with multiple sclerosis with inadequate response to ≥2 drugs because of severe adverse reactions

CONTRAINDICATIONS: HIV

DOSAGE AND ROUTES

Adult: IV 12 mg/day for 5 consecutive days (total 60 mg) for a first treatment course; follow 12 mo later with 12 mg/day for 3 consecutive days (total 36 mg) for a second treatment course

RARELY USED

antihemophilic factor Fc fusion protein

(an-tee-hee-moe-fil'ik fak'tor)
Eloctate
Func. class.: Hemostatic

USES: Hemophilia A (congenital factor VIII deficiency), control/prevention of bleeding, perioperative management of surgical bleeding

CONTRAINDICATIONS: Bleeding

DOSAGE AND ROUTES

Hemophilia A (congenital factor VIII deficiency)

Adult, adolescent, child, infant, and neonate: IV Infusion: Infuse dose ≤10 ml/min; Dose (IU) = body weight (kg) × desired factor VIII increase (IU/dl or % of normal) × 0.5 (IU/kg per IU/dl) OR estimated increment of factor VIII (IU/dl or % of normal) = [total dose (IU)/body weight (kg)] × 2 (IU/dl per IU/kg)

Control/prevention of bleeding

Adult, adolescent, child, infant, neonate: Dose and duration of treatment depend on the severity of the factor VIII deficiency, the location and extent of bleeding, and the patient's clinical condition

Perioperative management of surgical bleeding

Adult, adolescent, child, infant, and neonate: Dose and duration of treatment depend on the severity of the factor VIII deficiency, the location and extent of bleeding, and the patient's clinical condition

Routine bleeding prophylaxis to prevent/reduce the frequency of bleeding episodes: IV Initially, 50 IU/kg q4d; adjust dose based on response

apremilast

(a-pre'mi-last)
Otezla
Func. class.: Musculoskeletal agent: disease-modifying antirheumatic drug (DMARD)
Pregnancy category C

ACTION: A phosphodiesterase-4 (PDE4) inhibitor specific for cyclic adenosine monophosphate (cAMP). Inhibition of PDE4 results in an increase in intracellular concentration of cAMP, with a partial inhibition of proinflammatory mediators and an increase in the production of some antiinflammatory mediators

Therapeutic outcome: Resolution of symptoms of psoriatic arthritis or plaque psoriasis

USES: Treatment of active psoriatic arthritis; severe plaque psoriasis (in those not a candidate for phototherapy)

CONTRAINDICATIONS: Hypersensitivity

Precautions: Pregnancy **C**, breastfeeding, depression/suicidal, renal disease (CCr <30 ml/min)

DOSAGE AND ROUTES

Treatment of active psoriatic arthritis/severe plaque psoriasis

Adult: PO To reduce the risk for gastrointestinal symptoms, titrate to a final dose of 30 mg bid; day 1: 10 mg PO AM; day 2: 10 mg AM and PM; day 3: 10 mg AM and 20 mg PM; day 4: 20 mg AM and PM; day 5: 20 mg AM and 30 mg PM; day 6 and thereafter: 30 mg bid

Renal dose

Adult: PO CCr ≥30 ml/min: no change; CCr <30 ml/min: 30 mg every day. Initially, 10 mg AM days 1-3; 20 mg AM days 4 and 5; 30 mg every day for day 6 and thereafter

Available forms: Tab 30 mg; starter pack

Adverse effects: *italics* = common; **bold** = life-threatening

Implementation
Give whole, do not crush, break, or chew; give without regard to meals

ADVERSE EFFECTS
CNS: *Headache,* depression, suicidal ideation, fatigue, insomnia
GI: Diarrhea, nausea, vomiting, abdominal pain, frequent bowel movements, dyspepsia, weight loss
MS: Back pain
RESP: URI, pharyngitis, bronchitis
SYST: Hypersensitivity reactions

Pharmacokinetics

Absorption	Unknown
Distribution	68% bound to plasma proteins
Metabolism	Liver, metabolized by CYP3A4
Excretion	Urine (58%), feces (39%)
Half-life	6-9 hr

Pharmacodynamics

Onset	Unknown
Peak	2.5 hr
Duration	Unknown

INTERACTIONS
Drug classifications
CYP3A4 inducers (rifampin, isoniazid, pyrazinamide, barbiturates, phenytoin, carbamazepine, enzalutamide), avoid concurrent use; decreased effect of apremilast

Drug/herb
CYP3A4 inducers (St. Johns' wort), avoid concurrent use: decreased effect of apremilast

NURSING CONSIDERATIONS
Assessment
• **Psoriatic arthritis/severe plaque psoriasis:** assess for hypersensitivity reactions
• **Pregnancy and breastfeeding:** if used during pregnancy, call 1-877-311-8972; avoid use in breastfeeding
• Assess for depression and suicidal ideation, mood changes; for renal failure or severe renal impairment (CCr <30 ml/min), dosage reduction is required

Patient/family education
• Teach Patient to report rash, hypersensitivity reactions

• Teach patient to avoid use in pregnancy and breastfeeding; if used during pregnancy, call 1-877-311-8972
• Advise patient to be alert for depression and suicidal ideation, mood changes; if these occur, notify prescriber immediately

Evaluation
Positive therapeutic outcome
• Resolution of symptoms of psoriatic arthritis or plaque psoriasis

---

⚠ HIGH ALERT

belinostat
(beh-lih'noh-stat')
Beleodaq
Func. class.: Antineoplastic-biologic response modifier
Chem. class.: Histone deacetylase inhibitors

Pregnancy category D

ACTION: A class I and II inhibitor of the histone deacetylase (HDAC) enzymes. Overexpression of HDACs is present in some cancer cells. HDAC inhibitors have been shown to activate differentiation, inhibit the cell cycle, and induce apoptosis

Therapeutic outcome: Prevention of spread of disease

USES: For the treatment of relapsed or refractory peripheral T-cell lymphoma (PTCL)

CONTRAINDICATIONS: Hypersensitivity, pregnancy **D**

Precautions: Hematologic toxicity (thrombocytopenia, leukopenia, neutropenia, lymphopenia, anemia), serious infections (pneumonia, sepsis), fatal hepatic toxicity, tumor lysis syndrome (TLS), breastfeeding

DOSAGE AND ROUTES
Adult: IV 1000 mg/m^2 over 30 min on days 1-5 q21d. Reduce the dose to 750 mg/m^2 in those who are homozygous for the UGT1A1*28 allele. Cycles should be repeated until disease progression or unacceptable toxicity.

Available forms: Powder for injection 500 mg

⚠ Nurse Alert

Implementation
Intermittent IV route
• Reconstitution: Add 9 ml of sterile water for injection/500 mg, swirl until there are no visible particles in the solution (50 mg/ml); stable at room temperature for up to 12 hr
• Withdraw the appropriate amount from the reconstituted vial and further dilute in 250 ml 0.9% sodium chloride for injection; the final solution is stable at room temperature for up to 36 hr, including infusion time; use a 0.22-micron in-line filter; give over 30 min; if pain occurs at infusion site, run over 45 min

Dose adjustments due to treatment-related toxicity

Hematologic toxicities:
• Do not begin the next cycle of treatment until the absolute neutrophil count (ANC) is ≥1000/mm³ and platelet count ≥50,000/mm³
• ANC nadir ≥500/mm³ and platelet count nadir ≥25,000/mm³: no dose adjustment
• ANC nadir <500/mm³ (any platelet count): begin next cycle of treatment at a reduced dose of 750 mg/m². For the second occurrence of an ANC nadir <500/mm³, reduce the dose of the next cycle to 500 mg/m², if the ANC nadir is <500/mm³ after 2 dose reductions, discontinue therapy
• Platelet nadir <25,000/mm³ (any ANC): begin next cycle of treatment at a reduced dose of 750 mg/m². For the second occurrence of a platelet nadir <25,000/mm³, reduce the dose of the next cycle to 500 mg/m². If the platelet nadir is <25,000/mm³ after 2 dose reductions, discontinue therapy

Nonhematologic toxicities:
• Grade 3 or 4 nausea, vomiting, or diarrhea for >7 days with supportive management, or other grade 3 or 4 toxicity of any duration: hold treatment. When toxicity resolves to grade ≤2, restart the next cycle at a reduced dose of 750 mg/m². For the second occurrence of grade 3 or 4 toxicity (for a duration >7 days with supportive management for GI toxicities), resume therapy at 500 mg/m² upon resolution to grade ≤2. If the grade 3 or 4 toxicity recurs after 2 dose reductions, discontinue therapy

ADVERSE EFFECTS
CNS: Fatigue headache dizziness, fever, chills
CV: Hypotension, QT prolongation
GI: *Constipation, anorexia, abdominal pain, nausea, vomiting, diarrhea,* hepatotoxicity
HEMA: Anemia, thrombocytopenia, neutropenia

INTEG: Injection-site reactions, rash, phlebitis,
MISC: Hypokalemia
RESP: Dyspnea, cough
SYST: Multi-organ failure, TLS, serious infections

Pharmacokinetics

Absorption	Unknown
Distribution	92.9%-95.8% protein bound
Metabolism	80%-90% metabolized by hepatic UGT1A1; liver
Excretion	40% excreted renally, primarily as metabolites
Half-life	1.1 hr

Pharmacodynamics

Onset	Unknown
Peak	Unknown
Duration	Unknown

INTERACTIONS
Drug classifications
Strong UGT1A1 inhibitors: increased belinostat

NURSING CONSIDERATIONS
Assessment
• Hematologic toxicity (thrombocytopenia, leukopenia, neutropenia, lymphopenia, anemia): Monitor CBC before starting therapy and then every week. Dose modifications may be necessary in patients with bone marrow suppression and should be determined by the ANC and platelet count nadirs of the previous cycle of therapy. Platelet counts should be ≥50,000/mm³ and ANC >1000/mm³ before starting each cycle
• Serious infections (pneumonia, sepsis): May be fatal. Do not use in those with an active infection. Use caution in patients with a history of extensive or intensive chemotherapy, as they may be at higher risk for life-threatening infections.
• Fatal hepatic toxicity: Monitor LFTs before the start of each cycle. Those with signs of hepatic disease may require dose modification or discontinuation
• TLS: Those with high tumor burden or advanced stage disease are at greater risk for development of TLS; consider tumor lysis prophylaxis with antihyperuricemic agents and hydration beginning 12-24 hr before treatment; for TLS treatment, administer aggressive IV hydration, antihyperuricemic

agents, correct electrolyte abnormalities, and monitor renal function
• **Pregnancy (D) and breastfeeding:** Consider discontinuing breastfeeding, identify whether the patient is pregnant before using
• **Renal studies:** Monitor BUN/creatinine periodically

Patient/family education
• **Teach patient to avoid use in breastfeeding, and not to use in pregnancy (D)**
• Advise patient to report infusion-site reactions, rash, severe constipation or diarrhea, abdominal pain

Evaluation
Positive therapeutic outcome
• Prevention of spread of disease

---

dalbavancin
(dal-ba-van'sin)
Dalvance
Func. class.: Antiinfective-glycopeptide
Pregnancy category C

ACTION: Binds to the bacterial cell walls, inhibiting their synthesis

Therapeutic outcome: Decreased symptoms of infection, negative C&S

USES: Treatment of acute bacterial skin and skin structure infections caused by gram-positive organisms, (cellulitis, major abscess, wound infections)

CONTRAINDICATIONS: Hypersensitivity

Precautions: Antimicrobial resistance, breastfeeding, colitis, diarrhea, GI disease, inflammatory bowel disease, infusion-related reactions, pregnancy, pseudomembranous colitis, ulcerative colitis, vancomycin hypersensitivity, viral infection

DOSAGE AND ROUTES
Adult: **IV** 1000 mg once, then 500 mg **IV** 1 wk later

Available forms: Powder for injection 500 mg

Implementation
IV infusion route
• Visually inspect parenteral products for particulate matter and discoloration
• **Reconstitution:** Reconstitute each 500 mg/25 ml sterile water for injection; to avoid foaming, alternate between gentle swirling and inversion until completely dissolved, do not shake; further dilution is required
• **Storage:** Refrigerate or store at room temperature. Do not freeze. Total time from reconstitution to dilution to use should not exceed 48 hr
• **Dilution:** Transfer the dose of reconstituted solution from the vial(s) to an IV bag or bottle containing D_5W (1-5 mg/ml)
Intermittent IV INF
• Give over 30 min, do not infuse with other medications or electrolytes
• Saline-based infusion solutions may cause precipitation and should not be used
• If a common IV line is being used to administer other drugs, the line should be flushed before and after each dose

ADVERSE EFFECTS
CNS: Dizziness, headache, flushing
GI: Nausea, vomiting, **pseudomembranous colitis, GI bleeding,** abdominal pain, diarrhea
HEMA: Thrombocytopenia, neutropenia, leukopenia, anemia
INTEG: Rash, urticaria, **infusion-related reactions,** pruritus
SYST: Red man syndrome, hypersensitivity reactions

Pharmacokinetics
Absorption	Unknown
Distribution	Protein binding 93%, primarily to albumin
Metabolism	Decreased in renal disease
Excretion	Feces and urine
Half-life	Unknown

Pharmacodynamics
Onset	Unknown
Peak	Unknown
Duration	Unknown

INTERACTIONS

Drug classifications
Oral contraceptives: decreased with prolonged use

Drug/lab test
Increased: LFTs

NURSING CONSIDERATIONS
Assessment
• Assess: BUN/creatinine, lower dose may be required in severe renal disease
• Pseudomembranous colitis: bowel pattern daily, if severe diarrhea occurs, product should be discontinued
• IV site for INF-site reactions
• Anaphylaxis: rash, urticaria, pruritus, wheezing, may occur a few days after administration
• Red man syndrome: flushing, rash over upper torso and neck, may occur after a few minutes of infusion, may be treated with antihistamines and a slower infusion

Patient/family education
• Teach patient to report sore throat, bruising, bleeding, joint pain (blood dyscrasias); diarrhea with mucus, blood (pseudomembranous colitis)
• Advise patient to use nonhormonal contraceptive if on long-term therapy (controversial)

Evaluation
Positive therapeutic outcome
• Decreased symptoms of infection, negative C&S

---

droxidopa
(drox'-i-doe'-pa)
Northera
Func. class.: Cardiovascular agent-vasopressor
Pregnancy category C

ACTION: A synthetic amino acid precursor of norepinephrine. It is used to increase blood pressure with symptomatic neurogenic orthostatic hypotension (NOH) caused by primary autonomic failure (e.g., Parkinson's disease, multiple system atrophy, and pure autonomic failure), dopamine β-hydroxylase deficiency, or nondiabetic autonomic neuropathy

Therapeutic outcome: Decreased B/P

USES: Increased B/P

CONTRAINDICATIONS: Hypersensitivity

Precautions: Angina, breastfeeding, cardiac arrhythmias, cardiac disease, children, coronary artery disease, heart disease, hyperthermia, infants, mental status changes, myocardial infarction, neonates, pregnancy, salicylate/tartrazine dye hypersensitivity

> **BLACK BOX WARNING:** Hypertension

DOSAGE AND ROUTES
Adult: **PO** 100 mg tid: upon arising in the morning, at midday, and in the late afternoon at least 3 hr before bedtime; titrate to response, by 100 mg tid q24-48hr up to a dose of 600 mg PO tid, max 1800 mg/day

Available forms: Caps 100, 200, 300 mg

Implementation
• Give tid at the following times: upon arising in the morning, at midday, and in the late afternoon at least 3 hr before bedtime (to reduce the potential for supine hypertension during sleep)
• Use without regard to food, but should be taken consistently in regard to food to ensure consistent absorption
• Swallow capsules whole

ADVERSE EFFECTS
CNS: Headache, dizziness, fatigue
CV: Supine hypertension, arrhythmia exacerbation, chest pain
MISC: Urinary tract infection, **neuroleptic malignant syndrome**

Pharmacokinetics
Absorption	Unknown
Distribution	Unknown
Metabolism	Unknown
Excretion	Unknown
Half-life	Unknown

Pharmacodynamics
Onset	Unknown
Peak	Unknown
Duration	Unknown

INTERACTIONS
Drug classifications
Serotonin receptor agonists, sympathomimetics, carbidopa: Increased droxidopa effects
MAOIs: Increased hypertensive crisis

NURSING CONSIDERATIONS
Assessment
• Monitor supine B/P before and at every dosage increase, assess response periodically. Advise to elevate the head of the bed when resting or sleeping to lessen the risk for supine hypertension. B/P should be monitored, in supine

---

position and the recommended head-elevated sleeping position. Reduce or discontinue if supine hypertension persists
• **Neuroleptic malignant syndrome: Hyperthermia, severe extrapyramidal dysfunction, alterations in consciousness, mental status changes, and autonomic instability (tachycardia, blood pressure fluctuations, diaphoresis). In those with Parkinson's disease, this condition may occur with abrupt reduction of products with dopaminergic properties**
• **Arrhythmia exacerbation: exacerbation of existing ischemic cardiac disease (coronary artery disease, angina, myocardial infarction, CHF); consider the potential risk before initiating therapy; if chest pain occurs during use, assess cardiac status**

Patient/family education
• Instruct patients to rest and sleep in an upper-body-elevated position and to monitor B/P (to reduce the potential for supine hypertension)

Evaluation
Positive therapeutic outcome
• Increased B/P

---

empagliflozin
(em-pa-gli-floe′zin)
Jardiance
Func. class.: Antidiabetic
Chem. class.: Sodium-glucose cotransporter 2 (SGLT2) inhibitors
Pregnancy category C

ACTION: An inhibitor of sodium-glucose cotransporter 2 (SGLT2), the transporter responsible for reabsorbing the majority of glucose filtered by the tubular lumen in the kidney

Therapeutic outcome: Decreased blood glucose, A1c

USES: Type 2 diabetes mellitus with diet and exercise

CONTRAINDICATIONS: Hypersensitivity, dialysis, renal failure

Precautions: Adrenal insufficiency, breastfeeding, children, dehydration, diabetic ketoacidosis, fever, geriatric patients, hypercholesterolemia, hypercortisolism, hyperglycemia, hyperthyroidism, hypoglycemia, hypotension, hypothyroidism, hypovolemia, malnutrition, pituitary insufficiency, pregnancy, renal impairment, type 1 diabetes mellitus, vaginitis

DOSAGE AND ROUTES
Adult: **PO** 10 mg daily, may increase to 25 mg daily

Available forms: Tabs 10, 25 mg

Implementation
• Give every day without regard to food in the AM

ADVERSE EFFECTS
CNS: Syncope
CV: Hypotension, orthostatic hypotension
ENDO: Hypercholesterolemia, hyperlipidemia, hypoglycemia
GU: Increased urinary frequency, nocturia, polyuria, cystitis, dehydration, diuresis
GI: Nausea
MISC: Infection
MS: Arthralgia

Pharmacokinetics
Absorption	Unknown
Distribution	Protein binding 82.6%,
Metabolism	Unknown
Excretion	Unknown
Half-life	Terminal elimination half-life 12.4 hr

Pharmacodynamics
Onset	Unknown
Peak	1.5 hr
Duration	Unknown

INTERACTIONS
Individual drugs
Alcohol, bortezomib, clonidine, lithium: increased/decreased hypoglycemic effect
Baclofen, cyclosporine, dexfenfluramine, dextrothyroxine, ethotoin, fenfluramine, fosphenytoin, glucagon, phenytoin, tacrolimus, tobacco: decreased hypoglycemic effect
Fluoxetine, octreotide, olanzapine: Increased hypoglycemic effect
Gatifloxacin: do not use concurrently

Drug classifications
Androgens, sulfonamides: increase/decreased hypoglycemic effect
Angiotensin II receptor antagonists, angiotensin-converting enzyme (ACE) inhibitors, β-blockers, fibric acid derivatives, loop diuretics, MAOIs type A, thiazide diuretics: increased hypoglycemic effect

Atypical antipsychotics, carbonic anhydrase inhibitors, corticosteroids, estrogens, oral contraceptives, phenothiazines, progestins, salicylates: decreased hypoglycemic effect

Thyroid hormones: do not use concurrently

Drug/herb

Chromium, horse chestnut: increased hypoglycemia

Green tea: decreased hypoglycemia

Niacin: increased/decreased hypoglycemia

NURSING CONSIDERATIONS

Assessment

• Diabetes: Monitor blood glucose, glycosylated hemoglobin A1c (HbA1c), serum cholesterol profile, serum creatinine/BUN, assess for polydipsia, other products taken by patient

Patient/family education

• Teach patient how to check blood glucose, to continue with diet and exercise changes, to avoid smoking, alcohol

• Instruct patient to avoid other products unless approved by prescriber

Evaluation

Positive therapeutic outcome

• Decreased blood glucose, A1c

RARELY USED

factor IX Fc fusion protein, recombinant

(fak'tor nine')

Alprolix

Func. class.: Hemostatic

Pregnancy category C

USES: Hemophilia B, surgical bleeding

CONTRAINDICATIONS: Bleeding disorders

DOSAGE AND ROUTES

Hemophilia B

Adult, adolescent, child, infant, and neonate: **IV** INF Infuse dose ≤10 ml/min dose (IU) = body weight (kg) × desired factor IX increase (IU/dl or % of normal) × reciprocal of recovery (IU/kg per IU/dl) *OR* IU/dl (or % of normal) = [total dose (IU)/body weight (kg)] × recovery (IU/dl per IU/kg)

Surgical bleeding control, prevention

Adult, adolescent, child, infant, and neonate: Dose and duration of treatment depend on the severity of the factor IX deficiency, the location and extent of bleeding, and the patient's clinical condition. Refer to hemophilia B for dosage formula

Routine bleeding prophylaxis to prevent/reduce frequency of bleeding episodes

Adult, adolescent, child, infant, and neonate: **IV** INF Initially, 50 IU/kg every week or 100 IU/kg q10d

---

idelalisib

(eye-del'a-lis'ib)

Zydelig

Func. class.: Antineoplastic-biologic response modifier

Chem. class.: Signal transduction inhibitor (STI)

Pregnancy category D

ACTION: Selective, small-molecule inhibitor of one kinase (expressed in both normal and malignant B-cells). Induces apoptosis and inhibited proliferation, inhibits several cell signaling pathways

Therapeutic outcome: Decreased disease progression

USES: Treatment of relapsed chronic lymphocytic leukemia (CLL), in combination with rituximab, in those whom rituximab alone should not be used; non-Hodgkin's lymphoma (NHL), relapsed follicular B-cell NHL in those who have received at least 2 prior systemic therapies

CONTRAINDICATIONS: Infusion-related reaction, serious rash, pregnancy **D**

Precautions: Serious allergic reactions, grade 3 or 4 neutropenia, breastfeeding, hyperglycemia/hypoglycemia

---

BLACK BOX WARNING: Serious hepatotoxicity, grade 3 or higher diarrhea or colitis, fatal/serious pneumonitis

---

Adverse effects: *italics* = common; **bold** = life-threatening

DOSAGE AND ROUTES

Treatment of relapsed chronic lymphocytic leukemia (CLL)
Adult: PO 150 mg bid until disease progression or unacceptable toxicity, with 8 doses of rituximab (given as 375 mg/m² IV on day 1, then 2 wk later rituximab 500 mg/m² IV q2wk × 3 more doses, followed by rituximab 500 mg/m² IV q4wk × 4 doses)

Treatment of small lymphocytic lymphoma (SLL) in those who have received at least 2 prior systemic therapies
Adult: PO 150 mg bid until disease progression or unacceptable toxicity

Hepatic dose
• AST/ALT >3-5 × ULN: No change; monitor AST/ALT at least every week until ≤1 × ULN
• AST/ALT >5-20 × ULN: Hold doses, monitor AST/ALT at least every week, when AST/ALT are ≤1 × ULN, resume at 100 mg bid
• AST/ALT >20 × ULN: Permanently discontinue
• Bilirubin >1.5-3 × ULN: No change; monitor bilirubin at least every week until ≤1 × ULN
• Bilirubin >3-10 × ULN: Hold treatment; monitor bilirubin at least every week; when bilirubin is ≤1 × ULN, resume treatment at 100 mg bid
• Bilirubin >10 × ULN: Permanently discontinue

Available forms: Tabs 100, 150 mg

Implementation
• Take without regard to food, do not crush or dissolve tabs
• Do not take 2 doses at the same time, if a dose is missed by <6 hr, take the dose, take next dose at usual time
Therapeutic drug monitoring: dosage adjustments due to treatment-related toxicity
• Moderate diarrhea (4-6 stools/day over baseline): Continue current dosing; monitor at least every week until diarrhea is resolved
• Severe diarrhea (≥7 stools/day over baseline) or diarrhea requiring hospitalization: Hold treatment, and monitor at least every week for resolution. When diarrhea has resolved, resume with 100 mg bid
• Life-threatening diarrhea: Permanently discontinue treatment

• Neutropenia: ANC 1000-1499 cells/mm³: no change; ANC 500-999 cells/mm³: continue current dosing; monitor ANC at least every week; ANC <500 cells/mm³: hold treatment and monitor ANC at least every week, when ANC ≥500 cells/mm³, resume treatment at 100 mg bid
• Thrombocytopenia: Platelet count 50,000-75,000 cells/mm³: no change; platelet count 25,000-49,000 cells/mm³: continue dose; monitor platelet count at least every week; platelet count <25,000 cells/mm³: hold treatment, monitor platelet count at least every week, when platelet count ≥25,000 cells/mm³, resume treatment at 100 mg bid
• Symptomatic pneumonitis (any severity): Discontinue treatment
• Other severe or life-threatening toxicities: Hold until toxicity is resolved; if resuming treatment, reduce the dose to 100 mg bid; permanently discontinue treatment for any recurrence of severe or life-threatening toxicity after rechallenge

ADVERSE EFFECTS
CNS: Insomnia, fatigue, fever, headache
EENT: Sinusitis
ENDO: Hypoglycemia, hyperglycemia, hyponatremia
GI: Nausea, vomiting, hepatic failure, GI perforation, stomatitis, colitis, diarrhea, anorexia, abdominal pain
HEMA: Thrombocytopenia, neutropenia, anemia
INTEG: Rash
RESP: Pneumonitis, dyspnea, cough
SYST: Serious/fatal rashes

Pharmacokinetics

Absorption	Unknown
Distribution	84% protein binding
Metabolism	Unknown
Excretion	Unknown
Half-life	Half-life 8.2 hr

Pharmacodynamics

Onset	Unknown
Peak	1.5 hr
Duration	Unknown

INTERACTIONS

Drug classifications:
CYP3A4 inhibitors, inducers, substrates: avoid concurrent use

---

⚠ Nurse Alert

Drug/lab test:
Increase: LFTs

NURSING CONSIDERATIONS

Assessment
• **Hepatic failure:** Increased LFTs generally occurred within the first 12 wk of treatment and were reversible with dose interruption. Monitor LFTs q2wk × 3 mo of treatment, then q4wk for 3 mo, and q1-3 mo thereafter; monitor weekly if AST or ALT are >3 times the upper limit of normal (ULN) or bilirubin >1.5 × ULN. Hepatotoxicity may require treatment interruption, dose reduction, or discontinuation of therapy
• **Severe diarrhea/GI perforation:** Generally responds poorly to antimotility agents. The occurrence of ≥7 stools/day over baseline or hospitalization due to diarrhea may result in interruption of therapy, dose reduction, or permanent discontinuation. Assess for new or worsening abdominal pain, chills, fever, or nausea/vomiting. If intestinal perforation occurs, permanently discontinue treatment
• **Pneumonitis:** Monitor for cough, dyspnea, hypoxia, and bilateral interstitial infiltrates, or a decline in oxygen saturation by >5%. If pneumonitis is suspected, hold therapy. Permanently discontinue treatment for pneumonitis and consider treatment with corticosteroids.

Patient/family education
• Instruct patient to report planned or suspected pregnancy (D), use effective contraception during treatment and for at least 1 month after the last dose
• Instruct patient to avoid breastfeeding
• Instruct patient to report new or worsening side effects

Evaluation
Positive therapeutic outcome
• Decreased disease progression

insulin, inhaled
(in'su-lin)
Afrezza
Func. class.: Antidiabetic—insulin
Pregnancy category C

ACTION: Endogenous insulin regulates carbohydrate, fat, and protein metabolism by the storage of and inhibiting the breakdown of glucose, fat, and amino acids. Insulin decreases glucose concentrations by the uptake of glucose in muscle and adipose tissue, and by inhibiting hepatic glucose production. Insulin also regulates fat metabolism by the storage of fat and inhibiting the mobilization of fat for energy in adipose tissues (lipolysis and free fatty acid oxidation).

Therapeutic outcome: Decrease in blood glucose levels

USES: Diabetes mellitus types 1 and 2

CONTRAINDICATIONS: Hypersensitivity, lung cancer, asthma, COPD, hypoglycemia, smoking

Precautions: Hepatic disease, renal impairment, renal failure, diabetic ketoacidosis (DKA), hypokalemia, pregnancy **C,** breastfeeding, child <18 yr

DOSAGE AND ROUTES
Adult: INH: (type 1) the average initial dose is 0.5-0.6 unit/kg/day, usually ≥3 administrations/day; (type 2) the average initial dose is 0.2-0.6 unit/kg/day. When used in combination with oral hypoglycemic agents, may only need a single dose of a longer-acting insulin at a dosage of 10 units or 0.2 units/kg/day

Available forms: Inhalation 0.35 powder

Implementation
• Give by inhalation only; use at beginning of a meal; (blue cartridge = 4 units of regular insulin, green cartridge = 8 units of regular insulin), multiple cartridges may be needed, for single-use only, inhaler should be discarded after 15 days; store unopened cartridge packages in refrigerator, if not refrigerated, use within 10 days
• Sealed (unopened) blister cards and strips must be used within 10 days. Cartridges left over in an opened strip must be used within 3 days. Remove a blister card from the foil package. Tear along a perforation to remove one strip. Press the clear side of the strip to push the cartridge out. To load the cartridge, hold the inhaler level in one hand with the white mouthpiece on the top and purple base on the bottom; open the inhaler by lifting the white mouthpiece to a vertical position. Before placing the cartridge in the inhaler, both the cartridge and the inhaler should be at room temperature for 10 minutes. Hold the cartridge with the cup facing down, and line up the cartridge with the opening in the inhaler. The pointed end of the

cartridge should line up with the pointed end in the inhaler. The cartridge can be placed into the inhaler; ensure that the cartridge lies flat in the inhaler. Once the cartridge is loaded, keep level
• Remove the purple mouthpiece cover. Hold the inhaler away from the mouth and fully exhale. While keeping the head level, place the mouthpiece in the mouth and tilt the inhaler down toward the chin. Close lips around the mouthpiece to form a seal. Inhale deeply through the inhaler. Hold breath for as long as is comfortable, and at the same time remove the inhaler from the mouth. Exhale and continue to breathe normally

ADVERSE EFFECTS

CNS: Headache, fatigue
ENDO: Hypoglycemia
GI: Nausea, diarrhea
MISC: Urinary tract infection, weight gain, hypokalemia, peripheral edema
RESP: Cough, throat irritation/pain, productive cough, decreased pulmonary function tests, bronchitis, **acute bronchospasm**

Pharmacokinetics

Absorption	Unknown
Distribution	Unknown
Metabolism	Unknown
Excretion	Unknown
Half-life	Unknown

Pharmacodynamics

Onset	Unknown
Peak	Unknown
Duration	Unknown

INTERACTIONS

Drug classifications

ACE inhibitors, angiotensin II receptor antagonists, β-blockers: increased hypoglycemia
Bronchodilators, other inhaled products, agonists, MAOIs, salicylates: Increased inhaled insulin effect
Testosterone derivatives, or anabolic steroids: Increased or decreased hypoglycemic effects
Thiazide diuretics; thyroid hormones, estrogens, progestins, or oral contraceptives, corticosteroids: Decreased hypoglycemic effects

Individual drugs

Alcohol, fenfluramine: increased inhaled insulin effect
Bumetanide, furosemide, niacin (nicotinic acid), torsemide: increased hyperglycemia

Clonidine, metoclopramide, tegaserod: increased or decreased hypoglycemic effects
Danazol, dextrothyroxine, epinephrine, triamterene: decreased hypoglycemic effects
Disopyramide, guanethidine, octreotide: increased hypoglycemia
Pioglitazone, troglitazone: increased heart failure, ischemic events

NURSING CONSIDERATIONS

Assessment

• Monitor fasting blood glucose, A1c may be drawn to identify treatment effectiveness
• Monitor urine ketones during illness, insulin requirements may increase during times of stress, trauma, illness, surgery
• Assess for hypoglycemic reaction; can occur during peak times (sweating, weakness, dizziness, chills, confusion, headache, nausea, rapid, weak pulse)
• Assess for hyperglycemia: acetone breath, polyuria, fatigue, polydipsia, flushed dry skin, lethargy

Patient/family education

• Teach patient that blurred vision occurs; patient should not operate machinery until effect is known and should not change corrective lens for at least 1 mo
• Teach patient to keep all insulin equipment available at all times
• Inform patient that product does not cure, but controls symptoms
• Advise patient to carry ID as diabetic
• Teach patient about the symptoms of hypoglycemia, hyperglycemia, ketoacidosis
• Teach patient about dosage and how to use product, that the rest of the plan must be followed

Evaluation

Positive therapeutic outcome
• Decrease in blood glucose levels

⚠ HIGH ALERT

ledipasvir/sofosbuvir
(le-dip′as-vir/soe-fos′bue-veer)
Harvoni
Func. class.: Antiviral antihepatitis agent
Pregnancy category B

ACTION: A combination product with a HCV NS5A inhibitor (ledipasvir) and a nucleotide analog HCV NS5B polymerase inhibitor (sofosbuvir)

Therapeutic outcome: Hepatitis C RNA reduction

USES: Chronic hepatitis C virus (HCV) genotype 1 infection in patients with compensated liver disease

CONTRAINDICATIONS: Hypersensitivity

Precautions: Decompensated hepatic disease, decompensated cirrhosis, severe renal impairment (eGFR <30 ml/min/1.73 m²), end-stage renal failure requiring dialysis, pregnancy (B), breastfeeding

DOSAGE AND ROUTES
Adults with or without cirrhosis who are treatment-naive: **PO** One tab (90 mg ledipasvir; 400 mg sofosbuvir) every day with or without food for 12 wk; 8 wk can be considered for those patients with a baseline HCV RNA <6 million IU/ml
Adults without cirrhosis who are treatment-experienced: **PO** One tablet (90 mg ledipasvir; 400 mg sofosbuvir) every day with or without food for 12 wk; 8 wk can be considered for those patients with a baseline HCV RNA <6 million IU/ml
Adults with cirrhosis who are treatment-experienced: **PO** One tablet (90 mg ledipasvir; 400 mg sofosbuvir) every day with or without food for 24 wk

Available forms: Tab 90/400 mg

Implementation
• Without regard to food

ADVERSE EFFECTS
CNS: Fatigue, headache, insomnia
GI: Nausea, vomiting, diarrhea

Pharmacokinetics

Absorption	Unknown
Distribution	Ledipasvir: >99.8% protein binding, Sofosbuvir: 61%-65% protein binding
Metabolism	Unknown
Excretion	Ledipasvir: biliary; Sofosbuvir: kidneys 80% recovered in the urine
Half-life	Terminal half-life 47 hr

Pharmacodynamics

Onset	Unknown
Peak	Ledipasvir peak 4-5 hr, Sofosbuvir peak 0.8-1 hr
Duration	Unknown

INTERACTIONS
Drug classifications
Avoid use with products that increase P-glycoprotein

Drug/lab test
Increased: bilirubin

NURSING CONSIDERATIONS
Assessment
• Hepatitis C: monitor hepatitis C RNA, serum bilirubin, creatinine

Patient/family education
• Instruct patient to report effects to the prescriber

Evaluation
Positive therapeutic outcome
• Hepatitis C RNA reduction

RARELY USED

olaparib
(oh-lap′a-rib)
Lynparza
Func. class.: Antineoplastic-PARP
Pregnancy category D

USES: Treatment of deleterious or suspected deleterious germline BRCA-mutated advanced ovarian cancer in patients who have not responded successfully to ≥3 prior courses of chemotherapy, as monotherapy

CONTRAINDICATIONS: Hypersensitivity, pregnancy **D**

DOSAGE AND ROUTES
Adult female: **PO** 400 mg bid until disease progression or unacceptable toxicity. Avoid use of concomitant strong and moderate CYP3A4 inhibitors if possible

Available forms: Cap 50 mg

oritavancin

(or-it′a-van′sin)

Orbactive

Func. class.: Antiinfective agent

Chem. class.: Glycopeptide

Pregnancy category C

ACTION: Inhibits bacterial cell-wall biosynthesis by preventing transglycosylation (polymerization) by binding to precursors, as well as preventing cross-linking by binding to the peptide bridging segments of the cell wall; also disrupts the bacterial cell membrane integrity, resulting in depolarization, increased permeability, and eventual cell death

Therapeutic outcome: Resolution of infection

USES: *Enterococcus faecalis, Enterococcus faecium, Staphylococcus aureus* (MRSA), *Staphylococcus aureus* (MSSA), *Streptococcus agalactiae* (group B streptococci), *Streptococcus anginosus, Streptococcus constellatus, Streptococcus dysgalactiae, Streptococcus intermedius, Streptococcus pyogenes* (group A β-hemolytic streptococci); treatment of acute bacterial skin and skin structure infections (ABSSSI) due to gram-positive organisms, including cellulitis/erysipelas, major cutaneous abscesses, and wound infections

CONTRAINDICATIONS: Hypersensitivity

Precautions: Anticoagulant therapy, antimicrobial resistance, breastfeeding, colitis, diarrhea, inflammatory bowel disease, infusion reactions, pregnancy, pseudomembranous colitis, vancomycin hypersensitivity, viral infection

DOSAGE AND ROUTES

Adult: IV 1200 mg once

Available forms: Powder for injection: 400 mg

Implementation

• Visually inspect for particulate matter and discoloration beforehand, the reconstituted solution is clear, colorless to pale yellow

• Reconstitution: Reconstitute each 400-mg vial with 40 ml sterile water for injection. Three vials are necessary for a single dose; gently swirl until dissolved

• Dilution: Withdraw and discard 120 ml from a 1000-ml intravenous bag of D_5W, transfer 40 ml solution from each of the 3 reconstituted vials to the D_5W IV bag (1.2 mg/mg)

• Storage: Refrigerate or store at room temperature. The combined storage time (from reconstitution to dilution) and 3-hour infusion time should not exceed 6 hr at room temperature or 12 hr if refrigerated

Intermittent IV INF

• Infuse over 3 hr, do not infuse with other medications or electrolytes, do not use saline-based solution

ADVERSE EFFECTS

CNS: Dizziness, flushing, headache

CV: Sinus tachycardia, phlebitis

GI: Nausea, vomiting, diarrhea

HEMA: Anemia, eosinophilia

INTEG: Rash, vasculitis, pruritus, angioedema, infusion-related reaction

MISC: Wheezing, bronchospasm

MS: Myalgia, osteomyelitis

Pharmacokinetics

Absorption	Unknown
Distribution	85% protein binding
Metabolism	Unknown
Excretion	Unknown
Half-life	Terminal half-life 245 hr

Pharmacodynamics

Onset	Unknown
Peak	Unknown
Duration	Unknown

INTERACTIONS

Drug classifications

Products metabolized by CYP2D6 and CYP3A4: Increased toxicity

Drug/lab test

Increased: LFTs

NURSING CONSIDERATIONS

Assessment

• Monitor CBC and differential

• Assess for diarrhea, bloody stools, cramping

Patient/family education

• Teach patient reason for product, expected result

• Advise patient product is used only once to resolve infection

Evaluation

Positive therapeutic outcome

• Resolution of infection

⚠ **Nurse Alert**

⚠ HIGH ALERT

palbociclib
(pal-boe-sye'klib)
Ibrance
Func. class.: Antineoplastic
Chem. class.: Signal transduction inhibitor
Pregnancy category Unknown

ACTION: Inhibits progression of the cell cycle from G_1 into S phase, decreased proliferation of ER-positive breast cancer cell lines. When combined with antiestrogen therapy (letrozole), decreases retinoblastoma protein (Rb) phosphorylation, reducing E2F expression and signaling, and increasing growth arrest

Therapeutic outcome: Decreased progression of disease

USES: Treatment of estrogen receptor (ER)–positive, HER2-negative advanced breast cancer in postmenopausal women, in combination with letrozole as initial endocrine-based therapy

CONTRAINDICATIONS: Hypersensitivity

Precautions: Breastfeeding, children, fungal/viral infection, infants, infertility, neutropenia, pregnancy, testicular failure, thromboembolic disease

DOSAGE AND ROUTES
Adult female: PO 125 mg daily with food × 21 days, followed by 7 days off, repeat q28 days with letrozole 2.5 mg daily, given continuously through each 28-day cycle until progressive disease or unacceptable toxicity occurs

Available forms: Caps 75, 100, 125 mg

Implementation
Treatment-related hepatotoxicity:
• **Grade 1 or 2 hepatotoxicity: No dosage change**
• **Grade ≥3 hepatotoxicity (AST or ALT >5 × ULN or total bilirubin >3 × ULN) that persists despite medical treatment: Hold until toxicity resolves to grade ≤2 (AST or ALT ≤5 × ULN or total bilirubin ≤3 × ULN), resume treatment at the next lower dose level if not considered a safety risk for the patient; discontinue if grade ≥3 toxicity occurs at a dose of 75 mg/day**

Treatment-related nephrotoxicity:
• **Grade 1 or 2 nephrotoxicity: No change**
• **Grade ≥3 nephrotoxicity (CCr >3 × baseline or >4 mg/dl, or requiring hospitalization or dialysis) that persists despite medical treatment: Hold therapy. When toxicity resolves to grade ≤2 (CCr <3 × baseline or <4 mg/dl), resume at the next lower dose level if not considered a safety risk for the patient, discontinue if grade ≥3 toxicity occurs at a dose of 75 mg/day**
Other dosage adjustments
• **Strong CYP3A4 inhibitors: Avoid concomitant use. If a strong CYP3A4 inhibitor is needed, consider reducing the dose to 75 mg daily, if the strong CYP3A4 inhibitor is discontinued, increase the dose upward to the previously tolerated/recommended dose after a washout period of 3-5 half-lives of the inhibitor**
• **Strong CYP3A4 inducers: Avoid use**

ADVERSE EFFECTS
CNS: Weakness, fever, fatigue
EENT: Stomatitis, oral ulceration, glossitis, pharyngitis, sinusitis, epistaxis
GI: Vomiting, nausea, anorexia, diarrhea,
HEMA: Thrombocytopenia, neutropenia, leukopenia, lymphopenia, anemia
MISC: Peripheral neuropathy, alopecia, **infection, pulmonary embolism, thromboembolism**

Pharmacokinetics

Absorption	Unknown
Distribution	85% protein bound
Metabolism	Metabolized by CYP3A
Excretion	Unknown
Half-life	Elimination half-life was 24-34 hr

Pharmacodynamics

Onset	Unknown
Peak	Peak 6-12 hr
Duration	Unknown

INTERACTIONS
Drug classifications
CYP3A inhibitors and inducers: avoid concurrent use

Drug/herb
St. John's wort: Avoid concurrent use

Drug/food
Avoid use with grapefruit juice

NURSING CONSIDERATIONS
Assessment
• Pregnancy: Product can cause fetal harm; identify if the patient is pregnant or if pregnancy is planned
• Pulmonary embolism/thromboembolic events: Assess for dyspnea/shortness of breath, chest pain, arm or leg swelling, sudden numbness or weakness, severe headache or confusion, or problems with vision, speech, or balance
• Blood dyscrasias: Monitor CBC/differential

Patient/family education
• Identify if pregnancy is planned or suspected. Discuss the need for contraception due to possible fetal harm; avoid breastfeeding
• Advise patient laboratory testing will be needed during treatment
• Pulmonary/thromboembolic events: Instruct patient to seek medical attention if dyspnea/shortness of breath, chest pain, arm or leg swelling, sudden numbness or weakness, severe headache or confusion, or problems with vision, speech, or balance develop

Evaluation
Positive therapeutic outcome
• Decreased progression of disease

⚠ HIGH ALERT

pembrolizumab
(pem'broe-liz'ue-mab)
Keytruda
Func. class.: Antineoplastic, biologic response modifier
Chem. class.: Monoclonal antibody
Pregnancy category D

ACTION: A human monoclonal antibody that binds to the programmed death receptor-1 (PD-1) found on T-cells and blocks the interaction of PD-1 with its ligands, PD-L1 and PD-L2, on the tumor cell

Therapeutic outcome: Decreased progression of multiple myeloma

USES: Treatment of unresectable or metastatic malignant melanoma in those who have disease progression after ipilimumab or in BRAF V600 mutation–positive patients who have disease progression after ipilimumab and a BRAF inhibitor

CONTRAINDICATIONS: Hypersensitivity, pregnancy **D**, breastfeeding

Precautions: Immune-mediated colitis, immune-mediated hepatitis, immune-mediated hyperthyroidism/hypothyroidism; immune-mediated nephritis, acute interstitial nephritis, and renal failure; immune-mediated pneumonitis, adrenocortical insufficiency, arthritis, exfoliative dermatitis, hemolytic anemia, hypophysitis, myasthenia syndrome, myositis, optic neuritis, pancreatitis, partial seizures after inflammatory foci identified in brain parenchyma, rhabdomyolysis, uveitis, incidence of abortion/stillbirths

DOSAGE AND ROUTES
Adult: IV infusion: 2 mg/kg over 30 min q3wk until disease progression

Available forms: Powder for injection 50 mg

Implementation
IV INF route
• Add 2.3 ml of sterile water for injection, 50-mg vial (25 mg/ml); inject sterile water along the walls of the vial and not directly on the powder
• Gently swirl and allow up to 5 min for bubbles to clear, do not shake, solution will be clear to slightly opalescent, colorless to slightly yellow
• Add the required amount of product to a bag of normal saline (0.9% sodium chloride injection) to a final diluted concentration between 1 and 10 mg/ml; mix by gentle inversion
• Discard any unused solution left in the vial
• Storage after reconstitution and dilution: Store at room temperature up to 4 hr or refrigerate up to 24 hr (includes reconstitution, dilution, and administration time). If refrigerated, allow the diluted solution to warm to room temperature before use, give over 30 min
• Use a sterile, nonpyrogenic, low-protein binding 0.2- to 5-micron in-line or add-on filter
• Do not use with other drugs through the same infusion line
• Grade 2 or 3 toxicity: Withhold and give corticosteroids; resume when the adverse event recovers to grade ≤1. Permanently discontinue if there is no recovery within 12 wk, if the corticosteroid dose cannot be reduced to ≤10 mg/day of prednisone (or equivalent) within 12 wk, or for recurrent severe or grade 3 colitis

---

• Grade 4 toxicity: Permanently discontinue, give corticosteroids
Hepatitis:
• Grade 2 toxicity (AST or ALT >3-5 × upper limit of normal [ULN] or total bilirubin >1.5-3 × ULN): Withhold and give corticosteroids; resume when adverse event recovers to grade 1 or less. Permanently discontinue if there is no recovery within 12 wks or if the corticosteroid dose cannot be reduced to ≤10 mg/day of prednisone (or equivalent) within 12 wks.
• Grade 3 or 4 toxicity (AST or ALT >5 × ULN or total bilirubin >3 × ULN): Permanently discontinue, give corticosteroids
• Liver metastases and grade 2 elevated transaminase levels at baseline: Permanently discontinue if AST/ALT levels increase by ≥50% over baseline and transaminase level elevations persist for at least 1 wk

ADVERSE EFFECTS

CNS: *Seizures,* myasthenia, headache, fever, insomnia, chills, dizziness, fatigue
EENT: Optic neuritis
ENDO: Hyponatremia, hypothyroidism/hyperthyroidism, hyperglycemia, hypocalcemia
GI: Nausea, vomiting, abdominal pain, **pancreatitis,** colitis, diarrhea, **hepatitis,** constipation
GU: Interstitial nephritis, renal failure
INTEG: Rash, pruritus, skin discoloration
MS: Myalgia, **rhabdomyolysis**
RESP: Cough, dyspnea, pneumonitis
SYST: Exfoliative dermatitis

Pharmacokinetics

Absorption	Unknown
Distribution	Unknown
Metabolism	Unknown
Excretion	Unknown
Half-life	Unknown

Pharmacodynamics

Onset	Unknown
Peak	Unknown
Duration	Unknown

INTERACTIONS

Drug/lab test
Increased: LFTs, renal function studies

NURSING CONSIDERATIONS

Assessment

• For hyperthyroidism/hypothyroidism, renal function studies baseline, periodically during therapy, temporarily withheld or permanently discontinued
• For pneumonitis (new or worsening cough, chest pain, shortness of breath), confirm with radiographic imaging
• **Liver function tests and hepatitis (e.g., jaundice, severe nausea/vomiting, easy bleeding or bruising; withhold and give corticosteroids if grade 2 hepatitis (AST or ALT >3-5 × ULN or total bilirubin >1.5-3 × ULN)**

Patient/family education

• **Instruct patient to use highly effective contraceptive methods during and for 4 months after treatment, to contact their health care provider if pregnancy is suspected or confirmed (pregnancy D)**

Evaluation

Positive therapeutic outcome
• Decreased progression of multiple myeloma

peramivir
(per-am′i-vir)
Rapivab
Func. class.: Antiviral
Pregnancy category C

ACTION: Competitively binds to the active site of the influenza virus, inhibits the activity of strains of influenza A and B viruses:

Therapeutic outcome: Absence of developing influenza A or B

USES: Treatment of uncomplicated acute influenza (seasonal influenza A virus infection or seasonal influenza B virus infection)

Unlabeled uses: Treatment of H1N1 influenza A virus (swine influenza) infection in pediatric patients requiring hospitalization

CONTRAINDICATIONS: Hypersensitivity

Precautions: Breastfeeding, children, dialysis, infants, infection, pregnancy, psychosis, renal impairment

DOSAGE AND ROUTES

Influenza
Adult: **IV** 600 mg as a single dose infused over 15-30 min, give within 48 hr of onset of influenza symptoms

Available forms: Solution for injection 200 mg/20 ml

Implementation
• For IV use only, do not give IM, visually inspect parenteral products for particulate matter and discoloration
• Dilute the 10 mg/ml to a max volume of 100 ml, use only 0.9% or 0.45% NaCl, 5% dextrose, or LR
• Storage of diluted solution: Use immediately or refrigerate up to 24 hr. Refrigerated solution should be allowed to reach room temperature before administration. Discard any unused diluted solution after 24 hr
• Give over 15-30 min, do not mix or coadminister with other IV products

ADVERSE EFFECTS
CNS: Delirium, psychosis, hallucinations, insomnia
GI: Constipation, diarrhea, vomiting
MISC: Rash, **Stevens-Johnson syndrome**

Pharmacokinetics

Absorption	Unknown
Distribution	Protein binding <30%
Metabolism	Unknown
Excretion	Unknown
Half-life	Unknown

Pharmacodynamics

Onset	Unknown
Peak	Unknown
Duration	Unknown

INTERACTIONS

Drug classifications:
Intranasal influenza vaccines, H1N1 vaccines: avoid concurrent use

NURSING CONSIDERATIONS

Assessment
• Assess for hypersensitivity reactions/Stevens-Johnson syndrome
• Neuropsychiatric reactions: Assess for delirium, psychosis, hallucinations

Patient/family education
• Teach patient that product is only for use within 48 hr of infection

Evaluation
Therapeutic response
Absence of developing influenza A or B

RARELY USED

pirfenidone
(pir-fen′i-done)
Esbriet
Func. class.: Respiratory agent
Pregnancy category C

USES: Pulmonary fibrosis

CONTRAINDICATIONS: Hypersensitivity

DOSAGE AND ROUTES
Adult: **PO** Titrate over 2 wk to a maintenance dose of 801 mg tid. Give 267 mg tid on days 1-7, 534 mg tid on days 8-14, and 801 mg tid from day 15 onward

Available forms: Cap 267 mg

---

suvorexant
(soo′voe-rex′ant)
Belsomra
Func. class.: Psychotropic—sedative/hypnotic, anxiolytic
Chem. class.: Orexin receptor antagonist
Pregnancy category C

ACTION: Alters the signaling of neurotransmitters called orexins, which are responsible for regulating the sleep–wake cycle

Therapeutic outcome: Normalized sleeping patterns

USES: The treatment of insomnia characterized by difficulties with sleep onset and/or sleep maintenance

CONTRAINDICATIONS: Narcolepsy, hypersensitivity

Precautions: Preexisting respiratory disease, COPD, breastfeeding, pregnancy **C**, labor, geriatrics, hepatic disease, sleep apnea, substance abuse, alcohol use, suicidal ideation, mental changes, depression

---

DOSAGE AND ROUTES

Adult: **PO** 10 mg every night within 30 min of going to bed, and with ≥7 hr remaining before the planned time of awakening, may increase to maximum 20 mg every night

Available forms: Tabs 5, 10, 15, 20 mg

Implementation

- Give 30 min before bedtime
- Effect may be delayed if taken with food, take on empty stomach for faster effect

ADVERSE EFFECTS

CNS: Amnesia, **suicidal ideation,** anxiety, dizziness, drowsiness, hallucinations, headache, memory impairment
GI: Diarrhea

Pharmacokinetics

Absorption	Unknown
Distribution	High-protein binding
Metabolism	Unknown
Excretion	Feces (66%), urine (23%)
Half-life	Terminal half-life 12 hr

Pharmacodynamics

Onset	Unknown
Peak	2 hr
Duration	Unknown

INTERACTIONS

Drug classifications

CNS depressants: increased effects of both products
CYP3A inducers: decreased suvorexant effect
CYP3A inhibitors: avoid concurrent use

Drug/herb

Kava kava, melatonin, valerian: increased suvorexant effect

NURSING CONSIDERATIONS

Assessment

- Sleeping patterns: waking in the night, inability to fall asleep, stay asleep, amnesia

Patient/family education

- Advise patient to use on an empty stomach for faster effect
- **Teach patient to report suicidal thoughts/ behaviors immediately**
- Teach patient to avoid use with other products unless approved by prescriber

Evaluation

Therapeutic response

- Normalized sleeping patterns

---

tasimelteon

(tas'i-mel'tee-on)
Hetlioz
Func. class.: Anxiolytic/sedative/hypnotic
Pregnancy category C

USES: Sleep-wake disorder in the blind

CONTRAINDICATIONS: Hypersensitivity

DOSAGE AND ROUTES

Adult: **PO** 20 mg before bedtime at the same time every night; take without food

vedolizumab

(ve'-doe-liz'ue-mab)
Entyvio
Func. class.: Immunosuppressive, biologic response modifier
Pregnancy category B

ACTION: A specific integrin receptor antagonist that inhibits the migration of specific memory T-lymphocytes across the endothelium into inflamed gastrointestinal parenchymal tissue. The action reduces the chronic inflammatory process present in both ulcerative colitis and Crohn's disease

Therapeutic outcome: Lessening of ulcerative colitis and Crohn's disease

USES: For moderately to severely active ulcerative colitis/Crohn's disease to reduce signs and symptoms, and to induce and maintain clinical remission in patients who have an inadequate response to conventional therapy

CONTRAINDICATIONS: Hypersensitivity

Precautions: Hepatic disease, infections, progressive multifocal leukoencephalopathy (PML), pregnancy **B,** breastfeeding

DOSAGE AND ROUTES

Adult: **IV** INF 300 mg; give over 30 min at weeks 0, 2, and 6 as induction therapy, then 300 mg q8wk

Available forms: Powder for injection 30 mg

Implementation

• Full response is usually observed by 6 wk; those who do not respond by week 14 are unlikely to respond
• Give as IV infusion only, do not use as an IV push or bolus
• Make sure all immunizations are up to date
• Reconstitute with 4.8 ml of sterile water for injection, using a syringe with a 21- to 25-gauge needle
• Insert the syringe needle into the vial and direct the stream of sterile water for injection to the glass wall of the vial; gently swirl the solution for 15 sec; do not shake
• Allow the solution to stand for up to 20 min at room temperature to allow for reconstitution and for any foam to settle
• Once dissolved, product should be clear or opalescent, colorless to light brownish yellow, and free of visible particulates. Discard if discolored or if foreign particles are present
• Before withdrawing solution from vial, gently invert vial 3 times. Withdraw 5 ml (300 mg) of reconstructed product using a 21- to 25-gauge needle. Discard remaining product
• Add the 5 ml (300 mg) of reconstituted product to 250 ml of sterile 0.9% sodium chloride and gently mix infusion bag. Do not mix with other medications. Administer solution as soon as possible; if necessary, solution may be stored for up to 4 hr refrigerated; do not freeze. Infuse over 30 min; after infusion, flush line with 30 ml of sterile 0.9% sodium chloride injection. Discard any unused infusion solution

ADVERSE EFFECTS:

CNS: Headache, fatigue, dizziness
GI: Nausea, vomiting
MISC: Rash, pruritus, infusion-related reactions
MS: Arthralgia, back pain
SYST: Anaphylaxis, progressive multifocal leukoencephalopathy (PML)

Pharmacokinetics

Absorption	Unknown
Distribution	Unknown
Metabolism	Unknown
Excretion	Unknown
Half-life	Unknown

Pharmacodynamics

Onset	Unknown
Peak	Unknown
Duration	Unknown

INTERACTIONS

Drug classifications
Antineoplastics, immunosuppressives: increased infection risk
Do not use with tumor necrosis factor (TNF) modifiers
Toxoids, vaccines: decreased immune response

NURSING CONSIDERATIONS

Assessment
• Ulcerative colitis/Crohn's disease: Monitor symptoms before and after treatment
• **Liver dysfunction: Monitor for elevated hepatic enzymes, jaundice, malaise, nausea, vomiting, abdominal pain, and anorexia; these signs are predictive of severe liver injury that may be fatal or may require a liver transplant in some patients; if hepatic dysfunction is suspected, discontinue**
• **Tuberculosis (TB) latent/active: Obtain TB skin test both before and during treatment. Do not give in active infection such as influenza or sepsis**
• **Progressive multifocal leukoencephalopathy (PML): Assess for increased weakness on one side of the body or clumsiness of limbs, visual disturbance, and changes in thinking, memory, and orientation leading to confusion and personality changes; severe disability or death can come over weeks or months**

Patient/family education
• Teach patient about the symptoms of infection and to report to health care provider immediately
• Advise patient to report planned or suspected pregnancy, or if breastfeeding

Evaluation
Positive therapeutic response
• Lessening of ulcerative colitis and Crohn's disease

---

vorapaxar
(vor′a-pax′ar)
Zontivity
Func class.: Platelet inhibitor
Pregnancy category B

ACTION: Antagonizes the protease-activated receptor-1 (PAR-1) expressed on platelets

Therapeutic outcome: Absence of MI, stroke

USES: Secondary myocardial infarction prophylaxis or stroke prophylaxis or thrombosis prophylaxis for reduction of thrombotic cardiovascular events in patients with a history of myocardial infarction or with peripheral arterial disease

CONTRAINDICATIONS:

> **BLACK BOX WARNING:** Bleeding, intracranial bleeding, stroke

Precautions: Breastfeeding, coronary artery bypass graft surgery (CABG), geriatric patients, hepatic disease, labor, obstetric delivery, pregnancy **B**, renal impairment, surgery

DOSAGE AND ROUTES
Adult: **PO** 2.08 mg once daily with aspirin and/or clopidogrel

Available forms: Tab 2.08 mg

Implementation
• May be administered without regard to food

ADVERSE EFFECTS:
CNS: Depression
EENT: Diplopia, retinopathy
HEMA: Anemia, bleeding
MISC: Rash

Pharmacokinetics

Absorption	Unknown
Distribution	Within 1 week of treatment reaches ≥80% inhibition of thrombin receptor; protein binding 99%
Metabolism	Unknown
Excretion	Primarily feces
Half-life	3-4 days, terminal approximately 8 days

Pharmacodynamics

Onset	Unknown
Peak	1 hr
Duration	Unknown

INTERACTIONS
Drug classifications
Beers Criteria
CYP3A inducers: Decreased vorapaxar effect
Other platelet inhibitors, anticoagulants, calcium channel blockers, CYP3A inhibitors, estradiols, NSAIDs, rifampins, salicylates, SNRIs, SSRIs, thrombolytics: increased bleeding risk

NURSING CONSIDERATIONS
Assessment

> **BLACK BOX WARNING:** Assess for bleeding, including intracranial bleeding and stroke during treatment

• Bleeding should be suspected in any patient presenting with hypotension who has recently undergone surgery, coronary angiography, percutaneous coronary intervention (PCI), or CABG

Patient/family education
• Advise patient to report any unusual bruising, bleeding to prescriber; that it may take longer to stop bleeding
• Teach patient to take without regard to food

Evaluation
Positive therapeutic outcome
• Absence of MI, stroke